The Treatment of Epilepsy

PRINCIPLES & PRACTICE

FOURTH EDITION

The Treatment of Epilepsy

PRINCIPLES & PRACTICE

FOURTH EDITION

EDITOR-IN-CHIEF
ELAINE WYLLIE, MD
Head, Section of Pediatric Neurology
Department of Neurology
The Cleveland Clinic Foundation
Cleveland, Ohio

ASSOCIATE EDITORS
Ajay Gupta, MD
Department of Neurology
The Cleveland Clinic Foundation
Cleveland, Ohio

Deepak K. Lachhwani, MBBS, MD
Department of Neurology
The Cleveland Clinic Foundation
Cleveland, Ohio

LIPPINCOTT WILLIAMS & WILKINS
A **Wolters Kluwer** Company
Philadelphia • Baltimore • New York • London
Buenos Aires • Hong Kong • Sydney • Tokyo

Acquisitions Editor: Fran DeStefano
Managing Editor: Leah Hayes
Project Manager: Nicole Walz
Senior Manufacturing Manager: Ben Rivera
Associate Director of Marketing : Adam Glazer
Designer Coordinator: Terry Mallon
Cover Designer: Andrew Gatto
Compositor: TechBooks
Printer: Quebecor World- Taunton

Library of Congress Catalogue-in-Publication Data

The treatment of epilepsy: principles and practice.—4th ed. / editor-in-chief, Elaine
  Wyllie; associate editors, Ajay Gupta, Deepak K. Lachhwani.
    p. ; cm.
  Includes bibliographical references and index.
  ISBN 0-7817-4995-6 (alk. paper)
  1. Epilepsy. I. Wyllie, Elaine. II. Gupta, Ajay, 1965-   III. Lachhwani, Deepak K.
  [DNLM: 1. Epilepsy–therapy. 2. Epilepsy–diagnosis. WL 385 T7833 2006]
  RC372.T68 2006 616.8'53–dc22

                                                                        2005022784

Care has been taken to confirm the accuracy of the information presented and to describe generally accepted practices. However, the authors, editors, and publisher are not responsible for errors or omissions or for any consequences from application of the information in this book and make no warranty, expressed or implied, with respect to the currency, completeness, or accuracy of the contents of the publication. Application of this information in a particular situation remains the professional responsibility of the practitioner.

The authors, editors, and publisher have exerted every effort to ensure that drug selection and dosage set forth in this text are in accordance with current recommendations and practice at the time of publication. However, in view of ongoing research, changes in government regulations, and the constant flow of information relating to drug therapy and drug reactions, the reader is urged to check the package insert for each drug for any change in indications and dosage and for added warnings and precautions. This is particularly important when the recommended agent is a new or infrequently employed drug.

Some drugs and medical devices presented in this publication have Food and Drug Administration (FDA) clearance for limited use in restricted research settings. It is the responsibility of the health care provider to ascertain the FDA status of each drug or device planned for use in their clinical practice.

To purchase additional copies of this book, call our customer service department at (800) 638-3030 or fax orders to (301) 223-2320. International customers should call (301)223-2300.

Visit Lippincott Williams & Wilkins on the Internet: at LWW.com. Lippincott Williams & Wilkins customer service representatives are available from 8:30 am to 6 pm, EST.

10 9 8 7 6 5 4 3 2

Cover: Brain MRI showing left hemispheric malformation of cortical development, and FDG-PET showing left hemispheric hypermetabolism, in a 2-month-old infant with catastrophic epilepsy. The child is free of seizures following left hemispherectomy.

To my father, Jim Rees, and our renewed relationship; to Amy, who honored us by marrying our son Jim and embracing our family; to Betsy, our son Bob's fiancé, who joins our family in love; to our two sons, aforementioned, who make us proud; and once again, to Bob, my partner in life.

–E.W.

To my wife, Vishali, and our children Isha and Nalin, for their love, inspiration, and joyful support for this project; and to my parents, who encouraged me to go the next mile.

–A.G.

To my parents Krishan and Hansa, my wife Pilar and our children Neel and Karishma, and my family, who are requisite for joy in every endeavor.

–D.L.

Contents

Foreword by Daniel H. Lowenstein, MD xi
Preface xiii
Contributing Authors xv

PART I: PATHOLOGIC SUBSTRATES AND MECHANISMS OF EPILEPTOGENESIS 1

Section A: Neurodevelopment and Pathological Substrates of Epilepsy

1. Atlas of Pathologic Substrates of Epilepsy 3
   Richard A. Prayson and Ajay Gupta
2. Human Nervous System Development and Malformations 13
   Harvey B. Sarnat and Laura Flores-Sarnat
3. Malformations of Cortical Development and Epilepsy 37
   William B. Dobyns and Ruben Kuzniecky
4. Hippocampal Anatomy and Hippocampal Sclerosis 55
   Imad Najm, Henri Duvernoy, and Stephan Schuele

Section B: Cellular Aspects of Epileptogenesis

5. Basic Cellular Neurophysiology 69
   Stephen W. Jones
6. Mechanisms of Epileptogenesis and Experimental Models of Seizures 91
   Imad Najm, Gabriel Möddel, and Damir Janigro

Section C: Genetics and Epidemiology

7. Genetic Aspects of Epilepsy and Genetics of Idiopathic Generalized Epilepsy 103
   Ajay Gupta and Ingrid E. Scheffer
8. Epidemiologic Aspects of Epilepsy 109
   Anne T. Berg
9. The Natural History of Seizures 117
   W. Allen Hauser

PART II: BASIC PRINCIPLES OF ELECTROENCEPHALOGRAPHY 125

10. Neurophysiologic Basis of the Electroencephalogram 127
    Erwin-Josef Speckmann, Christian E. Elger, and Ulrich Altrup

11. Localization and Field Determination in Electroencephalography and Magnetoencephalography 141
    Richard C. Burgess, Masaki Iwasaki, and Dileep Nair
12. Application of Electroencephalogrphy in the Diagnosis of Epilepsy 169
    David R. Chabolla and Gregory D. Cascino
13. Electroencephalographic Atlas of Epileptiform Abnormalities 183
    Soheyl Noachtar and Elaine Wyllie

PART III: EPILEPTIC SEIZURES AND SYNDROMES 215

Section A: Epileptic Seizures

14. Classification of Seizures 217
    Christoph Kellinghaus, Hans O. Lüders, and Elaine Wyllie
    Appendix: Proposal for Revised Clinical and Electrographic Classification of Epileptic Seizures: *Commission on Classification and Terminology of the International League Against Epilepsy (1981)* 222
15. Epileptic Auras 229
    Norman K. So
16. Focal Seizures With Impaired Consciousness 241
    Prakash Kotagal and Tobias Loddenkemper
17. Focal Motor Seizures, Epilepsia Partialis Continua, and Supplementary Sensorimotor Seizures 257
    Andreas V. Alexopoulos and Dudley S. Dinner
18. Generalized Tonic-Clonic Seizures 279
    Bruce J. Fisch and Piotr W. Olejniczak
19. Absence Seizures 305
    Selim R. Benbadis and Samuel F. Berkovic
20. Atypical Absence, Myoclonic, Tonic, and Atonic Seizures 317
    William O. Tatum IV and Kevin Farrell
21. Epileptic Spasms 333
    W. Donald Shields and Susan Koh

Section B: Epilepsy Syndromes: Diagnosis and Treatment

22. Classification of the Epilepsies 347
    Tobias Loddenkemper, Hans O. Lüders, Imad M. Najm, and Elaine Wyllie

Appendix: Proposal for Revised Classification of Epilepsies and Epileptic Syndromes: *Commission on Classification and Terminology of the International League Against Epilepsy (1989)* 354

23. **Symptomatic Focal Epilepsies** 365
Nancy Foldvary-Schaefer

24. **Idiopathic and Benign Partial Epilepsies of Childhood** 373
Elaine C. Wirrell, Carol S. Camfield, and Peter R. Camfield

25. **Idiopathic Generalized Epilepsy Syndromes of Childhood and Adolescence** 391
Tobias Loddenkemper, Selim R. Benbadis, Jose M. Serratosa, and Samuel F. Berkovic

26. **The Myoclonic Epilepsies** 407
Renzo Guerrini, Paolo Bonanni, Carla Marini, and Lucio Parmeggiani

27. **Encephalopathic Generalized Epilepsy and Lennox-Gastaut Syndrome** 429
Kevin Farrell and William O. Tatum IV

28. **Rasmussen's Encephalitis (Chronic Focal Encephalitis)** 441
François Dubeau

29. **Continuous Spike Wave of Slow Sleep and Landau-Kleffner Syndrome** 455
Brian Neville and J. Helen Cross

30. **Epilepsy with Reflex Seizures** 463
Benjamin G. Zifkin and Frederick Andermann

31. **Less Common Epilepsy Syndromes and Epilepsy Associated with Chromosomal Abnormalities** 477
Sophia Varadkar and J. Helen Cross

Section C: Diagnosis and Treatment of Seizures in Special Clinical Settings

32. **Neonatal Seizures** 487
Robert R. Clancy and Eli M. Mizrahi

33. **Febrile Seizures** 511
Michael Duchowny

34. **Posttraumatic Epilepsy** 521
Jayanthi Mani and Elizabeth Barry

35. **Epilepsy in the Setting of Cerebrovascular Disease** 527
Bernd Pohlmann-Eden, Martin Del Campo, Neil R. Friedman, and Deepak K. Lachhwani

36. **Epilepsy in the Setting of Neurocutaneous Syndromes** 537
Prakash Kotagal and Deepak K. Lachhwani

37. **Epilepsy in the Setting of Inherited Metabolic and Mitochondrial Disorders** 547
Linda D. Leary, Douglas R. Nordli, Jr., and Darryl C. De Vivo

38. **Seizures Associated with Nonneurologic Medical Conditions** 571
Stephan Eisenschenk and Robin L. Gilmore

39. **Epilepsy in Patients with Multiple Handicaps** 585
John M. Pellock

40. **Epilepsy in the Elderly** 593
Ilo E. Leppik and Angela K. Birnbaum

41. **Status Epilepticus** 605
James J. Riviello, Jr.

Section D: Differential Diagnosis of Epilepsy

42. **Psychogenic Nonepileptic Seizures** 623
Selim R. Benbadis

43. **Other Nonepileptic Paroxysmal Disorders** 631
John M. Pellock

PART IV: ANTIEPILEPTIC MEDICATIONS 643

Section A: General Principles of Antiepileptic Drug Therapy

44. **Antiepileptic Drug Development and Experimental Models** 645
Jacqueline A. French

45. **Pharmacokinetics and Pharmacodynamics of Antiepileptic Drugs** 655
Blaise F.D. Bourgeois
Appendix: Selected Drug Interactions Between Antiepileptic Drugs and Other Types of Medications 665
Kay C. Kyllonen and Ajay Gupta

46. **Pharmacokinetics of Antiepileptic Drugs in Infants and Children** 671
Gail D. Anderson and Jong M. Rho

47. **Initiation and Discontinuation of Antiepileptic Drugs** 681
Varda Gross Tsur, Christine O'Dell, and Shlomo Shinnar

48. **Hormones, Catamenial Epilepsy, and Reproductive and Bone Health in Epilepsy** 695
Martha J. Morrell

49. **Treatment of Epilepsy During Pregnancy** 705
Nancy Foldvary-Schaefer

50. **Treatment of Epilepsy in the Setting of Renal and Liver Disease** 719
Jane G. Boggs, Elizabeth Waterhouse, and Robert J. DeLorenzo

51. **Monitoring for Adverse Effects of Antiepileptic Drugs** 735
L. James Willmore, Andrew Pickens IV, and John M. Pellock

52. **Pharmacogenetics of Antiepileptic Medications** 747
Tracy A. Glauser and Diego A. Morita

Section B: Specific Antiepileptic Medications and Other Therapies

53. **Carbamazepine and Oxcarbazepine** 761
Carlos A. M. Guerreiro and Marilisa M. Guerreiro

54. **Valproate** 775
Blaise F. D. Bourgeois

55. Phenytoin and Fosphenytoin 785
Diego A. Morita and Tracy A. Glauser

56. Phenobarbital and Primidone 805
Blaise F. D. Bourgeois

57. Ethosuximide 817
Tracy A. Glauser and Diego A. Morita

58. Benzodiazepines 829
L. John Greenfield, Jr., Howard C. Rosenberg, and Richard W. Homan

59. Gabapentin and Pregabalin 855
Michael J. McLean and Barry E. Gidal

60. Lamotrigine 869
Frank G. Gilliam and Barry E. Gidal

61. Topiramate 877
Michael D. Privitera

62. Zonisamide 891
Timothy E. Welty

63. Levetiracetam 901
Joseph I. Sirven and Joseph F. Drazkowski

64. Tiagabine 907
Steven C. Schachter

65. Felbamate 913
R. Edward Faught

66. Vigabatrin 921
Elinor Ben-Menachem

67. Adrenocorticotropin and Steroids 931
Melinda A. Nolan and O. Carter Snead III

68. Newer Antiepileptic Drugs 939
Norman Delanty and Jacqueline A. French

69. Less Commonly Used Antiepileptic Drugs 947
Basim M. Uthman and Ahmad Beydoun

70. The Ketogenic Diet 961
Douglas R. Nordli, Jr. and Darryl C. De Vivo

71. Vagus Nerve Stimulation Therapy 969
James W. Wheless

PART V: EPILEPSY SURGERY 981

Section A: Identification of Candidates and Presurgical Evaluation

72. Issues of Medical Intractability for Surgical Candidacy 983
Patrick Kwan and Martin J. Brodie

73. Recognition of Potential Surgical Candidates and Video-Electroencephalographic Evaluation 993
Gregory D. Cascino

74. Magnetic Resonance Imaging Techniques in the Evaluation for Epilepsy Surgery 1009
Susanne Knake and P. Ellen Grant

75. The Intracarotid Amobarbital Procedure 1031
Max R. Trenerry and David W. Loring

76. Metabolic and Functional Neuroimaging 1041
William D. Gaillard

77. Intracranial Electroencephalography and Localization Studies 1059
Selim R. Benbadis, Elaine Wyllie, and William E. Bingaman

Section B: Epilepsy Surgery in Specific Settings

78. Hippocampal Sclerosis and Dual Pathology 1069
Evan J. Fertig and Susan S. Spencer

79. Resection for Uncontrolled Epilepsy in the Setting of Focal Lesions on MRI: Tumor, Vascular Malformation, Trauma, and Infarction 1087
Dennis D. Spencer and Alexandre C. Carpentier

80. Epilepsy Surgery in Focal Malformations of Cortical Development 1103
Jorge A. González-Martinez, Imad M. Najm, William E. Bingaman, and Paul M. Ruggieri

81. Hemispherectomy: Medications, Technical Approaches, and Results 1111
José Luis Montes, Jean-Pierre Farmer, Frederick Andermann, and Chantal Poulin

82. Epilepsy Surgery in the Absence of a Lesion on Magnetic Resonance Imaging 1125
Elson L. So

83. Epilepsy Surgery in Infants and Children 1143
Ajay Gupta, Elaine Wyllie, and William E. Bingaman

84. Corpus Callosotomy and Multiple Subpial Transections 1159
Michael C. Smith, Richard Byrne, and Andres M. Kanner

85. Newer Operative and Stereotactic Techniques and Their Application to Hypothalamic Hamartoma 1169
A. Simon Harvey and Jeremy L. Freeman

86. Outcome and Complications of Epilepsy Surgery 1175
Deepak K. Lachhwani and Elaine Wyllie

PART VI: PSYCHOSOCIAL ASPECTS OF EPILEPSY 1183

87. Cognitive Effects of Epilepsy and of Antiepileptic Medications 1185
Kimford J. Meador

88. Psychiatric Comorbidity of Epilepsy 1197
Steven C. Schachter

89. Driving and Social Issues in Epilepsy 1201
Joseph F. Drazkowski and Joseph I. Sirven

Appendix: Indications for Antiepileptic Drugs Sanctioned by the United States Food and Drug Administration 1211
Kay C. Kyllonen

Foreword

Few would argue with the proposition that these are extraordinary times in the world of epilepsy research and clinical epileptology. In the past decade, we have witnessed the identification of single gene mutations responsible for relatively pure forms of inherited epilepsy, the deciphering of network properties that underlie absence epilepsy, and remarkable advances in developmental neurobiology that have a direct bearing on the nature of brain malformations observed in patients with epilepsy. On the clinical side, there has been a flood of new pharmacologic therapies and a huge increase in awareness of the importance of early identification of patients with medically refractory epilepsy; advances in neuroimaging have fundamentally altered diagnostic evaluation; and patients are now having devices implanted into epileptogenic foci—devices that are designed to detect the onset of electrographic seizures and deliver a focal electrical stimulus or drug dose that will abort the progression of the seizure. And all this is but a small sampling of the progress being made!

These advances signify major contributions to the knowledge base and skill set that are required for the effective care of patients with epilepsy, and it is no wonder that epileptology has matured into a distinct subspecialty—one that must address the needs of patients of all ages and cuts across the disciplines of adult and pediatric neurology, neurosurgery, psychiatry, nursing, neuroradiology, neuropharmacology, and neuropsychiatry, among others. "Keeping up" with the knowledge and skills in these fields that are relevant to epilepsy is an increasingly impossible task. The very nature of the methods we use to access this information is changing almost daily. But one thing remains unchanged—the need for a sourcebook that is a reasonable balance between encyclopedic coverage and a judicious, succinct overview of a field. In this, the fourth edition of *The Treatment of Epilepsy: Principles & Practice*, Dr. Wyllie and her colleagues have once again provided us an essential tool for our trade. The intellectual firepower behind the creation of the chapters of this book is staggering, equaled only by the care and intensity of effort required by the editors to bring it all together into one very readable volume. Knowing the editors as I do, I suspect the motivation behind their effort was very simple: to help us in our work. As someone who has had this book within close reach since the first edition, I am grateful for the editors' continued success.

Daniel H. Lowenstein, MD
Professor of Neurology
University of California, San Francisco

Preface

Since starting work on the first edition of this book in 1989, it has been my privilege to assemble and weave together the work of hundreds of dedicated and talented authors, each of whom gave many hours of their time to provide chapters for these collections. The authors' efforts have been appreciated by physicians all over the world who care for adults and children with epilepsy. I know this for certain, because it has been my honor to meet many of these readers over the years. Their expressions of appreciation for the book have been a wellspring of inspiration to me, and I wish to pass them along to all of the contributors to this volume.

With this fourth edition, I was privileged to have the help of two associate editors, Ajay Gupta and Deepak Lachhwani, whose energy and hard work were important to bringing the project to fruition.

Also critical to the project were Dayle Nolan and the team at IntraMed Scientific and Leah Hayes and Charles Mitchell at Lippincott Williams & Wilkins.

Glaxo Welcome provided a generous educational grant that will enable this book to be available to a wider readership, including physicians in training.

The purpose of the book is to help us all do our best to care for our patients and their families. With the addition of sections on new developments in the diagnosis and treatment of epilepsy, we sincerely hope that this volume will meet the goal.

Elaine Wyllie

Contributing Authors

ANDREAS ALEXOPOULOS, MD Department of Neurology, The Cleveland Clinic Foundation, Cleveland, Ohio

ULRICH ALTRUP, MD Department of Neurology, Institute for Experimental Epilepsy Research, Muenster, Germany

FREDERICK ANDERMANN, MD, FRCPC Professor, Department of Neurology and Pediatrics, McGill University, Director, Epilepsy Service, Montreal Neurological Hospital & Institute, Montreal, Quebec, Canada

GAIL D. ANDERSON, PhD Department of Pharmacy, University of Washington, Seattle, Washington

ELIZABETH BARRY, MD Department of Neurology, University of Maryland, Baltimore, Maryland

SELIM R. BENBADIS, MD Associate Professor, Departments of Neurology and Neurosurgery, University of South Florida, Comprehensive Epilepsy Program, Tampa General Hospital, Tampa, Florida

ELINOR BEN-MENACHEM, MD, PhD Associate Professor, Department of Neurology, Sahlgrenska University Hospital, Goteborg , Sweden

ANNE T. BERG, PhD Department of Biological Sciences, Northern Illinois University, DeKalb, Illinois

SAMUEL F. BERKOVIC, MD Department of Medicine, University of Melbourne, Melboure, Australia

AHMAD BEYDOUN, MD Associate Professor, Department of Neurology, Clinical Neurophysiology Laboratories and Epilepsy Program, University of Michigan Hospital, Ann Arbor, Michigan

WILLIAM E. BINGAMAN, MD Head, Section of Epilepsy Surgery, Department of Neurosurgery, The Cleveland Clinic Foundation, Cleveland, Ohio

ANGELA K. BIRNBAUM, MD College of Pharmacy, University of Minnesota, Minneapolis, Minnesota

JANE BOGGS, MD Orlando Regional Healthcare, Epilepsy Services, Orlando, Florida

PAOLO BONANNI, MD Division of Child Neurology and Psychiatry, University of Pisa, IRCCS Foundazione Stella Maris, Pisa, Italy

BLAISE F. D. BOURGEOIS, MD Professor, Department of Neurology, Harvard Medical School, Division of Epilepsy and Clinical Neurophysiology, Harvard Medical School, Children's Hospital, Boston, Massachusetts

MARTIN J. BRODIE, MD Epilepsy Unit, Western Infirmary, Glasgow, Scotland

RICHARD C. BURGESS, MD Head, Section of Neurological Computing, Department of Neurology, The Cleveland Clinic Foundation, Cleveland, Ohio

RICHARD BYRNE, MD Department of Neurosurgery, Rush Medical College, Rush University Medical Center, Chicago, Illinois

CAROL S. CAMFIELD, MD, FRCPC Professor, Department of Pediatrics, Division of Child Neurology, Dalhousie University, Halifax, Nova Scotia, Canada

PETER R. CAMFIELD, MD Professor and Chair, Department of Pediatrics, Dalhousie University, Chief, Department of Pediatrics, IWK Grace Health Centre, Halifax, Nova Scotia, Canada

ALEXANDRE C. CARPENTIER, MD, PhD Resident, Department of Neurosurgery, Pitie-Salpetriere Hospital, University of Paris IV, Paris, France

GREGORY D. CASCINO, MD Professor, Department of Neurology, Mayo Medical School, Chair, Division of Epilepsy, Department of Neurology, Mayo Clinic, Rochester, Minnesota

DAVID R. CHABOLLA, MD Assistant Professor, Department of Neurology, Mayo College of Medicine, Mayo Clinic, Jacksonville, Florida

ROBERT CLANCY, MD Division of Neurosurgery, Children's Hospital of Philadelphia, Philadelphia, Pennsylvania

J. HELEN CROSS, MD Neurosciences Unit, The Wolfson Center, London, United Kingdom

NORMAN DELANTY, MD, MRCPI Consultant Neurologist, Departments of Clinical Neurological Sciences and Neurology, Royal College of Surgeons in Ireland, Consultant Neurologist, Beaumont Hospital, Dublin, Ireland

MARTIN DEL CAMPO, MD Department of Neurology and Electroencephalography, Toronto Western Hospital, Toronto, Ontario, Canada

ROBERT J. DELORENZO, MD, PhD, MPH George B. Blilty Professor of Neurology, Department of Neurology, Virginia Commonwealth University, Medical College of Virginia Hospital, Richmond, Virginia

DARRYL C. DE VIVO, MD Departments of Pediatrics and Neurology, Columbia University Medical Center, The Neurological Institute, New York, New York

DUDLEY DINNER, MD Department of Neurology, The Cleveland Clinic Foundation, Cleveland Ohio

WILLIAM DOBYNS, MD Professor, Departments of Human Genetics, Neurology and Pediatrics, University of Chicago, Chicago, Illinois

JOSEPH F. DRAZKOWSKI, MD Department of Neurology, Division of Epilepsy, Mayo Clinic Hospital, Phoenix, Arizona

FRANÇOIS DUBEAU, MD, FRCPC Montreal Neurological Hospital & Institute, Montreal, Quebec, Canada

MICHAEL DUCHOWNY, MD Clinical Professor, Departments of Neurology and Pediatrics, University of Miami School of Medicine, Director, Comprehensive Epilepsy Program, Department of Neurology, Miami Children's Hospital, Miami, Florida

HENRI M. DUVERNOY, MD Professor Emeritus, Department of Anatomy, University of France, Besangon, France

STEPHAN EISENSCHENK, MD Assistant Professor, Department of Neurology, University of Florida, Gainesville, Florida, Assistant Professor, Department of Neurology, Shands Hospital, Gainesville, Florida

CHRISTIAN E. ELGER, MD Department of Epileptology, University of Bonn, Bonn Germany

JEAN-PIERRE FARMER, MD, CM, FRCSC Director, Neuro-surgery Training Program, Pediatric Neurosurgeon, Department of Neurology, The Montreal Children's Hospital, McGill University Health Centre, Montreal, Quebec, Canada

KEVIN FARRELL, MD Professor, Division of Neurology, Department of Pediatrics, University of British Columbia, Director, Epilepsy Service, Children's and Women's Hospital, Vancouver, British Columbia, Canada

R. EDWARD FAUGHT, MD Professor and Vice Chairman, Department of Neurology, University of Alabama School of Medicine, University of Alabama at Birmingham Epilepsy Center, Birmingham, Alabama

EVAN J. FERTIG, MD Yale University School of Medicine, Department of Neurology, New Haven, Connecticut

BRUCE J. FISCH, MD Professor, Department of Neurology, Comprehensive Epilepsy Center, Louisiana State University School of Medicine, University, Memorial, and Children's Hospitals, New Orleans, Louisiana

LAURA FLORES-SARNAT, MD Head, Neurology Service, Instituto Nacional de Pediatría, Mexico City, Mexico, Professor of Pediatric Neurology at the Universidad Nacional Autónoma de Mexico, Falcultad de Medicina, Mexico.

NANCY FOLDVARY-SCHAEFER, DO Department of Neurology, The Cleveland Clinic Foundation, Cleveland, Ohio,

NEIL R. FRIEDMAN, MD Dept. of Neurology, Cleveland Clinic Foundation, Cleveland, Ohio

JEREMY L. FREEMAN, MD Children's Epilepsy Program, Department of Neurology, Murdoch Children's Research Institute, University of Melbourne, Department of Paediatrics, Royal Children's Hospital, Comprehensive Epilepsy Programme, Department of Neurology, Epilepsy Research Institute and Brain Research Institute, Austin Hospital, Melbourne, Australia

JACQUELINE A. FRENCH, MD Associate Professor, Department of Neurology, Associate Director, Penn Epilepsy Center, University of Pennsylvania, Philadelphia, Pennsylvania

WILLIAM D. GAILLARD, MD Associate Professor Departments of Pediatrics and Neurology, The George Washington University School of Medicine, Director, Comprehensive Pediatric Epilepsy Program, Children's National Medical Center, Washington, DC

BARRY E. GIDAL, PHARMD Associate Professor, Department of Neurology, School of Pharmacy, University of Wisconsin, Madison, Wisconsin

FRANK G. GILLIAM, MD MPH Neurological Institute, Columbia University, New York, New York

ROBIN L. GILMORE, MD Professor, Department of Neurology, University of Florida Brain Institute, Shands Hospital, Gainesville, Florida

TRACY A. GLAUSER, MD Associate Professor, Departments of Neurology and Pediatrics, University of Cincinnati School of Medicine, Director, Comprehensive Epilepsy Program, Cincinnati Children's Hospital Medical Center, Cincinnati, Ohio

JORGE A. GONZÁLEZ-MARTINEZ, MD, PhD Department of Neuro-surgery, The Cleveland Clinic Foundation, Cleveland, Ohio

P. ELLEN GRANT, MD Division Head, Pediatric Radiology, Massachusetts General Hospital for Children, Assistant Professor, Harvard Medical School, Athinoula A. Martinos Center for Biomedical Imaging, Boston, Massachusetts

L. JOHN GREENFIELD JR, MD, PhD Department of Neurology, Medical College of Ohio, Ruppert Health Center, Toledo, Ohio

CARLOS A. M. GUERREIRO, MD Department of Neurology, University of Campinas, Campinas, Brazil

MARILISA GUERREIRO, MD, PhD Department of Neurology, University of Campinas, Campinas, Brazil

RENZO GUERRINI, MD University of Pisa & IRCCS Fondazione, Stella Maris via dei Giacinti, Pisa, Italy

AJAY GUPTA, MD Department of Neurology, The Cleveland Clinic Foundation, Cleveland, Ohio

A. SIMON HARVEY, MD Royal Children's Hospital, Children's Epilepsy Program, Melbourne, Australia

W. ALLEN HAUSER, MD Professor, Department of Neurology, School of Public Health, Sergievsky Center, Columbia University College of Physicians and Surgeons, Department of Neurology, New York Presbyterian Hospital, New York, New York

RICHARD W. HOMAN, MD (DECEASED) Institute for Medical Humanities, University of Texas Medical Branch, Galveston, Texas

MASAKI IWASAKI, MD Department of Neurosurgery, Tohoku University, Aoba-ku, Japan

DAMIR JANIGRO, MD Department of Neurosurgery, The Cleveland Clinic Foundation, Cleveland, Ohio

STEPHEN W. JONES, PhD Associate Professor, Departments of Physiology and Biophysics, Case Western Reserve University, Cleveland, Ohio

CHRISTOPH KELLINGHAUS, MD Department of Neurology, University of Münster, Münster, Germany

SUSANNE KNAKE, MD Department of Neurology, Section of Epilepsy, Philipps-University, Marburg Germany

SUSAN KOH, MD Division of Pediatric Neurology, David Geffen School of Medicine at UCLA, University of California, Los Angeles, California

PRAKASH KOTAGAL, MD Department of Neurology, Head, Section of Pediatric Epilepsy, The Cleveland Clinic Foundation, Cleveland, Ohio

RUBEN KUZNIECKY, MD Professor and Director, Epilepsy Center, Department of Neurology, University of Alabama at Birmingham, Birmingham, Alabama

PATRICK KWAN, MD Department of Medicine, United Christian Hospital, Kwun Tong, Hong Kong

KAY C. KYLLONEN, MD Department of Pharmacy, The Cleveland Clinic Foundation, Cleveland, Ohio

DEEPAK LACHHWANI, MD Department of Neurology, The Cleveland Clinic Foundation, Cleveland, Ohio

LINDA D. LEARY, MD Department of Neurology, Columbia University College of Physicians and Surgeons, New York Presbyterian Hospital, New York, New York

ILO E. LEPPIK, MD MINCEP Epilepsy Care, Minneapolis, College of Pharmacy and Department of Neurology, University of Minnesota, Minneapolis, Minnesota

TOBIAS LODDENKEMPER, MD Department of Neurology, The Cleveland Clinic Foundation, Cleveland, Ohio

DAVID W. LORING, MD Professor, Department of Neurology, Medical College of Georgia, Augusta, Georgia

HANS O. LÜDERS, MD, PhD Chairman, Department of Neurology, The Cleveland Clinic Foundation, Cleveland, Ohio

JAYANTHI MANI, MD, DM Consultant Neurologist and Epileptologist, Bombay Hospital, Mumbai, India

CARLA MARINI, MD Division of Child Neurology and Psychiatry, University of Pisa, IRCCS Foundazione Stella Maris, Pisa, Italy

MICHAEL J. MCLEAN, MD, PhD Associate Professor, Departments of Neurology and Pharmacology, Vanderbilt University Medical Center, Nashville, Tennessee

KIMFORD J. MEADOR, MD Department of Neurology, University of Florida, Gainesville, Florida

ELI M. MIZRAHI, MD Department of Neurology, Baylor College of Medicine, Houston, Texas

GABRIEL MÖDDEL, MD Department of Neurology, Münster University Clinic (UKM), Münster, Germany

JOSE L. MONTES, MD Associate Professor, Departments of Neurosurgery and Oncology,

McGill University, Director, Division of Neurosurgery, The Montreal Children's Hospital, McGill University Health Centre, Montreal, Quebec, Canada

DIEGO A. MORITA, MD Cincinnati Children's Hospital, Cincinnati Ohio

MARTHA MORRELL, MD Clinical Professor of Neurology, Department of Neurology, Stanford University School of Medicine, Stanford, California, Chief Medical Officer, NeuroPace, Inc., Mountain View, California

DILEEP NAIR, MD Department of Neurology, The Cleveland Clinic Foundation, Cleveland, Ohio

IMAD M. NAJM, MD Department of Neurology, The Cleveland Clinic Foundation, Cleveland, Ohio

BRIAN G. R. NEVILLE, MD, FRCP, FRCPCH Neurosciences Unit, The Wolfson Center, London, United Kingdom

SOHEYL NOACHTAR, MD Associate Professor, Department of Neurology, University of Munich, Head, Section of Epilepsy and Sleep Disorders, Klinikum Grosshadern, Munich, Germany

MELINDA A. NOLAN, MD Division of Neurology, University of Toronto, Toronto, Ontario, Canada

DOUGLAS R. NORDLI JR, MD Associate Professor, Department of Neurology, Director, Children's Epilepsy Center, Children's Memorial Hospital, Chicago, Illinois

CHRISTINE O'DELL, RN Albert Einstein College of Medicine, Montefiore Medical Center, Bronx, New York

PIOTR W. OLEJNICZAK, MD Epilepsy Center of Excellence, Louisiana State University Health Sciences Center, New Orleans, Louisiana

LUCIO PARMEGGIANI, MD Division of Child Neurology and Psychiatry, University of Pisa, IRCCS Foundazione Stella Maris, Pisa, Italy

JOHN M. PELLOCK, MD Professor, Department of Neurology, Pediatrics, and Pharmacy and Pharmaceutics, Chairman, Child Neurology, Department of Neurology, Medical College of Virginia, Virginia Commonwealth University, Richmond, Virginia

ANDREW PICKENS IV, MD Saint Louis University School of Medicine, St. Louis, Missouri

BERND POHLMANN-EDEN, MD Professor, Chefarzt des Epilepsie-Zentrums Bethel, Bielefeld, Germany

CHANTAL POULIN, MD Division of Neurology, Montreal Children's Hospital, Montreal Neurological Hospital/Institute, McGill Univeristy Health Centre, Montreal, Quebec, Canada

RICHARD PRAYSON, MD Department of Anatomic Pathology, The Cleveland Clinic Foundation, Cleveland, Ohio

MICHAEL D. PRIVITERA, MD Professor and Vice Chair Neurology, Director, Cincinnatti Epilepsy Center, University of Cincinnati Medical Center, Cincinnati, Ohio

JAMES J. RIVIELLO JR, MD Professor of Neurology Harvard Medical School. Division of Epilepsy and Clinical Neurophysiology, Critical Care Neurology Service, Department of Neurology, Children's Hospital, Boston, Massachusetts

JONG M. RHO, MD Barrow Neurological Institute, St. Joseph's Hospital and Medical Center, Phoenix, Arizona

HOWARD C. ROSENBERG, MD, PhD Professor and Chair, Department of Pharmacology and Therapeutics, Medical College of Ohio, Toledo, Ohio

PAUL M. RUGGIERI, MD Head, Section of MRI, Department of Radiology, The Cleveland Clinic Foundation, Cleveland, Ohio

HARVEY B. SARNAT, MD, FRCPC Division Chief, Paediatric Neurology, Calgary Health Region,

Alberta Children's Hospital, Calgary, Alberta, Canada

JOSE M. SERRATOSA, MD   Epilepsy Unit, Fundacion Jimenez Diaz Hospital, Madrid, Spain

STEVEN C. SCHACHTER, MD   Director of Research, Department of Neurology, Beth Israel Deaconess Medical Center, Boston, Massachusetts

INGRID SCHEFFER, MD   Department of Neurology, Austin and Repatriation Medical Centre, Melbourne, Australia

STEPHAN SCHUELE, MD   Department of Neurology, The Cleveland Clinic Foundation, Cleveland, Ohio

W. DONALD SHIELDS, MD   Division of Pediatric Neurology, Mattel Children's Hospital at UCLA, University of California, Los Angeles, California

SHLOMO SHINNAR, MD, PhD   Professor, Department of Neurology and Pediatrics, Albert Einstein College of Medicine, Director, Comprehensive Epilepsy Management Center, Montefiore Medical Center, Bronx, New York

JOSEPH I. SIRVEN, MD   Department of Neurology, Mayo Clinic Hospital, Phoenix, Arizona

MICHAEL C. SMITH, MD   Associate Professor, Department of Neurology, Rush Medical College, Director, Rush Epilepsy Center, Department of Neurology, Rush-Presbyterian-St. Luke's Medical Center, Chicago, Illinois

O. CARTER SNEAD III, MD   Professor, Departments of Pediatrics, Medicine, and Neurology, Head, Division of Neurology, University of Toronto, Department of Neurology, Hospital for Sick Children, Toronto, Ontario, Canada

NORMAN K. SO, MD   Medical Director, Department of Neurology, Oregon Comprehensive Epilepsy Program, Legacy Good Samaritan Hospital, Portland, Oregon

ELSON L. SO, MD   Director, Section of Electroencephalography, Mayo Clinic and Mayo Medical School, Rochester, Minnesota

ERWIN-JOSEF SPECKMANN, DR MED   Professor and Head, Institute of Physiology, Department of Neurophysiology, University of Muenster, Muenster, Germany

DENNIS D. SPENCER, MD   Professor and Chair, Department of Neurosurgery, Yale University School of Medicine, Neurosurgeon-in-Chief, Yale-New Haven Hospital, New Haven, Connecticut

SUSAN S. SPENCER, MD   Department of Neurology, Yale University School of Medicine, Yale-New Haven Hospital, New Haven, Connecticut

WILLIAM O. TATUM IV, DO   Clinical Associate Professor, Department of Neurology, University of South Florida, Vice-Chief, Department of Neurology, Tampa General Hospital, Tampa, Florida

MAX R. TRENERRY, MD, PhD   Department of Psychology, Mayo Clinic, Rochester, Minnesota

VARDA GROSS TSUR, MD   Neuropediatric Unit, Shaare Zedek Hospital, Jerusalem, Israel

BASIM M. UTHMAN, MD   Associate Professor, Departments of Neurology and Neuroscience, University of Florida College of Medicine, Assistant Chief, Neurology Service, Malcom Randall Veterans Affairs Medical Center, Gainesville, Florida

SOPHIA VARADKAR, MD   Institute for Child Health, London, United Kingdom

ELIZABETH WATERHOUSE, MD   Department of Neurology, Virginia Commonwealth University, Medical College of Virginia Hospital, Richmond, Virginia

TIMOTHY E. WELTY, PHARMD, BCPS   Associate Professor, Department of Pharmacy Practice, McWhorter School of Pharmacy, Stanford University, Clinical Pharmacy Specialist,

Department of Neurology, The Kirklin Clinic, Birmingham, Alabama

JAMES W. WHELESS, MD Professor and Chief of Pediatric Neurology, Le Bonheur Chair in Pediatric Neurology, University of Tennessee Health Science Center, Memphis, Tennessee

L. JAMES WILLMORE, MD Associate Dean and Professor of Neurology, St. Louis University, School of Medicine, St. Louis, Missouri

ELAINE WIRRELL, MD Alberta Children's Hospital, Calgary, Alberta, Canada

ELAINE WYLLIE, MD Head, Section of Pediatric Neurology, Department of Neurology, The Cleveland Clinic, Cleveland, Ohio

BENJAMIN G. ZIFKIN, MD, CM, FRCPC Hôpital du Sacre-Coeur de Montreal, Epilepsy Clinic, Montreal Neurological Hospital, Montreal, Quebec, Canada

The Treatment of Epilepsy

PRINCIPLES & PRACTICE

FOURTH EDITION

Part I

Pathologic Substrates and Mechanisms of Epileptogenesis

Section A NEURODEVELOPMENT AND PATHOLOGICAL SUBSTRATES OF EPILEPSY 3
1. Atlas of Pathologic Substrates of Epilepsy 3
2. Human Nervous System Development and Malformations 13
3. Malformations of Cortical Development and Epilepsy 37
4. Hippocampal Anatomy and Hippocampal Sclerosis 55

Section B CELLULAR ASPECTS OF EPILEPTOGENESIS 69
5. Basic Cellular Neurophysiology 69
6. Mechanisms of Epileptogenesis and Experimental Models of Seizures 91

Section C GENETICS AND EPIDEMIOLOGY 103
7. Genetic Aspects of Epilepsy and Genetics of Idiopathic Generalized Epilepsy 103
8. Epidemiologic Aspects of Epilepsy 109
9. The Natural History of Seizures 117

Atlas of Pathologic Substrates of Epilepsy

1

Richard A. Prayson   *Ajay Gupta*

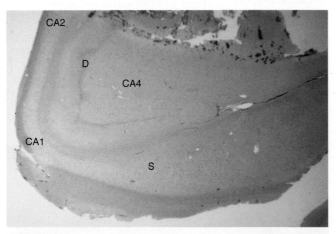

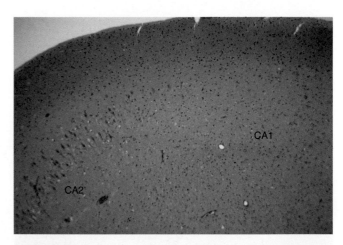

Figure 1.1 Low-magnification appearance of hippocampus in a patient with **hippocampal sclerosis (HS)**. An adult patient who underwent anterior temporal lobectomy for treatment of intractable temporal lobe epilepsy. HS is the most common cause of intractable partial epilepsy in adults. The disorder is generally marked by preferential loss of neurons in the dentate (D), CA4 region, CA1 region, and subiculum (S). A lesser degree of neuronal loss may be observed in the CA3 and CA2 regions. Loss of neurons is accompanied by **gliosis** and, in severe cases, by grossly evident atrophy.

Figure 1.2 Higher-magnification appearance of the hippocampus in **hippocampal sclerosis (HS)** at the interface between the CA2 and CA1 regions. There is a marked loss of neurons in the CA1 region with gliosis.

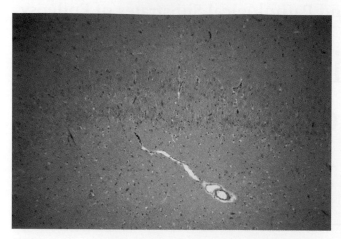

Figure 1.3 Histologic appearance of **double dentate,** marked by two bands of neurons in the hippocampus. This represents a form of hippocampal dysplasia, an infrequent cause of temporal lobe epilepsy that may be seen as a dysmorphic hippocampal formation on high-definition, three-dimensional, volume acquisition sequences on brain magnetic resonance imaging (MRI).

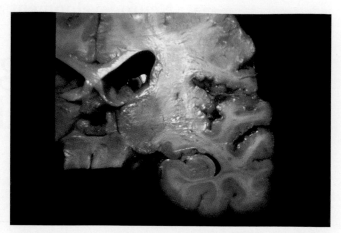

Figure 1.5 Gross appearance of **perisylvian polymicrogyria (micropolygyria),** marked by the focal presence of small, irregular gyri separated by shallow sulci. The cortex is often thinned and microscopically consists of two to four layers. The **leptomeninges** overlying polymicrogyria may be abnormally hypervascular because of a persistence of fetal leptomeningeal vascularization. (Photograph courtesy of Dr. Bette Kleinschmidt-DeMasters.) C congenital bilateral perisylvian polymicrogyria (CBPP) usually presents with seizures during childhood. Other clinical findings in patients with CBPP include pseudobulbar paresis, dysarthria, swallowing difficulties, and tongue paresis accompanied by the inability to protrude the tongue and perform lateral tongue movements.

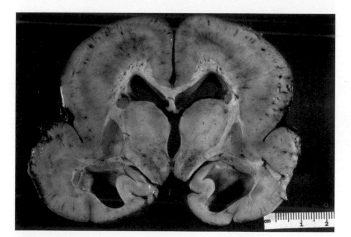

Figure 1.4 The gross appearance of **lissencephaly (agyria),** characterized by a lack of gyral formation and a decreased number of sulci. Note the enlargement of the ventricles, suggesting parenchymal volume loss. The cortex is usually thickened on cross section. Microscopically, an abnormally layered cortex is seen, typically three to five layers. Children with lissencephaly usually present with epileptic spasms, severe global developmental delay, microcephaly, and marked hypotonia during early infancy.

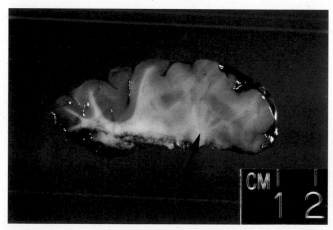

Figure 1.6 Gross appearance of **cortical dysplasia,** marked by an indistinct gray/white interface (right portion of cross section *[arrow]*) with evidence of gray matter tissue abnormally placed in the white matter (**nodular heterotopia**). Most of the focal cortical dysplasias are sporadic congenital malformations and, as a group, are an important cause of intractable epilepsy that is surgically remediable.

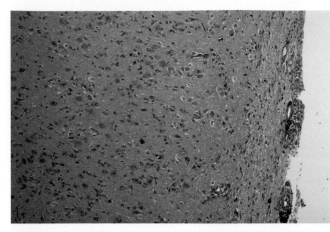

Figure 1.7 Histologic appearance of **cortical dysplasia,** marked by a loss of normal cortical lamination, increased cellularity, and malpositioning of neurons within the cortex. Neurons normally have their apical dendrites oriented perpendicular with respect to the surface of the brain.

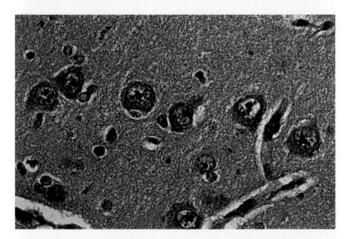

Figure 1.8 High-magnification appearance of neurons in cortical layer two of the parietal lobe in a patient with cortical dysplasia. The neurons are abnormally enlarged in size (**neuronal cytomegaly**), with no further evidence of dysmorphic features.

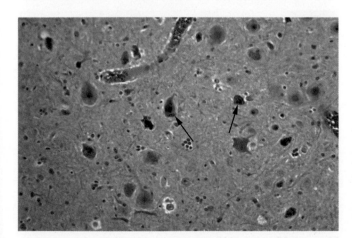

Figure 1.9 Histologic appearance of neurons in cortical layer three of the temporal lobe in a patient with cortical dysplasia. The neurons are marked by an abnormal cytologic appearance (**dysmorphic neurons**) (*arrows*), including abnormal nuclear morphology and atypical distribution of Nissl substance. In addition, neurons are haphazardly arranged within the cortex.

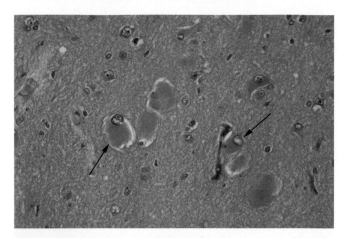

Figure 1.10 Histologic appearance of **balloon cells** (*arrows*) in the setting of cortical dysplasia. Balloon cells are marked histologically by the presence of abundant eosinophilic cytoplasm and eccentrically placed nuclei. **Multinucleation** may be observed. The derivation of these cells is still debated. A subset of balloon cells stain with markers of both glial differentiation (glial fibrillary acidic protein) and neural differentiation (neuron-specific enolase).

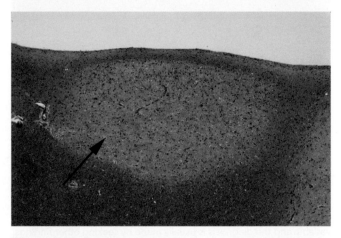

Figure 1.11 Microscopic appearance of a **subependymal nodular heterotopia** of gray matter (*arrow*). Microscopically, the nodule is marked by a mixture of neural and glial cells arranged in a disorganized fashion. Heterotopias are collections of mostly normal-appearing neurons in an abnormal location, presumably as a result of a disturbance in migration.

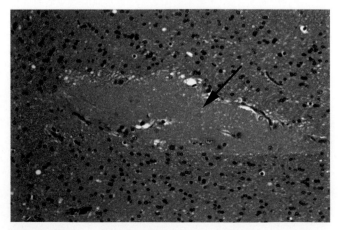

Figure 1.12 Small focus of **heterotopic gray matter** situated in the deep white matter of the frontal lobe region (*arrow*).

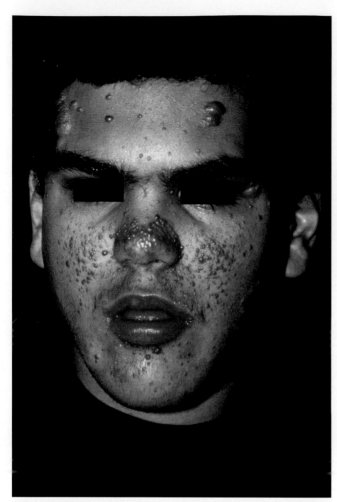

Figure 1.13 A patient with facial adenoma sebaceum, a diagnostic finding in **tuberous sclerosis (TS)**. TS is an autosomal dominant condition that involves multiple organs and systems, including the central nervous system (CNS). The clinical spectrum is highly variable and the diagnosis is usually made by seeking other findings, such as hypomelanotic skin patches, fibromatous skin plaques, dental pits, **ungual fibromas, retinal hamartomas,** cardiac rhabdomyomata, and renal cysts. TS is caused by mutations in the *TSC1* (hamartin) and *TSC2* (tuberin) genes located on chromosomes 9 and 16, respectively. The phenotype attributable to *TSC1* and *TSC2* mutations is generally difficult to distinguish clinically.

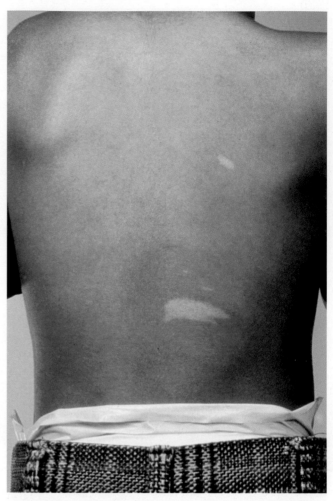

Figure 1.14 "Ash-leaf" macule in a patient with tuberous sclerosis. **Hypopigmented macules** may only be visible under ultraviolet light in patients with fair skin.

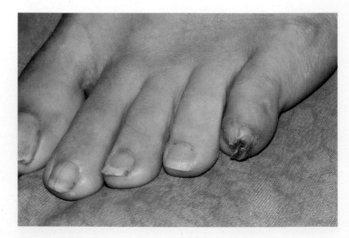

Figure 1.15 Ungual fibroma involving the little toe.

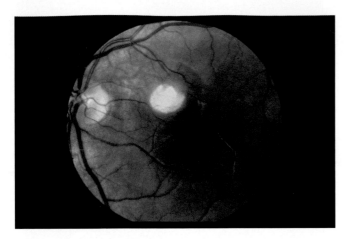

Figure 1.16   Retinal hamartoma seen on funduscopic examination.

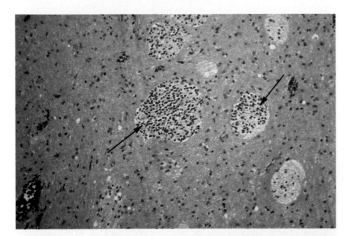

Figure 1.17   Histologic appearance of **hamartia** (arrows), characterized by an aggregation of small, immature-appearing neurons. This lesion most likely represents a form of cortical dysplasia and is seen in patients with tuberous sclerosis.

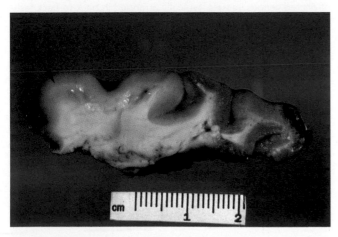

Figure 1.18   Gross appearance of a **cortical tuber,** marked by obliteration of the gray/white interface (leftmost gyrus [arrow]). Cortical tubers often have a firm consistency related to gliosis and **microcalcifications**. Other pathologic findings in the brains of patients with tuberous sclerosis include subependymal nodules and **giant cell astrocytomas,** typically located at the **foramen of Monro** and leading to obstructive **hydrocephalus** in some patients.

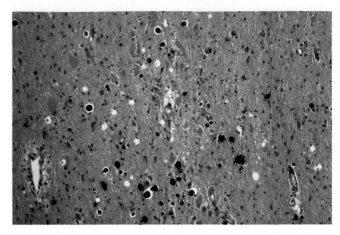

Figure 1.19   Histologic appearance of parenchyma from a **cortical tuber** in a patient with tuberous sclerosis. The histologic findings, which are generally those associated with cortical dysplasia, are marked by abnormal cortical lamination, a malorientation of neurons within the cortex, and dysmorphic neurons frequently accompanied by balloon cells. Microcalcifications are also prominently noted in this particular microscopic field.

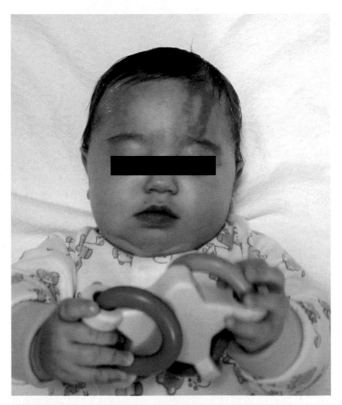

Figure 1.20   A child with **Sturge-Weber syndrome**. The presence of **nevus flammeus** in the distribution of the first division (ophthalmic) of the trigeminal nerve correlates highly with central nervous system involvement.

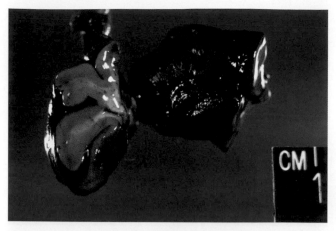

Figure 1.21 Cross sectional *(left)* and external *(right)* views from a resection in a patient with Sturge-Weber disease. The leptomeninges appear hemorrhagic because of a proliferation of vessels.

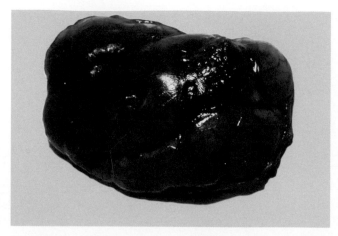

Figure 1.24 Gross appearance of a circumscribed hemorrhagic-appearing lesion situated in the temporal lobe, corresponding to a **cavernous angioma** *(arrow).*

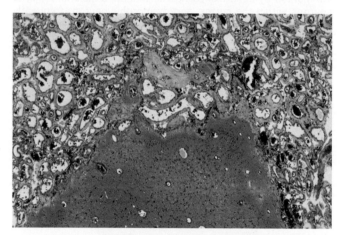

Figure 1.22 Histologic appearance of the leptomeninges in the setting of Sturge-Weber disease. The leptomeninges are marked by a proliferation of venous and capillary vessels arranged in a hemangiomatous configuration. There is no malignant potential to the lesion. The underlying cortex often demonstrates gliosis, with prominent microcalcifications.

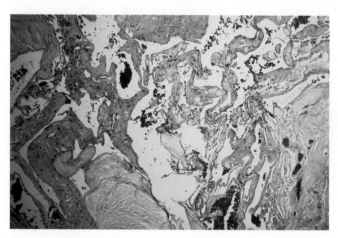

Figure 1.25 Microscopic appearance of the cavernous angioma in Figure 1.24. Cavernous angiomas are marked by a proliferation of dilated venous vessels, typically arranged in back-to-back fashion, without intervening neural parenchyma. Thickening of venous vessel walls may be observed. The lesions are often accompanied by adjacent gliosis and hemosiderin deposition.

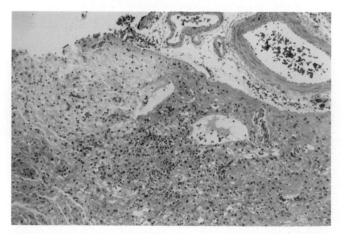

Figure 1.23 Histologic appearance of a **remote infarct,** resulting in chronic epilepsy. The parenchyma is marked by cystic degeneration accompanied by macrophages and gliosis. Note the relative sparing of the molecular layer, which is more commonly observed with infarcts versus contusions.

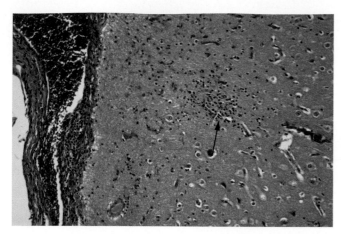

Figure 1.26 The histopathologic findings of **Rasmussen encephalitis** often resemble those of viral encephalitis. The findings that are illustrated here include leptomeningeal chronic inflammation, perivascular parenchymal inflammation with microglial nodule formation *(arrow)*, and gliosis. Rasmussen encephalitis typically presents with intractable partial seizures (usually focal motor seizures and epilepsia partialis continua), progressive hemiparesis, cognitive decline, and unilateral cerebral atrophy with early and prominent involvement of the insular region.

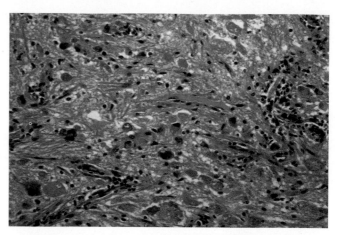

Figure 1.28 Histologic appearance of a **ganglioglioma**. The tumor represents a low-grade neoplasm (World Health Organization grade I). It is marked by a proliferation of atypical ganglion cells intermixed with an atypical gliomatous component, most commonly resembling a low-grade astrocytoma. Gangliogliomas arise most often in the temporal lobe, often in childhood, and are associated with cortical dysplasia. Perivascular chronic inflammation and eosinophilic granular bodies are also common features of this tumor type. This photomicrograph shows rare, atypical, large neuronal cells intermixed with a more spindle-cell glioma component.

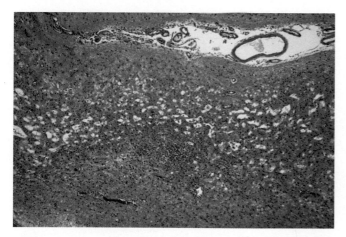

Figure 1.27 Many patients with Rasmussen encephalitis demonstrate cortical atrophy, which is seen here microscopically, and is marked by prominent gliosis, inflammation, and vacuolar degenerative changes in the cortex.

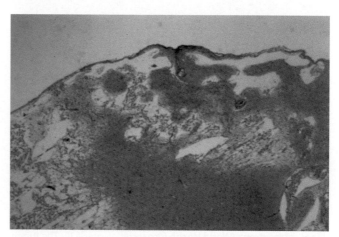

Figure 1.29 Low-magnification appearance of a temporal lobe **dysembryoplastic neuroepithelial tumor**. These World Health Organization grade I lesions arise most commonly in the temporal lobe and are predominantly cortical-based. Typically, they have a multinodular architectural pattern and a microcystic appearance, as seen in this photomicrograph.

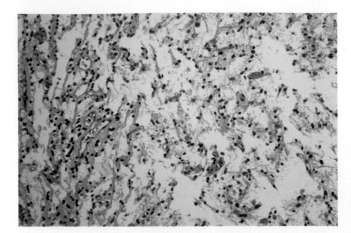

Figure 1.30 Higher-magnification appearance of a **dysembryoplastic neuroepithelial tumor** showing a proliferation of predominantly oligodendroglial-like rounded cells arranged against a mucoid background. Intermixed with these cells are smaller numbers of major-appearing neuronal cells and astrocytic cells. Dysembryoplastic neuroepithelial tumors are also frequently accompanied by adjacent cortical dysplasia.

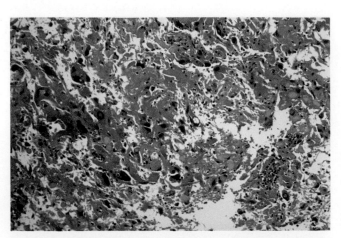

Figure 1.32 **Pleomorphic xanthoastrocytomas** are generally low-grade astrocytic tumors (World Health Organization grade II), marked by prominent hypercellularity and nuclear pleomorphism, lipidized astrocytic cells, perivascular lymphocytes, and increased reticulin staining between individual tumor cells. In contrast to high-grade astrocytic tumors, most pleomorphic xanthoastrocytomas lack appreciable mitotic activity or necrosis. The majority of these tumors arise either in the temporal or parietal lobe region in younger patients.

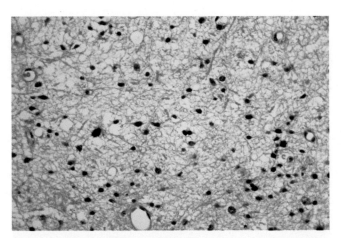

Figure 1.31 Histologic appearance of a **low-grade diffuse fibrillary astrocytoma** (World Health Organization grade II). The tumor is marked by a mildly hypercellular parenchyma and cytologic atypia, as evidenced by nuclear enlargement, and hyperchromasia and angularity to the nuclear contours. Areas of ganglioglioma may resemble low-grade astrocytoma, underscoring the importance of tissue sampling for identifying the atypical ganglion cell component that helps define ganglioglioma. This tumor has the potential of degenerating into a higher-grade lesion over time (**glioblastoma multiforme**).

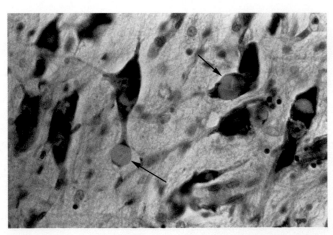

Figure 1.33 **Lafora bodies** (arrows) are intracytoplasmic neuronal polyglucosan structures that are seen in **Lafora disease,** which is an inherited, progressive myoclonic epilepsy syndrome. It is an autosomal-recessive disorder with onset in late childhood and in adolescence. Characteristic seizures include myoclonic and occipital lobe epilepsies with visual hallucinations, scotomata, and photoconvulsions. The disease leads to an inexorable decline in cognitive and neurologic functions, resulting in dementia and death, usually within 10 years of onset.

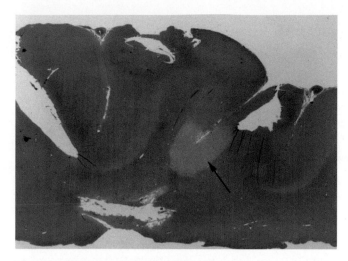

Figure 1.34 Invasive seizure monitoring with depth electrodes may occasionally result in infarcts associated with disruption of vessels. This low-magnification photomicrograph shows a pale zone of cortex *(arrow)* representing an acute infarct caused by placement of electrodes (**electrode-related infarct**).

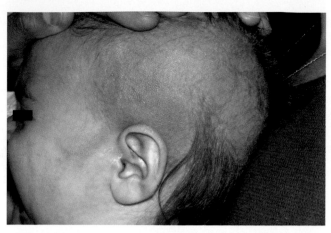

Figure 1.36 A child with a nevus on the cheek and left temple, extending onto the scalp with loss of hair. She presented with partial seizures. Her brain magnetic resonance image showed an extensive malformation of cortical development in the left temporoparietooccipital region. The constellation of findings suggests **epidermal nevus syndrome,** which is a sporadic condition.

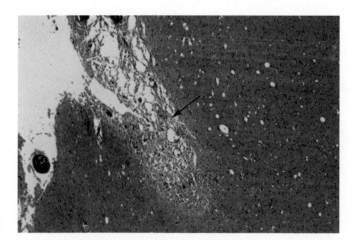

Figure 1.35 The tract along which a depth electrode was placed is observed. Evidence of **infarct/contusion along the electrode tract** as marked by vacuolated changes, surrounding gliosis, and a macrophage infiltrate *(arrow).*

Human Nervous System Development and Malformations

2

Harvey B. Sarnat   *Laura Flores-Sarnat*

Development of the brain, both normal and abnormal, is the result of genetically determined events that occur sequentially but often with so much overlap as to be almost simultaneous. At times, abnormal development may be the residual of acquired, nongenetic lesions of the brain, such as infarcts or hemorrhages, that interfere with processes still incomplete during fetal life, but this pathogenesis of cerebral malformations is less frequent (1).

The scope of modern embryology encompasses both classical descriptive morphogenesis and molecular genetic programming of ontogenesis. The term *maturation* implies both *growth*, a measurement of physical characteristics over time, and *development*, the acquisition of metabolic functions, synaptic circuits, reflexes, secretory and other cellular functions, sensory awareness, motor skills, language, and intellect. For neurons, maturation includes the development of an energy production system to actively maintain a resting membrane potential, the synthesis of neurotransmitters, and the formation of membrane receptors responsive to those molecules. Membrane receptors respond to various transmitters at synapses, to a variety of trophic and adhesion molecules, and, during development, to substances that either attract or repel growing axons in their intermediate and final trajectories. Molecular genetic data are accumulating rapidly because of intense interest in this key to understanding neuroembryology, including *neural induction*, the influence of one immature cell or tissue on another in development (2,3).

This chapter provides an overview of development in general, with a focus on the cerebral cortex and the ontogenetic processes that may lead to abnormal architecture, or *cerebral dysgenesis*, which may be expressed clinically and electrographically in part as epilepsy.

NORMAL ONTOGENESIS

Maturation progresses predictably and precisely. Insults that adversely affect maturational events occur at a particular time. Some insults are brief (e.g., a single exposure to a toxin), whereas others, such as congenital infections, diabetes mellitus, and genetic or chromosomal defects, act over many weeks or throughout gestation. Even genetic disorders may be timed, however, because genetic expression is not constant throughout ontogenesis and many genes change function between early and later periods of embryonic and fetal development. Maturation of the nervous system may be summarized as a genetically programmed series of anatomic and physiologic events: gastrulation; neurulation; segmentation; neural crest separation and migration; mitotic proliferation; apoptosis; neuroblast and glioblast migration; axonal pathfinding; dendritic ramification and synaptogenesis; membrane excitability; membrane receptors; biosynthesis and secretion of neurotransmitters; myelination.

In addition to the architectural organization of the tissue in each part of the neural tube, each cell derived from neuroepithelium—neurons, glial cells, and ependymal cells—also matures and undergoes further specialization. A *neuroepithelial cell*, even though still in the mitotic cycle, may already have a genetic program to differentiate as a particular cellular type even before the last division has occurred, although this program may be mutable in some circumstances. A *neuroblast* is a postmitotic cell too immature to be considered a neuron but committed to neuronal lineage. In this context, it differs from the term *blast* as it is used in the hematopoietic system, for example, in which the blast cells may still be in the mitotic cycle, unlike neuroblasts. For a neuroblast to become a neuron requires an electrically polarized membrane with an energy-producing system to maintain a resting membrane potential; synthesis of a secretory product (neurotransmitter); and membrane receptors to respond to extrinsic molecules not produced by this cell itself or to receive afferent innervation at synapses. Migratory neuroblasts to the cerebral cortex are still differentiating and may already project early axons even before migration is completed; however, because they do not yet have dendrites, synapses, polarized membranes, or secretory function, they are not yet neurons. The common term *neuronal migration* is technically incorrect because mature neurons do not migrate. The correct term is *neuroblast migration*.

Gastrulation and Formation of the Neural Placode

Gastrulation is the "birthday" of the nervous system, the earliest time that a neuroepithelium can be distinguished. It occurs in the human embryo when the primitive streak and Henson node form. The axes of the vertebrate body are established with bilateral symmetry—rostral and caudal (i.e., anterior and posterior) ends, dorsal and ventral surfaces, and medial and lateral aspects relative to the midline. These axes also subserve gradients of genetic expression for further development.

Neurulation

The bending of the neural placode to form a neural groove and, eventually, a neural tube depends for closure on external forces from both surrounding mesodermal tissues and surface ectoderm (4–7), as well as an intrinsic component within the neural placode itself. The floor plate in the ventral midline is the first neuroepithelial region to differentiate, induced by the *Sonic hedgehog (SHH)* gene from the notochord (1,8). Floor plate cells assume a pyramidal or wedge shape, with a broad base ventrally and a narrow apex dorsally which faces the cavity that will become the central canal in the spinal cord; the wedge shape of each floor plate ependymal cell causes a physical bending of the two sides of the neural placode toward the midline to form a U-shaped structure and later a tube (4,8). Mechanical resistance by adhesion molecules outside the neuroepithelium also contribute to the fusion of the neural folds into a tube. The neural tube does not close at the two extremes of the placode but at some distance from each end. Beginning in the cervical region and extending both rostrally and caudally, the anterior neuropore closes at 24 days' and the posterior neuropore at 28 days' gestation. Located at the site of the lamina terminalis, the anterior neuropore is the origin of the telencephalon. The posterior neuropore is in the lumbosacral region; the lowest sacral and caudal sections of the future spinal cord form posterior to this site. Closure of the neural tube is not the simple bidirectional "zipperlike" mechanism once thought; several sites at each neuropore close separately (9–13).

The rostral end of the neural tube becomes the brain, but at no time in embryonic development is it a "cephalic ganglion." It fulfills the criteria of a true brain from the beginning, with a bilaterally symmetric architecture, a rostral midline position, somatotopic organization of its tissue, connections with other parts of the nervous system, and a predominance of intrinsic connections by interneurons rather than external connections of primary sensory or motor neurons (14).

Cleavage of forebrain occurs at about 5 weeks gestation. This process involves a midsagittal cleft to create two telencephalic hemispheres from the single prosencephalon (cerebral vesicle) that proceded them.

Segmentation of the Neural Tube

The embryonic neural tube is genetically programmed by several families of genes (e.g., *HOX, PAX, WNT, EN*) to divide into compartments, or *neuromeres*, by physical and chemical barriers that limit the longitudinal cellular migration and facilitate the aggregation of a particular type of neuron to form nuclei or a cortex (15–18). The boundaries of these neuromeres are formed by cellular processes that resemble radial glial processes and produce secretory products that repel migratory cells; mitotic activity at the boundaries of neuromeres also is less than within the neuromeres. The mesencephalic neuromere, the first distinct neuromere to appear, is sometimes regarded as a "master" that initiates the programming of other neuromere formation both rostral and caudal to the embryonic midbrain. The embryonic hindbrain divides into eight *rhombomeres*. Rhombomere 1 (r1), together with a posterior portion of the mesencephalic neuromere, forms the entire cerebellum except for the deep nuclei that are derived from r2. The most caudal rhombomere, r8, forms the most caudal part of the medulla oblongata and the entire spinal cord. The spinal cord only seems to be a highly segmented structure because its paired nerve roots are grouped by the segmentation of surrounding mesodermal tissues of the somites. The spinal cord is actually columnar, although there is somatotopic regionalization of neurons that is a secondary form of segmentation (19). Rhombomere 8 is also subdivided because each portion of the spinal cord is different than other regions in giving origin to either sympathetic or parasympathetic preganglionic neurons.

Rostral to the mesencephalic neuromere are six forebrain *prosomeres*: three diencephalic and three telencephalic (20). These six prosomeres form the various structures of the hypothalamus, thalamus, epithalamus, basal forebrain, deep telencephalic nuclei, and cerebral cortex.

The boundaries that identify neuromeres disappear after embryonic life. Neuromeres are important in the genetic programming of the central nervous system (CNS) because genes are expressed in some, but not all, of them and mediate the development of specific structures of the brain in those neuromeres. For example, in the brainstem, the human gene *ERG2* (*Krox20* in rodents) is expressed only in r3 and r5, the only hindbrain segments from which no neural crest tissue migrates. *HOXA1* (*HOX 1.6*) is expressed only in r4 to r7 and *HOX2.1* only in r8. *GBX2* is expressed only in r1 to r3. *WNT1*, *EN1*, and *EN2* are expressed only in the mesencephalic neuromere and r1. In the telencephalon, *EMX1* is expressed in the basal prosomere that forms the basal ganglia, but not in the one that forms the cerebral cortex. *EMX2*, by contrast, is expressed in the latter but not in the former. The selective neuromeric expression of the organizer genes is important to the normal ontogenesis of the CNS and also to its malformation. The ectopic expression of genes in neuromeres may be induced in animals by upregulation and is the basis of some dysgeneses. An example is retinoic acid (vitamin A), which upregulates certain genes; an excess produces neural tube defects and other malformations in animals and may be teratogenic in early human embryogenesis. The mutation or deletion of some genes also causes abnormal segmentation and malformation. A controversial example is the mutation of human *EMX2*, which results in schizencephaly (see Schizencephaly).

Neural Crest Separation and Migration

Almost immediately after neurulation, the tissue formed at the dorsal midline of the neural tube, shortly after closure, separates and migrates ventrally on either side of the neural tube from all rhombomeres except r3 and r5 (21–24). Except for the axons themselves, this neural crest tissue forms the peripheral nerves, including the Schwann cells, dorsal root ganglia, autonomic nerves and ganglia, melanocytes, and adipose tissue. It therefore becomes the entire peripheral nervous system, including the autonomic nervous system, and differentiates into a variety of cells of both ectodermal and mesodermal germ layer origin. An important rostral neural crest migration is from the midbrain neuromere; a small prosencephalic neural crest also contributes. The prosencephalic neural crest migrates as a vertical sheet in the midline of the head. The mesencephalic neural crest tissue migrates in waves as streams of cells. These cephalic neural crest tissues form the cranial vault, facial cartilage and bone, connective tissue, blood vessels, nerve investments, and the globes of the eyes except for the retina, lens, choroid, and iris, as well as strictly neural structures such as the ciliary ganglion. The rhombencephalic neural crest migrates in streams as well, but more as blocks of cells. Many inductive genetic and growth factors are essential to neural crest development and migration, including the SHH gene, bone morphogenetic proteins (BMPs), glial cell-derived growth factor, and transforming growth factor-β (22).

Mitotic Proliferation of Neuroblasts (Neuronogenesis)

After the neural tube closes, neuroepithelial cells proliferate exponentially in the ventricular zone, with most mitotic activity occurring at the ventricular surface (Fig. 2.1). The rate of division is greatest during the early first trimester in the spinal cord and brainstem and during the late first and early second trimester in the forebrain. Within the ventricular zone of the human fetal telencephalon, approximately 33 mitotic cycles provide the total number of neurons required for the mature cerebral cortex (25). The orientation of the mitotic spindle determines the immediate fate of the daughter cells. If the cleavage plane is perpendicular to the ventricular surface, the two daughter cells become equal neuroepithelial cells preparing for further mitosis. If the cleavage is parallel to the ventricular surface, the two daughter cells are unequal (asymmetric cleavage). The daughter cell at the ventricular surface becomes another neuroepithelial cell; the other separates from its ventricular attachment and becomes a postmitotic neuroblast ready to migrate to the cortical plate. Furthermore, the products of two genes that determine cell fate, called *numb* and *notch*, are on different sides of the neuroepithelial cell. With symmetric cleavage, both daughter cells receive the same amount of each; with asymmetric cleavage, the cells receive unequal ratios of each, which also influences their subsequent development (26–28). The transcription product of *numb* and a related protein, *numblike*, maintains self-renewal properties of neural progenitor cells to generate the correct number of cells for the mature brain (29,30). Other genes influence mitotic cycling as well, and their mutation accounts for some cases of primary microcephaly and a thin cerebral mantle (see Disorders of Mitotic Proliferation and Apoptosis).

Active mitoses cease well before birth in most parts of the human nervous system, but retaining a potential for postnatal mitoses of neuroblasts are the periventricular region of the cerebral hemispheres (31) and, the best-documented site, the external granular layer of the cerebellar cortex, where mitoses persist until 1 year of age. Postnatal regeneration of these neurons, after most are destroyed by irradiation or cytotoxic drugs, is well documented in animals and probably occurs in humans as well. Primary olfactory receptor neurons also can regenerate. If they did not do so throughout life, the individual would become anosmic after a few upper respiratory infections, which transiently denude the nasal mucosa. Some undifferentiated neuroepithelial stem cells persist in the periventricular region of the mature brain, especially in the hippocampus, and might be induced to proliferate to replace neurons lost under pathologic conditions (32,33).

Apoptosis

Excessive neuroblasts are formed in every proliferative part of the embryonic, fetal, and, to some extent, the postnatal nervous system. *Apoptosis*, programmed cell death, restricts this overabundance until the definitive number of immature neurons is achieved (34). Apoptosis differs from necrosis, which might occur in infarcts. The many factors that arrest programmed cell death in the fetus are partly genetically determined and partly influenced by acquired events affecting the brain or spinal cord. Cells that do not match with targets are more vulnerable to degeneration than are those that achieve synaptic contact with other cells. Endocrine hormones and neuropeptides modulate apoptosis, as do the *c-FOS* gene and suppressor genes such as *BCL2*, which inhibit the expression of apoptotic genes. Growth factors—particularly four structurally related proteins: nerve growth factor (NGF), brain-derived neurotrophic factor (BDNF), neurotrophin-3 (NT3), and neurotrophin-4 (NT4)—modulate neural activity-dependent competition (35,36). NGF and BDNF are thus able to protect the neonatal brain against hypoxic/ischemic injury, an activity unique to the immature nervous system (37,38).

Apoptosis has two phases. The first phase involves undifferentiated neuroepithelial cells or neuroblasts with incomplete differentiation (first and second trimesters); the second phase involves fully differentiated neurons of the fetal brain and spinal cord (third trimester and postnatal period) that account for some progressive degenerative diseases such as spinal muscular atrophy. In normal development as well, mature neurons are eliminated to correct topographic targeting errors (39).

Neuroblast Migration

Neurons of the mature human brain occupy a different site from where they were generated, migrating to that site to establish synaptic connections with appropriate neighboring neurons and to send their axons in short or long trajectories to predetermined targets. The embryonic telencephalon consists of concentric layers. The subventricular zone ("germinal matrix") contains postmitotic, premigratory neuroblasts and glioblasts that are the source of radial migration. In general, maturing nerve cells move centrifugally, toward the brain surface. The cerebellar cortex is exceptional in that external granule cells first spread over the surface of the cerebellum and then migrate deep into the folia. Neuroblast migration begins at about 6 weeks' gestation in the human cerebrum and is not completed until at least 34 weeks of fetal life, although after midgestation most germinal matrix cells are glioblasts. Glioblasts continue to migrate until early in the postnatal period. Within the brainstem, neuroblast migration is complete by 2 months' gestation. Cerebellar external granule cells, by contrast, continue migrating until 18 months of age (40).

Most neuroblasts of the subventricular zone or germinal matrix reach the cerebral cortical plate by traveling radially along long, slender, centrifugal processes of specialized astrocytes of the subventricular zone called radial glial cells; the neuroblasts glide on the outside of these radial glial fibers as if they were on a monorail (Fig. 2.1). Facilitating gliding of neuroblasts along a radial glial fiber are specialized proteins such as astrotactin that are secreted by the neuroblast itself (41). The L1-CAM neural cell adhesion molecule is produced in the glial cell (42); other adhesion

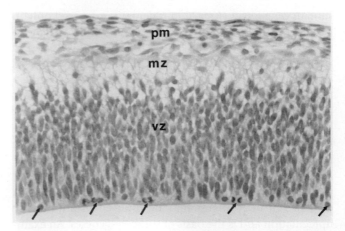

Figure 2.1   Cerebrum of a normal 6-week human fetus. Only two layers are recognized: an inner ventricular zone (vz), a neuroepithelium of undifferentiated cells undergoing mitotic proliferation at the ventricular surface, and an outer marginal zone (mz) containing the preplate plexus of neurons and their processes awaiting the arrival of the first wave of radial neuroblast migration. *Arrows* indicate neuroepithelial cells in active mitosis (hematoxylin and eosin stain).

molecules also facilitate gliding (43). Fetal ependymal cells have radiating processes that resemble those of the radial glial cell but do not extend beyond the germinal matrix and do not guide neuroblasts, although they do secrete molecules into the extracellular matrix (44,45). Some adhesion molecules of uncertain origin also reside in the extracellular matrix (46) where they serve as lubricants and adhesive factors between the membranes of the neuroblast and those of the radial glial fiber and also perhaps as nutritive and growth factors. The mechanism by which they stimulate cell movement is incompletely understood. Deficient molecules lead to defective migration. For example, *L1-CAM* is the defective genetic program in X-linked hydrocephalus accompanied by polymicrogyria and pachygyria (42).

The transformation of radial glial cells into astrocytes and ependymal cells begins during the first half of gestation and ends postnatally. During peak neuronal migration at midgestation, many radial glial cells remain attached to the ventricular and pial surfaces, lengthening and curving with the expansion and convolution of the cerebral wall. From 28 weeks' gestation to 6 years of age, astrocytes of the frontal lobe shift from the periventricular to the subcortical region. The centrifugal movement of this band of normal gliosis marks the end of neuronal migration in the cerebral mantle. Ependyma does not completely cover the surface of the lateral ventricles until 22 weeks' gestation (44).

Although the number of neuroblasts is far smaller, tangential migration also occurs (47,48) perpendicular to the radial fibers. The use of axonal rather than glial guides for migratory neuroblasts explains in part why all cells in a given region of cortex are not from the same clone or vertical column (49). Most tangentially migrating neuroblasts in the cerebral cortex originate from the ganglionic eminence, a large mass of neuroepithelial cells at the base of the telencephalon that later contribute to the basal ganglia.

Tangential migrations also occur in the brainstem, olfactory bulb, and subpial region.

Growth of Axons and Dendrites

During neuroblast migration, neurons remain largely undifferentiated, and the embryonic cerebral cortex at midgestation consists of vertical columns of tightly packed cells between radial blood vessels and extensive extracellular spaces. Cytodifferentiation begins with a proliferation of mainly endoplasmic reticulum and mitochondria in the cytoplasm and clumping of condensed nuclear chromatin at the inner margin of the nuclear membrane. Rough endoplasmic reticulum swells, and ribosomes proliferate.

The outgrowth of the axon precedes the development of dendrites, and the axon forms connections before dendrites begin to differentiate. The projection of the axon toward its destination was first recognized by Ramón y Cajal, who called it *cône d'accroissement* (growth cone). The chemical, endocrine, or electrotactic factors that guide the growth cone to its specific terminal synapse have long been a focus of controversy; however, growth cones are now known to be guided by diffusible molecules secreted along their pathway, such as netrins and semaphorins, and others attached to the cell surface, such as ephrins (50). Diffusible molecules are secreted by the processes of fetal ependymal cells and perhaps of glial cells (51–53). Some molecules, such as BDNF, netrin, and S-100β protein, attract growing axons, whereas the glycosaminoglycan *keratan sulfate* (not to be confused with the protein *keratin*) and the protein products of the gene *Slit* strongly repel them, preventing aberrant decussations and other deviations (51,54). Growth cone repulsion is sometimes called "collapsing" of the growth cone. Matrix proteins, such as laminin and fibronectin, also provide a substrate for axonal guidance. Proteins within the axonal growth cone itself, such as GAP43, may serve as intrinsic signal transduction in axonal guidance (55). Cell-to-cell attractions operate as the axon approaches its final target. Axonal transport, a later stage in axonogenesis, is regulated by phosphorylation of neurofilaments, a characteristic of neurofilament maturation (56). Genetic expression of several genes influences axonal growth cone projection; one of the most important is the *Wingless* (*WNT*) family (57).

Despite the long delay between the migration of an immature nerve cell and the beginning of dendritic growth, dendritic branching eventually accounts for more than 90% of the synaptic surface of the mature neuron and is specific for each type of neuron. Spines form on the dendrites as short protrusions with expanded tips, providing sites of synaptic membrane differentiation. Neurotrophins and calcium regulation are important for synaptic plasticity (58,59).

Electrical Polarity of the Cell Membrane

Membrane excitability is an important marker of neuronal maturation, but information is incomplete about its exact timing and duration. Membrane polarity is established before synaptogenesis and before the initiation of neurotransmitter biosynthesis. Because maintenance of a resting membrane potential requires continuous energy expenditure to fuel the sodium-potassium adenosine triphosphatase (ATPase) pump, it is beyond the capability of an undifferentiated neuroblast. The formation of ion channels within the neural membrane also enables the maintenance of a constant resting membrane potential.

Synaptogenesis

Synapses form after the development of dendritic spines and the polarization of the cell membrane. The relation of synaptogenesis to neuroblast migration differs in different parts of the nervous system. In the cerebral cortex, synaptogenesis always follows neuroblast migration. In the cerebellar cortex, however, the external granule cells develop axonal processes that become the long parallel fibers of the molecular layer and make synaptic contact with Purkinje cell dendrites before migrating through the molecular and Purkinje cell layer to their mature position within the folium. Afferent nerve fibers reach the neocortex early, before lamination occurs in the cortical plate. The first synapses are axodendritic and occur both external to and beneath the cortical plate in the future layers I and VI, the latter containing the first neurons of radial migration (see Ontogeny of Cerebral Neocortex).

An excessive number of synapses form on each neuron, with subsequent elimination of redundant ones. Outside the CNS, muscle fibers also receive multiple sources of innervation, later retaining only one. Transitory synapses also form at sites on neurons where they are not found at maturity. For example, the spinal motor neurons of newborn kittens display prominent synapses on their initial axonal segment, where they are never found in adult cats. Somatic spines are an important synaptic site on the embryonic Purkinje cell, but they and their synapses disappear as the dendritic tree develops.

A structural–functional correlation may be made in the developing visual cortex. In preterm infants of 24 to 25 weeks' gestation, the visual evoked potentials recorded at the occiput exhibit an initial long-latency negativity, but by 28 weeks' gestation, a small, positive wave precedes this negativity. This change corresponds to dendritic arborization and the formation of dendritic spines at that time. In the development of thalamocortical connections, major synaptic rearrangements are possible only during a critically defined period and not later (60).

The electroencephalogram (EEG) of the premature infant follows a predictable and time-linked progression in maturation that has been extensively studied. Reflecting synaptogenesis more closely than any other feature of cerebral maturation, the EEG provides a convenient, bedside, clinically useful measure of neurologic (i.e., electrocerebral) maturation in the preterm infant (1,61–63).

Biosynthesis and Release of Neurotransmitters and Formation of Transmitter Receptors

The synthesis of neurotransmitters and neuromodulating chemicals is based on the secretory character of the neuron, without which synaptic transmission is impossible. Several substances serve as transmitters: acetylcholine, monoamines (dopamine, norepinephrine, epinephrine, and serotonin), neuropeptides (substance P, somatostatin, and opioid-containing peptide chains such as the enkephalins), and simple amino acids (glutamic acid, aspartic acid, γ-aminobutyric acid [GABA], and glycine). Some transmitters (glycine, GABA, and acetylcholine in the CNS) are inhibitory. Each neuronal type produces a characteristic transmitter (motor neurons produce acetylcholine, cerebellar Purkinje cells, synthesize GABA; and granule cells produce glutamic acid in the adult). Neuropeptides may coexist with other types of transmitters in some neurons. Calcium ions are a strong trigger of neurotransmitter release, regardless of the transmitter's identity, and some synaptic vesicle proteins, such as synaptotagmin, serve as calcium sensors for this purpose (64).

In some parts of the brain, transitory fetal transmitters may appear during development and then disappear. Substance P and somatostatin are present in the fetal cerebellum at midgestation but are never found in the mature cerebellum. In the cerebral cortex of the frontal lobe, laminar distribution of cholinergic muscarinic receptors of the mature brain is the inverse of the fetal pattern. The functions of these transitory transmitter systems are unknown. Some act as trophic molecules rather than transmitters in early development. Even amino acid transmitters like GABA may have mainly a trophic function early in development. *In situ* hybridization and new immunocytochemical techniques demonstrate neurotransmitters in neurons of the developing brain of experimental animals, and these techniques also can be applied to human tissue (65). The ontogeny of neurotransmitter systems depends not only on the synthetic mechanisms of the specific chemical transmitters but also on the development of highly specific receptors of these chemical signals. That such receptors can modify the excitability of neuronal membranes and trigger action potentials after the recognition of specific molecules represent equally important components of the system of neurotransmission (66–68).

The development of receptors for neurotransmitters and specializations of the synaptic membrane are other important maturational processes of the neuron. Glutamate receptor expression and exact subunit composition, for example, are unique in each cell population and influence the cells' selective vulnerability during development (36).

Myelination

Myelin insulates individual axons and greatly increases speed of conduction. It is not essential in all nerves, and many autonomic fibers of the peripheral nervous system remain unmyelinated throughout life. Conduction velocity in central pathways coordinates time-related impulses from different centers that converge on a distant target and ensures that action potentials are not lost by synaptic block. The nervous system functions on the basis of temporal summation of impulses to relay messages across synapses.

Myelination of CNS pathways occurs in a predictable spatial and temporal sequence. Some tracts myelinate as early as 14 weeks' gestation and complete their cycle in a few weeks. Examples include the spinal roots, medial longitudinal fasciculus, dorsal columns of the spinal cord, and most cranial nerves. Between 22 and 24 weeks' gestation, myelination progresses in the olivary and cerebellar connections, the ansa lenticularis of the globus pallidus, the sensory trigeminal nerve, the auditory pathways, and the acoustic nerve, as well as in the trapezoid body, lateral lemniscus, and brachium of the inferior colliculus. By contrast, the optic nerve and the geniculocalcarine tract (i.e., optic radiations) do not begin to acquire myelin until near term. Some pathways have myelination cycles measured in years. The corpus callosum begins myelinating at 2 months postnatally, and the cycle is not complete until midadolescence. Some ipsilateral association fibers that connect the frontal with the temporal and parietal lobes do not achieve full myelination until about 32 years of age (69).

Myelination can now be accurately measured in specific central pathways of the living patient with the use of T2-weighted magnetic resonance imaging (MRI) sequences, albeit at a somewhat later time than with traditional myelin stains of brain tissue sections, such as Luxol fast blue. Newer neuropathologic methods that use gallocyanin and immunoreactivity to myelin basic protein may detect myelination even earlier than the traditional stains in postmortem tissue or in brain biopsy samples. Electron microscopy remains the most sensitive way to demonstrate the earliest myelination in tissue sections. Immunocytochemical markers of oligodendrocyte precursor cells provide another means of studying early myelination in the fetal brain (70).

SPECIAL FEATURES OF CEREBRAL CORTICAL DEVELOPMENT

What Is a Cortex?

Nuclear and *cortical* types of architecture characterize the vertebrate CNS. Neither pattern corresponds to the architecture of a ganglion in the peripheral nervous system (14). Nuclear organization is most common in the brainstem, most of the thalamus, and in the deep telencephalic nuclei (i.e., basal ganglia). It consists of aggregates of one or two types of neurons that often appear homogeneous and without special histologic arrangement but that actually have a highly defined somatotopic arrangement of synaptic relations. Scattered neurons along tracts, such as the fasciculus solitarius, the diagonal band of Broca, or the bed nucleus of the stria terminalis, also are regarded as nuclear architecture, even though not all neurons are in compact aggregates with sharply demarcated borders on histologic examination. Neuroanatomic nuclei may contain more than one type of neuron, either mixed together or segregated into clusters. Examples are the magnocellular and parvocellular parts of the red nucleus of the midbrain and the mixed large and small neurons comprising the caudate nucleus.

Cortical organization is a *laminated* architecture, with layers of neurons generally of the same type forming synaptic circuits with those of other layers. As a result, the synaptic architecture is columnar or perpendicular to the surface, whereas the histologic laminae are horizontal or parallel to the surface. Cortical architecture is just as early an evolutionary development as nuclear architecture, even though the mammalian cerebral neocortex is more recent. Cortical architecture is found in the cerebellar cortex of all vertebrates that possess a cerebellum; in many parts of the visual system, including the optic tectum (superior colliculus) of the midbrain, the lateral geniculate body of the thalamus, and the retina itself; and in the hippocampus or paleocortex, including both the dentate nucleus and the cornu ammonis. Many additional, small, inconspicuous brain regions also exhibit cortical lamination. An example is the islands of Calleja, which lie against the paraolfactory area of the basal forebrain. In these cup-shaped masses of neurons and polymorphic layers of pyramidal cells, fibers enter and leave at the opening of the cup or at the periphery. A cortex is defined, therefore, as a concentric laminar arrangement of neurons forming a band of gray matter with perpendicular columns of synaptic circuitry.

Ontogeny of the Cerebral Neocortex

The embryonic prosencephalon or cerebral vesicle "cleaves" sagittally in the midline at 33 days' gestation to form two symmetric telencephalic hemispheres. In the human fetus at 6 weeks' gestation, these consist of large ventricles not yet lined by ependyma that are surrounded by two concentric layers: a wide inner layer of neuroepithelium forming the ventricle wall, the *ventricular zone*, and an outer layer called the *marginal zone* (Fig. 2.2). The ventricular zone is a pseudostratified columnar epithelium in which every cell has a long cytoplasmic process; the proximal end is attached to the ventricular wall, and the distal end extends to the outer surface of the ventricular zone. The nucleus moves to and from within its own process, with a mitotic phase near the ventricular wall and a resting phase (S-phase) at the junctions with the marginal zone when DNA is being replicated in preparation for another mitosis (71,72).

The marginal zone, already a primordial cerebral cortex, has a plexus of bipolar neurons with long processes that extend in either direction parallel to the surface of the hemisphere. By 8 weeks' gestation, the cerebrum is more complex with more concentric zones (Fig. 2.3). The ventricular zone

persists, but peripheral to it is a *subventricular zone* of postmitotic, premigratory neuroblasts and radial glial cells; these specialized fetal astrocytes are not attached to the ventricular surface but have long processes extending to the pial surface of the brain to guide migratory neuroblasts and later glioblasts to the cortical plate. The next concentric zone is the *intermediate zone* of migrating neuroblasts and radial glial processes; it will later become the subcortical white matter. The former outermost or marginal zone, or the two-layer cerebrum, is no longer recognized as a single zone because it is divided by a cortical plate within its center as more neurons complete their journey from the subventricular zone. As the cortical plate forms, the outer portion of the marginal zone remains cell sparse, except for scattered Cajal-Retzius neurons, and is now called the *molecular layer*; the innermost part of the marginal zone beneath the cortical plate becomes the *subplate zone*. The cerebral cortex at this stage is said to be a four-layer structure, the outer layer being the molecular zone that will become layer 1 of the mature cortex. The second layer is the densely cellular cortical plate that corresponds to layers 2 through 6 of the mature cortex. The third layer is the subplate zone derived from the inner part of the previous marginal zone, and the fourth or deepest layer consists of still migrating neuroblasts within the intermediate zone. Arrest at this stage of development may result in malformations like some polymicrogyria and lissencephaly type 1 that have a four-layer cortex on histologic examination.

The radial neuroblast migration to the cortical plate occurs in waves and has an inside-out arrangement: the first wave becomes layer 6 because subsequent waves reach the cortical surface, displacing earlier arrivals into deeper positions. Layer 2 thus contains the most recently arrived neuroblasts. Layer 1 remains the oldest layer because it existed before radial migration began. Tangential migration occurs during all stages of radial migration, but particularly in the early stages. Before 22 weeks' gestation, the cerebral cortex appears histologically to be arranged as vertical columns of neurons rather than as horizontal layers and, indeed, the intracortical synaptic connections are columnar, more between than within layers (Fig. 2.4).

Further histogenesis of the cerebral cortical plate consists of the separation of the tightly packed individual neuroblasts by neuropil. This tissue is derived from the growth of dendritic processes and axons, synapse formation, and the addition of astrocytes migrating from the subventricular zone (i.e., germinal matrix), mostly during the second half of gestation, to become the protoplasmic astrocytes of the mature cerebral cortex. Lamination of the cortical plate is present from the onset, even if not yet evident histologically because of the tightly packed small cortical neurons, but becomes apparent as the neuropil increases and neurons grow (Fig. 2.3). The size of each layer is characteristic of the regional development of the neocortex. In the frontal lobe, the large pyramidal cells of layers 5 and 6 are prominent and numerous, but layer 4 is thin; in the occipital lobe,

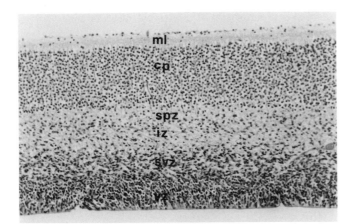

Figure 2.2 Cerebrum of a normal 10-week human fetus. A cortical plate (cp) is forming in the middle of the marginal zone, separating the superficial part that becomes the molecular layer (ml) and later layer 1 of the mature cortex from the deeper part of the former marginal zone, which is called the subplate zone (spz) and is later incorporated into layer 6. The intermediate zone (iz) contains radial glial processes with their migratory neuroblasts attached. The subventricular zone (svz) is the "germinal matrix" and contains postmitotic, premigratory neuroblasts and radial glial cell bodies, whereas the ventricular zone (vz) of neuroepithelium persists until the ependyma differentiates and stops all mitotic activity. The cortical plate consists of tightly packed immature neurons with little cytoplasm and little intervening neuropil, so that the layers of cortex and different types of cortical neurons are not yet histologically distinguished (hematoxylin and eosin stain; original magnification ×400).

layer 4 is most prominent and is even subdivided, whereas the large pyramidal cells of deeper layers are fewer. Radial glial cells are most prominent from 8 to 20 weeks' gestation and are fewer in the second half of gestation. The radial glial fibers are retracted and their specialized cells become fibrillary astrocytes in the white matter.

More than one type of neuron may appear in a particular layer at times, especially in restricted regions of cortex, and new neuronal types are still being discovered. Large spindle neurons appear after 4 months of age in the anterior cingulate gyrus (Brodmann area 24) and frontoinsular cortex. As much as four times larger than the large pyramidal neurons that populate most of layer 5, these bipolar cells have their axis perpendicular to the surface of the brain, large dendritic trees at either end, and a robust axon hillock. Like the neurons of the islands of Calleja, they exhibit serotonin-B and dopamine-D3 membrane receptors, but their origin and function are unknown (J. Allman, personal communication).

The ganglionic eminence is a densely cellular part of the subventricular zone of the early fetal forebrain that forms part of the deep telencephalic nuclei and contributes some neuroblasts to the cortex by tangential migration (Fig. 2.5).

Cajal-Retzius Neurons

These first mature neurons of the cerebral cortex are already secretory and functional before the first wave of

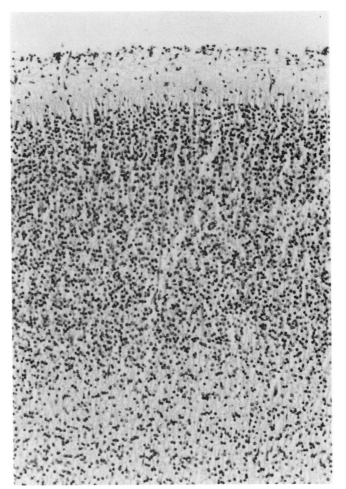

Figure 2.3 Cerebral cortex of a normal 22-week human fetus. Incipient cortical lamination is evident, although not as distinct as at older ages and considerable neuropil separates individual neurons (compare with the cortical plate in Fig. 2.2). This neuropil is mostly dentritic processes, axons, and some glial cells and their processes. Neurons of the cortex have more cytoplasm, and larger pyramidal cells of layers 3, 5, and 6 are distinguished from the smaller, rounder granule cells of layers 2 and 4. The cortical architecture is histologically transitional from a vertically columnar to a horizontally laminar appearance (hematoxylin and eosin stain; original magnification ×250).

radial migration of neuroblasts from the subventricular zone (73,74). Cajal-Retzius neurons form a plexus in the marginal zone, and, after the cortical plate begins to form, they make the initial intrinsic synaptic circuits of the primordial cerebral cortex, synapsing with neurons of layer 6 and eventually with neurons of all layers (73). Their bipolar long processes, which run parallel to the cortical surface, have numerous collateral axons that branch perpendicular to the main axon and plunge into the cortical plate; however, dendrites growing toward the cortical surface of deep cells also meet Cajal-Retzius axons in synaptic relation. As the cortex grows, Cajal-Retzius neurons become increasingly sparse in the molecular layer because no new ones are produced. They were thought to disappear at maturity by apoptosis, but they persist, albeit so diluted by the expansion of the cortex that only occasional examples are

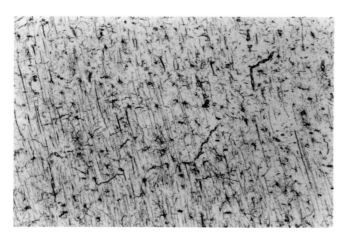

Figure 2.4 Radial glial fibers spanning the intermediate zone (future subcortical white matter) guiding migratory neuroblasts to the cortical plate as a "monorail." Their cells originate in the subventricular zone. (Vimentin immunoreactivity, original magnification ×250.)

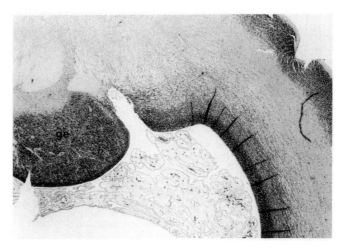

Figure 2.5 Parasagittal section through the ganglionic eminence (ge) in the subventricular zone of the telencephalon in a human fetus of 12 weeks' gestation. This aggregate of neuroepithelium contributes neuroblasts to the cerebral cortex by tangential migration and also provides cells for the development of the deep telencephalic nuclei (basal ganglia) (hematoxylin and eosin stain; original magnification ×100).

found in layer 1 of the neonatal brain and even rarer cells in the adult.

Cajal-Retzius neurons produce GABA, the first neurons of the cerebral cortex to do so. They also cosynthesize several calcium-binding proteins that act as secondary transmitters, including calbindin, parvalbumin, and possibly calretinin. Because neurons arising in the ganglionic eminence are GABAergic, this site has been proposed as the origin of these neurons of the marginal zone. The mesencephalic neuromere is another strong candidate site of origin, but where these early neurons actually come from remains uncertain. It is unlikely that they originate *in situ* from the molecular zone of the telencephalon, and they are not part of even the earliest radial migration from the subventricular zone.

Beyond helping to establish early intracortical synaptic circuitry and being an intrinsic part of the cortex, Cajal-Retzius neurons express several genes important in corticogenesis, including *Reelin* (*RLN*), *LIS1*, *EMX2*, and *DS-CAM*. These neurons also may have a role in cortical repair, particularly in fetal life and early infancy (75).

Subplate Neurons

Located deep in the marginal zone, these neurons are present before the first wave of radial neuroblast migration, similar to Cajal-Retzius neurons of the superficial aspect of the marginal zone (73). With maturation of the cerebral cortex, subplate neurons are incorporated into layer 6 and participate in mature synaptic networks within the cortex (76), but the subplate zone is a transitory fetal feature not present at term, unlike the molecular layer at the surface (77). The subplate zone at midgestation is cell sparse relative to the densely cellular cortical plate. Subplate neurons project descending *pioneer axons* to form the initial internal capsule as a template for the

large pyramidal cells of the deep cortical plate layers, whose long axons project through this provisional capsule as the permanent corticobulbar and corticospinal tracts (78). They also form the earliest commissural connections of the hippocampi.

Subplate neurons are involved in the formation of area-specific thalamocortical connections (79) and, by modulating BDNF and thalamocortical connectivity, of ocular dominance columns of the striate cortex (80,81). Subplate neuronal ablation in animals disrupts functional maturation in the visual cortical columns, including ocular dominance and orientation selectivity (80,82,83).

Gyration of the Cerebral Cortex

Folding tissue is an efficient way to increase surface area without concomitantly increasing its mass. The villi of the intestinal mucosa, the alveoli of lungs, and the gills of fishes are examples of absorptive and gas-exchange surfaces. Laminar architecture of neural tissue does not require a large surface area for absorption; it requires a large surface area to enable as much synaptic diversity as possible with the greatest number of ascending synaptic columns. For this reason, convolutions form in the cortex of many mammals. Rodents and rabbits retain a smooth cerebrum because the limited number of neurons does not require folding to achieve synaptic diversity. The degree of gyration does not, however, correspond to intelligence. The cow has as highly convoluted a brain as does the human, and the whale brain is even more convoluted. Among nonplacental mammals, the opossum and kangaroo have smooth brains, whereas in the more primitive egg-laying monotremes, such as the platypus, the cortex is convoluted.

Abnormalities in gyration are often associated with disturbances in neuroblast migration (see Disorders of Neuroblast Migration), but the abnormal migration itself does not cause normal gyration to fail. More than 90% of neuroblast migration is complete by midgestation, but the brain is still a relatively smooth cortex with only the sylvian and calcarine fissures evident at 20 weeks. Gyri and sulci form in the second half of human gestation in response to the expansion of the neuropil between neurons (i.e., the ramification of dendrites and growth of axons), the addition of glial cells migrating from the germinal matrix (subventricular zone), and the growth in size of all cells. Gyration of the cerebral cortex is as precise and time linked as other genetically programmed developmental processes of the nervous system, and the external examination of the fetal or premature neonatal brain at autopsy allows determination of gestational age within a 2-week period.

Development of Forebrain Commissures

The corpus callosum is the largest interhemispheric commissure. Its axons arise mainly from the small pyramidal neurons of layer 3, from all parts of the neocortex. The first callosal axons traverse the midline at 74 days, almost 3 weeks after formation of the two smaller forebrain commissures—the anterior commissure and psalterium or hippocampal commissure—at 54 days' gestation (1). The corpus callosum develops with a gradient, so that the rostrum forms earlier than the splenium.

Callosal axons initially have many collateral axons that project diffusely; with maturation, however, many collaterals retract, leaving fewer, but more specific, projections. Myelination of the corpus callosum does not begin until about 4 months postnatally and is completed in midadolescence. Callosal fibers are mainly inhibitory, an important consideration in their role in the propagation of epileptic activity, kindling, and the effects of corpus callosotomy. The anterior commissure mainly interconnects the anterior temporal lobes.

Ontogeny of the Paleocortex (Hippocampus)

The dentate gyrus and cornu ammonis are the earliest regions of the telencephalic cortex to differentiate. They develop within the dorsomedial wall of the cerebral hemisphere adjacent to the lamina terminalis at about 37 days postovulation. The cornu ammonis precedes, but the dentate gyrus follows, the formation of the olfactory bulbs (40,84,85). The hippocampal complex later rotates into a ventromedial position as the lateral ventricles and corpus callosum form, leaving as remnants a trail of unmigrated neurons at the dorsal surface of the corpus callosum, the *indusium griseum*, and the *septohippocampal nucleus* beneath the corpus callosum. The characteristic "sea horse" shape of the hippocampal complex becomes evident at 14 to 15 weeks' gestation.

At 9 weeks, the hippocampus consists of four layers: a ventricular zone of undifferentiated neuroepithelium, an intermediate zone of migratory neuroblasts, a homogeneous-appearing plate of bipolar neurons, and a wide marginal zone. By 15 to 19 weeks, individual subfields may be distinguished with a distal-to-proximal gradient of architectural and neuronal maturity. The radial migratory pattern from the ventricular zone is not the inside-out arrangement seen in the neocortex; the most superficial neurons of both the cornu ammonis and the dentate gyrus are from the earliest wave of migration and the deepest layer is the last migration. Three, rather than six, layers of neurons comprise the mature cornu ammonis and also the dentate gyrus, but the lamination is not as distinct as in the neocortex.

The subiculum, a transitional neocortical zone adjacent to the cornu ammonis, appears more advanced in development than the ammonic subfields, and the CA1 region of the cornu ammonis, next to the subiculum, is still less mature than other ammonic parts in the term neonate. The first ammonic subfield to mature is CA2 (Sommer sector), followed by CA4 (endplate neurons). The dentate gyrus assumes a mature cytoarchitecture only after 34 weeks; full adult maturity is not achieved until the second year of life. In young infants, immature neurons in the cornu ammonis are sometimes misinterpreted as resulting from hypoxic/ischemic injury in brain tissue for epilepsy surgery or at autopsy (40). Gradients of early to late maturation of dentate gyrus neurons are external to internal, suprapyramidal to infrapyramidal, and caudal to rostral in rats and humans.

GENETIC PROGRAMMING OF ONTOGENESIS

Organizer and Regulator Genes

All genes that program development can be broadly categorized as *organizers* or *regulators* (1–3). Organizer genes initiate and determine the fundamental axes of the body, segmentation, and the differentiation of tissues. Acting later, regulator genes determine differentiation of specific cellular types, secretory functions, and details of tissue architecture. These genes continue to act in adult life, conserving the identity of tissues and specific cellular characteristics. Many genes are antagonistic to others, and loss of this balance because of a defective genetic expression may result in apparent overexpression. For example, *SHH* has a strong ventralizing influence in the neural tube and is in equilibrium with genes exerting a strong dorsalizing influence, such as those of the BMP and some of the *paired homeobox (PAX)* families.

Organizer and regulator genes frequently are the same gene that serves one function early in ontogenesis and a different function later in development. Each has its period of expression and reexpression and also may activate, inhibit, or antagonize the expressions of other genes. Most genes that program neural development are not specific to the nervous system but program the development of other tissues and body systems as well.

Developmental defects of genetic expression involve a subtle but important semantic distinction between *overexpression* versus *upregulation* and *underexpression* versus *downregulation*. Overexpression and underexpression describe a genetic influence that appears too strong or too weak and that might be the result of a defective gene or loss of equilibrium with an antagonistic gene. Upregulation and downregulation, by contrast, indicate an increased or decreased transcription of a particular gene's messenger RNA, not simply the result of loss of antagonism.

Gradients of Genetic Expression in the Neural Tube

In addition to being temporally specific for the period of their expression, genes show spatial expression in some neuromeres and in some parts of neuromeres or specific cells. Most genes also show a gradient of descending expression in one or more of the three axes of the neural tube, being strongest at one site and showing extension to more distant areas, though of weaker expression. This phenomenon is illustrated in *holoprosencephaly*, in which the severity of the malformation is determined, in part, by the extent of the gradient of defective genetic expression in the vertical, rostrocaudal, and the mediolateral axes. These gradients can be recognized in this malformation regardless of which of the six identified genes is involved and even when the genetic defect is not yet demonstrated.

In the context of abnormal development of the neural tube, overexpression in the vertical axis (dorsoventral and ventrodorsal gradients) generally results in duplication or hyperplasia of structures, whereas underexpression results in noncleavage in the midline ("fusion") or hypoplasia of structures. Disorders of segmentation are related to disturbances of the genetic gradients of expression of certain genes—upregulation, downregulation, or ectopic expression.

CEREBRAL DYSGENESIS

No two cases of nervous system malformations are anatomically identical, even if both can be similarly categorized on brain MRI as in alobar holoprosencephaly, agenesis of the corpus callosum, or type 2 lissencephaly (1,86). Functional expression of anatomically similar cases also may vary widely. The anatomic defect does not always predict the clinical manifestations, such as the presence, type, or severity of epilepsy, mental retardation, cognitive deficits, visual impairment, or neuroendocrine dysfunction. Brain malformations could be ascribed to different

stages of development. Some genetic malformations, such as holoprosencephaly, begin much earlier in gestation (4–5 weeks) than others, such as lissencephaly (8–10 weeks).

Disorders of Gastrulation and Neurulation

Disturbances involving the zygote before or at gastrulation usually result in spontaneous abortion, although some early genes, if upregulated, may lead to duplication of structures and be one cause of conjoined twinning. Defects of neurulation are not usually lethal in the embryo or fetus and are a major cause of meningomyelocele and encephalocele with their attendant hydrocephalus and neurogenic bladder. Because epilepsy does not directly result from these types of neural tube defects, this topic is not discussed further in this chapter. Affected children have a higher incidence of epilepsy, however, because of secondary disturbances in ontogenesis.

Disorders of Neural Crest Separation and Migration

Many diseases of neural crest formation or migration are known as *neurocristopathies*. Two such examples, aganglionic megacolon (Hirschsprung disease) and familial dysautonomia (Riley-Day syndrome), are beyond the scope of this chapter. Hirschsprung disease associated with agenesis of the corpus callosum involves a mutation of *SIP1* (87). Abnormalities of mesencephalic neural crest may be associated with midfacial hypoplasia, hypotelorism, and cerebral malformations of midline cleavage, such as holoprosencephaly. Epilepsy is another complication in some cases. Disturbances in prosencephalic and mesencephalic neural crest migrations explain many cutaneous lesions and dysmorphic facial features of children with certain neurocutaneous syndromes, such as epidermal nevus and Waardenburg syndromes (88), as well as the hypo- and hypertelorism that occur in major cerebral dysgeneses (89–91).

Disorders of Segmentation

There are many murine models of ectopic genetic expression, reversal of rhombomeres, and hypoplasia or aplasia of certain neuromeres, but information on human disorders of neural tube segmentation mostly involves the hindbrain rhombomeres. A molecular genetic explanation of the Chiari II malformation is proposed on this basis (92), and congenital absence of the midbrain and metencephalon (rostral pons) with cerebellar hypoplasia in the human neonate closely resembles the mouse model of *En2* deletion (93). These disorders do not primarily involve the prosomeres, but congenital agenesis of the basal ganglia might be caused by mutation in candidate genes *EMX1*, *MASH1*, or *DLX* (94). These disorders are not discussed further.

Disorders of Mitotic Proliferation and Apoptosis

Any pathologic condition in the fetus that precociously arrests neuroepithelial cell proliferation and reduces the number of mitotic cycles needed to achieve the normal complement of neurons in the cerebral cortex results in micrencephaly (1). In severe cases, the brain may be very small and lack normal gyration or be totally lissencephalic (95,96) (Fig. 2.6). Further mitoses may be stopped by a genetic mutation or by an acquired condition, such as a congenital viral infection or teratogen inducing premature differentiation of the ependyma of the lateral ventricles (1).

Theoretically, a disease that accelerates apoptosis also could reduce the number of cerebral cortical neurons, but no disease of this type has been recognized. Spinal muscular atrophy is a prototype of apoptosis of motor neurons continuing beyond the time when it should have stopped (97); hence, a hypothetical disorder affecting cerebral cortical apoptosis is not without precedent in another part of the CNS. Several genes and proteins associated with primary hereditary microcephaly appear to act by regulating mitotic proliferation in the neuroepithelium, so that their downregulation or mutation results in an inadequate number of neurons in the cerebral cortex (98–100). Sotos syndrome, associated with macrocephaly and too many neurons, may be a disorder of insufficient

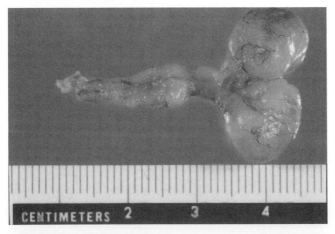

Figure 2.6 Global cerebral hypoplasia in a 20-week fetus. The cerebral hemispheres are tiny, and the entire brain weighs 2.3 g (expected weight for gestational age, 50 g). If this fetus had survived and been born at term, he would have been severely micrencephalic and the cortex would have remained lissencephalic. The etiology may be the result of a faulty gene that modulates mitotic proliferation and neuronogenesis, of excessive apoptosis in the neuroepithelium, or of an infection or toxin that induces precocious differentiation of the ependyma that arrests mitotic activity in the ventricular zone before the requisite number of neuroblasts are produced. (From Sarnat HB. *Cerebral dysgenesis. Embryology and clinical expression* p. 103. New York: Oxford University Press, 1992, with permission.)

apoptosis of cerebral cortical precursor cells (1). Despite a surplus of cortical neurons, affected children are mentally retarded.

Disorders of Neuroblast Migration

Nearly all brain malformations result from either faulty neuroblast migration or secondarily impaired migration. Imperfect cortical lamination, abnormal gyral development, subcortical heterotopia, and other focal dysplasias are related to some factor in fetal life—whether genetic, vascular, traumatic, metabolic, or infectious—that interferes with neuroblast migration. Disturbances in neuroblast migration represent the most important group of dysgeneses that affect the cerebral cortex, with epilepsy as one of the major clinical neurologic expressions.

The most severe migratory defects are often associated with early events in the gross formation of the neural tube and cerebral vesicles. Heterotopia of brainstem nuclei also occur. Later defects are expressed as generalized disorders of cortical lamination or gyration, such as lissencephaly, pachygyria, and cerebellar dysplasias. Insults in the third trimester cause more subtle or focal abnormalities of cerebral architecture. The genetic basis of hereditary migration disorders is better known than that of most disturbances in other developmental processes, such as neurulation and midline cleavage.

Disorders of neuroblast migration may be divided into anatomic groups corresponding to the stage during which the arrest occurred:

- Arrests before migration is initiated, with heterotopia in the subventricular zone, (e.g., periventricular nodular heterotopia)
- Arrests in the middle of migration, with heterotopia in the intermediate zone of subcortical white matter (e.g., subcortical laminar "band" heterotopia)
- Disturbances in arrangement of neurons within the cortical plate at the end of migration (e.g., lissencephaly)
- Overmigration beyond the limits of the pia mater (e.g., glioneuronal heterotopia in the leptomeninges)

None of the disorders is necessarily exclusive, however, so that primary disturbances of cortical lamination and architecture also may leave heterotopia in the white matter or overmigrated neurons in the meninges. The most frequent genetic forms of cerebral cortical dysgenesis are each associated with a particular single-gene mutation or deletion (Table 2.1) (101).

Heterotopia is a term derived from Greek that refers to cells abnormally displaced within their organ of origin, such as the brain. In the nervous system, heterotopic cells usually result from incomplete or arrested neuroblast migration along their migratory pathway. They may be single, apparently isolated neurons or nodules of gray matter within the white matter, often large enough to be demonstrated by

TABLE 2.1

LOCI AND GENES ASSOCIATED WITH CNS MALFORMATIONS THAT ARE NOT PRIMARY DISORDERS OF NEUROBLAST MIGRATION

Malformation	Trait	Locus	Gene or Transcription Factor
Holoprosencephaly	AD, AR	7q36-qter	Sonic hedgehog (*SHH*)
	AR; sporadic	13q32	*ZIC2*
	AR; sporadic	2q21	*SIX3*
	AR; sporadic	18p11.3	*TGIF*
	AR; sporadic	9q22.3	Patched (*PTCH*; an *SHH* receptor)
	AR; sporadic	10q11.2	*DKK* (head inducer)
Kallmann syndrome	XR	Xp22.3	*KAL1*; *EMX2*
Microcephaly, primary	AR	1q25-q32	*MCPH5*
Midbrain agenesis Cerebellar hypoplasia	?AR; sporadic	—	Engrailed 2 (*EN2*)
Rett syndrome	XD	Xq28	*MECP2*
Schizencephaly	AR	10q26.1	*EMX2*
Septo-optic-pituitary dysplasia	AR; sporadic	3p21.1-p21.2	*HESX1*; *PAX3*
Tuberous sclerosis	AD	9q34.3	*TSC1 hamartin*
	AD	16p13.2	*TSC2 tuberin*
X-linked hydrocephalus with pachygyria	XR	Xq28	*L1-CAM*

AD, autosomal dominant; AR, autosomal recessive; XD, X-linked dominant; XR, X-linked recessive
From Sarnat HB. Central nervous system malformations: gene locations of known human mutations. *Eur J Paediatr Neurol* 2003;7:43–45, with permission. See also Chapter 3 and Table 3.2 for genetic basis of primary neuroblast migratory disorders.

MRI, although the single neurons in white matter cannot be resolved by present imaging techniques. *Ectopia* refers to cells or whole tissues displaced outside their organ of origin. Ectopic neurons may occur in the leptomeninges, but within the brain they are heterotopic.

Abnormal convolutions or lack of gyration characterize many disturbances of neuroblast migration, but, as discussed, nearly all of that migration to the cortical plate occurs in the first half of gestation. Gyration occurs in the second half of gestation, influenced greatly by the formation of neurites and glia within the cortical plate that increases its volume. Lissencephaly is a smooth cerebral cortex without convolutions. At midgestation, the brain is essentially smooth; only the interhemispheric, sylvian, and calcarine fissures are formed. Gyri and sulci develop between 20 and 36 weeks' gestation. The mature pattern of gyration is evident at term, although parts of the cerebral cortex, such as the frontal lobes, are still relatively small. In lissencephaly type 1 (Miller-Dieker syndrome), the cerebral cortex remains relatively smooth or has only shallow grooves that do not correspond to normal sulci and are not evident on imaging. The histopathologic pattern is of a four-layer cortex in which the outermost layer 1 is the molecular layer, as in the normal six-layer neocortex. Layer 2 corresponds to layers 2 through 6 of normal neocortex; layer 3 is cell sparse as a persistent fetal subplate zone; and

layer 4 consists of incompletely migrated neurons in the subcortical intermediate zone. In lissencephaly type 2 (Walker-Warburg syndrome), a poorly laminated cortex with disorganized and disoriented neurons is seen histologically; the gross appearance is of a smooth brain or a few poorly formed sulci. The thin cerebral mantle suggests a disturbance of cell proliferation as well as of neuroblast migration. Malformations of the brainstem and cerebellum often are present. Lissencephalies (Walker-Warburg syndrome, Fukuyama-type muscular dystrophy, muscle-eye-brain disease of Santavuori) are genetic diseases with recently demonstrated specific mutations in genes responsible for glycosylation of α-dystroglycan at the plasma membrane of the cell (102). However, they also may be secondary to nongenetic disturbances of neuroepithelial proliferation or neuroblast migration. These include destructive encephaloclastic processes, such as congenital infections during fetal life, that markedly reduce the number of surviving cortical neurons.

Other abnormal gyral patterns also result from neuroblast migratory disorders (1,86). *Pachygyria* signifies abnormally large, poorly formed gyri, and may be present in some regions of cerebral cortex with lissencephaly in others. *Polymicrogyria* refers to excessively numerous and abnormally small gyri that similarly may coexist with pachygyria; it does not necessarily denote a primary migratory disorder of genetic origin. Small, poorly formed gyri may occur in zones of fetal ischemia, and they regularly surround porencephalic cysts caused by middle cerebral artery occlusion in fetal life. These disorders are discussed in more detail in Chapter 5.

Disorders of Neurite Growth

If a neuron faces the wrong direction in its final site, its axon is capable of reorienting itself as much as 180 degrees after emerging from the neuronal cell body. Dendrites, by contrast, conform strictly to the orientation of the cell body and do not change their axis. The dendritic tree becomes stunted if axodendritic synapses are not established.

Because so much dendritic differentiation and growth occurs during the last third of gestation and the first postnatal months, the preterm infant is particularly vulnerable to noxious influences that interfere with maturation of dendrites. Extraordinarily long dendrites of dentate granule cells and prominent basal dendrites of pyramidal cells have been described in term infants on life-support systems. Retardation of neuronal maturation in terms of dendrite development and spine morphology has been seen in premature infants, compared with term infants of the same conceptional age, possibly as a result of asphyxia. Infants with fetal alcohol syndrome also have a reduced number and abnormal geometry of dendritic spines of cortical neurons.

Traditional histologic examination of the brains of mentally retarded children often shows remarkably few alterations to account for a profound intellectual deficit. The study of dendritic morphology by the Golgi technique has revealed striking abnormalities in some of these cases. The alterations are best documented in chromosomal diseases, such as trisomy 13 and Down syndrome. Long, thin, tortuous dendritic spines and the absence of small, stubby spines are common. Children with unclassified mental retardation but normal chromosome numbers and morphology also exhibit defects in the number, length, and spatial arrangement of dendrites and synapses.

Cactus-like thickenings and loss of branchlet spines of cerebellar Purkinje cell dendrites occur in cerebellar dysplasias and hypoplasias. Abnormal development of the dendritic tree is also common in many metabolic encephalopathies, including Krabbe disease and other leukodystrophies, Menkes kinky-hair disease, gangliosidoses, ceroid lipofuscinosis, and Sanfilippo syndrome. Among genetically determined cerebral dysgeneses, aberrations in the structure and number of dendrites and spines are reported in cerebrohepatorenal (Zellweger) syndrome and in tuberous sclerosis.

Disorders of Myelination

Many metabolic diseases impede the rate of myelination. However, most genetic diseases that predominantly affect myelination also cause concurrent gray matter damage.

Examples are hypothyroidism and Menkes kinky-hair disease, a disorder of copper absorption and metabolism. Aminoacidurias, including phenylketonuria, are also associated with delayed myelination. The neuropathologic findings of Zellweger syndrome include disorders of neuroblast migration and of myelination. Krabbe disease and perinatal sudanophilic leukodystrophy are already expressed in fetal life with defective myelination.

Chronic hypoxia in premature infants is probably the most common cause of delayed myelination and contributes to the delay in clinical neurologic maturation. Acute, severe hypoxia in the fetus may delay myelination because oligodendrocyte precursor cells are particularly vulnerable to injury of this type and require time to replenish their number after massive loss (70). Myelination also depends on fatty acids that must be supplied by the maternal and infant diet; nutritional deficiencies during gestation or postnatally may result in delayed myelination and are clinically expressed as developmental delay. Unlike disorders of neuronal migration, delay in myelination is not necessarily irreversible; if the insult is removed, myelination may catch up to reach the appropriate level of maturity.

SELECTED CEREBRAL MALFORMATIONS PRIMARILY AFFECTING TELENCEPHALON

The following summary concerns developmental genetics of malformations affecting the cerebral cortex and highly associated with epilepsy. Many of these diseases also are expressed in subcortical structures, including the diencephalon, brainstem, and cerebellum. Dandy-Walker malformation, Chiari malformations (92), Joubert syndrome (103), midbrain-pontine agenesis (93), pontocerebellar hypoplasia (104), diplomyelia, and myelomeningocele, which primarily affect the brainstem, cerebellum, and spinal cord, are beyond the scope of this volume and are not discussed, but many of them also affect supratentorial structures, including the cerebral cortex. Brain MRI findings, a different classification scheme for brain malformations, natural history of epilepsy, and genetic testing/counseling for several of these dysgeneses are discussed in Chapter 5.

Holoprosencephaly

Holoprosencephaly, a malformation of cerebral midline noncleavage, occurs in 1 of 15,000 live births and in 1 of 250 spontaneous first-trimester abortuses, making it one of the most frequent malformations. The embryonic prosencephalon does not "cleave" into two distinct telencephalic hemispheres, and the frontal neocortex and hippocampus are continuous across the midline, with a single monoventricle instead of two lateral ventricles (1,86,105,106). Agenesis of the corpus callosum and of the olfactory bulbs and tracts are present in all but the mildest cases. Alobar, semilobar, and lobar variants have been described; a middle interhemispheric variant has recently been recognized (105–109). Each form has distinct imaging features. In the most severe, alobar form, a large "dorsal cyst" occupies the posterior half of the supratentorial intracranial space and sometimes expands through the anterior fontanelle to form a unique vertex encephalocele (110).

Six distinct genetic mutations have been demonstrated in various cases of holoprosencephaly (Table 2.1) (111–116), and each mutation is associated with each anatomic variant, so that the latter represents only an end-stage severity. Some genes, such as *SHH* and its receptor *PTCH*, have a strong ventrodorsal gradient of expression. Others, such as the zinc finger transcription factor gene *(ZIC2)*, have a dorsoventral gradient in the vertical plane. All have expression gradients in the longitudinal (rostrocaudal) and horizontal (mediolateral) axes as well, which determine many features of clinical presentation. At least 12 additional genetic loci are linked to a high incidence of holoprosencephaly, but the precise gene in these loci has not yet been identified. The six known genes together represent only approximately 20% of holoprosencephaly cases that have been studied by genetic methods. Holoprosencephaly occurs in children with Smith-Lemli-Opitz syndrome, an inborn metabolic disorder of cholesterol metabolism that affects the expression of *SHH* (117).

Some infants have a normal face. In others, midfacial hypoplasia ranges from mild hypotelorism with or without aplasia of the premaxilla and vomer bones, producing a unique midline cleft lip and palate, to cebocephaly with a single naris but preservation of the premaxilla, to cyclopia with a single median eye, a dorsal proboscis instead of a nose, a small mouth, and preserved premaxilla. These anomalies prompted DeMyers et al. to observe, "The face predicts the brain" (118), although exceptions abound. These facial features are probably related to the rostrocaudal gradient of genetic expression. If the gradient reaches the diencephalon, noncleavage of the thalamus and atresia of the third ventricle occur; if the gradient extends to involve the mesencephalic neuromere, there is noncleavage of the quadrigeminal plate and oculomotor nuclei as well as aqueductal atresia. Neural crest migration is affected, and the face does not form properly (110). Facial involvement is found in all anatomic variants of holoprosencephaly and often does not correlate with the severity of cerebral involvement. *ZIC2* and other genes expressed in dorsal regions are less associated with midfacial hypoplasia than those expressed in ventral regions of the vertical axis, such as *SHH* (119).

Children with holoprosencephaly have mental retardation, and more than 65% have diabetes insipidus as a result of posterior pituitary insufficiency; disturbances of anterior pituitary hormonal secretion are much less frequent (108). The olfactory bulbs and tracts, and sometimes the trigones, are aplastic (arhinencephaly) but may be only severely hypoplastic and fused at the base of the entorhinal cortex (1).

To exclude this anomaly, neurologic examination of the neonate should include testing of the olfactory reflex for cranial nerve I (120).

The severity of epilepsy varies. Of two infants with nearly identical morphologic forms of holoprosencephaly by imaging, or even by postmortem neuropathologic examination, one may have intractable seizures and the other no seizures or mild seizures easily controlled with a single medication. The difference may lie in the extent of the mediolateral gradient of genetic expression, as the parasagittal cortex is more severely disorganized than progressively more lateral regions, and the most lateral regions may show normal cortical lamination and architecture. Epilepsy also may be related to the degree of synaptic disorganization in the cortex (110). Overmigrated ectopic neurons in the leptomeninges and glioneuronal heterotopia extending beyond the pial membrane but still attached to the brain by a stalk are common in holoprosencephaly. These overmigrations may be related to absence of the external granular layer of Brun, a glial layer at the surface of the cerebral cortex in fetal life that disappears with maturation (1).

Septo-optic-Pituitary Dysplasia (De Morsier Syndrome)

In this disorder of midline noncleavage milder than holoprosencephaly, the septum pellucidum is absent, the optic nerves are hypoplastic, and the corpus callosum may be thin. The anterior pituitary is insufficient, with manifestations ranging from isolated growth hormone deficiency to panhypopituitarism. Patients may have normal intelligence, learning disabilities, or mental retardation. Visual impairment and endocrinopathies are common. Epilepsy is not universal, but the incidence of seizures is higher than normal. Several cases of this dysplasia have been linked to mutation in the gene *HESX1* (121), others to a *PAX3* mutation (122).

Periventricular Nodular Heterotopia

In this malformation, neuroepithelial cells in the subventricular zone mature *in situ* without migrating and form nodules of gray matter that may project into the ventricular lumen while retaining their ependymal lining. The nodules cannot establish their normally intended synaptic relations with the superficial cortex; however, in mice, and probably in humans, long axons of neurons in these nodules project radially to reach the cortex and thus influence electrocerebral activity (123). Axons also interconnect the subependymal nodules. The subependymal nodules occur in the walls of the lateral ventricles but not the third or fourth ventricles.

Whether these heterotopia are unilateral or bilateral, patients nearly always have seizure disorders that resist pharmacologic control. The multiple subependymal nodules are intrinsically epileptogenic, as shown by depth electrode recordings in humans (124). Nevertheless, the epileptic foci of clinical importance are not primarily in the heterotopic subependymal nodules but rather in the associated foci of dysplastic cerebral cortex; hence, they are accessible to surgical treatment if a strong focus is identified in a low-risk part of the cortex (125,126). Not all patients are epileptic, however. Micropolygyria and focal pachygyria sometimes are demonstrated, and there may be dysgenesis, but usually not total agenesis, of the corpus callosum. Hippocampal sclerosis is identified by MRI in some patients. Mental retardation is common in patients with severe epilepsy.

One well-defined form of bilateral periventricular nodular heterotopia occurs only in females and is transmitted as an X-linked dominant trait that usually is incompatible with male fetal survival. The locus is at Xq28, the site of many other, unrelated hereditary neurologic diseases, and the defective gene is *Filamin-A* (*FLN-A*, previously *Filamin-1*) (127,128). These girls and adult women usually have intractable seizure disorders. Other forms occur in both sexes and may be unilateral or bilateral; the genetic basis has not yet been demonstrated (128). Case reports describe patients with congenital nephrosis, gastrointestinal dysmotility, Ehlers-Danlos syndrome, and frontonasal dysplasia as variants, often in males (128). Tuberous sclerosis should be excluded in a child with periventricular gray matter nodules. Multiple subependymal nodules of hamartomas or even astrocytomas occur, but tuberous sclerosis has many cutaneous and other manifestations not found in periventricular nodular heterotopia. The subependymal nodules in tuberous sclerosis also tend to calcify, another feature that helps distinguish this disease. All forms of periventricular nodular heterotopia are well demonstrated by MRI and often can be recognized by computed tomography (CT) scans as well; the latter technique also distinguishes the calcified lesions of tuberous sclerosis.

Subcortical Laminar Heterotopia (Band Heterotopia; "Double Cortex")

This disorder represents an arrest of migratory neuroblasts in the subcortical white matter to form a band, sheet, or continuous nodules beneath the cerebral cortex. The subcortical sheet of gray matter heterotopia appears as a band on two-dimensional sections by imaging or histopathologic examination and has been called "double cortex" (Fig. 2.7). This term is misleading, because the subcortical sheet is neither a true cortex nor laminated, although the larger pyramidal cells tend to lie deeply. Whether early formation of the sheet physically obstructs passage of the next wave of neuroblasts or whether the abnormal genetic influence arrests migration is uncertain. Some neuroblasts reach the surface of the brain because a true cortex is formed. Areas of dysplasia and poor lamination are seen, but other regions appear histologically normal. Extensive

subcortical laminar heterotopia is generally an X-linked recessive trait found only in females that is caused by a defective gene named *doublecortin* (*DCX*) (129,130). A few males with the same genetic defect have survived postnatally, but they have more severe cerebral malformations, such as lissencephaly and microcephaly, than do the females. The females are mentally retarded and usually have severe epilepsy.

Many disorders of neuroblast migration have subcortical white matter heterotopia in the form of neuronal "nests" of gray matter or individual isolated neurons; the latter cannot be demonstrated during life with current imaging techniques. Even though individual neurons may appear isolated on tissue sections stained with hematoxylin and eosin, Nissl, or other histologic stains, special immunocytochemical techniques that demonstrate synaptic vesicle proteins show that these single neurons in white matter do have synaptic relations with other neurons and

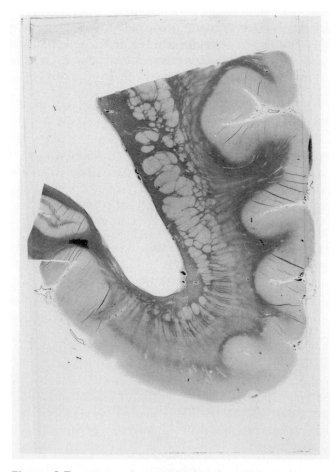

Figure 2.7 Section of occipital lobe of an adult woman with microcephaly, mental retardation, and intractable epilepsy since infancy, showing subcortical laminar heterotopia within the white matter between the surface cortical gray matter and the ventricular surface. This condition also is called "band heterotopia" and "double cortex," although the abnormal heterotopic layer is not a true cortex because it lacks the architectural organization implicit in the term *cortex*. (Luxol fest blue/periodic acid-Schiff (PAS) stain; original magnification ×40).

with the cortex. Therefore, they are not really isolated and may contribute to epileptogenic circuits (131).

Lissencephaly Type 1 (Miller-Dieker Syndrome)

Type 1 or "classic" lissencephaly is caused by a microdeletion at the 17p13.3 locus and mutation of the gene *LIS1* (132–134). This *LIS* family is normally expressed in both the primitive neuroepithelium and Cajal-Retzius neurons of the preplate plexus and layer 1 of the early fetal telencephalon, as well as in late fetal life (135).

The brain has characteristic neuropathologic features (1,86). Gross findings are best demonstrated by MRI. The entire cerebral cortex is smooth without gyration. Coronal sections show an abnormally thick cortex and thin white matter. Histologically, the cortex resembles the four-layer arrangement of the fetal cortical plate stage. A dysplastic or thin corpus callosum and hypoplasia of the cerebellar vermis are less constant features.

Lissencephaly Type 2 (Walker-Warburg Syndrome, Fukuyama Muscular Dystrophy, Muscle-Eye-Brain Disease of Santavuori, Meckel-Grüber Syndrome)

Type 2 lissencephaly is sometimes called "cobblestone lissencephaly" because the shallow, wandering grooves in the surface of the cortex resemble cobblestones and do not correspond to normal sulci. Numerous neuroblast migratory disorders accompany this malformation. The microscopic architecture of the cortex differs from that of type I because the lamination of the cortical plate is indistinct and neurons are disoriented and displaced into the wrong layers (1,86,136,137). Some pyramidal neurons are upside-down in relation to the cortical surface, and their axons must turn 180 degrees before descending. Many heterotopic neurons are found in the subcortical white matter, and overmigrated ectopic neurons in the leptomeninges also are seen. Migratory abnormalities in the brainstem and cerebellum are much more frequent than in lissencephaly type 1, and the brainstem and cerebellum often appear hypoplastic on MRI.

Dysmyelination or delayed myelination also are demonstrated by MRI or neuropathologic examination, and white matter may contain microcystic changes. In all types of lissencephaly, the ependyma of the lateral ventricles shows discontinuities, duplications, and many subventricular rosettes and clusters, as well as immunocytochemical immaturity (138). Because the ependyma is neurodevelopmentally important during fetal life (45), the abnormal ependyma may play an active role in abnormal neuroblast migration, though more evidence is needed.

Many syndromes of lissencephaly type 2 are associated with congenital muscular dystrophy, and sometimes the hypotonia, weakness, and developmental delay first bring attention to the abnormality rather than CNS symptoms such as seizures. Muscle biopsy confirms the diagnosis, and MRI of the brain is indicated if congenital muscular dystrophy is demonstrated. Conversely, the imaging demonstration of lissencephaly might provide justification for a muscle biopsy. Mental retardation is almost universal and profound. Multiple seizure types, including infantile spasms, occur from early infancy. Because retinal dysplasias and other ocular lesions are frequent, ophthalmologic evaluation is indicated.

Many lissencephaly/pachygyria disorders are associated with neurocutaneous syndromes and genetically determined inborn metabolic diseases that are sometimes called "syndromic lissencephaly." Other nonlissencephalic "syndromic cortical dysplasias" also occur. Most lissencephalies are transmitted as an autosomal recessive trait (139), but an X-linked recessive form also is known (140). Lissencephaly and cerebellar hypoplasia (141) result from mutation of *RENL*, a gene of the Cajal-Retzius neurons and of cerebellar granule cells that is essential to lamination and organization of the cerebral cortical plate and the cerebellar cortex. The gene *Fukutin* (*FKN*) is mutated in Fukuyama muscular dystrophy and associated with pachygyria/lissencephaly (142). Neuropathologic evidence of cortical dysplasia is seen as early as 23 weeks' gestation, before much gyration normally occurs (143). In type 2 lissencephaly, the genetic mutations have recently been identified as causing defective glycolysation (102). Merosin-deficient congenital muscular dystrophy also fails to express merosin in the developing brain, but the role of merosin in neuroblast migration remains unclear.

Schizencephaly

Schizencephaly is a unilateral or bilateral deep cleft in the general position of (but is not) the sylvian fissure, but it is not a true sylvian fissure. This cleft is the full thickness of the hemispheric wall, and no cerebral tissue remains between the meninges and the lateral ventricle (the pial-ependymal seam) (144). If the cerebral cortical walls on either side of the cleft are touching, the condition is called *closed lips*; if a wide subarachnoid space separates the two walls, it is known as *open lips*. These two variants do not provide a clue to pathogenesis. Schizencephaly occurs as a genetic trait associated with the gene *EMX2* (145,146), but the association and role of this gene, which is expressed in the Cajal-Retzius neuron, are incompletely understood. The clinical features are mental retardation, motor deficits with spastic diplegia or hemiplegia, and epilepsy of various types including partial and generalized major motor and infantile spasms. In some cases, surgical resection may be an effective treatment of an intractable epilepsy (147).

Schizencephaly also occurs sporadically as an acquired lesion associated with porencephaly caused by fetal cerebral infarction or congenital infection. The porencephalic cyst is surrounded by a ring of polymicrogyria. Bilateral perisylvian syndrome is sometimes confused with schizencephaly, but may be acquired (148). Hemiparesis or diparesis, frequent seizures, and mental retardation are common if the lesions are bilateral.

X-Linked Hydrocephalus with Pachygyria/Polymicrogyria

This disorder is a common cause of congenital hydrocephalus in boys and is associated with aqueductal stenosis. Abnormalities in cerebral gyration frequently accompany the hydrocephalus and may be expressed as cognitive and intellectual deficits and epilepsy (149). A mutation in *L1-CAM* has been demonstrated in some cases (150).

Focal Cortical Dysplasias

In most focal cortical dysplasias, no genetic basis is known and the family history is negative (151,152). Surgically resected tissue often shows "balloon cells," large swollen neurons with immunocytochemical markers of mixed neuronal and glial lineage, similar to those seen in hemimegalencephaly and tuberous sclerosis (153,154). These lesions are sometimes called focal cortical dysplasia of the Taylor type, and mutational analysis of the *TSC1* gene of tuberous sclerosis in the balloon cells suggests a pathogenic relation (154).

Agenesis and Dysgenesis of the Corpus Callosum

Agenesis, hypoplasia, and abnormal forms of portions or all of the corpus callosum are found in many unrelated cerebral dysgeneses with various genetic defects. These anomalies are also common in many systemic malformations involving multiple organ systems, in chromosomal diseases, and in many inborn errors of metabolism. The form, thickness, and shape of the corpus callosum vary greatly in these entities. In some, aberrant callosal axons that cannot cross the midline form a large fasciculus, the *bundle of Probst*, in the dorsomedial wall of the cerebral hemisphere. In malformations such as holoprosencephaly, the corpus callosum is not only absent but also its constituent axons cannot be identified as a fasciculus despite the small pyramidal neurons in layer 3 whose axons normally provide most callosal fibers (1,155–157). Some cases of callosal agenesis are associated with other, seemingly unrelated defects in the nervous system, such as disturbances of neural crest migration that form Hirschsprung disease (87) and with hereditary motor and sensory peripheral neuropathy (158).

Isolated agenesis of the corpus callosum characteristically features hypertelorism, a higher-than-expected incidence of epilepsy, and either normal intelligence or psychomotor retardation. In older children, faulty interhemispheric transfer of information can be demonstrated by careful testing of epicritic senses, such as naming objects placed in the left hand (perceived in the right hemisphere but requiring callosal transfer to the left to speak its name). The degree of deficit is an indirect measure of how completely the passage of axons across the midline is lacking.

The diagnosis can be confirmed by almost any imaging technique, including prenatal ultrasonography. CT and MRI scans show that the lateral ventricles are parallel rather than curved toward the midline, as seen in axial views, with the large bundle of Probst interposed between them and the medial border of the hemisphere. Colpocephaly often is present because of loss of the posterior fornix of white matter (splenium) that interconnects the occipital lobes. The third ventricle rises higher than expected in the vertical plane because expansion of its roof is not limited by the corpus callosum. The fornix is displaced. The septum pellucidum is absent or displaced. The anterior commissure is two to four times larger than expected, a finding confirmed by neuropathologic examination. The large anterior commissure undoubtedly carries some aberrant fibers that normally would cross in the corpus callosum; other aberrant axonal paths to the other hemisphere include the psalterium (hippocampal commissure) and a variety of small paths, even for individual axons in heterotopic sites. In rare cases, the ventral corticospinal tracts in the spinal cord may be greatly enlarged and probably carry aberrant callosal axons that join the normal descending motor fibers; in these brains studied postmortem, the internal capsule, midbrain cerebral peduncles, and medullary pyramids also are excessively thick, representing the more proximal corticospinal axons plus aberrant callosal axons.

The EEG shows asynchrony of sleep spindles and posterior rhythms and epileptic foci. The cause of epilepsy in callosal agenesis is not certain, as more than 80% of callosal fibers are inhibitory. Small focal cortical dysplasias, evident microscopically in acallosal brains, may be epileptogenic but are too small to be resolved by imaging. Agenesis of corpus callosum in a child with epilepsy should serve as a marker for further genetic and metabolic workup and genetic counseling.

Tuberous Sclerosis

This autosomal dominant disease has two separate genetic loci on different chromosomes, at 9q34.3 and 16p13.3; the respective genes and their transcription products are *TSC1*, hamartin (159,160), and *TSC2*, tuberin (161,162). Despite these two distinct genetic etiologies, the clinical manifestations are indistinguishable without phenotype/genotype correlation (163,164). Tuberous sclerosis has a reported prevalence ranging from 1:17,000 to 1:125,000; all racial and ethnic populations are involved (165). The hamartomas of the brain justify its classification as a cerebral dysgenesis. See chapter 36 for a detailed discussion.

Hemimegalencephaly

This disorder uniquely involves overgrowth of only one cerebral hemisphere, it does not correspond to any normal stage of embryonic or fetal cerebral development. Most cases involve only the cerebrum, but a minority also affect the ipsilateral cerebellum and brainstem. Hemifacial lipoma or hemicorporal hypertrophy of the body may be present (166,167). This hamartomatous malformation is not a primary disorder of neuroblast migration as is frequently said, but rather is a disturbance in cellular lineage, differentiation, and growth (168). Cells are morphologically abnormal and exhibit immunocytochemical features of mixed glial and neuronal derivation, including balloon cells (168,169). Several genes of corporal symmetry have

been proposed as playing a role in pathogenesis (166,167). The *L1-CAM* gene product is overexpressed in some cases (170). The winged helix transcription factor *FoxG1* plays multiple roles in the proliferation and differentiation of the telencephalon, and its overexpression in mice causes overgrowth of the neural tube (171).

Hemimegalencephaly may be either an isolated disorder, usually sporadically without an obvious hereditary trait, or part of a syndrome. The syndromic form is associated with several neurocutaneous syndromes, most frequently epidermal nevus, Proteus, and Klippel-Trenaunay-

---

TABLE 2.2

ETIOLOGIC CLASSIFICATION OF HUMAN NERVOUS SYSTEM MALFORMATIONS AS PATTERNS OF GENETIC EXPRESSION

I. Genetic mutations expressed in the primitive streak or node
  A. Upregulation of organizer genes
    1. Duplication of neural tube
  B. Downregulation of organizer genes
    1. Agenesis of neural tube
II. Disorders of ventralizing gradient in the neural tube
  A. Overexpression of ventralizing genes
    1. Duplication of spinal central canal
    2. Duplication of ventral horns of spinal cord
    3. Diplomyelia (and diastematomyelia?)
    4. Duplication of neural tube
    5. Ventralizing induction of somite
      a. Segmental amyoplasia
  B. Underexpression of ventralizing genes
    1. Fusion of ventral horns of spinal cord
    2. Sacral (thoracolumbosacral) agenesis
    3. Arrhinencephaly
    4. Holoprosencephaly
III. Disorders of dorsalizing gradient of the neural tube
  A. Overexpression of dorsalizing genes
    1. Duplication of dorsal horns of spinal cord
    2. Duplication of dorsal brainstem structures
  B. Underexpression of dorsalizing genes
    1. Fusion of dorsal horns of spinal cord
    2. Septooptic dysplasia
IV. Disorders of the rostrocaudal gradient and/or segmentation
  A. Increased homeobox domains and/or ectopic expression
    1. Chiari II malformation
  B. Decreased homeobox domains and/or neuromere deletion
    1. Agenesis of mesencephalon and metencephalon (*EN2*)
    2. Global cerebellar aplasia or hypoplasia
    3. Agenesis of basal telencephalic nuclei (*EMX1, MASH1?*)
V. Aberrations in cell lineages by genetic mutation
  A. Nonneoplastic
    1. Striated muscle in the central nervous system (CNS)
    2. Dysplastic gangliocytoma of the cerebellum (Lhermitte-Duclos)
    3. Tuberous sclerosis
    4. Hemimegalencephaly (also VIII. Disorders of symmetry)
  B. Neoplastic
    1. Myomedulloblastoma
    2. Dysembryoplastic neuroepithelial tumors

  3. Gangliogliomas and other mixed neural tumors
VI. Disorders of secretory molecules and genes that mediate migrations
  A. Neuroblast migrations
    1. Initial course of neuroblast migration
      a. *Filamin-1* (X-linked dominant periventricular nodular heterotopia)
    2. Middle course of neuroblast migration
      a. Doublecortin (*DCX*; X-linked dominant subcortical laminar heterotopia or band heterotopia)
      b. *LIS1* (type I lissencephaly or Miller-Dieker syndrome)
      c. Fukutin (type II lissencephaly; Fukuyama muscular dystrophy)
      d. Empty spiracles (*EMX2*; schizencephaly)
      e. Astrotactin
    3. Late course of neuroblast migration; architecture of cortical plate
      a. *Reelin* (pachygyria and cerebellar hypoplasia)
      b. *Disabled-1* (*DAB1*; also *VLDL*/Apoe2R? App receptor defect; downstream of reelin, *EMX2* and *DCX*)
      c. *L1-NCAM* (X-linked hydrocephalus and pachygyria with aqueductal stenosis)
  B. Glioblast migration
  C. Focal migratory disturbances due to acquired lesions of the fetal brain
VII. Disorders of secretory molecules and genes that attract or repel axonal growth cones
  A. Netrin downregulation
  B. Keratan sulfate and other glycosaminoglycan downregulations
  C. S-100β protein downregulation or upregulation (?)
VIII. Disorders of symmetry
  A. Hemimegalencephaly (also see V. Aberrations of cellular lineages)
    1. Isolated hemimegalencephaly
    2. Syndromic hemimegalencephaly
      a. Epidermal nevus syndrome
      b. Proteus syndrome
      c. Klippel-Trenaunay-Weber syndrome
      d. Hypomelanosis of Ito
    3. Hemicerebellar megalencephaly

From Sarnat HB, Flores-Sarnat L. Integrative classification of morphology and molecular genetics in central nervous system malformations. *Am J Med Genet* 2004;126A:386–392, with permission.

Weber syndromes (166,172). Hypomelanosis of Ito and neurofibromatosis I have been reported rarely (173). The imaging findings are diagnostic and consist of not only the enlargement of the hemisphere but also abnormalities of cerebral convolutions with pachygyria and lissencephaly, colpocephaly, and the "occipital sign," a shift across the midline of the occipital lobe (166). Most affected children have severe epilepsy, including infantile spasms, that often is refractory to pharmacologic treatment and requires hemispherectomy (174).

Neither the imaging nor the neuropathologic features distinguish the isolated from the syndromic form of hemimegalencephaly. This distinction is based on cutaneous lesions, multisystemic involvement (e.g., Proteus syndrome), and family history.

CHALLENGES IN THE CLASSIFICATION OF BRAIN MALFORMATIONS

Traditional classifications of cerebral malformations have been based on morphologic characteristics, with attempts to relate these features to anatomic and physiologic processes of development. This approach served well throughout the late 19th and 20th centuries, and it remains a valid and useful way to distinguish categories of developmental aberration and to interpret imaging and neuropathologic lesions on anatomic and histologic grounds. New data about genetic programming of the nervous system and the discovery of specific genetic mutations underlying many malformations have made it clear that classifications based on descriptive morphogenesis alone are no longer adequate. Lissencephaly and holoprosencephaly are examples of limitations of the traditional morphologic schemes. Multiple genetic causes have been identified for each syndrome, but the anatomic features of the brain may be difficult or impossible to distinguish and the clinical phenotype/ genotype correlation is ambiguous as well.

A classification scheme based exclusively on genetic mutations and deletions, without consideration of morphologic features, is impractical for clinicians, radiologists, and pathologists, and might not even be possible. Many genes are expressed several times in ontogenesis with different functions at each stage; some genes activate or inhibit others in a cascade, resulting in multiple genetic expressive defects; and only a fraction of the genes causing malformations are known. For these reasons, a scheme that integrates both traditional descriptive morphogenesis and molecular genetic programming as *patterns of genetic expression* may be both scientifically correct and clinically practical (94,175) (Table 2.2). In addition, each gene need not be known to enable the malformation to be classified. Finally, nongenetic disturbances in ontogenesis, such as those caused by fetal cerebral infarcts, also can be classified within the framework of the scheme.

Scales for the type of disturbances of neuroblast migration, based on morphologic features rather than genetics, have been proposed (139). Although such scales have a practical value for the clinician and radiologist, they do not provide an etiologic classification. Some authors attempt to restrict classification schemes to certain parts of the nervous system, such as the cerebral cortex, as described in Chapter 5 (176). However well-intentioned, such schemes exclude important dysgeneses of the cerebellum and brainstem that might result from downregulation of the same gene or of a downstream gene. The faulty genetic expression in subcortical structures or an extensive gradient in the longitudinal axis is variable but equally important. An example is Walker-Warburg syndrome with type 2 lissencephaly of the cerebral cortex but also with neuroblast migratory disorders in the brainstem. Similarly, classifications restricted to cerebellar malformations are inherently incomplete because many also involve other parts of the brain or spinal cord. Any consideration in neuroembryology must guard against a temptation to focus narrowly on the one brain region of primary interest to the exclusion of other neural tube derivatives. The global perspective of the scheme of development is no longer evident in fragmented classifications that impede, rather than enhance, comprehension.

REFERENCES

1. Sarnat HB. *Cerebral dysgenesis. Embryology and clinical expression.* New York: Oxford University Press, 1992.
2. Bronner-Fraser M, Fraser SE. Differentiation of the vertebrate neural tube. *Curr Opin Cell Biol* 1997;9:885–891.
3. Sarnat HB, Menkes JH. How to construct a neural tube. *J Child Neurol* 2000;15:110–124.
4. Jacobson AG. Experimental analysis of the shaping of the neural plate and tube. *Am Zool* 1991;31:628–643.
5. Álvarez IS, Schoenwolf GC. Expansion of surface epithelium provides the major extrinsic force for bending of the neural tube. *J Exp Zool* 1992;261:340–348.
6. van Straaten HWM, Hekking JWM, Consten C, et al. Intrinsic and extrinsic factors in the mechanism of neurulation: effect of curvature of the body axis on closure of the posterior neuropore. *Development* 1993;117:1163–1172.
7. Jacobson AG, Moury JD. Tissue boundaries and cell behavior during neurulation. *Dev Biol* 1995;171:98–110.
8. Smith J, Schoenwolf GC. Notochordal induction of cell wedging in the chick neural plate and its role in neural tube formation. *J Exp Zool* 1989;25:49–62.
9. O'Rahilly R, Müller F. Bidirectional closure of the rostral neuropore in the human embryo. *Am J Anat* 1989;184:259–268.
10. Golden JA, Chernoff GF. Intermittent pattern of neural tube closure in two strains of mice. *Teratology* 1993;47:73–80.
11. Busam KJ, Roberts DJ, Golden JA. Clinical teratology counseling and consultation case report: two distinct anterior neural tube defects in a human fetus: evidence for an intermittent pattern of neural tube closure. *Teratology* 1993;48:399–403.
12. Van Allen MI, Kalousek DK, Chernoff GF, et al. Evidence for multi-site closure of the neural tube in humans. *Am J Med Genet* 1993;47:723–743.
13. van Stratten HWM, Janssen HCJP, Peeters MCE, et al. Neural tube closure in the chick embryo is multiphasic. *Dev Dyn* 1996;207:309–318.
14. Sarnat HB, Netsky MG. When does a ganglion become a brain? Evolutionary origin of the central nervous system. *Semin Pediatr Neurol* 2002;9:240–253.

15. Keynes RJ, Lumsden A. Segmentation and the origin of regional diversity in the vertebrate central nervous system. *Neuron* 1990; 2:1–9.
16. Wilkinson DG, Krumlauf R. Molecular approaches to the segmentation of the hindbrain. *Trends Neurosci* 1990;13:335–339.
17. McGinnis W, Krumlauf R. Homeobox genes and axial patterning. *Cell* 1992;68:283–302.
18. Guthrie S, Lumbsden A. Formation and regeneration of rhombomere boundaries in the developing chick hindbrain. *Development* 1991;112:221–229.
19. Tsering C. Demonstration of segmental arrangement of thoracic spinal motor neurons using lipophilic dyes. *Dev Neurosci* 1992; 14:308–311.
20. Puelles L, Rubinstein JL. Forebrain gene expression domains and the evolving prosomeric model. *Trends Neurosci* 2003;26: 469–476.
21. Hall BK. *The neural crest in development and evolution.* New York: Springer-Verlag, 1999.
22. Le Dourarin NM, Kalcheim C. *The neural crest*, 2nd ed. Cambridge, UK: Cambridge University Press, 1999.
23. García-Castro M, Bronner-Fraser M. Induction and differentiation of the neural crest. *Curr Opin Cell Biol* 1999;11:695–698.
24. Young HM, Newgreen D. Enteric neural crest-derived cells: origin, identification, migration and differentiation. *Anat Rec* 2001;262:1–15.
25. Caviness VS Jr, Takahashi T, Nowakowski RS. Numbers, time and neocortical neurogenesis: a general developmental and evolutionary model. *Trends Neurosci* 1995;18:379–383.
26. Chenn A, McConnell SK. Cleavage orientation and the asymmetrical inheritance of notch 1 immunoreactivity in mammalian neurogenesis. *Cell* 1995;82:631–641.
27. Mione MC, Cavanagh JFR, Harris B, et al. Cell fate specification and symmetrical/asymmetrical divisions in the developing cerebral cortex. *J Neurosci* 1997;17:2018–2029.
28. Zhong W, Feder JN, Jiang M-M, et al. Asymmetric localization of mammalian numb homolog during mouse cortical neurogenesis. *Neuron* 1996;17:43–53.
29. Petersen PH, Zou K, Hwang JK, et al. Progenitor cell maintenance requires *numb* and *numblike* during mouse neurogenesis. *Nature* 2002;419:929–934.
30. Johnson JE. *Numb* and *numblike* control cell number during vertebrate neurogenesis. *Trends Neurosci* 2003;26:395–396.
31. Kendler A, Golden JA. Progenitor cell proliferation outside the ventricular and subventricular zones during human brain development. *J Neuropathol Exp Neurol* 1996;55:1253–1258.
32. Johansson CB, Momma S, Clarke DL, et al. Identification of a neural stem cell in the adult mammalian central nervous system. *Cell* 1999;96:25–34.
33. Schuldiner M, Figes R, Eden A, et al. Induced neuronal differentiation of human embryonic stem cells. *Brain Res* 2001;913: 201–205.
34. Blaschke AJ, Weiner JA, Chun J. Programmed cell death is a universal feature of embryonic and postnatal neuroproliferative regions throughout the central nervous system. *J Comp Neurol* 1998;396:39–50.
35. Bonhoeffer T. Neurotrophins and activity-dependent development of the neocortex. *Curr Opin Neurobiol* 1996;6:119–126.
36. McQuillen PS, Ferriero DM. Selective vulnerability in the developing central nervous system. *Pediatr Neurol* 2004;30:227–235.
37. Holzman DM, Sheldon RA, Jaffe W, et al. Nerve growth factor protects the neonatal brain against hypoxic-ischemic injury. *Ann Neurol* 1996;39:114–122.
38. Cheng Y, Gidday JM, Yan Q, et al. Marked age-dependent neuroprotection by brain-derived neurotrophic factor against neonatal hypoxic-ischemic brain injury. *Ann Neurol* 1997;41:521–529.
39. O'Leary DD, Fawcett JW, Cowan WM. Topographic targeting errors in the retinocollicular projection and their elimination by selective ganglion cell death. *J Neurosci* 1986;6:3692–3705.
40. Sarnat HB. Microscopic criteria to determine gestational age of the fetal and neonatal brain. In: García JH, ed. *Neuropathology. The diagnostic approach.* St. Louis: Mosby, 1997:529–540.
41. Zheng C, Heintz N, Hatten ME. CNS gene encoding astrotactin, which supports neuronal migration along glial fibers. *Science* 1996;272:417–419.

42. Jouet M, Kenwrick S. Gene analysis of L1 neural cell adhesion molecule in prenatal diagnosis of hydrocephalus. *Lancet* 1995; 345:161–162.
43. Herman J-P, Victor JC, Sanes JR. Developmentally regulated and spatially restricted antigens of radial glial cells. *Dev Dyn* 1993; 197:307–318.
44. Sarnat HB. Regional differentiation of the human fetal ependyma: immunocytochemical markers. *J Neuropathol Exp Neurol* 1992; 51:58–75.
45. Sarnat HB. Role of human fetal ependyma. *Pediatr Neurol* 1992;8:163–178.
46. Thomas LB, Gates MA, Steindler DA. Young neurons from the adult subependymal zone proliferate and migrate along an astrocyte, extracellular matrix-rich pathway. *Glia* 1996;17:1–14.
47. O'Rourke NA, Sullivan DP, Kaznowski CE, et al. Tangential migration of neurons in the developing cerebral cortex. *Development* 1995;121:2165–2176.
48. Rakic P. Radial versus tangential migration of neuronal clones in the developing cerebral cortex. *Proc Natl Acad Sci U S A* 1995;92: 11323–11327.
49. McManus MF, Nasrahhah IM, Gopal PP, et al. Axon mediated interneuron migration. *J Neuropathol Exp Neurol* 2004;63: 932–941.
50. Chisholm A, Tessier-Lavigne M. Conservation and divergence of axon guidance mechanisms. *Curr Opin Neurobiol* 1999;9: 603–615.
51. Snow DM, Steindler DA, Silver J. Molecular and cellular characterization of the glial roof plate of the spinal cord and optic tectum: a possible role for a proteoglycan in the development of an axon barrier. *Dev Biol* 1990;138:359–376.
52. McFarlane S. Attraction vs. repulsion: the growth cone decides. *Biochem Cell Biol* 2000;78:563–568.
53. Jacob J, Hacker A, Guthrie S. Mechanisms and molecules in motor neuron specification and axon pathfinding. *Bioessays* 2001;23:582–595.
54. Van Vactor D, Flanagan JG. The middle and the end: slit brings guidance and branching together in axon pathway selection. *Neuron* 1999;22:649–652.
55. Irwin N, Madsen JR. Molecular biology of axonal outgrowth. *Pediatr Neurosurg* 1997;27:113–120.
56. Shea TB, Jung C, Pant HC. Does neurofilament phosphorylation regulate axonal transport? *Trends Neurosci* 2003;26:397–400.
57. Zou Y. *Wnt* signaling in axon guidance. *Trends Neurosci* 2004; 27:528–532.
58. Schinder AF, Poo M-M. The neurotrophin hypothesis for synaptic plasticity. *Trends Neurosci* 2000;23:639–645.
59. Kasai H, Matsuzaki M, Noguchi J, et al. Structure-stability-function relationships of dendritic spines. *Trends Neurosci* 2003;26: 360–368.
60. Berardi N, Pizzorusso T, Mafei L. Critical periods during sensory development. *Curr Opin Neurobiol* 2000;10:138–145.
61. Dreyfus-Brisac C, Flescher J, Plassart E. L'électroencéphalogramme. Critère d'âge conceptionnel du nouveau-né à terme et prematuré. *Biol Neonat* 1962;4:154–173.
62. Lombroso CT. Quantified electrographic scales on 10 premature healthy newborns followed up to 40–43 weeks of conceptional age by serial polygraphic recordings. *Electroencephalogr Clin Neurophysiol* 1979;46:460–474.
63. Vecchierini M-F, d'Allest A-M, Verpillat P. EEG patterns in 10 extreme premature neonates with normal neurological outcome: qualitative and quantitative data. *Brain Dev* 2003;25: 330–337.
64. Koh T-W, Bellen HJ. Synaptotagmin I, a Ca^{2+} sensor for neurotransmitter release. *Trends Neurosci* 2003;26:413–422.
65. Dupuy S, Houser CR. Developmental changes in GABA neurons of the rat dentate gyrus: an *in situ* hybridization and birth dating study. *J Comp Neurol* 1997;389:402–418.
66. Rho JM, Storey TW. Molecular ontogeny of major neurotransmitter receptor systems in the mammalian central nervous system: norepinephrine, dopamine, serotonin, acetylcholine and glycine. *J Child Neurol* 2001;16:271–281.
67. Simeone TA, Donevan SD, Rho JM. Molecular biology and ontogeny of $GABA_A$ and $GABA_B$ receptors in the mammalian central nervous system. *J Child Neurol* 2003;18:39–48.

68. Wong CGT, Bottiglieri T, Snead OC III. GABA, γ-hydroxybutyric acid and neurological disease. *Ann Neurol* 2003;54(Suppl 6): S3–S12.

69. Yakovlev PI, Lecours A-R. The myelination cycles of regional maturation of the brain. In: Minkowski A, ed. *Regional development of the brain in early life.* Philadelphia: FA Davis 1967:3–70.

70. Back SA, Han BH, Luo NL, et al. Selective vulnerability of late oligodendrocyte progenitors to hypoxia-ischemia. *J Neurosci* 2002;22:455–463.

71. Smart IHM. Differential growth of the cell production systems in the lateral wall of the developing mouse telencephalon. *J Anat* 1985;141:219–229.

72. Takahashi T, Nowakowski RS, Caviness VS. The cell cycle of the pseudostratified ventricular epithelium of the embryonic murine cerebral wall. *J Neurosci* 1995;15:6046–6057.

73. Marín-Padilla M. Cajal-Retzius cells and the development of the neocortex. *Trends Neurosci* 1998;21:64–71.

74. Sarnat HB, Flores-Sarnat L. Cajal-Retzius and subplate neurons: their role in cortical development. *Eur J Paediatr Neurol* 2002;6: 91–97.

75. Takano T, Takikita S, Takeuchi Y. Role of Cajal-Retzius cells in ibotenate-induced cortical malformations in hamsters. *Eur J Paediatr Neurol* 2001;5:A118.

76. Friauf E, Shatz CJ. Changing patterns of synaptic input to subplate and cortical plate during development of visual cortex. *J Neurophysiol* 1991;66:2059–2071.

77. Ulfig N, Neudörfer F, Bohl J. Transient structures of the human fetal brain: subplate, thalamic reticular complex, ganglionic eminence. *Histol Histopathol* 2000;15:771–790.

78. McConnell SK, Ghosh A, Shatz CJ. Subplate pioneers and the formation of descending connections from the cerebral cortex. *J Neurosci* 1994;14:1892–1907.

79. McQuillen PS, DeFreitas MF, Zada G, et al. A novel role for p75NTR in subplate growth cone complexity and visual thalamocortical innervation. *J Neurosci* 2002;22:3580-3593.

80. Ghosh A, Shatz CJ. A role for subplate neurons in the patterning of connections from thalamus to neocortex. *Development* 1993;117:1031–1047.

81. Lein ES, Finney EM, McQuillen PS, et al. Subplate neuron ablation alters neurotrophin expression and ocular dominance column formation. *Proc Natl Acad Sci U S A* 1999;96:13491–13495.

82. Ghosh A, Shatz CJ. Involvement of subplate neurons in the formation of ocular dominance columns. *Science* 1992;255: 1441–1443.

83. Kanold PO, Kara P, Reid RC, et al. Role of subplate neurons in functional maturation of visual cortical columns. *Science* 2003; 301:521–525.

84. Humphrey T. The development of the human hippocampal fissure. *J Anat* 1967;101:655–676.

85. O'Rahilly R, Müller F. *The embryonic human brain. An atlas of developmental stages.* New York: Wiley-Liss, 1994.

86. Norman MG, McGillivray B, Kalousek DK, et al. *Congenital malformations of the brain. Pathological, embryological, radiological and genetic aspects.* New York: Oxford University Press, 1995.

87. Cacheux V, Dastot-Le Moal F, Kaariainen H, et al. Loss-of-function mutations in *SIP1 Smad* interacting protein 1 result in a syndromic Hirschsprung disease. *Hum Mol Genet* 2001;10:1503–1510.

88. Sarnat HB, Flores-Sarnat L. Embryology of neural crest and its inductive role in neurocutaneous syndromes. *J Child Neurol* 2005. In press.

89. Carstens MH. Development of the facial midline. *J Craniofac Surg* 2002;13:129–187.

90. Carstens M. Neural tube programming and craniofacial cleft formation. *Eur J Paediatr Neurol* 2004;8:160–178.

91. Sarnat HB, Flores-Sarnat L, Carstens MH. Mechanisms of hypotelorism and hypertelorism. *J Child Neurol* 2005. In press.

92. Sarnat HB. Regional ependymal upregulation of vimentin in Chiari II malformation, aqueductal stenosis, and hydromyelia. *Pediatr Dev Pathol* 2004;7:48–60.

93. Sarnat HB, Benjamin DR, Siebert JR, et al. Agenesis of the mesencephalon and metencephalon with cerebellar hypoplasia: putative mutation in the *EN2* gene: report of 2 cases in early infancy. *Pediatr Dev Pathol* 2002;5:54–68.

94. Sarnat HB. Molecular genetic classification of central nervous system malformations. *J Child Neurol* 2000;15:675–687.

95. Barth PG, Mullaart R, Stam FC, et al. Familial lissencephaly with extreme neopallial hypoplasia. *Brain Dev* 1982;4:145–151.

96. Barth PG. Fetal disruption as a cause of neuronal migration defects. In: Barth PG, ed. *Disorders of neuronal migration.* London: Mac Keith Press, 2003:182–194.

97. Roy N, Mahedevan N, McLean M, et al. The gene for neuronal apoptosis inhibitory protein is partially deleted in individuals with spinal muscular atrophy. *Cell* 1995;80:167–178.

98. Jamieson CR, Fryns JP, Jacobs J, et al. Primary autosomal recessive microcephaly: *MCPH5* maps to 1q25-q32 *Am J Hum Genet* 2000;67:1575–1577.

99. Bond J, Roberts E, Mochida GH, et al. ASPM is a major determinant of cerebral cortical size. *Nat Genet* 2002;32:316–320.

100. Jackson AP, Eastwood H, Bell SM, et al. Identification of microcephalin, a protein implicated in determining the size of the human brain. *Am J Hum Genet* 2002;71:136–142.

101. Sarnat HB. Central nervous system malformations: gene locations of known human mutations. *Eur J Paediatr Neurol* 2003; 7:43–45.

102. Yamamoto T, Kato Y, Karita M, et al. Expression of genes related to muscular dystrophy with lissencephaly. *Pediatr Neurol* 2004; 31:183–190.

103. Rivero-Martínez E, Pascual-Castroviejo I. Joubert syndrome. Report of four cases with a favourable evolution [in Spanish]. *Rev Neurol* 2002;35:918–921.

104. Barth PG. Pontocerebellar hypoplasias. An overview of a group of inherited neurodegenerative disorders with fetal onset. *Brain Dev* 1993;15:411–422.

105. Siebert JR, Cohen MM Jr, Sullik KK, et al. *Holoprosencephaly. An overview and atlas of cases.* New York: Wiley-Liss, 1990.

106. Golden JA. Holoprosencephaly. A defect in brain patterning. *J Neuropathol Exp Neurol* 1998;57:991–999.

107. Simon EM, Hevner RF, Pinter JD, et al. The middle interhemispheric variant of holoprosencephaly. *Am J Neuroradiol* 2002;23: 151–156.

108. Plawner LL, Delgado MR, Miller VS, et al. Clinical spectrum of holoprosencephaly: a clinical-neuroradiological analysis. *Neurology* 2002;59:1058–1066.

109. Hahn JS, Pinter JD. Holoprosencephaly: genetic, neuroradiological and clinical advances. *Semin Pediatr Neurol* 2002;9:309–319.

110. Sarnat HB, Flores-Sarnat L. Neuropathologic research strategies in holoprosencephaly. *J Child Neurol* 2001;16:918–931.

111. Brown SA, Warburton D, Brown LY, et al. Holoprosencephaly due to mutations in *Zic2*, a homologue of *Drosophila* odd-paired. *Nat Genet* 1998;20:180–183.

112. Roessler E, Belloni E, Gaudenz K, et al. Mutations in the human *Sonic hedgehog* gene cause holoprosencephaly. *Nat Genet* 1996; 14:357–360.

113. Wallis DE, Roessler E, Hehr U, et al. Mutations in the homeodomain of the human *SIX3* gene cause holoprosencephaly. *Nat Genet* 1999;22:196–198.

114. Gripp KW, Wotton D, Edwards MC, et al. Mutations in *TGIF* cause holoprosencephaly and link *NODAL* signalling to human neural axis determination. *Nat Genet* 2000;25:205–208.

115. Ming JE, Kaupas ME, Roessler E, et al. Mutations in *PATCHED-1*, the receptor for *Sonic Hedgehog*, are associated with holoprosencephaly. *Hum Genet* 2002;110:297–301.

116. Roessler E, Du Y, Glinka A, et al. The genomic structure, chromosome location and analysis of the human *DKK1* head inducer gene as a candidate for holoprosencephaly. *Cytogenet Cell Genet* 2000;89:220–224.

117. Kelley RL, Roessler E, Hennekam RC, et al. Holoprosencephaly in RSH/Smith-Lemli-Opitz syndrome: does abnormal cholesterol metabolism affect the function of *Sonic hedgehog*? *Am J Med Genet* 1996;66:78–84.

118. DeMyer W, Zeman W, Palmer GG. The face predicts the brain. Diagnostic significance of median facial anomalies for holoprosencephaly (arhinencephaly). *Pediatrics* 1964;34:256–263.

119. Brown LY, Odent S, Blayau M, et al. Holoprosencephaly due to mutations in *ZIC2*: alanine tract expansion mutations may be caused by parental somatic recombination. *Hum Mol Genet* 2001;10:791–796.

120. Sarnat HB. Olfactory reflexes in the newborn infant. *J Pediatr* 1978;92:624–626.

121. Dattani MT, Martínez-Barera JP, Thomas PQ, et al. *HESX1*: a novel gene implicated in a familial form of septo-optic dysplasia. *Acta Paediatr* 1999;88(Suppl):49–54.

122. Carey ML, Friedman TB, Asher JH Jr, et al. Septo-optic dysplasia and WS1 in the proband of a WS1 family segregating for a novel mutation in *PAX3* exon 7. *J Med Genet* 1998;35:248–250.

123. Colacitti C, Sancini G, DeBiasi S, et al. Prenatal methyla-zoxymethanol treatment in rats produces brain abnormalities with morphological similarities to human developmental brain dysgeneses. *J Neuropathol Exp Neurol* 1999;58:92–106.

124. Kothare SV, Van Landingham K, Armon C, et al. Seizure onset from periventricular nodular heterotopias; depth-electrode study. *Neurology* 1998;51:1723–1727.

125. Eksioğlu YZ, Scheffere IE, Cardenas P, et al. Periventricular heterotopia: an X-linked dominant epilepsy locus causing aberrant cerebral cortical development. *Neuron* 1996;16:77–87.

126. Battaglia G, Granata T, Farina L, et al. Periventricular nodular heterotopia: epileptogenic findings. *Epilepsia* 1997;38:1173–1182.

127. Fox JW, Lamperti ED, Eksioglu YZ, et al. Mutations in *filamin 1* prevent migration of cerebral cortical neurons in human periventricular heterotopia. *Neuron* 1998;21:1315–1325.

128. Leventer RJ, Dobyns WB. Periventricular gray matter heterotopias: a heterogeneous group of malformations of cortical development. In: Barth PG, ed. *Disorders of neuronal migration*. London: Mac Keith Press, 2003:72–82.

129. Pinard J-M, Motte J, Chiron C, et al. Subcortical laminar heterotopia and lissencephaly in two families: a single X-linked dominant gene. *J Neurol Neurosurg Psychiatry* 1994;57:914–920.

130. Gleeson JG, Minnerath SH, Fox JW, et al. Characterization of mutations in the gene *doublecortin* in patients with double cortex syndrome. *Ann Neurol* 1999;45:146–153.

131. Sarnat HB, Born DE. Synaptophysin immunocytochemistry with thermal intensification: a marker of terminal axonal maturation in the human fetal nervous system. *Brain Dev* 1999;21:41–50.

132. Dobyns WB, Reiner O, Carrozzo R, et al. Lissencephaly: a human brain malformation associated with deletion of the *LIS1* gene located at chromosome 17p13. *JAMA* 1993;270:2838–2842.

133. Chong SS, Pack SD, Roschke AV, et al. A revision of the lissencephaly and Miller-Dieker syndrome critical regions in chromosome 17p13.3. *Hum Mol Genet* 1997;6:147–155.

134. Lo Nigro C, Chong SS, Smith ACM, et al. Point mutations and an intragenetic deletion in *LIS1*, the lissencephaly causative gene in isolated lissencephaly sequence and Miller-Dieker syndrome. *Hum Mol Genet* 1997;6:157–164.

135. Clark DC, Mizuguchi M, Antalffy B, et al. Predominant localization of the *LIS* family of gene products to Cajal-Retzius cells and ventricular neuroepithelium in the developing human cortex. *J Neuropathol Exp Neurol* 1997;56:1044–1052.

136. Towfighi J, Sassani JW, Suzuki K, et al. Cerebro-ocular dysplasia-muscular dystrophy (COD-MD) syndrome. *Acta Neuropathol* 1984;65:110–123.

137. Squier MV. Development of the cortical dysplasia of type II lissencephaly. *Neuropathol Appl Neurobiol* 1993;19:209–213.

138. Sarnat HB, Darwish HZ, Barth PG, et al. Ependymal abnormalities in lissencephaly/pachygyria. *J Neuropathol Exp Neurol* 1993;52:525–541.

139. Dobyns WB, Leventer RJ. Lissencephaly: the clinical and molecular genetic basis of diffuse malformations of neuronal migration. In: Barth PG, ed. *Disorders of neuronal migration*. London: Mac Keith Press, 2003:24–57.

140. Uyanik G, Aigner L, Martin P, et al. X-linked lissencephaly with abnormal genitalia. *Neurology* 2003;61:232–235.

141. Hong SE, Shugart YY, Huang DT, et al. Autosomal recessive lissencephaly with cerebellar hypoplasia is associated with human *RELN* mutations. *Nat Genet* 2000;26:93–96.

142. Topaloğlu H, Brockington M, Yuva Y, et al. *FKRP* gene mutations cause congenital muscular dystrophy, mental retardation and cerebellar cysts. *Neurology* 2003;60:988–992.

143. Takada K, Nakamura H, Suzumori K, et al. Cortical dysplasia in a 23-week fetus with Fukuyama congenital muscular dystrophy (FCMD). *Acta Neuropathol* 1987;74:300–306.

144. Battaglia G, Granata T. Schizencephaly. In: Barth PG, ed. *Disorders of neuronal migration*. London: Mac Keith Press, 2003:127–134.

145. Brunelli S, Faiella A, Capra V, et al. Germline mutations in the homeobox gene *EMX2* in patients with severe schizencephaly. *Nat Genet* 1996;12:94–96.

146. Granata T, Farina L, Faiella A, et al. Familial schizencephaly associated with *EMX2* mutation. *Neurology* 1997;48:1403–1406.

147. Leblanc R, Tampieri D, Robitaille Y, et al. Surgical treatment of intractable epilepsy associated with schizencephaly. *Neurosurgery* 1991;29:421–429.

148. Kuznieckcy R, Andermann F. Congenital bilateral perisylvian syndrome: imaging findings in a multicenter study. *Am J Neuroradiol* 1994;15:139–144.

149. Graf WE, Born DE, Sarnat HB. The pachygyria-polymicrogyria spectrum of cortical dysplasia in X-linked hydrocephalus. *Eur J Pediatr Surg* 1998;8(Suppl 1):10–14.

150. Jouet M, Kenwrick S. Gene analysis of L1 neural cell adhesion molecule in prenatal diagnosis of hydrocephalus. *Lancet* 1995;345:161–162.

151. Palmini A, Andermann F, Olivier A, et al. Focal neuronal migration disorders and intractable partial epilepsy: a study of 30 patients. *Ann Neurol* 1991;30:742–749.

152. Kuznieckcy R, García JH, Faught E, et al. Cortical dysplasia in temporal lobe epilepsy: MRI correlations. *Ann Neurol* 1991;29:293–298.

153. Meagher-Villemure K, Gebhard S, Willemure J-G. Balloon cells in different pathological entities. *Can J Neurol Sci* 2001;28:369–375.

154. Becker AJ, Urbach H, Scheffler B, et al. Focal cortical dysplasia of Taylor's balloon cell type: mutational analysis of the *TSC1* gene indicates a pathogenic relationship to tuberous sclerosis. *Ann Neurol* 2002;52:29–37.

155. Bodensteiner JB, Schaefer GB, Breeding L, et al. Hypoplasia of the corpus callosum: a study of 445 consecutive MRI scans. *J Child Neurol* 1994;9:47–49.

156. Dávila-Gutiérrez G. Agenesis and dysgenesis of the corpus callosum. *Semin Pediatr Neurol* 2002;9:292–301.

157. Barkovich AJ. Anomalies of the corpus callosum and cortical malformations. In: Barth PG, ed. *Disorders of neuronal migration*. London: Mac Keith Press, 2003:83–103.

158. Dupré N, Howard HC, Mathieu J, et al. Hereditary motor and sensory neuropathy with agenesis of the corpus callosum. *Ann Neurol* 2003;54:9–18.

159. van Slegtenhorst M, de Hoogt R, Hermans C, et al. Identification of the tuberous sclerosis gene *TSC1* on chromosome 9q34. *Science* 1997;277:805–808.

160. Ali JB, Sepp T, Ward S, et al. Mutations in the *TSC1* gene account for a minority of patients with tuberous sclerosis. *J Med Genet* 1998;35:969–972.

161. Menchine M, Emeline JK, Mischel PS, et al. Tissue and cell-type specific expression of the tuberous sclerosis gene *TSC2* in human tissues. *Mod Pathol* 1996;9:1071–1080.

162. Au KS, Rodríguez JA, Finch JL, et al. Germ-line mutational analysis of the *TSC2* gene in 90 tuberous sclerosis patients. *Am J Hum Genet* 1998;62:286–294.

163. Gómez MR, Sampson JR, Whittemore VH, eds. *Tuberous sclerosis complex*, 3rd ed. New York: Oxford University Press, 1999.

164. Curatolo P, ed. *Tuberous sclerosis complex*. London: Mac Keith Press, 2003.

165. Kwiatkowska J, Jozwiak S, Hall J, et al. Comprehensive mutational analysis of the *TSC1* gene: observations on frequency of mutation, associated features and nonpenetrance. *Ann Hum Genet* 1998;62:277–285.

166. Flores-Sarnat L. Hemimegalencephaly: part 1. Genetic, clinical and imaging aspects. *J Child Neurol* 2002;17:373–384.

167. Flores-Sarnat L, Sarnat HB. Hemimegalencephaly. In: Barth PG, ed. *Disorders of neuronal migration*. London: Mac Keith Press, 2003:104–126.

168. Takashima S, Chan F, Becker LE, et al. Aberrant neuronal development in hemimegalencephaly: immunohistochemical and Golgi studies. *Pediatr Neurol* 1991;7:275–280.

169. Flores-Sarnat L, Sarnat HB, Dávila-Gutiérrez G, et al. Hemimegalencephaly: part 2. Neuropathology suggests a disorder of cellular lineage. *J Child Neurol* 2003;18:776–785.

170. Tsuru A, Mizuguchi M, Uyemura K, et al. Immunohistochemical expression of cell adhesion molecule L1 in hemimegalencephaly. *Pediatr Neurol* 1997;16:45–49.

171. Ahlgren S, Vogt P, Bronner-Fraser M. Excess *FoxG1* causes overgrowth of the neural tube. *J Neurobiol* 2003;57:337–349.

172. Pavone L, Curatolo P, Rizzo R, et al. Epidermal nevus syndrome: a neurologic variant with hemimegalencephaly, gyral malformation, mental retardation, seizures and facial hemihypertrophy. *Neurology* 1991;41:266–271.

173. Tagawa T, Futagi Y, Arai H, et al. Hypomelanosis of Ito associated with hemimegalencephaly. A clinicopathological study. *Pediatr Neurol* 1997;17:180–184.

174. Di Rocco C, Iannelli A. Hemimegalencephaly and intractable epilepsy: complications of hemispherectomy and their correlations with the surgical technique. A report of 15 cases. *Pediatr Neurosurg* 2000;33:198–207.

175. Sarnat HB, Flores-Sarnat L. Integrative classification of morphology and molecular genetics in central nervous system malformations. *Am J Med Genet* 2004;126A:386–392.

176. Barkovich AJ, Kuzniecky RI, Jackson GD, et al. Classification system for malformations of cortical development: update 2001. *Neurology* 2001;57:2168–2178.

Malformations of Cortical Development and Epilepsy

3

William B. Dobyns   *Ruben Kuzniecky*

Development of the human brain is a complex process that begins with appearance of the notochord and continues long after birth (1,2). Any disruption of this process, whether by genetic or environmental factors, may result in malformations, including those of the cerebral cortex (3). Until the advent of high-resolution neuroimaging, these disorders were the domain of the pathologist. Magnetic resonance imaging (MRI) has allowed malformations of cortical development to be identified in life, leading to improved diagnosis, knowledge of their clinical consequences, and rapid progress in understanding their pathogenesis. This chapter reviews common cortical malformations associated with epilepsy.

EPIDEMIOLOGY

The incidence of malformations of cortical development has not been adequately studied, but 15% of adults and 25% of children referred to epilepsy centers for intractable partial-onset seizures have focal cortical dysplasia (4,5). The most severe cortical malformations are less common, but current estimates are probably too low, as most data predated MRI. A case ascertainment study of lissencephaly in the Netherlands showed a prevalence of 11.7 per million births (6). Data from metropolitan Atlanta from 1994 through 1999 show rates of 0.04 per 1000 for lissencephaly and 0.01 per 1000 for polymicrogyria (Birth Defects and Genetic Diseases Branch personnel, Metropolitan Atlanta Congenital Defects Program, Centers for Disease Control and Prevention, Atlanta, GA, personal communication, 2002). No data were available for other malformations of cortical development.

CLASSIFICATION

Many different malformations of cortical development, including misplaced cortical elements such as heterotopia, have been recognized. Periventricular nodular heterotopia, lissencephaly, and focal cortical dysplasia are widely known; however, other major types exist, and many new syndromes have been described.

The nomenclature and classification of these disorders continue to evolve. Although often called neuronal migration disorders, many of these malformations involve abnormal cell formation in the ventricular zone before migration or abnormal cortical organization after migration has been largely completed. A classification system (Table 3.1) was devised and subsequently modified based on fundamental embryologic and genetic principles supplemented by gross pathologic, histologic, and neuroimaging criteria (7,8). The classification system will likely change further as the diagnoses and pathogenetic mechanisms of these malformations of cortical development are refined.

MALFORMATIONS OF CORTICAL DEVELOPMENT

Accurate diagnosis relies on recognition of the malformation on brain imaging studies; assessment of the prognosis and genetic counseling both depend on the specific diagnosis. In the following sections the major groups are reviewed, including some specific syndromes (Table 3.2) with their causative genes (2,4,9–119).

TABLE 3.1
CLASSIFICATION OF BRAIN MALFORMATIONS[a]

I. Malformations caused by abnormal neuronal and glial proliferation or apoptosis
  A. Decreased proliferation or increased apoptosis—microcephalies
    1. Microcephaly with normal to thin cortex
    2. Microlissencephaly (extreme microcephaly with thick cortex)
    3. Microcephaly with polymicrogyria or other cortical dysplasia
  B. Increased proliferation or decreased apoptosis (normal cell types)—megalencephalies
  C. Abnormal proliferation (abnormal cell types)
    1. Nonneoplastic
      a. Cortical hamartomas of tuberous sclerosis
      b. Cortical dysplasia with balloon cells
      c. Hemimegalencephaly
    2. Neoplastic (associated with disordered cortex)
      a. Dysembryoplastic neuroepithelial tumor
      b. Ganglioglioma
      c. Gangliocytoma
II. Malformations caused by abnormal neuronal migration
  A. Lissencephaly and subcortical band heterotopia spectrum
  B. Cobblestone brain malformation with congenital muscular dystrophy
  C. Heterotopia
    1. Subependymal (periventricular) heterotopia
    2. Subcortical heterotopia (other than band heterotopia)
    3. Marginal glioneuronal heterotopia
III. Malformations caused by abnormal cortical organization (including late neuronal migration)
  A. Polymicrogyria and schizencephaly
    1. Bilateral polymicrogyria syndromes
    2. Schizencephaly (polymicrogyria with clefts)
    3. Polymicrogyria with other brain malformations or abnormalities
    4. Polymicrogyria or schizencephaly as part of multiple congenital anomaly/mental retardation syndromes
  B. Cortical (architectural) dysplasia without balloon cells
  C. Microdysgenesis
IV. Malformations of cortical development, not otherwise classified
  A. Malformations secondary to inborn errors of metabolism
    1. Mitochondrial and pyruvate metabolic disorders
    2. Peroxisomal disorders
  B. Other unclassified malformations
    1. Sublobar dysplasia
    2. Others

[a]Each main category is expanded in additional tables in Reference 8.

MALFORMATIONS OF NEURONAL AND GLIAL PROLIFERATION WITH ABNORMAL CELL TYPES

Malformations in this group are characterized by abnormal neurons and, often, glia. Increased cell numbers further support abnormal proliferation early in development. All of these are localized malformations; in some, abnormal cell types have been classified as neoplastic, although the malig-

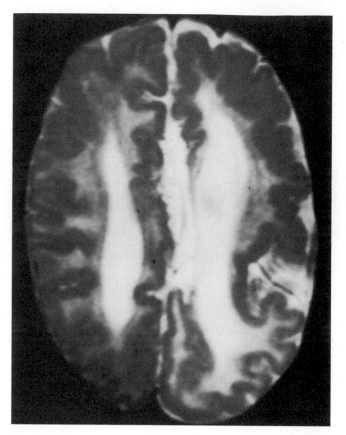

Figure 3.1 Hemimegalencephaly. Axial T2-weighted MRI shows hemimegalencephaly associated with an irregular surface and apparent pachygyria (probably fused polymicrogyria) of the entire left hemisphere and part of the right frontal region. White matter signal is strikingly increased on both sides, although more severe on the left. This child was reported previously. (From Dodge NN, Dobyns WB. Agenesis of the corpus callosum and Dandy-Walker malformation associated with hemimegalencephaly in the sebaceous nevus syndrome. *Am J Med Genet* 1995;56:147–150, with permission.)

nant potential is low. The most common of these is tuberous sclerosis, which is reviewed in chapter 36.

Hemimegalencephaly

Patients with hemimegalencephaly have mental retardation and, typically, intractable epilepsy. The overgrowth may involve part of one hemisphere, an entire hemisphere, or an entire hemisphere and part of the other side. Pathologic changes include those seen in cortical dysplasias occurring elsewhere in the brain, white matter abnormalities, and abnormal cell types. Although most patients have no other congenital anomalies, hemimegalencephaly has been observed in several sporadic neurocutaneous syndromes and rarely in tuberous sclerosis, an autosomal dominant disorder (Table 3.2). Recurrence in families has never been reported.

The clinical presentation almost always includes seizures that usually start within the first 6 months of life and arise from the enlarged and dysplastic hemisphere (120). The seizures are typically partial, with secondary generalization, and often intractable to medical therapy. Infantile spasms

TABLE 3.2

KNOWN CORTICAL MALFORMATION SYNDROMES, GENES, AND LOCI

Malformations and Syndromes	Genes, Loci	Malformations and Syndromes	Genes, Loci
Hemimegalencephaly (HMEG)		Heterotopia, other types	
• HMEG, isolated	None known	• Periventricular laminar heterotopia (unpublished data)	None known
• Epidermal nevus syndrome (9,10)	None known		
• Hypomelanosis of Ito (11)	None known	• Subcortical nodular heterotopia (63)	None known
• Klippel-Trenaunay syndrome	None known	Classic lissencephaly	
• Neuromelanosis (12)	None known	• Baraitser-Winter syndrome, a>p (64–67)	None known
• Proteus syndrome (13)	None known	• Miller-Dieker syndrome a=p (44,68,69)	LIS1, 14-3-3ε
Tuberous sclerosis (14–17)	TSC1, TSC2	• Isolated LIS sequence, a=p, a>p (70,71)	DCX
Focal cortical dysplasia (FCD) with balloon cells (18–20)	None known	• Isolated LIS sequence, a=p, p>a (70–75)	LIS1
Focal transmantle dysplasia	None known	• Subcortical band heterotopia a=p, a>p (76–80)	DCX
Megalencephaly (MEG)		• Subcortical band heterotopia, p>a (66,68,70,71,79)	LIS1
• MEG, isolated (21)	None known	LIS with cerebellar hypoplasia (LCH)	
• Macrocephaly-CMTC syndrome (22,23)	None known	• LCH group a, a=p, a>p, p>a (81)	LIS1, DCX
• MEG with mega-corpus callosum (24)	None known	• LCH group b, a>p (81–83)	RELN
• MEG-PMG-polydactyly-hydrocephalus (unpublished data) (200)	None known	• LCH group d, a=p (81)	None known
Microcephaly (MIC), moderate phenotype		LIS with agenesis of the corpus callosum (ACC)	
• MIC group 1 (25–34)	ASPM, MCPH1, 9q34, 15q, 19q13	• X-linked LIS with abnormal genitalia (XLAG), p>a (84–86)	ARX
MIC, severe phenotype		• LIS with ACC, other types, a=p (87, unpublished data)	None known
• Amish lethal MIC (35,36)	SLC25A19	Cobblestone malformations	
• MIC with heterotopia (37,38)	ARFGEF2	• Fukuyama congenital muscular dystrophy (88–91)	FCMD
• MIC group 2, other types (39–42)	None known		
• Seckel syndrome (43)	ATR	• Muscle-eye-brain disease, a>p (92–96)	POMGnT1, FKRP, LARGE
Microlissencephaly (MLIS)			
• MLIS group a, a=p (44–46)	None known	• Walker-Warburg syndrome, a=p (97–99)	POMT1, FCMD
• Barth MLIS syndrome (group b), a=p (45,47,48)	None known	Excessive neurons in white matter (100,101)	None known
Periventricular nodular heterotopia (PNH)		Polymicrogyria (PMG), regional	
• X-linked PNH (females) (49–51)	FLN1	• Frontal PMG (102)	None known
• PNH with agenesis corpus callosum (males) (52,53)	None known	• Frontoparietal PMG (103–105)	GPR56
		• Parasagittal PMG (unpublished data)	None known
• PNH with Ehlers-Danlos syndrome (females) (54,55)	None known	• Perisylvian PMG (106–113)	1p36, 1q44, 22q11, Xq28
• PNH with frontonasal malformation (males) (56,57)	None known	• Medial parietooccipital PMG (114)	None known
		• Generalized PMG (115)	None known
• PNH with mental retardation (males) (58,59)	None known	Polymicrogyria (PMG), others	
• PNH with nephrosis (males) (60)	None known	• PMG with abnormal white matter (unpublished data)	None known
• PNH with short gut syndrome (males) (2,61)	Xq28 (?)	• Schizencephaly (116)	None known
• PNH with frontoperisylvian PMG (unpublished data)	None known	• Septooptic dysplasia-schizencephaly (117–119)	None known
• PNH with posterior-inferior PMG (unpublished data)	None known	FCD and related	
• PNH with mental retardation and duplication 5p (62)	5p15.1, 5p15.33	• FCD without balloon cells (20)	None known
		• Microdysgenesis (4)	None known

a=p, Anterior equals posterior gradient; a>p, anterior more severe than posterior gradient; p>a, posterior more severe than anterior gradient; CMTC, cutis marmorata telangiectatica congenita.

and drop attacks may present in early childhood. Unilateral neurologic signs, such as hemiparesis and hemianopia, are common. Minimal neurologic dysfunction with normal cognitive abilities has been reported in some patients, when less than a full hemisphere is involved.

The appearance on MRI is characteristic (Fig. 3.1). Enlargement of at least one lobe that may range from mild to severe is present in all patients. In more than one half of

the patients, the entire hemisphere appears to be enlarged, but in some, enlargement may be localized to the frontal or temporoparietal regions. Careful review of the underlying gray matter reveals thick, broad, and flat gyri and shallow sulci. The underlying hemispheric white matter is usually abnormal, with abnormal signal characteristics and/or alteration in volume (increased or decreased) in some individuals. Heterotopia are commonly seen, and the ventricular system is enlarged in most patients, with the frontal horn typically straight. Electroencephalographic (EEG) abnormalities are often extensive throughout the abnormal hemisphere. Severity of hemiparesis, smoothness of the cortical surface on MRI, and abnormal activity on EEG predict a poor outcome. Both the epilepsy and the cognitive deficits may be improved in selected patients by timely hemispherectomy (121,122).

Focal Cortical Dysplasia and Transmantle Dysplasia with Abnormal but Nonneoplastic Cells

Focal cortical dysplasia with balloon cells has been observed in patients with tuberous sclerosis and in those with no other anomalies (123). The balloon cells are probably the result of proliferation of abnormal cells in the germinal zone rather than local effects on migrating cells within the intermediate zone. The appearance is similar to the changes in tuberous sclerosis, and a genetic relationship is possible (18). Focal transmantle dysplasia consists of a streak of abnormal cells extending from the ependyma to the pial surface, but the pathologic appearance is identical to that of focal cortical dysplasia with balloon cells (7).

Focal cortical dysplasia is probably the most common form of focal developmental disorder diagnosed in patients with intractable focal epilepsy. The characteristic pathologic abnormalities consist of disruption of cortical lamination with poorly differentiated glial cell elements. Since its original description, focal cortical dysplasia has been recognized to encompass a spectrum of pathologic changes ranging from mild cortical disruption, without apparent giant neurons, to the most severe forms, with cortical dyslamination, large bizarre cells, and astrocytosis. The presence of balloon cells differentiates type I (without balloon cells) and type II (with balloon cells) (4,19,124,125).

The clinical manifestations are variable (5,20,126). Seizures usually begin in the first or, less often, second decade of life, usually after age 2 to 3 years, but they sometimes appear shortly after birth. An improved ability to recognize subtle focal cortical dysplasia on brain MRI has permitted uncommon diagnosis in epilepsy of adult onset. The seizures may be partial simple motor, partial complex, or secondary generalized. The location of the lesion often dictates the clinical presentation (4,5). Most patients have extratemporal cortical dysplasia, most commonly in the frontal lobes. Involvement of precentral and postcentral gyri may lead to cortical motor and sensory abnormalities. MRI findings include abnormal gyral thickening with underlying T2-weighted white matter changes (Fig. 3.2) that are often circumscribed. Interictal EEG may show frequent spikes or even localized subclinical EEG seizures. Focal cortical dysplasia of the temporal lobe has also been

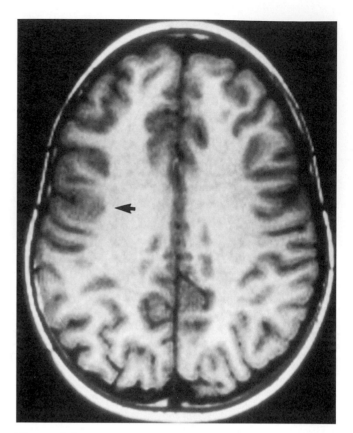

Figure 3.2 Focal cortical dysplasia. Axial T1-weighted MRI demonstrates a focal malformation in the right central region in a child with intractable epilepsy (*arrow*).

reported with involvement of mesial and lateral neocortical structures (4,125). The seizures and clinical course are similar to those of temporal lobe epilepsy caused by hippocampal sclerosis, but the EEG abnormalities are usually less circumscribed. MRI shows cortical thickening of temporal convolutions associated with poor differentiation of the gray-white junction. The association of hippocampal sclerosis with dysplastic cortex in the temporal lobe (dual pathology) is well known.

Cortical Dysplasia with Neoplastic Changes

Several low-grade primarily neuronal neoplasms are associated with cortical dysplasia, including dysembryoplastic neuroepithelial tumors, ganglioglioma, and gangliocytoma. Controversy continues over their proper classification. Their frequency in epilepsy surgical series is approximately 5% to 8%, and they occur most often in children or young adults. The tumors are most often located in the temporal lobes, where residual heterotopic neurons in the white matter are also common (100,101), but can also be seen elsewhere. Patients usually present with partial seizures that are difficult to control with anticonvulsant drugs. Surgical treatment is highly effective in most cases if the lesion is completely resected.

MALFORMATIONS OF NEURONAL AND GLIAL PROLIFERATION WITH NORMAL CELL TYPES

Malformations in this group are characterized by an increase or decrease in the number of neurons and glia with secondary changes in brain size, designated as either megalencephaly or microcephaly. No abnormal cell types are seen. The most common types of megalencephaly and microcephaly are not typically included under brain malformations, because brain structure appears grossly normal, although detailed studies of neuronal cell types have not been described.

Megalencephaly Syndromes

Megalencephaly, or enlarged brain, occurs as a mild familial variant with normal brain structure but otherwise is an uncommon malformation that may be associated with developmental and neurologic problems (127). The clinical findings have been variable but are usually mild to moderate, particularly with the familial form. A subset of patients has severe mental retardation, intractable epilepsy, and other neurologic abnormalities (127); however, the basis for this difference is not clear and few distinct subtypes have been described. Several megalencephaly syndromes with cortical malformations and severe epilepsy are likely underrecognized (Table 3.2 and Fig. 3.3).

Microcephaly Syndromes

Defining microcephaly as head circumferences of 2 standard deviations or more below the mean (128) results in almost 400 syndromes identified in a database search (Online Mendelian Inheritance in Man [OMIM]); therefore, −3 standard deviations is a more useful cutoff as a primary abnormality. When congenital microcephaly is the only abnormality on evaluation, the disorder is called primary microcephaly or microcephalia vera (128,129), but these terms are often little understood.

Most of these children fall into two groups (40). The first group comprises children with extreme microcephaly but only moderate neurologic problems, usually only moderate mental retardation without spasticity or epilepsy. Several genes associated with this phenotype have been identified (Table 3.2).

The second and more important group from an epilepsy perspective consists of primary microcephaly with severe spasticity and epilepsy (39–42). Abnormal reflexes and generalized spasticity are evident neonatally. Subsequent poor feeding and recurrent vomiting lead to poor weight gain, severe developmental delay with consequent profound mental retardation, and spastic quadriparesis. Early onset intractable epilepsy is common. In addition to a simplified gyral pattern, MRI of the brain may show enlarged extra-axial spaces, delayed myelinization, agenesis of the corpus callosum, or severe hypoplasia of the brainstem and cerebellum (Fig. 3.4). This clinical spectrum suggests pathogenetically heterogeneous conditions, and several genes have been identified (Table 3.2).

Children with severe congenital microcephaly are often incorrectly diagnosed as having lissencephaly because of a reduced number of broad gyri; however, the cortex is not thick as in true lissencephaly, and genetic tests for lissencephaly are always normal. A few patients with severe congenital microcephaly and a thick cortex

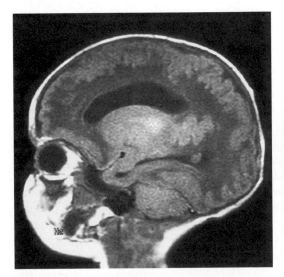
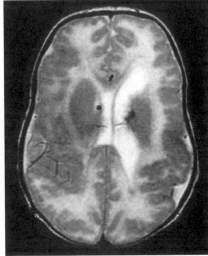

Figure 3.3 Megalencephaly and perisylvian polymicrogyria in a patient with severe mental retardation, hypotonia, mild distal spasticity, and epilepsy. Sagittal T1- and axial T2-weighted images show a large head and brain, thick, irregular cortex in the perisylvian and parietal regions, mildly enlarged lateral ventricles, and persistent cavum vergae.

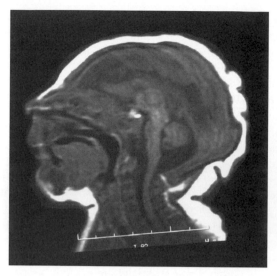
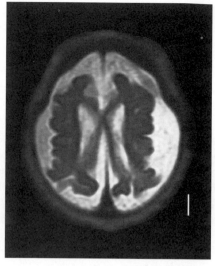

Figure 3.4 Severe congenital microcephaly in a patient with severe spasticity and mental retardation. Sagittal T1- and axial T2-weighted MRI show a low sloping forehead, mild cerebellar hypoplasia, enlarged extra-axial space, reduced number of gyri, and mildly enlarged lateral ventricles. The cortex is not seen well enough to determine whether it is dysplastic or not.

are designated as having microlissencephaly (45); these children also have intractable epilepsy. Most syndromes with severe congenital microcephaly have autosomal recessive inheritance.

MALFORMATIONS OF NEURONAL MIGRATION

The true malformations caused by deficient neuronal migration all have gray matter in the subependymal or subcortical regions. Location and extent vary remarkably from focal subcortical or subependymal heterotopia to lissencephaly.

Heterotopia

Periventricular nodular heterotopia are masses of gray matter that diffusely line the ventricular walls and protrude into the lumen, producing an irregular outline (130,131). Bilateral forms are contiguous and symmetric (Fig. 3.5), although occasionally they are noncontiguous and asymmetric. They may be associated with hypoplasia of the corpus callosum or cerebellum, especially if the nodules are diffuse and contiguous, and have accompanied polymicrogyria. Unilateral periventricular nodular heterotopia are usually noncontiguous.

Patients with unilateral or bilateral periventricular nodular heterotopia usually present with seizures that may be difficult to control. The EEG manifestations are less specific, with infrequent interictal abnormalities that may be generalized, focal, or multifocal. Pseudotemporal lobe localization has also been reported (132,133). A few

patients have had headache or other incidental symptoms, whereas others discovered during family evaluations are asymptomatic. Most females have normal intelligence; affected males often have mental retardation.

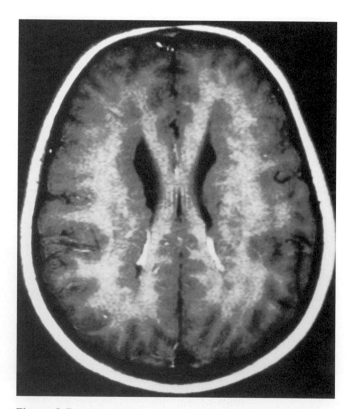

Figure 3.5 Bilateral periventricular nodular heterotopia. Sagittal T1-weighted MRI shows confluent nodules with the signal characteristics of gray matter surrounding the lateral borders of both lateral ventricles. The overlying cortex appears normal.

X-Linked Periventricular Nodular Heterotopia

The most common type of periventricular nodular heterotopia syndrome is X-linked and causes typical bilateral periventricular nodular heterotopia in females and prenatal lethality in males. Several observations contributed to the recognition of this syndrome, including a skewed sex ratio toward females among sporadic patients, reports of several families with multiple affected females, and a decrease in the number of sons born to affected women (130,134). The gene was mapped to Xq28 and identified as *FLNA* (49,135). Subsequent studies demonstrated mutations in patients with typical brain-imaging characteristics (136) and occurrence in both sexes (50,51).

Periventricular Nodular Heterotopia Syndromes

Periventricular nodular heterotopia with severe mental retardation or with frontonasal malformation have been described. Data from more than 20 patients with periventricular nodular heterotopia and overlying polymicrogyria have been reviewed. Most of these syndromes have been observed predominantly or exclusively in males, suggesting possible X-linked inheritance (Table 3.2). No mutations of *FLNA* have been identified in these cases.

Other Heterotopia

Subcortical nodular heterotopia typically consist of a large mass of heterotopia expanding a portion of one cerebral hemisphere. Rarely, if ever, bilateral, they are often associated with ipsilateral periventricular nodular heterotopia, agenesis of the corpus callosum, and cerebellar vermis hypoplasia. Overlying cortical dysplasia may occur (63,137). Despite the large size of these malformations, development is often normal or near normal, and seizures may not begin until the third decade. Patients with overlying cortical dysplasia have more severe problems including mental retardation.

Periventricular laminar heterotopia are rare and differ from periventricular nodular heterotopia in the lack of nodularity. Imaging studies from several patients have been reviewed, but no review has been published because of the paucity of cases at any single center. The cause is unknown.

Lissencephaly and Subcortical Band Heterotopia

Lissencephaly, or agyria-pachygyria, is a severe, diffuse brain malformation manifested by a smooth cerebral surface and an abnormally thick cortex with four abnormal layers, including a deep zone of diffuse neuronal heterotopia and enlarged, dysplastic ventricles (138–140). Subcortical band heterotopia consists of symmetric and circumferential bands of gray matter located just beneath the cortex and separated from it by a thin band of white matter. The inner margin of the band is usually smooth; the outer margin may be smooth or follow interdigitations of the true cortex and white matter. This appearance led to the alternative, although incorrect, term *double cortex* for this malformation. The overlying cortex appears normal or mildly simplified because of abnormally shallow sulci (63,130,141). Lissencephaly and subcortical band heterotopia comprise a single malformation. This conclusion is based on observations of rare patients with areas of lissencephaly that merge into subcortical band heterotopia and of multiple families with X-linked lissencephaly in males and subcortical band heterotopia in females (80,142–144).

The most common type, known as classic lissencephaly (previously type I), has a 10- to 20-mm cortex and no other major brain malformations; this is the only type associated with subcortical band heterotopia (130). Less common types involve an intermediately thick 8- to 12-mm cortex, agenesis of the corpus callosum, or severe cerebellar hypoplasia (81,83,84,139,145).

Lissencephaly and subcortical band heterotopia are distinguished by both the pattern and severity of the malformation. The pattern or gradient can be anteriorly more severe than posteriorly (a>p), posteriorly more severe than anteriorly (p>a), or anteriorly similar to posteriorly (a=p) (Fig. 3.6). These distinctions have become important in identifying the different syndromes and their associated genes (see below) (70,71).

Clinical Manifestations

Children with classic lissencephaly or other diffuse cortical malformations often appear normal as newborns but sometimes have apnea, poor feeding, or hypotonia. Seizures are uncommon during the first days of life, but they typically begin sometime before 6 months of age. The epileptic spectrum is homogeneous. In the first year of life, approximately 80% of children with lissencephaly present with infantile spasms, often appearing initially as hypsarrhythmia on scalp EEG. The infantile spasms respond at first to corticotropin or other anticonvulsants in a majority of children, but in the long-term, almost all of these children will have frequent seizures and severe mental retardation. Typical seizure types include myoclonic, tonic, and tonic-clonic; many meet criteria for Lennox-Gastaut syndrome. Profound mental retardation, early hypotonia, mild spastic quadriplegia, and opisthotonus also are seen. Many patients require a gastrostomy because of poor nutrition and repeated episodes of aspiration pneumonia (146).

In contrast, most patients with subcortical band heterotopia and the rare patients with partial lissencephaly have mild to moderate mental retardation (although normal intelligence and severe mental retardation occur), minimal pyramidal signs, and dysarthria (76,130,141). Seizures usually begin in childhood but may appear much later, and multiple types occur that may be difficult to control; however, frequency and severity vary. Cognitive development may slow after onset of seizures. EEG investigations

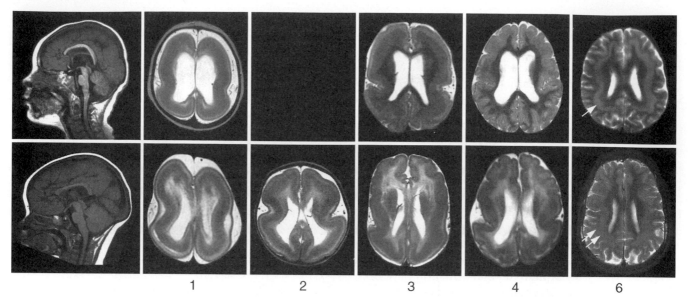

1   2   3   4   6

Figure 3.6   The patterns of lissencephaly associated with *DCX* mutations *(top row)* and *LIS1* mutations *(bottom row)* are different (70,71). Midline sagittal images show normal *(bottom left)* or minimally small *(top left)* cerebellar vermis for both, with vermis hypoplasia more common with *DCX* mutations. Axial T2 images show variable severity with grades listed below each column consisting of complete agyria (grade 1), mixed agyria-pachygyria (grade 4), generalized or partial pachygyria (grade 4), and subcortical band heterotopia (grade 6, *arrows* in far-right column). In lissencephaly grade 1 and diffuse subcortical band heterotopia *(top right)*, the malformation is too severe for a gradient to be detected. In the remainder, *DCX* mutations are consistently more severe anteriorly and *LIS1* mutations more severe posteriorly. The cortex is always very thick (12 to 20 mm).

usually demonstrate generalized spike-wave discharges or multifocal abnormalities (76,147,148). The neurologic outcome depends on the thickness of the heterotopic band as seen on MRI.

Lissencephaly Syndromes and Genes

The most common lissencephaly syndromes include isolated lissencephaly sequence, subcortical band heterotopia, Miller-Dieker syndrome, several types of lissencephaly with cerebellar hypoplasia, and X-linked lissencephaly with abnormal genitalia (Table 3.2). The approach to genetic testing and genetic counseling is detailed below.

Isolated lissencephaly sequence consists of classic lissencephaly with a normal facial appearance except for mild bitemporal hollowing and small jaw (44,146). Mutations of *DCX* and *LIS1* result in somewhat different patterns of lissencephaly. Isolated lissencephaly sequence associated with mutations of the X-linked *DCX* gene is characterized by either severe lissencephaly with no apparent gradient or lissencephaly with a clear a>p gradient and normal facial appearance (70,71). Mutations or deletions of the *LIS1* gene produce lissencephaly with a p>a gradient, although in rare patients, lissencephaly is too severe for the gradient to be detected. Facial appearance may be normal or have subtle dysmorphism similar to Miller-Dieker syndrome but much milder (68,146). The different lissencephaly patterns are readily distinguishable in most patients (Fig. 3.6).

Miller-Dieker syndrome consists of classic lissencephaly, characteristic facial abnormalities, and variable other birth defects such as heart malformations or omphalocele. The facial changes include prominent forehead, bitemporal hollowing, short nose with upturned nares, protuberant upper lip with thin vermilion border, and small jaw. The brain malformation consists of severe lissencephaly with no apparent gradient, although rare patients may have the same p>a gradient seen in isolated lissencephaly sequence with *LIS1* mutations (68,69). All patients with Miller-Dieker syndrome have large deletions of chromosome 17p13.3 that include *LIS1*, *14-3-3ε*, and all intervening genes. Approximately 60% to 70% of the deletions are visible during a routine karyotype; the remainder, though submicroscopic, are detectable by fluorescence *in situ* hybridization (FISH) (68,69).

With very rare exceptions, subcortical band heterotopia are an isolated malformation. Its observation predominantly in females suggests X-linked inheritance (130), although many affected males have also been reported (76). Mutations of *DCX* and *LIS1* result in somewhat different patterns of malformation. Subcortical band heterotopia associated with mutations of *DCX* is characterized by diffuse thick subcortical band heterotopia with no apparent gradient, or partial frontal, thin subcortical band heterotopia with an obvious a>p gradient (79,149). Mutations or deletions of the *LIS1* gene cause a rare subcortical band heterotopia with partial, posterior, thin or intermediate bands with an obvious p>a gradient. Most patients have mosaic mutations of *LIS1* (76,80,150) or deletions of 17p13.3 (W.B. Dobyns, unpublished data, 2004).

Lissencephaly with cerebellar hypoplasia affects a small percentage of patients with lissencephaly syndromes (81). Group a, the most common type, resembles isolated lissencephaly syndrome but with the addition of mild cerebellar vermis hypoplasia. Indeed, some patients have mutations of *DCX* or *LIS1*, although much less frequently than patients with typical isolated lissencephaly syndrome (Table 3.3). Group b consists of moderate lissencephaly with an a>p gradient, moderate 8- to 10-mm cortical thickness, a globular hippocampus, and a small, afoliar cerebellum. Some patients with this imaging appearance have had mutations of *RELN* (82,83,145), but in most patients with lissencephaly with cerebellar hyperplasia, mutation analysis of *DCX* and *LIS1* is normal (81).

X-linked lissencephaly with abnormal genitalia consists of variant lissencephaly in genotypic males with p>a gradient and intermediate 8- to 10-mm cortical thickness, usually complete agenesis of the corpus callosum, often cavitated or indistinct basal ganglia, severe postnatal microcephaly, and ambiguous or severely hypoplastic genitalia. Affected children have profound mental retardation, hypothalamic dysfunction with poor temperature regulation, intractable epilepsy typically beginning on the first day of life, infancy-onset dyskinesia that may be difficult to distinguish from seizures, and chronic diarrhea (84,85). Female relatives, including some mothers, have isolated agenesis of the corpus callosum. Mutations of the *ARX* gene have been found in almost all patients (85,86). Other syndromes with lissencephaly and agenesis of the corpus callosum appear to be very rare.

Less severe mutations of *ARX* have been found in males with cryptogenic infantile spasms, infancy-onset dyskinesia,

TABLE 3.3

FREQUENCY OF MUTATIONS IN LISSENCEPHALY AND SUBCORTICAL BAND HETEROTOPIA SYNDROMES

Syndrome	Gene or Locus				
	ARX	*DCX*	*LIS1*	*del 17p*	*RELN*
ILS	0	~12	~24	~40	0
LCH	Rare	~25	~15	0[a]	Rare
MDS	0	0	0	All[b]	0
SBH	0	~80	Rare	Rare	0
XLAG	95	0	0	0	0

ILS, isolated lissencephaly sequence; LCH, lissencephaly with cerebellar hypoplasia; MDS, Miller-Dieker syndrome; SBH, subcortical band heterotopia; XLAG, X-linked lissencephaly with abnormal genitalia.
[a]Deletion of 17p13.3 could be seen in lissencephaly group a (mild vermis hypoplasia).
[b]Miller-Dieker syndrome is partly defined by the deletion.

and some less specific mental retardation and epilepsy syndromes (151–158).

Cobblestone Brain Malformations (Cobblestone Complex)

Cobblestone complex (previously type 2 or cobblestone lissencephaly) is a severe brain malformation consisting of cobblestone cortex (a term proposed by Haltia), abnormal white matter, enlarged ventricles often with hydrocephalus, small brainstem, and small, dysplastic cerebellum (159–164). In the most severely affected patients, the brain surface is smooth, which led to the designation as lissencephaly, although less severe cobblestone malformations have an irregular, pebbled, rather than smooth, surface. The cortical changes consist of atypical agyria, pachygyria, and polymicrogyria with an unusual pebbled surface caused by leptomeningeal neuronal and glial heterotopia. Severe expression may include progressive hydrocephalus, large posterior fossa cysts (atypical for Dandy-Walker malformation), and occipital cephaloceles. Eye malformations are frequent, and congenital muscular dystrophy is probably always present.

The cobblestone malformation has been observed in three genetic syndromes, although they clearly overlap: Fukuyama congenital muscular dystrophy, muscle-eye-brain disease, and Walker-Warburg syndrome. All share a clinical course of severe to profound mental retardation, severe hypotonia, mild distal spasticity, and often poor vision. Walker-Warburg syndrome has the most severe brain malformations, with survival beyond 3 years a rarity. Fukuyama congenital muscular dystrophy, the least-severe form, results in moderate to severe mental retardation, only minor eye abnormalities, and survival well into the second decade. Muscle-eye-brain disease is the most variable—sometimes almost as severe as Walker-Warburg syndrome and at other times with survival into the third or fourth decade. This likely represents a semantic issue, as muscle-eye-brain disease is applied to any intermediate phenotype. All of these syndromes are autosomal recessive and have a recurrence risk of 25%.

Fukuyama congenital muscular dystrophy consists of relatively mild cobblestone complex, moderate to severe mental retardation and epilepsy, and severe congenital muscular dystrophy with progressive weakness, joint contractures, and elevated serum levels of creatine kinase (91,165). The causative *FCMD* gene was identified, as well as a common founder mutation of this gene in the Japanese population (89,90).

Muscle-eye-brain disease consists of moderate cobblestone dysplasia with moderate to severe mental retardation, epilepsy, complex eye abnormalities (including retinal and choroidal hypoplasia, optic nerve pallor, high-grade myopia, anterior chamber-angle abnormalities, glaucoma, iris hypoplasia, cataracts, and rare colobomas [166]), and congenital muscular dystrophy or myopathy with weakness, contractures, and elevated serum levels of creatine kinase. Mutations of three genes, *FKRP, LARGE,* and *POMGnT1* have been found; *POMGnT1* is associated with the classic Finnish form of the disease (92–96,167,169). Biochemical deficiency has been demonstrated in muscle (168).

Walker-Warburg syndrome includes lissencephaly and the most severe brainstem and cerebellar malformations of any of the cobblestone group. Most patients have hydrocephalus, and approximately 25% have occipital cephaloceles (159,160). All patients have profound mental retardation, epilepsy, and eye abnormalities similar to those of muscle-eye-brain disease and the same congenital muscular dystrophy or myopathy with elevated serum levels of creatine kinase and contractures. Mutations of *POMGnT1* do not appear to cause Walker-Warburg syndrome (40,169). However, mutations of *POMT1* and *FCMD* have been found in a few patients (97–99).

All of the genes that cause cobblestone complex malformation code for proteins known or suspected to be involved with glycosylation, particularly protein O mannosylation, of α-dystroglycan (170,171). Homozygous null mutations of α-dystroglycan cause embryonic lethality in mice, but a brain-specific mouse knockout resulted in a brain malformation that closely resembles the cobblestone malformation (172).

Excessive Single Ectopic White-Matter Neurons

Excessive white-matter neurons have been reported in patients undergoing epilepsy surgery and in postmortem studies. Observed most often in the temporal lobe, these abnormalities are also seen in frontal lobe specimens. Isolated heterotopic neurons in the white matter in normal brains are also most numerous in the temporal lobes (100,101). The clinical correlates of the pathologic disorder are not well understood. One study (125) found a statistically significantly increased number of neurons in the white matter in the temporal lobe of patients undergoing temporal resections for seizures. MRI studies may show an abnormal white-gray matter junction if the number of ectopic cells is large. No familial recurrence or specific sex or racial predominance has been observed.

MALFORMATIONS OF CORTICAL ORGANIZATION

This group includes malformations in which neurons reach the cortex but do not form normal cortical layers or intracortical connections. These malformations are characterized by an abnormal gyral pattern with moderately increased thickness of the cortex, typically 5 to 10 mm (the normal thickness is 3 to 4 mm in most regions). This group excludes heterotopia, which are classified as a true

migration disorder. The classic malformations in this category are four-layered and unlayered polymicrogyria, schizencephaly, focal cortical dysplasia with normal cell types, and microdysgenesis.

Polymicrogyria

Polymicrogyria is characterized by many small gyri separated by shallow sulci, slightly thick cortex, neuronal heterotopia, and enlarged ventricles. A simplified four-layered cortex consists of a superficial cellular zone continuous with normal layers II to IV, a deeper cellular zone continuous with layers V and VI that merges imperceptibly into the white matter, and a cell-sparse zone between them. The cortex is thinner than normal but appears thickened owing to infolding or festooning of the cortical ribbon, which in more severely affected areas gives the appearance of columns (173–175). The walls of the shallow sulci are fused in their deeper portions and have small penetrating blood vessels. The small, tightly packed microgyri mimic the appearance of pachygyria, leading to frequent misdiagnosis.

MRI shows loss of the normal gyral pattern, an irregular or pebbled brain surface, increased numbers of approximately 2- to 5-mm gyri, and an irregular border between the cortex and underlying white matter (Fig. 3.7).

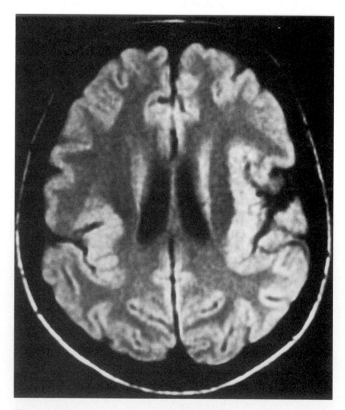

Figure 3.7 Congenital bilateral perisylvian syndrome. Axial T2-weighted MRI shows bilateral opercular abnormalities with thick cortex representing (fused) polymicrogyria. The abnormalities are asymmetric in location and extent.

Whenever the perisylvian region is involved, the sylvian fissures extend farther posteriorly to the parietal convexity. The cortex is usually 5 to 10 mm thick. Patients with schizencephaly have deep clefts extending down to the lateral ventricles that are lined by polymicrogyria and may appear as a column of gray matter with narrow clefts (116). Thus, these two malformations are closely related.

The clinical presentation is variable, except in perisylvian polymicrogyria. The major prognostic factors across all types are head size at birth, extent of polymicrogyria, and findings on the motor examination. The most unfavorable prognostic factors are severe congenital microcephaly, extensive involvement of the brain, especially the frontal lobes, and spastic quadriparesis. Involvement of the primary motor cortex is typically associated with spasticity.

Atypical absences, tonic-atonic attacks, and generalized tonic-clonic seizures occur in more than 80% of patients; most have severe epilepsy. The EEG shows generalized spike-wave or multifocal abnormalities. A syndrome consisting of unilateral central polymicrogyria and transient nonconvulsive status epilepticus has been reported (176). Epilepsy is relatively amenable to medical treatment until puberty, when seizures become intractable. In many adults, the seizures remain under relatively good control and may abate with adjustments of antiepileptic medications.

Perisylvian Polymicrogyria

Also known as congenital bilateral perisylvian syndrome (117), perisylvian polymicrogyria is the most common subtype, with a highly variable severity that depends largely on the extent of the polymicrogyria. Patients have prominent pseudobulbar paresis, in the form of swallowing difficulties and aspiration, inability to protrude the tongue, and dysarthria, as well as a moderate to severe developmental delay. The syndrome probably overlaps with congenital suprabulbar palsy, also known as Worster-Drought syndrome (177,178). Seizures occur in more than 80% of patients. Unique perioral seizures with bilateral facial involvement have been described.

Schizencephaly is included in the same category as polymicrogyria because the cortex around the lips of the cleft is polymicrogyric. Moreover, schizencephaly probably represents a severe form of polymicrogyria (116). Isolated schizencephaly and schizencephaly associated with absent septum pellucidum, optic nerve hypoplasia, or both, collectively have been designated the septooptic dysplasia-schizencephaly syndrome (117,118), and some of these patients have had polymicrogyria rather than schizencephaly, again demonstrating the relationship between these malformations (119). Polymicrogyria and schizencephaly belong to the same spectrum of malformation in some instances, as with twinning and septooptic dysplasia, but not in others. Schizencephaly has not been observed in the established regional polymicrogyria syndromes or periventricular nodular heterotopia-polymicrogyria syndromes (Table 3.2).

The clinical manifestations of schizencephaly are related to the type of defect, with type 2 open clefts often associated with severe, contralateral pyramidal signs and mental retardation. Callosal agenesis is also a marker for poor outcome. Seizures are usually focal and often intractable, but clinical variability is observed. Despite gross structural lesions, EEG localization is often regional rather than focal. The central location of the lesions and widespread areas of epileptogenic activity often render surgery impossible.

Vascular Causes

Many early studies concluded that polymicrogyria and schizencephaly were caused by an injury occurring soon after the last major wave of migration ends, as neurons of all six normal layers reach the cortical plate, but with apparent destruction of normal lamina IV to V, which appear continuous with the cell-sparse zone of polymicrogyria. The proposed extrinsic cause is placental perfusion failure, associated with intrauterine infections such as cytomegalovirus infection (179–181), twinning (182–184), or as maternal use of warfarin (175,185,186).

Genetic Polymicrogyria

Early reports of polymicrogyria and schizencephaly did not suspect a genetic basis. During the past decade, numerous papers have described familial recurrence of either condition (187–192), including reports of multiple families consistent with X-linked inheritance that led to mapping of a locus in Xq28 (111,191). This may explain the skewing of the sex ratio toward males among patients with polymicrogyria (193). Chromosome abnormalities, especially deletions of 22q11.2 (106–108,112) and of 1p36 (110), have also been described. We do not consider the report of *EMX2* mutations in schizencephaly to be reliable (194).

Polymicrogyria Syndromes

Numerous other recognizable polymicrogyria syndromes have been described (Table 3.2), although the perisylvian form accounts for approximately 60% of all patients (19). The recently described "bilateral generalized" polymicrogyria (115) appears to be a mixture of several different disorders including more severe perisylvian polymicrogyria, generalized polymicrogyria with macrocephaly, and Adams-Oliver syndrome. We have also evaluated patients with microcephaly and generalized polymicrogyria. A few syndromes with multiple congenital anomalies associated with polymicrogyria have been reported, including Adams-Oliver syndrome (195).

Focal Cortical Dysplasia without Balloon Cells and Microdysgenesis

Focal cortical dysplasia without balloon cells and cortical microdysgenesis usually require histopathologic confirmation before a final classification is established. For this reason, the clinical manifestations have not been well described. Cortical dysplasia without balloon cells and milder forms of microdysgenesis have been reported in patients with epilepsy (4). As for focal dysplasias associated with balloon cells, the clinical abnormalities correlate with location of the lesions. They are more frequent in the frontal lobes, followed by the temporal regions. In most individuals, the malformations do not follow any boundaries between various regions, usually involve more than a single gyrus or lobe, and are sporadic.

GENETIC TESTING AND GENETIC COUNSELING

Although many genes associated with malformations of cortical development have been identified (Table 3.2), only the causative genes for tuberous sclerosis, lissencephaly, and subcortical band heterotopia are available for clinical testing. Nonetheless, epileptologists must provide accurate information to families and consider referral to a genetics clinic.

Most malformations of neuronal and glial proliferation with abnormal cell types, such as megalencephaly and hemimegalencephaly, are sporadic, with the important exception of tuberous sclerosis. Tuberous sclerosis is autosomal dominant with high penetrance but variable expressivity, so the recurrence risk is 50% and multiple generations are in jeopardy. No familial recurrence has ever been reported for hemimegalencephaly, focal cortical dysplasia with balloon cells, transmantle dysplasia, or the cortical dysplasias with neoplastic changes such as dysembryoplastic neuroepithelial tumors. In light of observations in neurocutaneous syndromes with hemimegalencephaly, these are still likely to be genetic but caused by postzygotic mosaicism. The mild form of familial megalencephaly is often found in relatives, with apparent autosomal dominant inheritance; the rare and more severe syndromes have not recurred in families, although data are very limited.

In contrast, severe congenital microcephaly is usually genetic. When the head circumference at birth is at or below 3 standard deviations below the mean, counseling for autosomal recessive inheritance is prudent, given the 25% recurrence risk. When the birth head circumference is between 2 and 3 standard deviations below the mean, autosomal recessive inheritance is still possible, although heterogeneity is much greater. No adequate studies have been conducted, and a 10% to 25% risk for recurrence seems reasonable.

The true malformations of neuronal migration are probably all genetic, except for some sporadic, isolated heterotopia. Typical periventricular nodular heterotopia in females with normal development or mild cognitive deficiency is most likely caused by FLNA mutations, although other loci doubtless exist. Counseling for X-linked inheritance should be provided. The same phenotype in males or

multiple other syndromes with mental retardation in males (Table 3.2) may be X-linked as well, but current knowledge is limited. Periventricular nodular heterotopia with severe congenital microcephaly is autosomal recessive, and other autosomal recessive periventricular nodular heterotopia syndromes are known. Counseling for both X-linked and autosomal recessive inheritance should be reviewed when classification is not certain. The recurrence risk for unilateral or isolated single periventricular nodular heterotopia is probably much lower, but recurrences are known and experience is limited. We are aware of no recurrences of subcortical nodular heterotopia.

Genetic testing is available for at least 80% of patients with lissencephaly or subcortical band heterotopia, although the percentage varies with the specific phenotype. When either is suspected but the exact syndrome diagnosis is uncertain, the most productive order of testing is chromosomal analysis and FISH, followed by sequencing, in this order, of LIS1, DCX, and ARX; however, knowledge of the phenotype can be helpful. When the facial appearance is abnormal, this order should be followed, as many patients will have Miller-Dieker syndrome or isolated lissencephaly sequence because of smaller deletions of 17p13. In males with lissencephaly and normal facies, and in all females with subcortical band heterotopia, the mutation analysis may start with DCX. Brain imaging studies will usually demonstrate either a p>a or a>p gradient, which may be used to choose the testing order. Imaging results should generally not alter the testing sequence, however, except for clinicians with extensive experience. The X-linked lissencephaly with abnormal genitalia phenotype associated with ARX mutations is striking, and testing should begin with ARX.

Genetic testing for lissencephaly and subcortical band heterotopia is important, as several syndromes are associated with very high risks of recurrence. This is especially true for parents who are carriers of a rearrangement of chromosome 17 and for mothers who carry ARX or DCX mutations.

Chromosomal analysis in Miller-Dieker syndrome shows visible deletions of 17p13.3 in approximately 60% to 70% of patients, and FISH reveals deletions in the remaining patients. In approximately 30% of families, one parent carries a balanced chromosome rearrangement; the recurrence risk is approximately 33% (196).

Parents should be tested for isolated lissencephaly sequence whenever mutations or small deletions of LIS1 have been found. Normal results predict a low recurrence risk (we have not seen recurrence in more than 100 families). Because recurrence is possible owing to mosaicism in one parent, prenatal diagnosis for future pregnancies is suggested. Mutations of DCX warrant carrier testing in the mother, and we test fathers of female probands as well, having found one father who was a mosaic carrier for the mutation in his affected daughter. When the mother is a carrier, a rather frequent occurrence, the risk of recurrence is 50% (79), although this does vary somewhat according to the phenotype in the affected child. The frequency of mosaicism in carrier mothers appears to be high (78,79). In the absence of testing, counseling is more difficult. Recurrences in siblings have been noted (197,198), and counseling for a 10% to 25% recurrence risk is recommended.

For subcortical band heterotopia, the same rules apply as for isolated lissencephaly sequence, except that the large majority of subcortical band heterotopia is associated with mutations of *DCX*; most individuals need counseling for X-linked inheritance. When mutations of *LIS1* are found, testing is the same as for isolated lissencephaly sequence; however, the greater likelihood of mosaicism indicates a much lower risk of recurrence in siblings. Negative test results should prompt counseling for a 10% to 25% recurrence risk, as both autosomal dominant and recessive inheritance have been seen (199).

Because almost all patients with X-linked lissencephaly with abnormal genitalia have mutations of *ARX*, counseling for X-linked inheritance and testing are indicated. Many mothers are carriers. Counseling for autosomal recessive inheritance of the rare Baraitser-Winter syndrome and lissencephaly with cerebellar hypoplasia is suggested because of recurrence in several types of the latter, although this may not be correct for all types. Testing of *RELN* is not available clinically.

All of the syndromes associated with the cobblestone malformation have autosomal recessive inheritance, but testing of the identified genes (Table 3.2) is available only in a few research laboratories. However, biochemical testing of *POMGnT1*, and possibly *POMT1*, is possible (168). A clinical test for prenatal diagnosis is not available. Prenatal ultrasonography should detect most fetuses with cobblestone malformations, especially muscle-eye-brain disease and Walker-Warburg syndrome, which typically feature hydrocephalus.

All patients with polymicrogyria should undergo chromosomal analysis and FISH for deletions of 22q11.2, the DiGeorge syndrome region, even if this syndrome or velocardiofacial syndrome appears unlikely based on the clinical examination. FISH is also ordered for a subtelomeric probe set, as polymicrogyria has been observed with deletions of both telomeres of chromosome 1.

Several families with perisylvian polymicrogyria in multiple individuals have been reported; most have been consistent with X-linked inheritance but some with autosomal dominant or autosomal recessive inheritance (191). These observations and the preponderance of affected males suggest a recurrence risk of 15% to 20% for families with male probands and approximately 10% for families with female probands. The frontoparietal form of atypical polymicrogyria has autosomal recessive inheritance (104). Data on other types are too sparse, although some are certainly genetic (115).

Schizencephaly is common, but reports of familial occurrence are few. The recurrence risk is less than 5%. No instances of familial recurrence are known for focal cortical dysplasia with normal cells or for microdysgenesis; however, these diagnoses require brain biopsy for confirmation.

REFERENCES

1. Barkovich AJ, Gressens P, Evrard P. Formation, maturation, and disorders of brain neocortex. *Am J Neuroradiol* 1992;13:423–446.
2. Evrard P. Normal and abnormal development of the brain. In: Rapin I, Segalowitz S, eds. *Handbook of neuropsychology*. Amsterdam: Elsevier, 1992:11–44.
3. Rakic P. Mode of cell migration to the superficial layers of fetal monkey neocortex. *J Comp Neurol* 1972;145:61–84.
4. Kuzniecky R, Garcia JH, Faught E, et al. Cortical dysplasia in temporal lobe epilepsy: magnetic resonance imaging correlations. *Ann Neurol* 1991;29:293–298.
5. Kuzniecky R, Morawetz R, Faught E, et al. Frontal and central lobe focal dysplasia: clinical, EEG and imaging features. *Dev Med Child Neurol* 1995;37:159–166.
6. de Rijk-van Andel JF, Arts WFM, Hofman A, et al. Epidemiology of lissencephaly type I. *Neuroepidemiology* 1991;10:200–204.
7. Barkovich AJ, Kuzniecky RI, Dobyns WB, et al. A classification scheme for malformations of cortical development. *Neuropediatrics* 1996;27:59–63.
8. Barkovich AJ, Kuzniecky RI, Jackson GD, et al. Classification system for malformations of cortical development: update 2001. *Neurology* 2001;57:2168–2178.
9. Dodge NN, Dobyns WB. Agenesis of the corpus callosum and Dandy-Walker malformation associated with hemimegalencephaly in the sebaceous nevus syndrome. *Am J Med Genet* 1995;56:147–150.
10. Pavone L, Curatolo P, Rizzo R, et al. Epidermal nevus syndrome: a neurological variant with hemimegalencephaly, gyral malformation, mental retardation, seizures and facial hemihypertrophy. *Neurology* 1991;41:266–271.
11. Ross DL, Liwnicz BH, Chun RWM, et al. Hypomelanosis of Ito (incontinentia pigmenti achromians)—a clinicopathologic study: macrocephaly and gray matter heterotopias. *Neurology* 1982;32:1013–1016.
12. Wieselthaler NA, van Toorn R, Wilmshurst JM. Giant congenital melanocytic nevi in a patient with brain structural malformations and multiple lipomatosis. *J Child Neurol* 2002;17:289–291.
13. Ahmetoglu A, Isik Y, Aynaci O, et al. Proteus syndrome associated with liver involvement: case report. *Genet Couns* 2003;14:221–226.
14. Dabora SL, Jozwiak S, Franz DN, et al. Mutational analysis in a cohort of 224 tuberous sclerosis patients indicates increased severity of TSC2, compared with TSC1, disease in multiple organs. *Am J Hum Genet* 2001;68:64–80.
15. Jones AC, Shyamsundar MM, Thomas MW, et al. Comprehensive mutation analysis of TSC1 and TSC2-and phenotypic correlations in 150 families with tuberous sclerosis. *Am J Hum Genet* 1999;64:1305–1315.
16. Langkau N, Martin N, Brandt R, et al. TSC1 and TSC2 mutations in tuberous sclerosis, the associated phenotypes and a model to explain observed TSC1/TSC2 frequency ratios. *Eur J Pediatr* 2002;161:393–402.
17. Niida Y, Lawrence-Smith N, Banwell A, et al. Analysis of both TSC1 and TSC2 for germline mutations in 126 unrelated patients with tuberous sclerosis. *Hum Mutat* 1999;14:412–422.
18. Becker AJ, Urbach H, Scheffler B, et al. Focal cortical dysplasia of Taylor's balloon cell type: mutational analysis of the TSC1 gene indicates a pathogenic relationship to tuberous sclerosis. *Ann Neurol* 2002;52:29–37.
19. Taylor DC, Falconer MA, Bruton CJ, et al. Focal dysplasia of the cerebral cortex in epilepsy. *J Neurol Neurosurg Psychiatry* 1971;34:369–387.
20. Wyllie E, Baumgartner C, Prayson R, et al. The clinical spectrum of focal cortical dysplasia and epilepsy. *J Epilepsy* 1994;7:303–317.
21. DeMyer W. Microcephaly, micrencephaly, megalocephaly and megalencephaly. In: Swaimann KF, ed. *Pediatric neurology*. St. Louis: Mosby, 1999:301–311.

22. Giuliano F, David A, Edery P, et al. Macrocephaly-cutis marmorata telangiectatica congenita: seven cases including two with unusual cerebral manifestations. *Am J Med Genet* 2004;126A: 99–103.

23. Moore CA, Toriello HV, Abuelo DN, et al. Macrocephaly-cutis marmorata telangiectatica congenita syndrome: a distinct disorder with developmental delay and connective tissue abnormality. *Am J Med Genet* 1997;70:67–73.

24. Gohlich-Ratmann G, Baethmann M, Lorenz P, et al. Megalencephaly, mega corpus callosum, and complete lack of motor development: a previously undescribed syndrome. *Am J Med Genet* 1998;79:161–167.

25. Bond J, Roberts E, Mochida GH, et al. ASPM is a major determinant of cerebral cortical size. *Nat Genet* 2002;32:316–320.

26. Bond J, Scott S, Hampshire DJ, et al. Protein-truncating mutations in ASPM cause variable reduction in brain size. *Am J Hum Genet* 2003;73:1170–1177.

27. Jackson AP, McHale DP, Campbell DA, et al. Primary autosomal recessive microcephaly (MCPH1) maps to chromosome 8P22-PTER. *Am J Hum Genet* 1998;63:541–546.

28. Jackson AP, Eastwood H, Bell SM, et al. Identification of microcephalin, a protein implicated in determining the size of the human brain. *Am J Hum Genet* 2002;71:136–142.

29. Jamieson CR, Govaerts C, Abramowicz MJ. Primary autosomal recessive microcephaly: homozygosity mapping of MCPH4 to chromosome 15 [letter]. *Am J Hum Genet* 1999;65:1465–1469.

30. Jamieson CR, Fryns JP, Jacobs J, et al. Primary autosomal recessive microcephaly: MCPH5 maps to 1Q25-Q32. *Am J Hum Genet* 2000;67:1575–1577.

31. Moynihan L, Jackson AP, Roberts E, et al. A third novel locus for primary autosomal recessive microcephaly maps to chromosome 9Q34. *Am J Hum Genet* 2000;66:724–727.

32. Pattison L, Crow YJ, Deeble VJ, et al. A fifth locus for primary autosomal recessive microcephaly maps to chromosome 1Q31. *Am J Hum Genet* 2000;67:1578–1580.

33. Roberts E, Jackson AP, Carradice AC, et al. The second locus for autosomal recessive primary microcephaly (MCPH2) maps to chromosome 19Q13.1-13.2. *Eur J Hum Genet* 1999;7:815–820.

34. Roberts E, Hampshire DJ, Pattison L, et al. Autosomal recessive primary microcephaly: an analysis of locus heterogeneity and phenotypic variation. *J Med Genet* 2002;39:718–721.

35. Kelley RI, Robinson D, Puffenberger EG, et al. Amish lethal microcephaly: a new metabolic disorder with severe congenital microcephaly and 2-ketoglutaric aciduria. *Am J Med Genet* 2002;112:318–326.

36. Rosenberg MJ, Agarwala R, Bouffard G, et al. Mutant deoxynucleotide carrier is associated with congenital microcephaly. *Nat Genet* 2002;32:175–179.

37. Sheen VL, Topcu M, Berkovic S, et al. Autosomal recessive form of periventricular heterotopia. *Neurology* 2003;60:1108–1112.

38. Sheen VL, Ganesh VS, Topcu M, et al. Mutations in ARFGEF2 implicate vesicle trafficking in neural progenitor proliferation and migration in the human cerebral cortex. *Nat Genet* 2004;36: 69–76.

39. Barkovich AJ, Ferriero DM, Barr RM, et al. Microlissencephaly: a heterogeneous malformation of cortical development. *Neuropediatrics* 1998;29:113–119.

40. Dobyns WB. Primary microcephaly: new approaches for an old disorder. *Am J Med Genet* 2002;112:315–317.

41. Sztriha L, Al-Gazali LI, Varady E, et al. Autosomal recessive micrencephaly with simplified gyral pattern, abnormal myelination and arthrogryposis. *Neuropediatrics* 1999;30:141–145.

42. ten Donkelaar HJ, Wesseling P, Semmekrot BA, et al. Severe, non X-linked congenital microcephaly with absence of the pyramidal tracts in two siblings. *Acta Neuropathol (Berl)* 1999;98:203–211.

43. O'Driscoll M, Ruiz-Perez VL, Woods CG, et al. A splicing mutation affecting expression of ataxia-telangiectasia and rad3-related protein (ATR) results in Seckel syndrome. *Nat Genet* 2003;33: 497–501.

44. Dobyns WB, Stratton RF, Greenberg F. Syndromes with lissencephaly, I: Miller-Dieker and Norman-Roberts syndromes and isolated lissencephaly. *Am J Med Genet* 1984;18:509–526.

45. Dobyns WB, Barkovich AJ. Microcephaly with simplified gyral pattern (oligogyric microcephaly) and microlissencephaly: reply. *Neuropediatrics* 1999;30:104–106.

46. Norman MG, Roberts M, Sirois J, et al. Lissencephaly. *Can J Neurol Sci* 1976;3:39–46.

47. Barth PG, Mullaart R, Stam FC, et al. Familial lissencephaly with extreme neopallial hypoplasia. *Brain Dev* 1982;4:145–151.

48. Kroon AA, Smit BJ, Barth PG, et al. Lissencephaly with extreme cerebral and cerebellar hypoplasia. A magnetic resonance imaging study. *Neuropediatrics* 1996;27:273–276.

49. Fox JW, Lamperti ED, Eksioglu YZ, et al. Mutations in Filamin 1 prevent migration of cerebral cortical neurons in human periventricular heterotopia. *Neuron* 1998;21:1315–1325.

50. Guerrini R, Mei D, Sisodiya S, et al. Germline and mosaic mutations of *FLN1* in men with periventricular heterotopia. *Neurology* 2004;63:51–56.

51. Sheen VL, Dixon PH, Fox JW, et al. Mutations in the X-linked Filamin 1 gene cause periventricular nodular heterotopia in males as well as in females. *Hum Mol Genet* 2001;10: 1775–1783.

52. Vles JSH, Fryns JP, Folmer K, et al. Corpus callosum agenesis, spastic quadriparesis and irregular lining of the lateral ventricles on CT-scan. A distinct X-linked mental retardation syndrome? *Genet Couns* 1990;38:97–102.

53. Vles JSH, De Die-Smulders C, Van der Hoeven M, et al. Corpus callosum agenesis in two male infants of a heterozygotic triplet pregnancy. *Genet Couns* 1993;4:239–240.

54. Cupo LN, Pyeritz RE, Olson JL, et al. Ehlers-Danlos syndrome with abnormal collagen fibrils, sinus of Valsalva aneurysms, myocardial infarction, panacinar emphysema and cerebral heterotopia. *Am J Med* 1981;71:1051–1058.

55. Thomas P, Bossan A, Lacour JP, et al. Ehlers-Danlos syndrome with subependymal periventricular heterotopias. *Neurology* 1996;46:1165–1167.

56. Guerrini R, Dobyns WB. Bilateral periventricular nodular heterotopia with mental retardation and frontonasal malformation. *Neurology* 1998;51:499–503.

57. Guion-Almeida ML, Richieri-Costa A. Frontonasal dysplasia, macroblepharon, eyelid colobomas, ear anomalies, macrostomia, mental retardation, and CNS structural anomalies. A new syndrome? *Clin Dysmorphol* 1999;8:1–4.

58. Dobyns WB, Guerrini R, Czapansky-Beilman DK, et al. Bilateral periventricular nodular heterotopia (BPNH) with mental retardation and syndactyly in boys: a new X-linked mental retardation syndrome. *Neurology* 1997;49:1042–1047.

59. Fink JM, Dobyns WB, Guerrini R, et al. Identification of a duplication of XQ28 associated with bilateral periventricular nodular heterotopia. *Am J Hum Genet* 1997;61:379–387.

60. Palm L, Hagerstrand I, Kristoffersson U, et al. Nephrosis and disturbances of neuronal migration in male siblings—a new hereditary disorder? *Arch Dis Child* 1986;61:545–548.

61. Nezelof C, Jaubert F, Lyon G. Familial syndrome combining short small intestine, intestinal malrotation, pyloric hypertrophy and brain malformation. 3 anatomoclinical case reports [in French]. *Ann Anat Pathol (Paris)* 1976;21:401–412.

62. Sheen VL, Wheless JW, Bodell A, et al. Periventricular heterotopia associated with chromosome 5p anomalies. *Neurology* 2003;60: 1033–1036.

63. Barkovich AJ. Morphologic characteristics of subcortical heterotopia: MR imaging study. *Am J Neuroradiol* 2000;21:290–295.

64. Baraitser M, Winter RM. Iris coloboma, ptosis, hypertelorism, and mental retardation: a new syndrome. *J Med Genet* 1988; 25:41–43.

65. Ramer JC, Mascari MJ, Manders E, et al. Trigonocephaly, pachygyria, retinal coloboma, and cardiac defect: a distinct syndrome. *Dysmorphol Clin Genet* 1992;6:15–20.

66. Ramer JC, Lin AE, Dobyns WB, et al. Previously apparently undescribed syndrome: shallow orbits, ptosis, coloboma, trigonocephaly, gyral malformations, and mental and growth retardation. *Am J Med Genet* 1995;57:403–409.

67. Rossi M, Guerrini R, Dobyns WB, et al. Characterization of brain malformations in the Baraitser-Winter syndrome and review of the literature. *Neuropediatrics* 2003;34:287–292.

68. Cardoso C, Leventer RJ, Ward HL, et al. Refinement of a 400-kb critical region allows genotypic differentiation between isolated lissencephaly, Miller-Dieker syndrome, and other phenotypes secondary to deletions of 17p13.3. *Am J Hum Genet* 2003;72: 918–930.

69. Dobyns WB, Curry CJR, Hoyme HE, et al. Clinical and molecular diagnosis of Miller-Dieker syndrome. *Am J Hum Genet* 1991;48: 584–594.

70. Dobyns WB, Truwit CL, Ross ME, et al. Differences in the gyral pattern distinguish chromosome 17-linked and X-linked lissencephaly. *Neurology* 1999;53:270–277.

71. Pilz DT, Matsumoto N, Minnerath S, et al. LIS1 and XLIS (DCX) mutations cause most classical lissencephaly, but different patterns of malformation. *Hum Mol Genet* 1998;7:2029–2037.

72. Cardoso C, Leventer RJ, Matsumoto N, et al. The location and type of mutation predict malformation severity in isolated lissencephaly caused by abnormalities within the LIS1 gene. *Hum Mol Genet* 2000;9:3019–3028.

73. Cardoso C, Leventer RJ, Dowling JJ, et al. Clinical and molecular basis of classical lissencephaly: mutations in the LIS1 gene (PAFAH1B1). *Hum Mutat* 2002;19:4–15.

74. Leventer RJ, Cardoso C, Ledbetter DH, et al. LIS1 missense mutations cause milder lissencephaly phenotypes including a child with normal IQ. *Neurology* 2001;57:416–422.

75. Pilz DT, Macha ME, Precht KS, et al. Fluorescence in situ hybridization analysis with *LIS1* specific probes reveals a high deletion mutation rate in isolated lissencephaly sequence. *Genet Med* 1998;1:29–33.

76. D'Agostino MD, Bernasconi A, Das S, et al. Subcortical band heterotopia (SBH) in males: clinical, imaging and genetic findings in comparison with females. *Brain* 2002;125(Pt 11):2507–2522.

77. Gleeson JG, Minnerath SR, Fox JW, et al. Characterization of mutations in the gene doublecortin in patients with double cortex syndrome [see comments]. *Ann Neurol* 1999;45:146–153.

78. Gleeson JG, Minnerath S, Kuzniecky RI, et al. Somatic and germline mosaic mutations in the doublecortin gene are associated with variable phenotypes. *Am J Hum Genet* 2000;67:574–581.

79. Matsumoto N, Leventer RJ, Kuc JA, et al. Mutation analysis of the DCX gene and genotype/phenotype correlation in subcortical band heterotopia. *Eur J Hum Genet* 2001;9:5–12.

80. Pilz DT, Kuc J, Matsumoto N, et al. Subcortical band heterotopia in rare affected males can be caused by missense mutations in DCX (XLIS) or LIS1. *Hum Mol Genet* 1999;8:1757–1760.

81. Ross ME, Swanson K, Dobyns WB. Lissencephaly with cerebellar hypoplasia (LCH): a heterogeneous group of cortical malformations. *Neuropediatrics* 2001;32:256–263.

82. Hong SE, Shugart YY, Huang DT, et al. Autosomal recessive lissencephaly with cerebellar hypoplasia is associated with human RELN mutations. *Nat Genet* 2000;26:93–96.

83. Kato M, Takizawa N, Yamada S, et al. Diffuse pachygyria with cerebellar hypoplasia: a milder form of microlissencephaly or a new genetic syndrome? *Ann Neurol* 1999;46:660–663.

84. Dobyns WB, Berry-Kravis E, Havernick NJ, et al. X-linked lissencephaly with absent corpus callosum and ambiguous genitalia. *Am J Med Genet* 1999;86:331–337.

85. Kato M, Das S, Petras K, et al. Mutations of ARX are associated with striking pleiotropy and consistent genotype-phenotype correlation. *Hum Mutat* 2004;23:147–159.

86. Kitamura K, Yanazawa M, Sugiyama N, et al. Mutation of ARX causes abnormal development of forebrain and testes in mice and X-linked lissencephaly with abnormal genitalia in humans. *Nat Genet* 2002;32:359–369.

87. Sztriha L, Al-Gazali L, Dawodu A, et al. Agyria-pachygyria and agenesis of the corpus callosum: autosomal recessive inheritance with neonatal death. *Neurology* 1998;50:1466–1469.

88. Fukuyama Y, Osawa M, Suzuki H. Congenital progressive muscular dystrophy of the Fukuyama type—clinical, genetic and pathological considerations. *Brain Dev* 1981;3:1–29.

89. Kobayashi K, Nakahori Y, Miyake M, et al. An ancient retrotransposal insertion causes Fukuyama-type congenital muscular dystrophy. *Nature* 1998;394:388–392.

90. Kondo-Iida E, Kobayashi K, Watanabe M, et al. Novel mutations and genotype-phenotype relationships in 107 families with Fukuyama-type congenital muscular dystrophy (FCMD). *Hum Mol Genet* 1999;8:2303–2309.

91. Osawa M, Arai Y, Ikenaka H, et al. Fukuyama type congenital progressive muscular dystrophy. *Acta Paediatr Jpn* 1991;33: 261–269.

92. Beltran-Valero de Bernabe D, Voit T, Longman C, et al. Mutations in the FKRP gene can cause muscle-eye-brain disease and Walker-Warburg syndrome. *J Med Genet* 2004;41:e61.

93. Longman C, Brockington M, Torelli S, et al. Mutations in the human large gene cause MDC1D, a novel form of congenital muscular dystrophy with severe mental retardation and abnormal glycosylation of alpha-dystroglycan. *Hum Mol Genet* 2003; 12:2853–2861.

94. Taniguchi K, Kobayashi K, Saito K, et al. Worldwide distribution and broader clinical spectrum of muscle-eye-brain disease. *Hum Mol Genet* 2003;12:527–534.

95. Topaloglu H, Brockington M, Yuva Y, et al. FKRP gene mutations cause congenital muscular dystrophy, mental retardation, and cerebellar cysts. *Neurology* 2003;60:988–992.

96. Yoshida A, Kobayashi K, Manya H, et al. Muscular dystrophy and neuronal migration disorder caused by mutations in a glycosyltransferase, POMGNT1. *Dev Cell* 2001;1:717–724.

97. Beltran-Valero De Bernabe D, Currier S, Steinbrecher A, et al. Mutations in the *O*-mannosyltransferase gene POMT1 give rise to the severe neuronal migration disorder Walker-Warburg syndrome. *Am J Hum Genet* 2002;71:1033–1043.

98. Beltran-Valero de Bernabe D, van Bokhoven H, van Beusekom E, et al. A homozygous nonsense mutation in the Fukutin gene causes a Walker-Warburg syndrome phenotype. *J Med Genet* 2003;40:845–848.

99. Silan F, Yoshioka M, Kobayashi K, et al. A new mutation of the Fukutin gene in a non-Japanese patient. *Ann Neurol* 2003;53: 392–396.

100. Emery JA, Roper SN, Rojiani AM. White matter neuronal heterotopia in temporal lobe epilepsy: a morphometric and immunohistochemical study. *J Neuropathol Exp Neurol* 1997;56:1276–1282.

101. Rojiani AM, Emery JA, Anderson KJ, et al. Distribution of heterotopic neurons in normal hemispheric white matter: a morphometric analysis. *J Neuropathol Exp Neurol* 1996;55:178–183.

102. Guerrini R, Barkovich AJ, Sztriha L, et al. Bilateral frontal polymicrogyria: a newly recognized brain malformation syndrome. *Neurology* 2000;54:909–913.

103. Chang BS, Piao X, Bodell A, et al. Bilateral frontoparietal polymicrogyria: clinical and radiological features in 10 families with linkage to chromosome 16. *Ann Neurol* 2003;53:596–606.

104. Piao X, Basel-Vanagaite L, Straussberg R, et al. An autosomal recessive form of bilateral frontoparietal polymicrogyria maps to chromosome 16Q12.2-21. *Am J Hum Genet* 2002;70:1028–1033.

105. Piao X, Hill RS, Bodell A, et al. G protein-coupled receptor-dependent development of human frontal cortex. *Science* 2004;303:2033–2036.

106. Bingham PM, Lynch D, McDonald-McGinn D, et al. Polymicrogyria in chromosome 22 deletion syndrome. *Neurology* 1998;51:1500–1502.

107. Ghariani S, Dahan K, Saint-Martin C, et al. Polymicrogyria in chromosome 22Q11 deletion syndrome. *Eur J Paediatr Neurol* 2002;6:73–77.

108. Kawame H, Kurosawa K, Akatsuka A, et al. Polymicrogyria is an uncommon manifestation in 22Q11.2 deletion syndrome [letter]. *Am J Med Genet* 2000;94:77–78.

109. Kuzniecky RI, Andermann F, Guerrini R. The congenital bilateral perisylvian syndrome: study of 31 patients. *Lancet* 1993;341: 608–612.

110. Shapira SK, Heilstedt HA, Starkey DE, et al. Clinical and pathological characterization of epilepsy in patients with monosomy 1P36 and the search for candidate genes [abstract 564]. *Am J Hum Genet* 1999;65(4 Suppl):A107.

111. Villard L, Nguyen K, Cardoso C, et al. A locus for bilateral perisylvian polymicrogyria maps to XQ28. *Am J Hum Genet* 2002;70: 1003–1008.

112. Worthington S, Turner A, Elber J, et al. 22Q11 Deletion and polymicrogyria—cause or coincidence? *Clin Dysmorphol* 2000;9: 193–197.

113. Zollino M, Colosimo C, Zuffardi O, et al. Cryptic t(1;12)(q44; p13.3) translocation in a previously described syndrome with polymicrogyria, segregating as an apparently X-linked trait. *Am J Med Genet* 2003;117A:65–71.

114. Guerrini R, Dubeau F, Dulac O, et al. Bilateral parasagittal parietooccipital polymicrogyria and epilepsy. *Ann Neurol* 1997;41: 65–73.

115. Chang BS, Piao X, Giannini C, et al. Bilateral generalized polymicrogyria (BGP): a distinct syndrome of cortical malformation. *Neurology* 2004;62:1722–1728.

116. Barkovich AJ, Kjos BO. Schizencephaly: correlation of clinical findings with MR characteristics. *Am J Neuroradiol* 1992;13: 85–94.

117. Aicardi J, Goutieres F. The syndrome of absence of the septum pellucidum with porencephalies and other developmental defects. *Neuropediatrics* 1981;12:319–329.

118. Kuban KC, Teele RL, Wallman J. Septo-optic-dysplasia-schizencephaly. Radiographic and clinical features [see comments]. *Pediatr Radiol* 1989;19:145–150.

119. Miller SP, Shevell MI, Patenaude Y, et al. Septo-optic dysplasia plus: a spectrum of malformations of cortical development. *Neurology* 2000;54:1701–1703.

120. Vigevano F, Bertini E, Boldrini R, et al. Hemimegalencephaly and intractable epilepsy: benefits of hemispherectomy. *Epilepsia* 1989;30:833–843.

121. Devlin AM, Cross JH, Harkness W, et al. Clinical outcomes of hemispherectomy for epilepsy in childhood and adolescence. *Brain* 2003;126(Pt 3):556–566.

122. Maher CO, Cohen-Gadol AA, Raffel C. Cortical resection for epilepsy in children with linear sebaceous nevus syndrome. *Pediatr Neurosurg* 2003;39:129–135.

123. Guerrini R, Carrozzo R. Epileptogenic brain malformations: clinical presentation, malformative patterns and indications for genetic testing. *Seizure* 2002;11(Suppl A):532–543.

124. Crino PB, Miyata H, Vinters HV. Neurodevelopmental disorders as a cause of seizures: neuropathologic, genetic, and mechanistic considerations. *Brain Pathol* 2002;12:212–233.

125. Hardiman O, Burke T, Phillips J, et al. Microdysgenesis in resected temporal neocortex: incidence and clinical significance in focal epilepsy. *Neurology* 1988;38:1041–1047.

126. Colombo N, Tassi L, Galli C, et al. Focal cortical dysplasias: MR imaging, histopathologic, and clinical correlations in surgically treated patients with epilepsy. *Am J Neuroradiol* 2003;24:724–733.

127. DeMyer W. Megalencephaly in children. Clinical syndromes, genetic patterns, and differential diagnosis from other causes of megalocephaly. *Neurology* 1972;22:634–643.

128. Opitz JM, Holt MC. Microcephaly: general considerations and aids to nosology. *J Craniofac Genet Dev Biol* 1990;10:175–204.

129. Tolmie JL, McNay M, Stephenson JBP, et al. Microcephaly: genetic counseling and antenatal diagnosis after the birth of an affected child. *Am J Med Genet* 1987;27:583–594.

130. Dobyns WB, Andermann E, Andermann F, et al. X-linked malformations of neuronal migration. *Neurology* 1996;47:331–339.

131. Dubeau F, Tampieri D, Lee N, et al. Periventricular and subcortical nodular heterotopia: a study of 33 patients. *Brain* 1995;118: 1273–1287.

132. Battaglia G, Granata T, Farina L, et al. Periventricular nodular heterotopia: epileptogenic findings. *Epilepsia* 1997;38:1173–1182.

133. Sisodiya SM, Free SL, Thom M, et al. Evidence for nodular epileptogenicity and gender differences in periventricular nodular heterotopia. *Neurology* 1999;52:336–341.

134. Huttenlocher PR, Taravath S, Mojtahedi S. Periventricular heterotopia and epilepsy. *Neurology* 1994;44:51–55.

135. Eksioglu YZ, Scheffer IE, Cardenas P, et al. Periventricular heterotopia: an X-linked dominant epilepsy locus causing aberrant cerebral cortical development. *Neuron* 1996;16:77–87.

136. Poussaint TY, Fox JW, Dobyns WB, et al. Periventricular nodular heterotopia in patients with Filamin-1 gene mutations: neuroimaging findings. *Pediatr Radiol* 2000;30:748–755.

137. Barkovich AJ, Kjos BO. Gray matter heterotopias: MR characteristics and correlation with developmental and neurological manifestations. *Radiology* 1992;182:493–499.

138. Barkovich AJ, Koch TK, Carrol CL. The spectrum of lissencephaly: report of ten patients analyzed by magnetic resonance imaging. *Ann Neurol* 1991;30:139–146.

139. Dobyns WB, Truwit CL. Lissencephaly and other malformations of cortical development: 1995 update. *Neuropediatrics* 1995;26: 132–147.

140. Norman MG, McGillivray BC, Kalousek DK, et al. *Congenital malformations of the brain: pathological, embryological, clinical, radiological and genetic aspects.* New York: Oxford University Press, 1995:452.

141. Barkovich AJ, Guerrini R, Battaglia G, et al. Band heterotopia: correlation of outcome with magnetic resonance imaging parameters. *Ann Neurol* 1994;36:609–617.

142. des Portes V, Pinard JM, Smadja D, et al. Dominant X linked subcortical laminar heterotopia and lissencephaly syndrome (XSCLH/LIS): evidence for the occurrence of mutation in males and mapping of a potential locus in XQ22. *J Med Genet* 1997;34:177–183.

143. Matell M. Ein Fall von Heterotopie der frauen Substanz in den beiden Hemispheren des Grosshirns. *Arch Psychiatr Nervenkr* 1893;25:124–136.

144. Ross ME, Allen KM, Srivastava AK, et al. Linkage and physical mapping of x-linked lissencephaly/sbh (XLIS): a gene causing neuronal migration defects in human brain. *Hum Mol Genet* 1997;6:555–562.

145. Hourihane JOB, Bennett CP, Chaudhuri R, et al. A sibship with a neuronal migration defect, cerebellar hypoplasia and lymphedema. *Neuropediatrics* 1993;24:43–46.

146. Dobyns WB, Elias ER, Newlin AC, et al. Causal heterogeneity in isolated lissencephaly. *Neurology* 1992;42:1375–1388.

147. Battaglia A. Seizures and dysplasias of cerebral cortex in dysmorphic syndromes. In: Guerrini R, Andermann F, Canapicchi R, et al, eds. *Dysplasias of cerebral cortex and epilepsy.* Philadelphia: Lippincott-Raven, 1996:199–209.

148. Palmini A, Andermann F, Aicardi J, et al. Diffuse cortical dysplasia, or the "double cortex" syndrome: the clinical and epileptic spectrum in 10 patients. *Neurology* 1991;41:1656–1662.

149. Gleeson JG, Luo RF, Grant PE, et al. Genetic and neuroradiological heterogeneity of double cortex syndrome. *Ann Neurol* 2000;47:265–269.

150. Sicca F, Kelemen A, Genton P, et al. Mosaic mutations of the LIS1 gene cause subcortical band heterotopia. *Neurology* 2003;61: 1042–1046.

151. Bienvenu T, Poirier K, Friocourt G, et al. ARX, a novel prd-class-homeobox gene highly expressed in the telencephalon, is mutated in X-linked mental retardation. *Hum Mol Genet* 2002;11: 981–991.

152. Kato M, Das S, Petras K, et al. Polyalanine expansion of ARX associated with cryptogenic West syndrome. *Neurology* 2003;61: 267–276.

153. Scheffer IE, Wallace RH, Phillips FL, et al. X-linked myoclonic epilepsy with spasticity and intellectual disability: mutation in the homeobox gene ARX. *Neurology* 2002;59:348–356.

154. Stromme P, Mangelsdorf ME, Scheffer IE, et al. Infantile spasms, dystonia, and other X-linked phenotypes caused by mutations in aristaless related homeobox gene, ARX. *Brain Dev* 2002;24: 266–268.

155. Stromme P, Mangelsdorf ME, Shaw MA, et al. Mutations in the human ortholog of aristaless cause X-linked mental retardation and epilepsy. *Nat Genet* 2002;30:441–445.

156. Stromme P, Bakke SJ, Dahl A, et al. Brain cysts associated with mutation in the aristaless related homeobox gene, ARX. *J Neurol Neurosurg Psychiatry* 2003;74:536–538.

157. Turner G, Partington M, Kerr B, et al. Variable expression of mental retardation, autism, seizures, and dystonic hand movements in two families with an identical ARX gene mutation. *Am J Med Genet* 2002;112:405–411.

158. Wellington C. A spectrum of neurological phenotypes caused by mutations in the X-linked aristaless-related homeobox gene, ARX. *Clin Genet* 2003;63:177–179.

159. Dobyns WB, Kirkpatrick JB, Hittner HM, et al. Syndromes with lissencephaly, II: Walker-Warburg and cerebro-oculo-muscular syndromes and a new syndrome with type II lissencephaly. *Am J Med Genet* 1985;22:157–195.

160. Dobyns WB, Pagon RA, Armstrong D, et al. Diagnostic criteria for Walker-Warburg syndrome. *Am J Med Genet* 1989;32: 195–210.

161. Dubowitz V. 22nd ENMC-sponsored workshop on congenital muscular dystrophy, Baarn, the Netherlands; May 14–16, 1993. *Neuromusc Disord* 1994;4:75–81.

162. Haltia M, Leivo I, Somer H, et al. Muscle-eye-brain disease: a neuropathological study. *Ann Neurol* 1997;41:173–180.

163. Takada K, Nakamura H, Takashima S. Cortical dysplasia in Fukuyama congenital muscular dystrophy (FCMD): a Golgi and angioarchitectonic analysis. *Acta Neuropathol* 1988;76: 170–178.

164. Walker AE. Lissencephaly. *Arch Neurol Psychiatry* 1942;48: 13–29.

165. Fukuyama Y, Osawa M. A genetic study of the Fukuyama type congenital muscular dystrophy. *Brain Dev* 1984;6:373–390.

166. Santavuori P, Somer H, Sainio K, et al. Muscle-eye-brain disease (MEB). *Brain Dev* 1989;11:147–153.

167. Diesen C, Saarinen A, Pihko H, et al. *POMGNT1* mutation and phenotype spectrum in muscle-eye-brain disease. *J Med Genet* 2004;41(10):e115.

168. Zhang W, Vajsar J, Cao P, et al. Enzymatic diagnostic test for muscle-eye-brain type congenital muscular dystrophy using commercially available reagents. *Clin Biochem* 2003;36: 339–344.

169. Cormand B, Pihko H, Bayes M, et al. Clinical and genetic distinction between Walker-Warburg syndrome and muscle-eye-brain disease. *Neurology* 2001;56:1059–1069.

170. Hewitt JE, Grewal PK. Glycosylation defects in inherited muscle disease. *Cell Mol Life Sci* 2003;60:251–258.

171. Ross ME. Full circle to cobbled brain. *Nature* 2002;418:376–377.

172. Moore SA, Saito F, Chen J, et al. Deletion of brain dystroglycan recapitulates aspects of congenital muscular dystrophy. *Nature* 2002;418:422–425.

173. Crome L. Microgyria. *J Pathol Bacteriol* 1952;64:479–495.

174. Ferrer I. A Golgi analysis of unlayered polymicrogyria. *Acta Neuropathol* 1984;65:69–76.

175. Levine DN, Fisher MA, Caviness VS Jr. Porencephaly with microgyria: a pathologic study. *Acta Neuropathol* 1974;29:99–113.

176. Caraballo R, Cersosimo R, Fejerman N. A particular type of epilepsy in children with congenital hemiparesis associated with unilateral polymicrogyria. *Epilepsia* 1999;40:865–871.

177. Clark M, Carr L, Reilly S, et al. Worster-Drought syndrome, a mild tetraplegic perisylvian cerebral palsy: review of 47 cases. *Brain* 2000;123(Pt 10):2160–2170.

178. Nevo Y, Segev Y, Gelman Y, et al. Worster-Drought and congenital perisylvian syndromes—a continuum? *Pediatr Neurol* 2001; 24:153–155.

179. Barkovich AJ, Lindan CE. Congenital cytomegalovirus infection of the brain: imaging analysis and embryologic considerations. *Am J Neuroradiol* 1994;15:703–715.

180. Hayward JC, Titelbaum DS, Clancy RR, et al. Lissencephaly-pachygyria associated with congenital cytomegalovirus infection. *J Child Neurol* 1991;6:109–114.

181. Iannetti P, Nigro G, Spalice A, et al. Cytomegalovirus infection and schizencephaly: case reports. *Ann Neurol* 1998;43:123–127.

182. Barth PG, van der Harten JJ. Parabiotic twin syndrome with topical isocortical disruption and gastroschisis. *Acta Neuropathol* 1985;67:345–349.

183. Norman MG. Bilateral encephaloclastic lesions in a 26 week gestation fetus: effect on neuroblast migration. *Can J Neurol Sci* 1980;7:191–194.

184. Sugama S, Kusano K. Monozygous twin with polymicrogyria and normal co-twin. *Pediatr Neurol* 1994;11:62–63.

185. Barth PG. Migrational disorders of the brain. *Curr Opin Neurol Neurosurg* 1992;5:339–343.

186. Pati S, Helmbrecht GD. Congenital schizencephaly associated with in utero warfarin exposure. *Reprod Toxicol* 1994;8:115–120.

187. Bartolomei F, Gavaret M, Dravet C, et al. Familial epilepsy with unilateral and bilateral malformations of cortical development. *Epilepsia* 1999;40:47–51.

188. Borgatti R, Triulzi F, Zucca C, et al. Bilateral perisylvian polymicrogyria in three generations. *Neurology* 1999;52:1910–1913.

189. Caraballo RH, Cersosimo RO, Mazza E, et al. Focal polymicrogyria in mother and son. *Brain Dev* 2000;22:336–339.

190. Ferrie CD, Jackson GD, Giannakodimos S, et al. Posterior agyria-pachygyria with polymicrogyria: evidence for an inherited neuronal migration disorder. *Neurology* 1995;45:150–153.

191. Guerreiro MM, Andermann E, Guerrini R, et al. Familial perisylvian polymicrogyria: a new familial syndrome of cortical maldevelopment. *Ann Neurol* 2000;48:39–48.

192. Hilburger AC, Willis JK, Bouldin E, et al. Familial schizencephaly. *Brain Dev* 1993;15:234–236.

193. Leventer RJ, Lese CM, Cardoso C, et al. A study of 220 patients with polymicrogyria delineates distinct phenotypes and reveals genetic loci on chromosomes 1p, 2p, 6q, 21q and 22q [abstract]. *Am J Hum Genet* 2001;69(4 Suppl):177.

194. Brunelli S, Faiella A, Capra V, et al. Germline mutations in the homeobox gene EMX2 in patients with severe schizencephaly. *Nature Genet* 1996;12:94–96.

195. Amor DJ, Leventer RJ, Hayllar S, et al. Polymicrogyria associated with scalp and limb defects: variant of Adams-Oliver syndrome. *Am J Med Genet* 2000;93:328–334.

196. Pollin TI, Dobyns WB, Crowe CA, et al. Risk of abnormal pregnancy outcome in carriers of balanced reciprocal translocations involving the Miller-Dieker syndrome (MDS) critical region in chromosome 17p13.3. *Am J Med Genet* 1999;85:369–375.

197. Kuzniecky R. Familial diffuse cortical dysplasia. *Arch Neurol* 1994;51:307–310.

198. Ramirez D, Lammer EJ, Johnson CB, et al. Autosomal recessive frontotemporal pachygyria. *Am J Med Genet* 2004;124A: 231–238.

199. Deconinck N, Duprez T, des Portes V, et al. Familial bilateral medial parietooccipital band heterotopia not related to DCX or LIS1 gene defects. *Neuropediatrics* 2003;34:146–148.

200. Mirzaa G, Dodge NN, Glass I, et al. Megalencephaly and perisylvian polymicrogyria with postaxial polydactyly and hydrocephalus: a rare brain malformation syndrome associated with mental retardation and seizures. *Neuropediatr* 2004;35: 353–359.

Hippocampal Anatomy and Hippocampal Sclerosis

Imad Najm   Henri Duvernoy   Stephan Schuele

HIPPOCAMPAL ANATOMY

Because the hippocampal formation is frequently involved in patients with focal epilepsy, a thorough knowledge of this structure and its connections is critical to an understanding of the pathology and clinical semiology of temporal lobe epilepsy caused by hippocampal disease. The first part of this chapter reviews the anatomy of the hippocampal formation, its relation to surrounding structures, and its histology and connections (pathways). The reader is referred to *The Human Hippocampus* (1) for a comprehensive review. A brief review of the histopathologic changes, mechanisms of epileptogenesis, and neurophysiologic findings in hippocampal sclerosis follows.

The Limbic System

The limbic system is formed by the limbic lobe and associated subcortical structures: amygdala, habenula, mamillary bodies, septal nuclei, and portions of the thalamus, hypothalamus, and midbrain (2–5). The hippocampus is part of the limbic lobe and is situated on the inferomedial aspect of the hemisphere (Fig. 4.1). The limbic lobe is divided into two gyri (limbic and intralimbic) (6) and is separated from the surrounding cortical structures by the discontinuous limbic fissure, which is composed of cingulate, subparietal, anterior calcarine, collateral, and rhinal sulci. The limbic gyrus consists of the subcallosal, cingulate, and parahippocampal gyri. The latter can be divided into two segments: a narrow posterior segment and a more voluminous anterior segment called the piriform lobe, which comprises the uncus and the entorhinal area. The intralimbic gyrus arches within the limbic gyrus and is

composed of two main connected structures: a less developed, narrow, neuronal lamina, which is situated in the anterior (prehippocampal rudiment) and superior surface of the corpus callosum (indusium griseum), and the more developed posterior and ventral hippocampus.

The amygdala is a large nuclear complex in the dorsomedial part of the temporal lobe. It overhangs the hippocampal head along most of its surface and limits the ventral, superior, and medial walls of the temporal horn of the lateral ventricle. The amygdala is continuous with the parahippocampal gyrus caudally and is divided into two major masses of nuclei: the small corticomedial and the well-differentiated basolateral nuclear groups (3). The amygdala is part of the olfactory centers and the limbic system through its connections with both of them.

Hippocampal Anatomy

The hippocampus has the appearance of a sea horse: it bulges into the temporal horn of the lateral ventricle and is arched around the mesencephalon. It is divided into three anatomic segments: the head, which is a transversally oriented segment with prominent digitations (digitationes hippocampi); the body, which is a sagittally oriented segment; and the tail, which is narrow and transversally oriented. The tail disappears beneath the splenium of the corpus callosum posteriorly (Fig. 4.2). The total range of the hippocampus is between 4 and 4.5 cm, the width of the head is between 1.5 and 2 cm, and the width of the body is between 1 and 1.5 cm (7–9).

The Hippocampal Head

The hippocampal head includes intraventricular and extraventricular (uncal) parts. The intraventricular segment is

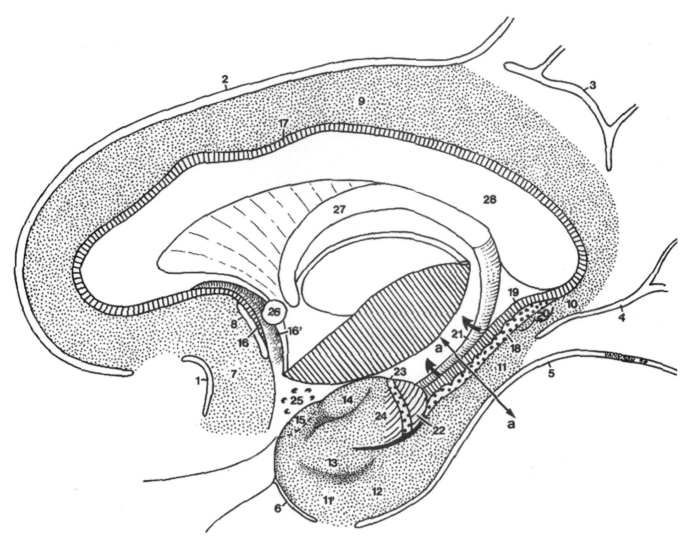

Figure 4.1 Dissection showing a sagittal section of the right hemisphere. The limbic lobe is separated from the isocortex by the limbic fissure and may be divided into two gyri: the limbic and intralimbic gyri. The line (*a-a*) indicates the plane of the section. Limbic fissure: *1*, anterior paraolfactory sulcus (subcallosal sulcus); *2*, cingulated sulcus; *3*, subparietal sulcus; *4*, anterior calcarine sulcus; *5*, collateral sulcus; *6*, rhinal sulcus. Limbic gyrus: *7*, subcallosal gyrus; *8*, posterior paraolfactory sulcus; *9*, cingulate gyrus; *10*, isthmus; *11*, parahippocampal gyrus, posterior part; *11′*, parahippocampal gyrus, anterior part (piriform lobe). Piriform lobe: *12*, entorhinal area; *13*, ambient gyrus; *14*, semilunar gyrus; *15*, prepiriform cortex. Intralimbic gyrus: *16*, prehippocampal rudiment; *16′*, paraterminal gyrus; *17*, indusium griseum. Hippocampus: *18*, gyrus dentatus; *19*, cornu ammonis; *20*, gyri of Andreas Retzius; *21*, fimbria (displaced upward, *arrows*); *22*, uncal apex; *23*, band of Giacomini; *24*, uncinate gyrus; *25*, anterior perforated substance; *26*, anterior commissure; *27*, fornix; *28*, corpus callosum.

anterior within the hippocampus and contains the hippocampal (or internal) digitations.

The Hippocampal Body

The hippocampal body, like the hippocampal head, is divided into intraventricular and extraventricular segments. It is bordered medially by the fimbria and laterally by the collateral eminence, which marks the intraventricular protrusion of cortex covering the collateral sulcus (Fig. 4.3). With the exception of the hippocampal head, the entire intraventricular hippocampal surface is covered by the choroid plexus. The extraventricular part of the hippocampus is limited to the dentate gyrus, fimbria, and superficial hippocampal sulcus (Fig. 4.1).

The Hippocampal Tail

The intraventricular part of the hippocampal tail is a transverse bulge. Digitations similar to those of the head are present on the tail's internal surface, but they are not typically found on its intraventricular surface.

HISTOLOGY OF THE HIPPOCAMPUS

The hippocampus is a bilaminar archicortical (allocortex) structure consisting of Ammon horn (hippocampus proper) and the dentate gyrus, with one lamina rolled up inside the other (Fig. 4.3). The two internal structures are interlocked forming two U-shaped laminae that are separated from each

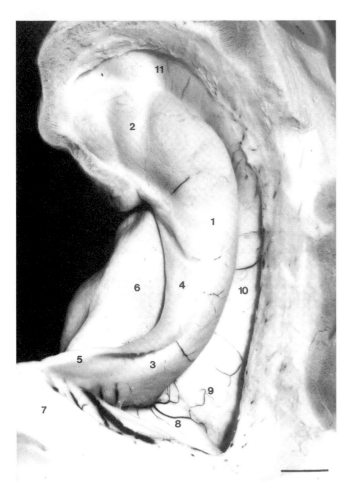

Figure 4.2 Intraventricular aspect of the hippocampus. The temporal horn has been opened and the choroid plexuses removed. *1*, Hippocampal body; *2*, head and digitationes hippocampi (internal digitations); *3*, hippocampal tail; *4*, fimbria; *5*, crus of fornix; *6*, subiculum; *7*, splenium of the corpus callosum; *8*, calcar avis; *9*, collateral trigone; *10*, collateral eminence; *11*, uncal recess of the temporal horn. Scale bar: 6.5 mm.

other by the hippocampal sulcus (Fig. 4.4), which is divided into a vestigial (deep) sulcus (10) and a superficial sulcus that is clearly visible on the mesial temporal lobe surface.

Hippocampal Layers

Ammon horn (cornu ammonis [CA]) may be divided into six layers: alveus, stratum oriens, stratum pyramidale, stratum radiatum, stratum lacunosum, and stratum moleculare (Fig. 4.5). These six layers are grouped into three allocortex layers: stratum oriens, stratum pyramidale, and stratum moleculare, which contains the last three layers (11,12).

The *alveus* covers the intraventricular surface and contains efferent hippocampal and subicular axons that enter the fimbria (Fig. 4.6), as well as afferent fibers mainly from the septum.

The *stratum oriens,* which has poorly defined borders, contains basket cells and is crossed by axons of pyramidal neurons to the alveus.

The *stratum pyramidale* contains the pyramidal cells, which are the major neurons of the hippocampus. From the base of these cells, axons connecting to the septal nuclei or association fibers traverse the stratum oriens toward the alveus. Pyramidal neurons have basal and apical dendrites (13). The basal dendrites arborize in the stratum oriens, whereas the apical dendrites traverse the cornu ammonis to reach the stratum moleculare in the proximity of the vestigial hippocampal sulcus. The pyramidal cells are surrounded by dense arborizations originating from basket cells in the stratum oriens (Fig. 4.7). The stratum pyramidale contains scattered basket cells (interneurons) and stellate cells (14).

The *stratum radiatum* contains mainly pyramidal cell apical dendrites that in CA1 are connected by the axons of the Schaffer collaterals, as well as septal and commissural fibers (Fig. 4.7).

The *stratum lacunosum* contains primarily perforant fibers from the entorhinal cortex and a lesser number of Schaffer collaterals (Fig. 4.7).

The *stratum moleculare* contains fewer interneurons and has broad arborizations of the apical dendrites from the pyramidal cells. It fuses with the stratum moleculare of the dentate gyrus as the vestigial hippocampal sulcus disappears during development.

Hippocampal Subfields

The CA contains four subfields, CA1 through CA4 (12), which are categorized according to the shape and location of the pyramidal neurons (Fig. 4.8).

CA1 neurons are triangular and multilayered and vary in sizes. CA1 (Sommer sector) (15) neurons continue into the five-layered subicular complex. *CA2 neurons* are larger, densely packed pyramidal cells. *CA3 neurons* are similar to CA2 neurons but are less densely packed. The CA3 subfield constitutes the genu of the CA. The CA3 subfield contains the mossy fibers, which are fine nonmyelinated fibers that originate from the granule neurons in the dentate gyrus and synapse with the *stratum lucidum* of CA3. *CA4 neurons* are large and triangular. Few in number, they are interspersed between the mossy fibers.

Dentate Gyrus (Fascia Dentata)

A concave structure on coronal sections that engulfs the CA4 subfield (Fig. 4.6), the dentate gyrus is separated from the hippocampal subfields by the vestigial hippocampal sulcus. It contains three layers that are more clearly identified that those of the CA: the stratum moleculare (long dendrites), stratum granulosum (granule cells), and the polymorphic layer or the subgranular zone, which contains mostly inhibitory interneurons of varied sizes (Figs. 4.7 and 4.8).

The *polymorphic layer* contains crossing axons that unite the neurons of the granular layer with those of CA4 and with interneurons in the polymorphic and CA4 regions.

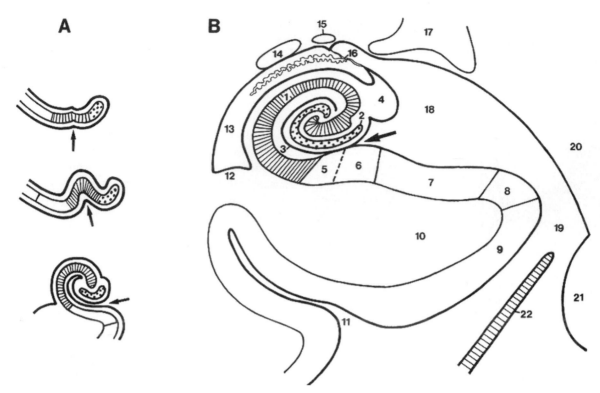

Figure 4.3   A: Development of the gyrus dentatus (*dotted area*) and of the cornu ammonis (*hatched area*) toward **(B)**, their definitive disposition. *Arrows* indicate the hippocampal sulcus (superficial part). *1*, Cornu ammonis; *2*, gyrus dentatus; *3*, hippocampal sulcus (deep or vestigial part); *4*, fimbria; *5*, prosubiculum; *6*, subiculum proper; *7*, presubiculum; *8*, parasubiculum; *9*, entorhinal area; *10*, parahippocampal gyrus; *11*, collateral sulcus; *12*, collateral eminence; *13*, temporal (inferior) horn of the lateral ventricle; *14*, tail of caudate nucleus; *15*, stria terminalis; *16*, choroid fissure and choroid plexuses; *17*, lateral geniculate body; *18*, lateral part of the transverse fissure (wing of ambient cistern); *19*, ambient cistern; *20*, mesencephalon; *21*, pons; *22*, tentorium cerebelli. (Adapted from Duvernoy HM. *The human hippocampus: functional anatomy, vascularization and serial sections with MRI.* Berlin: Springer-Verlag, 1998, with permission.)

The *stratum granulosum* is the main layer of the dentate gyrus and contains densely packed, small, round neurons. The *stratum moleculare* contains dendrites extending to the hippocampal fissure and a few interneurons. The outer and middle molecular zones receive fibers from the perforant pathway.

Parahippocampal Structures

The subiculum is the continuation of the hippocampus from CA1. It is divided into the prosubiculum, subiculum proper, presubiculum, and parasubiculum.

HIPPOCAMPAL CONNECTIONS

The entorhinal area is the principal input to the hippocampus (Fig. 4.7). Composed of the periallocortex, it is divided into deep and superficial layers (16,17). The intrahippocampal circuits are divided into the polysynaptic and direct intrahippocampal pathways.

The Polysynaptic Pathway

The polysynaptic pathway (perforant pathway) originates in the layer II stellate neurons of the entorhinal cortex. Large pyramidal cells also contribute to the granular aspect of the cortical surface (Fig. 4.6) (18). Excitatory (glutamatergic) fibers reach the stratum moleculare of the dentate gyrus where they synapse with the dendrites of the granule cells (19). The axons of the granule cells (mossy fibers) project to the dendrites of the CA4 and CA3 neurons (20), but do not extend into CA2. These axons contain a high concentration of zinc (21,22). The axons of CA3 and CA4 cells project as the Schaffer collaterals to the apical dendrites of CA2 and CA1 cells (Fig. 4.7). A small number of axons project rostrally to the septal nuclei (Fig. 4.6). The main output of the hippocampus occurs caudally through CA1 axons that may directly project to the alveus and fimbria or indirectly project to the subiculum, and from there to the alveus and fimbria. The subiculum is the major hippocampal output relay area. All the neurons of the polysynaptic pathways are excitatory (glutamatergic) (23).

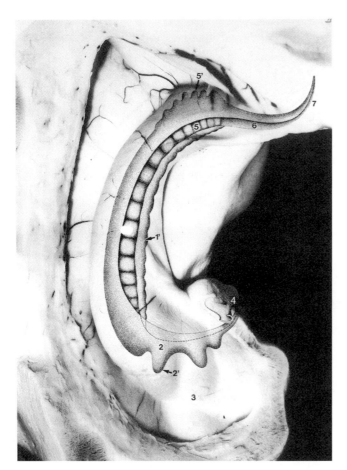

Figure 4.4 Gyrus dentatus seen through the hippocampus (transparent). *1*, Gyrus dentatus in the hippocampal body; *1*, margo denticulat us; *2*, gyrus dentatus in the hippocampal head; *2'*, digital extensions of the gyrus dentatus; *3*, digitationes hippocampi; *4*, band of Giacomini and terminal part of the gyrus dentatus in the medial surface of the uncus; *5*, gyrus dentatus in the hippocampal tail; *5'*, digital extensions of the gyrus dentatus; *6*, fasciola cinerea; *7*, terminal part of the fasciola cinerea.

The rostral output of the polysynaptic pathway to the cortex is through the fornix to the mamillary bodies, reaching the anterior thalamic nucleus (directly or indirectly through the mamillary bodies) (24). The cingulate area and the retrosplenial cortex are reached from the thalamus (Fig. 4.9).

The input to the polysynaptic pathway is through fibers that originate in the parietal association area (area 7) and surrounding temporal and occipital areas (areas 40, 39, and 22). These fibers project to the entorhinal cortex through the parahippocampal gyrus. The polysynaptic pathway may be involved in episodic and spatial memory, the most primitive memory types (25).

Direct Intrahippocampal Pathway

The direct intrahippocampal pathway originates in layer III of the entorhinal gyrus. These fibers reach directly to the pyramidal neurons of CA1, from which axons project

directly to the subiculum and then to the deep layers of the entorhinal cortex (Fig. 4.10) (26,27). The input to the direct intrahippocampal pathway is from the inferior temporal association cortex. The output of the pathway is to the temporal association cortex, the temporal pole, and the prefrontal cortex (Fig. 4.11). The direct pathway may be involved in semantic memory (25).

Other Hippocampal Connections

The septal nuclei are directly connected to the hippocampus. Axons of hippocampal and subicular pyramidal cells are the origin of these connections. The efferent hippocampal fibers reach the lateral septal nucleus through the precommissural fornix. Thereafter, fibers from the lateral septal nucleus connect with the medial septal nucleus, which constitutes the origin of the afferent hippocampal pathway from the septal nucleus. The septal nuclei are cholinergic and are thought to facilitate memory functions of the hippocampus (28,29). Moreover, the septal projections may control the characteristic hippocampal slow-wave rhythmic theta activity (30).

Commissural fibers joining the two hippocampi through the fornices are present in rodents. However, these fibers are few in primates and only reach limited regions of the hippocampi (31). Other direct cortical connections among the cingulate gyrus, temporal lobes, and prefrontal lobes have been described (32).

HIPPOCAMPAL SCLEROSIS

Bouchet and Cazauvieilh in 1825 first described a visible or palpable atrophy of the autopsied hippocampi of patients who died after decades of "mental alienation" seizures; they considered the abnormalities in the hippocampi as the likely cause of the seizures (33). With the advent of electroencephalography (EEG), it became clear that so-called psychomotor seizures originated from the temporal lobe and could potentially be cured with temporal lobe resection (34–36). Temporal lobe epilepsy associated with hippocampal sclerosis remains the most common presentation for epilepsy surgery in adolescents and adults, accounting for 70% of cases of intractable temporal lobe epilepsy (37). As is true for most of the focal epilepsies, the symptomatogenic area is in proximity to, although not identical with, the epileptogenic zone. The abdominal aura typical of mesial temporal lobe epilepsy is most probably determined by spreading of the epileptogenic discharge to the closely adjacent insular cortex, and fear is most probably produced by activation of the amygdala (38). Ictal symptoms and lateralizing signs in epilepsy from the mesial temporal region are an expression of seizure spread to adjacent brain regions. Mesial temporal sclerosis represents a distinct entity with a characteristic pathology and unique mechanisms of epileptogenesis and electrophysiologic findings.

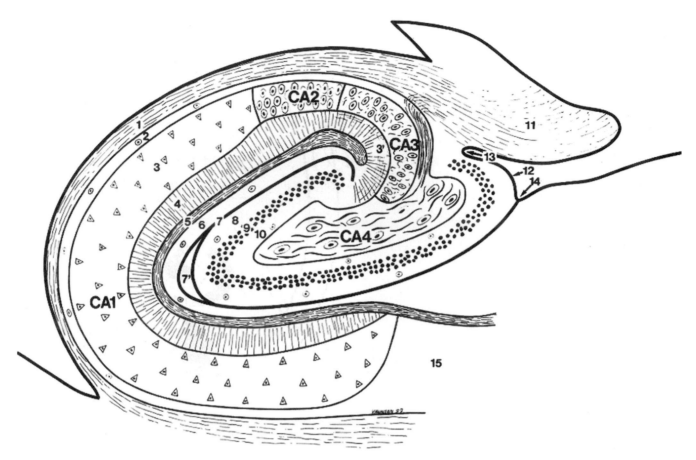

Figure 4.5 Structure of the hippocampus, coronal section. CA1 to CA4, fields of the cornu ammonis. Cornu ammonis: *1*, alveus; *2*, stratum oriens; *3*, stratum pyramidale; *3'*, stratum lucidum; *4*, stratum radiatum; *5*, stratum lacunosum; *6*, stratum moleculare; *7*, vestigial hippocampal sulcus (note a residual cavity, *7'*). Gyrus dentatus: *8*, stratum moleculare; *9*, stratum granulosum; *10*, polymorphic layer; *11*, fimbria; *12*, margo denticulatus; *13*, fimbriodentate sulcus; *14*, superficial hippocampal sulcus; *15*, subiculum.

Anatomic Pathology

Probably the first microscopic description of hippocampal sclerosis was in 1880 (15), when Sommer noted a specific pattern of neuron loss. The pyramidal neurons of the Ammon horn were largely destroyed, especially in the portion of the hippocampus, later labeled CA1 by Lorento de Nó, and in the prosubiculum (12). Sommer also described other hippocampal damage involving the granule cells and hilar neurons of the fascia dentata. Two decades later, Bratz gave a detailed histologic description of hippocampal sclerosis, differentiating the findings from those of other hippocampal pathologies (39). Hippocampal sclerosis is characterized by marked neuronal loss in the CA1 subfield of the hippocampus, with a lesser degree of cell loss in the CA3/CA4 subfields and relative sparing of the CA2 region. The severity of the cell loss in the CA1 and CA3 subfields is variable. Recent data suggest that the pattern of cell loss in the hippocampus is distinct in hippocampal sclerosis associated with other neocortical temporal lobe pathologies (so-called dual-pathology cases) (40). This pattern of cell loss is distinct from the classic forms of hippocampal sclerosis in that there is a trend toward more diffuse and homogenous neuronal loss in all hippocampal subfields, including the CA1 area.

Evidence that hippocampal sclerosis contributes to or causes chronic seizures in patients with temporal lobe epilepsy can be derived from outcome studies showing that inclusion of the hippocampal structures in the surgical resection is paramount for a good outcome (41). Patients with pathologic findings for hippocampal sclerosis do better than patients with no such pathologic findings (42). Furthermore, seizure control after resection was better in patients with regional ictal onset and focal anterior pathology than in patients with diffuse hippocampal damage, thus linking the cell loss to epileptogenicity (43). In addition, damage and neuronal loss that do not follow the pattern consistent with hippocampal sclerosis, such as end folium and amygdalar sclerosis, most likely do not contribute to temporal lobe epilepsy and probably are the consequence of repeated seizures from extrahippocampal sources (44,45).

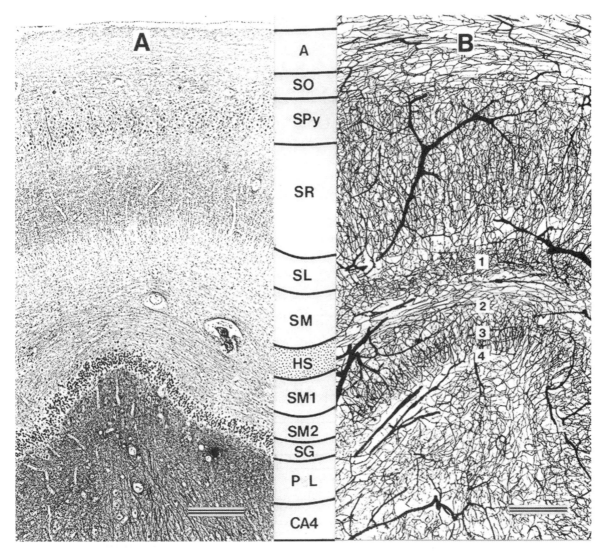

Figure 4.6   A and **B:** Structure of the hippocampus: **A:** Silver impregnation (Bodian). **B:** Intravascular India ink injection, showing the varying density of the vascular network in different hippocampal layers. Note the high vascular density in the stratum moleculare of the cornu ammonis (*1*). Cornu ammonis: *A*, alveus; *SO*, stratum oriens; *SPy*, stratum pyramidale; *SR*, stratum radiatum; *SL*, stratum lacunosum; *SM*, stratum moleculare; *HS*, vestigial hippocampal sulcus. Gyrus dentatus: *SM1*, stratum moleculare, external two thirds; *SM2*, stratum moleculare, inner third; *SG*, stratum granulosum; *PL*, polymorphic layer; *CA4*, field of the cornu ammonis. *1*, Stratum moleculare; *2*, external part of stratum moleculare of the gyrus dentatus; *3*, inner part, highly vascularized; *4*, stratum granulosum, poorly vascularized. Scale bar: 600 μm.

Pathogenesis of Hippocampal Sclerosis

There is a long-standing debate about whether hippocampal sclerosis is a cause or an effect of seizures. Spielmeyer introduced the hypothesis that hippocampal sclerosis is generated by repeated temporal lobe seizures and, hence, is the consequence and not the cause of the chronic epilepsy (46). He postulated that transient hippocampal ischemia led to the pathologic changes, although this could not account for the distinct pattern of neuronal loss and the often bilateral nature of changes seen in patients with hippocampal sclerosis. The clinical history of patients who underwent temporal lobe resections allowed identification

of a variety of precipitating injuries, including a history of status epilepticus, cerebral trauma, febrile convulsions, birth complications, meningitis/encephalitis, and cerebral hypoxia (47). Febrile seizures in childhood, particularly prolonged or focal seizures, are especially common in epileptic patients with hippocampal sclerosis (48). Studies suggest that the hippocampus is particularly susceptible to the excitotoxic effects of seizures in children younger than 5 years of age, corresponding with a period during which the hippocampus grows rapidly and therefore may be particularly vulnerable (49). The selective vulnerability of the hippocampal subfields can be reproduced by electrical stimulation of afferents to the hippocampus or by injection

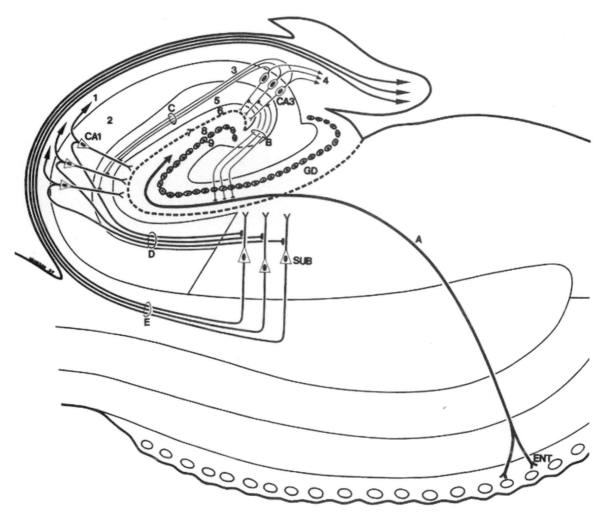

Figure 4.7 Polysynaptic intrahippocampal pathway. Parts of the neural chain (*A* though *E*) form the polysynaptic intrahippocampal pathway. Layer II of the entorhinal area (*ENT*) is the origin of this chain; its large pyramidal neurons are grouped in clusters, giving a granular aspect at the entorhinal surface. Cornu ammonis: *1*, alveus; *2*, stratum pyramidale; *3*, Schaffer collaterals; *4*, axons of pyramidal neurons (mainly to septal nuclei); *5*, strata lacunosum and radiatum; *6*, stratum moleculare; *7*, vestigial hippocampal sulcus. Gyrus dentatus *(GD): 8,* stratum moleculare; *9,* stratum granulosum *CA1* and *CA3* fields of the cornu ammonis; *SUB*, subiculum.

of excitatory amino acid analogues such as kainic acid (50). Patients with mesial temporal tumors or hamartomas usually have a mild degree of mesial temporal neuronal loss, attributed to the excitotoxic effect of hippocampal seizures. Generalized or focal status in adults may induce hippocampal swelling and eventually may lead to mesial temporal sclerosis (51). It seems likely, therefore, that hippocampal sclerosis represents merely the final pathologic common pathway from a variety of noxious stimuli.

Mechanisms of Epileptogenesis in Hippocampal Sclerosis

There are several hypotheses to explain how the selective neuronal cell loss seen in hippocampal sclerosis might lead to chronic epileptogenicity, including findings of aberrant mossy-fiber sprouting and synaptic reorganiza-

tion. The dentate gyrus can be considered the gatekeeper of excitability in the hippocampus (52). Excitatory input to the dentate granule cells comes through the polysynaptic pathway. Normally, mossy fibers sprouting from the granule cells connect with pyramidal cells as part of the hippocampal output pathway. In hippocampal sclerosis, however, these cells sprout mossy-fiber axons that are directed back into the inner molecular layer, possibly because the neurons to which they usually extend have been lost. There is some evidence that these aberrant mossy fibers instigate a recurrent excitatory circuit by forming synapses on the dendrites of neighboring dentate granule cells. Compared with normal hippocampus (Fig. 4.12A), in epileptic hippocampus, the granule cell axons (the excitatory mossy fibers) project back into the proximal granule cell dendrites (i.e., the inner molecular layer [Fig. 4.12B and C]), where they synapse on densely upregulated α-amino-3-

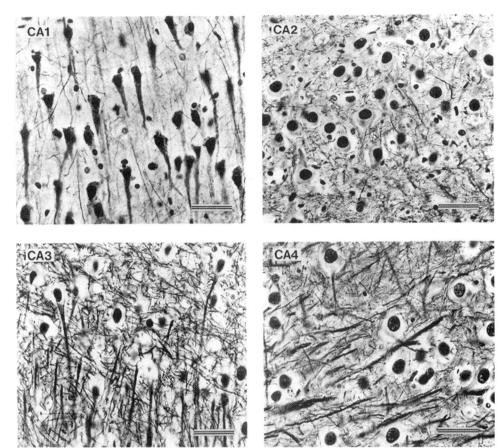

Figure 4.8 Neuronal types in the cornu ammonis (silver impregnation, Bodian). *CA1* through *CA4* are fields of the cornu ammonis. Scale bar: 52 μm.

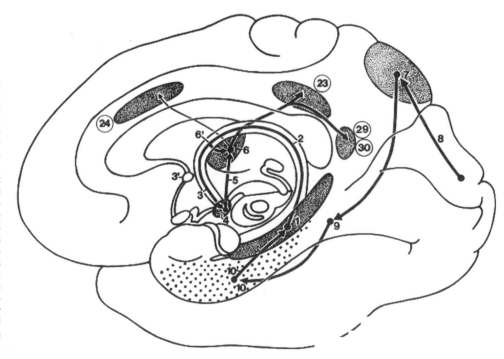

Figure 4.9 Cortical connections of the polysynaptic intrahippocampal pathway. Hippocampal output fibers to the cortex: arising from the hippocampus *(1)*, fibers successively reach the body *(2)* and column *(3)* of fornix *(3', anterior commissure)*, the mamillary body *(4)*, and then, by the mamillothalamic tract *(5)*, the anterior thalamic nucleus, the main cortical projections are the posterior cingulate (area *23)* and retrosplenial (areas *29* and *30)* cortices; some fibers may project to the anterior cingulate cortex (area *24)*. Input fibers from the cortex to hippocampus: the posterior parietal association cortex *(7)* in relation to the superior visual system *(8)* projects by means of the parahippocampal gyrus *(9)* to the entorhinal area *(10)*; 10', perforant path.

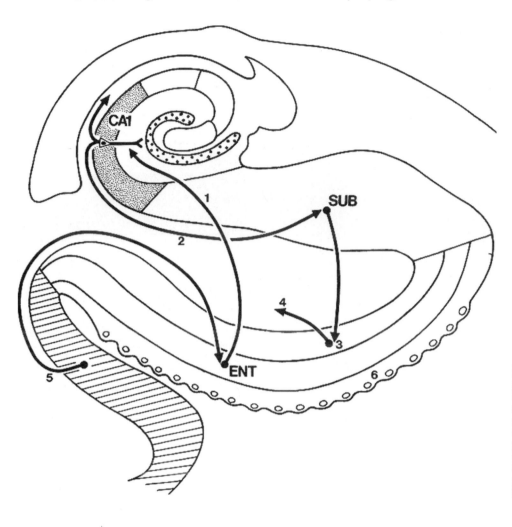

Figure 4.10 Direct intrahippocampal pathway. The entorhinal area *(ENT)* (layer III) projects directly *(1)* onto CA1 pyramidal neurons, which innervate *(2)* the subiculum *(SUB)*. Subicular axons project back to the deep layers of the cortex *(4)*. The direct pathway receives inputs through the perirhinal cortex *(5)*. *6*, Layer II of the entorhinal cortex.

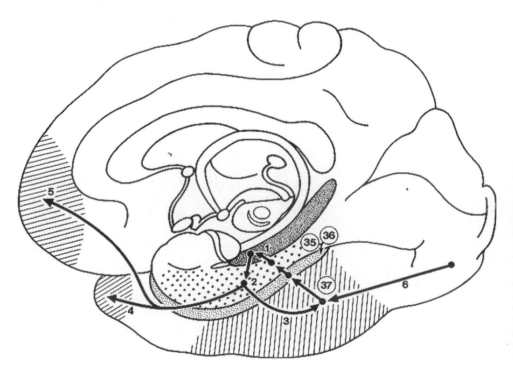

Figure 4.11 Cortical connections of the direct intrahippocampal pathway. *1*, Intrahippocampal circuitry. Hippocampal output fibers to the cortex: from the deep layers of the entorhinal cortex *(2)* fibers reach the inferior temporal association cortex *(3)*, the temporal pole *(4)*, and the prefrontal cortex *(5)*. Input fibers from the cortex to hippocampus: the main origin of these fibers is the inferior temporal association cortex (area *37*) in relation to the inferior visual system *(6)*, reaching the entorhinal cortex through the perirhinal cortex (areas *35* and *36*).

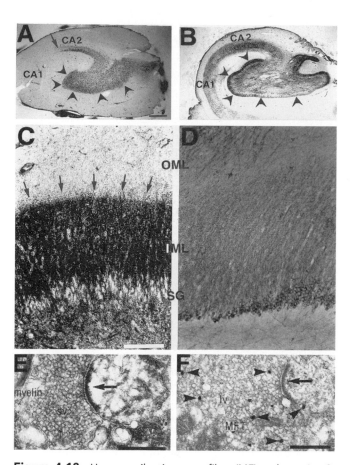

Figure 4.12 Human epileptic mossy fiber (MF) and α-amino-3-hydroxyl-5-methyl-4-isoxazolepropionic acid (AMPA) receptor synaptic reorganizations. Timm-stained autopsy of normal hippocampus (**A**), compared with epileptic hippocampus (**B**), showing (1) the normal distribution of MFs ending at the CA2 subfield (**A**, *arrow*) and having no supragranular inner molecular layer (IML) MFs (**B**, *arrowheads*) and extensive feedforward MF projections into the region superior to Ammon horn (**B**, CA2, CA1). **C:** The higher magnification of the Timm stain shows that in the fascia dentata all supragranular MFs are in the IML (*arrows*) and none in the outer molecular layer (OML) above. **D:** The AMPA receptor protein densities are greater in the IML but also are denser than normal in the OML. **E** and **F:** Timm-stained electron micrographs of human epileptic fascia dentata. OML axodentritic synapse (**E**, *arrow* within cross section of the dendrite) has the asymmetric profile and small-clustered vesicles typical of perforant path excitatory synapses from the entorhinal cortex. Notice the myelin in the upper left corner (in OML, not in IML). Timm granules (**F**, *black dots, arrowheads*) of a typically large MF terminal having large vesicles and an asymmetric excitatory synaptic profile (*arrow*). Scale bars: 1.0 mm (**A** and **B**); 200 μm (**C** and **D**); 0.5 μm (**E** and **F**). (**A** Adapted from Babb TL, Pretorius JK, Kupfer WR, et al. Aberrant synaptic reorganization in human epileptic hippocampus: evidence for feedforward excitation. *Dendron* 1992;7:7–25, with permission. **B** adapted from Babb TL, Pretorius JK, Mello LE, et al. Synaptic reorganization in epileptic human and rat kainite hippocampus may contribute to feedback and feedforward excitation. In: Engel J, Wasterlain C, Cavalheiro EA, et al., eds. *Molecular neurobiology of epilepsy.* Amsterdam: Elsevier Science, 1992:193–203, with permission. **E** and **F** adapted from Babb TL. Research on the anatomy and pathology of epileptic tissue. In: Lüders H, ed. *Epilepsy surgery.* New York: Lippincott-Raven Press, 1991:719–727, with permission.)

hydroxy-5-methyl-4-isoxazolepropionic acid receptors (Fig. 4.12D) (53–55). The Timm-stained electron micrograph (Fig. 4.12F, *arrowheads*) verifies that these mossy fibers terminate on inner molecular layer dendrites with asymmetric (excitatory type) synaptic profiles. In contrast, there are no mossy-fiber terminals in the outer molecular layer, where entorhinal cortex axons make excitatory synaptic (asymmetric) connections (Fig. 4.12E, *arrow*). This epileptic circuit would be a monosynaptic feedback excitation. Figure 4.12B shows that the mossy fibers also project past CA3 to all dendritic regions of CA2, CA1, and beyond, because these dendrites would be denervated by the extensive cell loss in all regions of the hippocampus and thereby provide feedforward excitation.

Progenitor cells in the dentate gyrus of the hippocampus preserve the capability of neurogenesis. Seizures appear to trigger mitotic activity and lead to differentiation of new dentate cells. There is evidence that these new granule cells may be also aberrantly integrated into the neuronal circuits, possibly contributing to an imbalance of excitation and inhibition (56). Mossy fibers in the hilum of the dentate gyrus provide excitatory feedback to γ-aminobutyric acid (GABA)-ergic interneurons and create a surround inhibition, thereby preventing hyperexcitability. In hippocampal sclerosis, sprouting and synaptic reorganization of mossy fibers lead to a loss of this spatially organized inhibition, although the absolute number of inhibitory GABA ergic synapses in the hippocampus may actually be increased (57). Figure 4.13 demonstrates that GABA neurons are well preserved and that reorganization by GABA ergic axons occurs in epileptic hippocampus (58). A glutamate decarboxylase immunohistochemistry (GAD-ICC) stain shows the dense GABA terminals in the granule cells of the inner molecular layer (Fig. 4.13B, *arrow*) and on the dendrites and pyramidal cell bodies (Fig. 4.13C, *arrowheads*); these are denser than with normal GABAergic innervation. GAD-positive inhibitory synapses and GAD-negative excitatory synapses are seen on the same proximal dendrite in epileptic hippocampus (Fig. 4.13D, *small arrowheads*).

Neurophysiology of Hippocampal Sclerosis

In vivo neurophysiologic studies consistently demonstrate enhanced inhibition in epileptic hippocampus in animals. Single-cell recordings reveal a higher degree of neuronal synchrony in the epileptic hippocampus compared with the contralateral side (59). Enhanced inhibition has the capability to synchronize the membrane potentials of a greater number of neurons, and the abnormal hypersynchrony may be a mechanism for ictal generation (60). Depth electrode studies reveal that patients with mesial temporal epilepsy tend to show a hypersynchronous ictal onset in contrast to patients with neocortical epilepsy, who more commonly demonstrate the buildup of low-voltage fast or recruiting rhythms (61). Intracranially recorded

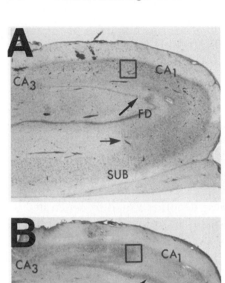

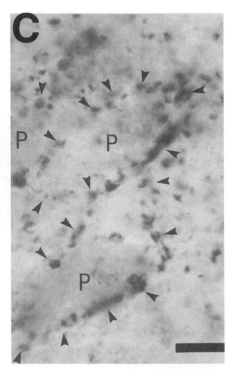

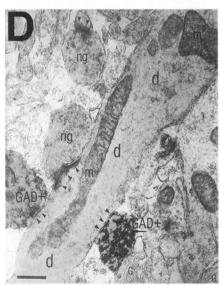

Figure 4.13 Cresyl-violet stain **(A)** of a typically sclerotic hippocampus, 60 μm adjacent to the glutamate decarboxylase immunohistochemistry (GAD-ICC) stain **(B)**, which shows aberrant "inhibitory" GABA-axon projections into the fascia dentata inner molecular layer (IML) (*arrow*), where mossy fiber terminals also aberrantly innervate the epileptic hippocampus. GABA-axon densities also are greater on cell bodies and in the dendritic junctions of CA2, CA1, and subiculum. **C:** GAD-ICC stain of pyramidal *(P)* cells in CA2 (boxed area of **B**) shows dense GABAergic terminals (*arrowheads*) around the somata and dendrites. This degree of epileptic hippocampal GABA hyperinnervation was found throughout Ammon horn and the fascia dentata. **D:** GAD-labeled electron micrograph of a typical proximal dendrite in an epileptic hippocampus shows inhibitory (GAD$^+$, symmetric profile) synapses next to non-GAD excitatory (ng, asymmetric profile) synapse. Both types synapse on the same dendrite *(d)*. Scale bars: 1.0 mm **(A and B)**; 15 μm **(C)**; 1 μm **(D)**. (**A** and **B** adapted from Babb TL, Pretorius JK, Kupfer WR, et al. Glutamate decarboxylase-immunoreactive neurons are preserved in human epileptic hippocampus. *J Neurosci* 1989;9:2562–2574, with permission.)

seizures precede the onset on scalp EEG and the appearance of clinical symptoms by 10 seconds to more than 1 minute (62). Despite this delay, findings on scalp EEG are relatively specific for temporal lobe epilepsy, and a rhythmic temporal theta activity at onset virtually excludes extratemporal seizure origin (63,64). However, the presence of this pattern requires the synchronous recruitment of adjacent inferolateral temporal neocortex, and ictal scalp EEG usually does not allow a distinction between mesial and neocortical temporal lobe epilepsy. Interictal epileptiform activity is thought to provide more accurate localization of the epileptogenic zone than do ictal patterns. Interictal epileptiform activity over the anterior temporal region was seen in 94% of patients with temporal lobe epilepsy (65). An amplitude maximum at the sphenoidal electrode alone appears to be significantly more frequent in patients with hippocampal sclerosis than in patients with medial temporal lobe tumors (66). Chapter 78 addresses issues related to epilepsy surgery for patients with hippocampal sclerosis.

REFERENCES

1. Duvernoy HM. *The human hippocampus: functional anatomy, vascularization and serial sections with MRI.* Berlin: Springer-Verlag, 1998.

2. Bronen RA. Hippocampal and limbic terminology. *J Neuroradiol* 1992;13:943–945.
3. Carpenter MB, Sutin J. *Human neuroanatomy,* 8th ed. Baltimore: Williams & Wilkins, 1983.
4. Kretschmann H-J, Weinricj W. *Cranial neuroimaging and clinical neuroanatomy,* 2nd ed. New York: Thieme, 1992.
5. Mark LP, Daniels DL, Naidich TP, et al. Limbic system anatomy: an overview. *Am J Neuroradiol* 1993;14:349–352.
6. Broca P. Anatomie comparée des circonvolutions cérébrales. Le grand lobe limbique et la scissure limbique dans la serie des mammiferes. *Rev Anthropol* 1878;1:385–498.
7. Poirier P, Charpy A. *Traité d'anatomie humaine,* vol 3, parts 1 and 2. Paris: Masson, 1921.
8. Testut L, Latarjet A. *Traité d'anatomie humaine,* 9th ed. *Angeiologie, systeme nerveux central.* Vol 2. Paris: Doin, 1948.
9. Déjerine J. *Anatomie des centres nerveux,* vol 1. Paris: Masson, 1980.
10. Humphrey T. The development of the human hippocampal fissure. *J Anat* 1967;101:655–676.
11. Ramon Y, Cajal S. *The structure of Ammon's horn.* Springfield, IL: Charles C Thomas, 1968.
12. Lorente de No R. Studies on the structure of the cerebral cortex, II: continuation of the study of the Ammonic system. *J Psychol Neurol* 1934;46:113–177.
13. Isaacson RL. *The limbic system.* New York: Plenum, 1974.
14. Olbrich HG, Braak H. Ratio of pyramidal cells versus non-pyramidal cells in sector CA1 of the human Ammon's horn. *Anat Embryol* 1985;173:105–110.
15. Sommer W. Erkrankung des Ammonshorns als aetiologisches Moment der Epilepsie. *Arch Psychiatr* 1880;10:631–675.
16. Hevner RF, Wong-Riley MT. Entorhinal cortex of the human, monkey, and rat: metabolic map as revealed by cytochrome oxidase. *J Comp Neurol* 1992;326:451–469.
17. Insausti R, Tunon T, Sobreviela T, et al. The human entorhinal cortex: a cytoarchitectonic analysis. *J Comp Neurol* 1995;355:171–198.
18. Amaral DG, Insausti R. Hippocampal formation. In: Praxinos G, ed. *The human nervous system.* San Diego, CA: Academic Press, 1990:711–755.
19. Cerbone A, Patacchioli FR, Sadile AG. A neurogenetic and morphogenetic approach to hippocampal functions based on individual differences and neurobehavioral co-variations. *Behav Brain Res* 1993;55:1–16.
20. Treves A. Quantitative estimate of the information relayed by the Schaffer collaterals. *J Comput Neurosci* 1995;2:259–272.
21. McLardy T. Zinc enzymes and the hippocampal mossy fiber system. *Nature* 1962;194:300–302.
22. Frederikson CJ, Klitenick MA, Manton WI, et al. Cytoarchitectonic distribution of zinc in the hippocampus of man and the rat. *Brain Res* 1983;273:335–339.
23. Francis PT, Cross AJ, Bowen DM. Neurotransmitters and neuropeptides. In: Terry RD, Katzman R, Bick KL, eds. *Alzheimer disease.* New York: Raven, 1994:247–261.
24. Devinsky O, Luciano D. The contributions of cingulate cortex to human behavior. In: Vogt BA, Gabriel M, eds. *Neurobiology of cingulated cortex and limbic thalamus.* Boston: Birkhauser, 1993:527–556.
25. Squire LR, Zola-Morgan S, Alvarez P. Functional distinctions within the medial temporal lobe memory system: what is the evidence. *Behav Brain Sci* 1994;17:495–496.
26. Du F, Whetsell WO, Abou-Khalil B, et al. Preferential neuronal loss in layer III of the entorhinal cortex in patients with temporal lobe epilepsy. *Epilepsy Res* 1993;16:223–233.
27. MacLean PD. The limbic system concept. In: Trimble MR, Bolwig TG, eds. *The temporal lobes and the limbic system.* Petersfield, UK: Wrightson Biomedical, 1992:1–265.
28. Stackman RW, Walsh TJ. Distinct profile of working memory errors following acute or chronic disruption of the cholinergic septohippocampal pathway. *Neurobiol Learn Mem* 1995;64: 226–236.
29. Alonso JR, Hoi Sang U, Amaral DG. Cholinergic innervation of the primate hippocampal formation, II. effects of the fimbria/fornix transection. *J Comp Neurol* 1996;375:527–551.
30. Vanderwolf CH, Leung LWS, Stewart DJ. Two afferent pathways mediating hippocampal rhythmical slow activity. In: Buzsaki G, Vanderwolf CH, eds. *Electrical activity of the archicortex.* Budapest, Hungary: Akademiai Kiado, 1985:47–66.
31. Amaral DG, Insausti R, Cowan WM. The commissural connections of the monkey hippocampal formation. *J Comp Neurol* 1984;224:307–336.
32. Schwerdtfeger WK. Direct efferent and afferent connections of the hippocampus with the neocortex in the marmoset monkey. *Am J Anat* 1979;156:77–82.
33. Bouchet C, Cazauvieilh JB. De l'épilepsie considerée dans ses rapports avec l'alienation mentale. *Arch Gen Med* 1825;9:510–542.
34. Bailey P, Gibbs FA. The surgical treatment of psychomotor epilepsy. *JAMA* 1951;145:365–370.
35. Jasper HH. Electroencephalography. In: Penfield W, Erickson TC, eds. *Epilepsy and cerebral localization.* Springfield, IL: Charles C Thomas, 1941:380–454.
36. Penfield W, Baldwin M. Temporal lobe seizures and the technic of subtotal temporal lobectomy. *Ann Surg* 1952;136:625–634.
37. Babb TL, Brown WJ. Pathological findings in epilepsy. In: Engel J Jr, ed. *Surgical treatment of the epilepsies.* New York: Raven Press, 1987:511–540.
38. Lüders HO. Symptomatic areas and electrical cortical stimulation. In: Lüders HO, Noachtar S, eds. *Epileptic seizures. Pathophysiology and clinical semiology.* Philadelphia: Churchill Livingstone, 2000:131–140.
39. Bratz E. Ammonshornbefunde der epileptischen. *Arch Psychiatr Nervenkr* 1899;31:820–836.
40. Diehl B, Najm I, Mohamed A, et al. Interictal EEG, hippocampal atrophy, and cell densities in hippocampal sclerosis and hippocampal sclerosis associated with microscopic cortical dysplasia. *J Clin Neurophysiol* 2002;19:157–162.
41. Green JR, Duisberg RE, McGrath WB. Focal epilepsy of psychomotor type; a preliminary report of observations on effect of surgical therapy. *J Neurosurg* 1951;8:157–172.
42. Mathern GW, Babb TL, Vickrey BG, et al. The clinical-pathogenic mechanisms of hippocampal neuron loss and surgical outcomes in temporal lobe epilepsy. *Brain* 1995;118:105–118.
43. Babb TL, Lieb JP, Brown WJ, et al. Distribution of pyramidal cell density and hyperexcitability in the epileptic human hippocampal formation. *Epilepsia* 1984;25:721–728.
44. Mathern GW, Babb TL, Vickrey BG, et al. Traumatic compared to non-traumatic clinical-pathologic associations in temporal lobe epilepsy. *Epilepsy Res* 1994;19:129–139.
45. Mathern GW, Pretorius JK, Babb TL. Influence of the type of initial precipitating injury and at what age it occurs on course and outcome in patients with temporal lobe seizures. *J Neurosurg* 1995;82:220–227.
46. Spielmeyer W. Die Pathogenese des epileptischen Krampfes. *Z Gesamte Neurol Psychiatr* 1927;109:501–520.
47. Falconer MA, Serfetinides EA, Corsellis JA. Etiology and pathogenesis of temporal lobe epilepsy. *Arch Neurol* 1964;10:233–248.
48. Kuks JB, Cook MJ, Fish DR, et al. Hippocampal sclerosis in epilepsy and childhood febrile seizures. *Lancet* 1993;342:1391–1394.
49. Marks DA, Kim J, Spencer DD, et al. Characteristics of intractable seizures following meningitis and encephalitis. *Neurology* 1992;42:1513–1518.
50. Westbrook GL. Seizures and epilepsy. In: Kandel ER, Schwartz JH, Jessell TM, eds. *Principles of neural science.* New York: McGraw-Hill, 2000:911–935.
51. Tien RD, Felsberg GJ. The hippocampus in status epilepticus: demonstration of signal intensity and morphologic changes with sequential fast spin-echo MR imaging. *Radiology* 1995;194:249–256.
52. Sloviter RS. Permanently altered hippocampal structure, excitability, and inhibition after experimental status epilepticus in the rat: the "dormant basket cell" hypothesis and its possible relevance to temporal lobe epilepsy. *Hippocampus* 1991;1:41–66.
53. Babb TL, Pretorius JK, Kupfer WR, et al. Aberrant synaptic reorganization in human epileptic hippocampus: evidence for feedforward excitation. *Dendron* 1992;7:7–25.
54. Babb TL, Pretorius JK, Mello LE, et al. Synaptic reorganization in epileptic human and rat kainite hippocampus may contribute to feedback and feedforward excitation. In: Engel J, Wasterlain C, Cavalheiro EA, et al, eds. *Molecular neurobiology of epilepsy.* Amsterdam: Elsevier Science, 1992:193–203.
55. Babb TL. Research on the anatomy and pathology of epileptic tissue. In: Lüders H, ed. *Epilepsy surgery.* New York: Lippincott-Raven Press, 1991:719–727.

56. Scharfman HE, Goodman JH, Sollas AL. Granule-like neurons at the hilar/CA3 border after status epilepticus and their synchrony with area CA3 pyramidal cells: functional implications of seizure-induced neurogenesis. *J Neurosci* 2000;20:6144–6158.

57. Nusser Z, Hajos N, Somogyi P, et al. Increased number of synaptic GABA(A) receptors underlies potentiation at hippocampal inhibitory synapses. *Nature* 1998;395:172–177.

58. Babb TL, Pretorius JK, Kupfer WR, et al. Glutamate decarboxylase-immunoreactive neurons are preserved in human epileptic hippocampus. *J Neurosci* 1989;9:2562–2574.

59. Isokawa-Akesson M, Wilson CL, Babb TL. Inhibition in synchronously firing human hippocampal neurons. *Epilepsy Res* 1989; 3:236–247.

60. Engel J Jr, Dichter M, Schwartzkroin P. Basic mechanisms of human epilepsy. In: Engel J Jr, Pedley TA, eds. *Epilepsy: a comprehensive textbook.* Philadelphia: Lippincott-Raven, 1997:499–512.

61. Spencer SS, Guimaraes P, Katz A, et al. Morphological patterns of seizures recorded intracranially. *Epilepsia* 1992;33:537–545.

62. Pacia SV, Ebersole JS. Intracranial EEG substrates of scalp ictal pattern from temporal foci. *Epilepsia* 1997;38:642–654.

63. Foldvary N, Klem G, Hammel J, et al. The localizing value of ictal EEG in focal epilepsy. *Neurology* 2001;57:2022–2028.

64. Risinger MW, Engel J Jr, Van Ness PC, et al. Ictal localization of temporal lobe seizures with scalp/sphenoidal recordings. *Neurology* 1989;39:1288–1293.

65. Williamson PD, French JA, Thadani VM, et al. Characteristics of medial temporal lobe epilepsy, II: interictal and ictal scalp electroencephalography, neuropsychological testing, neuroimaging, surgical results, and pathology. *Ann Neurol* 1993;34:781–787.

66. Hamer HM, Najm I, Mohamed A, et al. Interictal epileptiform discharges in temporal lobe epilepsy due to hippocampal sclerosis versus medial temporal lobe tumors. *Epilepsia* 1999;40: 1261–1268.

Basic Cellular Neurophysiology

5

Stephen W. Jones

ION CHANNELS AND INTRINSIC MEMBRANE PROPERTIES

Basis of Electrical Activity

The activity of ion channels is fundamental to signaling in the nervous system. Synaptic potentials and action potentials, the basic electrical signals, result directly from the movement of ions through channels. In past decades, patch clamp recording and molecular biology have identified a variety of ion channel types and have begun to clarify the mechanisms underlying channel activity.

The electrical activity of a biologic membrane can be represented as an equivalent circuit consisting of a resistor, a capacitor, and a battery (Fig. 5.1A). This corresponds physically to ion channels, the lipid bilayer, and ion gradients (Fig. 5.1B). The properties of the bilayer and the ion gradients are essentially constant, with the important exception of the Ca^{2+} gradient. In contrast, ion channels vary dramatically among cell types and can open or close in response to physiologic stimuli. The intrinsic membrane properties of a cell and its moment-to-moment electrical activity depend primarily on the types and numbers of ion channels that the cell expresses.

How do the channels, bilayer, and ion gradients work together to produce a membrane potential? A pure lipid bilayer is an excellent insulator, because its hydrophobic interior renders it essentially impermeable to ions. Movement of ions across the membrane (electrically, a current) occurs primarily through ion channels. Because an open ion channel catalyzes the flux of ions down a concentration gradient, it is more intuitive to think in terms of conductance rather than resistance: an increase in the number of open channels produces a higher electrical conductance. The energy source for ion flow through a channel is an ion gradient, resulting from the activity of pumps and carriers,

such as the Na^+ ,K^+ adenosine triphosphatase (ATPase). Ion flow changes the charge distribution across the membrane. Because like charges repel each other, the presence of net charge in bulk solution is an unstable situation (i.e., principle of electroneutrality). The lipid bilayer is extremely thin (7 nm), allowing strong attractive forces between positively and negatively charged ions on opposite sides of the membrane. This allows the bilayer to act as a capacitor to store charge. The separation of charge across the membrane is the source of the membrane potential (V_M): $V_M = Q/C$, where Q is the amount of charge, and C is the capacitance of the membrane. Biologic membranes have an essentially constant capacitance, approximately 1 µF/cm2.

The membrane potential depends primarily on the selectivity of the ion channels that are open at a given time. Ion channels can be highly selective for particular ions. For example, many K^+ channels are more than 100-fold more selective for K^+ than for Na^+. For a cell with only K^+ channels open (i.e., an approximation of a real neuron at its resting potential), a chemical or diffusional force allows K^+ to diffuse down the concentration gradient and out of the cell. As K^+ ions flow, however, the outside (o) of the cell becomes electrically positive with respect to the inside (i). Convention defines the voltage outside a cell as zero, so the membrane potential resulting from outward movement of K^+ ions is said to be negative. That voltage produces an electrical force that prevents further efflux of K^+ ions, as the excess of positive charge outside the cell repels the positively charged K^+. If no other ions can cross the membrane, a state of equilibrium is rapidly reached in which the outward diffusional force equals the inward electrical force. That would be a true thermodynamic equilibrium, stable indefinitely without input of metabolic energy. There would be no net flux of K^+ through an open K^+ channel. The voltage across the membrane would be the equilibrium potential for K^+ (E_K), as given by the Nernst

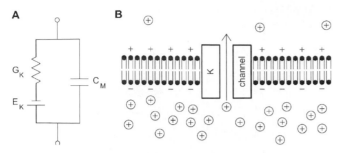

Figure 5.1   Electrical (**A**) and physical (**B**) views of a K$^+$-selective membrane.

equation for a battery: at 37°C, $E_K = 61.5 \log([K^+]_o/[K^+]_i)$. E_K is near -90 mV for a physiologic K$^+$ gradient.

By the same argument, if only Na$^+$-selective channels are open, the membrane potential would be E_{Na}, or about $+60$ mV. That is a first approximation to a neuron at the peak of the action potential.

In reality, the situation is more complex, because multiple channel types are open simultaneously. There is no generally valid way to calculate the membrane potential in that case, although two equations are commonly used. The more familiar is the Goldman equation:

$$V_M = 61.5 \log \{(P_K [K^+]_o + P_{Na} [Na^+]_o) / (P_K [K^+]_i + P_{Na} [Na^+]_i)\}$$

in which P_K and P_{Na} are the permeabilities of the membrane to K$^+$ and Na$^+$ (permeabilities are related to conductances). The derivation of the Goldman equation uses some assumptions that are not realistic for ion channels, particularly that ions move independently of one another, but it is a useful approximation and often serves as an empirical definition of ion permeability.

In another approach, Ohm's law is used to define the conductance for each ion: for K$^+$, $I_K = G_K (V_M - E_K)$. The "driving force," the difference between the membrane potential and the equilibrium potential, is used rather than the absolute voltage, because the current through an open K$^+$ channel goes to zero at the equilibrium potential. If the membrane potential is constant, there must be no net ionic current: $I_K + I_{Na} = 0$ (considering only K$^+$ and Na$^+$). That leads to the "parallel batteries" equation:

$$V_M = G'_K E_K + G'_{Na} E_{Na}$$

The equation uses normalized conductances $G'_K = G_K/(G_K + G_{Na})$ and $G'_{Na} = G_{Na}/(G_K + G_{Na})$. Qualitatively, the Goldman equation and the parallel batteries equation say that the membrane potential is a compromise among the equilibrium potentials for the individual ions. The higher the conductance (or permeability) for an ion, the closer the membrane potential is to that ion's equilibrium potential. This allows a better approximation to the situation at rest: the membrane potential is much closer to E_K than to E_{Na} because many more K$^+$ channels are open than Na$^+$ channels. The converse is true at the peak of the action

potential. For completeness, there is also a delay between channel opening and a change in voltage, because time is required for ion flow to change the net distribution of charge across the membrane (i.e., to charge the membrane capacitance).

General Properties of Ion Channels

Until 25 years ago, ion channels were considered hypothetical entities. The most direct demonstration of discrete ion channels came from patch clamp recording (Fig. 5.2A). When a glass electrode with an opening of about 1 µm is pressed onto a cell surface, gentle suction often forms a seal between the glass and the cell membrane that is tight electrically, chemically, and physically. The resistance of the seal is typically about 10 GΩ (10^{10} Ω). That extremely low rate of ion leakage under the seal implies molecular tightness. The high resistance of the seal gives very low levels of current noise, so that the tiny currents resulting from activity of individual ion channels in the "patch" of membrane directly under the electrode can be resolved. This was one of the first scientific techniques by which the behavior of a single molecule in real time could be observed.

Two types of information can be obtained from single-channel records (Fig. 5.2B): gating (i.e., when is a channel open?) and permeation (i.e., how does current flow through an open ion channel?). A channel's permeation properties determine its ion selectivity. The absolute amplitude of single-channel currents is also instructive. A typical 2-pA

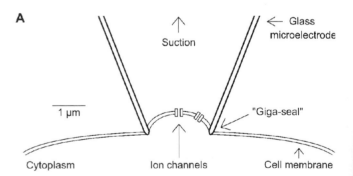

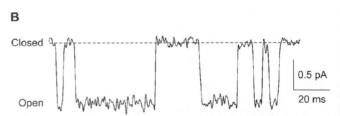

Figure 5.2   The patch clamp technique. **A:** A patch electrode is sealed onto a cell. This cell-attached configuration records the activity of individual ion channels located in the patch of membrane under the electrode. **B:** Example of ion channel gating for an L-type calcium channel from a smooth-muscle cell. (Courtesy of Dr. Carlos A. Obejero-Paz, Case Western Reserve University, Cleveland, OH.)

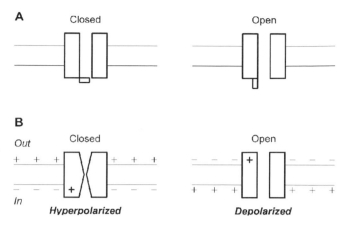

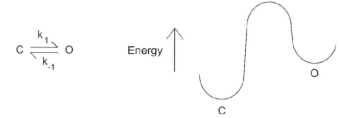

Figure 5.4 The simplest model for channel gating. Two conformational states of the protein (closed [*C*] and open [*O*]) spontaneously interconvert according to first-order rate constants k_1 and k_{-1}. The right-hand diagram shows the energy levels of the closed and open states, which determine the equilibrium, and the height of the energy barrier, which determines the rates.

Figure 5.3 Two possible mechanisms of channel gating. **A:** Movement of a "gate" can cause the channel pore to be open or blocked at one end, as is thought to occur for rapid inactivation of A-type potassium channels. **B:** Channel opening also may result from a concerted conformational change involving the entire protein. This diagram shows net outward movement of positive charges within the channel protein as the channel opens, which would produce a voltage-dependent channel that opens on depolarization.

current may seem inconsequential, but it translates into a flux of 10^7 ions per second through the channel pore. That simple calculation remains one of the strongest pieces of evidence that an ion channel is a channel, because that transport rate is orders of magnitude higher than the turnover number of even the fastest enzymes and carriers, and the only known mechanism that could produce such a rate is diffusion through a pore, with movement at a rate nearly as fast as if the ions were in bulk water. The combination of high flux and high selectivity among chemically similar ions remains an interesting puzzle.

Channel gating is crucial, because the opening and closing of ion channels in response to physiologic stimuli is the fundamental mechanism underlying signals such as synaptic potentials and action potentials. What is gating? Some general conclusions can be drawn from records of single channels (Fig. 5.2B). Channels switch between open and closed states, apparently at random. Under fixed recording conditions, the current observed when a channel is open generally is constant, implying a constant rate of ion movement through the pore. The current through a closed channel is almost undetectable. The transition between the open and closed states is too fast to measure, implying a completed conformational change in a few microseconds or less. Two extreme physical pictures can be used to illustrate gating: literal movement of a *gate*, a part of the channel protein that can occlude the pore or move out of the way (Fig. 5.3A), or a global conformational change in the protein (Fig. 5.3B). Both mechanisms probably occur.

The observed random opening and closing of channels are precisely what would be expected when a chemical reaction is viewed one molecule at a time (Fig. 5.4). The simplest possible reaction scheme, the closed-open (C–O)

model, with first-order transitions linking closed and open states, predicts that the channel will be open a particular fraction of the time, depending on the equilibrium constant for the reaction. The average amount of time that the channel stays in the closed state depends on the rate constant for the C → O reaction. The closed times are highly variable, because the channel must "wait" until thermal energy "pushes" it over the barrier linking the two states. Random does not mean causal, however. Although the duration of any individual closing event is unpredictable, the average behavior of the channel is determined by the rate constants in the kinetic scheme. Real ion channels can exist in considerably more than two states, but the simple two-state C–O model is the starting point for discussion of channel kinetics.

Although useful information can be obtained by recording channel behavior under fixed conditions, the response of channels to changes in conditions allows signaling in the nervous system. Two main factors affect the rates of channel opening and closing: binding of ligands (e.g., neurotransmitters) and voltage. *Ligand-gated channels* and *voltage-dependent channels* are functionally and molecularly distinct. The simplest scheme for a ligand-gated channel is a bimolecular binding reaction (Fig. 5.5), in which binding and channel opening are considered to be a single step. This model makes firm predictions: the channel never opens in the absence of ligand, and the channel's opening rate increases linearly with the ligand concentration. The channel's mean closed time (for this scheme, the reciprocal of the opening rate) decreases with concentration, and its mean open time does not depend on concentration. As the concentration of ligand increases, the time that the channel has to wait before a ligand binds decreases, enhancing the probability that the channel is open. At very high concentrations, channel closings are extremely brief. These predictions can be tested experimentally. If the tests fail, more states are added to the model, with the ultimate goal being to gain physical insight into the mechanism of channel activation.

Why ion channel gating would depend on voltage is less obvious. Typical membrane potentials are a few tens of

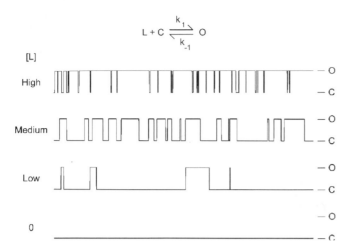

Figure 5.5 Simulation of a ligand-gated channel exhibiting two-state (C–O) gating. The channel-opening step is a bimolecular reaction between the ligand (e.g., neurotransmitter) and the channel. The probability that the channel is open increases with concentration, because the pseudo–first-order rate constant for channel opening (k_1) is proportional to the ligand concentration.

millivolts, but the voltage drop occurs across the extremely thin lipid bilayer. A 70-mV voltage for a 7-nm-thick membrane produces an electrical field of 10^7 V/m, nearly enough to electrolytically break down even as good a capacitor as a lipid bilayer. The electrical forces on any charged groups in a membrane protein are extremely strong if those charges are in the membrane's electrical field. That suggests a simple mechanism for voltage dependence. If the closed and open states of a channel differ in their distribution of charge across the membrane (Fig. 5.3B), the equilibrium between the two states will depend on voltage. Only a small number of charges have to move to change the open probability of a channel from near 0 to near 1 over the physiologic range of membrane potentials.

When the voltage changes, voltage-dependent channels do not instantly change from one state to another. Consider the two-state C–O channel (Fig. 5.6A). Suppose that at a negative voltage the rate constants are such that the channel spends 99% of its time closed. For the numbers given, on average, the channel would remain closed for 1 second, and then open for 10 milliseconds before closing again. Suppose that at a more positive voltage the rate constant for channel opening increases and that for closing decreases by 100-fold (for a voltage-dependent channel, both opening and closing rates usually change). The channel will spend 99% of its time open at equilibrium. If the voltage is changed instantly from negative to positive, the rate constants will change instantly, but the channel will require some time to open, as determined by the "new" rate constant. Figure 5.6A illustrates a simulated voltage clamp experiment in which a patch containing a single channel is repeatedly depolarized. At the negative voltage, the channel is nearly always closed at equilibrium. On depolarization, the channel waits a random time (mean, 10 milliseconds)

before accumulating enough energy to navigate the barrier to the open state. At equilibrium, the channel is nearly always open at the depolarized voltage. If the experiment is repeated many times, or if an analogous voltage clamp experiment is done on all of the cell's channels, an exponential relaxation from a p(open) of 0.01 to 0.99 will result, with a time constant of 10 milliseconds. This is a first approximation to the behavior of a voltage-dependent K^+ channel of the type involved in the action potential. The rates of channel opening and closing depend on the

A

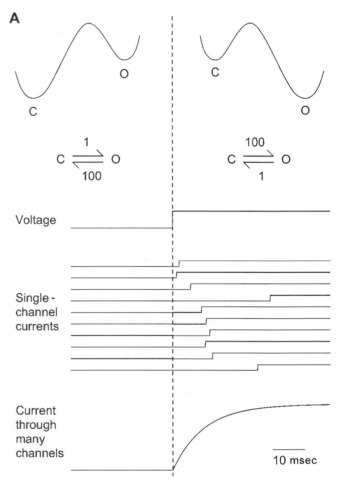

Figure 5.6 Simulation of channel gating for simplified K^+ and Na^+ channels. **A:** Response of a two-state K^+ channel to depolarization. The rate constants favor the closed state at negative voltages and the open state at depolarized voltages. The latency to first opening of a channel is the reciprocal of the opening rate constant (here, 10 milliseconds). The traces labeled *single-channel currents* show 10 simulated responses of a channel to depolarization; the *current through many channels* shows the predictable macroscopic behavior of a cell containing many thousands of channels. **B:** Response of a three-state Na^+ channel to depolarization. All the voltage dependence of the channel is assumed to be in the opening and closing rates. For such a model, the apparent voltage dependence of inactivation comes from kinetic coupling between the activation and inactivation steps. This adequately describes the channel's response to depolarization but not the recovery from inactivation. For these parameters, the channels usually open only once during a brief depolarization and occasionally fail to open at all, because there is a small probability that the channel will be inactivated (*I*) at the hyperpolarized holding potential.

B

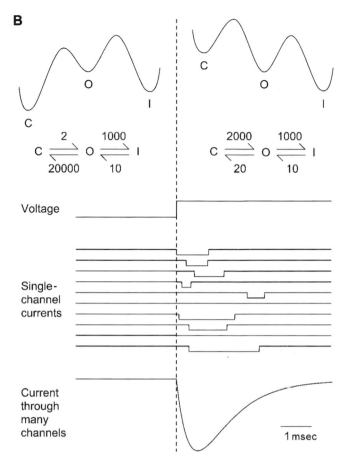

Voltage

Single-channel currents

Current through many channels

1 msec

Figure 5.6   (Continued)

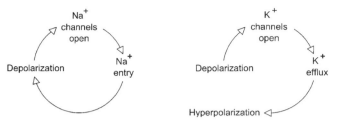

Figure 5.7   Positive and negative feedback resulting from opening of voltage-dependent channels. If enough Na$^+$ channels open to produce net inward current (i.e., more inward Na$^+$ current than outward K$^+$ current), the resulting depolarization will open even more Na$^+$ channels, and an action potential will result. In contrast, K$^+$ channel opening hyperpolarizes a cell.

height of the energy barriers at each voltage. The absolute rates vary widely among channel types.

The gating of a voltage-dependent Na$^+$ channel differs in two crucial ways from that of a K$^+$ channel. First, although it also opens on depolarization, the rate constant for opening is approximately 10-fold faster than for the K$^+$ channel. Second, during a maintained depolarization, the Na$^+$ channel does not remain open. Because this cannot be explained by the C–O model, at minimum, a third inactivated (I) state must be added to the kinetic scheme (Fig. 5.6B). That state is also closed in the sense that no ions go through the channel, but the closed and inactivated states are distinct conformational states of the channel protein.

The next step is to explain how channel opening and closing result in electrical signals. A discussion of the mechanism of the action potential follows.

Action Potential

When a cell with Na$^+$ and K$^+$ channels is depolarized, both types of channels open, but Na$^+$ channels open more rapidly. The influx of Na$^+$, net inward movement of positive charge, makes the interior of the cell more positive than before; it depolarizes the cell. The depolarization

opens more Na$^+$ channels, giving more Na$^+$ entry and causing more depolarization (Fig. 5.7). This positive feedback cycle initiates the action potential and is responsible for its all-or-none character. If the cell has sufficient Na$^+$ channels, the current generated greatly exceeds the stimulus necessary to trigger the action potential. Once initiated, the action potential is independent of the stimulus.

Termination of the action potential, called *repolarization*, involves two simultaneous processes. Na$^+$ channels inactivate, and K$^+$ channels open. Opening of K$^+$ channels provides negative feedback (Fig. 5.7); efflux of K$^+$ from the cell makes the inside more negative, which tends to close K$^+$ channels. The negative feedback contributes to repolarization.

The resting K$^+$ conductance of the membrane stabilizes the resting potential. Very small depolarizations do not trigger an action potential. They do not open a large number of Na$^+$ channels but increase the driving force on K$^+$ (because a depolarized membrane is further from E_K) and decrease the driving force on Na$^+$. The net effect of a small depolarization is to increase K$^+$ efflux, which leads to hyperpolarization. A sharp boundary, the threshold, exists between small depolarizations that produce only a subthreshold response and slightly larger depolarizations that trigger a full-sized action potential. *Threshold* is the point at which inward Na$^+$ current exceeds outward K$^+$ current; the net inward current produces an active depolarization, which initiates further Na$^+$ channel opening and the rest of the positive feedback cycle.

The kinetic differences between voltage-dependent Na$^+$ and K$^+$ channels are crucial to the action potential. During repolarization, K$^+$ channel opening and Na$^+$ channel inactivation cooperate. Because K$^+$ channels also close slowly, the K$^+$ conductance of the membrane immediately after repolarization is higher than at rest. The membrane potential is very close to E_K, producing an afterhyperpolarization (AHP).

Hodgkin-Huxley Experiments and Model

Our detailed understanding of the mechanism of the action potential is based on the classic experiments of Hodgkin and Huxley on the giant axon of the squid (1). Current views of the mechanisms of channel gating owe much to the kinetic models they proposed in 1952. That is remarkable, given that the structure of biologic membranes was then poorly understood. Although lipids and proteins were known to be involved, the idea of transmembrane proteins was yet to come. Nevertheless, their descriptions of "permeability changes" can be translated directly into the opening and closing of ion channels. As discussed later, contemporary views of channel gating differ from these original models, but the similarities are impressive.

The Hodgkin-Huxley experimental protocols are the foundation for analysis of ion channel gating to this day. Their basic experiment was to give step changes in voltage (Fig. 5.6). That makes perfect sense now: if a channel is voltage dependent, the first step toward understanding it is to control the relevant variable, the membrane potential. They first defined two kinetically distinct and independent pathways for ion movement, which we now interpret as Na^+ and K^+ channels. Ion substitutions played a major role in their separation of Na^+ and K^+ currents. For example, Hodgkin and Huxley demonstrated that the Na^+ current reversed from an inward flow of Na^+ to an outward current when the axon was depolarized beyond the expected E_{Na}. That "reversal potential" shifted, as predicted by the Nernst equation, when E_{Na} was changed by replacing some of the extracellular Na^+ with an impermeant cation. The reversal potential remains the primary criterion for determining ion channel selectivity. Hodgkin and Huxley also characterized the kinetics of channel opening and closing over the physiologic voltage range. They discovered that Na^+ channels inactivate and described the voltage dependence of that process.

Figure 5.8 summarizes much of their experimental data. Because conductance is roughly proportional to the probability that a channel is open, their data on Na^+ and K^+ conductance as a function of voltage and time reflect the kinetics of channel gating. In some ways, the K^+ and Na^+

conductances behaved as expected from the previously discussed C–O and C–O–I models (Fig. 5.6), but there were complications. In particular, the time course of activation of the currents was not exponential but showed a sigmoid delay, necessitating more complex kinetic models. No general strategy was available to translate data into a model, and computational limitations encouraged keeping the models as simple as possible.

Hodgkin and Huxley modeled Na^+ and K^+ channels as containing four independent gates (1). Each gate behaves kinetically like a C–O channel, but the channel is assumed to be open if and only if all four gates are open simultaneously. The K^+ channel model is simpler because it is assumed that the four gates are identical. The assumption that the gates are independent simplifies matters, because independent probabilities multiply. If the probability that one gate is open is n, then the probability that a channel is open is n^4. The requirement for all four gates to open produces the sigmoid delay in the time course of activation of the K^+ channel (Fig. 5.8).

To explain Na^+ inactivation, Hodgkin and Huxley assumed that one of the four Na^+ channel gates is an inactivation gate, with a reverse voltage dependence; it is open at negative voltages and closes at depolarized voltages. The three activation gates open on depolarization, more rapidly than the gates controlling a K^+ channel. In their equations, m is the probability that a Na^+ activation gate is open and h the probability that the inactivation gate is open, so that the probability that a Na^+ channel is open is m^3h. The Hodgkin-Huxley model included empirical equations for the voltage dependence of the rate constants for each gate's opening and closing. That allowed calculation of m, h, and n (and from them, the probabilities that Na^+ and K^+ channels are open) as functions of voltage and time. Their model reproduced the experimental data obtained under voltage clamp conditions and generated an action potential when the membrane voltage was not controlled. Like a real action potential, the computed action potential had a threshold, the ability to propagate, and a refractory period.

CONTEMPORARY WORK ON VOLTAGE-DEPENDENT ION CHANNELS

Since 1952, we have relearned something that Hodgkin and Huxley recognized, that different neurons can have dramatically different patterns of electrical excitability. One striking example is in leech sensory neurons (2). Three types of cells—called T, P, and N—can be identified from animal to animal on the basis of their anatomy and receptive field properties. They can also be distinguished by the shape of their action potentials. Their responses to a maintained depolarization differ systematically; for example, the N (nociceptive) cells have higher thresholds and less of a tendency to fire repetitively. These differences presumably stem from the numbers and types of ion channels

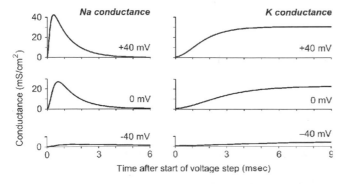

Figure 5.8 The time course for opening of Na^+ and K^+ channels, as calculated from the Hodgkin-Huxley model (1). The conductance is proportional to the number of channels open and is expressed (per cm^2 of membrane) in units of Siemens (S), or reciprocal ohms (Ω^{-1}). Notice that stronger depolarization activates more Na^+ and K^+ channels and that the channels open more rapidly.

expressed in each cell. Similar differences exist among cell types in the mammalian central nervous system. Although the methods and concepts of Hodgkin-Huxley remain relevant, it is incorrect to use the precise formulations of their models to describe electrical activity in other cell types.

The intrinsic electrical properties of neurons make major contributions to their characteristic patterns of electrical activity. Neurons need not passively await synaptic inputs but can generate spontaneous activity and shape the response to inputs from other cells. The diversity of neuronal electrical phenotypes is based on the selective expression of a subset of the many known ion channels. Instead of two active channel types (as in the Hodgkin-Huxley model for the squid axon), a typical neuron contains a dozen or more voltage-dependent channels.

Identification of Ion Channels

The diversity of electrical activity patterns is matched or exceeded by the diversity of ion channel types (3). Channels were initially distinguished electrophysiologically at the level of whole-cell currents or single-channel gating, but it is now evident that considerable molecular diversity exists among voltage-dependent ion channels. Major goals today are to correlate the different ion channel types identified by physiologic and molecular techniques and to determine how their functions relate to their structures. Ion channels are classified by ion selectivity, kinetics of channel gating, pharmacology, and molecular characteristics.

Ion Selectivity

Perhaps the most fundamental distinction among channels is their ion selectivity. The physical properties of a channel determine which ions flow through its pore. Ion selectivity is determined by measuring the reversal potential (i.e., the voltage at which no current flows through an open channel) and any shifts in reversal potential when ion concentrations are changed.

Kinetics

Channel types vary in their response to voltage, raising several questions. At what voltages does the channel activate? How rapid is activation in response to voltage changes? How rapid is deactivation on return to a voltage at which the channel is normally closed? How rapid are inactivation and recovery from inactivation? How do the speeds of activation, deactivation, and inactivation vary with voltage? Is the time course of the current exponential, sigmoid, or something else?

Pharmacology

Drugs and toxins have been extremely valuable in channel characterization. Familiar examples are channel blockers, such as tetrodotoxin (TTX) for Na^+ channels and tetraethylammonium (TEA) for K^+ channels. Nevertheless, some Na^+ channels (especially in the heart and in peripheral neurons) are TTX resistant, and the sensitivity of K^+ channels to TEA varies widely. Moreover, TEA can block certain chloride channels (4,5) and ganglionic nicotinic acetylcholine receptors. At high concentrations, TEA and choline are muscarinic antagonists (6). Pharmacologic criteria rarely define a channel type convincingly, but in combination with kinetic approaches, they can be powerful. Hodgkin and Huxley rigorously distinguished Na^+ and K^+ currents by ion selectivity and kinetics and without the use of TTX or TEA (1). Initial interpretation of the effects of TTX and TEA relied on the knowledge that Na^+ and K^+ channels were distinct.

Molecular Biology

Several molecular differences are possible between functionally different channel types: different gene products, subunit composition, alternative splicing, and posttranslational modifications such as phosphorylation.

Channel Structure

Information is available on the amino acid sequence, higher-order structure, and transmembrane topology of numerous channels (Fig. 5.9). Difficulties in obtaining structural data on membrane proteins have prevented atomic-level resolution of the structure of most channels. One spectacular exception is the crystal structures of bacterial K^+ channels (7–9). Those channels are members of a large superfamily of channel proteins with deep evolutionary roots (3,10) that has diverged to produce voltage-dependent

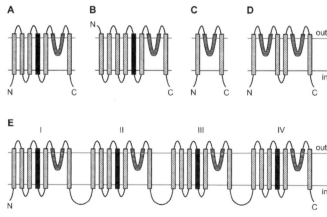

Figure 5.9 The proposed transmembrane architecture of the main (α) subunits of voltage-dependent channels. **A:** Kv, Eag, KCNQ, and SK K^+ channels. **B:** Slo (high-conductance Ca^{2+}-dependent K^+) channels. Notice the additional "S0" transmembrane region and extracellular N terminus. **C:** Inward-rectifier K^+ channels. **D:** K^+ channels with two P domains. **E:** A Na^+ or Ca^{2+} channel $α_1$ subunit, which resembles four Kv channels spliced together. Regions of known functional importance include the P loop (*vertical hatching*), which forms the outer portion of the channel pore, including the selectivity filter; the S4 voltage sensors (*solid bars*); and the N terminus, which forms a "ball" that can inactivate some Kv channels by occluding the pore. The cytoplasmic and extracellular regions vary in length.

K^+, Na^+, and Ca^{2+} channels, among others. The bacterial K^+ channels share a P loop with voltage-dependent channels, which forms the selectivity filter near the extracellular side of the pore. The structures are likely to be applicable to many other channel types and have implications for mechanisms of permeation (11) and gating (12,13). Unfortunately, the crystal structure of a bacterial voltage-dependent K^+ channel (14) places the voltage sensor in a location that seems inconsistent with a variety of functional data (15,16), so a molecular understanding of voltage-dependent gating remains a goal for the future.

Potassium Channels

K^+ channels are remarkably diverse. Physiologically, perhaps a dozen kinetically or pharmacologically distinct types are known, and more than 70 genes produce K^+ channels when expressed *in vitro* (17,18) (Table 5.1). To some extent, this makes sense, because K^+ channels perform a variety of physiologic functions. They set the resting potential, repolarize the action potential, affect the threshold for generation of the action potential, and regulate a cell's ability to fire repetitively. K^+ channels can sense metabolic activity by way of Ca^{2+} or adenosine triphosphate (ATP). K^+ channels can be modulated, often through G-protein–coupled receptors for hormones and neurotransmitters, by direct interaction with G-protein subunits or by phosphorylation (19,20).

Delayed Rectifiers

Many K^+ channels activate within milliseconds on depolarization and inactivate within hundreds of milliseconds or seconds. These channels, which resemble the K^+ channel of the squid axon, are often called *delayed rectifiers*, because the time course of activation typically has a sigmoid delay (Fig. 5.8). Ubiquitous in neurons, delayed rectifiers repolarize the action potential and contribute to the fast AHP after repolarization of an action potential. Hippocampal neurons have an I_D current that resembles the delayed rectifier but inactivates somewhat more strongly even at the resting potential (17). Some delayed rectifiers inactivate rapidly in response to repetitive-action-potential–like depolarizations, instead of the maintained depolarizations typically used in experimental models (21,22).

A large family of genes produces delayed-rectifier K^+ channels (but sometimes also A current) (18,23,24). The channels contain four α subunits (25) that can be identical, although heteromeric channels exist. Each subunit (Fig. 5.9A) includes six predicted transmembrane regions, S1 through S6, plus a P region between S5 and S6 that contributes much of the ion permeation pathway (26–28). The S4 region contains mostly hydrophobic amino acids, as expected for a transmembrane domain, but every third position can contain a positively charged amino acid (arginine or lysine), for a total of five to seven charges per subunit. This structure suggests that S4 is involved in voltage sensing, moving outwardly on depolarization (29,30). Activation of a K^+ channel is associated with movement of 12 to 16 positive charges (31,32); three to four charges per subunit move all the way across the cell plasma membrane. The structural basis of S4 movement remains controversial (14–16).

Four distinct but related gene families produce delayed-rectifier K^+ channels (Kv), with two to eight known members per family (3,24). The genes for channels Kv1 through Kv4 (designated *KCNA*, *KCNB*, *KCNC*, and *KCND*) correspond

TABLE 5.1

TYPES OF VOLTAGE-DEPENDENT CATION CHANNELS

	Channel Name	Number of Genes[a]	Physiologically Defined Currents
K^+	Kv	27	Neuronal delayed rectifier; A current
	KCNQ	5	M current; cardiac slow-delayed rectifier
	Eag	8	Cardiac fast-delayed rectifier
	SK	4	Ca^{2+}-dependent; low conductance
	Slo	4	Ca^{2+}- and voltage-dependent; high conductance
	Kir	15	Inward rectifiers; G-protein–activated; ATP-dependent
	2P	15	Leakage (resting potential)
Na^+	TTX-sensitive	6	Neurons, adult skeletal muscle, glia
	TTX-resistant	4	Cardiac muscle, some sensory neurons
Ca^{2+}	S, C, D, F	4	L-type (high-voltage–activated; Ca_V1)
	A, B, E	3	N, P, Q, R-types (high-voltage–activated; Ca_V2)
	G, H, I	3	T-type (low-voltage–activated; Ca_V3)
Cation	Pacemaker	4	Cardiac muscle, some neurons
	CNG	6	Cyclic nucleotide-gated
	Trp	20	Capacitative Ca^{2+} entry; capsaicin receptor; etc.

ATP, adenosine triphosphate.
[a]2004 values for the human genome. Most channels have been cloned, but surprises are always possible.

to the *Shaker, Shab, Shaw,* and *Shal* genes of the fruit fly *Drosophila.* For example, the gene for Kv1.1 (*KCNA1*) is a member of the K$^+$ channel family that is most closely related to the *Shaker* gene. The Kv5 (*KCNF*), Kv6 (*KCNG1*), Kv8 (*KCNB3*), and Kv9 (*KCNS*) gene families do not produce K$^+$ channels when expressed alone, but do modify the properties of other Kv channels (22,33–36). The Kv channel classification (23) is now widely accepted, but trivial names abound in earlier papers.

A Current

Also called transient outward current, the A current is a K$^+$ current that inactivates fairly rapidly (time constant, 10 to 100 milliseconds). In many cells, A channels are activated at somewhat more negative voltages than are delayed rectifiers, but a substantial fraction may be inactivated at the normal resting potential. The A current may be involved in low-frequency repetitive firing (37). An AHP can remove inactivation from the A current, and the channels then open as the AHP decays. The A current eventually inactivates, however, allowing the cell to fire the next action potential. Because it activates rapidly on depolarization, the A current can repolarize the action potential in cells where it is available at the resting potential (17). The A current is also important for the electrical activity of dendrites (38).

The first K$^+$ channel to be cloned was an A channel from *Drosophila,* whose *Shaker* mutant has a defect in the structural gene for a K$^+$ channel (39,40). Several channels can be produced from the *Drosophila Shaker* locus by alternative splicing, differing mainly in the N- and C-terminal regions outside the core that specifies the transmembrane regions (S1 through S6). The channels have surprisingly diverse kinetics, ranging from rapidly inactivating A currents to delayed-rectifier–like slow inactivation. Rapid inactivation can be removed by deletion of the N-terminal region and can be restored by addition of a synthetic peptide with the N-terminal sequence. This N-type inactivation is believed to occur by a ball and chain mechanism, in which the N-terminal "ball" (attached to the rest of the protein by a flexible "chain") plugs the channel's inner mouth (41–43).

Most mammalian *Shaker*-related K$^+$ channels are delayed rectifiers, but a few have rapid A-current–like inactivation. An accessory β subunit has been identified that confers rapid inactivation on channels that would otherwise inactivate only slowly. Inactivation mediated by the β subunit seems to occur by the ball-and-chain mechanism (44). Two lessons from the molecular biology of *Shaker*-related K$^+$ channels are that closely related gene products can have very different kinetic properties, but distantly related genes can produce similar K$^+$ currents. This complicates correlations between physiologic and molecular K$^+$ channel classifications.

Eag and Related K$^+$ Channels

The *Drosophila Eag* (*ether-à-go-go*) locus encodes a K$^+$ channel, and mammalian homologues have been discovered

(45). *Eag*-encoded channels contain S1 through S6 and P regions distantly related to those of the Kv channels and a long C-terminal region. The C-terminal region has some resemblance to cyclic nucleotide-gated channels, which are involved in retinal and olfactory signal transduction. The kinetics resemble those of neuronal delayed rectifiers in some respects, but one related channel, HERG, has an unusually rapid inactivation process that causes it to pass only small outward currents (46). HERG is responsible for a fast component ($I_{K,r}$) of the cardiac "delayed rectifier" (47).

M Current and Slow, Delayed Rectifiers

The M current was originally identified as a potassium current activated by slow, weak depolarizations in sympathetic neurons (48). Similar currents are present in many brain neurons, including hippocampal pyramidal cells (49). The M current limits repetitive firing during maintained depolarization (50), because it is activated in the critical region between the resting potential and threshold for generation of an action potential (half-maximal activation near −40 mV, τ about 100 milliseconds). It was named the M current because it is inhibited by activation of muscarinic receptors on sympathetic neurons, allowing those normally phasically firing neurons to fire in a more sustained manner (48). Its molecular basis is a gene family distantly related to those for the Kv channels but with the same transmembrane architecture (51).

Cardiac cells contain a K$^+$ current that activates extremely slowly on depolarization, with activation incomplete even after many seconds ($I_{K,s}$). It results from coexpression of an M-like channel (52) together with a completely different protein that contains a single transmembrane domain (53).

Ca^{2+}-Dependent K$^+$ Channels

One class of K$^+$ channel is activated synergistically by binding of intracellular Ca^{2+} and by depolarization (54). Increases in [Ca^{2+}]$_i$ allow the channel to activate at more negative voltages; strong depolarization allows activation at relatively low [Ca^{2+}]$_i$ (55–58). The source of Ca^{2+} is often Ca^{2+} entry through voltage-dependent Ca^{2+} channels. Ca^{2+} channels can be colocalized with Ca^{2+}-dependent K$^+$ channels, which sense the relatively high [Ca^{2+}]$_i$ transiently present near the cell membrane rather than bulk cytoplasmic [Ca^{2+}]$_i$ (59). In some neurons, Ca^{2+}-dependent K$^+$ channels can activate fast enough to repolarize the action potential and contribute to the fast AHP (17,60). This channel has an unusually high single-channel conductance of 100 to 250 pS (61), compared with 5 to 30 pS for Kv family K$^+$ channels.

Ca^{2+}-dependent K$^+$ channels with similar properties have been cloned from *Drosophila* (the *Slowpoke,* or *slo,* mutant) and mammalian sources (62,63). They share the S1 to S6 transmembrane architecture with the Kv family of K$^+$ channels, plus an additional S0 domain (Fig. 5.9B) (64), and they are homologous but distantly related. The C-terminal region of *slo* channels is much longer than that of Kv channels and may contain the Ca^{2+} binding site (65). Among the β subunits is one that induces rapid inactivation (66).

A second class of Ca^{2+}-dependent K^+ channels is not voltage dependent and is activated by modest increases in $[Ca^{2+}]_i$ (67). After a brief pulse of Ca^{2+} entry, this channel turns off slowly (hundreds of milliseconds to seconds), reflecting the return of bulk $[Ca^{2+}]_i$ to normal and intrinsically slow channel closing (68). These channels are responsible for slow AHPs in many neurons (69–72). They have a relatively low single-channel conductance (67) and are encoded by yet another family of genes distantly related to Kv channels (73) (Fig. 5.9A).

Inward Rectifier K⁺ Channels

Several unusual physiologic and molecular properties mark this class (74–76). These channels pass only small outward currents under physiologic conditions but produce large inward currents at voltages negative to E_K, hence the designation *inward rectifier*. That was surprising because the higher $[K^+]$ inside the cell should make it easier for a K^+ channel to pass outward current than inward current (for a given amount of driving force), and such outward rectification is observed for most other K^+ channels. With the explanation for inward rectification long elusive, the leading suggestions were gating (i.e., channel closing or inactivation on depolarization) and permeation (i.e., asymmetric pore structure). The primary cause appears to be blockade of inward rectifier channels by Mg^{2+} (77) and polyamines, probably spermine or spermidine (78,79), that bind in a voltage-dependent manner, with stronger blocking at more depolarized voltages. This suggests that the binding site is within the membrane's electrical field, presumably within the normal permeation pathway for K^+.

Despite their name, the physiologic role of inward rectifiers is to pass outward current, as for any K^+ channel. Because the membrane potential is rarely negative to E_K under physiologic conditions, any net K^+ flux through an open K^+ channel must be outward. Inward rectifiers pass some amount of outward current at the cell's resting potential, but depolarization reduces the current amplitude because blockade by Mg^{2+} or polyamines increases. That property allows inward rectifiers to contribute significantly to the resting K^+ conductance, but they are essentially inactive during depolarizations (e.g., action potentials). As a result, the ion flux during the action potential is reduced because the inward current need not continually fight the resting K^+ current to maintain the depolarization. That is particularly important during long action potentials, as in the heart. Inward rectifiers are major contributors to the resting potential of skeletal and cardiac muscle and are also present in some neurons (80,81).

Cloned inward-rectifier channels exhibit distant homology to "standard" K^+ channels in the S5 to S6 region, especially in the P loop, but lack the S1 through S4 transmembrane regions entirely (74,75) (Fig. 5.9C), which explains the lack of activation by depolarization. A region weakly resembling S4 is present but, on hydrophobicity analysis, is not transmembrane. A relatively large C-terminal region may contribute to the pore (82) and contains other functional domains. At least 15 different inward rectifiers have been cloned. In addition to the classic inward rectifier of muscle, this channel family includes G-protein–activated K^+ channels (responsible for many slow inhibitory synaptic potentials) and ATP-regulated K^+ channels. The inward rectification is weaker for the ATP-regulated channels, mainly as the result of a single amino acid in the second transmembrane region (i.e., equivalent to S6 in other K^+ channels) (83,84). Crystal structures are known for a bacterial inward rectifier (85) and for the cytoplasmic domain of a mammalian inward rectifier (82).

Resting Leakage Current

The dependence of the resting potential of neurons on selective permeability to K^+ has been known for more than a half century, but the molecular nature of the underlying channels is poorly understood. Inward rectifiers (and possibly M current) can contribute to the resting potential in some cells, but often a voltage-independent K^+-selective current is active around the resting potential (17,86). The current is small compared with the voltage-dependent currents in other voltage ranges and difficult to separate from artifactual leakage produced by cell damage. One molecular basis of resting K^+ conductance is a family of channels with two P regions, each flanked by transmembrane domains that resemble two inward rectifiers in tandem (87–90) (Fig. 5.9D).

Sodium Channels

Considerably less molecular and functional diversity exists among voltage-dependent Na^+ than K^+ channels. Presumably, the primary function of Na^+ channels is to generate the action potential, and diversity in threshold and ability to fire repetitively results mainly from the diversity of K^+ channels. Separate genes have been identified for Na^+ channels of adult skeletal and cardiac muscle, with several closely related genes known from brain (91–94). Cardiac muscle, denervated skeletal muscle, and some peripheral neurons contain a TTX-resistant Na^+ current (95) whose activation and inactivation kinetics are qualitatively similar to those of the TTX-sensitive Na^+ currents that dominate in brain neurons.

The main subunit of Na^+ channels is a large protein with four homologous domains, each resembling one Kv-type subunit (Fig. 5.9E), consistent with the tetrameric structure of K^+ channels. There is some sequence conservation between K^+ and Na^+ channels, especially in regions S1 through S6. Na^+ channels also have a P region in each of the four domains, with little similarity to K^+ channels. Mutations in the predicted extracellular portion of P can strongly affect TTX binding (96). Mutations in the linker between domains III and IV can dramatically slow inactivation, suggesting that the region acts analogously to the ball and chain of an inactivating K^+ channel (97).

In addition to the classic Na^+ channel, which rapidly activates and inactivates on strong depolarization, several reports have described non-inactivating Na^+ currents, often active near the resting potential (98,99), that may reflect novel Na^+ channel types or possibly "window currents." At weakly depolarized voltages, some normal Na^+ channels are activated, but incomplete inactivation allows a steady-state Na^+ current. Non-inactivating (or slowly inactivating) TTX-resistant Na^+ currents have also been reported (100), but they may be carried through K^+ channels that become nonselective in the absence of K^+ ions (101,102).

Calcium Channels

"Without Ca^{2+} channels, our nervous system would have no outputs" (3). Hille's statement emphasizes the vital role of voltage-dependent Ca^{2+} channels in neurotransmitter release. Ca^{2+} channels play electrical and metabolic roles in excitable cells. The inward current through Ca^{2+} channels can depolarize a cell, and action potentials can result from voltage-dependent opening of Ca^{2+} channels, as for Na^+. In neurons, however, the electrical role of Ca^{2+} channels is usually secondary. Influx of a relatively small amount of Ca^{2+} can raise $[Ca^{2+}]_i$ from the normal value of 10^{-7} M to nearly 10^{-6} M. $[Ca^{2+}]_i$ near the membrane is transiently much higher, and $[Ca^{2+}]_i$ near the mouth of an open Ca^{2+} channel can approach millimolar levels (59,103). The change in $[Ca^{2+}]_i$ can then exert a variety of metabolic effects by regulating enzymes and ion channels.

Because of their diverse functional roles, the different types of Ca^{2+} channels have attracted considerable attention (104–111). The primary distinction is between rapidly inactivating channels that are activated by relatively weak depolarization (low-voltage–activated [LVA] channels) and more slowly inactivating channels that require strong depolarization (high-voltage–activated [HVA] channels). LVA channels are thought to be involved in low-threshold spikes and pacemaker activity, whereas HVA channels are responsible for neurotransmitter release and most other Ca^{2+} channel functions.

Some technical problems should be kept in mind when data on Ca^{2+} channels are being reviewed. In whole-cell recording, neuronal Ca^{2+} currents generally are much smaller than Na^+ and K^+ currents, and rather nonphysiologic conditions are used to isolate Ca^{2+} currents: blocking Na^+ and K^+ channels, "starving" them of permeant ions, or both. Ba^{2+} often is used as the charge carrier instead of Ca^{2+} for several reasons. Currents carried by Ba^{2+} are larger than with Ca^{2+} (at least for HVA channels); Ba^{2+} blocks some potassium channels; and intracellular Ba^{2+} activates Ca^{2+}-dependent intracellular processes, such as Ca^{2+}-dependent currents, weakly or not at all. At the single-channel level, small current amplitudes and rapid gating make channel

behavior difficult to resolve except when approximately 100 mmol/L of Ba^{2+} is the charge carrier. As a result, comparison of single-channel with whole-cell data and extrapolation to physiologic conditions are difficult. Consider also shifts in surface potential. Channels appear to sense a negative surface charge—resulting from negative charges on phospholipids or the channel protein itself—that affects the electrical field in the immediate vicinity of the channel's voltage sensors. High concentrations of divalent cations effectively neutralize that surface charge by nonspecific screening and by binding to the negative charges. Ca^{2+} generally produces larger changes in surface potential than does Ba^{2+}, presumably reflecting stronger binding of Ca^{2+} to surface charges. Nevertheless, changes in Ba^{2+} can cause surface potential shifts greater than 30 mV from typical whole-cell conditions (2 mmol/L Ba^{2+}) to typical single-channel conditions (100 mmol/L Ba^{2+}) (112,113). Surface potential effects have been known for decades, but it has been recognized only recently how serious a problem they can be for interpretation of data on Ca^{2+} channels. Even classification of a channel as LVA or HVA requires evaluation of surface potentials.

High-Voltage–Activated Calcium Channels: L Current

The first calcium channel type to be well characterized for vertebrate cells has a "large" single-channel current and is sensitive to dihydropyridines (DHPs). DHP antagonists block the current, binding with higher affinity to open and/or inactivated states than to closed states, whereas the chemically similar DHP agonists favor channel opening. L channels normally open for about 1 millisecond or less, so induction of long openings by DHP agonists is a diagnostic test (114). L channels are the dominant type in muscle and are present also in neurons.

Two fundamentally different mechanisms account for inactivation of L channels (115). In cardiac and smooth muscle, rapid (about 20 milliseconds) Ca^{2+}-dependent inactivation results from local accumulation of Ca^{2+} in the immediate vicinity of the Ca^{2+} channel (116). Ca^{2+}-dependent inactivation involves calmodulin, which is bound to a cytoplasmic domain of the L channel (117–119). Ca^{2+}-dependent inactivation of neuronal L current can either be rapid (120,121) or slow, consequent to accumulation of bulk cytoplasmic Ca^{2+} (122). This may result from different L channel subtypes (123,124) or from differences in Ca^{2+} metabolism among cells. With Ba^{2+} as the charge carrier, inactivation is slower—approximately 300 milliseconds in muscle and virtually nil in some neurons. Inactivation with Ba^{2+} is generally voltage (not current) dependent, and a similar slow voltage-dependent inactivation can be observed with Ca^{2+} (115,125).

As in Na^+ channels, the primary (α_1) subunit of L channels has four internally homologous domains, each containing the S1 to S6 transmembrane regions and a P region (110) (Fig. 5.9E). Ca^{2+} channels normally select for Ca^{2+} over monovalent cations not by molecular sieving but by high-affinity (1 μmol/L) binding of Ca^{2+} within the pore (126–128). If two Ca^{2+} ions are in the pore simultaneously, electrostatic repulsion lowers the affinity at least 1,000-fold, allowing rapid exit of Ca^{2+} from the pore and Ca^{2+} permeation. Each P region contains a negatively charged glutamate or aspartate, which is crucial to formation of high-affinity sites (129). The α_1 subunit contains the DHP binding site. Additional subunits (α_2–δ, β, and γ) also can modulate channel function (130–133). Four α_1 genes produce DHP-sensitive L currents (104,109): α_{1S}, in skeletal muscle; α_{1C}, in cardiac muscle and neurons; α_{1D}, in neurons and endocrine cells, and α_{1F}, in the retina (134). Molecularly, α_{1D} is clearly a member of the family of HVA channels, but it activates at relatively negative voltages (135,136).

High-Voltage–Activated Calcium Channels: N Current

Soon after the distinction between HVA and LVA channels was made, it was proposed that two distinct HVA calcium channels, L and N, exist in neurons. The novel N channels were initially described as DHP resistant and rather rapidly inactivating (137). However, N channel inactivation is slow and incomplete in many cells (114,138,139). Inactivation of N current can change spontaneously for a single channel (140) and can be enhanced by phosphorylation (141). The β subunit strongly affects inactivation of N channels (142,143). Although N channels can undergo Ca^{2+}-dependent inactivation (144,145), in most cases voltage-dependent inactivation is the predominant mechanism (108,146).

Today, the defining characteristic of N channels is a combination of DHP resistance and high sensitivity to a peptide toxin isolated from predatory cone snails, ω-conotoxin GVIA (ωCgTx) (114). Activation kinetics between L and N channels differ subtly. Expression of one Ca^{2+} channel clone, α_{1B}, produces N-like currents with appropriate pharmacology and inactivation (147,148). However, some L currents and the α_{1D} clone are blocked weakly by ωCgTx (149). Biochemical studies have identified a receptor for ωCgTx (150).

Other High-Voltage–Activated Calcium Channels

While the distinction between L and N channels was being debated, some HVA current was found to be highly resistant to DHPs and ωCgTx (151). An extreme example was cerebellar Purkinje cells, in which virtually all HVA current was resistant. Toxins have helped to distinguish Purkinje cell-like "P" current from L and N currents. A peptide toxin from a spider, ωAgaIVA, blocks P current with high affinity, essentially complete blockade at 100 nmol/L (152). The voltage-dependent blockade permits little recovery except at extreme depolarized voltages (153). In several other cell types, a fraction of the HVA current is highly sensitive to ωAgaIVA, suggesting the presence of P channels (154).

The α_{1A} clone is expressed strongly in Purkinje cells, but in *Xenopus* oocytes it produces currents with only moderate sensitivity to ωAgaIVA. It also inactivates more rapidly than the cerebellar P current (155). Part of the HVA current in cerebellar granule cells resembles the α_{1A} channels in those respects. It has been proposed that the α_{1A} channel and the granule cell current represent a Q current that differs from P current by an approximately 10-fold higher affinity for another cone snail toxin, ω-conotoxin MVIIC (156,157). Much of this diversity, especially in inactivation rates and sensitivity to ωAgaIVA, may result from alternative splicing of α_{1A} (158). Many studies refer to a P/Q current.

A component of the HVA current, called R, is resistant to a combination of all blockers mentioned so far (159). The R current in cerebellar granule cells resembles channels expressed from the α_{1E} clone (157). Initial reports that α_{1E} encodes an LVA current (160–162) have not been generally accepted (163–166). Currents expressed from α_{1E} are more sensitive to Ni^{2+} than most other HVA currents, but unlike LVA currents, they are also blocked potently by Cd^{2+} (159). Some R currents have similar pharmacology and may activate at voltages intermediate between classic HVA and LVA currents (112,167).

Although there are multiple HVA currents beyond L and N, the separation into P, Q, and R should be considered a working hypothesis. First, it is based on the actions of drugs and toxins untested in a large number of cell types. Second, comparison of different experimental situations (e.g., naturally expressed channels in neurons versus cloned channels in oocytes) is complicated by the use of Ca^{2+} or Ba^{2+} at different concentrations, which affects surface potentials and the affinity of blockers (i.e., toxins and divalent cations). Third, not all HVA channels resistant to DHPs and toxins have identical properties. In particular, a toxin (SNX-482) that potently blocks α_{1E} channels expressed in *Xenopus* oocytes (168) has variable effects on R currents in native neurons (169–171).

High-Voltage–Activated Calcium Channels and Neurotransmitter Release

The N channel was initially thought to be specialized for mediation of rapid neurotransmitter release. It made sense that muscle contraction (involving L channels) and transmitter release might require Ca^{2+} channels with fundamentally different behaviors. It now seems likely that all pharmacologically defined classes of HVA Ca^{2+} channel, including L channels (172), can participate in neurotransmitter release (106). This belief is supported by the similarity in activation kinetics among HVA Ca^{2+} channels, all of which turn on rapidly enough to be partially activated by a single, brief neuronal action potential, with rapid closing at hyperpolarized voltages (173).

Why are there several kinds of HVA Ca^{2+} channels? First, there are far fewer than the number of K^+ channels and about the same number as Na^+ channels (Table 5.1). Second, the diversity of HVA Ca^{2+} channels may reflect a need for differential regulation, including expression and short-term regulation. In many cells, HVA currents are inhibited through G-protein–coupled receptors, a likely mechanism for presynaptic inhibition (20,174–176). That effect is not limited to one HVA channel type, but it can be selective. For example, in frog and rat sympathetic neurons, N current is inhibited with little or no effect on L current (114,177). P channels are also inhibited (178), as are some splice variants of R channels (179).

Low-Voltage–Activated Calcium Channels

Also called T channels for their tiny single-channel currents and transient kinetics, LVA channels inactivate more rapidly and at more negative voltages than other Ca^{2+} channels (137,180,181). In many cells, substantial inactivation of LVA channels occurs at the resting potential. Hyperpolarization (e.g., an AHP) can remove that inactivation. When LVA channels are available, weak depolarization can produce a low-threshold spike lasting several milliseconds that can trigger a burst of Na^+-dependent action potentials. LVA channels are central to burst generation and pacemaking in many neurons and may play a role in absence seizures (182–185).

LVA channels are also called slowly deactivating (SD) channels because, on repolarization, they close approximately 10 times more slowly than HVA channels (181). Unlike HVA channels, LVA channels show little difference in current amplitudes between Ca^{2+} and Ba^{2+} (182). Three α_1 subunits (α_{1G}, α_{1H}, and α_{1I}) produce LVA currents in *Xenopus* oocytes or mammalian cell lines (186–188). These LVA channels are differentially expressed in the nervous system and elsewhere (189). This molecular diversity may explain some subtle differences among LVA currents recorded from different cells (190,191). High sensitivity to blockade by Ni^{2+} (192) is observed for α_{1H} but not for α_{1G} or α_{1I} (193). The slowly inactivating LVA currents of thalamoreticular neurons (194) may result from expression of α_{1I} (188).

Gating of Voltage-Dependent Channels: Models and Mechanisms

Physiologic and molecular studies (32,195–200) have extended and, to some extent, transformed the concepts of channel gating based on the Hodgkin-Huxley (1) model. Two new principles are considered here. First, Na^+ channel inactivation is not independent (as assumed by the m^3h formulation) but is coupled to activation (201,202). Second, channel opening may be a concerted process involving all four subunits (or all four domains for a Na^+ or Ca^{2+} channel), distinct from voltage sensing itself (57,190,203–205).

Na+ Channel Inactivation

Two possibilities have been proposed to explain how inactivation of a Na^+ channel could be related to activation: the two processes are controlled by independently acting gates, as in the Hodgkin-Huxley model; or inactivation requires prior activation, as in the C–O–I model (Fig. 5.6B). In the second scheme, activation and inactivation are linked, because the channel must open before it can inactivate and must recover from inactivation through the open state. Both mechanisms can produce Na^+ currents that behave correctly. How can these alternatives be distinguished?

The first clear test was based on gating currents (201). If activation of a Na^+ channel involves movement of charged groups in the channel protein through the membrane's electrical field (Fig. 5.3B), that movement could be detected as a gating current. Gating currents (a few charges per channel) are tiny compared with the ionic currents carried by Na^+ flow through the open channel, but they can be recorded and provide complementary kinetic information. The Hodgkin-Huxley model makes two definite predictions for gating currents. First, they should be associated with both activation and inactivation. Because in that model both processes are voltage dependent, both involve charge movement and gating currents. Second, the total amount of charge moved on depolarization (i.e., channel opening and inactivation) should equal the total amount moved on repolarization (i.e., channel closing and recovery from inactivation). The charge moved by m gates that open and h gates that close on depolarization should be matched by m gate closing and h gate reopening on hyperpolarization.

Neither prediction was met experimentally (201). No detectable gating current was associated with inactivation. Instead, some of the m gates that opened during depolarization seemed to be "immobilized" during long depolarizations. The immobilization of gating charge had kinetics indistinguishable from inactivation of the Na^+ ionic current and suggested that inactivation prevents closing of the m gates, meaning that inactivation and activation are coupled. Qualitatively, that can be explained by the C–O–I model (Fig. 5.6B). If the m and h gates move sequentially, rather than independently, the m gate cannot close until the h gate reopens. Quantitatively, a more complex model is necessary (Fig. 5.10A). First, the C–O–I model predicts that all of the gating charge would be immobilized, but full inactivation produced approximately 70% immobilization, suggesting that some m gates can close while the channel is still inactivated. Second, although the O → I step has little or no voltage dependence, recovery from inactivation is voltage dependent (1). Third, most channels do not go back through the open state as they recover from inactivation (206,207). Fourth, some channels may inactivate without opening during a depolarization (208). These considerations require a "back door" connecting the inactivated state to one or more closed states. The modern view is that channel opening is coupled to inactivation, but the coupling is not absolute (202).

The modern convention is to express a kinetic model for channel gating as a Markov chain, in which different channel states are connected by first-order rate constants. The simplest versions of such models have been discussed

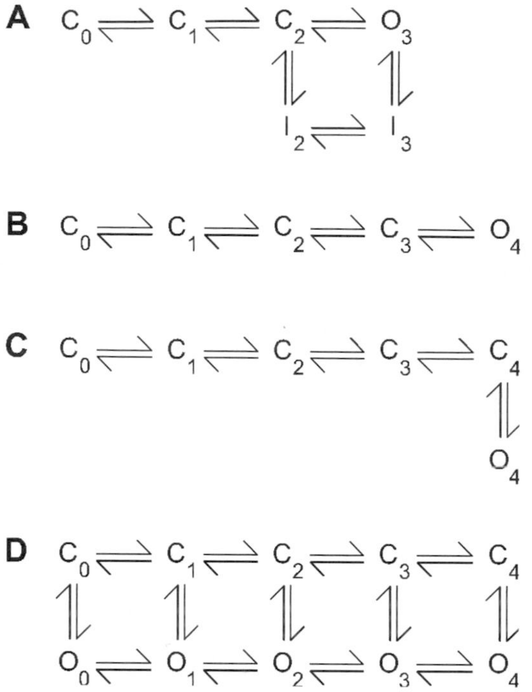

A
$$C_0 \rightleftharpoons C_1 \rightleftharpoons C_2 \rightleftharpoons O_3$$
$$\qquad\qquad\quad \updownarrow \qquad \updownarrow$$
$$\qquad\qquad\quad I_2 \rightleftharpoons I_3$$

B
$$C_0 \rightleftharpoons C_1 \rightleftharpoons C_2 \rightleftharpoons C_3 \rightleftharpoons O_4$$

C
$$C_0 \rightleftharpoons C_1 \rightleftharpoons C_2 \rightleftharpoons C_3 \rightleftharpoons C_4$$
$$\qquad\qquad\qquad\qquad\qquad\quad \updownarrow$$
$$\qquad\qquad\qquad\qquad\qquad\quad O_4$$

D
$$C_0 \rightleftharpoons C_1 \rightleftharpoons C_2 \rightleftharpoons C_3 \rightleftharpoons C_4$$
$$\updownarrow \quad\; \updownarrow \quad\; \updownarrow \quad\; \updownarrow \quad\; \updownarrow$$
$$O_0 \rightleftharpoons O_1 \rightleftharpoons O_2 \rightleftharpoons O_3 \rightleftharpoons O_4$$

Figure 5.10 Contemporary models for gating of voltage-dependent channels. **A:** Model for Na^+ channel inactivation, which allows some inactivation (and recovery) to bypass the open state (201,202). **B:** The Hodgkin-Huxley model for K^+ channel gating (1). Each transition is a movement of one n gate or voltage sensor. **C:** Sequential model for channel gating in which Hodgkin-Huxley–like voltage sensor movement is followed by a separate channel opening reaction (190,203,204). **D:** Generalization (205) of the model in **C** equivalent to the Monod-Wyman-Changeux model (209) for activation of an allosteric enzyme. For movement of the voltage sensors to be coupled to channel opening, the equilibrium for the C_0–O_0 reaction must favor the closed state, but as more voltage sensors activate, the C–O equilibrium shifts in favor of the open state.

(Fig. 5.6). Figure 5.10 illustrates more complex, but probably more realistic, models.

Allosteric Mechanisms for Activation

The observation that voltage-dependent K^+ channels have four possibly identical subunits (25) immediately suggested that the n^4 model for a Hodgkin-Huxley K^+ channel could be taken literally as a model for the molecular process underlying channel activation. An ion channel is analogous to an allosteric enzyme. How are the (presumably) local changes resulting from voltage sensor movement related to the (presumably) global change resulting in channel opening? According to the Hodgkin-Huxley model, the channel is open only if all four voltage sensors are in the activated position. The n^4 model can be expressed as a Markov model (Fig. 5.10B). Its five states appear complex, but the entire model is defined at a particular voltage by only two rate constants, those for opening and closing of a single n gate.

One prediction of the n^4 model is that channel closing should be voltage dependent, because the rate constant for

closing an n gate depends on voltage. For several different types of voltage-dependent channels, however, the mean open time shows little or no dependence on voltage (190, 203–205). That finding suggests a voltage-independent step distinct from voltage sensor movement, possibly a conformational change associated with channel opening itself. In the simplest model, activation of all four voltage sensors is necessary, but insufficient, for channel opening, with a voltage-independent channel-opening step after voltage sensor movement (203,204) (Fig. 5.10C). Figure 5.10C is a special case of the classic Monod-Wyman-Changeux model (209) for an allosteric enzyme (Fig. 5.10D), with enzyme activation considered analogous to channel opening and ligand binding analogous to voltage sensor movement. In that model, the channel can open with any number of voltage sensors activated, but opening is more likely and closing less likely as more voltage sensors activate.

Studies suggest two additional complications for K^+ channel gating: a possible additional source of cooperativity, in which movement of one voltage sensor favors movement of additional sensors (210), and evidence that movement of each voltage sensor occurs in two steps (211), producing an impressive number of states when expressed as a Markov model (32,195,212). This work is based on structure-function studies of cloned channels, in which mutations (e.g., in the S4 region) provide clues to gating mechanisms. The challenges are to extract a physically plausible mechanism from the wealth of empirical data and to interpret structure-function relations in the absence of a defined structure at atomic resolution.

Allosteric Mechanisms for Inactivation

In a model such as that illustrated in Figure 5.10A, inactivation depends primarily on the state of the channel, rather than directly on voltage. If activation of voltage sensors (left-to-right transitions) favors inactivation (top-to-bottom transitions), depolarization would indirectly favor inactivation, even if the rate constants for inactivation and recovery are voltage independent. A more general model including I_0 and I_1 states (21,206,213,214) predicts several inactivation features common to voltage-dependent channels. First, the inactivation rate is voltage dependent for weak depolarizations, in which voltage sensor movement is slow and rate limiting, but inactivation reaches a limiting voltage-independent rate at strong depolarization ($O_3 \rightarrow I_3$). Second, repolarization allows some channels to deactivate while still inactivated (e.g., $I_3 \rightarrow I_2$), although strong hyperpolarization is often necessary (215), making recovery from inactivation voltage dependent. Finally, recovery should approach a voltage-insensitive rate at extreme negative potentials, as observed for T-type Ca^{2+} (190,213,214) and some Na^+ channels (206).

Modulation of Channels and Electrical Activity

The tremendous diversity of voltage-dependent ion channels allows neurons to generate many different patterns of spontaneous and evoked electrical activity. Conversely, to generate appropriate electrical activity, a neuron must express the proper subset of properly functioning ion channels. Two aspects of ion channel regulation are discussed: short-term modulation of ion channels through G-protein–coupled receptors and diseases resulting from mutations in ion channel proteins.

Classic electrophysiology distinguished between ligand-gated ion channels, activated by binding of neurotransmitters, and voltage-gated channels, activated by changes in membrane potential. Contemporary studies confirm that both types are molecularly distinct gene families. However, many voltage-gated channels can be regulated indirectly by neurotransmitters, acting through G-protein–coupled receptors (19,20,174–176).

Neurotransmitter actions on ligand-gated channels have fairly simple mechanisms and functional consequences. Transmitter binding directly opens a channel, because the same protein molecule is a neurotransmitter receptor and an ion channel. The cell then depolarizes or hyperpolarizes, depending on the ion selectivity of the open channel. These 1- to 100-millisecond signals are highly localized, with the transmitter often acting within 1 μm of the release site, resulting in rapid, point-to-point transmission of information between neurons.

Signaling pathways involving G proteins involve several protein molecules, minimally including the receptor, the G protein, and the effector (e.g., channel), typically requiring 0.1 to 1 second (216). If the G protein activates an enzymatic cascade such as protein phosphorylation, the effect is slowed further (seconds to minutes) (217). The transmitter can also act over relatively large distances. For example, in the autonomic nervous system, nerve terminals are often several micrometers from the postsynaptic targets on end organs. In the heart, muscarinic receptors are located diffusely on atrial cells rather than being concentrated near nerve terminals (218). In sympathetic ganglia, peptides can diffuse to cells away from the synaptic contacts, and their action can last several minutes before termination (19).

G-protein–mediated pathways exert various effects on ion channels. Most simply, receptor activation can open a channel, as in the slow inhibitory postsynaptic potentials that are mediated by opening of inwardly rectifying K^+ channels by γ-aminobutyric acid (GABA$_B$) receptors (219). G-protein activation can also prevent channel activity, as in muscarinic inhibition of the M-type K^+ channel (19). More subtle effects are possible, as in the inhibition of N and P/Q Ca^{2+} channels by neurotransmitters (175,176). Although a reduction in channel activity is the most immediately obvious effect, closer examination reveals that the channels can still open, although only in response to longer or stronger depolarizations, as though the channels are "reluctant" to open (220). Perhaps the G protein binds more strongly to the closed state, and opening favors dissociation of the G protein and a return to normal channel gating (221).

G-protein–coupled pathways can dramatically affect the electrical activity of cells. Even simple activation of K^+ channels during slow inhibitory postsynaptic potentials is not exclusively inhibitory, because a postinhibitory rebound can favor repetitive activity (222). Inhibition of the M-type K^+ channel can switch a phasically firing neuron into a nearly tonic firing pattern (19). Inhibition of presynaptic Ca^{2+} channels can inhibit neurotransmitter release, although the voltage dependence of the inhibition potentially allows frequency-dependent reversal (221,223). In light of these complexities, most G-protein–coupled responses are best classified as modulatory, rather than simply excitatory or inhibitory.

Ion Channel Diseases and Electrical Activity Patterns

Molecular, physiologic, genetic, and clinical research has converged to identify channelopathies that result from inherited defects in genes coding for ion channels (224–230). Knowledge in this field is advancing rapidly, thanks largely to the human genome project and other approaches. Rather than attempt a comprehensive review, this chapter focuses on mutations of voltage-dependent cation channels that affect the electrical activity of neurons. Ion channel defects can cause abnormal electrical activity in other excitable cells, including myotonia and periodic paralysis of skeletal muscle (231) and cardiac arrhythmias (232,233). Several mutant mice with underlying ion channel defects are useful models for human disease (234–236).

A mutation in the gene coding for an ion channel can produce deleterious effects through several mechanisms, familiar in principle from classic genetics. A frameshift mutation or a point mutation in a crucial functional region can effectively knock out a channel. For most genes, a heterozygote with one copy of a gene can function almost normally, but that need not be true for ion channels. The approximately 100 genes coding for voltage-dependent cation channels (Table 5.1) reflect the diversity of channel function but also a degree of redundancy. In some cases, reduction in one particular channel is not critical; in others, small changes may be significant.

For channels that are multisubunit proteins, a coassembling mutant subunit that blocks function of the oligomeric channel is a dominant negative. If this occurs in a typical four-subunit K^+ channel, a heterozygote would have only one-sixteenth of the normal number of functional channels.

Gain-of-function mutations may be dramatic or subtle. Channels must open when they should, but not otherwise. Mutations that lead to tonic activation of channels or to changes in ion selectivity of open channels can be dysfunctional (234). Some mutations, however, may produce a shift of only a few millivolts in the voltage dependence of channel activation or inactivation.

A mutation identified from genetic studies can be introduced into a cloned ion channel and the effects on channel behavior examined in expression systems, such as *Xenopus* oocytes or mammalian cell lines. This approach can accurately reveal changes in channel behavior that are independent of the cellular environment and developmental history, perhaps most likely to be true for the fundamental processes underlying channel permeation and gating. Many mutations, however, affect expression of the channel, such as the fraction of channels targeted to the plasma membrane, which can vary between an expression system and an entire organism. The effects of a mutation *in vivo* can be affected by developmental processes: reduced by compensatory mechanisms (e.g., upregulation of one channel subunit to replace another) or increased by secondary effects (e.g., cell death). Excitement about molecular and physiologic insights must be balanced against these realities.

Kv1.1 and Episodic Ataxia Type 1

Several point mutations in the Kv1.1 delayed-rectifier K$^+$ channel are associated with episodic ataxia with myokymia, a rare dominant disorder (237). The mutations tend to occur in functionally significant sites in the channel protein, such as the highly conserved transmembrane domains. Some act as functional knockouts, whereas others reduce current amplitudes or modify channel gating (238,239). Mice lacking Kv1.1 exhibit spontaneous epileptiform seizures as well as hyperexcitability in hippocampal slices and peripheral nerve (240). Introduction of a human episodic ataxia mutation (V408A) into a mouse produces motor deficits (241).

It is not surprising that reduction in a K$^+$ current can induce repetitive firing. For example, in the original Hodgkin-Huxley model (1) of the action potential of the squid giant axon, a 50% reduction in the voltage-dependent K$^+$ current destabilizes the resting potential, producing spontaneous repetitive firing. However, the phenotype of Kv1.1 mutations depends on the details, because many other K$^+$ channels are capable of repolarizing neuronal action potentials.

KCNQ2/3 K$^+$ Channels and Benign Familial Neonatal Convulsions

Genetic studies of this rare dominant disorder identified two novel K$^+$ channel genes, *KCNQ2* and *KCNQ3* (242, 243), that act as a heteromultimer and underlie the slowly activating M current (51) found in sympathetic neurons and hippocampal pyramidal cells (19). Studies of these mutant channels expressed in *Xenopus* oocytes predict that the disorder results from quite small reductions in the M current (244).

Compared with delayed-rectifier K$^+$ channels, the M current is well designed to regulate repetitive firing (19), being activated more slowly (100 milliseconds) and at more negative voltages, between the resting potential and the threshold for generation of an action potential (50). Cells with an active M current tend to fire phasically, even in response to a maintained depolarization, but activation of various

G-protein–coupled receptors can inhibit the M current and allow repetitive firing (19). Genetic disruption of the M channel could easily disturb normal regulation of neuronal excitability.

Two other members of the KCNQ channel family are also mutated in human diseases. Mutations in *KCNQ1* (also called *KVLQT1*) cause long QT syndrome type 1, a potentially fatal cardiac arrhythmia (232), and mutations in *KCNQ4* can produce dominant deafness (245). This five-member channel family serves critical functions, with little redundancy.

P/Q-Type Ca^{2+} Channels: Familial Hemiplegic Migraine, Episodic Ataxia Type 2, and Spinocerebellar Ataxia Type 6

A variety of dominant conditions can result from mutations in the primary (α_{1A}) subunit of P/Q-type Ca^{2+} channels (230,246–248). Point mutations, which have disparate effects on channel gating (249–251), are linked to migraine. Mutations associated with episodic ataxia type 2 are severe and usually produce nonfunctional channels (248,252–254). One splice variant of the α_{1A} channel contains a polyglutamine repeat in the C-terminal region, and relatively short expansions of this repeat give rise to spinocerebellar ataxia type 6 (255). Truncation of the C-terminal region of α_{1A} can produce absence seizures (256). Several mouse mutants with defects in α_{1A} exhibit ataxia and, in some cases may experience absence seizures (230,246–248).

In many neurons, N channels participate in neurotransmitter release, possibly limiting the consequences of damage to the P/Q channels that dominate in that role. The Ca^{2+} current of cerebellar Purkinje neurons is almost exclusively (90%) the P type (152), however, making the sole output of the cerebellum unusually vulnerable. Ataxia is not unexpected. In general, it is difficult to relate defects in the α_{1A} protein to the specific resulting phenotypes. Few would have predicted that mutations in a Ca^{2+} channel could produce a symptom as specific as migraine. Nevertheless, these rare disorders offer fascinating insights into the complex relationship between ion channel physiology and human disease.

SUMMARY

Much is known about the molecular mechanisms underlying electrical excitability, including intrinsic electrical properties and synaptic signaling. This information has modified early views of neuronal computation based on model systems, such as the squid axon and the neuromuscular junction. In addition to the familiar fast synaptic potentials that last milliseconds, most neurotransmitters produce slow actions mediated through G-protein–coupled receptors that can modify the input-output relationships of neurons for seconds to minutes. Moreover, the surprising diversity of voltage-dependent ion channels leads to major differences in the intrinsic electrical properties of neurons. A postsynaptic neuron need not wait passively, adding excitatory postsynaptic potentials and subtracting inhibitory postsynaptic potentials, but can actively process synaptic inputs. These nonclassic mechanisms allow neurons and neuronal circuits to integrate information in complex and flexible ways. Disruption of the normal behavior of ion channels can produce abnormal patterns of electrical activity, including epilepsy.

REFERENCES

1. Hodgkin AL, Huxley AF. A quantitative description of membrane current and its application to conduction and excitation in nerve. *J Physiol* 1952;117:500–544.
2. Kuffler SW, Nicholls JG. *From neuron to brain.* Sunderland, MA: Sinauer Associates, 1976:486.
3. Hille B. *Ion channels of excitable membranes,* 3rd ed. Sunderland, MA: Sinauer, 2001:814.
4. Sanchez DY, Blatz AL. Voltage-dependent block of fast chloride channels from rat cortical neurons by external tetraethylammonium ion. *J Gen Physiol* 1992;100:217–231.
5. Sanchez DY, Blatz AL. Block of neuronal fast chloride channels by internal tetraethylammonium ions. *J Gen Physiol* 1994;104:173–190.
6. Caulfield MP. Muscarinic receptor-mediated inhibition of voltage-activated Ca current in neuroblastoma x glioma hybrid (NG 108-15) cells—reduction of muscarinic agonist and antagonist potency by tetraethylammonium (TEA). *Neurosci Lett* 1991;127: 165–168.
7. Doyle DA, Cabral JM, Pfuetzner RA, et al. The structure of the potassium channel: molecular basis of K^+ conduction and selectivity. *Science* 1998;280:69–77.
8. Jiang Y, Lee A, Chen J, et al. Crystal structure and mechanism of a calcium-gated potassium channel. *Nature* 2002;417:515–522.
9. Jiang Y, Lee A, Chen J, et al. X-ray structure of a voltage-dependent K^+ channel. *Nature* 2003;423:33–41.
10. MacKinnon R, Cohen SL, Kuo AL, et al. Structural conservation in prokaryotic and eukaryotic potassium channels. *Science* 1998; 280:106–109.
11. Zhou Y, MacKinnon R. The occupancy of ions in the K^+ selectivity filter: charge balance and coupling of ion binding to a protein conformational change underlie high conduction rates. *J Mol Biol* 2003;333:965–975.
12. Jiang Y, Lee A, Chen J, et al. The open pore conformation of potassium channels. *Nature* 2002;417:523–526.
13. MacKinnon R. Potassium channels. *FEBS Lett* 2003;555:62–65.
14. Jiang Y, Ruta V, Chen J, et al. The principle of gating charge movement in a voltage-dependent K^+ channel. *Nature* 2003;423: 42–48.
15. Cohen BE, Grabe M, Jan LY. Answers and questions from the KvAP structures. *Neuron* 2003;39:395–400.
16. Horn R. How S4 segments move charge. Let me count the ways. *J Gen Physiol* 2004;123:1–4.
17. Storm JF. Potassium currents in hippocampal pyramidal cells. *Prog Brain Res* 1990;83:161–187.
18. Chandy KG, Gutman GA. Voltage-gated potassium channel genes. In: Peroutka SJ, ed. *Handbook of receptors and channels.* Boca Raton, FL: CRC Press, 1994:1–71.
19. Adams PR, Jones SW, Pennefather P, et al. Slow synaptic transmission in frog sympathetic ganglia. *J Exp Biol* 1986;124: 259–285.
20. Hille B. Modulation of ion-channel function by G-protein-coupled receptors. *Trends Neurosci* 1994;17:531–536.
21. Klemic KG, Shieh C-C, Kirsch GE, et al. Inactivation of Kv2.1 potassium channels. *Biophys J* 1998;74:1779–1789.
22. Kramer JW, Post MA, Brown AM, et al. Modulation of potassium channel gating by coexpression of Kv2.1 with regulatory Kv5.1 or Kv6.1 α-subunits. *Am J Physiol* 1998;274:C1501–C1510.
23. Chandy KG, Gutman GA. Nomenclature for mammalian potassium channel genes. *Trends Pharmacol Sci* 1993;14:434.

24. Gutman GA, Chandy KG, Adelman JP, et al. International Union of Pharmacology. XLI. Compendium of voltage-gated ion channels: potassium channels. *Pharmacol Rev* 2003;55:583–586.
25. MacKinnon R. Determination of the subunit stoichiometry of a voltage-activated potassium channel. *Nature* 1991;350:232–235.
26. MacKinnon R, Yellen G. Mutations affecting TEA blockade and ion permeation in voltage-activated K^+ channels. *Science* 1990; 250:276–279.
27. Yellen G, Jurman ME, Abramson T, et al. Mutations affecting internal TEA blockade identify the probable pore-forming region of a K^+ channel. *Science* 1991;251:939–942.
28. Hartmann HA, Kirsch GE, Drewe JA, et al. Exchange of conduction pathways between two related K^+ channels. *Science* 1991; 251:942–944.
29. Mannuzzu LM, Moronne MM, Isacoff EY. Direct physical measure of conformational rearrangement underlying potassium channel gating. *Science* 1996;271:213–216.
30. Yang N, Horn R. Evidence for voltage-dependent S4 movement in sodium channels. *Neuron* 1995;15:213–218.
31. Schoppa NE, McCormack K, Tanouye MA, et al. The size of gating charge in wild-type and mutant *Shaker* potassium channels. *Science* 1992;255:1712–1715.
32. Sigworth FJ. Voltage gating of ion channels. *Q Rev Biophys* 1994; 27:1–40.
33. Post MA, Kirsch GE, Brown AM. Kv2.1 and electrically silent Kv6.1 potassium channel subunits combine and express a novel current. *FEBS Lett* 1996;399:177–182.
34. Hugnot JP, Salinas M, Lesage F, et al. Kv8.1, a new neuronal potassium channel subunit with specific inhibitory properties towards *Shab* and *Shaw* channels. *EMBO J* 1996;15:3322–3331.
35. Salinas M, Duprat F, Heurteaux C, et al. New modulatory α subunits for mammalian *Shab* K^+ channels. *J Biol Chem* 1997;272: 24371–24379.
36. Kerschensteiner D, Stocker M. Heteromeric assembly of Kv2.1 with Kv9.3: effect on the state dependence of inactivation. *Biophys J* 1999;77:248–257.
37. Connor JA, Stevens CF. Voltage clamp studies of a transient outward membrane current in gastropod neural somata. *J Physiol* 1971;213:21–30.
38. Johnston D, Christie BR, Frick A, et al. Active dendrites, potassium channels and synaptic plasticity. *Philos Trans R Soc Lond B Biol Sci* 2003;358:667–674.
39. Kamb A, Iverson LE, Tanouye MA. Molecular characterization of *Shaker,* a *Drosophila* gene that encodes a potassium channel. *Cell* 1987;50:405–413.
40. Timpe LC, Schwarz TL, Tempel BL, et al. Expression of functional potassium channels from *Shaker* cDNA in *Xenopus* oocytes. *Nature* 1988;331:143–145.
41. Hoshi T, Zagotta WN, Aldrich RW. Biophysical and molecular mechanisms of *Shaker* potassium channel inactivation. *Science* 1990;250:533–538.
42. Zagotta WN, Hoshi T, Aldrich RW. Restoration of inactivation in mutants of *Shaker* potassium channels by a peptide derived from ShB. *Science* 1990;250:568–571.
43. Zhou M, Morais-Cabral JH, Mann S, et al. Potassium channel receptor site for the inactivation gate and quaternary amine inhibitors. *Nature* 2001;411:657–661.
44. Rettig J, Heinemann SH, Wunder F, et al. Inactivation properties of voltage-gated K^+ channels altered by presence of β-subunit. *Nature* 1994;369:289–294.
45. Ludwig J, Terlau H, Wunder F, et al. Functional expression of a rat homologue of the voltage gated *ether à go-go* potassium channel reveals differences in selectivity and activation kinetics between the *Drosophila* channel and its mammalian counterpart. *EMBO J* 1994;13:4451–4458.
46. Smith PL, Baukrowitz T, Yellen G. The inward rectification mechanism of the HERG cardiac potassium channel. *Nature* 1996; 379:833–836.
47. Sanguinetti MC, Jiang C, Curran ME, et al. A mechanistic link between an inherited and an acquired cardiac arrhythmia: HERG encodes the I_{Kr} potassium channel. *Cell* 1995;81:299–307.
48. Brown DA, Adams PR. Muscarinic suppression of a novel voltage-sensitive K^+ current in a vertebrate neurone. *Nature* 1980;283: 673–676.

49. Halliwell JV, Adams PR. Voltage-clamp analysis of muscarinic excitation in hippocampal neurons. *Brain Res* 1982;250:71–92.

50. Adams PR, Brown DA, Constanti A. M-currents and other potassium currents in bullfrog sympathetic neurones. *J Physiol* 1982; 330:537–572.

51. Wang HS, Pan ZM, Shi WM, et al. KCNQ2 and KCNQ3 potassium channel subunits: molecular correlates of the M-channel. *Science* 1998;282:1890–1893.

52. Wang Q, Curran ME, Splawski I, et al. Positional cloning of a novel potassium channel gene: KVLQT1 mutations cause cardiac arrhythmias. *Nat Genet* 1996;12:17–23.

53. Sanguinetti MC, Curran ME, Zou A, et al. Coassembly of K_VLQT1 and minK (IsK) proteins to form cardiac I_{Ks} potassium channel. *Nature* 1996;384:80–83.

54. Kaczorowski GJ, Knaus HG, Leonard RJ, et al. High-conductance calcium-activated potassium channels; structure, pharmacology, and function. *J Bioenerg Biomembr* 1996;28:255–267.

55. Barrett JN, Magleby KL, Pallotta BS. Properties of single calcium-activated potassium channels in cultured rat muscle. *J Physiol* 1982;331:211–230.

56. Moczydlowski E, Latorre R. Gating kinetics of Ca^{2+}-activated K^+ channels from rat muscle incorporated into planar lipid bilayers. Evidence for two voltage-dependent Ca^{2+} binding reactions. *J Gen Physiol* 1983;82:511–542.

57. Jones SW. Commentary. A plausible model. *J Gen Physiol* 1999; 114:271–275.

58. Magleby KL. Gating mechanism of BK (Slo1) channels: so near, yet so far. *J Gen Physiol* 2003;121:81–96.

59. Roberts WM, Jacobs RA, Hudspeth AJ. Colocalization of ion channels involved in frequency selectivity and synaptic transmission at presynaptic active zones of hair cells. *J Neurosci* 1990;10: 3664–3684.

60. Adams PR, Constanti A, Brown DA, et al. Intracellular Ca^{2+} activates a fast voltage-sensitive K^+ current in vertebrate sympathetic neurones. *Nature* 1982;296:746–749.

61. Pallotta BS, Magleby KL, Barrett JN. Single channel recordings of Ca^{2+}-activated K^+ currents in rat muscle cell culture. *Nature* 1981;293:471–474.

62. Adelman JP, Shen KZ, Kavanaugh MP, et al. Calcium-activated potassium channels expressed from cloned complementary DNAs. *Neuron* 1992;9:209–216.

63. Butler A, Tsunoda S, McCobb DP, et al. mSlo, a complex mouse gene encoding "maxi" calcium-activated potassium channels. *Science* 1993;261:221–224.

64. Meera P, Wallner M, Song M, et al. Large conductance voltage- and calcium-dependent K^+ channel, a distinct member of voltage-dependent ion channels with seven transmembrane segments (S0-S6), an extracellular N terminus, and an intracellular (S9-S10) C terminus. *Proc Natl Acad Sci U S A* 1997;94:14066–14071.

65. Wei A, Solaro C, Lingle C, et al. Calcium sensitivity of BK-type KCa channels determined by a separable domain. *Neuron* 1994; 13:671–681.

66. Wallner M, Meera P, Toro L. Molecular basis of fast inactivation in voltage and Ca^{2+}-activated K^+ channels: a transmembrane β-subunit homolog. *Proc Natl Acad Sci U S A* 1999;96:4137–4142.

67. Blatz AL, Magleby KL. Ion conductance and selectivity of single calcium-activated potassium channels in cultured rat muscle. *J Gen Physiol* 1984;84:1–23.

68. Sah P, Clements JD. Photolytic manipulation of $[Ca^{2+}]_i$ reveals slow kinetics of potassium channels underlying the afterhyperpolarization in hippocampal pyramidal neurons. *J Neurosci* 1999;19:3657–3664.

69. Pennefather P, Lancaster B, Adams PR, et al. Two distinct Ca-dependent K currents in bullfrog sympathetic ganglion cells. *Proc Natl Acad Sci U S A* 1985;82:3040–3044.

70. Lancaster B, Adams PR. Calcium-dependent current generating the afterhyperpolarization of hippocampal neurons. *J Neurophysiol* 1986;55:1268–1282.

71. Sah P. Ca^{2+}-activated K^+ currents in neurones: types, physiological roles and modulation. *Trends Neurosci* 1996;19:150–154.

72. Vogalis F, Storm JF, Lancaster B. SK channels and the varieties of slow after-hyperpolarizations in neurons. *Eur J Neurosci* 2003;18: 3155–3166.

73. Koehler M, Hirschberg B, Bond CT, et al. Small-conductance, calcium-activated potassium channels from mammalian brain. *Science* 1996;273:1709–1714.

74. Kubo Y. Towards the elucidation of the structural-functional relationship of inward rectifying K^+ channel family. *Neurosci Res* 1994;21:109–117.

75. Doupnik CA, Davidson N, Lester HA. The inward rectifier potassium channel family. *Curr Opin Neurobiol* 1995;5:268–277.

76. Bichet D, Haass FA, Jan LY. Merging functional studies with structures of inward-rectifier K^+ channels. *Nat Rev Neurosci* 2003;4: 957–967.

77. Vandenberg CA. Inward rectification of a potassium channel in cardiac ventricular cells depends on internal magnesium ions. *Proc Natl Acad Sci U S A* 1987;84:2560–2564.

78. Ficker E, Taglialatela M, Wible BA, et al. Spermine and spermidine as gating molecules for inward rectifier K^+ channels. *Science* 1994;266:1068–1072.

79. Lopatin AN, Makhina EN, Nichols CG. Potassium channel block by cytoplasmic polyamines as the mechanism of intrinsic rectification. *Nature* 1994;372:366–369.

80. Stanfield PR, Nakajima Y, Yamaguchi K. Substance P raises neuronal membrane excitability by reducing inward rectification. *Nature* 1985;315:498–501.

81. Reimann F, Ashcroft FM. Inwardly rectifying potassium channels. *Curr Opin Cell Biol* 1999;11:503–508.

82. Nishida M, MacKinnon R. Structural basis of inward rectification. Cytoplasmic pore of the G protein-gated inward rectifier GIRK1 at 1.8 Å resolution. *Cell* 2002;111:957–965.

83. Lu Z, MacKinnon R. Electrostatic tuning of Mg^{2+} affinity in an inward-rectifier K^+ channel. *Nature* 1994;371:243–246.

84. Wible BA, Taglialatela M, Ficker E, et al. Gating of inwardly rectifying K^+ channels localized to a single negatively charged residue. *Nature* 1994;371:246–249.

85. Kuo A, Gulbis JM, Antcliff JF, et al. Crystal structure of the potassium channel KirBac1.1 in the closed state. *Science* 2003;300: 1922–1926.

86. Jones SW. On the resting potential of isolated frog sympathetic neurons. *Neuron* 1989;3:153–161.

87. Ketchum KA, Joiner WJ, Sellers AJ, et al. A new family of outwardly rectifying potassium channel proteins with two pore domains in tandem. *Nature* 1995;376:690–695.

88. Lesage F, Guillemare E, Fink M, et al. TWIK-1, a ubiquitous human weakly inward rectifying K^+ channel with a novel structure. *EMBO J* 1996;15:1004–1011.

89. Millar JA, Barratt L, Southan AP, et al. A functional role for the two-pore domain potassium channel TASK-1 in cerebellar granule neurons. *Proc Natl Acad Sci U S A* 2000;97:3614–3618.

90. Goldstein SA, Bockenhauer D, O'Kelly I, et al. Potassium leak channels and the KCNK family of two-P-domain subunits. *Nat Rev Neurosci* 2001;2:175–184.

91. Plummer NW, Meisler MH. Evolution and diversity of mammalian sodium channel genes. *Genomics* 1999;57:323–331.

92. Goldin AL, Barchi RL, Caldwell JH, et al. Nomenclature of voltage-gated sodium channels. *Neuron* 2002;28:365–368.

93. Catterall WA, Goldin AL, Waxman SG. International Union of Pharmacology. XXXIX. Compendium of voltage-gated ion channels: sodium channels. *Pharmacol Rev* 2003;55:575–578.

94. Yu FH, Catterall WA. Overview of the voltage-gated sodium channel family. *Genome Biol* 2003;4:207.

95. Yoshida S. Tetrodotoxin-resistant sodium channels. *Cell Mol Neurobiol* 1994;14:227–244.

96. Terlau H, Heinemann SH, Stuhmer W, et al. Mapping the site of block by tetrodotoxin and saxitoxin of sodium channel II. *FEBS Lett* 1991;293:93–96.

97. West JW, Patton DE, Scheuer T, et al. A cluster of hydrophobic amino acid residues required for fast Na^+-channel inactivation. *Proc Natl Acad Sci U S A* 1992;89:10910–10914.

98. French CR, Sah P, Buckett KJ, et al. A voltage-dependent persistent sodium current in mammalian hippocampal neurons. *J Gen Physiol* 1990;95:1139–1157.

99. Magistretti J, Alonso A. Biophysical properties and slow voltage-dependent inactivation of a sustained sodium current in entorhinal cortex layer-II principal neurons. A whole-cell and single-channel study. *J Gen Physiol* 1999;114:491–509.

100. Hoehn K, Watson TWJ, MacVicar BA. A novel tetrodotoxin-insensitive, slow sodium current in striatal and hippocampal neurons. *Neuron* 1993;10:543–552.

101. Callahan MJ, Korn SJ. Permeation of Na^+ through a delayed rectifier K^+ channel in chick dorsal root ganglion neurons. *J Gen Physiol* 1994;104:747–771.

102. Korn SJ, Ikeda SR. Permeation selectivity by competition in a delayed rectifier potassium channel. *Science* 1995;269:410–412.

103. Ríos E, Stern MD. Calcium in close quarters: microdomain feedback in excitation-contraction coupling and other cell biological phenomena. *Annu Rev Biophys Biomol Struct* 1997;26:47–82.

104. Birnbaumer L, Campbell KP, Catterall WA, et al. The naming of voltage-gated calcium channels. *Neuron* 1994;13:505–506.

105. Olivera BM, Miljanich GP, Ramachandran J, et al. Calcium channel diversity and neurotransmitter release: the ω-conotoxins and ω-agatoxins. *Annu Rev Biochem* 1994;63:823–867.

106. Dunlap K, Luebke JI, Turner TJ. Exocytotic Ca^{2+} channels in mammalian central neurons. *Trends Neurosci* 1995;18:89–98.

107. Tsien RW, Lipscombe D, Madison D, et al. Reflections on Ca^{2+}-channel diversity, 1988–1994. *Trends Neurosci* 1995;18:52–54.

108. Jones SW. Overview of voltage-dependent calcium channels. *J Bioenerg Biomembr* 1998;30:299–312.

109. Ertel EA, Campbell KP, Harpold MM, et al. Nomenclature of voltage-gated calcium channels. *Neuron* 2000;25:533–535.

110. Catterall WA. Structure and regulation of voltage-gated Ca^{2+} channels. *Annu Rev Cell Dev Biol* 2000;16:521–555.

111. Catterall WA, Striessnig J, Snutch TP, et al. International Union of Pharmacology. XL. Compendium of voltage-gated ion channels: calcium channels. *Pharmacol Rev* 2003;55:579–581.

112. Elmslie KS, Kammermeier PJ, Jones SW. Reevaluation of Ca^{2+} channel types and their modulation in bullfrog sympathetic neurons. *Neuron* 1994;13:217–228.

113. Zhou W, Jones SW. Surface charge and calcium channel saturation in bullfrog sympathetic neurons. *J Gen Physiol* 1995;105:441–462.

114. Plummer MR, Logothetis DE, Hess P. Elementary properties and pharmacological sensitivities of calcium channels in mammalian peripheral neurons. *Neuron* 1989;2:1453–1463.

115. Eckert R, Chad JE. Inactivation of Ca channels. *Prog Biophys Mol Biol* 1984;44:215–267.

116. Yue DT, Backx PH, Imredy JP. Calcium-sensitive inactivation in the gating of single calcium channels. *Science* 1990;250:1735–1738.

117. Peterson BZ, DeMaria CD, Adelman JP, et al. Calmodulin is the Ca^{2+} sensor for Ca^{2+}-dependent inactivation of L-type calcium channels. *Neuron* 1999;22:549–558.

118. Qin N, Olcese R, Bransby M, et al. Ca^{2+}-induced inhibition of the cardiac Ca^{2+} channel depends on calmodulin. *Proc Natl Acad Sci U S A* 1999;96:2435–2438.

119. Zühlke RD, Pitt GS, Deisseroth K, et al. Calmodulin supports both inactivation and facilitation of L-type calcium channels. *Nature* 1999;399:159–162.

120. Kohr G, Mody I. Endogenous intracellular calcium buffering and the activation/inactivation of HVA calcium currents in rat dentate gyrus granule cells. *J Gen Physiol* 1991;98:941–967.

121. Naegerl UV, Mody I. Calcium-dependent inactivation of high-threshold calcium currents in human dentate gyrus granule cells. *J Physiol* 1998;509:39–45.

122. Von Gersdorff H, Matthews G. Calcium-dependent inactivation of calcium current in synaptic terminals of retinal bipolar neurons. *J Neurosci* 1996;16:115–122.

123. Baumann L, Gerstner A, Zong X, et al. Functional characterization of the L-type Ca^{2+} channel $Ca_V1.4\alpha1$ from mouse retina. *Invest Ophthalmol Vis Sci* 2004;45:708–713.

124. McRory JE, Hamid J, Doering CJ, et al. The CACNA1F gene encodes an L-type calcium channel with unique biophysical properties and tissue distribution. *J Neurosci* 2004;24:1707–1718.

125. Giannattasio B, Jones SW, Scarpa A. Calcium currents in the A7r5 smooth muscle-derived cell line. Calcium-dependent and voltage-dependent inactivation. *J Gen Physiol* 1991;98:987–1003.

126. Almers W, McCleskey EW. Non-selective conductance in calcium channels of frog muscle: calcium selectivity in a single-file pore. *J Physiol* 1984;353:585–608.

127. Hess P, Tsien RW. Mechanism of ion permeation through calcium channels. *Nature* 1984;309:453–456.

128. Sather WA, McCleskey EW. Permeation and selectivity in calcium channels. *Annu Rev Physiol* 2003;65:133–159.

129. Yang J, Ellinor PT, Sather WA, et al. Molecular determinants of Ca^{2+} selectivity and ion permeation in L-type Ca^{2+} channels. *Nature* 1993;366:158–161.

130. Birnbaumer L, Qin N, Olcese R, et al. Structures and functions of calcium channel β subunits. *J Bioenerg Biomembr* 1998;30:357–375.

131. Dolphin AC. β Subunits of voltage-gated calcium channels. *J Bioenerg Biomembr* 2003;35:599–620.

132. Klugbauer N, Marais E, Hofmann F. Calcium channel $\alpha_2\delta$ subunits: differential expression, function and drug binding. *J Bioenerg Biomembr* 2003;35:639–647.

133. Black JL III. The voltage gated calcium channel γ subunits: a review of the literature. *J Bioenerg Biomembr* 2003;35:649–660.

134. Strom TM, Nyakatura G, Apfelstedt-Sylla E, et al. An L-type calcium-channel gene mutated in incomplete X-linked congenital stationary night blindness. *Nat Genet* 1998;19:260–263.

135. Xu W, Lipscombe D. Neuronal $Ca_V1.3\alpha_1$ L-type channels activate at relatively hyperpolarized membrane potentials and are incompletely inhibited by dihydropyridines. *J Neurosci* 2001;21:5944–5951.

136. Koschak A, Reimer D, Huber IG, et al. α_{1D} ($Ca_V1.3$) subunits can form L-type Ca^{2+} channels activating at negative voltages. *J Biol Chem* 2001;276:22100–22106.

137. Nowycky MC, Fox AP, Tsien RW. Three types of neuronal calcium channel with different calcium agonist sensitivity. *Nature* 1985;316:440–443.

138. Jones SW, Marks TN. Calcium currents in bullfrog sympathetic neurons, II: inactivation. *J Gen Physiol* 1989;94:169–182.

139. Artalejo CR, Perlman RL, Fox AP. Omega-conotoxin GVIA blocks a Ca^{2+} current in bovine chromaffin cells that is not of the "classic" N type. *Neuron* 1992;8:85–95.

140. Plummer MR, Hess P. Reversible uncoupling of inactivation in N-type calcium channels. *Nature* 1991;351:657–659.

141. Werz MA, Elmslie KS, Jones SW. Phosphorylation enhances inactivation of N-type calcium channel current in bullfrog sympathetic neurons. *Pflügers Arch* 1993;424:538–545.

142. Patil PG, Brody DL, Yue DT. Preferential closed-state inactivation of neuronal calcium channels. *Neuron* 1998;20:1027–1038.

143. Cahill AL, Hurley JH, Fox AP. Coexpression of cloned α_{1B}, β_{2a}, and α_2/δ subunits produces non-inactivating calcium currents similar to those found in bovine chromaffin cells. *J Neurosci* 2000;20:1685–1693.

144. Cox DH, Dunlap K. Inactivation of N-type calcium current in chick sensory neurons: calcium and voltage dependence. *J Gen Physiol* 1994;104:311–336.

145. Liang H, DeMaria CD, Erickson MG, et al. Unified mechanisms of Ca^{2+} regulation across the Ca^{2+} channel family. *Neuron* 2003;39:951–960.

146. Jones SW. Inactivation of N-type Ca^{2+} channels: Ca^{2+} vs. voltage. *J Physiol* 1999;518:630.

147. Fujita Y, Mynlieff M, Dirksen RT, et al. Primary structure and functional expression of the ω-conotoxin-sensitive N-type calcium channel from rabbit brain. *Neuron* 1993;10:585–598.

148. Williams ME, Brust PF, Feldman DH, et al. Structure and functional expression of an ω-conotoxin-sensitive human N-type calcium channel. *Science* 1992;257:389–395.

149. Williams ME, Feldman DH, McCue AF, et al. Structure and functional expression of α_1, α_2, and β subunits of a novel human neuronal calcium channel subtype. *Neuron* 1992;8:71–84.

150. McEnery MW, Snowman AM, Sharp AH, et al. Purified ω-conotoxin GVIA receptor of rat brain resembles a dihydropyridine-sensitive L-type calcium channel. *Proc Natl Acad Sci U S A* 1991;88:11095–11099.

151. Regan LJ, Sah DW, Bean BP. Ca^{2+} channels in rat central and peripheral neurons: high-threshold current resistant to dihydropyridine blockers and ω-conotoxin. *Neuron* 1991;6:269–280.

152. Mintz IM, Venema VJ, Swiderek KM, et al. P-type calcium channels blocked by the spider toxin ω-Aga-IVA. *Nature* 1992;355:827–829.

153. McDonough SI, Mintz IM, Bean BP. Alteration of P-type calcium channel gating by the spider toxin ω-Aga-IVA. *Biophys J* 1997;72: 2117–2128.

154. Mintz IM, Adams ME, Bean BP. P-type calcium channels in rat central and peripheral neurons. *Neuron* 1992;9:85–95.

155. Sather WA, Tanabe T, Zhang JF, et al. Distinctive biophysical and pharmacological properties of class A (BI) calcium channel α_1 subunits. *Neuron* 1993;11:291–303.

156. Randall A, Tsien RW. Pharmacological dissection of multiple types of Ca^{2+} channel currents in rat cerebellar granule neurons. *J Neurosci* 1995;15:2995–3012.

157. Zhang JF, Randall AD, Ellinor PT, et al. Distinctive pharmacology and kinetics of cloned neuronal Ca^{2+} channels and their possible counterparts in mammalian CNS neurons. *Neuropharmacology* 1993;32:1075–1088.

158. Bourinet E, Soong TW, Sutton K, et al. Splicing of α_{1A} subunit gene generates phenotypic variants of P- and Q-type calcium channels. *Nat Neurosci* 1999;2:407–415.

159. Ellinor PT, Zhang JF, Randall AD, et al. Functional expression of a rapidly inactivating neuronal calcium channel. *Nature* 1993; 363:455–458.

160. Soong TW, Stea A, Hodson CD, et al. Structure and functional expression of a member of the low voltage-activated calcium channel family. *Science* 1993;260:1133–1136.

161. Bourinet E, Zamponi GW, Stea A, et al. The α_{1E} calcium channel exhibits permeation properties similar to low-voltage-activated calcium channels. *J Neurosci* 1996;16:4983–4993.

162. Meir A, Dolphin AC. Known calcium channel α_1 subunits can form low threshold small conductance channels with similarities to native T-type channels. *Neuron* 1998;20:341–351.

163. Randall AD, Tsien RW. Contrasting biophysical and pharmacological properties of T-type and R-type calcium channels. *Neuropharmacology* 1997;36:879–893.

164. Bean BP, McDonough SI. Two for T. *Neuron* 1998;20:825–828.

165. Lambert RC, McKenna F, Maulet Y, et al. Low-voltage-activated Ca^{2+} currents are generated by members of the Ca_VT subunit family (α_1G/H) in rat primary sensory neurons. *J Neurosci* 1998; 18:8605–8613.

166. Nakashima YM, Todorovic SM, Pereverzev A, et al. Properties of Ba^{2+} currents arising from human α_{1E} and $\alpha_{1E}\alpha_3$ constructs expressed in HEK293 cells: physiology, pharmacology, and comparison to native T-type Ba^{2+} currents. *Neuropharmacology* 1998; 37:957–972.

167. Liang H, Elmslie KS. E_f-current contributes to whole-cell calcium current in low calcium in frog sympathetic neurons. *J Neurophysiol* 2001;86:1156–1163.

168. Newcomb R, Szoke B, Palma A, et al. Selective peptide antagonist of the class E calcium channel from the venom of the tarantula *Hysterocrates gigas*. *Biochemistry* 1998;37:15353–15362.

169. Tottene A, Volsen S, Pietrobon D. α_{1E} Subunits form the pore of three cerebellar R-type calcium channels with different pharmacological and permeation properties. *J Neurosci* 2000;20:171–178.

170. Wilson SM, Toth PT, Oh SB, et al. The status of voltage-dependent calcium channels in α_{1E} knock-out mice. *J Neurosci* 2000;20: 8566–8571.

171. Sochivko D, Pereverzev A, Smyth N, et al. The $Ca_V2.3$ Ca^{2+} channel subunit contributes to R-type Ca^{2+} currents in murine hippocampal and neocortical neurones. *J Physiol* 2002;542:699–710.

172. Heidelberger R, Matthews G. Calcium influx and calcium current in single synaptic terminals of goldfish retinal bipolar neurons. *J Physiol* 1992;447:235–256.

173. Jones SW. Calcium channels: unanswered questions. *J Bioenerg Biomembr* 2003;35:461–475.

174. Dolphin AC. G protein modulation of voltage-gated calcium channels. *Pharmacol Rev* 2003;55:607–627.

175. Jones SW, Elmslie KS. Transmitter modulation of neuronal calcium channels. *J Membr Biol* 1997;155:1–10.

176. Elmslie KS. Neurotransmitter modulation of neuronal calcium channels. *J Bioenerg Biomembr* 2003;35:477–489.

177. Elmslie KS, Kammermeier PJ, Jones SW. Calcium current modulation in frog sympathetic neurones: L-current is relatively insensitive to neurotransmitters. *J Physiol* 1992;456:107–123.

178. Mintz IM, Bean BP. $GABA_B$ receptor inhibition of P-type Ca^{2+} channels in central neurons. *Neuron* 1993;10:889–898.

179. Qin N, Platano D, Olcese R, et al. Direct interaction of $G\beta\gamma$ with a C-terminal $G\beta\gamma$-binding domain of the Ca^{2+} channel α_1 subunit is responsible for channel inhibition by G protein-coupled receptors. *Proc Natl Acad Sci U S A* 1997;94:8866–8871.

180. Carbone E, Lux HD. A low voltage-activated, fully inactivating Ca channel in vertebrate sensory neurones. *Nature* 1984;310:501–502.

181. Armstrong CM, Matteson DR. Two distinct populations of calcium channels in a clonal line of pituitary cells. *Science* 1985; 227:65–67.

182. Huguenard JR. Low-threshold calcium currents in central nervous system neurons. *Annu Rev Physiol* 1996;58:329–348.

183. Perez-Reyes E. Molecular physiology of low-voltage-activated T-type calcium channels. *Physiol Rev* 2003;83:117–161.

184. Yunker AMR, McEnery MW. Low voltage-activated ("T-type") calcium channels in review. *J Bioenerg Biomembr* 2003;35:533–575.

185. Destexhe A, Sejnowski TJ. Interactions between membrane conductances underlying thalamocortical slow-wave oscillations. *Physiol Rev* 2003;83:1401–1453.

186. Perez-Reyes E, Cribbs LL, Daud A, et al. Molecular characterization of a neuronal low-voltage-activated T-type calcium channel. *Nature* 1998;391:896–900.

187. Cribbs LL, Lee JH, Yang J, et al. Cloning and characterization of α_{1H} from human heart, a member of the T-type Ca^{2+} channel gene family. *Circ Res* 1998;83:103–109.

188. Lee JH, Daud AN, Cribbs LL, et al. Cloning and expression of a novel member of the low voltage-activated T-type calcium channel family. *J Neurosci* 1999;19:1912–1921.

189. Talley EM, Cribbs LL, Lee JH, et al. Differential distribution of three members of a gene family encoding low voltage-activated (T-type) calcium channels. *J Neurosci* 1999;19:1895–1911.

190. Chen CF, Hess P. Mechanism of gating of T-type calcium channels. *J Gen Physiol* 1990;96:603–630.

191. Todorovic SM, Lingle CJ. Pharmacological properties of T-type Ca^{2+} current in adult rat sensory neurons: effects of anticonvulsant and anesthetic agents. *J Neurophysiol* 1998;79:240–252.

192. Narahashi T, Tsunoo A, Yoshii M. Characterization of two types of calcium channels in mouse neuroblastoma cells. *J Physiol* 1987;383:231–249.

193. Lee JH, Gomora JC, Cribbs LL, et al. Nickel block of three cloned T-type calcium channels: low concentrations selectively block α_{1H}. *Biophys J* 1999;77:3034–3042.

194. Huguenard JR, Prince DA. A novel T-type current underlies prolonged Ca^{2+}-dependent burst firing in GABAergic neurons of rat thalamic reticular nucleus. *J Neurosci* 1992;12:3804–3817.

195. Bezanilla F, Stefani E. Voltage-dependent gating of ionic channels. *Ann Rev Biophys Biomol Struct* 1994;23:819–846.

196. Keynes RD. The kinetics of voltage-gated ion channels. *Q Rev Biophys* 1994;27:339–434.

197. Yellen G. The moving parts of voltage-gated ion channels. *Q Rev Biophys* 1998;31:239–295.

198. Bezanilla F. The voltage sensor in voltage-dependent ion channels. *Physiol Rev* 2000;80:555–592.

199. Yellen G. The voltage-gated potassium channels and their relatives. *Nature* 2002;419:35–42.

200. Bezanilla F, Perozo E. The voltage sensor and the gate in ion channels. *Adv Protein Chem* 2003;63:211–241.

201. Armstrong CM, Bezanilla F. Inactivation of the sodium channel, II: gating current experiments. *J Gen Physiol* 1977;70:567–590.

202. Patlak J. Molecular kinetics of voltage-dependent Na^+ channels. *Physiol Rev* 1991;71:1047–1080.

203. Koren G, Liman ER, Logothetis DE, et al. Gating mechanism of a cloned potassium channel expressed in frog oocytes and mammalian cells. *Neuron* 1990;4:39–51.

204. Zagotta WN, Aldrich RW. Voltage-dependent gating of *Shaker* A-type potassium channels in *Drosophila* muscle. *J Gen Physiol* 1990;95:29–60.

205. Marks TN, Jones SW. Calcium currents in the A7r5 smooth muscle-derived cell line. An allosteric model for calcium channel activation and dihydropyridine agonist action. *J Gen Physiol* 1992;99:367–390.

206. Kuo C-C, Bean BP. Na^+ channels must deactivate to recover from inactivation. *Neuron* 1994;12:819–829.

207. Raman IM, Bean BP. Resurgent sodium current and action potential formation in dissociated cerebellar Purkinje neurons. *J Neurosci* 1997;17:4517–4526.

208. Bean BP. Sodium channel inactivation in the crayfish giant axon. Must channels open before inactivating? *Biophys J* 1981;35:595–614.

209. Monod J, Wyman J, Changeux J-P. On the nature of allosteric transitions: a plausible model. *J Mol Biol* 1965;12:88–118.

210. Tytgat J, Hess P. Evidence for cooperative interactions in potassium channel gating. *Nature* 1992;359:420–423.

211. Baker OS, Larsson HP, Mannuzzu LM, et al. Three transmembrane conformations and sequence-dependent displacement of the S4 domain in *Shaker* K$^+$ channel gating. *Neuron* 1998;20:1283–1294.

212. Zagotta WN, Hoshi T, Aldrich RW. *Shaker* potassium channel gating, III: evaluation of kinetic models for activation. *J Gen Physiol* 1994;103:321–362.

213. Serrano JR, Perez-Reyes E, Jones SW. State-dependent inactivation of the α_{1G} T-type calcium channel. *J Gen Physiol* 1999;114:185–201.

214. Frazier CJ, Serrano JR, George EG, et al. Gating kinetics of the α_{1I} T-type calcium channel. *J Gen Physiol* 2001;118:457–470.

215. Shirokov R, Levis R, Shirokova N, et al. Two classes of gating current from L-type Ca channels in guinea pig ventricular myocytes. *J Gen Physiol* 1992;99:863–895.

216. Breitwieser GE, Szabo G. Mechanism of muscarinic receptor-induced K$^+$ channel activation as revealed by hydrolysis-resistant GTP analogues. *J Gen Physiol* 1988;91:469–493.

217. Frace AM, Mery P-F, Fischmeister R, et al. Rate-limiting steps in the β-adrenergic stimulation of cardiac calcium current. *J Gen Physiol* 1993;101:337–353.

218. Hartzell HC. Distribution of muscarinic acetylcholine receptors and presynaptic nerve terminals in amphibian heart. *J Cell Biol* 1980;86:6–20.

219. Andrade R, Malenka RC, Nicoll RA. A G protein couples serotonin and GABA$_B$ receptors to the same channels in hippocampus. *Science* 1986;234:1261–1265.

220. Bean BP. Neurotransmitter inhibition of neuronal calcium currents by changes in channel voltage dependence. *Nature* 1989;340:153–156.

221. Elmslie KS, Zhou W, Jones SW. LHRH and GTP-γ-S modify calcium current activation in bullfrog sympathetic neurons. *Neuron* 1990;5:75–80.

222. Ulrich D, Huguenard JR. γ-Aminobutyric acid type B receptor-dependent burst-firing in thalamic neurons: a dynamic clamp study. *Proc Natl Acad Sci U S A* 1996;93:13245–13249.

223. Brody DL, Patil PG, Mulle JG, et al. Bursts of action potential waveforms relieve G-protein inhibition of recombinant P/Q-type Ca^{2+} channels in HEK 293 cells. *J Physiol* 1997;499:637–644.

224. Doyle JL, Stubbs L. Ataxia, arrhythmia and ion-channel gene defects. *Trends Genet* 1998;14:92–98.

225. Lehmann-Horn F, Jurkat-Rott K. Voltage-gated ion channels and hereditary disease. *Physiol Rev* 1999;79:1317–1372.

226. Sanguinetti MC, Spector PS. Potassium channelopathies. *Neuropharmacology* 1997;36:755–762.

227. Benatar M. Neurological potassium channelopathies. *Q J Med* 2000;93:787–797.

228. Lerche H, Jurkat-Rott K, Lehmann-Horn F. Ion channels and epilepsy. *Am J Med Genet* 2001;106:146–159.

229. Kullmann DM. The neuronal channelopathies. *Brain* 2002;125:1177–1195.

230. Pietrobon D. Calcium channels and channelopathies of the central nervous system. *Mol Neurobiol* 2002;25:31–50.

231. Cannon SC. Sodium channel defects in myotonia and periodic paralysis. *Annu Rev Neurosci* 1996;19:141–164.

232. Kirsch GE. Ion channel defects in cardiac arrhythmia. *J Membr Biol* 1999;170:181–190.

233. Marban E. Cardiac channelopathies. *Nature* 2002;415:213–218.

234. Navarro B, Kennedy ME, Velimirovic B, et al. Nonselective and Gβγ-insensitive *weaver* K$^+$ channels. *Science* 1996;272:1950–1953.

235. Lorenzon NM, Lutz CM, Frankel WN, et al. Altered calcium channel currents in Purkinje cells of the neurological mutant mouse leaner. *J Neurosci* 1998;18:4482–4489.

236. Felix R. Insights from mouse models of absence epilepsy into Ca^{2+} channel physiology and disease etiology. *Cell Mol Neurobiol* 2002;22:103–120.

237. Browne DL, Gancher ST, Nutt JG, et al. Episodic ataxia/myokymia syndrome is associated with point mutations in the human potassium channel gene, KCNA1. *Nat Genet* 1994;8:136–140.

238. Zerr P, Adelman JP, Maylie J. Episodic ataxia mutations in Kv1.1 alter potassium channel function by dominant negative effects or haploinsufficiency. *J Neurosci* 1998;18:2842–2848.

239. Rea R, Spauschus A, Eunson LH, et al. Variable K$^+$ channel subunit dysfunction in inherited mutations of KCNA1. *J Physiol* 2002;538:5–23.

240. Smart SL, Lopantsev V, Zhang CL, et al. Deletion of the Kv1.1 potassium channel causes epilepsy in mice. *Neuron* 1998;20:809–819.

241. Herson PS, Virk M, Rustay NR, et al. A mouse model of episodic ataxia type-1. *Nat Neurosci* 2003;6:378–383.

242. Singh NA, Charlier C, Stauffer D, et al. A novel potassium channel gene, KCNQ2, is mutated in an inherited epilepsy of newborns. *Nat Genet* 1998;18:25–29.

243. Charlier C, Singh NA, Ryan SG, et al. A pore mutation in a novel KQT-like potassium channel gene in an idiopathic epilepsy family. *Nat Genet* 1998;18:53–55.

244. Schroeder BC, Kubisch C, Stein V, et al. Moderate loss of function of cyclic-AMP-modulated KCNQ2/KCNQ3 K$^+$ channels causes epilepsy. *Nature* 1998;396:687–690.

245. Kubisch C, Schroeder BC, Friedrich T, et al. KCNQ4, a novel potassium channel expressed in sensory outer hair cells, is mutated in dominant deafness. *Cell* 1999;96:437–446.

246. Fletcher CF, Copeland NG, Jenkins NA. Genetic analysis of voltage-dependent calcium channels. *J Bioenerg Biomembr* 1998;30:387–398.

247. Ophoff RA, Terwindt GM, Frants RR, et al. P/Q-type Ca^{2+} channel defects in migraine, ataxia and epilepsy. *Trends Pharmacol Sci* 1998;19:121–127.

248. Jen J. Calcium channelopathies in the central nervous system. *Curr Opin Neurobiol* 1999;9:274–280.

249. Kraus RL, Sinnegger MJ, Glossmann H, et al. Familial hemiplegic migraine mutations change α_{1A} Ca^{2+} channel kinetics. *J Biol Chem* 1998;273:5586–5590.

250. Hans M, Luvisetto S, Williams ME, et al. Functional consequences of mutations in the human α_{1A} calcium channel subunit linked to familial hemiplegic migraine. *J Neurosci* 1999;19:1610–1619.

251. Tottene A, Fellin T, Pagnutti S, et al. Familial hemiplegic migraine mutations increase Ca^{2+} influx through single human Ca$_V$2.1 channels and decrease maximal Ca$_V$2.1 current density in neurons. *Proc Natl Acad Sci U S A* 2002;99:13284–13289.

252. Wappl E, Koschak A, Poteser M, et al. Functional consequences of P/Q-type Ca^{2+} channel Ca$_V$2.1 missense mutations associated with episodic ataxia type 2 and progressive ataxia. *J Biol Chem* 2002;277:6960–6966.

253. Guida S, Trettel F, Pagnutti S, et al. Complete loss of P/Q calcium channel activity caused by a CACNA1A missense mutation carried by patients with episodic ataxia type 2. *Am J Hum Genet* 2001;68:759–764.

254. Denier C, Ducros A, Durr A, et al. Missense CACNA1A mutation causing episodic ataxia type 2. *Arch Neurol* 2001;58:292–295.

255. Zhuchenko O, Bailey J, Bonnen P, et al. Autosomal dominant cerebellar ataxia (SCA6) associated with small polyglutamine expansions in the α_{1A}-voltage-dependent calcium channel. *Nat Genet* 1997;15:62–69.

256. Jouvenceau A, Eunson LH, Spauschus A, et al. Human epilepsy associated with dysfunction of the brain P/Q-type calcium channel. *Lancet* 2001;358:801–807.

Mechanisms of Epileptogenesis and Experimental Models of Seizures

6

Imad Najm   Gabriel Möddel   Damir Janigro

The term *epileptogenesis* refers to abnormal firing of neurons sufficient to produce episodic epileptiform electrophysiologic activity that is detected as electroencephalographic (EEG) seizure activity with or without clinical manifestations. Such electric discharges may start in small neuronal populations (focal epilepsy), or in the entire brain simultaneously (generalized epilepsy). These epilepsies may be congenital or acquired.

The availability of resected focal epileptic tissue from patients with medically intractable focal epilepsy and the development and characterization of animal models for various types of epilepsies have enabled a better understanding of some of the cellular and electrophysiologic mechanisms of epileptogenesis. At the single cell or local circuitry levels, *in vitro* models of hyperexcitability/synchronization have provided additional insight into the various mechanisms of epileptogenicity.

Multiple factors contribute to the expression of epileptogenesis, such as intracellular, intrinsic membrane, and extracellular mechanisms. Based on animal data, Prince and Connors (1) hypothesized that three key elements contribute to the hyperexcitability needed for the expression of epileptogenesis: (a) the capability of membranes in pacemaker neurons to develop intrinsic burst discharges; (b) reduction of γ-aminobutyric acid (GABA) inhibition; and (c) enhancement of synaptic excitation through recurrent excitatory circuits (e.g., mossy fiber sprouting in hippocampal sclerosis). Although intrinsic membrane hyperexcitability provides a substrate for epileptogenesis, circuit dynamics are more important for the expression of paroxysmal electrophysiologic tendencies. Multicellular synchronization is necessary for the EEG and behavioral seizure expression, and is critical for the expression of interictal and ictal activities, as well as for the generation of cellular paroxysmal depolarization shifts. Whereas hyperexcitability may be easily reconciled with changes in neuronal circuitry, synchronization may involve other cell types (e.g., glia) and changes in the composition and size of the extracellular space.

This chapter reviews recent findings on the cellular mechanisms of hyperexcitability and data on the mechanisms of hypersynchrony in patients with focal epilepsies. A brief review of some animal models of epilepsies and their relevance and contribution to the investigation of epileptogenicity is presented at the end of the chapter.

HYPEREXCITABILITY

Two complementary mechanisms determine neuronal excitability: intrinsic membrane properties of neurons and ratio of inhibitory versus excitatory synapses (2). Consequently, extracellular levels of membrane-permeant ions and molecules available for neurotransmission also play a role. The control of neuronal excitability thus depends on numerous factors, including gating properties and voltage-dependency of ion channels, density of functional synapses, concentrations of ions, and availability of mechanisms to clear ions and neurotransmitters from the extracellular space. Neuronal cells use a single type of signaling based on all-or-nothing action potentials. Sodium action potentials, such as those recorded in axons or cell bodies, are relatively invariant in normal tissue, and thus the shape and duration of these electrical signals do not vary significantly within the nervous system. Calcium action potentials are similarly predictable, but the underlying ionic mechanism can be rather complex, depending on the cell type, and on the topographic location within the cell. The terms *sodium action potential* and *calcium action potential* refer only to the initial (depolarizing) phase of these rapid membrane polarity changes. Although genetic or molecular alteration of I_{Na} and I_{Ca} can significantly affect neuronal firing and, ultimately, the neurophysiology of a given region, gross changes in neuronal excitability may also result by alteration of the *repolarization* phase of individual action potentials. Given these considerations, it is not surprising that agents that prolong action potential duration (typically, potassium-channel blockers such as tetraethylammonium or tetraethyl barium) are proepileptogenic, while blockers of I_{Na} and I_{Ca} are used in the pharmacotherapy of epilepsy (e.g., phenytoin, valproic acid, and ethosuximide).

The mechanisms of epilepsy and of normal brain function are interlinked. Seizures result from excessive excitation or, in the case of absence seizures, from disordered inhibition. We summarize here some of the synaptic adjustments that may underlie these proepileptogenic changes in focal epilepsies.

AMPA and NMDA Glutamate Receptors

Glutamate is an amino acid neurotransmitter that mediates synaptic excitation in a large number of synapses in the central nervous system (CNS). The postsynaptic excitation induced by glutamate release depends largely on the specific receptor stimulated, but the overall effect on population behavior depends on the cellular target of excitatory input (i.e., principal vs. interneurons). On the basis of their pharmacologic and physiologic properties, the neuronal glutamate receptors are organized into two classes: ionotropic and metabotropic. The ionotropic receptors can be divided into two subpopulations, those that respond to α-amino-3-hydroxyl-5-methyl-4-isoxazolepropionic acid (AMPA) and/or kainic acid (KA) and those that respond to N-methyl-D-aspartate (NMDA) (3,4). Excitatory transmission appears to involve actions mediated by one or more combinations of these receptors. AMPA receptor channels are responsible for fast excitatory neurotransmission by the sodium-potassium channel and coexist with NMDA receptors in all synapses (3). NMDA receptor channels display slow opening and closing kinetics, and are permeated to both sodium and calcium. At normal resting membrane potential, the channel pore is obstructed by a magnesium ion ("magnesium block"). Depolarization of the postsynaptic membrane (e.g., by activation of AMPA receptors

and subsequent sodium influx) releases the magnesium block, and NMDA channels open to Na$^+$ and Ca^{2+} entry and provide the prolonged phase of the excitatory neurotransmission (5,6).

In 1973, Bliss and Lomo (7) demonstrated that relatively brief (millisecond) bursts of high-frequency stimulation induced long-lasting changes—enhancement, hence the term *long-term potentiation* (LTP)—of postsynaptic responses in the hippocampus. Owing to the enduring nature of this response and the relatively physiologic nature of the stimuli used, it has been suggested that LTP may constitute the synaptic mechanism of learning and memory. More recently, the flip side of LTP [i.e., long-term depression (LTD)] has been described, whereby synapses are "depotentiated" or partially silenced when long-lasting (minutes), low-frequency (1 Hz) stimuli are applied. Again, the original discovery of LTD was made in the hippocampal slice preparation, but LTP and LTD have been described in a variety of CNS synapses.

Both LTP and LTD share common features and can be elicited at the same synapse. Two forms of LTP have been described in the hippocampus (8). First, a Hebbian postsynaptic NMDA receptor-dependent form is seen in the CA1 region at the Schaffer collaterals-commissural axons and CA1 pyramidal cells; to trigger this form of LTP, several concomitant factors must be present. In addition, depending on the magnitude of these factors, either LTP or LTD occurs. The whole process is initiated by increases in presynaptic calcium concentration, triggered by presynaptic excitation; release of transmitter (glutamate) ensues, and activation of postsynaptic receptors initiates changes in the target cell. The magnitude of postsynaptic changes in intracellular calcium will determine whether LTP or LTD will be induced. Of relevance activation of postsynaptic, calcium-permeant NMDA receptors is essential for either process. As the NMDA receptor channel is voltage-dependently blocked by extracellular magnesium ions, one of the essential steps in this process involves removal of Mg^{2+} blockade (6). Physiologically, this occurs with depolarization of the postsynaptic membrane. Under experimental conditions, this can also be achieved by alteration of extracellular ion concentrations (i.e., removal of magnesium from the bathing medium). Hence (a) quasi-simultaneous depolarization by post- and presynaptic terminals is required for induction and maintenance of this form of synaptic plasticity, and (b) the resulting form of plasticity (LTP or LTD) depends on changes in [Ca^{2+}]$_{in}$.

The second form of hippocampal LTP is found at the mossy fiber (axon terminal of the dentate gyrus pyramidal cells)-CA3 pyramidal cell synapses. In contrast to its CA1 counterpart, this form of synaptic plasticity does not require postsynaptic depolarization, activation of NMDA receptors, or postsynaptic changes in [Ca^{2+}]$_{in}$, but depends rather on changes in presynaptic terminals. In spite of the numerous studies of LTP and LTD in preparations as diverse as isolated cells, cultured brain slices, and acutely isolated brain slices, and biochemical/molecular studies of subcellular fragments, a compelling demonstration of the physiologic relevance of LTP or LTD is still lacking. In particular, and relevant to the neurologic-neurosurgical practitioner, it is not clear whether loss of these forms of synaptic plasticity affects cognitive brain function or formation-retention of memory. Supporting a physiologic role for LTP are studies demonstrating that posttraumatic changes in cognitive function are paralleled by loss of measurable hippocampal LTP (9,10). Interestingly, whereas LTP was affected both *in vivo* and *in vitro*, LTD was spared and could be elicited in the same cells in which LTP was lacking (9), suggesting that the underlying pathologic changes did not imply cell loss or gross impairment of synaptic transmission. A possible mechanism of selective loss of LTP may depend on the facts that induction of LTP is a saturable phenomenon and that only a certain level of potentiation can be achieved at any given synapse. It was proposed that trauma may produce a nonspecific potentiation of synapses, impeding further LTP induced by physiologic stimuli. How traumatic brain injury may potentiate synaptic transmission remains unclear, but it is possible that changes in extracellular potassium, such as those seen after traumatic brain injury (9,11), may cause sufficient depolarization of pre- and postsynaptic terminals leading to $[Ca^{2+}]_{in}$ rises comparable to those normally achieved by physiologic action potential progression through presynaptic axons. Given the consideration listed above, this hypothesis predicts that the non-Hebbian form of LTP at the mossy fiber-CA3 interface should not be affected. Because several aspects of LTP-LTD partially overlap those believed to be involved in epileptogenesis (role of NMDA receptors; synaptic rearrangement; role of $[K^+]_{out}$; posttraumatic changes in excitability; similarities between kindling and LTP), it is possible that excessive LTP (or LTD?) may play a role in seizure disorders.

NMDA receptors are unique among glutamate receptors because of their voltage dependence and high permeability to Ca^{2+}. Molecular studies show that the NMDA receptor is composed of subunits from two gene families designated NR1 and NR2 (12–15). There are four NR2 gene products (NR2A-D) and a single NR1 gene product that can be expressed in eight different splice variants, which arise from different combinations of a single 5-prime terminal exon insertion or two 3-prime exons deletion (13,16). The NR1 subunits form a functional multimeric channel and show all the characteristic properties of an NMDA receptor (14). In contrast to NR1, members of the NR2 family expressed by themselves, or in combination with other NR2 members, never yield functional channels. However, the combined expression of individual NR2 subunits with NR1 markedly potentiates channel opening and current responses to NMDA or glutamate (14). All of these *in vitro* studies suggest that, at individual NMDA receptor channels, NR1 subunits serve as the general component of NMDA receptors and are essential for receptor function

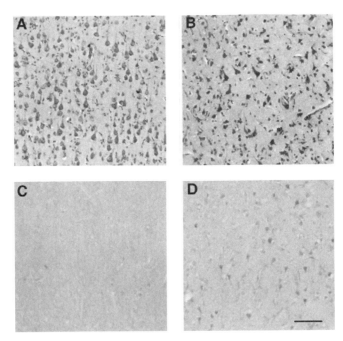

Figure 6.1 High-magnification photomicrographs of layers 3 to 5 from the superior frontal gyrus of a patient with intractable seizures arising from the same region (as confirmed by extraoperative prolonged subdural electrocorticographic recordings) showing two adjacent sections from EEG nonactive area (**A** and **C**) and two other adjacent sections from ictal EEG onset area (**B** and **D**). Note the CV darkly stained dysplastic neurons with various cellular and dendritic orientations and lack of normal columnar and horizontal lamination patterns (**B**) as compared to a section from an EEG non-active area (**A**) where the neurons are less darkly stained, show a much better lamination pattern, and do not exhibit extensive dendritic branching. Note the intensity and the distribution of NR2 A/B ICC staining (**D**) in an EEG active area (ictal EEG onset) as compared to the almost absent staining in a non-EEG active area (**C**). Scale bar: 120 μm.

and that NR2 subunits potentiate the channel activities to yield an increased ionic current.

Owing to the powerful influence of glutamatergic neurotransmission and the quasi-ubiquitous expression of glutamate receptors in the mammalian brain, it has been proposed that glutamatergic neurotransmission may play an important role in the pathogenesis of a variety of CNS disorders such as ischemic insults, neurodegenerative diseases, and epilepsy (17–20). Because acute activation of NMDA receptors plays a role in the neuronal cell loss seen in some forms of focal epilepsy (e.g., mesial temporal lobe epilepsy as a result of hippocampal sclerosis), what could be the link between epileptogenesis and glutamate receptors?

The cellular mechanisms underlying epileptogenicity in cortical dysplasia, particularly the role of AMPA/NMDA receptors in seizure expression, was investigated in dysplastic cortex resected from patients suffering from medically intractable epilepsy. A correlation was found between cytoarchitectural abnormalities and specific NMDA (NR1 and NR2A/B) and AMPA (GluR2-3) receptor subunits (21). These studies offered indirect evidence of a differential expression of some NMDA/AMPA receptor subunits in dysplastic neurons. The degree of NR1 and NR2A/B receptor expression in focal epileptogenicity has been assayed (22). The densities of NR2A/B, but not NR1, subunits are higher in resected cortical areas with EEG-proven epileptogenicity as compared to neighboring nonepileptic cortex (Fig. 6.1). The NR2 subunit is colocalized with NR1 protein expression, providing evidence of a potential functional substrate for a hyperexcitable NMDA receptor. Moreover, recent evidence suggests a differential expression of the NR1-NR2B receptor complex in the postsynaptic region in epileptic dysplastic tissue increased association of the NR1-NR2b complex with the postsynaptic density protein PSD-95 (23).

In patients with temporal lobe epilepsy caused by hippocampal sclerosis, AMPA receptors are denser in both the internal and external molecular layers of the fascia dentata than in normal fascia dentata (24). The cause(s) of increases in AMPA receptor densities in human epilepsy are unknown; the increases may be a result of mossy fiber synapse ingrowth or may precede the sprouting.

Metabotropic Glutamate Receptors

Metabotropic glutamate receptors (mGluRs) are second-messenger–coupled receptors that have diverse effects on the cellular and synaptic properties of nerve cells. Recent evidence suggests that mGluRs may play a role in the production of neuronal plasticity and epilepsy (25–27). The activation of mGluRs on astrocytes induces the release of glutamate through a calcium-dependent process, which reveals a pathway of regulated transmitter release from astrocytes and outlines the existence of an integrated glutamatergic crosstalk between neurons and astrocytes *in situ* that may play a critical role in epileptogenicity (28–30).

The mGluRs include at least eight receptor subtypes. These subtypes are grouped into three subclasses based on similarities in amino acid sequences, signal transduction mechanisms, and agonist selectivities (31). Various studies show evidence that activation of mGluR I subtype has proconvulsant effects and that activation of mGluR II and III subtypes results in anticonvulsant actions (25–27). Although the marked effects of mGluRs group I on epileptiform activity have been demonstrated experimentally, the relevance of these observations to seizure generation and epileptogenesis requires further studies in both animal models of seizures and epileptic human tissue.

GABA Receptors

In general, activation of the GABAergic system causes neuronal inhibition and prevents epileptiform activity. The GABA receptors are divided into two subtypes: $GABA_A$ and $GABA_B$.

$GABA_A$

In the CNS, the mature $GABA_A$ receptors are responsible for fast synaptic inhibition. Activation of the $GABA_A$ receptor opens a chloride channel, causing hyperpolarizing potentials. The abundance of excitatory synapses is paralleled by an impressive array of inhibitory cell-to-cell contacts. At least in cortical structures, inhibitory neurotransmission is mediated predominantly by the amino acid GABA release by different classes of interneurons on strategically localized postsynaptic structures. Thus, inhibitory inputs are found at the axodendritic, axosomatic, and even axoaxonic segments (32). Although most excitatory neurotransmission is meant to link relatively distant regions, most of the interneuronal networks belong to the so-called local circuitry (2). In neocortical and hippocampal structures of primates and rodents, the relatively repetitive morphologic appearance of principal cells differs from the cellular, morphologic, and structural diversity of GABAergic interneurons (32). In addition to modulating inhibition, GABA may act as a trophic factor (33) and excitatory neurotransmitter during early brain prenatal development.

The excitatory activity is related to the fact that resting membrane potentials are more negative than the average $GABA_A$ reversal potential (that is more positive during embryonic and early postnatal periods) (34–37). The GABA potential results in the depolarization of the cell, leading to the activation of the voltage-gated calcium channels with increased Ca^{2+} in immature neurons (37–39). The depolarizing effects of GABA-receptor activation have been reported in immature cells from a number of brain regions, including the neocortex (37,40) and hippocampus (34–36,41). These results suggest that depolarizing GABA-mediated synaptic activity may act synergistically with NMDA receptor activation by providing the depolarization necessary to relieve the Mg^{2+} block of the NMDA channel. The presence of this synergistic effect during the early postnatal period and/or its persistence during the late postnatal period may provide a synaptic substrate for the neuronal hyperexcitability seen in early life or later-onset epileptogenicity. Age-dependent predisposition to epilepsy results in a variety of pediatric neurologic conditions associated with seizures, which may influence or determine the appearance of epileptic disorders later in life. Maturational changes in neurotransmitter and channel function should be taken into account in the process of identification of the cellular mechanisms of seizure initiation.

Considerable evidence suggests that impaired GABA function can cause seizures and may be implicated in some types of epilepsies. Altered $GABA_A$ receptor function may contribute to inherited or acquired epilepsies. Epilepsy may result from genetic predisposition that leads to a decrease in GABA-mediated inhibition (42). Recent studies on tissue resected from patients with mesial temporal lobe and neocortical epilepsy showed reductions in the $GABA_A$ receptors (43–46). These results are discordant with those of other studies on human hippocampi resected from patients with temporal lobe epilepsy, which showed that GABA neurons are relatively preserved and their axons sprout into the supragranular layer for aberrant innervation of the fascia dentata (47). Moreover, the postsynaptic GABA receptor protein densities were increased throughout the extent of the fascia dentata molecular layer as compared to normal controls (47).

GABA$_B$

GABA$_B$ is a G-protein–coupled receptor that can open potassium or close calcium channels (48,49). GABA$_B$ receptors are presynaptic or postsynaptic. GABA$_B$-receptor activation may result in different effects depending on location. Activation of the GABA$_B$-receptor–linked potassium channels results in prolonged hyperpolarization and leads to postsynaptic inhibition. On the other hand, the long duration of the GABA$_B$-mediated potentials may be responsible for some epileptic effects, as GABA$_B$ agonists, such as baclofen, are reported to exacerbate the spike-wave discharges in generalized epilepsies. Absence seizures are believed to be generated by the interaction between the T-type (transient) calcium current (T-current), the GABA$_B$-induced hyperpolarization, and the intrinsic bursting activities of the relay cells (50).

Acetylcholine Receptors

Cholinergic inputs may help trigger epileptiform activity. Studies show that cholinergic agonists such as pilocarpine can cause severe seizures in animals. These seizures may progress into status epilepticus (SE) and produce permanent neuronal loss and synaptic reorganization (51). The possible role of the acetylcholine receptor was illustrated by the description of an Australian family in which a missense mutation in one subunit of brain acetylcholine receptor is associated with nocturnal frontal lobe epilepsy (52,53).

Adenosine Receptors

Adenosine is an endogenous neuromodulator that generally has inhibitory effects on brain function. One of the most important actions of the adenosine receptor (mainly the A1 receptor) is a reduction in excitatory transmission and in postsynaptic excitability. During seizures, brain adenosine concentrations rise markedly. This increase may play a role in the termination of seizures and may lead to the postictal depression of neural activity (54).

HYPERSYNCHRONY

The alteration of physiologic mechanisms of neuronal communication may mediate synchronization of neuronal activity leading to proepileptic conditions. One of the most important issues in epilepsy is to understand the mechanisms underlying the hypersynchrony and the possible role(s) of hypersynchronization between various neuronal populations in increased seizure susceptibility in patients with epilepsy.

Chemical synapses are implicated in the hyperexcitability and hypersynchrony during seizure activity: blockade of inhibitory circuits induces paroxysmal depolarization shifts. Recurrent synaptic excitation is usually masked by recurrent inhibition (55). The recurrent inhibition may be compromised under pathologic conditions, leading to multisynaptic excitatory-induced synchronization of neurons and to the generation of prolonged bursts and afterdischarges (55). Although chemical synapses contribute to synchronization of cortical neurons during seizures, nonsynaptic mechanisms can synchronize hippocampal neurons when chemical synapses are inoperative.

Role of Chemical and Electrical Interactions

Recurrent excitation between pyramidal cells is a fundamental mechanism of synchronization. Previous work suggested that the paroxysmal depolarization shifts generated when synaptic inhibitory mechanisms are inhibited (penicillin and picrotoxin models) are caused by intense synaptic excitation that probably arises, at least in part, from the interconnections of the pyramidal cells (56). The role of collateral or recurrent excitation may be less important in the hippocampus, as previous work showed that only 8% of the pyramidal cells in CA3 had recurrent local axonal excitation (57).

Electrical interactions between neurons have been extensively studied, but their role(s) in the synchronization of epileptic events remains controversial. Two possible mechanisms for neuronal synchronization are considered: electrotonic coupling of cortical neurons through the intermembranous channels (gap junctions) and current flow through the extracellular space that creates electrical field effects and may synchronize hippocampal pyramidal cells ("ephaptic interactions") (55).

Role of Changes in Extracellular Space and Ion Concentrations

Reductions in extracellular space induce seizure-like activity that is independent of chemical synaptic mechanisms (57–59). Treatment with furosemide that blocks activity-induced cell swelling and a decrease in extracellular space desynchronizes neuronal activity in a variety of seizure models (60). The repetitive synaptic activation of cortical neurons and the intense synchronous activity during epileptic events are associated with an increase in extracellular potassium and a decrease in extracellular calcium. Increased $[K^+]_o$ induces interictal spikes in the CA3 region that leads to seizure activity in CA1 area (61). On the other hand, decreases in $[Ca^{2+}]_o$ increases membrane excitability. Simultaneous occurrence of these two phenomena significantly increases seizure susceptibility in the hippocampus (62,63).

Role of Glial Cells in Epileptogenicity

There is growing evidence that a failure in glial protective mechanisms may signal the ictal transformation and

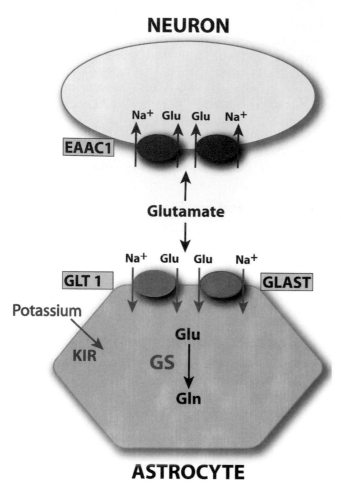

Figure 6.2 Clearance mechanisms of glutamate and the role of glial cells in the regulation of epileptogenicity. EAAC1, neuronal specific excitatory amino acid transporter; Glu, glutamate; GLT1, glial glutamate transporter; GLAST, glial glutamate transporter; GS, glutamine synthethase; KIR, potassium inward rectifier.

secondary generalization of a focal discharge (64,65). As Figure 6.2 illustrates, glial cells are involved in various interactive roles with the closely adjacent neuronal populations: (a) Glia play a role in synaptic neurotransmission through the expression of glial glutamate receptors, uptake of excitatory neurotransmitters (glutamate transporters, GLT-1) (66), and release of facilitatory substances (65); (b) the presence of gap junctions between mature glial cells enables the voltage to spread over 100 μm through the Ca^{2+} (67,68) and/or K^+ fluxes. Adenosine triphosphate (ATP) may also spread between cells. Moreover, there may be direct gap junction connection between glial cells and neurons (69); (c) release of glutamate by glia (27–29,70); and (d) the active K^+ uptake by glia after the significant increase in extracellular K^+ concentrations during neuronal activation.

CNS astrocytes are strategically located in proximity to excitable neurons and are sensitive to changes in extracellular ion composition that follow neuronal activity (71–75). Several lines of evidence suggest that brain glial cells support the homeostatic regulation of the neuronal

microenvironment. In cortical regions, glial cells participate in the genesis of the extracellular field potential changes associated with neuronal depolarization and efflux of potassium in the extracellular space. Neuronal excitability is regulated by a complex interaction of excitatory and inhibitory potentials. In pyramidal neurons, depolarizing ion conductances involved in action potential generation are regulated primarily by the voltage-dependent activation/inactivation properties of Na^+ and Ca^{2+} channels; in addition, inward Na^+ and Ca^{2+} currents underlie the generation of excitatory postsynaptic potentials (EPSPs). Termination of these depolarizing potentials occurs by the voltage- and calcium-dependent activation of intrinsic potassium conductances, and by activation of interneurons that release inhibitory neurotransmitters to produce inhibitory postsynaptic potentials (IPSPs); the latter are mediated by postsynaptic activation of chloride and potassium currents. Although I_{Na}, I_{Ca}, and I_{EPSP} are, under physiologic conditions, relatively independent of modest changes in the driving force for the permeant ions (because E_{Na} and E_{Ca} are remote with respect to cell resting potential), both repolarizing potassium and IPSP conductances are critically affected by even modest changes in cell resting membrane potential (RMP), $[K^+]_o$, and $[Cl]_i/[Cl]_o$. Because neuronal RMP depends significantly, albeit not exclusively, on $[K^+]_o$, the maintenance of homeostatic control for extracellular potassium plays a crucial role in the regulation of neuronal firing. The concentration of potassium in the extracellular space (K_{ecs}) in the mammalian CNS increases measurably (from 3 to about 4 mM) during physiologic stimulation; to a larger extent (up to 12 mM) during seizures or direct, synchronous stimulation of afferent pathways; and to exceedingly high values (>30 mM) during anoxia or spreading depression. In spite of these rapid and large changes in K_{ecs}, K^+ values return to normal levels in a relatively short time.

Several mechanisms have been suggested to explain the rapid clearance of K^+ from the extracellular space, including uptake by glia, passive diffusion, and neuronal reuptake. Experiments have suggested that glial uptake plays a pivotal role under conditions in which there is massive K_{out} accumulation. $[K]_{out}$ can also be redistributed through active removal by blood flow or by passive diffusion through the extracellular space; however, these mechanisms alone are not fast enough to account for rapid K^+ removal from the extracellular space seen under experimental conditions. The combination of potassium uptake into glial cells immediately followed by redistribution through electronically coupled glial gap junctions ("spatial buffering") provides a valid working hypothesis to explain some of the features of K^+ movements in the extracellular space.

Potassium ions play a fundamental role in the control of neuronal excitability. Action potential repolarization is curtailed by increased $[K^+]_{out}$, and elevated potassium causes a dramatic decrease of some inhibitory potentials. The most direct effect of elevated extracellular potassium,

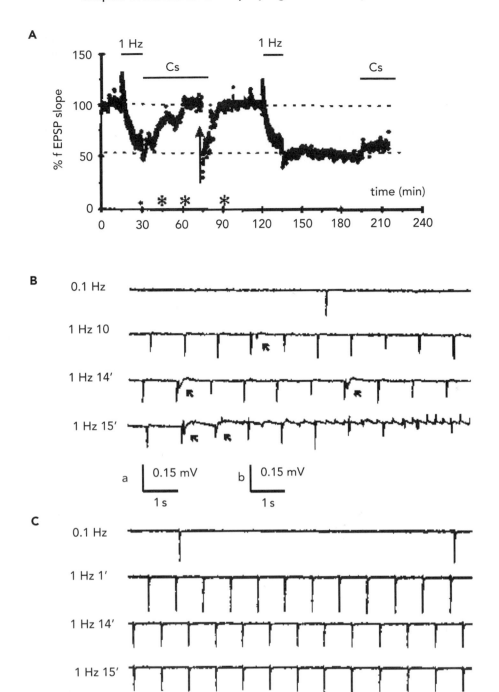

Figure 6.3 Blockade of glial potassium uptake by Cs^+ affects neuronal plasticity (long-term depression) and excitability synchronization. **A:** Cesium prevents maintenance of LTD. LTD was induced by orthodromic stimulation of the Schaffer collaterals at 1 Hz for 15 minutes. Field excitatory postsynaptic potentials (fEPSPs) were evoked and recorded by the extracellular pipette. Note the marked decrease in the fEPSP slope that occurred during 1 Hz stimulation **(A)**. At the end of the first 15 minutes of 1-Hz stimulation, cesium was added to the bath solution. This procedure reduced the synaptic depression. Note that the effects of cesium on spontaneous activity were not reversed by cesium washout. Following washout of cesium, LTD could be induced and maintained in the same slice. Cesium application following LTD induction effectively reduced the synaptic depression only if cesium actions were time-locked to LTD. Application of cesium 1 hour following LTD failed to induce any significant change in LTD maintenance or cause neuronal synchronization. The lack of effect was not because of the shorter exposure time to cesium, as similar results were obtained following prolonged perfusions. **B:** The effects of cesium are not mediated by neuronal currents because the neuronal blocker Zeneca ZD7288 fails to reproduce cesium actions. The effects on field potentials of cesium and Zeneca ZD7288 applications paired to 1-Hz stimulation were as follows: At low (0.1-Hz) stimulation frequency, cesium 3 mM failed to induce any effects on the evoked fEPSP even after prolonged perfusion (*top trace,* 15 minutes following Cs^{2+} 0.1-Hz stimuli). Similarly, brief episodes of stimulation at 1 Hz also left the fEPSP response unchanged. However, following protracted (10 minutes) exposure to cesium while stimulating at 1 Hz, afterdischarge activity became evident (*arrows*). The latter outlasted the wash out of cesium (not shown). **C:** In contrast to cesium, the neuronal I_h-specific blocker Zeneca ZD7288 (10 μM) did not cause the insurgence of spontaneous afterdischarge-like activity during 15 minutes of orthodromic stimulation used to elicit LTD. (Reproduced from Janigro D, Gasparini S, D'Ambrosio R, McKhann GM, DiFrancesco D. Reduction of K+ uptake in glia prevents LTD maintenance and causes epileptiform activity. *J Neuroscience* 1997;17:2813–2824, with permission.)

however, consists of its direct depolarizing effects on neurons and neuronal terminals. Experimentally, synaptic changes normally obtained by direct stimulation of presynaptic fibers (e.g., LTP) can be mimicked by small increases in potassium, while synchronous firing of thousands of cortical or hippocampal pyramidal cells is observed when $[K^+]_{out}$ is slightly elevated. The latter is commonly referred to as potassium-induced epileptogenesis (76,77). During low-frequency, unstimulated, asynchronous neuronal activity, potassium buildup is buffered independently from glial depolarizations (78). However, electrical stimulation at frequencies as low as 0.2 Hz is sufficient to cause glial depolarizations in the hippocampus. These depolarizing responses are concomitant with increased $[K^+]_{in}$ in glial cells resulting from uptake from the extracellular space (79) aimed at reestablishing physiologic $[K^+]_{out}$. When these homeostatic mechanisms fail, abnormal accumulation of potassium occurs, resulting in neuronal synchronous burst firing (Fig. 6.3) (11,80,81).

In summary, glial cells may play important roles in the expression of epileptogenicity through different mechanisms in different types of focal epilepsies (e.g., hippocampal sclerosis, cortical dysplasia, tumor, or vascular malformation-induced focal epilepsies). Increased glial cell connectivity through gap junctions and/or dysfunction through the loss of their buffering capacity or glutamate clearance may facilitate hypersynchrony. Moreover, an increased glial response may lead to an increased release of glutamate in the synaptic regions. Further work is still needed to clarify these issues.

ANIMAL MODELS OF EPILEPSY

Experimental models of seizures are an essential part of research into the pathophysiology of epilepsy and epileptic seizures. Epileptic animal models are generally used (a) to investigate neural physiology, (b) to screen new potential antiepileptic drugs, and (c) to investigate putative basic mechanisms of human epilepsy. In this chapter, we limit our discussion to the most widely used animal models. We briefly describe these potentially valuable models for the investigation of epileptogenesis and its molecular and electrophysiologic substrates.

Kainic Acid-Induced Seizures

KA injection (parenteral or intracerebral)-induced SE eventually represents a model of acute and chronic experimentally induced epilepsy (reactive seizures) (82). It is a model for focal seizures that arise from the limbic lobe. KA is a potent neurotoxic agent that mainly stimulates a subtype of the excitatory glutamate receptors and leads to a cascade of electrical, behavioral, and histopathologic changes in the rat brain (83–87). The areas commonly affected by KA-induced SE include the hippocampus, entorhinal cortex, and amygdala (83–87). The histopathologic lesions after both focal and systemic KA administration resemble the hippocampal sclerosis often found in patients with complex partial seizures of temporal lobe origin (88,89). Animals commonly used for KA injection include rats and mice.

Treatment with *cycloheximide*, a protein synthesis inhibitor, before KA injection significantly protects against seizure-induced neuronal damage without affecting the behavioral or electrical seizures (90,91). This model has been used to identify specific markers of prolonged seizures and seizure-induced cell damage (91).

Pilocarpine Model

Pilocarpine is used in another model of temporal lobe epilepsy or SE, and in a model of chronic epileptogenesis (92). After SE and a latent period that may last between 2 and 3 weeks, spontaneous recurrent seizures appear (93). Pilocarpine treatment in rats leads to seizures and cell losses of varying degrees in the hilus of the hippocampus and CA3 region (94). However, with higher doses of pilocarpine and associated increase in the severity and duration of the initial induced seizure episode, substantial neuronal loss occurs also in the CA1 subfield (95).

Bicuculline-Induced Seizures

The bicuculline-induced SE model was among the first experimental epilepsy models to be used for the assessment of magnetic resonance spectroscopy changes associated with seizures. It serves as a model of acute partial epilepsy. Bicuculline is a convulsant alkaloid that acts as a postsynaptic GABA$_A$-receptor antagonist and induces severe and long-lasting tonic-clonic seizures following either intravenous or intraperitoneal injections in paralyzed and ventilated animals (96,97). These seizures are associated with diffuse neuropathologic changes that predominantly involve the outer cortical layers (I–III) and CA1 area of the hippocampus (97). This model is used in dogs, rabbits, and rats.

Electroshock Model

Maximal electroshock-induced seizure is a model of acute generalized SE (98) and is commonly used for screening potential antiepileptic drugs. A brief electrical stimulation (about 10 milliseconds) induces a generalized tonic-clonic seizure of short duration.

Kindling Model

Amygdaloid and hippocampal kindling are used in a model of chronic partial seizures and have been well studied for limbic seizures in both rats and cats. Kindling is a phenomenon in which brief afterdischarges evoked by initially periodic subconvulsive electrical stimulations produce limbic and clonic motor seizures of progressively increasing severity. Once present, the enhanced sensitivity to electrical stimulation is lifelong.

The kindling phenomenon is a manifestation of the fact that "epilepsy induces epilepsy." It is one of the most popular models for the study of long-term plastic changes in brain excitability believed to participate in epileptogenesis and in learning and memory (99,100). Although there is some evidence for neuronal degeneration in the region of the mirror focus, morphologic damage has been difficult to document in kindled animals (101).

Penicillin Model

The focal cortical administration of penicillin to induce seizures is a model of acute partial (focal) epilepsy. It has been extensively used to study ictal and interictal electrical changes and the susceptibility of various brain areas to epileptogenesis secondary to the local application of penicillin, a specific blocker of postsynaptic $GABA_A$ receptors. However, whether any chronic pathologic changes are caused by local penicillin application is unknown (101,102). The intramuscular administration of penicillin in cats leads to generalized synchronous spike-wave discharges associated with staring, eye blinking, and myoclonus (103–106). This model is exacerbated by pentylenetetrazol and photic stimulation (107,108).

Aluminum Hydroxide Model

The aluminum hydroxide model of either simple motor (cortical application) (109) or limbic (hippocampal application) (110) seizures is one of the most validated models in monkeys. This model produces different pathologic changes; that is, there is severe necrosis at the injection site and a large granuloma walling off the alumina in cortical or hippocampal foci (101,102,110).

Pentylenetetrazol-Induced Seizures

Pentylenetetrazol or metrazol is a convulsant agent classified as a GABA antagonist, but it does not seem to act as a GABA receptor blocker (111,112). The parenteral administration of a large dose leads to a short episode of generalized tonic-clonic seizure in rats, with no subsequent significant histologic damage. This model represents a good means for the identification of possible specific changes associated with the seizure phenomenon.

Animal Models of Cortical Dysplasias

Over the past 10 years, there has been an increase in the number of patients diagnosed and operated on for medically refractory focal epilepsy. However, the postsurgical seizure-free outcome in these patients is still less favorable than in those patients with hippocampal sclerosis or tumor-induced epilepsy. Consequently, increased research efforts have been directed at better understanding the pathophysiology of seizures and the preoperative delineation of the area of epileptogenicity. To date, several animal models of genetic and induced focal cortical dysplasias have been described, including the tish mutant model, the reeler model, Ihara mutant rats (113), focal cold (freeze) injury model (114–116), the *in utero* treatment with an alkylating agent model (117–119), and the *in utero* radiation-induced model (120).

The freeze lesion model mimics the human layered microgyria (121). These lesions are characterized by dysmorphic neurons in the areas immediately adjacent to the lesion (122). The *in utero* methylazoxymethanol and irradiation models are characterized by histopathologic changes that are similar to those observed in some forms of human cortical dysplasias. These changes consist of partial or complete absence of the corpus callosum and multifocal cortical and subcortical clustering of dysmorphic neurons. Recent studies of the *in utero*-radiated offspring from our group and other groups showed evidence of both *in vitro* and *in vivo* (spontaneous and drug-induced) epileptogenicity arising from both neocortical and hippocampal structures (120,123). The EEG changes in the radiated rats are correlated with multifocal neocortical and hippocampal evidence of dyslamination, neuronal dispersion, and dysmorphic cells (123). Moreover, these areas show differential expression of the NR2 B subunit of the NMDA receptor that is similar to that seen in epileptogenic tissue resected from patients with medically intractable focal epilepsy due to cortical dysplasia (12,21,22).

CONCLUSIONS

Both synaptic and nonsynaptic mechanisms have been proposed as playing critical roles in seizure generation and spread. Changes in excitatory and/or inhibitory receptors and imbalance between excitation and inhibition constitute the most important factors underlying synaptic mechanisms of epileptogenicity. On the other hand, specific changes in the extracellular space, extracellular ion concentrations, and glial cell dysfunctions are additional factors that should be considered during the investigation of epileptogenesis. A better knowledge of the molecular mechanisms of seizure susceptibility, genesis, and spread will lead to the design of specific imaging markers to directly visualize epileptogenicity, rather than the indirect identification of possible anatomic substrates. Moreover, a rational drug design of blockers to specific subunits of the excitatory amino acid receptors may provide a therapeutic action without the side effects of the nonspecific blockers. Further identification of the possible roles and molecular changes initiated by nonneuronal and extracellular mechanisms of epileptogenesis may provide new therapeutic targets to control various types of epilepsies. Unique mechanisms may underlie different types of epilepsies that may be caused by dysfunction(s) in neuronal and/or non-neuronal mechanisms. These issues need to be studied and proper therapeutic strategies tailored to address specific dysfunctions. The use of animal models together with the availability of epileptic human tissue resected from patients with medically intractable epilepsy will provide the opportunity to test various hypotheses on the mechanisms of epileptogenicity.

ACKNOWLEDGMENTS

This chapter was prepared with support from the National Institutes of Health, with grants NS-02046 and NS-42354 to Dr. Najm, and ES-07033, NS-38195, and HL-51614 to Dr. Janigro, and from the "Zentrum Für innovative medizinische Forschung" (IMF), University of Münster, Germany (scholarship MO 62020 to Dr. Möddel).

REFERENCES

1. Prince DA, Connors BW. Mechanisms of interictal epileptogenesis. *Adv Neurol* 1986;44:275–300.
2. Schwartzkroin PA. Local circuit considerations and intrinsic neuronal properties involved in hyperexcitability and cell synchronization. In: Jasper HH, van Gelder NM, eds. *Basic mechanisms in neuronal hyperexcitability*. New York: Alan R. Liss, 1983:75–108.
3. Seeburg PH. The molecular biology of mammalian glutamate receptor channels. *Trends Neurosci* 1993;16:359–365.
4. Westbrook GL. Glutamate receptor update. *Curr Opin Neurobiol* 1994;4:337–346.
5. Collingridge GL, Lester RA. Excitatory amino acid receptors in the vertebrate central nervous system. *Pharmacol Rev* 1989;40:145–165.
6. Collingridge GL, Watkins JC. *The NMDA receptor*, 2nd ed. Oxford, England: Oxford University Press, 1994.
7. Bliss TV, Lomo T. Long lasting potentiation of synaptic transmission in the dentate area of the anesthetized rabbit following stimulation of the perforant path. *J Physiol (Lond)* 1973;232: 331–356.
8. Malenka RC. Synaptic plasticity in the hippocampus: LTP and LTD. *Cell* 1994;78:535–538.
9. D'Ambrosio R, Maris DO, Grady MS, et al. Selective loss of long-term synaptic potentiation, but not depression, following fluid percussion injury. *Brain Res* 1998;786:64–79.
10. Reeves TM, Lyeth BG, Povlishock JT. Long-term potentiation deficits and excitability changes following traumatic brain injury. *Exp Brain Res* 1995;106:248–256.
11. D'Ambrosio R, Maris DO, Grady MS, et al. Impaired K homeostasis and altered electrophysiological properties of post-traumatic hippocampal glia. *J Neurosci* 1999;19:8152–8162.
12. Mikuni N, Ying Z, Babb T, et al. NMDA receptor 1 and 2A/B coassembly increases in human epileptic focal cortical dysplasia. *Epilepsia* 1999;40:1683–1687.
13. Moriyoshi K, Masu M, Ishii T, et al. Molecular cloning and characterization of the rat NMDA receptor [see comments]. *Nature* 1991;354:31–37.
14. Monyer H, Sprengel R, Schoepfer R, et al. Heteromeric NMDA receptors: molecular and functional distinction of subtypes. *Science* 1992;256:1217–1221.
15. Akazawa C, Shigemoto R, Bessho Y, et al. Differential expression of five N-methyl-D-aspartate receptor subunit mRNAs in the cerebellum of developing and adult rats. *J Comp Neurol* 1994; 347:150–160.
16. Mikuni N, Najm I, Babb TL, et al. Pre and postnatal development of NMDA receptors 1 and 2A/B subunit protein expressions in rat cortical neurons. *Epilepsia* 1998;39:23.
17. Choi DW, Rothman SM. The role of glutamate neurotoxicity in hypoxic-ischemic neuronal death. *Annu Rev Neurosci* 1990;13: 171–182.
18. Cha JH, Kosinski CM, Kerner JA, et al. Altered brain neurotransmitter receptors in transgenic mice expressing a portion of an abnormal human Huntington disease gene. *Proc Natl Acad Sci U S A* 1998;95:6480–6485.
19. He XP, Patel M, Whitney KD, et al. Glutamate receptor GluR3 antibodies and death of cortical cells. *Neuron* 1998;20:153–163.
20. Lin CL, Bristol LA, Jin L, et al. Aberrant RNA processing in a neurodegenerative disease: the cause for absent EAAT2, a glutamate transporter, in amyotrophic lateral sclerosis. *Neuron* 1998;20: 589–602.
21. Ying Z, Babb T, Comair Y, et al. Induced expression of NMDAR2 proteins and differential expression of NMDAR1 splice variants in dysplastic neurons of human epileptic neocortex. *J Neuropathol Exp Neurol* 1998;57:47–62.
22. Najm I, Ying Z, Babb T, et al. NMDA receptor 2A/B subtype differential expression in human cortical dysplasia: correlation with in situ epileptogenicity. *Epilepsia* 2000;41:971–976.
23. Ying Z, Bingaman W, Najm I. Increased numbers of coassembled PSD-95 to NMDA-receptor subunits NR2B and NR1 in human epileptic cortical dysplasia. *Epilepsia* 2004;45:314–321.
24. Babb TL, Mathern GW, Leite GP, et al. Glutamate AMPA receptors in the fascia dentata of human and kainate rat hippocampal epilepsy. *Epilepsy Res* 1996;26:193–205.
25. Cartmell J, Curtic AR, Kemp JA, et al. Subtypes of metabotropic excitatory amino acid receptor distinguished by stereoisomers of the rigid glutamate analogue, 1-aminocyclopentane-1, 3-di-carboxylate. *Neurosci Lett* 1993;153:107–110.
26. Merlin LR, Taylor GW, Wong RKS. Role of metabotropic glutamate receptor subtypes in the patterning of epileptiform activities *in vitro*. *J Neurophysiol* 1995;74:896–900.
27. Taylor GW, Merlin LR, Wong RKS. Synchronized oscillations in hippocampal CA3 neurons induced by metabotropic glutamate receptor activation. *J Neurosci* 1995;15:8039–8052.
28. Carmignoto G, Pasti L, Pozzan T. On the role of voltage-dependent calcium channels in calcium signaling of astrocytes in situ. *J Neurosci* 1998;18:4637–4645.
29. Pasti L, Pozzan T, Carmignoto G. Long-lasting changes of calcium oscillations in astrocytes. A new form of glutamate-mediated plasticity. *J Biol Chem* 1995;270:15203–15210.
30. Bezzi P, Armignoto G, Pasti L, et al. Prostaglandins stimulate calcium-dependent glutamate release in astrocytes. *Nature* 1998; 391:281–285.
31. Nakanishi S. Metabotropic glutamate receptors: synaptic transmission, modulation, and plasticity. *Neuron* 1994;13:1031–1037.
32. Morin F, Beaulieu C, Lacaille JC. Alterations of perisomatic GABA synapses on hippocampal CA1 inhibitory interneurons and pyramidal cells in the kainate model of epilepsy. *Neuroscience* 1999;93:457–467.
33. Berninger B, Marty S, Zafra F, et al. GABAergic stimulation switches from enhancing to repressing BDNF expression in rat hippocampal neurons during maturation *in vitro*. *Development* 1995;121:2327–2335.
34. Janigro D, Schwartzkroin PA. Dissociation of the IPSP and response to GABA during spreading depression-like depolarizations in hippocampal slices. *Brain Res* 1987;404:189–200.
35. Janigro D, Schwartzkroin PA. Effects of GABA and baclofen on pyramidal cells in the developing rabbit hippocampus: an "in vitro" study. *Brain Res* 1988;469:171–184.
36. Janigro D, Schwartzkroin PA. Effects of GABA on CA3 pyramidal cell dendrites in rabbit hippocampal slices. *Brain Res* 1988;453: 265–274.
37. Owens DF, Boyce LH, Davis MBE, et al. Excitatory GABA responses in embryonic and neonatal cortical slices demonstrated by gramicidin perforated patch recordings and calcium imaging. *J Neurosci* 1996;16:6414–6423.
38. Lin M-H, Takahashi MP, Takahashi Y, et al. Intracellular calcium increase induced by GABA in visual cortex of fetal and neonatal rats and its disappearance with development. *Neurosci Res* 1994;20:85–94.
39. Yutse R, Katz LC. Control of postsynaptic Ca^{++} influx in developing neocortex by excitatory and inhibitory neurotransmitters. *Neuron* 1991;6:333–344.

40. Luhman HJ, Prince DA. Postnatal maturation of the GABAergic system rat neocortex. *J Neurophysiol* 1991;65:247–263.
41. Cherubini E, Rovira C, Gaiarsa JL, et al. GABA mediated excitation in immature rat CA3 hippocampal neurons. *Int J Dev Neurosci* 1990;8:481–490.
42. Olsen RW, Avoli M. GABA and epileptogenesis. *Epilepsia* 1997; 38:399–407.
43. McDonald J, Garofalo E, Hood T, et al. Altered excitatory inhibitory amino acid receptor binding in hippocampus of patients with temporal lobe epilepsy. *Ann Neurol* 1991;29: 529–541.
44. Johnson EW, deLanorelle NC, Kim JH, et al. Central and peripheral benzodiazepine receptors: opposite changes in human epileptogenic tissue. *Neurology* 1992;42:811–815.
45. Olsen RW, Bureau M, Houser CR, et al. GABA-benzodiazepine receptors in human epilepsy. *Epilepsy Res* 1992;8(Suppl): 389–397.
46. Savic I, Roland P, Sedvall F, et al. *In vivo* demonstration of reduced benzodiazepine receptor binding in human epileptic foci. *Lancet* 1988;15:863–866.
47. Babb TL, Pretorius JK, Kupfer WR, et al. Glutamate decarboxylase-immunoreactive neurons are preserved in human epileptic hippocampus. *J Neurosci* 1989;9:2562–2574.
48. Mott DD, Lewis DV. The pharmacology and function of central GABA$_B$ receptors. *Int Rev Neurobiol* 1994;36:97–223.
49. Ogata N. Pharmacology and physiology of GABA$_B$ receptors. *Gen Pharmacol* 1990;21:395–402.
50. Crunelli V, Leresche N. A role for GABA$_B$ receptors in excitation and inhibition of thalamocortical cells. *Trends Neurosci* 1991;14: 16–21.
51. Okazaki MM, Evenson DA, Nadler JV. Hippocampal mossy fiber sprouting and synapse formation after status epilepticus in rats: visualization after retrograde transport of biocytin. *J Comp Neurol* 1995;352:515–534.
52. Steinlein OK, Mulley JC, Propping P, et al. A missense mutation in the neuronal nicotinic acetylcholine receptor alpha-4-subunit is associated with autosomal dominant nocturnal frontal lobe epilepsy. *Nat Genet* 1995;11:201–210.
53. Weiland S, Witzemann V, Villaroel A, et al. An amino acid exchange in the second transmembrane segment of a neuronal nicotinic receptor causes partial epilepsy by altering its desensitization kinetics. *FEBS Lett* 1996;398:91–96.
54. Dunwiddie TV. Adenosine and suppression of seizures. In: Delgado-Escueta AV, Wilson WA, Olsen RW, Porter RJ, eds. *Jasper's basic mechanisms of the epilepsies. Advances in neurology,* vol 79, 3rd ed. Philadelphia: Lippincott Williams & Wilkins, 1999: 1001–1010.
55. Dudek FE, Patrylo PR, Wuarin J-P. Mechanisms of neuronal synchronization during epileptiform activity. In: Delgado-Escueta AV, Wilson WA, Olsen RW, Porter RJ, eds. *Jasper's basic mechanisms of the epilepsies. Advances in neurology,* vol 79, 3rd ed. Philadelphia: Lippincott Williams & Wilkins, 1999:699–708.
56. Ayala GF, Dichter M, Gumnit RJ, et al. Genesis of epileptic interictal spikes: new knowledge of cortical feedback systems suggests a neurophysiological explanation of brief paroxysms. *Brain Res* 1973;52:1–17.
57. Dudek FE, Obenaus A, Tasker JG. Osmolality-induced changes in extracellular volume alter epileptiform bursts independent of chemical synapses in the rat: importance of non-synaptic mechanisms in hippocampal epileptogenesis. *Neurosci Lett* 1990;120: 267–270.
58. Roper SN, Obenaus A, Dudek FE. Lowered osmolality causes non-synaptic epileptiform bursts in rat dentate gyrus: a comparison with area CA1. *Ann Neurol* 1992;31:81–85.
59. Andrew RD, Fagan M, Ballyk BB, et al. Seizure susceptibility and the osmotic state. *Brain Res* 1989;498:175–180.
60. Hochman DW, Baraban SC, Owens JWM, et al. Dissociation of synchronization and excitability in furosemide blockade of epileptiform activity. *Science* 1996;270:99–102.
61. Traynelis SF, Dingledine R. Potassium-induced spontaneous electrographic seizures in the rat hippocampal slice. *J Neurophysiol* 1988;59:259–276.
62. Schweitzer JS, Patrylo RR, Dudek FE. Prolonged field bursts in the dentate gyrus: dependence on low calcium, high potassium and nonsynaptic mechanisms. *J Neurophysiol* 1992;68:2016–2025.
63. Schweitzer JS, Williamson A. Relationship between synaptic activity and prolonged field bursts in the dentate gyrus of the rat hippocampal slice. *J Neurophysiol* 1995;74:1947–1952.
64. Delgado-Escueta AV. Introduction. In: Delgado-Escueta AV, Wilson WA, Olsen RW, Porter RJ, eds. *Jasper's basic mechanisms of the epilepsies. Advances in neurology,* vol 79, 3rd ed. Philadelphia: Lippincott Williams & Wilkins, 1999:561–564.
65. Kettenmann H. Physiology of cells. In: Delgado-Escueta AV, Wilson WA, Olsen RW, Porter RJ, eds. *Jasper's basic mechanisms of the epilepsies. Advances in neurology,* vol 79, 3rd ed. Philadelphia: Lippincott Williams & Wilkins, 1999:79:565–571.
66. Tanaka K, Watase K, Manabe T, et al. Epilepsy and exacerbation of brain injury in mice lacking the glutamate transporter GLT-1. *Science* 1997;276:1699–1702.
67. Dani JW, Chernjavsky A, Smith SJ. Neuronal activity triggers calcium waves in hippocampal astrocyte networks. *Neuron* 1992;3:429–440.
68. Finkbeiner SM. Modulation and control of intracellular calcium. In: Kettenmann H, Ransom BR, eds. *Neuroglial cells.* New York: Oxford University Press, 1995:273–288.
69. Nedergaard M. Direct signaling from astrocytes to neurons in cultures of mammalian brain cells. *Science* 1994;263: 1768–1771.
70. Parpura V, Basarsky TA, Liu F, et al. Glutamate-mediated astrocyte-neuron signaling. *Nature* 1994;369:744–747.
71. Lux HD, Heinemann U, Dietzel I. Ionic changes and alterations in the size of extracellular space during epileptic activity. In: Delgado-Escueta AV, Ward AA, eds. *Advances in neurology.* New York: Raven Press, 1986:619–639.
72. Ransom BR, Sontheimer H. The neurophysiology of glial cells. *J Clin Neurophysiol* 1992;9:224–251.
73. Ransom BR, Carlini WG. Electrophysiological properties of astrocytes. In: Fedoroff S, Vernadakis A, eds. *Astrocytes.* Orlando, FL: Academic Press, 1986:1–49.
74. Keyser DO, Pellmar TC. Synaptic transmission in the hippocampus: critical role for glial cells. *Glia* 1994;10:237–243.
75. Dietzel I, Heinemann U, Lux HD. Relations between slow extracellular potential changes, glial potassium buffering, and electrolyte and cellular volume changes during neuronal hyperactivity in cat brain. *Glia* 1989;2:25–44.
76. McBain CJ. Hippocampal inhibitory neuron activity in the elevated potassium model of epilepsy. *J Neurophysiol* 1995;72: 2853–2863.
77. Traynelis SF, Dingledine R. Potassium-induced spontaneous electrographic seizures in rat hippocampal slices. *J Neurophysiol* 1988;59:259–276.
78. Casullo J, Krnjevic K. Glial potentials in hippocampus. *Can J Physiol Pharmacol* 1987;65:847–855.
79. Ballanyi K, Grafe P, Bruggencate GT. Ion activities and potassium uptake mechanisms of glial cells of guinea-pig olfactory cortex slices. *J Physiol (Lond)* 1987;382:159–174.
80. D'Ambrosio R, Wenzel J, Schwartzkroin PA, et al. Functional specialization and topographic segregation of hippocampal astrocytes. *J Neurosci* 1998;18:1–14.
81. Janigro D, Gasparini S, D'Ambrosio R, et al. Reduction of K$^+$ uptake in glia prevents LTD maintenance and causes epileptiform activity. *J Neurosci* 1997;17:2813–2824.
82. Engel J Jr. Experimental animal models of epilepsy: classification and relevance to human epileptic phenomena. *Epilepsy Res Suppl* 1992;8:9–20.
83. Falconer MA, Serafetinides EA, Corsellis JAN. Etiology and pathogenesis of temporal lobe epilepsy. *Arch Neurol* 1964;10: 233–248.
84. Schwob JE, Fuller T, Price JL, et al. Widespread patterns of neuronal damage following systemic or intracerebral injections of kainic acid: a histological study. *Neuroscience* 1980;5:991–1014.
85. Lothman EW, Collins RC. Kainic acid induced limbic seizures: metabolic, behavioral, electroencephalographic and neuropathological correlates. *Brain Res* 1981;218:299–318.
86. Nitecka LE, Tremblay G, Charton JP, et al. Maturation of kainic acid seizure brain damage syndrome in the rat, II: histopathological sequelae. *Neuroscience* 1984;13:1073–1094.
87. Ben-Ari Y, Represa A, Tremblay E, et al. Selective and non-selective seizure related brain damage produced by kainic acid. *Adv Exp Med Biol* 1986;203:647–657.

88. Brown WJ. Structural substrate of seizures foci in the human temporal lobe. In: Brafier M, ed. *Epilepsy: its phenomenon in man.* New York: Academic Press, 1973:339–347.

89. Vinters HV, Armstrong DL, Babb TL, et al. The neuropathology of human symptomatic epilepsy. In: Engel J Jr, ed. *Surgical treatment of the epilepsies.* New York: Raven Press, 1993:593–608.

90. Schreiber SS, Tocco G, Najm I, et al. Cycloheximide prevents kainate-induced neuronal death and c-fos expression in adult rat brain. *J Mol Neurosci* 1993;4:149–159.

91. Najm I, Wang Y, Lüders H, et al. MRS metabolic markers of seizures and seizure-induced neuronal damage. *Epilepsia* 1998;39:244–250.

92. Turski WA, Cavalheiro EA, Schwartz M, et al. Limbic seizures produced by pilocarpine in rats: behavioral, electroencephalographic and neuropathological study. *Behav Brain Res* 1983;9:315–335.

93. Cavalheiro EA, Leite JP, Bartolotto ZA, et al. Long-term effects of pilocarpine in rats: structural damage of the brain triggers kindling and spontaneously recurrent seizures. *Epilepsia* 1991;32:778–782.

94. Obenaus A, Esclapez M, Houser CR. Loss of glutamate decarboxylase mRNA-containing neurons in the rat dentate gyrus following pilocarpine-induced seizures. *J Neurosci* 1993;13: 4470–4485.

95. Liu Z, Nagao T, Desjardin GC, et al. Quantitative evaluation of neuronal loss in the dorsal hippocampus in rats with long-term pilocarpine seizures. *Epilepsy Res* 1994;17:237–247.

96. Meldrum BS, Nilsson B. Cerebral blood flow and metabolic rate early and late in prolonged epileptic seizures induced in rats by bicuculline. *Brain* 1976;99:523.

97. Blennow G, Brierley JB, Meldrum BS, et al. Epileptic brain damage: the role of systemic factors that modify cerebral energy metabolism. *Brain* 1978;101:687–700.

98. Prichard JW, Petroff OAC, Ogino T, et al. Cerebral lactate elevation by electroshock: a 1H-magnetic resonance study. *Ann N Y Acad Sci* 1987;508:54.

99. Goddard GV, Douglas RM. Does the engram of kindling model the engram of long-term daily memory? *Can J Neurol Sci* 1975;2:385–394.

100. Fisher RS. Animal models of the epilepsies. *Brain Res Rev* 1989;14:245.

101. Engel J Jr. Basic mechanisms of epilepsy. In: *Seizures and epilepsy.* Philadelphia: FA Davis, 1989:71.

102. Prince DA. The depolarization shift in "epileptic" neurons. *Exp Neurol* 1968;21:467–485.

103. Gloor P. Electrophysiology of generalized epilepsy. In: Schwartzkroin PA, Wheal H, eds. *Electrophysiology of epilepsy.* New York: Academic Press, 1984:107–136.

104. Fisher RS, Prince DA. Spike-wave rhythms in cat cortex induced by parenteral penicillin, II: cellular features. *Electroencephalogr Clin Electrophysiol* 1977;42:625–639.

105. Taylor-Courval D, Gloor P. Behavioral alterations associated with generalized spike and wave discharges in the EEG of the cat. *Exp Neurol* 1984;83:167–186.

106. Guberman A, Gloor P, Sherwin AL. Response of generalized penicillin epilepsy in the cat to ethosuximide and diphenylhydantoin. *Neurology* 1975;25:758–674.

107. Gloor P, Testa G. Generalized penicillin epilepsy in the cat: effects of intracarotid and intravertebral pentylenetetrazol and amobarbital injections. *Electroencephalogr Clin Electrophysiol* 1974;36:499–515.

108. Quesney LP. Pathophysiology of generalized photosensitive epilepsy in the cat. *Epilepsia* 1984;25:61–69.

109. Westrum LE, White LE, Ward AA Jr. Morphology of the experimental epileptic focus. *J Neurosurg* 1964;21:1033–1046.

110. Soper HV, Strain GM, Babb TL, et al. Chronic alumina temporal lobe seizures in monkeys. *Exp Neurol* 1978;62:99–121.

111. Marangos PJ, Paul SM, Parma AM, et al. Purinergic inhibition of diazepam binding to rat brain *(in vitro). Life Sci* 1979;24: 851–857.

112. Simmons MA. Leptazol as GABA antagonist. *Br J Pharmacol* 1980;70:75.

113. Chevassus-au-Louis N, Baraban SC, Gaiarsa J-L, et al. Cortical malformations and epilepsy: new insights from animal models. *Epilepsia* 1999;40:811–821.

114. Humphreys P, Rosen GD, Press DM, et al. Freezing lesion of the developing rat brain: a model for cerebrocortical microgyria. *J Neuropathol Exp Neurol* 1991;50:145–160.

115. Rosen GD, Galaburda AM, Sherman GF. Cerebrocortical microdysgenesis with anomalous callosal connections: a case study in the rat. *Int J Dev Neurosci* 1989;47:237–247.

116. Holmes GL, Sarkisian MS, Ben-Ari Y, et al. Consequences of cortical microdysgenesis during development. *Epilepsia* 1999;40: 537–544.

117. Germano IM, Zhang YF, Sperber EF, et al. Neuronal migration disorders increase susceptibility to hyperthermia induced seizures in developing rats. *Epilepsia* 1996;37:902–910.

118. Germano IM, Sperber EF. Transplacentally induced neuronal migration disorders: an animal model for the study of the epilepsies. *J Neurosci Res* 1998;15:473–488.

119. Baraban SC, Schwartzkroin PA. Flurothyl seizure susceptibility in rats following prenatal methylazoxymethanol treatment. *Epilepsy Res* 1996;23:189–194.

120. Roper SN, Gilmore RL, Houser CR. Experimentally induced disorders of neuronal migration produce an increased propensity for electrographic seizures. *Epilepsy Res* 1995;21:205–219.

121. MacBride M, Temper T. Pathogenesis of four-layered microgyric cortex in man. *Acta Neuropathol* 1982,57:93–98.

122. Dvorak K, Feit J, Jurankova Z. Experimentally induced focal microgyria and status verrucosus deformis in rats: pathogenesis and interrelation. Histological and autoradiographical study. *Acta Neuropathol* 1978,44:121–129.

123. Roper SN, King MA, Abraham LA, et al. Disinhibited in vitro neocortical slices containing experimentally induced cortical dysplasia demonstrate hyperexcitability. *Epilepsy Res* 1997;26:443–449.

Genetics Aspects of Epilepsy and Genetics of Idiopathic Generalized Epilepsy

Ajay Gupta   *Ingrid E. Scheffer*

Epilepsy, defined by the recurrence of unprovoked seizures, is a complex disorder. Complex inheritance refers to the interaction of a number of genes with or without an environmental contribution and underlies the majority of idiopathic epilepsies in which seizures occur as the only symptom with no other neurologic or systemic abnormalities. On the simplest and purest level of genetic contribution, epilepsy may follow single-gene inheritance in a family. One example of this is autosomal dominant nocturnal frontal lobe epilepsy (ADNFLE), which manifests as motor seizures in sleep in an otherwise normal individual (1). In some families, ADNFLE may be a result of mutations in either the α_4 or the β_2 subunit of the neuronal nicotinic acetylcholine receptor (2,3). On the most complex level, the study of genetic influences may involve determining multiple genes (such as ion channel and neurotransmitter receptor genes) that interact with one another and with environmental factors, leading to epilepsy in some patients with underlying lesions, such as a brain tumor or remote intracranial trauma. Between the simplest and the most complex levels is a huge spectrum of disorders in which epilepsy is one, and sometimes the predominant, symptom (diagnosis) in the multifaceted neurologic and/or systemic expression of a disease. Examples include epilepsy seen in single-gene mendelian disorders with dysmorphic and/or neurocutaneous features (Chapters 36 and 37), heritable or sporadic brain malformations (Chapters 4 and 5), inborn errors of metabolism (Chapters 26 and 37), chromosomal aberrations and microdeletion chromosomal

disorders (Chapter 31), and mitochondrial disorders (Chapters 26 and 37).

A search of the online database of inheritable mendelian human diseases (OMIM [Online Mendelian Inheritance in Man (www.ncbi.nlm.nih.gov)]) with the keyword "epilepsy," reveals 299 hits from a total of 15,547 entries (2%) at this time. A search with the keyword "seizures" shows 645 hits (4%). This suggests an approximately 4% to 6% frequency ("epilepsy" and "seizures" are used mutually exclusively in OMIM) of epilepsy in human genetic disorders with mendelian inheritance, not including the chromosomal abnormalities and many sporadic conditions of presumed genetic etiology that are not part of the OMIM database. A recent review estimated a genetic contribution to etiology in approximately 40% of patients with epilepsy (4). Researchers are now studying genetic influences at the level of epilepsy treatment by focusing on genes that may influence intractability of seizures, drug transport, and metabolism (Chapter 52). Genetics, therefore, is of paramount importance in the study of epilepsy, and we are only beginning to understand the vast ways in which genes influence the expression of seizures and the success of epilepsy treatment.

This chapter discusses two genetic aspects of epilepsy: (a) when to suspect a genetic etiology and why the patient should be evaluated for a genetic cause, and (b) the complex genetics of idiopathic generalized epilepsies. The reader is referred to additional chapters (noted above) that include discussions of other genetic disorders that cause, or are associated with, epilepsy.

WHEN TO SUSPECT A GENETIC ETIOLOGY IN A PATIENT WITH EPILEPSY

Usually, a patient with idiopathic epilepsy has no family history of epilepsy or febrile seizures. Nevertheless, it is always essential to take a detailed family history, which, if positive, can provide important clues to the type of epilepsy affecting the family. A cursory history in a busy clinic setting may miss important pointers to a genetic etiology unless the extended family history is taken in detail and a pedigree is routinely constructed. It is unusual to obtain a strong family history of epilepsy affecting many members across multiple generations that unequivocally suggests a single-gene inheritance pattern. Much more common is when the patient reports a few distant relatives (such as a skipped generation or once-removed cousins or uncles or aunts) with a diagnosis of epilepsy. These affected family members illustrate how genetic factors may be relevant to the patient's epilepsy. It is often difficult to obtain detailed electroclinical data about affected relatives, but in some instances, such as ADNFLE, these data may be key to making the diagnosis. In other cases, the family history is not relevant, and epilepsy could be a result of "acquired factors." When these acquired factors are explored, however, they may not be convincing and the genetic etiology may not have been appreciated (or was denied); therefore, it is always helpful to obtain as much information as possible. Furthermore, investigations to uncover a genetic etiology may be hampered by the family's reluctance to cooperate owing to the stigma attached to the diagnosis of epilepsy and the potential of having inherited this disorder. On the other hand, when five or six family members over multiple generations report seizures, the possibility of single-gene disorders should not be dismissed if a few key individuals are unaffected, as they may be nonpenetrant carriers of a genetic mutation (5). Incomplete penetrance is usual in autosomal dominant disorders.

In all cases, a pedigree will highlight the degree of relationship between affected family members. A pedigree should identify the index patient, or proband, and clearly show the proband's relationship to affected and unaffected members on both the maternal and paternal sides. The clinician should always ask about parental consanguinity, which is vital in determining inheritance patterns. It is also good practice to obtain the names and dates of birth of affected individuals, any consanguinity elsewhere in the family, and obstetric history (miscarriages, stillbirths, neonatal deaths). The presence of multiple miscarriages may suggest X-linked dominant inheritance or other genetic causes. The clinician should always specifically inquire about a family history of epilepsy and febrile convulsions because, not recognizing that these two entities may be related genetically, many families will fail to mention febrile seizures. Obtaining age of seizure onset, course, semiology, and provoking factors in affected family members is helpful, and it is worth asking whether precise data can be secured from other family members. It is also important to update the pedigree as new information on family members becomes available at future consultations (5).

A genetic etiology is suspected in a patient with epilepsy who has multiple congenital anomalies with a known cytogenetic abnormality, imaging data and/or a clinical phenotype suggestive of a known single-gene disorder such as tuberous sclerosis or Rett syndrome, or clinical and laboratory findings of a genetically determined inborn error of metabolism or a mitochondrial cytopathy. In most of these instances, however, epilepsy is only one component of several complicated medical issues these patients and families face.

WHY EVALUATE FOR A GENETIC ETIOLOGY IN A PATIENT WITH EPILEPSY?

Accurate diagnosis of an underlying genetic etiology is of paramount importance for the patient with epilepsy and the family. A specific diagnosis often carries implications for appropriate antiepileptic drug (AED) selection, prognosis, and genetic counseling. In terms of the idiopathic epilepsies, clinical genetic factors may guide diagnosis and thus management. An example is a child presenting with nocturnal frontal lobe epilepsy and a normal magnetic resonance imaging scan of the brain. If that child has three other family members with nocturnal frontal lobe epilepsy that follows an autosomal dominant inheritance pattern, a diagnosis of ADNFLE can be made and guide AED selection based on the previous experience (6). Genetic counseling could also be performed in view of the clinical genetics of this disorder. Because the genes currently known for ADNFLE account for only a small proportion of families, the diagnosis more frequently relies on the clinical genetics and seizure semiology than on a molecular defect (7). Similarly, clinical genetics guides recognition of generalized epilepsy with febrile seizures plus (GEFS+) (8). Although a number of genes have been identified for GEFS+, they relate to only a minority of patients and families with this disorder. Diagnosis of a mild phenotype such as febrile seizures plus helps the clinician predict a good prognosis and potentially opt for no AED treatment for an 8-year-old child who continues to have a few febrile seizures.

Just as important, but to date relatively infrequent, genetic mutations have major implications for management. At present, there are two main situations in which a genetic defect will significantly influence clinical care. The first is the mild disorder of benign familial neonatal convulsions (BFNC) (see below). This idiopathic epilepsy is the only autosomal dominant epilepsy syndrome in which most families have mutations of the potassium-channel gene *KCNQ2*. The finding of a mutation in a neonate with seizures guides prognosis and reassures the family about the likely good outcome (9). The first molecular lesion to have major diagnostic implications for a patient with a severe epileptic encephalopathy is represented by mutations in the sodium-channel α_1 subunit gene *SCN1A* in severe myoclonic epilepsy of infancy (SMEI) (see below) (10). *SCN1A* mutations arise *de novo* in approximately 70% of patients with SMEI and, if considered pathogenic, mean that the clinician does not need to pursue other invasive diagnostic tests; confirmation of diagnosis by DNA tests, however, does not influence the choice of AEDs at this time (11).

Accurate genetic diagnosis also helps in the management of patients by timely investigation, treatment, and institution of surveillance for anticipated involvement of other organs and systems, particularly when symptomatic epilepsy occurs as part of a multisystem disorder. For example, in patients with tuberous sclerosis, surveillance and treatment are indicated for hydrocephalus, renal cysts or tumors, cardiac rhabdomyomas, cardiac conduction defects, ocular abnormalities, and pulmonary involvement (12,13). Precise genetic testing and counseling of family members at risk are also possible when an accurate genetic diagnosis is made. Furthermore, new epilepsy syndromes and brain malformations of genetic origin will be recognized only if families and patients with familial disorders are identified.

Sometimes, a genetic etiology has implications for the treatment of epileptic seizures. For example, in several genetically determined disorders, specific metabolic therapy is indicated: lifelong oral pyridoxine for B_6-dependent seizures (14), the ketogenic diet for glucose transporter defects (15), biotin supplementation in biotinidase deficiency-related seizures (16), and folinic acid for folinic acid-responsive seizures (17). In other situations, a specific AED may show superior efficacy in treating the seizures of a genetic condition, as, for example, vigabatrin for infantile spasms caused by tuberous sclerosis (18). New trials of drugs designed to ameliorate a genetically determined channel dysfunction are also on the horizon; an example is the potassium-channel drug retigabine for benign neonatal febrile convulsions caused by mutations in a potassium-channel gene(s) (19).

GENETICS OF IDIOPATHIC GENERALIZED EPILEPSIES

Epilepsies Linked to Voltage-Gated Sodium Channels

Mutations in three voltage-gated sodium-channel genes have been reported in patients with epilepsy. The voltage-gated sodium channel is composed of a pore-forming α subunit and regulatory β subunits (20). The three voltage-gated sodium-channel genes so far implicated encode the α_1 (*SCN1A*) (21,22), the α_2 (*SCN2A*) (23), and the β_1 (*SCN1B*) (24). Most families with several members affected

as a result of mutations in one of these three genes have an autosomal dominant pattern of inheritance with variable penetrance associated with GEFS+ (8). GEFS+ families with the same mutation in a single gene typically have a variable phenotype in different family members. While some family members have typical febrile seizures that they outgrow by 6 years of age, other individuals may have febrile and afebrile seizures that persist longer (febrile seizures plus). Still other family members have tonic-clonic seizures with other generalized or focal seizure types, while some may have severe epileptic encephalopathies such as myoclonic-astatic epilepsy of Doose and SMEI (8,22,25,26). Less frequently, mutations in a γ-aminobutyric acid (GABA)-receptor gene that encodes the γ_2 of the $GABA_A$ receptor (*GABRG2*) have also been reported in families with GEFS+ (27,28).

Mutations of *SCN1A* are also described in some patients with SMEI (10,29,30). SMEI typically begins with hemiclonic or generalized febrile status epilepticus at about 6 months of age. Between 1 and 4 years of age, other seizure types emerge, including partial, absence, atonic, and myoclonic. Cognitive decline follows normal early development in the first year of life; pyramidal features and ataxia may evolve (31). The majority of mutations in SMEI patients are *de novo*, which does not explain the family history of GEFS+ that is observed in 50% of SMEI patients (32–34). In general, the reported *SCN1A* gene mutations are more severe, often leading to protein truncation (10). It is believed that GEFS+ and SMEI represent a spectrum of phenotypes associated with mutations in the *SCN1A* gene (33).

Epilepsies Linked to Voltage-Gated Potassium Channels

Potassium channels in the brain are critical for maintaining neuronal resting membrane potential and rapid repolarization after action potentials. Two voltage-gated potassium-channel genes, *KCNQ2* and *KCNQ3*, are associated with the autosomal dominant syndrome of BFNC (35–37). *KCNQ2* and *KCNQ3* form a multimeric potassium channel responsible for the M current that is important in stabilizing the resting membrane potential. BFNC is characterized by unprovoked seizures beginning in the first week of life that usually resolve spontaneously by a few weeks to months of age (9,38–40). Only in a minority of patients (~10% to 20%) do seizures continue beyond infancy. A *KCNQ2* mutation has been reported in a family with BFNC and myokymia in later life (41).

Epilepsies Linked to Voltage-Gated Calcium Channels

Neuronal voltage-gated calcium channels of P/Q type are important for neurotransmitter release. Mutations in several types of voltage-gated calcium-channel genes in mice are associated with cortical epileptic discharges and absence epilepsy and are potentially considered models of human absence epilepsy (42,43). However, these murine models differ from human absence epilepsies in that they follow recessive inheritance and involve a more severe course, often with ataxia. The most important neuronal calcium-channel gene that causes human neurologic diseases is the one that encodes the pore-forming α-subunit gene (*CACNA1A*). *CACNA1A* mutations are described in several families with nonepileptic paroxysmal disorders like episodic ataxias, familial hemiplegic migraine, and certain types of spinocerebellar ataxia. Recently, however, different types of childhood epilepsy have been reported in association with other paroxysmal phenomena in several families with *CACNA1A* mutations (44–46). Another anecdotal report implicated the β₄ (*CACNB4*) in an individual with juvenile myoclonic epilepsy, but this case requires confirmation (47). A Chinese study found mutations in *CACNA1H*, a gene encoding a subunit of the T-type calcium channel, in childhood absence epilepsy (48). Attempts to replicate this finding demonstrated different mutations in other forms of idiopathic generalized epilepsy, suggesting that *CACNA1H* may be a susceptibility gene for idiopathic generalized epilepsy (49).

Epilepsies Linked to Voltage-Gated Chloride Channels

Mutations in *CLCN2*, a gene encoding a chloride-transporting protein, were associated with epilepsy in three families with idiopathic generalized epilepsy inherited as a dominant disorder (50). Affected family members had a variety of phenotypes, including juvenile myoclonic epilepsy, juvenile absence epilepsy, childhood absence epilepsy, and epilepsy with grand mal seizures on awakening.

Epilepsies Linked to Ligand-Gated GABA Receptors

As a major inhibitory neurotransmitter in the human central nervous system, GABA has been a target of intensive scrutiny for its role in human epilepsy. Type A GABA receptors (GABA_A) are ligand-gated chloride channels that mediate inhibitory neural activity. In a healthy postnatal brain, GABA_A receptors trigger chloride influx, leading to hyperpolarization of the postsynaptic membrane. The state of hyperpolarization opposes any excitatory synaptic inputs (40). GABA_A receptors are composed of five subunits encoded by multiple different gene families. Mutations in two genes coding for the α₁ subunit (*GABRA1*) and γ₂ subunit (*GABRG2*) are associated with idiopathic generalized epilepsy in humans (27,28,51). A *GABRA1* mutation was described in a family with juvenile myoclonic epilepsy inherited in a pattern suggestive of autosomal dominance (51). *GABRG2* is associated with a spectrum of phenotypes in families that suggests typical febrile seizures, GEFS+

syndrome, and childhood absence epilepsy (27,28,52,53). More recently, the GABA D subunit gene (*GABRD*) was associated with GEFS+ and idiopathic generalized epilepsy (54).

Epilepsies Linked to Ligand-Gated Nicotinic Acetylcholine Receptors

Located predominantly in the presynaptic membranes of the cerebral cortex, ligand-gated nicotinic acetylcholine (nACh) receptors are widely expressed in human brain. These pentameric complexes differ in their subunit composition. Mutations in two genes encoding for the α₄ subunit (CHRNA4) and β₂ subunit (CHRNB4) of neuronal nACh receptors have been reported in families with epilepsy (2,3). Mutations in both genes cause the clinically indistinguishable phenotype ADNFLE (6,55). ADNFLE presents near the end of the first decade of life in otherwise healthy children. Seizures are mostly nocturnal, with a variety of motor manifestations that may be mistaken for sleep-related parasomnias. Seizure manifestations include a nonspecific aura described as fear or vague feelings in the body, followed by stiffening, thrashing, and violent motor movements. Seizures are typically brief and occur in clusters during the night. The penetrance of ADNFLE is approximately 70% (6).

SUMMARY AND CONCLUSIONS

Neuronal ion channels play an important role in human epilepsies. Monogenic epilepsies with a clear pattern of inheritance are rare and perhaps represent "the tip of the iceberg." It is more likely that most idiopathic generalized epilepsies occur as a result of a complex inheritance in which a number of "susceptibility genes" interact with one another to produce the epilepsy syndrome (clinical phenotype) (1). Furthermore, the relationship between genotype and phenotype is heterogeneous, even in the same family with a monogenic channelopathy, and to date defies a clear explanation. As we discover more genes and gain a better understanding of their function and interactions with one another, genetics will likely have a major impact on the diagnosis and treatment of human idiopathic generalized epilepsies.

REFERENCES

1. Durner M, Keddache MA, Tomasini L, et al. Genome scan of idiopathic generalized epilepsy: evidence for major susceptibility gene and modifying genes influencing the seizure type. *Ann Neurol* 2001;49:328–335.
2. Steinlein OK, Mulley JC, Propping P, et al. A missense mutation in the neuronal nicotinic acetylcholine receptor alpha 4 subunit is associated with autosomal dominant nocturnal frontal lobe epilepsy. *Nat Genet* 1995;11:201–203.
3. De Fusco M, Becchetti A, Patrignani A, et al. The nicotinic receptor beta 2 subunit is mutant in nocturnal frontal lobe epilepsy. *Nat Genet* 2000;26:275–276.

4. Gardiner RM. Impact of our understanding of the genetic aetiology of epilepsy. *J Neurol* 2000;247:327–334.

5. Scheffer IE, Berkovic SF. Rational diagnosis of genetic epilepsies. In: Schmidt D, Schachter SC, eds. *Epilepsy: problem solving in clinical practice.* London: Martin Dunitz, 2000:111–131.

6. Scheffer IE, Bhatia KP, Lopes-Cendes I, et al. Autosomal dominant nocturnal frontal lobe epilepsy. A distinctive clinical disorder. *Brain* 1995;118(Pt 1):61–73.

7. Scheffer IE, Berkovic SF. The genetics of human epilepsy. *Trends Pharmacol Sci* 2003;24:428–433.

8. Scheffer IE, Berkovic SF. Generalized epilepsy with febrile seizures plus. A genetic disorder with heterogeneous clinical phenotypes. *Brain* 1997;120(Pt 3):479–490.

9. Singh NA, Westenskow P, Charlier C, et al. KCNQ2 and KCNQ3 potassium channel genes in benign familial neonatal convulsions: expansion of the functional and mutation spectrum. *Brain* 2003;126(Pt 12):2726–2737.

10. Claes L, Del Favero J, Ceulemans B, et al. De novo mutations in the sodium-channel gene SCN1A cause severe myoclonic epilepsy of infancy. *Am J Hum Genet* 2001;68:1327–1332.

11. Guerrini R, Dravet C, Genton P, et al. Lamotrigine and seizure aggravation in severe myoclonic epilepsy. *Epilepsia* 1998;39(Suppl):508–512.

12. Roach ES, DiMario FJ, Kandt RS, et al. Tuberous Sclerosis Consensus Conference: recommendations for diagnostic evaluation. *J Child Neurol* 1999;14:401–407.

13. Hyman MH, Whittemore VH. National Institutes of Health Consensus Conference: tuberous sclerosis complex. *Arch Neurol* 2000;57:662–665.

14. Coker SB. Postneonatal vitamin B_6-dependent epilepsy. *Pediatrics* 1992;90(2 Pt 1):221–223.

15. Brockmann K, Wang D, Korenke CG, et al. Autosomal dominant glut-1 deficiency syndrome and familial epilepsy. *Ann Neurol* 2001;50:476–485.

16. Bressman S, Fahn S, Eisenberg M, et al. Biotin-responsive encephalopathy with myoclonus, ataxia, and seizures. *Adv Neurol* 1986;43:119–125.

17. Hyland K, Buist NR, Powell BR, et al. Folinic acid responsive seizures: a new syndrome? *J Inherit Metab Dis* 1995;18:177–181.

18. Mackay MT, Weiss SK, Adams-Webber T, et al. Practice parameter: medical treatment of infantile spasms: report of the American Academy of Neurology and the Child Neurology Society. *Neurology* 2004;62:1668–1681.

19. Cooper EC. Potassium channels: how genetic studies of epileptic syndromes open paths to new therapeutic targets and drugs. *Epilepsia* 2001;42(Suppl 5):49–54.

20. Isom LL. The role of sodium channels in cell adhesion. *Front Biosci* 2002;7:12–23.

21. Wallace RH, Scheffer IE, Barnett S, et al. Neuronal sodium-channel alpha$_1$-subunit mutations in generalized epilepsy with febrile seizures plus. *Am J Hum Genet* 2001;68:859–865.

22. Escayg A, MacDonald BT, Meisler MH, et al. Mutations of SCN1A, encoding a neuronal sodium channel, in two families with GEFS+2. *Nat Genet* 2000;24:343–345.

23. Sugawara T, Tsurubuchi Y, Agarwala KL, et al. A missense mutation of the Na$^+$ channel alpha II subunit gene Na(v)1.2 in a patient with febrile and afebrile seizures causes channel dysfunction. *Proc Natl Acad Sci U S A* 2001;98:6384–6389.

24. Wallace RH, Wang DW, Singh R, et al. Febrile seizures and generalized epilepsy associated with a mutation in the Na$^+$-channel beta$_1$ subunit gene SCN1B. *Nat Genet* 1998;19:366–370.

25. Singh R, Scheffer IE, Crossland K, et al. Generalized epilepsy with febrile seizures plus: a common, childhood onset, genetic epilepsy syndrome. *Ann Neurol* 1999;45:75–81.

26. Abou-Khalil B, Ge Q, Desai R, et al. Partial and generalized epilepsy with febrile seizures plus and a novel SCN1A mutation. *Neurology* 2001;57:2265–2272.

27. Wallace RH, Marini C, Petrou S, et al. Mutant GABA(A) receptor gamma$_2$-subunit in childhood absence epilepsy and febrile seizures. *Nat Genet* 2001;28:49–52.

28. Baulac S, Huberfeld G, Gourfinkel-An I, et al. First genetic evidence of GABA(A) receptor dysfunction in epilepsy: a mutation in the gamma$_2$-subunit gene. *Nat Genet* 2001;28:46–48.

29. Sugawara T, Mazaki-Miyazaki E, Fukushima K, et al. Frequent mutations of SCN1A in severe myoclonic epilepsy in infancy. *Neurology* 2002;58:1122–1124.

30. Claes L, Ceulemans B, Audenaert D, et al. De novo SCN1A mutations are a major cause of severe myoclonic epilepsy of infancy. *Hum Mutat* 2003;21:615–621.

31. Dravet C, Bureau M, Oguni H, et al. Severe myoclonic epilepsy in infancy (Dravet syndrome). In: Roger J, Bureau M, Dravet C, et al., eds. *Epileptic syndromes in infancy, childhood and adolescence,* 3rd ed. Eastleigh, UK: John Libbey, 2002:81–103.

32. Scheffer IE. Severe infantile epilepsies: molecular genetics challenge clinical classification. *Brain* 2003;126:513–514.

33. Singh R, Andermann E, Whitehouse WP, et al. Severe myoclonic epilepsy of infancy: extended spectrum of GEFS+? *Epilepsia* 2001;42:837–844.

34. Fujiwara T, Sugawara T, Mazaki-Miyazaki E, et al. Mutations of sodium channel alpha subunit type 1 (SCN1A) in intractable childhood epilepsies with frequent generalized tonic-clonic seizures. *Brain* 2003;126(Pt 3)531–546.

35. Biervert C, Schroeder BC, Kubisch C, et al. A potassium channel mutation in neonatal human epilepsy. *Science* 1998;279:403–406.

36. Singh NA, Charlier C, Stauffer D, et al. A novel potassium channel gene, KCNQ2, is mutated in an inherited epilepsy of newborns. *Nat Genet* 1998;18:25–29.

37. Charlier C, Singh NA, Ryan SG, et al. A pore mutation in a novel KQT-like potassium channel gene in an idiopathic epilepsy family. *Nat Genet* 1998;18:53–55.

38. Rett A, Teubel R. Neugeborenenkrämpfe im Rahmen einer epileptisch belasteten familie. *Wien Klin Wochenschr* 1964;76:609–613.

39. Plouin P, Anderson VE. Benign familial and non-familial neonatal seizures. In: Roger J, Bureau M, Dravet C, et al, eds. *Epileptic syndromes in infancy, childhood and adolescence,* 3rd ed. Eastleigh, UK: John Libbey, 2002:3–13.

40. George AL Jr. Molecular basis of inherited epilepsy. *Arch Neurol* 2004;61:473–478.

41. Dedek K, Kunath B, Kananura C, et al. Myokymia and neonatal epilepsy caused by a mutation in the voltage sensor of the KCNQ2 K$^+$ channel. *Proc Natl Acad Sci U S A* 2001;98:12272–12277.

42. Meisler MH, Kearney J, Ottman R, et al. Identification of epilepsy genes in human and mouse. *Annu Rev Genet* 2001;35:567–588.

43. Burgess DL, Noebels JL. Single gene defects in mice: the role of voltage-dependent calcium channels in absence models. *Epilepsy Res* 1999;36:111–122.

44. Kors EE, Melberg A, Vanmolkot KR, et al. Childhood epilepsy, familial hemiplegic migraine, cerebellar ataxia, and a new CACNA1A mutation. *Neurology* 2004;63:1136–1137.

45. Beauvais K, Cave-Riant F, De Barace C, et al. New CACNA1A gene mutation in a case of familial hemiplegic migraine with status epilepticus. *Eur Neurol* 2004;52:58–61.

46. Imbrici P, Jaffe SL, Eunson LH, et al. Dysfunction of the brain calcium channel CaV2.1 in absence epilepsy and episodic ataxia. *Brain* 2004; 127;2682–2692.

47. Escayg A, De Waard M, Lee DD, et al. Coding and noncoding variation of the human calcium-channel beta$_4$-subunit gene CACNB4 in patients with idiopathic generalized epilepsy and episodic ataxia. *Am J Hum Genet* 2000;66:1531–1539.

48. Chen Y, Lu J, Pan H, et al. Association between genetic variation of CACNA1H and childhood absence epilepsy. *Ann Neurol* 2003;54:239–243.

49. Heron SE, Phillips HA, Mulley JC, et al. Genetic variation of CACNA1H in idiopathic generalized epilepsy. *Ann Neurol* 2004;55:595–596.

50. Haug K, Warnstedt M, Alekov AK, et al. Mutations in CLCN2 encoding a voltage-gated chloride channel are associated with idiopathic generalized epilepsies. *Nat Genet* 2003;33:527–532.

51. Cossette P, Liu L, Brisebois K, et al. Mutation of GABRA1 in an autosomal dominant form of juvenile myoclonic epilepsy. *Nat Genet* 2002;31:184–189.

52. Kananura C, Haug K, Sander T, et al. A splice-site mutation in GABRG2 associated with childhood absence epilepsy and febrile convulsions. *Arch Neurol* 2002;59:1137–1141.

53. Harkin LA, Bowser DN, Dibbens LM, et al. Truncation of the GABA(A)-receptor gamma$_2$ subunit in a family with generalized epilepsy with febrile seizures plus. *Am J Hum Genet* 2002;70: 530–536.

54. Dibbens LM, Feng HJ, Richards MC, et al. GABRD encoding a protein for extra- or peri-synaptic GABA$_A$ receptors is a susceptibility locus for generalized epilepsies. *Hum Mol Genet* 2004;13: 1315–1319.

55. McLellan A, Phillips HA, Rittey C, et al. Phenotypic comparison of two Scottish families with mutations in different genes causing autosomal dominant nocturnal frontal lobe epilepsy. *Epilepsia* 2003;44:613–617.

Epidemiologic Aspects of Epilepsy

8

Anne T. Berg

Until the 1960s, the prevailing view about epilepsy was captured by the words of Sir William Gowers: "The tendency of the disease is toward self-perpetuation; each attack facilitates the occurrence of another by increasing the instability of the nerve elements. . . . The spontaneous cessation of the disease is an event too rare to be reasonably anticipated" (1). Epilepsy was considered a progressive, nonremitting disease. Gowers, who studied and characterized patients seen in the early tertiary referral centers of the late 1800s, was extremely observant, however. In the same text, he noted that ". . . the cases in which the best results are obtained, in which no more fits occur, are precisely those who are never heard of again. Such cases are, assuredly, far more numerous than imagined. The few which are incidentally heard of at a subsequent time make it quite certain that they represent a much larger number of whom no trace is obtained." In this brief comment, Gowers identified what would help pave the way for the important role played by epidemiology in the study of seizures: to obtain those traces and to study not only those patients in need of continuous care, but those whose seizures resolved as well.

Early epidemiologic studies provided the basis for at least two major contributions to the understanding of epilepsy and seizures in the general population. These studies demonstrated that seizures are relatively common. The cumulative lifetime risk of the occurrence of any type seizure may reach as high as 10%, possibly higher (2,3). These early studies also provided a better basis for understanding the prognosis of epilepsy and for distinguishing the disorder from other conditions in which seizures might occur. In short, these studies showed that the majority of individuals with epilepsy fared very well (4). Contrary to Gowers' characterization (although not inconsistent with his subsequent comment), the majority of patients became completely seizure-free for extended periods and often for the rest of their lives. The early epidemiologic studies also provided some impetus and data for distinguishing situational-related seizures and single seizures from epilepsy proper (5). This led to substantial changes in clinical practice, in counseling, and, most likely, in the lives of individuals affected by seizures.

Since these studies in the 1960s and 1970s, epidemiologic investigations have become more sophisticated and more informative, having incorporated new knowledge and distinctions about seizure disorders. This chapter discusses the current definitions and distinctions used in epidemiologic research, as well as some of the more recent and challenging aspects of epidemiologic studies of seizure disorders, especially as they affect comparative work and investigations in developing countries.

CURRENT DEFINITIONS AND DISTINCTIONS USED IN EPIDEMIOLOGIC EPILEPSY RESEARCH

Epilepsy (recurrent, unprovoked seizures) is now distinguished from many other conditions and situations in which seizures may occur. The following accepted definitions are in current use and are used throughout this chapter.

Epileptic Seizure

An epileptic seizure is characterized by the clinical manifestation of a discrete, abnormal discharge of neurons in a part of the brain or throughout the brain. Epileptic seizures must be distinguished from nonepileptic seizures and from other conditions that can produce clinical manifestations that are highly similar to those caused by epileptic seizures (6).

Acute Provoked Seizure

An acute provoked seizure is one that occurs in the context of an acute brain insult or systemic disorder, such as, but not limited to, stroke, head trauma, a toxic or metabolic insult, or an intracranial infection (7).

Unprovoked Seizure

A seizure that occurs in the absence of an acute provoking event is considered unprovoked (7).

Epilepsy

Epilepsy is generally diagnosed after the occurrence of at least two unprovoked seizures on separate days, at least 24 hours apart. An individual with a single unprovoked seizure or with two or more unprovoked seizures within a 24-hour period is not considered to have epilepsy per se (7), although it is still entirely reasonable to identify the underlying form of the epileptic disorder at the time of the initial seizure (8).

Etiology

Etiology is considered symptomatic if there is an antecedent condition that is causally related to an increased risk of developing epilepsy. Symptomatic factors include, but are not limited to, history of stroke, brain malformation, clear neurodevelopmental abnormality such as cerebral palsy, history of bacterial meningitis or viral encephalitis, a variety of genetic conditions, and tumors. Epilepsy in the context of a progressive condition (e.g., neurodegenerative disease or an aggressive tumor) is often considered a subgroup within symptomatic epilepsy. In contrast, epilepsy is considered nonsymptomatic in the absence of such antecedent factors. The nonsymptomatic epilepsies are further divided into idiopathic (i.e., those in which other clinical evidence including electroencephalograms [EEGs] indicates that the individual has a form of idiopathic epilepsy) and cryptogenic (in which the underlying cause remains unclear). Recently, the distinction between these two designations has become blurred by the realization that there may be some commonalities between syndromes traditionally considered idiopathic and others considered cryptogenic (9,10).

Gray Areas

Neonatal seizures (i.e., those occurring in an infant <28 days old) are usually differentiated from epilepsy for a variety of reasons; however, several specific forms of epilepsy have been reported in this age group (11). Febrile seizures are a well-described and recognized seizure disorder that, for historical reasons, has been distinguished (both clinically and in research) from epilepsy. This has had important clinical implications for the treatment of children with such seizures. From a scientific standpoint, however, this may obscure significant aspects of the genetics and underlying neurophysiologic mechanisms of seizure-related disorders.

Epilepsy Syndromes

Epilepsy syndromes are presented in greater detail in subsequent chapters of this book; however, they are important to modern epidemiologic endeavors and thus merit mention in this context. As with cancer, epilepsy is not a single disease. In theory, epilepsy syndromes represent forms of epilepsy that have different causes, different manifestations, different implications for short- and long-term management and treatment, and different outcomes. The classification of epileptic syndromes was first proposed more than 30 years ago. The current version, which was published in 1989, is undergoing major restructuring and revision (12–17).

EPIDEMIOLOGY

As already mentioned, early epidemiologic studies were key to understanding the frequency of seizures in the population and to providing the initial impetus for some of the distinctions previously outlined. Prior to the advent of epidemiology, one could say that "the forest had been lost for the trees"—and the most intractable trees at that! Epidemiology provided the context, the forest, and a bit about what was in that forest. Many of the distinctions described above cannot be made without considering diagnostic technologies and capabilities.

Diagnostic Technology and Expertise

Seizures and epilepsy present a complex situation because the diagnosis is not based on a single source or type of information. Rather, epilepsy is a clinical diagnosis supported to a greater or lesser extent by a wide range of data obtained from several sources: the medical history, the history (both from the patient and witnesses) of the events believed to be seizures, a neurologic examination, a reliable EEG, and sometimes neuroimaging (18). To have a valid diagnosis, one must also be able to rule out many other conditions that mimic seizures. These disorders include, but are not limited to, movement disorders, parasomnias, attention deficit hyperactivity disorder (ADHD), pseudo- or nonepileptic seizures, transient ischemic attacks, and syncope. In addition to the simple diagnosis of epilepsy, adequate information is needed to identify as accurately as possible the specific syndrome and its underlying cause. In turn, this depends largely on clinical features and on the EEG, and often on neuroimaging.

Screening questionnaires have been used in epidemiologic studies for the purpose of obtaining a rough estimate of the frequency of seizure disorders (19–21). Their diagnostic specificity, however, can be quite poor (i.e., they identify individuals as having epilepsy who, in fact, do not have the disorder). Individuals identified via such an approach are then evaluated more thoroughly by physicians. Unfortunately, the training of these physicians or other health care professionals and the access to such basic diagnostic tools as EEGs are often less than ideal.

The importance of professional training has been highlighted in several studies. The British National General Practice Study of Epilepsy (NGPSE) included all individuals referred by general practitioners. Of these patients, only 71% were confirmed by an expert as having epilepsy (22). The Dutch study of epilepsy in childhood reported that greater than 25% of children referred for epilepsy consultation by general practitioners and pediatricians did not have the disorder (23). By contrast, the epidemiologic study of incident epilepsy in the Gironde region of France (EPIGIR), which identified patients through hospital neurology services and EEG laboratories, excluded only about 10% of patients (24). In the Connecticut study, only about 2% of referrals from child neurologists were not confirmed (by the research team) as having epilepsy (25). Finally, the Coordination Active du Réseau Observatoire Longitudinal de L'Epilepsie (CAROLE) study, which also relied on referral after diagnosis by a network of neurologists, did not exclude any patients because of an unconfirmed diagnosis (8). In all these studies, epileptologists reviewed the medical data; however, the level of expertise of the individual(s) who collected the initial information and how that information was interpreted and recorded varied.

Health care systems vary enormously in terms of (a) sophistication of care, (b) access to that care, and (c) use of available care. These differences affect how the same study might be conducted in different settings. To obtain adequate evaluations and diagnostic accuracy, either the study itself must provide all of the evaluations, or the evaluations must depend on the health care system. The first approach can be prohibitively expensive, and the feasibility of the second approach depends on where the study is conducted. In health care systems that rely heavily on specialist care, new-onset seizures are often evaluated by a specialist (26–29). In settings that rely on general practitioners, on the other hand, only the more difficult cases tend to be seen by a specialist with the necessary expertise to render an accurate diagnosis (30). In many developing nations, there is no system in place for epilepsy care and for most other medical needs (31–35).

Considerations in Ascertaining Cases

Epidemiologic studies often focus on a disorder as it occurs in a defined population, with the goal of determining the incidence or prevalence of the disorder and of its subtypes. This requires that a complete ascertainment method be used or that the sampling fraction be known. Even when complete ascertainment or systematic partial sampling is not feasible, a sample that is representative of the patients in the general population from which it was drawn allows one to make inferences regarding the relative significance of various causes and the frequency of particular types of epilepsy. There are several biases to avoid.

Prevalence Bias

Prevalent cases refer to individuals who, at a given time, carry a diagnosis of epilepsy or are under the care of a health care professional for epilepsy. In a disorder with a relatively low mortality rate, prevalent cases are overrepresented compared with those who remit courses (Fig. 8.1) (36). Gowers' comment is a prime example of an erroneous conclusion based on prevalent samples. As another example, Viani and colleagues reported the distribution of syndromes in a newly diagnosed versus a prevalent sample (37). Benign rolandic epilepsy accounted for 8.3% of newly diagnosed cases but only 2.3% of prevalent cases. Lennox-Gastaut syndrome accounted for 5% of newly diagnosed cases but 17% of prevalent cases. When mortality is high, prevalent samples tend to underestimate the number of severe cases (who die early) in favor of survivors. Although prevalent samples provide some relevant information for health care services, for the purposes of understanding the occurrence, causes, and outcomes of a disorder, they are methodologically inappropriate and prone to bias because they selectively emphasize the ongoing cases of a disease. Incident cases are generally preferred.

Ascertainment Bias

Poor response rate, inadequate ascertainment methods, and other problems that decrease the proportion of eligible cases recruited into a particular study can all affect the generalizability of the results of that study. This is because

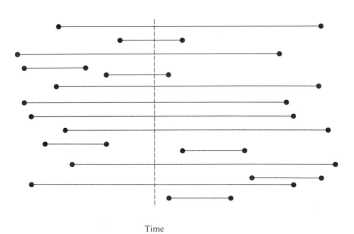

Time

Figure 8.1 Prevalence bias. Each horizontal line represents a case with active disease (i.e., a prevalent case). The length of the line represents the time of the active disease, with onset to the left and offset or death to the right. The dashed vertical line represents the day on which prevalence is measured. Long-duration cases are oversampled (eight of eight are ascertained on the prevalence day) relative to short-duration cases (two of seven are ascertained on the prevalence day).

those who do not participate or who are not included are often systematically different from those who are included.

Referral Center Bias

Recruitment through a specialty center biases a study group toward more extreme, difficult-to-diagnose and difficult-to-treat cases. This was demonstrated with febrile seizures in relation to the risk of epilepsy (38). Children with febrile seizures studied in population-based or near population-based cohorts had a uniformly low risk of subsequent epilepsy. In contrast, the estimated risks of epilepsy in studies that recruited children from special referral centers were very inconsistent, with many exceeding 30%.

To avoid these and related biases requires an understanding of the typical process by which persons with epilepsy are diagnosed and a concerted effort to identify and recruit all potentially eligible individuals in a population during a specified time frame. In developed nations, these issues may seem relatively trivial. In developing nations, however, they can pose tremendous challenges to the researcher. Pal and associates eloquently describe their experiences and observations from studies they conducted on childhood epilepsy in rural India (39–42). The paucity of health care services, the expenses and difficulties involved in using those services, the mistrust of westernized medicine, local beliefs about healers, and the stigma associated with epilepsy were just some of the factors that had to be addressed in order to proceed with their research.

Diagnostic Accuracy Versus Representativeness

Ideally, specialists should routinely and uniformly evaluate all individuals with a suspected diagnosis of epilepsy. This could, however, limit studies to wealthy, developed nations, whereas epilepsy is a global problem that is of pressing concern in developing nations (43). The requirements of diagnostic accuracy and representativeness of the sample are inherently in conflict with each other. This discord is accentuated in settings in which specialists do not routinely diagnose individuals with seizures. Generally, a clear statement of the research purpose will go a long way toward indicating where compromises may be made and where one must insist on certain standards or approaches.

Frequency Measures in Populations— Incidence and Prevalence

Incidence is expressed as the number of new cases of disease in a standard-sized population per unit of time—for example, the number of cases per 100,000 population per year. Prevalence, which measures the total number of persons with a particular disease at a specified time, is expressed as the number of persons per some standard-sized population. For example, in epilepsy, prevalence is usually expressed as the number of persons per 1000 population. Active prevalence, often preferred in epilepsy terminology,

includes only patients who are currently being treated or have had a seizure within a specified time period (e.g., the last 5 years). Patients with a remote history (more than 5 years ago) who are not treated are not counted in active prevalence figures.

Table 8.1 provides results from several studies conducted throughout the world that have estimated the incidence, prevalence, or both of epilepsy in defined populations. Active prevalence estimates typically range from 4 to 7 per 1000 population. Incidence rates for epilepsy are typically between 30 and 50 per 100,000 population per year, although several estimates are in the 60- to 80-per-100,000-per-year range.

Several studies have examined the relative, if not absolute, frequency of different forms of epilepsy in well-characterized series of incident patients who were reasonably representative of the populations from which they were drawn (Table 8.2) (8,24,25,69–71). In children, approximately 50% to 60% of all epilepsy is localization related or unclassified (frequently, epilepsy that is initially unclassified turns out to be localization related) (72). This contrasts with adults, in whom approximately 90% of all epilepsy cases are localization related or initially unclassified. In children, approximately 30% to 40% of all newly diagnosed epilepsy is idiopathic, either localization related (approximately 10%) or generalized (20% to 30%). By contrast, in adults, only about 5% of all epilepsy cases are idiopathic (apparently all generalized). In children, only about 10% of new cases have symptomatic localization-related epilepsy, compared with close to 30% in adults.

Aside from methodologic issues, other factors, particularly age and etiology, influence the frequency of epilepsy in and across populations.

Age

Two similarly designed studies in Geneva, Switzerland, and the island of Martinique demonstrated the bimodal incidence of unprovoked seizures, with children and adults older than 55 years of age having relatively higher incidence rates than younger adults (20 to 55 years of age) (47,73). Because the overall incidence rate (or prevalence) in a population is the weighted average of the age-specific figures, the age structure of the population influences the overall incidence and prevalence of epilepsy.

Age structures differ across populations. In postindustrialized nations, the infant mortality rate is typically less than or equal to 5 per 1,000, with the average life expectancy in the upper seventies and often close to 80 years. In these settings, epilepsy, which has often been considered a childhood disorder, is now also becoming known as a disorder of the elderly, perhaps secondary to neurodegenerative and neurovascular causes (50). By contrast, in many developing nations, infant mortality rates can run as high as 5% to 10% and life expectancy is typically less than or equal to 60 years of age. The large number of elderly cases with

TABLE 8.1

INCIDENCE AND PREVALENCE OF EPILEPSY AS REPORTED IN SELECTED POPULATION-BASED STUDIES THROUGHOUT THE WORLD

First Author/Year	Country/Region	Age-Group (Years)	Incidence/ 100,000/Year	Prevalence/ 1000
Annegers, 1999 (44)	Texas, USA	All ages	35.5	—
Beilmann, 1999 (45)	Estonia	0–19	—	3.6
Karaağaç, 1999 (46)	Silivri, Turkey	All ages	—	10.2
Jallon, 1998 (47)	Martinique	All ages	64.1	—
Jallon, 1997 (48)	Geneva, Switzerland	All ages	45.6	—
Camfield, 1996 (49)	Nova Scotia, Canada	<16	41	—
de la Court, 1996 (50)	Rotterdam, Netherlands	55–95	—	9.0
Mendizabal, 1996 (51)	Guatemala	All ages	—	5.8
Olafsson, 1996 (52)	Iceland	All ages	47	—
Sidenvall, 1996 (53)	Northern Sweden	0–16	—	4.2
Braathen, 1995 (54)	Stockholm, Sweden	0–16	53	—
Aziz, 1994 (55)	Karachi, Pakistan	All ages	—	10.1 (total) 14.8 (rural) 7.4 (urban)
Snow, 1994 (56)	Kilifi, Kenya	All ages	—	4.0 (total) 2.5 (females) 5.9 (males)
Attia-Romdhane, 1993 (57)	Kelibia, Tunisia	All ages	—	4.0
Sidenvall, 1993 (58)	Västerbotten, Sweden	0–15	78.5	—
Loiseau, 1990 (59)	Gironde, France	All ages	24–42	—
Forsgren, 1990 (60)	Västerbotten, Sweden	≥17	33.6	—
Bharucha, 1988 (61)	Bombay, India	All ages		4.7
Koul, 1988 (62)	Kashmir, India	<14 ≥14	—	3.8 2.0
Osuntokun, 1987 (32)	Igbo-Ora, Nigeria	All ages	—	5.3
Joensen, 1986 (63)	Faroe Islands	All ages	42	7.6
Li, 1985 (64)	Urban China	All ages	—	4.4
Granieri, 1983 (65)	Copparo, Italy	All ages	33.1	6.2
Juul-Jensen, 1983 (66)	Great Aarhus, Denmark	All ages	—	12.7
Shamansky, 1979 (67)	Connecticut, USA	<15	73	—
Hauser, 1975 (3)	Minnesota, USA	All ages	—	5.4
Stanhope, 1972 (68)	Guam, Mariana Islands	All ages	—	5.3

epilepsy secondary to neurodegenerative conditions does not occur. Instead, causes of epilepsy that affect children predominate. Age standardization is often used to adjust for these differences in age structure and to provide a basis for meaningful comparisons across populations (74).

Etiology

The CAROLE study provides a glimpse at the underlying causes of epilepsy in a Western European nation (8). Of all epilepsy cases in that cohort, half had forms of epilepsy with cryptogenic etiology and another third had idiopathic

forms of epilepsy. In the remaining 18%, a remote symptomatic cause was found. In 88% of these cases, the remote symptomatic cause was a static disorder or insult. Head trauma, cerebral vascular accident, and pre- or perinatal insults were the most common. In the other 12%, there was a progressive lesion or process, most frequently a tumor.

These data represent the current situation in France. They probably also represent what one would find throughout much of Western Europe but not necessarily in other parts of the world. The underlying cause of epilepsy can vary between populations and over time. For example, neurocysticercosis is almost nonexistent in the northern regions

TABLE 8.2

DISTRIBUTION OF EPILEPSY SYNDROMES IN NEWLY DIAGNOSED PATIENTS FROM FOUR DIFFERENT COUNTRIES

Syndrome	Connecticut* (25) Children <16 Years Old		CAROLE[†] (8) Children <14 Years Old		Adults ≥25 Years Old		Netherlands (69) Children <16 Years Old		Italy[‡] (37) Children	
	No. of Patients	%	No. of Patients	%	No. of Patients	%	No. of Patients	%	No. of Patients	%
Benign partial	61	10.0	47	9.4	1	0.3	31	6.7	21	8.7
Symptomatic partial	71	11.6	34	6.8	81	26.6	74	16.0	92	38.2
Cryptogenic partial	227	37.0	121	24.2	107	35.1	87	18.8	0	0
Idiopathic generalized	126	20.6	199	39.7	15	4.9	195	42.2	67	27.8
Cryptogenic/ symptomatic generalized	43	7.0	39	7.8	0	0	29	6.3	50	20.7
Symptomatic generalized	9	1.5	14	2.8	7	2.3	41	8.9	1	0.4
Generalized and focal features	5	0.8	13	2.6	0	0	1	0.2	1	0.4
Unclassified	71	11.6	34	6.8	94	30.1	2	0.4	19	7.7
Total number of patients	613		501		305		462		251	

*The cryptogenic and symptomatic localization-related categories were redefined to be consistent with the interpretation of other authors and to facilitate comparisons.
[†]Limited to children younger than 14 years of age. CAROLE, Coordination Active du Réseau Observatoire Longitudinal de L'Epilepsie study.
[‡]Pediatric epilepsy center (referral) in Milan; published prior to 1989.

of North America and Northern Europe, although in the southwest regions of the United States, it may be more common than previously thought (75). In some countries it is actually a very common cause of epilepsy. In Ecuador, neurocysticercosis is implicated in 20% of cases of adult-onset epilepsy (76). The acquired immune deficiency syndrome (AIDS) epidemic has brought its own changes to the face of epilepsy, as cerebral complications of AIDS can result in seizures and epilepsy. In many African nations, diseases such as AIDS and malaria are endemic, and access to modern health care is extremely limited, if not entirely absent.

In developed nations, public health and primary care initiatives have greatly improved birth weight and infant survival. Decreases in the incidence of serious infections that can cause meningitis and subsequent symptomatic epilepsy, decreases in hypertension and resulting stroke, and possible changes in the occurrence of head injury and resulting posttraumatic epilepsy, are some of the factors that have influenced the frequency of epilepsy. The presence of these problems and the interventions used to correct them vary from one country to another and change over time (77).

Genetic variation across populations may also influence the frequency of epilepsy and of specific forms of epilepsy. Febrile seizures, for example, occur in two to four times as many individuals in Japan as in Europe and North America (78). Whether this represents geographic variations in genetic influences or necessary environmental cofactors is a matter that warrants further investigation.

SUMMARY

Epidemiology has been key in demonstrating the relatively high frequency of seizures in the population and in challenging long-held beliefs about the uniformly poor outcomes associated with seizures. Research pursuits within the epidemiology of epilepsy have come a long way from the days of simply counting how many people in a given population had seizures. As diagnostic technology has become increasingly sophisticated, the methods used for ascertaining cases in a population have become increasingly complex. Representativeness and diagnostic accuracy are increasingly at odds, especially in underdeveloped areas. Once these issues are appropriately addressed, or at least acknowledged, cross-regional or cross-national comparisons of similarly conducted studies may help identify forms of epilepsy and causes of epilepsy that are unusually common in certain areas. In turn, this may lead to insights into prevention. Combining the strengths of epidemiologic methods with the sophistication of new medical diagnostic technology and our growing understanding of epilepsy has the promise of advancing our knowledge of the causes, consequences, and possibly prevention of this common set of disorders.

REFERENCES

1. Gowers WR. *Epilepsy and other chronic convulsive disorders: their causes, symptoms and treatment.* London: J&A Churchill, 1881.
2. Kurland LT. The incidence and prevalence of convulsive disorders in a small urban community. *Epilepsia* 1959;1:143–161.
3. Hauser WA, Kurland LT. The epidemiology of epilepsy in Rochester, Minnesota, 1935 through 1967. *Epilepsia* 1975;16:1–66.
4. Annegers JF, Hauser WA, Elveback LR. Remission of seizures and relapse in patients with epilepsy. *Epilepsia* 1979;20:729–737.
5. Nelson KB, Ellenberg JH. Predictors of epilepsy in children who have experienced febrile seizures. *N Engl J Med* 1976;295:1029–1033.
6. Commission on Classification and Terminology of the International League Against Epilepsy. Proposal for revised clinical and electroencephalographic classification of epileptic seizures. *Epilepsia* 1981;22:489–501.
7. Commission on Epidemiology and Prognosis, International League Against Epilepsy. Guidelines for epidemiologic studies on epilepsy. *Epilepsia* 1993;34:592–596.
8. Jallon P, Loiseau P, Loiseau J. Newly diagnosed unprovoked epileptic seizures: presentation at diagnosis in CAROLE study. *Epilepsia* 2001;42:464–475.
9. Singh R, Andermann E, Whitehouse WPA, et al. Severe myoclonic epilepsy of infancy: extended spectrum of GEFS+? *Epilepsia* 2001;42:837–844.
10. Staden U, Isaacs E, Boyd SG, et al. Language dysfunction in children with Rolandic epilepsy. *Neuropediatrics* 1998;29:242–248.
11. Plouin P, Raffo E, de Oliveira T. Prognosis of neonatal seizures. In: Jallon P, Berg AT, Dulac O, et al., eds. *Prognosis of epilepsies.* Montrouge, France: John Libbey Eurotext, 2003:199–209.
12. Engel J Jr. Classifications of the International League Against Epilepsy: time for reappraisal. *Epilepsia* 1998;39:1014–1017.
13. Engel J Jr. A proposed diagnostic scheme for people with epileptic seizures and with epilepsy: report of the ILAE Task Force on Classification and Terminology. *Epilepsia* 2001;42:796–803.
14. Engel J. Reply to "Of cabbages and kings: some considerations on classifications and diagnostic schemes, semiology, and concepts." *Epilepsia* 2003;44:4–6.
15. Wolf P. Of cabbages and kings: some considerations on classifications, diagnostic schemes, semiology, and concepts. *Epilepsia* 2003;44:1–4.
16. Avanzini G. Of cabbages and kings: do we really need a systematic classification of epilepsies? *Epilepsia* 2003;44:12–13.
17. Berg AT, Blackstone NW. Of Cabbages and kings: perspectives on classification from the field of systematics. *Epilepsia* 2003;44:8–11.
18. Hirtz D, Ashwal S, Berg AT, et al. Practice parameter: evaluating a first nonfebrile seizure in children: report of the quality standards committee of the American Academy of Neurology, the Child Neurology Society, and the American Epilepsy Society. *Neurology* 2000;55:616–623.
19. Placencia M, Suarez J, Crespo F, et al. A large-scale study of epilepsy in Ecuador: methodological aspects. *Neuroepidemiology* 1992;11:74–84.
20. Osuntokun B, Schoenberg B, Nottidge V, et al. Research protocol for measuring the prevalence of neurologic disorders in developing countries. *Neuroepidemiology* 1982;1:143–153.
21. Aziz H, Guvener A, Akhtar SW, et al. Comparative epidemiology of epilepsy in Pakistan and Turkey: population-based studies using identical protocols. *Epilepsia* 1997;38:716–722.
22. Cockerell OC, Johnson AL, Sander JW, et al. Prognosis of epilepsy: a review and further analysis of the first nine years of the British National General Practice Study of Epilepsy, a prospective population-based study. *Epilepsia* 1997;38:31–46.
23. Arts WFM, Geerts AT, Brouwer OF, et al. The early prognosis of epilepsy in childhood: the prediction of a poor outcome. The Dutch study of epilepsy in childhood. *Epilepsia* 1999;40:726–734.
24. Loiseau J, Loiseau P, Guyot M, et al. Survey of seizure disorders in the French southwest. I. Incidence of epileptic syndromes. *Epilepsia* 1990;31:391–396.
25. Berg AT, Shinnar S, Levy SR, et al. Newly diagnosed epilepsy in children: presentation at diagnosis. *Epilepsia* 1999;40:445–452.
26. Gram L. Perspectives on epilepsy care in Denmark. *Neurology* 1997;48(Suppl 8):S16–S19.
27. Dulac O, Jallon P. Patterns of care for patients with epilepsy in France. *Neurology* 1997;48(Suppl 8):S30–S32.
28. Schmidt D. Epilepsy care in Germany: a clinical perspective. *Neurology* 1997;48(Suppl 8):S25–S29.
29. Henriksen O. Perspectives of epilepsy care in Norway. *Neurology* 1997;48(Suppl 8):S20–S24.
30. Chadwick D, Reynolds EH. Services for epilepsy in the United Kingdom. *Neurology* 1997;48:S3–S7.
31. Placencia MS, Sander JW, Roman M, et al. The characteristics of epilepsy in a largely untreated population in rural Ecuador. *J Neurol Neurosurg Psychiatry* 1994;57:320–325.
32. Osuntokun BO, Adeuja AOG, Nottidge VA, et al. Prevalence of the epilepsies in Nigerian Africans: a community-based study. *Epilepsia* 1987;28:272–278.
33. Watts AE. The natural history of untreated epilepsy in a rural community in Africa. *Epilepsia* 1992;33:464–468.
34. Feksi AT, Kaamugisha J, Sander JW, et al. Comprehensive primary health care antiepileptic drug treatment programme in rural and semi-urban Kenya. ICEBERG (International Community-based Epilepsy Research Group). *Lancet* 1991;337:406–409.
35. Shorvon SD, Farmer PJ. Epilepsy in developing countries: a review of epidemiological, sociocultural, and treatment aspects. *Epilepsia* 1988;29(Suppl 1):S36–S54.
36. Sackett DL. Bias in analytic research. *J Chronic Dis* 1979;32:51–63.
37. Viani F, Beghi E, Atza MG, et al. Classifications of epileptic syndromes: advantages and limitations for evaluation of childhood epileptic syndromes in clinical practice. *Epilepsia* 1988;29:440–445.
38. Ellenberg JH, Nelson KB. Sample selection and the natural history of disease: studies of febrile seizures. *JAMA* 1980;243:1337–1340.
39. Pal DK, Das T, Sengupta S. Comparison of key informant and survey methods for ascertainment of childhood epilepsy in West Bengal, India. *Int J Epidemiol* 1998;27:672–676.
40. Pal DK, Das T, Sengupta S. Case-control and qualitative study of attrition in a community epilepsy programme in rural India. *Seizure* 2000;9:119–123.
41. Pal DK, Das T, Sengupta S, et al. Help-seeking patterns for children with epilepsy in rural India: implications for service delivery. *Epilepsia* 2002;43:904–911.
42. Pal DK. *Shadows and light,* 2002. Available at: http://www.ich.ucl.ac.uk/ich/html/academicunits/int_P_C/pdfs/Shadows&Light.pdf. Accessed September 24, 2003.
43. Jallon P. Epilepsy in developing countries. *Epilepsia* 1997;38:1143–1151.
44. Annegers JF, Dubinsky S, Coan SP, et al. The incidence of epilepsy and unprovoked seizures in multiethnic, urban health maintenance organizations. *Epilepsia* 1999;40:502–506.
45. Beilmann A, Napa A, Hamarik M, et al. Incidence of childhood epilepsy in Estonia. *Brain Dev* 1999;21:166–174.
46. Karaağaç N, Yeni SN, Senocak M, et al. Prevalence of epilepsy in Silivri, a rural area of Turkey. *Epilepsia* 1999;40:637–642.
47. Jallon P, Smadja D, Cabre P, et al. Epileptic seizures, epilepsy and risk factors: experiences with an investigation in Martinique. Epimart Group. *Rev Neurol (Paris)* 1998;154:408–411.
48. Jallon P, Goumaz M, Haenggeli C, et al. Incidence of first epileptic seizures in the canton of Geneva, Switzerland. *Epilepsia* 1997;38:547–552.

49. Camfield CS, Camfield PR, Gordon K, et al. Incidence of epilepsy in childhood and adolescence: a population-based study in Nova Scotia from 1977 to 1985. *Epilepsia* 1996;37: 19–23.

50. de la Court A, Breteler MMB, Meinardi H, et al. Prevalence of epilepsy in the elderly: the Rotterdam Study. *Epilepsia* 1996;37: 141–147.

51. Mendizabal JE, Salguero LF. Prevalence of epilepsy in a rural community of Guatemala. *Epilepsia* 1996;37:373–376.

52. Olafsson E, Hauser WA, Ludvigsson P, et al. Incidence of epilepsy in rural Iceland: a population-based study. *Epilepsia* 1996;37: 951–955.

53. Sidenvall R, Forsgren L, Heijbel J. Prevalence and characteristics of epilepsy in children in northern Sweden. *Seizure* 1996;5: 139–146.

54. Braathen G, Theorell K. A general hospital population of childhood epilepsy. *Acta Paediatr* 1995;84:1143–1146.

55. Aziz H, Ali SM, Frances P, et al. Epilepsy in Pakistan: a population-based epidemiologic study. *Epilepsia* 1994;35:950–958.

56. Snow R, Williams R, Rogers J, Mung'ala V, Peshu N. The prevalence of epilepsy among a rural Kenyan population: its association with premature mortality. *Trop Geogr Med* 1994;46: 175–179.

57. Attia-Romdhane N, Mrabet A, Ben Hamida M. Prevalence of epilepsy in Kelibia, Tunisia. *Epilepsia* 1993;34:1028–1032.

58. Sidenvall R, Forsgren L, Blomquist HR, et al. A community-based prospective incidence study of epileptic seizures in children. *Acta Paediatr* 1993;82:60–65.

59. Loiseau P, Duche B. Stopping antiepileptic treatment. *Rev Neurol (Paris)* 1990;146:380–382.

60. Forsgren L. Prospective incidence study and clinical characterization of seizures in newly referred adults. *Epilepsia* 1990;31:292–301.

61. Bharucha NE, Bharucha EP, Bharucha AE, et al. Prevalence of epilepsy in the Parsi community of Bombay. *Epilepsia* 1988;29: 111–115.

62. Koul R, Razdan S, Motta A. Prevalence and pattern of epilepsy (Lath/Mirgi/Laran) in rural Kashmir, India. *Epilepsia* 1988;29: 116–122.

63. Joensen P. Prevalence, incidence, and classification of epilepsy in the Faroes. *Acta Neurol Scand* 1986;74:150–155.

64. Li SC, Schoenberg BS, Wand C, et al. Epidemiology of epilepsy in urban areas of the People's Republic of China. *Epilepsia* 1985;26: 391–394.

65. Granieri E, Rosati G, Tola R, et al. A descriptive study of epilepsy in the District of Copparo, Italy, 1964–1978. *Epilepsia* 1983;24: 502–514.

66. Juul-Jensen P, Foldspang A. Natural history of epileptic seizures. *Epilepsia* 1983;24:297–312.

67. Shamansky SL, Glaser GH. Socioeconomic characteristics of childhood seizure disorders in the New Haven area: an epidemiologic study. *Epilepsia* 1979;20:457–474.

68. Stanhope JM, Brody JA, Brink E. Convulsions among the Chamorro people of Guam, Mariana Islands. I. Seizure disorders. *Am J Epidemiol* 1972;95:292–298.

69. Callenbach PM, Geerts AT, Arts WF, et al. Familial occurrence of epilepsy in children with newly diagnosed multiple seizures: Dutch Study of Epilepsy in Childhood. *Epilepsia* 1998;39:331–336.

70. Shinnar S, O'Dell C, Berg AT. Epilepsy syndromes in children identified at the time of their first unprovoked seizure. *Epilepsia* 1998;39(Suppl 6):148.

71. Epilepsies and time to diagnosis. Descriptive results of the CAROLE survey. *Rev Neurol (Paris)* 2000;156:481–490.

72. Berg AT, Shinnar S, Levy SR, et al. How well can epilepsy syndromes be identified at diagnosis? A reassessment 2 years after initial diagnosis. *Epilepsia* 2000;41:1269–1275.

73. Jallon P, Goumaz M, Morabia A. First epileptic seizures in Geneva County: incidence rate and epidemiological classification of the risk factors. *Epilepsia* 1994;35(Suppl 8):110.

74. Selvin S. *Statistical analysis of epidemiologic data*. New York: Oxford University Press, 1991.

75. Ong S, Talan DA, Moran GJ, et al. Neurocysticercosis in radiographically imaged seizures patients in U.S. emergency departments. *Emerg Infect Dis* 2002;8:608–613.

76. Carpio A, Escobar A, Hauser WA. Cysticercosis and epilepsy: a critical review. *Epilepsia* 1998;39:1025–1040.

77. Berg AT, Testa FM, Levy SR, et al. The epidemiology of epilepsy: past, present, and future. *Neurol Clin* 1996;14:383–398.

78. Stafstrom CE. The incidence and prevalence of febrile seizures. In: Baram TZ, Shinnar S, eds. *Febrile seizures*. San Diego: Academic Press, 2001;1–26.

The Natural History of Seizures

9

W. Allen Hauser

Descriptive epidemiologic studies provide information about the frequency of epilepsy and other convulsive disorders in the population. Individuals identified in these cohorts form an unselected group in which to evaluate the natural history and prognosis of convulsive disorders. Prognosis may cover a number of concepts. The clinician is interested in prognosis primarily for seizure control, because this is the most obvious assessment of the success or failure of a treatment regimen. Nevertheless, mortality, comorbidity for other disease, and the likelihood of normal intellectual and social functioning are important when natural history is considered. Because seizures distinguish the person with epilepsy from the rest of the population, it is possible to think that seizure control will affect other potential outcomes. Although this assumption may not be valid, most of this discussion deals with prognosis in terms of seizure control, remission, likelihood of successful withdrawal of medication, and likelihood of intractability, as these are of greatest interest to physicians and patients.

As recently as 35 years ago, studies of highly selected populations with epilepsy drawn from tertiary-care centers suggested that epilepsy was predominantly a lifelong condition with little likelihood of seizure control, much less remission of the illness (1). Today, the prognosis for most people with epilepsy is excellent in terms of likelihood of seizure control, remission, and eventual medication withdrawal. This major departure from these long-held attitudes resulted largely from epidemiologic studies undertaken in the past three decades (2–7). Population-based studies consistently indicate that 60% to 70% of individuals with a new diagnosis of epilepsy ultimately become seizure free on medication. Most of those achieving complete control can successfully discontinue medication (2,8–10).

Seizure remission can be evaluated at several points during the clinical course of epilepsy. Studies provide data on differential risks for recurrence after a first seizure; predictors, at the initial diagnosis, of subsequent course and remission; predictors of remission after diagnosis but during active epilepsy; predictors of successful medication withdrawal in patients who have achieved total seizure control; and factors associated with relapse after long-term remission. Nevertheless, these estimates of overall remission and the factors that alter the likelihood of remission are invariably based on prior probability and therefore cannot be applied with certainty to an individual patient.

Many studies estimate the frequency of remission of epilepsy in groups defined by specific clinical characteristics. Although these characteristics are at times imprecisely determined, some consistency exists in predictors of remission at each point of evaluation. Obviously, inconsistent or imprecise definition of these variables may preclude direct comparisons across specific studies.

Predictive factors of continued seizure control or subsequent relapse are discussed in Chapter 47. However, aspects relevant to the natural history of seizures are summarized here.

LIKELIHOOD OF REMISSION FROM TIME OF FIRST SEIZURE

Epilepsy is generally defined as a condition in which an individual tends to experience recurrent unprovoked seizures (11). A person with only one unprovoked seizure does not, by definition, have epilepsy but clearly differs from the general population in terms of risk to develop the illness.

Several studies have attempted to evaluate predictors of recurrence after a first seizure. Although estimates of the total proportion of patients who will experience recurrent seizures vary substantially across studies, much of the variation

TABLE 9.1

SEIZURE RECURRENCE AFTER A FIRST UNPROVOKED SEIZURE: AN EXTENDED FOLLOW-UP

Risk Factor	Recurrence in Subgroups, % Months of Follow-up		
	12 mo	24 mo	36 mo
Baseline (N = 78)	7.0	13.0	16.7
Idiopathic or cryptogenic with an affected sibling (N = 10)	20.0	20.0	31.0
Idiopathic or cryptogenic with a generalized spike-and-wave EEG pattern (N = 10)	10.0	55.0	55.0
Idiopathic or cryptogenic with prior acute seizures (all febrile) (N = 7)	0.0	14.0	28.6
Idiopathic or cryptogenic with abnormal neurologic examination (N = 13)	9.3	15.4	20.3
Idiopathic or cryptogenic with abnormal examination and additional feature (N = 23)	14.3	14.3	22.7
Idiopathic or cryptogenic with two or more features and normal examination (N = 5)	40.0	40.0	70.0
Remote symptomatic with no other features (N = 32)	15.9	15.9	24.8
Remote symptomatic with Todd's paresis (N = 4)	0.0	25.0	50.0
Remote symptomatic with prior acute symptomatic seizures (N = 3)	100.0	100.0	100.0
Remote symptomatic with multiple seizures or status epilepticus at presentation (N = 8)	25.0	37.5	37.5
Remote symptomatic with two or more risk factors (N = 12)	41.7	75.0	75.0

Abbreviation: EEG, electroencephalogram.
From Hauser WA, Rich SS, Annegers JF, et al. Seizure recurrence after a first unprovoked seizure: an extended follow-up. *Neurology* 1990;40:1163–1170, with permission.

seems related, in part, to differences in methodology. Prospective follow-up studies of individuals identified at their first seizure suggest that only approximately 25% experience a second episode within the next 2 years (12,13); this contrasts considerably with the overall recurrence risk of 70% or more reported in retrospective studies (14). Also influencing the reported variation is the heterogeneous nature of clinical epilepsy. For example, when several factors were assessed in a single study, recurrence risk at 2 years varied from less than 15% in those with no identified risk factors to 100% in those with a combination of two or more risk factors (Table 9.1) (12). Although multiple factors appear to influence recurrence risk after a first unprovoked seizure, and not all studies have identified the same predictors, a meta-analysis of studies performed through 1990 suggests some consistency in predictors and in recurrence risk after controlling for these factors (15).

A prior neurologic insult, such as neurologic deficits from birth (mental retardation, cerebral palsy), is the most powerful and consistent predictor of recurrence after a first seizure (12,13,15–18). Moreover, the likelihood of a second seizure is increased by partial seizure type, abnormal electroencephalogram (EEG) (in some studies specific epileptiform EEG patterns) (12,13,16,18,19), prior acute seizures including febrile seizures (12,13), status epilepticus or multiple seizures at the index episode (12,20), and Todd's paralysis (12,13).

In these descriptive studies, the risk for seizure recurrence has been consistently higher in patients for whom antiepileptic drugs (AEDs) have been prescribed (but not necessarily used by the patient), even after controlling for the other identified risk factors (12,13). Results from such descriptive studies may be confounded by poor compli-

ance or failure to achieve therapeutic doses. It is reassuring, although not surprising, that in two randomized clinical trials (21,22), use of AEDs in doses to maintain serum levels in the therapeutic range was associated with a reduction in the proportion of patients who experienced seizure recurrence after a first seizure.

PREDICTORS OF REMISSION FROM TIME OF DIAGNOSIS

Individuals with multiple unprovoked seizures (epilepsy) differ clinically from those with one unprovoked seizure, and the risk for additional seizures is substantial (11). Even so, approximately 75% of all patients with a diagnosis of epilepsy enter remission (i.e., become seizure free for 5 or more years) (2). More than one half of those who enter remission do so during the first year after diagnosis (Fig. 9.1) (2).

Although predictors of seizure remission at the time of diagnosis of epilepsy may vary from those identified in association with seizure recurrence after a first seizure, some consistency is evident. Features predicting remission at initial diagnosis include young age at onset, young age at diagnosis, generalized-onset seizures, normal neurologic examination, and idiopathic or cryptogenic cause (2,23–28). Few multivariate analyses have been performed, but these factors probably are independent. In one multivariate analysis of data from 613 children with newly diagnosed epilepsy, age (onset between 5 and 9 years of age) and a generalized idiopathic syndrome were associated with remission (29).

Conversely, a known cause, partial seizure type, neurologic deficit from birth (mental retardation or cerebral

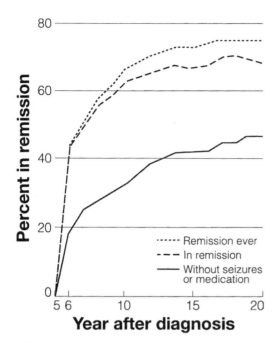

Figure 9.1 Remission of seizures and relapse in people with epilepsy. (From Annegers JF, Hauser WA, Elveback LR. Remission of seizures and relapse in patients with epilepsy. *Epilepsia* 1979;20:729–737, reprinted by permission of the International League Against Epilepsy.)

palsy), occurrence of a primary or secondarily generalized seizure, and abnormal EEG findings—particularly a generalized spike-and-wave pattern (18,26)—are linked to a reduced likelihood of remission. The number and duration of seizures prior to diagnosis are inversely proportional to the likelihood of remission (30,31). On multivariate analysis, remote symptomatic cause, family history of epilepsy, seizure frequency, and slowing on the initial EEG were independent predictors of a reduced likelihood of remission (29). In some studies, remission was less likely in children whose epilepsy began before age 1 year, but when syndrome was taken into account, early age of onset was not a factor (32,33). Numerous seizures before initiation of treatment negatively impacted chances for remission in other studies (29,30).

PROGNOSTIC PREDICTORS DURING EPILEPSY

During the course of epilepsy, the presence of multiple seizure types (e.g., generalized onset and partial onset) and frequent generalized tonic-clonic seizures portend a lower likelihood of remission (22,34). The duration of active epilepsy before achieving control has been thought to be the most important clinical predictor of remission (2,33). In children, failure to attain control in the first 3 months predicted a poor outcome (34,35), as did the use of multiple medications (36–38). In a study involving primarily adults (31), the total number of seizures in the first 6 months after

treatment began was inversely correlated with likelihood of remission. If seizures are not controlled in the first year after diagnosis or if multiple medications are needed in the first year, only approximately 60% of patients can be expected to achieve remission (2,34,36). If seizures remain uncontrolled for more than 4 years after diagnosis, only approximately 10% of the initial cohort can be expected to enter remission after that time (2). Fewer than 5% of patients with epilepsy who continue to have seizures 10 or more years after diagnosis ever achieve total seizure control.

Early use of anticonvulsant medication does not influence the prognosis for seizure control. Randomized clinical trials from Kenya and Ecuador (39,40) indicate that 50% of patients with long-standing epilepsy achieve control if expeditiously treated with carbamazepine or phenobarbital. Presumably missing from this population are the individuals who enter remission shortly after onset. These cases probably represent the 20% of patients who fail to achieve remission early after onset of disease. In these studies, neither the duration of epilepsy nor the lifetime number of seizures affected the outcome.

PREDICTORS OF SUCCESSFUL MEDICATION WITHDRAWAL AFTER REMISSION

Among the 60% to 70% of patients with epilepsy who enter long-term remission, 40% to 90% can have AEDs withdrawn without seizure recurrence (2,13,24,31,34,35, 41–47). Factors associated with the success or failure of AED withdrawal are familiar, being largely the same as those previously identified from initial diagnosis. Predictors of relapse after medication withdrawal include an abnormal examination in children (generally an indicator of mental retardation or cerebral palsy) (2,9,10,17,24,25,32–34,46,48); a presumed cause for the epilepsy (8,34,44,46–48); abnormal EEG findings at diagnosis (10,41,46,49), particularly a spike-wave pattern (43); worsening or persistence of an abnormal pattern (6,43); need for multiple medications to achieve control (44,50); and occurrence of many generalized seizures before control (24,25,39). In contrast, continued seizure freedom after medication withdrawal is predicted by control of seizures with monotherapy and with low serum drug concentrations, few seizures before control, and a brief interval between onset of seizures and initial control (2,24,33, 34,51). Seizure type is not a consistent predictor of relapse, although partial or secondarily generalized seizures are associated with a higher relapse rate (33,47). Young age at onset predicts successful AED withdrawal in studies of adults (52) and children (24,25,32,46,47). Family history, rate of AED withdrawal, and age at AED withdrawal (9,33,34) have been evaluated but have not been shown to influence seizure recurrence. Duration of seizure freedom may not predict successful withdrawal (33,47).

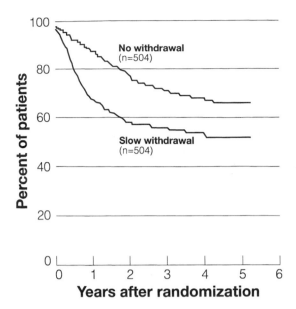

Figure 9.2 Seizure relapse in patients in remission who were withdrawn from medication. (From Medical Research Council Antiepileptic Drug Withdrawal Study Group. Randomized study of antiepileptic drug withdrawal in patients in remission. *Lancet* 1991;337:1175–1180, with permission.)

The most ambitious and comprehensive study of AED withdrawal was conducted by the Medical Research Council Antiepileptic Drug Withdrawal Study Group (33). The study is unique by virtue of its size (more than 1000 subjects) and the randomization of subjects to continuation or cessation of medication. By 4 years after entry, seizures had recurred in approximately 45% of previously seizure-free patients undergoing medication withdrawal, compared with 25% of those who continued treatment for the entire study period (Fig. 9.2). The study used a multivariate model to identify predictors of recurrence and found that a history of partial seizures without secondary generalization, myoclonic seizures, and any generalized seizures increased the risk for relapse after withdrawal. Seizures after treatment initiation, long duration of treatment (more than 20 years), use of multiple AEDs at randomization, and onset of seizures as an adolescent or adult were associated with an increased risk of seizure recurrence. This study provided two additional useful pieces of information: 25% of patients whose treatment was maintained experienced seizure recurrence, indicating that further seizures cannot be attributed solely to medication withdrawal, and even though a substantial proportion of patients remained seizure free after medication withdrawal, no powerful predictors allowed identification of these individuals.

RELAPSE AFTER REMISSION

After successful medication withdrawal or a prolonged period of seizure freedom, relapse is more likely in patients with complex partial seizures and in those with older age at diagnosis (53). Some may be seizure free for many years after withdrawal before a recurrent episode. It is not known whether this represents recurrence of the initial condition or the manifestation of a new convulsive disorder related to a new insult in a susceptible individual. It appears that people who are unsuccessfully withdrawn from medication after a prolonged seizure-free period generally achieve full control after reinstitution of medication (3,10,32).

ARE THERE PREDICTORS OF INTRACTABLE EPILEPSY?

Only 5% to 10% of all incidence cases of epilepsy (10,000 to 15,000 new cases annually in the United States in 2005) ultimately result in truly intractable disease. In these patients, however, seizures are sufficiently frequent or severe despite optimal AED therapy that alternative treatments, including surgery, may need to be considered. Although the number each year is small, such cases probably account for one half of the prevalence cases of epilepsy.

All the studies discussed have addressed the outcome of total seizure control. This wealth of information comes about in part because control (the absence of seizures) is relatively easy to define. Intractability of epilepsy is not, however, the converse of seizure freedom, and predictors of intractability may differ from those of seizure control or remission. Moreover, the definition of drug resistance may vary, depending on the investigator's interest and available procedures (10,32,36,54). Older age of onset, evidence of an abnormal neurologic state based on history or examination, abnormal or worsening EEG findings, and the presence of multiple seizure types seem to be consistent predictors of reduced probability of remission. Even in combination, however, these factors lack specificity for the identification of intractability at the time of diagnosis. Cause, younger age at onset (younger than age 1 year), high initial seizure frequency, and mental retardation are predictors of intractability among children (54,55). Type of syndrome—cryptogenic or symptomatic generalized epilepsies—has predicted intractability in multivariate analyses. After adjustment for syndrome, initial seizure frequency, focal EEG slowing, and acute symptomatic or neonatal status epilepticus ($p = 0.001$) also involved an increased risk (29,32). Other studies of intractability excluded these cases, presumably on the assumption that prognosis was poor (23,54).

Approximately 60% of patients with intractable epilepsy can be expected to suffer from partial seizures. Although all of these individuals with partial epilepsy may require expert care and possibly presurgical evaluation, only about 3000 patients each year with newly diagnosed epilepsy become candidates for a standard surgical procedure based on present criteria. An additional small number may be considered for alternative surgical procedures such as corpus callosotomy. This leaves an accumulating pool of candidates for new medication or for interventions such as vagal nerve stimulation.

OTHER MEASURES OF NATURAL HISTORY

Mortality

Few studies of mortality or survivorship have been performed in people with epilepsy, and it is impossible to determine a referent population for autopsy studies. Death certificates have little value in the study of mortality in epilepsy; in fewer than 10% of patients is the condition mentioned. Moreover, a substantial misclassification of deaths attributed to epilepsy frequently occurs (56). Even when review of the medical records is possible, no evidence of a convulsive disorder can be identified for many individuals with seizures or epilepsy recorded on a death certificate. When deaths from epilepsy are identified from death certificates, deaths of institutionalized individuals and those neurologically handicapped from birth are disproportionately represented. Life insurance data are flawed because insured individuals are likely to be in higher socioeconomic strata and unrepresentative of the general population with epilepsy. Conversely, studies of clinic populations are likely to include people with more severe epilepsy or low socioeconomic status, or both; such groups are unrepresentative. If clinic data are compared with life insurance actuarial information, a further inflation of differences in mortality is expected, because life insurance policyholders have better survivorship than does the general population.

Despite differences in populations studied and in measures used to determine mortality, increased mortality of patients with epilepsy has been consistently reported (8,49,56–63). The excess risk is greater in men than in women, is seen in all age groups, and is highest in individuals whose epilepsy has an identified cause. In younger age groups, the excess mortality occurs primarily for those with mental retardation, cerebral palsy, or congenital malformations of the central nervous system. In older age groups, mortality is increased for individuals with brain tumors or cerebrovascular disease. Much of the excess mortality is related to the underlying or associated cause of the epilepsy rather than to the epilepsy per se.

When survivorship analysis is restricted to those with idiopathic or cryptogenic epilepsy, mortality is increased for adults (49,56) but not children (56). In this group with epilepsy of unknown cause, increased mortality can be identified for patients with generalized tonic-clonic and myoclonic seizures but not for those with absence or complex partial seizures. In Denmark, mortality was greater for persons with "moderate or severe" epilepsy than for seizure-free individuals or those with "infrequent" seizures

(48). Mortality was not increased for persons with a single idiopathic seizure in studies conducted in the United States and Iceland (49,56).

Mortality from epilepsy seems to increase with the severity of the disease, and it continues to be high in patients who underwent unsuccessful epilepsy surgery, even if postoperatively their condition improved. The risk of dying is lowered only for people who have no seizures (64,65).

In community-based studies, altered mortality varied with duration of illness. Among idiopathic cases, the difference in observed and expected numbers of deaths was most striking in the first year after diagnosis. In patients surviving more than 10 years after diagnosis, no increased mortality was identified (5,56,66). In population-based studies in Iceland, people with idiopathic epilepsy had a significant increase in mortality 25 years after diagnosis (49).

When specific causes of death in patients with epilepsy were examined for incidence cohorts (56), an increased mortality attributable to neoplasms was identified even after exclusion of brain tumors. In most cases, the malignancy had been identified before the diagnosis of epilepsy. In cases in which the diagnosis of malignancy was made after the diagnosis of epilepsy, the question of the association with epilepsy or its correlates, such as prolonged exposure to antiseizure medication, remained unanswered. Consistent with clinical studies, an increased risk of death was attributed to accidents, particularly drowning. This cause of death also may be linked to the neurologic handicaps that accompany the development of epilepsy (67). Mortality is higher, but causes are similar among prevalence cohorts (60).

On the basis of information from clinical and surgical series and studies in hospitals and institutions, patients with epilepsy may have an increased risk for suicide (68). The highest risk has been reported from clinical or surgical series of "temporal lobe" epilepsy (59,69). Population-based data from Rochester, Minnesota, found no evidence of an increased risk for suicide among people with epilepsy (56), although studies in Iceland did report an increased cause-specific mortality attributable to suicide (61).

Data from postmortem studies, as well as clinical impressions, have led to the suggestion that individuals with epilepsy are at increased risk for sudden death (70–72), perhaps as a result of cardiac arrhythmia associated with seizures, reduction in AED dose, or pulmonary complications linked to seizures. Heart disease mortality and, specifically, the frequency of sudden death in epilepsy patients (SUDEP) have been explored in one population-based study (73). The risk of sudden death was twice as frequent for the group with epilepsy as for the general population (standardized mortality ratio = 2.3; 95% confidence interval, 1.2 to 3.9), but this increase was accounted for by patients with remote symptomatic epilepsy—primarily epilepsy attributed to cerebrovascular disease (standardized mortality ratio = 3.9; confidence interval, 1.7 to 7.7).

Later studies suggest that SUDEP occurs in about 5 of 10,000 people with epilepsy per year among incidence cohorts (73,74); this rate is similar to that in the general population. Sudden death occurs in a substantially greater proportion of people with chronic epilepsy. The frequency is 2 to 5 deaths per 1000 per year for patients seen in epilepsy centers or enrolled in clinical trials (75,76) and increases to 1% to 1.5% per year in people being evaluated for surgery or in whom surgery has failed (65,77). Factors associated with increased risk for SUDEP include long duration of epilepsy, high seizure frequency, increased number of medications, and etiology of epilepsy (78). SUDEP is rare in children (57), but so is sudden death, accounting for the high risk elevation. Adults with SUDEP generally have frequent seizures, are receiving polytherapy, and have epilepsy of long duration, frequently starting in childhood (79).

Comorbidity

Repeated seizures may lead to intellectual deterioration, but few studies have evaluated this topic. In the National Perinatal Collaborative Project (80), no significant difference in mental performance could be identified when children with epilepsy were compared with nonepileptic siblings. Only a small proportion of these children might be expected to develop "intractable" epilepsy. Studies of children with febrile seizures indicate that intellectual deterioration may be attributable to the use of phenobarbital rather than to the seizures themselves (81). One report (82) suggested that the occurrence of status epilepticus rather than seizure frequency may be associated with reduced intellectual function and impaired social adjustment.

As reflected in the mortality studies, people with epilepsy appear to be at increased risk for some cancers. Brain tumors occur with increased frequency, but it is not clear that they are a specific factor in children. Accidents are also increased, although not only episodes associated with seizures are accounted for. There is an increase in risk for osteoporosis, probably attributable to the long-term effects of antiseizure medication (83). An increase in the incidence of hip fracture has been reported, although this has not been consistently linked to use of antiseizure medication (84–86). Even when epilepsy is in remission, social difficulties seem to persist (6,7,87). People with epilepsy have lower education levels, lower marriage rates, and higher unemployment rates. They also seem to have altered reproductive function (88,89), although as with other conditions (e.g., SUDEP), the phenomenon seems limited to people with chronic epilepsy.

SUMMARY

The natural history of patients with epilepsy generally is favorable. Most patients can expect complete seizure control, and the majority of seizure-free individuals can discontinue medication. The increased risk for mortality, although real, occurs predominantly in those with symptomatic epilepsy and probably is related to the underlying condition rather than to epilepsy itself. An increased risk for accidental death has been detected for persons with epilepsy, and selected subgroups may have an enhanced risk of suicide. No studies convincingly demonstrate an adverse effect on intellectual function in most patients. Reproductive function may be altered, although this seems to be associated with the severity of epilepsy. The reasons for differences in the impact of transient compared with persistent seizures is a fertile area for future investigation.

ACKNOWLEDGMENT

This work was funded, in part, by grants NS0764312 and NS3266305 from the National Institute of Neurological Disorders and Stroke (NINDS).

REFERENCES

1. Rodin E. *The prognosis of patients with epilepsy.* Springfield, Ill: Charles C Thomas, 1968.
2. Annegers JF, Hauser WA, Elveback LR. Remission of seizures and relapse in patients with epilepsy. *Epilepsia* 1979;20:729–737.
3. Casetta I, Granieri E, Monetti VC, et al. Prognosis of childhood epilepsy: a community-based study in Copparo, Italy. *Neuroepidemiology* 1997;16:22–28.
4. Goodrich DMG, Shorvon SD. Epileptic seizure in a population of 6000, II: treatment and prognosis. *BMJ* 1983;287:645–647.
5. Hauser WA, Kurland LT. The epidemiology of epilepsy in Rochester, Minnesota, 1935–1968. *Epilepsia* 1975;1:1–66.
6. Sillanpää M. Remission of seizures and predictors of intractability in long-term follow-up. *Epilepsia* 1993;34:930–936.
7. Sillanpää M, Jalava M, Kaleva O, et al. Long-term prognosis of seizures with onset in childhood. *N Engl J Med* 1998;338:1715–1722.
8. Brorson LO, Wranne L. Long-term prognosis in childhood epilepsy: survival and seizure prognosis. *Epilepsia* 1987;28:324–330.
9. Callaghan N, Garrett A, Googin T. Withdrawal of anticonvulsant drugs in patients free of seizures for two years. *N Engl J Med* 1988;318:942–946.
10. Shinnar S, Berg AT, Moshe SL, et al. Discontinuing antiepileptic drugs in children with epilepsy: a prospective study. *Ann Neurol* 1994;35:534–545.
11. Hauser WA, Rich SS, Lee JR, et al. Risk of recurrent seizures after two unprovoked seizures. *N Engl J Med* 1998;338:429–434.
12. Hauser WA, Rich SS, Annegers JF, et al. Seizure recurrence after a first unprovoked seizure: an extended follow-up. *Neurology* 1990;40:1163–1170.
13. Shinnar S, Berg D, Moshe SL, et al. The risk of seizure recurrence following a first unprovoked seizure in childhood: a prospective study. *Pediatrics* 1990;85:1076–1085.
14. Elwes RDC, Chesterman P, Reynold SEH. Prognosis after a first untreated tonic-clonic seizure. *Lancet* 1985;2:752–753.
15. Berg AT, Shinnar S. The risk of seizure recurrence following a first unprovoked seizure: a quantitative review. *Neurology* 1991;41:965–972.
16. Annegers JF, Shirts SB, Hauser WA, et al. Risk of recurrence after an initial unprovoked seizure. *Epilepsia* 1986;27:43–50.
17. Hopkins A, Garman A, Clarke C. The first seizure in adult life. *Lancet* 1988;1:721–726.
18. Stroink H, Brouwer OF, Arts WF, et al. The first unprovoked, untreated seizure in childhood: a hospital based study of the

accuracy of the diagnosis, rate of recurrence, and long term outcome after recurrence. Dutch Study of Epilepsy in Childhood. *J Neurol Neurosurg Psychiatry* 1998;64:595–600.

19. van Donselaar CA, Gertz AT, Schumsheimer RJ. Idiopathic first seizure in adult life. Who should be treated? *BMJ* 1991;302:620–623.
20. Camfield P, Camfield C. Epilepsy can be diagnosed when the first two seizures occur on the same day. *Epilepsia* 2000;41:1230–1233.
21. Camfield P, Camfield C, Dooley J, et al. A randomized study of carbamazepine versus no medication after a first unprovoked seizure in childhood. *Neurology* 1989;39:851–852.
22. Mussico M, First Seizure Trial Group (FIRST Group). Randomized clinical trial on the efficacy of antiepileptic drugs in reducing the risk of relapse after a first unprovoked tonic-clonic seizure. *Neurology* 1993;43:478–483.
23. Camfield C, Camfield P, Gordon K, et al. Outcome of childhood epilepsy: a population-based study with a simple predictive scoring system for those treated with medication. *J Pediatr* 1993;122:861–868.
24. Overweg J, Binnie CD, Oosting J, et al. Clinical and EEG prediction of seizure recurrence following antiepileptic drug withdrawal. *Epilepsy Res* 1987;1:272–283.
25. Sakarnoto Y, Kasahara M, Satouchi H. Long-term prognosis on recurrence of seizures among children with epilepsy after drug withdrawal-elimination. *Folio Psychiatr Neurol Jpn* 1978;321:435–437.
26. Shafer SQ, Hauser WA, Annegers JF, et al. EEG and other early predictors of epilepsy remission: a community study. *Epilepsia* 1988;29:580–600.
27. Sofijanov NG. Clinical evolution and prognosis of childhood epilepsies. *Epilepsia* 1982;21:61–69.
28. Rantala H, Ingalsuo H. Occurrence and outcome of epilepsy in children younger than 2 years. *J Pediatr* 1999;135:761–764.
29. Berg AT, Shinnar S, Levy SR, et al. Two-year remission and subsequent relapse in children with newly diagnosed epilepsy. *Epilepsia* 2001;42:1553–1562.
30. Camfield C, Camfield P, Gordon K, et al. Does the number of seizures before treatment influence ease of control or remission of childhood epilepsy? Not if the number is 10 or less. *Neurology* 1996;46:41–44.
31. MacDonald BK, Johnson AL, Goodridge DM, et al. Factors predicting prognosis of epilepsy after presentation with seizures. *Ann Neurol* 2000;48:833–841.
32. Berg AT, Shinnar S, Levy SR, et al. Early development of intractable epilepsy in children: a prospective study. *Neurology* 2001;56:1430–1431.
33. Medical Research Council Antiepileptic Drug Withdrawal Study Group. Randomized study of antiepileptic drug withdrawal in patients in remission. *Lancet* 1991;337:1175–1180.
34. Arts WF, Geerts AT, Brouwer OF, et al. The early prognosis of epilepsy in childhood: the prediction of a poor outcome. The Dutch Study of Epilepsy in Childhood. *Epilepsia* 1999;40:726–734.
35. Wakamoto H, Nagao H, Hayashi M, et al. Long-term medical, educational, and social prognoses of childhood-onset epilepsy: a population-based study in a rural district of Japan. *Brain Dev* 2000;22:246–255.
36. Camfield PR, Camfield CS, Gordon K, et al. If a first antiepileptic drug fails to control a child's epilepsy, what are the chances of success with the next drug? *J Pediatr* 1997;131:821–824.
37. Carpay HA, Arts WF, Geerts AT, et al. Epilepsy in childhood: an audit of clinical practice. *Arch Neurol* 1998;55:668–673.
38. Kwan P, Brodie MJ. Early identification of refractory epilepsy. *N Engl J Med* 2000;342:314–319.
39. Feksi AT, Kaarnugisha J, Sander JWAS, et al. Comprehensive primary health care antiepileptic drug treatment programme in rural and semi-urban Kenya. *Lancet* 1991;337:406–409.
40. Placencia M, Sander JWAS, Shorvon SD, et al. Antiepileptic drug treatment in a community health care setting in northern Ecuador: a prospective 12-month assessment. *Epilepsy Res* 1993;14:237–244.
41. Arts WFM, Visser LH, Loonen MCB, et al. Follow-up of 146 children with epilepsy after withdrawal of antiepileptic therapy. *Epilepsia* 1988;29:244–250.
42. Bouma PAD, Peters ABC, Marts RJH, et al. Discontinuation of antiepileptic therapy: a prospective study in children. *J Neurol Neurosurg Psychiatry* 1987;50:1579–1583.
43. Braathen G, Melander H. Early discontinuation of treatment in children with uncomplicated epilepsy: a prospective study with a model for prediction of outcome. *Epilepsia* 1997;38:561–569.
44. Juul-Jensen P. Frequency of seizure recurrence after discontinuance of anticonvulsant medication in patients with epileptic seizures. *Epilepsia* 1964;5:352–363.
45. Matricardi M, Brinciotti M, Benedetti P. Outcome after discontinuation of antiepileptic drug therapy in children. *Epilepsia* 1989;30:582–589.
46. Todt H. The late prognosis of epilepsy in childhood: results of a prospective follow-up study. *Epilepsia* 1984;25:137–144.
47. Peters AC, Brouwer OF, Geerts AT, et al. Randomized prospective study of early discontinuation of antiepileptic drugs in children with epilepsy. *Neurology* 1998;50:724–730.
48. Juul-Jensen P, Foldspang A. Natural history of epileptic seizures. *Epilepsia* 1983;24:297–312.
49. Olafsson E, Gudmundson G, Hauser WA. Long term survival of people with unprovoked seizures. A population-based study. *Epilepsia* 1998;39:89–92.
50. Schmidt D, Tsai B, Janz D. Generalized tonic-clonic seizures in patients with complex partial seizures: natural history and prognostic relevance. *Epilepsia* 1983;24:43–48.
51. Emerson R, D'Souza BJ, Vining EP, et al. Stopping medication in children and epilepsy predictors of outcome. *N Engl J Med* 1981;304:1125–1129.
52. Sillanpää M. Social functioning and seizure status of young adults with onset of epilepsy in childhood. An epidemiological 20 year follow-up study. *Acta Neurol Scand* 1983;68(Suppl 96):1–81.
53. Chadwick D, Taylor J, Johnson T. Outcomes after seizure recurrence in people with well-controlled epilepsy and the factors that influence it. The MRC Antiepileptic Drug Withdrawal Group. *Epilepsia* 1996;37:1043–1050.
54. Casetta I, Granieri E, Monetti VC, et al. Early predictors of intractability in childhood epilepsy: a community-based case-control study in Copparo, Italy. *Acta Neurol Scand* 1999;99:329–333.
55. Berg AT, Novotny EJ, Levy SR, et al. Predictors of intractable epilepsy in children: a case-control study. *Epilepsia* 1996;37:24–30.
56. Hauser WA, Annegers JF, Elveback LR. Mortality in patients with epilepsy. *Epilepsia* 1980;21:339–412.
57. Camfield C, Camfield P, Veugelers PJ. Death in children with epilepsy: a population-based study. *Lancet* 2002;359:1891–1895.
58. Henriksen B, Juul-Jensen P, Lund M. The mortality of epileptics. In: Brackenridge RDC, ed. *Proceedings of the 10th International Congress of Life Assurance Medicine*. London: Pitman Medical, 1970:139–148.
59. Loiseau J, Picot MC, Loiseau P. Short-term mortality after a first epileptic seizure: a population-based study. *Epilepsia* 1999;40:1388–1392.
60. Nilsson L, Tomson T, Farahmand BY, et al. Cause-specific mortality in epilepsy: a cohort study of more than 9,000 patients once hospitalized for epilepsy *Epilepsia* 1997;38:1062–1068.
61. Rafnsson V, Olafsson E, Hauser WA, et al. Cause-specific mortality in adults with unprovoked seizures. A population-based incidence cohort study. *Neuroepidemiology* 2001;20:232–236.
62. Singer RD, Levinson L, eds. *Medical risks: patterns of mortality and survival. Neuropsychiatric disorders*. Toronto: Lexington Books, 1976:248–249.
63. Zielinski JJ. Epilepsy and mortality rate and cause of death. *Epilepsia* 1974;15:191–201.
64. Sperling MR, O'Connor MJ, Saykin AJ, et al. Temporal lobectomy for refractory epilepsy. *JAMA* 1996;276:470–475.
65. Sperling MR, Feldman H, Kinman J, et al. Seizure control and mortality in epilepsy. *Ann Neurol* 1999;46:45–50.
66. Cockerell OC, Johnson AL, Sander JWAS, et al. Mortality from epilepsy: results from a prospective population-based study. *Lancet* 1994;344:918–921.
67. Davis S, Ledman J, Kilgore J. Drownings of children and youths in a desert state. *West J Med* 1985;143:196–201.
68. Matthews WS, Barabas G. Suicide and epilepsy: a review of the literature. *Psychosomatics* 1981;22:515–524.

69. Barraclough BM. The suicide rate of epilepsy. *Acta Psychiatr Scand* 1987;76:339–345.
70. Jay GW, Leestma JE. Sudden death in epilepsy: a comprehensive review of the literature and proposed mechanisms. *Acta Neurol Scand* 1981;82(Suppl):1–66.
71. Leestma JE, Kelelkar MB, Teas SS, et al. Sudden unexpected death associated with seizures: analysis of 66 cases. *Epilepsia* 1984;25:84–88.
72. Neuspiel DR, Kuller LH. Sudden and unexpected natural death in childhood and adolescence. *JAMA* 1985;254:1321–1325.
73. Annegers JF, Hauser WA, Shirts SB. Heart disease mortality and morbidity in patients with epilepsy. *Epilepsia* 1984;25:699–704.
74. Ficker DM, So EL, Shen WK, et al. Population-based study of the incidence of sudden unexplained death in epilepsy. *Neurology* 1998;51:1270–1274.
75. Leestma JE, Annegers JF, Brodie MJ, et al. Sudden unexplained death in epilepsy: observations from a large clinical development program. *Epilepsia* 1997;38:47–55.
76. Leppik IE. Tiagabine: the safety landscape. *Epilepsia* 1995;36 (Suppl 6):S10–S13.
77. Dasheiff RM, Dickinson LJ. Sudden unexpected death of epileptic patient due to cardiac arrhythmia after seizure. *Arch Neurol* 1991; 8:216–222.
78. Nilsson L, Farahmand BY, Persson PG, et al. Risk factors for sudden unexpected death in epilepsy: a case-control study. *Lancet* 1999;353:888–893.
79. Walczak TS, Leppik IE, D'Amelio M, et al. *Neurology* 2001;56:519–525.
80. Ellenberg JH, Hirtz DG, Nelson KB. Do seizures cause intellectual deterioration? *N Engl J Med* 1986;314:1085–1088.
81. Farwell JR, Lee HJ, Hirtz DG, et al. Phenobarbital for febrile seizures: effects on intelligence and on seizure recurrence. *N Engl J Med* 1990;322:364–369.
82. Dodrill CS. Correlates of generalized tonic-clonic seizures with intellectual, neuropsychological, emotional and social function in patients with epilepsy. *Epilepsia* 1986;27:399–411.
83. Vestergaard P, Tigaran S, Rejnmark L, et al. Fracture risk is increased in epilepsy. *Acta Neurol Scand* 1999;99:269–275.
84. Annegers JF, Melton LJ, Sun CA, et al. Risk of age-related fractures in patients with unprovoked seizures. *Epilepsia* 1989;30:348–355.
85. Cummings SR, Nevitt MC, Browner WS, et al. Risk factors for hip fracture in white women. Study of Osteoporotic Fractures Research Group. *N Engl J Med* 1995;332:767–773.
86. Nilsson OS, Lindholm TS, Elmstedt E, et al. Fracture incidence and bone disease in epileptics receiving long-term anticonvulsant drug treatment. *Arch Orthop Trauma Surg* 1986;105:146–149.
87. Jacoby A. Felt versus enacted stigma: a concept revisited. Evidence from a study of people with epilepsy in remission. *Soc Sci Med* 1994;38:269–274.
88. Schupf N, Ottman R. Reproduction among individuals with idiopathic/cryptogenic epilepsy: risk factors for reduced fertility in marriage. *Epilepsia* 1996;37:833–840.
89. Webber MP, Hauser WA, Ottman R, et al. Fertility in persons with epilepsy in Rochester, Minnesota, 1935–1974. *Epilepsia* 1986;27:746–752.

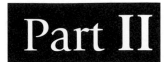

Basic Principles of Electroencephalography

10. Neurophysiologic Basis of the Electroencephalogram   127
11. Localization and Field Determination in Electroencephalography and Magnetoencephalography   141
12. Application of Electroencephalography in the Diagnosis of Epilepsy   169
13. Electroencephalographic Atlas of Epileptiform Abnormalities   183

Neurophysiologic Basis of the Electroencephalogram

Erwin-Josef Speckmann   *Christian E. Elger*   *Ulrich Altrup*

Field potentials appear and are detectable in the space surrounding cellular elements of the nervous system. They comprise rapid waves and baseline shifts; the former correspond to the conventional electroencephalogram (EEG), and both phenomena are included in the so-called direct current (DC) potential. Field potentials are essential in the diagnosis and classification of epileptic seizures as well as in the control of antiepileptic therapy. This chapter describes the elementary mechanisms underlying the generation of field potentials and the special functional situations leading to "epileptic" field potentials.

BIOELECTRICAL ACTIVITY OF NEURONAL AND GLIAL CELLS

The cells of the nervous system are generally differentiated into neurons and glial cells, whose processes intermingle and form a dense, highly complex matrix (Fig. 10.1). Because the actual interactions of these cellular elements are barely recognizable in spatiotemporal dimensions, principles of their structure and function inevitably are taken into account.

Neurons

A typical neuron consists of a soma (body, perikaryon) and fibers (dendrites and axons). In functional terms, with respect to information input, the relatively short and highly arborized dendrites can be considered extensions of the soma, as reflected in their being covered by thousands of synaptic endings. Axons are relatively long and, especially in their terminal regions, branch into collaterals. These neuronal output structures carry information into the terminal regions. Information is transferred to other neurons by way of synaptic endings (1–9).

Neuronal function is closely correlated with bioelectrical activity, which can be studied with intracellular microelectrode recordings. When a neuron is impaled by a microelectrode, a membrane potential of approximately 70 mV with negative polarity in the intracellular space becomes apparent. This resting membrane potential, existing in the soma and all its fibers, is based mainly on a potassium-outward current through leakage channels. If the resting membrane potential is critically diminished, that is, if a threshold is surpassed, an action potential (AP) is triggered, which is based on sodium-inward and potassium-outward currents through voltage-dependent membrane channels. APs are conducted along the axons to the terminations, where they lead to a release of transmitter substances. These transmitters open another class of membrane channels in the postsynaptic neuron. Dependent on the ionic composition of the currents flowing through the transmitter (ligand)-operated channels, two types of membrane potential changes, commonly called postsynaptic potentials (PSPs), are induced in the postsynaptic neuron. When a sodium-inward current prevails, depolarization of the postsynaptic neuron occurs. This synaptic depolarization is called an excitatory postsynaptic potential (EPSP) because it increases the probability that an AP will be triggered. When a potassium-outward current or a chloride-inward current prevails, hyperpolarization of the postsynaptic neuron occurs. Because hyperpolarization increases

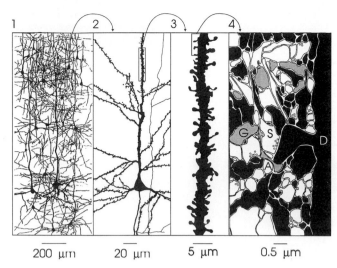

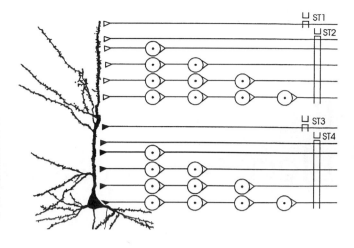

200 μm   20 μm   5 μm   0.5 μm

Figure 10.1 Morphology and histology of neuronal and glial elements in the neocortex. *Rectangles* and *arrows* indicate extended sections. In section 1, only a minor portion of the neurons is stained. A, axon; D, dendrite; G, glial cell; S, synapse. (Modified from references Gaze RM. *The Formation of nerve connections.* New York: Academic Press, 1970; Purpura DP. Dendritic differentiation in human cerebral cortex: normal and aberrant developmental patterns. In: Kreutzberg GW, ed. *Advances in neurology,* vol 12. New York: Raven Press, 1975:91–116; Valverde F. The organization of area 18 in the monkey: a golgi study. *Anat Embryol* 1978;154: 305–334; and Westrum LE, Blackstad TW. An electromicroscopic study of the stratum radiatum of the rat hippocampus (regio superior, CA1) with particular emphasis on synaptology. *J Comp Neurol* 1962;113:281–293, with permission.)

the distance between membrane potential and threshold, the synaptic hyperpolarization is called an inhibitory postsynaptic potential (IPSP) (10–12).

The EPSPs and IPSPs can interact with each other (Fig. 10.2). Electrical stimulation of an axon (ST1 in Fig. 10.2A) forming an excitatory synapse on a postsynaptic neuron can induce an AP at the site of stimulation. Conducted along the axon, the AP finally induces an EPSP in the postsynaptic neuron (ST1 in Fig. 10.2B). When only one synapse separates the site of stimulation from the site of EPSP generation, a monosynaptic EPSP appears. One way in which a summation of EPSP takes place is when the stimulation is repeated with an interstimulus interval shorter than the duration of the EPSP. With this temporal summation, the second EPSP can surpass the threshold and induce an AP (ST1 in Fig. 10.2B). A summation of EPSPs also can occur when monosynaptic EPSPs are evoked simultaneously at several locations on the postsynaptic neuron (spatial summation). Temporal and spatial summations are often combined with each other and are essential for information processing in the central nervous system, as when the AP reaches the target neuron by different ways. With stimulation at ST2 in Figure 10.2A, the triggered APs pass through varying numbers of relays before reaching their target. As APs are delayed with each synaptic transmission, they appear with temporal dispersion at the postsynaptic neuron and induce a long-lasting depolarization

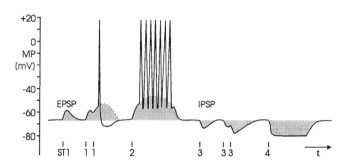

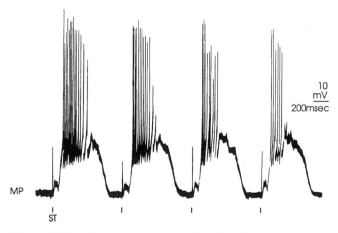

Figure 10.2 Bioelectrical activity of neuronal elements: membrane potential (MP), action potential (AP), excitatory postsynaptic potential (EPSP), and inhibitory postsynaptic potential (IPSP). **A:** Indicated are stimulation sites and the pyramidal neuron from which the recording was made. Open symbols represent excitatory synapses and filled symbols inhibitory synapses. Up to four interneurons are schematically drawn between stimulation sites (ST1 to ST4) and the neuron. **B:** Intracellular recording from the pyramidal neuron in **A** is shown. Single electrical stimuli applied at ST1 and ST3 evoked monosynaptic EPSP and IPSP, respectively. Paired stimulation at ST1 and ST3 led to a summation of the corresponding monosynaptic responses. After stimulation at ST2 and ST4, polysynaptic EPSP and IPSP, respectively, were elicited. **C:** Original tracing of synaptically mediated neuronal depolarizations in a spinal motoneuron of the cat is shown. Stimulation (ST) of pathways oligosynaptically and polysynaptically linked to the neuron led to early (oligosynaptic) and late (polysynaptic) potentials. (**A** and **B** adapted from Speckmann E-J. *Experimentelle epilepsieforschung.* Darmstadt, Germany: Wissenschaftliche Buchgesellschaft, 1986:13, with permission.)

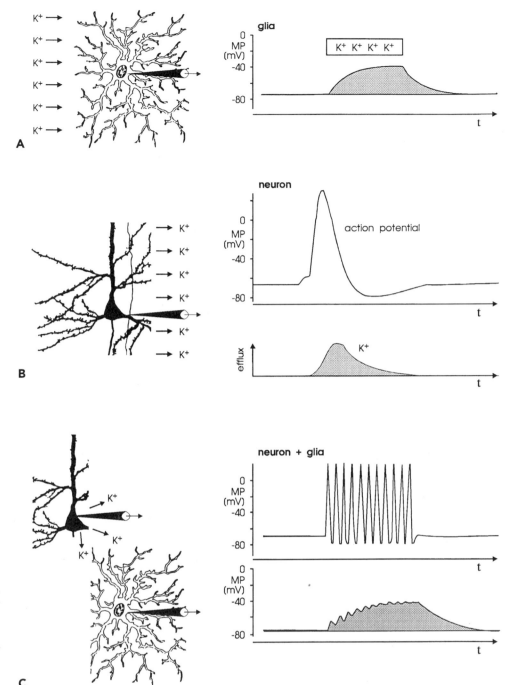

Figure 10.3 Changes in membrane potential (MP) of a glial cell induced by an increase in extracellular potassium concentration (**A**) and functional linkage between neuronal and glial activity (**B**) and (**C**). **A:** The increased extracellular concentration of K$^+$ led to a sustained depolarization of the glial cell. **B:** During a neuronal action potential, an efflux of K$^+$ occurred. **C:** The K$^+$ concentration in the extracellular space close to the glial cell was raised during the repetitive firing of a neuron. This led to sustained depolarization of the neighboring glial cell. (**A** and **C** adapted from Zenker W. Feinstruktur des Nervengewebes. In: Zenker W, ed. *Makroskopische und mikroskopische anatomie des menschen*, vol 3. Munich, Germany: Urban & Schwarzenberg, 1985: 3–55, and **B** and **C** adapted from Valverde F. The organization of area 18 in the monkey: a golgi study. *Anat Embryol* 1978;154: 305–334, with permission.)

(ST2 in Fig. 10.2B). Because many synapses are involved, such a depolarization is called a polysynaptic EPSP. When a polysynaptic network is activated repeatedly, EPSPs of considerable amplitude and duration can appear, as demonstrated by the original recording in Figure 10.2C. As with EPSPs, IPSPs can be induced both monosynaptically and polysynaptically and also are subject to temporal and spatial summation (ST3 and ST4 in Fig. 10.2A and B) (5,11,12).

In complex neuronal systems, EPSPs and IPSPs are often superimposed and induce long-lasting sequences of fluctu-

ations of the membrane potential. These kinds of postsynaptic responses play a prominent role in the generation of extracellular potential fields, such as the EEG.

Glial Cells

Consisting of a soma and fibers, glial cells intermingle with the neuronal structures. Glial cell fibers are electrically coupled, building up an extended functional network (3,8,13).

Glial cells also show a membrane potential (Fig. 10.3A). Unlike neurons, glial cells do not generate APs and PSPs.

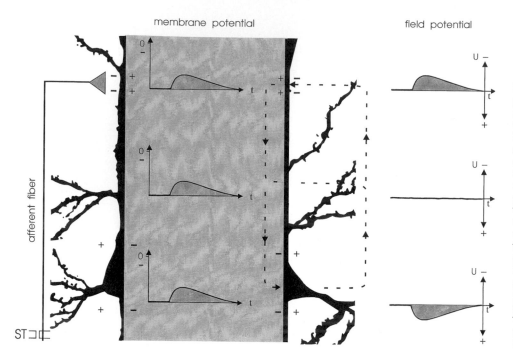

membrane potential

field potential

afferent fiber

ST

Figure 10.4 Principles of field potential generation in the neocortex. A perpendicular pyramidal neuron with an extended intracellular space (*hatched area*) is shown. An afferent fiber (*left*) formed an excitatory synaptic contact at the superficial aspect of the apical dendrite. Changes in membrane potential and in corresponding field potential are given in the intracellular and extracellular spaces, respectively. After stimulation of the afferent fiber (ST), an excitatory postsynaptic potential developed in the upper part of the dendrite and spread electrotonically to the lower parts. The local excitation (+ and −) led to tangential current flows (*broken lines*) and to the field potential changes in the extracellular space.

Because their resting membrane potential is based exclusively on potassium-outward current through leakage channels, its value is close to the potassium equilibrium potential. With an increase and a subsequent decrease in extracellular potassium concentration, glial cells depolarize and repolarize, respectively (Fig. 10.3A). Changes in the extracellular concentration of other cations have only small effects on the membrane potential of glial cells (14,15).

Glial cells and neurons are functionally linked by way of the extracellular potassium concentration (Fig. 10.3B and C). As mentioned, neuronal APs are associated with an outflow of potassium ions (Fig. 10.3B). Thus, with an increase in the repetition rate of neuronal APs, the extracellular potassium concentration increases, resulting in depolarization of glial cells adjacent to the active neurons (Fig. 10.3C) (11,14–16).

PRINCIPLES OF FIELD POTENTIAL GENERATION

Changes in membrane potential of neurons and glial cells are the basis of changes in extracellular field potential. The mechanisms involved can be described as follows: (a) primary transmembranous ion fluxes at a restricted membrane area of cells and consequent localized membrane potential changes; (b) development of potential gradients between sites of primary events and the remaining areas of the membrane; and (c) secondary ion currents because of the potential gradient along the cell membrane in the intracellular and extracellular spaces. The secondary current flowing through the extracellular space is directly

responsible for the generation of field potentials (9,17). Because EPSPs and IPSPs are important in the generation of the EEG findings, the processes are explained in greater detail using the examples of an excitatory synaptic input (2,12,18,19).

A vertically oriented neuronal element, shown schematically in Figure 10.4, is impinged on by a single excitatory synapse whose afferent fiber can be stimulated. The resulting net influx of cations leads to depolarization of the membrane, that is, to an EPSP. Consequently, a potential gradient exists along the neuronal membrane and evokes an intracellular and extracellular current flow. As a result of the intracellular current, the EPSP spreads electrotonically; the extracellular current induces field potentials. The polarity depends on the site of recording. The electrode near the synapse "sees" the inflow of cations (a negativity), whereas the electrode distant from the synapse "sees" the outflow of cations (a positivity). Between the two electrodes is the reversal point of the field potentials (12,20).

Corresponding effects occur with the generation of IPSPs. Activation of an inhibitory synapse induces an outflow of cations or an inflow of anions at the synaptic site. In this way, the membrane potential is increased at the synaptic site, and a potential gradient develops along the cell membrane, similar to that described for EPSPs. The potential gradient evokes a current flow from the synaptic site to the surrounding regions of the membrane. Compared with EPSPs, the extracellular current flow is inverted, as is the polarity of field potentials. Thus, the electrode near the synapse "sees" a positivity and the electrode distant from the synapse a negativity.

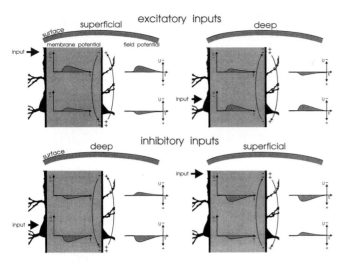

Figure 10.5 Generation of field potential in the neocortex by excitatory and inhibitory synaptic inputs reaching the superficial and deep parts of perpendicular pyramidal neurons. The intracellular space is extended (*hatched areas*). Changes in membrane potential and in the corresponding field potential are given in the intracellular and extracellular spaces, respectively. Locations of active inputs are indicated (*heavy arrows*). EPSP and IPSP, excitatory and inhibitory postsynaptic potentials, respectively. Excitatory inputs: With superficial excitation, an inward current generated an EPSP in upper and lower regions. Because of the direction of the extracellular current flow (*light arrows*), the field potential had negative polarity at the surface and positive polarity in the deep recording (*cf.* Fig. 10.4). With deep excitation, the current flow—and the field potentials—had inverse direction to that elicited by superficial excitation. Inhibitory inputs: With deep inhibition, an outward current generated an IPSP in lower and upper regions. Because of the direction of the extracellular current flow (*arrows*), the field potential had positive polarity in the deep recording and negative polarity at the surface. With superficial inhibition, the direction of current flow was inverse to that seen with deep inhibition; the field potentials were inverted as well. Differences in the shape of the various potentials were caused by the electrical properties of the tissue.

Field potentials are generated by extracellular currents, and their polarity depends on the direction of the current as well as on the positions of the extracellular electrodes. Figure 10.5 illustrates the generation and polarity of field potentials, as elicited by excitatory and inhibitory inputs to superficial and deep regions of vertical neuronal elements. Negative field potentials at the cortical surface may be based on superficial EPSPs as well as on deep IPSPs, and positive field potentials at the surface may be based on superficial IPSPs as well as on deep EPSPs (Fig. 10.6) (12,19,20).

POTENTIAL FIELDS IN NEURONAL NETWORKS

Many neuronal elements contribute to the extracellular currents that generate field potentials recorded at the surface of central nervous system structures. The spatial arrangement of the neuronal elements and the positions of the recording electrodes play an essential role in estab-

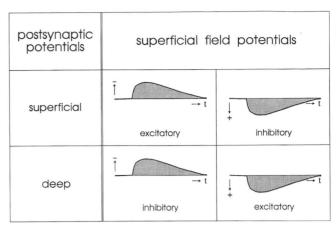

Figure 10.6 Synopsis of the synaptic processes underlying the generation of superficial field potentials in the cerebral cortex. Different mechanisms may lead to uniform superficial field potentials.

lishing and detecting extracellular potential fields (2,12,21).

Two principal types of neuronal arrangements can be identified (Fig. 10.7). In the parallel type, the somata are in one layer and the dendrites are in opposite layers (Fig. 10.7A). In the other type, the somata are in the center of a pool and the dendrites extend to its periphery (Fig. 10.7B). The first arrangement is realized in the cortex and the second in brainstem nuclei.

The two neuronal arrangements build up the so-called open and closed fields. In open fields, one electrode (E2 in Fig. 10.7A) largely integrates the potentials of the population (i.e., it is near the zero potential line), and the other electrode (E1 in Fig. 10.7A) sees only the positive or negative field, permitting the recording of a field potential. In closed fields, external electrodes do not see significant potential differences because the current flows within the pool compensate for each other (Fig. 10.7B) (2,21).

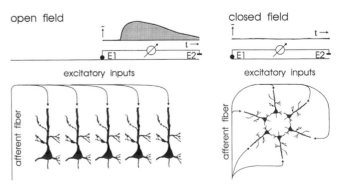

Figure 10.7 Neurons arranged to give open (**A**) and closed (**B**) fields. Field potentials are present (**A**) or missing (**B**) during excitatory inputs by way of afferent fibers. E1 and E2 indicate different and reference electrodes.

TYPES OF FIELD POTENTIAL CHANGES

With respect to the time course, two types of field potentials can be differentiated, depending on the time constant of the amplifying recording device. The conventional EEG is recorded with a time constant of 1 second or less. Amplification with an infinite time constant, that is, by a DC amplifier, permits additional recording of baseline shifts and wave-like potentials (EEG/DC) (22–24).

Wave Generation (Conventional Electroencephalogram)

The generation of wave-like potentials is described in Figure 10.8, a representation of a column of neocortex. In its upper dendritic region, the neuron is activated by an afferent fiber by way of an excitatory synapse. The superficial EEG and the membrane potentials of the dendrite and afferent fiber are recorded. The afferent fiber shows grouped, followed by regular, discharges. With grouped discharges prominent, summated EPSPs occur in the dendrite; with sustained regular activity, a depolarizing shift of the membrane potential appears. The changes in membrane potential in the upper dendrite lead to field potentials. When amplifiers with a finite time constant are used, only fluctuations in field potential are recorded, corresponding to findings on conventional EEG. The shift of the membrane potential is not reflected (21,25).

Baseline Shifts (Electroencephalogram/Direct Current)

The generation of baseline shifts is described in Figures 10.9 and 10.10. In a column of the neocortex (Fig. 10.9), a neuron is activated in its upper dendritic region by an afferent fiber by way of an excitatory synapse. In this case, the afferent fiber displays three levels of sustained activity. Medium regular activity is interrupted by periods of high repetition and silence. Consequently, owing to facilitation, the upper dendrite is depolarized during the high discharge in the afferent fiber and is hyperpolarized in the silent period because of disfacilitation. This results in corresponding field potential shifts. When amplifiers with an infinite time constant are used, these baseline shifts, which reflect sustained values of the membrane potential of neuronal elements, are recorded. With a sufficiently high upper-frequency limit, the DC recording comprises conventional EEG waves as well as slow potential deviations (26–32).

Glial cells also are involved in the generation of baseline shifts (Figs. 10.10 and 10.11). As noted, a functional coupling between neurons and glial cells exists (Fig. 10.3). Figure 10.10 shows a neuron in deep cortical layers and a network of electrically coupled glial cells extending to the surface. The superficial EEG/DC and the membrane potentials of a glial cell and the neuron are recorded. With increased discharge frequency of the neuron, extracellular potassium concentration rises, evoking a depolarization of the adjacent glial cell. The potassium-induced depolarization is conducted electrotonically within the

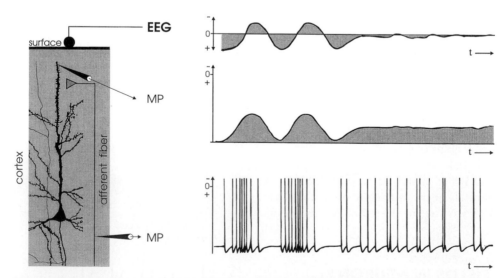

Figure 10.8 Wave generation in the electroencephalogram (EEG) at the surface of the cerebral cortex. A perpendicular pyramidal neuron is shown. An afferent fiber formed an excitatory synaptic contact at the superficial part of the apical dendrite. Simultaneous recordings of the membrane potentials (MPs) of the afferent fiber and the dendritic element, as well as of the EEG, are displayed. Groups of action potentials in the afferent fiber generate wave-like excitatory postsynaptic potentials (EPSPs) in the dendritic region and corresponding waves in the EEG recording. Tonic activity in the afferent fiber results in long-lasting EPSP with only small fluctuations. The long-lasting depolarization is not reflected on the conventional EEG recording.

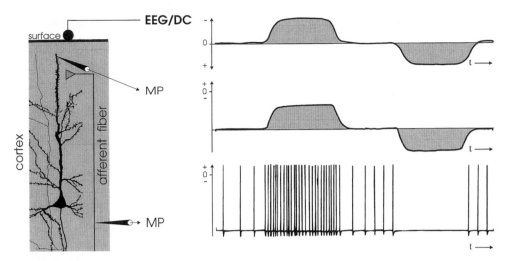

Figure 10.9 Sustained shifts in the electroencephalogram (EEG) at the surface of the cerebral cortex resulting from sustained neuronal activities. If recordings are performed with a direct-current (DC) amplifier (EEG/DC), sustained potentials can also be recorded at the surface. In the perpendicular pyramidal neuron depicted, an afferent fiber formed an excitatory synaptic contact at the superficial part of the apical dendrite. The membrane potentials (MPs) of the afferent fiber and the dendritic element were recorded simultaneously, as was the EEG/DC. Increased and decreased sustained activity in the afferent fiber generated sustained depolarizations and hyperpolarizations of the dendritic region and corresponding negative and positive shifts of the EEG/DC recording.

glial network. A functional situation is present similar to that in a perpendicular neuron with a deep excitatory synaptic input (Figs. 10.5 and 10.6). The superficial EEG/DC electrode sees a long-lasting positivity because of an outflow of cations from the glial cells in the upper layers. In other respects, this corresponds to the well-known spatial buffering of potassium. In principle, the aforementioned mechanism can make visible the activity of closed fields (Fig. 10.7B) in baseline shifts of field potentials (31,33,34).

Glial cells contribute to the generation of field potentials, although this mechanism is not dominant. Thus, the original recordings of cortical EEG/DC and membrane potentials of cortical glial cells demonstrate that glial depolarization occurs parallel to negative (Fig. 10.11A and B) and positive (Fig. 10.11C) baseline shifts of field potentials.

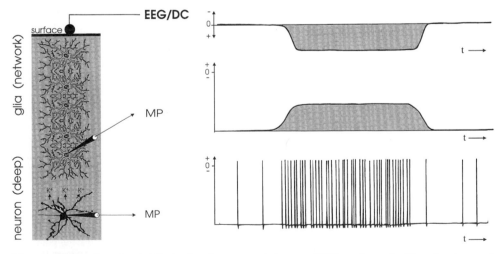

Figure 10.10 Sustained shifts in the electroencephalogram (EEG) performed with a direct-current (DC) amplifier (EEG/DC) at the surface of the cerebral cortex generated by neuronal activity and mediated by a glial network. If recordings are performed with a DC amplifier, sustained potentials can also be recorded. A deep neuron functionally coupled to a perpendicularly oriented glial network is shown. The membrane potentials (MPs) of the deep neuron and of a glial cell as well as the EEG/DC were recorded simultaneously. Sustained increased activity of the deep neuron induced an increase in extracellular K^+ concentration and a corresponding depolarization of the glial cells. Because of the electrotonically coupled network of glial cells, a sustained positive potential was induced in the surface EEG/DC recording.

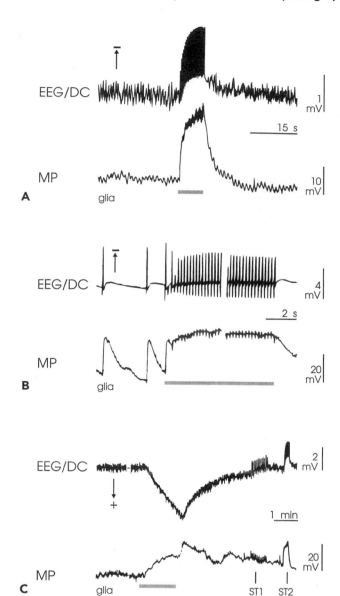

On the whole, field potential changes can be thought to be generated primarily by neuronal structures (16,31).

BASICS OF EPILEPTIC FIELD POTENTIALS

As described, field potentials recorded during epileptic activity are based on changes in neuronal membrane potential. The amplitudes of field potentials exceed those of nonepileptic potentials because the underlying neuronal activity is highly synchronized. As a result of the synchronization, the activity of a single element represents that of the entire epileptic population. On that basis, changes in field potentials and neuronal membrane potential can clearly be related to one another (12,35–39).

Figure 10.10 shows typical recordings of epicortical EEG and of the membrane potential of a neuron in upper cortical layers. During the development of epileptic activity, flat depolarizations superimposed by APs appear first. These membrane potential changes evolve into typical paroxysmal depolarizations that consist of a steep depolarization triggering a burst of APs, a plateau-like diminution of the membrane potential, and a steep repolarization followed by an afterhyperpolarization or an afterdepolarization. With the appearance of the epileptic neuronal depolarizations, negative fluctuations of the local field potential develop. As Figure 10.12 shows, a close temporal relationship exists

Figure 10.11 Simultaneous recordings of the electroencephalogram (EEG) potential performed with a direct-current (DC) amplifier (EEG/DC) at the surface of the cerebral cortex and of the membrane potential (MP) of glial cells in an anesthetized and artificially ventilated rat. **A:** High-frequency electrical stimulation of the cortical surface (*horizontal bar*) is indicated. **B:** Focal epileptic activity induced by penicillin is indicated. Repetitive cortical stimulation (*horizontal bar*) increased the frequency of epileptic discharges (interruption, approximately 5 seconds). **C:** Increase of the local partial pressure of carbon dioxide (PCO_2) during apnea (*horizontal bar*) is shown. ST1 and ST2, low- and high-frequency electrical stimulation of the cerebral cortex, respectively. Depolarization of glial cells can be associated with both a positive (**C**) and a negative (**A** and **B**) shift in the EEG/DC. (**A** adapted from Caspers H, Speckmann E-J, Lehmenkühler A. DC potentials of the cerebral cortex. Seizure activity and changes in gas pressures. *Rev Physiol Biochem Pharmacol* 1987;106:127–178; **B** adapted from Speckmann E-J. *Experimentelle epilepsieforschung.* Darmstadt, Germany: Wissenschaftliche Buchgesellschaft, 1986; and **C** adapted from Caspers H, Speckmann E-J, Lehmenkühler A. Electrogenesis of slow potentials of the brain. In: Elbert T, Rockstroh B, Lutzenberger W, et al., eds. *Self-regulation of the brain and behavior.* New York: Springer, 1984:26–41, with permission.)

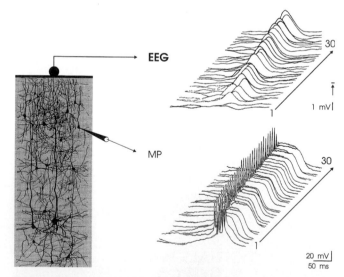

Figure 10.12 Simultaneous establishment of paroxysmal depolarizations of a neuron in superficial cortical layers and of sharp waves in the electroencephalogram at the cortical surface during development of an epileptic focus. Focal epileptic activity was induced by local penicillin application. MP, membrane potential. Graphic superposition of 30 successive potentials with the commencement of focal epileptic activity is shown. (Adapted from Elger CE, Speckmann E-J. Vertical inhibition in motor cortical epileptic foci and its consequences for descending neuronal activity to the spinal cord. In: Speckmann E-J, Elger CE, eds. *Epilepsy and motor system.* Baltimore, Md: Urban & Schwarzenberg, 1983: 152–160, with permission.)

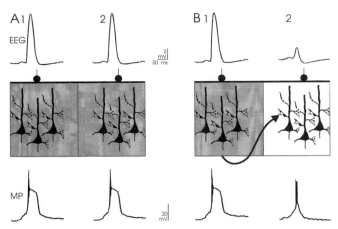

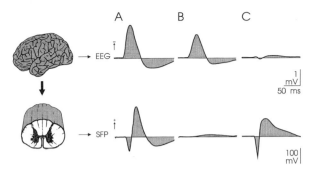

Figure 10.14 Dissociation in occurrence of epileptiform potentials on the surface electroencephalogram and of spinal field potentials (SFPs). Focal epileptiform activity was restricted to motor cortical layers. **A:** Simultaneous appearance of cortical and spinal activity is indicated. **B:** Presence of cortical activity and failure of spinal activity are shown. **C:** Failure of cortical activity and presence of spinal activity are shown. [Adapted from Elger CE, Speckmann E-J, Prohaska O, et al. Pattern of intracortical potential distribution during focal interictal epileptiform discharges (FIED) and its relation to spinal field potentials in the rat. *Electroencephalogr Clin Neurophysiol* 1981;51:393–402, with permission.]

Figure 10.13 Electroencephalographic waves at the cortical surface representing locally generated (A1 and 2 and B1) and synaptically transmitted (B2) epileptiform neuronal discharges. Cortical columns with (*hatched areas*) and without (*open area*) locally generated epileptic activity are shown. Both A1 and A2 potentials represent directly epileptiform neuronal depolarizations. The potential in B1 represents directly epileptiform neuronal discharges, and that in B2 represents indirectly epileptiform discharges in the primary nonepileptic neighboring column, that is, a potential synaptically evoked by the epileptically active neurons (*arrow*). MP, membrane potential.

between development of the intracellularly recorded membrane potential and the extracellularly generated field potentials. Later the duration and amplitude of the neuronal depolarizations and of the negative field potentials increase and reach a final level. The transition from epileptic to normal activity is also associated with a parallelism between field potentials and membrane potential changes. Thus, the epileptic negative field potentials represent the activity of an epileptic neuronal network (35–37,39).

Epileptic foci can induce evoked potentials in nonepileptic areas (Fig. 10.13). In Figure 10.13A, two cortical columns generate epileptic activity, as indicated by the neuronal paroxysmal depolarizations and the concomitant negative spikes in the EEG. The epileptic activities at both sites are not necessarily synchronous. In Figure 10.13B, only one column is epileptically active. The epileptic discharges elicit synaptic potentials in the neighboring nonepileptic area. The synchronized burst discharges induced in the nonepileptic column then give rise to "epileptic evoked potentials."

FIELD POTENTIALS WITH FOCAL EPILEPTIC ACTIVITY

For practical reasons, the description of field potential generation with focal epileptic activity takes into account the functional significance of an epileptic focus, especially motor phenomena (12,35,38,40,41).

The relationship between epileptic field potentials in motor cortical areas and their output to the spinal cord is detailed in Figure 10.14. In Figure 10.14A, the epicortical EEG spike is associated with a defined high-amplitude

spinal field potential, indicating synchronized descending neuronal activity. These events result finally in muscular clonus. Superficial EEG potentials and spinal output are not always closely related, however. Each of these motor phenomena may be present without the other (Fig. 10.14B and C) (42–47).

The aforementioned discrepancies between superficial EEG potentials and cortical output can be clarified by

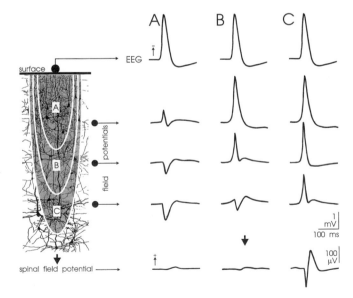

Figure 10.15 Epicortical (electroencephalogram), intracortical, and spinal field potentials during focal epileptiform activity. The actual vertical extension of the focus is indicated on the left and related to the tracings by letters. The occurrence of synchronized spinal field potentials is linked to the appearance of negative field potentials in lamina V (**A–C**). (Adapted from Elger CE, Speckmann E-J, Caspers H, et al. Focal interictal epileptiform discharges in the cortex of the rat: laminar restriction and its consequences for activity descending to the spinal cord. In: Klee MR, Lux HD, Speckmann E-J, eds. *Physiology and pharmacology of epileptogenic phenomena.* New York: Raven Press, 1982:13–20, with permission.)

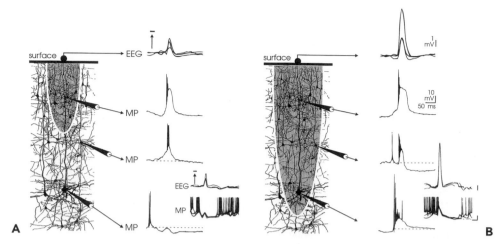

Figure 10.16 Membrane potential (MP) changes of single neurons in layers of the motor cortex during focal epileptic activity with different vertical extensions. Epileptic activity was recorded 5 (**A**) and 15 (**B**) minutes after local application of penicillin to the cortical surface. The drawings indicate vertical extension of the focus. The MP changes were recorded simultaneously with the electroencephalographic changes, which are superimposed to show the relationship of the curves to each other. **Insets:** Shown are three superimposed superficial electroencephalographic and deep MP recordings. (Adapted from Speckmann E-J. *Experimentelle epilepsieforschung.* Darmstadt, Germany: Wissenschaftliche Buchgesellschaft, 1986:122, with permission.)

recording field potentials from within the cortex. In Figure 10.15, the superficial EEG was recorded simultaneously with intracortical field potentials at three depths, including layer V, and with spinal field potentials. With positive field potentials in layer V, spinal field potentials are missing (Fig. 10.15A and B). Synchronized motor output appears only when the typical epileptic negative spike occurs in

layer V (Fig. 10.15C). In all these cases, the EEG spikes at the cortical surface are identical (42–44,46,47).

The situations presented in Figure 10.15A and C are shown at the level of intracellular recordings in Figure 10.16. The positive field potentials in layer V parallel long-lasting and highly effective neuronal inhibitions, and the negative field potentials at the same site are based on typical neuronal paroxysmal depolarization shifts. Thus, the synchronized excitation of pyramidal neurons in layer V is a prerequisite for epileptic motor output. This excitation is not necessarily reflected in the superficial EEG, however (Fig. 10.14C). Epileptic motor reactions based on a cortical focus may occur without appropriate signs on such a recording (43,44,46–48).

The difference between bioelectrical activity at the cortical surface and in deeper cortical layers becomes very clear when voltage-sensitive dyes are used instead of field potential recordings (49–51). With this technique, neuronal activity can be seen, although the requirements for the generation of field potentials are not fulfilled (see above).

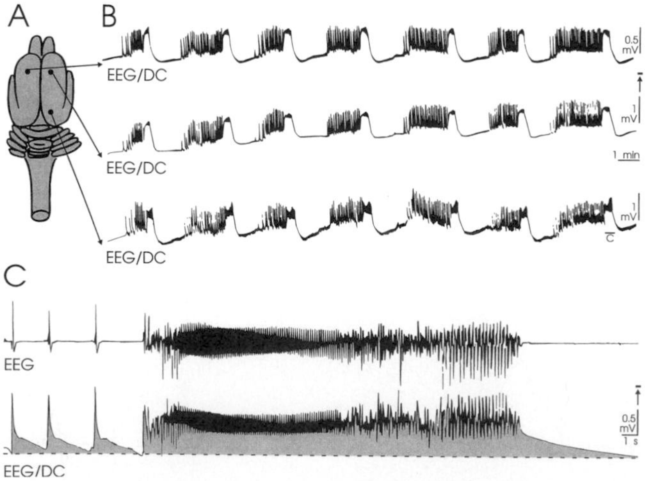

FIELD POTENTIALS WITH GENERALIZED TONIC-CLONIC ACTIVITY

Figure 10.17 Experimental animal model of generalized tonic-clonic seizures elicited by repeated systemic administration of pentylenetetrazol. **A:** The recording arrangement is shown. **B:** Simultaneous recordings of the epicortical direct current (DC) potential from the motor regions of both hemispheres and from an occipital area are presented. **C:** Part C in B is displayed as a conventional electroencephalogram (EEG) and EEG/DC potential with an extended time scale. (Adapted from Speckmann E-J. *Experimentelle epilepsieforschung.* Darmstadt, Germany: Wissenschaftliche Buchgesellschaft, 1986:69, with permission.)

Observations made during tonic-clonic seizures in experimental animal studies are used to explain the generation of field potentials during generalized seizures. After repeated injections of pentylenetetrazol, typical tonic-clonic seizures appear (Fig. 10.17) accompanied by field potential changes consisting of baseline shifts and superimposed rapid waves. The latter allow the differentiation between tonic and clonic phases (Fig. 10.17C) (12,35–38,41).

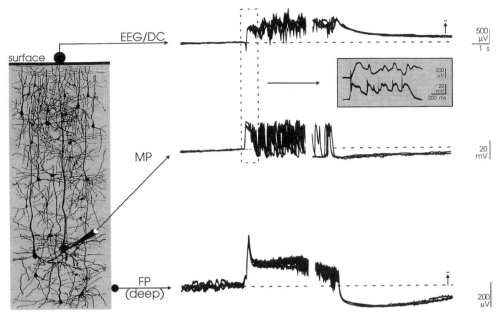

Figure 10.18   Relationship between shifts of the epicortical [electroencephalogram (EEG) performed with a direct-current (DC) amplifier (EEG/DC)] and laminar field potentials (FPs) and changes in the membrane potential (MP) of a pyramidal tract cell during tonic-clonic seizures (inkwriter recordings with graphic superpositions). Epileptic activity was elicited by repeated systemic administrations of pentylenetetrazol. Interruptions were 30 to 60 seconds. **Inset:** Shown are parts of the EEG/DC and MP recordings displayed on an oscilloscope with an extended time scale.

Baseline Shifts (Electroencephalogram/ Direct Current)

Figure 10.18 shows the relationship between baseline shifts of field potentials, from both surface and deep recordings, and membrane potential changes of pyramidal neurons in layer V. During tonic-clonic seizures, a series of paroxysmal depolarizations occurs in pyramidal tract neurons. This means that neuronal depolarization parallels a negative shift of the baseline of field potentials on superficial and deep recordings. The close temporal relationship can be discerned also on recordings with an extended time scale. Although the bioelectrical events are similar, discrepancies exist in the commencement of seizures and in the postictal phase. With seizure onset, a monophasic negative shift always occurs on deep recordings of field potentials. In contrast, the superficial EEG/DC findings can start with a monophasic negative or positive as well as a biphasic negative-positive fluctuation. In the postictal period, deep recordings always show a positive displacement of the baseline of field potentials and superficial recordings a negative displacement. Comparison of the different simultaneous recordings of field potentials and membrane potential reveals the following findings. The initial negative fluctuation and the postictal positive displacement of the field potential in deeper layers correspond, respectively, to the initial highly synchronized depolarization and to the postictal hyperpolarization of pyramidal tract neurons. This close correspondence is missing when superficially recorded EEG/DC shifts and neuronal membrane potential changes are compared. Thus, the mean neuronal activity is well represented in the baseline shift of deep field potentials. As far as the superficial field potentials are concerned, additional generators, for example, glial networks, must be taken into account (14–16,18,52–54).

Waves (Conventional Electroencephalogram)

The rapid waves superimposed on the baseline shifts of the EEG/DC can best be interpreted when the afferent impulse inflow to the upper cortical layers is evaluated. Figure 10.19 represents a cortical column with a perpendicularly oriented neuron. An afferent fiber forms an excitatory synapse in upper dendritic regions. The discharge frequency of the afferent fiber was recorded simultaneously with the surface EEG/DC. For further description, three types of waves were selected: monophasic negative (Fig. 10.19A), monophasic positive (Fig. 10.15C), and biphasic positive-negative (Fig. 10.19B) waves. With the commencement of negative waves, the discharge rate increased from a low initial level (Fig. 10.15A and B); during positive waves, the discharge rate decreased from a high level (Fig. 10.19C). Thus, the generation of superficial waves can be explained as resulting from facilitation (negative waves) and disfacilitation (positive waves) of neuronal structures in upper cortical layers (20,22–24, 40,46,47).

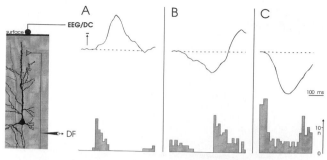

Figure 10.19 Relationship between different patterns of fluctuations of the epicortical field potential [electroencephalogram (EEG) performed with direct-current (DC) amplifier (EEG/DC)] and changes in discharge frequency (DF) of neuronal elements in superficial cortical layers during tonic-clonic seizures. Epileptic activity was elicited by repeated systemic administrations of pentylenetetrazol. Up to 16 single events were averaged: monophasic negative (**A**) and positive (**C**), as well as biphasic positive-negative (**B**), fluctuations of EEG/DC. N, number of action potentials. (Adapted from Speckmann E-J. *Experimentelle epilepsieforschung.* Darmstadt, Germany: Wissenschaftliche Buchgesellschaft, 1986:143, with permission.)

CONCLUSION

Changes of neuronal activity associated with net current flows in the extracellular space produce field potentials. In clinical practice, a synchronization of the activity of neuronal elements is needed to recognize signals. As seen in superficial and deep potential fields, field potentials are generated in functionally different structures and may be based on different elementary mechanisms. Field potentials at the cortical surface, for example, can be interpreted in a variety of ways because they are not constantly related to neuronal activity in deep cortex.

REFERENCES

1. Gaze RM. *The Formation of nerve connections.* New York: Academic Press, 1970.
2. Hubbard JI, Llinas R, Quastel DMJ. *Electrophysiological analysis of synaptic transmission.* London: Edward Arnold, 1969.
3. Palay SL, Chan-Palay V. General morphology of neurons and neuroglia. In: Kandel ER, ed. *Handbook of physiology, the nervous system,* vol 1. Bethesda, Md: American Physiological Society, 1977: 5–37.
4. Purpura DP. Dendritic differentiation in human cerebral cortex: normal and aberrant developmental patterns. In: Kreutzberg GW, ed. *Advances in neurology,* vol 12. New York: Raven Press, 1975: 91–116.
5. Shepherd GM. *The Synaptic organization of the brain.* London: Oxford University Press, 1974.
6. Valverde F. The organization of area 18 in the monkey: a golgi study. *Anat Embryol* 1978;154:305–334.
7. Westrum LE, Blackstad TW. An electromicroscopic study of the stratum radiatum of the rat hippocampus (regio superior, CA1) with particular emphasis on synaptology. *J Comp Neurol* 1962; 113:281–293.
8. Zenker W. Feinstruktur des Nervengewebes. In: Zenker W, ed. *Makroskopische und mikroskopische anatomie des menschen,* vol 3. Munich, Germany: Urban & Schwarzenberg; 1985:3–55.
9. Zschocke ST. *Klinische elektroenzephalographie.* Berlin: Springer, 1995.
10. Eccles JC. *The physiology of synapses.* Berlin: Springer, 1964.
11. Rall W. Core conductor theory and cable properties of neurons. In: Kandel ER, ed. *Handbook of physiology. The nervous system,* vol 1. Bethesda, Md: American Physiological Society, 1977:39–97.
12. Speckmann E-J. *Experimentelle epilepsieforschung.* Darmstadt, Germany: Wissenschaftliche Buchgesellschaft, 1986.
13. De Robertis EDP, Carrea R, eds. *Biology of neuroglia.* New York: Elsevier, 1965:15.
14. Kuffler SW, Nicholls JG. The physiology of neuroglial cells. *Erg Physiol* 1966;57:1–90.
15. Kuffler SW, Nicholls JG, Orkand RK. Physiological properties of glial cells in the central nervous system of amphibia. *J Neurophysiol* 1966;29:768–780.
16. Somjen GG, Trachtenberg M. Neuroglia as generator of extracellular current. In: Speckmann E-J, Caspers H, eds. *Origin of cerebral field potentials.* Stuttgart, Germany: Thieme, 1979:21–32.
17. Speckmann E-J, Bingmann D. Komplexe Hirnfunktionen im Spiegel des EEG. In: Deetjen P, Speckmann E-J, eds. *Physiologie,* vol 5.1. Munich, Germany: Urban & Fischer, 1999:225–232.
18. Speckmann E-J, Caspers H, Janzen RWC. Laminar distribution of cortical field potentials in relation to neuronal activities during seizure discharges. In: Brazier MAB, Petsche H, eds. *Architectonics of the cerebral cortex,* vol 3. New York: Raven Press, 1978: 191–209.
19. Speckmann E-J, Walden J. Mechanisms underlying the generation of cortical field potentials. *Acta Otolaryngol Suppl* 1991;491:17–24.
20. Speckmann E-J, Caspers H, Elger CE. Neuronal mechanisms underlying the generation of field potentials. In: Elbert T, Rockstroh B, Liitzenberger W, et al., eds. *Self-regulation of the brain and behavior.* New York: Springer; 1984:9–25.
21. Creutzfeldt O, Houchin J. Neuronal basis of EEG waves. In: Remond A, ed. *Handbook of electroencephalography and clinical neurophysiology,* vol 2. Amsterdam: Elsevier, 1974:71–79.
22. Speckmann E-J, Caspers H. The effect of O_2- and CO_2-tensions in the nervous tissue on neuronal activity and DC potentials. In: Remond A, ed. *Handbook of electroencephalography and clinical neurophysiology,* vol 2. Amsterdam: Elsevier, 1974:71–89.
23. Speckmann E-J, Caspers H. Cortical field potentials in relation to neuronal activities in seizure conditions. In: Speckmann E-J, Caspers H, eds. *Origin of cerebral field potentials.* Stuttgart, Germany: Thieme, 1979:205–213.
24. Speckmann E-J, Caspers H, eds. *Origin of cerebral field potentials.* Stuttgart, Germany: Thieme, 1979.
25. Andersen P, Andersson SA. *Physiological basis of the alpha rhythm.* New York, NY: Meredith Corp.; 1968.
26. Caspers H. Relations of steady potential shifts in the cortex to the wakefulness-sleep spectrum. In: Brazier MAB, ed. *Brain function.* Berkeley: University of California Press, 1963:177–200.
27. Caspers H. DC potentials recorded directly from the cortex. In: Remond A, ed. *Handbook of electroencephalography and clinical neurophysiology,* vol 10. Amsterdam: Elsevier, 1974:3.
28. Caspers H, Speckmann E-J. DC potential shifts in paroxysmal states. In: Jasper HH, Ward AA Jr, Pope A, eds. *Basic mechanisms of the epilepsies.* Boston: Little, Brown, 1969:375–395.
29. Caspers H, Speckmann E-J. Cortical DC shifts associated with changes of gas tensions in blood and tissue. In: Remond A, ed. *Handbook of electroencephalography and clinical neurophysiology,* vol 10. Amsterdam: Elsevier, 1974:41–65.
30. Caspers H, Speckmann E-J, Lehmenkühler A. Effects of CO_2 on cortical field potentials in relation to neuronal activity. In: Speckmann E-J, Caspers H, eds. *Origin of cerebral field potentials.* Stuttgart, Germany: Thieme, 1979:151–163.
31. Caspers H, Speckmann E-J, Lehmenkühler A. DC potentials of the cerebral cortex. Seizure activity and changes in gas pressures. *Rev Physiol Biochem Pharmacol* 1987;106:127–178.
32. Goldring S. DC shifts released by direct and afferent stimulation. In: Remond A, ed. *Handbook of electroencephalography and clinical neurophysiology,* vol 10. Amsterdam: Elsevier, 1974:12–24.
33. Caspers H, Speckmann E-J, Lehmenkühler A. Electrogenesis of cortical DC potentials. In: Kornhuber HH, Deecke L, eds. *Motivation, motor and sensory processes of the brain: electrical potentials, behaviour and clinical use,* vol 54. New York: Elsevier, 1980:3–15.
34. Caspers H, Speckmann E-J, Lehmenkühler A. Electrogenesis of slow potentials of the brain. In: Elbert T, Rockstroh B, Lutzenberger W, et al., eds. *Self-regulation of the brain and behavior.* New York: Springer, 1984:26–41.
35. Jasper HH, Ward AA, Pope A, eds. *Basic mechanisms of the epilepsies.* Boston: Little, Brown, 1969.

36. Klee MR, Lux HD, Speckmann E-J, eds. *Physiology and pharmacology of epileptogenic phenomena.* New York: Raven Press, 1982.

37. Klee MR, Lux HD, Speckmann E-J, eds. *Physiology, pharmacology and development of epileptogenic phenomena.* Berlin: Springer, 1991:20.

38. Purpura DP, Penry JK, Tower DE, et al., eds. *Experimental models of epilepsy.* New York: Raven Press, 1972.

39. Speckmann E-J, Elger CE. The neurophysiological basis of epileptic activity: a condensed review. In: Degen R, Niedermeyer E, eds. *Epilepsy, sleep and sleep deprivation.* Amsterdam: Elsevier, 1984:23–34.

40. Speckmann E-J, Elger CE, eds. *Epilepsy and motor system.* Baltimore, MD: Urban & Schwarzenberg, 1983.

41. Wieser HG. *Electroclinical features of the psychomotor seizure. A stereoencephalographic study of ictal symptoms and chronotopographical seizure patterns including clinical effects of intracerebral stimulation.* New York: Gustav Fischer, 1983.

42. Elger CE, Speckmann E-J. Focal interictal epileptiform discharges (FIED) in the epicortical EEG and their relations to spinal field potentials in the rat. *Electroencephalogr Clin Neurophysiol* 1980;48:447–460.

43. Elger CE, Speckmann E-J. Vertical inhibition in motor cortical epileptic foci and its consequences for descending neuronal activity to the spinal cord. In: Speckmann E-J, Elger CE, eds. *Epilepsy and motor system.* Baltimore, MD: Urban & Schwarzenberg, 1983:152–160.

44. Elger CE, Speckmann E-J, Caspers H, et al. Focal interictal epileptiform discharges in the cortex of the rat: laminar restriction and its consequences for activity descending to the spinal cord. In: Klee MR, Lux HD, Speckmann E-J, eds. *Physiology and pharmacology of epileptogenic phenomena.* New York: Raven Press, 1982:13–20.

45. Elger CE, Speckmann E-J, Prohaska O, et al. Pattern of intracortical potential distribution during focal interictal epileptiform discharges (FIED) and its relation to spinal field potentials in the rat. *Electroencephalogr Clin Neurophysiol* 1981;51:393–402.

46. Petsche H, Müller-Paschinger IB, Pockberger H, et al. Depth profiles of electrocortical activities and cortical architectonics. In: Brazier MAB, Petsche H, eds. *Architectonics of the cerebral cortex,* vol 3. New York: Raven Press, 1978:257–280.

47. Petsche H, Pockberger H, Rappelsberger P. Current source density studies of epileptic phenomena and the morphology of the rabbit's striate cortex. In: Klee MR, Lux HD, Speckmann E-J, eds. *Physiology and pharmacology of epileptogenic phenomena.* New York: Raven Press, 1981:53–63.

48. Elger CE, Speckmann E-J. Penicillin-induced epileptic foci in the motor cortex: vertical inhibition. *Electroencephalogr Clin Neurophysiol* 1983;56:604–622.

49. Köhling R, Höhling J-M, Straub H, et al. Optical monitoring of neuronal activity during spontaneous sharp waves in chronically epileptic human neocortical tissue. *J Neurophysiol* 2000;84: 2161–2165.

50. Köhling R, Reindel J, Vahrenhold J, et al. Spatio-temporal patterns of neuronal activity: analysis of optical imaging data using geometric shape matching. *J Neurosci Meth* 2002;114:17–23.

51. Straub H, Kuhnt U, Höhling J-M, et al. Stimulus induced patterns of bioelectric activity in human neocortical tissue recorded by a voltage sensitive dye. *Neuroscience* 2003;121:587–604.

52. Gumnit RJ, Matsumoto H, Vasconetto C. DC activity in the depth of an experimental epileptic focus. *Electroencephalogr Clin Neurophysiol* 1970;28:333–339.

53. Gumnit RJ. DC shifts accompanying seizure activity. In: Remond A, ed. *Handbook of electroencephalography and clinical neurophysiology,* vol 10. Amsterdam: Elsevier, 1974:66–77.

54. Speckmann E-J, Caspers H, Janzen RWC. Relations between cortical DC shifts and membrane potential changes of cortical neurons associated with seizure activity. In: Petsche H, Brazier MAB, eds. *Synchronization of EEG activity in epilepsies.* New York: Springer, 1972:93–111.

11

Localization and Field Determination in Electroencephalography and Magnetoencephalography

Richard C. Burgess   *Masaki Iwasaki*   *Dileep Nair*

LOCALIZATION AND MAPPING

The word electroencephalogram (EEG) was derived from Greek roots to create a term meaning an electrical picture of the brain. While interpreting an EEG, electroencephalographers maintain a three-dimensional picture of the brain/head in their minds. In principle, there are an infinite number of different source configurations of an electrical event within the head that may give rise to the same electrical and magnetic field distribution at the scalp. Despite this theoretical constraint, one of the key functions of the electroencephalographer is to conceptualize the generators in relationship to this vision and to build an increasingly clear mental image of the foci of these generators. Methods for localization and field determination are tools to help the electroencephalographer infer the location, strength, and orientation of generator sources within the cortex, based on their manifestation at 21 or more EEG recording sites. The same generators that originate and spread their activity for measurement by EEG also produce magnetic fields that can be picked up by extremely sensitive detectors—that is, magnetoencephalography (MEG).

Scalp electrical activity arises from both physiologic and pathologic brain generators. Localization of epileptiform potentials from scalp EEG is critically important for pinpointing the epileptic focus and identifying the region of brain pathology (1). Many electroencephalographers take a simplistic approach, assuming that the generator source must be close to the point where the maximum voltage is recorded. Attempts to systematize the localization of specific EEG activity date back to the early years of electroencephalography. In the mid-1930s, Adrian and Matthews (2), as well as Adrian and Yamagiwa (3), used phase-reversal techniques to localize normal rhythms, and Walter (4) used phase reversals for localization of abnormal EEG activity, as did Gibbs and Gibbs (5) in 1941 in their classic atlas. More recently, a variety of reviews have outlined general principles for the use of polarity, montages, and localization (5–11). It should be emphasized that phase reversals are not inherently an indicator of abnormality. Phase reversals occur as a result of both normal and abnormal activity. Phase reversals are most obvious in sharply contoured transient activity and, therefore, provide a dramatic visual clue in the case of epileptiform abnormalities.

Despite the critical importance of accuracy in localization, there has been an absence in the literature of descriptions of systematic methods for accomplishing this localization in a simple, manual fashion (12,13). Most textbooks emphasize the distribution that would occur as a result of an assumed generator (i.e., the "forward" problem). With the evolution of digital EEG (14), a variety of methods for computerized source localization have become available (15,16) at the push of a button within the EEG machine itself or as stand-alone software (17,18). These techniques are primarily model-based and have significant limitations; they have generally not been used in routine clinical practice. A practical guide for the step-by-step identification of the origin of epileptiform activity was developed at the

Cleveland Clinic Foundation (19) and is discussed in detail in this chapter. This review concentrates primarily on defining the electrophysiologic origin of epileptiform activity.

New imaging techniques have decreased the importance of EEG for many neurologic disorders, but EEG is still the *sine qua non* for the diagnosis of epilepsy. Although sometimes marketed as an "imaging" tool, MEG senses brain electrical behavior in a way similar to that of conventional scalp EEG (20). With MEG as well, a systematic way to arrive at the sources of the observed magnetic fields is required, quite analogous to that with EEG. Despite the relatively high equipment cost, MEG possesses a number of inherent advantages: (a) It requires simpler forward modeling, resulting in an inherently higher source resolution; (b) recordings are reference-free; (c) signals are not attenuated by bone and scalp; and (d) it is easy to obtain multichannel, whole-head, high spatial-density recordings. As MEG becomes increasingly available, it may play a more important role in the localization of epileptic discharges.

There are two steps in the interpretation of epileptiform discharges: surface field determination and source localization. Proper determination of the field distribution, based on the manifestations detected by either electrical or magnetic sensors, results from correct interpretation or calculations, and there is only one answer. Accurate field determination is essential not only for accurate source localization, but also for discrimination of epileptic activity from other nonepileptic transients. For source localization, on the other hand, no single unique solution exists. To arrive at a plausible solution for the source location, several assumptions are useful. In this chapter, practical neurophysiologic concepts that relate the generator to the surface electrical fields are described in the first section. The next three sections describe important conventions used in visual interpretation of EEG regarding instrumentation, field determination, and source localization. Last, the principles of MEG recording and its complementary perspective on source localization of the very same signals are reviewed.

PRACTICAL CONCEPTS OF ELECTRICAL FIELDS APPLIED TO BRAIN GENERATORS

Sources

The electrical sources seen at the scalp arise from intracranial focal dipoles or sheets of dipoles. These dipoles represent the postsynaptic potentials originating from vertically oriented neurons. A unit current dipole is created by the intercellular laminar currents in the apical dendrites arising from the pyramidal cells in the outer layer of the cerebral cortex. Specifically, superficial excitatory postsynaptic potentials and deep inhibitory postsynaptic potentials gen-

erate almost all spontaneous EEG activity (21), particularly the epileptogenic abnormalities. When populations of neurons are more or less synchronously activated for relatively long durations, the activity can be macroscopically recorded from a certain distance as a linear summation of the unit dipoles (22–24). This summated activity may also be represented as a dipole or sheet of dipoles along the cortex. Thus, the generator of epileptic activity can be explained by a single or multiple equivalent current dipoles (8,13,25,26). The surface potential can be thought of as a two-dimensional projection, or shadow, of a complex three-dimensional electrical object residing inside the head.

Fundamental to scalp localization is the concept of the "inverse" problem, which entails an estimate, based on surface data, of the magnitude, location, and distribution of electrical fields throughout the brain. Whereas the forward problem is solvable with unique solutions, the inverse problem is not. Nunez (9) described the mathematical representation of the biophysics underlying volume conduction.

The forward problem can be stated as follows: Given known charge distributions and volume conductor geometries and properties, predict the resulting surface potential distribution. The solution involves applying numerical or analytical methods for any known set of geometries and boundary conditions (9,27) to solve Poisson's equation:

$$\nabla^2 \Phi = -\rho/\varepsilon$$

In this equation, ∇^2 is the second spatial gradient operator, Φ is the scalar potential in volts, ρ is the free charge density, and ε is the permittivity of the mass of tissue. Multiple sources can be shown to combine linearly, so that a combination of sources results in the arithmetic sum of the potential distributions that each would produce individually.

The corresponding inverse problem can be stated as follows: Given a surface potential distribution and the volume conductor geometries and properties, determine the underlying charge distribution. Unfortunately, a given surface map can be produced by any of an infinite number of possible source distributions. EEG and MEG record at a distance from the sources, and they use only a limited number of sensors—typically, 20 to 100 for scalp EEG and 100 to 300 for whole-head MEG. Therefore, this problem generally has no unique solution (28). Nevertheless, simplifying assumptions are possible.

The single-dipole solution is the most frequently sought interpretation of scalp potential distributions and is the solution produced by most "dipole localization" systems in current use. Such a solution should account for a maximum amount of the observed map, but a residual "error" term may remain. In addition, the following assumptions are made: (a) the source dipole is near the surface; (b) the source dipole is perpendicular to the surface; (c) the head is a uniform, homogeneous volume conductor; (d) at least

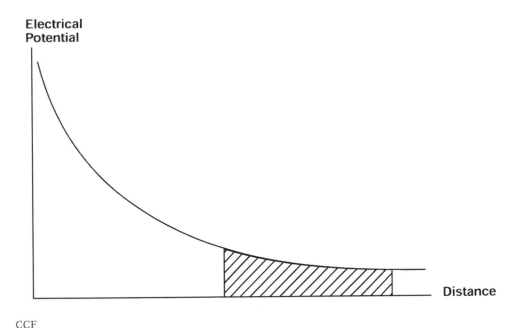

Figure 11.1 The electrical potential recorded by an electrode decreases in a parabolic fashion the farther away it is from the source. The difference recorded between two electrodes close to the source (near-field potentials) will be greater than the differential recordings from the tail of the curve. These far-field potentials (in the *shaded region*) are also lower in absolute amplitude.

one recording electrode is essentially over the source; and (e) the reference is not contained in the active region.

On the basis of these assumptions, one generally looks for a single predominating potential maximum on the surface, with the source lying directly below it; however, a variety of nondipolar source configurations could produce the same observation. For example, a simple monopolar charge buildup, a curved dipole sheet, or a finite-thickness dipole "pancake" would produce a single well-defined maximum. In addition, signals originating from confined, but deep-seated, generators are broadly distributed when recorded from the surface (29,30), and cannot be reliably distinguished from more superficial, but widespread, epileptic regions.

In addition to these "equivalent" source possibilities, others are physiologically similar but generate very different surface maps. Through variations in orientation and shape, dipole sheets can produce charge reorientation and cancellation. The resultant range of possible scalp distributions serves as a reminder that observed scalp maxima do not necessarily lie directly above maximal brain activity. Jayakar and colleagues (31) pointed out the difficulties involved in localizing epileptic foci on the basis of simple models, owing to effects from dipolar orientation, anatomic variations, and inhomogeneities, among other factors.

Volume Conduction

In a volume conductor, the electrical field spreads instantaneously over an infinite number of pathways between the positive and negative ends of the dipole. Outside the neuron, the circuit is completed by the current flowing through the extracellular fluid in a direction opposite to the intracellular current. Through the process of volume conduction, electrical activity originates from a generator and spreads through a conductive medium to be picked up by a distant recording electrode. Volume conduction is passive—that is, it does not involve active regeneration of the signal by intervening neurons or synaptic relays—and occurs as easily through saline as it does through brain parenchyma. Potentials recorded by way of volume conduction are picked up synchronously and at the speed of light at all recording electrodes. Although attenuated with distance by the medium, volume-conducted components preserve their original polarity and morphology.

The attenuation factor is defined by the inverse square law—that is, the recorded electrical potential falls off in direct proportion to the square of the distance from the generator (32,33). For example, a 100-mV potential seen at the electrode directly overlying a cortical generator (assume a distance of 1 cm away) will be reflected as a 4-mV potential at an electrode that is 5 cm away and as only a 1-mV potential at 10 cm away. The rapidity of this falloff is a function of the depth of the generator, with more superficial generators falling off much more rapidly. Distant generators have a "flat" falloff, one of the hallmarks of a "far-field" potential (Fig. 11.1).

The medium through which current travels to reach the recording electrode is not homogeneous, but rather exhibits a variety of conductivities (34). As the current attempts to complete its circuit by following the path of least resistance, these differences in conductivities, especially differences among cerebrospinal fluid (CSF), skull, and scalp, and their associated boundaries, affect the electrical potential recorded on the scalp. The signal is not only altered in amplitude, but also low-pass filtered during its passage to the surface because of the capacitive and shunting effects of the intervening layers. In the skull, the conductivity in a tangential direction is higher than that in a direction perpendicular to the surface. This produces a "smearing effect" on the surface potential distribution (35). Although the current tends to flow along the path of least resistance, there is still some flow throughout the volume conductor, thereby permitting recording of the electrical potential at all sites on the volume conductor, albeit with the amplitude inversely related to the square of the distance from the source (Fig. 11.1).

The head also contains normal or abnormal openings that present low-resistance paths to conducted currents. The current tends to flow toward skull defects, whether physiologic (such as foramina) or acquired through trauma or surgery, and around cavities (such as the ventricles), markedly distorting the field in the region of the defect. The resistivity of scalp or brain tissue is many times smaller than that of bone (36–38). As a result, surface potentials near these openings will be unusually high, and the largest potentials can be seen at the location of the defect even when the source is several centimeters away from the defect (35,39,40). MEG signals are less distorted by these heterogeneities in conductivity.

Surface Electrical Manifestations

A variety of real-world considerations complicate the interpretation of surface recordings. Because the dipoles measured at the scalp are ordinarily oriented radially, scalp electrodes "see" primarily the positive or the negative pole. Although generators located at the apex of a gyrus lie perpendicular to the scalp (i.e., vertical dipoles), any generator within a cortical fissure will present a dipole at an angle to the scalp. Nearly 70% of the cortical surface lies within the sulcal depths (41). In addition, many brain areas—most notably, the mesial frontal, parietal, occipital, and basal temporal cortex—are diversely oriented and lie at varying distances from surface electrodes. Hence, it is not sufficient to assume that the generator must be close to the point where the maximum potential is recorded (7). Finally, the choice of reference affects the form of the EEG measurements.

When a generator dipole is oblique or parallel to the scalp, the resulting surface potentials can lead to false localization of the potential maximum. The typical bell-shaped distribution of the electrical field is replaced by one shaped like a sideways "S." Because both the positive and the negative ends of the dipole may be recorded at the scalp, the surface potential can exhibit two "maxima" of opposite polarity. Between the two ends is a zero isopotential boundary where the generator will not be picked up at all.

It is important to distinguish true horizontal dipoles, such as those arising at a sulcus or the interhemispheric fissure, from field distributions resulting from widely separated activity but giving rise to distinct negative and positive maxima. For example, bisynchronous temporal spikes differing slightly in phase, such that the negative component

on the left aligns with the positive component on the right, may appear to represent huge transverse dipoles (31); however, careful evaluation with an alternative reference (or the demonstration that the spikes also occur asynchronously) can prove that the fields represent not the source and sink of a single dipole, but rather two generators (42) linked by corticocortical propagation.

When a source lies deeper in the brain, two changes occur: the surface potential becomes smaller, and the field becomes more widespread relative to the surface maximum (29,30,42). Although the shape of the electrical field gradient can indicate the type of field and the distance of the generator, identifying the source on the basis of the potential difference between any scalp electrodes becomes increasingly more difficult. When the potential field gradient is relatively flat, as is the case in the far-field potential from a deep-seated source, a bipolar montage will display the waveform at relatively smaller amplitude (Fig. 11.1). Diffuse discharges may be better appreciated on referential montages, assuming that the reference is not involved. An adequate "vantage point" may be impossible with surface electrodes when a focus is deep. It may be impossible to find a scalp electrode reference that is not electrically involved in the active region, and some cases can only be resolved by invasive electrode placements that can monitor more limited areas (30,44–47).

The combination of multiple sources can produce a variety of results. A superficial source can overshadow a deep one, distorting or even hiding it. Because the amplitude of a measured potential is inversely proportional to the square of the distance from the recording electrode, nearby sources can appear disproportionally higher at the recording electrodes. A given electrode thus has a "view" of the nearby generators, such that dipoles that combine to reinforce each other will have a large net effect, whereas those that cancel will produce a smaller or null potential (48).

Complicating this problem is the fact that the equivalent dipole is an abstraction. In reality, only sources that extend over multiple layers of several square centimeters of cortical tissue have sufficient energy to generate detectable scalp discharges (43,49). An epileptogenic zone almost always consists of a continuum of dipoles, resulting in a sheet, or "patch" (50), dipole. Such a source may cover an extended brain region, with the constituent areas lying at various depths and orientations. Again, it is possible for both reinforcement and cancellation to produce a variety of surface potential distributions. Overall, the conduction phenomena leading to surface potentials follow the "solid-angle" rule (51)—that is, the net surface potential is proportional to the solid angle subtended by the recording electrode. Unless a dipole sheet parallels the surface, the maximum surface potential may be somewhere other than directly over the affected area, as illustrated in Figure 11.2. The solid-angle theorem helps to explain the results of multiple synchronously discharging pyramidal neurons arrayed over a cortical region containing both sulci and gyri.

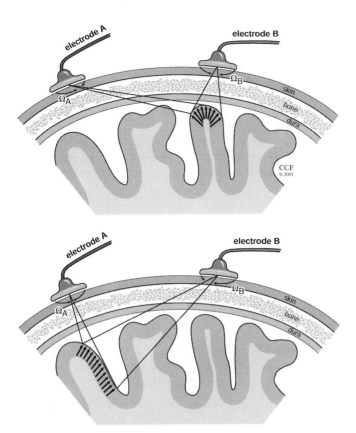

Figure 11.2 Use of the solid-angle rule to ascertain the signal measured on the scalp surface relative to the orientation of the dipole. *Top:* Surface electrode B sees a large electrical potential because of the orientation and proximity of the dipole layer, as borne out by the solid angle ΩB. *Bottom:* In this case, the potential seen by electrode A is actually lower than that measured by the more distant electrode B, because of the arrangement of the dipoles in the discharging region. The smaller solid angle, ΩA, is proportional to the voltage measured on the scalp.

In the same way that opposing dipoles can cancel each other relative to a distant electrode, a sheet of nonparallel dipoles can produce a "closed" field (52) whose potential contributions will cancel, resulting in a negligible potential at the surface (53). These generators, usually not visible on scalp EEG, are observed primarily on invasive recordings (48). Even when not a completely closed field, multipolar source-sink configurations tend both to produce more cancellation than dipolar generators and to attenuate more quickly as a function of distance (9). This irregular structure is particularly likely in the basal and mesial areas of the temporal cortex and the hippocampus, where cortical infolding is so prevalent (54).

The head consists of a series of roughly concentric layers that separate the brain from the scalp surface. Each of these layers—CSF, meninges, bone, and skin—presents different electrical characteristics to the currents that conduct the EEG to the surface. These layers occasion considerable current spreading, which causes the potential for localized foci to appear in a much broader scalp area (9,55). Spreading in itself is not an insurmountable problem, because it is theoretically possible to recover deep dipole sources based

on observed surface potentials, using appropriate mathematical transformations. Such recovery, however, is guaranteed only in a perfectly spherical concentric conductor, onto which electrodes can be placed in any location. The head is not a perfect globe, however, and significant constraints disqualify the face or neck, which may be preferred for certain sources, as electrode sites.

Electrode Placement as Spatial Sampling

Placement of scalp electrodes should be considered an exercise in spatial sampling. Electrode density must be generous enough to capture the available information but not so closely spaced as to overwhelm with redundant data. Inability to precisely locate a cortical generator may be the result of spatial undersampling (i.e., "aliasing"). The assumption that a potential will decrease monotonically as distance increases from the involved electrode is based not only on an uncomplicated electrical field—that is, a monopole—but also on an electrode placement sufficiently dense to accurately represent the spatial contours of the field. Cooper and associates (49) suggested that 6 cm^2 or more of cortex discharging simultaneously is required to reflect a visible potential on the scalp surface. Because most epileptogenic potentials seen on the scalp are visible at multiple electrodes, a considerably larger cortical area must be synchronously discharging to produce these potentials. The widely accepted International 10–20 Electrode Placement System (56), although relatively easy to apply reproducibly, has some inherent limitations in terms of the accuracy of localization (57). When more precise localization is indicated to avoid spatial aliasing, scalp electrodes should be placed at least once every 2.5 cm (58). The maximum spacing can be determined theoretically (59) as well as experimentally, and as many as 128 electrodes (spaced approximately 2 cm apart) is sometimes necessary (60).

Boundary Problems

Regardless of the fineness of the scalp electrode grid, boundary effects will occur at the edges of the array. The maximum potential must be well within the scope of the recording electrodes to ascertain that a physiologic gradient exists away from the electrode. For example, epileptic sharp waves arising from mesial temporal structures are frequently localized outside the area covered by the 10–20 Electrode Placement System (61–64). It is impossible to determine the complete extent of the maximum fields unless the area is surrounded by regions of lesser activity. Recordings in which the activity is large all the way to the boundary of the region defined by the montage must be "remontaged" to include, if possible, all the relevant electrodes, or further recording must be done with additional electrodes. This may be especially complicated when it is difficult to position electrodes inferior to the customary borders of scalp coverage.

A significant portion of the head cannot be practically surveyed, and important brain areas, such as the basomesial temporal cortex and other deep sources, are only indirectly accessible with standard scalp electrodes. Additional electrodes inferior to the 10–20 Electrode Placement System (56) must be used to provide a better view. In certain circumstances, the information obtained from a combination of closely spaced scalp electrodes, such as the International 10–10 Electrode Placement System (65–67), and sphenoidal electrodes can obviate the need for more invasive recordings (68).

ELECTROENCEPHALOGRAM INSTRUMENTATION CONSIDERATIONS RELATED TO LOCALIZATION

Differential Amplifiers

Amplifiers used in clinical neurophysiology measure the difference between two potentials at the inputs to the amplifier and provide an amplified version of this difference at the output. These devices, called differential amplifiers, eliminate unwanted signals that are identical at both inputs, called common mode signals. The two terminals at the input to a differential amplifier are sometimes labeled

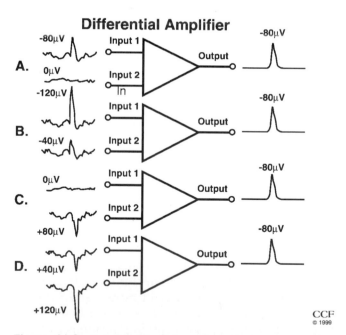

Differential Amplifier

Figure 11.3 **A** and **B:** Illustrations of a surface-negative spike. Input 1 is more negative than input 2. Because a differential amplifier responds only to the difference between the two inputs (input 1 − input 2), the spikes illustrated will yield identical output voltages; (−80) − (0) is the same as (−120) − (−40). Because it is more widespread than the spikes and therefore almost the same at both inputs, the background electroencephalographic activity is largely canceled out. **C** and **D:** The spike is surface-positive, that is, input 2 is more positive than input 1. The calculations (0) − (+80) and (+40) − (+120) both result in an answer of −80, and the background is still canceled out. All four circumstances yield identical outputs despite the differing amplitudes and polarities.

G1 and G2, recalling when a grid within the vacuum tube amplifier controlled the flow of electrons from cathode to plate. Modern operational amplifier (op-amp)-based differential amplifiers use complex integrated circuits, and the terms "input 1" and "input 2" are used throughout this chapter.

The amplifier itself has no concept of polarity; it simply does the subtraction and the gain multiplication, and then provides an output voltage that is a linear function of the input voltages, according to the following equation:

$$V_{output}(t) = G \times [V_{input1}(t) - V_{input2}(t)]$$

In this equation, $V_{output}(t)$ and $V_{inputN}(t)$ are the output and input voltages, respectively, and G is the gain of the amplifier. It is only during interpretation of the EEG waveform in the context of the underlying generators that the concept of polarity has any meaning. Inexperienced electroencephalographers often mistakenly ascribe a polarity at the input to a specific pen deviation at the output (12). It should be remembered that there are no positive deflections and no negative deflections; there are only upward and downward deflections (12). Figure 11.3 illustrates four different input conditions that give rise to exactly the same deflection.

Polarity Conventions

Deflection refers to the direction on the page or display screen in which the waveform component under study appears to go, and it is a function only of the display instrumentation. By EEG convention, upward deflections are caused by input 1 being more negative than input 2. Downward deflections are caused by input 1 being more positive than input 2. These relationships imply nothing about the underlying polarity of the signals at inputs 1 and 2, only about the polarity of their differences. When the name of the electrode connected to input 1 is written above the deflection and the name of input 2 below, the deflection will point to the electrode with the "relative" negativity, as in Figure 11.4.

If the difference between the two signals at the input is zero, no deflection will occur. When two electrodes (no matter how close to the source of the sharp wave or spike) that lie along the same isopotential line (typically at the same distance from the generator) are input to a differential amplifier, the output will reflect no activity, even though both electrodes may be measuring high amplitudes in an absolute sense. Some amplifiers used in basic neurophysiology research and in clinical evoked potentials use another convention, designed to display positive input 1 as an upward deflection.

Derivations and Montages

A derivation describes the connections of the electrodes to the amplifier inputs. A montage is a combination of

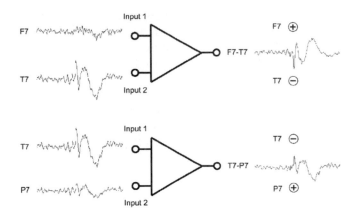

Differential amplifiers and polarity convention

Figure 11.4 Differential amplifier and polarity conventions. The differential amplifier is designed to amplify only the difference between the signals at the two inputs. An upward deflection appearing at the output is caused by input 1 being more negative than input 2. A downward deflection results from input 1 being more positive than input 2. This convention is common to all clinical electroencephalograph machines. When the name of the electrode (i.e., its "derivation") connected to input 1 is written above the waveform and input 2 written below, as in this figure, the deflection always points to the electrode of higher "relative" negativity.

derivations arranged down the EEG page to display many amplifier channels simultaneously in a way that aids in the identification and localization of abnormalities (69). Each amplifier could be connected to any pair of available electrodes. Likewise, these amplifier outputs could be arranged in any fashion on the screen; the arrangement in chains assists our visual localization capabilities.

The arrangement of derivations into a montage determines whether it is called bipolar or referential. Derivations in bipolar montages are established between neighboring electrodes to emphasize focal activity. They take advantage of the subtractive nature of differential amplifiers to effect a high degree of cancellation. Any montage can be analyzed to locate the maximum of a sharp wave or spike, provided that the montage has a logical order (6,70,71).

ELECTRICAL FIELD DETERMINATION ON THE SCALP

Identification of Peaks and Measurement of the Amplitude

Interictal epileptiform abnormalities are recognized by their morphology—an impression of "standing out" from the background—and by their electrical field distribution, which must demonstrate a realistic relationship between the electrical potentials at topographically associated electrode positions. In choosing an abnormality to localize, the peak selected must be representative of the patient's population of spikes, and the sample must be as clean as possible.

It is assumed that an activity starts from zero and reaches its maximum after a certain time. The amplitude of the activity is measured between the zero and the maximum peak. However, it is often difficult to identify the level of the "zero" in each EEG channel correctly, because the activity is superimposed on the background, arises from the noise level, or continues from the preceding activity. Sometimes sharp activity can be separated from a slower background, provided the frequency of the epileptic activity is clearly different, by using filtering.

Practically, the amplitude is measured as peak-to-peak or baseline-to-peak. Identification of the baseline and peak may be particularly troublesome in the case of polyphasic discharges, in which each phase is brief and difficult to line up temporally. When analyzing a peak, the maximum value in each EEG channel should be identified at exactly the same time point. During visual analysis of a waveform, the montage selected will influence identification of the peak, resulting in different, or sometimes erroneous, field determinations. Multiple peaks or phase reversals with small time shifts reflect a sequential change in the location of the maximum. In the EEG tracings shown in Figure 11.5, note that the peaks of several of the channels were reached on different phases of the waveform, giving the erroneous appearance of a phase reversal. Computerized source localization techniques are especially sensitive to the selection of the appropriate time frame. Errors in identifying the peaks that are to be mapped can cause extraordinary displacements in the apparent localization of the sources (72,73).

The peak of the sharp wave (i.e., the negative extrema) generally has the highest amplitude at the electrode closest to the involved cortical epileptogenic neurons (7). The main component of an epileptic discharge may be preceded by a smaller deflection of the opposite polarity. Early components show a more localized field than do later ones (74,75), and they are more synchronous than the slow wave that frequently follows a spike. Thus, the initial deflection probably contains more localizing information (31), and using the lower-frequency waves for localization may not always represent the epileptogenic region.

Mapping the Electrical Field

Two-dimensional display of the scalp regions involved in epileptiform or other activity is called mapping. Isopotential lines are drawn on a representation of the scalp to specify the topography of equivalent electrical potentials, similar to the isocontour lines drawn by a surveyor on a land map.

The potential fields of spikes and sharp waves can be mapped even without electronic assistance by tracking the relationships of the electrical potential level between electrodes. As the initial step, a longitudinal or transverse chain of the electrodes is used to map the one-dimensional relationship of voltage level to electrode position, as illustrated in Figure 11.6 (*top*). Then two chains are connected to each other through a common electrode to obtain the

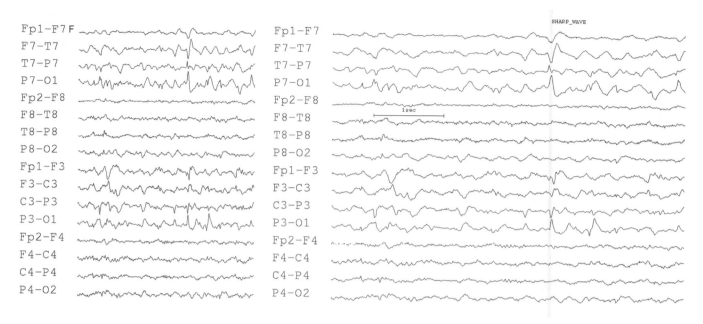

Figure 11.5 Phase reversals: choosing the same component. Be certain to select the proper phase of the discharge. On first glance, the electroencephalogram on the left appears to show a confusing distribution, with phase reversals at multiple sites. On the right, the time scale of the same epoch was doubled. The vertical marker reveals that the discharge actually consists of three phases, with each peak at a slightly different time. The phase reversal at T_7–P_7 occurs prior to the phase reversal at P_3.

two-dimensional relationship. To create an isopotential contour map, a 100% value is assigned to the maximum and a 0% value to the minimum. However, as discussed (in source localization choosing between two possibilities) the polarity of the maximum depends on an assumption about the generator. The maximum may be the highest negative point or the highest positive point. Similarly, the minimum may be negative or positive, or may have a mid-curve value when two maxima of opposite polarities are assumed—for example, a horizontal dipole generator. Depending on the polarity of the maximum—that is, the point given a 100% value—at least two different isocontour maps can be obtained, as shown in Figure 11.6. To make the correct choice, some assumptions must be introduced, as is described in source localization assumptions.

The ideal situation in referential recording occurs when the reference electrode is totally inactive or picks up activity of negligible amplitude. In this situation, those channels showing some activity will deflect in one direction only, as illustrated in Figure 11.7 (*bottom*). The electrode closest to the generator will show the largest deflection, with the amplitude of the deflection in all the other channels directly proportional to the magnitude of activity recorded from each of those electrodes. This situation makes it especially easy to find the maximum and to assess the extent of the field distribution (Fig. 11.7). To achieve this ideal situation, an alert technologist will recognize a contaminated reference and construct a "distribution montage," typically with a reference electrode from the other hemisphere (Fig. 11.8).

In mapping potentials measured from a bipolar recording, the bipolar measurements first must be converted to voltages relative to a selected "reference" electrode. The wisest choice usually is to select the least involved electrode at the beginning or end of the chains, taking advantage of the fact that certain electrodes are common to more than one chain. For instance, in the "double-banana" longitudinal montage, the frontal polar and occipital electrodes occur in both ipsilateral chains. These common electrodes provide an electrical connection between chains and allow an algebraic determination of the potential gradient of the electrical field over the entire area covered by the two chains. Because all the electrodes in both chains are related to each other by a sequence of subtractions, one can determine the relative amplitude at any electrode to the reference electrode. Of course, the exact amplitude (in absolute terms) at any scalp electrode is unknown. However, electrodes relatively distant from the site of maximum activity "see" a negligible potential, hence the assumption that the potential of the particular transient under study at these uninvolved electrodes is zero. The fact that the potential at this uninvolved electrode may not be exactly zero is unimportant because the relative differences between electrodes will be appropriately preserved.

Although it is possible to localize a spike or sharp wave from a single montage if electrical connections between the chains (or appropriate assumptions) exist, recording from multiple montages, especially "crisscrossing" montages, will help to confirm the topography of the discharge and can better define the topographic distribution. When the amplitudes of the potential distribution do not match exactly between chains or montages, the discrepancies most likely arise from errors in visual measurement,

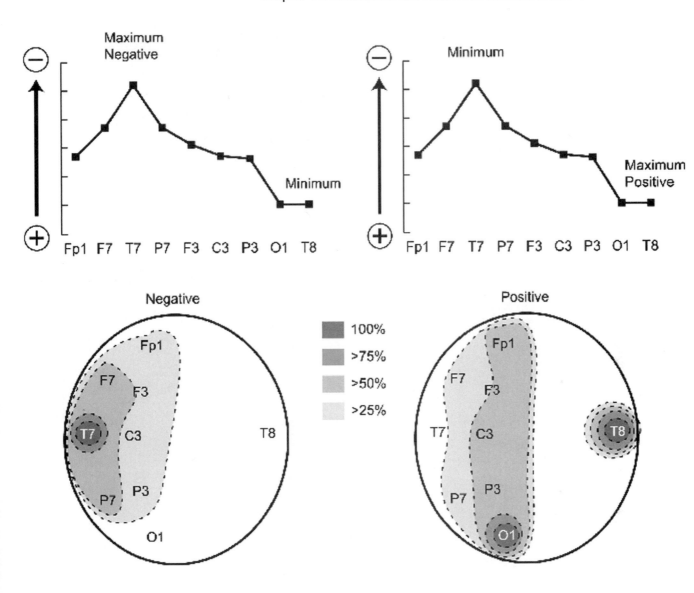

Iso-potential map

Figure 11.6 Isopotential contour map. As in Figure 11.1, the vertical axis of the top figures represents electrical potential, and the horizontal axis shows electrode location. A 100% value is assigned to the maximum and a 0% value is assigned to the minimum. Depending on the polarity of the maximum, at least two different maps can be obtained, illustrated in the bottom row. In the map on the left side, the maximum is assumed to be negative, and the falloff of potential with distance is physiologic. On the right, the opposite assumption was made—that is, that the maximum is a positive potential—resulting in a very nonphysiologic distribution. Thus, it was deduced that this spike has maximum negativity from the left temporal area.

erroneous assumptions of zero potential, or difficulty recognizing the same waveform in different montages. Generally, referential montages with uninvolved references are better able to map the distribution of the activity.

The procedure for mapping the potential field, illustrated in Figures 11.6 and 11.7, can be summarized as follows:

1. Measure the amplitude of the component of interest in each channel.
2. Select an electrode that appears to be uninvolved. Assume a value of zero for that electrode.

3. Calculate the amplitude of all the electrodes relative to the selected electrode based on the algebraic relationship established by the montage.
4. Follow this procedure for all the chains connected by common electrodes.
5. Assume another zero electrode to calculate the distribution in chains not connected by a common electrode.
6. If the resulting distribution has potentials both above and below zero, start with another "zero" electrode.
7. Draw isopotential contours around the resulting distribution.

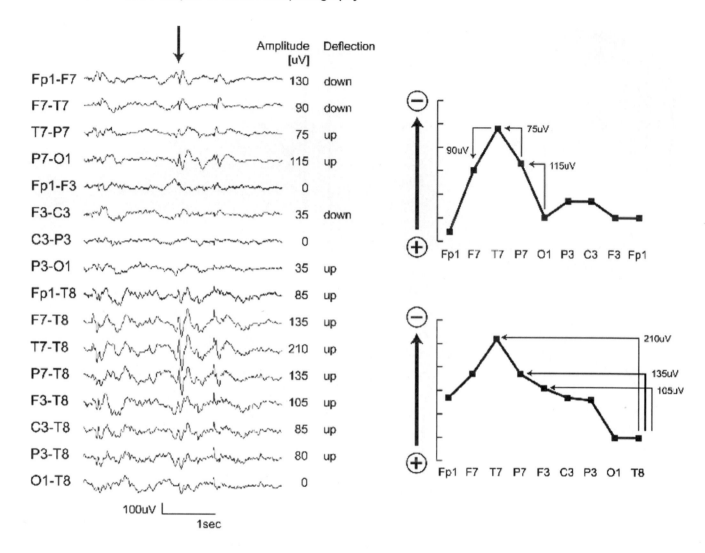

Voltage / Electrode map

Figure 11.7 Voltage/electrode map. The electroencephalogram shows the same activity in two different montages: a bipolar montage in the top eight traces and a referential montage in the bottom eight. Two voltage/electrode maps for the spike indicated by the *arrow* are reconstructed manually from the two montages, respectively. In the bipolar montage, the difference of the potential level (amplitude) and relative polarity (deflection) between neighboring electrodes is sequentially tracked along the "chain" of the montage. Here, the potential mapping was started from a common electrode, O_1, with a value of 0 μV assumed. Using the algebraic relationships between the electrode derivations, the calculated amplitudes at each individual electrode are graphed. The resulting voltage level at Fp_1 differed slightly between the two bipolar chains, owing to minor differences in manual measurement of the amplitudes. For the referential montage, the measured amplitudes are written down directly, as no calculations are necessary. If all the deflections are in the same direction and the reference electrode (input 2) is located at the minimum, as seen in this example, then the amplitude of the deflection simply reflects the voltage level of the electrode. No matter which montage is used, the field determination should be the same in terms of location of the maximum. The voltage/electrode maps may differ in detail, however, reflecting a varying degree of visibility of the spike between montages.

8. If the topographic distribution is unphysiologic, assume the opposite polarity for the waveform.

These principles can be applied most profitably when electrode montages are simple and systematic, as recommended by the American Clinical Neurophysiology Society (69).

Rules for Field Identification

Table 11.1 outlines a practical set of rules for identification of the electrical fields seen on the EEG. These rules assume that the field in question is reflected at the scalp as a monopole and not a dipole, as described in "Source Localization: Assumptions."

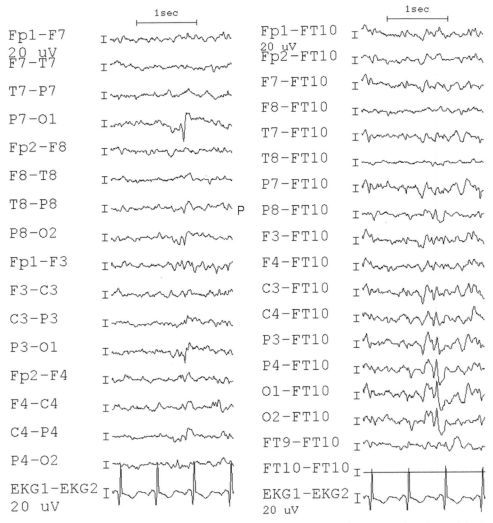

Figure 11.8 On the *left*, a bipolar montage with no phase reversal suggests that the activity is either at the beginning or the end of the chain. The same time period is shown on the *right*, and the distribution montage to an uninvolved contralateral electrode confirms the left posterior maximum of this surface-negative discharge.

The following sections provide more detailed instructions for the application of these rules.

Bipolar Montage

Derivations in a bipolar montage are customarily arranged in chains (6,69,70)—that is, the electrode connected to input 2 of one channel is also connected to input 1 of the next channel. Electrode chains are usually parallel, along transverse or sagittal axes, and contain no single electrode common to all channels.

When the deflections of two channels move simultaneously in opposite directions, this defines a "phase reversal." The presence or absence of phase reversals provides useful and immediate clues to localize maxima and minima. Whether the montage is bipolar or referential radically alters the meaning of the phase reversal (Table 11.1). In bipolar montages, there are two types of phase reversals:

TABLE 11.1

RULES FOR POTENTIAL DISTRIBUTION OF MONOPOLAR FIELDS

Montage Type	Phase Reversal	Conclusion
Bipolar	No	Maximum or minimum is located at the end of the chain
Bipolar	Yes	Maximum or minimum is located at the electrode of the phase reversal
Referential	No	Reference electrode is either maximum or minimum
Referential	Yes	Reference electrode is neither maximum nor minimum

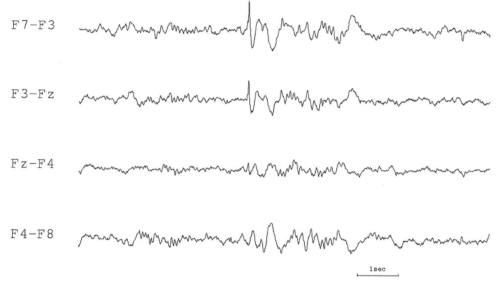

Figure 11.9 Bipolar montage with no phase reversal. Electroencephalographers are used to looking for phase reversals in a bipolar montage. In this tracing there is no phase reversal; consequently, the discharge must be coming from either the beginning or the end of the chain. If the sharp wave is negative, implying that the activity is at the beginning of the chain (F_7), the distribution has a much more realistic falloff (i.e., it has a single peak with a monotonic decline). If the sharp wave is assumed to be positive, then the maximum would have to be at the end of the chain (F_8), with an oddly flat distribution on the right and a rapid falloff on the left.

negative phase reversals (wherein the deflections point toward each other) and positive phase reversals (wherein they point away from each other).

If there is a phase reversal, the electrode where it occurs is either the minimum or the maximum of the electrical field. The location of the maximum depends on the assumed polarity of the generator. Phase reversals involving surface-negative activity generate a negative phase reversal, in which the deflections "point" toward each other. However, the same picture theoretically could result from a positive electrical field that is minimum at the site of the phase reversal and larger at the ends of the chain. Conversely, a positive potential maximum at an electrode in the middle of a bipolar chain will cause the deflections to point away from each other—that is, positive phase reversal.

If there is no phase reversal, then the electrical field maximum must be located under either the first or the last electrode of the chain (Fig. 11.9). The potential field minimum must then be at the opposite end of the chain. Because the potential gradient for each pair of electrodes in the chain is in the same direction, the potential decreases progressively from the electrode with the highest potential to the one with the lowest potential.

In a bipolar montage, the amplitude may be misleading because it indicates differences in electrical potential and not the electrode of maximal involvement (Fig. 11.10). Because the gradients tend to be steeper in regions of highest activity, the electroencephalographer may habitually, but unwisely, determine the maximum on the basis of amplitude.

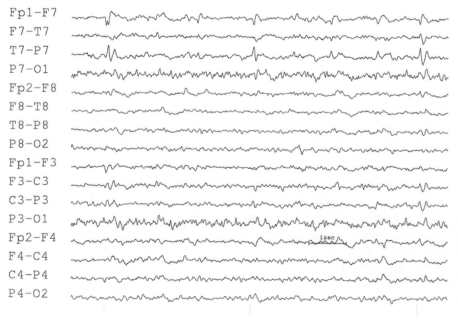

Figure 11.10 Bipolar montage with phase reversal. The amplitudes of the differences between the voltages at input 1 and input 2 do not indicate the maximum of the electrical field. In this circumstance, the amplitude of the sharp wave is actually maximum at F_7 and T_7, but approximately equal in those two adjacent electrodes, so the discharge is localized to both electrodes.

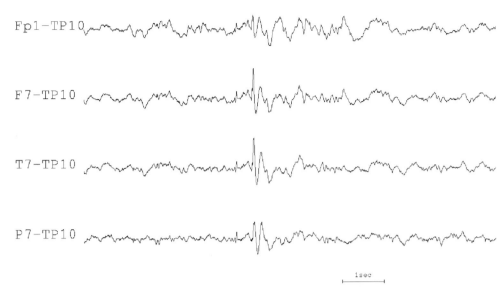

Figure 11.11 Referential montage without phase reversal. This montage, which uses a contralateral reference chosen because it appeared to be uninvolved in the discharge, helps to clarify the location of a spike widely distributed across the left temporal region.

Referential Montage

All derivations in a referential montage connect the same electrode (or electrode combination) to input 2. If some derivations within a given montage use one reference electrode (e.g., the left ear) whereas others use a different reference (e.g., the right ear), only those sets of channels with a common reference should be analyzed together.

If there is no phase reversal (as shown in Fig. 11.11), the reference electrode (i.e., the one connected to input 2) is either the minimum or the maximum of the electrical field. If the reference electrode is the minimum of the electrical field, the maximum will be at the electrode with the largest amplitude. This situation is the easiest to analyze, because the amplitude of the deflection in each channel directly reflects the level of activity in input 1 of the channel.

If the reference is maximum, the electrode at input 1 of the largest-amplitude channel is at the minimum of the electrical field. If the reference is maximum and some

channels show no deflection, the electrodes connected to input 1 of those channels are also maximum.

If there is a phase reversal, then the reference electrode is neither the minimum nor the maximum of the electrical field (Fig. 11.12). Hence, the reference is "involved"—that is, at some intermediate potential. This indicates that some electrodes connected to input 1 have a greater potential and some a lower potential than the reference. If, for instance, the polarity of the discharge is negative, those electrodes connected to input 1 that have a higher potential than the reference will point upward, whereas those less negative than the reference will point downward. The channels that show no activity (i.e., isopotential with the reference) measure a negativity at input 1 equal to that at the reference. If the recorded potential has two maxima of opposite polarity, such as seen in tangential dipole sources, then referential montages will show phase reversals even if the reference is the minimum.

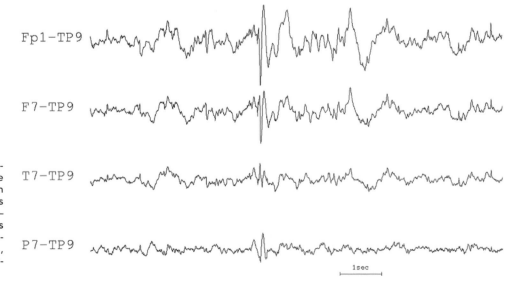

Figure 11.12 Referential montage with phase reversal. Because there is a phase reversal between channels 2 and 3, the reference is neither minimum nor maximum—that is, it must be "involved." This tracing is actually of the same discharge shown in Figure 11.11, using a less-wisely chosen reference.

Choice of a Reference

In a referential montage, any electrode may be the reference, but ordinarily it is one uninvolved in the electrical field. The voltage difference between any pair of electrodes is entirely unrelated to the choice of reference (76,77); subtracting the voltage measured referentially at electrode B from that measured referentially at electrode A will produce exactly the voltage measured bipolarly from the AB derivation, regardless of the reference chosen. This is true for a single electrode or a mathematically calculated one, such as the average reference (78–80) and is the principle of computer-aided montage reformatting.

The amplifiers in a reference montage perform their differential function exactly as in a bipolar montage. Referential recordings do not measure the absolute potential under the various scalp electrodes, but rather the potential difference, as do bipolar recordings. Specifically, however, they measure the difference between each electrode and a chosen common reference. Instead of chains of electrodes, with each succeeding amplifier sharing one input from the previous amplifier, all the amplifiers share a common input 2. What the amplifier "sees" depends on the electrical relationship between the reference and the field of the waveform. The reference may be completely uninvolved in the field (a minimum), it may be in an area that picks up a higher value of the waveform than any of the other electrodes (a maximum), or it may lie somewhere in between (neither a maximum nor a minimum).

When mapping the distribution of a particular wave, the choice of reference electrode will affect the appearance of the traces, as well as the electroencephalographer's ability to localize. For evaluating epileptic foci, the reference is normally chosen to be completely uninvolved in the electrical field distribution of the spike or sharp wave (all deflections should point in the same direction). Typically, the electrode most distant from the activity of interest will be the least involved reference. "Standard" referential montages occasionally include the reference in the field distribution (some deflections pointing upward, some downward). An electrode at the vertex (C_z) is an excellent reference for displaying temporal spikes but may be a poor choice during sleep, when it is very active. In the linked-ears reference (81) (frequently used to decrease electrocardiographic artifact), the reference electrode (A_1 connected to A_2) connects the two brain regions. This electrical shunt changes the field generated (82), decreasing, for example, asymmetries between the temporal regions (9) and producing other distortions (83). The "weighting" applied to activity from each side will depend entirely on the electrode impedances, with the ear having the lower impedance predominating. When temporal lobe epileptiform activity spreads to the ipsilateral ear, the linked-ear reference will inappropriately reveal spikes in both hemispheres.

A common average reference has been advocated (79) to avoid the problem of an "active reference." Using passive summing networks, active amplifier configurations, or combinatorial software, it is possible to devise a reference that combines all the electrodes applied to the head, the so-called common average reference (78,79). The disadvantages of this system are threefold: (a) The common average reference is, by definition, contaminated because the abnormal potential will influence all of the channels (84); (b) depending on the number of electrodes included in the average, the potential under study will be reduced by a small proportion; and (c) large-amplitude focal pathologic activities will be reflected proportionally in all the inactive channels as well, albeit with apparently opposite polarity.

A variety of calculated references and transformations are available, but these must be used with caution. The "source derivation" provides useful "deblurring" by arithmetically estimating the cortical sources that generate a scalp distribution; however, this method gives increasing weight to distant electrodes and can produce erroneous results when these sites are active (31,33,85,86). Because there is no ideal reference for all cases, it is usually best to distribute the electrical field potentials by manual selection of an uninvolved and quiet electrode as a reference.

SOURCE LOCALIZATION

Assumptions

After determination of the electrical field, the sources responsible for the production of the field can be localized with the aid of a number of simplifications. The procedure for determining the polarity and location of the generator is based on the following four specific assumptions:

1. Epileptogenic sources are simple dipoles or sheets of dipoles obeying a simple principle of superposition (43).
2. Dipoles are fundamentally oriented perpendicularly and can be treated as if they were monopoles. When both the positive and the negative poles are recorded from the surface, the localization system outlined in the next two subsections will not apply.
3. Epileptiform discharges are chiefly surface-negative phenomena. In the absence of a skull defect, a transversely-lying dipole (as in benign focal epileptiform discharges of childhood) or other evidence of an unusual discharge, the assumption of surface negativity will usually result in the proper distribution. (The term "maximum" denotes absolute value, not necessarily maximum negativity.)
4. The head is essentially a uniform, homogeneous volume conductor.

Choosing Between Two Possibilities

The application of the rules above yields two possible hypotheses in each case. In a bipolar chain, for example, a downward deflection with no phase reversals may be

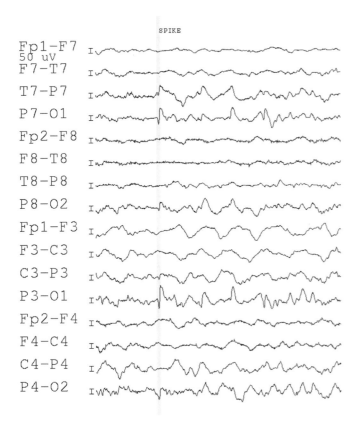

SPIKE

Fp1–F7
50 uV
F7–T7
T7–P7
P7–O1
Fp2–F8
F8–T8
T8–P8
P8–O2
Fp1–F3
F3–C3
C3–P3
P3–O1
Fp2–F4
F4–C4
C4–P4
P4–O2

Figure 11.13 Bipolar montage with maximum negativity at the end of the chain. The marker brackets the downward negative component.

generated by either a negativity maximum at the last electrode of the chain (Fig. 11.13) or a positivity maximum at the first electrode of the chain. To choose between the two possibilities in any given case, one must guess about the polarity of the source generator or the relative likelihood of one of two electrodes being the more active.

Because the localization of a transient will depend on a correct assumption about its polarity, all possible clues must be used to make an educated guess about polarity. For example, if the transient appears to be epileptiform, it is most likely to be surface negative, whereas if morphology and location suggest a positive occipital sharp transient (POST), it can be expected to be surface positive (Fig. 11.14). The best strategy is to see if the distribution based on the assumed polarity makes physiologic sense; if not, the opposite polarity has to be tried. In Figure 11.7, the isopotential map based on an assumption that the polarity of the maximum is negative displays a more logical potential falloff for focal activity than the opposite assumption. Therefore, it is most likely that this activity has negative polarity with a maximum at electrode T_7.

Determination of the electrical field of a discharge may help to differentiate artifacts or extracortical physiologic activity from abnormal brain activity (Fig. 11.15). Because the electrical gradient is steepest at the electrodes closest to the source, the electrical potential difference between

inputs 1 and 2 becomes smaller as one moves farther away from the generator source (87). For this reason, the steepest potential gradient and the largest deflection will most often appear in the channels nearest the source.

When dealing with an invariant spike, as observed in various chains and montages, analyses based on any of the multiple electrode chains or montages should all reach the same conclusion (Figs. 11.6 and 11.16). Corroborating a potential localized on a longitudinal montage by using a transverse montage (i.e., montages that are at right angles to each other), for example, can be helpful. If different conclusions result from the analysis of different montages, the assumptions about polarity or location were probably incorrect on one of the montages. Nevertheless, consistent conclusions across montages do not prove that the assumptions were correct, as the same error about polarity or location may have been made throughout the analysis.

Localization Rules: Cautions and Limitations

The simple rules and procedures for manual localization of electrical activity on the basis of bipolar or referential montages, outlined above, are valid only for single sources; that is, they presuppose a single monopolar generator. Regional abnormalities such as those encountered in focal epilepsy quite frequently satisfy this assumption as an approximation. Some EEG patterns, however, are produced by two or more generators of the same or different polarity acting simultaneously. When multiple sources or horizontal dipoles are involved, even highly sophisticated mathematical source localization techniques may not enable us to identify the exact composition of such generators.

Although both poles of the dipolar generator must be present by definition, one of them is oriented deep within the head, allowing assumption of a monopole. On occasion, however, both poles may be represented on the scalp surface, precluding the use of these rules. This occurs, for example, in the case of an epileptogenic focus originating from the superior mesial portion of the motor strip (88). Cortical regions involving the interhemispheric fissure, such as the foot area or the calcarine cortex, are especially likely to produce these horizontal dipoles. Specifically, the end of the dipole traditionally at the surface will be buried within the fissure with its maximum seen on the contralateral scalp, and what ordinarily would be the deep end of the dipole may be close to the scalp surface on the ipsilateral side. Because of their location, horizontal dipoles also can be seen in benign focal epileptiform discharges of childhood (89).

The electrical fields resulting from these transverse dipoles are characterized by a simultaneous surface-negative and surface-positive potential seen at different electrodes on the scalp or by a double-phase reversal (13,90). Note that when double-phase reversals or other factors indicate, for example, a huge anteroposterior dipole or a transverse dipole extending from one hemisphere to

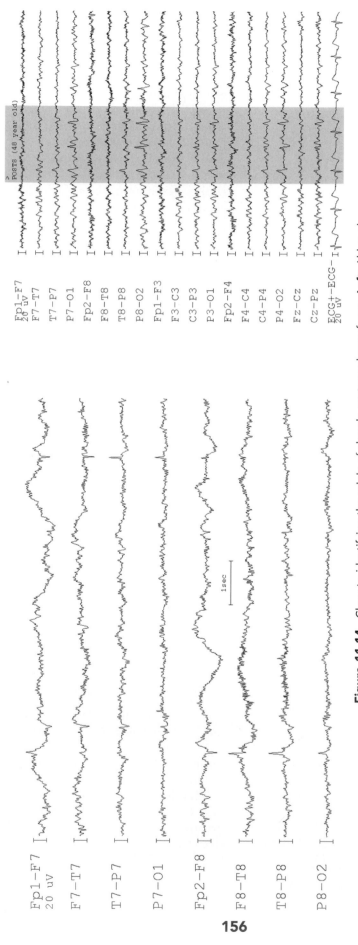

Figure 11.14 Clues to identifying the origin of sharply contoured waveforms. **Left:** Although these discharges stand out dramatically from the background, their presence during sleep and their very brief duration suggest that the transients here are benign epileptiform transients of sleep (BETS). BETS are often multiphasic, but the predominant component is negative, as in this example. **Right:** The electrical field distribution of these sharply contoured waves is consistent with positive occipital sharp transients (POSTs)—that is, a positivity at the end of the chain. If the electroencephalographer assumed instead that the waveforms were negative, suggesting epileptiform discharges, their distribution across the entire head would have been more difficult to explain physiologically.

156

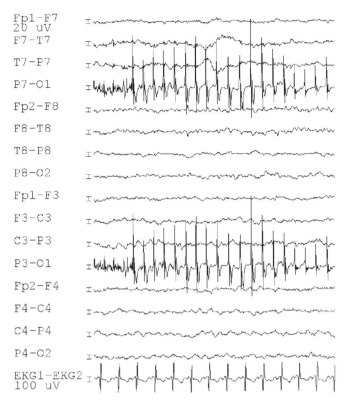

Fp1—F7
20 uV
F7—T7

T7—P7

P7—O1

Fp2—F8

F8—T8

T8—P8

P8—O2

Fp1—F3

F3—C3

C3—P3

P3—O1

Fp2—F4

F4—C4

C4—P4

P4—O2

EKG1—EKG2
100 uV

Figure 11.15 Artifacts. The sharply contoured discharges emanating from the left posterior region cannot be dismissed as artifacts on the basis of morphology alone, nor do they match up with the electrocardiogram artifact. However, because they appear only in channels 4 and 12, they must be arising solely from electrode O_1. If these large-amplitude occipital "spikes" were epileptogenic, electrical field theory would dictate a much more gradual falloff. Because the field shows a precipitous, and therefore impossible, distribution, these discharges must be artifacts.

the other (42), the physiologic meaning of such an unusual field must be questioned. A horizontal dipole should not be the first consideration when an electroencephalographer confronts deflections pointing in opposite directions. An involved reference, the most common cause for this phenomenon, must first be excluded.

As noted, in a bipolar montage, the channels of highest amplitude must not be confused with the area of greatest activity. This mistake is most likely to occur when the chain has no phase reversals, indicating that the maximum of the discharge originates from either the beginning or the end of the chain, or when the maximum is broadly distributed across several channels (Fig. 11.17). A greater amplitude seen in one or more channels is solely a manifestation of a greater potential *difference*.

Obviously, determining whether a phase reversal is present is a key aspect of the localization procedure. Multiple fast components may be confusingly mixed when viewed from a bipolar montage and are more accurately represented in a referential montage that identifies the individual components that are phase-reversing across channels. A discharge with an extremely broad field can result in rather tiny differences between adjacent electrodes.

Because the brain, skull, and scalp do not have homogeneous conductivity, current pathways from active epileptogenic areas can vary dramatically among the recording sites. This variability may lead to a site of maximal scalp activity considerably distant from the fundamental generator (91).

Although general physiologic and physical principles can explain the phenomena involved, clinical interpretation of a particular set of measurements often has to be based on experience and information that is not easily derivable from first principles. Nevertheless, by remaining aware of alternative possibilities, the electroencephalographer can avoid misinterpreting unusual recordings.

COMPUTER-AIDED METHODOLOGY FOR LOCATING ELECTROENCEPHALOGRAM SOURCES

Topographic Mapping of Voltage and Other Parameters

Topographic EEG mapping is the generation of a pictorial representation based on measurements obtained from multichannel EEG analysis—usually simultaneous, instantaneous amplitudes of some parameter. Computer-aided mapping can accurately summarize the field distribution and may help to highlight locally originating activity (92). Computed topographic maps can be used to (a) describe an already known localization (perhaps for communication with nonneurophysiologists); (b) confirm a conventionally determined localization; (c) identify changes not detected in the original interpretation; and (d) display statistical differences among patient populations (so-called *z* scores [93]). These maps should always be used in conjunction with the raw EEG data (94,95).

Automated mapping can be used to represent the topographic distribution of any variable, whether derived from complex calculations or simply displaying electrical field distributions, as shown in Figure 11.18, depending on the application. In the evaluation of patients with epilepsy, the topographic distribution of sharp waves may present a valuable display, once their characteristics have been reduced to a metric (96). It is important to remember that a computerized system is unlikely to perform the measurement in every case as would have been done manually, so that visual inspection of the waveform is essential for each map (94).

When used to map the amplitude of the EEG or evoked potential at a specific point in time, interpolation between the voltages measured at the electrodes must be carried out to present a smooth contour on the map. The most practical interpolation method is one based on spherical splines (97). Unlike magnetic resonance imaging (MRI) and computerized tomography, in which the intensity of every pixel is based on a measurement, topographic maps are derived

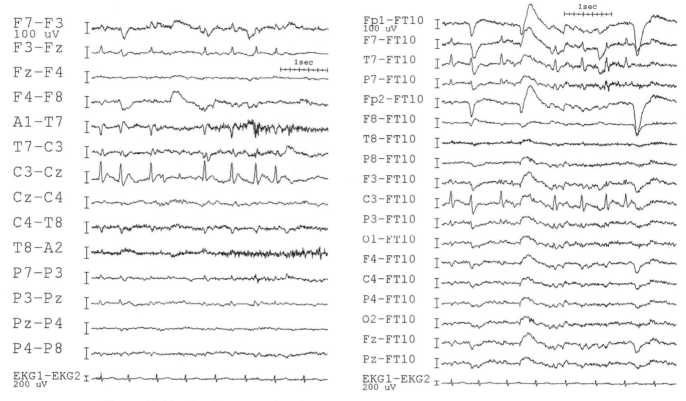

Figure 11.16   The phase reversals in the transverse montage shown on the *left* suggest the possibility of benign rolandic spikes. On the *right*, an ad hoc distribution montage using a contralateral electrode clearly shows a typical centrotemporal distribution. In this montage, it is also easier to distinguish the eye movement artifacts from the sharp waves.

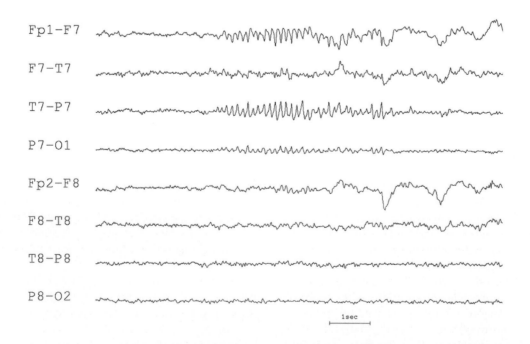

Figure 11.17   Bipolar montage with phase reversal. Phase reversals need not always occur in adjacent channels. This electroencephalogram shows the phenomenon for some normal activity, rather than the abnormal discharges seen in Figure 11.10. The phase reversal of this arciform activity spans the isoelectric channels, consistent with the broad distribution of a wicket rhythm.

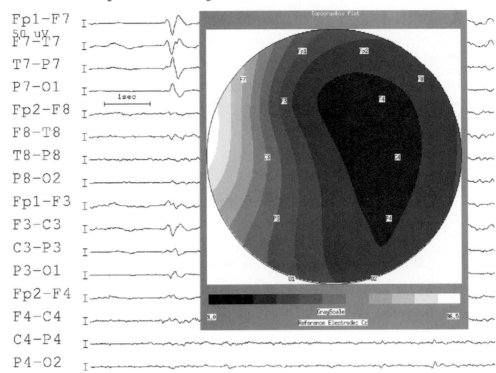

Left Temporal Sharp Wave

Figure 11.18 Topographic mapping. Digitization of the electroencephalogram (EEG) offers the opportunity for interactive postprocessing that may help to convey location in an easy-to-understand way. In this figure, the electrical field of the sharp wave seen phase-reversing at T_7 in the EEG was automatically mapped onto a top view of a spherical model of the head. Using baseline-to-peak amplitude measurements from a C_z reference, interpolating the amplitudes at every scalp location between electrodes, and dividing into 10 isocontours, the amplitude map has been plotted as a grayscale intensity. Koszer and associates (103) demonstrated relatively good congruence between the manual process carried out by electroencephalographers described in the text and computerized topographic mapping methods.

from measurements at only 16 to 32 points, with the balance obtained via interpolation, creating the illusion of a higher resolution than actually exists.

Once the computer has associated the amplitude information with its topographic location, mathematical techniques even more powerful than electrical field mapping can be brought to bear. As a result of volume conduction, potentials generated within a small brain region will be seen over a wide area of the scalp. The spreading of the field to the scalp can be mathematically reduced by current source derivation methods (92,98). These spatial deblurring techniques, such as the Laplacian operator (99), can narrow the apparent distribution of the electrical field, thereby emphasizing discrete foci (84). The Laplacian operator supplies information about the locally occurring activity in a "reference-free" manner (71), taking into account the direction of the field along the scalp to define the differences between adjacent electrodes.

Commercial instrumentation for topographic mapping is relatively easy to use. Although much attention has been paid to the algorithms for generating and presenting these displays, the possibility exists that the relatively complex calculations involved in generating these maps will lead to gross misinterpretation because of the wide range of variables (91,95,100,101). There are a number of pitfalls and caveats associated with topographic mapping (101,102) that have prevented widespread acceptance of this technique for most clinical applications (91). Jayakar and colleagues (31) described several limitations of these methods.

Computer-aided topographic mapping is actually not well suited to display epileptiform EEG elements, owing to their rapid time course. Because all the channels may not be at their peak simultaneously, the maps may show an unexpected result; that is, the maps may demonstrate spike progression but will not necessarily reflect the manually determined localization (103). Moreover, computer topographic mapping of the amplitude of the EEG signal (or of evoked potentials, spectral measurements, or statistical analyses) provides no new information and cannot be used to make classifications not apparent in the raw data. Even with sophisticated enhancements, such as the Laplacian operator or spatial deblurring, topographic mapping techniques do not provide any conclusive three-dimensional information about the source of scalp-recorded signals (104). Nevertheless, they can make it easier to grasp the special relationships existing among electrodes in various neighborhoods of the scalp. To decrease errors, several restrictions imposed by the interpolation methods and the boundary value problem dictate the use of more electrodes than are conventionally placed. Indeed, adding closely spaced electrodes alone may reveal new information.

Dipole Modeling and Source Localization

Because three-dimensional localization of the generator of a transient is a key objective of electroencephalography, computerized "source analysis" was applied, beginning in the mid-1980s, to identify single or multiple foci (105,106).

Dipole source localization is an attempt to identify the origin of electrical potentials seen on the scalp by solving the inverse problem. Source analysis is carried out by postulating a single or multiple spatiotemporal dipole model chosen to account for the surface signals and their timing relationships (107). Although the sources of electrical activity recorded by the EEG are actually folded sheets of dipolar pyramidal neurons, the traditional computer model is only a single dipole with no spatial extent. To explain a widespread scalp distribution, the computer model tends to find these dipoles deep in the actual cortical location. Solutions to the inverse problem involve simplifications and approximations and, even when well-defined dipoles using implanted sources in the human brain are used, often produce errors of a few centimeters (108,109). Although it is not possible to uniquely identify the positions of the electrical sources in the brain from the scalp electrodes (110), appropriate assumptions can yield useful information in some cases (16,111). Localization using dipole source analysis has been the subject of many validation (112) and comparison studies (113). Even though the modeling results are not always accurate, they can be useful for separating different sources.

MAGNETOENCEPHALOGRAPHY

Instrumentation: Magnetometers and Gradiometers

Recording of weak magnetic fields generated by the brain became practical after the introduction of the superconducting quantum interference device (SQUID) technique (114). The SQUID is a transducer that converts magnetic flux into an electrical signal. Whole-head MEG systems have a cylinder-shaped Dewar vessel with a helmet-shaped concavity on one end, into which the subject's head is placed for measurement (115,116). Typically, 100 to 300 channels of magnetic sensors with SQUID are arrayed over the inner surface of the concavity, immersed in the liquid helium within the Dewar vessel, and maintained at a temperature of 4.2° kelvin ($-268.95°C$; $-452.11°F$). The helmet-shaped concavity of a whole-head MEG system has a coverage similar to that of scalp EEG with the standard 10–20 Electrode Placement System. The magnetic field distribution originating from the lowest part of the brain—for example, the basal temporal cortex—might not be fully depicted (117).

There are two types of magnetic sensors: magnetometers and gradiometers (115). Both use pickup coils arranged parallel to the head surface, thereby measuring magnetic flux emerging from or penetrating the surface. The magnetometer, consisting of a single pickup coil, measures magnetic flux penetrating the coil. The gradiometer, consisting of a pick-up coil and a compensation coil, measures the gradient of magnetic flux between the two coils.

The gradiometer configuration is used to cancel out the influence of environmental magnetic noise originating from a distance. Regardless of the sensor type, isocontour magnetic field maps will be reconstructed automatically by a computer-aided calculation for display and interpretation. In contrast to EEG, MEG is inherently reference free (59).

To limit interference from external environmental magnetic noise, MEG is measured in a magnetically shielded room. Because the patient must remain motionless during MEG recording, duration is limited and generally confined to the interictal state (118). Typical MEG monitoring times for patients with epilepsy range from 10 minutes to a few hours. Patients with frequent seizures may undergo ictal MEG, but the success rate for capturing seizures on MEG is as low as 30% (119,120).

MEG can be recorded simultaneously with scalp EEG. Because EEG and MEG record the same phenomenon—for example, epileptic spikes—reports should include the results of MEG localization, along with interpretation of the simultaneous EEG. Interpretation of these two complementary techniques may help clinicians understand the results.

MAGNETOENCEPHALOGRAPHY WAVEFORMS

A current dipole generated in the cerebral cortex produces both electrical and magnetic, fields (121–123). The magnetic field is formed around the current dipole with the magnetic flux perpendicular to and oriented clockwise to the current (116), as shown in Figure 11.19. Hence, the measurement of magnetic fields provides information about both the amplitude and the orientation of the current. As noted above, the sensors used in commercial MEG systems are sensitive to a size and distribution of the brain volume that is similar to that of neighboring pairs of scalp EEG electrodes if applied with an electrode spacing given by the standard 10–20 Electrode Placement System (20). Because MEG and EEG both pick up regional brain electrical activity as a sum of dipolar generators contained in a brain volume of similar size, the waveform characteristics of epileptic phenomena and other spontaneous activities recorded by EEG and MEG are similar (124). The strength of the magnetic field decreases in proportion to the square of the distance from the current dipole, according to the Bio-Savart law. Therefore, the sensitivity of MEG to deep sources is similar to that of scalp EEG; certainly, the depth capability does not exceed that of EEG (20).

Because MEG is a relatively new and clinically uncommon technique, criteria for waveform interpretation, field determination, and source localization are not yet fully established. However, it is important to recognize that MEG waveforms first appear as "brain waves" to the interpreter. They are directly analogous to the EEG, and *the fundamental concepts of field determination and source localization, previously*

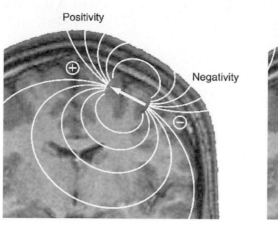
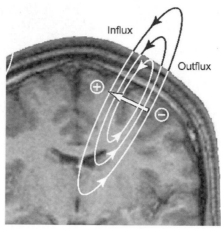

Electric and magnetic fields due to a current dipole

Figure 11.19 Electrical fields and magnetic fields produced by a current dipole generator (*white arrow*). On the *left*, the *white lines* show volume-conducted current paths arising from the positive pole of the dipole and returning back to the negative pole. The electroencephalograph detects the electrical potentials on the scalp surface, which can be negativity or positivity. If the dipole is oriented tangentially, as in this figure, two field maxima of both polarities appear on the surface. If the dipole is oriented vertically to the surface, the electroencephalograph detects one of the poles exclusively. The right-hand figure illustrates how magnetic fields are formed perpendicular to the current dipole in a clockwise direction to the dipole orientation. If the dipole is oriented tangentially, as in this figure, a pair of magnetic field maxima consisting of the influx and outflux will be observed on the scalp surface. Magnetometers and gradiometers detect the magnetic flux perpendicular to the scalp surface. If the dipole is oriented vertically, the magnetic flux does not enter and exit perpendicular to the surface, so the contribution to the surface magnetic field distribution is minimal.

described for EEG, are also similarly applied to MEG interpretation. The principles of visual identification of abnormal and normal waveforms on the basis of morphology are also probably transferable from EEG to MEG. However, studies on this issue are very scarce, and most available articles are focused on source localization of acquired abnormal or physiologic waveforms (117,125). Generally, reliable identification of epileptic spikes or other abnormalities in MEG is performed with the assistance of simultaneously recorded EEG (126–128). However, epileptic spikes are rarely seen in MEG alone (126,129,130).

Volume Conduction in MEG

The skull and other extracerebral tissues are practically transparent to magnetic fields. MEG measures magnetic fields coming out of or going into the surface of a head sphere, typically generated by a tangential current dipole source. In a spherical homogeneous volume conductor, the radial current dipole does not produce a magnetic field outside the sphere (115).

It is volume conduction of the current from a dipole—that is, secondary current—that produces measurable EEG activity. The volume current also produces magnetic fields. In a spherical homogeneous volume conductor, those magnetic fields produced by volume currents are totally

canceled out, making no contribution to the extracranial magnetic field (115). Even in a realistic (i.e., nonspherical and nonhomogeneous) situation, their contribution to the extracranial magnetic field is still practically negligible (35). In the presence of a skull defect or large structural lesion close to the generator, however, there may be asymmetry in the volume conduction, producing a small effect on the magnetic field distribution (35,39). Magnetic fields arising from volume conduction may also be significant in anatomical regions that deviate largely from a spherical volume, such as the basal brain area.

The magnetic field pattern outside the head is much less distorted by the inhomogeneity of the tissue conductivity than is the electrical field. This is because the field pattern depends largely on the primary current, and contribution of the secondary current becomes increasingly small as the sensor is moved away from the generator. Therefore, forward modeling of the MEG is simpler than that of EEG, which makes computerized source estimation feasible in MEG (116).

Field Determination

Magnetic field distribution is usually displayed as an isofield contour map with the aid of computerized calculation. The field distribution produced by a single current

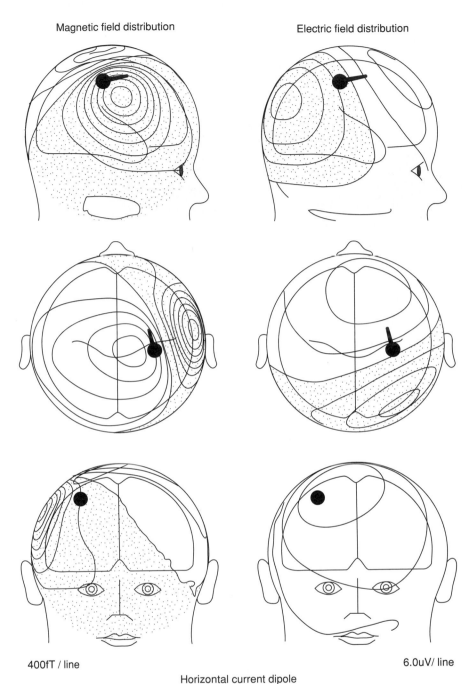

Magnetic field distribution

Electric field distribution

400fT / line

6.0uV/ line

Horizontal current dipole

Figure 11.20 The difference of the field patterns between electroencephalography and magnetoencephalography. The electrical and magnetic field distribution are simulated in a spherical volume conductor head model. A tangentially oriented dipole is placed in the right central area. The position (*black dot*), strength, and orientation (indicated by the *line originating from the dot*) of the dipole are the same for both electroencephalography and magnetoencephalography. The "sink" for both fields (i.e., magnetic field influx and negative electrical potentials) is shown by the *dotted area*. The magnetic field produces two strong focal maxima lateral to the dipole. In contrast, the electrical field maxima appear anterior and posterior to and along the same axis as the dipole, and with a broader distribution.

dipole is observed as a pair of influx and outflux field maxima distributed on each side of the dipole location (116). The typical "dipolar pattern" shown in Figure 11.20 is produced by a dipole tangential to the scalp surface. Radially oriented dipoles produce minimal contribution to the field, as shown in Figure 11.21. Dipoles of real generators, however, are rarely exactly perpendicular, and obliquely oriented dipoles, even at an angle of 80 to 90 degrees to the surface, can have a clearly observed dipolar field distribution, because MEG detects the tangential vector component of the dipole (116).

This dipolar field pattern is a good indicator of the location and orientation of the generator, as long as an interpreter assumes a single dipolar source for the observed distribution. However, multiple dipolar sources or extended sources can produce complicated field patterns, or a single maximum of either influx or outflux magnetic fields.

Localization

Assuming a single dipolar generator for a typical dipolar field distribution, an equivalent current dipole is localized below the middle point of both influx and outflux field maxima (Fig. 11.22). The orientation of the dipole can also be determined from the field (116).

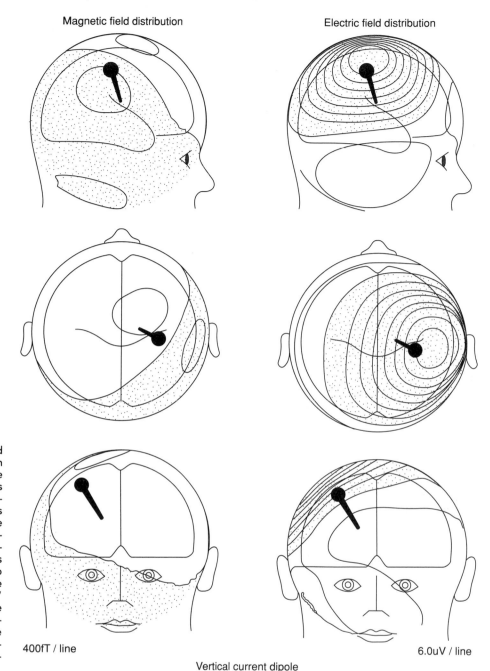

Magnetic field distribution   Electric field distribution

400fT / line   6.0uV / line

Vertical current dipole

Figure 11.21 The magnetic and electrical field patterns associated with a vertically oriented dipole. This dipole has the same position and strength as in the previous figure, but the orientation is different. The electrical fields show a single focal maximum above the dipole. This falloff of potential with distance is commonly observed in epileptic spikes. The vertical dipole produces very weak magnetic fields on the scalp surface. Though weak, note that the magnetic fields still show a "dipolar" distribution similar to that seen with the tangential dipole, because magnetoencephalography is sensitive only to the vector dipole components that are tangential (this vertical dipole is not completely normal to the surface).

Computerized source estimation is more feasible in MEG than in EEG, because of the relatively simpler source and volume conductor models. In the EEG forward calculation, the volume conduction model consists of three or four shells, each layer of which represents the differences in electrical conductivity of the brain, CSF, bone, and skin. MEG, on the other hand, usually uses a single shell volume conductor model of the brain, thereby significantly decreasing the computational complexity and the error of the forward calculation in MEG (131).

The most popular MEG method is a single or multiple dipole model with a least-square approach (116) (Fig. 11.22). A nonlinear algorithm searches for the optimal location, orientation, and strength of the dipoles. With this method, an interpreter has to provide a starting point for the dipole search, based on an "initial guess" of approximate source location and orientation. The computer then calculates via forward modeling an expected magnetic field distribution for the initially chosen dipole in a given head conductor model, compares it with the measured data, and quantifies the error between the two. The dipole is shifted in position, orientation, and strength, and the forward calculation is then repeated. This fitting procedure is reiterated up to hundreds of times in different combinations in order to approach a minimum error between the forward model and the measurement (115). The remaining error is

C. Dipole source co-registration to MRI

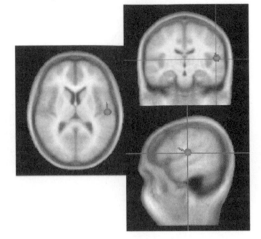

A. MEG waves

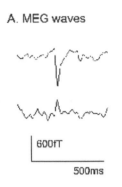

600fT

500ms

B. MEG field distribution

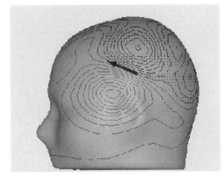

D. Minimum norm estimation

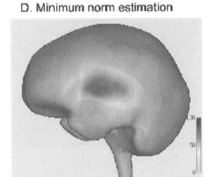

Figure 11.22 A: The raw magnetoencephalographic waveform arises from the same source that generates the electroencephalogram and therefore appears as "brain waves." After visual analysis, this activity was interpreted as an epileptiform spike. **B:** Magnetic field distribution at the time of spike peak. The isocontour map depicts the outflux and influx (*shaded area*) of the magnetic fields. This pair of opposite field maxima is recognized as a "dipolar field pattern." Assuming that this is produced by a single dipolar generator, the approximate location of the dipole is estimated between the two maxima, as indicated by the *dark arrow*. **C:** A dipole search was performed for this activity. The best fit for the dipole was achieved at the location (*circle*) and orientation (*bar*) shown on the magnetic resonance image, leaving a goodness-of-fit value of 85%. **D:** Minimum-norm estimation (MNE) for the same activity. Current strength of a number of distributed sources are projected onto the brain surface in a percentage scale. Although the maximum activity is estimated in the same region, the location indicated by the MNE method is more distributed, while the dipole analysis provides a focal answer.

usually quantified as a "goodness-of-fit" value or residual variance. Dipole modeling provides a reliable solution for known regional sources, such as somatosensory evoked responses. However, for sources of unknown origin like epileptic spikes, the solution can be significantly biased by the interpreter's assumptions (initial guess) on the number of dipoles and starting point of the search, and even by acceptance or denial of the search results. Several automated approaches have been proposed to avoid such biases (132–134).

In contrast to EEG electrodes, MEG sensors are not attached to the scalp. The spatial relationships of the sensor locations to the brain are obtained indirectly based on three-dimensional digitization of several anatomical landmarks—for example, nasion and preauricular points. These anatomic landmarks are acquired during each MEG recording session in relation to the sensor location. Using these landmarks to coregister the MEG fields with the anatomy, the location and orientation of the equivalent current dipole solution is displayed graphically on the patient's MRI. For epileptiform discharges, dipole locations of one or a few representative spikes are shown (117,126,128,130,135). Some authors try to superimpose as many as 100 dipoles on one image in an effort to convey the extent or variability of spike distribution (127).

The result of dipole modeling is always a "point" solution. However, the underlying phenomenon is not point activation, but rather distributed to a greater or lesser extent within the cerebral cortex (136). These dipole sheets are represented by an equivalent current dipole, which is a linear summation over the cortex. The dipole location may represent the center of the activity but has an unknown spatial accuracy. Dipole displays do not usually convey the dipole's probability of correctness or other accuracy information. Reliability is especially problematic in the case of extended sources, which tend to be represented as excessively deep dipoles (116,127).

The so-called minimum-norm estimation (MNE) of source currents takes a different approach (132,137–139). This method provides the most probable current distribution in the brain. The orientation and strength of a number (~10,000) of current sources assigned in the brain conductor model are approximated to the measured data to minimize the norm (length) of the current vector. This procedure assumes a seemingly "natural" current distribution. To overcome a potentially ill-posed condition, the minimum-norm solution uses several constraints based on known brain anatomy, physiology, and mathematical regularization. In contrast to dipole modeling, this procedure does not require an initial guess by the interpreter. The images resulting from MNE, displayed as "current density maps," tend to show a "smeared" distribution of the current strength. Figure 11.22 illustrates the two methods— single equivalent dipole and MNE— for an epileptiform transient.

Dipole sources in sulci or fissures generate tangential currents and may be major contributors to the activity recorded by MEG, resulting in several favorable brain areas for MEG source localization. Temporal lobe spikes are largely classified into two dipole locations: temporal pole and superior temporal plane (126,136,140). Both of these regions contain a large cortical area perpendicular to the head surface. Theoretically, basal temporal cortex, opercular area, mesial frontoparietal cortex, and deep sulcus, such as the central sulcus, are also favorable areas for MEG source generators.

REFERENCES

1. Engel J. Approaches to localization of the epileptogenic lesion. *Surgical treatment of the epilepsies.* New York: Raven Press, 1987: 75–95.
2. Adrian ED, Matthews BHC. The Berger rhythm: potential changes from the occipital lobes in man. *Brain* 1934;57: 355–385.
3. Adrian ED, Yamagiwa K. The origin of the Berger rhythm. *Brain* 1935;58:351.
4. Walter WG. The localization of cerebral tumours by electroencephalography. *Lancet* 1936;2:305–308.
5. Gibbs FA, Gibbs EL. *Atlas of electroencephalography.* Reading, MA: Addison-Wesley, 1941.
6. Gloor P. Application of volume conduction principles to montage design. *Am J EEG Technol* 1977;17:520.
7. Gloor P. Neuronal generators and the problem of localization in electroencephalography: application of volume conductor theory to electroencephalography. *J Clin Neurophysiol* 1985;2: 327–354.
8. Magnus O. On the technique of location by electroencephalography. *Electroencephalogr Clin Neurophysiol* 1961;19(Suppl):135.
9. Nunez PL. *Electrical fields of the brain.* New York: Oxford University Press, 1981.
10. Osselton JW. Bipolar, unipolar and average reference recording methods, I: mainly theoretical considerations. *Am J EEG Technol* 1966;5:53–64.
11. Osselton JW. Bipolar, unipolar and average reference recording methods, II: mainly practical considerations. *Am J EEG Technol* 1969;9:117–133.
12. Knott JR. Further thoughts on polarity, montages, and localization. *J Clin Neurophysiol* 1985;2:63–75.
13. Lesser RP, Luders H, Dinner DS, Morris H. An introduction to the basic concepts of polarity and localization. *J Clin Neurophysiol* 1985;2:45–61.
14. Burgess RC. Design and evolution of a system for long-term electroencephalographic and video monitoring of epilepsy patients. *Methods* 2001;25:231–248.
15. Scherg M, Ebersole JS. Models of brain sources. *Brain Topogr* 1993;5:419–423.
16. Scherg M, Ebersole JS. Brain source imaging of focal and multifocal epileptiform EEG activity. *Neurophysiol Clin* 1994;24: 51–60.
17. Lantz G, Holub M, Ryding E, Rosen I. Simultaneous intracranial and extracranial recording of interictal epileptiform activity in patients with drug-resistant partial epilepsy: patterns of conduction and results from dipole reconstructions. *Electroencephalogr Clin Neurophysiol* 1996;99:69–78.
18. Santiago-Rodriguez E, Harmony T, Fernandez-Bouzas A, et al. EEG source localization of interictal epileptiform activity in patients with partial complex epilepsy: comparison between dipole modeling and brain distributed source models. *Clin Electroencephalogr* 2002;33:42–47.
19. Hamer HM, Luders H. Electrode montages and localization of potentials in clinical electroencephalography. In: Levin KH, Luders H, eds. *Comprehensive clinical neurophysiology.* Philadelphia: Lippincott Williams & Wilkins, 2000:358–387.
20. Malmivuo J, Suihko V, Eskola H. Sensitivity distributions of EEG and MEG measurements. *IEEE Trans Biomed Eng* 1997;44: 196–208.
21. Okada Y. Neurogenesis of evoked magnetic fields. In: Williamson RJ, Romani GL, Kaurman L, eds. *Biomagnetism, an interdisciplinary approach.* New York: Plenum Press, 1983:399–408.
22. Creutzfeldt OD, Watanabe S, Lux HD. Relations between EEG phenomena and potentials of single cortical cells. I. Evoked responses after thalamic and epicortical stimulation. *Electroencephalogr Clin Neurophysiol* 1966;20:1–18.
23. Creutzfeldt OD, Watanabe S, Lux HD. Relations between EEG phenomena and potentials of single cortical cells. II. Spontaneous and convulsoid activity. *Electroencephalogr Clin Neurophysiol* 1966;20:19–37.
24. Elul R. The genesis of the EEG. *Int Rev Neurobiol* 1971;15:227–272.
25. Brazier MAB. A study of the electrical fields at the surface of the head. *Electroencephalogr Clin Neurophysiol* 1951;2:38–52.
26. Shaw JC, Roth M. Potential distribution analysis. I and II. *Electroencephalogr Clin Neurophysiol* 1955;7:273–292.
27. Plonsey R. *Bioelectric phenomena.* New York: McGraw-Hill, 1969.
28. Helmholtz. Ueber einige Gesetze der Vertheilung elektrischer Strome in korperlichen Leitern mit Anwendung. *Ann Physik und Chemie* 1853;9:211–377.
29. Ludwig BI, Marsan CA. Clinical ictal patterns in epileptic patients with occipital electroencephalographic foci. *Neurology* 1975;25:463–471.
30. Olivier A, Gloor P, Andermann F, Ives J. Occipitotemporal epilepsy studied with stereotaxically implanted depth electrodes and successfully treated by temporal resection. *Ann Neurol* 1982;11:428–432.
31. Jayakar P, Duchowny M, Resnick TJ, Alvarez LA. Localization of seizure foci: pitfalls and caveats. *J Clin Neurophysiol* 1991;8: 414–431.
32. Brazier MAB. The electrical fields at the surface of the head during sleep. *Electroencephalogr Clin Neurophysiol* 1949;1:195–204.
33. Nunez PL, Pilgreen KL. The spline-Laplacian in clinical neurophysiology: a method to improve EEG spatial resolution. *J Clin Neurophysiol* 1991;8:397–413.
34. Nicholson PW. Specific impedance of cerebral white matter. *Exp Neurol* 1965;13:386–401.
35. van den Broek SP, Reinders F, Donderwinkel M, Peters MJ. Volume conduction effects in EEG and MEG. *Electroencephalogr Clin Neurophysiol* 1998;106:522–534.
36. Nunez PL. An overview of electromyogenic theory. In: Nunez PL, ed. *Electrical fields of the brain.* New York: Oxford University Press, 1981:42–74.
37. Goncalves SI, de Munck JC, Verbunt JP, et al. *In vivo* measurement of the brain and skull resistivities using an EIT-based method and realistic models for the head. *IEEE Trans Biomed Eng* 2003;50:754–767.
38. Hoekema R, Wieneke GH, Leijten FS, et al. Measurement of the conductivity of skull, temporarily removed during epilepsy surgery. *Brain Topogr* 2003;16:29–38.
39. Haueisen J, Ramon C, Eiselt M, et al. Influence of tissue resistivities on neuromagnetic fields and electric potentials studied with a finite element model of the head. *IEEE Trans Biomed Eng* 1997;44:727–735.
40. Heasman BC, Valentin A, Alarcon G, et al. A hole in the skull distorts substantially the distribution of extracranial electrical fields in an *in vitro* model. *J Clin Neurophysiol* 2002;19:163–171.
41. Carpenter MB. *Core text of neuroanatomy,* 4th ed. Philadelphia: Lippincott Williams & Wilkins, 1991:210.
42. Ebersole JS, Wade PB. Intracranial EEG validation of single versus dual dipolar sources for temporal spikes in presurgical candidates. *Epilepsia* 1990;31:621.
43. Lutzenberger W, Elbert T, Rockstroh B. A brief tutorial on the implications of volume conduction for the interpretation of the EEG. *J Psychophysiol* 1987;1:81–89.

44. Awad IA, Luders H, Burgess RC. Epidural pegs and foramen ovale electrodes: a new class of electrodes of intermediate invasiveness for the mapping of seizure foci. *J Clin Neurophysiol* 1989;6:338.

45. Erenberg G. Localization of epileptogenic spike foci: comparative study of closely spaced scalp electrodes, nasopharyngeal, sphenoidal, subdural, and depth electrodes. In: Akimoto H, Kazamatsuri H, Seino M, eds. *Advances in epileptology: XIIIth International Symposium.* New York: Raven Press, 1982:185–189.

46. Friedman L, Skipper G, Wyllie E. Commentary: chronic intracranial recording and stimulation with subdural electrodes. In: Engel JP, ed. *Surgical treatment of the epilepsies.* New York: Raven Press, 1987: 297–321.

47. Wyllie E, Luders H, Morris HH III, et al. Subdural electrodes in the evaluation for epilepsy surgery in children and adults. *Neuropediatrics* 1988;19:80–86.

48. Gregory DL, Wong PKH. Clinical and EEG features of "tripole" spike discharges in children. *Epilepsia* 1986;27:605.

49. Cooper R, Winter AL, Crow HJ, Walter WG. Comparison of subcortical, cortical and scalp activity using chronically indwelling electrodes in man. *Electroencephalogr Clin Neurophysiol* 1965;18: 217–228.

50. Ebersole JS, Hanes-Ebersole S. EEG dipole patch: a realistic extended source model for spikes and seizures. *Muscle and Nerve* 2003(Suppl 12):S37.

51. Woodbury JW. Potentials in volume conductor. In: Ruch TC, Fulton JF, eds. *Medical physiology and biophysics.* Philadelphia: WB Saunders, 1960:83–91.

52. Klee M, Rall W. Computed potentials of cortically arranged populations of neurons. *J Neurophysiol* 1977;40:647–666.

53. Lorente De No R. Correlation of nerve activity with polarization phenomena. *Harvey Lect* 1947;42:43–105.

54. Gloor P, Vera CL, Sporti L. Electrophysiological studies of hippocampal neurons. I. Configuration and laminar analysis of the "resting" potential gradient, of the main transient response to perforant path, fimbrial and mossy fiber volleys and of "spontaneous" activity. *Electroencephalogr Clin Neurophysiol* 1963;15: 353–378.

55. Neshige R, Luders H, Shibasaki H. Recording of movement-related potentials from scalp and cortex in man. *Brain* 1988; 111(pt 3):719–736.

56. Jasper HH. The Ten Twenty Electrode System of the International Federation. *Electroencephalogr Clin Neurophysiol* 1958;10: 371–375.

57. Myslobodsky MS, Coppola R, Bar-Ziv J, Weinberger DR. Adequacy of the International 10–20 electrode system for computed neurophysiologic topography. *J Clin Neurophysiol* 1990;7: 507–518.

58. Gevins AS. Analysis of the electromagnetic signals of the human brain: milestones, obstacles, and goals. *IEEE Trans Biomed Eng* 1984;31:833–850.

59. Lopes da Silva FH, van Rotterdam A. Biophysical aspects of EEG and magnetoencephalogram generation. In: Niedermeyer E, ed. *EEG basic principles, clinical applications and related fields.* Baltimore, MD: Lippincott Williams & Wilkins; 1999:93–109.

60. Gevins AS, Bressler SL. Functional topography of the human brain. *Functional brain imaging.* Toronto: Hans Huber, 1988: 99–116.

61. Gibbs EL, Gibbs FA, Fuster B. Psychomotor epilepsy. *Arch Neurol Psychiatry* 1948;60:331–339.

62. Luders H, Hahn J, Lesser RP, et al. Basal temporal subdural electrodes in the evaluation of patients with intractable epilepsy. *Epilepsia* 1989;30:131–142.

63. Rovit RL, Gloor P, Henderson LR. Temporal lobe epilepsy—a study using multiple basal electrodes, I: description of method. *Neurochirurgia* 1960;3:634.

64. Sperling MR, Engel J Jr. Electroencephalographic recording from the temporal lobes: a comparison of ear, anterior temporal, and nasopharyngeal electrodes. *Ann Neurol* 1985;17:510–513.

65. Chatrian GE, Lettich E, Nelson PL. Ten percent electrode system for topographic studies of spontaneous and evoked EEG activities. *Am J Electroencephalogr Clin Neurophysiol* 1985;25:83–92.

66. Morris HH III, Luders H, Lesser RP, et al. The value of closely spaced scalp electrodes in the localization of epileptiform foci: a study of 26 patients with complex partial seizures. *Electroencephalogr Clin Neurophysiol* 1986;63:107–111.

67. Nuwer MR. Recording electrode site nomenclature. *J Clin Neurophysiol* 1987;4:121–133.

68. Morris HH III, Kanner A, Luders H, et al. Can sharp waves localized at the sphenoidal electrode accurately identify a mesiotemporal epileptogenic focus? *Epilepsia* 1989;30:532–539.

69. Klass DW, Bickford RG, Ellingson RJ. A proposal for standard EEG montages to be used in clinical electroencephalography. In: *Guidelines in EEG.* Atlanta, GA: American Electroencephalography Society, 1980.

70. MacGillivray BB, Binnie CD, Osselton JW. Traditional methods of examination in clinical EEG. Derivations and montages. In: Delucchi MR, ed. *Handbook of electroencephalography and clinical neurophysiology, III.* Amsterdam: Elsevier Scientific, 1974: C22–C57.

71. Sharbrough FW. The mathematical logic for the design of montages. *Am J EEG Technol* 1977;17:73–83.

72. Merlet I, Paetau R, Garcia-Larrea L, et al. Apparent asynchrony between interictal electric and magnetic spikes. *Neuroreport* 1997;8:1071–1076.

73. Minami T, Gondo K, Yamamoto T, et al. Magnetoencephalographic analysis of rolandic discharges in benign childhood epilepsy. *Ann Neurol* 1996;39:326–334.

74. Takahashi H, Yasue M, Ishijima B. Dynamic EEG topography and analysis of epileptic spikes and evoked potentials following thalamic stimulation. *Appl Neurophysiol* 1985;48:418–422.

75. Thickbroom GW, Davies HD, Carroll WM, Mastaglia FL. Averaging, spatio-temporal mapping and dipole modelling of focal epileptic spikes. *Electroencephalogr Clin Neurophysiol* 1986;64:274–277.

76. Lehmann D, Skrandies W. Reference-free identification of components of checkerboard-evoked multichannel potential fields. *Electroencephalogr Clin Neurophysiol* 1980;48:609–621.

77. Walter DO, Etevenon P, Pidoux B, et al. Computerized topo-EEG spectral maps: difficulties and perspectives. *Neuropsychobiology* 1984;11:264–272.

78. Goldman D. The clinical use of the "average" electrode in monopolar recording. *Electroencephalogr Clin Neurophysiol* 1950; 2:211–214.

79. Lehmann D, Michel CM. Intracerebral dipole sources of EEG FFT power maps. *Brain Topogr* 1989;2:155–164.

80. Osselton JW. Acquisition of EEG data by bipolar, unipolar and average reference methods: a theoretical comparison. *Electroencephalogr Clin Neurophysiol* 1965;19:527–528.

81. John ER, Prichep LS, Fridman J, Easton P. Neurometrics: computer-assisted differential diagnosis of brain dysfunctions. *Science* 1988;239:162–169.

82. Katznelson RD. EEG recording, electrode placement, and aspects of generator localization. In: Nunez PL, Katznelson RD, eds. *Electric fields of the brain: the neurophysics of EEG.* London: Oxford University Press, 1981:176–213.

83. Fisch BJ, Pedley TA. The role of quantitative topographic mapping or "neurometrics" in the diagnosis of psychiatric and neurological disorders: the cons. *Electroencephalogr Clin Neurophysiol* 1989;73:5–9.

84. Lopes da Silava FH. A critical review of clinical applications of topographic mapping of brain potentials. *J Clin Neurophysiol* 1990;7:535–551.

85. Burgess RC. Editorial: localization of neural generators. *J Clin Neurophysiol* 1991;8:369.

86. van Oosterom A. History and evolution of methods for solving the inverse problem. *J Clin Neurophysiol* 1991;8:371–380.

87. Morris HH III, Luders H. Electrodes. *Electroencephalogr Clin Neurophysiol* 1985;37(Suppl):3–26.

88. Lueders H, Dinner DS, Lesser RP, Klem G. Origin of far-field subcortical-evoked potentials to posterior tibial and median nerve stimulation. A comparative study. *Arch Neurol* 1983;40:93–97.

89. Luders H, Lesser RP, Dinner DS. Benign focal epilepsy of childhood. In: Luders H, Lesser RP, eds. *Epilepsy: electroclinical syndromes.* Berlin: Springer-Verlag, 1987:303–346.

90. Adelman S, Lueders H, Dinner DS, Lesser RP. Paradoxical lateralization of parasagittal sharp waves in a patient with epilepsia partialis continua. *Epilepsia* 1982;23:291–295.

91. Perrin F, Bertrand O, Giard MH, Pernier J. Precautions in topographic mapping and in evoked potential map reading. *J Clin Neurophysiol* 1990;7:498–506.
92. Hjorth B. Principles for transformation of scalp EEG from potential field into source distribution. *J Clin Neurophysiol* 1991;8:391–396.
93. Duffy FH, Bartels PH, Burchfiel JL. Significance probability mapping: an aid in the topographic analysis of brain electrical activity. *Electroencephalogr Clin Neurophysiol* 1981;51:455–462.
94. American Electroencephalography Society. Statement on the clinical use of quantitative EEG. *J Clin Neurophysiol* 1987;4:197.
95. Nuwer MR. Frequency analysis and topographic mapping of EEG and evoked potentials in epilepsy. *Electroencephalogr Clin Neurophysiol* 1988;69:118–126.
96. Collura TF, Vuong TA. An integrated computer graphics system for clinical EEG. Seattle, WA: IEEE, 1989.
97. Perrin F, Pernier J, Bertrand O, Echallier JF. Spherical splines for scalp potential and current density mapping. *Electroencephalogr Clin Neurophysiol* 1989;72:184–187.
98. Rodin E, Cornellier D. Source derivation recordings of generalized spike-wave complexes. *Electroencephalogr Clin Neurophysiol* 1989;73:20–29.
99. Babiloni F, Babiloni C, Carducci F, et al. High resolution EEG: a new model-dependent spatial deblurring method using a realistically shaped MR-constructed subject's head model. *Electroencephalogr Clin Neurophysiol* 1997;102:69–80.
100. Herrman WM, Kubicki ST, Kunkel H. Empfehlungen der deutschen EEG-gesellschaft fur das mapping von EEG-parametern. *EEG-EMG Z* 1989;20:125–132.
101. Kahn EM, Weiner RD, Brenner RP, Coppola R. Topographic maps of brain electrical activity—pitfalls and precautions. *Biol Psychiatry* 1988;23:628–636.
102. Duffy FH. Brain electrical activity mapping: issues and answers. *Topographic mapping of brain electrical activity*. Boston: Butterworth-Heinemann, 1986:401–418.
103. Koszer S, Moshe SL, Legatt AD, et al. Surface mapping of spike potential fields: experienced EEGers vs. computerized analysis. *Electroencephalogr Clin Neurophysiol* 1996;98:199–205.
104. Gevins A, Le J, Leong H, et al. Deblurring. *J Clin Neurophysiol* 1999;16:204–213.
105. Scherg M, Von Cramon D. Evoked dipole source potentials of the human auditory cortex. *Electroencephalogr Clin Neurophysiol* 1986;65:344–360.
106. Scherg M. Fundamentals of dipole source potential analysis. In: Gradori F, Hoke M, Romani GL, eds. *Auditory evoked magnetic fields and electric potentials*. Basel: Karger, 1990:40–69.
107. Scherg M, Bast T, Berg P. Multiple source analysis of interictal spikes: goals, requirements, and clinical value. *J Clin Neurophysiol* 1999;16:214–224.
108. Cuffin BN, Cohen D, Yunokuchi K, et al. Tests of EEG localization accuracy using implanted sources in the human brain. *Ann Neurol* 1991;29:132–138.
109. Smith DB, Sidman RD, Flanigin H, et al. A reliable method for localizing deep intracranial sources of the EEG. *Neurology* 1985;35:1702–1707.
110. Regan D. *Human brain electrophysiology: evoked potentials and evoked magnetic fields in science and medicine*. New York: Elsevier Science, 2003.
111. Scherg M. Functional imaging and localization of electromagnetic brain activity. *Brain Topogr* 1992;5:103–111.
112. Cohen D, Cuffin BN, Yunokuchi K, et al. MEG versus EEG localization test using implanted sources in the human brain. *Ann Neurol* 1990;28:811–817.
113. Sutherling WW, Levesque MF, Crandall PH, Barth DS. Localization of partial epilepsy using magnetic and electric measurements. *Epilepsia* 1991;32(Suppl 5):S29–S40.
114. Cohen D. Magnetoencephalography: detection of the brain's electrical activity with a superconducting magnetometer. *Science* 1972;175:664–666.
115. Hamalainen M, Hari R, Ilmoneimi RJ. Magnetoencephalography—theory, instrumentation, and applications to noninvasive studies of the working brain. *Rev Mod Phys* 1993;65:413–497.
116. Hari R. Magnetoencephalography as a tool of clinical neurophysiology. In: Niedermeyer E, ed. *EEG, basic principles, clinical applications and related fields*. Baltimore, MD: Lippincott Williams & Wilkins, 1999:1107.
117. Leijten FS, Huiskamp GJ, Hilgersom I, Van Huffelen AC. High-resolution source imaging in mesiotemporal lobe epilepsy: a comparison between MEG and simultaneous EEG. *J Clin Neurophysiol* 2003;20:227–238.
118. Barkley GL, Baumgartner C. MEG and EEG in epilepsy. *J Clin Neurophysiol* 2003;20:163–178.
119. Eliashiv DS, Elsas SM, Squires K, et al. Ictal magnetic source imaging as a localizing tool in partial epilepsy. *Neurology* 2002;59:1600–1610.
120. Tilz C, Hummel C, Kettenmann B, Stefan H. Ictal onset localization of epileptic seizures by magnetoencephalography. *Acta Neurol Scand* 2002;106:190–195.
121. Barth DS, Sutherling W. Current source-density and neuromagnetic analysis of the direct cortical response in rat cortex. *Brain Res* 1988;450:280–294.
122. Barth DS. Empirical comparison of the MEG and EEG: animal models of the direct cortical response and epileptiform activity in neocortex. *Brain Topogr* 1991;4:85–93.
123. Okada YC, Wu J, Kyuhou S. Genesis of MEG signals in a mammalian CNS structure. *Electroencephalogr Clin Neurophysiol* 1997;103:474–485.
124. Salmelin R, Hari R. Characterization of spontaneous MEG rhythms in healthy adults. *Electroencephalogr Clin Neurophysiol* 1994;91:237–248.
125. Zijlmans M, Huiskamp GM, Leijten FS, et al. Modality-specific spike identification in simultaneous magnetoencephalography/electroencephalography: a methodological approach. *J Clin Neurophysiol* 2002;19:183–191.
126. Baumgartner C, Pataraia E, Lindinger G, Deecke L. Neuromagnetic recordings in temporal lobe epilepsy. *J Clin Neurophysiol* 2000;17:177–189.
127. Iwasaki M, Nakasato N, Shamoto H, et al. Surgical implications of neuromagnetic spike localization in temporal lobe epilepsy. *Epilepsia* 2002;43:415–424.
128. Knowlton RC, Laxer KD, Aminoff MJ, et al. Magnetoencephalography in partial epilepsy: clinical yield and localization accuracy. *Ann Neurol* 1997;42:622–631.
129. Iwasaki M, Nakasato N, Shamoto H, Yoshimoto T. Focal magnetoencephalographic spikes in the superior temporal plane undetected by scalp EEG. *J Clin Neurosci* 2003;10:236–238.
130. Stefan H, Hummel C, Scheler G, et al. Magnetic brain source imaging of focal epileptic activity: a synopsis of 455 cases. *Brain* 2003;126(Pt 11):2396–2405.
131. Hamalainen MS, Sarvas J. Realistic conductivity geometry model of the human head for interpretation of neuromagnetic data. *IEEE Trans Biomed Eng* 1989;36:165–171.
132. Fuchs M, Wagner M, Kohler T, Wischmann HA. Linear and nonlinear current density reconstructions. *J Clin Neurophysiol* 1999;16:267–295.
133. Jeffs B, Leahy R, Singh M. An evaluation of methods for neuromagnetic image reconstruction. *IEEE Trans Biomed Eng* 1987;34:713–723.
134. Mosher JC, Leahy RM. Recursive MUSIC: a framework for EEG and MEG source localization. *IEEE Trans Biomed Eng* 1998;45:1342–1354.
135. Otsubo H, Ochi A, Elliott I, et al. MEG predicts epileptic zone in lesional extrahippocampal epilepsy: 12 pediatric surgery cases. *Epilepsia* 2001;42:1523–1530.
136. Ebersole JS. Defining epileptogenic foci: past, present, future. *J Clin Neurophysiol* 1997;14:470–483.
137. Uutela K, Hamalainen M, Somersalo E. Visualization of magnetoencephalographic data using minimum current estimates. *Neuroimage* 1999;10:173–180.
138. Wang JZ, Williamson SJ, Kaufman L. Magnetic source images determined by a lead-field analysis: the unique minimum-norm least-squares estimation. *IEEE Trans Biomed Eng* 1992;39: 665–675.
139. Gorodnitsky IF, George JS, Rao BD. Neuromagnetic source imaging with FOCUSS: a recursive weighted minimum norm algorithm. *Electroencephalogr Clin Neurophysiol* 1995;95:231–251.
140. Pataraia E, Baumgartner C, Lindinger G, Deecke L. Magnetoencephalography in presurgical epilepsy evaluation. *Neurosurg Rev* 2002;25:141–159.

Application of Electroencephalography in the Diagnosis of Epilepsy

12

David R. Chabolla   Gregory D. Cascino

The electroencephalogram (EEG) is the most frequently performed neurodiagnostic study in patients with a seizure disorder (1) and, despite its introduction more than 60 years ago (2), still has important clinical and research applications. Because of the paroxysmal nature of epilepsy (1,3), an EEG is usually obtained between seizure episodes. The interictal EEG may be useful in confirming the diagnosis of epilepsy, classifying seizure type, and monitoring and predicting response to treatment (1,4–13). Localized electrographic alterations such as continuous focal slowing and certain epileptiform discharges may even "suggest" the presence of underlying pathology (14,15). Correlation of the ictal and interictal EEG changes with ictal semiology underlie the current classification of seizures (1,16).

When routine interictal EEG recordings prove diagnostically inadequate (14,17), long-term EEG studies may be used to improve the yield of EEG abnormalities and to localize the epileptogenic zone (14,17).

This chapter discusses the relationship between extracranial EEG studies and epilepsy and the clinical applications of interictal and ictal EEG recordings.

HISTORICAL PERSPECTIVE

In 1933, Berger (18) published his observations of EEG changes in patients during "convulsions" but failed to recognize the tremendous potential of these studies in epilepsy. EEG findings appeared to validate Jackson's earlier hypothesis that epilepsy was caused by a "discharging lesion" (19). In 1935, Gibbs and colleagues (20) documented the association of specific interictal and ictal EEG alterations in patients with seizures. They also indicated that interictal EEG findings may localize the epileptogenic zone (21). Various interictal EEG patterns in patients with partial and generalized epilepsy were subsequently recognized, and attempts were made to classify seizures according to electroclinical correlations (20). Penfield and Jasper (9) later revealed the importance of electrocorticography in recording interictal EEG abnormalities during focal cortical resective surgery for intractable partial epilepsy.

CLINICAL APPLICATIONS

Rationale

Despite impressive technical advances, the purpose of the EEG has not changed since the days of Gibbs and Gibbs (21). As the cornerstone of the evaluation of patients with episodic symptoms and recurrent behavioral alterations (1,16), the EEG identifies specific interictal or ictal abnormalities that are associated with an increased epileptogenic potential and correlate with a seizure disorder (16). A persistently normal EEG recording does not exclude the diagnosis of epilepsy (3), and epileptiform alterations may occur without a history of seizures (22), although this happens rarely. Ultimately, EEG findings must be correlated with the clinical history.

The patient with recurrent clinical symptoms, for example, staring spells with behavioral arrest, presents a diagnostic challenge. A variety of physiologic and psychological disorders may mimic epileptic seizure activity (1). The sensitivity and specificity of the EEG in this setting depends on the classification of the seizure disorder, seizure type and frequency, and localization of the epileptic brain tissue (3,17). Epileptiform discharges are usually highly specific in the patient with episodic behavioral alterations; unfortunately, the EEG has variable sensitivity in epilepsy (3), and identification of the ictal patterns may be needed to clarify the underlying etiology. The absence of interictal epileptiform alterations does not distinguish a nonepileptic disorder from epilepsy, and false interpretation of nonspecific changes with hyperventilation or drowsiness may lead to an error in diagnosis and treatment. In patients who present with a behavior consistent with epilepsy, an EEG can elucidate the classification of a partial or generalized disorder that often cannot be determined by ictal semiology alone. The appropriate classification affects subsequent diagnostic evaluation and therapy, and may have prognostic importance. For example, recurrent secondarily generalized tonic-clonic seizures and anterior temporal lobe interictal spike discharges would be classified as a partial seizure disorder and set the stage for magnetic resonance imaging and antiseizure drug therapy.

The EEG has fundamental value in evaluating surgical candidacy and determining operative strategy (23) in selected patients with intractable partial epilepsy (24). In these individuals, interictal epileptiform alterations identified on EEG provide only limited information about lateralization and localization of the epileptic brain tissue (3,14,17), as the diagnostic yield depends on the site of seizure onset (3,17,25). Identification of ictal EEG patterns, performed in an inpatient unit with concomitant video recordings (3,14,17,23,25,26), is necessary to localize the epileptogenic zone preoperatively.

Methods

Recordings should be performed according to the methodology established by the American Clinical Neurophysiology Society (formerly the American Electroencephalography Society) (27). Standard activation procedures such as hyperventilation and photic stimulation should be included. The recording of drowsiness and nonrapid eye movement (NREM) sleep, facilitated by sleep deprivation, may increase the sensitivity of the EEG to demonstrate interictal epileptiform alterations, especially in patients with partial epilepsy (28,29). Adequate levels of sleep may be attained after administration of chloral hydrate. Benzodiazepines should not be used as a sedative because of their associated increase in β activity and the possible masking of epileptiform alterations. During the recording, the EEG technologist should obtain information about seizure manifestations, time of the latest seizure, current medications and antiepileptic drug levels, and precipitating events.

Interictal Recording

The recording of interictal epileptiform activity depends on the seizure type, localization of the epileptogenic zone, recording methodology, age at seizure onset, and frequency of seizure activity (1,10,28–32). The diagnostic yield of the interictal EEG can be increased by performing multiple EEG recordings (30), increasing the duration of the EEG, and timing a study shortly after a seizure, because interictal epileptiform discharges may be potentiated following an attack (31–33).

Ictal Recording

Recognition of ictal EEG patterns is indicated in patients with medically refractory partial epilepsy being considered for surgical treatment. The effectiveness of scalp-recorded ictal EEG for identifying the seizure onset zone may be enhanced by altering the recording technique (3,6,14–17, 23,26,34,35). Closely spaced scalp electrodes increase the diagnostic accuracy of such monitoring (36). With application of the standard extension of the 10–20 Electrode Placement System, as outlined in the American Clinical Neurophysiology Society guidelines, inferolateral temporal electrode positions, namely, F_9, F_{10}, T_9, and T_{10}, may be used to record epileptiform activity of anterior temporal lobe origin (34). Special extracranial electrodes also may improve diagnostic effectiveness. Sphenoidal electrodes may reveal the topography of interictal and ictal epileptiform discharges in patients with temporal lobe seizures and indicate the mesial temporal localization of the epileptogenic region (14). Supraorbital electrodes, which record from the orbitofrontal region, may be useful in patients with partial epilepsy of frontal lobe origin (3). Digital EEG acquisition and storage in a format suitable for subsequent remontaging and filtering have improved the speed with which interpretable ictal recordings may be obtained over paper recordings.

Limitations of Extracranial Recordings

Several limitations of scalp-recorded, or extracranial, EEG affect the interpretation of these studies in patients with epilepsy (8). Epileptiform activity generated in cortex remote from the surface electrodes, for example, amygdala and hippocampus, may not be associated with interictal extracranial EEG alterations (8). Attenuation of spike activity by the dura, bone, and scalp also limits the sensitivity of these recordings (1), which may be degraded further by muscle artifacts. Approximately 20% to 70% of cortical spikes are recorded on the scalp EEG (37). Patients with seizure disorders may have repetitively normal interictal EEG studies (1,8,30). Extracranial EEG recordings may also inaccurately localize the epileptogenic zone (17). For example, interictal scalp EEG may fail to detect specific alterations arising from the amygdala only to reveal distant, more widespread cortical excitability (8,17). Localization of the epileptogenic zone as suggested by interictal specific EEG patterns may also be discordant with ictal extracranial or long-term intracranial monitoring (17,38).

Pitfalls in Interpretation

Differentiating artifact from electrical activity of cerebral origin is challenging (1), and both the EEG technologist and the electroencephalographer must be constantly alert. Various types of artifacts can superficially mimic interictal and ictal epileptiform patterns. Artifacts can be related to *extrinsic* factors (such as the electrical interference generated by power cables and fluorescent lights), *biologic* factors (for example, myogenic and eye movement artifacts), and *technological* factors (such as poor electrical impedance causing an electrode "pop"). Changes during drowsiness, hyperventilation, photic stimulation, and arousal from sleep can be particularly confounding in pediatric patients. Thus, knowledge of the normal EEG background for age is critical to appropriate interpretation.

Some EEG patterns—such as small sharp spikes (see Fig. 13.4), 14- and 6-Hz positive bursts (see Fig. 13.5), 6-Hz spike and wave (see Fig. 13.6), wicket waves, rhythmic temporal θ activity of drowsiness, psychomotor variant pattern, and subclinical rhythmic epileptiform discharges of adults—are not associated with increased epileptogenic potential (11,29,39–43).

SPECIFIC INTERICTAL EPILEPTIFORM PATTERNS IN PARTIAL EPILEPSIES

EEG abnormalities in patients with seizure disorders may be categorized as *specific* or *nonspecific*. Specific patterns, that is, the spike, sharp wave, spike-wave complex, temporal intermittent rhythmic delta activity (TIRDA), and periodic epileptiform discharges (PLEDs), are potentially epileptogenic and provide diagnostically useful information (8,44). Nonspecific changes, such as generalized or focal slow-wave activity and amplitude asymmetries, are not unique to epilepsy and do not indicate an increased

epileptogenic potential (8). Potentially epileptogenic EEG alterations identified in patients with seizure disorders are rarely detected in nonepileptic patients (22,45). Interictal epileptiform alterations identify the irritative zone that may mark the epileptic brain tissue (46). Patients with seizures beginning in childhood typically display a higher incidence of EEG abnormalities than do those with adult-onset epilepsy (30).

Spikes and Sharp Waves

The main types of epileptiform discharges are spikes and sharp waves, occurring either as single potentials or with an after-following slow wave, that is, a spike-and-wave complex. Spike discharges are predominantly negative transients easily recognized by their characteristic steep ascending and descending limbs and duration of 20 to 70 msec (47). Sharp-wave discharges are broader potentials with a pointed peak that last between 70 and 200 msec (47). These abnormalities should have a physiologic potential field and should involve more than one electrode to exclude electrode artifact. Spike-and-wave complexes consist of a spike followed by a slow wave in an isolated or repetitive fashion. The mechanisms of epileptogenesis (Chapter 6), atlas of pathologic substrates (Chapter 1), and the neurophysiologic bases of the EEG (Chapter 10) are discussed elsewhere in this volume. The morphology and localization of specific EEG epileptiform patterns may provide useful information on the predictability of seizure recurrence and may influence the selection of antiepileptic drug therapy. Unfortunately, interictal EEG may produce variable results, and during brief recording periods, specific abnormalities may not be seen despite repetition of several EEGs (30). The frequency of spiking may not be a good predictor of the seizure activity and is independent of antiepileptic drug levels (31,32).

Temporal Intermittent Rhythmic Delta Activity

The interictal potentially epileptogenic pattern TIRDA (Fig. 12.1) has been identified in patients with partial epilepsy of temporal lobe origin (11,44) and has the same epileptogenic

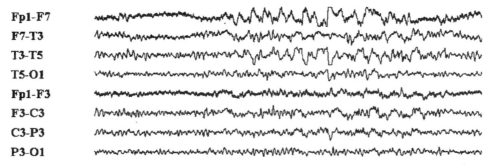

Figure 12.1 Temporal intermittent rhythmic delta activity (TIRDA) appears to increase in amplitude, slow in frequency, and spread slightly in distribution (note the late development of rhythmic slowing over the frontocentral region) over 3 to 4 seconds.

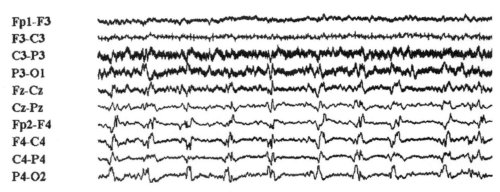

Figure 12.2 Periodic lateralizing epileptiform discharges (PLEDs), maximum over the right centroparietal region, with some spread to the left posterior head regions.

significance as temporal lobe spike or sharp-wave discharges (44). This pattern, most prominent during drowsiness and NREM sleep, consists of rhythmic trains of low- to moderate-amplitude δ frequency slow waves over the temporal region, unilaterally or bilaterally, without apparent clinical accompaniment (11,44). Persistent polymorphic δ frequency activity over the temporal region due to a focal structural brain lesion may not be potentially epileptogenic and should be differentiated from TIRDA.

Periodic Lateralized Epileptiform Discharges

The focal or lateralized sharp-wave discharges called PLEDs may have a wide field of distribution and occur in a periodic or quasi-periodic fashion (Fig. 12.2) (48). Typically occurring at 0.5 to 2.0 Hz, they vary in amplitude and duration (100 to 200 msec) and most commonly appear as broad diphasic or triphasic waves (11,49), although complexes of repetitive discharges also may be seen (50). This EEG pattern is not specific for any one pathologic lesion and is usually transient (11); however, chronic, persistent PLEDs have been reported (51). Alteration of consciousness, focal or secondarily generalized seizures, and acute or subacute neurologic dysfunction may be associated with PLEDs (11). The prognosis depends mainly on the underlying etiology.

Ictal Patterns in Partial Epilepsies

Partial, or localization-related, epilepsy implies seizure activity of focal onset (1,8,13,52,53). The electrographic onset of a seizure is characterized by a sudden change of frequency and the appearance of a new rhythm. The initial change may be desynchronization or attenuation of EEG activity in the ictal onset zone (25). An aura preceding impairment of consciousness may be without obvious electrographic accompaniment, and the new EEG rhythm may be intermittent at first but evolve into more distinct patterns. Seizure activity of δ, θ, α, or β frequency typically shifts from one frequency to another, slowing with increasing amplitudes and developing more distinct rhythmic waves.

Focal onset of the electrographic seizure evolves through several phases: (a) focal attenuation of EEG activity; (b) focal, rhythmic, low-voltage, fast-activity discharge; and (c) progressive increase in amplitude with slowing that spreads to a regional anatomic distribution. Focal epileptiform discharges, such as repetitive spikes or fast activity recorded at a single electrode, are a relatively rare but important first change localizing the epileptogenic zone, provided an electrode artifact is ruled out (25).

Most patients with partial epilepsy experience complex partial seizures (13), with onset commonly in the anterior temporal region and emanating from the medial temporal lobe (amygdala or hippocampus) or the lateral temporal neocortex (54). Results of extracranial EEG monitoring may be unremarkable in most patients experiencing simple partial seizures (55). A localized epileptiform abnormality on interictal scalp EEG may aid in the diagnostic classification of simple partial seizures; however, those associated with transient psychic or visual experiential phenomena rarely occur with a precise, focal, epileptiform discharge during extracranial EEG recording. In one series (55), approximately 80% of patients had no definite extracranial EEG alteration when evaluated by simultaneous intracranial and extracranial recordings. Therefore, the lack of EEG changes alone should not be used to establish the diagnosis of nonepileptic clinical behavior.

CLINICAL USE OF THE ELECTOENCEPHALOGRAPH IN THE PARTIAL EPILEPSIES

Various areas of the brain differ significantly in their susceptibility to epilepsy. The temporal lobe has the lowest threshold for seizures, followed by the rolandic motor strip area and portions of the frontal lobe. The parietal and occipital lobes have the lowest degree of epileptogenicity. Focal epileptiform discharges may occur over any location on the scalp and depend on the age of the individual and the site of the pathologic lesion. This is particularly important in newborns and infants, whose brain maturation is

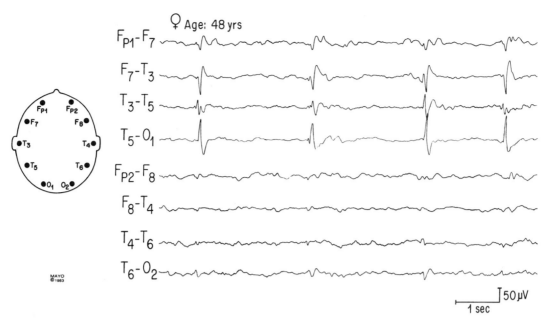

Figure 12.3   Left temporal spikes. Characteristic interictal left temporal spike discharges. (Courtesy of B.F. Westmoreland, Mayo Clinic, Rochester, MN.)

incomplete or abnormal. Epileptiform discharges may appear to be generalized or multiregional (hypsarrhythmia) even in the presence of a focal brain lesion on magnetic resonance imaging (see Chapter 83).

Temporal Lobe Epilepsy

Temporal spikes are highly epileptogenic and represent the most common interictal EEG alteration in adults with partial epilepsy (Fig. 12.3) (29,33). This spike discharge has a maximum amplitude over the anterior temporal region (in contrast to the centrotemporal spike) and may prominently involve the ear leads. Sleep markedly potentiates the presence of temporal spikes; approximately 90% of patients with temporal lobe seizures show spikes during sleep (11,20). Most patients with independent bilateral and bisynchronous temporal spikes are ultimately demonstrated to have unilateral temporal lobe seizures (3). The morphology of interictal spikes in the temporal lobe is clearly distinct from the ictal pattern (6,10,11).

Sphenoidal and inferolateral temporal scalp (T_1, T_2, F_9, F_{10}) electrodes, as well as closely placed scalp electrodes,

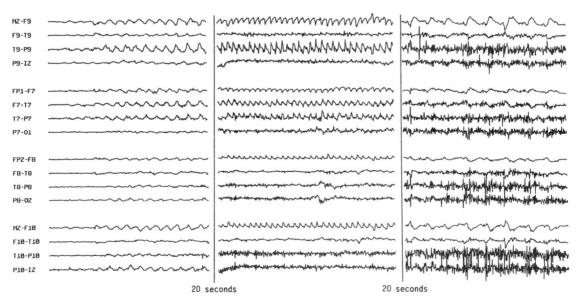

Figure 12.4   Scalp-recorded left temporal lobe seizure showing θ-, α-, and δ-frequency activity during consecutive phases.

can be useful in delineating the topography of the interictal activity (3,10,17,25,34,35). Sphenoidal electrodes record epileptiform activity emanating from the mediobasal limbic region and help to localize the epileptogenic zone prior to an anterior temporal lobectomy (3). In patients with temporal lobe epilepsy, the sensitivity of sphenoidal electrodes compared with scalp electrodes is unclear (10). Nasopharyngeal electrodes are artifact prone and poorly tolerated (which may interfere with a sleep recording) and have not demonstrated more sensitivity or specificity than lateral inferior scalp electrodes (37).

Patients with complex partial seizures of anterior temporal lobe origin may demonstrate localized, lateralized, or generalized ictal scalp EEG patterns (6,15–17,56–58). Prior to the seizure, an increase in interictal temporal lobe (or bitemporal) spiking may be evident; however, robust interictal spike discharges must be distinguished from electrographic seizure activity (15). Simple partial seizures or auras of mesial temporal lobe origin commonly show no seizure pattern on scalp EEG.

Lobar onset of a seizure is the most common scalp-recorded alteration in complex partial seizures of anterior temporal lobe origin (Fig. 12.4). A lateralized moderate- to high-amplitude rhythmic paroxysm of activity is most prominent in the temporal scalp electrodes and may progress to generalized rhythmic slowing maximal on the side of seizure onset. Focal temporal lobe or generalized arrhythmic slow-wave activity may occur postictally. Interictal temporal lobe spiking may increase at the termination of the seizure (32).

The sensitivity and specificity of ictal extracranial EEG have been analyzed in patients with partial seizures of temporal lobe origin (3,13,14,17,59,60). The localizing value of scalp EEG has ranged from approximately 40% to 90% in reported patient series (3,17,59,60). This variability may depend on the timing of the predominant ictal EEG change related to the clinical seizure; that is, initial focal epileptiform discharges as opposed to subsequent focal rhythmic abnormalities. Sphenoidal electrodes have been shown to increase the diagnostic yield of ictal extracranial EEG (14). In a study performed between 1978 and 1980 at the Montreal Neurological Institute, 311 seizures were recorded in 30 patients with "mostly" temporal lobe epilepsy and complex partial seizures (3,17) by means of long-term EEG monitoring with supplementary (sphenoidal or nasopharyngeal) electrodes. Focal or lobar-restricted paroxysmal events characterized 40.7% of seizures and a lateralized seizure onset an additional 9.4%. Bilateral or generalized alteration was identified in another 22.8% of complex partial seizures. The extracranial EEG recordings were uninterpretable in 27.4%. All patients in this series had an ictal electrographic alteration. Ictal extracranial EEG in patients with large destructive temporal lobe lesions may incorrectly lateralize seizure onset (26).

Frontal Lobe Epilepsy

The second most common site of seizure onset in partial epilepsy is the frontal lobe (16,17,54). This region presents difficult challenges in attempts to localize the epileptogenic zone with interictal scalp EEG recordings (3,17,25, 59,61). The interictal EEG is not as sensitive and specific in frontal lobe epilepsy as it is in temporal lobe epilepsy (3,59,61). Interictal EEG activity recorded by way of prolonged extracranial monitoring in 34 patients who remained seizure free following frontal corticectomy identified a localized specific EEG pattern in the frontal lobe in only 9% (17). A lateralized, but not localized, interictal abnormality was noted in 59% of patients. No interictal abnormality was observed in 11.7% of those studied. Epileptogenic zones in the frontal lobe remote from scalp electrodes (orbitofrontal and mesiofrontal regions) may not be associated with interictal activity despite multiple or prolonged EEG recordings (17).

Supraorbital surface electrodes may increase the sensitivity and specificity of EEG scalp recordings in patients with frontal lobe epilepsy associated with seizures originating from the orbitofrontal region (3,17). These electrodes are preferred for nocturnal recordings because of the artifact generated by eye movement and blinking (3).

In frontal lobe epilepsy, seizures may begin in the dorsolateral frontal cortex, orbitofrontal region, cingulate gyrus, supplementary cortex, or frontal pole (13,61–64). Interictal frontal lobe epileptogenic discharges may be associated with simple partial, complex partial, atonic, or secondarily generalized tonic-clonic seizures (11,20). Ictal behavior in frontal lobe epilepsy is highly variable, and establishing the diagnosis based on ictal semiology alone may be difficult (13,62,65). Frontal lobe seizures, especially those arising from the supplementary sensorimotor region, may be confused with nonepileptic behavioral events (13,61).

Occipital Lobe Epilepsy

Occipital spike activity occurs less frequently than does epileptiform activity that emanates from the temporal or frontal regions (Fig. 12.5). Interictal occipital epileptiform activity is most common in children and indicates only moderate epileptogenicity; approximately 40% to 50% of patients with occipital spikes have seizures (5,11). Occipital "needle-sharp spikes" may also occur in congenitally blind individuals (usually children) who do not have epilepsy (66). Interictal occipital spikes may be unilateral or bilateral and may be associated with simple or complex partial seizures (5,7,11).

As described by Gastaut in 1982 (52), occipital spikes also may occur in patients with idiopathic age-related occipital epilepsy, a less common variant of benign rolandic epilepsy. The seizures begin with a visual phenomenon and

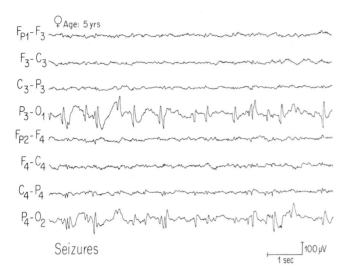

Figure 12.5 Occipital spikes. Bilateral occipital lobe interictal spiking in a child with a seizure disorder. (Courtesy of B.F. Westmoreland, Mayo Clinic, Rochester, MN.)

may be followed by generalized tonic-clonic episodes (52). Headache may occur during or after the seizures (52). The typical interictal occipital spikes attenuate with eye opening (52). Patients with this "benign partial" disorder have an excellent prognosis, and the seizures usually do not persist into adulthood (7,11,52).

Perirolandic Epilepsy

The most common cause of perirolandic epilepsy is benign focal epilepsy of childhood, although not all patients with seizures and centrotemporal spike discharges have benign

rolandic epilepsy. The interictal EEG pattern in benign focal epilepsy of childhood is a high-voltage diphasic or polyphasic spike followed by a slow wave with a duration of 200 to 300 msec (Fig. 12.6) (1,7,11). Scalp EEG spike activity appears to be maximal over the lower rolandic and midtemporal regions (67). The discharges may be unilateral or bilateral and shift from side to side, and may not correspond to the hemisphere associated with ictal symptoms (11). Spiking is usually more abundant during drowsiness and sleep and is not a good predictor of the severity of seizure activity (11). The central midtemporal spike may exhibit a surrounding region of positivity, suggesting a tangential dipole source (1,7). Central spikes have a moderate degree of epileptogenicity, with approximately 40% to 60% of patients having clinical seizures (2,11,67,68).

Benign childhood epilepsy with centrotemporal spikes, or "rolandic epilepsy," is a common and distinct seizure disorder. Seizure onset is typically between 2 and 12 years of age, and seizures disappear between 15 and 18 years of age (5). Antiepileptic drug therapy can usually be deferred, although the seizures typically respond well if treatment is elected. The ictal behavior includes focal motor or sensory seizures with frequent secondary generalization, excessive salivation and drooling, and motor speech arrest (4).

ELECTROENCEPHALOGRAPHY IN THE PRIMARY GENERALIZED EPILEPSIES

The specific interictal patterns associated with generalized epilepsies are easily distinguishable from normal background activity and include 3-Hz generalized spike and

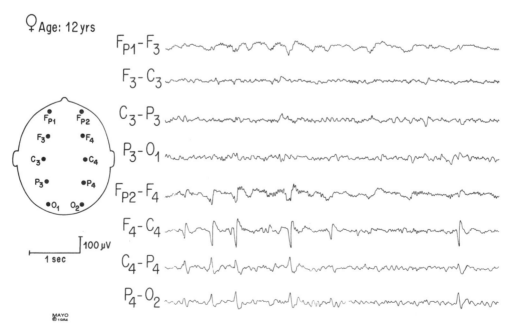

Figure 12.6 Right central spikes. Bipolar electroencephalogram (EEG) tracing shows interictal spiking in the right central region in a patient with benign rolandic epilepsy. Note normal background EEG activity. (Courtesy of B.F. Westmoreland, Mayo Clinic, Rochester, MN.)

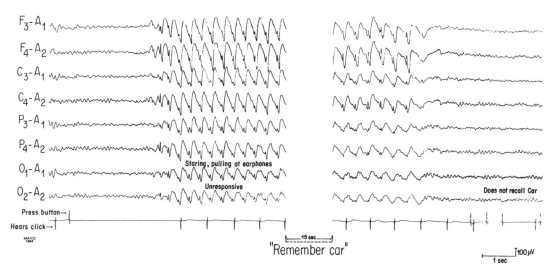

Figure 12.7 Absence seizure (hyperventilation: 80 seconds). Electrographic correlate of a typical absence seizure precipitated by hyperventilation. Response testing during the seizure shows that the patient stopped pressing the button when a clicking sound was made in his ear. (Courtesy of J.D. Grabow, Mayo Clinic, Rochester, MN.)

wave, slow spike and wave, atypical generalized spike and wave, and generalized paroxysmal fast activity. Generalized epilepsies are classified further as symptomatic or idiopathic, depending on etiology, seizure activity, and EEG alterations (4). Seizure types include absence, generalized tonic-clonic, atonic, myoclonic, tonic, clonic-tonic-clonic, and atypical absence (4). Experimental models of generalized epilepsy indicate pathologic cortical hyperexcitability as the basic mechanism for epileptogenesis (11,69). Thalamocortical connections are necessary for the development of typical spike-and-wave epileptiform activity (11,69).

SPECIFIC PATTERNS

3-Hz Spike and Wave

This morphologic pattern of the spike-and-wave complexes is similar in both interictal and ictal recordings. The EEG alteration consists of generalized, often anterior predominant, repetitive, bisynchronous, symmetric spike- and slow-wave discharges occurring at approximately 3 Hz (Fig. 12.7) (1,7,8,11,70,71). The typical pattern often varies, however. The frequency may be faster than 4.0 Hz at the beginning of the discharge and slower than 2.5 Hz at the end (72). Shifting minor asymmetries may occur over homologous head regions and, at times, double spikes associated with an aftercoming slow wave (70). Hyperventilation, hypoglycemia, drowsiness, and eye closure may potentiate the generalized spike-and-wave discharge (2,70). During sleep, the morphology of the interictal abnormality may appear as fragmented or asymmetric spike-and-wave bursts (29,70). Background activities are usually normal; however, some intermittent, rhythmic, bisynchronous slow waves may be present over the posterior head regions (70).

This highly epileptogenic pattern occurs typically in children 3 to 15 years old with idiopathic generalized epilepsy and absence seizures (29,70). Absence seizures are more frequent in girls and display a strong genetic predisposition. They usually occur frequently (multiple daily) as brief absences that typically last less than 30 seconds. Staring, automatisms, rapid eye blinking, and myoclonic movements of the extremities are closely correlated to the EEG recording and may occur when EEG changes persist for more than 3 to 4 seconds (16,56).

Multiple Spike and Wave

The multiple spike-and-wave pattern (also called atypical spike and wave and fast spike and wave) consists of a generalized mixture of intermittent brief spike and polyspike complexes associated with slow waves of variable frequency (3.5 to 6 Hz), morphology, and spatial distribution (Fig. 12.8) (73). The usually 1- to 3-second bursts are mostly subclinical. The background between bursts may be normal or contain focal or generalized slow irregularities.

This pattern is associated with generalized tonic-clonic, clonic, atonic, myoclonic, and atypical absence seizures (8). In a generalized tonic-clonic seizure, the ictal EEG alterations at onset are bilateral, symmetric, and synchronous. The tonic phase begins with generalized, low-voltage, fast activity (the "epileptic recruiting rhythm") that progresses to a generalized spike and polyspike burst (Fig. 12.9) (16,56). The spike discharges gradually slow in frequency as they increase in amplitude. The clonic phase is associated with muscular relaxation and generalized EEG suppression with intermixed generalized spike and polyspike discharges. Postictally, at the termination of the

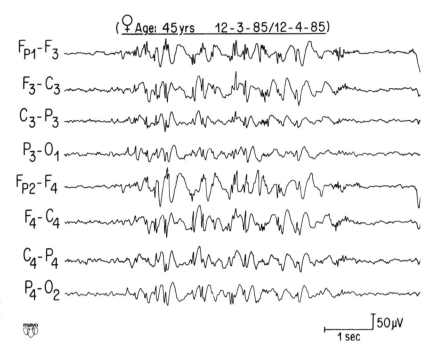

Figure 12.8 Generalized atypical spike and wave in an adult patient with a mixed seizure disorder that includes atypical absence seizures. (Courtesy of F.W. Sharbrough, Mayo Clinic, Rochester, MN.)

seizure, prominent generalized background slowing gradually returns to baseline.

Slow Spike and Wave

The slow spike-and-wave pattern (see Fig. 13.24) consists of generalized, repetitive, bisynchronous, sharp-wave or spike discharges occurring at 1.5 to 2.5 Hz (1,7,8,52,73) and is electrographically and clinically distinct from the 3-Hz pattern (2). The interictal and ictal EEG alterations are

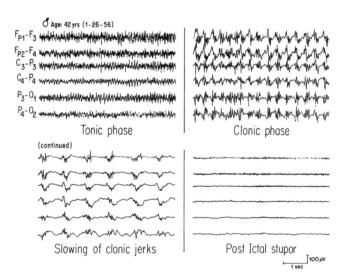

Figure 12.9 Multiple scalp-recorded electroencephalogram phases of a generalized tonic-clonic seizure. (From Westmoreland BF. The electroencephalogram in patients with epilepsy. In: Aminoff MJ, ed. *Neurology clinics.* Philadelphia: WB Saunders, 1985:599–613, by permission of Mayo Foundation for Medical Education and Research.)

widely distributed, may occur asymmetrically with a shifting focal emphasis (74), and may be prolonged. Often, no clinical manifestations are apparent, although appropriate testing may disclose some alteration in psychomotor performance. Focal spikes and focal or generalized background slowing between the spike-and-wave bursts may also be present (74). Slow spike-and-wave discharges are less likely than the 3-Hz discharge to be activated by hyperventilation and hypoglycemia (73). Sleep recordings may show generalized spikes and multiple spike-and-wave discharges (29,73). The unusual similarity of the ictal and interictal EEG patterns may complicate the assessment of epilepsy in a child with severe cognitive impairment and reported frequent staring.

Seizures in these patients can vary but usually consist of tonic-clonic, tonic, atonic, atypical absences, and myoclonic types. The slow spike-and-wave pattern is most common in children with mental retardation and may persist into adulthood (73,75). Compared with the 3-Hz spike and wave, which rarely is present before the child is 4 years of age, the slow discharge may begin as early as age 6 months (75). Slow spike-and-wave discharges, mental retardation, and multiple generalized seizure types make up Lennox-Gastaut syndrome (74).

Paroxysmal or Rhythmic Fast Activity

This pattern of repetitive spike discharges with a frequency of 8 to 20 Hz often occurs at the onset of generalized tonic-clonic seizures, in association with tonic seizures, and during sleep recordings in patients with generalized seizures. The ictal scalp EEG reveals a generalized, synchronous, symmetric alteration, usually in the form of low-voltage

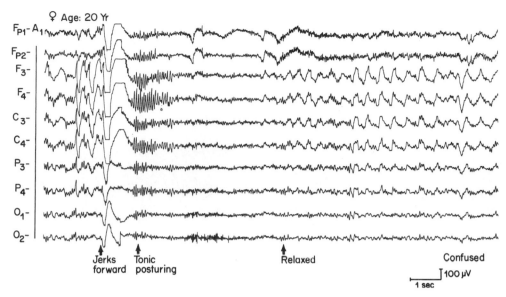

Figure 12.10 High-amplitude generalized sharp wave followed by desynchronization and generalized paroxysmal fast activity during a tonic seizure. (Courtesy of F.W. Sharbrough, Mayo Clinic, Rochester, MN.)

fast-frequency (approximately 20- to 25-Hz) activity that progressively increases in amplitude (Fig. 12.10).

Electrodecremental Response

This ictal EEG pattern, seen mostly with tonic and atonic seizures and with infantile spasms, consists of an abrupt generalized "flattening" or desynchronization of activity, usually arising from an abnormal background (Fig. 12.11). The EEG desynchronization may last longer than the clinical seizure (56). The degree of EEG suppression may depend on the duration of the seizure and the alteration in mentation. Muscle artifact may make identification difficult when the seizure is brief (16,56).

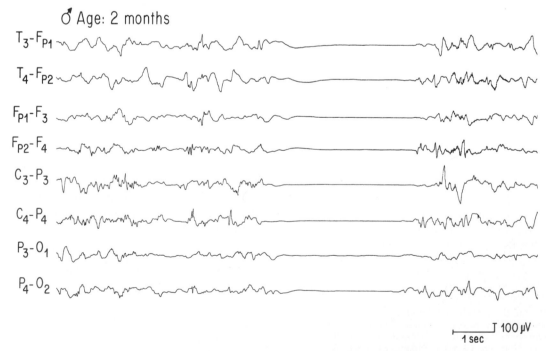

Figure 12.11 Electrodecremental episode associated with infantile spasms (onset 3 weeks, cause unknown). (Courtesy of D.W. Klass, Mayo Clinic, Rochester, MN.)

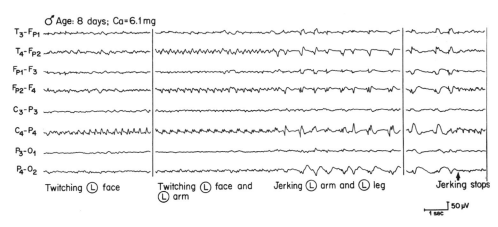

Figure 12.12   Scalp-recorded right hemisphere seizure in a neonate with hypocalcemia. (Courtesy of B.F. Westmoreland, Mayo Clinic, Rochester, MN.)

Photoparoxysmal Response

This abnormal cerebral response to photic stimulation consists of generalized multiple spike-and-wave complexes and is likely a variant of the atypical spike and wave (76). It is best seen at flash frequencies between 10 and 20 Hz, and the resulting seizure discharge may outlast the stimulus by a few seconds; however, frequencies shift and generally become slower as the amplitude increases. The response may be accompanied by brief body jerks or impaired consciousness (77,78). Photoparoxysmal responses may be seen at any age, as a familial trait or an acquired phenomenon (76–78), but maximal expression is between ages 8 and 20 years. Acquired photoparoxysmal responses may be seen following withdrawal from various medications and alcohol and in metabolic derangements (77,78).

The photoparoxysmal response must be contrasted with the noncerebral, nonepileptogenic, photomyogenic response to photic stimulation. Brief muscle spikes and eye movement artifacts are time-locked to the photic flashes that cease when the stimulus is discontinued (79). Again, this response is best seen at flash frequencies of 8 to 15 Hz. The EEG artifacts may show recruitment, that is, become more prominent as the stimulus continues, and may be attenuated with eye opening. Myoclonic or oscillatory movements of the eyes may accompany the photomyogenic response, which is seen mainly in adults and is related to nervousness, as well as to drug and alcohol withdrawal (79).

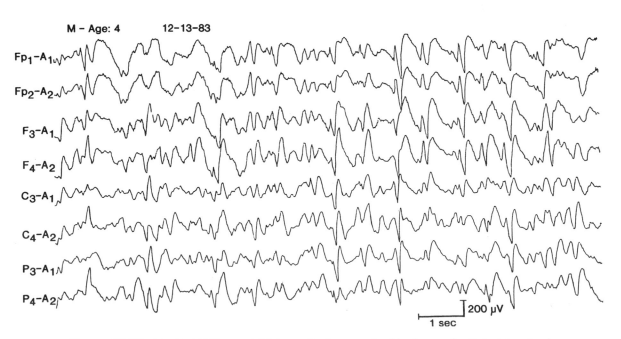

Figure 12.13   Interictal EEG reveals high-amplitude generalized background activity intermixed with multifocal spike discharges (hypsarrhythmia) in a child with infantile spasms. (Courtesy of B.F. Westmoreland, Mayo Clinic, Rochester, MN.)

SPECIAL ELECTROENCEPHALOGRAPHIC PATTERNS IN NEWBORNS AND INFANTS

Neonatal Recording

Ictal EEG seizure discharges in neonates may vary in frequency, amplitude, morphology, and duration. These paroxysms of rhythmic sharp-wave discharges or rhythmic activity in the θ-, α-, or β-frequency ranges may occur in a focal or multifocal distribution (Fig. 12.12). The seizure discharges may shift from one location to another. The epileptiform activity may be associated with clinical seizures; however, subclinical EEG phenomena without an observed clinical accompaniment are common. The interictal background activity is prognostically important in this population. Neonatal seizures associated with symptomatic neurologic disease such as anoxic encephalopathy may feature a low-voltage background abnormality or a burst-suppression pattern indicative of a poor prognosis.

Hypsarrhythmia

Hypsarrhythmia is a chaotic mixture of high-amplitude (exceeding 300 mV), generalized, continuous, arrhythmic slow-wave activity intermixed with spike and multifocal spike discharges (Fig. 12.13) (29,74,80). Nearly continuous during wakefulness, it becomes more discontinuous during NREM sleep, with high-voltage spikes and sharp waves alternating with lower-voltage irregular slow-wave activity (80). Epileptiform activity decreases during rapid eye movement sleep (81). The specific interictal EEG alteration usually resolves between 2.5 and 3 years of age and may not predict neurologic outcome (80,81). Hypsarrhythmia occurs most commonly from 4 months to 5 years of age in children with infantile spasms (West syndrome). Nevertheless, not all patients with infantile spasms have this EEG alteration, and not all patients with hypsarrhythmia have infantile spasms. Infantile spasms may be symptomatic (cause can be determined) or cryptogenic (cause is unknown); however, the EEG cannot distinguish one etiology from another (80,81). The hypsarrhythmic pattern likely represents a response of the immature brain to a variety of disturbances in cerebral function.

REFERENCES

1. Daly DD. Epilepsy and syncope. In: Pedley TA, Daly DD, eds. *Current practice of clinical electroencephalography*. New York: Raven Press, 1990:269–334.
2. Gibbs FA, Gibbs EL, Lennox WG. Epilepsy: a paroxysmal cerebral dysrhythmia. *Brain* 1937;60:377–388.
3. Quesney LF. Extracranial EEG evaluation. In: Engel J Jr, ed. *Surgical treatment of the epilepsies*. New York: Raven Press, 1987:129–166.
4. Gastaut H. Clinical and electroencephalographic classification of epileptic seizures. *Epilepsia* 1970;11:102–113.
5. Kellaway P. The incidence, significance and natural history of spike foci in children. In: Henry CE, ed. *Current clinical neurophysiology. Update of EEG and evoked potentials*. New York: Elsevier, 1980:151–175.
6. King DW, Ajmone-Marsan C. Clinical features and ictal patterns in epileptic patients with EEG temporal lobe foci. *Ann Neurol* 1977;2:138–147.
7. Niedermeyer E, da Silva FL. Abnormal EEG patterns (epileptic and paroxysmal). In: *Electroencephalography: basic principles, clinical applications, and related fields*, 2nd ed. Baltimore, MD: Urban & Schwarzenberg, 1987:183–207.
8. Pedley TA. Interictal epileptiform discharges: discriminating characteristics and clinical correlations. *Am J EEG Technol* 1980;20:101–119.
9. Penfield W, Jasper H, eds. *Epilepsy and the functional anatomy of the brain*. Boston: Little, Brown, 1954.
10. Sharbrough FW. Commentary: extracranial EEG monitoring. In: Engel J Jr, ed. *Surgical treatment of the epilepsies*. New York: Raven Press, 1987:167–171.
11. Westmoreland BF. The electroencephalogram in patients with epilepsy. In: Aminoff MJ, ed. *Neurology clinics*. Philadelphia: WB Saunders, 1985:599–613.
12. Williamson PD, Spencer DD, Spencer SS. Complex partial seizures of frontal lobe origin. *Ann Neurol* 1985;18:497–504.
13. Williamson PD, Weiser H-G, Delgado-Escueta AV. Clinical characteristics of partial seizures. In: Engel J Jr, ed. *Surgical treatment of the epilepsies*. New York: Raven Press, 1987:101–120.
14. Risinger MW, Engel J Jr, Van Ness PC, et al. Ictal localization of temporal lobe seizures with scalp-sphenoidal recordings. *Neurology* 1989;39:1288–1293.
15. Sharbrough FW. Complex partial seizures. In: Lüders H, Lesser RP, eds. *Epilepsy: electroclinical syndromes*. Berlin: Springer-Verlag, 1987:279–302.
16. Engel J Jr. Epileptic seizures. In: Engel J Jr, ed. *Seizures and epilepsy*. Philadelphia: FA Davis, 1989:137–178.
17. Quesney LF, Gloor P. Localization of epileptic foci. *Electroencephalogr Clin Neurophysiol* 1985;37(Suppl):165–200.
18. Berger H. Uber das Elektrenkephalogram des menschen. *Arch Psychiatry* 1933;100:301–320.
19. Jackson JH. In: Taylor J, ed. *Selected writings of John Hughlings Jackson on epilepsy and epileptiform conditions, I*. London: Hodder and Stoughton, 1931.
20. Gibbs FA, Davis H, Lennox WG. The electroencephalogram in epilepsy and in conditions of impaired consciousness. *Arch Neurol Psychiatry* 1935;34:1133–1148.
21. Gibbs EL, Gibbs FA. Diagnostic and localizing value of electroencephalographic studies in sleep. *Res Publ Assoc Res Nerv Ment Dis* 1947;23:366–376.
22. Zivin L, Ajmone-Marsan C. Incidence and prognostic significance of epileptiform activity in the EEG of nonepileptic subjects. *Brain* 1969;91:751–778.
23. Gloor P. Postscript: when are noninvasive tests enough? In: Engel J Jr, ed. *Surgical treatment of the epilepsies*. New York: Raven Press, 1987:259–261.
24. Andermann FA. Identification of candidates for surgical treatment of epilepsy. In: Engel J Jr, ed. *Surgical treatment of the epilepsies*. New York: Raven Press, 1987:51–70.
25. Quesney LF, Constain M, Fish DR, et al. Frontal lobe epilepsy: a field of recent emphasis. *Am J EEG Technol* 1990;30:177–193.
26. Gloor P. Preoperative electroencephalographic investigation in temporal lobe epilepsy: extracranial and intracranial recordings. *Can J Neurol Sci* 1991;18:554–558.
27. Guidelines in electroencephalography, evoked potentials and polysomnography. *J Clin Neurophysiol* 1994;2:1.
28. Ellingson RJ, Wilken K, Beenet DR. Efficacy of sleep deprivation as an activation procedure in epilepsy patients. *J Clin Neurophysiol* 1984;2:83–101.
29. Gibbs FA, Gibbs EL. *Atlas of electroencephalography, II*, 2nd ed. Cambridge, MA: Addison-Wesley, 1952.
30. Ajmone-Marsan C, Zivin LS. Factors related to the occurrence of typical paroxysmal abnormalities in the EEG records of epileptic patients. *Epilepsia* 1970;11:361–381.
31. Gotman J, Koffler DJ. Interictal spiking increases after seizures but does not after decrease in medication. *Electroencephalogr Clin Neurophysiol* 1989;72:7–15.
32. Gotman J, Marciani MG. Electroencephalographic spiking activity, drug levels, and seizure occurrence in epileptic patients. *Ann Neurol* 1985;17:597–603.

33. Gotman J, Gloor P. Automatic recognition and quantification of interictal epileptic activity in the human scalp EEG. *Electroencephalogr Clin Neurophysiol* 1976;41:513–529.
34. Sharbrough FW. Electrical fields and recording techniques. In: Daly D, Pedley TA, eds. *Current practice of clinical electroencephalography*. New York: Raven Press, 1990:29–49.
35. Sperling MR, Engel J Jr. Comparison of nasopharyngeal with scalp electrodes including ear and true temporal electrodes in the detection of spikes. *Electroencephalogr Clin Neurophysiol* 1984;58:39.
36. Lüders H, Hahn J, Lesser RP, et al. Localization of epileptogenic spike foci: comparative study of closely spaced scalp electrodes, nasopharyngeal, sphenoidal, subdural and depth electrodes. In: Akimoto H, Kazamatsuri H, Seino M, et al, eds. *XIIIth epilepsy international symposium*. New York: Raven Press, 1984:185–189.
37. Abraham D, Ajmone-Marsan C. Patterns of cortical discharges and their relation to routine scalp electroencephalography. *Electroencephalogr Clin Neurophysiol* 1958;10:447–461.
38. Ojemann GA, Engel J Jr. Acute and chronic intracranial recording and stimulation. In: Engel J Jr, ed. *Surgical treatment of the epilepsies*. New York: Raven Press, 1987:263–288.
39. Maulsby RL. EEG patterns of uncertain diagnostic significance. In: Klass DW, Daly DD, eds. *Current practice of clinical electroencephalography*. New York: Raven Press, 1979:411–419.
40. Reiher J, Beaudry M, Leduc CP. Temporal intermittent rhythmic delta activity (TIRDA) in the diagnosis of complex partial epilepsy: sensitivity, specificity, and predictive value. *Can J Neurol Sci* 1989;16:389–401.
41. Reiher J, Lebel M. Wicket spikes: clinical correlates of a previously undescribed EEG pattern. *Can J Neurol Sci* 1977;4:39–47.
42. Thomas JE, Klass DW. Six-per-second spike and wave pattern in the electroencephalogram. *Neurology* 1968;18:587–593.
43. White JC, Langston JW, Pedley TA. Benign epileptiform transients of sleep: clarification of the "small sharp spike" controversy. *Neurology* 1977;27:1061–1068.
44. Reiher J, Lebel M, Klass DW. Small sharp spikes (SSS): reassessment of electroencephalographic characteristics and clinical significance [abstract]. *Electroencephalogr Clin Neurophysiol* 1977;23:755.
45. Eeg-Olofson O, Petersen I, Sellden V. The development of the electroencephalogram in normal children from the age of one through fifteen years. *Neuropaediatrie* 1971;4:375–404.
46. Schwartzkroin PA, Wyler AR. Mechanisms underlying epileptiform burst discharges. *Ann Neurol* 1980;7:95–107.
47. International Federation of Society for Electroencephalography and Clinical Neurophysiology. *Electroencephalography and clinical neurophysiology*. New York: Elsevier, 1974.
48. de la Paz D, Brenner RP. Bilateral independent periodic epileptiform discharges. *Arch Neurol* 1981;38:713–715.
49. Chatrian GE, Shaw CM, Leffman H. The significance of periodic, lateralized epileptiform discharges in EEG: an electrographic, clinical and pathological study. *Electroencephalogr Clin Neurophysiol* 1964;17:177–193.
50. Reiher J, Rivest J, Grand'Maison F, et al. Periodic lateralized epileptiform discharges with transitional rhythmic discharges: association with seizures. *Electroencephalogr Clin Neurophysiol* 1991;78:12–17.
51. Westmoreland BF, Klass DW, Sharbrough FW. Chronic periodic lateralized epileptiform discharges. *Arch Neurol* 1986;43:494–496.
52. Gastaut H. A new type of epilepsy: benign partial epilepsy of childhood with occipital spike-waves. *Clin Electroencephalogr* 1982;13:13–22.
53. Sperling MR, Sutherling WW, Nuwer MR. New techniques for evaluating patients for epilepsy surgery. In: Engel J Jr, ed. *Surgical treatment of the epilepsies*. New York: Raven Press, 1987:235–257.
54. Williamson PD, Spencer SS. Clinical and EEG features of complex partial seizures of extratemporal origin. *Epilepsia* 1986;27(Suppl 2):S46–S63.
55. Devinsky O, Sato S, Kufta CV, et al. Electroencephalographic studies of simple partial seizures with subdural electrode recordings. *Neurology* 1989;39:527–533.
56. Gastaut H, Broughton R. Epileptic seizures: clinical features and pathophysiology. In: Gastaut H, Broughton R, eds. *Epileptic seizures*. Springfield, IL: Charles C Thomas, 1972:25–140.
57. Gabor AJ, Ajmone-Marsan C. Coexistence of focal and bilateral diffuse paroxysmal discharge in epileptics. *Epilepsia* 1969;29 (Suppl 2):S15–S34.
58. Klass DW. Electroencephalographic manifestations of complex partial seizures. *Adv Neurol* 1975;11:113–140.
59. Swartz BE, Walsh GO, Delgado-Escueta AV, et al. Surface ictal electroencephalographic patterns in frontal vs temporal lobe epilepsy. *Can J Neurol Sci* 1991;18:649–662.
60. Wyllie E, Lüders H, Morris HH, et al. Clinical outcome after complete or partial resection for intractable partial epilepsy. *Neurology* 1987;33:1634–1641.
61. Williamson PD. Intensive monitoring of complex partial seizures: diagnosis and classification. *Adv Neurol* 1987;46:69–84.
62. Rasmussen T. Characteristics of a pure culture of frontal lobe epilepsy. *Epilepsia* 1983;24:482–493.
63. Tharp BR. Orbital frontal seizures. A unique electroencephalographic and clinical syndrome. *Epilepsia* 1972;13:627–642.
64. Tukel K, Jasper H. The electroencephalogram in parasagittal lesions. *Electroencephalogr Clin Neurophysiol* 1952;4:481–494.
65. Fegersten L, Roger A. Frontal epileptogenic foci and their clinical correlations. *Electroencephalogr Clin Neurophysiol* 1961;13:905–913.
66. Gibbs FA, Gibbs EL. *Atlas of electroencephalography, IV*. Reading, MA: Addison-Wesley, 1978.
67. Lombroso CT. Sylvian seizures and midtemporal spike foci in children. *Arch Neurol* 1967;17:52–59.
68. Beaussart M. Benign epilepsy of children with rolandic (centrotemporal) paroxysmal foci. A clinical entity. Study of 221 cases. *Epilepsia* 1972;13:795–811.
69. Avoli M, Gloor P. Interaction of cortex and thalamus in spike and wave discharges of feline generalized penicillin epilepsy. *Exp Neurol* 1982;64:155–173.
70. Dalby MA. Epilepsy and 3 per second spike and wave rhythms. *Acta Neurol Scand* 1969;45(Suppl 40):1–180.
71. Sato S, Dreifuss FE, Penry JK. The effect of sleep on spike-wave discharges in absence seizures. *Neurology* 1973;23:1335–1345.
72. Gibbs FA, Gibbs EL. *Atlas of electroencephalography, III*, 2nd ed. Reading, MA: Addison-Wesley Publishing, 1964.
73. Blume WT, David RB, Gomez MR. Generalized sharp and slow wave complexes—associated clinical features and long-term follow-up. *Brain* 1973;289:306.
74. Gastaut H, Roger J, Soulayrol R, et al. Childhood epileptic encephalography with diffuse slow spike-waves (otherwise known as "petit mal variant") or Lennox syndrome. *Epilepsia* 1966;7:139–179.
75. Markand O. Slow spike and wave activity in EEG and associated clinical features: often called "Lennox-Gastaut" syndrome. *Neurology* 1977;25:463–471.
76. Newmark ME, Penry KJ. *Photosensitivity and epilepsy. A review*. New York: Raven Press, 1979.
77. Fisch BJ, Hauser WA, Brust JCM, et al. The EEG response to diffuse and patterned photic stimulation during acute untreated alcohol withdrawal. *Neurology* 1989;39:434–436.
78. Jeavons PM, Harding GFA. *Photosensitive epilepsy. A review of the literature and a study of 460 patients*. London: Heinemann, 1975.
79. Meier-Ewert K, Broughton RJ. Photomyoclonic response of epileptic and nonepileptic subjects during wakefulness, sleep, and arousal. *Electroencephalogr Clin Neurophysiol* 1976;23:301–304.
80. Hrachovy RA, Frost JD Jr, Kellaway P. Hypsarrhythmia: variations on a theme. *Epilepsia* 1984;35:317–325.
81. Hrachovy RA, Frost JD Jr, Kellaway P. Sleep characteristics in infantile spasms. *Neurology* 1981;31:688–694.

Electroencephalographic Atlas of Epileptiform Abnormalities

13

Soheyl Noachtar   Elaine Wyllie

Electroencephalography (EEG) is generally considered the single most important laboratory tool in the evaluation of patients with epilepsy. This atlas of material from patients seen at the Cleveland Clinic Foundation illustrates some of the EEG findings discussed throughout this book. Additional EEG atlases and textbooks are listed in the bibliography at the end of this chapter.

METHODS

These tracings were made following American Electroencephalographic Society guidelines (1), with electrodes placed according to the International 10–20 Electrode Placement System (2). Additional closely spaced electrodes (Fig. 13.1) were used in some cases to better define a focal epileptogenic zone. The combinatorial electrode nomenclature used here is that recently proposed by the American Electroencephalographic Society (3) and the International Federation of Clinical Neurophysiology (4).

For consistency and ease of interpretation, we displayed most tracings with the same longitudinal bipolar montage (Fig. 13.2). Occasionally, the activity was best shown with a transverse bipolar montage (Fig. 13.3), a longitudinal bipolar montage with anterior temporal or sphenoidal electrodes (Fig. 13.2), or a referential montage.

PART I: NORMAL EEG PATTERNS AND VARIANTS SOMETIMES CONFUSED WITH EPILEPTIFORM ACTIVITY

For epileptologists to fulfill the basic obligation to "do no harm," they must avoid "overreading" normal variants on EEG (5,6). This section includes several normal patterns that may be easily mistaken for epileptiform discharges, resulting in an incorrect diagnosis of epilepsy and inappropriate recommendations for antiepileptic medication.

Small sharp spike	Figure 13.4
14- and 6-Hz positive spikes	Figure 13.5
6-Hz "phantom" spike and wave	Figure 13.6
Wicket spikes	Figure 13.7
Subclinical rhythmical electrographic discharges of adults	Figure 13.8
Rhythmic temporal theta bursts of drowsiness	Figure 13.9
Hypnagogic hypersynchrony	Figure 13.10
V-waves and positive occipital sharp transients (POSTS)	Figure 13.11
Sleep spindle	Figure 13.12
Hyperventilation effect	Figure 13.13
Photic driving	Figure 13.14
Breach rhythm	Figure 13.15

PART II: ELECTROENCEPHALOGRAM ABNORMALITIES OF THE GENERALIZED EPILEPSIES

Childhood Absence Epilepsy

Absence seizure	Figures 13.16 and 13.17
Absence status epilepticus	Figures 13.18 and 13.19

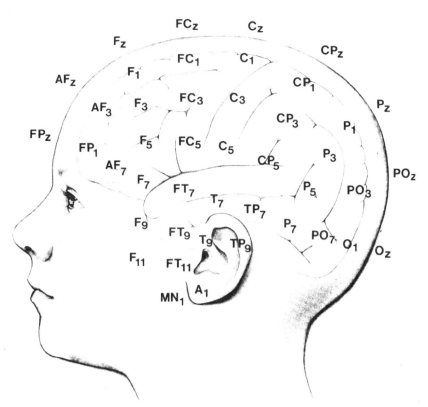

Figure 13.1 Electrode positions and nomenclature of the combinatorial system proposed by the American Electroencephalographic Society. (Adapted from Sharbrough F, Chatrian GE, Lesser RP, et al. American EEG Society: Guidelines for standard electrode position nomenclature. *J Clin Neurophysiol* 1991;8:200–202, with permission.)

Juvenile Myoclonic Epilepsy

Myoclonic jerk with photic stimulation	Figure 13.20
Cluster of myoclonic jerks	Figure 13.21

Infantile Spasms

Hypsarrhythmia	Figure 13.22
Seizure	Figure 13.23

Lennox-Gastaut Syndrome

Generalized sharp- and slow-wave complexes	Figure 13.24

Generalized paroxysmal fast and polyspikes in sleep	Figure 13.25
Atonic seizures	Figure 13.26

Intractable Epilepsy with Multifocal Spikes

Intractable epilepsy with multifocal spikes	Figure 13.27

Stimulation-Related Epilepsy

Reading-induced spike-and-wave complexes	Figure 13.28

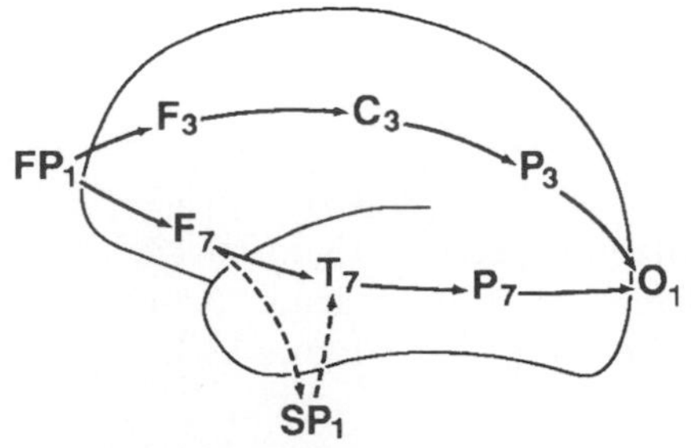

Figure 13.2 Longitudinal bipolar montages, left-sided electrodes. The "double-banana" montage used for almost all the tracings in this atlas includes the channels shown with *filled arrows*, ordered as follows: left temporal chain, right temporal chain, left parasagittal chain, and right parasagittal chain. The "anterior temporal" montage used in some of the tracings is modified to include the channels shown with *broken arrows* to reflect anterior, basal, or mesial temporal discharges.

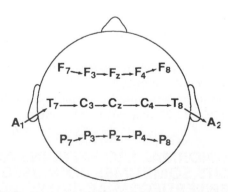

Figure 13.3 Transverse bipolar montage, vertex view. Channels are arrayed in order, as follows: frontal chain, temporocentral chain, and parietal chain.

PART III: ELECTROENCEPHALOGRAM ABNORMALITIES OF THE FOCAL EPILEPSIES

Localization-related (partial, focal, or local) epilepsies (7) involve seizures arising from a cortical region within one hemisphere. The first several illustrations are from children who had benign epileptiform discharges of childhood on EEG, with or without clinical seizures. The rest of the figures are from patients with symptomatic epilepsy and focal seizures arising from specific cortical regions, grouped by location of the epileptogenic zone. For most of the titles and legends, we use terminology from the most recent seizure and epilepsy classification systems of the International League Against Epilepsy (7,8). Some additional terms are also used here, such as "aura" instead of "simple partial seizure with special sensory symptoms" and "focal clonic seizure" instead of "simple partial seizure with focal motor signs." Some newer terms were also included; these are discussed further in Chapter 14.

Benign Focal Epileptiform Discharges of Childhood

Centrotemporal sharp waves	Figure 13.29
Dipole potential	Figure 13.30
Occipital sharp waves	Figure 13.31
Left and right central sharp waves	Figure 13.32

Temporal Lobe Epilepsy

Temporal sharp wave	Figure 13.33
Complex partial ("hypomotor") seizure	Figure 13.34
Bitemporal sharp waves	Figures 13.35 and 13.36
Complex partial seizure with automatisms	Figures 13.37 and 13.38

Frontal Lobe Epilepsy

Frontal sharp waves	Figure 13.39
Secondary bilateral synchrony	Figure 13.40
Subclinical EEG seizure	Figures 13.41 and 13.42

Occipital Lobe Epilepsy

Visual aura and focal clonic seizure	Figures 13.43 and 13.44

Supplementary Motor Area Epilepsy

Sharp waves at vertex	Figure 13.45
Tonic seizure	Figure 13.46

Perirolandic Epilepsy

Focal clonic seizure	Figures 13.47 and 13.48
Right frontocentral sharp waves	Figure 13.49
Left arm tonic seizure	Figure 13.50
Epilepsia partialis continua	Figure 13.51

PART IV: ELECTROENCEPHALOGRAPH FINDINGS IN NONEPILEPTIC PAROXYSMAL DISORDERS

The differential diagnosis of epilepsy includes a wide variety of paroxysmal disorders (see Chapter 43). During a clinical episode, the EEG recording may be crucial to clarifying the exact nature of the spells. In most of these disorders, the ictal electroencephalogram is normal. Three nonepileptic paroxysmal disorders with abnormal EEG findings are syncope, breath-holding spells, and sleep attacks caused by narcolepsy.

Pallid infantile syncope	Figures 13.52 and 13.53
Cyanotic breath-holding spell	Figures 13.54 and 13.55
Narcolepsy	Figure 13.56

SMALL SHARP SPIKE

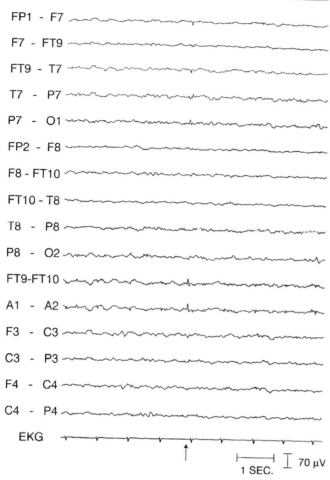

EKG

↑

1 SEC.   70 μV

Figure 13.4 Thirty-five-year-old woman, otherwise normal, with chronic headache. Note the low-amplitude monophasic sharp transient (*arrow*) followed by a minimal slow wave, maximum negativity in the left temporal region, undisturbed background rhythms, and occurrence during light sleep. Small, sharp spikes have also been called benign epileptiform transients of sleep (9).

14-HZ AND 6-HZ POSITIVE SPIKES

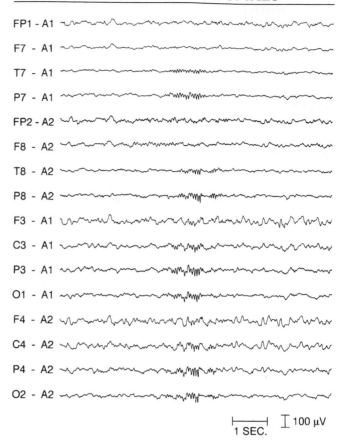

1 SEC.   100 μV

Figure 13.5 Fourteen-year-old boy, otherwise normal, with nonepileptic episodes of dizziness. Note the burst of sharply contoured 14-Hz activity with maximum positivity posteriorly, occurring in light sleep (10,11). Elsewhere in the recording were similar bursts with predominantly 6-Hz frequency. Positive spikes of 14- and 6-Hz have also been called ctenoids.

6-HZ "PHANTOM" SPIKE AND WAVE

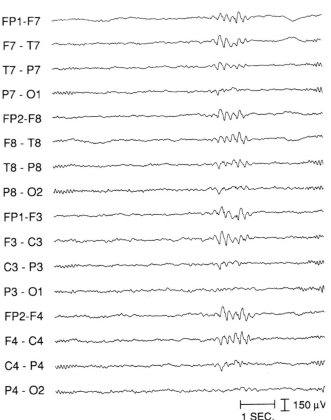

Figure 13.6 Fourteen-year-old boy with muscle contraction headaches, dizziness, and syncope. Note the generalized burst of 6-Hz low-amplitude spikes with prominent slow waves occurring during drowsiness (6).

WICKET SPIKES

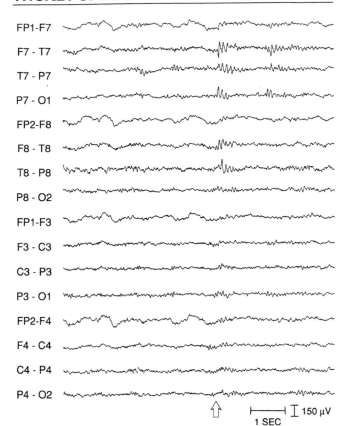

Figure 13.7 Seventy-five-year-old woman with gait disturbance and no seizures. Note the 9-Hz, rhythmic, sharply contoured waves with maximum negativity in midtemporal regions, occurrence during drowsiness, and undisturbed background rhythms. The typical frequency of wicket spikes is 6- to 11-Hz (12).

SUBCLINICAL RHYTHMICAL ELECTROGRAPHIC DISCHARGES OF ADULTS

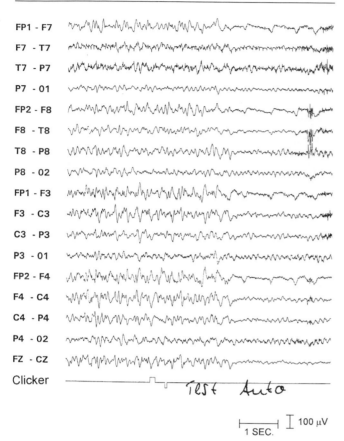

| FP1 - F7 |
| F7 - T7 |
| T7 - P7 |
| P7 - 01 |
| FP2 - F8 |
| F8 - T8 |
| T8 - P8 |
| P8 - 02 |
| FP1 - F3 |
| F3 - C3 |
| C3 - P3 |
| P3 - 01 |
| FP2 - F4 |
| F4 - C4 |
| C4 - P4 |
| P4 - 02 |
| FZ - CZ |
| Clicker |

1 SEC.   100 µV

Figure 13.8 Sixty-one-year-old woman with depression. Note the diffuse frontal-maximum, rhythmic, sharply contoured theta and delta activity (13) that ended after 34 seconds and was immediately followed by a normal posterior-dominant alpha rhythm. During the rhythmic activity, the patient responded appropriately to an auditory stimulus (clicker). In the last channel, the upward deflection was from the technician's sound stimulus, and the subsequent downward deflection was from the button pressed by the patient in response. The patient remained awake and responsive throughout the recording and afterward recalled the test word ("auto").

RHYTHMICAL TEMPORAL THETA BURSTS OF DROWSINESS

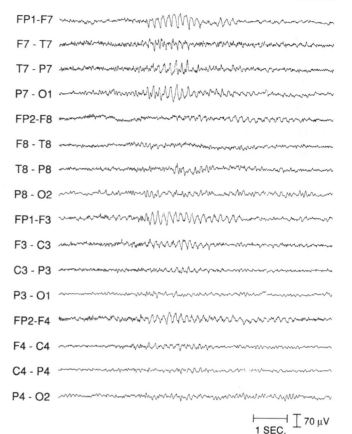

| FP1-F7 |
| F7 - T7 |
| T7 - P7 |
| P7 - O1 |
| FP2-F8 |
| F8 - T8 |
| T8 - P8 |
| P8 - O2 |
| FP1-F3 |
| F3 - C3 |
| C3 - P3 |
| P3 - O1 |
| FP2-F4 |
| F4 - C4 |
| C4 - P4 |
| P4 - O2 |

1 SEC.   70 µV

Figure 13.9 Sixty-year-old man with a single transient ischemic attack involving the right hemisphere. This rhythmic theta activity during drowsiness, with sharply contoured waves maximal in the left midtemporal region, has also been called psychomotor variant (6,14).

HYPNAGOGIC HYPERSYNCHRONY

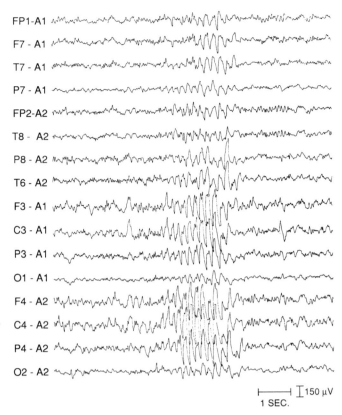

Figure 13.10 One-and-a-half-year-old normal boy. Note the generalized, rhythmic, high-amplitude theta activity with intermixed sharp transients during drowsiness.

V-WAVES AND POSITIVE OCCIPITAL SHARP TRANSIENTS

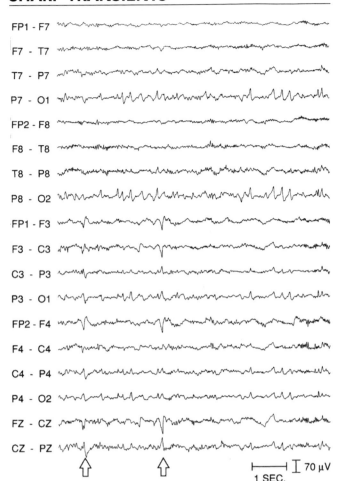

Figure 13.11 Sixteen-year-old girl with vasovagal syncope. Note the central vertex waves (*arrows*) and runs of positive occipital sharp transients (channels 4 and 8), both normal features of stage I or II nonrapid eye movement sleep.

SLEEP SPINDLE

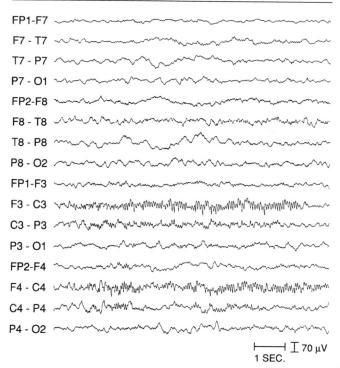

Figure 13.12 Two-month-old normal infant. Prolonged spindles with 12-Hz mu-like waveforms are common in infants during stage II nonrapid eye movement sleep and may be asynchronous over the right and left hemispheres.

HYPERVENTILATION EFFECT

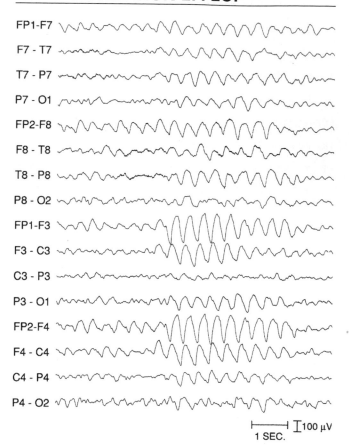

Figure 13.13 Eight-year-old girl with school problems. She was misdiagnosed as having absence epilepsy because of hyperventilation-induced high-amplitude rhythmic slowing. The girl was alert and responsive during this tracing, which was obtained after 2 minutes of hyperventilation.

PHOTIC DRIVING

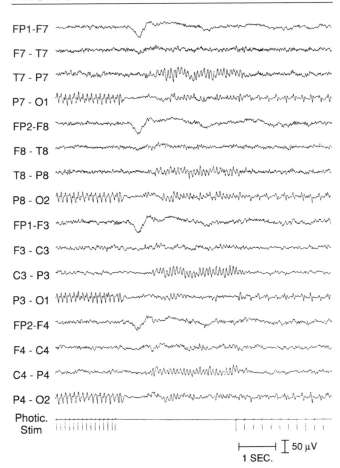

FP1-F7

F7 - T7

T7 - P7

P7 - O1

FP2-F8

F8 - T8

T8 - P8

P8 - O2

FP1-F3

F3 - C3

C3 - P3

P3 - O1

FP2-F4

F4 - C4

C4 - P4

P4 - O2

Photic. Stim

1 SEC.   50 µV

Figure 13.14 Twelve-year-old boy with childhood absence epilepsy since 4 years of age, seizure free on medication for the last 1.5 years. Note the time-locked, unsustained, bioccipital response to 8- and 4-Hz photic stimulation, separated by normal posterior background activity.

BREACH RHYTHM

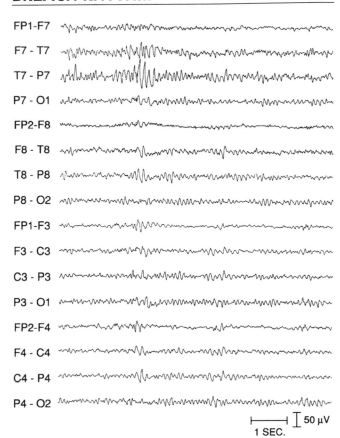

FP1-F7

F7 - T7

T7 - P7

P7 - O1

FP2-F8

F8 - T8

T8 - P8

P8 - O2

FP1-F3

F3 - C3

C3 - P3

P3 - O1

FP2-F4

F4 - C4

C4 - P4

P4 - O2

1 SEC.   50 µV

Figure 13.15 Twenty-one-year-old woman with trigeminal neuralgia, status after left parietotemporal craniotomy for vascular decompression. Note the asymmetry of background rhythms owing to the skull defect (15), maximum at the T_7 electrode.

CHILDHOOD ABSENCE EPILEPSY: ABSENCE SEIZURE

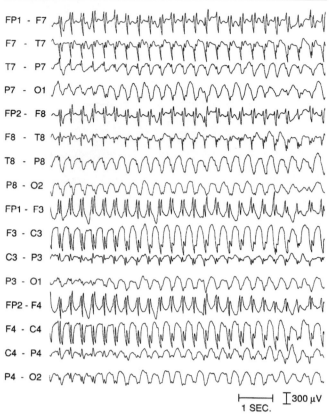

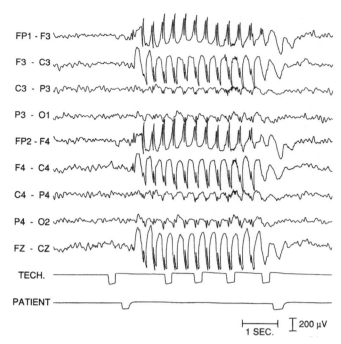

Figure 13.16 Eight-year-old girl, otherwise normal, with recent onset of absence seizures. This seizure with generalized 3-Hz spike-and-wave complexes was precipitated by hyperventilation and lasted for 25 seconds, with staring and unresponsiveness.

Figure 13.17 Fifteen-year-old girl with absence and rare generalized tonic-clonic seizures since age 10 years. Note the patient's unresponsiveness until the end of the 4-second burst, demonstrated by failure to respond to auditory stimuli from a clicker.

ABSENCE STATUS EPILEPTICUS: GENERALIZED POLYSPIKE-AND-WAVE COMPLEXES

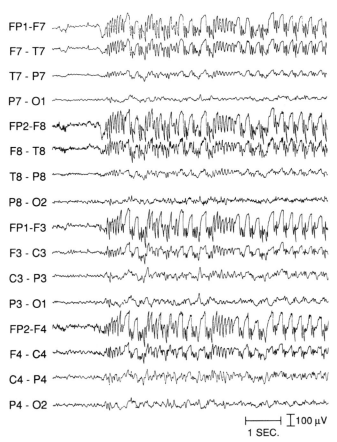

Figure 13.18 Forty-three-year-old woman with absence seizures during childhood. She was seizure free throughout adulthood until absence status epilepticus began during chemotherapy for breast cancer. During this episode, with generalized polyspike-and-wave complexes, she had unresponsiveness and eyelid fluttering. Electroencephalographic findings and behavior returned to normal after intravenous injection of diazepam.

ABSENCE STATUS EPILEPTICUS: GENERALIZED SHARP AND SLOW WAVE COMPLEXES

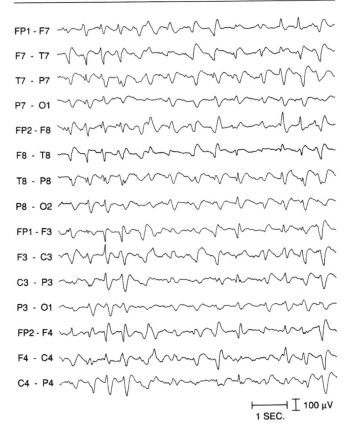

Figure 13.19 Fifty-eight-year-old woman with a 3-day history of confusion and agitation prior to this electroencephalogram (EEG). She had no previous history of seizures, and this was her first manifestation of generalized absence epilepsy. EEG findings and behavior returned to normal after intravenous injection of diazepam.

JUVENILE MYOCLONIC EPILEPSY: MYOCLONIC JERK WITH PHOTIC STIMULATION

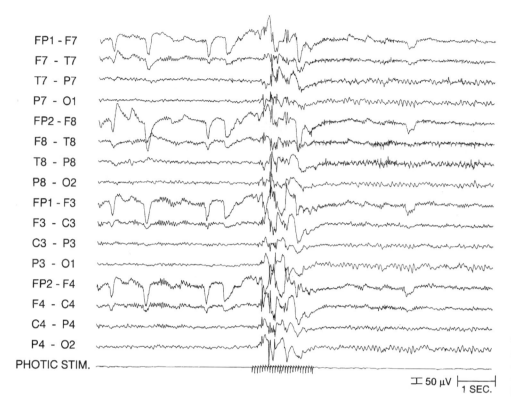

Figure 13.20 Fifteen-year-old boy with an 8-month history of myoclonic jerks of the upper extremities in the morning after awakening. A generalized tonic-clonic seizure occurred in the morning 2 weeks before this electroencephalogram. Note the poly-spike component of the spike-and-wave complexes during the myoclonic jerk precipitated by photic stimulation.

JUVENILE MYOCLONIC EPILEPSY: CLUSTER OF MYOCLONIC JERKS

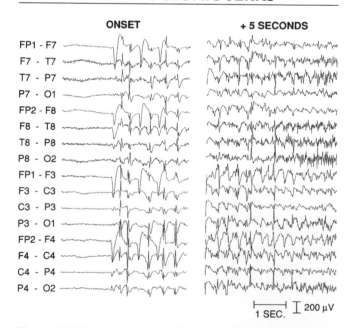

Figure 13.21 Thirty-two-year-old woman, otherwise normal, with myoclonic and generalized tonic-clonic seizures on awakening since adolescence. This episode began with repeated myoclonic jerks of the arms and upper body synchronous with the generalized spike-and-wave complexes. This flurry evolved after 20 seconds into a generalized tonic-clonic convulsion ("clonic-tonic-clonic seizure").

INFANTILE SPASMS: HYPSARRHYTHMIA

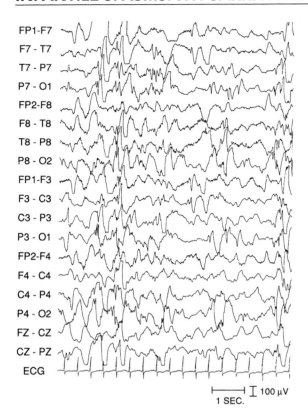

Figure 13.22   Eight-month-old boy with infantile spasms and developmental delay. Awake electroencephalographic record showed disorganized background rhythms dominated by multifocal spikes and high-amplitude slowing.

INFANTILE SPASMS: SEIZURE

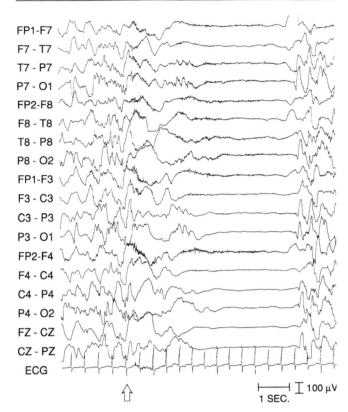

Figure 13.23   EEG during a spasm (*arrow*), from the same infant as in Figure 13.22. Note the generalized high-amplitude slow transient followed by a generalized electrodecremental pattern for 3 seconds. The spasm involved tonic abduction and extension of both arms with flexion of the trunk and neck.

LENNOX-GASTAUT SYNDROME: GENERALIZED SHARP- AND SLOW-WAVE COMPLEXES

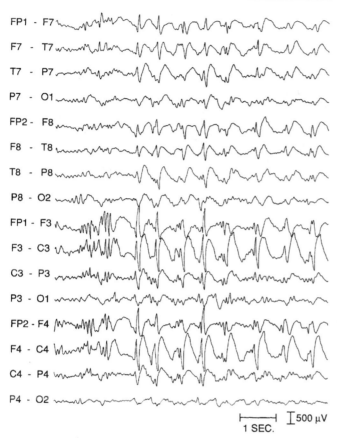

Figure 13.24 Six-year-old girl with developmental delay and intractable generalized tonic, tonic-clonic, and atypical absence seizures since age 3 years. Note the bifrontal polyspikes preceding the generalized sharp- and slow-wave complexes (5), also called slow spike-and-wave complexes.

LENNOX-GASTAUT SYNDROME: GENERALIZED PAROXYSMAL FAST AND POLYSPIKES IN SLEEP

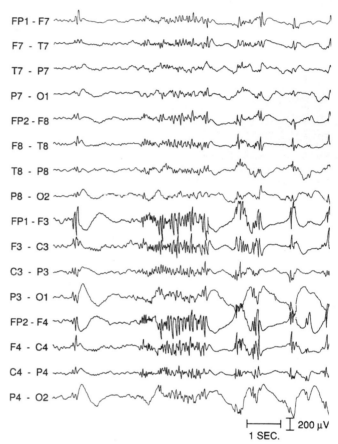

Figure 13.25 Eleven-year-old boy with moderately severe mental retardation and intractable generalized tonic, atonic, myoclonic, and atypical absence seizures since age 4 years. Awake EEG showed generalized sharp- and slow-wave complexes.

LENNOX-GASTAUT SYNDROME: ATONIC SEIZURES

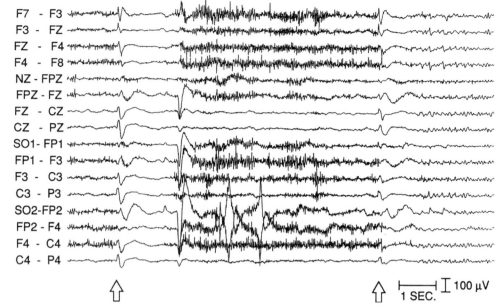

Figure 13.26 Forty-one-year-old man with borderline intelligence and intractable generalized tonic, atonic, generalized tonic-clonic, and atypical absence seizures since age 3 years. Interictal electroencephalogram showed generalized sharp- and slow-wave complexes, are recorded here, with limp head nodding plus tonic stiffening and elevation of both arms. Each seizure began with a generalized sharp wave (*arrows*) followed by attenuation of electroencephalograph activity and cessation of muscle artifact.

INTRACTABLE EPILEPSY WITH MULTIFOCAL SPIKES

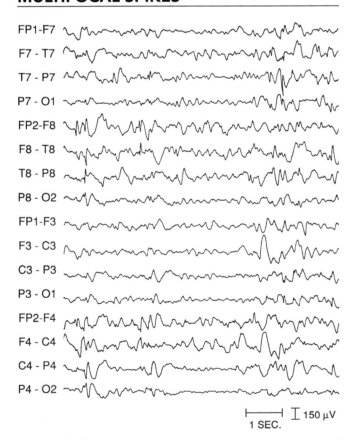

Figure 13.27 Three-year-old boy with developmental delay and intractable clusters of generalized tonic, myoclonic, and atypical absence seizures. This electroencephalographic pattern is not uncommon in children with clinical features similar to those of Lennox-Gastaut syndrome (16).

STIMULATION-RELATED EPILEPSY: READING-INDUCED SPIKE-AND-WAVE COMPLEXES

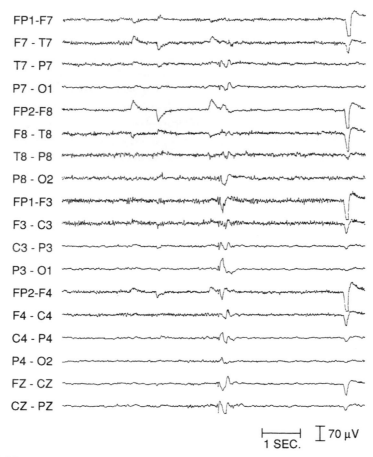

Figure 13.28 Twenty-seven-year-old woman with reading-induced brief myoclonic or (rarely) generalized tonic-clonic seizures since age 12 years (17). During this electroencephalography, the patient was reading; note the horizontal eye movement artifact. She consistently reported a feeling of "jerking" in her body and eyelids and "loss of function" in her arms whenever the electroencephalograph recorded an isolated spike-and-wave discharge, as shown here.

BENIGN FOCAL EPILEPTIFORM DISCHARGES OF CHILDHOOD: CENTROTEMPORAL SHARP WAVES

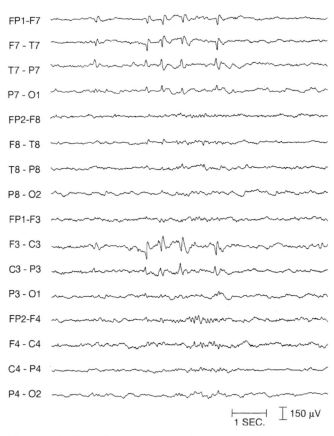

Figure 13.29 Eight-year-old boy with attention deficit hyperactivity disorder and no history of seizures. Awake electroencephalogram showed normal findings, but recording during drowsiness and light sleep showed left centrotemporal sharp waves (benign focal epileptiform discharges of childhood) (18). Many children with benign focal epileptiform discharges of childhood do not have seizures (18), and the finding may be incidental.

BENIGN FOCAL EPILEPTIFORM DISCHARGES OF CHILDHOOD: DIPOLE POTENTIALS

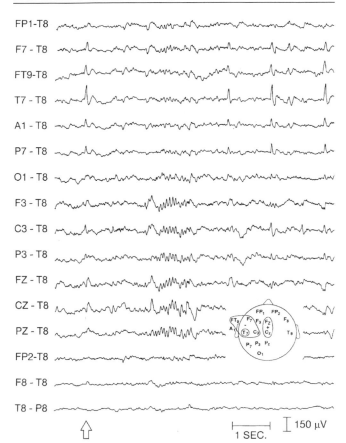

Figure 13.30 This referential electroencephalogram was from the patient described in Figure 13.29. Note that the sharp waves were reflected at the scalp as dipoles, with maximum negativity over the left centrotemporal region and maximum positivity over the vertex. Dipole potentials are typical of benign focal epileptiform discharges of childhood, possibly as a result of horizontal orientation along banks of the sylvian or rolandic fissures (18).

BENIGN EPILEPTIFORM DISCHARGES OF CHILDHOOD: OCCIPITAL SHARP WAVES

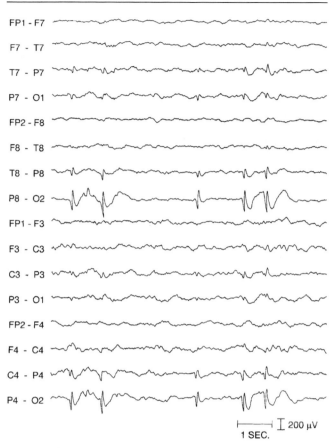

Figure 13.31 Eight-year-old boy with mild language delay and no history of seizures. The right occipital sharp waves with typical morphology of benign focal epileptiform discharges of childhood (18) were abundant in light sleep but rare during wakefulness.

BENIGN FOCAL EPILEPTIFORM DISCHARGES OF CHILDHOOD: LEFT AND RIGHT CENTRAL SHARP WAVES

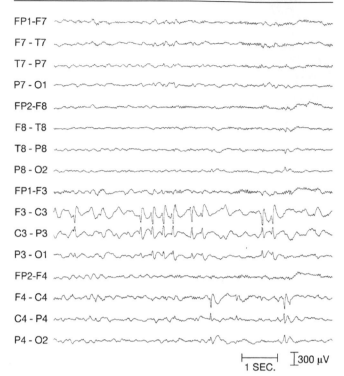

Figure 13.32 Eight-year-old boy, otherwise normal, with rare nocturnal generalized tonic-clonic convulsions since age 4 years. Benign focal epileptiform discharges of childhood are commonly bifocal or multifocal, often from homologous areas of both hemispheres (18).

TEMPORAL LOBE EPILEPSY: TEMPORAL SHARP WAVE

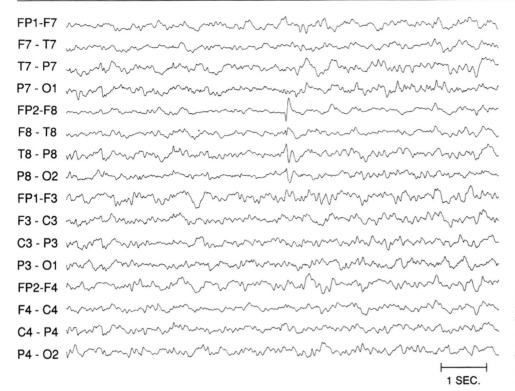

Figure 13.33 Twenty-three-year-old woman with complex partial seizures with automatisms since age 15. Interictal electroencephalogram showed sharp waves from the right anterior temporal region, with maximum amplitude at electrode F_8.

TEMPORAL LOBE EPILEPSY: COMPLEX PARTIAL ("HYPOMOTOR") SEIZURE

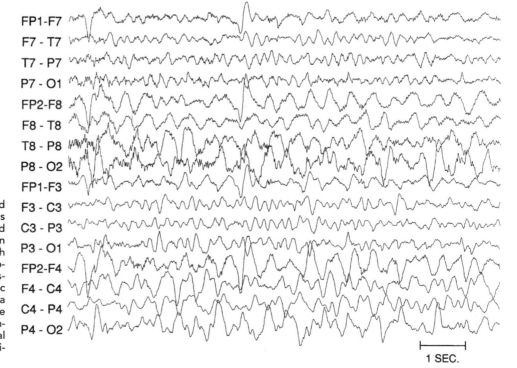

Figure 13.34 Sixteen-month-old girl with complex partial seizures since age 6 years. Episodes involved a subtle change of facial expression and decreased responsiveness with minimal or no automatisms ("hypomotor" symptomatology, as discussed in Chapter 14). Magnetic resonance imaging disclosed a large cystic ganglioglioma in the right temporal lobe. Ictal electroencephalogram showed paroxysmal delta activity in the right hemisphere.

TEMPORAL LOBE EPILEPSY: BITEMPORAL SHARP WAVES

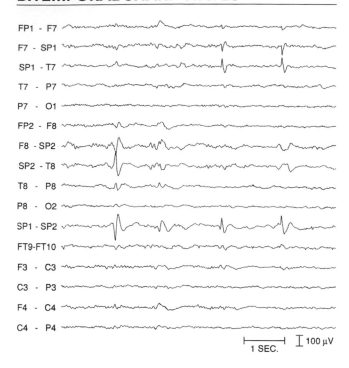

FP1 - F7
F7 - SP1
SP1 - T7
T7 - P7
P7 - O1
FP2 - F8
F8 - SP2
SP2 - T8
T8 - P8
P8 - O2
SP1 - SP2
FT9-FT10
F3 - C3
C3 - P3
F4 - C4
C4 - P4

1 SEC.   ⊥ 100 μV

Figure 13.35 Thirty-seven-year-old man with adult-onset complex partial seizures with automatisms. Interictal sharp waves were left or right temporal, maximal at sphenoidal electrodes. All recorded seizures were from the right temporal lobe.

BITEMPORAL SHARP WAVES

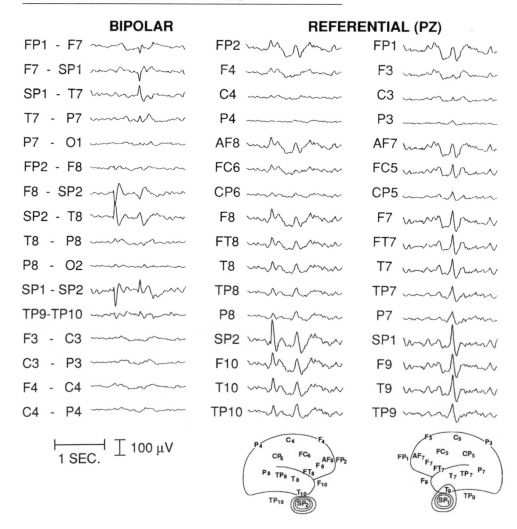

BIPOLAR

FP1 - F7
F7 - SP1
SP1 - T7
T7 - P7
P7 - O1
FP2 - F8
F8 - SP2
SP2 - T8
T8 - P8
P8 - O2
SP1 - SP2
TP9-TP10
F3 - C3
C3 - P3
F4 - C4
C4 - P4

1 SEC.   ⊥ 100 μV

REFERENTIAL (PZ)

FP2   FP1
F4   F3
C4   C3
P4   P3
AF8   AF7
FC6   FC5
CP6   CP5
F8   F7
FT8   FT7
T8   T7
TP8   TP7
P8   P7
SP2   SP1
F10   F9
T10   T9
TP10   TP9

Figure 13.36 Two-second sample of electroencephalogram from the patient in Figure 13.35, showing the distribution of the left and right temporal sharp waves.

TEMPORAL LOBE EPILEPSY: COMPLEX PARTIAL SEIZURE WITH AUTOMATISMS

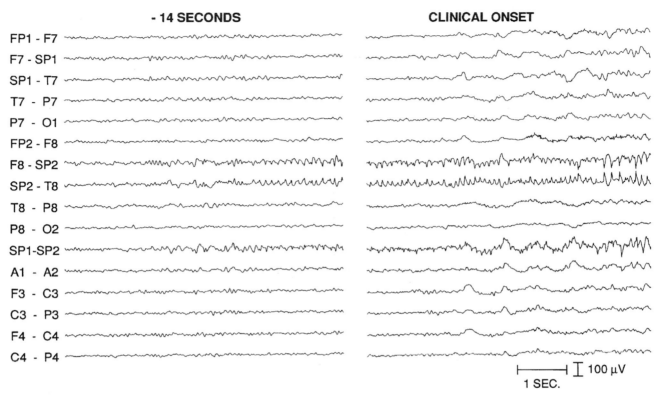

Figure 13.37 Thirty-one-year-old woman with complex partial seizures with automatisms since age 5 years. Fourteen seconds before clinical onset, an electroencephalographic seizure pattern was maximal at the right sphenoidal electrode.

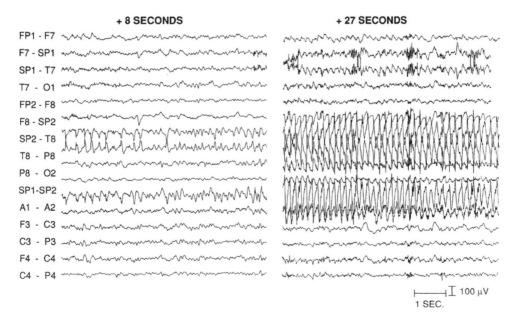

Figure 13.38 Continuation of the seizure shown in Figure 13.37. Clinical features included staring, unresponsiveness, and oral automatisms.

FRONTAL LOBE EPILEPSY: FRONTAL SHARP WAVES

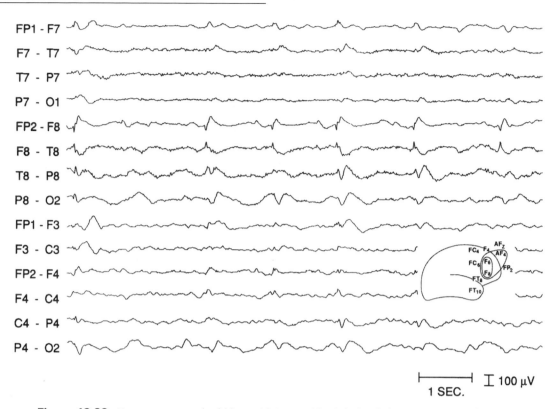

FP1 - F7

F7 - T7

T7 - P7

P7 - O1

FP2 - F8

F8 - T8

T8 - P8

P8 - O2

FP1 - F3

F3 - C3

FP2 - F4

F4 - C4

C4 - P4

P4 - O2

1 SEC.   100 μV

Figure 13.39 Twenty-one-month-old boy with intractable daily focal clonic seizures involving the left side of the body. Interictal electroencephalogram showed nearly continuous periodic sharp waves from the right frontal lobe, with the distribution shown in the inset. MRI disclosed an area of increased signal in the same area, and histologic examination of resected tissue showed cortical dysplasia.

FRONTAL LOBE EPILEPSY: FRONTAL SHARP WAVES WITH 2-DEGREE BILATERAL SYNCHRONY

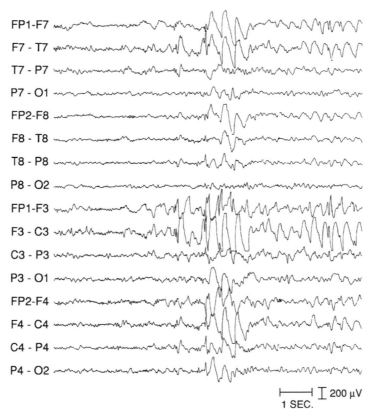

Figure 13.40 Seventeen-year-old boy with intractable complex partial and generalized tonic-clonic seizures and extensive encephalomalacia of the left frontal lobe as a result of head trauma at age 13 years. Interictal sharp waves were maximum in the left frontal region but frequently showed secondary bilateral synchrony with generalization.

FRONTAL LOBE EPILEPSY: SUBCLINICAL ELECTROENCEPHALOGRAPHIC SEIZURE, ONSET

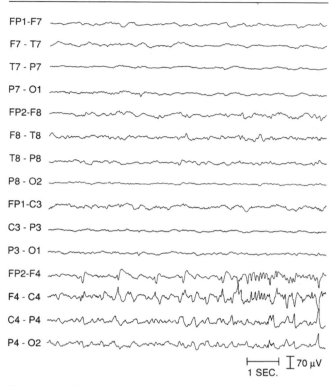

Figure 13.41 Fifty-year-old man with focal clonic seizures involving the left face and arm. Seizures began after right frontotemporal craniotomy and evacuation of right frontal intracerebral hemorrhage. The electroencephalographic seizure pattern begins in the region of the F_4 electrode.

FRONTAL LOBE EPILEPSY: SUBCLINICAL EEG SEIZURE, +50 SECONDS

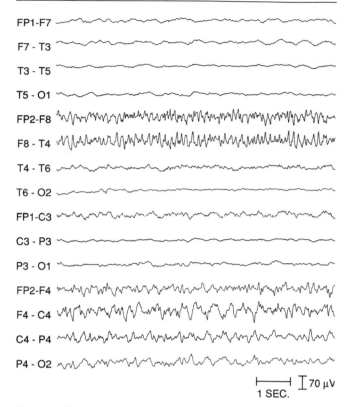

Figure 13.42 Evolution of the subclinical seizure in Figure 13.41. The seizure pattern has spread to involve more widespread frontal and central regions of the right hemisphere.

OCCIPITAL LOBE EPILEPSY: VISUAL AURA AND FOCAL CLONIC SEIZURE, −10 SECONDS

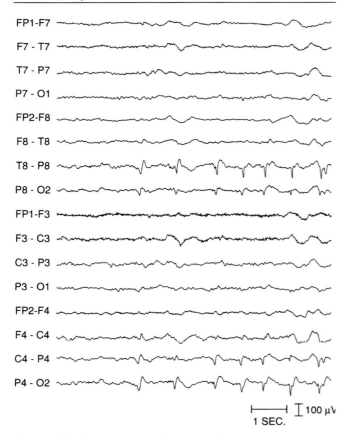

Figure 13.43 Sixty-year-old woman with recent onset of visual aura of flashing lights followed by version of eyes to the left and clonic jerking of the left face and arm. Ictal electroencephalogram showed repetitive sharp waves in the right occipitoparietal area.

OCCIPITAL LOBE EPILEPSY: VISUAL AURA FOCAL CLONIC SEIZURE, CLINICAL ONSET

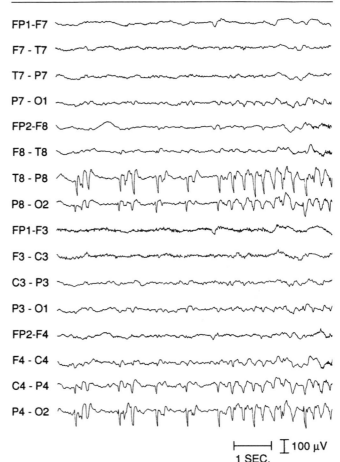

Figure 13.44 Evolution of the electroencephalographic seizure pattern in Figure 13.43.

SUPPLEMENTARY MOTOR AREA EPILEPSY: SHARP WAVES AT VERTEX

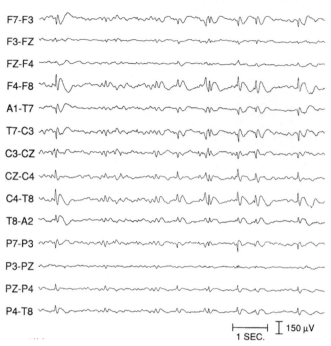

Figure 13.45   Seventeen-year-old woman with a low-grade astrocytoma in the left mesial frontal lobe (paracentral lobule). Intractable seizures involved brief tonic abduction of both arms, version of head and eyes to the right, and falling backward without loss of consciousness.

SUPPLEMENTARY MOTOR AREA EPILEPSY: TONIC SEIZURE

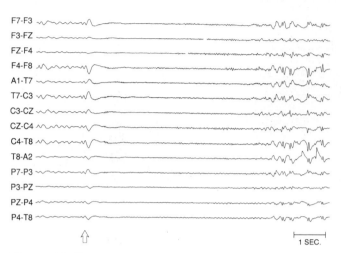

Figure 13.46   Electroencephalogram during a typical seizure from the patient described in Figure 13.45. At clinical onset (*arrow*), a vertex slow transient and then a generalized electrodecremental pattern with paroxysmal fast activity were recorded, followed by paroxysmal vertex sharp waves.

PERIROLANDIC EPILEPSY: FOCAL CLONIC SEIZURE, CLINICAL ONSET

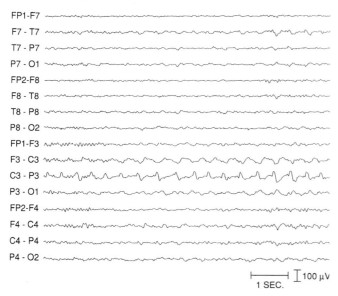

Figure 13.47 Four-year-old girl with frequent nocturnal focal clonic seizures with jacksonian spread. Seizures began with twitching of the right shoulder and thoracic wall, followed by version of the head to the right and clonic jerking of the right arm and leg without loss of consciousness. Seizure pattern on electroencephalogram was maximum at the left central region.

PERIROLANDIC EPILEPSY: FOCAL CLONIC SEIZURE, +10 SECONDS

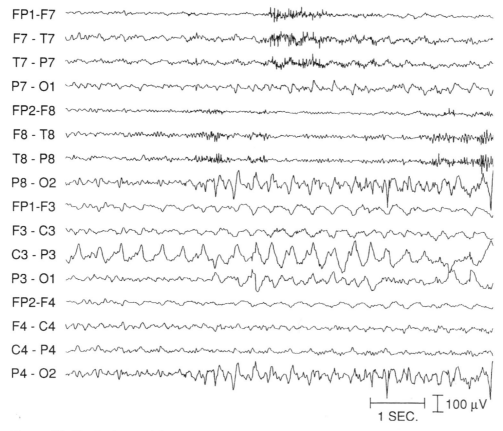

Figure 13.48 Evolution of the seizure in Figure 13.47, with spread of the ictal discharge into left parietal and occipital regions.

PERIROLANDIC EPILEPSY: RIGHT FRONTOCENTRAL SHARP WAVES

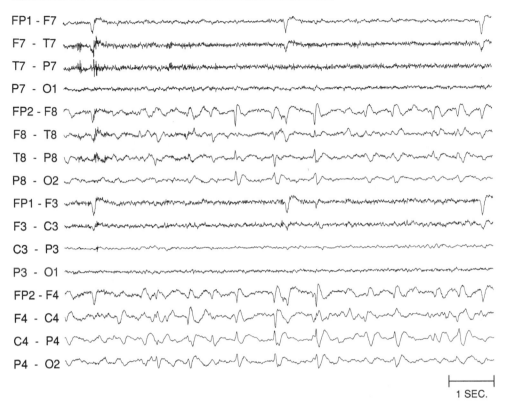

Figure 13.49 Eight-year-old boy with left hemiparesis and post-traumatic encephalomalacia in the right frontocentral white matter as a result of a motor vehicle accident at age 3 months. Interictal electroencephalogram showed right hemisphere slowing with sharp waves over the right frontocentral region (maximum at the C_4 electrode).

PERIROLANDIC EPILEPSY: LEFT ARM TONIC SEIZURE

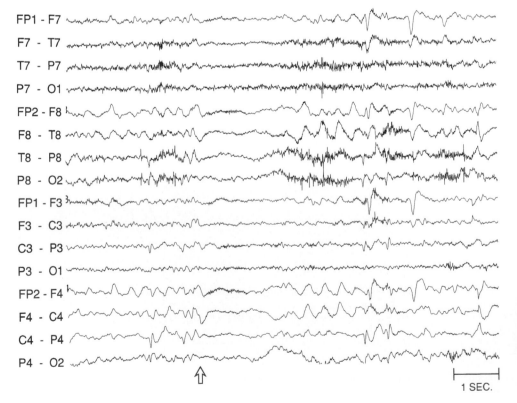

Figure 13.50 Same patient as in Figure 13.49. Electroencephalography showed diffuse electrodecrement during brief tonic seizures with stiffening and extension of the left arm and leg. Seizures ceased after right frontocentral resection.

PERIROLANDIC EPILEPSY: EPILEPSIA PARTIALIS CONTINUA

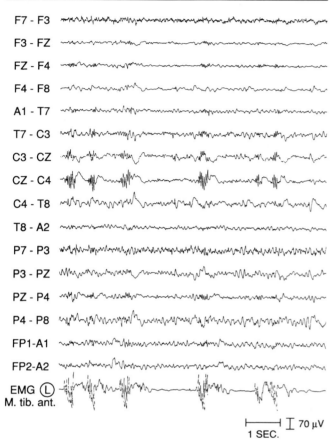

Figure 13.51 Sixty-nine-year-old man with continual jerking of the left foot and leg for 6 weeks, without loss of consciousness. Electromyography from the left tibialis anterior muscle showed that jerks occurred synchronously with each burst of polyspikes on electroencephalogram. Polyspikes were maximum at left vertex electrodes, presumably as a result of paradoxical lateralization of the discharge from the right interhemispheric region (19).

PALLID INFANTILE SYNCOPE: OCULAR COMPRESSION TEST

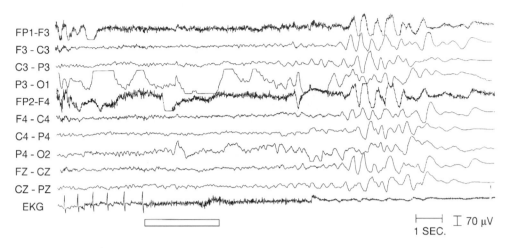

Figure 13.52 Two-year-old boy with pallid infantile syncope. Ocular compression (20,21) (*bar*), a controversial provocative maneuver, resulted in syncope with cardiac asystole for 12.5 seconds. Electroencephalography showed diffuse high-amplitude slowing followed by cerebral suppression as a result of global cerebral ischemia.

PALLID INFANTILE SYNCOPE: OCULAR COMPRESSION TEST, CONTINUED

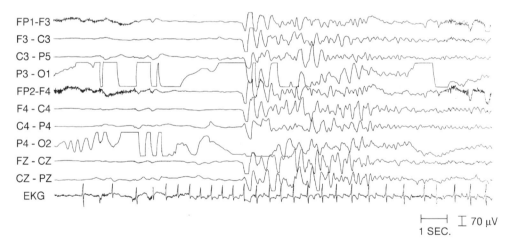

Figure 13.53 With recovery of the patient shown in Figure 13.52, electroencephalogram showed high-amplitude slowing followed by normal rhythms. Asystole with ocular compression may be caused by activation of the oculocardiac reflex (trigeminal afferent, vagal efferent pathways) (20,21).

CYANOTIC BREATH-HOLDING SPELL

+10 SECONDS   +25 SECONDS

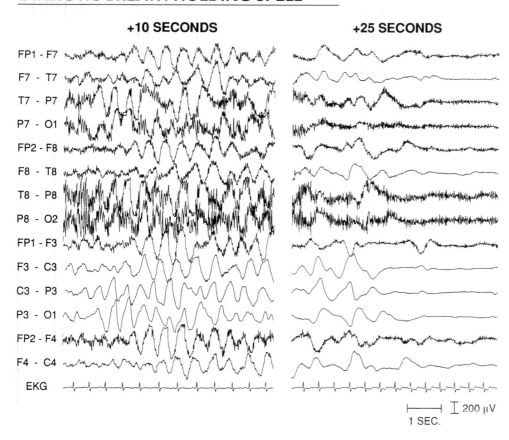

Figure 13.54 Two-year-old boy with cyanotic breath-holding spells sometimes followed by generalized tonic-clonic seizures. This episode occurred during crying and involved cessation of respiration for 40 seconds, oxygen desaturation to 73%, cyanosis, loss of consciousness, opisthotonic posturing, and urinary incontinence.

CYANOTIC BREATH-HOLDING SPELL

+31 SECONDS   +43 SECONDS

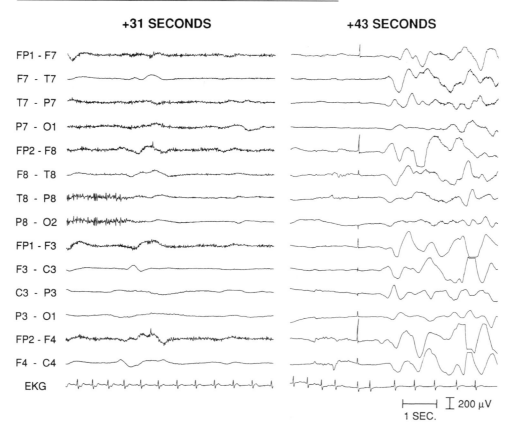

Figure 13.55 As the episode continued in the patient shown in Figure 13.54, electroencephalographic activity was similar to that during the syncopal attack in Figures 13.52 and 13.53, but the electroencephalogram showed tachycardia instead of asystole.

NARCOLEPSY

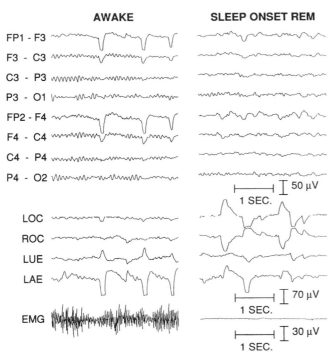

Figure 13.56 Fifty-six-year-old man with episodes of loss of consciousness (sleep attacks) and automatic behavior (minisleeps). Multiple sleep latency test gave evidence of narcolepsy with short sleep latency (2 minutes) and sleep-onset rapid eye movement periods (REM latency, 1 minute). Typical features during rapid eye movement sleep included rapid eye movements, absent muscle artifact, and drowsy electroencephalographic pattern. LOC and ROC, left and right outer canthus; LUE and RUE, left and right under eye. Ocular electrodes were referential to A_1A_2.

ACKNOWLEDGMENTS

The EEG tracings in this atlas were prepared by Diana Roth, R EEGT, and Jim Reed.

REFERENCES

1. American Electroencephalographic Society. Guidelines in EEG, 1–7 (revised 1985). *J Clin Neurophysiol* 1986;3: 133–168.
2. Jasper HH. The ten-twenty electrode system of the International Federation. *Electroencephalogr Clin Neurophysiol* 1958;10: 371–375.
3. Sharbrough F, Chatrian GE, Lesser RP, et al. American EEG Society: guidelines for standard electrode position nomenclature. *J Clin Neurophysiol* 1991;8: 200–202.
4. Klem G, Lüders H, Jasper HH, Elger C. The ten-twenty electrode system of the International Federation. The International Federation of Clinical Neurophysiology. *Clin Neurophysiol Suppl* 1999;52: 3–6.
5. Daly DD. Epilepsy and syncope. In: Daly DD, Pedley TA, eds. *Current practice of clinical electroencephalography*, 2nd ed. New York: Raven Press, 1990: 306–310.
6. Klass DW, Westmoreland BF. Nonepileptogenic epileptiform electroencephalographic activity. *Ann Neurol* 1985;18: 627–635.
7. Commission on Classification and Terminology of the International League against Epilepsy. Proposal for revised clinical and electroencephalographic classification of epileptic seizures. *Epilepsia* 1981;22: 489–501.
8. Commission on Classification and Terminology of the International League against Epilepsy. Proposal for revised classification of epilepsies and epileptic syndromes. *Epilepsia* 1989;30: 389–399.
9. White JC, Langston JW, Pedley TA. Benign epileptiform transients of sleep. *Neurology* 1977;27: 1061–1068.
10. Eeg-Olofsson O. The development of the electroencephalogram in normal children from age 1 through 15 years: 14- and 6-Hz positive spike phenomena. *Neuropaediatrie* 1971;2: 405–427.
11. Lombroso CT, Schwartz IH, Clark DM, et al. Ctenoids in healthy youths. Controlled study of 14- and 6-per-second positive spiking. *Neurology* 1966;16: 1152–1158.
12. Reiher J, Lebel M. Wicket spikes: clinical correlations of a previously undescribed EEG pattern. *Can J Neurol Sci* 1977;4: 39–47.
13. Westmoreland BF, Klass DW. A distinctive rhythmic EEG discharge of adults. *Electroencephalogr Clin Neurophysiol* 1981;51: 186–191.
14. Gibbs FA, Rich CL, Gibbs EL. Psychomotor variant type of seizure discharge. *Neurology* 1963;13: 991–998.
15. Cobb WA, Guiloff RF, Cast J. Breach rhythm: the EEG related to skull defects. *Electroencephalogr Clin Neurophysiol* 1979;47: 251–271.
16. Kotagal P. Multifocal independent spike syndrome: relationship to hypsarrhythmia and the slow spike-wave (Lennox-Gastaut) syndrome. *Clin Electroencephalogr* 1995;26: 23–29.
17. Bickford RG, Whelan JL, Klass DW, et al. Reading epilepsy: clinical and electroencephalographic studies of a new syndrome. *Trans Am Neurol Assoc* 1956;81: 100–102.
18. Lüders H, Lesser RP, Dinner DS, et al. Benign focal epilepsy of childhood. In: Lüders H, Lesser RP, eds. *Epilepsy: electroclinical syndromes*. London: Springer-Verlag, 1987: 303–346.
19. Adelman S, Lüders H, Dinner DSD, et al. Paradoxical lateralization of parasagittal sharp waves in a patient with epilepsia partialis continua. *Epilepsia* 1982;23: 291–295.
20. Lombroso CT, Lerman P. Breath-holding spells (cyanotic and pallid infantile syncope). *Pediatrics* 1967;39: 563–581.
21. Stephenson JBP. Two types of febrile seizures: anoxic (syncopal) and epileptic mechanisms differentiated by oculocardiac reflex. *Br Med J* 1978;2: 726–729.

BIBLIOGRAPHY

Blume WT, Kaibara M. *Atlas of adult electroencephalography*. New York: Raven Press, 1995.
Blume WT, Kaibara M. *Atlas of pediatric electroencephalography*, 2nd ed. Philadelphia: Lippincott-Raven, 1999.
Ebersole JS, Pedley TA, eds. *Current practice of clinical electroencephalography*, 3rd ed. Philadelphia: Lippincott Williams & Wilkins, 2003.
Gubermann A, Couture M. *Atlas of electroencephalography*. Boston: Little Brown, 1989.
Lüders H, Noachtar S. *Atlas and classification of electroencephalography*. Philadelphia: WB Saunders, 2000.
Niedermeyer E, Lopez da Silva FH, eds. *Electroencephalography: basic principles, clinical applications and related fields*, 3rd ed. Baltimore, MD: Urban & Schwarzenberg, 1993.
Osselton R, Cooper JW, Shaw JC. *EEG technology*, 3rd ed. London: Butterworths, 1980.
Spehlmann E. *EG primer*, 2nd ed. Amsterdam: Elsevier, 1991.
Stockard-Pope JE, Werner SS, Bickford RG. *Atlas of neonatal electroencephalography*, 2nd ed. New York: Raven Press, 1992.
Tyner FS, Knott JR, Mayer WB Jr. *Fundamentals of EEG technology*, vol 1. *Basic concepts and methods*. New York: Raven Press, 1983.

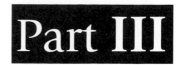

Epileptic Seizures and Syndromes

Section A EPILEPTIC SEIZURES 217

 14. Classification of Seizures 217
   Appendix: Proposal for Revised Clinical and Electrographic Classification of
   Epileptic Seizures: Commission on Classification and Terminology of the
   International League Against Epilepsy (1981) 222
 15. Epileptic Auras 229
 16. Focal Seizures with Impaired Consciousness 241
 17. Focal Motor Seizures, Epilepsia Partialis Continua, and Supplementary
   Sensorimotor Seizures 257
 18. Generalized Tonic-Clonic Seizures 279
 19. Absence Seizures 305
 20. Atypical Absence, Myoclonic, Tonic, and Atonic Seizures 317
 21. Epileptic Spasms 333

Section B EPILEPSY SYNDROMES: DIAGNOSIS AND TREATMENT 347

 22. Classification of the Epilepsies 347
   Appendix: Proposal for Revised Classification of Epilepsies and Epileptic
   Syndromes: Commission on Classification and Terminology of the
   International League Against Epilepsy (1989) 354
 23. Symptomatic Focal Epilepsies 365
 24. Idiopathic and Benign Partial Epilepsies of Childhood 373
 25. Idiopathic Generalized Epilepsy Syndromes of Childhood and Adolescence 391
 26. The Myoclonic Epilepsies 407
 27. Encephalopathic Generalized Epilepsy and Lennox-Gastaut Syndrome 429
 28. Rasmussen's Encephalitis (Chronic Focal Encephalitis) 441
 29. Continuous Spike Wave of Slow Sleep and Landau Kleffner Syndrome 455
 30. Epilepsy with Reflex Seizures 463
 31. Less Common Epilepsy Syndromes and Epilepsy Associated with
   Chromosomal Abnormalities 477

continued

Section C DIAGNOSIS AND TREATMENT OF SEIZURES IN SPECIAL CLINICAL SETTINGS 487

32. Neonatal Seizures   487
33. Febrile Seizures   511
34. Posttraumatic Epilepsy   521
35. Epilepsy in the Setting of Cerebrovascular Disease   527
36. Epilepsy in the Setting of Neurocutaneous Syndromes   537
37. Epilepsy in the Setting of Inherited Metabolic and Mitochondrial Disorders   547
38. Seizures Associated with Nonneurologic Medical Conditions   571
39. Epilepsy in Patients with Multiple Handicaps   585
40. Epilepsy in the Elderly   593
41. Status Epilepticus   605

Section D DIFFERENTIAL DIAGNOSIS OF EPILEPSY   623

42. Psychogenic Nonepileptic Seizures   623
43. Other Nonepileptic Paroxysmal Disorders   631

Classification of Seizures

14

Christoph Kellinghaus   *Hans O. Lüders*   *Elaine Wyllie*

Efforts to categorize epileptic seizures and syndromes date to classic medical literature (1). Various classifications were developed for different purposes (2–11), so that by the middle of the twentieth century, a profusion were in active use. As more diagnostic and treatment modalities became available, the resulting confusion pointed to the need for a widely accepted system.

The classification system currently used most extensively is the International Classification of Epileptic Seizures (ICES). First articulated by the Commission on Classification and Terminology of the International League Against Epilepsy (ILAE) in 1964 (12), the system was revised in 1981 (13). The current ICES is used worldwide and is reproduced in its entirety as an appendix immediately following this chapter. In light of still unresolved issues and controversies, however, the ILAE's Commission on Classification and Terminology is currently further revising its seizure classification system (14).

EVOLUTION OF THE CURRENT SYSTEM

Early observers of epileptic seizures noted that seizure symptomatology could shed some insight into the underlying epileptic process, with focal seizures (e.g., right arm clonic jerking) tending to occur in patients with focal lesions (e.g., remote traumatic injury to the left perirolandic region) and bilateral or generalized seizures (generalized myoclonic jerks) being associated with more generalized processes. These observations suggested a strong correlation between the clinical features of seizures and the underlying epileptic process or syndrome. With the advent of electroencephalography (EEG) in the 1930s, however, it became clear that similar or identical clinical seizure types could be present in patients with either generalized or focal EEG abnormalities.

For example, episodes of staring and loss of consciousness could occur with either generalized 3-Hz spike-wave complexes or anterior temporal sharp waves.

Continued research identified various electroclinical syndromes considered essential for diagnosis of the epilepsy syndrome. This philosophy dominated during the development of the 1964 ICES, which used terms derived from descriptions of symptomatology to characterize electroclinical syndromes. The 1981 ICES added new terminology that divided seizures into focal or generalized types on the basis of electroclinical features. For example, seizures characterized by staring and impaired consciousness were called "absence" if the patient's EEG features were generalized and "complex partial" if the EEG features were focal. This approach reflected the assumption that a strict one-to-one relationship exists between the electroclinical syndromes and the corresponding epilepsy syndromes.

LIMITATIONS OF THE ELECTROCLINICAL APPROACH TO SEIZURE CLASSIFICATION

Although EEG features are an integral part of the 1981 ICES, they are not always available in clinical practice. Routine interictal EEG may not be revealing, and only a small minority of patients with epilepsy undergo prolonged video-EEG recording. In these cases, assumptions are often based on other lines of evidence. In a patient with no interictal epileptiform discharges on EEG, for example, episodes of loss of consciousness are assumed to be complex partial seizures if magnetic resonance imaging (MRI) shows a temporal lobe tumor. If neither test is revealing, or before any test has been performed (as may be the case at a patient's initial visit), the focal or generalized nature of the epilepsy may not be apparent solely from a description of the seizures. In this situation, precise use of the 1981 ICES is not possible.

Moreover, the electroclinical approach does not allow for easy expression of many potentially important seizure signs and symptoms. By focusing heavily on the presence or absence of altered consciousness as the key distinction between complex or simple types of focal seizures, the 1981 ICES deemphasizes much of the rich symptomatology that may carry localizing or lateralizing significance. The ictal level of consciousness may be difficult to determine and offers little localizing information, because seizures with or without loss of consciousness may arise from any region of the brain. Other seizure signs or symptoms may greatly enhance epileptogenic localization, but they are not easily expressed in the 1981 ICES. For example, the 1981 classification offers "simple partial seizure with focal motor signs," whereas a clearer and more informative description might be "left arm clonic seizure." A classification system encompassing a broad range of seizure symptomatology would be especially valuable to neurologists evaluating patients for epilepsy surgery, because convergence of data from different lines of testing is key to localization of the epileptogenic zone.

Recently, it has become clear that a strict one-to-one relationship between electroclinical syndromes and the corresponding epilepsy syndromes does not exist. Modern neuroimaging has allowed neurologists to identify important etiologies *in vivo*, such as cortical dysplasia and hippocampal sclerosis, that were previously often found only on histopathologic analysis. Correlation of neuroimaging and video-EEG results demonstrates the variable relationship between an electroclinical syndrome and the underlying epileptogenic process (15), especially among infants (16) in whom interrater agreement for seizure classification according to the 1981 ICES proved to be poor (17). Whereas focal epilepsy in children and adolescent seems to present with features commonly associated with focal seizure onset—for example, auras and clonic jerking of one extremity—infants frequently exhibit either subtle motor signs only or symmetric tonic movements commonly thought to be associated with generalized epileptogenicity (18,19). Infantile spasms and hypsarrhythmia, traditionally thought to correspond to a generalized epilepsy syndrome, may be due to a focal brain lesion identified on MRI (20–22). At this point, assumption of a one-to-one relationship, as in the 1981 ICES, leads to confusion between the classification of epileptic seizures and epilepsy syndromes.

ADVANTAGES OF A SEIZURE CLASSIFICATION SYSTEM BASED SOLELY ON SYMPTOMATOLOGY

In an effort to avoid these limitations, Lüders and colleagues (16,23–27) have proposed a seizure classification

system based solely on the main signs and symptoms of the seizures identified by a patient or by a direct observer, or by analysis of ictal videotapes. This system, which has been used at selected epilepsy centers for more than 10 years, has several advantages.

"Unbundling" the signs and symptoms of seizures from EEG, neuroimaging, and other clinical information allows them to contribute independently to the diagnosis of an epilepsy syndrome. The assignment to generalized or focal pathophysiology is thus deferred until the entire clinical picture—available results from family history, a patient's past and present history, neurologic and physical examination, seizure symptomatology, EEG, neuroimaging, and genetic testing—can be considered together. This system emphasizes the importance of a diagnosis of epilepsy syndrome in every case, because symptomatology alone provides limited information about the best choice of antiepileptic drugs, prognosis, need for neuroimaging, and other therapeutic considerations. This type of seizure classification is similar to classification systems used in other fields of neurology. For example, in a patient with tremor, the movement disorder syndrome is the essential diagnostic end point, not the tremor itself.

Keeping seizure symptomatology separate from other clinical and laboratory features eliminates the current confusion between electroclinical complexes and epilepsy syndromes, thus emphasizing the importance of symptoms and focusing attention on their role in a diagnosis of epileptic syndrome. Such a system, which encourages research into the types of ictal signs and symptoms observed in different epilepsy syndromes and vice versa, can be applied in the absence of MRI or EEG abnormalities.

A PROPOSAL

The seizure classification system proposed by Lüders and colleagues places ictal signs and symptoms into one of four domains: sensation, consciousness, autonomic function, or motor function (Table 14.1).

Seizures characterized by sensory or psychic disturbances without loss of consciousness or other features are called auras; seizures characterized by abnormal movements, with or without loss of consciousness, are known as motor seizures; seizures with predominantly autonomic (i.e., involuntary) features are considered autonomic seizures; and seizures in which prominent feature is loss of consciousness are referred to as absence, or dileptic, seizures. Knowledge of the focal or generalized nature of the epilepsy is not required for this classification. For example, absence (or dileptic) seizures characterized by quiet unconsciousness may be seen in childhood absence epilepsy, as well as in some cases of frontal or temporal lobe epilepsy. The neutral but unfamiliar term "dileptic" was proposed to avoid confusion with the traditional use of "absence" as an electroclinical syndrome.

TABLE 14.1

CLASSIFICATION OF EPILEPTIC SEIZURES BASED SOLELY ON SYMPTOMATOLOGY

Aura	
Somatosensory	Visual
Auditory	Gustatory
Olfactory	Autonomic
Abdominal	Psychic
Motor	
Simple motor seizure	
Clonic	Myoclonic
Tonic	Versive
Tonic-clonic	Epileptic spasm
Complex motor seizure	
Automotor	
Hypermotor	
Gelastic	
Dialeptic seizure	
Autonomic seizure	
Special seizure	
Atonic	Akinetic
Astatic	Negative myoclonic
Hypomotor	Aphasic

From Lüders H, Acharya J, Baumgartner C, et al. A new epileptic seizure classification based exclusively on ictal semiology. *Acta Neurol Scand* 1998;98:1–5, with permission.

Motor seizures are subdivided into simple and complex types. In simple motor seizures, unnatural and apparently involuntary motor movements are similar to those elicited by electrical stimulation of the primary motor areas. Simple motor seizures may be further subdivided into clonic, tonic, tonic-clonic, myoclonic, and versive seizures, and epileptic spasms. In complex motor seizures, the relatively complicated movements simulate natural movements but are inappropriate for the situation. The term "complex" here does not mean that the patient necessarily loses awareness during the seizures, although impaired consciousness is common. Complex motor seizures may be further subdivided into automotor seizures with repetitive oral or gestural automatisms, often seen in temporal lobe epilepsy; hypermotor seizures with dramatically increased behavioral movements, which sometimes occur in seizures arising from mesial or orbitofrontal regions; and gelastic seizures with inappropriate or mirthless laughter, typically seen with hypothalamic hamartoma.

Seizures that do not fit into other categories, including those characterized by "negative" or "inhibitory" features, are classified as special. Atonic seizures involve loss of postural tone, resulting in head drops or limp falling. Astatic seizures consist of epileptic falls. Videopolygraphic studies show that these may be caused by pure atonia, atonia following a myoclonic jerk, or pure tonic stiffening, but in clinical practice, the exact pathogenesis is often unclear. Hypomotor seizures are characterized by decreased or absent behavioral motor activity without the emergence of new motor manifestations; this descriptive term is useful

for infants or severely mentally impaired individuals, in whom it is not possible to test consciousness directly (16,28). Akinetic seizures are characterized by the inability to perform voluntary movements despite preserved consciousness, as may occur with activation of the negative motor areas in the mesial frontal and inferior frontal gyri. Negative myoclonic seizures consist of a brief interruption of tonic muscle activity caused by an epileptiform discharge; the resulting brief, sudden movement is caused by loss of muscle tone. During aphasic seizures, the patient cannot speak and often cannot understand spoken language. Aphasic seizures may be a negative phenomenon induced by the epileptic activation of a cortical language center, similar to that induced by electrical stimulation of cortical language areas.

Modifiers may be added to express the somatotopic distribution of ictal signs and symptoms, as, for example, "left-hand clonic seizure" or "generalized clonic seizure." Modifiers refer to the part(s) of the body involved in the seizure, not to the side or lobe of the brain generating the ictal discharge. To express the evolution of symptoms that occurs as the seizure discharge spreads to new cortical areas, the components can be listed in order of appearance and linked by arrows (see examples below).

Examples:

- left visual aura → left versive seizure (loss of consciousness) → generalized tonic-clonic seizure
- abdominal aura → automotor seizure; lateralizing sign: left arm dystonic posturing

Verification of the state of consciousness is necessary only for some specific seizure types, such as dileptic seizures, in which loss of consciousness is the predominant symptom, and auras, in which consciousness is always preserved. However, the state of consciousness may be an important semiological variable. The semiological seizure classification allows for the specification at which point in the sequence of symptoms the patient lost consciousness by inserting the expression "loss of consciousness" (LOC) after the seizure component during which consciousness was lost.

There are several semiological features of the ictal or postictal state that are not necessarily the main element of a seizure component, but have been established as reliably lateralizing the hemisphere of seizure onset—for example, dystonic posturing (29), ictal speech (30), or postictal weakness (31). These lateralizing signs can be listed following the seizure sequence.

This system permits classification of seizures with different degrees of precision to match the available information. If information is limited, as in the absence of a witness or a complete or accurate history, a less detailed classification may be appropriate (e.g., "motor seizure"). Progressively greater amounts of information may permit further categorization of the seizure as "simple motor," "right arm motor," or "right arm clonic."

CONCLUSIONS

The 1981 ICES, which defines epileptic syndromes on the basis of electroclinical syndromes, has provided a common language for the advancement of patient care and research. However, the authors of the 1981 ICES revision expected (and actually hoped for) further revisions of the classification, as they were aware that increasing knowledge would lead to modification of their approaches and concepts (13). Recent advances in neuroimaging and molecular biology have revolutionized the definition of epileptic syndromes, providing insights beyond those obtained from EEG alone and demonstrating that a strict one-to-one relationship between electroclinical syndromes and the underlying epileptic processes does not exist. In addition, an alternative seizure classification system based solely on symptomatology has been proposed by Lüders and colleagues (23–26). As a result of those developments, the Commission on Classification and Terminology of the ILAE is revising the classification (14).

Recently, a proposal for a five-axis diagnostic scheme has been put forth by the ILAE Task Force on Classification and Terminology (32). This proposal uses the strictly descriptive terminology of the semiological seizure classification, but categorizes it as a glossary (33). The second axis contains the epileptic seizure types "that present diagnostic entities with physiologic, therapeutic, and/or prognostic implications" (32). In this axis, the ICES dichotomy of focal and generalized seizures remains essentially unchanged, complemented by some semiological details, as well as by status epilepticus types and reflex seizure types. This approach, with its imminent redundancy of information as well as the whole proposal of the diagnostic scheme, has been hotly debated (34–38) and remains controversial (see also Chapter 22). On the other hand, the semiological seizure classification has been used successfully in the clinical management of patients, as well as in the scientific investigation of epilepsy in various settings and age-groups (18,39,40). In addition, two independent studies (41,42) have compared the semiological seizure classification with the current ILAE seizure classification and have found it to be more useful particularly in localized epilepsies. Regardless of the seizure classification system that is used, one must bear in mind that in every case the seizure classification must be complemented by an epilepsy syndrome classification that integrates all available clinical information from history, examination, and laboratory testing.

REFERENCES

1. Wolf P. *Epileptic seizures and syndromes: terms and concepts*. London: Libbey, 1994:3–7.
2. Gastaut H. Classification of the epilepsies. Proposal for an international classification. *Epilepsia* 1969;10(Suppl):14–21.
3. Gastaut H. Clinical and electroencephalographical classification of epileptic seizures. *Epilepsia* 1969;10(Suppl):2–13.
4. Gastaut H. Clinical and electroencephalographical classification of epileptic seizures. *Epilepsia* 1970;11:102–113.
5. Gastaut H. *Dictionary of epilepsy*. Geneva: World Health Organization, 1973.
6. Masland RL. Classification of the epilepsies. *Epilepsia* 1959;1:512–520.
7. Masland RL. Comments on the classification of epilepsy. *Epilepsia* 1969;10(Suppl):22–28.
8. Masland RL. The classification of the epilepsies. A historical review. In: Vinken PJ, Bruyn GW, eds. *Handbook of clinical neurology, XV*. Amsterdam: Elsevier, 1974;1–29.
9. McNaughton FL. The classification of the epilepsies. *Epilepsia* 1952;1:7–16.
10. Merlis JK. Proposal for an international classification of the epilepsies. *Epilepsia* 1970;11:114–119.
11. Merlis JK. Treatment in relation to classification of the epilepsies. *Acta Neurol Latinoam* 1972;18:42–51.
12. Commission on Classification and Terminology of the International League Against Epilepsy. A proposed international classification of epileptic seizures. *Epilepsia* 1964;5:297–306.
13. Commission on Classification and Terminology of the International League Against Epilepsy. Proposal for revised clinical and electroencephalographic classification of epileptic seizures. *Epilepsia* 1981;22:489–501.
14. Engel J Jr. Classifications of the International League Against Epilepsy: time for reappraisal. *Epilepsia* 1998;39:1014–1017.
15. Manford M, Fish DR, Shorvon SD. An analysis of clinical seizure patterns and their localizing value in frontal and temporal lobe epilepsies. *Brain* 1996;119(Pt 1):17–40.
16. Acharya JN, Wyllie E, Lüders HO, et al. Seizure symptomatology in infants with localization-related epilepsy. *Neurology* 1997;48:189–196.
17. Nordli DR Jr, Bazil CW, Scheuer ML, et al. Recognition and classification of seizures in infants. *Epilepsia* 1997;38:553–560.
18. Hamer HM, Wyllie E, Lüders HO, et al. Symptomatology of epileptic seizures in the first three years of life. *Epilepsia* 1999;40:837–844.
19. Nordli DR Jr, Kuroda MM, Hirsch LJ. The ontogeny of partial seizures in infants and young children. *Epilepsia* 2001;42:986–990.
20. Chugani HT, Shields WD, Shewmon DA, et al. Infantile spasms: I. PET identifies focal cortical dysgenesis in cryptogenic cases for surgical treatment. *Ann Neurol* 1990;27:406–413.
21. Chugani HT, Shewmon DA, Shields WD, et al. Surgery for intractable infantile spasms: neuroimaging perspectives. *Epilepsia* 1993;34:764–771.
22. Wyllie E, Comair YG, Kotagal P, et al. Epilepsy surgery in infants. *Epilepsia* 1996;37:625–637.
23. Lüders H, Acharya J, Baumgartner C, et al. Semiological seizure classification. *Epilepsia* 1998;39:1006–1013.
24. Lüders H, Acharya J, Baumgartner C, et al. A new epileptic seizure classification based exclusively on ictal semiology. *Acta Neurol Scand* 1999;99:137–141.
25. Lüders HO, Noachtar S. *Atlas und Klassifikation der Elektroenzephalographie. Einführung in die EEG-Auswertung*. Wehr, Germany: Ciba-Geigy Verlag, 1994.
26. Lüders HO, Noachtar S. *Atlas und Video epileptischer Anfälle und Syndrome*. Wehr, Germany: Ciba-Geigy Verlag, 1995.
27. Bautista JF, Lüders HO. Semiological seizure classification: relevance to pediatric epilepsy. *Epileptic Disord* 2000;2:65–72.
28. Kallen K, Wyllie E, Lüders HO, et al. Hypomotor seizures in infants and children. *Epilepsia* 2002;43:882–888.
29. Bleasel A, Kotagal P, Kankirawatana P, et al. Lateralizing value and semiology of ictal limb posturing and version in temporal lobe and extratemporal epilepsy. *Epilepsia* 1997;38:168–174.
30. Marks WJ Jr., Laxer KD. Semiology of temporal lobe seizures: value in lateralizing the seizure focus. *Epilepsia* 1998;39:721–726.
31. Kellinghaus C, Kotagal P. Lateralizing value of Todd's palsy in patients with epilepsy. *Neurology* 2003;60(Suppl 1):A355.
32. Engel J Jr. A proposed diagnostic scheme for people with epileptic seizures and with epilepsy: report of the ILAE Task Force on Classification and Terminology. *Epilepsia* 2001;42:796–803.
33. Blume WT, Lüders HO, Mizrahi E, et al. Glossary of descriptive terminology for ictal semiology: report of the ILAE Task Force on Classification and Terminology. *Epilepsia* 2001;42:1212–1218.
34. Avanzini G. Of cabbages and kings: do we really need a systematic classification of epilepsies? *Epilepsia* 2003;44:12–13.

35. Berg AT, Blackstone NW. Of cabbages and kings: perspectives on classification from the field of systematics. *Epilepsia* 2003;44:8–11.

36. Engel J. Reply to "Of cabbages and kings: some considerations on classifications, diagnostic schemes, semiology, and concepts." *Epilepsia* 2003;44:4–5.

37. Lüders H, Najm I, Wyllie E. Reply to "Of cabbages and kings: some considerations on classifications, diagnostic schemes, semiology, and concepts." *Epilepsia* 2003;44:6–7.

38. Wolf P. Of cabbages and kings: some considerations on classifications, diagnostic schemes, semiology, and concepts. *Epilepsia* 2003;44:1–3.

39. Henkel A, Noachtar S, Pfander M, et al. The localizing value of the abdominal aura and its evolution: a study in focal epilepsies. *Neurology* 2002;58:271–276.

40. Werhahn KJ, Noachtar S, Arnold S, et al. Tonic seizures: their significance for lateralization and frequency in different focal epileptic syndromes. *Epilepsia* 2000;41:1153–1161.

41. Benbadis SR, Thomas P, Pontone G. A prospective comparison between two seizure classifications. *Seizure* 2001;10:247–249.

42. Parra J, Augustijn PB, Geerts Y, et al. Classification of epileptic seizures: a comparison of two systems. *Epilepsia* 2001;42:476–482.

Proposal for Revised Clinical and Electrographic Classification of Epileptic Seizures

Commission on Classification and Terminology of the International League Against Epilepsy (1981)

PART I: PARTIAL (FOCAL, LOCAL) SEIZURES

Partial seizures are those in which, in general, the first clinical and electroencephalographic changes indicate initial activation of a system of neurons limited to part of one cerebral hemisphere. A partial seizure is classified primarily on the basis of whether or not consciousness is impaired during the attack (Table 14A.1). When consciousness is not impaired, the seizure is classified as a simple partial seizure. When consciousness is impaired, the seizure is classified as a complex partial seizure. Impairment of consciousness may be the first clinical sign, or simple partial seizures may evolve into complex partial seizures. In patients with impaired consciousness, aberrations of behavior (automatisms) may occur. A partial seizure may not terminate, but instead progress to a generalized motor seizure. Impaired consciousness is defined as the inability to respond normally to exogenous stimuli by virtue of altered awareness and/or responsiveness (see "Definition of Terms").

There is considerable evidence that simple partial seizures usually have unilateral hemispheric involvement and only rarely have bilateral hemispheric involvement; complex partial seizures, however, frequently have bilateral hemispheric involvement.

Partial seizures can be classified into one of the following three fundamental groups:

A. Simple partial seizures
B. Complex partial seizures
   1. With impairment of consciousness at onset
   2. Simple partial onset, followed by impairment of consciousness
C. Partial seizures evolving to generalized tonic-clonic convulsions (GTCs)
   1. Simple evolving to GTC
   2. Complex evolving to GTC (including those with simple partial onset)

PART II: GENERALIZED SEIZURES (CONVULSIVE OR NONCONVULSIVE)

Generalized seizures are those in which the first clinical changes indicate initial involvement of both hemispheres (Table 14A.2). Consciousness may be impaired and this impairment may be the initial manifestation. Motor

From *Epilepsia* 1981;22:489–501, with permission.

TABLE 14A.1
CLASSIFICATION OF PARTIAL SEIZURES

Clinical Seizure Type	EEG Seizure Type	EEG Interictal Expression

A. *Simple partial seizures* (consciousness not impaired)
  1. With minor signs
    (a) Focal motor without march
    (b) Focal motor with march (jacksonian)
    (c) Versive
    (d) Postural
    (e) Phonatory (vocalization or arrest of speech)
  2. With somatosensory or special-sensory symptoms (simple hallucinations, e.g., tingling, light flashes, buzzing)
    (a) Somatosensory
    (b) Visual
    (c) Auditory
    (d) Olfactory
    (e) Gustatory
    (f) Vertiginous
  3. With autonomic symptoms or signs (including epigastric sensation, pallor, sweating, flushing, piloerection, and pupillary dilation)
  4. With psychic symptoms (disturbance of higher cerebral function); these symptoms rarely occur without impairment of consciousness and are much more commonly experienced as complex partial seizures
    (a) Dysphasic
    (b) Dynamic (e.g., déjà vu)
    (c) Cognitive (e.g., dreamy states, distortions of time sense)
    (d) Affective (fear, anger, etc.)
    (e) Illusions (e.g., macropsia)
    (f) Structured hallucinations (e.g., music, scenes)
	Local contralateral discharge starting over the corresponding area of cortical representation (not always recorded on the scalp)	Local contralateral discharge

B. *Complex partial seizures* (with impairment of consciousness; may sometimes begin with simple symptomatology)
  1. Simple partial onset followed by impairment of consciousness
    (a) With simple partial features (A.1–A.4.) followed by impaired consciousness
    (b) With automatisms
  2. With impairment of consciousness at onset
    (a) With impairment of consciousness only
    (b) With automatisms
	Unilateral or, frequently, bilateral discharge, diffuse or focal in temporal or frontotemporal regions	Unilateral or bilateral generally asynchronous focus; usually in temporal or frontal regions

C. *Partial seizures evolving to secondarily generalized seizures* (may be generalized tonic-clonic, tonic, or clonic)
  1. Simple partial seizures (A) evolving to generalized seizures
  2. Complex partial seizures (B) evolving to generalized seizures
  3. Simple partial seizures evolving to complex partial seizures evolving to generalized seizures
	Above discharges become secondarily and rapidly generalized	

manifestations are bilateral. The ictal electroencephalographic patterns initially are bilateral, and presumably reflect neuronal discharge, which is widespread in both hemispheres.

PART III: UNCLASSIFIED EPILEPTIC SEIZURES

Includes all seizures that cannot be classified because of inadequate or incomplete data and some that defy classification in hitherto described categories. This includes some neonatal seizures, for example, rhythmic eye movements, chewing, and swimming movements.

PART IV: ADDENDUM

Repeated epileptic seizures occur under a variety of circumstances: (1) as fortuitous attacks, coming unexpectedly and without any apparent provocation; (2) as cyclic attacks, at more or less regular intervals (e.g., in relation to

TABLE 14A.2
CLASSIFICATION OF GENERALIZED SEIZURES

Clinical Seizure Type	EEG Seizure Type	EEG Interictal Expression
A. 1. *Absence seizures* (a) Impairment of consciousness only (b) With mild clonic components (c) With atonic components (d) With tonic components (e) With automatism (f) With autonomic components (*b* through *f* may be used alone or in combination)	Usually regular and symmetrical 3 Hz but may be 2- to 4-Hz spike-and-slow-wave complexes and may have multiple spike-and-slow-wave complexes; abnormalities are bilateral	Background activity usually normal, although paroxysmal activity (such as spikes or spike-and-slow-wave complexes) may occur; this activity is usually regular and symmetric
2. *Atypical absence* May have: (a) Changes in tone that are more pronounced than in A.1 (b) Onset and/or cessation that is not abrupt	EEG more heterogeneous: may include irregular spike-and-slow-wave complexes, fast activity, or other paroxysmal activity, abnormalities are bilateral but often irregular and asymmetric	Background usually abnormal; paroxysmal activity (such as spikes or spike-and-slow-wave complexes) frequently irregular and asymmetric
B. *Myoclonic seizures* Myoclonic jerks (single or multiple)	Polyspike and wave, or sometimes spike and wave or sharp and slow waves	Same as ictal
C. *Clonic seizures* Myoclonic jerks (single or multiple)	Fast activity (10 Hz or more) and slow waves: occasional spike-and-wave patterns	Spike-and-wave or polyspike-and-wave discharges
D. *Clonic seizures*	Low voltage, fast activity or a fast rhythm of 9–10 Hz or more, decreasing in frequency and increasing in amplitude	More or less rhythmic discharges of sharp and slow waves, sometimes asymmetric, background often abnormal for age
E. *Tonic-clonic seizures*	Rhythm at 10 Hz or more, decreasing in frequency and increasing in amplitude during tonic phase, interrupted by slow waves during clonic phase	Polyspikes and waves or spike and wave or, sometimes, sharp and slow-wave discharge
F. *Atonic seizures* (Astatic) Combinations of the above may occur, e.g., B and F, B and D	Polyspikes and wave or flattening or low-voltage fast activity	Polyspikes and slow wave

the menstrual cycle, or the sleep-waking cycle); and (3) as attacks provoked by: (a) nonsensory factors (fatigue, alcohol, emotion, etc.) or (b) sensory factors, sometimes referred to as reflex seizures.

Prolonged or repetitive seizures (status epilepticus). The term status epilepticus is used whenever a seizure persists for a sufficient length of time or is repeated frequently enough that recovery between attacks does not occur. Status epilepticus may be divided into partial (e.g., jacksonian) or generalized (e.g., absence status or tonic-clonic status). When very localized motor status occurs, it is referred to as epilepsia partialis continua.

PART V: DEFINITION OF TERMS

Each seizure type will be described so that the criteria used will not be in doubt.

Partial Seizures

The fundamental distinction between simple partial seizures and complex partial seizures is the presence or the impairment of the fully conscious state.

Consciousness has been defined as "that integrating activity by which Man grasps the totality of his phenomenal field" (21) and incorporates it into his experience. It corresponds to "Bewusstsein" and is thus much more than "Vigilance," for were it only vigilance (which is a degree of clarity) then only confusional states would be representative of disordered consciousness.

Operationally in the context of this classification, *consciousness* refers to the degree of awareness and/or responsiveness of the patient to externally applied stimuli. *Responsiveness* refers to the ability of the patient to carry out simple commands of willed movement; *awareness* refers to the patient's contact with events during the period in question and its recall. A person aware and unresponsive will be able to recount the events that occurred during an attack and his or her inability to respond by movement or speech. In this context, unresponsiveness is other than the result of paralysis, aphasia, or apraxia.

With Motor Signs

Any portion of the body may be involved in focal seizure activity depending on the site of origin of the attack in the motor strip. Focal motor seizures may remain strictly focal or they may spread to contiguous cortical areas producing a sequential involvement of body parts in an epileptic "march." The seizure is then known as a jacksonian seizure. Consciousness is usually preserved; however, the discharge may spread to those structures whose participation is likely to result in loss of consciousness and generalized convulsive movements. Other focal motor attacks may be versive with head turning to one side, usually contraversive to the discharge. If speech is involved, this is either in the form of speech arrest or, occasionally, vocalization. Occasionally, a partial dysphasia is seen in the form of epileptic palilalia with involuntary repetition of a syllable or phrase.

Following focal seizure activity, there may be a localized paralysis in the previously involved region. This is known as Todd's paralysis and may last from minutes to hours.

When focal motor seizure activity is continuous it is known as epilepsia partialis continua.

With Autonomic Symptoms

Vomiting, pallor, flushing, sweating, piloerection, pupil dilatation, borborygmi, and incontinence may occur as simple partial seizures.

With Somatosensory or Special Sensory Symptoms

Somatosensory seizures arise from those areas of cortex subserving sensory function, and they are usually described as pins-and-needles or a feeling of numbness. Occasionally, a disorder of proprioception or spatial perception occurs. Like motor seizures, somatosensory seizures also may march and also may spread at any time to become complex partial or generalized tonic-clonic seizures as in A.1. Special sensory seizures include visual seizures varying in elaborateness and depending on whether the primary or association areas are involved, from flashing lights to structured visual hallucinatory phenomena, including persons, scenes, etc. Like visual seizures, auditory seizures may also run the gamut from crude auditory sensations to such highly integrated functions as music. Olfactory sensations, usually in the form of unpleasant odors, may occur.

Gustatory sensations may be pleasant or odious taste hallucinations. They vary in elaboration from crude (salty, sour, sweet, bitter) to sophisticated. They are frequently described as "metallic."

Vertiginous symptoms include sensations of falling in space and floating, as well as rotatory vertigo in a horizontal or vertical plane.

With Psychic Symptoms (Disturbance of Higher Cerebral Function)

These usually occur with impairment of consciousness (i.e., complex partial seizures).

Dysphasia
This was referred to earlier.

Dysmnesic Symptoms
A distorted memory experience such as distortion of the time sense, a dreamy state, a flashback, or a sensation as if a naïve experience had been experienced before, known as déjà vu, or as if a previously experienced sensation had not been experienced, known as jamais-vu, may occur. When this refers to auditory experience, these are known as déjà-entendu or jamais-entendu. Occasionally, as a form of forced thinking, the patient may experience a rapid recollection of episodes from his or her past life, known as panoramic vision.

Cognitive Disturbances
These include dreamy states; distortions of the time sense; and sensations of unreality, detachment, or depersonalization.

With Affective Symptomatology
Sensation of extreme pleasure or displeasure, as well as fear and intense depression with feelings of unworthiness and rejection may be experienced during seizures. Unlike those of psychiatrically induced depression, these symptoms tend to come in attacks lasting for a few minutes. Anger or rage is occasionally experienced, but unlike temper tantrums, epileptic anger is apparently unprovoked, and abates rapidly. Fear or terror is the most frequent symptom; it is sudden in onset, usually unprovoked, and may lead to running away. Associated with the terror, there are frequently objective signs of autonomic activity, including pupil dilatation, pallor, flushing, piloerection, palpitation, and hypertension.

Epileptic or gelastic seizure laughter should not, strictly speaking, be classed as an affective symptom because the laughter is usually without affect and hollow. Like other forms of pathologic laughter it is often unassociated with true mirth.

Illusions

These take the form of distorted perceptions in which objects may appear deformed. Polyoptic illusions such as monocular diplopia and distortions of size (macropsia or micropsia) or of distance may occur. Similarly, distortions of sound, including microacusia and macroacusia, may be experienced. Depersonalization, as if the person were outside his or her body, may occur. Altered perception of size or weight of a limb may be noted.

Structured Hallucinations

Hallucinations may occur as manifestations or perceptions without a corresponding external stimulus and may affect somatosensory, visual, auditory, olfactory, or gustatory senses. If the seizure arises from the primary receptive area, the hallucination would tend to be rather primitive. In the case of vision, flashing lights may be seen; in the case of auditory perception, rushing noises may occur. With more elaborate seizures involving visual or auditory association areas with participation of mobilized memory traces, formed hallucinations occur, and these may take the form of scenery, persons, spoken sentences, or music. The character of these perceptions may be normal or distorted.

Seizures with Complex Symptomatology

Automatisms

(These may occur in both partial and generalized seizures. They are described in detail here for convenience.) In the *Dictionary of Epilepsy* (5), automatisms are described as "more or less coordinated adapted (eupractic or dyspractic) involuntary motor activity occurring during the state of clouding of consciousness either in the course of, or after, an epileptic seizure, and usually followed by amnesia for the event. The automatism may be simply a continuation of an activity that was going on when the seizure occurred, or, conversely, a new activity developed in association with the ictal impairment of consciousness. Usually, the activity is commonplace in nature, often provoked by the subject's environment, or by his sensations during the seizure; exceptionally, fragmentary, primitive, infantile, or antisocial behavior is seen. From a symptomatological point of view, the following are distinguished: (a) eating automatisms (chewing, swallowing); (b) automatisms of mimicry, expressing the subject's emotional state (usually of fear) during the seizure; (c) gestural automatisms, crude or elaborate, directed toward either the subject or his environment; (d) ambulatory automatisms; and (e) verbal automatisms."

Ictal epileptic automatisms usually represent the release of automatic behavior under the influence of clouding of consciousness that accompanies a generalized or partial epileptic seizure (confusional automatisms). They may occur in complex partial seizures, as well as in absence seizures. Postictal epileptic automatisms may follow any severe epileptic seizure, especially a tonic-clonic one, and are usually associated with confusion.

While some regard masticatory or oropharyngeal automatisms as arising from the amygdala or insular and opercular regions, these movements are occasionally seen in the generalized epilepsies, particularly absence seizures, and are not of localizing help. The same is true of mimicry and gestural automatisms. In the latter, fumbling of the clothes, scratching, and other complex motor activity may occur both in complex partial and absence seizures. Ictal speech automatisms are occasionally encountered. Ambulatory seizures again may occur either as prolonged automatisms of absence, particularly prolonged absence continuing, or of complex partial seizures. In the latter, a patient may occasionally continue to drive a car, although may contravene traffic light regulations.

There seems to be little doubt that automatisms are a common feature of different types of epilepsy. While they do not lend themselves to simple anatomic interpretation, they appear to have in common a discharge involving various areas of the limbic system. Crude and elaborate automatisms do occur in patients with absence, as well as complex partial seizures. Of greater significance is the precise descriptive history of the seizures; the age of the patient; and the presence or absence of an aura and of postictal behavior, including the presence or absence of confusion. The EEG [electroencephalogram] is of cardinal localizational importance here.

Drowsiness or Somnolence

Drowsiness or somnolence implies a sleep state from which the patient can be aroused to make appropriate motor and verbal responses. In stupor, the patient may make some spontaneous movement and, by painful or other vigorously applied stimuli, can be aroused to make avoidance movements. The patient in confusion makes inappropriate responses to his or her environment and is disoriented with regard to place or time or person.

Aura

A frequently used term in the description of epileptic seizures is aura. According to the *Dictionary of Epilepsy*, this term was introduced by Galen to describe the sensation of a breath of air felt by some subjects prior to the onset of a seizure. Others have referred to the aura as the portion of a seizure experienced before loss of consciousness occurs. This loss of consciousness may be the result of secondary generalization of the seizure discharge or of alteration of consciousness imparted by the development of a complex partial seizure.

The aura is that portion of the seizure that occurs before consciousness is lost and for which memory is retained afterwards. It may be that, as in simple partial seizures, the aura is the whole seizure. Where consciousness is subsequently lost, the aura is, in fact, the signal symptom of a complex partial seizure.

An aura is a retrospective term that is described after the seizure has ended.

Generalized Seizures: Absence Seizures

The hallmark of the absence attack is a sudden onset, interruption of ongoing activities, a blank stare, possibly a brief upward rotation of the eyes. If the patient is speaking, speech is slowed or interrupted; if walking, he or she stands transfixed; if eating, he or she will stop the food on the way to the mouth. Usually the patient will be unresponsive when spoken to. In some, attacks are aborted when the patient is spoken to. The attack lasts from a few seconds to half a minute and evaporates as rapidly as it commenced.

Absence with Impairment of Consciousness Only

The above description fits the description of absence simple in which no other activities take place during the attack.

Absence with Mild Clonic Components

Here, the onset of the attack is indistinguishable from the above, but clonic movements may occur in the eyelids, at the corner of the mouth, or in other muscle groups, which may vary in severity from almost imperceptible movements to generalized myoclonic jerks. Objects held in the hand may be dropped.

Absence with Atonic Components

Here, there may be a diminution in tone of muscles subserving posture, as well as in the limbs, leading to drooping of the head, occasionally slumping of the trunk, dropping of the arms, and relaxation of the grip. Rarely, tone is sufficiently diminished to cause one to fall.

Absence with Tonic Components

Here, during the attack, tonic muscular contraction may occur, leading to an increase in muscle tone, which may affect the extensor muscles or the flexor muscles symmetrically or asymmetrically. If the patient is standing, the head may be drawn backward and the trunk may arch. This may lead to retropulsion. The head may tonically draw to one or another side.

Absence with Automatisms

(See also prior discussion on automatisms.) Purposeful or quasi-purposeful movements occurring in the absence of awareness during an absence attack are frequent and may range from lip licking and swallowing to clothes fumbling or aimless walking. If spoken to, the patient may grunt or turn to the spoken voice, and when touched or tickled, may rub the site. Automatisms are quite elaborate and may consist of combinations of the above-described movements or may be so simple as to be missed by casual observation. Mixed forms of absence frequently occur.

Tonic-Clonic Seizures

The most frequently encountered of the generalized seizures are the generalized tonic-clonic seizures, often known as grand mal. Some patients experience a vague ill-described warning, but the majority lose consciousness without any premonitory symptoms. There is a sudden, sharp tonic contraction of muscles, and when this involves the respiratory muscles, there is stridor, a cry or moan, and the patient falls to the ground in the tonic state, occasionally injuring him or herself. The patient lies rigid, and during this stage, tonic contraction inhibits respiration and cyanosis may occur. The tongue may be bitten and urine may be passed involuntarily. This tonic stage then gives way to clonic convulsive movements lasting for a variable period of time. During this stage, small gusts of grunting respiration may occur between the convulsive movements, but usually the patient remains cyanotic and saliva may froth from the mouth. At the end of this stage, deep respiration occurs and all the muscles relax, after which the patient remains unconscious for a variable period of time and often awakes feeling stiff and sore all over. He or she then frequently goes into a deep sleep and when awakened feels quite well apart from soreness and, frequently, headache. GTCs may occur in childhood and in adult life; they are not as frequent as absence seizures, but vary from one a day to one every 3 months and occasionally to one every few years. Very short attacks without postictal drowsiness may occur on occasion.

Myoclonic Seizures

Myoclonic jerks (single or multiple) are sudden, brief shock-like contractions that may be generalized or confined to the face and trunk or to one or more extremities or even to individual muscles or groups of muscles. Myoclonic jerks may be rapidly repetitive or relatively isolated. They may occur predominantly around the hours of going to sleep or awakening from sleep. They may be exacerbated by volitional movement (action myoclonus). At times they may be regularly repetitive.

Many instances of myoclonic jerks and action myoclonus are not classified as epileptic seizures. The myoclonic jerks of myoclonus due to spinal cord disease, dyssynergia cerebellaris myoclonica, subcortical segmental myoclonus, paramyoclonus multiplex, and opsoclonus-myoclonus syndrome must be distinguished from epileptic seizures.

Clonic Seizures

Generalized convulsive seizures occasionally lack a tonic component and are characterized by repetitive clonic jerks. As the frequency diminishes, the amplitude of the jerks do not. The postictal phase is usually short. Some generalized convulsive seizures commence with a clonic phase passing into a tonic phase, as described below, leading to a "clonic-tonic-clonic" seizure.

Tonic Seizures

To quote Gowers, a tonic seizure is "a rigid, violent muscular contraction, fixing the limbs in some strained position. There is usually deviation of the eyes and of the head toward one side, and this may amount to rotation involving the whole body (sometimes actually causing the patient to turn around, even two or three times). The features are distorted; the color of the face, unchanged at first, rapidly becomes pale and then flushed and ultimately livid as the fixation of the chest by the spasms stops the movements of respiration. The eyes are open or closed; the conjunctiva is insensitive; the pupils dilate widely as cyanosis comes on. As the spasm continues, it commonly changes in its relative intensity in different parts, causing slight alterations in the position of the limbs." Tonic axial seizures with extension of head, neck, and trunk may also occur.

ATONIC SEIZURES

A sudden diminution in muscle tone occurs, which may be fragmentary, leading to a head drop with slackening of the jaw, the dropping of a limb or a loss of all muscle tone leading to a slumping to the ground. When these attacks are extremely brief, they are known as "drop attacks." If consciousness is lost, this loss is extremely brief. The sudden loss of postural tone in the head and trunk may lead to injury by projecting objects. The face is particularly subject to injury. In the case of more prolonged atonic attacks, the slumping may be progressive in a rhythmic, successive relaxation manner.

(So-called drop attacks may be seen in conditions other than epilepsy, such as brainstem ischemia and narcolepsy cataplexy syndrome.)

Unclassified Epileptic Seizures

This category includes all seizures that cannot be classified because of inadequate or incomplete data and includes some seizures that, by their natures, defy classification in the previously defined broad categories. Many seizures occurring in the infant (e.g., rhythmic eye movements, chewing, swimming movements, jittering, and apnea) will be classified here until such time as further experience with videotape confirmation and electroencephalographic characterization entitles them to subtyping in the extant classification.

Epilepsia Partialis Continua

Under this name have been described cases of simple partial seizures with focal motor signs without a march, usually consisting of clonic spasms, which remain confined to the part of the body in which they originate, but which persist with little or no intermission for hours or days at a stretch. Consciousness is usually preserved, but postictal weakness is frequently evident.

POSTICTAL PARALYSIS (TODD'S PARALYSIS)

This category refers to the transient paralysis that may occur following some partial epileptic seizures with focal motor components or with somatosensory symptoms. Postictal paralysis has been ascribed to neuronal exhaustion due to the increased metabolic activity of the discharging focus, but it may also be attributable to increased inhibition in the region of the focus, which may account for its appearance in nonmotor somatosensory seizures.

Epileptic Auras

15

Norman K. So

The word *aura* (from the Greek for "air," Latin for "breeze") was first applied to epilepsy by Galen's teacher, Pelops (1), who interpreted reports of altered sensations ascending to the head from an extremity as support for a humoral mechanism in which a vapor passed up the blood vessels. For many centuries, Galen's followers believed that somatosensory auras beginning in the extremities indicated a peripheral origin of epileptic seizures.

The aura, of course, is the start, not the cause, of a seizure, as Erastus pointed out around 1580. Jackson's systematic study of auras ushered in a new era, when he correlated the sensations with functional localization in the brain (2). The 1981 International Classification of Epileptic Seizures (3) defined an aura as "that portion of the seizure which occurs before consciousness is lost and for which memory is retained afterwards." An aura in isolation thus corresponds to a simple partial sensory seizure. Conventional usage further limits the word to the initial sensations of a seizure, without observable signs, that a patient is aware of and recollects. This definition specifically separates an aura from a focal motor seizure and is used in this chapter. Whether autonomic phenomena in seizures should be considered auras remains debatable. To the extent that patients can clearly recollect such symptoms as shivering with piloerection at seizure onset, autonomic phenomena can be experienced as an aura. However, when flushing or pupillary dilatation is reported by others without a patient's awareness, the term aura cannot be used.

PRODROMES AND PREMONITIONS

An aura usually lasts seconds to minutes and immediately precedes the signs of an attack. On occasion, auras can be long-lasting, continuous, or recurrent, with short intervening breaks. Intracranial electroencephalographic (EEG) studies show that prolonged auras (aura continua) can represent continuous or recurrent seizures, a form of focal status epilepticus (4). More frequently, for hours to days before attacks, patients may experience prodromal symptoms of nervousness, anxiety, dizziness, and headache that should not be regarded as auras. The prodrome may be evident on awakening and signals a seizure that will occur later in the day. Sometimes a patient may not be conscious of anything untoward, but family members or friends may describe irritability or "a mean streak." Such prodromal symptoms resemble those recounted by patients with migraine. Gowers' speculation (1) that the prodrome is "indicative of slight disturbance of the nerve centres" has not been improved on.

Less commonly, some patients with generalized epilepsy may experience stereotyped sensations before the occurrence of a generalized seizure. Like an aura, these premonitory symptoms immediately precede the seizure but are brief and nonspecific, lacking the features that suggest activation of a circumscribed area of the cortex. Sensations include dizziness, warmth, cold, generalized tingling, anxiety, and a spaced-out, or confused, feeling. Rarely, ill-formed visual imagery and abdominal sensations have been reported. Some of the sensations likely correspond to a buildup of absence (dizziness, lightheadedness, and confusion) or myoclonic seizures (anxiety, restlessness, jumpiness, and jerking).

AURA COMBINATIONS AND MARCH

Although an aura reflects activation of functional cortex by a circumscribed seizure discharge, the seizure discharge frequently spreads. When the seizure discharge spreads along a single functional area, such as the postcentral gyrus, the sensory equivalent of focal motor jacksonian march is seen. An aura can also spread across different functional regions. A seizure that begins in the primary visual area of the occipital lobe and spreads to the temporal limbic structures may present with initial transient blindness, followed by other sensations referable to the temporal lobe (5).

Multiple sensations can occur even when seizure activity is relatively confined to one region, as at the start of a temporal lobe seizure. In some cases, the multiple auras can be dissected out along a sequence, implying spread of the seizure discharge. Anxiety, epigastric, and "indescribable" sensations commonly precede the more complex phenomena of *déjà vu* and other illusions of vision or sound (6), although the sequence is not always stable in different attacks. In other cases, a time series cannot be discerned, and the multiple sensations seem to occur simultaneously. An alternative explanation for multiple auras could be that they are secondary to activation of a system with access to more than one functional region. The temporal limbic system, with extensive connections to the septum, hypothalamus, temporal neocortex, insula, and parietooccipital association cortex, is an example (7). In support of this hypothesis, electrical stimulation of temporal limbic structures by depth electrodes can produce different sets of sensations at different times, despite stimulation of the same contact (8).

PRESENCE AND ABSENCE OF AURAS

The incidence of auras in large populations is imprecise. In the 32-year epidemiologic study from Rochester, Minnesota (9), epilepsy with focal sensory seizures was reported in 3.7% of all patients. An additional 26.4% were classified as having temporal lobe epilepsy, but the incidence of aura in this group was not separately reported. In the two large series of clinic- and office-based patients with epilepsy studied by Gowers (1) and by Lennox and Cobb (10) (Table 15.1), an aura was present in 56% of patients. Although notable discrepancies exist between the two series with respect to relative frequencies of unilateral somatosensory auras, bilateral general sensations, and visual auras, other categories are remarkably consistent. Differences are most likely explained on the basis of definitions of aura type.

The findings in other series were more variable. In patients with complex partial seizures or temporal lobe epilepsy, the incidence of auras ranged between 22.5% and 83% (6,11–15). During long-term scalp and sphenoidal or intracranial EEG monitoring of seizures, 46% to 70% of patients reported auras, either independent of or as part of their habitual seizures (16–18).

Some patients who do not describe auras may have had them early in their illness. Anecdotal experience suggests that auras may disappear as the disease progresses, and as seizures cause increasingly profound loss of awareness and postictal confusion. As Lennox and Cobb (10) stated: "It is more accurate to speak of the recollection of aura(s) rather than of their presence." Young children may lack the verbal capacity to describe the sensations that herald a seizure, even though their actions indicate some awareness of the impending event. Similarly, adults who deny having any

TABLE 15.1

INCIDENCE OF AURAS IN TWO SERIES OF CLINIC- AND OFFICE-BASED PATIENTS WITH EPILEPSY

Aura	Gowers (1) % [a](n = 2,013)	Lennox and Cobb (10) % (n = 1,359)
Present	1,145 (57%)	764 (56%)
Somatosensory[b]	18.0	8.5
Bilateral sensations	4.5	38.0
Visceral/epigastric	18.0	14.5
Vertiginous	19.0	12.0
Cephalic	8.0	5.5
Psychical	8.0	11.0
Visual[c]	16.0	6.5
Auditory	6.0	2.0
Olfactory	1.0	1.0
Gustatory	1.5	0.1

[a]Percentages apply to patients with aura.
[b]Includes motor phenomena at onset.
[c]Includes illusions and hallucinations.
From Gowers WR. *Epilepsy and other chronic convulsive diseases: their causes, symptoms and treatment*, 2nd ed. London: J & A Churchill, 1901; and Lennox WG, Cobb S. Aura in epilepsy: a statistical review of 1,359 cases. *Arch Neurol Psychiatry* 1933;30:374–387, with permission.

warning, may nevertheless press the seizure alarm button during video-EEG monitoring but have no recollection of doing so. The seizure either induces an amnesia so immediate that there is no memory of a warning or causes retrograde amnesia. This is supported by a study that showed amnesia for auras depended on the severity of the seizure (19). An isolated aura is nearly always recollected and associated with either no ictal discharge or a unilateral EEG ictal discharge. The aura is more likely to be forgotten if the seizure becomes secondarily generalized and involves bilateral EEG ictal discharge.

The complete cessation of all seizures—the desired goal of successful epilepsy surgery—cannot always be achieved. Auras can persist as isolated phenomena following epilepsy surgery, when complex partial or secondarily generalized seizures no longer occur, and even after discontinuation of antiepileptic drugs. Isolated postoperative auras are often ignored and classified among the "seizure-free" outcomes. In a few studies, isolated postoperative auras occurred in 20% (20,21) to 35% (22) of patients following surgery for temporal lobe epilepsy and in 22% of patients after focal resective surgery unselected for location (23). Residual auras seem particularly common following temporal lobe surgery, and may be related to incomplete removal of the mesial temporal structures comprising the amygdala, hippocampus, and parahippocampal gyrus. The persistence of epigastric auras after functional hemispherectomy, in which the insula is the only cortical structure still functionally connected on the side of surgery, suggests that continuing seizure activity in that structure may be another mechanism. Postoperative auras commonly recurred within the first 6 months of surgery and tended to persist (22). Although isolated postoperative auras are widely regarded as being of little significance, they may accompany an increased risk for recurrence of complex partial seizures (22) and reduced quality of life on self-assessment (23).

A small number of patients may lose their auras following temporal lobectomy, even as they continue to have postoperative complex partial seizures; others may experience a different aura. Such alterations occurred in 55% of patients who had residual postoperative seizures (20).

INDIVIDUAL DETERMINANTS

A long duration of epilepsy correlates with an increased incidence of auras, which Lennox and Cobb (10) thought "presumably due to the greater total number of seizures and the greater likelihood of experiencing aura." Early onset epilepsy, lower intelligence quotient (IQ), male gender, and right temporal lobe focus are all associated with a higher incidence of "simple primitive" auras, whereas complex "intellectual" auras with illusions or hallucinations accompany male gender and a verbal IQ greater than 100 (24).

Aura content may be related to a patient's psychological makeup. Stimulation of various mesial limbic structures elicited auras with features that were intimately related to ongoing psychopathologic processes (25). Emotional responses and hallucinations produced by electrical stimulation were reported to depend on the background affective state (26,27). Similarly, patients who experienced anxiety or fear during temporal lobe electrical stimulation scored higher on the Psychasthenia scale of the Minnesota Multiphasic Personality Inventory, whereas those experiencing dreamlike or memory-like hallucinations scored higher on the Schizophrenia scale (8). The aura phenomena shown to be sensitive to personality factors are precisely those that comprise an individual's personality. Thus, the memory flashback that may be recalled in an aura is not a generic item, but rather an experience specific to a patient.

CLINICAL LOCALIZATION

An aura provides evidence of focal seizure onset. The nature of the symptoms may localize the epileptogenic zone. All sensations near the onset of seizures are not necessarily auras, however. It is important to differentiate auras from prodromes and from nonspecific premonitions before generalized seizures. Auras may vary in the same patient or occur in combination but should show a certain stereotypy and consistency. It may be particularly difficult to classify a first seizure based on the report of a preceding sensation. One study (28) noted poor interobserver agreement about the nature of such preceding sensations. In the same study, the incidence of generalized versus focal epileptiform EEG abnormalities and of structural abnormalities

on computed tomography was similar in the 67 patients with and the 82 patients without sensations preceding a generalized convulsion. At 1-year follow-up, seizures had recurred in 22 of the 67 patients with preceding sensations, but only 11 of these had clinical indications that the recurrences were of focal onset. Thus, self-report of a preceding sensation in an isolated first convulsion may not be a reliable indicator of focal epilepsy.

The sensation before an ictal event can be misleading in another situation. Sometimes, albeit rarely, patients have pseudoseizures beginning with an epileptic aura (29). The epileptic seizures often are well controlled except for the auras. Whether the pseudoseizure that follows the aura represents a learned response or occurs from other psychogenic mechanisms cannot be determined.

Current concepts of the localizing value of auras rely heavily on the pioneering studies of Penfield and Jasper (14), who correlated sensations and signs obtained through electrical stimulation of the awake patient with those of the patient's spontaneous seizures. Subsequent studies with long-term intracranial electrodes for the recording of spontaneous seizures and extraoperative electrical brain stimulation have extended early observations (30–34).

Although an aura may help to localize the epileptogenic zone, an important point must be kept in mind: The initial sensation of an aura is related to the first functional brain area activated by the seizure that has access to consciousness, but this may not be the site of seizure origin. A seizure starting in the posterior parietal region may be initially asymptomatic, until ictal activity spreads to adjacent functional areas. Spread to the postcentral gyrus may elicit a somatosensory sensation as the first warning; propagation to the parietooccipital association cortex may give rise to initial visual illusions or hallucinations. Furthermore, it remains unclear whether experience of an aura is contingent on direct ictal involvement of the cortical areas subserving those functions or whether an aura sensation may also be evoked by excitation at a distance, provided a pathway of projection or facilitation exists between the site of excitation and an eloquent cortical structure. Both mechanisms are probably operative in human epilepsy. A sensory jacksonian march cannot be explained other than by ictal spread along the somatosensory cortex. The indistinguishable auras found in patients with hippocampal sclerosis and temporal neocortical pathology underlie the distributed network that functionally links the limbic and neocortical structures in the temporal lobe. Cortical stimulation in patients with extratemporal epilepsy also showed that sites at which an aura is reproduced can extend well beyond the expected functional map for those sensations (33).

The localizing value of auras has been studied in a number of ways. Penfield and Kristiansen (35) recorded the initial seizure phenomenon in 222 patients with focal epilepsy and commented on the likely localization of different auras. Auras reported in patients with well-defined epileptogenic foci in different brain regions can be compared from different series (Table 15.2) or, better yet, prospectively (36) (Table 15.3). Data from patients (37,38) who become seizure free after localized brain resections are particularly important because their surgical outcome is absolute proof of the correct localization of the epileptogenic zone. Making comparisons from different series in the literature is hampered by several problems: Definitions of aura type are not uniform, data on different auras are often grouped in dissimilar ways, and classification rules may differ when multiple sensations occur in the same aura. In spite of the different approaches, however, retrospective and prospective series yielded a remarkably similar conclusion: Auras have localizing significance. Patients with temporal lobe epilepsy have the highest incidence of epigastric, emotional, and psychic auras (36,37). Frontal lobe epilepsy is distinguished by frequent reports of no aura (36,38). When an aura is present in a patient with frontal lobe epilepsy, cephalic and general body sensations predominate (36). Perirolandic epilepsy with centroparietal foci is most likely to involve somatosensory aura (39). Unsurprisingly, occipital lobe epilepsy is associated with the highest incidence of visual aura (36,40). No single aura sensation is necessarily restricted to a single lobe, however.

Except for unilateral somatosensory and visual auras contralateral to the site of seizure onset, the nature of an aura provides no reliable lateralizing information. Penfield and colleagues (14,41) reported that psychic illusions were lateralized mainly to the nondominant temporal lobe. Subsequently, these findings have been confirmed by some researchers (42) but refuted by others (6,12,16).

ELECTROENCEPHALOGRAPHIC LOCALIZATION

The EEG signature of an aura depends on the recording technique. An isolated aura is a focal seizure of restricted extent, with an intensity between that of a subclinical EEG seizure and a complex partial seizure. Because the success of an ictal EEG recording is determined by the proximity of the electrode(s) to the epileptogenic trigger zone, scalp EEGs frequently fail to detect any changes during an isolated aura and during the aura component of a complex partial seizure. In one study (43) of depth electrode-recorded temporal lobe seizures, only 19% of auras had surface ictal EEG changes. In the same study, 10% of subclinical EEG seizures and 86% of clinical (psychomotor) seizures were accompanied by surface changes. An EEG that incorporates sphenoidal electrodes may have a better chance (28%) of detecting an electrographic change during an aura (17). The surface EEG ictal pattern is often incomplete and subtle compared with that of a complex partial seizure and may appear as low-frequency rhythmic sharp waves, sudden attenuation of the ongoing background, or

TABLE 15.2

RELATIVE INCIDENCE OF AURAS IN PATIENTS WITH FOCAL EPILEPSIES (%)

	Temporal[a] Rasmussen (37) (n = 147)	Frontal[a] Rasmussen (38) (n = 140)	Centroparietal Ajmone-Marsan and Goldhammer (39) (n = 40)	Occipital Ludwig and Ajmone-Marsan (40) (n = 18)
Somatosensory	5	17.5	52[b]	0
Epigastric/emotional	52[b]	12.5	22	6
Cephalic	5	12.5	7	6
General body	8	12.5	7	6
Psychical	15	7.5	10	17
Visual	11	5.0	25	56[b]
Auditory	11	—	25	—
Olfactory	11	—	25	11
Gustatory	11	—	25	11
Vertiginous	11	2.5	—	—
None	15	42.5[b]	22	6

[a]Seizure free after surgery.
[b]Indicates highest incidence for location.
From Rasmussen T. Localizational aspects of epileptic seizure phenomena. In: Thompson RA, Green JR, eds. New perspectives in cerebral localization. New York: Raven Press; 1982:177–203; Rasmussen T. Characteristics of a pure culture of frontal lobe epilepsy. Epilepsia 1983;24:482–493; Ajmone-Marsan C, Goldhammer L. Clinical ictal patterns and electrographic data in cases of partial seizures of frontal-central-parietal origin. In: Brazier MAB, ed. Epilepsy: its phenomena in man. New York: Academic Press; 1973:235–259; and Ludwig BI, Ajmone-Marsan C. Clinical ictal patterns in epileptic patients with occipital electroencephalographic foci. Neurology 1975;25:463–471, with permission.

TABLE 15.3

FREQUENCY OF AURAS IN PATIENTS WITH FOCAL EPILEPSIES

	No. of Patients	Retrospective Series			Prospective Series		
		Temporal	Frontal	Posterooccipital	Temporal	Frontal	Posterooccipital
Somatosensory	32	1	8	15	0	1	7
Epigastric	47	20	3	3	20	0	1
Cephalic	22	5	13	1	3	0	0
Diffuse warm sensation	10	1	9	0	0	0	0
Psychic	51	27	2	2	19	0	1
Elementary visual	13	1	0	12	0	0	0
Elementary auditory	3	3	0	0	0	0	0
Vertiginous	7	0	1	2	1	1	2
Conscious confusion	11	4	3	1	2	1	0
Total	196	62	39	36	42	3	11

Adapted from Palmini A, Gloor P. The localizing value of auras in partial seizures: a prospective and retrospective study. *Neurology* 1992;42:801–808, with permission.

abrupt cessation of ongoing interictal spikes sometimes followed by rhythmic slow waves.

Depth electrodes targeted directly at mesial limbic structures (where the majority of temporal lobe seizures originate) have been more successful in demonstrating EEG ictal activity in temporal lobe auras than were simultaneous recordings from subdural electrodes over the lateral temporal convexity (44,45). Nevertheless, even in patients with seizure onset in one temporal lobe, localized by depth electrode recording, only about half of the isolated auras showed an ictal EEG correlate (18,46). In neurophysiologic terms, these observations support the belief that only a very small portion of the brain must be activated to produce aura sensations. On the basis of firing patterns of limbic neurons recorded by microelectrode techniques in patients with temporal lobe epilepsy, only 14% of neurons at the epileptogenic trigger zone are estimated to increase their firing rate in an aura. The corresponding estimate for a subclinical seizure is 7% and for a clinical complex partial seizure it is 36% (47). In the same patient, some auras may be associated with ictal EEG changes, whereas others show no change (46). This suggests that seizures may arise dynamically from different discrete areas within a larger epileptic zone. That identical auras may arise from sites remote from those where they were successfully recorded is unlikely. Patients who had electrodes implanted into homologous regions of the opposite hemisphere often became seizure free following temporal lobectomy (46).

SOMATOSENSORY AURAS

Tingling, numbness, and an electrical feeling are common manifestations of somatosensory auras, whereas absence of sensation or a sensation of movement is experienced less often. A sensation that begins focally or shows a sensory march, such as an ascent up the arm from the hand in the course of seconds, points to a seizure discharge in the primary somatosensory area of the contralateral postcentral gyrus. A primary somatosensory aura can be interrupted by clonic jerking, usually of the part with the abnormal sensation, which presumably reflects spread from the postcentral to the precentral gyrus. Occasionally, a seizure starting in the primary motor area of the precentral gyrus also causes a somatosensory aura, which is usually followed rapidly or simultaneously accompanied by clonic motor phenomena. A clinically identical seizure may have begun more posteriorly in the "silent" parietal cortex and caused symptoms only after it spread to the postcentral gyrus.

Somatic sensations with a wide segmental or bilateral distribution indicate seizure activity outside the primary somatosensory area. Seizures arising from or involving the second sensory area, situated in the superior bank of the sylvian fissure anterior to the precentral gyrus (14,48), evoke somatic sensations of the contralateral sides of the body, the ipsilateral sides of the body, or both. The sensation is often rudimentary, as in primary somatosensory auras; however, second sensory auras include pain, coldness, and a desire for movement (49). The sensation occasionally is followed by the inability to move or control the affected part, an example of a "sensory inhibitory seizure."

Seizures arising from the supplementary motor area were preceded by an aura in nearly half the patients in one study (50). Penfield and Jasper (14) elicited somatic sensations from the supplementary sensory area, a part of the mesial cortex in the interhemispheric fissure, posterior to the supplementary motor area. Recently, extraoperative stimulation using chronically implanted subdural electrodes not only confirmed the existence of supplementary sensory areas but also showed that they intermingle and overlap with the supplementary motor area, so that the two regions can best be regarded as a single functional entity (51,52). Auras from the supplementary motor and sensory areas include non-specific tingling, desire for or sensation of movement, and feelings of stiffness, pulling, pulsation, and heaviness. These sensations usually involve extensive areas of a contralateral extremity or side of the body or bilateral body parts. They may be perceived as a generalized body sensation as well. Penfield and Jasper (14) also elicited epigastric sensations on stimulation of the supplementary motor area.

Chronic recordings and stimulation studies of depth electrodes implanted into the posterior insular cortex revealed another brain region that can give rise to contralateral somatosensory sensations (34,53). The sensations include those of tingling, electrical shock, heat, and sometimes pain. They can involve more localized or more extensive regions on the contralateral side of the body.

As an aura, a general body sensation, including diffuse warm and cold thermal sensations, has little value in cortical localization, having been reported as seizure aura from all regions of the brain. Besides the supplementary motor area, the mesial temporal structures (54) have responded to stimulation with such diffuse sensations.

Ictal pain as an aura can be classified according to the affected parts: cephalic, abdominal, and somesthetic. Ictal headache will be discussed along with other cephalic auras, and abdominal pain along with epigastric aura. Painful body sensations may represent the initial aura or occur as a component of an aura or seizure. The pain may be sharp, burning, electric, cold, or cramplike and may be focally to diffusely distributed. Pain as an isolated symptom is much less common than it is as an association of paresthesia and other somatic sensations (55,56). Some patients experience cramp-like pain with tonic muscle spasm of an affected part. Well-localized and unilateral ictal pain generally occurs contralateral to an epileptic focus in the postcentral gyrus or neighboring parietal lobe (55–59). Electrical stimulation of the postcentral gyrus can elicit contralateral pain (57,60). Resection of the parietal cortex with the epileptic focus has successfully abolished painful seizures (56,57). Other areas reported to produce painful somesthetic auras are the second sensory area (14,48) and the insular cortex (53). The localization of heat, cold, warmth, and flushing is variable or poorly understood. When these sensations are focal and unilateral, the same cortical regions described above are likely responsible. When they are felt over wide segmental areas, on both sides of the body or in a generalized distribution, they lack reliable localizing value. Pharyngeal dysesthesias of tingling and burning are uncommon auras, sometimes reported in patients with temporal lobe epilepsy or seizures arising from the insula (53).

VISUAL AURAS

Spots, stars, blobs, bars, or circles of light that are monochromatic or variously colored, implicate seizure activity in the visual areas of the occipital lobes (14). These stationary or moving images may be lateralized to the visual field contralateral to the involved lobe, but they may also appear directly ahead. When they are lateralized and move across the field of vision, the patient's head may turn to follow them. Some patients describe darkness proceeding to blindness, which can also occur as a postictal phenomenon in those with visual auras. An occipital seizure may propagate to the temporal lobe or the parietal cortex. In the former instance, a visual aura may be followed by psychic experiences, epigastric aura, or emotional feelings, whereas a somatosensory aura may follow in the latter case. Auras with formed visual hallucinations are discussed under psychic auras, along with such visual illusions as macropsia and micropsia.

AUDITORY AURAS

The auditory area lies in the transverse gyrus of Heschl. Electrical stimulation there and in the adjacent superior temporal gyrus produces simple sounds variously described as ringing, booming, buzzing, chirping, or machine-like (14). A lateralized sound is usually contralateral to the side of stimulation. At other times, partial deafness may occur. Auras with such "unformed" auditory hallucinations suggest seizure activity in the superior temporal neocortex and temporal operculum (14,61). Because seizures can spread to other portions of the temporal lobe, auditory auras are frequently accompanied by other temporal lobe phenomena. Other auditory illusions and hallucinations are discussed later in this chapter.

VERTIGINOUS AURAS

Stimulation of the superior temporal gyrus can elicit feelings of displacement or movement, including rotatory sensations (14). True vertiginous auras are probably uncommon but may be localized to the posterior portion of the superior temporal neocortex (61). More frequently, patients report dizziness, which, on questioning, may be further clarified as a cephalic aura, blurring of vision, or knowledge of impending loss of awareness. Early reports of patients with so-called vertiginous seizures probably included a large number with nonspecific dizziness (62,63). Vertiginous auras usually form only one element of the sensations experienced before a seizure.

OLFACTORY AURAS

Jackson and Beevor (64) reported a "case of tumor of the right temporosphenoidal lobe bearing on the localization of the sense of smell and on the interpretation of a particular variety of epilepsy." The patient experienced a "very horrible smell which she could not describe." The term *uncinate fits* has been used to describe seizures with this aura, because pathologic lesions are frequently found in the medial temporal lobe. The smell of an olfactory aura is often unpleasant or disagreeable (14,65). Odors akin to burning rubber, sulfur, or organic solvents have been reported. In contrast, the smell can also be neutral or even pleasant (66). The incidence of olfactory aura is generally about 1% (Table 15.1). Whether patients with this symptom are disproportionately more likely to have temporal lobe tumor is open to debate (65,67), as nonneoplastic lesions such as mesial temporal sclerosis have also been responsible (66,68).

Other than the medial temporal lobe, the olfactory bulb is the only structure that can produce an olfactory sensation on electrical stimulation. It remains to be seen whether seizure activity beginning in the orbitofrontal region will cause an olfactory aura. Olfactory auras rarely occur in isolation; gustatory or other sensations referable to the temporal lobe also may be experienced.

GUSTATORY AURAS

Usually disagreeable, the taste experienced may be described as sharp, bitter, acid, or sickly sweet. The incidence is low (Table 15.1). Penfield and Jasper (14) ascribed the representation of taste deep in the sylvian fissure adjacent to and above the insular cortex. Hausser-Hauw and Bancaud (69) localized gustatory hallucinations to the parietal or rolandic operculum. They also recorded spontaneous and electrically induced seizures from the temporal limbic structures that were associated with gustatory phenomena, but believed that the aura resulted from seizure propagation to the opercular region. Temporal lobectomies failed to abolish the gustatory hallucinations in three of the patients in the study. The course of seizures with gustatory aura depends on the site of the epileptogenic zone (69). Suprasylvian seizures are likely to involve salivation, second sensory area sensations, and clonic facial contractions. Seizures of temporal origin may be accompanied by epigastric aura and may develop into typical psychomotor attacks.

EPIGASTRIC OR ABDOMINAL AURAS

Under this heading are various sensations localized to the abdomen or lower chest that may move to the throat and head, but rarely descend in the opposite direction. "Visceral," and "viscerosensory" are other terms used to describe this aura. Commonly characterized as a feeling of nausea, epigastric aura may also be like butterflies in the stomach, emptiness, "going over a hill," tightness, and churning; occasionally, it may be painful (58,70). This aura is frequently associated with or preceded or followed by other sensory, psychic, emotional, or autonomic phenomena (71). The sensation cannot be considered secondary to altered gastroesophageal function, as direct intraesophageal and intragastric pressure recordings showed its occurrence with and without peristalsis (71,72). Although epigastric aura is most common in patients with temporal lobe epilepsy, it has been associated with epilepsies from all lobes (Tables 15.2 and 15.3). Epigastric sensations can be elicited in epileptic and nonepileptic individuals by electrical stimulation of the amygdala, hippocampus, anteromedial temporal region, sylvian fissure, insula, supplementary motor area, pallidum, and centrum medianum of the thalamus (14,49,71).

CEPHALIC AURAS AND ICTAL HEADACHES

Cephalic auras include ill-defined sensations felt within the head, such as dizziness, electrical shock, tingling, fullness, or pressure. For this reason, a cephalic aura cannot be confused with a somatosensory aura arising from the primary sensory area. Moreover, electrical stimulation studies have provided no clear localization, and cephalic sensations have been reported as auras in focal seizures arising from all brain regions (Tables 15.2 and 15.3).

The relationship of headache to seizures is complex and still the subject of considerable scrutiny (73). Patients often experience a diffuse postictal headache that is generally related to the intensity of the seizure (74). Headaches may also occur as an epileptic prodrome. Some patients with migraines and epilepsy may note that their seizures seem to be triggered by their headaches. Other headaches of abrupt onset signal the beginning of a seizure and can be considered an aura or an ictal headache. An ictal headache can be pounding like a migraine, but also sharp and steady. The pain may build gradually, but several patients studied with scalp or intracranial recording showed abrupt pain onset and offset synchronous with EEG seizure activity (75,76).

An ictal headache is not well localized to any specific region and has been described in patients with generalized epilepsy (75). A lateralized headache is likely to be ipsilateral to the side of the epileptogenic focus (56,75). Many well-studied patients had temporal lobe epilepsy, probably reflecting the increased likelihood of intensive presurgical EEG monitoring in this group. Patients with occipital lobe epilepsy represent the other major population with ictal headache. In patients with classic migraine, the occipital cortex seems to be a primary site of dysfunction, as evidenced by early migrainous aura with visual phenomena and spreading oligemia that starts at the occipital pole (77). Ictal or postictal headache is often a striking symptom in benign epilepsy of childhood with occipital paroxysms (78), as well as in occipital seizures of patients with Lafora disease (79) and other progressive myoclonus epilepsies. The physiologic mechanism of ictal headaches remains unclear. It is possible that ictal headaches are often not auras at all in the ordinary sense of the term, but that many of them result "from an alteration in intracranial circulation either preceding the attack or coincidental with its onset" (14).

EMOTIONAL AURAS

Fear ranges from mild anxiety to intense terror and is "unnatural," out of proportion to, and separable from the understandable apprehension that accompanies the beginning of a seizure. In some patients, the fear resembles a real-life experience, such as suddenly finding a stranger standing close behind, and also may be associated with an unpleasant psychic hallucination of past events. Others seemingly localize the sensation to the chest or stomach, and fear is frequently associated with an epigastric aura (80). Ictal fear may be accompanied by symptoms and signs of autonomic activation, such as mydriasis, piloerection, tachycardia, and hyperventilation. On the basis of lesions in patients with epilepsy, an aura of fear has been linked to temporal lobe epilepsy (80,81). Fear has also been elicited on stimulation of the temporal lobe, particularly the mesial structures (31,82). An aura of fear must be distinguished from a panic attack, and correct identification as an epileptic aura is aided by subsequent ictal phenomena; however, the distinction may be difficult if an aura of fear occurs in isolation, as at the onset of epilepsy.

Elation and pleasure are infrequent auras. The preictal happiness and ecstasy reported by Dostoyevski have often been cited as examples. Pleasurable sensations have not been elicited by electrical stimulation in the vicinity of epileptogenic lesions (8,14,31) and are not considered to be of localizing value.

Depression as an aura or ictal phenomenon is rare. In the largest series, reported by Williams (80), many of the patients had depression that lasted for hours to days, making it likely that this state constituted a prodromal mood change rather than an aura. No consistent cortical localization has been demonstrated.

PSYCHIC AURAS

In 1880, Hughlings Jackson (2) described "certain psychical states during the onset of epileptic seizures" that included "intellectual aurae . . . reminiscence . . . dreamy feelings . . . dreams mixing up with present thoughts...double consciousness . . . 'as if I went back to all that occurred in my childhood.' These are all voluminous mental states and yet of different kinds. . . ." Admittedly, the range of experiences encompassed by the term "psychical auras" is imprecise. Both Gowers (1) and Penfield and Jasper (14) included emotional auras under this heading. Such states have also been called "experiential" phenomena, particularly those related to psychic hallucinations (31,82).

An illusion results from faulty interpretation of present experience in relation to the environment. Aware of the error in perception, the patient has "mental diplopia" in the jacksonian sense. A hallucination is a sensory lifelike experience unrelated to present environment and reality. Psychic hallucinations usually consist of dreamlike events or memory flashbacks that are complex and "formed," in contrast to the elementary "unformed" hallucinations that characterize excitation of the primary sensory areas. Nevertheless, patients with epilepsy invariably sense that the hallucinations are not real.

The nature of psychic auras is as varied as is their complexity. Many attempts at classification have been made (Table 15.4), but it may be fruitless to adhere to an overly rigid categorization of these rich phenomena that offer glimpses into the workings of the human consciousness. For example, *déjà vu* can be considered an illusion of familiar memory; the converse, when what should have been a familiar visual experience becomes unfamiliar, is called *jamais vu*. The corresponding auditory illusions are *déjà entendu* and *jamais entendu*. Autoscopy, a hallucination of self-image, is seeing oneself in external space, either as a "double" or as an external entity observed from a distance after the mind is felt to have left the body (83).

Despite reports that psychic auras can occur with focal seizures from elsewhere in the brain, the consensus ascribes them to epileptic activation of the temporal lobe. Penfield and Jasper's assertion (14) that "a psychical hallucination or dream is produced only by discharge in the temporal cortex" remains valid, based on the vast experience with intracranial electrical stimulation that has since accumulated. Penfield and Perot (41) found that the sites eliciting psychic phenomena were nearly all in the lateral temporal neocortex, particularly along its superior border, and only occasionally from basal or mesial temporal regions. In contrast, later studies from the same institution (31) identified the mesial temporal limbic structures, especially the amygdala, as the sites most frequently producing psychic

TABLE 15.4
PSYCHIC AURAS

	Illusion	Hallucination
Memory	*Déjà vu, jamais vu, déjà entendu, jamais entendu,* strangeness	Memory flashbacks, dreams of past
Vision	Macropsia, micropsia, objects nearer or farther, clearer or blurred	Objects, faces, scenes
Sound	Advancing or receding, louder or softer, clearer or fainter	Voices, music
Self-image	Mental diplopia, depersonalization, derealization, remoteness	Autoscopy
Time	Standing still, rushing, or slowing	—
Others	Increased awareness, decreased awareness	—

phenomena, even in the absence of an electrical after-discharge. Gloor (84) pointed to methodologic differences to account for the discrepant results: Penfield and colleagues (14,41) stimulated mainly the lateral neocortical surface intraoperatively, whereas Gloor and associates (31) based their observations on extraoperative stimulation in patients with chronically implanted depth electrodes to explore the temporal lobes. To reconcile these differences, Gloor (84) proposed a hypothesis based on the model of a neuronal network with reciprocal connections—in this case, between the limbic structures and the temporal isocortex. Psychic phenomena arising "from the activation of matrices in distributed neuronal networks could presumably be elicited from different locations within the temporal lobe, including temporal isocortex and various limbic structures."

Forced thinking refers to an awareness of intrusive stereotyped thoughts, a fixation on, or a crowding of thoughts. Penfield and Jasper (14) separated it from psychic auras and localized it to the frontal lobe.

AUTONOMIC AURAS

There is no consensus on the range of phenomena that should be included in this category. Epigastric sensations are considered an autonomic aura by some, although there is insufficient evidence for implication of autonomic afferent or efferent pathway activation.

A common sensation is that of palpitations. This can usually be verified by accompanying tachycardia on an electrocardiogram. Palpitations are usually associated with auras of fear, anxiety, or epigastric sensation. Such auras are often reported in patients with temporal lobe epilepsy. Tachycardia, of course, occurs not just with the aura, but even more frequently in patients with complex partial or generalized seizures.

Respiratory symptoms experienced as an aura include such sensations as not being able to breathe, a need to breathe more deeply, and of a breath filling the chest that would not expire. Alterations in respiratory rhythms have been reported on stimulation of temporal limbic structures and in seizures of insular origin (53).

Cold shivering and associated piloerection as auras are usually experienced over diffuse or extended areas, but can be localized as well. There are usually other auras associated with these phenomena. Such auras are probably not localized to a single cortical area, but seem most common in patients with temporal lobe epilepsy (85,86). With these auras, a left hemispheric predominance in lateralization has been observed.

Urinary urgency has been reported both at seizure onset or afterwards. The same can be said of the rectal sensation to defecate. The localization of these sensations is not clear.

SEXUAL AURAS

These uncommon erotic feelings may or may not be accompanied by genital sensations or signs or symptoms of sexual arousal. They are distinguished from the sometimes unpleasant superficial genital sensations without sexual content that arise from stimulation of the primary somatosensory area at the parasagittal convexity or interhemispheric fissure and possibly the perisylvian region. Sexual auras seem to arise most frequently from the temporal lobe (87), with other cases reported from the parasagittal area implicating the sensory cortex. The cases reported thus far show a female preponderance. Of those patients whose sexual aura resulted in orgasm, a right hemisphere lateralization was found in one review (88).

REFERENCES

1. Gowers WR. *Epilepsy and other chronic convulsive diseases: their causes, symptoms and treatment,* 2nd ed. London: J & A Churchill, 1901.
2. Jackson JH. On right or leftsided spasm at the onset of epileptic paroxysms, and on crude sensation warnings, and elaborate states. *Brain* 1880/1881;3:192–206.
3. Commission on Classification and Terminology of the International League Against Epilepsy. Proposal for revised clinical and electroencephalographic classification of epileptic seizures. *Epilepsia* 1981;22:489–501.
4. Wieser HG, Hailemariam S, Regard M, et al. Unilateral limbic epileptic status activity: stereo EEG, behavioral, and cognitive data. *Epilepsia* 1985;26:19–29.
5. Olivier A, Gloor P, Andermann F, et al. Occipitotemporal epilepsy studied with stereotaxically implanted depth electrodes and successfully treated by temporal resection. *Ann Neurol* 1982;11:428–432.
6. Kanemoto K, Janz D. The temporal sequence of aura-sensations in patients with complex focal seizures with particular attention to ictal aphasia. *J Neurol Neurosurg Psychiatry* 1989;52:52–56.
7. Gloor P. Physiology of the limbic system. In: Penry JK, Daly DD, eds. *Complex partial seizures and their treatment. Advances in Neurology.* New York: Raven Press; 1975;11:27–53.
8. Halgren E, Walter RD, Cherlow D, et al. Mental phenomena evoked by electrical stimulation of the human hippocampal formation and amygdala. *Brain* 1978;101:83–117.
9. Hauser EA, Kurland LT. The epidemiology of epilepsy in Rochester, Minnesota, 1935 through 1967. *Epilepsia* 1975;16:1–66.
10. Lennox WG, Cobb S. Aura in epilepsy: a statistical review of 1,359 cases. *Arch Neurol Psychiatry* 1933;30:374–387.
11. Gibbs FA, Gibbs EL. *Atlas of electroencephalography, II. Epilepsy,* 2nd ed. Cambridge, MA: Addison-Wesley Press, 1952.
12. Janati A, Nowack WJ, Dorsey S, et al. Correlative study of interictal electroencephalogram and aura in complex partial seizures. *Epilepsia* 1990;31:41–46.
13. King DW, Ajmone-Marsan C. Clinical features and ictal patterns in epileptic patients with EEG temporal lobe foci. *Ann Neurol* 1977;2:7.
14. Penfield W, Jasper H. *Epilepsy and the functional anatomy of the human brain.* Boston: Little, Brown, 1954.
15. Theodore WH, Porter RJ, Penry JK. Complex partial seizures: clinical characteristics and differential diagnosis. *Neurology* 1983;33:1115–1121.
16. Marks WJ Jr, Laxer KD. Semiology of temporal lobe seizures: value in lateralizing the seizure focus. *Epilepsia* 1998;39:721–726.
17. Sirven JI, Sperling MR, French JA, et al. Significance of simple partial seizures in temporal lobe epilepsy. *Epilepsia* 1996;37:450–454.
18. Sperling MR, O'Connor MJ. Auras and subclinical seizures: characteristics and prognostic significance. *Ann Neurol* 1990;28:320–329.

19. Schulz R, Lüders HO, Noachtar S, et al. Amnesia of the epileptic aura. *Neurology* 1995;45:231–235.
20. Blume WT, Girvin JP. Altered seizure patterns after temporal lobectomy. *Epilepsia* 1997;38:1183–1187.
21. Lund JS, Spencer SS. An examination of persistent auras in surgically treated epilepsy. *Epilepsia* 1992;33(Suppl 3):95.
22. Tuxhorn I, So N, Van Ness P, et al. Natural history and prognostic significance of auras after temporal lobectomy. *Epilepsia* 1992;33 (Suppl 3):95.
23. Vickrey BG, Hays RD, Engel J Jr, et al. Outcome assessment for epilepsy surgery: the impact of measuring health-related quality of life. *Ann Neurol* 1995;37:158–166.
24. Taylor DC, Lochery M. Temporal lobe epilepsy: origin and significance of simple and complex auras. *J Neurol Neurosurg Psychiatry* 1987;50:673–681.
25. Ferguson SM, Rayport M. Psychosis in epilepsy. In: Blumer D, ed. *Psychiatric aspects of epilepsy.* Washington, DC: American Psychiatric Press, 1984:229–270.
26. Mahl GF, Rothenberg A, Delgado JMR, et al. Psychological response in humans to intracerebral stimulation. *Psychosom Med* 1964;26: 337–368.
27. Rayport M, Ferguson SM. Qualitative modification of sensory responses to amygdaloid stimulation in man by interview content and context [abstract]. *Electroencephalogr Clin Neurophysiol* 1974;34:714.
28. Van Donselaar CA, Geerts AT, Schimsheimer RJ. Usefulness of an aura for classification of a first generalized seizure. *Epilepsia* 1990;31:529–535.
29. Kapur J, Pillai A, Henry TR. Psychogenic elaboration of simple partial seizures. *Epilepsia* 1995;36:1126–1130.
30. Bancaud J, Talairach J, Bonis A, et al. *La stéréo-électro-encéphalographie dans l'épilepsie.* Paris: Masson, 1965.
31. Gloor P, Olivier A, Quesney LF, et al. The role of the limbic system in experiential phenomena of temporal lobe epilepsy. *Ann Neurol* 1982;12:129–144.
32. Lüders H, Lesser R, Dinner DS, et al. Commentary: chronic intracranial recording and stimulation with subdural electrodes. In: Engel J Jr, ed. *Surgical treatment of the epilepsies.* New York: Raven Press, 1987:297–321.
33. Schulz R, Lüders HO, Tuxhorn I, et al. Localization of epileptic auras induced on stimulation by subdural electrodes. *Epilepsia* 1997;38:1321–1329.
34. Ostrowsky K, Isnard J, Guénot M, et al. Functional mapping of the insular cortex: clinical implication in temporal lobe epilepsy. *Epilepsia* 2000;41:681–686.
35. Penfield W, Kristiansen K. *Epileptic seizure patterns.* Springfield, L: Charles C. Thomas, 1951.
36. Palmini A, Gloor P. The localizing value of auras in partial seizures: a prospective and retrospective study. *Neurology* 1992;42:801–808.
37. Rasmussen T. Localizational aspects of epileptic seizure phenomena. In: Thompson RA, Green JR, eds. *New perspectives in cerebral localization.* New York: Raven Press, 1982:177–203.
38. Rasmussen T. Characteristics of a pure culture of frontal lobe epilepsy. *Epilepsia* 1983;24:482–493.
39. Ajmone-Marsan C, Goldhammer L. Clinical ictal patterns and electrographic data in cases of partial seizures of frontal-central-parietal origin. In: Brazier MAB, ed. *Epilepsy: its phenomena in man.* New York: Academic Press, 1973:235–259.
40. Ludwig BI, Ajmone-Marsan C. Clinical ictal patterns in epileptic patients with occipital electroencephalographic foci. *Neurology* 1975;25:463–471.
41. Penfield W, Perot P. The brain's record of auditory and visual experience: a final summary and discussion. *Brain* 1963;86:595–694.
42. Gupta K, Jeavons PM, Hughes RC, et al. Aura in temporal lobe epilepsy: clinical and electroencephalographic correlation. *J Neurol Neurosurg Psychiatry* 1983;46:1079–1083.
43. Lieb JP, Walsh GO, Babb TL, et al. A comparison of EEG seizure patterns recorded with surface and depth electrodes in patients with temporal lobe epilepsy. *Epilepsia* 1976;17:137–160.
44. Spencer SS, Spencer DS, Williamson PD, et al. Combined depth and subdural electrode investigation in uncontrolled epilepsy. *Neurology* 1990;40:74–79.
45. Sperling MR, O'Connor MJ. Comparison of depth and subdural electrodes in recording temporal lobe seizures. *Neurology* 1989;39: 1497–1504.
46. Sperling MR, Lieb JP, Engel J Jr, et al. Prognostic significance of independent auras in temporal lobe seizures. *Epilepsia* 1989; 30:322–331.
47. Babb TL, Wilson CL, Isokawa-Akesson M. Firing patterns of human limbic neurons during stereoencephalography (SEEG) and clinical temporal lobe seizures. *Electroencephalogr Clin Neurophysiol* 1987;66:467–482.
48. Woolsey CN, Erickson TC, Gilson WE. Localization in somatic sensory and motor areas of human cerebral cortex as determined by direct recording of evoked potentials and electrical stimulation. *J Neurosurg* 1979;51:476–506.
49. Penfield W, Rasmussen T. *The cerebral cortex of man.* New York: Macmillan, 1950.
50. Morris HH, Dinner DS, Lüders H, et al. Supplementary motor seizures: clinical and electroencephalographic findings. *Neurology* 1988;38:1075–1082.
51. Fried I, Katz A, Sass J, et al. Functional organization of supplementary motor cortex: evidence from electrical stimulation [abstract]. *Epilepsia* 1989;30:725.
52. Lim SH, Dinner DS, Pillay PK, et al. Functional anatomy of the human supplementary sensorimotor area: results of extraoperative electrical stimulation. *Electroencephalogr Clin Neurophysiol* 1994;91:179–193.
53. Isnard J, Guénot M, Ostrowsky K, et al. The role of the insular cortex in temporal lobe epilepsy. *Ann Neurol* 2000;48:614–623.
54. Weingarten SM, Cherlow DG, Halgren E. Relationship of hallucinations to the depth structures of the temporal lobe. In: Sweet WR, Obrador S, Martin-Rodriguez JG, eds. *Neurosurgical treatment in psychiatry, pain and epilepsy.* Baltimore, MD: University Park Press, 1976:553–568.
55. Mauguiere F, Courjon J. Somatosensory epilepsy. *Brain* 1978;101: 307–332.
56. Young GB, Blume WT. Painful epileptic seizures. *Brain* 1983;106: 537–554.
57. Lewin W, Phillips CG. Observations on partial removal of the postcentral gyrus for pain. *J Neurol Neurosurg Psychiatry* 1952;15: 143–147.
58. Siegel AM, Williamson PD, Roberts DW, et al. Localized pain associated with seizures originating in the parietal lobe. *Epilepsia* 1999;40:845–855.
59. Wilkinson HA. Epileptic pain: an uncommon manifestation with localizing value. *Neurology* 1973;23:518–520.
60. Hamby WB. Reversible central pain. *Arch Neurol* 1961;5:82–86.
61. Wieser HG. *Electroclinical features of the psychomotor seizure.* London: Butterworth, 1983.
62. Berman S. Vestibular epilepsy. *Brain* 1955;78:471–486.
63. Smith BH. Vestibular disturbances in epilepsy. *Neurology* 1960;10: 465–469.
64. Jackson JH, Beevor CE. Case of tumour of the right temporosphenoidal lobe bearing on the localization of the sense of smell and on the interpretation of a particular variety of epilepsy. *Brain* 1889;12:346–357.
65. Daly DD. Uncinate fits. *Neurology* 1958;8:250–260.
66. Acharya V, Acharya J, Lüders H. Olfactory epileptic auras. *Neurology* 1998;51:56–61.
67. Howe JG, Gibson JD. Uncinate seizures and tumors, a myth reexamined. *Ann Neurol* 1982;12:227.
68. Fried I, Spencer DD, Spencer SS. The anatomy of epileptic auras: focal pathology and surgical outcome. *J Neurosurg* 1995;83:60–66.
69. Hausser-Hauw C, Bancaud J. Gustatory hallucinations in epileptic seizures: electrophysiological, clinical and anatomical correlates. *Brain* 1987;110:339–359.
70. Nair DR, Najm I, Bulacio J, et al. Painful auras in focal epilepsy. *Neurology* 2001;57:700–702.
71. Van Buren JM. The abdominal aura: a study of abdominal sensations occurring in epilepsy produced by depth stimulation. *Electroencephalogr Clin Neurophysiol* 1963;15:1–19.
72. Van Buren JM, Ajmone-Marsan C. A correlation of autonomic and EEG components in temporal lobe epilepsy. *Arch Neurol* 1960;3: 683–693.
73. Andermann F, Lugaresi E, eds. *Migraine and epilepsy.* Boston: Butterworth, 1987.
74. Schon F, Blau JN. Postepileptic headache and migraine. *J Neurol Neurosurg Psychiatry* 1987;50:1148–1152.
75. Isler H, Wieser HG, Egli M. Hemicrania epileptica: synchronous ipsilateral ictal headache with migraine features. In: Andermann

F, Lugaresi E, eds. *Migraine and epilepsy.* Boston: Butterworth, 1987:249–264.

76. Laplante P, Saint-Hilaire JM, Bouvier G. Headache as an epileptic manifestation. *Neurology* 1983;33:1493–1495.

77. Olesen J, Larsen B, Lauritzen M. Focal hyperemia followed by spreading oligemia and impaired activation of rCBF in classic migraine. *Ann Neurol* 1981;9:344–352.

78. Gastaut H. A new type of epilepsy: benign partial epilepsy of childhood with occipital spike-waves. *Clin Electroencephalogr* 1982;13:13–22.

79. Kobayashi K, Iyoda K, Ohtsuka Y, et al. Longitudinal clinicoelectrophysiologic study of a case of Lafora disease proven by skin biopsy. *Epilepsia* 1990;31:194–201.

80. Williams D. The structure of emotions reflected in epileptic experiences. *Brain* 1956;79:29–67.

81. Macrae D. Isolated fear. A temporal lobe aura. *Neurology* 1954;4:479–505.

82. Mullan S, Penfield W. Illusions of comparative interpretation and emotion. *Arch Neurol Psychiatry* 1959;81:269–284.

83. Devinsky O, Feldmann E, Burrowes K, et al. Autoscopic phenomena with seizures. *Arch Neurol* 1989;46:1080–1088.

84. Gloor P. Experiential phenomena of temporal lobe epilepsy: facts and hypotheses. *Brain* 1990;113:1673–1694.

85. Green JB. Pilomotor seizures. *Neurology* 1984;34:837–839.

86. Stefan H, Pauli E, Kerling F, et al. Autonomic auras: left hemispheric predominance of epileptic generators of cold shivers and goose bumps? *Epilepsia* 2002;43:41–45.

87. Remillard GM, Andermann F, Testa GF, et al. Sexual ictal manifestations predominate in women with temporal lobe epilepsy: a finding suggesting sexual dimorphism in the human brain. *Neurology* 1983;33:323–330.

88. Janszky J, Szücs A, Halász P, et al. Orgasmic aura originates from the right hemisphere. *Neurology* 2002;58:302–304.

Focal Seizures with Impaired Consciousness

16

Prakash Kotagal   *Tobias Loddenkemper*

HISTORICAL BACKGROUND

From the earliest description of epileptic seizures, in a Babylonian medical text collection (1067–1046 BC), impaired consciousness has been a major defining symptom and an important factor in classifying severity of the seizure and predicting outcome (1). Although descriptions of seizures with loss of consciousness and automatisms suggesting focal origin date to the days of Hippocrates, Galen, and Areatus (2), Hughlings Jackson first suggested their origin in the temporal lobe and called them "uncinate fits" (3–6). The invention of the electroencephalogram (EEG) in 1929 made it possible to identify the characteristic interictal and ictal features of these seizures (7). In 1937, Gibbs, Gibbs, and Lennox proposed the term "psychomotor epilepsy" to describe a characteristic EEG pattern of temporal lobe seizures accompanied by mental, emotional, motor, and autonomic phenomena (8). Penfield and Kristiansen (9) and Penfield and Jasper (10) observed that some patients with seizures and loss of consciousness had extratemporal sharp waves. Jasper and colleagues (11,12) first pointed out that the localization of the EEG ictal discharge was more important than its actual pattern and that this pattern originated from "deep within the temporal lobes, near the midline" (12).

The early work of investigators at the Montreal Neurological Institute in Canada, and in Paris, France, contributed immensely to our understanding of various types of epilepsy, including temporal and extratemporal, and used information from multiple techniques: scalp recordings, invasive recordings from depth electrodes and intraoperative corticography, and cortical stimulation studies (9,10,13–16). Ajmone-Marsan and colleagues (17–20) used chemical activation with pentylenetetrazol to study partial seizures from various locations. The Paris group

(21–23) published a number of papers on frontal lobe epilepsy. Tharp (24) was the first to identify seizures with loss of consciousness arising from the orbitofrontal regions.

Early work on the symptomatology of focal seizures with impaired consciousness was based on eyewitness descriptions by family members, nurses, or physicians (14,16,25,26). Some studies employed cine film and analyzed photographs taken at three per second (19). The introduction of videotape technology provided an inexpensive and effective way to easily record and play back seizures as often as needed, resulting in a better grasp of phenomenology. The observations of Delgado-Escueta, Theodore, Williamson, Quesney, Bancaud, and others vastly improved our understanding of focal seizures with impaired consciousness (27–35). Crucial insights were provided by Gastaut (36), who proposed the first International Classification of Epileptic Seizures in 1970 (37).

In his 1983 monograph, *Electroclinical Features of the Psychomotor Seizure*, Wieser (38) described the order of symptom onsets and symptom clusters and attempted to correlate these clusters with electrographic activity recorded with depth electrodes. Maldonado and associates (39) also examined the sequences of symptoms in hippocampal-amygdalar–onset seizures. Using methods similar to those of Wieser, we examined temporal lobe psychomotor seizures in patients who were seizure free after temporal lobectomy (40). Similar methods also have been used to study frontal lobe seizures (41,42).

TERMINOLOGY

Complex partial seizure, as defined by the 1981 International Classification of Epileptic Seizures (43), refers to a focal seizure with impairment of consciousness.

Loss of consciousness either can occur at the onset of the seizure or the seizure can manifest with a "simple partial onset followed by impairment of consciousness." Therefore, the term covers a variety of seizure types that have little in common except for a presumably focal epileptogenic zone and impaired consciousness with or without secondary generalization (44). For example, partial seizures arising from the perirolandic region or supplementary motor area may involve impairment of consciousness but are very different from complex partial seizures arising from the mesial temporal lobe with an aura of *déjà vu*, staring, unresponsiveness, and stereotyped oroalimentary and hand automatisms. Because it mixes semiologic information with EEG data, the term *complex partial* is not always accurate and is often of limited clinical value.

The distinction between seizure semiology and EEG seizure localization is central to a new classification scheme, proposed by Lüders and colleagues (45–47), that groups seizures by semiology alone, without relying on the EEG. Seizures with impaired consciousness as the predominant feature are called dileptic (from the Greek word *dialepein*, which means "to stand still," "to interrupt," or "to pass out"). In seizures with reduction of activity, in which loss of consciousness cannot be documented (as in young infants), the term *hypomotor* is used (48). *Automotor* describes seizures with oroalimentary and manual automatisms and usually (but not always) impairment of consciousness. Seizures with vigorous body and limb movements are called hypermotor. The terms *dileptic, hypomotor, automotor,* and *hypermotor* convey much more useful information than complex partial. The significance of semiologic features has been recently recognized by the International League Against Epilepsy (ILAE), which included major parts of the semiologic seizure classification in its glossary of descriptive terminology for ictal semiology (49). The International Classification of Epilepsies uses this glossary as one of five classification axes and no longer includes the term complex partial (50) (see Chapter 22). Until the revision of this classification is complete, however, the 1989 ILAE version remains in place (44). Hence, the more widely used term *complex partial seizures* is used in this chapter, with the understanding that it will be replaced.

Focal seizures with loss of consciousness usually arise from the temporal or frontal lobes but may also start elsewhere and spread to the temporal lobes (51–53). Therefore, distinction between localization of the epileptogenic zone and seizure semiology is crucial. The following two sections define the constituting features of complex partial seizures: focal localization of the epileptogenic zone and clinical loss of consciousness.

Focal Epilepsy

The term *focal epilepsy* is used if delineation of the epileptogenic zone in one cerebral region is possible, as evidenced by data from the history, seizure semiology, EEG, and (functional) imaging (54). The more information available in each case, the more precise the localization of the epileptogenic zone. The epileptogenic zone includes not only the ictal-onset zone that generates the patient's typical seizures but also brain tissue that can induce seizures when the primary focus is removed (55).

Loss of Consciousness

Consciousness has different aspects such as perception, cognition, memory, affect, and voluntary motility (56). For practical purposes, ictal loss of consciousness is usually defined by unresponsiveness during a seizure, along with amnesia for events during the seizure and for a variable period before and after it. Consciousness may be difficult or impossible to assess during seizures in infants (48,57).

Unresponsiveness

To determine unresponsiveness—the inability to respond to external stimuli—the patient is tested during and after the seizure. In some laboratories, motor response to an auditory or visual stimulus is tested (29). A patient may not respond because the patient cannot comprehend the command; even if comprehension and consciousness are intact, the motor or verbal output may be blocked. In some patients, lack of responsiveness may be the result of a peculiar motivational state (as if the person were absorbed by a hallucination) (56). During the postictal interview, the patient is asked to recall test words or items given during the seizure. Language and praxis also should be evaluated at this time to identify any deficits. Preserved responsiveness associated with automatisms is noted in complex partial seizures arising from the nondominant temporal lobe (58).

Amnesia

Patients with complex partial seizures with automatisms are often unaware that they have just had a seizure and cannot recall activities engaged in before the seizure onset or events that occurred during the ictus. The degree of retrograde and anterograde amnesia is variable. Postictal amnesia probably results from bilateral impairment of hippocampal function. The patient is unable to form new memories, but previously established ones are intact. Bilateral stimulation of medial temporal lobe structures or unilateral medial temporal lobe stimulation that produces afterdischarges affects the formation and retrieval of long-term memories (59–61).

FOCAL SEIZURES WITH IMPAIRMENT OF CONSCIOUSNESS ARISING FROM DIFFERENT LOCATIONS

Research during the past two decades has advanced our understanding of the symptomatology of focal seizures with impairment of consciousness arising from various locations (30,39,40,62–64). Most such seizures arise in the temporal lobe; however, in at least 10% to 30% of patients evaluated in epilepsy surgery programs, the origin is extratemporal, most commonly the frontal lobe (65). Focal seizures with impairment of consciousness can present with or without an aura. The auras last from a few seconds to as long as 1 to 2 minutes before consciousness is actually lost. Impairment of consciousness is maximal initially. Partial recovery later in the seizure may allow the patient to look at an observer walking into the room or interact in some other way with the environment (40). Most of these seizures with automatisms last longer than 30 seconds—up to 1 to 2 minutes (sometimes as long as 10 minutes). Very few are briefer than 10 seconds, which helps distinguish them clinically from typical absence seizures (29).

Escueta and colleagues described three types of complex partial seizures (29). Type I begin with a motionless stare or behavioral arrest (seen in 24% to 30% of mesial temporal lobe seizures) that is not present at the beginning of type II attacks. Type III complex partial seizures, previously called temporal lobe syncope, begin with a drop attack, followed by confusion, amnesia, and gradual return of composure (29). The localizing value of the motionless stare was believed to indicate mesial temporal lobe epilepsy (29,62–64,66). However, behavioral arrest is also seen in 20% of patients with frontal lobe (67). Types II (68) and III are thought to be of extratemporal origin (68–70).

Different components of consciousness may be impaired depending on the location of the ictal seizure pattern. Frontal lobe seizures are more likely to manifest with loss of orientation behavior and expressive speech; left temporal lobe seizures lead to impairments of memory and expressive and receptive speech; and right temporal lobe seizures rarely involve impairment of consciousness (71).

Seizures of Frontal Lobe Origin

Seizures arising from the frontal lobes occur in up to 30% of patients with focal epilepsy are the second most common focal type after temporal lobe seizures (72,73). In 50% of patients with frontal lobe epilepsy, seizures are accompanied by loss of consciousness (74). Seizures with loss of consciousness can arise from various locations within the frontal lobe (except from the rolandic strip) (33,42,66,68,72,75,76). Semiologic features include occurrence in clusters, occurrence many times a day, brief duration (lasting about 30 seconds with a sudden onset), and minimal postictal confusion. Bizarre attacks with prominent motor automatisms involving the lower extremities (pedaling or bicycling movements), sexual automatisms, and prominent vocalizations are common, and the seizures are remarkably stereotyped for each patient (33,42,68,77,78). Identification of seizure onset within the frontal lobe by semiology alone and differentia-

tion of mesial temporal lobe epilepsy and frontal lobe epilepsy may be misleading and difficult (79); however, analysis of the earliest signs and symptoms, as well as their order of appearance, may allow this distinction in onset (41). Clonic seizures frequently arise from the frontal convexity, tonic seizures from the supplementary motor area, and automotor seizures from the orbitofrontal region (80). Seizures with "motor agitation" and hypermotor features are more likely to arise from the orbitofrontal and frontopolar regions (79). Up to 50% of patients develop complex partial status epilepticus (33,80,81).

The unique symptomatology of supplementary motor seizures includes an onset with abrupt tonic extension of the limbs that is often bilateral but may be asymmetric and is accompanied by nonpurposeful movements of uninvolved limbs and vocalizations (42,78,82,83). Typically, these occur out of sleep and recur many times a night. Because of their bizarre symptomatology, they are sometimes mistaken for pseudoseizures. Consciousness is often preserved in supplementary motor area seizures, and postictally baseline mentation returns quickly. Vigevano and Fusco (84) reported a familial form of supplementary motor area seizures in young children with good outcome.

Cingulate gyrus seizures, in addition to phenomena associated with supplementary motor seizures, such as asymmetric bilateral tonic posturing of the proximal limbs, may show complex behavior including oroalimentary, gestural, and sexual automatisms, mood changes, and urinary incontinence (23,85–88).

Orbitofrontal seizures manifest prominent autonomic phenomena, with flushing, mydriasis, vocalizations, and automatisms. The vocalizations may consist of unintelligible screaming or loud expletives of words or short sentences. Patients also may get up and run around the room (24).

Quesney and associates (78) reported that seizures of the anterolateral dorsal convexity seizures may manifest with auras (89) such as dizziness, epigastric sensation, or fear in 50% of patients, behavioral arrest in 20%, and speech arrest in 30%. One third of the patients exhibited sniffing, chewing or swallowing, laughing, crying, hand automatisms, or kicking. A tendency to partial motor activity in the form of tonic or clonic movements contralateral to the side of the focus was also noted. Bancaud and colleagues (90) described speech arrest, visual hallucinations, illusions, and forced thinking in some patients during seizures of dorsolateral frontal origin. These patients may also show contralateral tonic eye and head deviation or asymmetric tonic posturing of the limbs before contralateral clonic activity or secondary generalization. Other patients may have autonomic symptoms such as pallor, flushing, tachycardia, mydriasis, or apnea (90).

Seizures of Temporal Lobe Origin

Approximately 40% to 80% of patients with temporal lobe epilepsy have seizures with stereotyped automatisms of the mouth and hands and other motor manifestations (excluding focal clonic activity and version) that suggest a temporal lobe origin (29–32,38–40). Secondary generalization occurs in approximately 60% of temporal lobe seizures (91,92). Postically, gradual recovery follows several minutes of confusion; however, patients may carry out automatic behavior, such as getting up, walking about, or running, of which they have no memory. Attempts to restrain them may only aggravate matters. Violence, invariably nondirected, may be seen during this period (93,94). The patient is usually amnestic for the seizure but may be able to recall the aura. A few patients may exhibit retrograde amnesia for several minutes before the seizure. In young children, partial seizures of temporal lobe onset are characterized predominantly by behavioral arrest with unresponsiveness (48,57,95); automatisms are usually oroalimentary, whereas discrete manual and gestural automatisms tend to occur in children older than age 5 or 6 years (96–98). In younger children, symmetric motor phenomena of the limbs, postures similar to frontal lobe seizures in adults, and head nodding as in infantile spasms were typical (96). Because it is impossible to test for consciousness in infants, focal seizures with impairment of consciousness may manifest as hypomotor seizures, a bland form of complex partial seizure with none or only few automatisms (99). In very young infants, these may also occasionally be accompanied by central apnea (100).

Seizures of Parietal Lobe Origin

A few well-documented cases of complex partial seizures arising from the parietal lobes have been reported (101–103). Like seizures of occipital lobe onset, partial seizures from the parietal lobe manifest loss of consciousness and automatisms when they spread to involve the temporal lobe. Initial sensorimotor phenomena may point to onset in the parietal lobe, as do vestibular hallucinations such as vertigo, described in seizures beginning near the angular gyrus. Language dysfunction may occur in seizures arising from the dominant hemisphere. Also described in parietal lobe complex partial seizures have been auras including epigastric sensations, formed visual hallucinations, behavioral arrest, and panic attacks (18,27,103–106). In a study of patients with parietal lobe epilepsy as evidenced by ictal single-photon-emission computed tomography (SPECT) (7 of 14 patients with focal seizures with impairment of consciousness) (101), 6 had prominent staring and relative immobility (dileptic), and one patient had hypermotor features.

A limiting factor in many studies of seizure symptomatology is that relatively few reported patients with extratemporal complex partial seizures become seizure free after cortical resection. This casts some doubt on the localization of the epileptic focus (42,78,100, 107,108).

Seizures of Occipital Lobe Origin

The following features suggest the occipital lobe as the origin of a complex partial seizure: (a) Visual auras, usually of elementary sensations such as white or colored flashing lights, are often in the part of the visual field corresponding to the focus (20, 109,110); the visual phenomena may remain stationary or move across the visual field. (b) Ictal blindness in the form of a whiteout or blackout may be reported (111). (c) Version of the eyes and head to the opposite side is common and is a reliable lateralizing sign (65,112); patients may report a sensation of eye pulling to the opposite side even in the absence of eye deviation (20,113). (d) Rapid, forced blinking and oculoclonic activity also may be seen (114). Other symptoms may result from spread to the temporal or parietal lobes (19,53,103,115). Suprasylvian spread to the mesial or parietal cortex produces symptomatology similar to that in supplementary motor seizures, whereas spread to the lateral parietal convexity gives rise to sensorimotor phenomena. Spread to the lateral temporal cortex followed by involvement of the mesial structures may produce formed visual hallucinations followed by automatisms and loss of consciousness. Direct spread to the mesial temporal cortex may mimic mesial temporal epilepsy. The visual auras may be the only clue to recognizing the occipital lobe onset of these seizures; however, the patient may not recall them because of retrograde amnesia, if the aura was fleeting, or if the seizure is no longer preceded by the aura as it was in the past (110).

In a study of 42 patients with occipital lobe epilepsy, 73% experienced visual auras (116) frequently followed by loss of consciousness possibly as a consequence of ictal spread into the frontotemporal region. Vomiting is more common in benign than in symptomatic occipital lobe seizures and may also represent ictal spread to the temporal lobes (89,117).

SEMIOLOGIC FEATURES IN FOCAL EPILEPSY WITH SEIZURES CHARACTERIZED BY LOSS OF CONSCIOUSNESS

Auras

Auras have been reported in 20% to 93% of patients with temporal lobe seizures (26,29,31,118–121) and in approximately 50% to 67% of seizures arising from the frontal lobe (78–119). The auras may be similar in both groups. In the Cleveland Clinic series of patients with documented temporal lobe epilepsy (seizure free after temporal lobectomy), only 28% of seizures recorded in the laboratory were accompanied by a definite aura (40). Some patients who experience an aura cannot recall it after a focal seizure with impairment of consciousness. This is frequently observed during video-electroencephalography monitoring in which the patient may press a buzzer alarm at the onset of the seizure but cannot recall doing so subsequently (P. Kotagal, personal observation). Young children with auras (who are unable to verbalize them) may run to their mothers and cling to them (122).

Because aura is the first symptom of a seizure, several studies have evaluated its localizing value (6,26,83,88, 123–128). Gupta and colleagues (124) found that autonomic and psychic auras were most commonly associated with right-sided temporal lobe interictal abnormalities. Palmini and Gloor (129) noted the following auras to be significantly correlated with seizure localization: viscerosensory and experiential auras with temporal lobe seizures; somatosensory auras with frontal and parietal seizures; cephalic auras and diffuse warm sensation with frontal seizures; and visual auras with parietooccipital seizures.

Automatisms

Automatisms were described by Falret, who reported a type of epilepsy with "suspension of comprehension and convulsive phenomena consisting in successively repeated motions of swallowing with alternative elevation and lowering of the lower jaw" (2). Hughlings Jackson first introduced the term *mental automatisms* (6): "It is convenient to have one name for all kinds of doings after epileptic discharge from slight vagaries to homicidal actions. They have one thing in common—they are automatic. The mental automatism results, I consider, from overaction of the lower nervous structures, because the higher controlling centers have been put out of use."

Jasper (130) referred to this as "activation paralysis" of limbic and brainstem circuits. Automatic behavior for which the patient has no memory is common to any confusional state. Not everyone agrees that all automatic behavior during a seizure should be called automatisms or that the term should be reserved for those behaviors that are stereotyped and consistent from one seizure to the next (19,30), although it could be argued that the patient's behavior may change from seizure to seizure, depending on the immediate environment. Automatic behaviors occur not only during the seizure but also in the postictal period, although at times this distinction may be difficult to make clinically (19). Most authors agree that automatisms are usually accompanied by impaired consciousness and subsequent amnesia (17,19,102,130,131). Ebner and coworkers (58) found that 10% of patients with right temporal lobe epilepsy had automatisms with preservation of consciousness; this was never observed in those with left temporal lobe epilepsy. Other researchers have made similar observations (132).

As yet, no uniform classification of the various automatisms exists. Penry and Dreifuss (133) divided automatisms into *de novo* and perseverative types. *De novo* automatisms begin with or after onset of the ictus and do not persist beyond it. They are further classified as reactive automatisms, if they are in response to external or internal stimuli, and as release automatisms, which include actions that are normally socially inhibited. Perseverative automatisms are behaviors initiated before the ictus that are continued automatically during it. Gastaut and Broughton (134) listed five subclasses of automatisms: alimentary, mimetic, gestural, ambulatory, and verbal. This list does not include stereotyped bicycling or pedaling movements or sexual automatisms.

Of course, automatisms are not limited to temporal lobe complex partial seizures. Automatisms occur in complex partial seizures restricted to frontal lobe origin (20,51,53,115), as well as in parietal or occipital lobe seizures that spread to the temporal lobes. Automatisms are also found in atypical and typical absences, especially when they are prolonged (133,135). Although automatisms usually accompany impaired consciousness (4,7), this is not a prerequisite. Oroalimentary automatisms have been shown to occur without loss of consciousness in temporal lobe seizures in which the ictal discharge is confined to the amygdala and anterior hippocampus, without spread to the opposite temporal lobe or either frontal lobe (23,58,136,137). Perhaps it is best to reserve the term *automatisms* for stereotyped behavior during seizures and the term *automatic behavior* for all other activities that change from seizure to seizure depending on the environment (128).

Another controversial point is whether automatisms are simply release phenomena, as suggested by Jackson (6,119) and Jasper (130), or whether they result from ictal activation of specific brain structures. In this context, we have observed oroalimentary and hand automatisms occurring almost exclusively during the ictus and not in the postictal state, supporting the latter hypothesis (40,138). Some automatisms such as ictal speech, however, are probably caused by a release phenomenon when the nondominant hemisphere is inactivated by the ictal discharge (139). Iani and associates (140) reported a patient with multisystem atrophy who manifested staring and masticatory automatisms during postural hypotension without ictal activity noted on an electroencephalogram; they concluded that these automatisms resulted from a release phenomenon.

Specific Automatisms

Oroalimentary automatisms are repetitive, stereotyped movements of the mouth, involving the tongue, lips, and jaw, as though the individuals were chewing or smacking the lips. At times, gulping or swallowing movements may also be seen. Spitting may occur, without accompanying salivation (6,141,142). Oroalimentary automatisms tend to occur early in the seizure, often with hand automatisms, and may be elicited as well by electrical stimulation of the amygdala (73). They may occur without loss of consciousness in temporal lobe seizures when the ictal discharge is confined to the amygdala and anterior hippocampus (23,58,136,137). A complex automatism such as singing has been described (143).

Hand automatisms, also referred to as simple discrete movements by Maldonado and colleagues (39) or bimanual automatisms, are rapid, repetitive, pill-rolling movements of the fingers or fumbling, grasping movements in which the patient may pull at sheets and manipulate any object within reach. Searching movements may also be seen. Wada (144) believed that unilateral automatisms had lateralizing value. In our experience, they did not, unless accompanied by tonic/dystonic posturing in the opposite limb. In these patients, the seizures may begin with bilateral hand automatisms that are interrupted by dystonic posturing on one side while the automatisms continue on the other side (ipsilateral to the ictal discharge) (138) (Table 16.1). Like oroalimentary automatisms, the hand automatisms suggest onset from the mesial temporal region. In extratemporal seizures with unilateral tonic posturing, thrashing to-and-fro movements, which are more proximal and not discrete, are sometimes seen in the opposite limb.

Gestural automatisms of the hands may be seen with both frontal and temporal complex partial seizures but are believed to be more frequent in the former without necessarily spreading to the temporal lobe (23).

Eye blinking or fluttering may be observed. Although usually symmetric, unilateral blinking has been reported ipsilateral to the seizure focus (145,146). A mechanism similar to unilateral hand automatisms may be operative, but this has not been documented. Rapid, forced eye blinking when the seizure begins is thought to indicate occipital lobe onset (145). Seizures arising from the occipital region may produce version of the eyes to the opposite side (20,114).

Truncal or body movements may be seen, usually in the middle or late third of the seizure, when the patient attempts to sit up, turn over, or get out of bed (40). If standing, the person may run or walk, sometimes in a circle; this is called a versive seizure.

Bicycling or pedaling movements of the legs are more commonly observed in complex partial seizures arising from the mesial frontal and orbitofrontal regions (34,35,78,108) than in temporal lobe seizures (147). They are sometimes seen in temporal lobe seizures (148) but probably reflect spread of the ictal discharge to the mesial frontal cortex.

Mimetic automatisms, with changes in facial expression, grimacing, smiling, or pouting, are common in complex partial seizures (26,123,149). Ictal laughter may occur and has also been reported with generalized seizures associated with lesions in the third ventricle and hypothalamus (150). Crying has been noted in complex partial seizures arising from the nondominant temporal lobe (151).

Sexual or genital automatisms such as pelvic or truncal thrusting, masturbatory activity, or grabbing or fondling of the genitals are relatively uncommon during complex partial seizures. However, they have been reported in complex partial seizures of frontal lobe origin (152), as well as in those arising from the temporal lobes (153). Leutmezer and colleagues (153) postulate that discrete genital automatisms such as fondling or grabbing the genitals are seen in temporal lobe seizures, whereas hypermotoric sexual automatisms such as pelvic or truncal thrusting usually occur in frontal lobe seizures.

Motor Phenomena

Tonic posturing consists of simple flexion/extension of the extremity, often more proximal than distal; dystonic posturing involves an element of rotation of the limb with assumption of unnatural postures, affecting the distal

TABLE 16.1
USEFULNESS OF VARIOUS LATERALIZING SIGNS

Sign	Frequency of occurrence (%)	Interobserver agreement K[a]	Predictive value (%)
Version	45	0.76	94
Nonversive head turning	26	0.83	80
Dystonic posturing	37	0.47[b]	93
Mouth deviation	34	0.83	92
Postictal dysphasia	21	0.89	100
Ictal speech	16	0.75	83
Unilateral automatisms	21	0.65	100
Overall	78	0.68	94

[a]Interobserver reliability was assessed by the kappa statistic (see text for discussion).
[b]In a subsequent study from the same center (23), the kappa score for dystonic posturing was 0.68, with a similar predictive value.
Modified from Chee ML, Kotagal P, Van Ness PC, et al. Lateralizing value in intractable partial epilepsy; blinded multiple-observer analysis. Neurology 1993;43:2519-2525, with permission.

more than the proximal limbs (138,154,155). Tonic posturing is sometimes observed in complex partial seizures of temporal or extratemporal onset (18,51,68,138,156) and usually occurs contralateral to the ictal discharge, especially when accompanied by automatisms in the opposite limb. The arm is usually involved, although the leg also may be affected (138,154,155).

Dystonic posturing was observed in 15% of patients with temporal lobe seizures in one series (138), and usually involved the upper limb contralateral to the ictal discharge (rarely, the contralateral lower limb also was affected). An excellent lateralizing sign, it always occurred on the same side as version (40,138,157,158). It may be accompanied by unilateral automatisms in the opposite extremity (see above) and sometimes ipsilateral head deviation (159). Lateralized ictal paresis appears to be a related phenomenon, as some patients in the Cleveland Clinic series (154) went on to develop dystonic posturing in the same limb. Oestreich and colleagues (160), however, believe that ictal hemiparesis is unrelated to dystonic posturing. Dystonic posturing also has been reported during complex partial seizures arising from the frontal lobe (157,158), but the posturing in extratemporal seizures is usually tonic rather than dystonic and is probably caused by involvement of the supplementary motor area (138).

Subdural recordings during unilateral dystonic posturing showed no suprasylvian spread in the course of complex partial seizures of mesial basal temporal origin, suggesting perhaps a subcortical or basal ganglia origin of this phenomenon (138). Using ictal SPECT studies, Newton and associates (161) demonstrated hyperperfusion in the region of the basal ganglia and confirmed this hypothesis. Interictal (^{18}F)fluoro-2-deoxyglucose positron emission tomography (PET) has shown hypometabolism in the striatum in patients with ictal dystonia (162). Contrary to the experience of Bossi and coworkers (163), the Cleveland Clinic group did not find unilateral dystonic posturing to be a poor prognostic sign, as many patients in their series who underwent temporal lobectomy became seizure free (40). Clonic movements of the face or limbs occurred late in the seizure, after suprasylvian spread (10).

Other phenomena that have lateralizing value include postictal nose wiping or nose rubbing, in which the ipsilateral hand is used, presumably because of paresis or neglect of the contralateral hand (164,165). Ictal smiling has been noted in temporal or parietal lobe seizures arising from the nondominant hemisphere. Spitting has been observed during temporal lobe seizures arising from the nondominant hemisphere (142,166).

The lateralizing significance of head turning and version has been controversial. Although some authors use the terms interchangeably (31,39,167–169), these are most likely two different phenomena. Wyllie and colleagues (170) restricted the use of "version" to unquestionably forced and involuntary tonic or clonic deviation of the eyes and head to one side; "nonversive" indicated mild, seemingly voluntary turning of the head or eyes (or both) to one side in an unsustained, wandering fashion. Nonversive head turning has been elicited in animals through stimulation of the amygdala (contralateral to the side stimulated) (171,172) and the hippocampus (ipsilateral to the side stimulated) (171,173). Nonversive movements may occur early in the seizure (31).

Studies that used a stricter definition of version found it consistently contralateral to the side of ictal discharge (138,170). McLachlan (174) reported that head and eye turning was contralateral to the seizure focus in 90% of patients with frontal or temporal lobe seizures. Nonversive movements, on the other hand, have no lateralizing significance (170). Version has been elicited by stimulation of the frontal eye fields (Brodmann areas 6 and 8) as well as the occipital eye field (Brodmann area 19) (85,105, 175–177).

Version in temporal lobe complex partial seizures occurs late after suprasylvian spread, just before secondary generalization when the patient is unconscious (170). In some frontal lobe seizures from the precentral region, prominent head turning is seen, often ipsilateral to the side of onset; many of these patients are conscious of this movement (78). In these patients, unequivocal version may occur later (by which time the patient is unconscious), just before secondary generalization. Version immediately preceding generalization has been invariably correct in lateralization (138,154,155,170,178). Chee and colleagues (155) found that version occurred earlier in extratemporal seizures (usually within 18 seconds after clinical onset) than in temporal lobe seizures.

The interobserver reliability and positive predictive value of the various lateralizing signs were examined by the Cleveland Clinic group (154,155). Interobserver reliability was assessed by the kappa statistic: A kappa score of more than 0.75 indicated excellent agreement beyond chance, between 0.4 and 0.7 indicated fair agreement, and less than 0.4 was poor agreement. The positive predictive value indicated how well a given sign was correctly lateralizing (Table 16.1) (155).

Language Disturbances

Various types of speech disturbances have been described (155,179–182). Gabr and associates (139) classified speech manifestations as follows: Vocalizations are sustained or interrupted sounds of no speech quality—crying, grunting, moaning, whistling, or humming—without lateralizing or localizing value. Ictal speech, usually seen in complex partial seizures of temporal lobe origin, is clearly understandable and may be repetitive or nonrepetitive. It appears to have lateralizing value, as 10 of 12 patients with ictal speech in the Gabr series (139) had complex partial seizures arising from the nondominant hemisphere. Similar results were noted in a later study (182).

Other speech impairments may take the following forms: (a) speech arrest during the ictus, in which the patient is unable to talk and subsequently recalls being unable to do so (this usually indicates seizure onset from the parasagittal frontal convexity in the dominant hemisphere) (78); (b) dysarthria; and (c) dysphasia occurring both during and after a complex partial seizure and suggesting onset from the dominant hemisphere. An ictal SPECT scan performed in a patient with ictal aphasia showed hyperperfusion in the region of the frontal operculum (183).

Autonomic Phenomena

Several authors have noted autonomic changes, including elevation of blood pressure, tachycardia, sinoatrial arrest, anginal symptoms, decrease in skin galvanic resistance, esophageal peristalsis, inhibition of gastric motility, inhibition of respiration, pallor, pilomotor erection, mydriasis, and lacrimation (184), as well as urinary symptoms (104, 126,185–187). These changes are often difficult to identify on videotape and are overlooked (188). Occasionally, it may be difficult to determine whether the autonomic change is a primary seizure manifestation or a secondary manifestation related to an aura, such as fear, which could also lead to blood pressure elevation, tachycardia, mydriasis, or piloerection. Autonomic features are frequently seen in seizures arising from the orbitofrontal and opercular-insular regions (24,38).

Ictal vomiting is seen in focal seizures involving the opercular region and in benign occipital lobe epilepsy (whether it occurs postictally in the latter is unclear) (109,130,151,189–192). It has also been reported during nocturnal seizures in children with benign childhood partial epilepsies not of occipital onset (193). Ictal vomiting is often accompanied by impairment of consciousness and retching or drooling; oroalimentary automatisms may be present. The mechanism is unknown, but we have observed a significant correlation between ictal vomiting preceded by epigastric sensation and seizures of right temporal lobe origin (40). Using subdural electrodes, Kramer and coworkers (192) showed spread of the ictal discharge to the lateral temporal convexity at the time of vomiting. Ictal abnormalities in all nine of their patients were lateralized to the right hemisphere, suggesting an asymmetric representation of the gastrointestinal tract. Devinsky and colleagues (194) reported similar findings. Ictal SPECT studies in two patients with ictal vomiting showed hyperperfusion of the nondominant temporal lobe as well as the occipital region (195).

ELECTROENCEPHALOGRAPHIC FINDINGS

Interictal Electroencephalography

Most complex partial seizures with automatisms arise from the anterior temporal regions of one side or the other.

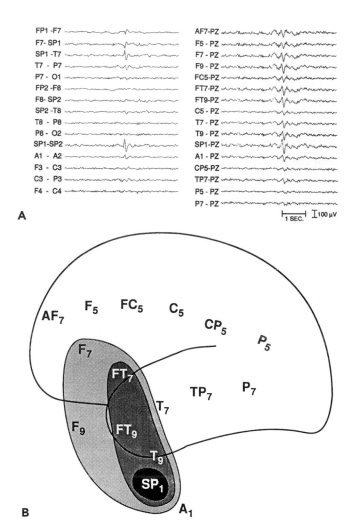

Figure 16.1   Left mesial temporal lobe. Interictal sharp wave focus (*left*). **A** and **B**: Distribution of the field of an interictal spike from a patient with temporal lobe epilepsy. The spike amplitude is maximal at SP_1 (measured on referential recordings), greater than 90% at T_9, FT_9, and FT_7 electrodes, and greater than 70% at F_7 and F_9.

Bitemporal sharp-wave foci are noted in 25% to 33% of patients and may be independent or synchronous (8). Mesial temporal spikes may not be well seen at the surface, and intermittent rhythmic slowing may be the only clue to deep-seated spikes (196). On a single routine EEG recording, 30% to 40% of patients may have normal interictal findings; activating techniques can reduce this to approximately 10% (8,197,198).

At the scalp, the field of mesial temporal spikes is often maximal at the anterior temporal electrodes (T_1 or T_2, FT_9 or FT_{10}). When nasopharyngeal or sphenoidal electrodes are used (especially in prolonged monitoring), the amplitude of the spike is usually maximal at these electrodes, consistent with their origin in the amygdalar-hippocampal region (52) (Fig. 16.1).

Less frequently, sharp-wave foci are seen in the midtemporal or posterior temporal region. Interictal foci may be

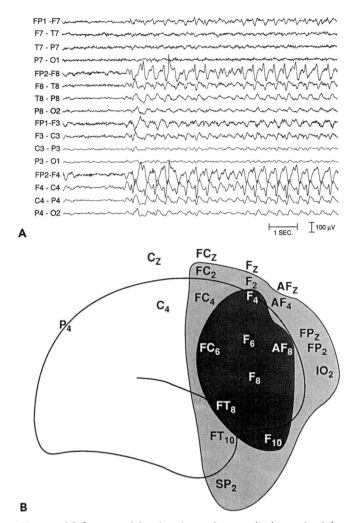

Figure 16.2 Run of focal spike and wave discharge in right frontal lobe with no clinical signs (*left*) and right frontal lobe, interictal spikes (*right*). **A** and **B:** Distribution of the field of interictal spikes occurring in runs from a patient with frontal lobe complex partial seizures. The field is widespread, involving most of the right frontal convexity.

mapped according to amplitude, and the relative frequency of various sharp-wave foci may be taken into account during monitoring of epilepsy surgery candidates. A fair degree of correlation is present between the predominant spike focus and side of ictal onset (63% in Wieser and coworkers' series of 133 patients [199]). Hyperventilation may activate focal temporal slowing or spikes and may provoke a clinical seizure.

In 10% to 30% of patients with complex partial seizures, an extratemporal focus is seen, usually in the frontal lobes (26,35) (Fig. 16.2). In some patients with mesial frontal foci, the interictal discharge may take the form of a bifrontal spike-and-wave discharge.

Care should be taken to exclude nonepileptiform sharp transients such as benign epileptiform transients of sleep or small sharp spikes, wicket spikes, complex partial variant, and 14- and 6-Hz spikes. Evidence suggests that when benign epileptiform transients of sleep occur in epileptic individuals, they do so frequently and in runs (200). Transients resembling benign epileptiform transients of sleep sometimes are found to be maximal at the sphenoidal electrode; such discharges should be interpreted cautiously.

Ictal Electroencephalography

Although interictal EEGs may show normal findings in some patients with complex partial seizures, ictal changes are seen in 95% of patients (except during isolated auras) (134). In frontal lobe seizures from the mesial frontal or orbitofrontal cortex, ictal and interictal activity may not be reflected at the surface or is often masked by electromyographic and movement artifacts (Fig. 16.3).

An electrodecremental pattern is seen at the onset of a complex partial seizure in about two thirds of patients (16). It is usually quite diffuse (perhaps owing to an associated arousal); if focal or accompanied by low-voltage fast activity, it has lateralizing significance (201). The low-voltage fast activity, best seen with depth electrodes, may appear only as flattening at the surface (19). Alternatively, diffuse bitemporal slowing, higher on one side, may occur (202).

Approximately 50% to 70% of patients with temporal lobe epilepsy exhibit a so-called prototype pattern (16,202) consisting of a 5- to 7-Hz rhythmic θ discharge in the temporal regions, maximum at the sphenoidal electrode (Fig. 16.4). This pattern may appear as the first visible EEG change or follow diffuse or lateralized slowing in the δ range (often within 30 seconds of clinical onset). Depth electrode studies have shown this pattern to have 80% accuracy in localizing the onset to the ipsilateral mesial temporal structures (203). Postictal slowing is also helpful in lateralization (204). In patients with unitemporal interictal spikes, the lateralizing value of the ictal data was excellent (205). Seizure rhythms at ictal onset confined to the sphenoidal electrode were seen only in patients with mesial temporal lobe epilepsy and not in those with non–temporal lobe epilepsy (206). Use of coronal transverse montages incorporating the sphenoidal electrodes may permit earlier identification of seizure onset (207).

Although previous reports described false lateralization on the basis of scalp EEG (208,209), subsequent systematic studies have shown this to be infrequent except in the presence of a structural lesion that may mask or attenuate the amplitude of the ictal discharge on that side (147). Although lateralization from scalp EEG is usually satisfactory (210), localization within a lobe is sometimes incorrect, because seizures from an extratemporal site may spread to the temporal lobe and produce similar EEG patterns. The ictal discharge may then propagate to the rest of the hemisphere, or it may propagate bilaterally. Spread to the opposite temporal lobe is common. With some frontal

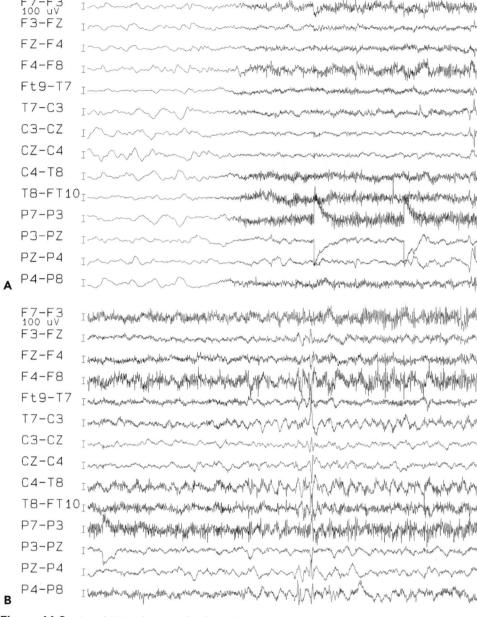

Figure 16.3   A and **B:** Ictal onset of a frontal lobe complex partial seizure arising out of sleep, beginning with low-amplitude fast rhythms, followed by rhythmic slowing near the vertex. The electroencephalographic seizure pattern cannot be lateralized.

lobe seizures, scalp ictal changes are difficult to appreciate because of electromyographic and movement artifacts. Occasionally, a generalized spike-and-wave discharge with a mesial frontal focus is seen.

TREATMENT OF PATIENTS WITH FOCAL EPILEPSY AND SEIZURES WITH IMPAIRED CONSCIOUSNESS

The diagnostic evaluation and treatment of complex partial seizures with automatisms are similar to those of other partial seizures. Details of the medical approach to partial seizures are discussed elsewhere in this book.

In patients with medically intractable focal seizures with impairment of consciousness who are being evaluated for epilepsy surgery, seizure semiology may give considerable lateralizing and localizing information about the seizure focus. An adequate presurgical evaluation of the patient with epilepsy should allow the clinician to answer the following questions: Does the patient have only one seizure type? How frequent are the seizures? Is there a consistent aura, which may have localizing significance? Where is the epileptogenic zone (e.g., in the temporal lobe

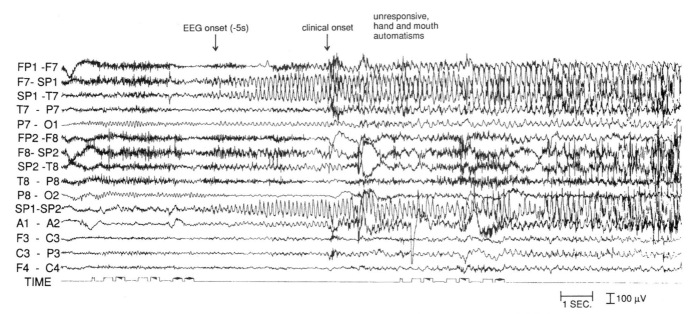

Figure 16.4 Ictal onset of a complex partial seizure (same patient as in Fig. 16.1). A brief electrodecremental response in the left temporal region is followed by the buildup of a rhythmic 5- and 6-Hz theta pattern, maximal at the left sphenoidal electrode. The electroencephalographic changes preceded the clinical onset by 5 seconds.

or in extratemporal regions)? Are there any lateralizing signs, namely, version of the eyes and head, tonic or dystonic posturing, unilateral automatisms, ictal vomiting, unilateral eye blinking, ictal speech, speech arrest, postictal dysphasia or anomia, or postictal Todd paralysis? Is the seizure semiology consistent with neuroimaging and EEG data? Are there any associated medical conditions?

Most epilepsy centers record spontaneous seizures after partial or complete drug withdrawal. Sleep deprivation is also used to elicit seizures; inducing seizures with pentylenetetrazol is rarely necessary. Pharmacologically induced seizures are usually representative of the patient's attacks (211), although atypical localizing features have been reported (34).

REFERENCES

1. Wilson JV, Reynolds EH. Texts and documents. Translation and analysis of a cuneiform text forming part of a Babylonian treatise on epilepsy. *Med Hist* 1990;34:185–198.
2. Temkin O. *The falling sickness: a history of epilepsy from the Greeks to the beginning of modern neurology.* Baltimore, MD: Johns Hopkins, 1971.
3. Jackson JH. On a particular variety of epilepsy "intellectual aura": one case with symptoms of organic brain disease. *Brain* 1888;11:179–207.
4. Jackson JH. On asphyxia in slight epileptic paroxysms—on the symptomatology of slight epileptic fits supposed to depend on discharge lesions of the uncinate gyrus. *Lancet* 1889;1:79–80.
5. Jackson JH, Stewart P. Epileptic attacks with a warning of crude sensation of smell and with the intellectual aura (dreamy state) in a patient who had symptoms pointing to gross organic disease of the right temporosphenoidal lobe. *Brain* 1889;22:534–549.
6. Taylor J. *Selected writings of John Hughlings Jackson.* London: Hodder & Stoughton, 1931.
7. Berger H. Uber das Elektroenzephalogram des Menschen. *Arch Psychiatrie* 1929;87:527–570.
8. Gibbs F, Gibbs E, Lennox W. Epilepsy: a paroxysmal cerebral dysrhythmia. *Brain* 1937;60:377–388.
9. Penfield W, Kristiansen K. *Epileptic seizure pattern.* Springfield, IL: Charles C Thomas, 1951.
10. Penfield W, Jasper H. *Epilepsy and the functional anatomy of the human brain.* Boston: Little, Brown, 1954.
11. Jasper HH, Hawke WA. Electroencephalography, IV: localization of seizure waves in epilepsy. *Arch Neurol Psychiatry* 1938;39:885–901.
12. Jasper HH, Kershman J. Electroencephalographic classification of seizures. *Arch Neurol Psychiatry* 1941;45:903–943.
13. Ballenger C, King D, Gallagher B. Partial complex status epilepticus. *Neurology* 1983;33:1545–1552.
14. Daly D. Ictal clinical manifestations of complex partial seizures. In: Penry J, Daly D, eds. *Complex partial seizures and their treatment,* vol II, *advances in neurology.* New York: Raven Press, 1975:57–82.
15. Feindel W, Penfield W. Localization of discharge in temporal lobe automatism. *Arch Neurol Psychiatry* 1954;72:605–630.
16. Gastaut H, Vigoroux M. Electroclinical correlations in 500 cases of psychomotor seizures. In: Baldwin M, Bailey P, eds. *Temporal lobe epilepsy.* Springfield, IL: Charles C Thomas, 1958:118–130.
17. Ajmone-Marsan C, Abraham K. A seizure atlas. *Electroencephalogr Clin Neurophysiol* 1960;15:12–15.
18. Ajmone-Marsan C, Goldhammer L. Clinical ictal patterns and electrographic data in cases of partial seizures of frontal-central-parietal origin. In: Brazier M, ed. *Epilepsy: its phenomena in man.* New York: Academic Press, 1973:235–258.
19. Ajmone-Marsan J, Ralston B. *The epileptic seizure. Its functional morphology and diagnostic significance.* Springfield, IL: Charles C Thomas, 1957.
20. Ludwig BI, Marsan CA. Clinical ictal patterns in epileptic patients with occipital electroencephalographic foci. *Neurology* 1975;25:463–471.
21. Geier S, Bancaud J, Talairach J, et al. Automatisms during frontal lobe epileptic seizures. *Brain* 1976;99:447–458.
22. Geier S, Bancaud J, Talairach J, et al. The seizures of frontal lobe epilepsy. A study of clinical manifestations. *Neurology* 1977;27:951–958.
23. Munari C, Stoffels C, Bossi L, et al. Automatic activities during frontal and temporal lobe seizures: are they the same? In: Dam

M, Gram L, Penry J, eds. *Advances in epileptology: XIIth Epilepsy International Symposium.* New York: Raven Press, 1981:287–291.

24. Tharp BR. Orbital frontal seizures. An unique electroencephalographic and clinical syndrome. *Epilepsia* 1972;13:627–642.

25. Daly D. Uncinate fits. *Neurology* 1958;8:250–260.

26. King D, Ajmone-Marsan C. Clinical features and ictal patterns in epileptic patients with EEG temporal lobe foci. *Ann Neurol* 1977;2:138–147.

27. Bancaud J. Epileptic attacks of temporal lobe origin in man. *Jpn J EEG-EMG* 1981;(Suppl):67–71.

28. Bancaud J. Clinical symptomatology of epileptic seizures of temporal origin [French]. *Rev Neurol* 1987;143:392–400.

29. Escueta AV, Kunze U, Waddell G, et al. Lapse of consciousness and automatisms in temporal lobe epilepsy: a videotape analysis. *Neurology* 1977;27:144–155.

30. Escueta AV, Bacsal FE, Treiman DM. Complex partial seizures on closed-circuit television and EEG: a study of 691 attacks in 79 patients. *Ann Neurol* 1982;11:292–300.

31. Quesney LF. Clinical and EEG features of complex partial seizures of temporal lobe origin. *Epilepsia* 1986;27(Suppl 2): S27–S45.

32. Theodore WH, Porter RJ, Penry JK. Complex partial seizures: clinical characteristics and differential diagnosis. *Neurology* 1983;33:1115–1121.

33. Williamson PD, Spencer DD, Spencer SS, et al. Complex partial seizures of frontal lobe origin. *Ann Neurol* 1985;18:497–504.

34. Williamson PD. Intensive monitoring of complex partial seizures: diagnosis and subclassification. In: Gumnit RJ, ed. *Intensive neurodiagnostic monitoring.* New York: Raven Press, 1986:69–84.

35. Williamson PD, Spencer SS. Clinical and EEG features of complex partial seizures of extratemporal origin. *Epilepsia* 1986;27 (Suppl 2):S46–S63.

36. Gastaut H. Clinical and electroencephalographical classification of epileptic seizures. *Epilepsia* 1970;11:102–113.

37. Merlis JK. Proposal for an international classification of the epilepsies. *Epilepsia* 1970;11:114–119.

38. Wieser HG. *Electroclinical features of the psychomotor seizure.* London: Butterworths, 1983.

39. Maldonado HM, Delgado-Escueta AV, Walsh GO, et al. Complex partial seizures of hippocampal and amygdalar origin. *Epilepsia* 1988;29:420–433.

40. Kotagal P, Luders HO, Williams G, et al. Psychomotor seizures of temporal lobe onset: analysis of symptom clusters and sequences. *Epilepsy Res* 1995;20:49–67.

41. Kotagal P, Arunkumar G, Hammel J, et al. Complex partial seizures of frontal lobe onset: statistical analysis of ictal semiology. *Seizure* 2003;12:268–281.

42. Salanova V, Morris HH, Van Ness P, et al. Frontal lobe seizures: electroclinical syndromes. *Epilepsia* 1995;36:16–24.

43. Dreifuss FE. Proposal for revised clinical and electroencephalographic classification of epileptic seizures. From the Commission on Classification and Terminology of the International League Against Epilepsy. *Epilepsia* 1981;22:489–501.

44. Commission on Classification and Terminology of the International League Against Epilepsy. Proposal for revised classification of epilepsies and epileptic syndromes. *Epilepsia* 1989;30:389–399.

45. Luders H, Acharya J, Baumgartner C, et al. Semiological seizure classification. *Epilepsia* 1998;39:1006–1013.

46. Luders H, Acharya J, Baumgartner C, et al. A new epileptic seizure classification based exclusively on ictal semiology. *Acta Neurol Scand* 1999;99:137–141.

47. Luders HO, Burgess R, Noachtar S. Expanding the international classification of seizures to provide localization information. *Neurology* 1993;43:1650–1655.

48. Acharya JN, Wyllie E, Luders HO, et al. Seizure symptomatology in infants with localization-related epilepsy. *Neurology* 1997;48: 189–196.

49. Blume WT, Luders HO, Mizrahi E, et al. Glossary of descriptive terminology for ictal semiology: report of the ILAE Task Force on Classification and Terminology. *Epilepsia* 2001;42:1212–1218.

50. Engel J Jr. A proposed diagnostic scheme for people with epileptic seizures and with epilepsy: report of the ILAE Task Force on Classification and Terminology. *Epilepsia* 2001;42:796–803.

51. Geier S, Bancaud J, Talairach J, et al. Ictal tonic postural changes and automatisms of the upper limb during epileptic parietal lobe discharges. *Epilepsia* 1977;18:517–524.

52. Morris HH III, Kanner A, Luders H, et al. Can sharp waves localized at the sphenoidal electrode accurately identify a mesio-temporal epileptogenic focus? *Epilepsia* 1989;30:532–539.

53. Williamson PD, Spencer SS, Spencer DD, et al. Complex partial seizures with occipital lobe onset. *Epilepsia* 1981;22:247–248.

54. Rosenow F, Luders H. Presurgical evaluation of epilepsy. *Brain* 2001;124:1683–1700.

55. Carreno M, Lüders H. General principles of presurgical evaluation. In: Luders HO, Coumair YG, eds. *Epilepsy surgery,* 2nd ed. Philadelphia: Lippincott, Williams & Wilkins, 2000:185–199.

56. Gloor P. Consciousness as a neurological concept in epileptology: a critical review. *Epilepsia* 1986;27(Suppl 2):S14–S26.

57. Nordli DR Jr, Bazil CW, Scheuer ML, et al. Recognition and classification of seizures in infants. *Epilepsia* 1997;38:553–560.

58. Ebner A, Dinner DS, Noachtar S, et al. Automatisms with preserved responsiveness: a lateralizing sign in psychomotor seizures. *Neurology* 1995;45:61–64.

59. Halgren E. Mental phenomena induced by stimulation in the limbic system. *Hum Neurobiol* 1982;1:251–260.

60. Halgren E, Wilson CL, Stapleton JM. Human medial temporal-lobe stimulation disrupts both formation and retrieval of recent memories. *Brain Cogn* 1985;4:287–295.

61. Halgren E, Wilson CL. Recall deficits produced by afterdischarges in the human hippocampal formation and amygdala. *Electroencephalogr Clin Neurophysiol* 1985;61:375–380.

62. Brey R, Laxer KD. Type I/II complex partial seizures: no correlation with surgical outcome. *Epilepsia* 1985;26:657–660.

63. Delgado-Escueta AV, Walsh GO. Type I complex partial seizures of hippocampal origin: excellent results of anterior temporal lobectomy. *Neurology* 1985;35:143–154.

64. Williams LB, Thompson EA, Lewis DV. Intractable complex partial seizures: the "initial motionless stare" and surgical outcome following temporal lobectomy. *Neurology* 1987;37: 1255–1258.

65. Olivier A. Extratemporal cortical resections: principles and methods. In: Lüders H, ed. *Epilepsy surgery.* New York: Raven Press, 1991:559–568.

66. Delgado-Escueta AV, Swartz BE, Maldonado HM, et al. Complex partial seizures of frontal lobe origin. In: Wieser H, Elger C, eds. *Presurgical evaluation of epileptics.* Berlin: Springer-Verlag, 1987: 267–299.

67. Quesney L, Krieger C, Leitner C, et al. Frontal lobe epilepsy. Clinical and electrographic presentation. In: Porter J, Mattson R, Ward AJ, et al, eds. *Advances in epileptology: XVth Epilepsy International Symposium.* New York: Raven Press, 1984:503–508.

68. Walsh GO, Delgado-Escueta AV. Type II complex partial seizures: poor results of anterior temporal lobectomy. *Neurology* 1984;34:1–13.

69. Gambardella A, Reutens DC, Andermann F, et al. Late-onset drop attacks in temporal lobe epilepsy: a reevaluation of the concept of temporal lobe syncope. *Neurology* 1994;44:1074–1078.

70. Pazzaglia P, D'Alessandro R, Ambrosetto G, et al. Drop attacks: an ominous change in the evolution of partial epilepsy. *Neurology* 1985;35:1725–1730.

71. Lux S, Kurthen M, Helmstaedter C, et al. The localizing value of ictal consciousness and its constituent functions: a video-EEG study in patients with focal epilepsy. *Brain* 2002;125:2691–2698.

72. Williamson PD. Frontal lobe seizures. Problems of diagnosis and classification. *Adv Neurol* 1992;57:289–309.

73. Bancaud J, Talairach J. Clinical semiology of frontal lobe seizures. *Adv Neurol* 1992;57:3–58.

74. Inoue Y, Mihara T. Awareness and responsiveness during partial seizures. *Epilepsia* 1998;39(Suppl 5):7–10.

75. Kotagal P, Arunkumar GS. Lateral frontal lobe seizures. *Epilepsia* 1998;39(Suppl 4):S62–S68.

76. Harvey AS, Hopkins IJ, Bowe JM, et al. Frontal lobe epilepsy: clinical seizure characteristics and localization with ictal ^{99m}Tc-HMPAO SPECT. *Neurology* 1993;43:1966–1980.

77. Kotagal P, Arunkumar G, Hammel J, et al. Complex partial seizures of frontal lobe onset: statistical analysis of ictal semiology. *Seizure* 2003;12:268–281.

78. Quesney LF, Constain M, Fish DR, et al. The clinical differentiation of seizures arising in the parasagittal and anterolaterodorsal frontal convexities. *Arch Neurol* 1990;47:677–679.
79. Manford M, Fish DR, Shorvon SD. An analysis of clinical seizure patterns and their localizing value in frontal and temporal lobe epilepsies. *Brain* 1996;119(Pt 1):17–40.
80. Jobst BC, Siegel AM, Thadani VM, et al. Intractable seizures of frontal lobe origin: clinical characteristics, localizing signs, and results of surgery. *Epilepsia* 2000;41:1139–1152.
81. Williamson PD, Spencer DD, Spencer SS, et al. Complex partial status epilepticus: a depth-electrode study. *Ann Neurol* 1985;18:647–654.
82. Morris HH III, Dinner DS, Luders H, et al. Supplementary motor seizures: clinical and electroencephalographic findings. *Neurology* 1988;38:1075–1082.
83. Waterman K, Purves SJ, Kosaka B, et al. An epileptic syndrome caused by mesial frontal lobe seizure foci. *Neurology* 1987;37:577–582.
84. Vigevano F, Fusco L. Hypnic tonic postural seizures in healthy children provide evidence for a partial epileptic syndrome of frontal lobe origin. *Epilepsia* 1993;34:110–119.
85. Crandall P. Developments in direct recordings from epileptogenic regions in the surgical treatment of partial epilepsies. In: Brazier M, ed. *Epilepsy: its phenomena in man.* New York: Academic Press, 1973:287–310.
86. Mazars G. Cingulate gyrus epileptogenic foci as origin for generalized seizures. In: Gastaut H, Jasper H, Bancaud J, et al, eds. *The physiopathogenesis of the epilepsies.* Springfield, IL: Charles C Thomas, 1969:186–189.
87. Stoffels C, Munari C, Bossi L. Seizures of anterior cingulate gyrus in man: a stereo-EEG study. In: Dam M, Gram L, Penry JK, eds. *Advances in epileptology: XIIth Epilepsy International Symposium.* New York: Raven Press, 1981:85–86.
88. Talairach J, Bancaud J, Geier S, et al. The cingulate gyrus and human behaviour. *Electroencephalogr Clin Neurophysiol* 1973;34:45–52.
89. Guerrini R, Ferrari AR, Battaglia A, et al. Occipitotemporal seizures with ictus emeticus induced by intermittent photic stimulation. *Neurology* 1994;44:253–259.
90. Bancaud J, Talairach J, Morrel P, et al. La corne d'Ammon et le noyau amygdalien: effects cliniques et électriques de leur stimulation chez l'homme. *Rev Neurol* 1966;115:329–352.
91. Currie S, Heathfield KW, Henson RA, et al. Clinical course and prognosis of temporal lobe epilepsy. A survey of 666 patients. *Brain* 1971;94:173–190.
92. Lennox W. Phenomena and correlates of the psychomotor triad. *Neurology* 1953;1:357–371.
93. Delgado-Escueta AV, Mattson RH, King L, et al. Special report. The nature of aggression during epileptic seizures. *N Engl J Med* 1981;305:711–716.
94. Treiman DM. Epilepsy and violence: medical and legal issues. *Epilepsia* 1986;27(Suppl 2):S77–S104.
95. Hamer HM, Wyllie E, Luders HO, et al. Symptomatology of epileptic seizures in the first three years of life. *Epilepsia* 1999;40:837–844.
96. Brockhaus A, Elger CE. Complex partial seizures of temporal lobe origin in children of different age groups. *Epilepsia* 1995;36:1173–1181.
97. Wyllie E, Chee M, Granstrom ML, et al. Temporal lobe epilepsy in early childhood. *Epilepsia* 1993;34:859–868.
98. Wyllie E. Developmental aspects of seizure semiology: problems in identifying localized-onset seizures in infants and children. *Epilepsia* 1995;36:1170–1172.
99. Kallen K, Wyllie E, Luders HO, et al. Hypomotor seizures in infants and children. *Epilepsia* 2002;43:882–888.
100. Watanabe K, Hara K, Hakamada S, et al. Seizures with apnea in children. *Pediatrics* 1982;70:87–90.
101. Ho SS, Berkovic SF, Newton MR, et al. Parietal lobe epilepsy: clinical features and seizure localization by ictal SPECT. *Neurology* 1994;44:2277–2284.
102. Salanova V, Andermann F, Rasmussen T, et al. Parietal lobe epilepsy. Clinical manifestations and outcome in 82 patients treated surgically between 1929 and 1988. *Brain* 1995;118(Pt 3):607–627.
103. Williamson PD, Boon PA, Thadani VM, et al. Parietal lobe epilepsy: diagnostic considerations and results of surgery. *Ann Neurol* 1992;31:193–201.
104. Bancaud J. *La stéréo-encéphalographie dans l'epilepsie.* Paris: Masson, 1965.
105. Rasmussen T, Penfield W. Movement of the head and eyes from stimulation of human frontal cortex. *Res Publ Assoc Res Nerv Ment Dis* 1947;27:346–361.
106. Alemayehu S, Bergey G, Barry E, et al. Panic attacks as ictal manifestations of parietal lobe seizures. *Epilepsia* 1995;36:824–830.
107. Trottier S, Chauvel P, Klieemann F, et al. Symptomatology of partial seizures of "proven" frontal lobe origin. *Epilepsia* 1989;30:664–664.
108. Williamson PD, Wieser HG, Delgado-Escueta AV. Clinical characteristics of partial seizures. In: Engel J Jr, ed. *Surgical treatment of the epilepsies.* New York: Raven Press, 1987:101–120.
109. Newton R, Aicardi J: Clinical findings in children with occipital spike-wave complexes suppressed by eye-opening. *Neurology* 1983;33:1526–1529.
110. Williamson PD, Thadani VM, Darcey TM, et al. Occipital lobe epilepsy: clinical characteristics, seizure spread patterns, and results of surgery. *Ann Neurol* 1992;31:3–13.
111. Huott AD, Madison DS, Niedermeyer E. Occipital lobe epilepsy. A clinical and electroencephalographic study. *Eur Neurol* 1974;11:325–339.
112. Russell W, Whitty C. Studies in traumatic epilepsy, III: visual fits. *J Neurol* 1954;18:79–86.
113. Holtzman RN. Sensations of ocular movement in seizures originating in occipital lobe. *Neurology* 1977;27:554–556.
114. Bancaud J. Les crises épileptiques d'origine occipitale (étude stéréoelectroencéphalographique). *Rev Otoneuroophthalmol* 1969;41:299–315.
115. Olivier A, Gloor P, Andermann F, et al. Occipitotemporal epilepsy studied with stereotaxically implanted depth electrodes and successfully treated by temporal resection. *Ann Neurol* 1982;11:428–432.
116. Salanova V, Andermann F, Olivier A, et al. Occipital lobe epilepsy: electroclinical manifestations, electrocorticography, cortical stimulation and outcome in 42 patients treated between 1930 and 1991. *Brain* 1992;115(Pt 6):1655–1680.
117. Kuzniecky R. Symptomatic occipital lobe epilepsy. *Epilepsia* 1998;39(Suppl 4):S24–S31.
118. Daly D. Ictal effect. *Am J Psychiatry* 1958;115:87–108.
119. Panayiotopoulos CP. Vomiting as an ictal manifestation of epileptic seizures and syndromes. *J Neurol Neurosurg Psychiatry* 1988;51:1448–1451.
120. Van Buren J, Ajmone-Marsan C, Mutsuga H, et al. Surgery of temporal lobe epilepsy. In: Purpura D, Penry JK, Walter R, eds. *Neurosurgical management of the epilepsies.* New York: Raven Press, 1975:155–196.
121. Wieser HG, Hailemariam S, Regard M, et al. Unilateral limbic epileptic status activity: stereo EEG, behavioral, and cognitive data. *Epilepsia* 1985;26:19–29.
122. Blume W. Temporal lobe seizures in childhood. Medical aspects. In: Blaw M, Rapin I, Kinsbourne M, eds. *Topics in childhood neurology.* New York: Spectrum, 1977:105–125.
123. Ajmone-Marsan C. Clinical-electrographic correlations of partial seizures. In: Wada J, ed. *Modern perspective in epilepsy. Proceedings of the Canadian League Against Epilepsy.* Montreal: Eden Press, 1978:76–98.
124. Gupta AK, Jeavons PM, Hughes RC, et al. Aura in temporal lobe epilepsy: clinical and electroencephalographic correlation. *J Neurol Neurosurg Psychiatry* 1983;46:1079–1083.
125. Maldonado HM, Delgado-Escueta A, Walsh G, et al. Initial warning symptoms or auras in partial seizures of medial temporal lobe origin (MTL). *Epilepsia* 1988;29:420–433.
126. Van Buren J, Ajmone-Marsan C. A correlation of autonomic and EEG components in temporal lobe epilepsy. *Arch Neurol* 1960;3:683–703.
127. Van Buren J, Ajmone-Marsan C. The abdominal aura. A study of abdominal sensations occurring in epilepsy and produced by depth stimulation. *Electroencephalogr Clin Neurophysiol* 1963; 15: 1–19.
128. Van der Waans P, Binnie C. Consistency of ictal signs in complex partial seizures. In: Wolf P, Dam M, Janz D, et al, eds. *Advances in*

epileptology. XVIth Epilepsy International Symposium. New York: Raven Press, 1987:217–219.

129. Palmini A, Gloor P. The localizing value of auras in partial seizures: a prospective and retrospective study. *Neurology* 1992; 42:801–808.

130. Jasper H. Some physiological mechanisms involved in epileptic automatisms. *Epilepsia* 1964;23:1–20.

131. Anderson J. On sensory epilepsy. A case of cerebral tumor affecting the left temporosphenoidal lobe and giving rise to a paroxysmal taste sensation and dreamy state. *Brain* 1886;9:385–395.

132. Alacron G, Elwes R, Polkey CE, et al. Ictal oroalimentary automatisms with preserved consciousness: implications for the pathophysiology of automatisms with relevance to the International Classification of Seizures. *Epilepsia* 1998;39:1119–1127.

133. Penry JK, Dreifuss FE. Automatisms associated with the absence of petit mal epilepsy. *Arch Neurol* 1969;21:142–149.

134. Gastaut H, Broughton R. *Epileptic seizures: clinical and electrographic features, diagnosis and treatment.* Springfield, IL: Charles C Thomas, 1972.

135. Penry JK, Porter RJ, Dreifuss RE. Simultaneous recording of absence seizures with video tape and electroencephalography. A study of 374 seizures in 48 patients. *Brain* 1975;98:427–440.

136. Munari C, Bancaud J, Stoffels C, et al. Manifestations automatiques dans les crises épileptiques partielles d'origine temporale. In: Cranger R, Avansini G, Tassinari C, eds. *Progressi in epilettologia.* Milan: Lega Italiana contro l'Epilepsia, 1980:115–117.

137. Munari C, Stoffels C, Bossi L, et al. Partial seizures with elementary or complex symptomatology: a valid classification for temporal lobe seizures? In: Akimoto H, Kazamatsuri H, Seino M, et al, eds. *Advances in epileptology. XIIIth Epilepsy International Symposium.* New York: Raven Press, 1982:25–27.

138. Kotagal P, Luders H, Morris HH, et al. Dystonic posturing in complex partial seizures of temporal lobe onset: a new lateralizing sign. *Neurology* 1989;39:196–201.

139. Gabr M, Luders H, Dinner D, et al. Speech manifestations in lateralization of temporal lobe seizures. *Ann Neurol* 1989;25:82–87.

140. Iani C, Attanasio A, Manfredi M. Paroxysmal staring and masticatory automatisms during postural hypotension in a patient with multiple system atrophy. *Epilepsia* 1996;37:690–693.

141. Hecker A, Andermann F, Rodin EA. Spitting automatism in temporal lobe seizures with a brief review of ethological and phylogenetic aspects of spitting. *Epilepsia* 1972;13:767–772.

142. Kellinghaus C, Loddenkemper T, Kotagal P. Ictal spitting: clinical and electroencephalographic features. *Epilepsia* 2003;44: 1064–1069.

143. Doherty MJ, Wilensky AJ, Holmes MD, et al. Singing seizures. *Neurology* 2002;59:1435–1438.

144. Wada JA. Cerebral lateralization and epileptic manifestations. In: Akimoto H, Kazamatsuri H, Seino M, et al., eds. *Advances in epileptology. XIIIth Epilepsy International Symposium.* New York: Raven Press, 1982:365–372.

145. Benbadis S, Kotagal P, Klem G. Unilateral blinking: a lateralizing sign in partial seizures. *Neurology* 1996;46:45–48.

146. Wada J. Unilateral blinking as a lateralizing sign of partial complex seizure of temporal lobe origin. In: Wada J, Penry JK, eds. *Advances in epileptology. Xth Epilepsy International Symposium.* New York: Raven Press, 1980:533.

147. Sammaritano M, de Lotbiniere A, Andermann F, et al. False lateralization by surface EEG of seizure onset in patients with temporal lobe epilepsy and gross focal cerebral lesions. *Ann Neurol* 1987;21:361–369.

148. Sussman NM, Jackel RA, Kaplan LR, et al. Bicycling movements as a manifestation of complex partial seizures of temporal lobe origin. *Epilepsia* 1989;30:527–531.

149. Molinuevo JL, Arroyo S. Ictal smile. *Epilepsia* 1998;39:1357–1360.

150. Gascon GG, Lombroso CT. Epileptic (gelastic) laughter. *Epilepsia* 1971;12:63–76.

151. Luciano D, Devinsky O, Perrine K. Crying seizures. *Neurology* 1993;43:2113–2117.

152. Spencer SS, Spencer DD, Williamson PD, et al. Sexual automatisms in complex partial seizures. *Neurology* 1983;33:527–533.

153. Leutmezer F, Serles W, Bacher J, et al. Genital automatisms in complex partial seizures. *Neurology* 1999;52:1188–1191.

154. Bleasel A, Kotagal P, Kankirawatana P, et al. Lateralizing value and semiology of ictal limb posturing and version in temporal and extratemporal epilepsy. *Epilepsia* 1997;38:168–174.

155. Chee MW, Kotagal P, Van Ness PC, et al. Lateralizing signs in intractable partial epilepsy: blinded multiple-observer analysis. *Neurology* 1993;43:2519–2525.

156. Berkovic S, Bladin P. An electroclinical study of complex partial seizures. *Epilepsia* 1984;25:668–669.

157. Varelas M, Wada J. Lateralizing significance of unilateral upper limb dystonic posturing in temporal/frontal seizures. *Neurology* 1988;38(Suppl 1):107.

158. Walker EB, Sharbrough FW. The significance of lateralized ictal paresis occurring during complex partial seizures. *Epilepsia* 1988; 28:665.

159. Fakhoury T, Abou-Khalil B. Association of ipsilateral head turning and dystonia in temporal lobe seizures. *Epilepsia* 1995;36: 1065–1070.

160. Oestreich LJ, Berg MJ, Bachmann DL, et al. Ictal contralateral paresis in complex partial seizures. *Epilepsia* 1995;36:671–675.

161. Newton M, Berkovic S, Reutens D, et al. Ictal dystonia: lateralizing value and mechanism revealed by ictal SPECT. *Epilepsia* 1991;32(Suppl 3):78.

162. Dupont S, Semah F, Baulac M, et al. The underlying pathophysiology of ictal dystonia in temporal lobe epilepsy: an FDG-PET study. *Neurology* 1998;51:1289–1292.

163. Bossi L, Munari C, Stoffels C, et al. Somatomotor manifestations in temporal lobe seizures. *Epilepsia* 1984;25:70–76.

164. Hirsch LJ, Lain AH, Walczak TS. Postictal nose wiping lateralizes and localizes to the ipsilateral temporal lobe. *Epilepsia* 1998;39: 991–997.

165. Leutmezer F, Serles W, Lehrner J, et al. Postictal nose wiping: a lateralizing sign in temporal lobe complex partial seizures. *Neurology* 1998;51:1175–1177.

166. Voss NF, Davies KG, Boop FA, et al. Spitting automatism in complex partial seizures: a nondominant temporal localizing sign? *Epilepsia* 1999;40:114–116.

167. Cotte-Ritaud M, Courjon J. Semiological value of adversive epilepsy. *Epilepsia* 1962;3:151–166.

168. Ochs R, Gloor P, Quesney F, et al. Does head-turning during a seizure have lateralizing or localizing significance? *Neurology* 1984;34:884–890.

169. Robillard A, Saint-Hilaire JM, Mercier M, et al. The lateralizing and localizing value of adversion in epileptic seizures. *Neurology* 1983;33:1241–1242.

170. Wyllie E, Luders H, Morris HH, et al. The lateralizing significance of versive head and eye movements during epileptic seizures. *Neurology* 1986;36:606–611.

171. Blum B, Liban E. Experimental basal temporal lobe epilepsy in the cat. *Neurology* 1960;10:544–546.

172. Vigoroux R, Gastaut H, Baldier M. Les formes expérimentales de l'épilepsie. Provocation des principales manifestations cliniques de l'épilepsie dite temporale par stimulation des structures rhinocéphaliques chez le chat no anesthésie. *Rev Neurol* 1951;85:505–508.

173. Green J, Clemente C, De Groot J. Experimentally induced epilepsy in the cat with injury of the cornu Ammonis. *Arch Neurol Psychiatry* 1957;78:259–263.

174. McLachlan RS. The significance of head and eye turning in seizures. *Neurology* 1987;37:1617–1619.

175. Foerster O. The cerebral cortex of man. *Lancet* 1931;2:309–312.

176. Penfield W. Somatic motor and sensory representation in the cerebral cortex in man as studied by electrical stimulation. *Brain* 1937;60:398–443.

177. Smith W. The frontal eye fields. In: Bucy P, ed. *The precentral motor cortex.* Urbana: University of Illinois Press, 1944: 308–342.

178. Marks WJ Jr, Laxer KD. Semiology of temporal lobe seizures: value in lateralizing the seizure focus. *Epilepsia* 1998;39: 721–726.

179. Alajouanine T, Sabourand O. Paroxysmal disturbances of speech in epilepsy (clinical study). *Encephale* 1960;49:95–133.

180. Hécacen H, Piercy M. Paroxysmal dysphasia and the problem of cerebral dominance. *J Neurol Neurosurg Psychiatry* 1956;19: 194–201.

181. Serafetinides EA, Falconer MA. Speech disturbances in temporal lobe seizures: a study in 100 epileptic patients submitted to anterior temporal lobectomy. *Brain* 1963;86:333–346.

182. Yen DJ, Su MS, Yiu CH, et al. Ictal speech manifestations in temporal lobe epilepsy: a video-EEG study. *Epilepsia* 1996;37:45–49.

183. Sakai K, Hidari M, Fukai M, et al. A chance SPECT study of ictal aphasia during simple partial seizures. *Epilepsia* 1997;38:374–376.

184. Dan B, Boyd SG. Dacrystic seizures reconsidered. *Neuropediatrics* 1998;29:326–327.

185. Brogna CG, Lee SI, Dreifuss FE. Pilomotor seizures. Magnetic resonance imaging and electroencephalographic localization of originating focus. *Arch Neurol* 1986;43:1085–1086.

186. Devinsky O, Price BH, Cohen SI. Cardiac manifestations of complex partial seizures. *Am J Med* 1986;80:195–202.

187. Marshall DW, Westmoreland BF, Sharbrough FW. Ictal tachycardia during temporal lobe seizures. *Mayo Clin Proc* 1983;58:443–446.

188. Baumgartner C, Lurger S, Leutmezer F. Autonomic symptoms during epileptic seizures. *Epileptic Disord* 2001;3:103–116.

189. Babb R, Echman P. Abdominal epilepsy. *JAMA* 1972;222:65–66.

190. Gastaut H. A new type of epilepsy: benign partial epilepsy of childhood with occipital spike-waves. *Clin Electroencephalogr* 1982;13:13–22.

191. Jacome DE, FitzGerald R. Ictus emeticus. *Neurology* 1982;32: 209–212.

192. Kramer RE, Luders H, Goldstick LP, et al. Ictus emeticus: an electroclinical analysis. *Neurology* 1988;38:1048–1052.

193. Panayiotopoulos CP. Extraoccipital benign childhood partial seizures with ictal vomiting and excellent prognosis. *J Neurol Neurosurg Psychiatry* 1999;66:82–85.

194. Devinsky O, Frasca J, Pacia SV, et al. Ictus emeticus: further evidence of nondominant temporal involvement. *Neurology* 1995; 45:1158–1160.

195. Baumgartner C, Olbrich A, Lindinger G, et al. Regional cerebral blood flow during temporal lobe seizures associated with ictal vomiting: an ictal SPECT study in two patients. *Epilepsia* 1999;40:1085–1091.

196. Marks DA, Katz A, Booke J, et al. Comparison and correlation of surface and sphenoidal electrodes with simultaneous intracranial recording: an interictal study. *Electroencephalogr Clin Neurophysiol* 1992;82:23–29.

197. Dinner DS, Luders H, Rothner AD, et al. Complex partial seizures of childhood onset: a clinical and encephalographic study. *Cleve Clin Q* 1984;51:287–291.

198. Klass D, Fischer-Williams M. Sensory stimulation, sleep and sleep deprivation. In: Naquet R, ed. *Activation and provocation methods in clinical neurophysiology: handbook of electroencephalography and clinical neurophysiology.* New York: Elsevier, 1976:5–73.

199. Wieser HG, Bancaud J, Talairach J, et al. Comparative value of spontaneous and chemically and electrically induced seizures in establishing the lateralization of temporal lobe seizures. *Epilepsia* 1979;20:47–59.

200. Molaie M, Santana HB, Otero C, et al. Effect of epilepsy and sleep deprivation on the rate of benign epileptiform transients of sleep. *Epilepsia* 1991;32:44–50.

201. Klass D. Electroencephalographic manifestations of complex partial seizures. In: Penry J, Daly D, eds. *Complex partial seizures and their treatment,* vol II, *Advances in Neurology.* New York: Raven Press, 1975:113–140.

202. Blume WT, Young GB, Lemieux JF. EEG morphology of partial epileptic seizures. *Electroencephalogr Clin Neurophysiol* 1984;57: 295–302.

203. Risinger MW, Engel J Jr, Van Ness PC, et al. Ictal localization of temporal lobe seizures with scalp/sphenoidal recordings. *Neurology* 1989;39:1288–1293.

204. Walczak TS, Radtke RA, Lewis DV. Accuracy and interobserver reliability of scalp ictal EEG. *Neurology* 1992;42:2279–2285.

205. Steinhoff BJ, So NK, Lim S, et al. Ictal scalp EEG in temporal lobe epilepsy with unitemporal versus bitemporal interictal epileptiform discharges. *Neurology* 1995;45:889–896.

206. Pacia SV, Jung WJ, Devinsky O. Localization of mesial temporal lobe seizures with sphenoidal electrodes. *J Clin Neurophysiol* 1998;15:256–261.

207. Ives JR, Drislane FW, Schachter SC, et al. Comparison of coronal sphenoidal versus standard anteroposterior temporal montage in the EEG recording of temporal lobe seizures. *Electroencephalogr Clin Neurophysiol* 1996;98:417–421.

208. Ebner A, Hoppe M. Noninvasive electroencephalography and mesial temporal sclerosis. *J Clin Neurophysiol* 1995;12:23–31.

209. Spencer SS, Williamson PD, Bridgers SL, et al. Reliability and accuracy of localization by scalp ictal EEG. *Neurology* 1985; 35:1567–1575.

210. Sharbrough FW. Scalp-recorded ictal patterns in focal epilepsy. *J Clin Neurophysiol* 1993;10:262–267.

211. Spencer SS, Spencer DD, Williamson PD, et al. Ictal effects of anticonvulsant medication withdrawal in epileptic patients. *Epilepsia* 1981;22:297–307.

Focal Motor Seizures, Epilepsia Partialis Continua, and Supplementary Sensorimotor Seizures

17

Andreas V. Alexopoulos   *Dudley S. Dinner*

HISTORY

Focal motor seizures have been recognized since the time of Hippocrates, who first observed seizures affecting the body contralateral to the side of head injury (1). Hughlings Jackson was the first to hypothesize that focal seizures are caused by "a sudden and excessive discharge of gray matter in some part of the brain" and that the clinical manifestations of the seizure depend on the "seat of the discharging lesion" (2,3).

During the second half of the 19th century, Fritsch and Hitzig pioneered stimulation of the brain in animals (4). They discovered that electrical stimulation of the exposed cerebral cortex produced contralateral motor responses in dogs (5,6). Experimental faradic stimulation of the human cerebral cortex was first performed by Bartholow in 1874 (7). In 1909. Cushing reported that faradic stimulation of the postcentral gyrus could be used to determine the anatomic relationship of the sensory strip to an adjacent tumor (8). Motor responses elicited by electrical stimulation in humans were first described by Krause in the beginning of the 20th century (9) and by Foerster more than 60 years ago (3). These early observations led to the fundamental work of Penfield and Brodley, who used electrical stimulation to describe the motor and sensory representation of the human cerebral cortex and pioneered the

techniques for the functional localization of the sensorimotor cortex during surgery (10).

FUNCTIONAL ANATOMY OF THE MOTOR CORTEX

Strictly speaking, the motor cortex (Fig. 17.1) consists of three motor areas: the primary motor cortex (PMA or M1) in the precentral gyrus, which houses a complete representation of body movements; the supplementary sensorimotor area (SSMA or SMA) on the mesial surface rostral to the PMA, also containing a complete motor representation (hence the term *supplementary*); and a more loosely defined premotor cortex (PMC) on the lateral cortical convexity (11).

The prefrontal and orbitofrontal cortex, as well as the dorsolateral and mesial frontal cortex anterior to the SSMA, are not considered part of the motor cortex. The term *prefrontal cortex* is used to define the extensive part of the frontal lobe that lies anterior to the motor and premotor zones (12). Recent studies in humans and primates challenge the traditional division of motor areas. For example, part of the cingulate motor cortex, which was previously linked to the limbic system, is now viewed as a potential fourth motor area. Moreover, the use of modern

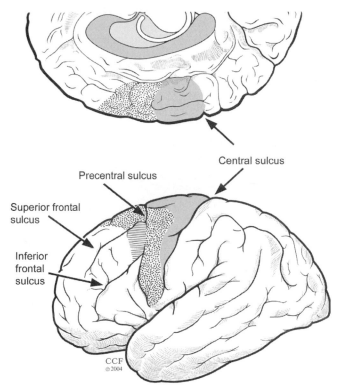

Figure 17.1 Mesial and lateral aspects of the left hemisphere: schematic representation of the three motor areas and their approximate relationship to the surface hemispheric anatomy. The *shaded area* corresponds to the primary motor cortex (Brodmann area 4). The *stippled area* illustrates the supplementary sensorimotor cortex on the mesial aspect. On the lateral view, the *stippled area* represents the premotor cortex. Also note the approximate location of the frontal eye field (*hatched area*).

anatomic and physiologic techniques has enabled researchers to explore and define additional subdivisions of motor areas in both humans and primates (13).

Activation studies using positron emission tomography (PET) or functional magnetic resonance imaging (fMRI) allude to the complex organization of the motor system. The breadth of cortical and subcortical areas activated with even the simplest movements attests to the wide distribution and extent of interconnected neural networks underlying motor control (14). Observed movements presuppose a series of parallel or sequential processes involving the selection, planning, preparation, and initiation of action (14,15).

Efferent and Afferent Connections

The familiar hierarchical model of motor control is based on the four levels of spinal cord, brainstem, PMA, and premotor cortex-SSMA. This concept has influenced our understanding of the various motor manifestations of seizures (16). Motor commands are organized hierarchically from the most automatic (e.g., deep tendon reflexes) to the least (e.g., skilled and precise voluntary movements). Each level of motor control retains a somatotopic

organization and receives peripheral sensory information that is used to modify the motor output at that level (17). The cerebral cortex exerts its motor control by way of the corticospinal and corticobulbar pathways. The cortex also modulates the action of motor neurons in the brainstem and spinal cord indirectly through its influence on the brain's various descending systems.

To this day, limited direct information exists about specific neuronal connections between functional brain regions of the human cortex (18). Our knowledge of detailed connectivities derives from studies of nonhuman primates using invasive tracer techniques. Such invasive studies, however, cannot be performed in humans, and animal results cannot always be extrapolated to human systems (19,20).

Brainstem Motor Efferents

The brainstem gives rise to several descending motor pathways, which are divided into ventromedial and dorsolateral groups (21,22). The ventromedial system sends fibers through the ventral columns of the spinal cord and terminates predominantly in the medial part of the ventral horn, which contains the motor nuclei controlling proximal limb and axial muscle groups. In contrast, the dorsolateral system descends in the lateral part of the spinal cord and terminates on the lateral motor cell complex (23), which innervates more distal limb muscles.

The rubrospinal tract comprises the main dorsolateral pathway and has its origin in the midbrain (in the magnocellular portion of the red nucleus). The red nucleus receives input from the motor cortex and cerebellum and provides an indirect route for these areas to influence the spinal cord.

The ventromedial system consists of four major descending tracts. Two arise from the midbrain—tectospinal tract (from the superior colliculus) and interstitiospinal tract (from the interstitial nucleus of Cajal in the rostral mesencephalon)—while the other two have their origin in the medulla and pons (vestibulospinal and reticulospinal tracts). The pontine and medullary vestibulospinal pathways play a role in extensor muscle control and maintenance of posture (24). Finally, the reticulospinal pathways modulate postural reflexes and crude voluntary movements. Their excitatory connections with spinal motor neurons innervating axial and proximal limb muscles are largely ipsilateral (23) and are implicated in the production of tonic and atonic motor phenomena (16).

Motor Cortex Efferents

The axons that project from layer V of the cortex to the spinal cord run together in the corticospinal tract (a massive bundle of fibers containing approximately 1 million axons). About one third of corticospinal and corticobulbar fibers arise from the PMA. Another third originate from the SSMA and PMC, and the rest have their origin in the parietal lobe (arising mainly from the somatosensory cortex of the postcentral gyrus) (17,22,25). The corticospinal fibers together with the corticobulbar fibers run through the posterior limb of the internal capsule to reach the ventral portion of the brainstem and send collaterals to the striatum, thalamus, red nucleus, and other brainstem nuclei (26). In the brainstem, the corticobulbar fibers terminate bilaterally in cranial nerve motor nuclei (either directly via a monosynaptic route or indirectly), with the exception of motor neurons innervating the lower face, which receive mostly contralateral corticobulbar input. About three-fourths of the corticospinal fibers cross the midline in the pyramidal decussation at the junction of the medulla and spinal cord and descend in the spinal cord as the lateral corticospinal tract (17). Uncrossed fibers descend as the ventral corticospinal tract. The lateral and ventral divisions of the corticospinal tract terminate in approximately the same regions of spinal gray matter along with corresponding brainstem-originating pathways. The majority of corticospinal tract terminals project on spinal interneurons. An estimated 5% of the fibers synapse directly on (both alpha and gamma) motor neurons (27).

These anatomic arrangements of descending tracts underlie the contralateral and/or bilateral motor manifestations of focal seizures arising from the motor cortex (16).

Motor Cortex Afferents

The major cortical inputs to the motor areas of cortex are from the prefrontal and parietal association areas (17). These are focused mainly on the PMC and the SSMA, whereas the PMA receives a large input from the primary somatosensory cortex (28). In addition, the PMA receives direct and indirect input from the PMC and the SSMA. In particular, the SSMA projects bilaterally to the primary motor cortex in a somatotopically organized manner. Other corticocortical inputs arrive from the opposite hemisphere through the corpus callosum, which interconnects heterotopic as well as homologous areas in the two hemispheres (29). The major subcortical input to the motor cortical areas comes from the thalamus, where separate nuclei convey modulating inputs from the basal ganglia and cerebellum (17,28).

Stimulation Studies

In clinical practice, insights into the functional anatomy of the motor cortex and other eloquent brain cortical areas are afforded by direct cortical stimulation. The development of subdural electrodes, which are implanted long term and allow recordings over several days or weeks in patients with epilepsy, has provided the opportunity to perform electrical stimulation studies of the cortex, including the PMA and SSMA, before surgery. At the same time, electrical stimulation of the human cortex provides an experimental model that can be used to reproduce the effects of cortical activation after an ictal discharge (30). In

fact, several groups have used cortical stimulation to trigger habitual auras and/or seizures, in an attempt to better delineate the ictal onset zone before epilepsy surgery.

In general, the observed clinical response is assumed to arise from cortex below the stimulated electrode or from the region between two closely spaced electrodes, given that the current density drops off rapidly with increasing distance from the tissue underlying the stimulated electrode (31,32). Electrical stimulation can elicit "positive" responses (such as localized movements resulting from activation of the PMA or SSMA cortex) or "negative" responses (such as inhibition of motor activity). The latter becomes apparent only if the patient engages in specific tasks during stimulation.

In areas such as the supplementary motor cortex, both positive responses in the form of bilateral motor movements and negative responses such as speech arrest can be demonstrated. The area of stimulation gives rise to distinctive patterns of motor activation of the PMA, SSMA, or premotor regions. In addition, however, overlapping clinical manifestations may be observed as a result of the highly developed interconnectivity between these regions (33).

Negative motor responses interfere with a person's ability to perform a voluntary movement or sustain a voluntary contraction when cortical stimulation is applied (34). The patient is unaware of the effects of stimulation unless asked to perform the specific function integrated by the stimulated cortical region. In a systematic review of 42 patients who had subdural electrodes implanted over the perirolandic area, the Cleveland Clinic group observed negative motor responses when stimulating the agranular cortex immediately in front of the primary and supplementary face areas. Negative motor responses were seen over both hemispheres (34). To distinguish the two negative motor areas, investigators proposed the terms *primary negative motor area* (PNMA, in regard to the region of the inferior frontal gyrus immediately in front of the face PMA) and *supplementary negative motor area* (SNMA, in reference to the mesial portion of the superior frontal gyrus immediately in front of the face SSMA).

The effects of electrical stimulation on the different components of the motor cortex are discussed below.

Primary Motor Area

The PMA resides in the anterior wall of the central sulcus (Fig. 17.1) and corresponds to Brodmann's area 4. On the basis of cytoarchitectonic criteria, area 4 is recognized primarily by the presence of Betz cells (giant pyramidal cells) in cortical layer V and the absence of a granular layer IV (35). The central sulcus marks the border between the agranular motor cortex and the granular somatosensory cortex (36).

The somatotopic organization of the PMA was elucidated by the pioneering work of Krause (9), Penfield and Jasper, and others (37,38) (Fig. 17.2). In this region of the

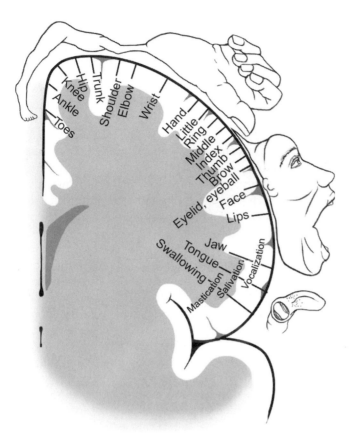

Figure 17.2 The motor homunculus after Penfield and Rasmussen (37), depicting the somatotopic arrangement of the primary motor cortex (PMA) (with the tongue and lips near the sylvian fissure and the thumb, fingers, arm, and trunk represented successively along the precentral gyrus ending with the leg, foot, and toes on the mesial surface). Muscle groups involved in fine movements feature a disproportionately large representation. (Adapted from Penfield W, Rasmussen T. *The cerebral cortex of man—a clinical study of localization of function.* New York: Macmillan, 1950 p. 57)

PMA, simple movements were elicited with the lowest intensity of electrical stimulation (39). The resulting motor maps show an orderly arrangement with the tongue and lips near the sylvian fissure and the thumb, digits, arm, and trunk represented successively along the central sulcus, ending with the leg, foot, and toes on the mesial surface. The layout of the motor homunculus (Fig. 17.2) is topographically similar to that of the somatosensory homunculus, which resides immediately behind the PMA. The somatotopic organization of the motor cortex is not fixed and can be altered during motor learning or after injury. Output of the PMA is directed to the corticospinal and corticobulbar tracts, as well as to the SSMA and homologous areas in the opposite hemisphere via the corpus callosum (40).

Stimulation Studies

In the PMA, single stimuli typically elicit single clonic movements of the contralateral somatic muscles represented by the area of the motor homunculus being stimulated. High-frequency (50 to 60 Hz) stimulus series result in slower,

tonic contralateral motor responses (41). Intraoperative application of electrical stimulation mapping provides the most direct and easy way to localize the somatosensory cortex (42). In most adults, motor responses can be evoked from the precentral rolandic cortex under local or general anesthesia. When local anesthesia is used, these effects are usually observed with currents of 2 to 4 mA. Sensory responses are elicited with stimulation of the postcentral gyrus, often at slightly lower thresholds (43). The threshold for eliciting a motor response in humans is lowest in the PMA.

Supplementary Sensorimotor Area

The SSMA is a distinct anatomic region located on the mesial surface of the superior frontal gyrus and its adjacent dorsal convexity (44). The cerebral cortex of the SSMA corresponds to the mesial portion of area 6 of Brodmann's cytoarchitectonic map of the brain (Fig. 17.1) (38,45). Similar to the PMA cortex, the SSMA is referred to as agranular cortex, because the internal granular layer (layer IV) is not prominent. In contrast to area 4, area 6 does not contain Betz cells (45). The medial precentral sulcus defines the border between the primary motor area for the foot and the posterior limit of the SSMA (13,46). No clear cytoarchitectonic or anatomic boundary separates the SSMA from the adjacent PMC (47).

The macaque and human mesial area 6 (SSMA) is further subdivided into pre-SSMA (rostrally) and SSMA proper (caudally) on the basis of comparable cytoarchitectonic and transmitter receptor studies (36). Studies in primates suggest that the pre-SSMA holds a hierarchically higher role in motor control. However, the functional properties of the SSMA subdivisions have not been detailed in humans (48). The border between the pre-SSMA and SSMA proper corresponds to the VCA line (the vertical line passing through the anterior commissure and perpendicular to the AC-PC line, which connects the anterior and posterior commissures). The border between SSMA proper and PMA corresponds approximately to the VCP line (the vertical line that traverses the posterior commissure and is perpendicular to the AC-PC line) (49).

Stimulation Studies

More than 60 years ago, Foerster was the first to describe motor responses in humans elicited by electrical stimulation of the mesial aspect of the superior frontal gyrus anterior to the primary motor representation for the lower extremity (3). Systematic study of this region with electrical stimulation was carried out at the Montreal Neurological Institute during the intraoperative evaluation of patients with intractable focal epilepsy preceding surgical resection (50,51).

This was the first group to use the term *supplementary motor area.* Direct electrical stimulation of the SMA produced vocalization, speech arrest, postural movements of all extremities, inhibition of voluntary movements, and autonomic changes. The Montreal studies demonstrated that both positive (such as bilateral motor movements) and negative responses (such as speech arrest) could be elicited by stimulating this region. Intraoperative studies of the SMA may be limited because of the restricted amount of time and relative difficulty of accessing the mesial aspect of the hemisphere and recognizing the specific gyral landmarks during surgery.

With the advent of subdural electrodes, the Cleveland Clinic series of extraoperative stimulation studies showed that positive motor responses were not restricted to the mesial aspect of the superior frontal gyrus, but could also be elicited from its dorsal convexity, the lower half of the paracentral lobule, and the precuneus (52). The same group confirmed the presence of sensory symptoms that were elicited along with the positive motor responses after stimulation of the SMA and coined the term *supplementary sensorimotor area* instead of SMA.

Using depth electrodes, Talairach and Bancaud were the first to describe a somatotopic organization within the SSMA (53). The Yale group confirmed the presence of somatotopic distribution in the SSMA, where the face, upper extremity, and lower extremity responses are oriented in a rostrocaudal direction, with the lower extremities represented posteriorly, head and face most anteriorly, and the upper extremities between these two regions (54). Likewise, studies of movement-related potentials (MRPs) using subdural electrodes implanted over the SSMA region demonstrated that the MRPs for different types of movements (of the finger, foot, and tongue as well as vocalization) also have a somatotopic distribution within the SSMA, which is consistent with the SSMA organization defined by electrical stimulation (55–57).

Premotor Cortex

Fulton coined the term *premotor cortex* in 1935 (58) to describe the third major component of the motor cortex. This area encompasses the more loosely defined agranular cortex of the lateral frontal convexity rostral to the PMA (11,22), which corresponds to the lateral portion of Brodmann's area 6 (Fig. 17.1). It is very difficult to define the anterior border of the agranular PMC in humans, where a broad zone of progressive transition exists between area 6 and the granular cortex of Brodmann's frontal area 9 (59). In the macaque, the PMC is further subdivided into a dorsal portion on the dorsolateral convexity and a ventral portion on the ventrolateral convexity (11). Despite the lack of direct correlation between microstructure and function in humans, the two subdivsions of the premotor area are considered to have homologous counterparts in the human brain.

The motor and premotor cortices, as well as the frontal eye fields and the anterior cingulate cortex of area 24, have reciprocal connections with the SSMA (45). Anatomic labeling experiments in the macaque have demonstrated that the more anterior dorsal premotor cortex projects to

the spinal cord, challenging the notion that the PMC, unlike the PMA and SSMA, lacks prominent corticospinal connections (22,60,61).

According to the classic schema, the PMC is responsible for the preparation and organization of movements (47). Several recent studies show that the PMC also plays a central role in nonmotor attentional and receptive domains. Therefore, our current understanding suggests a dual PMC function pertaining to motor and cognitive behavior (62).

Stimulation Studies

On the basis of early electrical stimulation studies of the monkey brain (63) the agranular lateral PMC (area 6) has been subdivided into a rostral (6aβ or 6r) and a caudal section (6aα or 6c). Recent quantitative architectonic and neurotransmitter studies have corroborated the presence of similar topographic boundaries in the human brain (36,59). The rostral subdivision covers the anterior part of the precentral gyrus, and its caudal counterpart resides in the posterior part of the superior and middle frontal gyri, in front of the precentral sulcus (64).

Eye movements can be electrically induced from a large area of the human dorsolateral frontal cortex and the precentral gyrus. These stimulation-elicited responses have been attributed to electrical interference with the human homologue of the monkey frontal eye field (65). Electrical cortical stimulation studies in epileptic patients undergoing presurgical evaluation have confirmed the functional location of the eye movement sites anterior to the motor representation of arm and face (65,66). However, some ambiguity exists as regards the exact location of the human frontal eye field within this rather extensive oculomotor region. The divergence is largely caused by the methodologic differences of neuroimaging and electrical cortical stimulation studies.

The electrically defined human frontal eye field is located in the posterior end of the middle frontal gyrus (Fig. 17.1) immediately anterior to the precentral sulcus (and in proximity to the superior frontal sulcus). Electrical cortical stimulation of this area produces constant oculomotor responses characterized by low stimulation thresholds (65).

Conversely, neuroimaging studies of cerebral blood flow (CBF) changes suggest that the homologous region for the human frontal eye field lies posterior to the electrically defined frontal eye field. Indeed, the CBF-defined frontal eye field is located between the central and precentral sulci in front of the primary hand representation, suggesting that the eye movement field lies in Brodmann area 6 (in the region of the PMC homologous to the ventral PMC) (67,68).

FOCAL MOTOR SEIZURES

Focal seizure is the term proposed by the Task Force of the International League Against Epilepsy (ILAE) to describe seizures in which the initial activation involves a limited number of neurons in part of one hemisphere (69). The terms *localization-related* or *partial* seizures have been used to describe the same seizure type. However, the more recently proposed diagnostic scheme of the ILAE Task Force prefers the less ambiguous term *focal* to partial or localization-related seizures (70).

Motor features constitute the main clinical manifestations of motor seizures. As a rule, consciousness is retained in the majority of seizures arising from discrete motor regions. It is possible, however, for an ictal discharge to remain localized and still produce alteration of consciousness. Furthermore, certain motor manifestations and a patient's anxious reaction to the seizure symptoms may prevent the patient from responding appropriately during seizures. It may therefore be difficult to ascertain the level of consciousness in several patients with focal motor seizures. In the past, the presence or absence of altered awareness was used to dichotomize seizures of focal onset into "simple partial" and "complex partial." It is now proposed to move away from this dichotomy, which seems to "have lost its meaningful precision" (70).

The established International Classification of Epileptic Seizures (69) divides focal motor seizures into those with or without a march, versive, postural, and phonatory seizures. The diagnostic scheme proposed in 2001 is based on the use of a system of five axes (levels) intended to provide a standardized description of individual patients (70). Axis 2 now defines the epileptic seizure type or types experienced by the patient. Hence, focal motor seizures may present with elementary clonic motor signs, with asymmetric tonic motor seizures (a term commonly used to describe seizures arising from the SSMA), typical automatisms (a term that refers to seizures arising from the temporal lobe), with hyperkinetic automatisms, with focal negative myoclonus, and, finally, with inhibitory motor seizures. The addition of axis 1 allows for the systematic description of ictal semiology observed during seizures utilizing a standardized glossary of descriptive terminology (71). Ictal motor phenomena may be subdivided into elementary motor manifestations (such as tonic, clonic, dystonic, versive) and automatisms. Automatisms consist of a more or less coordinated, repetitive motor activity (such as oroalimentary, manual or pedal, vocal or verbal, hyperkinetic or hypokinetic) (71). Somatotopic modifiers may be added to describe the body part producing motor activity during seizures.

Another recent seizure classification is based on clinical symptomatology and is independent of electroencephalogram (EEG), neuroimaging, and historical information (72). This classification uses terms such as *focal clonic*, *focal tonic*, or *versive*, and evolution during the seizure is indicated by arrows. For example: left hand somatosensory aura → left arm clonic seizure → left versive seizure.

Clinical Semiology

This section reviews the elementary motor phenomena resulting from a variety of focal motor seizures. These seizures typically present with clonic or tonic manifestations. Hyperkinetic manifestations are usually attributed to seizures arising from (or spreading to) the frontal lobe. Other complex motor automatisms seen with focal seizures (such as oroalimentary, mimetic, or gestural automatisms) are reviewed elsewhere.

In a population-based study conducted in Denmark of 1054 patients with epilepsy who were between the ages of 16 and 66 years, 18% had "simple partial" seizures (73). In a large series of patients admitted to a single hospital over a period of 10 years, Mauguiere and Courjon (74) reviewed the types of focal seizures defined in 8938 patients with focal and/or generalized seizures. They found that 1158 patients (12.9%) had focal tonic or clonic seizures without march; 582 (6.5%) presented with hemitonic or clonic seizures; 461 (5.2%) had adversive seizures; and only 199 (2.2%) had jacksonian seizures.

Perirolandic epileptogenic lesions often involve both the precentral and postcentral gyri, giving rise to both motor and sensory phenomena (in one study of 87 "simple partial" seizures in 14 patients studied by video-electroencephalography, sensory phenomena were observed in approximately one-third of patients with focal motor seizures [75]). In a study examining the relationship between early ictal motor manifestations and interictal abnormalities of cerebral glucose consumption, Shlaug and colleagues (76) analyzed 48 consecutive patients with neocortical seizures. Patients with unilateral clonic seizures primarily had a hypometabolic defect in the contralateral perirolandic region. Patients with predominantly focal tonic manifestations showed hypometabolism within the frontomesial and perirolandic regions, whereas patients with versive seizures showed contralateral hypometabolism without a consistent regional pattern. Finally, patients with hypermotor seizures had areas of depressed metabolism involving the frontomesial, perirolandic, anterior cingulate, and anterior insular regions.

Postictally, patients may experience a transient functional deficit, such as localized paresis (Todd paralysis), which may last for minutes or hours (up to 48 hours or longer). This interesting clinical phenomenon of "postepileptic paresis" is the signature of a focal seizure and bears the name of Dr. Bentley Todd, who first described it in the mid-19th century (77). Todd paralysis is believed to result from persistent focal dysfunction of the involved epileptogenic region. Postictal Todd paralysis is a clinical sign of substantial value in lateralizing the hemisphere of seizure onset (78).

Clonic Seizures

Clonic seizures consist of repeated, short contractions of various muscle groups characterized by rhythmic jerking or twitching movements (79). These movements recur at regular intervals of less than 1 to 2 seconds. Most clonic seizures are brief and last for less than 1 or 2 minutes. During this period, clonic movements may remain restricted to one region or spread in a jacksonian manner. The majority of focal motor seizures tend to involve the hand and face, although any body part may potentially be affected (80). Such predilection is attributed to the large cortical representation of the hand and face areas.

In accordance with the somatotopic arrangement within the precentral sulcus, clonic twitching of a corresponding group of muscles is the typical ictal manifestation of a localized discharge within the contralateral precentral gyrus. Penfield and Jasper (38) also noted that the angle of the mouth was involved first in seizures affecting the face; seizures of the upper extremity began in the thumb and index finger, whereas seizures of the lower extremity often began in the great toe.

The clonic movements are limited initially to the corresponding area of the body but may spread during the attack. Such a spread (e.g., from the muscles of the face to the ipsilateral hand or arm) is known as the "jacksonian march." In these "jacksonian attacks," the symptoms travel slowly from one territory to another, following the order of the corresponding somatotopic representation. The march usually starts from a distal body region (such as the thumb, fingers, great toe, or eyelids) and spreads toward a more proximal part. At times, the march may skip some areas, a phenomenon that may be related to different seizure thresholds in the symptomatogenic region. Holowach and associates (81) reported that 25 of 60 jacksonian seizures in children began in the face (8 in the periocular and 5 in the perioral region), 17 in the hand, 7 in the arm, 2 in the shoulder, and 9 in the leg and foot.

The term *jacksonian epilepsy* was proposed by Charcot in 1887 to describe seizures that begin and spread with a similar march of symptoms (82). Its continued use today serves to remind us of Hughlings Jackson's astute clinical observations, which provided the basis for his revolutionary principles of functional localization (83). In his own words:

> The part of the body where the convulsion begins indicates the part of the brain where the discharge begins and where the discharging lesion is situated. But from the focus discharging primarily the discharge spreads laterally to the adjacent "healthy" foci. One focus after the other is seized by the radiating waves of impulses. The march of the attack, the order in which the different parts of the body become involved, reveals the arrangement of the corresponding foci in the precentral convolution (3).

The term *hemiconvulsions* refers to unilateral clonic seizures (i.e., clonic activity affecting one side of the body). Prolonged unilateral convulsions followed by the onset of hemiparesis are described in the childhood syndrome of hemiconvulsion-hemiplegia-epilepsy (HHE), discussed briefly in the section on selected epilepsy syndromes at the end of this chapter.

A variety of myoclonic phenomena need to be differentiated from focal clonic seizures. Typically, myoclonic jerks are arrhythmic compared with clonic motor activity. Notable exceptions of more rhythmic motoric manifestations, which are usually discussed under the broad definition of myoclonus, include the terms *epilepsia partialis continua* (see below), *segmental myoclonus*, and *palatal myoclonus* (also called palatal tremor) (84). Many types of myoclonic phenomena (e.g., myoclonus caused by spinal cord disease or essential myoclonus) do not have an epileptic origin. In contrast, epileptic myoclonus is typically accompanied by an EEG correlate of spike or multispike-wave complexes (85,86). Therefore, the term *myoclonic seizure* is reserved for seizures whose main components are single or repeated epileptic myoclonias (87). Focal motor seizures are generally not considered to be myoclonic, although sometimes an accurate distinction may prove difficult (86). In fact, focal cortical myoclonus has been described in four children who had dysplastic lesions of the motor cortex and coexistent focal motor seizures (88). Finally, the paradoxic term *negative myoclonus* is reserved for cases of sudden, brief relaxations in tonic muscle contraction (84). Epileptic negative myoclonus can be seen in relationship with a number of heterogeneous epilepsy syndromes (89,90).

Tonic Seizures

Tonic seizures consist of sustained muscle contractions that usually last for more than 5 to 10 seconds (91) and result in posturing of the limbs or whole body. From the standpoint of clinical semiology, tonic seizures can be described according to the distribution and symmetry of tonic contractions with involvement of the axial (neck, trunk, and pelvis) and limb musculature. Generalized tonic seizures involve axial and limb muscles in a symmetric and synchronous fashion. Unequal or asynchronous contraction of muscle groups involving both sides of the body results in bilateral asymmetric tonic seizures. Finally, contraction may be restricted to a portion of the body on the left or right side, giving rise to focal tonic seizures (92).

In contrast to focal clonic seizures, which represent epileptic discharges in the corresponding region of the precentral gyrus, tonic motor seizures may implicate a wider area of motor cortex including the SSMA and PMC (16,93). Even though focal tonic seizures are attributed to activation of Brodmann area 6 (and the mesial frontal region in particular), some overlap in symptomatology occurs, with ictal involvement of the premotor and/or primary motor areas (94).

Stimulation of the SSMA elicits bilateral, asymmetric tonic contractions affecting primarily the more proximal muscles. Less frequently, focal tonic contractions may be seen. The symptomatogenic zone is less clear in cases of symmetric, bilateral tonic seizures. However, these seizures are believed to be generated by simultaneous activation of Brodmann area 6, rostral to the precentral region of both hemispheres (30). It is also possible that generalized tonic seizures result from direct activation of brainstem reticular-activating systems (95,96).

Nonepileptic focal tonic symptoms can result from subcortical pathology (e.g., spinal cord or brainstem dysfunction in the case of compression or multiple sclerosis). In addition, paroxysmal tonic phenomena may be seen as part of certain movement disorders (such as paroxysmal choreoathetosis or spasmodic torticollis) or other nonepileptic paroxysmal disorders (e.g., in the setting of convulsive syncope) (92).

Oculocephalic Deviation and Versive Seizures

Foerster and Penfield classically described versive seizures, which consist of a sustained, unnatural turning of the eyes and head to one side (97), in 1930. They are a manifestation of the predominantly tonic contraction of head and eye muscles. Although consciousness is often lost by the time a patient experiences version, at times patients may be aware of the forced eye and head deviation (40,98).

As discussed, electrical cortical stimulation studies using subdural electrodes in epileptic patients have confirmed the functional location of eye movement sites in proximity to the primary motor representation of the arm and face (66). On stimulating this region, Rasmussen and Penfield (99) reported that the more anterior points were responsible for contralateral rotation. Stimulation of more posterior points (closer to the central sulcus) elicited contralateral, ipsilateral, or upward eye movements. Head rotation was usually seen in conjunction with contralateral eye rotation.

The lateralizing significance of oculocephalic deviation has met with controversy. Indeed a number of authors use the terms *head turning* and *head version* interchangeably (100–102). This lexical ambiguity prompted Wyllie and colleagues to restrict the term *version* to unquestionably forced, involuntary head and eye deviation to one side resulting in sustained unnatural positioning of the head and eyes. The authors performed a retrospective review of lateral head and eye movements observed during 74 spontaneous seizures in 37 patients (97). Mild, unsustained, wandering, or seemingly voluntary head and eye movements were classified as "nonversive." Visual analysis of high-quality video recordings was performed without prior knowledge of EEG findings. In this study, adherence to the strict definition of "version" showed that the presence of contralateral versive head and eye movement can be a reliable lateralizing sign (especially when this movement precedes secondary generalization).

On the other hand, one should be cautious about interpreting the direction of eye and head turning if the seizure does not become secondarily generalized (103,104).

Version may result from seizures originating from various locations and spreading to the PMC. An important clinical observation is that extratemporal seizures give rise to version earlier in the seizure (within 18 seconds from seizure onset), compared with seizures of temporal lobe origin (in which version is usually seen after 18 seconds or later) (103).

Seizures Manifested by Vocalization or Arrest of Vocalization

Several types of utterances can occur during epileptic seizures (16). A prolonged continuous or interrupted vocalization may occur in seizures involving the SSMA or lower PMA on either hemisphere (53). Vocalization, when it occurs as part of SSMA seizures, tends to be more sustained (105). Penfield and Jasper (38) produced such phonatory phenomena in humans by stimulating the SSMA or the PMA below the lip or tongue area. Finally, the so-called epileptic cry is frequently seen at the onset of generalized tonic-clonic seizures.

Speech arrest, defined as inability to speak during the seizure despite conscious attempts by the patient (40), may result from involvement of the PMA (106) or SSMA (107) region in either the dominant or nondominant hemisphere. Electrical cortical stimulation studies suggest that the speech arrest observed in cases of SSMA stimulation represents a negative motor response (resulting from inhibition of tongue movement) (107).

Electroencephalographic Findings

The ability of scalp electroencephalography to detect interictal activity depends on the extent of the irritative zone and the orientation of the dipole. Special techniques may be required to demonstrate epileptiform activity in patients with focal seizures. Sleep recordings, for example, have been reported to increase the yield of interictal epileptiform abnormalities (108–111). Special electrodes (such as sphenoidal, anterior temporal, or ear electrodes) and closely spaced additional scalp electrodes (Fig. 17.3A) may help to distinguish temporal from frontal foci and determine whether the electrical field of a midline sharp wave is higher over the left or right hemisphere (112–114).

Small epileptogenic foci may be entirely missed with surface EEG recordings. On the other hand, epileptiform abnormalities may have a misleadingly widespread appearance because of the large distance and intervening cortical area that separates the epileptogenic zone from the scalp EEG electrodes (115).

Random EEG tracings in patients with focal epilepsy may not show evidence of focal epileptiform activity. In a case series of 19 patients with refractory frontal lobe epilepsy, Salanova and associates (116) reported absence of interictal sharp waves in 7 of 19 (37%) patients. Secondary bilaterally synchronous discharges may be seen in up to

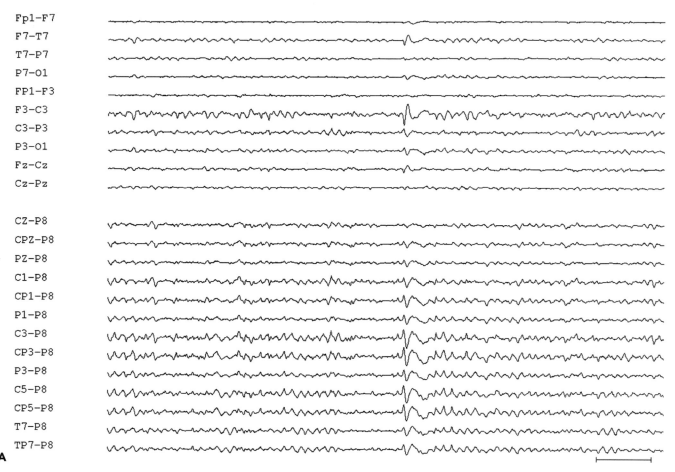

Figure 17.3 Scalp electroencephalogram tracings (A, B, and C) from a 41-year-old patient with medically intractable left perirolandic epilepsy of unknown etiology since age 11 years. He presented with daily focal motor seizures involving the right leg and shoulder sometimes preceded by a somatosensory aura (tingling sensation in the right foot) and rare secondarily generalized tonic-clonic seizures. **A:** Interictal left centroparietal sharp wave as seen on a longitudinal bipolar (*upper part*) and referential montage (*lower part*). The P8 reference derivation of the sharp wave shows maximum negativity at electrode CP3. The addition of closely spaced surface electrodes (placed according to the 10–10 Electrode Placement System) provides for a more accurate distribution map. In this instance, the potential amplitude at electrode C5 is 85% and at electrodes C3 and CP3 is 83% of the amplitude recorded at the maximally involved electrode CP3.

two thirds of patients with frontal lobe epilepsy (117). EEG interpretation should take into account the possibility of "secondary bilateral synchrony," a term introduced by Tükel and Jasper (118) to describe the bilateral discharges seen in patients with parasagittal epileptogenic lesions.

Functional neuroimaging with ^{18}FDG-PET (fluorodeoxyglucose positron emission tomography) may reveal hypometabolism in up to 60% of patients with frontal lobe epilepsy. Almost 90% of the patients with evidence of hypometabolism on PET have an underlying structural abnormality as shown with structural neuroimaging (119).

Ictal recordings may show regional seizure patterns (Fig. 17.3C) or may have limited localizing or lateralizing value. As a rule, the patterns are more widespread and more difficult to lateralize compared with those seen with seizures of temporal lobe origin. Studies show that ictal electroencephalography may be nonlocalizing in more than half of

patients with frontal lobe epilepsy (116,120). False localization may occur with an erroneous temporal ictal pattern on surface EEG as a result of underlying frontolimbic connections (115). Invasive recordings using subdural electrodes may only show evidence for a focal onset in a relatively small number of patients with frontal lobe epilepsy; often, a more diffuse "regional" pattern may be seen (121).

EPILEPSIA PARTIALIS CONTINUA

The *epileptic seizure types*, which constitute axis 2 of the recently proposed ILAE diagnostic scheme (70), have been divided into self-limited and continuous. The term *continuous seizure types* encompasses the diverse presentations of status epilepticus.

Status epilepticus could be broadly divided into status epilepticus with motor or without motor phenomena

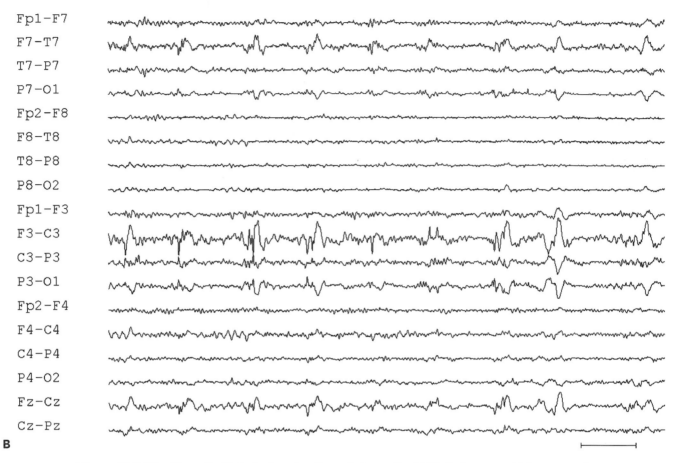

Figure 17.3 (Continued) **B:** Periodic epileptiform discharge-like (PLED-like) pattern of left centroparietal sharp waves and polyspikes. This interictal finding was present during the first 24 hours of admission for acute exacerbation of the patient's habitual focal motor seizures.

(122). Subcategories of motor status epilepticus include the generalized type as well as the secondarily generalized and focal motor status. *Focal motor status epilepticus* is characterized by repetitive typical somatomotor seizures with or without jacksonian march originating from the perirolandic region. This condition may occur at the onset or during epilepsies manifesting with focal motor seizures. Consciousness is usually preserved, and cerebral function of the uninvolved cortex remains intact. A variety of motor phenomena may be observed in the context of focal motor status. For example, epileptic nystagmus may be the manifestation of oculoclonic status epilepticus (123,124).

Epilepsia partialis continua of Kojevnikov (EPC or partial continuous epilepsy) constitutes one form of focal motor status epilepticus, characterized by localized unremitting myoclonus. The condition was first described by Kojevnikov in 1895 (125) as a disorder of persistent localized motor seizures (and can also found in the literature as Kojewnikow syndrome or Kozhevnikov syndrome).

Clinical Semiology

Epilepsia partialis continua is defined by the occurrence of almost continuous and rhythmic or semirhythmic muscular

contractions (myoclonic jerks) that remain localized to a limited area on one side of the body and persist for hours, days, or even years (126,127). The definition has undergone several revisions in the past, reflecting differences of opinion among various authors. In 1989, the ILAE Commission defined EPC as a specific form of continuous somatomotor seizures involving the rolandic cortex (128). Any muscle group may be involved, but distal musculature is more commonly affected. The myoclonic jerks may appear isolated or in clusters and usually have a frequency of 1 to 2 per second. In general, unilateral involvement with synchronous activation of agonists and antagonists is observed. By definition, the jerks are spontaneous, although they may be aggravated by action or sensory stimuli (129). In most cases, the jerks may be reduced in amplitude but persist during sleep (130,131). Other seizure types (such as jacksonian or generalized seizures) and a variety of neurologic deficits may be seen in these patients depending on the underlying etiology.

Bancaud and coworkers (127) divided epilepsia partialis continua into two broad categories based on the presence (type 2) or absence (type 1) of a progressive brain lesion: Type 1 was associated with a regional nonprogressive lesion in the sensorimotor cortex, whereas type 2 was

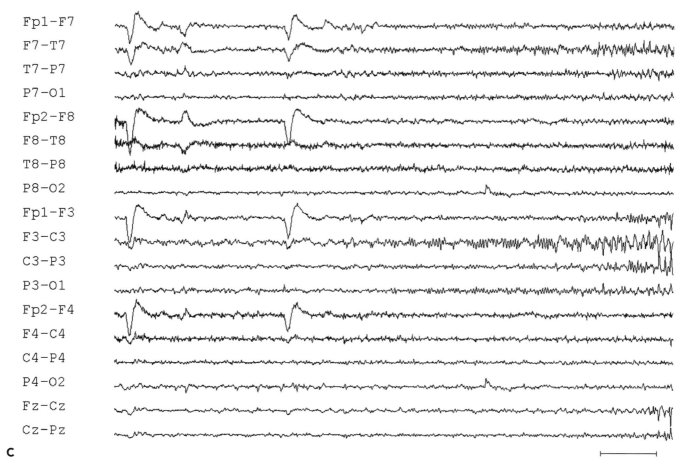

Figure 17.3 (Continued)   C: The ictal onset is punctuated by the appearance of evolving low- to higher-amplitude paroxysmal fast activity arising from the left centroparietal region.

typically seen in the setting of Rasmussen syndrome. This syndrome is briefly discussed in the section on selected epilepsy syndromes at the end of this chapter.

Epilepsia partialis continua may develop at any age. The usual etiology of EPC is a focal lesion involving the cortex (principally the sensorimotor cortex) that results from stroke, trauma, infection, metastasis, or primary tumor. A hypoxic, metabolic, or septic encephalopathy may predispose patients with a pre-existing focal lesion to develop epilepsia partialis continua. All patients presenting with EPC should be carefully evaluated for an underlying lesion that may be amenable to curative resective surgery.

Moreover, epilepsia partialis continua is a common manifestation of Rasmussen syndrome (observed in almost 50% of cases) (132). EPC and its variants have also been reported in the setting of multiple sclerosis (133), human immunodeficiency virus infection (134,135), Creutzfeldt-Jakob disease (136), and other neurodegenerative diseases (e.g., children with mitochondrial disorders [137,138], or Alpers syndrome [139]).

Focal motor seizures or epilepsia partialis continua, or both, may be the presenting feature of nonketotic hyperglycemia or may occur as a late complication especially in the presence of an underlying focal cerebral lesion (140). Hyperglycemia, hyponatremia, mild hyperosmolarity, and lack of ketoacidosis were found to contribute to the development of EPC predominantly in areas of pre-existing focal cerebral damage in 21 patients with evidence of nonketotic hyperglycemia (141). However, epilepsia partialis continua occurring in the setting of ketotic hyperglycemia has also been reported (126,142).

Depending on the etiology, EPC may be an early or late feature in the course of the underlying disease and may be seen either in isolation or in association with other seizure types (143). Similar to EPC, focal somatomotor status may reflect an underlying focal brain lesion (secondary to a vascular, neoplastic, traumatic, or infectious etiology) or may present in the context of toxic-metabolic abnormalities. In patients without pre-existing epilepsy, the onset of focal motor status may signify underlying "asymptomatic" ischemia or interterritorial cerebral infarction (infarction in watershed territories).

Subcortical or spinal myoclonus and certain forms of tremor and other extrapyramidal movement disorders should be considered in the differential diagnosis of EPC. Clinical differentiation is often challenging, and special neurophysiologic examinations may be necessary (143,144).

Electroencephalographic Findings

The conventional scalp EEG may be unrevealing or misleadingly normal. There may be very few or no paroxysmal abnormalities, and the background rhythm may be normal. In some cases, time-locked EEG events can be detected by back-averaging. In addition, special stereoencephalographic or electrocorticographic recordings may prove helpful in resolving the underlying spike focus.

In other cases, irregular 0.5- to 3-Hz slowing may be seen in the frontocentral region along with reduction of the beta activity in the same area (40). In a study of 32 cases (145), the most common EEG finding was regional spiking. Other abnormalities included bursts of sharp waves or spike-and-wave discharges and unilateral or bilateral runs of abnormal rhythms.

Rarely, periodic lateralized epileptiform discharges (PLEDs) that are time locked to the jerks are observed (146). PLEDs are usually viewed as a transient interictal pattern (Fig. 17.3B), which may last as long as 3 months or longer (147) and can occur in a variety of disorders (148). However, on rare occasions, PLEDs may actually represent an ictal EEG pattern. The most common seizure type seen in the presence of PLEDs is focal motor seizures affecting the contralateral body (149) often presenting as status epilepticus or as repetitive focal motor seizures (149–151).

In a single case report of an 11-year-old girl with Rasmussen syndrome and a 5-month history of epilepsia partialis continua, studies with FDG-PET revealed an area of hypermetabolism in the right central cortex and ipsilateral thalamus. A congruent sharp-wave focus was present in the same region on scalp EEG recordings. Using simultaneously recorded electromyography (EMG) of the left tibialis anterior muscle, the authors demonstrated regular jerks, time locked with the right central sharp waves (126,152).

SUPPLEMENTARY SENSORIMOTOR SEIZURES

Clinical Semiology

Seizures arising from the SSMA are of brief duration, usually lasting only 10 to 40 seconds. Rapid onset of asymmetric tonic posturing involving one or more extremities is characteristically observed (44,153). While it is common for both sides of the body to be affected simultaneously, unilateral tonic motor activity may occur (154). The typical seizure is frequently referred to as a *bilateral asymmetric tonic seizure*.

Speech arrest and vocalization are common. Somatosensory symptoms may precede the phase of tonic posturing (38); these body sensations are not well localized.

Common descriptions include a feeling of tension, pulling, or heaviness in an extremity or a sense that the extremity is "about to move" (155). Although consciousness is usually preserved, patients may not be able to respond verbally during the tonic phase of the seizure. Toward the end of the seizure, a few rhythmic clonic movements of the extremities may be observed (155). Postictal confusion is absent in the majority of SSMA seizures.

The asymmetric involvement of the upper extremities manifests with abduction at the shoulders, flexion of one elbow, and extension of the other upper extremity. As a rule, the lower extremities are also involved in the tonic posturing, with abduction at the hips and flexion or extension at the knees (44). Even patients, in whom tonic posturing appears to be unilateral, have bilaterally increased (or decreased) tone (33).

In their original report and illustrations of "somatic sensory seizures" arising from the SSMA, Penfield and Jasper (38) described head turning to the side of the flexed upper extremity. They observed that the head appears as if looking toward the flexed and raised arm with the patient adopting the so-called *fencing posture* (a motor response reminiscent of the asymmetric tonic neck reflex [33]). Ajmone Marsan and Ralston (156) subsequently coined the term *M2e* to describe the abduction and elevation of the contralateral arm with external rotation at the shoulder and slight flexion at the elbow. The patient's head and eyes deviate as if looking at the elevated arm, while both lower extremities remain extended or slightly flexed at the hips and knees.

In contrast to these early reports, further analysis of SSMA seizures showed that assumption of the classic fencing or M2e posture is not common (157,158). Among the less common motor manifestations, coarse movements of the tonic postured extremities may be observed (159). If present, vocalization may be prominent during the tonic phase (reflecting the tonic involvement of the diaphragm and laryngeal muscles, which contract against semiclosed vocal cords) (155,160).

Ictal activity may spread to involve the PMA of the face on the dorsolateral convexity, resulting in unilateral clonic movements or contralateral head version. Secondary generalization may lead to a generalized tonic-clonic seizure. Clonic movements have been described toward the end of the tonic seizure (155). Finally, writhing movements may be seen as some patients attempt to move around or sit up during the tonic seizure.

SSMA seizures may be frequent (up to 5 to 10 per day) and can occur in clusters. They tend to occur predominantly during sleep (155,161,162). In a systematic review of the relationship of sleep and SSMA seizures (163), almost two thirds of a total of 322 SSMA seizures, recorded during prolonged video-EEG evaluation in 24 patients, occurred during sleep (almost exclusively during nonrapid eye movement [NREM] sleep stages I and II).

Only a minority of patients with seizures displaying the clinical features of SSMA activation actually have SSMA

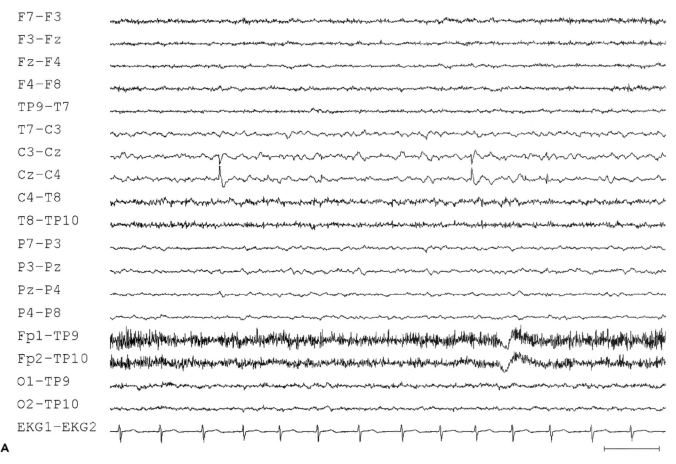

F7–F3
F3–Fz
Fz–F4
F4–F8
TP9–T7
T7–C3
C3–Cz
Cz–C4
C4–T8
T8–TP10
P7–P3
P3–Pz
Pz–P4
P4–P8
Fp1–TP9
Fp2–TP10
O1–TP9
O2–TP10
EKG1–EKG2

A

Figure 17.4 Interictal (**A**) and ictal (**B** and **C**) scalp electroencephalogram (EEG) tracings with a transverse bipolar montage from a 12-year-old girl with left SSMA epilepsy. Bilateral asymmetric tonic seizures arising from sleep and wakefulness were captured during video-electroencephalograph evaluation. **A:** This awake recording shows sharp waves at the vertex (virtually confined to the Cz electrode). Note that the potential amplitude is slightly higher on the left (C3) than on the right (C4) central electrode.

epilepsy (164). In most cases, the SSMA functions as the symptomatogenic zone: the observed seizures reflect the expression of ictal discharges originating from clinically silent regions near the SSMA (such as the basal frontal regions, the dorsolateral convexity of the frontal lobe, and the mesial parietal regions) (44).

The clinical picture of SSMA seizures with involvement of all four extremities and simultaneous preservation of awareness may be misleading, and it is not unusual for patients with this type of paroxysmal activity to be misdiagnosed as having psychogenic seizures (105).

Electroencephalographic Findings

Interictal sharp waves, when present, are usually found at the midline, maximum at the vertex, or just adjacent to the midline in the frontocentral region (Fig. 17.4A). Only 50% of 16 patients with supplementary sensorimotor seizures, who underwent evaluations with subdural electrodes, had shown scalp EEG evidence of midline frontocentral interictal epileptiform activity (160).

It is important to distinguish midline interictal epileptiform discharges from vertex sharp transients of sleep. This distinction may be impossible, when sharp waves are seen only during sleep. The presence of prominent aftergoing slow waves, polyspikes, and/or consistently asymmetric distribution of the electrical field may raise the suspicion of epileptiform activity (160,165). Normal sleep-related transients have a symmetric field, whereas midline sharp waves may be asymmetric. Certainly, the appearance of the same midline sharp waves or spikes during wakefulness (Fig. 17.4A) will lead to the correct diagnosis of underlying epilepsy. Furthermore, the possibility of paradoxic scalp EEG lateralization exists when the generator of sharp waves is situated in the interhemispheric fissure producing a transverse or oblique dipole orientation (166).

During seizures originating from the SSMA (Fig. 17.4B), the EEG is frequently obscured by prominent EMG artifact owing to the associated tonic activity and the midline location of the ictal EEG discharges. However, careful review of the vertex region with the appropriate (usually transverse bipolar) montage and use of closely spaced parasagittal

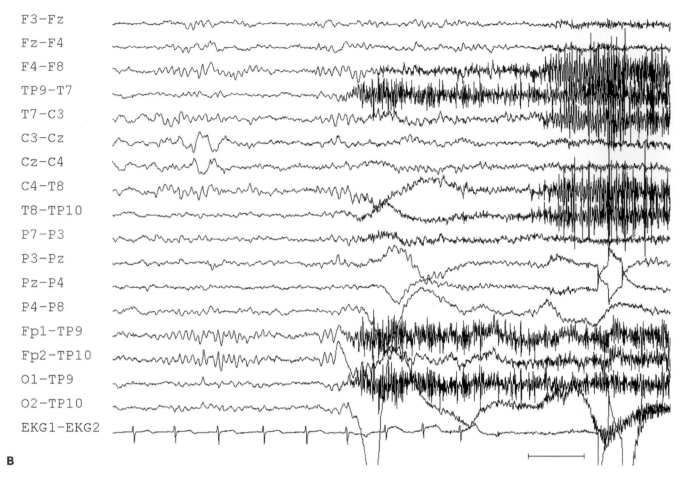

```
F3-Fz
Fz-F4
F4-F8
TP9-T7
T7-C3
C3-Cz
Cz-C4
C4-T8
T8-TP10
P7-P3
P3-Pz
Pz-P4
P4-P8
Fp1-TP9
Fp2-TP10
O1-TP9
O2-TP10
EKG1-EKG2
```

B

Figure 17.4   B: Clinical onset of typical seizure occurring out of sleep coincides with the appearance of bilateral electromyographic artifact. Scalp EEG does not reveal a clear ictal pattern at the time of clinical onset.

scalp electrodes may reveal the ictal EEG pattern despite considerable EMG artifact.

There is frequently an initial high-amplitude slow transient or sharp wave present at the vertex followed by midline low-amplitude fast activity or an electrodecremental pattern (155,165). These early changes are often followed by the development of high-amplitude rhythmic slowing distributed bilaterally in the frontocentral regions. Ictal activity may remain restricted to the vertex (Fig. 17.4C) or have a more widespread distribution. In general, the lateralizing value of such ictal EEG changes is rather limited. In addition, a small percentage of patients with SSMA epilepsy have no identifiable scalp EEG change during the ictus.

SELECTED EPILEPSY SYNDROMES

Benign Focal Epilepsy of Childhood

The benign focal epilepsies of childhood are idiopathic, localization-related epilepsies characterized by focal seizures and EEG abnormalities (128) in the absence of a demonstrable anatomic lesion. These age-related syndromes occur in neurologically normal children and are characterized by a tendency for spontaneous remission.

Benign childhood epilepsy with centrotemporal spikes (BCECTS), also known as benign rolandic epilepsy, is the most common syndrome, comprising 10% to 16% of all epileptic seizures before the age of 15 years (167–169). In comparison, other benign focal epilepsies of childhood, such as the syndromes of childhood occipital epilepsy (COE, known as childhood epilepsy with occipital spike waves), benign frontal epilepsy of childhood, and benign epilepsy with affective symptoms, are relatively rare.

The age of onset of BCECTS ranges from 2 to 13 years, with peak incidence at 9 years. Children usually experience sleep-related seizures, which typically occur during NREM sleep. It is thought that approximately 75% of the seizures in this syndrome manifest during sleep (170,171). Simple partial seizures with sensorimotor symptoms involving the face, tongue, mouth, chin and/or muscles of the oropharynx, hemiconvulsions, and generalized nocturnal tonic-clonic seizures followed by postictal Todd paralysis (suggesting focal onset with secondary generalization) are the most common manifestations. Nearly 80% of patients experience isolated or infrequent seizures (171). The genetic

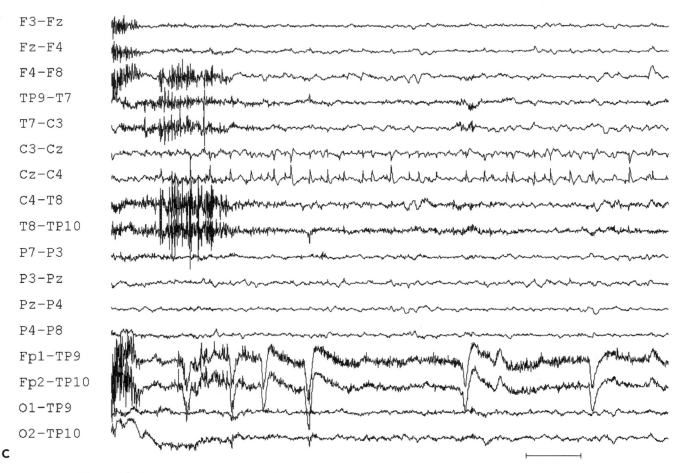

Figure 17.4   C: Rhythmic, repetitive sharp waves are present at the vertex within 15 seconds of clinical onset.

nature of the disease is supported by reports of BCECTS and benign focal epileptiform discharges of childhood in identical twins. It is important, however, to distinguish the EEG trait from the epilepsy phenotype, in that epileptic seizures appear in only 25% or fewer of individuals having the EEG trait (172).

The interictal sharp waves (described as benign focal epileptiform discharges of childhood) have an extremely stereotyped, diphasic morphology and occur in a focal distribution in the centrotemporal region superimposed on normal background activity (173). Centrotemporal spikes are characterized by a transverse dipole and are usually seen independently on both sides of the head. Frequently, these discharges may show a bifocal or multifocal distribution. In addition, epileptiform activity tends to be markedly enhanced during NREM sleep.

BCECTS can be distinguished from the symptomatic epilepsies by seizure semiology, EEG manifestations, response to antiepileptic drugs, and absence of abnormalities on neurologic examination and neuroimaging studies. Similar seizure patterns and electrographic features may be seen in patients with focal brain lesions involving the operculum and perirolandic cortex. The clinical semiology of BCECTS suggests that the origin of seizures lies in the lower

perirolandic cortex in the area representing the face and oropharynx. Penfield and Rasmussen (37) were able to reproduce the typical symptoms of BCECTS seizures by stimulating this cortical area.

The less common syndrome of COE has been divided into an early onset form presenting between 1 and 14 years of age with a peak at 4 to 5 years (early onset benign COE, also known as Panayiotopoulos type) and a late-onset variant (70) (late-onset COE, also known as Gastaut type) with onset between 3 and 15 years and a peak around 8 years (167). Nocturnal seizures with vomiting, tonic eye deviation and occasional involvement of the head and limbs are seen in the early onset variant (167). On the other hand, visual symptoms such as amaurosis and/or visual hallucinations are the characteristic manifestations of the late-onset variant of COE. Headache, nausea, and vomiting may be present postictally. Migraine and lesional occipital lobe epilepsy need to be considered in the differential diagnosis of common clinical conditions mimicking COE.

Rasmussen Syndrome

As mentioned, epilepsia partialis continua may occur in the setting of Rasmussen syndrome, a progressive condition that includes other types of pharmacoresistant focal seizures, abnormal movements, and evolving neurologic deficits such as hemiplegia, aphasia, and cognitive deterioration in a previously healthy child. More than half of these patients develop epilepsia partialis continua during the course of the disorder (174).

The onset of focal seizures occurs during childhood (median age of onset is 5 years, ranging from 14 months to 14 years in the series from the Montreal Neurologic Institute [174,175]). Seizures are typically focal motor events originating from the affected hemisphere, but complex partial or generalized tonic-clonic seizures may also occur. The progressive neurologic deterioration usually appears within the first year after seizure onset. Slowly evolving, predominantly unilateral brain atrophy and congruent EEG abnormalities (with persistent lateralized slow activity, ipsilateral loss of background features, and abundant epileptiform discharges) are typically present.

In most cases, medical treatment fails to control seizures or arrest the relentless disease progression. However, encouraging results have been reported after anatomic or functional hemispherectomy (174,176) (in the operative series from the Montreal Neurologic Institute, 52% of 21 patients were free of seizures after hemispherectomy, and another 24% of patients had fewer than two seizures per year [174]).

Hemiconvulsion-Hemiplegia-Epilepsy Syndrome

The term *hemiconvulsions* refers to unilateral clonic seizures (i.e., clonic activity affecting one side of the body) as observed by Gastaut and colleagues (123,177,178). Some of the reported cases had jacksonian spread of their seizures (including some with onset around the eye) (179) and often occurred in the setting of infantile hemiplegia (178,180).

The term *hemiconvulsion-hemiplegia-epilepsy syndrome* was first used by Gastaut in 1960 to describe the three phases of this uncommon syndrome. Typically, infants (ages 6 months to 2 years) develop hemiconvulsions in the course of a febrile illness. The initial phase of *hemiconvulsions* (exclusively or predominantly unilateral seizures) may have a long duration (which ranges from 1 hour to a few days and constitutes a particular form of focal somatomotor status epilepticus). The second phase of persistent *hemiplegia* (arbitrarily lasting more than 7 days in contradistinction to the transient nature of postictal Todd paralysis) usually leaves the patient with a permanent residual motor deficit. The third stage (*epilepsy*) is the final step in the temporal evolution of the syndrome leading to the eventual development of focal seizures (33).

Hemispheric Epilepsy

In 1998, Blume employed the term *hemispheric epilepsy* to describe an uncommon syndrome of "one-sided generalized epilepsy" (181). The author reviewed 13 neurologically normal patients with a seemingly "generalized" seizure disorder, whose interictal spike-wave discharges were consistently accentuated in one hemisphere. Blume postulated that this syndrome might represent a possible bridge between focal and generalized epilepsies.

Four major components defined this syndrome: interictal EEG characterized by diffuse unilateral spike waves, which appear consistently over the same hemisphere in a given patient; persistent (usually pharmacoresistant) seizures with both generalized (present in all patients) and focal ictal features (of note, focal features were present in most, but not all, patients); seizure onset during childhood or adolescence; and no apparent etiology or related structural abnormality. Nine of the 13 patients had seizure semiology suggestive of a focal origin (auras or unilateral motor phenomena), but only four of these nine patients had focal clinical features consistently occurring contralateral to the principal spike-wave focus (16,181).

DIFFERENTIAL DIAGNOSIS

The differential diagnosis of focal motor seizures includes tic disorders, nonepileptic myoclonus (182), nonepileptic seizures, and other paroxysmal movement disorders such as paroxysmal choreoathetosis and tremor.

As mentioned, the absence of abnormalities on routine electroencephalography does not exclude the possibility of focal motor seizures. When available, home videotape recordings can provide valuable diagnostic information by capturing the semiology of the episodes in question. Otherwise, prolonged inpatient video-electroencephalographic monitoring may be necessary. Patients who present with infrequent attacks of unclear etiology pose considerable diagnostic challenges, given the low diagnostic yield of prolonged EEG recordings. Ambulatory electroencephalography is not particularly helpful in this setting, especially if no ictal EEG patterns are seen during the paroxysmal behavior. Good-quality videotape recordings of the events are essential in making a diagnosis.

Seizures arising from the frontal lobe can be bizarre (such as seizures characterized by prominent thrashing movements and preserved consciousness) and may be misdiagnosed as nonepileptic seizures of psychogenic origin. The reverse can also be true. Saygi and coworkers (183) compared the ictal manifestations in 63 focal seizures of frontal lobe origin in 11 patients with the clinical presentation of 29 "psychogenic seizures" in 12 patients. The authors did not find any single clinical criterion that would sufficiently differentiate these two groups. In this study, seizure characteristics favoring an epileptic diagnosis included younger age at onset, stereotyped patterns of movements, turning to a prone position during seizures, shorter duration of seizures, nocturnal occurrence, and the presence of magnetic resonance imaging and EEG abnormality. In another study (105), which only compared the clinical features of SSMA and nonepileptic seizures, the duration of SSMA seizures was much shorter than that of psychogenic events. None of the SSMA seizures lasted longer than 38 seconds, whereas psychogenic seizures had a mean duration of 173 seconds. In addition, SSMA seizures occurred predominantly out of sleep, whereas psychogenic seizures usually occurred from the waking state.

Epileptic motor seizures may manifest themselves at any time of the day or night. However, a number of epilepsy syndromes (including SSMA epilepsy, frontal lobe epilepsy, benign focal epilepsy of childhood, generalized epilepsy, and autosomal dominant nocturnal frontal lobe epilepsy) tend to manifest with seizures occurring predominantly during sleep. In addition, sleep-related paroxysmal motor phenomena can be seen with various sleep disorders (including NREM arousal disorders, REM behavior disorder of sleep, and sleep-wake transition disorder). The differential diagnosis of such nocturnal paroxysmal events is broad and often challenging, given the frequently poor clinical description and overlap of clinical manifestations (184).

It is not understood why certain seizure types occur preferentially during sleep (185). Patients with frontal lobe epilepsy (including those with SSMA epilepsy and others whose epileptogenic zone is located outside the SSMA region) tend to manifest with seizures arising out of sleep (44). In a study of patients with intractable focal epilepsy (186), presurgical continuous video-electroencephalography and polysomnography were used to compare sleeping-waking distribution of seizures and quality of sleep organization in 15 patients with frontal lobe epilepsy and 15 patients with temporal lobe epilepsy. The authors showed that, in patients with pharmacoresistant focal epilepsy, seizures of frontal lobe origin occurred more frequently during the night compared with seizures arising from the temporal lobe.

Recently, autosomal dominant nocturnal frontal lobe epilepsy (ADNFLE) has been identified as a distinctive clinical syndrome (187,188). The disorder is characterized by clusters of brief nocturnal motor seizures with hyperkinetic or tonic manifestations. Stereotyped attacks are frequently seen in individual family members despite the significant intrafamilial variation. Interictal EEGs are frequently normal, and the diagnosis is established on a clinical basis. Seizures usually begin in childhood and may persist throughout life, although the overall seizure frequency tends to decrease over time (187). A strong linkage with the neuronal nicotinic acetylcholine receptor has been established in the years following initial descriptions of this syndrome (189,190).

Several case reports highlight the unusual occurrence of repetitive involuntary movements in the setting of transient cerebral ischemia (the so-called limb-shaking transient ischemic attacks or limb-shaking TIAs) that may be mistaken for focal motor seizures (191–195). These episodic attacks are often precipitated by standing up or walking and seem to involve only the limbs (hand-arm alone or hand-arm and ipsilateral leg) without spreading to the facial or truncal musculature (191,192). The need to recognize these paroxysmal positive motor manifestations as a sign of severe contralateral carotid occlusive disease is emphasized (191,194).

REFERENCES

1. Souques A. *Étapes de la neurologie dans l'antiquité grecque*. Paris: Masson et Cie, 1936.
2. Taylor J. *Selected writings of John Hughlings Jackson*. London: Hodder and Stoughton, 1931.
3. Foerster O. The motor cortex in man in the light of Hughlings Jackson's doctrines. *Brain* 1936;59:135–139.
4. Fritsch G, Hitzig E. Über die elektrische Erregbarkeit des Grosshirns. *Arch Anat Physiol Wiss Med* 1870;37:300–332.
5. Wieser HG. Historical review of cortical electrical stimulation. In: Lüders HO, Noachtar S, eds. *Epileptic seizures—pathophysiology and clinical semiology*. Philadelphia: Churchill Livingstone, 2000: 141–152.
6. Uematsu S, Lesser RP, Gordon B. Localization of sensorimotor cortex: the influence of Sherrington and Cushing on the modern concept. *Neurosurgery* 1992;30:904–912.
7. Bartholow R. Experimental investigations into functions of the human brain. *Am J Med Sci* 1874;67:305–313.
8. Cushing H. A note upon the faradic stimulation of the postcentral gyrus in conscious patients. *Brain* 1909;32:44–53.
9. Zimmerman M. Electrical stimulation of the human brain. *Hum Neurobiol* 1982;1:227–229.
10. Penfield W, Brodley E. Somatic motor and sensory representation in the cerebral cortex of man as studied by electrical stimulation. *Brain* 1937;60:389–443.
11. Geyer S, Matelli M, Luppino G, et al. Functional neuroanatomy of the primate isocortical motor system. *Anat Embryol (Berl)* 2000; 202:443–474.
12. Petrides M. Mapping prefrontal cortical systems for the control of cognition. In: Toga AW, Mazziotta JC, eds. *Brain mapping: the systems*. San Diego: Academic Press, 2000:159–176.
13. Roland PE, Zilles K. Functions and structures of the motor cortices in humans. *Curr Opin Neurobiol* 1996;6:773–781.
14. Fink GR, Frackowiak RS, Pietrzyk U, et al. Multiple nonprimary motor areas in the human cortex. *J Neurophysiol* 1997;77: 2164–2174.
15. Grafton ST, Hari R, Salenius S. The human motor system. In: Toga AW, Mazziotta JC, eds. *Brain mapping: the systems*. San Diego: Academic Press, 2000:331–363.
16. Blume W. Focal motor seizures and epilepsia partialis continua. In: Wyllie E, ed. *The treatment of epilepsy: principles & practice*, 3rd ed. Philadelphia: Lippincott Williams & Wilkins, 2001:329–343.
17. Ghez C, Krakauer J. The organization of movement. In: Kandel ER, Schwartz JH, Jessell TM, eds. *Principles of neural science*. New York: McGraw-Hill, 2000:653–673.
18. Crick F, Jones E. Backwardness of human neuroanatomy. *Nature* 1993;361:109–110.
19. Conturo TE, Lori NF, Cull TS, et al. Tracking neuronal fiber pathways in the living human brain. *Proc Natl Acad Sci U S A* 1999;96:10422–10427.
20. Passingham RE, Ramnani N, Rowe JB. The motor system. In: Frackowiak RSJ, Friston KJ, Frith CD, et al, eds. *Human brain function*. San Diego: Academic Press, 2004:5–32.
21. Kuypers HGJM. Anatomy of the descending pathways. In: Brookhart JM, Mountcastle VB, Brooks VB, et al., eds. *The nervous system, II. Motor control*. Bethesda, MD: American Physiological Society, 1981:597–666.
22. Blume WT. Motor cortex: anatomy, physiology and epileptogenesis. In: Wyllie E, ed. *The treatment of epilepsy: principles & practice*. Philadelphia: Lea & Febiger, 1993:16–25.
23. Carpenter MB. Tracts of the spinal cord. In: Carpenter MB, ed. *Human neuroanatomy*. Baltimore, MD: Williams & Wilkins, 1976:238–284.

24. Holstege G. The anatomy of the central control of posture: consistency and plasticity. *Neurosci Biobehav Rev* 1998;22:485–493.

25. Galea MP, Darian-Smith I. Multiple corticospinal neuron populations in the macaque monkey are specified by their unique cortical origins, spinal terminations, and connections. *Cereb Cortex* 1994;4:166–194.

26. Arslan O. Motor neurons. In: *Neuroanatomical basis of clinical neurology.* New York: Parthenon, 2001:361–385.

27. Nauta WJ, Feirtag M. Descending paths; the motor system. In: *Fundamental neuroanatomy.* New York: WH Freeman, 1986: 91–107.

28. Passingham R. Lateral premotor cortex (area 6). In: *The frontal lobes and voluntary action.* Oxford: Oxford University Press, 1993: 38–68.

29. Goldman-Rakic PS. Anatomical and functional circuits in prefrontal cortex of nonhuman primates—relevance to epilepsy. *Adv Neurol* 1995;66:51–65.

30. Lüders HO. Symptomatogenic areas and electrical stimulation. In: Lüders HO, Noachtar S, eds. *Epileptic seizures—pathophysiology and clinical semiology.* Philadelphia: Churchill Livingstone, 2000: 131–140.

31. Nathan SS, Sinha SR, Gordon B, et al. Determination of current density distributions generated by electrical stimulation of the human cerebral cortex. *Electroencephalogr Clin Neurophysiol* 1993;86:183–192.

32. Lesser RP, Gordon B. Methodologic considerations in cortical electrical stimulation in adults. In: Lüders HO, Noachtar S, eds. *Epileptic seizures—pathophysiology and clinical semiology.* Philadelphia: Churchill Livingstone, 2000:153–165.

33. Arzimanoglou A, Guerrini R, Aicardi J. *Aicardi's epilepsy in children,* 3rd ed. Philadelphia: Lippincott Williams & Wilkins, 2004.

34. Luders H, Dinner D, Morris H, et al. Cortical electrical stimulation in humans. The negative motor areas. *Adv Neurol* 1995;67: 115–129.

35. White LE, Andrews TJ, Hulette C, et al. Structure of the human sensorimotor system, I: morphology and cytoarchitecture of the central sulcus. *Cereb Cortex* 1997;7:18–30.

36. Zilles K, Schlaug G, Matelli M, et al. Mapping of human and macaque sensorimotor areas by integrating architectonic, transmitter receptor, MRI and PET data. *J Anat* 1995;187(Pt 3):515–537.

37. Penfield W, Rasmussen T. *The cerebral cortex of man—a clinical study of localization of function.* New York: Macmillan, 1950.

38. Penfield W, Jasper H. *Epilepsy and the functional anatomy of the human brain.* Boston: Little, Brown, 1954.

39. Krakauer J, Ghez C. Voluntary movement. In: Kandel ER, Schwartz JH, Jessell TM, eds. *Principles of neural science.* New York: McGraw-Hill, 2000:756–781.

40. Kotagal P, Lüders HO. Simple motor seizures. In: Engel J, Pedley TA, eds. *Epilepsy: the comprehensive CD-ROM.* Philadelphia: Lippincott Williams & Wilkins, 1999.

41. Neuloh G, Schramm J. Intraoperative neurophysiological mapping and monitoring. In: Deletis V, Shils JL, eds. *Neurophysiology in neurosurgery—a modern intraoperative approach.* San Diego: Academic Press, 2002:339–401.

42. Wood CC, Spencer DD, Allison T, et al. Localization of human sensorimotor cortex during surgery by cortical surface recording of somatosensory evoked potentials. *J Neurosurg* 1988;68:99–111.

43. Toga AW, Ojemann GA, Ojemann JG, et al. Intraoperative brain mapping. In: Mazziotta JC, Toga AW, Frackowiak RSJ, eds. *Brain mapping: the disorders.* San Diego: Academic Press, 2000:77–105.

44. Dinner DS. Supplementary sensorimotor area epilepsy. In: Bazil CW, Malow BA, Sammaritano MR, eds. *Sleep and epilepsy: the clinical spectrum.* Amsterdam: Elsevier, 2002:223–236.

45. Wiesendanger M. Recent developments in studies of the supplementary motor area of primates. *Rev Physiol Biochem Pharmacol* 1986;103:1–59.

46. Zilles K, Schlaug G, Geyer S, et al. Anatomy and transmitter receptors of the supplementary motor areas in the human and nonhuman primate brain. *Adv Neurol* 1996;70:29–43.

47. Wise SP. The primate premotor cortex: past, present, and preparatory. *Annu Rev Neurosci* 1985;8:1–19.

48. Tanji J. New concepts of the supplementary motor area. *Curr Opin Neurobiol* 1996;6:782–787.

49. Vorobiev V, Govoni P, Rizzolatti G, et al. Parcellation of human mesial area 6: cytoarchitectonic evidence for three separate areas. *Eur J Neurosci* 1998;10:2199–2203.

50. Penfield W, Welch K. The supplementary motor area in the cerebral cortex of man. *Trans Am Neurol Assoc* 1949;74:179–184.

51. Penfield W, Welch K. The supplementary area of the cerebral cortex. A clinical and experimental study. *Arch Neurol Psychiatry* 1951;66:289–317.

52. Lim S, Dinner DS, Pillay P, et al. Functional anatomy of the human supplementary sensorimotor area: results of extraoperative electrical stimulation. *Electroencephalogr Clin Neurophysiol* 1994;91:179–193.

53. Talairach J, Bancaud J. The supplementary motor area in man (anatomo-functional findings by stereo-encephalography in epilepsy). *Int J Neurol* 1966;5:330–347.

54. Fried I, Katz A, McCarthy G, et al. Functional organization of human supplementary motor cortex studied by electrical stimulation. *J Neurosci* 1991;11:3656–3666.

55. Ikeda A, Luders HO, Burgess RC, et al. Movement-related potentials recorded from supplementary motor area and primary motor area. Role of supplementary motor area in voluntary movements. *Brain* 1992;115(Pt 4):1017–1043.

56. Ikeda A, Luders HO, Burgess RC, et al. Movement-related potentials associated with single and repetitive movements recorded from human supplementary motor area. *Electroencephalogr Clin Neurophysiol* 1993;89:269–277.

57. Ikeda A, Luders HO, Shibasaki H, et al. Movement-related potentials associated with bilateral simultaneous and unilateral movements recorded from human supplementary motor area. *Electroencephalogr Clin Neurophysiol* 1995;95:323–334.

58. Fulton JF. A note on the definition of the "motor" and "premotor" areas. *Brain* 1935;58:311–316.

59. Baleydier C, Achache P, Froment JC. Neurofilament architecture of superior and mesial premotor cortex in the human brain. *Neuroreport* 1997;8:1691–1696.

60. Schluter ND, Rushworth MF, Mills KR, et al. Signal-, set-, and movement-related activity in the human premotor cortex. *Neuropsychologia* 1999;37:233–243.

61. Dum RP, Strick PL. The origin of corticospinal projections from the premotor areas in the frontal lobe. *J Neurosci* 1991;11:667–689.

62. Schubotz RI, von Cramon DY. Functional-anatomical concepts of human premotor cortex: evidence from fMRI and PET studies. *Neuroimage* 2003;20(Suppl 1):S120–S131.

63. Vogt C, Vogt OJ. Allgemeinere Ergebnisse unserer Hirnforschung. *J Psychol Neurol* 1919;25(Suppl 1):279–462.

64. Duffau H, Capelle L, Denvil D, et al. The role of dominant premotor cortex in language: a study using intraoperative functional mapping in awake patients. *Neuroimage* 2003;20:1903–1914.

65. Blanke O, Spinelli L, Thut G, et al. Location of the human frontal eye field as defined by electrical cortical stimulation: anatomical, functional and electrophysiological characteristics. *Neuroreport* 2000;11:1907–1913.

66. Godoy J, Luders H, Dinner DS, et al. Versive eye movements elicited by cortical stimulation of the human brain. *Neurology* 1990;40:296–299.

67. Luna B, Thulborn KR, Strojwas MH, et al. Dorsal cortical regions subserving visually guided saccades in humans: an fMRI study. *Cereb Cortex* 1998;8:40–47.

68. Paus T. Location and function of the human frontal eye-field: a selective review. *Neuropsychologia* 1996;34:475–483.

69. Commission on Classification and Terminology of the International League Against Epilepsy. Proposal for revised clinical and electroencephalographic classification of epileptic seizures. *Epilepsia* 1981;22:489–501.

70. Engel J Jr. A proposed diagnostic scheme for people with epileptic seizures and with epilepsy: report of the ILAE Task Force on Classification and Terminology. *Epilepsia* 2001;42:796–803.

71. Blume WT, Luders HO, Mizrahi E, et al. Glossary of descriptive terminology for ictal semiology: report of the ILAE Task Force on Classification and Terminology. *Epilepsia* 2001;42:1212–1218.

72. Luders HO, Burgess R, Noachtar S. Expanding the international classification of seizures to provide localization information. *Neurology* 1993;43:1650–1655.

73. Wagner AL. A clinical and epidemiological study of adult patients with epilepsy. *Acta Neurol Scand Suppl* 1983;94:63–72.

74. Mauguiere F, Courjon J. Somatosensory epilepsy. A review of 127 cases. *Brain* 1978;101:307–332.

75. Devinsky O, Kelley K, Porter RJ, et al. Clinical and electroencephalographic features of simple partial seizures. *Neurology* 1988;38:1347–1352.

76. Schlaug G, Antke C, Holthausen H, et al. Ictal motor signs and interictal regional cerebral hypometabolism. *Neurology* 1997;49:341–350.

77. Todd RB. *Clinical lectures on paralysis, certain diseases of the brain, and other affections of the nervous system,* 2nd ed. London: John Churchill, 1856.

78. Kellinghaus C, Kotagal P. Lateralizing value of Todd's palsy in patients with epilepsy. *Neurology* 2004;62:289–291.

79. Noachtar S, Arnold S. Clonic seizures. In: Lüders HO, Noachtar S, eds. *Epileptic seizures: pathophysiology and clinical semiology.* Philadelphia: Churchill Livingstone, 2000:412–424.

80. Matsuo F. Partial epileptic seizures beginning in the truncal muscles. *Acta Neurol Scand* 1984;69:264–269.

81. Holowach J, Thurston D, O'Leary J. Jacksonian seizures in infancy and childhood. *J Pediatr* 1958;52:670–686.

82. Holmes G. Local epilepsy. *Lancet* 1927;1:957–962.

83. Sengoku A. The contribution of J. H. Jackson to present-day epileptology. *Epilepsia* 2002;43(Suppl 9):6–8.

84. Faught E. Clinical presentations and phenomenology of myoclonus. *Epilepsia* 2003;44(Suppl 11):7–12.

85. Hallett M. Myoclonus: relation to epilepsy. *Epilepsia* 1985;26(Suppl 1):S67–S77.

86. Leppik IE. Classification of the myoclonic epilepsies. *Epilepsia* 2003;44(Suppl 11):2–6.

87. Serratosa JM. Myoclonic seizures. In: Wyllie E, ed. *The treatment of epilepsy: principles and practice,* 3rd ed. Philadelphia: Lippincott Williams & Wilkins, 2001:395–404.

88. Kuzniecky R, Berkovic S, Andermann F, et al. Focal cortical myoclonus and rolandic cortical dysplasia: clarification by magnetic resonance imaging. *Ann Neurol* 1988;23:317–325.

89. Tassinari CA, Rubboli G, Gardella E. Negative myoclonus. *Clin Neurosci* 1995;3:209–213.

90. Tassinari CA, Rubboli G, Parmeggiani L, et al. Epileptic negative myoclonus. *Adv Neurol* 1995;67:181–197.

91. Lüders HO, Noachtar S, Burgess RC. Semiologic classification of epileptic seizures. In: Lüders HO, Noachtar S, eds. *Epileptic seizures—pathophysiology and clinical semiology.* Philadelphia: Churchill Livingstone, 2000:263–285.

92. Bleasel AF, Lüders HO. Tonic seizures. In: Lüders HO, Noachtar S, eds. *Epileptic seizures—pathophysiology and clinical semiology.* Philadelphia: Churchill Livingstone, 2000:389–411.

93. Geier S, Bancaud J, Talairach J, et al. The seizures of frontal lobe epilepsy. A study of clinical manifestations. *Neurology* 1977;27:951–958.

94. Chauvel P, Trottier S, Vignal JP, et al. Somatomotor seizures of frontal lobe origin. *Adv Neurol* 1992;57:185–232.

95. Egli M, Mothersill I, O'Kane M, et al. The axial spasm—the predominant type of drop seizure in patients with secondary generalized epilepsy. *Epilepsia* 1985;26:401–415.

96. Fromm GH. The brain-stem and seizures: summary and synthesis. In: Fromm GH, Feingold CL, Browning RA, eds. *Epilepsy and the reticular formation: the role of the reticular core in convulsive seizures.* New York: Alan R. Liss, 1987:203–218.

97. Wyllie E, Luders H, Morris HH, et al. The lateralizing significance of versive head and eye movements during epileptic seizures. *Neurology* 1986;36:606–611.

98. McLachlan RS. The significance of head and eye turning in seizures. *Neurology* 1987;37:1617–1619.

99. Rasmussen T, Penfield W. Movement of head and eyes from stimulation of the human frontal cortex. *Res Publ Assoc Res Nerv Ment Dis* 1947;27:346–361.

100. Robillard A, Saint-Hilaire JM, Mercier M, et al. The lateralizing and localizing value of adversion in epileptic seizures. *Neurology* 1983;33:1241–1242.

101. Ochs R, Gloor P, Quesney F, et al. Does head-turning during a seizure have lateralizing or localizing significance? *Neurology* 1984;34:884–890.

102. Quesney LF. Clinical and EEG features of complex partial seizures of temporal lobe origin. *Epilepsia* 1986;27(Suppl 2):S27–S45.

103. Chee MW, Kotagal P, Van Ness PC, et al. Lateralizing signs in intractable partial epilepsy: blinded multiple-observer analysis. *Neurology* 1993;43:2519–2525.

104. Kotagal P, Arunkumar GS. Lateral frontal lobe seizures. *Epilepsia* 1998;39(Suppl 4):S62–S68.

105. Kanner AM, Morris HH, Luders H, et al. Supplementary motor seizures mimicking pseudoseizures: some clinical differences. *Neurology* 1990;40:1404–1407.

106. Gabor AJ. *Physiological basis of electrical activity of cerebral origin.* Quincy, MA: Grass Instrument, 1978.

107. Dinner DS, Lüders H, Shih-Hui L. Electrical stimulation of the supplementary sensorimotor area. In: Lüders HO, Noachtar S, eds. *Epileptic seizures—pathophysiology and clinical semiology.* Philadelphia: Churchill Livingstone, 2000:192–198.

108. Martins DS, Aarts JH, Binnie CD, et al. The circadian distribution of interictal epileptiform EEG activity. *Electroencephalogr Clin Neurophysiol* 1984;58:1–13.

109. Rossi GF, Colicchio G, Pola P. Interictal epileptic activity during sleep: a stereo-EEG study in patients with partial epilepsy. *Electroencephalogr Clin Neurophysiol* 1984;58:97–106.

110. Frost JD Jr, Hrachovy RA, Glaze DG, et al. Sleep modulation of interictal spike configuration in untreated children with partial seizures. *Epilepsia* 1991;32:341–346.

111. Gibbs EL, Gibbs FA. Diagnostic and localizing value of electroencephalographic studies in sleep. *Proc Assoc Res Nerv Ment Dis* 2004;26:366–376.

112. Sperling MR, Engel J Jr. Electroencephalographic recording from the temporal lobes: a comparison of ear, anterior temporal, and nasopharyngeal electrodes. *Ann Neurol* 1985;17:510–513.

113. Morris HH III, Luders H, Lesser RP, et al. The value of closely spaced scalp electrodes in the localization of epileptiform foci: a study of 26 patients with complex partial seizures. *Electroencephalogr Clin Neurophysiol* 1986;63:107–111.

114. Kanner AM, Jones JC. When do sphenoidal electrodes yield additional data to that obtained with antero-temporal electrodes? *Electroencephalogr Clin Neurophysiol* 1997;102:12–19.

115. Pedley TA, Mendiratta A, Walczak TS. Seizures and epilepsy. In: Ebersole JS, Pedley TA, eds. *Current practice of clinical electroencephalography.* Philadelphia: Lippincott Williams & Wilkins, 2003:506–587.

116. Salanova V, Morris HH III, Van Ness PC, et al. Comparison of scalp electroencephalogram with subdural electrocorticogram recordings and functional mapping in frontal lobe epilepsy. *Arch Neurol* 1993;50:294–299.

117. Rasmussen T. Characteristics of a pure culture of frontal lobe epilepsy. *Epilepsia* 1983;24:482–493.

118. Tükel K, Jasper H. The electroencephalogram in parasagittal regions. *Electroencephalogr Clin Neurophysiol* 1952;4:481–494.

119. Duncan JS. The epilepsies. In: Mazziotta JC, Toga AW, Frackowiak RSJ, eds. *Brain mapping: the disorders.* San Diego: Academic Press, 2000:315–355.

120. Lee SK, Kim JY, Hong KS, et al. The clinical usefulness of ictal surface EEG in neocortical epilepsy. *Epilepsia* 2000;41:1450–1455.

121. Quesney LF, Constain M, Rasmussen T, et al. Presurgical EEG investigation in frontal lobe epilepsy. In: Theodore W, ed. *Surgical treatment of epilepsy.* Amsterdam: Elsevier, 1992:55–69.

122. Logroscino G, Hesdorffer DC, Cascino G, et al. Time trends in incidence, mortality, and case-fatality after first episode of status epilepticus. *Epilepsia* 2001;42:1031–1035.

123. Gastaut H, Roger A. Une forme inhabituelle de l'épilepsie: le nystagmus épileptique. *Rev Neurol (Paris)* 1954;90:130–132.

124. Kanazawa O, Sengoku A, Kawai I. Oculoclonic status epilepticus. *Epilepsia* 1989;30:121–123.

125. Kojewnikoff AY. Eine besondere form von corticaler epilepsie. *Neurol Zentralbl* 1895;14:47–48.

126. Cockerell OC, Rothwell J, Thompson PD, et al. Clinical and physiological features of epilepsia partialis continua. Cases ascertained in the UK. *Brain* 1996;119(Pt 2):393–407.

127. Bancaud J, Bonis A, Trottier S, et al. L'epilepsie partielle continue: syndrome et maladie. *Rev Neurol (Paris)* 1982;138:803–814.

128. Commission on Classification and Terminology of the International League Against Epilepsy. Proposal for revised classification of epilepsies and epileptic syndromes. *Epilepsia* 1989; 30:389–399.

129. Obeso JA, Rothwell JC, Marsden CD. The spectrum of cortical myoclonus. From focal reflex jerks to spontaneous motor epilepsy. *Brain* 1985;108(Pt 1):193–24.

130. Thomas JE, Reagan TJ, Klass DW. Epilepsia partialis continua. A review of 32 cases. *Arch Neurol* 1977;34:266–275.

131. Wieser HG, Graf HP, Bernoulli C, et al. Quantitative analysis of intracerebral recordings in epilepsia partialis continua. *Electroencephalogr Clin Neurophysiol* 1978;44:14–22.

132. Panayiotopoulos CP. Kozhevnikov-Rasmussen syndrome and the new proposal on classification. *Epilepsia* 2002;43:948–949.

133. Hess DC, Sethi KD. Epilepsia partialis continua in multiple sclerosis. *Int J Neurosci* 1990;50:109–111.

134. Bartolomei F, Gavaret M, Dhiver C, et al. Isolated, chronic, epilepsia partialis continua in an HIV-infected patient. *Arch Neurol* 1999;56:111–114.

135. Ferrari S, Monaco S, Morbin M, et al. HIV-associated PML presenting as epilepsia partialis continua. *J Neurol Sci* 1998;161: 180–184.

136. Lee K, Haight E, Olejniczak P. Epilepsia partialis continua in Creutzfeldt-Jakob disease. *Acta Neurol Scand* 2000;102:398–402.

137. Veggiotti P, Colamaria V, Dalla Bernardina B, et al. Epilepsia partialis continua in a case of MELAS: clinical and neurophysiological study. *Neurophysiol Clin* 1995;25:158–166.

138. Antozzi C, Franceschetti S, Filippini G, et al. Epilepsia partialis continua associated with NADH-coenzyme Q reductase deficiency. *J Neurol Sci* 1995;129:152–161.

139. Wilson DC, McGibben D, Hicks EM, et al. Progressive neuronal degeneration of childhood (Alpers syndrome) with hepatic cirrhosis. *Eur J Pediatr* 1993;152:260–262.

140. Schomer DL. Focal status epilepticus and epilepsia partialis continua in adults and children. *Epilepsia* 1993;34(Suppl 1): S29–S36.

141. Singh BM, Strobos RJ. Epilepsia partialis continua associated with nonketotic hyperglycemia: clinical and biochemical profile of 21 patients. *Ann Neurol* 1980;8:155–160.

142. Placidi F, Floris R, Bozzao A, et al. Ketotic hyperglycemia and epilepsia partialis continua. *Neurology* 2001;57:534–537.

143. Cock HR, Shorvon SD. The spectrum of epilepsy and movement disorders in EPC. In: Guerrini R, Aicardi J, Andermann F, et al., eds. *Epilepsy and movement disorders*. Cambridge, UK: Cambridge University Press, 2002:211–226.

144. Shorvon S. Clinical forms of status epilepticus. In: *Status epilepticus: its clinical features and treatment in children and adults*. Cambridge, U.K.: Cambridge University Press, 1994:34–138.

145. Thomas JE, Reagan TJ, Klass DW. Epilepsia partialis continua. A review of 32 cases. *Arch Neurol* 1977;34:266–275.

146. PeBenito R, Cracco JB. Periodic lateralized epileptiform discharges in infants and children. *Ann Neurol* 1979;6:47–50.

147. Westmoreland BF, Klass DW, Sharbrough FW. Chronic periodic lateralized epileptiform discharges. *Arch Neurol* 1986;43:494–496.

148. Lüders HO, Noachtar S. *Atlas and classification of electroencephalography*. Philadelphia: WB Saunders, 2000.

149. Garcia-Morales I, Garcia MT, Galan-Davila L, et al. Periodic lateralized epileptiform discharges: etiology, clinical aspects, seizures, and evolution in 130 patients. *J Clin Neurophysiol* 2002;19: 172–177.

150. Snodgrass SM, Tsuburaya K, Ajmone-Marsan C. Clinical significance of periodic lateralized epileptiform discharges: relationship with status epilepticus. *J Clin Neurophysiol* 1989;6:159–172.

151. Pohlmann-Eden B, Hoch DB, Cochius JI, et al. Periodic lateralized epileptiform discharges—a critical review. *J Clin Neurophysiol* 1996;13:519–530.

152. Hajek M, Antonini A, Leenders KL, et al. Epilepsia partialis continua studied by PET. *Epilepsy Res* 1991;9:44–48.

153. Laich E, Kuzniecky R, Mountz J, et al. Supplementary sensorimotor area epilepsy. Seizure localization, cortical propagation and subcortical activation pathways using ictal SPECT. *Brain* 1997;120(Pt 5):855–864.

154. Morris HH III. Supplementary motor seizures. In: Wyllie E, ed. *The treatment of epilepsy: principles & practice*. Philadelphia: Lea & Febiger, 1993:541–546.

155. Morris HH III, Dinner DS, Luders H, et al. Supplementary motor seizures: clinical and electroencephalographic findings. *Neurology* 1988;38:1075–1082.

156. Ajmone-Marsan C, Ralston BL. *The epileptic seizure: its functional morphology and diagnostic significance. A clinical-electroencephalographic analysis of metrazole-induced attacks*. Springfield, IL: Charles C Thomas, 1957.

157. Chauvel P, Kliemann F, Vignal JP, et al. The clinical signs and symptoms of frontal lobe seizures. Phenomenology and classification. *Adv Neurol* 1995;66:115–125.

158. Quesney LF, Constain M, Fish DR, et al. The clinical differentiation of seizures arising in the parasagittal and anterolaterodorsal frontal convexities. *Arch Neurol* 1990;47:677–679.

159. So NK. Mesial frontal epilepsy. *Epilepsia* 1998;39(Suppl 4): S49–S61.

160. Bleasel AF, Morris HH III. Supplementary sensorimotor area epilepsy in adults. *Adv Neurol* 1996;70:271–284.

161. Bass N, Wyllie E, Comair Y, et al. Supplementary sensorimotor area seizures in children and adolescents. *J Pediatr* 1995;126:537–544.

162. Wyllie E, Bass NE. Supplementary sensorimotor area seizures in children and adolescents. *Adv Neurol* 1996;70:301–308.

163. Anand I, Dinner DS. Relationship of supplementary motor area epilepsy and sleep. *Epilepsia* 1997;38(Suppl 8):48–49.

164. Luders HO. The supplementary sensorimotor area. An overview. *Adv Neurol* 1996;70:1–16.

165. Pedley TA, Tharp BR, Herman K. Clinical and electroencephalographic characteristics of midline parasagittal foci. *Ann Neurol* 1981;9:142–149.

166. Adelman S, Lueders H, Dinner DS, et al. Paradoxical lateralization of parasagittal sharp waves in a patient with epilepsia partialis continua. *Epilepsia* 1982;23:291–295.

167. Loiseau P. Idiopathic and benign partial epilepsies. In: Wyllie E, ed. *The treatment of epilepsy: principles & practice*, 3rd ed. Philadelphia: Lippincott Williams & Wilkins, 2001:475–484.

168. Berg AT, Shinnar S, Levy SR, et al. Newly diagnosed epilepsy in children: presentation at diagnosis. *Epilepsia* 1999;40:445–452.

169. Blom S, Heijbel J, Bergfors PG. Benign epilepsy of children with centro-temporal EEG foci. Prevalence and follow-up study of 40 patients. *Epilepsia* 1972;13:609–619.

170. Lerman P, Kivity S. Benign focal epilepsy of childhood. A follow-up study of 100 recovered patients. *Arch Neurol* 1975;32: 261–264.

171. Loiseau P, Orgogozo JM. An unrecognized syndrome of benign focal epileptic seizures in teenagers? *Lancet* 1978;2:1070–1071.

172. Lüders H, Lesser RP, Dinner DS, et al. Benign focal epilepsy of childhood. In: Lüders H, Lesser RP, eds. *Epilepsy: electroclinical syndromes*. Berlin: Springer-Verlag, 1987:303–346.

173. Lombroso CT. Sylvian seizures and midtemporal spike foci in children. *Arch Neurol* 1967;17:52–59.

174. Rasmussen T, Andermann F. Rasmussen's syndrome—symptomatology of the syndrome of chronic encephalitis and seizures: 35-year experience with 51 cases. In: Lüders HO, ed. *Epilepsy surgery*. New York: Raven Press, 1991:173–182.

175. Hart Y, Andermann F. Rasmussen's syndrome. In: Lüders HO, Comair YG, eds. *Epilepsy surgery*, 2nd ed. Philadelphia: Lippincott Williams & Wilkins, 2001:145–156.

176. Vining EP, Freeman JM, Brandt J, et al. Progressive unilateral encephalopathy of childhood (Rasmussen's syndrome): a reappraisal. *Epilepsia* 1993;34:639–650.

177. Gastaut H, Roger J, Faidherbe J, et al. Non-jacksonian hemiconvulsive seizures. One sided generalized epilepsy. *Epilepsia* 1962;3:56–68.

178. Gastaut H, Poirier F, Payan H, et al. H.H.E. syndrome. Hemiconvulsions, hemiplegia, epilepsy. *Epilepsia* 1960;1:418–447.

179. Lesser RP, Lüders H, Dinner DS, et al. Simple partial seizures. In: Lüders H, Lesser RP, eds. *Epilepsy: electroclinical syndromes*. Berlin: Springer-Verlag, 1987:223–278.

180. Gold AP, Carter S. Acute hemiplegia of infancy and childhood. *Pediatr Clin North Am* 1976;23:413–433.

181. Blume WT. Hemispheric epilepsy. *Brain* 1998;121(Pt 10): 1937–1949.

182. Plant G. Spinal meningioma presenting as focal epilepsy. *Br Med J* 1981;282:1974–1975.

183. Saygi S, Katz A, Marks DA, et al. Frontal lobe partial seizures and psychogenic seizures: comparison of clinical and ictal characteristics. *Neurology* 1992;42:1274–1277.

184. Vaughn BV. Differential diagnosis of paroxysmal nocturnal events in adults. In: Bazil CW, Malow BA, Sammaritano MR, eds. *Sleep and epilepsy: the clinical spectrum.* Amsterdam: Elsevier, 2002:325–338.

185. Sammaritano MR. Focal epilepsy and sleep. In: Dinner DS, Lüders HO, eds. *Epilepsy and sleep: physiologic and clinical relationships.* San Diego: Academic Press, 2001:85–100.

186. Crespel A, Baldy-Moulinier M, Coubes P. The relationship between sleep and epilepsy in frontal and temporal lobe epilepsies: practical and physiopathologic considerations. *Epilepsia* 1998;39:150–157.

187. Scheffer IE, Bhatia KP, Lopes-Cendes I, et al. Autosomal dominant nocturnal frontal lobe epilepsy. A distinctive clinical disorder. *Brain* 1995;118:61–73.

188. Scheffer IE, Bhatia KP, Lopes-Cendes I, et al. Autosomal dominant frontal epilepsy misdiagnosed as sleep disorder. *Lancet* 1994;343:515–517.

189. Bertrand D, Picard F, Le Hellard S, et al. How mutations in the nAChRs can cause ADNFLE epilepsy. *Epilepsia* 2002; 43(Suppl 5): 112–122.

190. Anderson E, Berkovic S, Dulac O, et al. ILAE Genetics Commission conference report: molecular analysis of complex genetic epilepsies. *Epilepsia* 2002;43:1262–1267.

191. Baquis GD, Pessin MS, Scott RM. Limb shaking—a carotid TIA. *Stroke* 1985;16:444–448.

192. Baumgartner RW, Baumgartner I. Vasomotor reactivity is exhausted in transient ischaemic attacks with limb shaking. *J Neurol Neurosurg Psychiatry* 1998;65:561–564.

193. Niehaus L, Neuhauser H, Meyer BU. Hemodynamically induced transitory ischemic attacks. A differential focal motor seizures diagnosis? *Nervenarzt* 1998;69:901–904.

194. Schulz UG, Rothwell PM. Transient ischaemic attacks mimicking focal motor seizures [German]. *Postgrad Med J* 2002;78:246–247.

195. Yanagihara T, Piepgras DG, Klass DW. Repetitive involuntary movement associated with episodic cerebral ischemia. *Ann Neurol* 1985;18:244–250.

Generalized Tonic-Clonic Seizures

18

Bruce J. Fisch   Piotr W. Olejniczak

Generalized tonic-clonic seizures (GTCSs) are the oldest known and most feared of all epileptic attacks. They are also the final common pathway in the ictal progression of other seizure types, and are the maximal behavioral and physiologic expression of epilepsy. All GTCSs share the following features: (a) loss of consciousness (onset may vary in relation to seizure progression), (b) a sequence of motor events that includes widespread tonic muscle contraction evolving to clonic jerking, (c) approximately symmetrical clinical and electroencephalographic manifestations (as implied by the term *generalized*), and (d) postictal cerebral metabolic and behavioral suppression (1). The duration and intensity of the attack, the muscle groups involved, the degree of autonomic activation, and the degree of bilateral synchrony of electroencephalographic and motor activity vary considerably (2). GTCSs may generalize behaviorally and electroencephalographically from the onset, may secondarily generalize from one cerebral hemisphere, or may evolve directly from another type of generalized seizure.

In humans, primary and secondary generalized seizures are differentiated by clinical and electroencephalographic phenomena. Whether the actual anatomic and physiologic substrate of the onset of primary generalized seizures is bilateral, subcortical, or widespread has not yet been determined in human epilepsy. Secondary GTCSs have an electroencephalographic onset in one hemisphere. Spread of the seizure may be extremely rapid, or it may begin more slowly as a well-defined partial seizure that evolves into the GTCS. In clinical practice, the diagnosis of secondary generalized seizures often depends on indirect evidence, including a history of partial seizures, focal brain lesion(s), or consistently localized electroencephalographic background abnormalities or focal interictal epileptiform activity. Even with indirect evidence, distinguishing between primary and secondary generalized seizures is not always straightforward. For example, an asymmetrical behavioral seizure onset or an electroencephalogram (EEG) with unilateral interictal epileptiform activity may be reported in patients with primary generalized seizures. Alternatively, secondary generalization may be missed because the scalp-recorded EEG fails to detect activity arising from a focal epileptogenic area, or the interhemispheric spread of the seizure discharge occurs so rapidly that secondary generalization cannot be appreciated. Because convincing seizure classification minimally requires electroencephalography and simultaneous clinical/behavioral video or cinematic monitoring, few large clinical studies clearly distinguish between primary and secondary GTCSs. Therefore, much of the following discussion, particularly regarding epidemiologic factors, applies to both.

CLASSIFICATION

Historical Overview

The earliest descriptions of tonic-clonic seizures appear in Egyptian hieroglyphics prior to 700 BC. Indeed, until the time of Hippocrates (400 BC), all seizures were considered "a convulsion of the whole body together with an impairment of leading functions" (3). From that time forward, a clear distinction between unilateral and generalized convulsive seizures is present in medical literature. Remarkably, another 2000 years passed before nonconvulsive ("de petits") seizures were widely recognized as epileptic events separate from convulsive ("grand acces") seizures (4). In the early 19th century, tonic-clonic seizures were grouped with other convulsive attacks, all referred to as "le grand mal" (5).

Terminology

The preferred description, *generalized tonic-clonic seizure*, is based on observations documented by closed-circuit television or cinematography with electroencephalographic monitoring (6). Although still used frequently, the term *grand mal* is now discouraged; it does not imply the presence or absence of a sequence of events that could help to distinguish clinically between primary and secondary generalized seizures or between GTCSs and other types of convulsive seizures. Other similarly ambiguous designations are "generalized convulsion" and "major motor seizure." Even "tonic-clonic" warrants further qualification, because a tonic-clonic sequence of motor events may be generalized, asymmetrical, unilateral, or focal.

The Commission on Classification and Terminology of the International League Against Epilepsy (ILAE) (6) defines seizures according to clinical and electroencephalographic criteria. Because GTCSs are described simply as a tonic phase followed by a clonic phase, future revisions likely will focus on the clinical description. For example, GTCSs are often preceded by one or more myoclonic jerks or a brief clonic seizure and may be followed by a prominent postictal phase of tonic contraction (7). The classification also describes known patterns of progression (e.g., a partial seizure secondarily generalizing to a tonic-clonic seizure). Further distinctions based on the precise sequence of clinical ictal events may be useful in the future for differentiating primary from secondary generalization, identifying specific epilepsy syndromes (8), or predicting therapeutic response.

Epilepsy Syndrome Classification

According to the Commission on Classification and Terminology of the ILAE (9), epilepsy syndromes with bilateral tonic-clonic seizures are divided into idiopathic (cryptogenic, essential, primary) and symptomatic (secondary) categories. This distinction is further discussed in Chapters 14 and 22. Symptomatic epilepsy syndromes have a presumed cause based on a known disturbance of brain function. Those syndromes currently classified as idiopathic that have the greatest number of specific defining criteria (e.g., age of onset, characteristic electroencephalographic expression, provoking factors) are now assumed to be specific genetic disorders.

As noted by Aicardi (10), GTCSs occur in so many different types of epilepsy that their diagnostic value is limited. However, other types of coexisting seizures are often useful for syndrome classification. The generalized idiopathic epilepsies (9) in which GTCSs occur along with other seizure types include benign myoclonic epilepsy in infancy (GTCSs in adolescence), childhood absence epilepsy (pyknoepilepsy; GTCSs in 40% to 60% of cases), juvenile absence epilepsy (GTCSs in 80% of cases), Lennox-Gastaut syndrome (idiopathic in 30% of patients;

GTCSs are infrequent), myoclonic astatic epilepsy (Doose syndrome; GTCS is the initial seizure type in >50% of cases), juvenile myoclonic epilepsy (impulsive petit mal; GTCSs in >90% of cases), and epilepsy with myoclonic-astatic seizures (which may also be symptomatic in some patients) (9). Partial idiopathic epilepsies (idiopathic focal epilepsies) in which GTCSs occur secondarily include benign childhood epilepsy with centrotemporal spikes and childhood epilepsy with occipital paroxysms (benign epilepsy of childhood with occipital spike-and-wave complexes) (11). In addition, there are some epilepsy syndromes in which GTCSs never occur, such as early infantile epileptic encephalopathy (Ohtahara syndrome) and early myoclonic encephalopathy, as well as those in which GTCSs are usually the only seizure type, such as grand mal seizures upon awakening. Seizures in otherwise normal individuals in which GTCSs are triggered by photic stimulation are almost always indicative of primary generalized epilepsy. Some epilepsy syndromes, such as Dravet syndrome, are typically associated with multiple seizure types, but occasionally with only GTCSs (12). Hot-water exposure and fever may trigger a variety of seizure types, particularly partial seizures. Hot-water exposure may also trigger seizures in patients with Dravet syndrome.

Some proposed syndromes of idiopathic epilepsy with GTCSs emphasize the presence, absence, or degree of associated generalized myoclonus (8) (see also juvenile myoclonic epilepsy versus epilepsy with GTCSs upon awakening). Although some syndromes are more widely accepted than others, evidence for each has been difficult to obtain for six reasons:

1. GTCSs, particularly primary generalized, regardless of cause, may begin with a succession of bilateral myoclonic jerks (7,13);
2. Myoclonic jerks occurring hours or days before a tonic-clonic seizure are considered a nonspecific prodrome (14);
3. Epidemiologic studies, which are typically based on information extracted from chart reviews or questionnaires, usually define tonic-clonic epilepsy without reference to either preictal myoclonus or consistent electroencephalographic information;
4. Because a history of myoclonus is often missed, even with repeated physician-patient interviews (15), frequent errors of omission are expected in epidemiologic studies;
5. Until recently, even nonepidemiologic investigations of epilepsy have not distinguished clearly among tonic-clonic, clonic-tonic-clonic, and other grand mal patterns; and
6. There is no consensus on the precise point at which GTCSs preceded by myoclonus become classified as clonic-tonic-clonic rather than tonic-clonic seizures.

The number of clinical and electroencephalographic features that overlap among some proposed syndromes with GTCSs, the limited number of diagnostic features for certain proposed syndromes, the phenotypic variation in seizure types that can occur with the same genetic abnormality, and the existence of patients who apparently have more than one syndrome all continue to make the electroclinical classification of some patients with GTCSs highly problematic. Although phenotypic classifications have necessarily preceded the development of genetic classifications, dramatic advances in molecular genetics promise to revolutionize the classification of the epilepsies. Currently, idiopathic epilepsies that are presumed to have a genetic basis are thought to account for up to 60% of all epilepsies (16).

Eisner and colleagues (17,18) provided early evidence for a genetic factor in GTCSs by demonstrating a significant familial aggregation in individuals whose seizures began before age 15 years, 6 months; this effect was even stronger among those whose seizures began before the age of 4 years. Tonic-clonic seizures occurred in 8.3% of probands' relatives, in contrast to 2.2% of relatives of the control population. Tsuboi and Endo (19) also found a clear genetic basis for idiopathic grand mal epilepsy. In their study, individuals with idiopathic GTCSs had the highest rate of offspring with either febrile or afebrile seizures (16.8%); a healthy control population was not studied. Genetic linkage studies by Greenberg and colleagues (20) and Durner and associates (21) showed a strong link between the seizures of juvenile myoclonic epilepsy and human leukocyte antigen (HLA) factors on chromosome 6 (see Chapters 7 and 25). Their work also supports the notion that generalized epileptiform activity on EEG readings is a subclinical electroencephalographic marker of the disorder in unaffected family members. More recently, Cossette and coworkers (22) described an Ala322Asp mutation in the γ-aminobutyric acid receptor α_1 subunit in a single pedigree with recognized juvenile myoclonic epilepsy. Indeed, it is now known that a variety of genetic-based abnormalities can give rise to epilepsy. These include abnormal ion channel function, neuronal nicotinic acetylcholine receptor (nAChR) site abnormalities, disordered brain development, progressive neurodegeneration, and disturbances of cerebral energy metabolism (23).

Idiopathic epilepsies inherited in a mendelian fashion in which GTCSs may occur include autosomal dominant nocturnal frontal lobe epilepsy mapped to chromosome 20q13-q13.3 with mutations in CHRNA4 (the gene encoding the α_4 subunit of the nAChR), benign familial neonatal convulsions (BFNC), generalized epilepsy with febrile seizures plus (GEFS+), and other rare disorders (23). BFNC is an autosomal dominant epilepsy of infancy, with loci mapped to human chromosomes 20q13.3 (EBN1) and 8q24 (EBN2) (24,25). BFNC is characterized by GTCSs starting on the second or third postnatal day and is considered a prototypic model of monogenic idiopathic generalized epilepsy (IGE) (26,27). Mutations in the voltage-gated potassium channel gene KCNQ2 and the homologous gene KCNQ3 have been found in cases linked to chromosome 20q13.3 (28,29).

GEFS+ is a genetic syndrome with heterogeneous phenotypes (30,31). The most common phenotype was described by the authors as "febrile seizures plus" (FS+), with febrile seizures occurring after 6 years of age with or without associated afebrile tonic-clonic seizures. The GEFS+ spectrum includes other seizure types, such as absence, myoclonic, and atonic, as well as myoclonic-astatic epilepsy. Inheritance is autosomal-dominant with linkage to chromosome 19q. A mutation has been identified in the α_1 subunit of the neuronal sodium channel in one family (SCNB1) (32). Recently, Baulac and colleagues (33) reported a GEFS+ family with the locus mapped to chromosome 2q21-q33, with genes coding for three isoforms of the brain sodium channel α subunit (SCN1A, SCN2A, and SCN3A) being strong candidates. Temporal lobe epilepsy may be an occasional late consequence of the GEFS+ syndrome (31). Two loci responsible for febrile seizures, FEB1 and FEB2, have been mapped on chromosomes 18q and 19p, respectively (33).

Idiopathic epilepsies with a complex mode of inheritance in which GTCSs occur are rarely, if ever, monogenic. Hoping to find one gene common to all IGEs, Durner and associates (34) performed a genome scan in 89 families chosen because a proband had adolescent-onset IGE. They found the strongest evidence for linkage to chromosome 18 when all families were analyzed together. In patients with juvenile myoclonic epilepsy, there was strong linkage on chromosome 6 near the HLA region. According to Sander and coworkers (35), three tentative loci predisposing individuals to juvenile myoclonic epilepsy have been mapped to the chromosomal segments 6p21.3, 6p11, and 15q14, but replication studies have failed to establish unequivocal linkage relationships. Other IGE families without myoclonus provide evidence for linkage to chromosome 8 in the area that encompasses the locus for the β_3 subunit of the nAChR (CHRNB3) (36,37). However, Sander and associates (35) failed to replicate evidence of a major locus for common familial IGEs in chromosome region 8q24. Furthermore, Durner and associates (34) found that if a family member had absence seizures (irrespective of the syndrome), there was strong linkage to two areas on chromosome 5. The investigators concluded that the most likely genetic model for IGE is oligogenic, with strong evidence for a locus common to all IGEs on chromosome 18 and differentiating loci for specific seizure types on chromosomes 5, 6, and 8. They recommended that further investigations be aimed at identifying individual genes for specific seizure types rather than epilepsy syndromes.

Genetic mapping of the progressive myoclonic epilepsies (see also discussion of zonisamide in "Therapy" below) now includes epilepsy of the Unverricht-Lundborg type (EPM1) mapped to the *cystatin B* gene on chromosome 21 band q22.3 and Lafora disease (EPM2) mapped to 6q23-q25 (38,39). Rapid progress has also been made in establishing the genetic basis of neuronal ceroid lipofuscinoses (40) and determining the mitochondrial abnormalities responsible for myoclonic epilepsy with ragged-red fibers (MERRF), mitochondrial encephalopathy with lactic acidosis and stroke-like episodes (MELAS), and Leigh disease (41).

Neuronal migration disorders associated with tonic-clonic seizures that have a known genetic basis include X-linked lissencephaly (X-linked dominant, male) and sub-cortical band heterotopia/double cortex (X-linked dominant, female), both of which are associated with a double cortin gene on chromosome Xq21-24 (23). Periventricular nodular heterotopia (X-linked dominant with male lethality) is ascribed to the defect of a gene coding for a filamin-1 actin-binding protein on chromosome Xq28 (23).

EPIDEMIOLOGIC FACTORS

Tonic-clonic seizures affect more patients than any other kind of generalized seizure. In their definitive study, Hauser and Kurland (42) found that more than half of all patients with epilepsy experienced one or more GTCSs, and the prevalence of patients presenting exclusively with GTCSs in their study was 20.6%. Patients with GTCSs also accounted for 23% of the overall yearly incidence of epilepsy. In contrast to other seizure types, the incidence among children and adults with GTCSs exclusively did not vary significantly with age. Juul-Jensen and Foldspang (43) noted that grand mal seizures accounted for 25.6% of all seizure types in a Danish population of 244,800 individuals. Tsuboi (44) studied 17,044 children from age 3 years onward who were monitored at a regional health center and found that 87% of those who developed IGE had GTCSs exclusively. Thus, GTCSs account for the majority of patients with idiopathic epilepsy who have only one seizure type.

Of patients with typical absence seizures, 37% also have GTCSs (45–49), as do 90% of patients with absence epilepsy of adolescence and more than half of those with clonic absences (10). About half of patients with absence seizures and GTCSs present with tonic-clonic seizures only (50), and most continue to have GTCSs into adulthood (49,50). No reliable method exists for predicting which patients with absence attacks will subsequently experience tonic-clonic seizures.

In the epilepsy clinic, the relative proportion of patients with GTCSs may vary considerably in comparison with general population studies. Gastaut and associates (51) conducted the largest clinical and electroencephalographic survey of a clinic population, enrolling 45,106 patients. In contrast to other investigators' findings (42,43), only 11.3% of patients had idiopathic (primary) generalized epilepsy characterized mainly or entirely by tonic-clonic seizures. Such differences might be expected considering the dissimilar methods of patient selection and classification. In the clinic population, patients with symptomatic (secondary) GTCSs were considered rare. Gastaut and

coworkers (52) also analyzed the features of a clinic population with idiopathic GTCSs, noting that 68% experienced seizure onset during puberty whereas 33% had isolated, bilateral, massive myoclonic jerks that might now be classified as juvenile myoclonic epilepsy. The majority of patients achieved complete remission, with the remainder experiencing a decline in seizure frequency.

The prevalence of symptomatic GTCSs among different disorders of the central nervous system (CNS) varies widely. For example, GTCSs are said to occur in 2% to 3% of patients with multiple sclerosis and in 5% of those with juvenile-onset Huntington disease (53), whereas they occur in virtually all cases of Lafora disease and MERRF. Any disorder that creates structural lesions involving the cerebral cortex (cerebrovascular disease, trauma, tumor, infection) substantially increases the likelihood of GTCS. Migraine also increases the risk for epilepsy, and in rare cases, migraine attacks with or without typical visual auras may trigger GTCSs (54), with intensification of the headache following the seizure. In a study (55) of autopsy-proven uncomplicated Alzheimer disease, 69 (15%) of 446 patients were reported to have developed new-onset GTCS. More-rigorous scrutiny may reveal that clinical attacks in some neurologic disorders are actually tonic, clonic, or myoclonic (56). In adults, particularly those with coexisting neurologic disorders, on a clinical basis, the great majority of GTCSs are undoubtedly secondarily generalized (57). GTCSs that take place almost exclusively during sleep are somewhat more likely to be idiopathic in nature (58).

Because GTCSs occur in so many neurologic disorders, they have little diagnostic specificity. A far greater number of patients without epilepsy experience GTCSs that are related to an acute illness, a toxic reaction, or in childhood as a response to febrile illnesses. Approximately one-third of patients with dialysis-dependent chronic renal failure will experience one or more GTCSs (53). Some medications can also precipitate seizures. According to Devinsky and Pacia (59), a cumulative 10% risk for GTCSs accompanies the use of clozapine for more than 3 years. For a more extensive list of various etiologic factors, see references 7, 56, 60, and 61.

CLINICAL AND PHYSIOLOGIC MANIFESTATIONS

Generalized tonic-clonic seizures do not occur in newborn infants and are rare in the first 6 months of life (62–64). Similar observations have been made in studies of experimentally induced cortical epileptogenic lesions in immature animals. Five factors explain the absence of GTCSs in this age group:

1. The immaturity of important pathways of propagation, including the corpus callosum and intracortical arcuate fibers, inhibits the elaboration of tonic-clonic activity (65);

2. Incomplete myelination impairs the rapidity and synchrony with which neuronal interactions can develop (66,67);
3. The normal relationship between excitatory and inhibitory synaptogenesis is not yet established (68–70);
4. The maximum spike frequency is reduced in immature neurons (71); and
5. Synaptic connections are impaired by structural immaturity (72).

The clinical manifestations of GTCSs can be divided into five main phases: premonitory signs and symptoms, immediate pretonic-clonic, tonic-clonic, immediate postictal, and postictal recovery. All may vary in duration within or among individuals. For secondary GTCSs, three additional phases, defined by Theodore and colleagues (2), precede the pretonic-clonic phase: simple partial; complex partial, atypical absence; and onset of generalization. As the severity and duration of GTCSs increase, the patient is less likely to remember auras or simple partial seizures (73). GTCSs may also be preceded by other generalized seizures, including clonic, tonic, or typical absence. Much of what is known about the clinical sequence of ictal events in GTCSs is based on the detailed observations of Gastaut and Broughton (7); more recent information on secondary GTCSs has come from videotape analyses by Bromfield and associates (74), Porter (75), and Theodore and coworkers (2). The mean duration of GTCSs is approximately 1 minute (2,76). Following generalization, secondary GTCSs rarely last longer than 2 minutes; GTCSs that persist beyond that time warrant immediate intravenous (IV) therapy (2). Given the growing number of video electroencephalographic studies (77–81), it is hoped that additional clinical investigations of GTCSs will be forthcoming.

Premonitory Symptoms and Precipitating Factors

A variety of symptoms may precede GTCSs by hours or even days (Table 18.1). These are thought to arise either directly from heightened cortical excitability (e.g., myoclonus or difficulty concentrating) or indirectly from the physiologic changes that alter the seizure threshold (e.g., mood change or headache). The physician should not be misled into thinking that these symptoms represent the auras of partial seizures, particularly in individuals who can reliably predict their seizures because of the regularity with which the symptoms occur. For the majority of patients with GTCSs, however, premonitory symptoms are absent.

The coexistence of generalized myoclonus supports a diagnosis of primarily generalized, as opposed to secondarily generalized, tonic-clonic seizures. Myoclonus of the arms and trunk occurs in approximately 10% to 50% of all patients with generalized convulsions (14), and myoclonus on awakening is a key feature in juvenile myoclonic epilepsy (impulsive petit mal). In addition to premonitory

TABLE 18.1
COMMON NEUROLOGIC PREMONITORY SYMPTOMS

Headache	Decreased concentration
Mood change	Sleep disturbance
Emotional instability	Unusual appetite
Anxiousness	Myoclonus, eyelid flutter
Irritability	Dizziness and light-headedness
Lethargy	Behavioral withdrawal

Data from Fisch BJ, Pedley TA. Generalized tonic-clonic epilepsies. In: Lüders IJ, Lesser RP, eds. *Epilepsy: electroclinical syndromes.* New York: Springer-Verlag, 1987:151–185.

symptoms, some seizures may be anticipated on the basis of known precipitating factors, such as sleep or photic stimulation (82). Nocturnal idiopathic GTCSs usually take place near the beginning or the end of sleep and only rarely during rapid eye movement (REM) sleep (83,84). Light-sensitive seizures are facilitated by sleep deprivation. Abrupt withdrawal of antiepileptic drugs (AEDs) in patients with established epilepsy may be more likely to trigger an isolated GTCS or, occasionally, life-threatening GTCS status epilepticus than other kinds of seizures. Malow and colleagues (85) found that rapid withdrawal of AEDs during monitoring resulted in the occurrence of significantly more GTCSs than did gradual tapering, whereas no apparent differential effect on the rate of complex partial seizures was reported. Fortunately, life-threatening status epilepticus is rare in epilepsy-monitoring units in which AEDs are routinely withdrawn, perhaps because of the dramatic reduction in the patient's level of activity produced by bed rest. If the purpose of monitoring is to localize seizure onset, it is preferable to record partial seizures (with or without secondary GTCSs) rather than rapidly evolving secondary GTCSs. In such circumstances, gradual withdrawal of AEDs before and during monitoring may reduce the likelihood of GTCSs.

Immediate Pre–Tonic-Clonic Phase

Idiopathic GTCSs may evolve directly from typical absence (86), clonic, or tonic seizures (7). Secondary GTCSs may evolve from partial seizures in individuals with idiopathic epilepsy (e.g., benign epilepsy with centrotemporal spikes) or symptomatic epilepsy. Generalization occurs during a brief period (up to 40 seconds) (2) between the end of the partial seizure and the beginning of the GTCS. This phase is often marked by versive (turning) head movements, body movements, or vocalization.

Clonic activity is the most common immediate precursor to the tonic-clonic phase. As Gastaut and Broughton (7) observed, idiopathic GTCSs are frequently preceded by several myoclonic jerks or a brief clonic seizure. Myoclonic or clonic activity also may occur during the transition from partial seizures to GTCSs (2,74). Analyzing videotapes of 32 secondary GTCSs in which all phases of GTCS (including generalization) were present, Theodore and coworkers (2) found that antecedent clonic activity lasted from 3 to 21 seconds. Our own experience indicates that generalized myoclonus at the onset of an unprovoked tonic-clonic seizure is practically pathognomonic for primary generalization.

Although GTCSs typically involve both sides of the body symmetrically, they may begin with versive movements of the head and eyes (87). The significance of these movements is controversial. In two studies (88,89), initial conjugate eye and head turning was noted in patients with either partial (e.g., frontal or temporal foci) or primary generalized seizures; in those with partial-onset seizures, ipsilateral head turning was as common as contralateral head turning. We have also observed head and eye deviation at the onset of primary generalized seizures evolving out of 3- to 4-Hz spike-and-wave activity. However, in a third study, Wyllie and associates (90) found that strongly versive head and eye movements consistently occurred in patients with secondary GTCSs arising from the contralateral hemisphere. Kernan and colleagues (91) also observed that forced head turning was contralateral to seizure onset greater than 85% of the time if it consisted of sustained, unnatural tonic or clonic movements that either occurred during the 10 seconds prior to generalization or continued through it. In this study, ipsilateral head turning almost always appeared to be volitional and ended before secondary generalization in more than 90% of cases. Although all authors noted exceptions to the localizing value of versive head movements, we agree with the latter two studies (90,91) that forceful involuntary movements at seizure onset with greater than 45 degrees of rotation, as distinguished from volitional movements or brief automatisms, have lateralizing value.

Tonic-Clonic Phase

The tonic-clonic convulsion begins with brief tonic flexion of the axial musculature, accompanied by upward eye deviation and pupillary dilatation. The tonic muscle contraction spreads quickly, elevating and abducting the arms. The elbows semiflex and the hands rotate with the palms forward. The lower extremities simultaneously assume a position of flexion, adduction, and external rotation. Muscular contraction in the limbs is greatest proximally. The mouth is characteristically held rigid and half open.

This brief flexor spasm is followed by a longer period of tonic extension, also beginning in the axial musculature; the tonic extension phase is heralded by forced closure of the mouth, which sometimes produces oral trauma. It also causes a forced expiration of air, sometimes resulting in a 2- to 12-second "epileptic cry." The arms then become semiflexed and abducted, with the forearms partially crossed in front of the chest. At the same time, the legs are adducted, extended, and fixed in internal rotation with the feet and toes in extension. During the tonic phase, heart rate and blood pressure may more than double, and intravesicular bladder pressure may increase to five times the normal value. Sweating is a regular occurrence and leads to a measurable drop in skin resistance (Fig. 18.1). The tonic phase may be as brief as 1 to 3 seconds or as long as 20 seconds (2,7). The transition from the tonic to the clonic phase is gradual. Referred to by Gastaut and Broughton (7) as the "intermediate vibratory period," it emerges from the tonic phase as an approximately 8-Hz diffuse tremor that

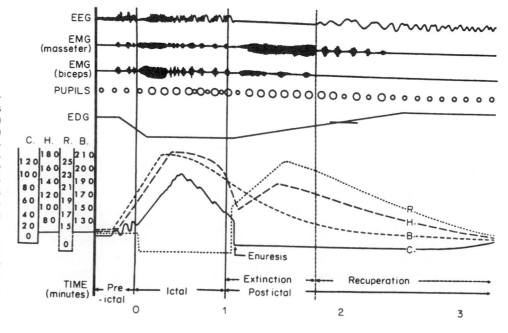

Figure 18.1 Generalized tonic-clonic seizure showing fluctuations in electroencephalographic (*EEG*) activity, electromyographic (*EMG*) activity, pupillary size, skin resistance, intravesicular bladder pressure (*C*), heart rate (*H*), respiratory rate (*R*), and systolic blood pressure (*B*). All autonomic changes except apnea reach their maximum at the end of the tonic phase and then progressively attenuate. EDG indicates electrodermogram. (From Gastaut H, Broughton R. *Epileptic seizures: clinical and electroencephalographic features, diagnosis and treatment.* Springfield, IL: Charles C Thomas, 1972, with permission.)

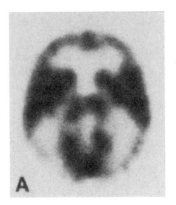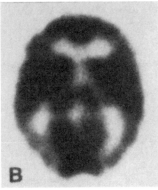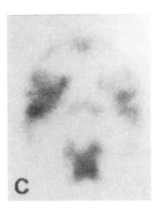

Figure 18.2   Control (A), ictal (B), and postictal (C) fluorodeoxyglucose positron emission tomography of a patient undergoing electroconvulsive shock treatment. B: Metabolic activity is increased because of a 20-second generalized tonic-clonic seizure, followed by 7.5 minutes of clinical postictal depression. C: Postictal metabolic depression followed injection of fluorodeoxyglucose in the immediate postictal period. (From Engel J Jr, Kuhl DE, Phelps ME. Patterns of human local cerebral glucose metabolism during epileptic seizures. *Science* 1982;218:64–66, with permission.)

gradually slows to 4 Hz as the clonic phase becomes established. This early clonic, or tremulous, phase lasts from 3 to 17 seconds (2).

When each recurrent inhibition of tetanic contraction produces complete atonia, the clonic phase appears as repeated, violent flexor spasms, each accompanied by pupillary contraction and dilatation. The intervals of atonia gradually become more prolonged and somewhat irregular until a final spasm occurs. The lengthening of the atonic intervals is independent of the absolute number of clonic contractions (75). Contraction of sphincter muscles blocks enuresis until the end of the clonic phase. In secondary generalized seizures, in which the frequency and duration of clonic jerking are uninterrupted, there is almost always a regular, gradual slowing of clonic jerks. In an uncomplicated secondary generalized seizure, the duration of clonic activity ranges widely from 3 to 65 seconds (2). Near the end of this phase, jerking slows to approximately 1 Hz.

In human electroconvulsive therapy-induced GTCSs, it has not been possible to dissociate the contribution of postictal hypometabolism from that of ictal hypermetabolism through the use of fluorodeoxyglucose positron emission tomography (PET) because of limitations in time resolution; however, the increase in cerebral blood flow during GTCSs is likely a result of increased cerebral glucose metabolism (Fig. 18.2).

Gastaut and Broughton (7) suggested that when convulsive activity on the two sides of the body is clearly asynchronous, the convulsion may be viewed as two independent unilateral seizures rather than as a single generalized one. Whether such seizures are more typical of secondary generalization is unclear.

Immediate Postictal Phase

Following the last clonic jerk, respiration returns within several seconds, and there is sustained pupillary dilatation.

In many cases, tonic activity returns, lasting from several seconds to minutes. Occasionally, postictal tonic activity is as intense as the initial tonic contraction and results in opisthotonos and trismus, which may cause tongue laceration. The activity usually has a rostral predominance, which in its most limited form appears only as jaw tetany (92), and may selectively affect the arms, the legs, or both. Because the tonic contraction involves predominantly extensor muscles and coexists with profound metabolic depression of cortical function, Ajmone-Marsan and Ralston (92) hypothesized that it represents a functional decerebrate state. This view is supported by postictal PET findings that show hypometabolism predominating in cortical structures (Fig. 18.2) (86,93). In approximately 50% of GTCSs, extensor plantar responses can be elicited postictally (94); in secondary generalized seizures, these are likely to be found contralateral to the hemisphere of onset. Incontinence occurs between the end of the clonic phase and the beginning of the postictal tonic phase. Ejaculation and fecal incontinence are rare in the immediate postictal period.

Postictal Recovery Phase

As the patient gradually awakens, a confusional state with automatic behavior may ensue. Often, the individual falls asleep directly and awakens feeling tired. Complaints of generalized muscle soreness and headache are common. Diffuse ictal skin color changes (probably from venous congestion as a result of impaired venous return or cyanosis caused by apnea-induced hypoxia) disappear quickly. Piloerection and petechial hemorrhages occasionally are seen. The actual ictus lasts 1 to 2 minutes, but patients often measure seizure duration through the initial part of the postictal period as lasting 5 to 15 minutes. During this time, cerebral hypometabolism resolves gradually (Fig. 18.2). In one of only a few studies of the postictal recovery of cognitive function, Helmstaedter and colleagues (95) found that complete reorientation (to person, location, and time) occurred at an average of 18 minutes following secondarily generalized seizures (range, 4 to 45 minutes; 1 standard deviation, 15 minutes; 18 seizures studied). This contrasted with an orientation recovery time of 1 to 10 minutes for complex partial seizures (1 standard deviation, 3 minutes; 13 seizures studied).

Immediately following the seizure, the arterial pH level is decreased to 7.14±0.06 (rarely to <7.0). Changes in mean levels of CO_2 (17.1±1.1) and venous lactate (12.7±1.0 mEq/L) also occur. The acid-base equilibrium is restored to normal within 60 minutes by the metabolism of lactic acid (96). Serum glucose increases transiently (usually <200 mg/dL) (97), although with recurrent seizures (status epilepticus), hypoglycemia is the rule. Cerebrospinal fluid (CSF) cell counts are usually normal following a single, uncomplicated GTCS, but in patients with idiopathic status epilepticus, a minor pleocytosis (5 to 30 cells/mm^3) is not unusual (98), and counts of up to 80 cells/mm^3 are seen occasionally (99). Regardless of the number of seizures, a cell count greater than 10 cells/mm^3 should be considered evidence of an intracranial inflammatory process until proven otherwise (17).

Transient fluctuations in endocrine function always follow a GTCS (Table 18.2; for review, see ref. 99). Most consistent and easily observable is an increase in prolactin level (present in >90% of GTCSs; Fig. 18.3) (100). Prolactin increases within 5 minutes, reaches a peak of 5 to

TABLE 18.2

POSTICTAL HORMONAL CHANGES IN GENERALIZED TONIC-CLONIC SEIZURES

Increased	Inconsistent	None
Prolactin	Thyroid-stimulating hormone	Melatonin
Corticotropin	Luteinizing hormone	
Plasma cortisol	Follicle-stimulating hormone	
Vasopressin		
4-Norepinephrine		
β-Endorphin		
β-Lipotropin		
Growth hormone		

30 times baseline levels in 19 to 20 minutes, and remains significantly elevated for 1 hour postictally (101,102). In multiple GTCSs, each successive seizure elicits a lower rise in prolactin level. In GTCS status epilepticus, the serum prolactin level is usually within normal range. This failure of prolactin to rise does not appear to be the result of simple depletion, because the injection of thyrotropin-releasing hormone under such conditions still results in a significant (twofold) increase (103). Although other hormones also may increase following GTCSs (Table 18.2), the relatively limited circadian variation of serum prolactin and the consistency of its increase make it the most useful clinical marker for sporadic seizures.

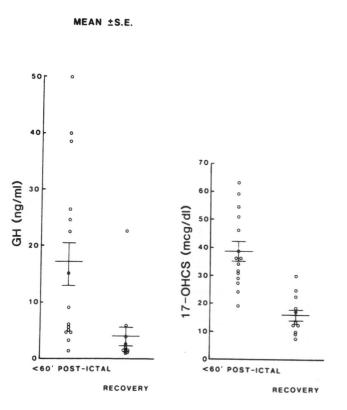

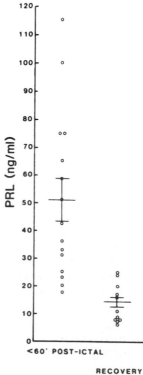

Figure 18.3 Comparison of early (≤60 minutes) postictal values with recovery (≥24 hours) for growth hormone (*GH*), cortisol (*17-OHCS*), and prolactin (*PRL*). All comparisons are significant. (From Culebras A, Miller M, Bertram L, et al. Differential response of growth hormone, cortisol, and prolactin to seizures and stress. *Epilepsia* 1987;28:564–570, with permission.)

Prolactin elevation also may help to distinguish GTCSs from psychogenic pseudoseizures or other nonepileptic events. For diagnostic purposes, a prolactin level should be measured within 60 minutes of the seizure, and a second level, to be used as a baseline for comparison, should be obtained at least 24 hours later. False-negative results have been reported in the settings of both electroconvulsive and spontaneous tonic-clonic seizures, although they are far more likely with simple or complex partial seizures (100,101,104,105). With the exception of one case report (106), psychogenic pseudoseizures have not been found to significantly increase prolactin levels in patients classified according to closed-circuit television /electroencephalographic findings (102,107). Absence and myoclonic seizures and absence status do not cause significant elevations in prolactin levels (108). Minor increases may occur during periods of stress (e.g., seriously ill patients in the emergency department) (109), but not of the magnitude seen with GTCSs.

The pattern of hormonal responses in GTCSs (Table 18.2) strongly suggests that the seizure directly activates the hypothalamus, either electrically or by changes in the release of neurotransmitters or other neuromodulators. The ictal release of β-endorphin probably contributes as well to the development of hyperprolactinemia (100). CSF levels of neuropeptides, cortisol, and amino acids determined through lumbar puncture before and after the occurrence of GTCSs do not show significant increases postictally (110).

Prolonged postictal elevations of skeletal muscle-derived creatine kinase (CK) may occur following GTCSs. Wyllie and colleagues found significant CK elevations (sometimes exceeding 19 times the baseline value) in 6 of 12 patients with GTCSs studied during video electroencephalographic recordings (111). Although significant elevations did not occur with every GTCS, none occurred following psychogenic seizures (6 patients studied) or complex partial, focal motor, or tonic seizures (15 patients studied). It appears that the degree of elevation of CK depends on the severity of muscle activity (111,112). Consequently, postictal CK, either alone or in combination with prolactin determinations, may be useful for distinguishing various forms of pseudoseizures from GTCS.

Complications

In order of likelihood, complications that may occur in the ictal or immediate postictal period following a single GTCS are oral trauma, significant head trauma, stress fractures, effects on pregnancy, aspiration pneumonia, pulmonary edema, diaphragmatic herniation, and sudden death. Status epilepticus increases the likelihood of all these complications. In addition, a variety of dermatologic changes may follow GTCSs. Finally, cognitive decline may be a direct result of GTCSs.

Oral Trauma

Oral trauma can include tongue, lip, or cheek laceration. In general, attempting to place an object in the patient's mouth to block the jaw open at the beginning of a seizure is not recommended. Mouth closure occurs so quickly that the insertion of objects often causes greater oral trauma than would have been produced by the seizure.

Head Trauma

Serious head trauma usually can be avoided if an observer can block the patient's fall or immediately place his or her hands between the patient's head and the floor or other hard surface. Skull fractures, contusions, and epidural or subdural hematomas may result from head injury during a GTCS.

Orthopedic Injury

Of the skeletal fractures caused by GTCSs, vertebral compression fractures are the most common, occurring in approximately 5% to 15% of all patients (113). Compared with compression fractures from external trauma, which are usually located near the thoracolumbar junction (114), compression fractures from seizures are usually more evenly distributed between the T3 and T8 vertebrae and the thoracolumbar area (113). Such fractures are more likely to occur during nocturnal seizures and in older individuals. Remarkably, they are asymptomatic in approximately 80% of patients.

In our experience, vertebral compression fractures are one of the more common complications seen during epilepsy monitoring when AEDs are withdrawn. However, we have also observed serious shoulder and knee joint injuries. GTCSs, which are rarely useful for seizure localization during presurgical evaluations, should be minimized during epilepsy monitoring by gradual drug withdrawal and frequent monitoring of AED levels. If a GTCS occurs during monitoring, all attempts to reposition the patient—especially pulling on the patient's arm—should be avoided until the seizure is complete. Otherwise, the risk for joint dislocation or joint strain is greatly increased.

Pregnancy

Although occasional GTCSs do not preclude a successful pregnancy, the risk for fetal injury increases as pregnancy progresses. The size of the fetus, reduced maternal ventilatory volume, increased maternal cardiac demand, and relative reduction in impact cushioning account for the increased risk in the latter half of pregnancy. This is fortuitous only to the extent that the teratogenicity of AEDs declines abruptly after the first trimester, when organogenesis ends. Thus, at the time when the risk for trauma is greatest, the risk from aggressive AED use is lowest. GTCS in late pregnancy should therefore be treated aggressively.

Aspiration Pneumonia

Pneumonia is a potentially life-threatening complication of GTCSs, caused by the aspiration of saliva and tracheobronchial secretions when the normal protective reflexes of the airway are inhibited postictally. Because aspiration also may result from the regurgitation of stomach contents early in the postictal phase, the observer should always attempt to place the patient in a lateral decubitus or prone position as quickly as possible. Aspiration pneumonia is more likely to occur in individuals with lowered resistance to infection or depressed airway reflexes from drug or alcohol abuse who remain supine during postictal recovery. The overwhelming majority of persons with GTCSs never experience aspiration pneumonia, whereas those who experience one episode commonly have recurrent episodes.

Pulmonary Edema

Pulmonary edema is an infrequent complication of single, uncomplicated GTCSs (115–117) but becomes more likely with repeated seizures (118). In most cases, it resolves rapidly with oxygen, independent of diuretic use. This complication often occurs in the setting of mild hypoxemia and usually is misdiagnosed as pneumonia. Diagnosis is complicated by the leukocytosis and low-grade fever that frequently accompany seizures. The radiographic diagnosis is certain when the findings are restricted to haziness of pulmonary markings and thickening of the interlobar septa. If the alveoli are involved, however, as evidenced by irregular, randomly distributed, patchy shadows primarily in the middle third of the lungs, or if pulmonary edema is unilateral (Fig. 18.4) (119,120), differentiation from aspiration pneumonia is difficult. The diagnosis is then made retrospectively with repeated chest radiographs. The electrocardiogram (ECG) is usually normal (115).

The pathophysiology of ictal pulmonary edema is not fully understood, although it may contribute to sudden unexplained death following seizures. Experimental animal studies demonstrate that elevations in intracranial pressure can increase pulmonary capillary permeability in the absence of other significant hemodynamic effects (121). Although pulmonary pressure probably becomes elevated during seizures, in part because of intense muscular contractions, animal studies show that pulmonary deterioration cannot be prevented by curarization (122). It is also unlikely that postictal pulmonary edema arises from the cardiac or vascular effects of systemic increases in epinephrine or norepinephrine, because adrenalectomy is not protective in animals (123). Instead, postictal pulmonary edema appears to be mediated by direct autonomic innervation of the pulmonary vascular bed. According to evidence derived from clinical and experimental studies, a central anatomic site of neurogenic pulmonary edema may exist in the nucleus tractus solitarius of the caudal brainstem (124).

Diaphragmatic Herniation

Although it is not extensively documented in the medical literature, we have observed unilateral transdiaphragmatic intestinal herniation following GTCSs.

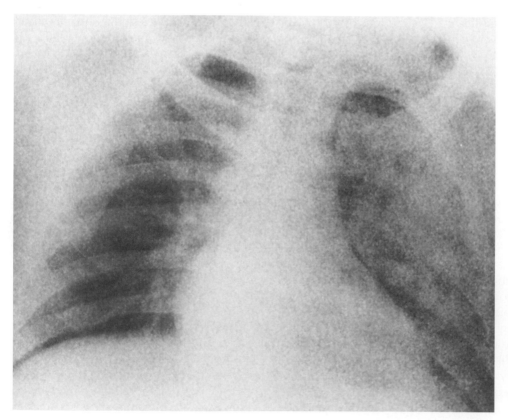

Figure 18.4 Unilateral interstitial pulmonary edema of the left lung (with normal heart size) in a 25-year-old following a single generalized tonic-clonic seizure. On other occasions, postictal bilateral pulmonary edema with transient cardiac enlargement occurred. (From Koppel BS, Pearl M, Perla E. Epileptic seizures as a cause of unilateral pulmonary edema. *Epilepsia* 1987;28:41–44, with permission.)

Sudden Death

The death rate for individuals with epilepsy is approximately twice that of the general population (125). This excess mortality is largely a result of accidental and nonaccidental deaths occurring during and immediately after seizures (126,127). Between 5% and 30% of deaths in persons with epilepsy have no apparent cause on postmortem examination (128,117). Most sudden unexpected deaths occur during sleep and affect mainly adults between 20 to 40 years of age who have long-standing epilepsy. The incidence of sudden unexpected death in patients with epilepsy (SUDEP) is estimated to be approximately 1 in 600 (129–132). In a population-based study conducted at the Mayo Clinic (133), the incidence of SUDEP was 0.35 per 1000 person-years. Although SUDEP remains rare, it exceeds the expected rate of sudden death in the general population by nearly 24-fold. Moreover, the risk of SUDEP is significantly higher in patients with GTCSs than in patients with other kinds of seizures (132). Proposed mechanisms include cardiac arrest (134), QT interval lengthening as shown on ECG (135), pulmonary edema (136), suffocation (134), and autonomic dysfunction (137). Ictal increases in plasma epinephrine levels sufficient to produce cardiac arrhythmias may account for some cases of sudden death (138,139), although this remains unproven; a study of 338 consecutive patients with epilepsy did not show an increased incidence of or tendency toward life-threatening cardiac arrhythmias (60). Cerebrovascular disease is an important risk factor for sudden cardiac death in patients with epilepsy (140). Possible iatrogenic causes, such as vagus nerve stimulation (141), or use of such newer AEDs as lamotrigine (142) have not been found to contribute to SUDEP. Derby and colleagues (143) concluded that the use of two or more AEDs actually decreases the probability of sudden death. This appears to be consistent with the observation by George and Davis (144) that poor compliance with AEDs increases the likelihood of SUDEP.

Dermatologic Signs

Abrasions, lacerations, ecchymoses, and scleral and petechial hemorrhages commonly occur following a single GTCS. All except scleral and petechial hemorrhages are usually caused by external trauma. Petechial hemorrhages caused by capillary bleeding from internal pressure changes typically occur over the face, neck, or chest, but rarely may appear only in a periocular distribution (145). When present on arising from sleep, they suggest a diagnosis of nocturnal GTCS. As with other skin changes, they resolve over a period of days and do not necessarily indicate a hematologic disorder.

Cognitive Decline

Cognitive decline is well known to occur following prolonged status epilepticus with GTCSs. Although a definitive study has not been conducted, existing studies of neuropsychological function and duration of epilepsy that compare the cumulative effect of different seizure types strongly suggest that GTCSs lead to gradual cognitive decline, particularly in individuals experiencing 100 or more GTCSs.

ELECTROENCEPHALOGRAPHIC MANIFESTATIONS

Nonepileptiform Activity

The EEG in uncomplicated idiopathic GTCSs typically contains normal background activity. When generalized slowing occurs, it usually results from the effects of such AEDs as phenytoin (which may selectively slow the alpha and mu rhythms), other psychotropic medications (such as phenothiazines and lithium carbonate), or postictal metabolic depression (Fig. 18.2). Paralleling the clinical course, postictal slowing resolves rapidly after a single, uncomplicated seizure. Barbiturate and benzodiazepine anticonvulsants increase beta activity, particularly in the 14- to 20-Hz range, and induce generalized slowing at toxic levels, as do phenytoin, valproic acid, and carbamazepine. Chloral hydrate, commonly used for sedation in electroencephalography laboratories, also may increase beta activity in children when administered in relatively high doses.

Certain nonepileptiform electroencephalographic findings occur more commonly in patients with idiopathic GTCSs and in clinically asymptomatic family members than in the general population. These findings can be divided into three categories: partial expressions of the patient's characteristic interictal epileptiform pattern, rhythmic delta activity, and rhythmic theta activity. Individuals who exhibit a typical 3-Hz spike-and-wave pattern may also have bursts or runs of 3-Hz frontal delta activity that otherwise resemble the spike-and-wave pattern. The delta activity likely represents a partial expression of the 3-Hz spike and wave. Similarly, patients with generalized atypical spike-and-wave activity often exhibit nonspecific paroxysmal bursts that closely resemble the interictal epileptiform activity but lack well-developed epileptiform spikes or sharp waves. In many cases, these nonspecific or "degraded" patterns are the only finding in an electroencephalographic recording.

Three typical EEG patterns of intermittent rhythmic activity may occur in patients with idiopathic GTCSs: bioccipital delta, frontal delta, and parietal theta activity. Bioccipital delta activity may be seen in patients with typical absence seizures and GTCSs (56), usually in children and adolescents. It tends to occur in prolonged runs (Fig. 18.5), and in some cases, may be consistently activated by eye closure. Occasionally it evolves directly into the frontal-dominant typical 3-Hz spike-and-wave pattern. Only one-third of those who exhibit this pattern have epilepsy. Also called the phi rhythm, bioccipital delta activity that lasts from 1 to 3 seconds and occurs only immediately following eye closure is less clearly related to epilepsy (146). Frontal intermittent delta activity may occur in brief runs over the anterior head in patients with either idiopathic or secondary GTCSs (Fig. 18.6A). Unlike the delta

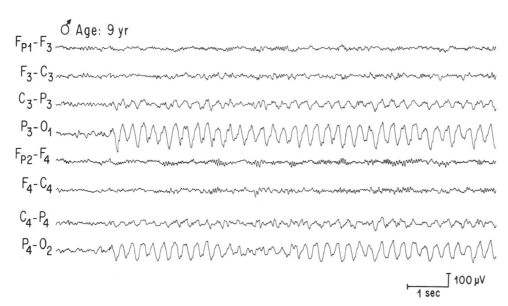

Figure 18.5 Bioccipital rhythmic delta activity in a patient with primary epilepsy. Prolonged runs of delta activity are often seen in association with typical absence seizures and generalized tonic-clonic seizures. (Courtesy of Barbara Westmoreland, M.D.)

waveforms of the 3-Hz spike-and-wave pattern, the repetition rate is slower and the pattern does not include epileptiform spikes. Frontal intermittent delta activity also may be seen in patients with diffuse cortical abnormalities or deep-seated midline lesions (e.g., tumors of the third ventricle). Finally, prolonged runs of parietal theta activity, varying from 4 to 7 Hz, have been identified as a nonspecific finding in patients with absence seizures and GTCSs (147).

In individuals with secondary GTCSs, nonspecific abnormalities, such as diffuse background slowing and disorganization, are far more common than in patients with idiopathic epilepsy. Therefore, in patients with an established seizure disorder, these findings provide electroencephalographic evidence for symptomatic epilepsy. Voltage asymmetries or focal slowing may help to identify an underlying structural lesion. In the absence of epileptiform abnormalities, intermittent focal rhythmic delta activity is the nonspecific finding most suggestive of epilepsy (Fig. 18.6B), particularly when it is localized to the temporal head regions (148).

Although these nonspecific findings by themselves have little diagnostic value (other than temporal rhythmic intermittent delta activity), they may help to distinguish between primary and secondary generalized seizure disorders when present in individuals with known epilepsy or when seen in association with clearly abnormal epileptiform patterns.

Interictal Epileptiform Activity

Approximately half of all patients with GTCSs have epileptiform activity on the first EEG. Ajmone-Marsan and Zivin (149) found epileptiform patterns on the initial EEG in 132 (58%) of 228 patients with GTCSs. On serial examinations, only 32% of all patients had epileptiform patterns on every recording. These authors also observed that recording the EEG within 5 days following a seizure increased the

likelihood of obtaining positive results. Gibbs and Gibbs (150) found epileptiform activity in 1191 (49%) of 2430 patients with a history of GTCSs. Generalized epileptiform activity is suppressed during REM sleep (151,152).

Interictal epileptiform patterns in patients with idiopathic epilepsy are almost always greatest in voltage over the anterior or frontocentral regions. Rarely, and more often in children, the spike and slow-wave complexes are posterior-dominant. Four main interictal epileptiform patterns occur in individuals with idiopathic GTCSs (Fig. 18.7):

1. *Typical 3-Hz spike-and-wave complexes (typical spike and wave)*, which is associated with idiopathic epilepsy and typical absence seizures with or without GTCSs;
2. *Irregular spike-and-wave complexes* that are irregular in frequency and amplitude; may be associated with idiopathic or symptomatic epilepsy; and also occur acutely in individuals experiencing drug withdrawal (e.g., anticonvulsants, primarily barbiturates) (153) and in certain toxic-metabolic encephalopathies, such as renal failure and toxic reactions to lithium;
3. *Four- to 5-Hz spike-and-wave complexes*, which are most often associated with idiopathic epilepsy; and
4. *Multiple-spike complexes* of short duration that are often associated with idiopathic epilepsy and myoclonus.

As a rule, generalized tonic-clonic, myoclonic, and clonic seizures become more likely as the generalized pattern deviates from 3-Hz spike-and-wave, although 3-Hz spike-and-wave occasionally may be seen in some individuals who clinically seem to have GTCSs only ("pure grand mal") (56). More than one generalized epileptiform pattern may occur in the same recording (Fig. 18.7).

A common pitfall in EEG interpretation is to regard an asymmetrical fragment of a generalized epileptiform burst as evidence of secondary generalized seizures or so-called secondary bilateral synchrony. Associated background

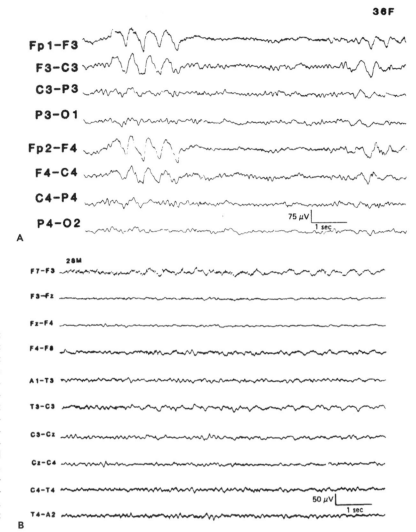

Figure 18.6 Nonspecific electroencephalographic findings in patients with generalized tonic-clonic seizures **(A)** and secondary generalized tonic-clonic seizures **(B)**. **A:** Frontal intermittent rhythmic delta activity, a nonspecific indication of dysfunction of thalamocortical interconnections, appears at the beginning and end of the epoch shown. B: Runs of focal, left temporal, rhythmic delta waves. Sphenoidal electrodes revealed coincident epileptiform spiking; however, even with closed-circuit television/electroencephalographic monitoring of seizures, no clinical findings suggested a focal origin. T3 is equal to T7, and T4 is equal to T8, as used elsewhere in this volume. (From Fisch BJ, Pedley TA. Generalized tonic-clonic epilepsies. In: Lüders H, Lesser RP, eds. *Epilepsy: electroclinical syndromes.* New York: Springer-Verlag, 1987:151–185, with permission).

abnormalities, such as focal delta activity, sometimes provide a basis for such conclusions, but in their absence, bilateral asymmetrical epileptiform activity, or even focal spikes with simultaneous regional background changes, should be interpreted with caution. Typical 3-Hz spike-and-wave patterns fragment during sleep, and atypical spike-and-wave patterns may have a more disorganized appearance at any time during wakefulness or sleep. Multiple spikes or focal or lateralized spikes are likely to occur, particularly during nonrapid eye movement sleep (151,154).

Interictal epileptiform responses to photic stimulation in idiopathic epilepsy have a prevalence of approximately 25% (155) and occur more often in children and adolescents than in adults. Although the exact incidence and electroencephalographic defining criteria vary from study to study, it is estimated that fewer than 2% of healthy adults with no family history of epilepsy have photoparoxysmal (photoconvulsive) responses (for a review, ref. 156). Epileptiform responses to photic stimulation appear to be under separate genetic control and therefore do not have the same significance as does spontaneous generalized epileptiform activity

(147,157). Most patients with photoparoxysmal responses do not have light-sensitive epilepsy (Fig. 18.8), but for those in whom seizures are activated by light, photic stimulation can induce GTCSs, absence seizures, or myoclonus. Spontaneous epileptiform activity is more highly correlated with epilepsy than is the photoparoxysmal response. Although photoparoxysmal responses are usually deemed suggestive of primary generalized seizures, most patients with consistently focal interictal epileptiform activity and photoparoxysmal responses have partial or secondary generalized seizures (158). Photic stimulation rarely activates focal epileptiform activity unless the epileptogenic zone is within or adjacent to the occipital lobe. Among patients with reflex epilepsy, photosensitivity accounts for approximately one-third of all cases (159).

Secondary Generalized Interictal Epileptiform Activity

Tükel and Jasper (160) introduced the concept of secondary bilateral synchrony to explain how a unilateral cortical

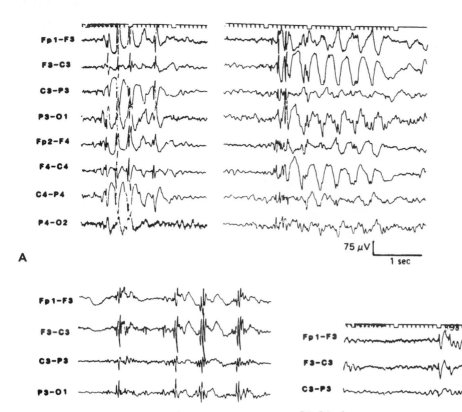

Figure 18.7 Interictal epileptiform patterns in different patients with generalized tonic-clonic seizures. **A:** Irregular spike-and-wave complexes, the most commonly encountered pattern. Note the asymmetry in the second epoch. Occasional asymmetries alone should not be considered an indication of secondary generalized seizures. **B:** Multiple spike complexes. Fragments or partial expressions of generalized bursts are common and occasionally more asymmetrical than the example shown in **C.** (From Fisch BJ, Pedley TA. Generalized tonic-clonic epilepsies. In: Lüders H, Lesser RP, eds. *Epilepsy: electroclinical syndromes.* New York: Springer-Verlag, 1987:151–185, with permission).

lesion can give rise to generalized epileptiform activity (Figs. 18.9 and 18.10). They hypothesized that a cortical epileptogenic focus stimulates a diffusely projecting system capable of inducing bilateral cortical epileptiform activity. This "centrencephalic system" was conceptualized as an epileptogenic pathway within which primary generalized seizures were initiated and propagated (a phenomenon they called primary bilateral synchrony). The seat of pathology for primary generalized seizure disorders was thought to lie within the brainstem reticular system and thalamus and its cortical projections. Although the cortex and certain brainstem structures, such as the substantia nigra, are now believed to play a key role in the pathophysiology of tonic-clonic seizures, recent PET scans from patients with primary GTCSs have shown reduced benzodiazepine receptor density mainly in the thalamus, but not in the cerebral cortex, basal ganglia, or cerebellar cortex. Similar receptor findings have also been demonstrated by PET scan within epileptogenic foci in patients with partial seizures (161).

The unilateral mesial frontal cortex is the epileptogenic zone most commonly implicated in the generation of bilaterally symmetrical epileptiform activity (162), although other cortical areas, including those in the temporal lobe (163), may evoke the same phenomenon. Electroencephalographic features consistent with secondary bilateral synchrony (Figs. 18.9 and 18.10) are repetitive spike-and-wave discharges of less than 3 Hz, considerable morphologic variability from complex to complex, consistently asymmetrical epileptiform activity, a single lateralized site of phase reversal in transverse bipolar montages, and unilateral focal spikes (164). Other findings that suggest secondary bilateral synchrony are those associated with cerebral lesions such as focal slowing, background disorganization, and attenuation. If on a single, routine EEG it is difficult to distinguish between secondary and primary generalized discharges, a more prolonged recording often provides the necessary electroencephalographic features.

Special noninvasive computerized techniques for EEG analysis have been used to study interhemispheric propa-

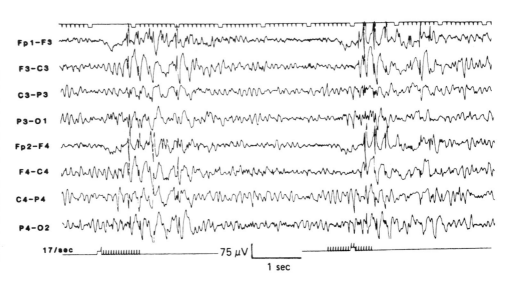

Figure 18.8 Photoparoxysmal response consistently elicited by intermittent flash frequencies in a patient with generalized tonic-clonic seizures but no clinical photosensitivity. Note that in contrast to a normal photomyogenic (photomyoclonic) response, the photoparoxysmal response is not time-locked to the stimulus and, as shown here, may outlast it. (From Fisch BJ, Pedley TA. Generalized tonic-clonic epilepsies. In: Lüders H, Lesser RP, eds. *Epilepsy: electroclinical syndromes.* New York: Springer-Verlag, 1987:151–185, with permission.)

gation in secondary bilateral synchrony (165,166). These studies show that secondary generalization is likely if a localized spike or sharp wave consistently precedes subsequent activity in the contralateral hemisphere by at least 20 milliseconds (163). Gotman (167) found that patients with idiopathic epilepsy had interhemispheric delays of less than 5 milliseconds, whereas those with symptomatic tonic-clonic epilepsies had interhemispheric delays between 10 and 30 milliseconds. Invasive methods for detecting secondary bilateral synchrony include the intracarotid amobarbital test (injection ipsilateral to the lesion selectively abolishes all activity) (168) and the IV thiopental test (following injection, only the unilateral focus remains electroencephalographically active) (169).

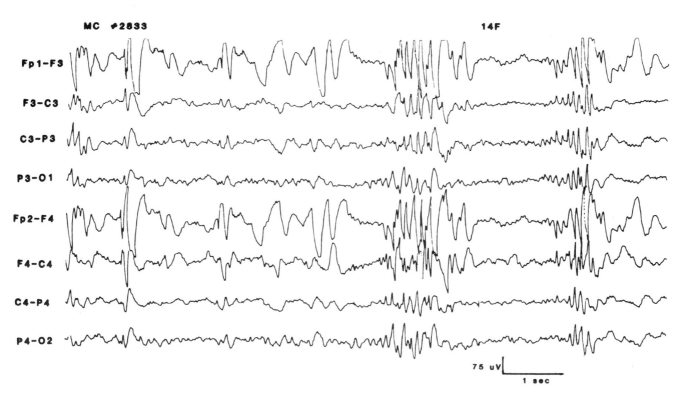

Figure 18.9 Secondary bilateral synchrony in a 14-year-old girl, arising from an epileptic zone adjacent to a right frontal cystic ganglioglioma. Slowing and the regional spread of epileptiform activity are somewhat greater on the right than on the left. Resection of the lesion and surrounding gliotic epileptogenic cortex eliminated the generalized spike bursts. (From Fisch BJ, Pedley TA. Generalized tonic-clonic epilepsies. In: Lüders H, Lesser RP, eds. *Epilepsy: electroclinical syndromes.* New York: Springer-Verlag, 1987:151–185, with permission.)

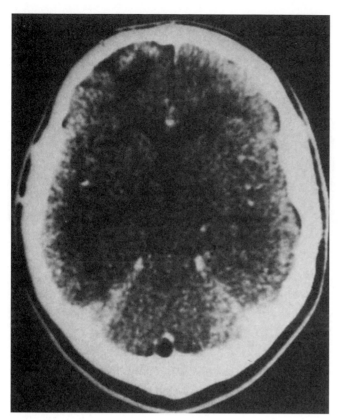

Figure 18.10 Computed tomography of the right frontal lesion described in Figure 18.9. (From Fisch BJ, Pedley TA. Generalized tonic-clonic epilepsies. In: Lüders H, Lesser RP, eds. *Epilepsy: electroclinical syndromes.* New York: Springer-Verlag, 1987:151–185, with permission.)

Incidental Interictal Epileptiform Activity

Generalized epileptiform patterns are more likely than focal epileptiform patterns to occur in persons without epilepsy. The generalized epileptiform patterns that are most likely to be encountered as the only EEG abnormality in individuals with no complaint of seizures who are undergoing electroencephalography include photoparoxysmal responses (light stimulation-induced) and occipital-dominant irregular spike and wave (170). Earlier studies examining the incidence of epileptiform patterns in large populations of unaffected individuals are generally viewed with some reservation, because the electroencephalographic criteria for epileptiform abnormalities continue to change and the interpretive skills of electroencephalographers vary widely. Indeed, subclinical rhythmic electroencephalographic discharges in adults, paroxysmal hypnagogic hypersynchrony, other paroxysmal patterns of drowsiness (171), prominent photic driving, and rhythmic temporal discharges during drowsiness (psychomotor variant) have only in the recent past become widely recognized as normal variants (for a review, see ref. 164). With these caveats in mind, the following information is provided.

Zivin and Ajmone-Marsan (172) found that only 45 (0.7%) of 6497 individuals without epilepsy had generalized epileptiform activity. Gerken and Doose (173) observed generalized spike-wave bursts in 12 (1.8%) of the EEGs of 685 normal children; however, if the child had a first-degree relative with spike-wave epilepsy, the incidence peaked at 12% to 13% at ages 3 to 6 years, fell to 1.4% at ages 9 to 10 years, and rose to 9.7% at age 15 years. Their data suggests that a "regular" spike-and-wave pattern was more likely than an "irregular" one if the child had an affected relative. Cavazzuti and associates (174) reported a 1.1% incidence of generalized spike-wave discharges among 3726 normal children, none of whom had a history of epilepsy.

Ictal Electroencephalogram Findings

Although the onset of ictal electroencephalographic activity in spontaneous idiopathic GTCSs is generalized on routine electroencephalographic examination, noninvasive computerized EEG analysis reveals that the ictal electroencephalographic pattern, like the interictal one, is rarely, if ever, truly bisynchronous (163,167,175). Instead, minor, shifting, interhemispheric asynchronies occur at the onset and during the seizure. Because a minority of patients with secondary GTCSs also may show the same slight degree of interhemispheric asynchrony, an electroencephalographic distinction between focal and generalized onset may not always be possible. According to the classification of seizures (6), in the absence of focal interictal epileptiform activity, such seizures are considered to be primary generalized. In contrast, the classification of epilepsies and epileptic syndromes (9) ultimately depends on additional findings from the neurologic examination and laboratory tests.

Immediately preceding the tonic phase, many patients experience one or more myoclonic jerks accompanied by synchronous, widespread muscle and head movement spikes on the EEG. Rarely, high-amplitude, anterior-dominant, epileptiform spikes occur with each body jerk. When the tonic-clonic seizure is not preceded by myoclonus or, more rarely, by an absence seizure (Fig. 18.11), the onset appears clearly as a generalized attenuation of all activity (Fig. 18.12), leaving only very low-voltage waveforms in the 20- to 40-Hz range (EEG desynchronization). Muscle and movement artifacts almost always obscure subsequent electroencephalographic activity. Accurate electroencephalographic information on GTCSs has therefore been derived largely from patients who were pharmacologically paralyzed at the time of the seizure (Fig. 18.12).

The patterns of primary and secondary generalized seizures are virtually indistinguishable once the tonic phase is established (Fig. 18.13). Three main electroencephalographic onset patterns of secondary generalized seizures have been identified: focal rhythmic or arrhythmic epileptiform spiking (Fig. 18.13); brief, localized voltage attenuation or low-voltage fast activity; and a buildup of focal rhythmic activity (176).

As the tonic phase continues, the electroencephalographic activity gradually increases in amplitude and slows

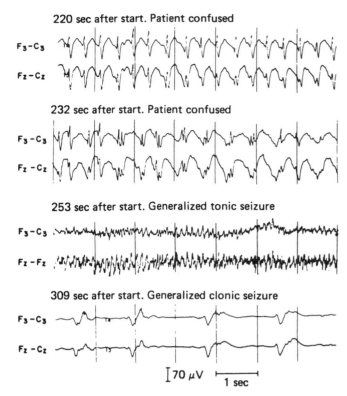

Figure 18.11   Seizure progression from an absence seizure to a generalized tonic-clonic seizure (12-year history). (From Lüders H, Lesser RP, Dinner DS, et al. Generalized epilepsies: a review. *Cleve Clin Q* 1984;1:205–226, with permission.)

to a sustained 10-Hz rhythm. Because it reminded Gastaut and Fischer-Williams (177) of the thalamic recruiting rhythm described by Dempsey and Morison (178), they referred to it as the "epileptic recruiting rhythm." A similar, if not identical, rhythm has been observed at the onset of other types of generalized convulsive seizures (56). This pattern lasts approximately 10 seconds before a slower 8-Hz activity emerges. The remnants of the recruiting rhythm and the slower activity combine with high-amplitude spikes to gradually form high-amplitude repetitive complexes that increase in amplitude and slow to 1 Hz. As the rhythmic slow waves decelerate through the 4-Hz range, tonic muscle contractions give way to interrupted muscle tone (the intermediate vibratory period). On further deceleration, these rhythmic inhibitory slow waves produce the longer intervals of muscle atonia that characterize the clonic phase.

After the final clonic jerk, the EEG may be isoelectric, or it may contain only low-amplitude (<20 mV) delta activity. At the cellular level, sustained depolarization during the clonic period is followed by postictal hyperpolarization that corresponds to the period of electroencephalographic depression (179,180). The duration of electroencephalographic suppression varies from several seconds to about 2 minutes. The immediate postictal EEG also may contain atypical features, such as a burst-suppression pattern (181) or a triphasic wave pattern (Fig. 18.14) (182).

Although postictal depression is proportional to the number of immediately preceding seizures (and is usually more prolonged in children), Robin and colleagues (183) found an inverse relationship between the degree and duration of the postictal electroencephalographic disturbance (in adults undergoing electroconvulsive therapy) and the duration of the seizure. They hypothesized that the early termination of a seizure requires more intense inhibition and is therefore associated with more severe postictal metabolic depression.

The return of the EEG to baseline parallels the patient's recovery, and is characterized by a gradual increase in frequency and amplitude of the ongoing activity. Secondary generalized seizures without localized interictal abnormalities or focal electroencephalographic features at onset are revealed occasionally by a prominent asymmetry of postictal slowing. Although baseline activity usually returns within 30 minutes or less, in practice it is best to accept mild degrees of slowing as a postictal effect for at least 24 hours following a single, uncomplicated GTCS (176).

PROGNOSIS

Substantial evidence from animal experimentation suggests that seizures, particularly generalized convulsive seizures, beget seizures. In humans, however, this phenomenon is not so clear. There is general agreement that provoked seizures rarely lead to further seizures if the provoking condition is reversible. In contrast, Hauser and Lee (184) found that the risk for additional seizures among patients with unprovoked seizures of unknown etiology increased incrementally with each subsequent seizure. Additional seizures in patients with unprovoked seizures with an identified etiology did not increase the risk for subsequent seizures. To our knowledge, there are no other human studies addressing the question of seizures begetting seizures. The investigators' findings seem to suggest that different pathologic epileptic processes affect the likelihood that seizures either predict or perhaps cause further seizures.

The prognosis of patients who have only idiopathic GTCSs is more favorable than that of patients with focal or secondary generalized seizures (Fig. 18.15) (63,125,185). Indeed, Elwes and coworkers (185) reported that among all patients with epilepsy, the probability of remission is greatest in those who have only GTCSs diagnosed before age 10 years. Approximately 95% of individuals with idiopathic GTCSs experience a 5-year continuous remission within the first 20 years after onset (125). Juul-Jensen and Foldspang (43) found that 47% of patients with grand mal epilepsy were seizure-free 2 years from the time of diagnosis. The chance of relapse in patients with idiopathic GTCSs who have been in remission for 5 years is 21% within 20 years (125). The exception is patients with juvenile myoclonic epilepsy, who experience a very low rate of spontaneous remission (see Chapter 25).

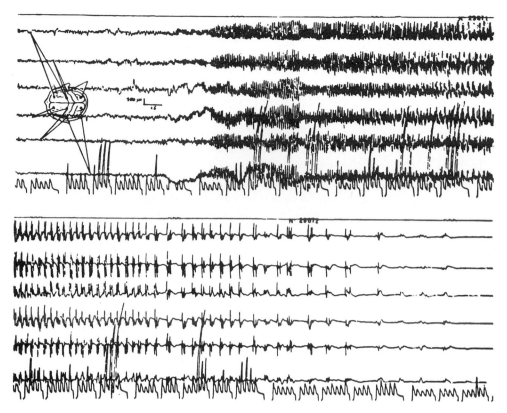

Figure 18.12 Electroencephalographic recording of a generalized tonic-clonic seizure in a patient in whom partial curarization prevented cerebral activity from being obscured by artifact. (From Gastaut H, Broughton R. *Epileptic seizures: clinical and electroencephalographic features, diagnosis and treatment.* Springfield, IL: Charles C Thomas, 1972, with permission.)

The prognosis for individuals with secondary GTCSs is less favorable than that for patients with most types of idiopathic GTCSs (186). Although these findings are somewhat controversial (187,188), a particularly poor prognosis has been reported in patients with complex partial and secondary GTCSs (43,63,189). In two studies, the frequency of GTCSs was an important risk factor in individuals with complex partial seizures (188,190). Indeed, Emerson and colleagues (190) found the frequency of tonic-clonic seizures to be an important risk factor in the prognosis for all types of childhood epilepsy. Among patients who have both GTCSs and complex partial seizures, those who present with mainly GTCSs seem to have a better prognosis than do those who present with mainly complex partial seizures.

Neurologic impairment, particularly if present at birth, and onset in adult life reduce the possibility of seizure remission in all individuals with epilepsy (125). Among children who have only GTCSs, failure to enter remission within 2 years of diagnosis reduces the chance of a remission in the subsequent 3 years (185). Several studies also have shown that the presence of frequent seizures prior to treatment initiation adversely affects prognosis (63,185,191). The need for early intervention is underscored by the observation that in some patients the time intervals between GTCSs gradually shortens, as if an adverse process favoring progressive epileptogenesis were taking place (192,193).

THERAPY

Complete control with the use of AEDs can be achieved in approximately 45% to 55% of patients with secondary GTCSs and in more than 60% of those with primary generalized seizures. Although the therapy for GTCSs is primarily medical, surgery should be considered in patients with medically refractory seizures if the GTCSs are secondarily generalized and if corpus callosotomy (see also Chapter 84) or a safe resection of a localized epileptogenic zone (see also Chapters 78 to 80) can be performed. AEDs in combination with the ketogenic diet may be useful in children with multiple seizure types. Vagus nerve stimulation was approved by the U.S. Food and Drug Administration (FDA) in 1997 for the treatment of partial seizures, but recent studies and our own experience suggest that it can also be useful in a minority of cases of medication-resistant generalized epilepsy (194). Although it is not understood how the vagus nerve stimulator works, it does have a direct, frequency-dependent effect on human epileptiform discharges recorded from a hippocampal depth electrode (195). Investigational approaches include electrical stimulation of the centromedian thalamus (196).

In patients with GTCS who have undergone a thorough diagnostic evaluation, a monotherapeutic AED trial is the initial recommended approach. The use of a single AED reduces the risks for idiosyncratic and dose-related toxic reactions, the cost of medication and laboratory testing,

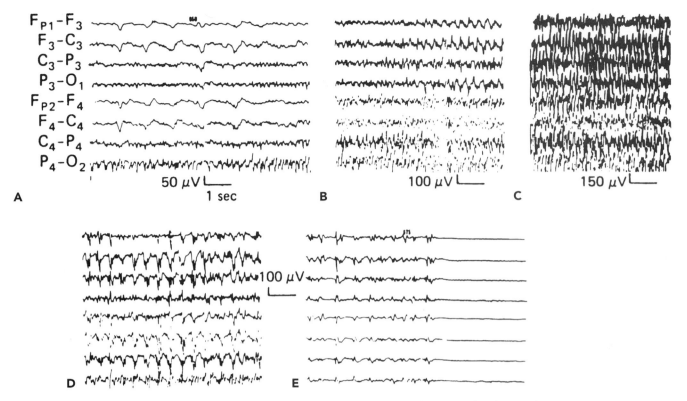

Figure 18.13 Electroencephalographic discharge from a secondary generalized tonic-clonic seizure. This patient had a right occipital metastatic lesion. The ictal episode began focally in the right occipital region, with subsequent ipsilateral and contralateral homologous spread. The tonic and clonic phases were identical to a primary generalized tonic-clonic convulsion. Because the patient was completely paralyzed with curare, no muscle artifact is present. (From Fisch BJ, Pedley TA. Generalized tonic-clonic epilepsies. In: Lüders H, Lesser RP, eds. *Epilepsy: electroclinical syndromes.* New York: Springer-Verlag, 1987:151–185, with permission.)

and the possibility of drug interactions, while substantially increasing the likelihood of compliance. Approximately 70% of patients with either primary or secondary GTCSs obtain excellent seizure control with one AED. In the past decade, rational selection of AEDs has been greatly facilitated by studies of the genetically transmitted epilepsies and results of several major monotherapy trials. However, not all patients respond to AEDs monotherapy.

The terms "rational polytherapy" and "rational polypharmacy" were introduced (197–199) in conjunction with the marketing of a series of newer AEDs that were approved by the FDA only as add-on medications (198). Following reports of a high incidence of life-threatening complications in patients taking felbamate (200,201), lamotrigine was the first AED to receive approval in the United States for conditional (add-on first) monotherapy status. It is clear, however, that most, if not all, of the newer AEDs are effective against both primary and secondary GTCSs.

The efficacy of valproate in absence seizures, myoclonic seizures, and GTCSs makes it the agent of choice for GTCSs with typical absence seizures or juvenile myoclonic epilepsy with GTCSs. Although typical absence seizures also respond to ethosuximide, GTCSs do not. Juvenile

myoclonic epilepsy with GTCSs may respond only to valproate. When GTCSs are the only seizure type or are accompanied by complex partial seizures, the recommended approach to treatment is based primarily on the results of two large AED trials (202–204): (a) The Veterans Administration (VA) Collaborative Group Study (203,204), which included only patients who had partial seizures, with or without secondary GTCSs, and (b) a recent trial from the United Kingdom, which enrolled only patients with new-onset epilepsy with either primary or secondary GTCSs (202).

For patients with only primary GTCSs, the UK study found that phenobarbital, phenytoin, carbamazepine, and valproic acid were approximately equal in efficacy (defined by time to first recurrence or time to achieve a 1-year remission). However, the toxicity profiles of the AEDs differed strikingly. Approximately 10% of all patients studied had to be withdrawn from medication because of toxic side effects. More than half of all cases of toxicity were caused by drowsiness or lethargy from phenobarbital. Carbamazepine was discontinued because of drowsiness or rash. The somewhat higher-than-expected incidence of drowsiness with carbamazepine occurred early in treatment and was probably

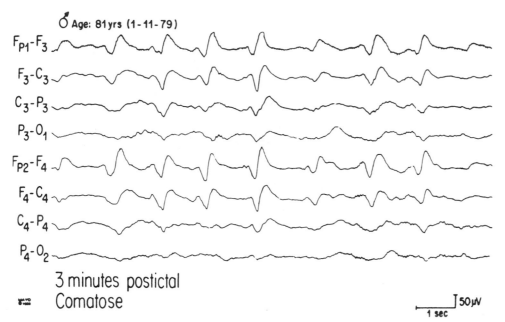

♂ Age: 81 yrs (1-11-79)

F_{P1}-F_3

F_3-C_3

C_3-P_3

P_3-O_1

F_{P2}-F_4

F_4-C_4

C_4-P_4

P_4-O_2

3 minutes postictal
Comatose

1 sec   50 μV

Figure 18.14 Triphasic waves in the immediate period following a generalized tonic-clonic seizure. (From Fisch BJ, Klass DW. The diagnostic specificity of triphasic wave patterns. *Electroencephalogr Clin Neurophysiol* 1988;70:18, with permission.)

attributable to the starting dosage of 400 mg/day. We found that this problem can be overcome by restarting carbamazepine at a low dosage—less than 200 mg/day, if necessary—with increases at 1- to 3-week intervals. The lowest rates of withdrawal because of toxic reactions in the UK study were reported with phenytoin and valproate. These results and those of other studies (203–208) indicate that for patients with new-onset GTCSs and no other seizure type, without signs of "valproate-sensitive" epilepsy syndrome and without either a progressive neurologic disorder or toxic exposure (e.g., alcohol-related seizures), the agent of choice for monotherapy should be limited to carbamazepine, valproate, or phenytoin. The initial selection is based on a consideration of potential side effects (e.g., cosmetic effects with phenytoin; weight gain or likelihood of serious hepatic injury, particularly in young children, with valproate) and cost (valproate is the most expensive of the three agents).

For patients with secondary GTCSs, with or without isolated partial seizures, drug selection is guided by the results of both the UK and VA studies, as well as other, somewhat more limited trials (202–208). Carbamazepine, phenytoin, or valproate is recommended as initial monotherapy. In the second VA study (203), carbamazepine was judged to be slightly more efficacious than valproate, particularly for associated complex partial seizures. In the first VA study (204), carbamazepine was the best-tolerated agent compared with primidone, phenobarbital, and phenytoin. Both VA studies used a higher range of doses than the UK study and noted a higher rate of withdrawals because of toxic reactions (20% versus 10%, respectively). Moreover, most patients in the VA studies had previously undergone treatment for epilepsy, whereas none of the patients enrolled in the UK study had received prior treatment. The

expected higher percentage of monotherapy failures in the VA patients never materialized; efficacy was comparable in both trials. Because of possible advantages in efficacy and the relatively low toxicity profile and cost, carbamazepine is generally considered the agent of first choice for the treatment of secondary GTCSs.

More recently, studies were performed documenting the efficacy of the newer AEDs, such as felbamate, lamotrigine, tiagabine, topiramate, gabapentin, zonisamide, and vigabatrin (209,210). Unfortunately, there are no direct comparative studies of the new AEDs that are similar to the VA cooperative trials. All of the new AEDs have unique characteristics and are structurally and mechanistically different from the standard AEDs. However, with the exception of gabapentin and perhaps levetiracetam, all are associated with some major safety concerns (118).

Felbamate was the first new AED to be approved in the United States in 15 years, following the introduction of valproate in 1978. In 1993, based on the effectiveness and safety of felbamate in clinical trials, the FDA approved the agent for monotherapy in the treatment of both partial (localization-related) and generalized epilepsies (201,211,212). In September 1994, the FDA issued a warning to all physicians because of a higher-than-expected incidence of aplastic anemia and hepatic failure among patients receiving felbamate (200,201,212). A practice advisory sponsored by the American Academy of Neurology and the American Epilepsy Society was published in 1999 to establish the current role of felbamate for the treatment of various types of intractable epilepsy (201). The risk-to-benefit ratio supports the use of felbamate in the following situations: (a) in patients with Lennox-Gastaut syndrome who are older than 4 years of age and are unresponsive to primary AEDs; (b) in patients with

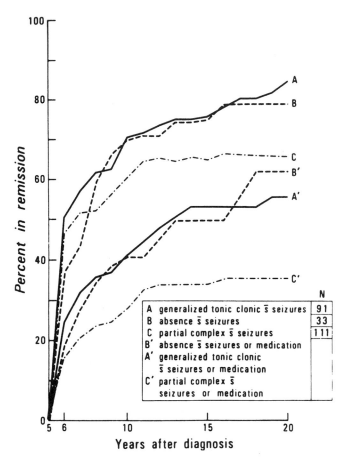

Figure 18.15 Percentage of patients with idiopathic seizures in remission, by seizure type and medication status. (From Annegers JF, Hauser WA, Elveback LR. Remission of seizures and relapse in patients with epilepsy. *Epilepsia* 1979;20:729–737, with permission.)

intractable partial seizures who are older than 18 years of age and have failed to respond to standard AEDs at therapeutic levels (data indicate a better risk-to-benefit ratio for felbamate used as monotherapy); and (c) continuing use in patients who have been taking felbamate for more than 18 months. A U.S. Felbamate Registry funded initially by Wallace Laboratories and now supported by MedPointe has been established (213). Upon patient entry, potential risk is assessed by HLA typing and a urine acid monocarbamate-to-mercapturate ratio.

Clinically, lamotrigine is effective for both partial and generalized seizures and is now considered by many to be the agent of second choice after valproate for the treatment of absence epilepsy and juvenile myoclonic epilepsy. Therapy with lamotrigine must be initiated slowly in adults, with initial doses of 25 mg/day without concomitant valproate or 12.5 mg/day with valproate; 25- and 12.5-mg/week increments, respectively, are recommended. Initial adult target doses of lamotrigine monotherapy range from 200 to 400 mg/day. With inducing agents, doses of 600 to 1000 mg/day or higher may be needed. In combination with valproate, doses of lamotrigine 100 to 200 mg are often sufficient (211). This slow rate of initial

dosing has been mandated by a relatively high incidence of dermatologic reactions (with progression to Stevens-Johnson syndrome), especially in children (incidence of rash, 1 in 50), prompting an FDA warning against the use of lamotrigine in children. Lamotrigine is effective for the treatment of generalized seizures associated with Lennox-Gastaut syndrome (214) and, as mentioned above, can also be an effective therapy for patients with juvenile myoclonic epilepsy (215,216). However, the agent is reported to aggravate myoclonus in some patients with severe myoclonic epilepsy of infancy and Lennox-Gastaut syndrome (217,218).

Tiagabine is effective in the treatment of partial-onset seizures (211). Its role in the treatment of generalized seizures remains to be established.

Topiramate appears to have multiple mechanisms of action that may contribute to its efficacy in several seizure types, including GTCSs. The agent received FDA approval for efficacy as add-on therapy to standard AEDs in patients with partial-onset seizures, with or without secondary generalized seizures (219). Biton and associates (219) conducted a randomized, placebo-controlled study of topiramate add-on therapy in 80 patients with primary GTCSs. The 56.7% median reduction from baseline in the average monthly primary GTCS rate in the topiramate-treated group was significantly greater than the 9% reduction in placebo-treated patients. In a double-blind, randomized trial of 98 patients with Lennox-Gastaut syndrome, topiramate adjunctive therapy was effective in reducing the number of drop attacks and major motor seizures (220). The current indications for the agent include adjunctive therapy for adults and pediatric patients 2 to 16 years of age with partial-onset seizures or primary generalized tonic-clonic seizures, and treatment of patients 2 years or older with seizures associated with Lennox-Gastaut syndrome. The most troubling side effects associated with topiramate use involve the CNS and include global cognitive changes (particularly dysphasia or speech apraxia) and psychological changes that are dose related and reversible in affected individuals. The occurrence of these side effects appears to be slightly lower with the recommended slow titration rate. Other serious, but rare, side effects include non-anion gap metabolic acidosis, acute myopia with secondary angle-closure glaucoma, and oligohidrosis with hyperthermia. It is important to consider the lattermost in warm climates in children and in physically active individuals. Although the recommended starting dose with topiramate is 25 mg/day with 25-mg/week increments to a target dose of approximately 200 to 400 mg/day in adults (221), most patients who respond achieve seizure control with 200 mg/day.

Like topiramate, zonisamide contains a sulfa group, which probably contributes to its similar side-effect profile, with reversible cognitive deficits and nephrolithiasis (222,223). In the United States, zonisamide is FDA approved as adjunctive therapy for the treatment of partial seizures in adults. As with topiramate, oligohidrosis with hyperthermia has been described in pediatric patients. Zonisamide has been found to be effective in a broad spectrum of partial and generalized seizures, including infantile spasms and idiopathic generalized seizures with myoclonus (224), and the agent appears to be particularly useful in patients with progressive myoclonus epilepsy (e.g., Unverricht-Lundborg syndrome).

In a series of large parallel-group studies, gabapentin has been found to be effective against simple partial, complex, and secondary generalized seizures (204,225,226). A study of patients with generalized seizures (227) was conducted in a heterogeneous population that included persons with both symptomatic and idiopathic generalized epilepsy. In that study, gabapentin reduced the frequency of generalized seizures to a greater degree than did placebo, but the difference failed to reach statistical significance. Gabapentin is generally well tolerated, with most side effects attributable to CNS toxicity (somnolence, vertigo, ataxia, fatigue). The agent is not metabolized by the liver, and it is not bound to plasma proteins. Thus, it does not display significant interactions with other drugs. Gabapentin is almost completely eliminated by renal clearance that is linearly related to creatinine clearance (211).

Vigabatrin has not been approved for use in the United States, mainly because of concerns about loss of peripheral vision. The agent can be effective against partial seizures with secondary generalization. Vigabatrin was found to be very effective against infantile spasms, especially those related to tuberous sclerosis; however, it can aggravate myoclonic and absence seizures (228).

New formulations of the standard AEDs have become important for the treatment of generalized seizures, including status epilepticus. Fosphenytoin sodium injection allows for faster and safer parenteral (IV and intramuscular) administration of phenytoin. Valproate sodium is also available as an injection and provides fast and effective replacement therapy or acute interventional therapy. Diazepam rectal gel has become a valuable tool for the management of recurrent seizure clusters in selected individuals. Intranasal midazolam can become a cheaper and more acceptable alternative to the rectal gel; however, more safety and efficacy studies are needed (229).

Oxcarbazepine is a keto analogue of carbamazepine, with an almost identical anticonvulsant profile. Its lower CNS toxicity is attributed to the fact that biotransformation of oxcarbazepine does not involve formation of an epoxide metabolite (210,230). The efficacy of oxcarbazepine in patients with IGE syndromes or symptomatic generalized epilepsy, including Lennox-Gastaut syndrome, has not been established (230).

According to Leppik and collaborators (231), levetiracetam, one of the last AEDs to become available in the United States, is successful as add-on therapy to other AEDs in reducing secondary generalized seizures. Levetiracetam also has the advantage of more rapid titration compared with such other new AEDs as topiramate and lamotrigine. Adverse behavioral effects, such as extreme irritability and difficulty sleeping, may occur in children and adults (232).

Whether newly introduced AEDs will become first-line agents for monotherapy of GTCSs will depend on the outcome of large, ongoing comparative clinical trials. The improved tolerability profiles of some new AEDs diminish the limitations of polytherapy, which is the only option when monotherapy fails. Unfortunately, the hierarchy of AEDs for combination therapy is far less certain than that for monotherapy. Some combinations should theoretically be avoided because of redundant mechanisms of action (e.g., primidone and phenobarbital) or the increased likelihood of toxicity (e.g., valproate and phenobarbital). Ultimately, combination preferences should be based on efficacy, cost, ease of introduction (including the rate of titration), and side effects, pending definitive study results. In the future, better drug delivery systems may increase the number of individuals who respond to AEDs. For example, it has been demonstrated that some individuals with drug-resistant epilepsy lack a glycoprotein transporter essential for the movement of medications across the blood-brain barrier (233). Direct drug delivery into the CNS might lead to seizure control in such individuals. Currently, in patients with secondary generalized seizures, failure of two or more appropriately chosen and adequately tried AEDs warrants consideration for epilepsy surgery (see also Chapter 73). Indeed, anyone who continues to experience GTCSs despite medical therapy should be referred without delay to a specialized epilepsy center.

REFERENCES

1. Merlis JK. Proposal for an international classification of the epilepsies. *Epilepsia* 1970;11:114–119.
2. Theodore WH, Porter RJ, Albert P, et al. The secondary generalized tonic-clonic seizure: a videotape analysis. *Neurology* 1994; 44:1403–1407.
3. Masland RL. The classification of the epilepsies: a historical review. In: Vinken PJ, Bruyn GW, eds. *The epilepsies. Handbook of clinical neurology,* vol 15. New York: American Elsevier, 1974:129.
4. Tissot SA. *Traite de l'epilepsie. Tome troisieme du traite des nerfs et de leurs maladies.* Paris: 1770.
5. Esquirol JED. *Des maladies mentales.* Paris: JB Bailliere, 1838.
6. Commission on Classification and Terminology of the International League Against Epilepsy. Proposal for revised clinical and electroencephalographic classification of epileptic seizures. *Epilepsia* 1981;22:489–501.
7. Gastaut H, Broughton R. *Epileptic seizures: clinical and electroencephalographic features, diagnosis and treatment.* Springfield, IL: Charles C Thomas, 1972.
8. Delgado-Escueta AV, Treiman DM, Walsh GO. The treatable epilepsies: parts 1 and 2. *N Engl J Med* 1983;308:1508–1514, 1576–1584.
9. Commission on Classification and Terminology of the International League Against Epilepsy. Proposal for classification of epilepsies and epileptic syndromes. *Epilepsia* 1985;26: 268–278.
10. Aicardi J. Epileptic syndromes in childhood. *Epilepsia* 1988; 29:S1–S5.
11. Gastaut H, Zifkin BG. Benign epilepsy of childhood with occipital spike and wave complexes. In: Andermann F, Lugaresi E, eds. *Migraine and epilepsy.* Stoneham, England: Butterworths, 1987: 47–82.

12. Bebek N, Gürses C, Gokyigit A, et al. Hot water epilepsy: clinical and electrophysiologic findings based on 21 cases. *Epilepsia* 2001;42:1180–1184.
13. Browne TR. Tonic-clonic (grand mal) seizures. In: Brown TR, Feldman RG, eds. *Epilepsy diagnosis and management.* Boston: Little, Brown, 1983:51–60.
14. Marsden CD, Reynolds EH. Neurology, Part 1. In: Laidlaw J, Richens A, eds. *A textbook of epilepsy.* Edinburgh: Churchill Livingstone, 1982:97–131.
15. Panayiotopoulos CP, Tahan R, Obeid T. Juvenile myoclonic epilepsy: factors of error involved in diagnosis and treatment. *Epilepsia* 1991;32:672–676.
16. Annegers JF, Rocca WA, Hauser WA. Causes of epilepsy: contributions of the Rochester epidemiology project. *Mayo Clin Proc* 1996;71:570–575.
17. Eisner V, Pauli LL, Livingston S. Hereditary aspects of epilepsy. *Bull Johns Hopkins Hosp* 1959;105:245–271.
18. Eisner V, Pauli LL, Livingston S. Epilepsy in the family of epileptics. *J Pediatr* 1960;56:347–354.
19. Tsuboi T, Endo S. Incidence of seizures and EEG abnormalities among offspring of epileptic patients. *Hum Genet* 1977;36:173–189.
20. Greenberg DA, Delgado-Escueta AV, Widelitz H, et al. Juvenile myoclonic epilepsy (JME) may be linked to the Bf and HLA loci on human chromosome 6. *Am J Med Genet* 1988;31:185–192.
21. Durner M, Sander T, Greenberg DA, et al. Localization of idiopathic generalized epilepsy on chromosome 6p in families of juvenile myoclonic epilepsy patients. *Ann Neurol* 1991;41: 1651–1655.
22. Cossette P, Liu L, Brisebois K, et al. Mutation of GABRA1 in an autosomal dominant form of juvenile myoclonic epilepsy. *Nat Genet* 2002;31:184–189.
23. Bate L, Gardiner M. Genetics of inherited epilepsies. *Epileptic Disord* 1999;1:7–19
24. Biervert C, Schroeder C, Kubisch C, et al. A potassium channel mutation in neonatal epilepsy. *Science* 1998;279:403–406.
25. Singh NA, Charlier C, Stauffer D, et al. A novel potassium channel KCNQ2 is mutated in an inherited epilepsy of newborns. *Nat Genet* 1998;18:25–29.
26. Steinlein OK. Gene defects in idiopathic epilepsy. *Rev Neurol* 1999;155:450–453.
27. Steinlein OK. Idiopathic epilepsies with a monogenic mode of inheritance. *Epilepsia* 1999;40(Suppl 3):9–11.
28. Hirsch E, de Saint-Martin A, Marescaux C. Benign familial neonatal convulsions: a model of idiopathic epilepsy [French]. *Rev Neurol* 1999;155:463–467.
29. Steinlein OK, Stoodt J, Biervert C, et al. The voltage gated potassium channel KCNQ2 and idiopathic generalized epilepsy. *Neuroreport* 1999;10:1163–1166.
30. Scheffer IE, Berkovic SF. Generalized epilepsy with febrile seizures plus: a genetic disorder with heterogenous clinical phenotypes. *Brain* 1997;1220:479–490.
31. Singh R, Scheffer IE, Crossland K, et al. Generalized epilepsy with febrile seizures plus: a common childhood-onset genetic epilepsy syndrome. *Ann Neurol* 1999;45:75–81.
32. Wallace RH, Wang DW, Singh R, et al. Febrile seizures and generalised epilepsy associated with a mutation Na$^+$-channel 1 subunit gene SCN1B. *Nat Genet* 1998;19:366–370.
33. Baulac S, Gourfinkel-An I, Picard F, et al. A second locus for familial generalized epilepsy with febrile seizures plus (GEFS+) maps to chromosome 2Q21-Q33. *Epilepsia* 1999;40(Suppl 9):S164.
34. Durner M, Greenberg DA, Shinnar S, et al. Genome search in idiopathic generalized epilepsy. *Epilepsia* 1999;40(Suppl 9):S164.
35. Sander T, Kretz R, Schulz H, et al. Replication analysis of a putative susceptibility locus (EGI) for idiopathic generalized epilepsy on chromosome 8q24. *Epilepsia* 1998;39:715–720.
36. Durner M, Zhou G, Fu D, et al. Evidence for linkage of adolescent-onset idiopathic generalized epilepsies to chromosome 8 and genetic heterogeneity. *Am J Hum Genet* 1999;64:1411–1419.
37. Mikami M, Yasuda T, Terao A, et al. Localization of a gene for benign adult familial myoclonic epilepsy to chromosome 8q23.3-q24.1. *Am J Hum Genet* 1999;65:745–751.
38. Lehesjoki AE, Koskiniemi M. Progressive myoclonus epilepsy of Unverricht-Lundborg type. *Epilepsia* 1999;40(Suppl 3):S23–S28.
39. Ziegler A. Basic mechanisms of monogenic inheritance. *Epilepsia* 1999;40(Suppl 3)S4–S8.
40. Mole S, Gardiner M. Molecular genetics of neuronal ceroid lipofuscinoses. *Epilepsia* 1999;40(Suppl 3):S29–S32.
41. Cock H, Schapira AHV. Mitochondrial DNA mutations and mitochondrial dysfunction in epilepsy. *Epilepsia* 1999;40(Suppl 3): S33–S40.
42. Hauser WA, Kurland LT. The epidemiology of epilepsy in Rochester, Minnesota, 1935 through 1967. *Epilepsia* 1975;16:1–66.
43. Juul-Jensen P, Foldspang A. Natural history of epileptic seizures. *Epilepsia* 1983;24:297–312.
44. Tsuboi T. Prevalence and incidence of epilepsy in Tokyo. *Epilepsia* 1988;29:103–110.
45. Charlton MH, Yahr MD. Long-term follow-up of patients with petit mal. *Arch Neurol* 1967;16:595–598.
46. Currier RD, Kooi KA, Saidman LJ. Prognosis of "pure" petit mal: a follow-up study. *Neurology* 1963;13:959–967.
47. Dalby MA. Epilepsy and 3 per second spike and wave rhythms: a clinical, electroencephalographic and prognostic analysis of 346 patients. *Acta Neurol Scand* 1969;45(Suppl 40):1–183.
48. Livingston S, Torres I, Pauli LL, et al. Petit mal epilepsy. Results of a prolonged follow-up study of 117 patients. *JAMA* 1965;194: 227–232.
49. Sato S, Dreifuss FE, Penry JK. Diagnostic factors in absence seizures. *Neurology* 1976;26:788–796.
50. Sato S, Dreifuss FE, Penry JK, et al. Long-term follow-up of absence seizures. *Neurology* 1983;33:1590–1595.
51. Gastaut H, Gastaut JL, Goncalves e Silva GE, et al. Relative frequency of different types of epilepsy: a study employing the classification of the International League Against Epilepsy. *Epilepsia* 1975;16:457–461.
52. Gastaut H, Gastaut JA, Gastaut J, et al. Epilepsie generalisée primaire grand mal. In: Lugaresi E, Pazzaglia P, Tassinari CA, eds. *Evolution and prognosis of the epilepsies.* Bologna: Aulo Gaggi, 1973.
53. Niedermeyer E. Epileptic seizure disorders. In: Niedermeyer E, Lopes da Silva F, eds. *Electroencephalography: basic principles, clinical applications and related fields.* Baltimore, MD: Urban & Schwarzenberg, 1987:405–510.
54. Niedermeyer E. Migraine-triggered epilepsy. *Clin Electroencephalogr* 1993;24:37–43.
55. Mendez MF, Catanzaro P, Doss RC, et al. Seizures in Alzheimer's disease: clinicopathologic study. *J Geriatr Psychiatry Neurol* 1994;7:230–233.
56. Gastaut H, Tassinari CA, eds. *Epilepsies. Handbook of electroencephalography and clinical neurophysiology,* vol 13. Amsterdam: Elsevier Science, 1975.
57. Porter RJ. Diagnosis: generalized seizures. In: Walton J, ed. *Epilepsy: 100 elementary principles,* 2nd ed. *Major problems in neurology,* vol 20. London: WB Saunders, 1989:39–41.
58. Engel J Jr. *Seizures and epilepsy.* Philadelphia: FA Davis, 1989:31.
59. Devinsky O, Pacia SV. Seizures during clozapine therapy. *J Clin Psychiatry* 1994;55(Suppl B):153–156.
60. Keilson MJ, Hauser WA, Magrill JP, et al. ECG abnormalities in patients with epilepsy. *Neurology* 1987;37:1624–1626.
61. Laidlaw J, Richens A. *A textbook of epilepsy.* Edinburgh: Churchill Livingstone, 1982.
62. Dreyfus-Brisac C, Monod N. Electroclinical studies of status epilepticus and convulsions in the newborn. In: Kellaway P, Petersen I, eds. *Neurological and electroencephalographic correlative studies in infancy.* New York: Grune & Stratton, 1964:250–271.
63. Gomez MR, Klass DW. Epilepsies of infancy and childhood. *Ann Neurol* 1983;13:113–124.
64. Niedermeyer E, Sakkubai N. Degenerative disorders of the central nervous system. In: Niedermeyer E, Lopes da Silva F, eds. *Electroencephalography: basic principles, clinical applications and related fields.* Baltimore, MD: Urban & Schwarzenberg, 1987:263–282.
65. Caveness WF. Ontogeny of focal seizures. In: Jasper H, Ward AA Jr, Pope A, eds. *Basic mechanisms of the epilepsies.* Boston: Little, Brown, 1969:517–534.
66. Hess A. Postnatal development and maturation of nerve fibers in the central nervous system. *J Comp Neurol* 1954;100:461–480.
67. Huttenlocher PR. Myelination and the development of function in immature pyramidal tract. *Exp Neurol* 1970;29:405–415.

68. Purpura DP. Stability and seizure susceptibility of immature brain. In: Jasper H, Ward AA Jr, Pope A, eds. *Basic mechanisms of the epilepsies.* Boston: Little, Brown, 1969:481–505.

69. Schwartzkroin PA. Development of rabbit hippocampus: physiology. *Dev Brain Res* 1982;2:469–486.

70. Schwartzkroin PA, Altschuler RJ. Development of kitten hippocampal neurons. *Brain Res* 1977;134:429–444.

71. Prince DA, Gutnick MJ. Neuronal activities in epileptogenic foci of the immature cortex. *Brain Res* 1972;45:455–468.

72. Dyson SE, Jones DG. The morphological categorization of developing synaptic junctions. *Cell Tissue Res* 1976;167:363–371.

73. Schulz R, Lüders HO, Noachtar S, et al. Amnesia of the epileptic aura. *Neurology* 1995;45:231–235.

74. Bromfield EB, Porter RJ, Kelley K, et al. Progression to generalized tonic-clonic seizures. *Epilepsia* 1989;30:724–725.

75. Porter RJ. Clinical phenomenology of seizure spread. *Epilepsia* 1990;31:617.

76. Kramer RE, Levisohn PM. The duration of secondary generalized tonic-clonic seizures [abstract]. *Epilepsia* 1983;24:43–48.

77. Agathonikou A, Panayiotopulos CP, Giannakodimos S, et al. Typical absence status in adults: diagnostic and syndromic considerations. *Epilepsia* 1998;39:1265–1276.

78. Bell WL, Walczak TS, Shin C, et al. Painful generalised clonic and tonic-clonic seizures with retained consciousness. *J Neurol Neurosurg Psychiatry* 1997;63:792–795.

79. Hamer HM, Wyllie E, Lüders HO, et al. Symptomatology of epileptic seizures in the first three years of life. *Epilepsia* 1999;40:837–844.

80. Marks WJ Jr, Laxer KD. Semiology of temporal lobe seizures: value in lateralizing the seizure focus. *Epilepsia* 1998;39:721–726.

81. Oguni H, Uehara T, Imai K, et al. Atonic epileptic drop attacks associated with generalized spike-and-slow wave complexes: video-polygraphic study in two patients. *Epilepsia* 1997;38:813–818.

82. Bickford RG, Klass DW. Sensory precipitation and reflex mechanisms. In: Jasper H, Ward AA Jr, Pope A, eds. *Basic mechanisms of the epilepsies.* Boston: Little, Brown, 1969:543–564.

83. Baldy-Moulinier M, Touchon J, Besset A, et al. Sleep architecture and epileptic seizures. In: Degen R, Niedermeyer E, eds. *Epilepsy, sleep and sleep deprivation.* Amsterdam: Elsevier Science, 1984:109–118.

84. Kawahara R, Umegawa Y, Fukuhara T, et al. Polygraphic study of the clinical seizures induced during nocturnal sleep. *Folia Psychiatr Neurol Jpn* 1977;31:429–435.

85. Malow BA, Blaxton TA, Stertz B, et al. Carbamazepine withdrawal: effects of taper rate on seizure frequency. *Neurology* 1993;43:2280–2284.

86. Engel J Jr, Ochs RF, Gloor P. Metabolic studies of generalized epilepsy. In: Avoli M, Gloor P, Kostopoulos G, et al., eds. *Generalized epilepsy: neurobiological approaches.* Boston: Birkhauser, 1990:387–396.

87. Penfield W, Jasper H. *Epilepsy and the functional anatomy of the human brain.* Boston: Little, Brown, 1954.

88. Ochs R, Gloor P, Quesney F, et al. Does head turning during a seizure have lateralization or localizing significance? *Neurology* 1984;34:884–890.

89. Robillard A, Saint-Hilaire JM, Mercier RFT, et al. The lateralizing and localizing value of adversion in epileptic seizures. *Neurology* 1983;33:1241–1242.

90. Wyllie E, Lüders H, Morris HH, et al. The lateralizing significance of versive head and eye movements during epileptic seizures. *Neurology* 1986;36:606–611.

91. Kernan JC, Devinsky O, Luciano DJ, et al. Lateralized significance of head and eye deviation in secondary generalized tonic-clonic seizures. *Neurology* 1993;43:1308–1310.

92. Ajmone-Marsan C, Ralston BL. *The epileptic seizure.* Springfield, IL: Charles C Thomas, 1971.

93. Engel J Jr, Kuhl DE, Phelps ME. Patterns of human local cerebral glucose metabolism during epileptic seizures. *Science* 1982; 218:64–66.

94. Walczak TS, Rubinsky M. Plantar responses after epileptic seizures. *Neurology* 1994;44:2191–2193.

95. Helmstaedter C, Elger CE, Lendt M. Postictal courses of cognitive deficits in focal epilepsies. *Epilepsia* 1994;35:1073–1078.

96. Orringer CE, Eustace JC, Wunsch CD, et al. Natural history of lactic acidosis after grand-mal seizures. A model for the study of an anion-gap acidosis not associated with hyperkalemia. *N Engl J Med* 1977;297:796–799.

97. Simon RP. Management of status epilepticus. In: Pedley TA, Meldrum BS, eds. *Recent advances in epilepsy,* 2nd ed. New York: Churchill Livingstone, 1985:137–160.

98. Fishman RA. *Cerebrospinal fluid in diseases of the nervous system.* Philadelphia: WB Saunders, 1980:322.

99. Schmidley JW, Simon RP. Postictal pleocytosis. *Ann Neurol* 1981;9:81–84.

100. Aminoff MJ, Simon RP, Weidemann E. The hormonal responses to generalized tonic-clonic seizures. *Brain* 1984;107:569–578.

101. Abbott RJ, Browning MCK, Davidson DLW. Serum prolactin and cortisol concentrations after grand mal seizures. *J Neurol Neurosurg Psychiatry* 1980;43:163–167.

102. Pritchard PB III, Wannamaker BB, Sagel J, et al. Serum prolactin and cortisol levels in evaluation of pseudoepileptic seizures. *Ann Neurol* 1985;18:87–89.

103. Lindbom U, Tomson T, Nilsson BY, et al. Serum prolactin response to thyrotropin-releasing hormone during status epilepticus. *Seizure* 1993;2:235–239.

104. Dana-Haeri J, Trimble MR, Oxley J. Prolactin and gonadotropin changes following generalized and partial seizures. *J Neurol Neurosurg Psychiatry* 1983;46:331–335.

105. Ohman R, Wallinder J, Balidin J, et al. Prolactin response to electroconvulsive therapy. *Lancet* 1976;2:936–937.

106. Oxley J, Roberts M, Dana-Haeri J, et al. Evaluation of prolonged 4-channel EEG taped recordings and serum prolactin levels in the diagnosis of epileptic and nonepileptic seizures. In: Dam M, Gram L, Penry JK, eds. *Advances in epileptology: XIIth International Symposium.* New York: Raven Press, 1981:343–355.

107. Rao ML, Stefan H, Bauer J. Epileptic but not psychogenic seizures are accompanied by simultaneous elevation of serum pituitary hormones and cortisol levels. *Neuroendocrinology* 1989;49:33–39.

108. Pritchard PB III. The effect of seizures on hormones. *Epilepsia* 1991;32(Suppl 6):S46–S50.

109. Culebras A, Miller M, Bertram L, et al. Differential response of growth hormone, cortisol, and prolactin to seizures and stress. *Epilepsia* 1987;28:564–570.

110. Devinsky O, Emoto S, Nadi NS, et al. Cerebrospinal fluid levels of neuropeptides, cortisol, and amino acids in patients with epilepsy. *Epilepsia* 1993;34:255–261.

111. Wyllie E, Lüders H, Pippenger C, et al. Postictal serum creatine kinase in the diagnosis of seizure disorders. *Arch Neurol* 1985;42:123–126.

112. Chesson AL, Kasarskis EJ, Small VW. Postictal elevation of serum creatine kinase level. *Arch Neurol* 1983;40:315–317.

113. Vasconcelos D. Compression fractures of the vertebrae during major epileptic seizures. *Epilepsia* 1973;14:323–328.

114. Worthing HS, Kalinowsky LW. The question of vertebral fractures in convulsive therapy and epilepsy. *Am J Psychiatry* 1942;98:533–537.

115. Archibald R, Armstrong J. Recurrent postictal pulmonary edema. *Postgrad Med* 1978;63:210–213.

116. Mulroy JJ, Mickell JJ, Tong TK, et al. Postictal pulmonary edema in children. *Neurology* 1985;35:403–405.

117. Terrence CF, Wisotzky HM, Perper JA. Unexpected, unexplained death in epileptic patients. *Neurology* 1975;15:594–598.

118. Darnell JC, Jay SJ. Recurrent postictal pulmonary edema: a case report and review of the literature. *Epilepsia* 1982;23:71–83.

119. Greene R, Platt R, Matz R. Postictal pulmonary edema. *N Y State J Med* 1975;75:1257–1261.

120. Koppel BS, Pearl M, Perla E. Epileptic seizures as a cause of unilateral pulmonary edema. *Epilepsia* 1987;28:41–44.

121. McClellan MD, Dauber IM, Weil JV. Elevated intracranial pressure increased pulmonary vascular permeability to protein. *J Appl Physiol* 1989;67:1185–1191.

122. Bean J, Zee D, Thorn B. Pulmonary changes with convulsions induced by drugs and oxygen at high pressure. *J Appl Physiol* 1966;21:865–872.

123. Simon RP. Physiological consequences of status epilepticus. *Epilepsia* 1985;26(Suppl 1):S58–S66.

124. Simon RP. Medullary lesion inducing pulmonary edema: a magnetic resonance imaging study. *Ann Neurol* 1991;30:727–730.

125. Annegers JF, Hauser WA, Elveback LR. Remission of seizures and relapse in patients with epilepsy. *Epilepsia* 1979;20:729–737.

126. Nashef L, Garner S, Sander JW, et al. Circumstances of death in epilepsy: interviews of bereaved relatives. *J Neurol Neurosurg Psychiatry* 1998;64:349–352.
127. Nashef L, Sander JW. Sudden unexpected death in epilepsy? Where are we now? *Seizure* 1996;5:235–238.
128. Leestma JE, Kalekar MB, Teas SS, et al. Sudden unexpected death associated with seizures: analysis of 66 cases. *Epilepsia* 1984;25:84–88.
129. Kirby S, Sadler RM. Injury and death as a result of seizures. *Epilepsia* 1995;36:25–28.
130. Leestma J, Walczak T, Hughes JR, et al. A prospective study on sudden unexpected death in epilepsy. *Ann Neurol* 1989;26:195–203.
131. Tennis P, Cole TB, Annegers JF, et al. Cohort study of incidence of sudden unexplained death in persons with seizure disorder treated with antiepileptic drugs in Saskatchewan, Canada. *Epilepsia* 1995;36:29–36.
132. Timmings PL. Sudden unexpected death in epilepsy: a local audit. *Seizure* 1993;2:287–290.
133. Ficker DM, So EL, Shen WK, et al. Population-based study of the incidence of sudden unexplained death in epilepsy. *Neurology* 1998;51:1270–1274.
134. Nashef L, Walker F, Allen P, et al. Apnoea and bradycardia during epileptic seizures: relation to sudden death in epilepsy. *J Neurol Neurosurg Psychiatry* 1996;60:297–300.
135. Tavernor SJ, Brown SW, Tavernor RM, et al. Electrocardiographic QT lengthening associated with epileptiform EEG discharges? A role in sudden unexplained death in epilepsy? *Seizure* 1996;5:79–83.
136. Wayne SL, O'Donovan CA, McCall WV, et al. Postictal neurogenic pulmonary edema: experience from ECT model. *Convuls Ther* 1997;13:181–184.
137. Drake ME Jr, Andrews JM, Castleberry CM. Electrophysiologic assessment of autonomic function in epilepsy. *Seizure* 1998;7:91–96.
138. Clutter WE, Bier DM, Shah SD, et al. Epinephrine plasma metabolic clearance rates and physiological thresholds for metabolic and hemodynamic actions in man. *J Clin Invest* 1980;66:94–101.
139. Simon RP, Aminoff MJ, Benowitz NL. Changes in plasma catecholamines after tonic-clonic seizures. *Neurology* 1984;34:255–257.
140. Annegers JF, Hauser WA, Shirts SB. Heart disease mortality and morbidity in patients with epilepsy. *Epilepsia* 1984;25:699–704.
141. Annegers JF, Coan SP, Hauser WA, et al. Epilepsy, vagal nerve stimulation by the NCP system, mortality, and sudden, unexpected, unexplained death. *Epilepsia* 1998;39:206–212.
142. Leestma JE, Annegers JF, Brodie MJ, et al. Sudden unexplained death in epilepsy: observations from a large clinical development program. *Epilepsia* 1997;38:47–55.
143. Derby LE, Tennis P, Jick H. Sudden unexplained death among subjects with refractory epilepsy. *Epilepsia* 1996;37:931–935.
144. George JR, Davis GG. Comparison of anti-epileptic drug levels in different cases of sudden death. *J Forensic Sci* 1998;43:598–603.
145. Bauer J, Guldenberg V, Elger CE. The "trout phenomenon": a rare symptom of epileptic seizures [German]. *Nervenarzt* 1993;64:394–395.
146. Silbert PL, Radhakrishnan K, Johnson J, et al. The significance of the phi rhythm. *Electroencephalogr Clin Neurophysiol* 1995;95:71–76.
147. Doose H, Gerken H, Horstmann T, et al. Genetic factors in spike-wave absences. *Epilepsia* 1973;14:57–75.
148. Normand MM, Wszolek ZK, Klass DW. Temporal intermittent rhythmic delta activity in electroencephalograms. *J Clin Neurophysiol* 1995;12:280–284.
149. Ajmone-Marsan C, Zivin LS. Factors related to the occurrence of typical paroxysmal abnormalities in the EEG records of epileptic patients. *Epilepsia* 1970;11:361–381.
150. Gibbs FA, Gibbs EL. *Epilepsy. Atlas of electroencephalography.* Cambridge, MA: Addison-Wesley, 1952:2.
151. Broughton RJ. Epilepsy and sleep: a synopsis and prospectus. In: Degen R, Niedermeyer E, eds. *Epilepsy, sleep and sleep deprivation.* Amsterdam: Elsevier Science, 1984:317–346.
152. Cadilhac J, Vlakovitch B, Delange-Walter MME. Considérations sur les modifications des décharges épileptiques au cours de la période des mouvements oculaires. In: Fischgold H, ed. *Le sommeil de nuit normal et pathologique. Etudes Electroencéphalographiques.* Paris: Masson et Cie, 1965:275–282.
153. Ludwig B, Ajmone-Marsan C. EEG changes after withdrawal of medication in epileptic patients. *Electroencephalogr Clin Neurophysiol* 1975;39:173–181.
154. Niedermeyer E. Generalized seizure discharges and possible precipitating mechanisms. *Epilepsia* 1966;7:23–29.
155. Binnie CD. Generalized epilepsy: ictal and interictal. In: Wada JA, Ellingson RJ, eds. *Clinical neurophysiology of epilepsy. Handbook of electroencephalography and clinical neurophysiology,* vol. 4. Revised series. Amsterdam: Elsevier Science, 1990:263–290.
156. Newmark ME, Penry JK. *Photosensitivity and epilepsy: a review.* New York: Raven Press, 1979.
157. Hauser WA, Anderson VE, Rich SS. Effect of photoconvulsive response on the occurrence of seizures and of generalized EEG patterns in siblings of generalized spike and wave probands [abstract]. *Electroencephalogr Clin Neurophysiol* 1983;56:27P.
158. Gilliam FG, Chiappa KH. Significance of spontaneous epileptiform abnormalities associated with a photoparoxysmal response. *Neurology* 1995;45:453–456.
159. Naquet R, Valin A. Focal discharges in photosensitive generalized epilepsy. In: Avoli M, Gloor P, Kostopoulos G, et al., eds. *Generalized epilepsy: neurobiological approaches.* Boston: Birkhauser, 1990:273–295.
160. Tükel K, Jasper H. The electroencephalogram in parasagittal lesions. *Electroencephalogr Clin Neurophysiol* 1952;4:481–494.
161. Savic I, Pauli S, Thorell JO, et al. In vivo demonstration of altered benzodiazepine receptor density in patients with generalised epilepsy. *J Neurol Neurosurg Psychiatry* 1994;57:797–804.
162. Pedley TA, Tharp BR, Herman K. Clinical and electroencephalographic characteristics of midline parasagittal foci. *Ann Neurol* 1981;9:142–149.
163. Klass DW. Electroencephalographic manifestations of complex partial seizures. *Adv Neurol* 1975;11:113–140.
164. Fisch BJ. *Spehlmann's EEG primer.* Amsterdam: Elsevier Science, 1991:384–402.
165. Daube JR, Groover RV, Klass DW. Detection of focally initiated paroxysmal abnormalities by computerized spatial display [abstract]. *Electroencephalogr Clin Neurophysiol* 1973;34:104.
166. Gotman J. Computer analysis in epilepsy. In: Lopes da Silva FH, Storm van Leeuwen W, Rèmond A, eds. *Clinical applications of computer analysis of EEG and other neurophysiological signals. Handbook of electroencephalography and clinical neurophysiology,* vol 2. Revised series. Amsterdam: Elsevier Science, 1986: 171–200.
167. Gotman J. Interhemispheric relations during bilateral spike and wave activity. *Epilepsia* 1981;22:453–466.
168. Rovit RL, Gloor P, Rasmussen T. Intracarotid amobarbital in epileptic patients: a new diagnostic tool in clinical electroencephalography. *Arch Neurol* 1961;5:606–626.
169. Lombroso CT, Erba G. Primary and secondary bilateral synchrony in epilepsy. *Arch Neurol* 1970;22:321–334.
170. Fisch BJ. Interictal epileptiform activity: diagnostic and behavioral implications. *J Clin Neurophysiol* 2003;20:155–162.
171. Santamaria J, Chiappa KH. *The EEG of drowsiness.* New York: Demos Publications, 1987.
172. Zivin L, Ajmone-Marsan C. Incidence and prognostic significance of "epileptiform" activity in the EEG of nonepileptic subjects. *Brain* 1978;91:751–778.
173. Gerken H, Doose H. On the genetics of EEG anomalies in childhood, III: spikes and waves. *Neuropadiatrie* 1973;4:88–97.
174. Cavazzuti GB, Capella L, Nalin A. Longitudinal study of epileptiform EEG patterns in normal children. *Epilepsia* 1980;21:43–55.
175. Lüders H, Daube J, Johnson J, et al. Computer analysis of generalized spike and wave complexes. *Epilepsia* 1980;21:183.
176. Fisch BJ, Pedley TA. Generalized tonic-clonic epilepsies. In: Lüders H, Lesser RP, eds. *Epilepsy: electroclinical syndromes.* New York: Springer-Verlag, 1987:151–185.
177. Gastaut H, Fischer-Williams M. The physiopathology of epileptic seizures. In: Field J, Magoun HW, Hall VE, eds. *Handbook of physiology,* vol 1. *Neurophysiology.* Baltimore, MD: Williams & Wilkins, 1959:329–364.
178. Dempsey EW, Morison RS. The production of rhythmically recurrent cortical potentials after localized thalamic stimulation. *Am J Physiol* 1942;135:293–300.
179. Oakley JC, Seypert GW, Ward AA Jr. Conductance changes in neocortical propagated seizures: seizure termination. *Exp Neurol* 1972;37:300–311.

180. Ward AA Jr. Physiological basis of chronic epilepsy and mechanisms of spread. *Adv Neurol* 1983;34:189–198.
181. Lüders H, Lesser RP, Dinner DS, et al. Generalized epilepsies: a review. *Cleve Clin Q* 1984;1:205–226.
182. Fisch BJ, Klass DW. The diagnostic specificity of triphasic wave patterns. *Electroencephalogr Clin Neurophysiol* 1988;70:1–8.
183. Robin A, Binnie CD, Copas JB. Electrophysiological and hormonal responses to three types of electroconvulsive therapy. *Br J Psychiatry* 1985;147:707–712.
184. Hauser WA, Lee JR. Do seizures beget seizures? In: Sutula T, Pitkanen A, eds. *Progress in brain research.* Amsterdam Elsevier, 2002:215–220.
185. Elwes RDC, Johnson AL, Shorvon SD, et al. The prognosis for seizure control in newly diagnosed epilepsy. *N Engl J Med* 1984;311:944–947.
186. Group for the Study of the Prognosis of Epilepsy in Japan. Natural history and prognosis of epilepsy: report of a multi-institutional study in Japan. *Epilepsia* 1981;22:35–53.
187. Currie S, Heathfield KWG, Henson RA, et al. Clinical course and prognosis of temporal lobe epilepsy, a survey of 666 patients. *Brain* 1971;44:173–190.
188. Schmidt D, Tsai JJ, Janz D. Generalized tonic-clonic seizures in patients with complex partial seizures: natural history and prognostic relevance. *Epilepsia* 1983;24:43–48.
189. Rodin EA. *The prognosis of patients with epilepsy.* Springfield, IL: Charles C Thomas, 1968.
190. Emerson R, D'Souza BJ, Vining EP, et al. Stopping medication in children with epilepsy. *N Engl J Med* 1981;304:1125–1129.
191. Holowach Thurston J, Thurston DL, Nixon BB, et al. Prognosis in childhood epilepsy. Additional followup of 148 children 15–33 years after withdrawal of anticonvulsant therapy. *N Engl J Med* 1982;306:831–836.
192. Reynolds EH. The initiation of anticonvulsant drug therapy. In: Pedley TA, Meldrum BS, eds. *Recent advances in epilepsy,* 2nd ed. Edinburgh: Churchill Livingstone, 1985:101–109.
193. Reynolds EH, Elwes RDC, Shorvon SD. Why does epilepsy become intractable? Prevention of chronic epilepsy. *Lancet* 1983;2:952–954.
194. Labar D, Murphy J, Tecoma E, and the E04 VNS Study Group. Vagus nerve stimulation for medication-resistant generalized epilepsy. *Neurology* 1999;52:1510–1512.
195. Olejniczak P, Fisch BJ, Carey M, et al. The effect of vagus nerve stimulation on epileptiform activity recorded from hippocampal depth electrodes. *Epilepsia* 2001;42:423–429.
196. Velasco F, Velasco M, Velasco AL, et al. Electrical stimulation of the centromedian thalamic nucleus in control of seizures: long term studies. *Epilepsia* 1995;36:63–71.
197. Guberman A. Monotherapy or polytherapy for epilepsy? *Can J Neurol Sci* 1998;25:S3–S8.
198. Leppik IE. Rational monotherapy for epilepsy. *Baillieres Clin Neurol* 1996;54:749–755.
199. Wilder BJ, Homan RW. Definition of rational antiepileptic polypharmacy. *Epilepsy Res* 1996;11(Suppl):253–258.
200. Cruzan S. *Suspension of Felbatol use urged.* Washington, DC: Press Office, Food and Drug Administration, United States Department of Health and Human Services: August 1, 1994.
201. French J, Smith M, Faught E, et al. Practice advisory: the use of felbamate in the treatment of patients with intractable epilepsy. Report of the Quality Standards Subcommittee of the American Academy of Neurology and the American Epilepsy Society. *Epilepsia* 1999;40:803–808.
202. Heller AJ, Chesterman P, Elwes RDC, et al. Phenobarbitone, phenytoin, carbamazepine, or sodium valproate for newly diagnosed adult epilepsy: a randomized comparative monotherapy trial. *J Neurol Neurosurg Psychiatry* 1995;58:44–50.
203. Mattson RH, Cramer JA, Collins JF. A comparison of valproate with carbamazepine for the treatment of complex partial seizures and secondary generalized tonic-clonic seizures in adults. *N Engl J Med* 1992;328:207–208.
204. Mattson RH, Cramer JA, Collins JF, et al. Comparison of carbamazepine, phenobarbital, phenytoin, and primidone in partial and secondary generalized tonic-clonic seizures. *N Engl J Med* 1985;313:145–151.

205. Callaghan N, Kenny RA, O'Neill B, et al. A prospective study between carbamazepine, phenytoin, and primidone in partial and secondary generalized tonic-clonic seizures. *N Engl J Med* 1985;313:145–151.
206. Ramsay RE, Wilder BJ, Berger JR, et al. A double-blind study comparing carbamazepine with phenytoin as initial seizure therapy in adults. *Neurology* 1983;33:904–910.
207. Turnbull DM, Howell D, Rawlins MD, et al. Which drug for the adult epileptic patient: phenytoin or valproate? *Br Med J* 1985;290:8150–8159.
208. Wilder BJ, Ramsay RE, Murphy JV, et al. Comparison of valproic acid and phenytoin in newly diagnosed tonic clonic seizures. *Neurology* 1983;33:1474–1476.
209. Cramer J, Fisher R, Ben-Menachem E, et al. New antiepileptic drugs: comparison of key clinical trials. *Epilepsia* 1999;40: 590–600.
210. White HS. Comparative anticonvulsant and mechanistic profile of the established and newer antiepileptic drugs. *Epilepsia* 1999;40(Suppl 5):S2–S10.
211. Leppik IE. Role of new and established antiepileptic drugs. *Epilepsia* 1998;39(Suppl 5):S2–S6.
212. Pellock JM. Felbamate. *Epilepsia* 1999;40(Suppl 5):S57–S62.
213. Cereghino JJ, Leppik IE. Felbamate registry: HLA typing and urine metabolite screening. *Epilepsia* 1999;40(Suppl 9):99.
214. Motte J, Trevathan E, Arvidsson JF, et al. Lamotrigine for generalized seizures associated with the Lennox-Gastaut syndrome. Lamictal Lennox-Gastaut Study Group. *N Engl J Med* 1997;337:1807–1812.
215. Buchanan N. The use of lamotrigine in juvenile myoclonic epilepsy. *Seizure* 1996;5:149–151.
216. Wallace SJ. Myoclonus and epilepsy in childhood: a review of treatment with valproate, ethosuximide, lamotrigine and zonisamide. *Epilepsy Res* 1998;29:147–154.
217. Guerrini R, Belmonte A, Parmeggiani L, et al. Myoclonic status epilepticus following high dosage lamotrigine therapy. *Brain Dev* 1999;21:420–424.
218. Guerrini R, Dravet C, Genton P, et al. Lamotrigine and seizure aggravation in severe myoclonic epilepsy. *Epilepsia* 1998;39: 508–512.
219. Biton V, Montouris GD, Ritter F, et al, and the Topiramate YTC Study Group. A randomized, placebo-controlled study of topiramate in primary generalized tonic-clonic seizures. *Neurology* 1999;52:1330–1337.
220. Sachdeo RC, Glauser TA, Ritter F, et al. A double blind, randomized trial of topiramate in Lennox-Gastaut syndrome. Topiramate YL Study Group. *Neurology* 1999;52:1882–1887.
221. Glauser TA. Topiramate. *Epilepsia* 1999;40(Suppl 5):S71–S80.
222. Ojemann LM, Crawford CA, Dodrill CB, et al. Language disturbances as a side effect of topiramate and zonisamide therapy. *Epilepsia* 1999;40(Suppl 7):66.
223. Oommen KJ, Mathews S. Zonisamide: a new antiepileptic drug. *Clin Neuropharmacol* 1999;22:192–200.
224. Leppik IE. Zonisamide. *Epilepsia* 1999;40(Suppl 5):S23–S29.
225. Chadwick D. Gabapentin: clinical use. In: Levy RH, Mattson RH, Meldrum BS, eds. *Antiepileptic drugs,* 4th ed. New York: Raven Press, 1995:915–923.
226. Morris GL. Gabapentin. *Epilepsia* 1999;40(Suppl 5):S63–S70.
227. Chadwick D, Leiderman DB, Sauermann W, et al. Gabapentin in generalized seizures. *Epilepsy Res* 1996;25:191–197.
228. French JA. Vigabatrin. *Epilepsia* 1999;40(Suppl 5):S11–S16.
229. Fisgin T, Gurer Y, Tezic T, et al. Effects of intranasal midazolam and rectal diazepam on acute convulsions in children: Prospective randomized study. *J Child Neurol* 2002;17: 123–126.
230. Tecoma ES. Oxcarbamazepine. *Epilepsia* 1999;40(Suppl 5): S37–S46.
231. Leppik I, Norhria V, French JA, et al. Levetiracetam is effective in reducing partial onset seizures that are secondary generalized. *Epilepsia* 1999;40(Suppl 7):S144.
232. Cramer J, De Rue K, Devinsky O, et al. A systematic review of the behavioral effects of levetiracetam in adults with epilepsy, cognitive disorders, or an anxiety disorder during clinical trials. *Epilepsy Behav* 2003;4:124–132.
233. Siddiqui A, Kerb R, Weale ME, et al. Association of multidrug resistance in epilepsy with a polymorphism in the drug-transporter gene ABCB1. *N Engl J Med* 2003;348:1442–1448.

Absence Seizures

19

Selim R. Benbadis Samuel F. Berkovic

Absence seizures are the most extensively studied type of epileptic seizure. The remarkable association of clinical absences with generalized spike-wave discharges was recognized soon after the advent of electroencephalography (1–3). The relatively stereotyped clinical manifestations, along with frequent occurrence, ease of precipitation in the laboratory, and obvious and consistent electroencephalographic (EEG) expression, made absences the paradigm for detailed electroclinical correlations (4–9).

As discussed in Chapter 19, the terms "absence seizure" and "dialeptic seizure" have been proposed in a semiologic classification based on signs and symptoms only, regardless of EEG findings. In contrast to a purely symptomatologic approach, this chapter discusses absence seizures as defined electroclinically by the International Classification of Epileptic Seizures.

CLINICAL FEATURES

The International League Against Epilepsy (ILAE) classification of epileptic seizures recognizes two major types of absences: typical and atypical (10). Typical absences are characteristic of the idiopathic ("primary") generalized epilepsies (11,12), especially childhood and juvenile absence epilepsy and, less frequently, juvenile myoclonic epilepsy. Atypical absences, which have been less intensively studied, are seen in patients with symptomatic or cryptogenic generalized epilepsies, particularly Lennox-Gastaut syndrome (13–15).

Typical Absences

The characteristic features of typical absences allowed their identification as early as 1705, when Poupart wrote the first description. In the 20th century, Sauer introduced the term "pyknolepsy," which Adie subsequently used in characterizing the syndrome of childhood absence epilepsy (16,17). Although typical absences generally manifest in childhood, persistence into adult life may occur (18,19), and occasionally they can present *de novo* in adulthood (20). Typical absences usually last about 10 seconds (5,7,21). In the study by Penry and associates (7) of 374 absence seizures in 48 patients, the mean duration was 9 seconds (range, 1 to 45 seconds). Postictal confusion is either absent or very brief, lasting 2 or 3 seconds. Video EEG monitoring has allowed a moment-by-moment analysis of the attacks.

The ILAE classification recognizes subtypes of typical absence seizures (10), and mixed forms with various combinations can be seen.

- Absence with impaired consciousness. Ongoing activities cease abruptly, and the patient is motionless with a fixed blank stare and loss of contact; the eyes may roll upward briefly. The attack ends suddenly, with the patient usually unaware of the episode, although the passage of time may be deduced. After the attack, activities resume.
- Absence with (mild) clonic components. Mild clonic activity involves the eyelids, corners of the mouth, and sometimes the upper extremities. These clonic jerks, usually at 3 per second, can be subtle.
- Absence with atonic components. Sudden hypotonia may cause the head or trunk to slump forward and objects to drop from the hand. Falling is rare.
- Absence with tonic components. Increased tone may affect the flexors or extensors and may be symmetrical or asymmetrical. A standing patient may be propelled backward, and an asymmetrical increase in tone may turn the head or trunk to one side. Tonic features are always relatively minor and should not lead to confusion with the movements of generalized tonic seizures.
- Absence with automatisms. When the absence attack is relatively prolonged, automatisms may resemble those of complex partial seizures. Automatisms evolve in a craniocaudal fashion, with elevation of the eyelids, licking and swallowing, and, finally, fiddling and scratching movements of the hands (8,9).

■ Absence with autonomic phenomenon. Perioral pallor, pupillary dilation, flushing, tachycardia, piloerection, salivation, and incontinence may occur.

The frequency of these various features depends on how carefully they are looked for and the referral base from which cases are drawn. On the basis of ordinary history taking, simple absences and absences with mild clonic phenomena are by far the most common, followed by absences with automatisms and decreased postural tone. Studies using videotapes increase the frequency of the less commonly identified types and mixed forms (7). The categorization of typical absences into the above subtypes, although useful descriptively, probably has no clinical or neurobiologic significance. Many authors now refer only to simple absences and complex absences, the latter describing attacks with any combination of clonic, atonic, tonic, automatic, or autonomic features (22,23).

In the electroencephalography laboratory, typical absences are precipitated by hyperventilation in virtually all untreated patients and by photic stimulation in approximately 15% of individuals. The level of hypocapnia that induces absence seizures appears to vary among individuals (24). In everyday life, absences often occur with tiredness or boredom and are generally suppressed by attention, although demanding tasks and, in some patients, specific mental activities, such as calculation, may precipitate absences (25). Overbreathing during physical exercise decreases the frequency of absences (26).

Atypical Absences

Atypical absences have not been studied as thoroughly as typical absences and have been distinguished from the latter mainly by EEG criteria (5,21). The clinical features of atypical absences have resisted easy recognition because the patients are often mentally retarded and exhibit multiple other seizure types, both features being typical of symptomatic or cryptogenic generalized epilepsies (see Chapter 22). In addition, onset and offset are not as crisply delineated as are those of typical absences, partly because polypharmacy in intellectually disabled patients makes detection of altered awareness difficult. Careful analysis of videotaped seizures, however, often shows a change in behavior when the ictal discharge terminates (21).

Atypical absences average about 5 to 10 seconds in length (5,21,27), although they can be prolonged to the extent of absence status. Minor myoclonic, tonic, atonic, and autonomic features, as well as automatisms, may accompany the altered awareness. Tonic seizures, characterized by rhythmic fast activity, frequently occur, and the clinical and EEG features merge into those of the atypical absence (21,23). Unlike typical absences, however, atypical absences are usually not precipitated by hyperventilation or photic stimulation (21,28).

Other Types of Absences

The relationship of absence and myoclonus is complex, and the nomenclature in the literature is confusing. Rhythmic jerking of the eyelids and facial muscles is common in typical absences, but more widespread myoclonus as part of absence seizures is rare. In some patients, however, discrete myoclonic seizures involving the extremities (without impairment of consciousness) occur independently of absences. In principle, the distinction between absences with myoclonus and independent absence with myoclonic seizures is obvious, being based on impaired consciousness with myoclonic movements. In practice, however, this distinction can be ill defined in some patients and may require video-EEG monitoring to establish.

Tassinari and colleagues (29,30) described the myoclonic absence. Not specifically identified in the ILAE classification, this seizure involves 10 to 60 seconds of rhythmic jerking of the shoulders, arms, and legs, with tonic contraction around the shoulders. It has a poor prognosis and appears to be specific to the syndrome of epilepsy with myoclonic absences (see causes). The myoclonic absence cannot be confused clinically with true absence because of its obvious convulsive features; the name derives from an association with typical 3-Hz spike-and-wave discharges.

At the onset of an attack, some patients with absences and photosensitivity have jerking of the eyelids with upward eye deviation. Some experts regard these seizures as a special type known as eyelid myoclonia with absences (19,31–33). Others believe that the so-called eyelid myoclonia represents voluntary (or subconscious) eye blinking that precipitated photosensitive absences (34–36). Characteristically, voluntary eye closure is followed by slow upward eye movement and rapid fluttering of the eyelids. Some patients continue to show eye blinking, without impaired consciousness, when the epileptiform discharges have been suppressed by medication. Thus, continued blinking must not be uncritically accepted as evidence of uncontrolled absences. Whether the clinical features and natural history of these patients warrant designation as a separate subgroup remains unproved. Similarly, the proposal to designate perioral myoclonia with absences as a distinct group requires further study (37).

Delgado-Escueta and associates (38) used the terms "myoclonus absence," "myoclonic absence with 4- to 6-Hz multispike-and-wave complexes," and "juvenile absence with 8- to 12-Hz rhythms" to denote other allegedly distinct types of absence. Although attacks resembling absences with unusual electroclinical features undoubtedly occur, we find this nomenclature unhelpful and unsubstantiated by published data.

In absences with focal features (39), cerebral damage is often present, and at least some of the attacks probably represent frontal lobe seizure mimicking absences (22,40).

ELECTROENCEPHALOGRAPHIC FEATURES

The EEG signature of an absence attack is a bilaterally synchronous spike-and-wave discharge at 2.5 to 4.0 Hz. So strong is the association of clinical absences with generalized spike-and-wave discharge that it is probably inappropriate to regard staring spells with any other type of epileptic discharge as absences. Some electroclinical observations (see other electroencephalographic patterns) suggest that other types of discharges may accompany clinical absences, but the classification of these events remains controversial. Because any epileptic spike is typically followed by a slow wave, a useful rule of thumb is to reserve the term spike-wave complexes for repetitive discharges of 3 or more seconds (41).

Typical Absences

Ictal Discharges

Typical absences show the classic 3-Hz spike-wave discharges (Fig. 19.1). The discharge begins suddenly without any preictal EEG disturbance. The frequency is usually about 3 to 4 Hz at onset and slows to 2.5 to 3.0 Hz toward the end of the discharge. A characteristic electrical field shows maximum negativity symmetrically at F_7/F_8 or F_3/F_4. A single spike is followed by a single wave ("dart and dome"); however, during sleep or in older patients, a double spike or, more rarely, multiple spikes may develop. Toward the end of the discharge, not only does the frequency decrease slightly, but the spikes may also become less apparent and drop out. The discharges are characteristically provoked by hyperventilation. Photic stimulation precipitates absence seizures in approximately 15% of patients (4,5,22,42–46).

Interictal Electroencephalography

Brief generalized 3-Hz spike-wave discharges occur without obvious clinical change. The distinction between interictal and ictal discharges in patients with typical absences is blurred and depends on the sophistication of testing. The morphology of the discharges does not differ, but the longer the discharge, the more likely it will have subtle or obvious clinical accompaniments. A generally accepted observation is that discharges lasting longer than 3 seconds can be noticed in everyday life by an attentive observer. Continuous response tasks show decreased performance during even briefer discharges and sometimes even slightly before the discharge. The background activity is normal, except for intermittent rhythmic posterior delta activity seen in some children.

During light sleep, the discharges increase in frequency and irregularity, and may develop into multiple spike discharges (Fig. 19.1). In stages III and IV of sleep, the number of spikes rises again, and the waves become longer and more distorted. The basic morphology during rapid eye movement sleep is similar to that during resting wakefulness. Polyspikes during sleep appear to be associated with a less favorable prognosis (47). This would make sense, because such cases would move closer toward the symptomatic

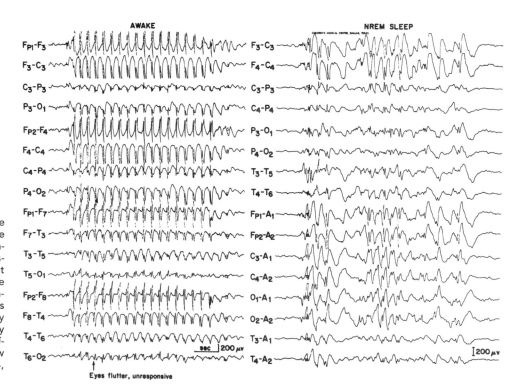

Figure 19.1 Typical absence recorded in a 7-year-old girl. The awake record shows a classic generalized 3-Hz spike-and-wave discharge. In nonrapid eye movement sleep, the discharges are more irregular, and the one-to-one relationship between spikes and waves is lost. (From Daly DD. Epilepsy and syncope. In: Daly DD, Pedley TA, eds. *Current practice of clinical electroencephalography.* New York: Raven Press, 1990:269–334, with permission.)

generalized epilepsy on the neurobiologic continuum described later in Figure 19.4.

The discharges in simple absences are characteristically bilateral and symmetrical, but varying degrees of asymmetry and occasional brief unilateral discharges can be present. In such electroencephalograms, the asymmetries typically change from side to side, and on evaluation of the whole record, the generalized process becomes clear. Exceptionally, persistently unilateral discharges may occur. Such asymmetries should not lead to an erroneous diagnosis of partial epilepsy (48,49).

Atypical Absences

Ictal Discharges

Generalized slow spike-wave discharges are usually far less regular (monomorphic) in morphology, lower in amplitude, and have broader and blunter spikes than those seen in typical absences (Fig. 19.2). The frequency is approximately 1.5 Hz (<2.5 Hz).

The discharges are distributed similarly to those of typical absences, but are more often asymmetrical and usually less perfectly monomorphic (i.e., more irregular). The asymmetry may correlate with focal neurologic signs or radiologic deficits on the affected side.

Interictal Electroencephalography

Brief bursts of slow spike and wave are superimposed on a diffusely slow background and focal or multifocal spikes. This combination of findings is characteristic of symptomatic or cryptogenic generalized epilepsies (see Chapter 22). The discharges are activated in sleep and interspersed with brief runs of generalized rapid spikes, with or without clinical tonic seizures (1,4,5,15,42,43,50,51).

Other Electroencephalographic Patterns

A number of other EEG patterns are associated with staring spells, but they are not clearly associated with absence seizures.

Generalized Rhythmic Delta Activity

Lee and Kirby (52) described seven children who experienced brief periods of loss of awareness associated with generalized high-amplitude rhythmic delta activity, without a spike component. Nearly all electroclinical observations were made during hyperventilation. The authors characterized these events as absences because of the consistent clinical features and the response to antiabsence medication. Our view, and that of others (28,53,54), is that such attacks represent hyperventilation-induced nonepileptic spells.

Low-Voltage Fast Rhythms

Gastaut and Broughton (5) described patterns of diffuse flattening, low-voltage fast activity at about 20 Hz, and rhythmic 10-Hz sharp waves associated with atypical absences, in addition to the classic slow spike-and-wave discharge. These patterns also typically accompany tonic seizures in patients with Lennox-Gastaut syndrome. It is therefore arguable whether staring spells associated with these faster EEG rhythms, and often with some increase in axial tone, should be regarded as atypical absences; they are probably better classified as tonic seizures (5,14). Similarly, staring spells with generalized fast rhythms or diffuse EEG flattening are occasionally observed without tonic seizures or Lennox-Gastaut syndrome (38,42). Some episodes represent partial seizures from occult frontal lobe foci, whereas others remain unclassified (46,55,56). Generalized fast activity has also been described during (clinically) typical absence seizures (57).

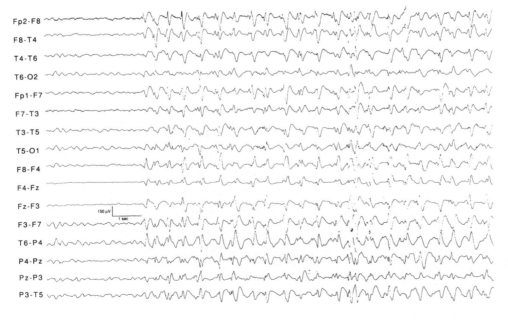

Figure 19.2 Slow spike-and-wave discharge (2 Hz) in an 18-year-old boy with atypical absences as a consequence of Lennox-Gastaut syndrome.

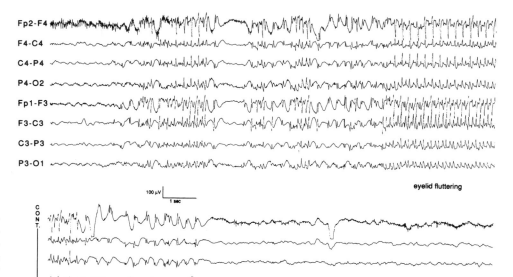

Figure 19.3 Staring spell associated with eyelid fluttering in a 45-year-old man with refractory generalized epilepsy since adolescence. Other family members had well-controlled generalized epilepsy. The clinical attack was associated with a complex generalized electroencephalographic abnormality comprising periods of 9- to 13-Hz spikes, intermingled with 2- to 4-Hz spike-and-wave discharges and periods of generalized flattening.

Mixed Patterns

Exceptional patients with staring spells show mixed slow and diffuse fast rhythms during attacks (Fig. 19.3), whose nosologic position is uncertain. The fast rhythms are likely caused by a neurophysiologic mechanism different from that of spike-and-wave discharges. Until the neurobiologic differences of these discharges are better understood, the value of classification will remain dubious.

DIAGNOSIS

Establishing the diagnosis of typical absences is usually not difficult. Staring spells reported by parents or schoolteachers and observation of attacks induced by hyperventilation raise the suspicion, which can be confirmed by a single electroencephalogram recording. Provided that hyperventilation is well performed, the lack of spike-and-wave discharges should cast serious doubt on the diagnosis of typical absence seizures. If 3 minutes of hyperventilation is ineffective, an extension to 5 minutes may be valuable. In adults, typical absences may be mild and inconspicuous, occurring infrequently with only incomplete loss of awareness. Momentary lack of concentration ("phantom absences") or experiential phenomena could be misinterpreted as complex partial seizures or psychogenic events (19).

Atypical absences rarely will be the sole clinical feature of an epileptic syndrome, but this eventuality can signal a more sinister disorder with mental retardation and multiple other seizure types, particularly tonic and atonic attacks (15,58).

Seizure Type Versus Epileptic Syndrome

Although interesting descriptively, the distinctions among multiple subtypes of typical absences likely have no clinical or neurobiologic significance (59). The important and practical diagnosis is that of idiopathic generalized epilepsy with absence seizures (60), as explained in Chapter 25. Similarly, atypical absence and its variants indicate a diagnosis of symptomatic or cryptogenic generalized epilepsy of the Lennox-Gastaut type. It is the syndromic diagnosis, not the identification of the seizure type, which is most useful for management (61).

Differential Diagnosis

Distinguishing absence seizures from simple daydreaming and inattentiveness is a common challenge in pediatrics. Many children are occasionally inattentive; this is a very common complaint in the outpatient setting. The family or teacher reports brief episodes of staring and unresponsiveness with no significant motor manifestations. Is the child having absence seizures or innocent nonepileptic staring spells? Based on a questionnaire given to parents, several features were identified that can help distinguish the two scenarios in otherwise normal children (62). Three features suggest *nonepileptic* events: (a) the events do not interrupt play; (b) the events were first noticed by a professional, such as a schoolteacher, speech therapist, occupational therapist, or physician (rather than by a parent); and (c) the staring child is responsive to touch, or "interruptible" by other external stimuli. These features each have approximately 80% specificity for suggesting nonepileptic staring episodes. Several factors are associated with an *epileptic* etiology, including twitches of the arms or legs, loss of urine, or upward eye movement. Thus, video-EEG monitoring may not be necessary in otherwise normal children with staring spells, a normal routine EEG, positive responses to the nonepileptic types of questions, and no positive responses to the epileptic types of questions. Other features that are suggestive of nonepileptic or behavioral, rather than epileptic, staring include lower age and lower frequency of episodes (63). Similarly, *sustained* inattention is more often associated with attention deficit hyperactivity disorder than with absence seizures (64).

Differentiating absences and brief complex partial seizures, particularly those of temporal lobe origin, is not usually difficult, but occasionally, brief temporal lobe seizures may be clinically indistinguishable from more prolonged absences that show automatisms. In general, however, complex partial seizures of temporal lobe origin have an aura, last longer than 30 seconds (compared with 20 seconds or less for absences), involve complex automatisms or postictal confusion, and are usually infrequent and clustered, rather than frequent and related to the time of day or fatigue (22,55). The interictal electroencephalogram may show focal temporal spikes instead of generalized discharges. Video-EEG monitoring (65) is occasionally required to make the distinction—a crucial one, because of the greatly different prognostic and therapeutic implications.

Less commonly, complex partial seizures of frontal lobe origin can mimic absences. Clinical, EEG, or radiologic features of a frontal focus usually lead to correct diagnosis (55,66–69); however, an occult frontal focus, especially on the mesial surface of one hemisphere, can sometimes cause brief seizures with generalized discharges (i.e., "secondary bilateral synchrony"), complicating the differentiation (40,56,70,71). Clues from the electroencephalogram include irregular epileptiform discharges, with a maximum field in or just adjacent to the midline, rather than the characteristic bilateral maximum field at F_7/F_8, and occasional focal discharges (43,72).

CAUSES

Typical absences are observed in the context of the idiopathic (genetic) generalized epilepsies, especially childhood and juvenile absence epilepsies, and juvenile myoclonic epilepsy (73–75). Atypical absences, on the other hand, are seen in patients with Lennox-Gastaut syndrome and other varieties of cryptogenic or symptomatic generalized epilepsy (14,22,50,55,58,76) (see Chapter 27).

As discussed, myoclonic absences are characteristic of and probably exclusive to the rare syndrome of epilepsy with myoclonic absences. Recognition of this syndrome is important because of its guarded prognosis in the presence of apparently "benign" EEG findings with 3-Hz spike-and-wave discharges (29,30,77).

In rare instances, absences can be symptomatic of specific diffuse cerebral disorders (40,55,78), such as subacute sclerosing panencephalitis (79,80), lysosomal storage disorders (81,82), and metabolic encephalopathies or benzodiazepine withdrawal (83), although in these settings, absence status is usually seen, rather than isolated absence seizures (46,84,85).

Exceptionally, diencephalic lesions have been associated with generalized spike-and-wave discharges, although other seizure patterns are more characteristic of these lesions than are absence attacks (46,86–88).

Brief staring attacks occur in patients with frontal epilepsy (66–68,70). When such attacks are associated with frontal damage and bilaterally synchronous epileptic discharges, it can be impossible to determine whether the case is a focal, multifocal, or secondarily generalized form of epilepsy (55,71,89,90). Such cases illustrate that although the distinction between focal and generalized epileptic processes is extremely valuable, it is not absolute.

PATHOGENESIS

Genetic and Acquired Factors

The inherited factor in human absences has long been recognized. In the 1960s, Metrakos and Metrakos (91–93) showed that the spike-and-wave trait was inherited with an age-dependent penetrance that was low at birth, rose to a maximum of approximately 40% at age 10 years, and gradually declined to near zero after age 40 years. Of the relatives who showed this trait, however, only about 20% experienced clinical generalized epilepsy. The authors suggested that the trait was autosomal dominant (91–93). Although it can be transmitted vertically through families, subsequent studies and reinterpretation of their original data suggest that a single autosomal dominant gene is less likely (55,94–100).

Twin studies provided strong evidence of the primacy of genetic factors in typical absences. Lennox and Lennox (101) observed that monozygotic twins have a 75% concordance for absence seizures and an 84% concordance for the 3-Hz spike-and-wave trait. Researchers obtained essentially identical findings in a contemporary series of twins with idiopathic generalized epilepsies, demonstrating that genetic factors are central to the etiology of the syndromes of childhood absence and juvenile absence epilepsies, but that inheritance was polygenic (102). The concordance in monozygotic twins does not reach 100%, however, suggesting a small role for acquired factors (55,89,101,102).

Acquired factors have major importance in the symptomatic generalized epilepsies (13,14,22,101). The slow spike-and-wave discharges, diffusely slow background, and association with intellectual disability suggest the presence of diffusely pathologic gray matter. A wide variety of prenatal, perinatal, and postnatal factors have been implicated, although a clear-cut cause is often not identifiable in individual patients (13,14,22,101). Defined genetic causes of these epilepsies (e.g., tuberous sclerosis, lipid storage disorders) are relatively rare, but additional cases provide some evidence that genetic factors are involved (15,22,44,51). Recent twin data indicate that the genetic influence in these epilepsies has been underestimated in the past (102).

Some cases do not fit easily into either idiopathic or symptomatic generalized epilepsies, and are best understood by regarding these epilepsies as a neurobiologic continuum (Fig. 19.4) comprising both genetic and acquired factors (55,89,90,94,103,104).

Genes responsible for common absence epilepsies have not yet been definitively identified. Two families with childhood absence epilepsy and mutations in the gamma-2 subunit gene of the γ-aminobutyric acid A (GABA$_A$) receptor have been described (105,106), but most patients with absence do not have mutations in this gene. A report from China described variations in the calcium channel gene *CACNA1H* in some subjects with childhood absence epilepsy (107), but this was not replicated in a white sample (108). Animal models of inherited generalized epilepsies offer the possibility of identifying genetic mechanisms relevant to human absence epilepsies. Some single-gene rodent models, however, have other major neurologic defects (109) and thus do not resemble human idiopathic generalized epilepsies. Rodent models more closely resembling human idiopathic absence epilepsies have now been identified, with genetic analysis suggesting that, like

human syndromes, these models also show polygenic inheritance, although specific genes have not yet been identified (110).

Anatomical Abnormalities

By definition, the brain in patients with typical absences due to idiopathic generalized epilepsies is anatomically normal on magnetic resonance imaging (MRI) or routine histologic examination. Some studies suggested minor morphologic changes (i.e., microdysgenesis) in patients with typical idiopathic generalized epilepsies, but these remain controversial (111–114). These changes, which would be expected to appear in the last trimester of intrauterine development, may represent the gross morphologic correlate of abnormal synaptic connectivity, due to genetic or acquired factors, that underlies diffuse cortical hyperexcitability (see below).

In atypical absences, the issue of structural abnormalities is more complicated. Some patients have obvious diffuse or focal cortical abnormalities on the basis of clinical signs, cognitive deficits, or radiologic studies. Histologic examination would be expected to show heterogeneous change (50). Other patients, however, display microdysgenesis similar to that observed in those with primary generalized epilepsy (112).

Neurophysiology

The striking electroclinical phenomenon of absence with generalized spike-and-wave discharge has intrigued neurophysiologists since its discovery in the 1930s (2,3,115,116). Gibbs and associates (1–3) first proposed that a diffuse cortical disturbance caused these discharges. Subsequently, Penfield and Jasper (45,117–119) proposed the centrencephalic hypothesis, in which a subcortical neuronal system centered on the midline structures of the upper brainstem and diencephalon (centrencephalic system) gives rise to discharges that synchronously entrain cortical regions in both hemispheres. This intuitively appealing hypothesis has been controversial (116).

An impressive body of data from human studies (46,56,70,71,120) points to the cerebral cortex as the site of the primary abnormality. Gloor's studies (90,121–124) in feline generalized penicillin epilepsy suggest that the basic disturbance is a diffuse moderate hyperexcitability of cortical neurons, which causes them to respond to thalamocortical volleys by inducing spike-and-wave discharges instead of spindles. However, Gloor has moved away from the view that the thalamus acts only as a source of thalamocortical impulses that trigger cortical spike-and-wave bursts (121). Rather, he believes that the thalamus becomes actively involved in and constitutes an essential component of the neuronal system sustaining these discharges (123,125).

Currently, generalized spike-and-wave discharges are believed to reflect a widespread phase-locked oscillation

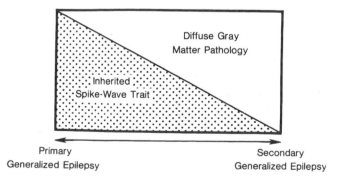

Figure 19.4 The spectrum of the generalized epilepsies. On one end, the primary (idiopathic) generalized epilepsies are largely determined by genetic factors. On the other end, the secondary (symptomatic) generalized epilepsies are associated with diffuse gray matter pathology. (From Berkovic SF, Andermann F, Andermann E, et al. Concepts of absence epilepsies: discrete syndromes or biological continuum? *Neurology* 1987;37:993–1000, with permission.)

between excitation (spike) and inhibition (wave) in mutually connected thalamocortical neuronal networks (123). Studies of spontaneous spike-and-wave discharges in the Wistar rat support data from the feline penicillin model suggestive of a tightly interlocked thalamocortical mechanism, although initiation of the discharge from the cortex does not seem to occur in this rat model (109).

The finding that the antiabsence drug ethosuximide specifically affects low-threshold calcium currents in thalamic neurons has again raised the question of the primacy of the thalamus in generating the seizures (126). A defect of the low-threshold calcium channels is unlikely to be the primary cause of absence seizures, however. Rather, the thalamocortical system must be viewed as an oscillating network generating a variety of physiologic and pathologic rhythms (127), which is also influenced by ascending projections to both cortex and thalamus. Thus, interference at many points in the network can precipitate or interrupt absence seizures (127,128).

Cerebral Blood Flow and Metabolism

Using positron emission tomography (PET), Engel and colleagues (129) noted a diffuse increase in cerebral glucose metabolism in children with typical absences during periods of prolonged spike-and-wave discharges, but this finding was not replicated in two other studies in older patients with more difficult types of epilepsy (130,131). Thus, the EEG spike-and-wave discharge appears to have no specific metabolic correlate (132). In a genetic model of absence seizures in rats, affected animals had an increased rate of glucose use in most cerebral structures compared with that in control animals (133), which would support the human data supplied by Engel and colleagues. A 15% increase in global cerebral blood flow with an additional increase in the thalamus on the left (134,135) was demonstrated by means of $H_2{}^{15}O$ and PET. Contrary data come from transcranial Doppler studies of the middle cerebral artery during absence seizures. Decreased blood flow velocities and increased pulsatility index indicated reduced cerebral blood flow (136). Recent transcranial Doppler data revealed that flow velocities increase just before and decrease immediately after the seizure (137). Some evidence, including data derived from ictal single-photon emission computed tomography, suggests that blood flow may be reduced in the cortex but increased in subcortical structures (138–140). A coherent synthesis of data on cerebral blood flow and metabolism therefore awaits the results of further studies (134).

Functional Magnetic Resonance Imaging

One patient with idiopathic generalized epilepsy and frequent absences was studied using EEG-correlated functional MRI (141). Four prolonged runs of generalized spike-wave discharges occurred during a 35-minute experiment. Time-locked activation was observed bilaterally within the thalami in conjunction with widespread, but symmetrical, cortical deactivation with a frontal maximum. This study suggests reductions in cortical blood flow in response to synchronized electroencephalogram activity.

Neurochemistry

Snead (128) reviewed the complex literature on neurochemical and neuropharmacologic findings in animal models of absence, including intensive investigations of the role of GABA, the major cerebral inhibitory transmitter. Although early studies raised the possibility that increased GABA activity might suppress absences (142) as it does major convulsive seizures (143), recent data clearly show that increased GABAergic inhibition potentiates experimental spike-and-wave discharges (128). The exacerbation of human absences by vigabatrin (47) and tiagabine (144) supports this conclusion. Moreover, $GABA_B$, but not $GABA_A$, antagonists block experimental absence seizures (128,145). $GABA_B$ receptors mediate long-lasting thalamic inhibitory postsynaptic potentials that are critical to the generation of normal thalamocortical rhythms. An inherited defect in the $GABA_B$ receptor could therefore underlie absence epilepsies, although the preponderance of experimental data does not favor this hypothesis (128). In humans with generalized epilepsy, the $GABA_A$-benzodiazepine receptor complex has been studied using the benzodiazepine antagonist $[{}^{11}C]$ flumazenil; no significant difference in receptor density was found between patients and control subjects in the interictal state (146,147) or during absences (134).

Other possible mechanisms of absence include the actions of γ-hydroxybutyric acid, a naturally occurring metabolic product of GABA that has its own specific binding sites and can cause absences experimentally (128). Modulation of glutamatergic, noradrenergic, dopaminergic, cholinergic, and opioid mechanisms also influences experimental absences (108,109,128). No evidence suggests that abnormalities in these systems are fundamental to the etiology of inherited absences, except in the tottering mouse mutant, which exhibits a proliferation of noradrenergic locus ceruleus axons in thalamocortical target regions (107). In humans, PET studies with the opiate ligand $[{}^{11}C]$diprenorphine showed no difference in receptor density compared with that in control subjects in the interictal state, although release of endogenous opioids was suggested during absences (134).

REFERENCES

1. Gibbs FA, Gibbs EL. *Atlas of electroencephalography, II.* Cambridge, MA: Addison-Wesley, 1952:9–10.
2. Gibbs FA, Gibbs EL, Lennox WG. The influence of blood sugar level on the wave and spike formation in petit mal epilepsy. *Arch Neurol Psychiatry* 1939;41:1111–1116.
3. Gibbs FA, Lennox WG, Gibbs EL. The electroencephalogram in diagnosis and in localization of epileptic seizures. *Arch Neurol Psychiatry* 1936;36:1225–1235.

4. Gastaut H. Clinical and electroencephalographic correlates of generalized spike-and-wave bursts occurring spontaneously in man. *Epilepsia* 1968;9:179–184.
5. Gastaut H, Broughton R. *Epileptic seizures: clinical and electroencephalographic features, diagnosis and treatment.* Springfield, IL: Charles C Thomas, 1972:64–85.
6. Panayiotopoulos CP, Obeid T, Waheed G. Differentiation of typical absences in epileptic syndromes: a video EEG study of 224 seizures in 20 patients. *Brain* 1989;112:1039–1056.
7. Penry JK, Porter RJ, Dreifuss FE. Simultaneous recording of absence seizures with videotape and electroencephalography. A study of 374 seizures in 48 patients. *Brain* 1975;98:427–440.
8. Stefan H. *Epileptische absencen.* Stuttgart, Germany: Georg Thieme, 1982.
9. Stefan H, Burr W, Hildenbrand K, et al. Basic temporal structure of absence symptoms. In: Akimoto H, Kazamatsuri H, Seino M, et al., eds. *Advances in epileptology: XIIIth Epilepsy International Symposium.* New York: Raven Press, 1982:55–60.
10. Commission on Classification and Terminology of the International League Against Epilepsy. Proposal for revised clinical and electroencephalographic classification of epileptic seizures. *Epilepsia* 1981;22:489–501.
11. Commission on Classification and Terminology of the International League Against Epilepsy. Proposal for revised classification of epilepsies and epileptic syndromes. *Epilepsia* 1989;30:389–399.
12. Roger J, Bureau M, Dravet C, et al., eds. *Epileptic syndromes in infancy, childhood and adolescence,* 2nd ed. London: John Libbey, 1992.
13. Dreifuss FE. Lennox-Gastaut syndrome. In: Dreifuss FE, ed. *Pediatric epileptology.* Boston: John Wright, 1983:121–127.
14. Erba G, Browne TR. Atypical absence, myoclonic, atonic and tonic seizures, and the "Lennox-Gastaut syndrome." In: Browne TR, Feldman RG, eds. *Epilepsy: diagnosis and management.* Boston: Little, Brown, 1983:75–94.
15. Gastaut H, Roger J, Soulayrol R, et al. Childhood epileptic encephalopathy with diffuse slow spike-waves (otherwise known as petit mal variant or Lennox syndrome). *Epilepsia* 1966;7:139–179.
16. Adie WJ. Pyknolepsy: a form of epilepsy occurring in children with a good prognosis. *Brain* 1924;47:96–102.
17. Drury I, Dreifuss FE. Pyknoleptic petit mal. *Acta Neurol Scand* 1985;72:353–362.
18. Gastaut H, Zifkin BG, Mariani E, et al. The long-term prognosis of primary generalized epilepsy with persisting absences. *Neurology* 1986;36:1021–1028.
19. Panayiotopoulos CP. The clinical spectrum of typical absences seizures and absence epilepsies. In: Malafosse A, Genton P, Hirsch E, et al, eds. *Idiopathic generalized epilepsies: clinical, experimental and genetic aspects.* London: John Libbey, 1994:75–85.
20. Thomas P, Beaumanoir A, Genton P, et al. "De novo" absence status of late onset: report of 11 cases. *Neurology* 1992;42:104–110.
21. Holmes GL, McKeever M, Adamson M. Absence seizures in children: clinical and electroencephalographic features. *Ann Neurol* 1987;21:268–273.
22. Aicardi J. *Epilepsy in children,* 2nd ed. New York: Raven Press, 1994:94–117.
23. Dreifuss FE. Absence epilepsies. In: Dam M, Gram L, eds. *Comprehensive epileptology.* New York: Raven Press, 1991:145–153.
24. Wirrell EC, Camfield PR, Gordon KE, et al. Will a critical level of hyperventilation-induced hypocapnia always induce an absence seizure? *Epilepsia* 1996;37:459–462.
25. Goossens LAZ, Andermann F, Andermann E, et al. Reflex seizures induced by calculation, card or board games, and spatial tasks: a review of 25 patients and delineation of the epileptic syndrome. *Neurology* 1990;40:1171–1176.
26. Esquivel E, Chaussain M, Plouin P, et al. Physical exercise and voluntary hyperventilation in childhood absence epilepsy. *Electroencephalogr Clin Neurophysiol* 1991;79:127–132.
27. Yagi K, Seino M, Fujiwara T. Typical and atypical epileptic absence seizures. In: Akimoto H, Kazamatsuri H, Seino M, et al., eds. *Advances in epileptology: XIIIth Epilepsy International Symposium.* New York: Raven Press, 1982:49–53.
28. Epstein MA, Duchowny M, Jayakar P, et al. Altered responsiveness during hyperventilation-induced EEG slowing: a non-epileptic phenomenon in normal children. *Epilepsia* 1994;35:1204–1207.
29. Tassinari CA, Bureau M. Epilepsy with myoclonic absences. In: Roger J, Dravet C, Bureau M, et al., eds. *Epileptic syndromes in infancy, childhood and adolescence.* London: John Libbey, 1985:121–129.
30. Tassinari CA, Lyagoubi S, Santos V, et al. Study on spike and wave discharges in man. II. Clinical and electroencephalographic aspects of myoclonic absences [French]. *Rev Neurol (Paris)* 1969;121:379–383.
31. Appleton RE. Eyelid myoclonia with absences. In: Duncan JS, Panayiotopoulos CP, eds. *Typical absences and related epileptic syndromes.* London: Churchill Communications, 1995:213–220.
32. Appleton RE, Panayiotopoulos CP, Acomb BA, et al. Eyelid myoclonia with typical absence: an epilepsy syndrome. *J Neurol Neurosurg Psychiatry* 1993;56:1312–1316.
33. Jeavons PM. Nosological problems of myoclonic epilepsies in childhood and adolescence. *Dev Med Child Neurol* 1977;19:3–8.
34. Binnie CD, Darby CE, de Corte RA, et al. Self-induction of epileptic seizures by eye closure: incidence and recognition. *J Neurol Neurosurg Psychiatry* 1980;41:386–389.
35. Darby CE, Wilkins AJ, Binnie CD, et al. The self-induction of epileptic seizures by eye closure. *Epilepsia* 1980;21:31–42.
36. Wilkins A, Lindsay J. Common forms of reflex epilepsy: physiological mechanisms and techniques for treatment. In: Pedley TA, Meldrum BS, eds. *Recent advances in epilepsy, II.* Edinburgh: Churchill Livingstone, 1985:239–271.
37. Panayiotopoulos CP, Ferrie CD, Giannakodimos S, et al. Perioral myoclonia with absences. In: Duncan JS, Panayiotopoulos CP, eds. *Typical absences and related epileptic syndromes.* London: Churchill Communications, 1995:221–230.
38. Delgado-Escueta AV, Treiman DM, Walsh GO. The treatable epilepsies: part 1. *N Engl J Med* 1983;308:1508–1514.
39. Dalby MA. Epilepsy and 3 per second spike-and-wave rhythm. *Acta Neurol Scand [Suppl]* 1969;45:1–183.
40. Ferrie CD, Giannakodimos S, Robinson RO, et al. Symptomatic typical absence seizures. In: Duncan JS, Panayiotopoulos CP, eds. *Typical absences and related epileptic syndromes.* London: Churchill Communications, 1995:241–252.
41. Benbadis SR, Wyllie E. Pediatric epilepsy syndromes. In: Levin KH, Lüders HO, eds. *Comprehensive clinical neurophysiology.* Philadelphia: WB Saunders, 2000:468–480.
42. Blume WT. *Atlas of pediatric electroencephalography.* New York: Raven Press, 1982:139–148.
43. Daly DD. Epilepsy and syncope. In: Daly DD, Pedley TA, eds. *Current practice of clinical electroencephalography.* New York: Raven Press, 1990:269–334.
44. Doose H. Myoclonic astatic epilepsy of early childhood. In: Roger J, Dravet C, Bureau M, et al. *Epileptic syndromes in infancy, childhood and adolescence.* London: John Libbey, 1985:78–88.
45. Jasper H, Kershman J. Electroencephalographic classification of the epilepsies. *Arch Neurol Psychiatry* 1941;45:903–943.
46. Niedermeyer E. *The generalized epilepsies.* Springfield, IL: Charles C Thomas, 1972.
47. Parker AP, Agathonikou A, Robinson RO, et al. Inappropriate use of carbamazepine and vigabatrin in typical absence seizures. *Dev Med Child Neurol* 1998;40:517–519.
48. Benbadis SR. Observations on the misdiagnosis of generalized epilepsy as partial epilepsy: causes and consequences. *Seizure* 1999;8:140–145.
49. Panayiotopoulos CP. Diagnosis in epilepsies: still a central problem. *Eur J Neurol* 1996;3(Suppl 3):3–8.
50. Gastaut H. The Lennox-Gastaut syndrome: comments on the syndrome's terminology and nosological position amongst the secondary generalized epilepsies of childhood. *Electroencephalogr Clin Neurophysiol [Suppl]* 1982;35:71–84.
51. Lennox WG, Davis JP. Clinical correlates of the fast and slow spike-wave electroencephalogram. *Pediatrics* 1950;5:626–644.
52. Lee SI, Kirby D. Absence seizure with generalized rhythmic delta activity. *Epilepsia* 1988;29:262–267.
53. Lafleur J, Reiher J. Pseudo-absences. *Electroencephalogr Clin Neurophysiol* 1977;43:279–280.

54. North K, Ouvrier RA, Nugent M. Pseudoseizures caused by hyperventilation resembling absence epilepsy. *J Child Neurol* 1990;5:288–294.

55. Berkovic SF, Andermann F, Andermann E, et al. Concepts of absence epilepsies: discrete syndromes or biological continuum? *Neurology* 1987;37:993–1000.

56. Niedermeyer E, Laws ER, Walker AE. Depth EEG findings in epileptics with generalized spike-wave complexes. *Arch Neurol* 1969;21:51–58.

57. Fakhoury T, Abou-Khalil B. Generalized absence seizures with 10–15 Hz fast discharges. *Clin Neurophysiol* 1999;110:1029–1035.

58. Chevrie JJ, Aicardi J. Childhood epileptic encephalopathy with slow spike-wave: a statistical study of 80 cases. *Epilepsia* 1972;13:259–271.

59. Reutens DC, Berkovic SF. Idiopathic generalized epilepsy of adolescence: are the syndromes clinically distinct? *Neurology* 1995;45:1469–1476.

60. Benbadis SR, Tatum WO 4th, Gieron M. Idiopathic generalized epilepsy and choice of antiepileptic drugs. *Neurology* 2003;61:1793–1795.

61. Benbadis SR, Lüders HO. Epileptic syndromes: an underutilized concept. *Epilepsia* 1996;37:1029–1034.

62. Rosenow F, Wyllie E, Kotagal P, et al. Staring spells in children: descriptive features distinguishing epileptic and nonepileptic events. *J Pediatr* 1998;133:660–663.

63. Carmant L, Kramer U, Holmes GL, et al. Differential diagnosis of staring spells in children: a video-EEG study. *Pediatr Neurol* 1996;14:199–202.

64. Williams J, Sharp GB, DelosReyes E, et al. Symptom differences in children with absence seizures versus inattention. *Epilepsy Behav* 2002;3:245–248.

65. So EL, King DW, Murvin AJ. Misdiagnosis of complex absence seizures. *Arch Neurol* 1984;41:640–641.

66. Geier S, Bancaud J, Talairach J, et al. Automatisms during frontal lobe epileptic seizures. *Brain* 1976;99:447–458.

67. Rasmussen T. Characteristics of a pure culture of frontal lobe epilepsy. *Epilepsia* 1983;24:482–493.

68. Tukel K, Jasper H. The electroencephalogram in parasagittal lesions. *Electroencephalogr Clin Neurophysiol* 1952;4:481–494.

69. Williamson PD, Spencer DD, Spencer SS, et al. Complex partial seizures of frontal lobe origin. *Ann Neurol* 1985;18:497–504.

70. Bancaud J, Talairach J, Morel P, et al. "Generalized" epileptic seizures elicited by electrical stimulation of the frontal lobe in man. *Electroencephalogr Clin Neurophysiol* 1974;37:275–282.

71. Gloor P, Rasmussen T, Altuzarra A, et al. Role of the intracarotid amobarbital-pentylenetetrazol EEG test in the diagnosis and surgical treatment of patients with complex seizure problems. *Epilepsia* 1976;17:15–31.

72. Blume WT, Pillay N. Electrographic and clinical correlates of secondary bilateral synchrony. *Epilepsia* 1985;26:636–641.

73. Bartolomei F, Roger J, Bureau M, et al. Prognostic factors for childhood and juvenile absence epilepsies. *Eur Neurol* 1997;37:169–175.

74. Janz D. Epilepsy with impulsive petit mal (juvenile myoclonic epilepsy). *Acta Neurol Scand* 1985;72:449–459.

75. Janz D, Christian W. Impulsive-petit mal. *Dtsch Z Nervenheilk* 1957;176:346–386.

76. Lugaresi E, Pazzaglia P, Roger J, et al. Evolution and prognosis of petit mal. In: Harris P, Mawdsley C, eds. *Epilepsy: proceedings of the Hans Berger Centenary Symposium.* Edinburgh: Churchill Livingstone, 1974:151–153.

77. Manonmani V, Wallace SJ. Epilepsy with myoclonic absences. *Arch Dis Child* 1994;70:288–290.

78. Olsson I, Hedstrom A. Epidemiology of absence epilepsy, II: typical absences in children with encephalopathies. *Acta Paediatr Scand* 1991;80:235–242.

79. Broughton R, Nelson G, Gloor P, et al. Petit mal epilepsy evolving to subacute sclerosing panencephalitis. In: Lugaresi E, Pazzaglia P, Tassinari CA, eds. *Evolution and prognosis of epilepsies.* Bologna, Italy: Aulo Gaggi, 1973:63–72.

80. Ishikawa A, Murayama T, Sakuma N, et al. Subacute sclerosing panencephalitis: atypical absence attacks as first symptom. *Neurology* 1981;31:311–315.

81. Andermann F. Absence attacks and diffuse neuronal disease. *Neurology* 1967;17:205–212.

82. Hodson A, Coleman R. Absence seizures in Farber's lipogranulomatosis. *Electroencephalogr Clin Neurophysiol* 1985;61(Suppl):S186.

83. Thomas P, Lebrun C, Chatel M. De novo absence status epilepticus as a benzodiazepine withdrawal syndrome. *Epilepsia* 1993;34:355–358.

84. Berkovic SF, Bladin PF. Absence status in adults. *Clin Exp Neurol* 1982;19:198–207.

85. Pritchard PB, O'Neal DB. Nonconvulsive status epilepticus following metrizamide myelography. *Ann Neurol* 1984;16:252–254.

86. Berkovic SF, Andermann F, Melanson D, et al. Hypothalamic hamartomas and associated ictal laughter: evolution of the characteristic epileptic syndrome and diagnostic value of magnetic resonance imaging. *Ann Neurol* 1988;23:429–439.

87. Diebler C, Ponsot G. Hamartomas of the tuber cinereum. *Neuroradiology* 1983;25:93–101.

88. Scherman RG, Abraham K. "Centrencephalic" electroencephalographic patterns in precocious puberty. *Electroencephalogr Clin Neurophysiol* 1963;15:559–567.

89. Berkovic SF, Reutens DC, Andermann E, et al. The epilepsies: specific syndromes or a neurobiological continuum? In: Wolf P, ed. *Epileptic seizures and syndromes.* London: John Libbey, 1994:25–37.

90. Gloor P. The EEG in seizure disorders: a neurobiological view and some new technological applications. In: Robb P, ed. *Epilepsy updated: causes and treatment.* Miami, FL: Symposia Specialists, 1980:31–50.

91. Metrakos JD, Metrakos K. Childhood epilepsy of subcortical ("centrencephalic") origin. *Clin Pediatr* 1966;5:536–542.

92. Metrakos K, Metrakos JD. Genetics of convulsive disorders, II: genetic and electroencephalographic studies in centrencephalic epilepsy. *Neurology* 1961;11:474–483.

93. Metrakos K, Metrakos JD. Genetics of epilepsy. In: Vinken PJ, Bruyn GW, eds. *Handbook of clinical neurology, XV.* Amsterdam: North-Holland Publishing, 1974:429–439.

94. Andermann E. Genetic aspects of the epilepsies. In: Sakai T, Tsuboi T, eds. *Genetic aspects of human behaviour.* Tokyo: Igaku-Shoin, 1985:129–145.

95. Doose H, Gerken H. On the genetics of EEG anomalies in childhood, IV: photoconvulsive reaction. *Neuropaediatrie* 1973;4:162–167.

96. Doose H, Gerken H, Horstmann T, et al. Genetic factors in spike-wave absences. *Epilepsia* 1973;14:57–75.

97. Gerken H, Doose H. On the genetics of EEG anomalies in childhood, III: spike and waves. *Neuropaediatrie* 1973;4:88–97.

98. Matthes A, Weber H. Clinical and electroencephalographic family studies on pyknolepsy [German]. *Dtsch Med Wochenschr* 1968;93:429–435.

99. Rabending G, Klepel H. Photoconvulsive and photomyoclonic reactions: age-dependent, genetically determined variants of enhanced photosensitivity [German]. *Neuropaediatrie* 1970;2:164–172.

100. Tsuboi T, Okada S. The genetics of epilepsy. In: Sakai T, Tsuboi T, eds. *Genetic aspects of human behavior.* Tokyo: Igaku-Shoin, 1985:113–127.

101. Lennox WG, Lennox MA. *Epilepsy and related disorders.* Boston: Little, Brown, 1960:548–574.

102. Berkovic SF, Howell RA, Hay DA, et al. Epilepsies in twins. In: Wolf P, ed. *Epileptic seizures and syndromes.* London: John Libbey, 1994:157–164.

103. Andermann E. Multifactorial inheritance of generalized and focal epilepsy. In: Anderson VE, Hauser WA, Penry JK, et al., eds. *Genetic basis of the epilepsies.* New York: Raven Press, 1982:355–374.

104. Gloor P, Metrakos J, Metrakos K, et al. Neurophysiological, genetic and biochemical nature of the epileptic diathesis. *Electroencephalogr Clin Neurophysiol [Suppl]* 1982;35:45–56.

105. Wallace RH, Marini C, Petrou S, et al. Mutant GABA$_A$ receptor γ$_2$-subunit in childhood absence epilepsy and febrile seizures. *Nat Genet* 2001;28:49–52.

106. Kananura C, Haug K, Sander T, et al. A splice-site mutation in GABRG2 associated with childhood absence epilepsy and febrile convulsions. *Arch Neurol* 2002;59:1137–1141.

107. Chen Y, Lu J, Pan H, et al. Association between genetic variation of CACNA1H and childhood absence epilepsy. *Ann Neurol* 2003;54:239–243.

108. Heron SE, Phillips HA, Mulley JC, et al. Genetic variation of *CACNA1H* in idiopathic generalised epilepsy. *Ann Neurol* 2004;55:595–596.

109. Steinlein OK, Noebels JL. Ion channels and epilepsy in man and mouse. *Curr Opin Genet Dev* 2000;10:286–291.

110. Rudolf G, Therese Bihoreau M, Godfrey R, et al. Polygenic control of idiopathic generalized epilepsy phenotypes in the genetic absence rats from Strasbourg (GAERS). *Epilepsia* 2004;45:301–308.

111. Meencke HJ. Neuron density in the molecular layer of the frontal cortex in primary generalized epilepsy. *Epilepsia* 1985;26:450–454.

112. Meencke HJ, Janz D. Neuropathological findings in primary generalized epilepsy: a study of eight cases. *Epilepsia* 1984;25:8–21.

113. Lyon G, Gastaut M. Considerations on the significance attributed to unusual cerebral histological findings recently described in eight patients with primary generalized epilepsy. *Epilepsia* 1985;26:365–367.

114. Opeskin K, Kalnins RM, Halliday G, et al. Idiopathic generalised epilepsy: lack of significant microdysgenesis. *Neurology* 2000;55:1101–1106.

115. Gloor P. Evolution of the concept of the mechanism of generalized epilepsy with bilateral spike-and-wave discharge. In: Wada JA, ed. *Modern perspectives in epilepsy.* Montreal, Canada: Eden Press, 1978:99–137.

116. Jasper HH. Current evaluation of the concepts of centrencephalic and cortico-reticular seizures. *Electroencephalogr Clin Neurophysiol* 1991;78:2–11.

117. Jasper HH, Droogleever-Fortuyn J. Experimental studies on the functional anatomy of petit mal epilepsy. *Assoc Res Nerv Ment Dis* 1947;26:272–298.

118. Penfield W, Jasper H. Highest level seizures. *Assoc Res Nerv Ment Dis* 1947;26:252–271.

119. Penfield W, Jasper H. *Epilepsy and the functional anatomy of the human brain.* Boston: Little, Brown, 1954.

120. Gloor P. Neurophysiological basis of generalized seizures termed centrencephalic. In: Gastaut H, Jasper H, Bancaud J, et al, eds. *The physiopathogenesis of the epilepsies.* Springfield, IL: Charles C Thomas, 1969:209–236.

121. Gloor P. Generalized epilepsy with spike-and-wave discharge: a reinterpretation of its electrographic and clinical manifestations. *Epilepsia* 1979;20:571–588.

122. Gloor P. Electrophysiology of generalized epilepsy. In: Schwartzkroin P, Wheal H, eds. *Electrophysiology of epilepsy.* London: Academic Press, 1984:107–136.

123. Gloor P, Avoli M, Kostopoulos G. Thalamocortical relationships in generalized epilepsy with bilaterally synchronous spike-and-wave discharge. In: Avoli M, Gloor P, Kostopoulos G, et al., eds. *Generalized epilepsy: neurobiological approaches.* Boston: Birkhauser, 1990:190–212.

124. Gloor P, Fariello RG. Generalized epilepsy: some of its cellular mechanisms differ from those of focal epilepsy. *Trends Neurosci* 1988;11:63–68.

125. Avoli M, Gloor P, Kostopoulos G, et al. An analysis of penicillin-induced generalized spike-and-wave discharge during simultaneous recordings of cortical and thalamic single neurons. *J Neurophysiol* 1983;50:819–837.

126. Coulter DA, Huguenard JR, Prince DA. Characterization of ethosuximide reduction of low-threshold calcium current in thalamic neurons. *Ann Neurol* 1989;25:582–593.

127. Steriade M, McCormick DA, Sejnowski TJ. Thalamocortical oscillations in the sleeping and aroused brain. *Science* 1993;262:679–685.

128. Snead OC. Basic mechanisms of generalized absence seizures. *Ann Neurol* 1995;37:146–157.

129. Engel J Jr, Lubens P, Kuhl DE, et al. Local cerebral metabolic rate for glucose during petit mal absences. *Ann Neurol* 1985;17:121–128.

130. Ochs RF, Gloor P, Tyler JL, et al. Effect of generalized spike-and-wave discharge on glucose metabolism measured by positron emission tomography. *Ann Neurol* 1987;21:458–464.

131. Theodore WH, Brooks R, Margolin R, et al. Positron emission tomography in generalized seizures. *Neurology* 1985;35:684–690.

132. Engel J Jr, Ochs RF, Gloor P. Metabolic studies of generalized epilepsy. In: Avoli M, Gloor P, Kostopoulos G, et al, eds. *Generalized epilepsy: neurobiological approaches.* Boston: Birkhauser, 1990:387–396.

133. Nehlig A, Vergnes M, Marescaux C, et al. Local cerebral glucose utilization in rats with petit mal-like seizures. *Ann Neurol* 1991;29:72–77.

134. Prevett MC, Duncan JS. Functional imaging studies in humans. In: Duncan JS, Panayiotopoulos CP, eds. *Typical absences and related epileptic syndromes.* London: Churchill Communications, 1995:83–91.

135. Prevett MC, Duncan JS, Jones T, et al. Demonstration of thalamic activation during typical absence seizures using H$_2$^{15}O and PET. *Neurology* 1995;45:1396–1402.

136. Sanada S, Murakami N, Ohtahara S. Changes in blood flow of the middle cerebral artery during absence seizures. *Pediatr Neurol* 1988;4:158–161.

137. De Simone R, Silvestrini M, Marciani MG, et al. Changes in cerebral blood flow velocities during childhood absence seizures. *Pediatr Neurol* 1998;18:132–135.

138. Benbadis SR, Pallagi J, Morris GL, et al. Ictal SPECT findings in typical absence seizures. *J Epilepsy* 1998;11:187–190.

139. Nehlig A, Vergnes M, Waydelich R, et al. Absence seizures induce a decrease in cerebral blood flow: human and animal data. *J Cereb Blood Flow Metab* 1996;16:147–155.

140. Sperling MR, Skolnick BE. Cerebral blood flow during spike-wave discharge. *Epilepsia* 1995;36:156–163.

141. Salek-Haddadi A, Lemieux L, Merschhemke M, et al. Functional magnetic resonance imaging of human absence seizures. *Ann Neurol* 2003;53:663–667.

142. Mirsky AF, Duncan CC, Myslobodsky MS. Petit mal epilepsy: a review and integration of recent information. *J Clin Neurophysiol* 1986;3:179–208.

143. Meldrum BS. GABAergic agents as anticonvulsants in baboons with photosensitive epilepsy. *Neurosci Lett* 1984;47:345–349.

144. Knake S, Hamer HM, Schomburg U, et al. Tiagabine-induced absence status in idiopathic generalized epilepsy. *Seizure* 1999;8:314–317.

145. Hosford DA, Clark S, Cao Z, et al. The role of GABA$_B$ receptor activation in absence seizures of lethargic (*lh/lh*) mice. *Science* 1992;257:398–401.

146. Prevett MC, Lammertsma AA, Brooks DJ, et al. Benzodiazepine-GABA$_A$ receptors in idiopathic generalized epilepsy measured with ^{11}C-flumazenil and positron emission tomography. *Epilepsia* 1995;36:113–121.

147. Savic I, Widen L, Thorell JO, et al. Cortical benzodiazepine receptor binding in patients with generalized and partial epilepsy. *Epilepsia* 1990;31:724–730.

Atypical Absence, Myoclonic, Tonic, and Atonic Seizures

20

William O. Tatum IV   *Kevin Farrell*

Atypical absence, myoclonic, tonic, and atonic seizures are all types of generalized seizures that occur when the initial clinical and ictal electroencephalographic changes arise from both hemispheres (1). Atypical absence, tonic, atonic and often myoclonic seizures are symptoms of an underlying disease process (1–4). Despite an apparent homogeneous classification, various pathophysiologies may occur. Conversely, although several seizure types can coexist, they may share a common epileptogenic substrate (5). Classification of symptomatic seizures has been recognized since 175 AD (6). Atypical absence, myoclonic, tonic, and atonic seizures are often associated with mental retardation, an abnormal electroencephalogram (EEG), a poor response to therapy, and typify patients with encephalopathic generalized epilepsy (7). Some seizures that appear generalized clinically may be focal on the ictal EEG (8), emphasizing the importance of both the clinical features of the seizure and the EEG in classification (8,9). Seizures may defy classification, because this population often has comorbid mental retardation and multiple handicaps that limit subjective reporting and objective behavioral description. Video-electroencephalographic monitoring has improved recognition, identification, and classification for patients with atypical absence, myoclonic, tonic, and atonic seizures (10), with revision of former classifications (11–13) and the development of newer semiologic-based classifications (14).

SEIZURE TYPES

Atypical Absence Seizures

Clinical Features

Absence seizures are subdivided into *typical* and *atypical* forms. The initial description of atypical absence seizures was in association with atypical, or slow spike-and-wave (SSW), EEG discharges that were less than 3 Hz (15,16). *Petit mal* is a colloquialism used to describe typical absence seizures (17), which may be either *simple* or *complex*. The semiology of atypical absences may resemble that of complex typical absence, although atypical absences are usually differentiated by the association with a severe epileptic encephalopathy, with mental retardation, multiple seizure types, neurologic disabilities, and EEG features (16,18). Atypical absence seizures may occur at any age, but they rarely begin before 2 years of age or after the teenage years (19). Such seizures may occur alone with brief staring and a variable degree of impaired consciousness, or may be prolonged with atypical absence status. Behaviorally, they are often associated with motor signs, particularly changes in muscle tone, but also including clonic components and autonomic features (16,19). Atypical absence seizures evolve gradually, with less abrupt onset and termination, more pronounced changes in tone, and durations that, unlike typical absence seizures, last longer than 5 to 10 seconds and possibly for minutes. Consciousness is variably impaired, and postictal confusion is brief when observed (2,16). Atypical absence seizures are most likely to occur in states of drowsiness, and do not show activation with hyperventilation and photic stimulation (18). Nonepileptic staring episodes may mimic atypical absence seizures in patients with Lennox-Gastaut syndrome (LGS) (20). In one study, episodes of staring were found to be epileptic in origin in only 27% of patients on video-electroencephalographic monitoring (21), with a more reliable diagnosis of seizures established when motor features were observed.

Electrophysiology

Atypical absence seizures have a characteristic pattern on electroencephalography (22), with interictal generalized SSW discharges that are often irregular, asymmetrical, and lower in amplitude, with spikes (or sharp waves) that repeat at approximately 1.5 to 2.5 Hz (Fig. 20.1). This is in contrast to the regular generalized 3-Hz SSW pattern associated with typical absence seizures. The EEG background is usually diffusely slow. Focal or multifocal independent epileptiform discharges or even generalized polyspike-and-wave activity may appear concomitantly. The individual SSW discharges may occur as single complexes or in bursts that are longer in duration and more blunted in morphology in encephalopathic generalized epilepsy (15,19). The SSW pattern on EEG is typically a malignant pattern, although the appearance is not always associated with a change in behavior. Patients with SSW discharges on EEG and a cryptogenic etiology are more likely to show bilaterally symmetrical SSW activity than those with lateralized structural abnormalities, who show asymmetrical EEGs with higher-amplitude SSW discharges over the unaffected hemisphere (23).

The ictal EEG associated with atypical absence seizures typically demonstrates diffuse, irregular SSW discharges with or without lateralization; however, irregular diffuse fast activity at 10 to 13 Hz, or a combination of fast spike wave or sharp waves of increasing amplitude, may also be seen (16). Forms of absence seizures "intermediate" between typical and atypical absences have been described, with cognitive impairment, social and learning handicaps, pharmacoresistance, poorer prognosis, and fast rhythmic discharges during sleep (similar to those seen in patients with LGS). Sleep may help identify rhythmic fast activity on EEG that is the marker for this transitional form (24).

Centromedian thalamic nuclei recording through implanted intracerebral electrodes during atypical absence seizures has shown simultaneous 1- to 2-Hz SSW complex discharges (25). Quantitative electroencephalography has elucidated interhemispheric asynchrony and morphologic asymmetries of SSW discharges to help differentiate generalized epilepsy from frontal lobe epilepsy with secondary bilateral synchrony (26). A selective effect on electroencephalography using antiepileptic drugs (AEDs) to modify the atypical SSW pattern underlying atypical absence seizures has been reported (27).

Clinical Correlation

A spectrum of clinical and electroencephalographic manifestations of absence seizures has been noted (28) and further delineated by video-electroencephalographic monitoring (29). Although atypical absences are one of the most common seizure types observed in patients with LGS, they have received considerably less attention than typical absence seizures (30). In studies of longer than 10 years' duration, patients with LGS and a predominance of atypical absence seizures have demonstrated a strong clinical correlation with poor seizure outcome (31). Patients with combined seizure types, including those with epilepsy who have myoclonic absences with a prominent myoclonic component to the absences, carry a guarded prognosis despite the associated 3-Hz SSW pattern that typically denotes a favorable prognosis. Distinguishing atypical absence from complex typical absence seizures may be challenging, although the clinical course and seizure types seen with encephalopathic generalized epilepsy, with a paucity of automatisms, tonal changes, and longer seizure duration, may help. Complex partial seizures may manifest as brief staring attacks and mimic atypical absences,

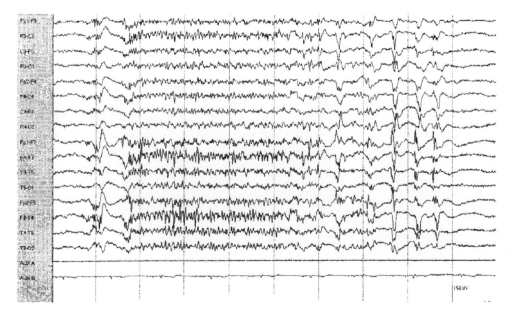

Figure 20.1 Generalized paroxysmal fast activity preceded by polyspike-and-wave discharges and followed by slow spike-wave activity in a 28-year-old male with secondary generalized epilepsy, mild static encephalopathy, and tonic seizures. The burst of 14 to 18 Hz, followed by slow spike-wave activity, was asymptomatic.

but the clinical course with focal clinical and EEG features should help distinguish the two (32). Secondary bilateral synchronous SSW discharges on EEG may occur with focal epilepsy of frontal lobe origin, yet even in the presence of a focal pathologic process, atypical absence seizures are characterized by their association with generalized clinical and electrographic abnormalities (33–35). Atypical absences may overlap with SSW complexes during slow sleep (36), and occur with the Landau-Kleffner syndrome, the syndrome of continuous spike waves during slow sleep, atypical benign partial epilepsy, and electroencephalographic status of benign Rolandic epilepsy (37).

Myoclonic Seizures

Clinical Features

A sudden, brief, involuntary, shock-like muscular contraction that results in a body movement is referred to as *myoclonus* (38,39) and may be epileptic (*myoclonic jerks*) or nonepileptic. Myoclonic seizures are generalized seizures (9,11) that occur either as part of an idiopathic epilepsy syndrome or in encephalopathic generalized epilepsy. When combined manifestations occur, such as myoclonic absence, semiology is identified by the primary component with absence the main seizure type. Four types of epilepsy with myoclonic components have been described (40)—combined myoclonic seizure types (Chapter 31), myoclonic seizures associated with encephalopathic generalized epilepsy syndromes (Chapter 26), myoclonic seizures associated with idiopathic generalized epilepsy syndromes (Chapter 25), and infantile spasms (Chapter 21)—and are discussed elsewhere in this text. Infantile spasms may have a shock-like appearance, although they have dissimilar EEG correlates than myoclonic seizures. *Massive* epileptic myoclonus implies that a bilateral jerk is large enough to create a fall. Whereas myoclonic seizures usually imply a generalized onset, *cortical reflex myoclonus* is a term that reflects a motor movement as a result of focal epilepsy (41), may appear segmental, and may originate in the regions of the brain responsible for motor activation. *Reticular reflex myoclonus*, on the other hand, occurs with generalized epilepsy but originates in subcortical structures of the brainstem.

Myoclonic seizures are characterized by sudden, involuntary, brief, muscle contractions of the head, trunk, or limbs. They usually occur without detectable loss of consciousness and may be generalized, regional (involving two adjacent areas), or focal (confined to one area). They may be regular or erratic, symmetrical or asymmetrical, synchronous or asynchronous, and positive or negative (41). Myoclonic seizures are often bilateral jerks that vary from subtle restricted twitches of the periocular or facial muscles to massive movements, with generalized involvement of the arms and legs accompanied by falling or retropulsion (2). They may occur singly or in repeated clusters, with some cognitive impairment noted during pro-

longed clusters or myoclonic status epilepticus (2). The associated features, rather than the semiology of the myoclonic seizures themselves, define the syndromes associated with myoclonic seizures.

Electrophysiology

In general, myoclonic jerks associated with encephalopathic generalized epilepsy have a high-amplitude, bisynchronous SSW or polyspike-and-wave discharge as the electrophysiologic correlate (Fig. 20.2). A brief latency between short bursts of synchronized electromyographic potentials in agonist and antagonist muscles, and that of the corresponding spikes, occurs. The spikes are time-locked events that are coupled with the myoclonic jerks that follow. By using back-averaging techniques, latencies are found to occur between 21 and 80 milliseconds (42,43). When a myoclonic jerk is generated by subcortical structures, a generalized spike discharge follows the first electromyographic sign of myoclonus; however, in this case, an epileptogenic phenomenon is disputed by some (43). Negative myoclonus caused by a lapse of tone, which can be seen only during antigravity posture, is coupled with either the slow wave or the second positive component of a polyspike-and-wave discharge (43). Myoclonic seizures have correlates with an electromyographic pattern, demonstrating a brief synchronous potential of less than 50 milliseconds that is seen simultaneously in the involved muscle groups (41). During the jerks, medium- to high-amplitude repetitive 16-Hz spikes are seen. (44,45). The background activity of the interictal EEG in patients with encephalopathic generalized epilepsy is characteristically diffusely slow. A unique EEG pattern is seen in early myoclonic encephalopathy and neonatal myoclonic seizures, with burst suppression or multiple paroxysmal abnormalities with random asynchronous attenuations (46). Recordings from thalamic nuclei during myoclonic seizures demonstrate subcortical slow polyspike-and-wave discharges that lead those recorded on the scalp surface in patients with LGS (25,47). Giant visual evoked potentials appearing as occipital high-amplitude polyphasic spikes may be observed during intermittent photic stimulation at less than 3 Hz in patients with neuronal ceroid lipofuscinosis of late infancy, in which myoclonic, as well as atypical absence and atonic, seizures are common (48).

Focal myoclonus is suspected to be derived from a hyperexcitable cortex responsible for corresponding motor activation. A recordable paroxysmal depolarizing shift in animal models may occur with cortical application of proconvulsants (49). Electrographic secondary bilateral synchrony has been reported in patients with myoclonic and partial seizures (50), with generalized epileptiform discharges showing a small delay in interhemispheric propagation as a function of coherence and phase analysis, suggesting frontal lobe onset (50).

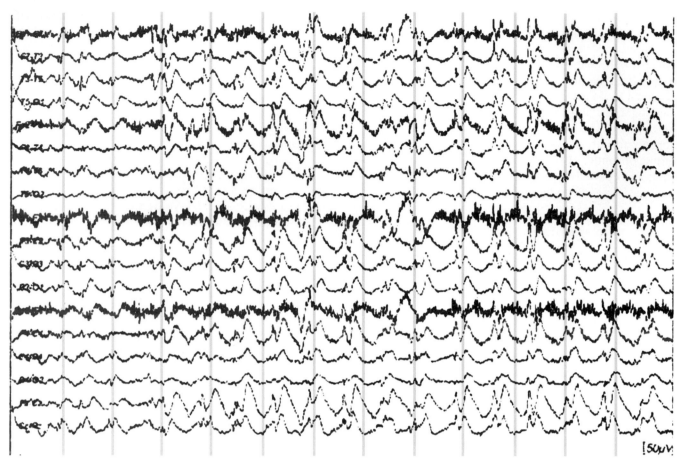

Figure 20.2 A burst of slow spike-and-wave discharges in a 9-year-old girl with secondary generalized epilepsy and atypical absence seizures. Note the 1.5-Hz frequency and intermittent left lateralization that is seen.

Clinical Correlation

Most epilepsies with myoclonic seizures begin during the first 5 years of life (51). They are clinically and etiologically heterogeneous, and represent a group of disorders that may occur in many epilepsy types and syndromes from early infancy into adulthood (52,53). Myoclonic seizures must be differentiated from infantile spasms, partial seizures with tonic posturing, and nonepileptic conditions (54), and difficulty may arise in differentiating massive myoclonic seizures from tonic and atonic seizures. Causes of myoclonic seizures vary greatly from acquired causes of almost any etiology to familial epilepsies with varied inheritance patterns (52,53). There are subgroups of patients with idiopathic generalized epilepsy with refractory myoclonic seizures and developmental delay, yet with a genetic component. Myoclonic-astatic epilepsy and severe myoclonic epilepsy in infancy represent the more severe phenotypes of *generalized epilepsy with febrile seizures plus (GEFS+),* which mimic patients with encephalopathic generalized epilepsy, but with no discernible etiology and a genetic foundation for expression (55). Epilepsy with myoclonic-astatic seizures is a syndrome intermediate between idiopathic and encephalopathic generalized epilepsy, with

febrile seizures and subsequent myoclonic jerks during childhood that involve mainly the axial muscles, more than the face, upper trunk, and arms with jerks strong enough to cause patients to fall (i.e., astatic seizures) (56,57). Similarly, epilepsy with myoclonic absences is characterized by prolonged absence seizures with prominent rhythmic generalized myoclonic jerks involving both shoulders, arms, and legs, which may repeat at 3 Hz during activation techniques, distinguishing myoclonic absence from childhood absence epilepsy (36,58).

A symptomatic or cryptogenic etiology is often found when myoclonic seizures begin before the age of 4 years (55). Early myoclonic encephalopathy manifests as neonatal-onset irregular myoclonic jerks. Severe myoclonic epilepsy of infancy (Dravet syndrome) occurs with myoclonic seizures following febrile seizures during the first year of life (59). Myoclonic seizures are common but least characteristic in patients with LGS, although a myoclonic variant that has a better prognosis for cognitive development has been noted (60). The progressive myoclonus epilepsies (see Chapter 26) are a rare but extremely debilitating and progressive heterogeneous subgroup of encephalopathic generalized epilepsy, with myoclonic seizures as the clinical marker (61). The presence of mental retardation and abnormal neurologic examination does not preclude an independent idiopathic generalized epilepsy (62), but severe myoclonic epilepsy of infancy, early myoclonic encephalopathy, LGS, the progressive myoclonus epilepsies, and mitochondrial encephalopathies are strongly associated with myoclonic seizures and portend an unfavorable prognosis. Myoclonic status epilepticus typically occurs in patients with encephalopathic generalized epilepsy (63,64), although it occurs less frequently during sleep (65).

Tonic Seizures

Clinical Features

Tonic seizures are generalized seizures (12,13,66) that are *convulsive* (13,67), but may be very brief, appear nonconvulsive, and are grouped with absence, myoclonic, and atonic seizures (2). The prevalence is inadequately represented, given the discrepancy between observed seizure incidence and seizures noted on electrographic recording during video-electroencephalographic monitoring (10). In an effort to distinguish different forms of tonic seizures, the taxonomy includes (a) *tonic axial seizures* with abrupt tonic muscular contraction and rigidity of the neck, facial, or masticatory muscles; (b) *global tonic seizures* involving widespread contraction of the axial and appendicular musculature; and (c) *tonic axorhizomelic seizures* as an intermediate form, with contraction of the upper limb muscles and deltoid muscles that leads to elevation of the shoulders. Partial seizures with asymmetrical tonic posturing are referred to as *tonic postural seizures. Short tonic seizures* have high-amplitude, rapid muscular contractions maximal in the neck and shoulder girdle, but involve mainly the axis of the body and trunk and last 500 to 800 milliseconds, with

forward leaning that resembles infantile spasms (68). When tonic posturing is observed in patients with West syndrome and infantile spasms, *tonic spasms* with massive flexion of the head, trunk, and extremities ("Jackknifing") is a term used to describe a seizure type that is refractory to treatment (69,70). Myoclonic jerks may appear to be brief tonic seizures but are actually single muscular contractions lasting less than 200 milliseconds. Tonic seizures, on the other hand, are more sustained, lasting seconds (71) with increasing intensity, although they may be associated with an atonic or myoclonic component (25). *Prolonged tonic seizures* with a vibratory component may resemble generalized tonic-clonic seizures (72), although tonic seizures are briefer, averaging 10 to 15 seconds (71).

Tonic seizures may vary, from a short, upward deviation of the eyeballs with or without oscillatory nystagmus to a more intense seizure, with generalized symmetrical or asymmetrical tonic stiffening, loss of consciousness, and falls and repeated injury (10,16). Falls may be forward or backward, depending on whether the axial and lower limb musculature are fixed in flexion, or less commonly with extension of the head and/or trunk (16). Scars from old injuries may be observed on the forehead (Fig. 20.3) and occipital regions, reflecting injury patterns associated with seizures. Contraction of the respiratory and abdominal muscles may create a high-pitched cry or period of hypopnea. Seizure intensities may vary among patients and individuals, and combined seizure types may occur (73). The duration of tonic seizures is several seconds to a minute, although most last for 5 to 20 seconds and are most common during stages I and II of nonrapid eye movement (NREM) sleep (10). Autonomic signs include respiratory, heart rate, or blood pressure increases; pupillary dilation; and facial flushing (10). Postictally, patients have variable degrees of cognitive and motor recovery (74), with the depth of the postictal

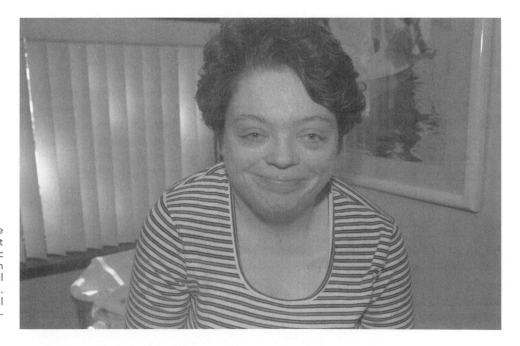

Figure 20.3 A 32-year-old female with cryptogenic Lennox-Gastaut syndrome and brief, massive tonic seizures. Note the large scar on her forehead from a propulsive fall associated with a tonic seizure. Also, note the left chest surgical scar at the site of vagus nerve stimulator placement.

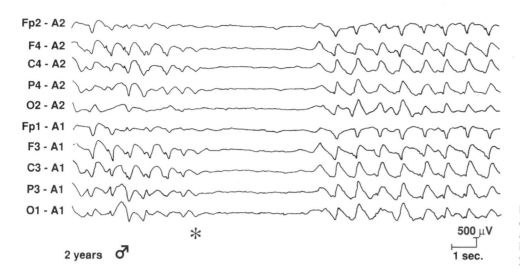

Figure 20.4 An electroencephalogram that demonstrates an abrupt, generalized "flattening" during a tonic seizure in a 2-year-old boy.

state proportional to the seizure intensity (10). In patients with LGS, tonic seizures are reported to occur in large numbers during NREM sleep (75). Tonic status epilepticus (75) may occur in 54% to 97% of patients with an insidious or brief initial tonic component (71).

Electrophysiology

Nonepileptic tonic posturing is readily distinguished by normal interictal and ictal EEGs (76,77). The interictal EEG characteristics seen with tonic seizures are dependent on the specific epileptic syndrome. In most patients, tonic seizures are associated with encephalopathic generalized epilepsy, and a diffusely slow background with multifocal spikes and sharp waves on EEG is suggested (78). In patients with LGS beginning before the age of 5 years, generalized SSW complexes may not appear until the onset of epilepsy is well established (79). The ictal EEG manifestations of tonic seizures associated with encephalopathic generalized epilepsy reveal a generalized frontally predominant initial attenuation of background activity that is associated with desynchronization (Fig. 20.4) and precedes the bilateral 10- to 25-Hz spikes, with the amplitude ranging from flattened scalp EEG to greater than 100 μV (80). Generalized paroxysmal fast activity (Fig. 20.5), which

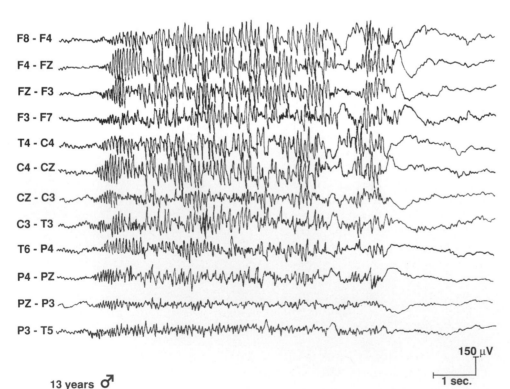

Figure 20.5 Generalized paroxysmal fast activity with bilateral 15 Hz of increasing amplitude during a tonic seizure in a 13-year-old girl.

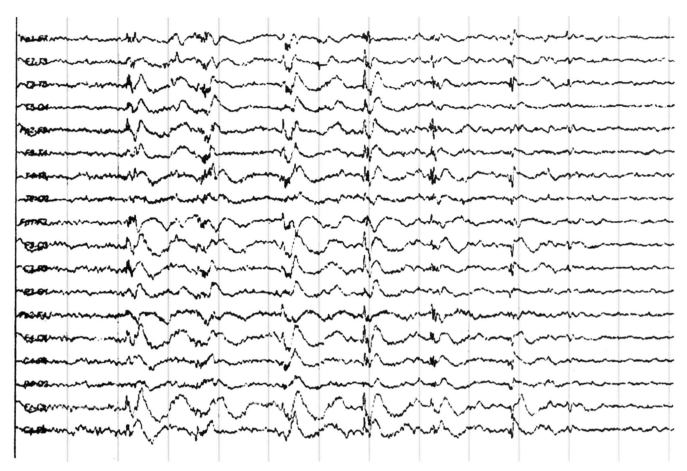

Figure 20.6 The electroencephalogram of a 27-year-old patient with secondary generalized epilepsy, static encephalopathy, and myoclonic seizures demonstrates generalized polyspike discharges with intermittent mild myoclonus of the neck and proximal upper limbs.

consists of diffuse, repetitive, medium- to high-amplitude spike discharges, occurs as the counterpart of tonic seizures during slow-wave sleep (81). Mixtures of clinical and electroencephalographic patterns may be seen, with tonic-absence seizures occurring with a tonic seizure and subsequent staring associated with generalized paroxysmal fast activity, followed by SSW, on EEG (Fig. 20.6) (73). Fast ictal spike discharges were noted in deeper centromedian thalamic nuclei, correlating bilaterally with the onset of tonic seizures and diffuse scalp EEG changes in patients with LGS (25). Rhythmic ictal theta and delta patterns that differ from the background activity have been described in patients with tonic status epilepticus (82), and nonconvulsive status is not an uncommon occurrence in patients with LGS (83).

Tonic postural seizures associated with focal epilepsy may have interictal midline spikes (84), although interictal epileptiform discharges may be notably absent. Because the ictal discharges in patients with tonic postural seizures may arise from "deep" in the mesial frontal cortex, scalp electroencephalography during the seizure may be unrevealing, resulting from a low-amplitude, regional,

high-frequency ictal discharge (85) or from diffuse attenuation of background, even in tonic seizures with a focal origin (77,86).

Clinical Correlation

Tonic seizures may present as either the initial (87) or the primary manifestation (80) of encephalopathic generalized epilepsy. Tonic seizures are associated with falls less consistently than atonic seizures, because the leg muscles are often not involved or have an increased extensor tone to maintain an upright posture (40). Tonic seizures have a rigid muscular extension, whereas atonic seizures manifest as an abrupt loss of muscle tone. Tonic seizures are the most common cause of sudden falls in children with LGS (71,88) and a major cause of morbidity and mortality with repeated injury, often necessitating the use of a protective helmet (89). Although tonic seizures are characteristic of LGS and affect between 74% and 90% of patients (71), they are notably absent in other encephalopathic generalized epilepsies, including atypical benign partial epilepsy of childhood (pseudo-Lennox syndrome) (90). Tonic, as well as myoclonic, seizures are clinical markers for medical intractability in patients with epilepsy (91,92). Mental retardation is less common when tonic seizures begin later in childhood or in adulthood, and is associated with a poor prognosis for seizure control and normal development with seizure onset before the age of 2 years (71).

The epileptic mechanism for generating tonic seizures is based on the clinical history and disease course (76,93). Generalized tonic seizures are reported most often in patients with encephalopathic generalized epilepsy and represent one of the cardinal seizure types in patients with LGS (2). Nonepileptic tonic or opisthotonic posturing should be considered when posturing occurs with pain or with the lack of epileptiform discharges during the event (94). When seizures are present during neonatal development, tonic seizures represent one of the earliest clinically identifiable forms (95). Although infantile spasms may appear to be clinically similar to tonic seizures, spasms are more rapid in onset (lasting for 1 to 2 seconds), peak more slowly than a myoclonic jerk (70), occur in clusters, and have unique EEG characteristics. Secondarily generalized seizures with asymmetrical tonic abduction and elevation of the arms may occur in patients with focal epilepsy and may mimic tonic seizures seen in patients with LGS (23), although they are differentiated by the presence of associated simple partial and/or complex partial seizures (84,96–99). Seizures are often frequent, nocturnal, and associated with episodes of status epilepticus (100).

Atonic Seizures

Clinical Features

Epilepsy received early distinction as "the falling sickness" (101). Atonic seizures are classified as generalized seizures with a sudden loss of postural tone that predispose an individual to epileptic falls, although the term has been incorrectly used synonymously with *drop attacks* (12,13). Limited uniformity of taxonomy exists, with attempts to categorize atonic seizures as drop attacks, astatic, or akinetic, and applying descriptive terminology worsens the difficulty with classification (72). Atonic seizures may be brief, lasting seconds (drop attack), or become prolonged, lasting 1 to several minutes (also known as akinetic seizures). Atonic seizures begin suddenly and without warning, with a loss of postural tone in the flexor and extensor muscles of the limbs, trunk, or neck. They range in severity, from a brief head nod to a sudden, intense loss of tone in the extensor and flexor postural muscles that leads to an abrupt fall straight downward (56). Brief atonic seizures can result in a fall within 1 to 2 seconds (16,71). An initial head drop lasting approximately 250 milliseconds is followed by truncal and leg collapse that occurs within 800 milliseconds (72,102). Video-electroencephalographic analysis of drop attacks with the patient in the standing position demonstrates the first manifestations to be flexion at the waist and

knees, followed by additional knee buckling leading to a fall straight downward, such that the individual lands on his or her buttocks (103). In contrast, tonic seizures occur with tonic flexion at the hips and propulsive or retropulsive falls. Consciousness is impaired during the fall. Postictal confusion is rare and recovery may vary, depending on the duration of the attack, with return of consciousness immediately to within several minutes and the patient resuming the standing position within a couple of seconds (72,88). A more prolonged atonic seizure precipitated by a febrile illness (104) and atonic seizures induced by startle (105) have been described. Pure atonia is unusual and seizures often appear along with other motor components, such as a myoclonic jerk (16,106). The atonic seizure component in patients with myoclonic-astatic epilepsy may have late motor features, with transient changes in facial expression or twitching of the extremities following the initial atonia making classification of the clinical features challenging (107).

Electrophysiology

In most patients with atonic seizures, a diffusely slow posterior dominant rhythm, with bursts of SSW or polyspike-and-wave complexes, is seen on the interictal EEG (16). Generalized SSW discharges occur most often in the first 5 years of life, waning with increasing age and rarely seen in patients older than age 40 years (71). Focal, lateralized, multifocal independent spikes, or diffuse irregular discharges, may also occur. During atonic seizures, scalp electroencephalography reveals generalized polyspike-and-wave discharges or, more infrequently, generalized irregular SSW discharges. The discharges are followed immediately by diffuse, generalized slow waves, maximal in the vertex and central regions, that correlate with the generalized atonia (71,102). During a prolonged atonic seizure, the diffuse, bilateral slow waves often mask an underlying discharge of bilateral, synchronous, symmetrical sharp waves recurring at approximately 10 Hz (104), with the morphology of the initial discharge characterized by a positive-negative-deep-positive wave, followed by a larger surface-negative after-going slow wave. Rarely, has a correlation between the intensity of the atonia and the depth of the positive components of the SSW complex been observed (56). Activation by intermittent photic stimulation is also not typically noted (71).

Patients with extratemporal epilepsy may have brief focal loss of postural tone lasting from 100 to 150 milliseconds, corresponding to low-voltage fast activity or repetitive spikes in the contralateral frontocentral region (108), though the relationship between EEG amplitude and intensity of the clinical features is inconsistent (109). Intraoperative electroencephalography during corpus callosotomy has been performed in patients with atonic-tonic seizures, with transformation of generalized to lateralized epileptiform discharges, although this did not always correlate clinically with the degree of seizure reduction (110).

Clinical Correlation

Seizures that result in falls are not synonymous with atonic seizures and may also occur with tonic, myoclonic, and partial seizures. Video-electroencephalographic monitoring may be necessary to classify the individual seizure type (Fig. 20.7) (111). Atonic seizures associated with an abrupt loss of brief postural tone are commonly observed in patients with encephalopathic generalized epilepsy, but they may also occur with atypical absences that have a prominent postural component (71,108). Because of the risk for falls and for seizure-related injury, atonic seizures are one of the most common and severe seizure types (112). Atonic seizures often occur as a combination of different seizure types (16). Myoclonic and atonic seizures often coexist during a single event or individually in the same patient (i.e., myoclonic-astatic epilepsy) (71). Partial seizures resulting in a fall may mimic the atonic seizures of encephalopathic generalized epilepsy, although this is uncommon. Ictal paresis from epileptic negative myoclonus may vary in intensity, with manifestations from transient unsteadiness to falls to the ground. When atonic seizures are observed in patients with focal epilepsy, they

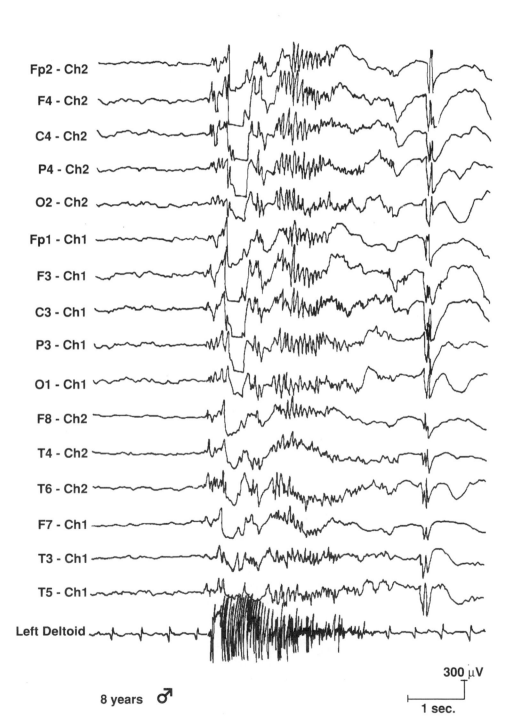

Figure 20.7 Ictal electroencephalography during a "drop attack" in an 8-year-old boy with Lennox-Gastaut syndrome. Note the muscle artifact on polygraphic recording depicting a component of tonic contraction with 15-Hz activity during video-electroencephalography.

8 years ♂

300 μV

1 sec.

are similar to asymmetrical tonic postural seizures and usually arise from the mesial frontal or parietal lobe (107,113).

PATHOPHYSIOLOGY

The pathophysiologic basis for atypical absence, myoclonic, tonic, and atonic seizures is poorly understood (45,114). Some anatomical substrates or neural connections have been elucidated with brain stimulation and seizure surgery in patients with refractory seizures, and the genetic basis for individuals with these seizure types is expanding (43,115,116). Various structural pathologies may underlie the ictal behavior associated with these seizure types (40,117–119).

Frontal lobe connections appear to play a role in the expression of the SSW pattern on EEG and may thus be operational in atypical absences (120), with the precise events that herald the transition from the interictal to ictal state yet to be fully defined. Genetic causes are infrequently associated with atypical absence seizures, although underlying developmental abnormalities associated with a disordered cerebral cortex may be influenced by inherited patterns (115,121) and are probably underestimated (122). The neurochemical mechanism of atypical absence seizures is incompletely delineated. However, increased γ-aminobutyric acid (GABA) antagonism potentiates SSW discharges and may play a central role (123), although the lack of an appropriate model has limited investigation (114).

It has been hypothesized that myoclonic seizures are produced by both a cortical and subcortical generator involving thalamocortical and reticular projections (42,43). Because of the wide variety of mechanisms associated with the clinical expression of myoclonic seizures, no single pathology has been identified. In patients with encephalopathic generalized epilepsy, a wide range of pathologic substrates may exist, although frontal lobe abnormalities may preferentially occur (124). Genetic predisposition and/or the presence of a structural lesion underpin the best-described pathophysiologic mechanism for myoclonic seizures with various modes of inheritance (125–127), and the progressive myoclonic epilepsy syndromes have isolated gene loci involved in the majority of the disorders (61). Myoclonic seizures associated with chromosomal abnormalities (128), mutant mitochondrial DNA (129), ion channelopathies (87), and defects of neurotransmitter systems (130) form a wide variety of the genetic influences that are reported.

Tonic seizures often have a cryptogenic etiology, although congenital brain malformation, hypoxic-ischemic encephalopathy, and central nervous system infections are the symptomatic causes most often found. Tonic seizures and LGS involve subcortical structures (68), whereas tonic postural seizures arise from the frontal or parietal cortex (98) via structural (97) or indirectly via a genetic means

(131,132). The maximal electroshock animal model for AED development produces generalized tonic extensor rigidity during electrical stimulation (133). Other animal models have shown that an intact brain stem is required to produce a tonic seizure that is not dependent on the frontal cortex (134). The reticular formation within the upper mid-brainstem is probably involved, given that electrical stimulation will reproduce similar behaviors whereas lesioning of the area will suppress them (135). Blocking extrapyramidal motor inhibition with tonic spasms occurring as a release phenomenon has been postulated (68). The GABA-chloride ionophore complex appears to play a role in the development of tonic seizures (81). Neuroimaging with magnetic resonance imaging (MRI) has demonstrated altered anatomical architecture near the red nucleus of the brainstem in patients with LGS and tonic seizures, providing further support for brainstem involvement (23), although neuronal migration disorders and cortical malformations may also occur (136).

Atonic seizures also have subcortical brain stem structures implicated in their pathophysiology (72). The reticular formation within the brainstem has efferent neuronal synaptic connections with the medial medulla reported to be involved in atonia during rapid eye movement (REM) sleep, and is suspected to play a central role in the atonia of cataplexy via motor inactivation, disturbed integration, or activation of inhibitory neural connections (137,138). When the fast-conducting corticoreticulospinal pathways are activated by subcortical brainstem inhibitory centers, bilateral atonia of axial postural muscles may occur (139). The motor cortex probably participates in production of some atonic seizures with negative motor features (i.e., "inhibitory seizures") (137,140), given the reproducible effect using electrical brain stimulation (139). Since inhibition of bilateral motor cortices in conjunction with bilateral SSW complexes on electroencephalography has been noted (141), a subcortical-cortical polysynaptic connection seems plausible, given the clinical observation that corpus callosotomy has a beneficial effect in patients with atonic seizures (142).

TREATMENT

The treatment of patients with atypical absence, myoclonic, tonic, and atonic seizures is predicated upon appropriate recognition and classification of the specific type of seizure, type of epilepsy, and epilepsy syndrome (143). Evidence-based medical and surgical outcome for these seizure types is limited (63,114). Divalproex sodium, lamotrigine, and ethosuximide, alone or in combination, are often used as first-line therapies for atypical absence seizures (144). Valproate is often recommended as initial treatment for patients, although rare cases of seizure aggravation have been reported with myoclonic absence seizures (144,145). A synergistic combination has been noted using valproate plus ethosuximide or valproate plus lamotrigine (146,147). Lamotrigine is effective for the treatment of absence seizures but has an inconsistent effect on myoclonic jerks (146,148–150). Clonazepam may also be useful, especially if absence seizures are combined with myoclonic components. Other AEDs not commonly available may be effective as well (151).

Some AEDs have antimyoclonic activity (53,152). Valproate has broad-spectrum efficacy, with patients with myoclonic seizures responding in the majority of cases (146). Valproate-resistance (153) or bizarre myoclonic seizures (154) may occur with seizures of frontal lobe origin. Lamotrigine has been used as an initial treatment approach in patients with LGS and in those with myoclonic-astatic epilepsy (155), although caution is advised because of the possibility of aggravating myoclonic seizures (148). Benzodiazepines, valproate, topiramate, zonisamide, and levetiracetam may all be effective AEDs in patients with myoclonic seizures (156), whereas phenytoin (157), carbamazepine (157,158), gabapentin (159), and vigabatrin (160) may aggravate these seizures (43,157,161). Lamotrigine may either be effective (156) or aggravate (148) myoclonic seizures. Other less commonly used agents including acetazolamide (162) and piracetam (163). The ketogenic diet should be considered if AEDs are ineffective for myoclonic seizures (164), although exacerbation of behavioral problems has been noted following successful treatment (165).

Phenytoin is an effective treatment for patients with tonic seizures and tonic status epilepticus (10). Valproate is a useful alternative, with an intravenous (IV) preparation available for rapid loading (10,166). Patients with LGS who have tonic seizures may respond to carbamazepine; however, the same agent can aggravate atypical absences in patients with encephalopathic generalized epilepsy (167). Lamotrigine, topiramate, zonisamide, and levetiracetam are evolving as broad-spectrum AEDs for the treatment of patients with mixed seizure types, including tonic seizures (166). Benzodiazepines may also be beneficial; however, tolerance limits long-term efficacy, and tonic seizures have occurred paradoxically from IV benzodiazepine administration (168).

Resective surgery may be an effective option for some patients in whom a focal structural lesion is responsible for the seizures (169–172), although it is rarely efficacious when mixed seizure types exist (173,174). Corpus callosotomy is an effective treatment for most patients with drop attacks caused by tonic or atonic seizures (142). Vagus nerve stimulation is a less-invasive adjunctive treatment (175), and deep brain stimulation may hold promise for patients with tonic seizures (25).

Valproate is often recommended as the initial treatment for patients with atonic seizures (144); other effective AEDs include felbamate, lamotrigine, topiramate, and benzodiazepines (63). Felbamate was the first new AED with class 1 evidence of efficacy as add-on therapy in patients with LGS, demonstrating the best response in patients with atonic seizures (176,177). Patients with atonic and absence seizures respond most favorably to lamotrigine therapy (149,178). Topiramate reduces the number of drop attacks in patients with LGS and also improves seizure severity (179). Atonic seizures were noted to decrease rapidly in children with LGS after fasting prior to introduction of the ketogenic diet (180). Children with atonic seizures respond quite favorably to vagal nerve stimulation (VNS) (181), and this procedure has been recommended prior to corpus callosotomy (173,175). In two studies, VNS was associated with a reduction in the number of atonic seizures and atypical absence seizures (181,182). Tolerance does not appear to develop (183,184) and drug reduction is possible (185,186), although children with swallowing problems should be monitored for potential aspiration (2,182). Corpus callosotomy renders few patients seizure free (140,142), but atonic seizures, followed by tonic, generalized tonic-clonic, and atypical absence seizures, are most improved, whereas myoclonic seizures and partial seizures are not (141,142). A palliative benefit is noted in most patients (142,187), and an improved response to AED therapy may follow (188). Radiosurgical corpus callosotomy may ultimately prove to be a promising alternative (189).

SUMMARY

Atypical absence, myoclonic, tonic, and atonic seizures in patients with encephalopathic generalized epilepsy are among the most difficult seizures to diagnose and treat accurately (190). Seizure identification directs not only the evaluation of an underlying condition or disease process, but also aids in facilitating appropriate treatment (6,7). The clinical and electroencephalographic manifestations of these seizure types are often syndrome-related, with genetic influences, associated developmental disorders, and multiple handicaps (63). The SSW pattern on EEG is typically an unfavorable one that is not specific for atypical absence seizures, and may also occur with atonic, tonic, myoclonic seizures, and even partial seizures (191). The long-term prognosis for patients with atypical absence, myoclonic, tonic, and atonic seizures seen in conjunction with encephalopathic generalized epilepsy and LGS is poor, often accompanied by uncontrolled seizures; cognitive, psychosocial, and physical consequences; and recurrent seizure-related injuries (192). Over time, the clinical course of an individual patient may change, losing the initial electroclinical features and evolving into different seizure manifestations or even different seizure semiologies. Recent advances in pharmacogenomics, new AEDs, and nonablative surgical techniques will provide greater hope for patients and family members of those with encephalopathic generalized epilepsy and LGS associated with refractory atypical absence, myoclonic, tonic, and atonic seizures (193,194).

REFERENCES

1. Engel J Jr. Epileptic seizures. In: Engel J Jr, ed. *Seizures and epilepsy*. Philadelphia: FA Davis, 1989:137–178.
2. Pellock JM. New delivery systems in the treatment of epilepsy: will they help promote compliance? *Hosp Med* 1999;8:43–49.
3. Mattson RH. Overview: idiopathic generalized epilepsies. *Epilepsia* 2003;44(Suppl 2):2–6.
4. Pedley TA. Overview: diseases associated with epilepsy. In: Engel J Jr, Pedley TA, eds. *Epilepsy: a comprehensive textbook*. Philadelphia: Lippincott-Raven, 1997:2515–2516.
5. Jallon P, Loiseau P, Loiseau J. Newly diagnosed unprovoked epileptic seizures: presentation at diagnosis in CAROLE study. Coordination Active du Reseau Observatoire Longitudinal de l'Epilepsie. *Epilepsia* 2001;42:464–475.
6. Galen, cited by Tempkin O. The falling sickness: a history of epilepsy from the Greeks to the beginnings of modern neurology. 2nd ed. Baltimore, MD: Johns Hopkins Press, 1971.
7. Sisodiya SM. Mechanisms of antiepileptic drug resistance. *Curr Opin Neurol* 2003;16:197–201.
8. Hamer HM, Wyllie E, Luders HO, et al. Symptomatology of epileptic seizures in the first three years of life. *Epilepsia* 1999;40:837–844.
9. Niaz FE, Abou-Khalil B, Fakhoury T. The generalized tonic-clonic seizure in partial versus generalized epilepsy: semiologic differences. *Epilepsia* 1999;40:1664–1666.
10. Vigevano F, Fusco L, Kazuichi Y, et al. Tonic seizures. In: Engel J Jr, Pedley TA, eds. *Epilepsy: a comprehensive textbook*. Philadelphia: Lippincott-Raven, 1997:617–625.
11. Bodensteiner JB, Brownsworth RD, Knapik JR, et al. Interobserver variability in the ILAE classification of seizures in childhood. *Epilepsia* 1988;29:123–128.
12. Proposal for revised clinical and electroencephalographic classification of epileptic seizures. From the Commission on Classification and Terminology of the International League Against Epilepsy. *Epilepsia* 1981;22:489–501.
13. Engel J Jr. A proposed diagnostic scheme for people with epileptic seizures and with epilepsy: report of the ILAE Task Force on Classification and Terminology. *Epilepsia* 2001;42:796–803.
14. Luders H, Acharya J, Baumgartner C, et al. Semiological seizure classification. *Epilepsia* 1998;39:1006–1013.
15. Lennox WG, Davis JP. Clinical correlates of the fast and slow spike-wave electroencephalogram. *Pediatrics* 1950;5:626–644.
16. Yaqub BA. Electroclinical seizures in Lennox-Gastaut syndrome. *Epilepsia* 1993;34:120–127.
17. Stefan H, Snead III OC. Absence seizures. In: Engel J Jr, Pedley TA, eds. *Epilepsy: a comprehensive textbook*. Philadelphia: Lippincott-Raven, 1997:579–590.
18. Epstein MA, Duchowny M, Jayakar P, et al. Altered responsiveness during hyperventilation-induced EEG slowing: a non-epileptic phenomenon in normal children. *Epilepsia* 1994;35:1204–1207.
19. Gastaut H, Roger J, Soulayrol R, et al. Childhood epileptic encephalopathy with diffuse slow spike-waves (otherwise known as "petit mal variant") or Lennox syndrome. *Epilepsia* 1966;7:139–179.
20. Carmant L, Kramer U, Holmes GL, et al. Differential diagnosis of staring spells in children: a video-EEG study. *Pediatr Neurol* 1996;14:199–202.
21. Bare MA, Glauser TA, Strawsburg RH. Need for electroencephalogram video confirmation of atypical absence seizures in children with Lennox-Gastaut syndrome. *J Child Neurol* 1998;13:498–500.
22. Holmes GL, McKeever M, Adamson M. Absence seizures in children: clinical and electroencephalographic features. *Ann Neurol* 1987;21:268–273.
23. Velasco AL, Boleaga B, Santos N, et al. Electroencephalographic and magnetic resonance correlations in children with intractable seizures of Lennox-Gastaut syndrome and epilepsia partialis continua. *Epilepsia* 1993;34:262–270.
24. Guye M, Bartolomei F, Gastaut JL, et al. Absence epilepsy with fast rhythmic discharges during sleep: an intermediary form of generalized epilepsy? *Epilepsia* 2001;42:351–356.
25. Velasco M, Velasco F, Alcala H, et al. Epileptiform EEG activity of the centromedian thalamic nuclei in children with intractable generalized seizures of the Lennox-Gastaut syndrome. *Epilepsia* 1991;32:310–321.
26. Matsuzaka T, Ono K, Baba H, et al. Quantitative EEG analyses and surgical outcome after corpus callosotomy. *Epilepsia* 1999;40:1269–1278.
27. Marciani MG, Spanedda F, Placidi F, et al. Changes of the EEG paroxysmal pattern during felbamate therapy in Lennox-Gastaut syndrome: a case report. *Int J Neurosci* 1998;95:247–253.
28. Gloor P. Generalized epilepsy with spike-and-wave discharge: a reinterpretation of its electrographic and clinical manifestations. *Epilepsia* 1979;20:571–588.
29. Penry JK, Porter RJ, Dreifuss RE. Simultaneous recording of absence seizures with video tape and electroencephalography. A study of 374 seizures in 48 patients. *Brain* 1975;98:427–440.
30. Goldsmith IL, Zupanc ML, Buchalter JR. Long-term seizure outcome in 74 patients with Lennox-Gastaut syndrome: effects of incorporating MRI head imaging in defining the cryptogenic subgroup. *Epilepsia* 2000;41:395–399.
31. Ogawa K, Kanemoto K, Ishii Y, et al. Long-term follow-up study of Lennox-Gastaut syndrome in patients with severe motor and intellectual disabilities: with special reference to the problem of dysphagia. *Seizure* 2001;10:197–202.
32. Rasmussen T. Characteristics of a pure culture of frontal lobe epilepsy. *Epilepsia* 1983;24:482–493.
33. Ohtahara S, Ohtsuka Y, Kobayashi K. Lennox-Gastaut syndrome: a new vista. *Psychiatry Clin Neurosci* 1995;49:S179–S183.
34. Chaix Y, Daquin G, Monteiro F, et al. Absence epilepsy with onset before age three years: a heterogeneous and often severe condition. *Epilepsia* 2003;44:944–949.
35. Barkovich AJ, Kuzniecky RI. Gray matter heterotopia. *Neurology* 2000;55:1603–1608.
36. Tatum WO IV, Genton P, Bureau M, et al. Less common epilepsy syndromes. In: Wyllie E, ed. *The treatment of epilepsy: principles & practice*, 3rd ed. Philadelphia: Lippincott Williams & Wilkins, 2001:551–575.
37. Aicardi J. Atypical semiology of rolandic epilepsy in some related syndromes. *Epileptic Disord* 2000;2(Suppl 1):S5–S9.
38. Fahn S, Marsden CD, Van Woert MH. Definition and classification of myoclonus. In: Fahn S, Marsden CD, Van Woert MH, eds. *Myoclonus. Advances in neurology*, vol 43. New York: Raven Press, 1986:1–5.
39. Marsden CD, Hallett M, Fahn S. The nosology and pathophysiology of myoclonus. In: Marsden CD, Fahn S, eds. *Movement disorders*. London: Butterworth, 1982:196–248.
40. Erba G, Browne TR. Atypical absence, myoclonic, atonic and tonic seizures, and the "Lennox-Gastaut syndrome." In: Browne TR, Feldman RG, eds. *Epilepsy: diagnosis and management*. Boston: Little, Brown, 1983:75–94.
41. Hallet M. Myoclonus: relation to epilepsy. *Epilepsia* 1985; 26(Suppl 1):S67–S77.
42. Oguni H, Mukahira K, Uehara T, et al. Electrophysiological study of myoclonic seizures in children. *Brain Dev* 1997;19:279–284.
43. Dulac O, Plouin P, Shewmon A. Myoclonus and epilepsy in childhood: 1996 Royaumont meeting. *Epilepsy Res* 1998;30:91–106.
44. Renganathan R, Delanty N. Juvenile myoclonic epilepsy: under-appreciated and under-diagnosed. *Postgrad Med J* 2003;79:78–80.
45. Gordon N. Review: juvenile myoclonic epilepsy. *Child Care Health Dev* 1994;20:71–76.
46. Wang PJ, Lee WT, Hwu WL, et al. The controversy regarding diagnostic criteria for early myoclonic encephalopathy. *Brain Dev* 1998;20:530–535.
47. Spiegel EA, Wycis HT. Thalamic recordings in man: special reference to seizure discharges. *Electroencephalogr Clin Neurophysiol* 1950;2:23–27.
48. Rapin I. Myoclonus in neuronal storage and Lafora diseases. In: Fahn S, Marsden CD, Van Woert MH, eds. *Myoclonus. Advances in neurology*, vol 43. New York: Raven Press, 1986:65–85.
49. Gioanni Y, Everett J, Lamarche M. The transcortical reflex triggered by cutaneous or muscle stimulation in the cat with a penicillin epileptic focus: relative importance of regions 3a and 4. *Exp Brain Res* 1983;51:57–64.
50. Kobayashi K, Maniwa S, Ogino T, et al. Myoclonic seizures combined with partial seizures and probable pathophysiology of

secondary bilateral synchrony. *Clin Neurophysiol* 2000;111: 1813–1816.

51. Aicardi J. Early myoclonic encephalopathy. In: Roger J, Bureau M, Dravet C, et al., eds. *Epileptic syndromes in infancy, childhood and adolescence,* 2nd ed. London: John Libbey, 1992:13–23.

52. Zara F, Gennaro E, Stabile M, et al. Mapping of a locus for a familial autosomal recessive idiopathic myoclonic epilepsy of infancy to chromosome 16p13. *Am J Hum Genet* 2000;66: 1552–1557.

53. Plaster NM, Uyama E, Uchino M, et al. Genetic localization of the familial adult myoclonic epilepsy (FAME) gene to chromosome 8q24. *Neurology* 1999;53:1180–1183.

54. Bauer J, Elger CE. Psychogenic seizures mimicking juvenile myoclonic epilepsy: case reports. *Seizure* 2001;10:208–211.

55. Scheffer IE, Wallace R, Mulley JC, et al. Clinical and molecular genetics of myoclonic-astatic epilepsy and severe myoclonic epilepsy in infancy (Dravet syndrome). *Brain Dev* 2001;23: 732–735.

56. Oguni H, Fukuyama Y, Tanaka T, et al. Myoclonic-astatic epilepsy of early childhood—clinical and EEG analysis of myoclonic-astatic seizures, and discussions on the nosology of the syndrome. *Brain Dev* 2001;23:757–764.

57. Doose H. Myoclonic astatic epilepsy of early childhood. In: Roger J, Bureau M, Dravet C, et al., eds. *Epileptic syndromes in infancy, childhood and adolescence,* 2nd ed. London: John Libbey, 1992:103–114.

58. Tassinari CA, Lyagoubi S, Santos V, et al. Study on spike and wave discharges in man. II. Clinical and electroencephalographic aspects of myoclonic epilepsy [French]. *Rev Neurol (Paris)* 1969;121:379–383.

59. Gennaro E, Veggiotti P, Malacarne M, et al. Familial severe myoclonic epilepsy of infancy: truncation of Nav1.1 and genetic heterogeneity. *Epileptic Disord* 2003;5:21 25.

60. Aicardi J, Chevrie JJ. Myoclonic epilepsies of childhood. *Neuropadiatrie* 1971;3:177–190.

61. Conry JA. Progressive myoclonic epilepsies. *J Child Neurol* 2002;17(Suppl 1):S80–S84.

62. Gelisse P, Genton P, Raybaud C, et al. Is it juvenile myoclonic epilepsy? *Epileptic Disord* 2000;2:27–32.

63. Bergin AM. Pharmacotherapy of paediatric epilepsy. *Expert Opin Pharmacother* 2003;4:421–431.

64. Tatum WO IV, French JA, Benbadis SR, et al. The etiology and diagnosis of status epilepticus. *Epilepsy Behav* 2001;2:311–317.

65. Froscher W. Sleep and prolonged epileptic activity (status epilepticus). *Epilepsy Res Suppl* 1991;2:165–176.

66. Proposal for revised classification of epilepsies and epileptic syndromes. Commission on Classification and Terminology of the International League Against Epilepsy. *Epilepsia* 1989;30:389–399.

67. Karbowski K. Developments in epileptology in the 18th and 19th century prior to the delineation of the Lennox-Gastaut syndrome. In: Niedermeyer E, Degen R, eds. *The Lennox-Gastaut syndrome.* New York: Alan R. Liss, 1988:1–8.

68. Egli M, Mothersill I, O'Kane M, et al. The axial spasm—the predominant type of drop seizure in patients with secondary generalized epilepsy. *Epilepsia* 1985;26:401–415.

69. Fusco L, Vigevano F. Ictal clinical electroencephalographic findings of spasms in West syndrome. *Epilepsia* 1993;34:671–678.

70. Pachatz C, Fusco L, Vigevano F. Epileptic spasms and partial seizures as a single ictal event. *Epilepsia* 2003;44:693–700.

71. Farrell K. Tonic and atonic seizures. In: Wyllie E, ed. *The treatment of epilepsy: principles & practice,* 3rd ed. Philadelphia: Lippincott Williams & Wilkins, 2001:405–413.

72. Tassinari CA, Michelucci R, Shigematsu H, et al. Atonic and falling seizures. In: Engel J Jr, Pedley TA, eds. *Epilepsy: a comprehensive textbook.* Philadelphia: Lippincott-Raven, 1997:605–616.

73. Shih TT, Hirsch LJ. Tonic-absence seizures: an underrecognized seizure type. *Epilepsia* 2003;44:461–465.

74. Ishida S, Kato M, Oonuma T, et al. Tonic-automatism complex: cases with violent gestural automatisms following a brief tonic seizure. *Jpn J Psychiatry Neurol* 1993;47:271–272.

75. Froscher W. Sleep and prolonged epileptic activity (status epilepticus). *Epilepsy Res Suppl* 1991;2:165–176.

76. Vigevano F, Lispi ML. Tonic reflex seizures of early infancy: an age-related non-epileptic paroxysmal disorder. *Epileptic Disord* 2001;3:133–136.

77. Bye A, Lamont P, Healy L. Commencement of a paediatric EEG-video telemetry service. *Clin Exp Neurol* 1990;27:83–88.

78. Burnstine TH, Vining EP, Uematsu S, et al. Multifocal independent epileptiform discharges in children: ictal correlates and surgical therapy. *Neurology* 1991;41:1223–1228.

79. Chevrie JJ, Aicardi J. Childhood epileptic encephalopathy with slow spike-wave. A statistical study of 80 cases. *Epilepsia* 1972;13:259–271.

80. Niedermeyer E. Lennox-Gastaut syndrome. Clinical description and diagnosis. *Adv Exp Med Biol* 2002;497:61–75.

81. Halasz P. Runs of rapid spikes in sleep: a characteristic EEG expression of generalized malignant epileptic encephalopathies. A conceptual review with new pharmacological data. *Epilepsy Res Suppl* 1991;2:49–71.

82. Gastaut H, Tassinari CA. Tonic seizures. In: Gastaut H, Tassinari CA, eds. *Handbook of electroencephalography and clinical neurophysiology,* vol 13, part A. Amsterdam: Elsevier, 1975:29–31.

83. Hoffmann-Riem M, Diener W, Benninger C, et al. Nonconvulsive status epilepticus—a possible cause of mental retardation in patients with Lennox-Gastaut syndrome. *Neuropediatrics* 2000;31: 169–174.

84. Kutluay E, Passaro EA, Gomez-Hassan D, et al. Seizure semiology and neuroimaging findings in patients with midline spikes. *Epilepsia* 2001;42:1563–1568.

85. Arroyo S, Lesser RP, Fisher RS, et al. Clinical and electroencephalographic evidence for sites of origin of seizures with diffuse electrodecremental pattern. *Epilepsia* 1994;35:974–987.

86. Ikeda A, Yazawa S, Kunieda T, et al. Scalp-recorded, ictal focal DC shift in a patient with tonic seizure. *Epilepsia* 1997;38: 1350–1354.

87. Claes L, Del-Favero J, Ceulemans B, et al. De novo mutations in the sodium-channel gene SCN1A cause severe myoclonic epilepsy of infancy. *Am J Hum Genet* 2001;68.1327–1332.

88. Ikeno T, Shigematsu H, Miyakoshi M, et al. An analytic study of epileptic falls. *Epilepsia* 1985;26:612–621.

89. Besag FM. Lesson of the week: tonic seizures are a particular risk factor for drowning in people with epilepsy. *BMJ* 2001;322: 975–976.

90. Hahn A, Pistohl J, Neubauer BA, et al. Atypical "benign" partial epilepsy or pseudo-Lennox syndrome. Part 1: symptomatology and long-term prognosis. *Neuropediatrics* 2001;32:1–8.

91. Ko TS, Holmes GL. EEG and clinical predictors of medically intractable childhood epilepsy. *Clin Neurophysiol* 1999;110: 1245–1251.

92. Aso K, Watanabe K. Limitations in the medical treatment of cryptogenic or symptomatic localization-related epilepsies of childhood onset. *Epilepsia* 2000;41(Suppl 9):18–20.

93. Libenson MH, Stafstrom CE, Rosman NP. Tonic "seizures" in a patient with brainstem demyelination: MRI study of brain and spinal cord. *Pediatr Neurol* 1994;11:258–262.

94. Okada S, Kinoshita M, Fujioka T, et al. Two cases of multiple sclerosis with painful tonic seizures and dysesthesia ameliorated by administration of mexiletine. *Jpn J Med* 1991;30: 373–375.

95. Scher MS, Aso K, Beggarly ME, et al. Electrographic seizures in preterm and full-term neonates: clinical correlates, associated brain lesions, and risk for neurologic sequelae. *Pediatrics* 1993;91:128–134.

96. Vigevano F, Fusco L. Hypnic tonic postural seizures in healthy children provide evidence for a partial epileptic syndrome of frontal lobe origin. *Epilepsia* 1993;34:110–119.

97. Chauvel P, Trottier S, Vignal JP, et al. Somatomotor seizures of frontal lobe origin. In: Chauvel P, Delgado-Escueta AV, Halgren E, et al., eds. *Frontal lobe seizures and epilepsies. Advances in neurology,* vol 57. New York: Raven Press, 1992:185–232.

98. Ikeda A, Matsumoto R, Ohara S, et al. Asymmetric tonic seizures with bilateral parietal lesions resembling frontal lobe epilepsy. *Epileptic Disord* 2001;3:17–22.

99. Werhahn KJ, Noachtar S, Arnold S, et al. Tonic seizures: their significance for lateralization and frequency in different focal epileptic syndromes. *Epilepsia* 2000;41:1153–1161.

100. Salanova V, Morris HH, Van Ness P, et al. Frontal lobe seizures: electroclinical syndromes. *Epilepsia* 1995;36:16–24.

101. Tempkin O. *The falling sickness.* Baltimore, MD: Johns Hopkins Press, 1945.

102. Gastaut H, Tassinari CA, Bureau-Paillas M. Polygraphic and clinical study of "epileptic atonic collapses" [French]. *Riv Neurol (Paris)* 1966;36:5–21.
103. Oguni J, Uehara T, Imai K, et al. Atonic epileptic drop attacks associated with generalized spike-and-slow wave complexes: video-polygraphic study in two patients. *Epilepsia* 1997;38:813–818.
104. Gastaut H, Broughton R. *Epileptic seizures.* Springfield, IL: Charles C Thomas, 1972:37–47.
105. Lin YY, Su MS, Yiu CH, et al. Startle epilepsy presenting as drop attacks: a case report. *Zhonghua Yi Xue Za Zhi (Taipei)* 1995;56:270–273.
106. Meletti S, Tinuper P, Bisulli F, et al. Epileptic negative myoclonus and brief asymmetric tonic seizures. A supplementary sensorimotor area involvement both for negative and positive motor phenomena. *Epileptic Disord* 2000;2:163–168.
107. Oguni H, Fukuyama Y, Imaizumi Y, et al. Video-EEG analysis of drop seizures in myoclonic astatic epilepsy of early childhood (Doose syndrome). *Epilepsia* 1992;33:805–813.
108. Satow T, Ikeda A, Yamamoto J, et al. Partial epilepsy manifesting atonic seizure: report of two cases. *Epilepsia* 2002;43:1425–1431.
109. Oguni H, Sato F, Hayashi K, et al. A study of unilateral brief focal atonia in childhood partial epilepsy. *Epilepsia* 1992;33:75–83.
110. Fiol ME, Gates JR, Mireles R, et al. Value of intraoperative EEG changes during corpus callosotomy in predicting surgical results. *Epilepsia* 1993;34:74–78.
111. Tatum WO IV. Long-term EEG monitoring: a clinical approach to electrophysiology. *J Clin Neurophysiol* 2001;18:442–455.
112. Nakken KO, Lossius R. Seizure-related injuries in multihandicapped patients with therapy-resistant epilepsy. *Epilepsia* 1993;34:836–840.
113. Pazzaglia P, D'Alessandro R, Ambrosetto G, et al. Drop attacks: an ominous change in the evolution of partial epilepsy. *Neurology* 1985;35:1725–1730.
114. Vergnes M, Marescaux C. Pathophysiological mechanism underlying genetic absence epilepsy in rats. In: Malafosse A, Genton P, Mirsch E, et al., eds. *Idiopathic generalized epilepsies: clinical, experimental, and genetic aspects.* London: John Libbey, 1994:151–168.
115. Kuzniecky R. Familial diffuse cortical dysplasia. *Arch Neurol* 1994;51:307–310.
116. Capovilla G, Rubboli G, Beccaria F, et al. A clinical spectrum of the myoclonic manifestations associated with typical absences in childhood absence epilepsy. A video-polygraphic study. *Epileptic Disord* 2001;3:57–62.
117. Gastaut H. The Lennox-Gastaut syndrome: comments on the syndrome's terminology and nosological position amongst the secondary generalized epilepsies of childhood. *Electroencephalogr Clin Neurophysiol Suppl* 1982;35:71–84.
118. Berkovic SF, Benbadis SR. Absence seizures. In: Wyllie E, ed. *The treatment of epilepsy: principles & practice,* 3rd ed. Philadelphia: Lippincott Williams & Wilkins, 2001:357–367.
119. Meencke HJ, Janz D. The significance of microdysgenesis in primary generalized epilepsy: an answer to the considerations of Lyon and Gastaut. *Epilepsia* 1985;26:368–371.
120. Pavone A, Niedermeyer E. Absence seizures and the frontal lobe. *Clin Electroencephalogr* 2000;31:153–156.
121. Metrakos K, Metrakos JD. Childhood epilepsy of subcortical ("centrencephalic") origin. Some questions and answers for the pediatrician. *Clin Pediatr (Phila)* 1966;5:537–542.
122. Berkovic SF, Howell RA, Hay DA, et al. Epilepsies in twins. In: Wolf P, ed. *Epileptic seizures and syndromes.* London: John Libbey, 1994:157–164.
123. Snead OC 3rd. Basic mechanisms of generalized absence seizures. *Ann Neurol* 1995;37:146–157.
124. Devinsky O, Gershengorn J, Brown E, et al. Frontal functions in juvenile myoclonic epilepsy. *Neuropsychiatry Neuropsychol Behav Neurol* 1997;10:243–246.
125. Sano A, Mikami M, Nakamura M, et al. Positional candidate approach for the gene responsible for benign adult familial myoclonic epilepsy. *Epilepsia* 2002;43(Suppl 9):26–31.
126. Zara F, Gennaro E, Stabile M, et al. Mapping of a locus for a familial autosomal recessive idiopathic myoclonic epilepsy of infancy to chromosome 16p13. *Am J Hum Genet* 2000;66:1552–1557.
127. Scheffer IE, Wallace RH, Phillips FL, et al. X-linked myoclonic epilepsy with spasticity and intellectual disability: mutation in the homeobox gene ARX. *Neurology* 2002;59:348–356.
128. Elia M, Guerrini R, Musumeci SA, et al. Myoclonic absence-like seizures and chromosome abnormality syndromes. *Epilepsia* 1998;39:660–663.
129. Fang W, Huang CC, Chu NS, et al. Myoclonic epilepsy with ragged-red fibers (MERRF) syndrome: report of a Chinese family with mitochondrial DNA point mutation in tRNA (Lys) gene. *Muscle Nerve* 1994;17:52–57.
130. Cossette P, Liu L, Brisebois K, et al. Mutation of GABRA1 in an autosomal dominant form of juvenile myoclonic epilepsy. *Nat Genet* 2002;31:184–189.
131. So NK. Mesial frontal epilepsy. *Epilepsia* 1998;39(Suppl 4):S49–S61.
132. Ito M, Kobayashi K, Fuji T, et al. Electroclinical picture of autosomal dominant frontal lobe epilepsy in a Japanese family. *Epilepsia* 2000;41:52–58.
133. Gale K. Animal models of generalized convulsive seizures: some neuroanatomical differentiations of seizure types. In: Avoli M, Gloor P, Kostopoulos G, et al., eds. *Generalized epilepsy. Neurobiological approaches.* Boston: Birkhauser, 1990:329–343.
134. Browning RA, Nelson DK. Modification of electroshock and pentylenetetrazol seizure patterns in rats after precollicular transections. *Exp Neurol* 1986;93:546–556.
135. Gale K. Subcortical structures and pathways involved in convulsive seizure generation. *J Clin Neurophysiol* 1992;9:264–277.
136. Ricci S, Cusmai R, Fariello G, et al. Double cortex. A neuronal migration anomaly as a possible cause of Lennox-Gastaut syndrome. *Arch Neurol* 1992;49:61–64.
137. So NK. Atonic phenomena and partial seizures: a reappraisal. In: Fahn S, Hallett M, Luders H, et al., eds. *Negative motor phenomena. Advances in neurology,* vol 67. Philadelphia: Lippincott-Raven, 1995:29–39.
138. Siegel JM, Nienhuis R, Fahringer HM, et al. Neuronal activity in narcolepsy: identification of cataplexy-related cells in the medial medulla. *Science* 1991;252:1315–1318.
139. Luders HO, Dinner DS, Morris HH, et al. Cortical electrical stimulation in humans. The negative motor areas. *Adv Neurol* 1995;67:115–129.
140. Andermann F, Tenembaum S. Negative motor phenomena in generalized epilepsies. A study of atonic seizures. *Adv Neurol* 1995;67:9–28.
141. Aihara M, Hatakeyama K, Koizumi K, et al. Ictal EEG and single photon emission computed tomography in a patient with cortical dysplasia presenting with atonic seizures. *Epilepsia* 1997;38:723–727.
142. Cendes F, Ragazzo PC, da Costa V, et al. Corpus callosotomy in treatment of medically resistant epilepsy: preliminary results in a pediatric population. *Epilepsia* 1993;34:910–917.
143. Chabolla DR. Characteristics of the epilepsies. *Mayo Clin Proc* 2002;77:981–990.
144. Guerrini R, Dravet C, Genton P, et al. Lamotrigine and seizure aggravation in severe myoclonic epilepsy. *Epilepsia* 1998;39:508–512.
145. Alvarez N, Besag F, Iivanainen M. Use of antiepileptic drugs in the treatment of epilepsy in people with intellectual disability. *J Intellect Disabil Res* 1998;42(Suppl 1):1–15.
146. Lerman-Sagie T, Watemberg N, Kramer U, et al. Absence seizures aggravated by valproic acid. *Epilepsia* 2001;42:941–943.
147. Panayiotopoulos CP. Treatment of typical absence seizures and related epileptic syndromes. *Paediatr Drugs* 2001;3:379–403.
148. Czuczwar SJ, Borowicz KK. Polytherapy in epilepsy: the experimental evidence. *Epilepsy Res* 2002;52:15–23.
149. Donaldson JA, Glauser TA, Olberding LS. Lamotrigine adjunctive therapy in childhood epileptic encephalopathy (the Lennox-Gastaut syndrome). *Epilepsia* 1997;38:68–73.
150. Carrazana EJ, Wheeler SD. Exacerbation of juvenile myoclonic epilepsy with lamotrigine. *Neurology* 2001;56:1424–1425.
151. Farwell JR, Anderson GD, Kerr BM, et al. Stiripentol in atypical absence seizures in children: an open trial. *Epilepsia* 1993;34:305–311.

152. Kanazawa O. Refractory grand mal seizures with onset during infancy including severe myoclonic epilepsy in infancy. *Brain Dev* 2001;23:749–756.

153. Fernando-Dongas MC, Radtke RA, VanLandingham KE, et al. Characteristics of valproic acid resistant juvenile myoclonic epilepsy. *Seizure* 2000;9:385–388.

154. Bassan H, Bloch AM, Mesterman R, et al. Myoclonic seizures as a main manifestation of Epstein-Barr virus infection. *J Child Neurol* 2002;17:446–447.

155. Dulac O, Kaminska A. Use of lamotrigine in Lennox-Gastaut and related epilepsy syndromes. *J Child Neurol* 1997;12(Suppl 1):S23–S28.

156. Chiron C, Marchand MC, Tran A, et al. Stiripentol in severe myoclonic epilepsy in infancy: a randomised placebo-controlled syndrome-dedicated trial. STICLO study group. *Lancet* 2000;356:1638–1642.

157. Perucca E, Gram L, Avanzini G, et al. Antiepileptic drugs as a cause of worsening seizures. *Epilepsia* 1998;39:5–17.

158. Berkovic SF. Aggravation of generalized epilepsies. *Epilepsia* 1998;39(Suppl 3):S11–S14.

159. Asconape J, Diedrich A, DellaBadia J. Myoclonus associated with the use of gabapentin. *Epilepsia* 2000;41:479–481.

160. Appleton RE. Vigabatrin in the management of generalized seizures in children. *Seizure* 1995;4:45–48.

161. Nieto-Barrera M, Candau R, Nieto-Jimenez M, et al. Topiramate in the treatment of severe myoclonic epilepsy in infancy. *Seizure* 2000;9:590–594.

162. Resor SR Jr, Resor LD. Chronic acetazolamide monotherapy in the treatment of juvenile myoclonic epilepsy. *Neurology* 1990;40:1677–1681.

163. Koskiniemi M, Van Vleymen B, Hakamies L, et al. Piracetam relieves symptoms in progressive myoclonus epilepsy: a multicentre, randomised, double-blind, crossover study comparing the efficacy and safety of three dosages of oral piracetam with placebo. *J Neurol Neurosurg Psychiatry* 1998;64:344–348.

164. Prasad AN, Stafstrom CE, Holmes GL. Alternative epilepsy therapies: the ketogenic diet, immunoglobulins, and steroids. *Epilepsia* 1996;37(Suppl 1):S81–S95.

165. Yamamoto T, Pipo JR, Akaboshi S, et al. Forced normalization induced by ethosuximide therapy in a patient with intractable myoclonic epilepsy. *Brain Dev* 2001;23:62–64.

166. Tatum WO IV, Galvez R, Benbadis S, et al. New antiepileptic drugs: into the new millennium. *Arch Fam Med* 2000;9:1135–1141.

167. Genton P. When antiepileptic drugs aggravate epilepsy. *Brain Dev* 2000;22:75–80.

168. DiMario FJ Jr, Clancy RR. Paradoxical precipitation of tonic seizures by lorazepam in a child with atypical absence seizures. *Pediatr Neurol* 1988;4:249–251.

169. Jobst BC, Siegel AM, Thadani VM, et al. Intractable seizures of frontal lobe origin: clinical characteristics, localizing signs, and results of surgery. *Epilepsia* 2000;41:1139–1152.

170. Lee SA, Ryu JY, Lee SK, et al. Generalized tonic seizures associated with ganglioglioma: successful treatment with surgical resection. *Eur Neurol* 2001;46:225–226.

171. Wiebe S, Blume WT, Girvin JP, et al. A randomized, controlled trial of surgery for temporal-lobe epilepsy. *N Engl J Med* 2001;345:311–318.

172. Bourgeois M, Sainte-Rose C, Lellouch-Tubiana A, et al. Surgery of epilepsy associated with focal lesions in childhood. *J Neurosurg* 1999;90:833–842.

173. Holmes GL. Overtreatment in children with epilepsy. *Epilepsy Res* 2002;52:35–42.

174. Wheless JW. The ketogenic diet: an effective medical therapy with side effects. *J Child Neurol* 2001;16:633–635.

175. Benbadis SR, Tatum WO, Vale FL. When drugs don't work: an algorithmic approach to medically intractable epilepsy. *Neurology* 2000;55:1780–1784.

176. Dodson WE. Felbamate in the treatment of Lennox-Gastaut syndrome: results of a 12-month open-label study following a randomized clinical trial. *Epilepsia* 1993;34(Suppl 7):S18–S24.

177. Felbamate Study Group in Lennox-Gastaut Syndrome. Efficacy of felbamate in childhood epileptic encephalopathy (Lennox-Gastaut syndrome). *N Engl J Med* 1993;328:29–33.

178. Mikati MA, Holmes GL. Lamotrigine in absence and primary generalized epilepsies. *J Child Neurol* 1997;12(Suppl 1):S29–S37.

179. Sachdeo RC, Glauser TA, Ritter F, et al. A double-blind, randomized trial of topiramate in Lennox-Gastaut syndrome. Topiramate YL Study Group. *Neurology* 1999;52:1882–1887.

180. Freeman JM, Vining EP. Seizures decrease rapidly after fasting: preliminary studies of the ketogenic diet. *Arch Pediatr Adolesc Med* 1999;153:946–949.

181. Patwardhan RV, Stong B, Bebin EM, et al. Efficacy of vagal nerve stimulation in children with medically refractory epilepsy. *Neurosurgery* 2000;47:1353–1357.

182. Frost M, Gates J, Helmers SL, et al. Vagus nerve stimulation in children with refractory seizures associated with Lennox-Gastaut syndrome. *Epilepsia* 2001;42:1148–1152.

183. Tatum WO IV, Benbadis SR, Vale FL. The neurosurgical treatment of epilepsy. *Arch Fam Med* 2000;9:1142–1147.

184. Hosain S, Nikalov B, Harden C, et al. Vagus nerve stimulation treatment for Lennox-Gastaut syndrome. *J Child Neurol* 2000;15:509–512.

185. Tatum WO, Johnson KD, Goff S, et al. Vagus nerve stimulation and drug reduction. *Neurology* 2001;56:561–563.

186. Morris GL III, Mueller WM. Long-term treatment with vagus nerve stimulation in patients with refractory epilepsy. The Vagus Nerve Stimulation Study Group E01-E05. *Neurology* 1999;53:1731–1735.

187. Maehara T, Shimizu H. Surgical outcome of corpus callosotomy in patients with drop attacks. *Epilepsia* 2001;42:67–71.

188. Vossler DG, Lee JK, Ko TS. Treatment of seizures in subcortical laminar heterotopia with corpus callosotomy and lamotrigine. *J Child Neurol* 1999;14:282–288.

189. Pendl G, Eder HG, Schroettner O, et al. Corpus callosotomy with radiosurgery. *Neurosurgery* 1999;45:303–307.

190. Dulac O, N'Guyen T. The Lennox-Gastaut syndrome. *Epilepsia* 1993;34(Suppl 7):S7–S17.

191. Martinez-Menendez B, Sempere AP, Mayor PP, et al. Generalized spike-and-wave patterns in children: clinical correlates. *Pediatr Neurol* 2000;22:23–28.

192. Hauser WA. The natural history of drug resistant epilepsy: epidemiologic considerations. *Epilepsy Res Suppl* 1992;5:25–28.

193. Thompson PJ, Upton D. The impact of chronic epilepsy on the family. *Seizure* 1992;1:43–48.

194. Nguyen DK, Spencer SS. Recent advances in the treatment of epilepsy. *Arch Neurol* 2003;60:929–935.

Epileptic Spasms

21

W. Donald Shields   *Susan Koh*

In 1841, James West wrote a letter to *Lancet* describing an infant with a "peculiar" seizure disorder (1). He gave a remarkably clear account of the characteristic clusters of brief flexor jerks that later became known as infantile spasms and, in honor of that initial description, West syndrome. The letter also described the distinctive developmental failure. Sadly, Dr. West's patient was his son.

In the past, spasms were believed to be limited to young children, hence the term *infantile*. In recent years, as it has become clear that older children and adults may have seizures that are clinically and electrographically indistinct from infantile spasms, the general term *epileptic spasms* is now sometimes employed (2). Juvenile spasms occur in older children, and infantile spasms manifest in younger children. Most research into epileptic spasms has focused on the infantile form, the primary topic of this chapter.

Until the advent of electroencephalography (EEG) (3), it was not obvious that West syndrome was an epileptic disorder. Since Gibbs' identification of hypsarrhythmia as a specific electroencephalographic pattern associated with infantile spasms (4), epileptic spasms have been further studied and classified. Whether infantile spasms are a generalized or partial epilepsy has depended on changes in classification. In 1970, the International League Against Epilepsy placed infantile spasms among the generalized seizure disorders, dropped spasms altogether from the 1981 revision, defined infantile spasms as an age-related generalized epilepsy in 1989, and concluded in 1991 that spasms should be classified as a syndrome whose etiology is either symptomatic or cryptogenic. The seizures associated with infantile spasms can be either generalized or occasionally localized or lateralized (i.e., hemihypsarrhythmia or hemi-infantile spasms). The spasms may be generalized even when the underlying lesion is localized—an important observation because such lesions may be amenable to surgical management even in patients with apparently generalized seizures.

EPIDEMIOLOGY

The incidence for epileptic spasms is approximately 2 to 5 per 10,000 live births worldwide (5–9), with an estimated lifetime prevalence by age 10 years of 1.5 to 2 per 10,000 children (6,10). The lower prevalence rates are a result of mortality, evolution of epileptic spasms into other seizure types, and incomplete determination in population-based studies of older children (11). A genetic predisposition may exist, as infantile spasms have been reported in both monozygotic and dizygotic twins (12,13). Sex differences are inconsistent (14), although some studies suggest a moderate male predominance (5,8).

CLINICAL PRESENTATION

West syndrome is a triad of epileptic spasms, hypsarrhythmia, and developmental failure or regression. Over the years, salaam seizures, jackknife seizures, axial spasms, periodic spasms, and serial spasms have been used to describe events that are not epileptic spasms (15).

Age of onset is typically between 4 and 8 months (16), but epileptic spasms can occur as early as 2 weeks or as late as 18 months of age (11,17) and, rarely, can begin in adulthood. In some studies (17), late-onset spasms were cryptogenic and occurred despite previously normal development; other studies (15) found that half were associated with cortical dysplasia, hypoxic-ischemic encephalopathy, or genetic anomalies and were refractory to medications (16). Late-onset spasms have been intermixed with atonic, tonic, partial, myoclonic, or generalized tonic-clonic seizures or atypical absences. The characteristic spasms generally resolve spontaneously or evolve into Lennox-Gastaut syndrome or intractable partial seizures. Spasms may persist in 15% to 23% of all patients beyond 3 to 7 years of age (18,19).

Epileptic spasms consist of clusters of seizures involving a flexion jerk of the neck, trunk, and extremities. The phasic contraction lasts for less than 2 seconds, the ensuing tonic contraction for 2 to 10 seconds, although only the phasic contraction may be present (16). Sometimes called tonic spasms, prolonged muscle or tonic contractions are seen in intractable cases (20). The three types of spasms—flexion, extension, and mixed—are classified by the type of contraction. In flexion spasms, the trunk, arms, legs, and head flex. In extension spasms, the back arches and arms and legs extend. Mixed spasms combine extension of the legs and flexion of the neck, trunk, and arms. The mixed type accounts for 42% of all epileptic spasms; extensor spasms, the least common, comprise 23% of all epileptic spasms (16). Many children have more than one type, even in the same cluster (21), often influenced by position. If the trunk remains vertical, the resemblance is to a flexion spasm; if the patient is horizontal, what looks like an extension spasm is seen (22). The contractions themselves also vary. Spasms can range from only a subtle head drop or shoulder shrug to more violent action (21). Subtle spasms usually occur at the onset or offset of the episode (23). Although videotelemetry alone reveals no electrographic difference in the spasm, electromyography (EMG) with videotelemetry shows that the first activated muscle can vary in the same patient between different clusters or even from spasm to spasm within the same cluster. Even if the same muscle were initially activated with every spasm, the ensuing sequence or pattern of muscle involvement may differ within the same cluster (24).

Eye deviation or nystagmus may occur in two-thirds of all infantile spasms (16). Eye movements may be independent of the spasm or may precede its development by weeks. Usually an aspect of typical spasms, eye movements may coexist with the spasm and represent variability or changes in consciousness (23). Decreased responsiveness may follow motor spasms or occur independently as a second seizure type (11). Between spasms, most children cry, although this is apparently not an ictal phenomenon (16) and may be a result of surprise or pain. Up to 60% of all patients have respiratory pauses. Pulse changes occur less often. Some spasms are induced by sound or touch, rarely by photic stimulation (21).

Rarely, one arm or leg is more extended or the head deviates to one side. Spasms are usually asymmetric on the side contralateral to a unilateral lesion such as hemimegalencephaly. Symmetric spasms and a symptomatic etiology usually indicate diffuse lesions, not lateralized as in Down syndrome or neurofibromatosis (25); however, some children with focal or unilateral lesions may have only symmetric spasms (21,25). Recently, videotelemetry has allowed more frequent detection of asymmetric spasms. These patients either have consistently asymmetric spasms or alternate between asymmetric or symmetric spasms.

Spasms may be intermixed with other seizure types in one-third to one-half of patients (18,19,26–28). The muscle contraction in spasms is faster than that in tonic seizures but slower than that in myoclonic seizures (29,30). Tonic seizures can occur simultaneously with or precede spasms and may be difficult to differentiate, requiring videotelemetry to define the seizure type. Tonic seizures last longer than spasms and lack the initial phasic component. Both may be generated by a similar mechanism or have a similar origin such as the brainstem (16).

Partial seizures may occur before, during, or after a spasm and frequently precede a cluster of spasms (22). Partial seizures suggest a symptomatic cortical lesion. Prenatal etiology is implied if the partial seizure precedes the spasms (31). Partial seizures occurring simultaneously with spasms may be a result of chance. Alternatively, partial seizures may induce the appearance of infantile spasms or may stem from a critical factor, such as arousal mechanism, that simultaneously affects a mechanism generating both partial seizures and spasms (16). If the partial seizure precedes the spasms themselves, the patient usually will have asymmetric spasms with the predominant side changing to conform to that of the preceding partial seizure. In a patient with partial seizures and symmetric spasms, the spasm following the seizure would be initially asymmetric but gradually become symmetric (22,25).

Spasms occur on awakening or after feeding, and less often during sleep (16). Most occur in clusters, although single spasms, lasting for less than 1 to 5 seconds, have been documented (16). Clusters consist of 3 to 20 spasms that occur several times a day (11). The spasms decrease in intensity at the end of longer clusters (16). In a 2-week comparison, the number and type of spasms varied markedly; day-to-day variation was less common (32).

Approximately 50% of patients have abnormal neurologic findings on presentation, including blindness, hemiparesis, or microcephaly (33), that help to identify the 85% to 90% of that group who will eventually have developmental delay (14,33,34). Other studies quote mental retardation in 75% and cerebral palsy in 50% of patients (10,18,19,27,28,35,36).

In many children, infantile spasms eventually evolve into Lennox-Gastaut syndrome. Tonic seizures usually coexist with and are more marked in that syndrome. Seizure clustering is seen in West syndrome, but infrequently in Lennox-Gastaut syndrome (25). Clusters of epileptic spasms will become the single spasms of Lennox-Gastaut syndrome concurrently with the change in interictal pattern from hypsarrhythmia to diffuse slow spike and wave at 1 to 2.5 Hz (37). Conversely, if the interictal background continues to show multifocal independent spike discharges, the seizure semiology may not change (37).

PATHOPHYSIOLOGY

Conclusive evidence as to the pathophysiology of epileptic spasms is lacking, perhaps because there are no good experimental models (38). Some believe that infantile spasms represent a nonspecific age-dependent reaction of the immature brain to injury involving subcortical structures (11) that acts diffusely on the cortex, leading to the hypsarrhythmic electroencephalogram pattern and the generalized spasms. Individual case reports have described abnormalities in the pons and involvement of the serotonergic, noradrenergic, or cholinergic neurons in the brainstem nuclei (39–41). Brainstem origin has also been postulated on the basis of abnormalities in brainstem auditory evoked responses in patients with spasms (42) and disruptions of rapid eye movement (REM) sleep (43,44). Because hypsarrhythmia occurs mainly during sleep and the brainstem controls sleep cycles, the sleep association suggests involvement of the brainstem in infantile spasms (44,45).

The frequent intermixture of partial seizures with generalized or asymmetric spasms suggests a cortical-subcortical interaction, a hypothesis supported by the effectiveness of cortical resection in controlling generalized infantile spasms (22). In other words, the cortical lesion interacts with developing brainstem pathways, causing motor spasms that are similar to startle or cortical reflex myoclonus (37,46).

Further supporting the brainstem hypothesis are results of positron emission tomography (PET) scans in patients with epileptic spasms showing hypermetabolism of the lenticular nuclei (47). That serotonergic ([^{11}C]-methyl-L-tryptophan) and γ-aminobutyric acid (GABA)-ergic ([^{11}C]-flumazenil) tracers may be more effective than fluorodeoxyglucose PET in defining a focus in patients with epileptic spasms also suggests brainstem involvement, because the raphe-cortical or striatal projections use serotonin as a neurotransmitter and these pathways cause the diffuse hypsarrhythmic patterns on EEG (48). On ictal single-photon-emission computed tomography studies, both subcortical and cortical structures were activated (49).

The response to corticotropin suggests involvement of the hypothalamus and pituitary-adrenal axis. Baram has proposed that a nonspecific stressor releases the proconvulsant corticotropin-releasing hormone (CRH) (50), which may be the final common pathway for the multitude of etiologies of infantile spasms. CRH causes severe seizures and death in neurons associated with learning and memory, and its effects are especially important in infants because CRH receptors are most abundant during the early developmental period (51). To support the hypothesis that corticotropin inhibits the release and production of CRH through a negative feedback mechanism, Nagamitsu and colleagues (52) measured cerebrospinal fluid (CSF) levels of β-endorphin (also derived from a common precursor of corticotropin), corticotropin, and CRH (which releases both corticotropin and β-endorphin) in 20 patients with spasms. The CSF levels of β-endorphin and corticotropin were lower than in controls, as was the CRH level, although not significantly. Riikonen observed that CSF corticotropin levels were higher in infants with cryptogenic than symptomatic spasms (53).

Because infantile spasms typically begin at the time when the first immunizations are administered, the question has been whether the association is causative or coincidental. Numerous anecdotal reports have noted the appearance of infantile spasms within a few hours to a few days after a diphtheria, pertussis, tetanus vaccination, although all controlled studies to date have failed to demonstrate any association (54–57). Some proposed immunologic mechanisms have been based on antibodies to brain tissue in blood samples from patients with infantile spasms (58,59), or increased numbers of activated B and T cells in the blood (60), or increased levels of HLA-DRw52 antigen (34). Finally, calcium-mediated models have been postulated, but no studies have yet been published (61).

ETIOLOGY

Many disorders can give rise to spasms, and correct identification of the cause often has therapeutic and prognostic implications. When the underlying cause cannot be identified, spasms are classified as cryptogenic and in the past accounted for up to 50% of cases. Since the advent of magnetic resonance imaging (MRI) and newer sequences, however, only 10% to 15% are cryptogenic (34,62–64). In fact, some imaging studies that were normal early in life may later demonstrate lesions on MRI as a result of progressive myelination (65). PET may also increase the chance of detecting a lesion in some cryptogenic patients. Spasms are symptomatic when a disorder can be identified by history, physical and neurologic examination, neuroimaging, and metabolic or genetic testing. Symptomatic patients account for 70% to 80% of all cases (8,28, 36,38,48) and generally have a poorer prognosis than cryptogenic children. Cryptogenic patients often are products of a normal pregnancy and birth, with normal development prior to the onset of spasms and normal findings on physical examination. The spasms begin abruptly without a background of previous partial seizures. Results of neuroimaging and laboratory evaluations are normal (66). Cryptogenic patients have higher levels of CSF corticotropin, serum progesterone, CSF GABA, and CSF nerve growth factor (53), but these may reflect brain damage from the spasms. Symptomatic patients usually have more focality on neurologic examination, a history of partial seizures evolving into spasms, or lateralization on EEG (67).

Watanabe (66) proposed a subset of the cryptogenic group with "idiopathic" West syndrome. These patients have normal development, and their spasms stop completely after a short time. Developmental regression and focal interictal EEG abnormalities are absent, and hypsarrhythmia disappears between each spasm, which is symmetric. A family history of seizures is common. This group may represent from 44% to 87% of all cryptogenic cases (30,68).

Although most children with spasms have no family history, a possible X-linked transmission has been mapped to regions Xp11.4-Xpter and Xp21.3-Xp22.1 that also is associated with mental retardation (69). One of these loci is implicated in neuroaxonal processing (radixin, RDXP2) (70).

The diseases associated with symptomatic epileptic spasms are classified as prenatal, perinatal, and postnatal. Prenatal causes include congenital malformation, TORCH (toxoplasmosis, other infections, rubella, cytomegalovirus, and herpes simplex) infections, neurocutaneous disorders, chromosomal abnormalities, metabolic disorders, and congenital syndrome. Prenatal etiologies account for 30% to 45%, perhaps as many as 50%, of all cases (26,35,71,72). Tuberous sclerosis causes from 10% to 30% of prenatal spasms (27,72,73). A comparatively large tuber burden is more likely to produce spasms rather than partial seizures (74). Although partial seizures are most common with focal cortical dysplasia, epileptic spasms can occur (75); PET scans may help to identify these patients (76). Occipital lesions are associated with earlier onset of epileptic spasms than are frontal lesions (77). Neurofibromatosis type I can also cause spasms, but these usually have a better prognosis than other symptomatic causes (78). Chromosomal abnormalities, most commonly Down syndrome (72,79), represent approximately 13% of prenatal etiology; these children usually do not have a poor prognosis compared to other symptomatic cases (68).

Perinatal causes account for 14% to 25% of spasms but may be decreasing in frequency (66), perhaps because of a lowered incidence of neonatal hypoglycemia (80). Perinatal causes include hypoxic ischemic encephalopathy and hypoglycemia. The difference may be relative, however, and reflect an increased survival in low-birth-weight infants rather than a true decrease in perinatal causes. Hypoxic-ischemic encephalopathy often involves severe neonatal electroencephalographic findings such as markedly or maximally depressed backgrounds in the first week of life (81). In children with cerebral palsy, deep white-matter injuries are not associated with West syndrome; therefore, spasms are less likely in premature infants (80). Spasms associated with periventricular leukomalacia are typically hypsarrhythmic and located more posteriorly than anteriorly (30,82).

Postnatal causes include meningoencephalitis and other types of infections, stroke and trauma, hypoxic ischemic insult such as near drowning and cardiac arrest, and tumors.

ELECTROPHYSIOLOGY

Hypsarrhythmia is the most common interictal electroencephalographic pattern (23), although diffuse slow, focal slow, multifocal independent spike discharges, generalized spike-and-slow discharges, and, rarely, normal interictal patterns are also seen (16). Hypsarrhythmia manifests as high-voltage (500 to 1000 mV), disorganized, asynchronous, multifocal, independent spike-and-wave discharges that wax and wane, with attenuation between the epileptiform activities (4). Generally considered pathognomonic for infantile spasms, it can, rarely, be found in other diseases (83). The interictal pattern often changes on serial electroencephalographies (84,85). Hypsarrhythmia is usually seen early in the disorder, but there can sometimes be a lag from clinical symptoms. Long-term monitoring has disclosed variable patterns throughout the day, with more hypsarrhythmia noted in slow-wave sleep and less in REM sleep (21). During arousal from sleep or during REM sleep, the background may look normal; this "pseudonormalization" may also immediately precede a cluster of spasms (86). Severity may vary from patient to patient and can decrease with corticotropin treatment (87). Hypsarrhythmia depends on the intensity of the spasms, not on the etiology (30,68).

Any variation in the characteristic pattern is called modified hypsarrhythmia and includes background synchronization, focal features, voltage asymmetries, generalized background burst suppression, and slow waves without spikes (16) (Fig. 21.1). Modified hypsarrhythmia is more frequent than typical hypsarrhythmia (21). In an analysis of precorticotropin electroencephalograms (88), the modified pattern occurred in up to 36 (69%) of 53 patients with spasms; cortical dysplasia was associated with hemihypsarrhythmia or burst suppression.

A burst-suppression pattern, as seen in children with Ohtahara syndrome, suggests a poor prognosis; a lower-voltage electroencephalogram may indicate a better outcome (87), as may preservation of hypsarrhythmia between spasms (30,68), faster background activity, and absence of electrodecremental response. However, less-typical features of hypsarrhythmia (such as disorganization, slowing, high amplitude, spike and electrodecremental response, absence sleep architecture, relative normalization, burst suppression, hemihypsarrhythmia, occipital hypsarrhythmia, interhemispheric asymmetry, and interhemispheric synchronization) would give a better prognosis (88). This view is controversial, however, as modified hypsarrhythmia has been linked to a worse prognosis than typical hypsarrhythmia (26). In late-onset epileptic spasms, a more organized electroencephalogram background correlated with better development; persistent hypsarrhythmia and a disorganized background worsened the prognosis (15).

The most common ictal discharge is a triphasic, positive, high-amplitude slow wave; a low-amplitude brief rapid discharge occurs less frequently (22,30) (Fig. 21.2). The generalized positive slow waves are followed by attenuation or an electrodecremental response (16), observed mainly at PZ (parietal midline), FZ/PZ, or FZ (frontal midline) with laterality (25). Because the decremental activity always follows the slow wave and clinical spasm, it is postictal (22,30). The slow wave corresponds to the actual spasm. An electrodecremental response can also be

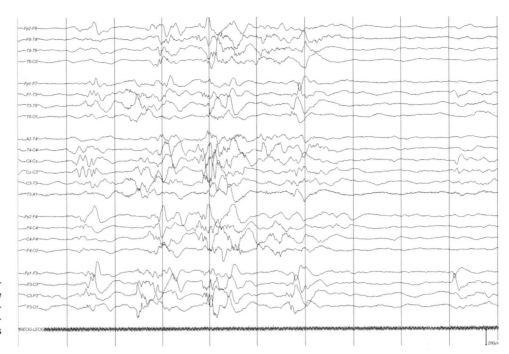

Figure 21.1 Modified hypsarrhythmia with high-amplitude multifocal spike discharges superimposed on a disorganized background and interspersed with areas of severe voltage attenuation.

seen without an obvious clinical seizure (11). Slow-sharp and slow-wave complexes, although less frequent with spasms, differ from the elongated appearance of those in myoclonic seizures (30). Diffuse attenuation, generalized spike wave, paroxysmal fast activity or fast frequencies, and slow wave are also associated with infantile spasms. There is no real difference between the semiology of the spasms and the different ictal patterns. The ictal pattern lasts for only 1 second; a 1-minute or longer pattern is associated with behavioral arrest (21). EMG shows that the axial

muscles contract earlier than the limb muscles and the head earlier than the arms (25). A review of the electroencephalographic and behavioral changes before and between the spasms (89) suggests that a cluster of spasms may represent a single sustained ictal event rather than brief, repetitive seizures. Pseudonormalization and high-amplitude slowing precede the spasms and are associated with decreased activity and interaction (90).

Fast-wave bursts were seen during REM sleep in 35% of patients with spasms, sometimes occurring periodically

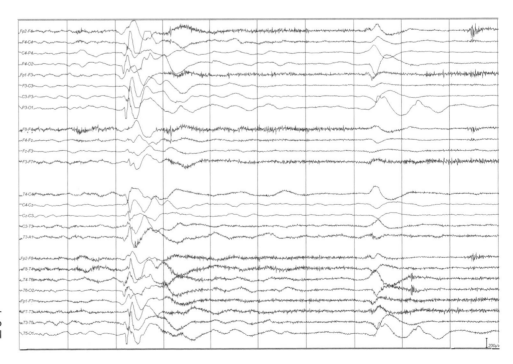

Figure 21.2 Electroencephalogram showing generalized sharp wave and electrodecremental response during a spasm.

until clinical spasms appeared and the patient awoke (25). Spasms start subclinically in REM sleep (90); subclinical discharges without clinical manifestations are also possible at the end of the spasm cluster. Surface EMG shows subclinical contractions without actual movement on video-EEG during the subclinical discharges (30,68).

Fast activity sometimes occurred either alone or following the high-amplitude slow wave, usually in the left or right occipital, posterior temporal, and parietal areas, and corresponded to the stare that preceded the spasms (25,46). Fast activity is often associated with tonic spasms with sustained tonic muscle contraction (90–92) and may be more common in asymmetric spasms (90,93), suggesting a cortical onset for spasms. Fast activity can also fade during repeated spasms or in partial seizures that occur with spasms (46).

The wide variety of diseases that can mimic infantile spasms and the underreporting or overreporting of spasms prompted by subtle semiology often necessitate videotelemetry for differentiation. Videotelemetry may also help to distinguish between concurrent tonic seizures and partial seizures intermixed in a spasm cluster.

DIFFERENTIAL DIAGNOSIS AND EVALUATION OF SUSPECTED INFANTILE SPASMS

Infantile spasms can occasionally be confused with other, less severe, epilepsy syndromes, particularly benign familial infantile convulsions (BFIC) (94,95) and benign myoclonic epilepsy of infancy (BMEI) (96). A firm diagnosis is necessary before initiation of therapy because many common medications (specifically corticotropin and vigabatrin) carry a higher risk of morbidity or mortality than most commonly used anticonvulsants. Like infantile spasms, BFIC and BMEI present in the first year of life. The seizures of BFIC are usually partial, but the electroencephalogram may be normal (95). Myoclonic seizures in BMEI can occur in clusters. The electroencephalogram may be normal or show generalized spike-and-wave discharges but not the hypsarrhythmia or multifocal independent spike discharges typical of infantile spasms. Because patients with infantile spasms may not display the distinguishing electroencephalographic abnormalities early in the disease, a normal or mildly abnormal record does not rule out infantile spasms at that stage; follow-up studies may be needed for clarification. Children with the benign syndromes are developmentally normal before seizures begin and continue to develop at a normal rate. In contrast, children with infantile spasms may or may not be normal at seizure onset but will invariably demonstrate either developmental regression or failure to achieve developmental milestones in a timely fashion.

Once the diagnosis of infantile spasms is established, attention shifts to etiology. In recent years, two developments have prompted a subtle, but significant, change in the focus of the evaluation. First, several underlying causes of the seizures have a specific therapy different from that of traditional medications (Table 21.1). Second, many underlying causes are genetic disorders, and correct identification will allow for appropriate family counseling, to prevent recurrences in other children.

Besides the division of etiologies into symptomatic and cryptogenic, subdivision of the symptomatic group reflects the issues noted above: [1] symptomatic with specific therapy: (a) with a genetic etiology, (b) without an identified genetic etiology; [2] symptomatic without specific therapy: (a) with a genetic etiology, (b) without an identified genetic etiology (Table 21.1).

As with all forms of epilepsy, the evaluation begins with the history and physical/neurologic examination. Table 21.2 lists the diagnoses that can be established from these initial findings. The skin should be examined for evidence of neurocutaneous disorders and the fundi for a cherry-red macula suggestive of a storage or mitochondrial disorder or for chorioretinitis indicating possible transplacental infection. Nearly half of all of the etiologic diagnoses are established or suspected by the historical and physical data. Many diagnoses, however, require confirmatory MRI, and once imaging is complete, approximately 70% of patients will have a confirmed etiologic diagnosis (Table 21.3) (97). In many cases, expensive and time-consuming laboratory studies can be avoided. In the remaining 30% of cases, an etiology will be established for no more than one third, leaving about 10% of cases in which a diagnosis is determined by results of lumbar puncture or metabolic or genetic testing.

Neuroimaging

Much of the decrease in cryptogenic cases is a result of the advances in MRI techniques of the past 10 to 15 years. Comparing etiologic categories of infantile spasms, Riikonen noted that identification of brain malformations increased from 10% between 1960 and 1977 to nearly 35% between 1977 and 1991 (97). Imaging should be considered essential to the evaluation. MRI is preferred to computed tomography (CT) scanning because of the greater sensitivity for brain malformations. CT, however, can show subtle calcifications caused by transplacental infections. In a study of 86 patients with infantile spasms, MRI assigned 91% to a symptomatic etiology, most commonly hypoxic-ischemic encephalopathy (30%) (98) characterized by diffuse atrophy and thinning of the corpus callosum. Delayed myelination in 27% of patients did not appear to be associated with any specific etiology.

Some MRI abnormalities suggest specific etiologies, many genetically based, that may require further workup

TABLE 21.1

SYMPTOMATIC INFANTILE SPASMS WITH POSSIBLE SPECIFIC THERAPY

Symptomatic, Treatable Disorder	Therapy
Pyridoxine-dependent seizures	Pyridoxine (1a)
Phenylketonuria	Diet (1a)
Maple-syrup urine disease	Diet (1a)
Glucose transporter defect	Ketogenic diet
Tumor	Surgery to remove tumor (1b)
Arteriovenous malformation	Surgery to treat the malformation (1b)
Sturge-Weber syndrome	Surgery if medications fail (1a)
Tuberous sclerosis	Vigabatrin, possible surgery if medications fail (1a)
Biotinidase deficiency	Biotin (1a)
Menkes disease	Copper histidinate (1a)
Hyperammonemia disorders	Possible diet, depending on the disorder (1a)
Nonketotic hyperglycinuria	Benzoate (1a)
Cortical dysplasias	Possible cortical resection if medications fail (1b)
Focal cortical dysplasia	
Hemimegalencephaly	

1a, Symptomatic with a specific therapy and a genetic etiology; 1b, symptomatic with a specific therapy without an identified genetic etiology.

(Table 21.4). Additional abnormalities will be added to this list as our understanding of genetics advances.

Metabolic Studies

Metabolic studies are indicated to identify the more than 50 disorders associated with infantile seizures (99–101). A trial of folinic acid is warranted (102), as is a 100-mg intravenous pyridoxine bolus to rule out pyridoxine-dependent seizures. Complete blood count, electrolytes (looking for an anion gap), and glucose determinations are appropriate. Measurements of uric acid, transaminases, lactate, pyruvate, ammonia, urine organic acids, and serum amino acids will identify the vast majority of inborn errors of metabolism linked to infantile spasms. In the past, phenylketonuria was a relatively common inborn error identified by testing that has been nearly eliminated by neonatal screening. Nevertheless, such screening is not

TABLE 21.2

ETIOLOGIC DIAGNOSES BASED ON HISTORY AND PHYSICAL/NEUROLOGIC EXAMINATION

History	Examination
Hypoxic-ischemic encephalopathy	Neurocutaneous disorders
Perinatal hypoxic-ischemic encephalopathy (2b)	Tuberous sclerosis (2a)
Near-miss sudden infant death syndrome (2b)	Neurofibromatosis (2a)
Cardiac arrest (2b)	Sebaceous nevus syndrome
Near drowning (2b)	Incontinentia pigmenti
Maternal toxemia (2b)	Sturge-Weber syndrome (2b)
Encephalitis (usually herpes) (2b)	Epidermal nevus syndrome
Meningitis (2b)	Hydrocephalus (+ imaging) (2b)
Cerebral abscess (2b)	Miller-Dieker syndrome (+ imaging) (2a)
Transplacental infections (2b)	Down syndrome (2b)
Trauma (2b)	
Postcardiac surgery (2b)	
Neonatal hypoglycemia	

2a, Symptomatic without a specific therapy but with a genetic etiology; 2b, symptomatic without a specific therapy and without an identified genetic etiology.

TABLE 21.3

ETIOLOGIC DIAGNOSES CONFIRMED OR ESTABLISHED BY MAGNETIC RESONANCE IMAGING

Tuberous sclerosis (2a)
Aicardi syndrome
Cortical dysplasias
    Lissencephaly (2a)
    Pachygyria
    Hemimegalencephaly
    Band heterotopia (2a)
    Focal cortical dysplasia
Porencephaly
Hypoxic-ischemic encephalopathy
Tumor
Arteriovenous malformation
Leigh disease (2a)
Hydranencephaly
Corpus callosum agenesis/dysgenesis (2a)
Septooptic dysplasia
Schizencephaly
Holoprosencephaly
Sturge-Weber syndrome
Multiple pineal cysts
Transplacental infections
Periventricular leukomalacia

2a, Symptomatic without a specific therapy but with a genetic etiology.

routine in all countries, and measurement of urine amino acid levels will detect phenylketonuria and maple-syrup urine disease, as well as other, rarer, metabolic diseases. Zellweger syndrome and neonatal adrenoleukodystrophy are other rare causes of hypsarrhythmia that can be diagnosed with the serum very-long-chain fatty acid test.

Lumbar Puncture

A few very rare disorders, such as nonketotic hyperglycinemia, may be detected only by study of the CSF (103). In addition to routine evaluations for glucose, protein, and cells, the CSF should be assessed for amino acids plus lactate and pyruvate to detect possible mitochondrial disorders.

TREATMENT

The purpose of James West's 1841 letter was to solicit recommendations for a cure. It would be more than a century before adrenocorticotropic hormone, or corticotropin, was recognized as the first effective therapy (104) and to date only two medications have class 1 evidence of efficacy: corticotropin and vigabatrin (105). Corticotropin is approved by the Food and Drug Administration for use in the United States. The ketogenic diet and high-dose intravenous gammaglobulin (IVIG), as well as surgical procedures, also can play a role.

Unlike most other seizure types in which a 50% or 90% reduction defines success, therapy for infantile spasms must completely eliminate both the spasms and the hypsarrhythmic electroencephalographic pattern.

For this reason, a timely diagnosis accelerates prompt identification of the most effective therapy, which allows the child's normal brain plasticity to bring about the best

TABLE 21.4

MAGNETIC RESONANCE IMAGING FINDINGS REQUIRING FURTHER EVALUATION

Abnormality	Possible Association
Lissencephaly	
• Posterior predominant lissencephaly or Miller-Dieker syndrome	LIS1 gene on chromosome 17
• Anterior predominant lissencephaly or band heterotopia	XLIS gene on X chromosome
• Lissencephaly with cerebellar hypoplasia	Reelin gene
Cortical tubers, periventricular nodules	Tuberous sclerosis; two genes identified; 75% to 85% are spontaneous mutations; parents should be evaluated
Perisylvian polymicrogyria	Some are familial; multiple associations X-linked recessive X-linked dominant Autosomal recessive 22q11.2 deletions
Cerebral calcifications	Transplacental infections
Loss of cerebral white matter	Pyruvate carboxylase deficiency
Hypoplasia of corpus callosum	Nonketotic hyperglycemia

possible developmental outcome. In many patients, however, underlying disorders, for example, lissencephaly concurrent with infantile spasms, preclude normal development regardless of seizure control. In the past, the effect of seizure control on development was debated. Infantile spasms caused by tuberous sclerosis have responded to vigabatrin, proving that, sometimes at least, seizure control can improve development (106).

The vast majority of patients eventually "outgrow" the seizures and either evolve to another type or stop having seizures. Persistent seizures usually evolve to either Lennox-Gastaut syndrome or a similar disorder or to partial seizures. In any case, if spasms are followed by other seizures, mental retardation is virtually a universal outcome. On the other hand, some patients who become free of spasms develop normal or near-normal intellect.

Corticotropin

In 1958, Sorel and colleagues administered 4 to 10 IU/day of corticotropin to seven patients (104), four of whom responded within a few days; therapy failed in only one patient. The effectiveness of corticotropin underscores how infantile spasms differ from all other epilepsy syndromes. In the 45 years since that report, efficacy has been repeatedly confirmed, but agreement is still lacking on the most appropriate dose and duration of treatment. Dosing is complicated by the existence of natural and synthetic forms of corticotropin. Studies of the synthetic product generally used much lower doses than studies of the natural product. It is estimated that 1 IU of synthetic corticotropin is equivalent to 40 IU of natural corticotropin. The synthetic version is used primarily in Japan where a low dose is 0.2 IU/kg/day and a high dose is 1 IU/kg/day. Even with the low dose, 75% of patients responded in one study (107). In contrast, natural corticotropin at doses up to 150 IU/m^2/day succeeded in 14 of 15 patients; 5 later had relapses, for a long-term response rate of 60% (108). A review of seven studies (19) did not confirm a better response with 150 IU/day than with 40 IU/day, a common dose. The overall long-term response rate ranged from 53% to 91%. Treatment often begins with 40 IU/day for 1 to 2 weeks and increases to 60 or even to 80 IU/day if the response is incomplete. If spasms are controlled and hypsarrhythmia disappears, the dose is tapered over 1 to 4 months. Failure mandates rapid tapering and discontinuation.

Despite its effectiveness for infantile spasms, no medication carries a higher potential for significant side effects. Most children develop cushingoid obesity and intense irritability. All are at risk for arterial hypertension, electrolyte imbalance, gastric ulcer, growth retardation, cardiomyopathy, or immunosuppression with increased risk of infection. In one study (5), the risk of serious side effects was 43% with 160 IU/day; the incidence was lower with lower doses. Death from infection and cardiomyopathy has ranged from 2% to 5% in some series. Corticotropin exacerbates the seizures in a few infants, and treatment for more than a few weeks leads to steroid insufficiency if the drug is stopped abruptly (109). Parents must be fully apprised of the morbidity and mortality risks before therapy begins, and these must be balanced against the virtual certainty of mental retardation if the spasms are not controlled. Careful follow-up with regular measurements of blood pressure and electrolytes is mandatory. The current risk-to-benefit assessment favors corticotropin, but if another, less hazardous medication proves to be as effective, it would be the drug of choice.

Vigabatrin

In 1991, 29 of 68 patients with medically refractory infantile spasms achieved complete resolution with vigabatrin as add-on therapy, as did 12 of 14 patients who had tuberous sclerosis (110). Vigabatrin also might be effective in Down syndrome (111).

Since 1997, four controlled trials have been reported. Vigevano and Cilio (112) administered either corticotropin 10 IU/day or vigabatrin 100 to 150 mg/kg/day to children with newly diagnosed infantile spasms. Eleven of 23 vigabatrin patients responded (one late relapse) compared with 14 of 19 corticotropin patients (six late relapses). Vigabatrin was more effective in patients with tuberous sclerosis or cerebral malformations; corticotropin was more effective in patients with perinatal hypoxic-ischemic encephalopathy. There was no difference in cryptogenic cases. Appleton and colleagues (113) used vigabatrin or placebo for 5 days, followed by open-label vigabatrin. Seven of 20 patients in the vigabatrin group were seizure free at the end of 5 days, as were two of 20 in the placebo group. For 14 days, Elterman and associates (114) treated 75 patients with 18 to 36 mg/kg/day (low dose) and 67 patients with 100 to 148 mg/kg/day (high dose) of vigabatrin. Eight low-dose patients and 24 high-dose patients achieved complete control. In a study involving underlying tuberous sclerosis, all 11 patients treated with vigabatrin responded, compared with only 5 of 11 patients treated with hydrocortisone (115).

Vigabatrin appears to be well tolerated. The reports of hypotonia, somnolence, or insomnia (110) are expected in a drug that enhances GABA activity. Constriction of peripheral visual fields, which substantially limits the drug's use, was not reported until 1997 (116) and now affects from 15% to 50% of patients. In one report (117), constriction occurred in more than 90% of patients who had been taking vigabatrin for a mean of 8.5 years. Foveal function also may be impaired (118). Most studies have suggested that the constriction is not reversible; however, 8 of 12 patients who underwent full withdrawal improved significantly; none of the 12 who continued taking the drug did so (117). The problem is mild enough that most patients are unaware of the disturbance, which becomes apparent only on perimetric studies.

Unfortunately, visual fields are virtually impossible to evaluate in these very young children, many with cortical visual impairment and visual inattention unrelated to vigabatrin therapy. Given the catastrophic nature of infantile spasms, visual-field constriction may be an acceptable price for seizure control and improved opportunity for normal development (119). Vigabatrin may be the drug of choice for children with infantile spasms caused by tuberous sclerosis.

Pyridoxine

Because pyridoxine (vitamin B_6) dependence is a rare cause of infantile spasms, a trial of 100 mg intravenously is appropriate for patients whose diagnosis remains in doubt after the initial history, physical examination, and MRI (120). Seizures caused by pyridoxine-dependent epilepsy cease immediately following intravenous administration of vitamin B_6. As early as 1968, however, long-term oral administration of high doses has been effective against non–pyridoxine-dependent seizures (121). In 1993, 5 of 17 patients treated with 100 to 300 mg/kg/day responded within 4 weeks—most within 1 week (122). In Japan, high-dose vitamin B_6 is the drug of choice (123,124), with reported response rates of 10% to 30%. Loss of appetite, irritability, and vomiting are modest compared with the side effects of corticotropin or vigabatrin. Pyridoxine has not found favor outside Japan and a few other epilepsy centers, but given its low-risk profile, a 1- to 2-week trial of 100 to 400 mg is reasonable before other therapy is started.

Valproic Acid

In a 1981 report (125), valproic acid produced an "excellent" response in 4 of 18 patients treated with 20 mg/kg/day. A year later, 7 of 19 patients achieved good control (11 had also been treated with corticotropin) (126). Seizures were controlled in 11 of 22 patients treated with up to 100 mg/kg/day for 4 weeks (127). Other patients later responded but also received dexamethasone or carbamazepine, so the effect of valproic acid was less clear. Prospective randomized studies of efficacy against infantile spasms are lacking. Because liver failure is a risk in children younger than 2 years of age (128), although none of the reported patients were affected, valproic acid should be used cautiously as therapy for infantile spasms.

Benzodiazepines

One of the earliest nonsteroid treatments for infantile spasms (129–131), the benzodiazepines succeed only occasionally but may be useful if more effective therapies have failed. Nitrazepam administered to 24 children controlled infantile spasms in 11 (132). A multicenter, randomized comparison of corticotropin and nitrazepam (133) demonstrated no statistical difference between the two medications in significantly reducing spasms. Side effects with corticotropin were more severe, leading to dis-

continuation in six patients. Many reports noted an increase in oral secretions and a higher incidence of aspiration and pneumonia with nitrazepam. Several deaths occurred in one series (134). The incidence of mortality was 3.98 deaths per 100 patient-years when young epilepsy patients were taking nitrazepam and 0.26 deaths per 100 patient-years if the medication had been discontinued (135).

Other Antiepileptic Drugs

None of the new anticonvulsants have enough evidence of efficacy to permit a recommendation. The Japanese experience suggests that zonisamide may be effective in about one-third of patients (136), but controlled and comparison trials are lacking. Five of 25 patients had a complete clinical and electrographic response to doses ranging from 8 to 32 mg/kg/day; most responses occurred in 1 to 2 weeks (137). Zonisamide was well tolerated, but 20% of the patients in one study experienced anorexia and 1 patient lost weight (138). If the more than 30% efficacy figures hold up in controlled studies, zonisamide could become a first-line therapy.

Topiramate up to 25 mg/kg/day was effective in 4 of 11 patients with intractable infantile spasms (139). Seizures decreased in 43% of 14 patients, but worsened in 29%; no patient became seizure free (140).

Before reports of aplastic anemia, 3 of 4 patients with medically intractable infantile spasms responded to felbamate as add-on therapy (141). Because aplastic anemia has not been noted in prepubertal patients, felbamate may be as safe as some other drugs and could be recommended if other medications have failed.

Anecdotal evidence, but no prospective controlled trials, supports the efficacy of lamotrigine. One report noted that 25 of 30 patients became seizure free (142). The usual dose is 6 to 10 mg/kg/day; however, three patients in whom vigabatrin and corticotropin had failed responded to less than 1 mg/kg/day (143). Use of a low dose is important because rash, the major side effect, depends to some extent on how rapidly the dose is increased. The usual recommendation is a slow rise over 2 months to the minimum expected therapeutic dose. Given the need to control infantile spasms as soon as possible, this 2-month requirement decreases the therapeutic value of lamotrigine. If the very low dose is effective, however, lamotrigine becomes a fallback drug.

Two nondrug approaches are possible options when other treatments have failed. The ketogenic diet is a decades-old therapy enjoying a resurgence of interest. Two retrospective reports of 40 children suggest control of spasms in 20% to 35% of patients with otherwise intractable disease (144,145). Children younger than 1 year of age can achieve ketosis and may benefit from the diet. Despite generally good tolerability, renal stones, gastritis, hyperlipidemia, and gastroesophageal reflux occurred. High-dose IVIG, the other nondrug therapy, is useful in a variety of seizure disorders. All six children with cryptogenic infantile spasms, but only 1 of 5 symptomatic patients, achieved complete remission (146). IVIG may also improve juvenile spasms (147). Doses range from 100 to 200 mg/kg administered every 2 to 3 weeks to 400 mg/kg/day for 5 consecutive days. Actual efficacy is unclear, however, and the most appropriate doses and duration have not been determined.

Some children with infantile spasms have a localized cortical abnormality, whose removal may control seizures and possibly improve developmental outcome (47,148). A history of partial seizures that preceded or accompanied infantile spasms, cortical disturbances on MRI, or localized EEG abnormalities that suggest a cortical defect should prompt referral to a pediatric epilepsy surgery center.

PROGNOSIS

Death, intractable epilepsy, mental retardation, and autism are possible consequences of infantile spasms. A 25- to 35-year follow-up of 214 patients (19,149) demonstrated that 31% died, many in the first 3 years of life. Eight of the 24 deaths by age 3 years were a consequence of complications of corticotropin therapy. The most common cause of death overall was infection. Of the 147 survivors, 25 (17%) had an intelligence quotient (IQ) of 85 or higher; 11 others (7%) were in the dull-normal range with IQs of 68 to 84; and 45% were retarded. Outcome depends on two factors. First is the underlying etiology. Some etiologies, such as severe hypoxic-ischemic encephalopathy and lissencephaly, will lead to death or mental retardation regardless of whether infantile spasms develop. However, children with cryptogenic spasms or spasms caused by focal cortical dysplasia may have a normal or near-normal developmental outcome if the second factor, seizure control, is achieved.

REFERENCES

1. West W. On a particular form of infantile convulsions. *Lancet* 1841;1:724–725.
2. Cerullo A, Marini C, Carcangiu R, et al. Clinical and video-polygraphic features of epileptic spasms in adults with cortical migration disorder. *Epileptic Disord* 1999;1:27–33.
3. Livingston S, Eisner V, Pauli V. Minor motor epilepsy: diagnosis, treatment and prognosis. *Pediatrics* 1958;21:916–928.
4. Gibbs F, Gibbs E. Atlas of electroencephalography. In: Gibbs F, Gibbs E, eds. *Epilepsy*. Reading, MA: Addison-Wesley, 1952.
5. Riikonen R, Donner M. Incidence and aetiology of infantile spasms from 1960 to 1976: a population study in Finland. *Dev Med Child Neurol* 1979;21:333–343.
6. Cowan LD, Hudson LS. The epidemiology and natural history of infantile spasms. *J Child Neurol* 1991;6:355–364.
7. Ludvigsson P, Olafsson E, Sigurthardottir S, et al. Epidemiologic features of infantile spasms in Iceland. *Epilepsia* 1994;35:802–805.
8. Sidenvall R, Eeg-Olofsson O. Epidemiology of infantile spasms in Sweden. *Epilepsia* 1995;36:572–574.
9. van den Berg B, Yerushalmy J. Studies on convulsive disorders in young children, I: incidence of febrile and nonfebrile convulsions by age and other factors. *Pediatr Res* 1969;3:298–304.
10. Trevathan E, Murphy C, Yeargin-Allsopp M. The descriptive epidemiology of infantile spasms among Atlanta children. *Epilepsia* 1999;40:748–751.
11. Wong M, Trevathan E. Infantile spasms. *Pediatr Neurol* 2001;24:89–98.
12. Pavone L, Mollica F, Incorpa G, et al. Infantile spasms syndrome in monozygotic twins. *Arch Dis Child* 1980;55:870–872.
13. Senga P, Mayanda H, Yidika M. Spasmes infantiles chez deux jumeaux monozygotiques: une novelle observation. *Presse Med* 1986;15:485.
14. Lacy J, Penry J. Infantile spasms. In: Lacy J, Penry J, eds. *Infantile spasms*. New York: Raven Press, 1976.
15. Sotero de Menezes M, Rho J. Clinical and electrographical features of epileptic spasms persisting beyond the second year of life. *Epilepsia* 2002;43:623–630.
16. Hrachovy R. West's syndrome (infantile spasm). Clinical description and diagnosis. *Adv Exp Med Biol* 2002;497:33–50.
17. Bednarek N, Motte J, Soufflet C, et al. Evidence of late-onset infantile spasms. *Epilepsia* 1998;39:55–60.
18. Jeavons P, Bower B, Dimitrakoudi M. Long-term prognosis of 150 cases of West syndrome. *Epilepsia* 1973;14:153–164.
19. Riikonen R. A long-term follow-up study of 214 children with syndrome of infantile spasms. *Neuropediatrics* 1982;13:14–23.
20. Fusco L, Vigevano F. Tonic spasm seizures: a particular and previously unreported type of seizure. *Epilepsia* 1994;35(Suppl 7):87.
21. Ohtahara S, Yamatogi Y. Severe encephalopathic epilepsy in infants: West syndrome. In: Pellock J, Dodson W, Bourgeois B, eds. *Pediatric epilepsy: diagnosis and therapy*. New York: Demos Medical, 2001:177–192.
22. Vigevano F, Fusco L, Pachatz C. Neurophysiology of spasms. *Brain Dev* 2001;23:467–472.
23. Donat J, Wright F. Seizures in series: similarities between seizures of the West and Lennox-Gastaut syndromes. *Epilepsia* 1991;32:504–509.
24. Bisulli F, Volpi L, Meletti S, et al. Ictal pattern of EEG and muscular activation in symptomatic infantile spasms: a videopolygraphic and computer analysis. *Epilepsia* 2002;43:1559–1563.
25. Watanabe K, Negoro T, Okumura A. Symptomatology of infantile spasms. *Brain Dev* 2001;23:453–466.
26. Lombroso C. A prospective study of infantile spasms: clinical and therapeutic correlations. *Epilepsia* 1983;24:135–158.
27. Matsumoto A, Watanabe K, Negoro T, et al. Infantile spasms: etiologic factors, clinical aspects and long term prognosis in 200 cases. *Eur J Pediatr* 1981;135:239–244.
28. Koo B, Hwang P, Logan W. Infantile spasms: outcome and prognostic factors of cryptogenic and symptomatic groups. *Neurology* 1993;43:2322–2327.
29. Holmes G, Vigevano F. Infantile spasms. In: Engel J Jr, Pedley T, eds. *Epilepsy: a comprehensive textbook*. Philadelphia: Lippincott Williams & Wilkins, 1998:627–660.
30. Vigevano F, Fusco L, Cusmai R, et al. The idiopathic form of West syndrome. *Epilepsia* 1993;34:743–746.
31. Dulac O. Infantile spasms and West syndrome. In: Engel J Jr, Pedley T, eds. *Epilepsy: a comprehensive textbook*. Philadelphia: Lippincott-Raven, 1997:2277–2283.
32. Hrachovy R, Frost J Jr. Intensive monitoring of infantile spasms. In: Schmidt D, Morselli P, eds. *Intractable epilepsy: experimental and clinical aspects*. New York: Raven Press, 1986:87–91.
33. Kellaway P. Neurologic status of patients with hypsarrhythmia. In: Gibbs F, ed. *Molecules and mental health*. Philadelphia, PA: JB Lippincott, 1959:134–149.
34. Hrachovy R, Frost JD Jr, Pollack MS, et al. Serologic HLA typing in infantile spasms. *Epilepsia* 1988;29:817–819.
35. Kurokawa T, Goya N, Fukuyama Y, et al. West syndrome and Lennox-Gastaut syndrome: A survey of natural history. *Pediatrics* 1980;65:81–88.
36. Rantala H, Putkonen T. Occurrence, outcome and prognostic factors of infantile spasms and Lennox-Gastaut syndrome. *Epilepsia* 1999;40:287–289.
37. Ohtsuka Y, Ohmori I, Oka E. Long-term follow-up of childhood epilepsy associated with tuberous sclerosis. *Epilepsia* 1998;39:1158–1163.
38. Carmant L. Infantile spasms: West syndrome. *Arch Neurol* 2002;59:317–318.

39. Morimatsu Y, Murofuchi K, Handa T. Pathology in severe physical and mental disabilities in children—with special reference to four cases of nodding spasms. *Adv Neurol Sci* 1972;20:465–470.

40. Satho J, Mizutani T, Morimatsu Y. Neuropathology of the brainstem in age dependent epileptic encephalopathy—especially in cases of infantile spasms. *Brain Dev* 1986;8:443–449.

41. Pranzatelli M. Putative neurotransmitter abnormalities in infantile spasms: cerebrospinal fluid neurochemistry and drug effects. *J Child Neurol* 1994;9:119–129.

42. Kaga K, Mark R, Fukuyama Y. Auditory brainstem responses in infantile spasms. *J Pediatr Otorhinolaryngol* 1982;4:57–67.

43. Fukuyama Y, Shionaga A, Idia Y. Polygraphic study during night sleep in infantile spasms. *Eur Neurol* 1979;18:302–311.

44. Hrachovy R, Frost J Jr, Kellaway P. Sleep characteristics in infantile spasms. *Neurology* 1981;31:688–694.

45. Hrachovy R, Frost J Jr. Infantile spasms: a disorder of the developing nervous system. In: Kellaway P, Noebels J, eds. *Problems and concepts in developmental neurophysiology.* Baltimore, MD: Johns Hopkins University Press, 1989:131–147.

46. Panzica F, Franceschetti S, Binelli S, et al. Spectral properties of EEG fast activity ictal discharges associated with infantile spasms. *Clin Neurophysiol* 1999;110:593–603.

47. Shields WD, Shewmon DA, Chugani HT, et al. Treatment of infantile spasms: medical or surgical? *Epilepsia* 1992;33(Suppl 4):S26–S31.

48. Juhasz C, Chugani HT, Muzik O, et al. Neuroradiological assessment of brain structure and function and its implication in the pathogenesis of West syndrome. *Brain Dev* 2001;23:488–495.

49. Haginoya K, Munakata M, Yokoyama H, et al. Mechanism of tonic spasms in West syndrome viewed from ictal SPECT findings. *Brain Dev* 2001;23:496–501.

50. Baram T. Pathophysiology of massive infantile spasms: perspective on the putative role of brain adrenal axis. *Ann Neurol* 1993;33:231–236.

51. Brunson K, Eghbal-Ahmadi M, Baram T. How do the many etiologies of West syndrome lead to excitability and seizures? The corticotropin releasing hormone excess hypothesis. *Brain Dev* 2001;23:533–538.

52. Nagamitsu S, Matsuishi T, Yamashita Y, et al. Decreased cerebrospinal fluid levels of beta-endorphin and ACTH in children with infantile spasms. *J Neural Transm* 2001;108:363–371.

53. Riikonen R. How do cryptogenic and symptomatic infantile spasms differ? Review of biochemical studies in Finnish patients. *J Child Neurol* 1996;11:383–388.

54. Bellman MH, Ross EM, Miller DL. Infantile spasms and pertussis immunisation. *Lancet* 1983;1:1031–1034.

55. Fukuyama Y, Tomori N, Sugitate M. Critical evaluation of the role of immunization as an etiological factor of infantile spasms. *Neuropadiatrie* 1977;8:224–237.

56. Melchior J. Infantile spasms and early immunization against whooping cough. Danish survey from 1970 to 1975. *Arch Dis Child* 1977;52:134–137.

57. Shields WD, Nielsen C, Buch D, et al. Relationship of pertussis immunization to the onset of neurologic disorders: a retrospective epidemiologic study. *J Pediatr* 1988;113:801–805.

58. Reinskov T. Demonstration of precipitating antibody to extract of brain tissue in patients with hypsarrhythmia. *Acta Paediatr Scand* 1963;(Suppl):140–173.

59. Mota N, Rezkallah-Iwasse MT, Peracoli MT, et al. Demonstration of antibody and cellular immune response to brain extract in West and Lennox-Gastaut syndromes. *Arq Neuropsiquiatr* 1984;42:126–131.

60. Hrachovy R, Frost J Jr, Shearer W. Immunological evaluation of patients with infantile spasms. *Ann Neurol* 1985;18:414.

61. Carmant L, Goodyear E, Sauerwein C. The use of calcium channel blockers in the treatment of West syndrome [abstract]. *Neurology* 2000;54(Suppl 3):A295.

62. Hrachovy RA, Frost JD Jr, Kellaway P, et al. A controlled study of prednisone therapy in infantile spasms. *Epilepsia* 1979;20:403–407.

63. Hrachovy R, Frost JD Jr, Kellaway P, et al. A controlled study of ACTH therapy in infantile spasms. *Epilepsia* 1980;21:631–636.

64. Hrachovy R, Frost JD Jr, Kellaway P, et al. Double-blind study of ACTH vs prednisone therapy in infantile spasms. *J Pediatr* 1983;103:641–645.

65. Sankar R, Curran JG, Kevill JW, et al. Microscopic cortical dysplasia in infantile spasms: evolution of white matter abnormalities. *Am J Neuroradiol* 1995;16:1265–1272.

66. Watanabe K. West syndrome: etiological and prognostic aspects. *Brain Dev* 1998;20:1–8.

67. Carranza E, Lombroso CT, Mikati M, et al. Facilitation of infantile spasms by partial seizures. *Epilepsia* 1993;34:94–109.

68. Silva M, Cieuta C, Guerrini R, et al. Early clinical and EEG features of infantile spasms in Down syndrome. *Epilepsia* 1996;37:977–982.

69. Claes S, Devriendt K, Lagae L, et al. The X-linked infantile spasms syndrome (MIM 308350) maps to Xp11.4-Xpter in two pedigrees. *Ann Neurol* 1997;42:360–364.

70. Brueyere H, Lewis S, Wood S, et al. Confirmation of linkage in X-linked infantile spasms (West syndrome) and refinement of the disease locus to Xp21.3-Xp22.1. *Clin Genet* 1999;55:173–181.

71. Watanabe K. Recent advance and some problems in the delineation of epileptic syndromes in children. *Brain Dev* 1996;18:423–437.

72. Ohtahara S, Ohtsuka Y, Yamatogi Y, et al. Prenatal etiologies of West syndrome. *Epilepsia* 1993;34:716–722.

73. Watanabe K, Matsumoto A, Maehara M. Epilepsy and perinatal brain damage [Japanese]. *Sinkei Kenkyu no Shinpo (Tokyo)* 1983;27:599–609.

74. Shephard C, Houser O, Gomez M. MR findings in tuberous sclerosis complex and correlation with seizure development and mental impairment. *Am J Neuroradiol* 1995;16:149–155.

75. Dulac O, Pinard J, Plouin P. Infantile spasms associated with cortical dysplasia and tuberous sclerosis. In: Guerrini R, ed. *Dysplasias of cerebral cortex and epilepsy.* Philadelphia: Lippincott-Raven, 1996:217–225.

76. Koo B, Hwang P. Localization of focal cortical lesions influences age of onset of infantile spasms. *Epilepsia* 1996;37:1068–1071.

77. Chugani H, Shewmon DA, Shields WD, et al. Surgery for intractable infantile spasms: neuroimaging perspectives. *Epilepsia* 1993;34:764–771.

78. Motte J, Billard C, Fejerman N, et al. Neurofibromatosis type one and West syndrome: a relatively benign association. *Epilepsia* 1993;34:723–726.

79. Mizukawa M, Ohtsuka Y, Murashima I, et al. West syndrome associated with chromosome abnormalities: clinicoelectrical study. *Jpn J Psychiatr Neurol* 1992;46:435–436.

80. Riikonen R. Decreasing perinatal mortality: unchanged infantile spasm morbidity. *Dev Med Child Neurol* 1995;37:232–238.

81. Yamamoto N, Watanabe K, Negoro T, et al. Long-term prognosis of tuberous sclerosis with epilepsy in children. *Brain Dev* 1987;9:292–295.

82. Okumura A, Hayakawa F, Kuno K, et al. Periventricular leucomalacia and West syndrome. *Dev Med Child Neurol* 1996;38:13–18.

83. Friedman E, Pampiglione G. Prognostic implications of electroencephalographic findings of hypsarrhythmia in first year of life. *Br Med J* 1971;4:323–325.

84. Watanabe K, Iwase K, Hara K. The evolution of EEG features in infantile spasms: a prospective study. *Dev Med Child Neurol* 1973;15:584–596.

85. Kotagal P. Multifocal independent spike syndrome: relationship to hypsarrhythmia and the slow spike-wave (Lennox-Gastaut) syndrome. *Clin Electroencephalogr* 1995;26:23–29.

86. Hrachovy R, Frost J Jr, Kellaway P. Hypsarrhythmia: variation on a theme. *Epilepsia* 1984;25:317–325.

87. Foley C, Bowens P, Riviello J. Low voltage EEG predicts the prognosis of infantile spasms [abstract]. *Epilepsia* 1989;30:654.

88. Kramer U, Sue W, Mikati M. Hypsarrhythmia: frequency of variant patterns and correlation with etiology and outcome. *Neurology* 1997;48:197–203.

89. Shewmon D. Ictal aspects with emphasis on unusual variants. In: Dulac O, Chugani H, Dalla Bernardina B, eds. *Infantile spasms and West syndrome.* London: WB Saunders, 1994:36–51.

90. Kellaway P, Hrachovy RA, Frost JD Jr, et al. Precise characterization and quantification of infantile spasms. *Ann Neurol* 1979;6:214–218.

91. Aicardi J. Infantile spasms and related syndromes. In: Aicardi J, ed. *Epilepsy in children.* New York: Raven Press, 1994:18–43.

92. Dulac O, Plouin P, Jambaque I, et al. Benign infantile spasms [French]. *Rev Electroencephalogr Neurophysiol Clin* 1986;16:371–382.

93. Gailey EK, Shewmon DA, Chugani HT, et al. Asymmetric and asynchronous infantile spasms. *Epilepsia* 1995;36:873–882.

94. Vigevano F, Fusco L, Di Capua M, et al. Benign infantile familial convulsions. *Eur J Pediatr* 1992;151:608–612.

95. Caraballo RH, Cersosimo RO, Amartino H, et al. Benign familial infantile seizures: further delineation of the syndrome. *J Child Neurol* 2002;17:696–699.

96. Dravet C, Giraud N, Bureau M, et al. Benign myoclonus of early infancy or benign non-epileptic infantile spasms. *Neuropediatrics* 1986;17:33–38.

97. Riikonen R. Epidemiological data of West syndrome in Finland. *Brain Dev* 2001;23:539–541.

98. Saltik S, Kocer N, Dervent A. Magnetic resonance imaging findings in infantile spasms: etiologic and pathophysiologic aspects. *J Child Neurol* 2003;18:241–246.

99. Nordli DR Jr, De Vivo DC. Classification of infantile seizures: implications for identification and treatment of inborn errors of metabolism. *J Child Neurol* 2002;17(Suppl 3):3S3–3S7; discussion 3S8.

100. Trasmonte JV, Barron TF. Infantile spasms: a proposal for a staged evaluation. *Pediatr Neurol* 1998;19:368–371.

101. Saudubray JM, Nassogne MC, de Lonlay P, et al. Clinical approach to inherited metabolic disorders in neonates: an overview. *Semin Neonatol* 2002;7:3–15.

102. Torres OA, Miller VS, Buist NM, et al. Folinic acid-responsive neonatal seizures. *J Child Neurol* 1999;14:529–532.

103. Dalla Bernardina B, Aicardi J, Goutieres F, et al. Glycine encephalopathy. *Neuropadiatrie* 1979;10:209–225.

104. Sorel L, Dusaucy-Bauloye A. A propos de 21 cas d'hyparythmie de Gibbes. Son traitement spectaculaire par l'ACTH. *Acta Neurol Belg* 1958;58:130–141.

105. Mackay M, Weiss S, Snead OC 3rd. Treatment of infantile spasms: an evidence-based approach. *Int Rev Neurobiol* 2002;49:157–184.

106. Jambaque I, Chiron C, Dumas C, et al. Mental and behavioural outcome of infantile epilepsy treated by vigabatrin in tuberous sclerosis patients. *Epilepsy Res* 2000;38:151–160.

107. Yanagaki S, Ogoni H, Hayashi K, et al. A comparative study of high-dose and low-dose ACTH therapy for West syndrome. *Brain Dev* 1999;21:461–467.

108. Snead OC 3rd, Benton JW Jr, Hosey LC, et al. Treatment of infantile spasms with high-dose ACTH: efficacy and plasma levels of ACTH and cortisol. *Neurology* 1989;39:1027–1031.

109. Perheentupa J, Riikonen R, Dunkel L, et al. Adrenocortical hyporesponsiveness after treatment with ACTH of infantile spasms. *Arch Dis Child* 1986;61:750–753.

110. Chiron C, Dulac O, Beaumont D, et al. Therapeutic trial of vigabatrin in refractory infantile spasms. *J Child Neurol* 1991;(Suppl 2):S52–S59.

111. Nabbout R, Melki I, Gerbaka B, et al. Infantile spasms in Down syndrome: good response to a short course of vigabatrin. *Epilepsia* 2001;42:1580–1583.

112. Vigevano F, Cilio MR. Vigabatrin versus ACTH as first-line treatment for infantile spasms: a randomized, prospective study. *Epilepsia* 1997;38:1270–1274.

113. Appleton RE, Peters AC, Mumford JP, et al. Randomised, placebo-controlled study of vigabatrin as first-line treatment of infantile spasms. *Epilepsia* 1999;40:1627–1633.

114. Elterman RD, Shields WD, Mansfield KA, et al. Randomized trial of vigabatrin in patients with infantile spasms. *Neurology* 2001;57:1416–1421.

115. Chiron C, Dumas C, Jambaque I, et al. Randomized trial comparing vigabatrin and hydrocortisone in infantile spasms due to tuberous sclerosis. *Epilepsy Res* 1997;26:389–395.

116. Eke T, Talbot JF, Lawden MC. Severe persistent visual field constriction associated with vigabatrin. *BMJ* 1997;314:180–181.

117. Fledelius HC. Vigabatrin-associated visual field constriction in a longitudinal series. Reversibility suggested after drug withdrawal. *Acta Ophthalmol Scand* 2003;81:41–46.

118. Banin E, Shelev RS, Obolensky A, et al. Retinal function abnormalities in patients treated with vigabatrin. *Arch Ophthalmol* 2003;121:811–816.

119. Shields WD, Sankar R. Vigabatrin. *Semin Pediatr Neurol* 1997;4:43–50.

120. Baxter P. Epidemiology of pyridoxine dependent and pyridoxine responsive seizures in the UK. *Arch Dis Child* 1999;81:431–433.

121. Hansson O, Hagberg B. Effect of pyridoxine treatment in children with epilepsy. *Acta Soc Med Ups* 1968;73:35–43.

122. Pietz J, Benninger C, Schafer H, et al. Treatment of infantile spasms with high-dosage vitamin B$_6$. *Epilepsia* 1993;34:757–763.

123. Ohtsuka Y, Matsuda M, Ogino T, et al. Treatment of the West syndrome with high-dose pyridoxal phosphate. *Brain Dev* 1987;9:418–421.

124. Watanabe K. Medical treatment of West syndrome in Japan. *J Child Neurol* 1995;10:143–147.

125. Pavone L, Incorpora G, La Rosa M, et al. Treatment of infantile spasms with sodium dipropylacetic acid. *Dev Med Child Neurol* 1981;23:454–461.

126. Bachman DS. Use of valproic acid in treatment of infantile spasms. *Arch Neurol* 1982;39:49–52.

127. Siemes H, Spohr HL, Michael T, et al. Therapy of infantile spasms with valproate: results of a prospective study. *Epilepsia* 1988.29:553–560.

128. Bryant AE 3rd, Dreifuss FE. Valproic acid hepatic fatalities. III. U.S. experience since 1986. *Neurology* 1996;46:465–469.

129. Hanson RA, Menkes JH. A new anticonvulsant in the management of minor motor seizures. *Neurology* 1970;20:379–380.

130. Jan JE, Riegl JA, Crichton JU, et al. Nitrazepam in the treatment of epilepsy in childhood. *Can Med Assoc J* 1971;104:571–575.

131. Gibbs FA, Anderson EM. Treatment of hypsarrhythmia and infantile spasms with a Librium analogue. *Neurology* 1965;15:1173–1176.

132. Volzke E, Doose H, Stephan F. The treatment of infantile spasms and hypsarrhythmia with Mogadon. *Epilepsia* 1967;8:64–70.

133. Dreifuss F, Farwell J, Holmes G, et al. Infantile spasms. Comparative trial of nitrazepam and corticotropin. *Arch Neurol* 1986;43:1107–1110.

134. Murphy JV, Sawasky F, Marquardt KM, et al. Deaths in young children receiving nitrazepam. *J Pediatr* 1987;111:145–147.

135. Rintahaka PJ, Nakagawa JA, Shewmon DA, et al. Incidence of death in patients with intractable epilepsy during nitrazepam treatment. *Epilepsia* 1999;40:492–496.

136. Glauser TA, Pellock JM. Zonisamide in pediatric epilepsy: review of the Japanese experience. *J Child Neurol* 2002;17:87–96.

137. Suzuki Y. Zonisamide in West syndrome. *Brain Dev* 2001;23:658–661.

138. Lotze TE, Wilfong AA. Zonisamide treatment for symptomatic infantile spasms. *Neurology* 2004;62:296–298.

139. Glauser TA, Clark PO, McGee K. Long-term response to topiramate in patients with West syndrome. *Epilepsia* 2000;41(Suppl 1):S91–S94.

140. Mikaeloff Y, de Saint-Martin A, Mancini J, et al. Topiramate: efficacy and tolerability in children according to epilepsy syndromes. *Epilepsy Res* 2003:53:225–232.

141. Hurst DL, Rolan TD. The use of felbamate to treat infantile spasms. *J Child Neurol* 1995;10:134–136.

142. Veggiotti P, Cieuta C, Rex E, et al. Treatment of infantile spasms with lamotrigine. *Lancet* 1994;344:1375–1376.

143. Cianchetti C, Pruna D, Coppola G, et al. Low-dose lamotrigine in West syndrome. *Epilepsy Res* 2002;51:199–200.

144. Kossoff EH, Pyzik PL, McGregan JR, et al. Efficacy of the ketogenic diet for infantile spasms. *Pediatrics* 2002;109:780–783.

145. Nordli DR Jr, Kureda MM, Carroll J, et al. Experience with the ketogenic diet in infants. *Pediatrics* 2001;108:129–133.

146. Ariizumi M, Baba K, Hibio S, et al. Immunoglobulin therapy in the West syndrome. *Brain Dev* 1987;9:422–425.

147. Bingel U, Pinter JD, Sotero de Menezes M, et al. Intravenous immunoglobulin as adjunctive therapy for juvenile spasms. *J Child Neurol* 2003;18:379–382.

148. Chugani HT, Shewmon DA, Sankar R, et al. Infantile spasms: II. Lenticular nuclei and brain stem activation on positron emission tomography. *Ann Neurol* 1992;31:212–219.

149. Riikonen R. ACTH therapy of West syndrome: Finnish views. *Brain Dev* 2001;23:642–646.

Classification of the Epilepsies

22

Tobias Loddenkemper   **Hans O. Lüders**   **Imad M. Najm**   **Elaine Wyllie**

The most widely used system for classification of epilepsies was proposed in 1989 by the Commission on Classification and Terminology of the International League Against Epilepsy (ILAE) (1). ILAE's 1981 seizure classification (2) and its 1989 classification of the epilepsies (1) have given physicians around the world a common language. The ILAE classifications were based mainly on two features: (a) distinction between generalized and focal seizure types and (b) etiologic considerations. This classification, like all other classification systems, is not without its shortcomings, and new approaches have been proposed.

THE 1989 ILAE CLASSIFICATION

The 1989 ILAE epilepsy classification is used worldwide and is reproduced in the appendix to this chapter. It was revised from proposals made in 1970 (3) and 1985 (4), and, like the 1981 ILAE seizure classification (2), is based primarily on the definition of electroclinical syndromes. In 1969, Henri Gastaut proposed the first classification of epilepsies (5), which was used as the basis of the first ILAE epilepsy classification system that was proposed 1 year later (3). This classification provided the major division between "partial" (focal) and generalized epilepsies. Each seizure type was grouped according to this dichotomy and associated with interictal and ictal electroencephalographic (EEG) findings, etiology and pathologic findings, and age of manifestation.

About 15 years later, a revision introduced the concept of epilepsy syndromes "defined as an epileptic disorder characterized by a cluster of signs and symptoms customarily occurring together. The signs and symptoms may be clinical (e.g., case history, seizure type, modes of seizure recurrence, and neurological and psychological findings) or as a result of findings detected by ancillary studies (e.g., EEG, x-ray, CT [computed tomography], and NMR [nuclear

magnetic resonance])" (4). This revision divided many specific epilepsy syndromes under the major dichotomy of generalized and "localization-related" (focal) epilepsies and associated them with clinical and EEG findings, etiologies, and disease severity.

The primary dichotomy of these classification systems was set between localization-related (focal) epilepsies, "in which seizure semiology or findings at investigation disclose a localized origin of the seizures" (1), and generalized epilepsies, characterized by "seizures in which the first clinical changes indicate initial involvement of both hemispheres...[and] the ictal encephalographic patterns initially are bilateral" (1). EEG findings are the laboratory results that carry the most weight for defining a focal epilepsy syndrome.

In addition to localizing information, previous epilepsy classifications also contained etiologic information. The 1970 epilepsy classification (3) further divided the generalized epilepsies into *primary*—those occurring in the setting of normal neurologic status, with seizures that begin in childhood or adolescence and lack any clear cause—and *secondary*—those involving abnormal neurologic or psychological findings and diffuse or multifocal brain lesions. Because the term *secondary generalized epilepsy* was sometimes confused with the different concept of "secondary" or "secondarily" generalized tonic-clonic seizures, it was abandoned in the 1985 (4) and 1989 (1) revisions. Primary and secondary were replaced with *idiopathic* and *symptomatic*. The 1970 classification (3) applied the etiologic dichotomy only to generalized epilepsies because all focal epilepsies were assumed to be associated with some type of brain lesion. This neglected the idiopathic syndrome of benign epilepsy of childhood with centrotemporal spikes, and therefore the 1985 (4) and 1989 (1) revisions applied idiopathic and symptomatic to the focal epilepsies as well. The term *cryptogenic* was added in the 1989 (1) classification to describe epilepsy syndromes that are presumed to be symptomatic but are of unknown cause in specific patients.

2001 ILAE PROPOSAL: A SYNDROME-ORIENTED CLASSIFICATION

To resolve existing controversies, the ILAE's Commission on Classification and Terminology published a common terminology for ictal semiology (6) and a revised five-axis classification scheme of epilepsies (7). This proposal (7) is again based on epilepsy syndromes that appeared in previous classifications. The author defines an epileptic syndrome as "[a] complex of signs and symptoms that define a unique epilepsy condition" (7). In this classification, the epilepsy syndrome represents the third of five axes of the ILAE proposal and is separated from the epileptic disease, which consists of "a pathologic condition with a single specific, well-defined etiology. Thus progressive myoclonic epilepsy is a syndrome, but Unverricht-Lundborg is a disease" (7).

Axes of the 2001 ILAE Proposal

The different axes in the 2001 ILAE proposal include seizure description (axis 1), seizure type (axis 2), epilepsy syndrome (axis 3), etiology (axis 4), and impairment (axis 5) (Table 22.1). Details are available online at http://www.epilepsy.org/ctf.

Axis 1 describes ictal seizure semiology through a standardized glossary of descriptive ictal terminology (6). This terminology is independent of pathophysiologic mechanisms, epilepsy focus, or seizure etiology.

Axis 2 is based on a list of accepted epileptic seizure types constructed by the task force. These seizure types are closely related to diagnostic epilepsy entities or indicate underlying mechanisms, pathophysiology, or etiology, or implicate related prognosis and therapy. The list is divided into continuous and self-limited seizure types and includes precipitating stimuli for reflex seizures. Self-limited and continuous seizure types are further divided into seizures of generalized and focal origin.

Axis 3 identifies the epilepsy syndrome diagnosis and separates epilepsy syndromes from entities with epileptic seizures. Epilepsy syndromes are divided into "syndromes in development" and fully characterized syndromes (7).

Axis 4 delineates the etiology of epilepsies, which includes pathologic and genetic causes as well as diseases frequently associated with epilepsy. The ILAE Task Force (7) is revising and updating this list of diseases.

Axis 5 will include an optional classification of the degree of disability and impairment caused by the epilepsy and will be based on the revised International Classification of Functioning, Disability and Health (ICIDH-2) (http://www.who.int/icidh).

Advantages of the 2001 ILAE Proposal

Diagnostic Scheme

Compared with the 1989 version of epilepsy classification, the diagnostic scheme of the 2001 proposal is an attempt to overcome shortcomings and confusion among EEG features, clinical seizure semiology, and syndromatic classification efforts. By dividing the seizure classification into several axes, the ILAE responds to the criticism that a strict one-to-one relationship is lacking between epilepsy syndromes and seizure types. The introduction of a multiaxial diagnostic scheme reflects the recognition of epilepsy as a clinical symptom that can manifest with different semiologic seizure types and be intertwined with different etiologies. Further disentanglement of clinical presentation, etiology, and disease severity is a long-anticipated milestone that will facilitate additional clinical and research applications of the proposed diagnostic scheme.

Emphasis on Seizure Semiology

By including an axis that is based solely on seizure semiology, the ILAE moves away from the electroclinical approach to epilepsy syndromes in the 1989 proposal. The diagnostic multiaxial scheme shifts focus from alteration of consciousness to other semiologic features, thus placing greater emphasis on the symptomatology of seizures that may carry localizing and lateralizing information.

Breaking Up the Dichotomy Between Generalized and Localization-Related Epilepsy

The diagnostic multiaxial scheme pays more attention to the spectrum between previously described "localization-related" epilepsies and generalized epilepsies. This is

TABLE 22.1

KEY FEATURES OF THE 2001 ILAE CLASSIFICATION AND THE PATIENT-ORIENTED EPILEPSY CLASSIFICATION

Five-Axial Syndrome-Oriented Diagnostic Scheme	Five-Dimensional Patient-Oriented Epilepsy Classification
Axis 1: Ictal seizure semiology	Dimension 1: Epileptogenic zone (epilepsy syndrome)
Axis 2: Epileptic seizure type	Dimension 2: Semiologic seizure classification
Axis 3: Epilepsy syndrome	Dimension 3: Etiology (multifaceted approach)
Axis 4: Etiology (single-etiology approach)	Dimension 4: Seizure frequency
Axis 5: Degree of impairment	Dimension 5: Related medical condition

reflected in the replacement of the expression "partial," which has been used for epilepsies as well as seizures and the never-really-established term *localization related*, by "focal." The regression to the older but more established terminology facilitates communication. The broadened meaning of focal will now involve more widespread areas of cortical dysfunction.

Syndromes Are Not Fixed Entities

Compared with the 1989 ILAE classification, the 2001 proposal's diagnostic scheme addresses the criticism that syndromes are not fixed entities and introduces the concept of accepted syndromes versus syndromes in development. This separation allows for the incorporation of new scientific findings and entities into the classification system.

Advances and Clarifications in Terminology

The expression *cryptogenic* is replaced by the more self-explanatory term *probably symptomatic*. Additionally, the avoidance of the word *convulsions* will decrease miscommunications and facilitate more exact seizure description.

Limitations of the 2001 ILAE Proposal

Epilepsy Syndrome Concept

The 2001 ILAE proposal (7) defines an epilepsy syndrome as "[a] complex of signs and symptoms that define a unique epilepsy condition. This must involve more than just the seizure type: thus frontal lobe seizures per se, for instance, would not constitute a syndrome." Syndromes variously combine a constellation of findings including seizure semiology, electrophysiologic ictal or interictal findings, pathologic-anatomic substrate, etiology, imaging findings, age of onset, related medical conditions, and medical history. Seizure types are not unique to etiologies and may be associated with many different clinical, radiologic, and electrophysiologic features leading to a wide variety of possible syndromic combinations. The 2001 proposal lists more than 50 epilepsy syndromes. The currently recognized syndromes provide the clinician with limited reliable information on prognosis, outcome, and etiology owing to heterogeneity within each syndrome. This can be attributed to the fact that syndromes are classified according to varying inclusion criteria.

Epilepsy Syndromes as a Function of Age

Gibbs, Gibbs, and Lennox (8) note in their historic article, "Epilepsy: A Paroxysmal Cerebral Dysrhythmia," that "[d]iseases change their names with increase, not of age (like Chinese children), but with the increase of medical knowledge. Most disorders begin life bearing the name of the man who first recognized them or else they are temporarily tagged with some purely descriptive term. When the etiology or pathology is discovered, the nomenclature is changed." According to the ILAE's syndrome-oriented classification, the same patient can bear several epilepsy syndrome diagnoses at different ages. Infants initially diagnosed with Ohtahara syndrome can later be described as having West syndrome, Lennox-Gastaut syndrome, and then undefined generalized epilepsy. If epilepsy syndromes reflect biologic entities, the diagnosis should be affected only by increase in medical knowledge and not by the patient's age.

Application of the ILAE Epilepsy Syndrome Classification

Studies indicate that in a general family practice, only 5% of all patients can be classified according to the ILAE syndromes (9); in a general neurology practice, 11% of all epilepsy patients can be classified according to the ILAE syndromes (10); and epileptologists can sort only 25% of all patients into ILAE epilepsy syndrome categories (11). These studies indicate that more patients can be classified as further information becomes available in each case and the more skilled the classifying physician is. Nevertheless, 75% of all patients are not classifiable according to the ILAE syndrome-oriented classification even by fully trained epileptologists, indicating that the majority of epilepsy patients do not fit any syndromic category. The 2001 ILAE proposal recognizes this flaw (7).

ILAE Classification Axes Overlap

Terminology in the first three axes of the ILAE proposal mingles seizure semiology and epilepsy syndromes, as demonstrated by the following example: A 3-year-old patient with daily myoclonic seizures (20 per day) followed by astatic seizures frequently triggered by light and photic stimulation would be classified according to the ILAE system as:

Axis 1 (ictal semiology)—myoclonic-astatic seizure
Axis 2 (pathophysiologic seizure types)—myoclonic-astatic seizure
Axis 3 (epilepsy syndrome)—epilepsy with myoclonic-astatic seizures
Axis 4 (etiology)
Axis 5 (impairment)

FIVE-DIMENSIONAL PATIENT-ORIENTED EPILEPSY CLASSIFICATION PROPOSAL

An alternative patient-oriented epilepsy classification (12) was developed in an effort to address some of the difficulties with the 2001 ILAE proposal (7). The five dimensions can be used to capture the critical features in patients with epilepsy. However, at the first encounter, it is sometimes difficult to determine whether a patient is suffering from epilepsy or is having nonepileptic seizures. Therefore, early in the investigation, the term *paroxysmal event* may be used to indicate the uncertainty of an epilepsy diagnosis. As more information becomes available (e.g., observations by witnesses, routine EEG recordings, magnetic resonance imaging [MRI] of the brain, and video-electroencephalography), the classification can become more specific. If these results indicate that the patient has nonepileptic seizures, other classification systems can further characterize the event (13).

Dimensions of the Patient-oriented Classification

Dimension 1: The Epileptogenic Zone

The first dimension characterizes the localization of the epileptogenic zone, as determined by all available clinical information (e.g., history, examination, electroencephalography, MRI). Classification is recognized as an ongoing interactive process with an increasing degree of precision as additional clinical data become available. If it is uncertain whether the patient has epilepsy or nonepileptic seizures, the term *paroxysmal event* is used. As further information becomes available (e.g., an electroencephalogram demonstrating left mesial temporal sharp waves, left temporal electroencephalographic seizures, and an MRI showing left hippocampal atrophy), the classification becomes more precise (left mesial temporal lobe epilepsy). If the patient has epilepsy but the epileptogenic zone cannot be determined further, the expression *unclassified epileptogenic zone* is used. If additional localizing evidence is available, a subcategory such as focal, multifocal, multilobar, generalized, or other is used. The categories focal, multilobar, and multifocal allow for further specification (Table 22.2) (14). Multifocal indicates more than one epileptogenic zone in different lobes. The term *generalized* is used if the cortex is diffusely epileptogenic without a localizable epileptogenic zone. Further characterization of the localization of the epileptogenic zone is possible by the addition of "left" or "right."

The traditional ILAE epilepsy syndrome (if applicable) can be added in parentheses after the epileptogenic zone (e.g., Rasmussen encephalitis) to provide clinicians with traditionally used key words. However, the five dimensions of this classification contain all the information necessary to identify ILAE syndromes.

Single seizures and situation-related seizures (e.g., febrile seizures and seizures induced by electrolyte or metabolic disturbances) can also be classified within certain limits by this system, but classification of these disorders is not the primary intention of this epilepsy classification.

Dimension 2: Seizure Classification

The clinical signs and symptoms are the most important pieces of information for localizing a lesion in the central nervous system. Seizures and seizure semiology are the clinical manifestation of epilepsy. A seizure classification based solely on this clinical presentation of the epilepsy has been used successfully at several centers (15–19).

TABLE 22.2

CLASSIFICATION OF THE EPILEPTOGENIC ZONE (FIVE-DIMENSIONAL EPILEPSY CLASSIFICATION)

Unclassified epileptogenic zone
Focal—if the epileptogenic zone can be localized to a single area within one lobe of the brain on the basis of findings from the history, semiology, electroencephalogram, and imaging, the category focal or the more specific characterizations, frontal, temporal, parietal, occipital, or perirolandic (central), are used

  Frontal
  Perirolandic (central)[a]
  Temporal
    • Neocortical temporal
    • Mesial temporal
  Parietal
  Occipital
  Other[b]
Multilobar—one extensive epileptogenic zone within two or more adjacent lobes of the same hemisphere
  Frontotemporal
  Temporoparietal
  Frontoparietal
  Temporoparietooccipital
  Other
Hemispheric—the epileptogenic zone involves the whole hemisphere; a distinction of noninvolved areas is not possible
Multifocal—multiple separate zones of epileptogenicity from distinct brain regions
  Bitemporal
  Other
  Other[c]
  Generalized

---

[a]The perirolandic (or central) area is defined as the precentral gyrus and the postcentral gyrus containing the primary motor and sensory areas. Anterior border to the frontal lobe is the precentral sulcus; posterior border to the parietal lobe is the postcentral sulcus; inferior border to the temporal lobe is the sylvian fissure (14).
[b]Other locations, such as subcortical regions (e.g., hypothalamus), are suspected to be capable of generating seizures and can be included in this category.
[c]Other multifocal epileptogenic zones can include multiple combinations of epilepsy locations, such as "left frontal and right parietooccipital" or "right and left parietooccipital."

This seizure classification uses only the clinical semiology and does not require any additional diagnostic techniques other than analysis of an observed or videotaped seizure. Information from MRI, EEG, or positron emission tomography (PET) is unnecessary. The semiologic seizure classification distinguishes among auras, autonomic seizures, dialeptic seizures (characterized primarily by loss of awareness), motor seizures, and special seizures such as atonic, hypomotor, and negative myoclonic seizures (17–19).

Seizures frequently consist of more than one clinical component and follow a certain time sequence (e.g., an aura of nausea and uprising epigastric discomfort can be followed by distal picking hand movements; this can evolve into generalized stiffening and generalized rhythmic jerking of the body). This sequential evolution is considered in the semiologic seizure classification through linkage of separate

TABLE 22.3
ETIOLOGIES (FIVE-DIMENSIONAL EPILEPSY CLASSIFICATION)

Hippocampal sclerosis
Tumor
- Glioma
- Dysembryoplastic neuroepithelial tumor
- Ganglioglioma
- Other

Malformation of cortical development
- Focal malformation of cortical development
- Hemimegalencephaly
- Malformation of cortical development with epidermal nevi (epidermal nevus syndrome)
- Heterotopic grey matter
- Hypothalamic hamartoma
- Hypomelanosis of Ito
- Other

Malformation of vascular development
- Cavernous angioma
- Arteriovenous malformation
- Sturge-Weber syndrome
- Other

CNS infection
- Meningitis
- Encephalitis
- Abscess
- Other

(Immune-mediated) CNS inflammation
- Rasmussen encephalitis
- Vasculitis
- Other

Hypoxic-ischemic brain injury
- Focal ischemic infarction
- Diffuse hypoxic-ischemic injury
- Periventricular leukomalacia
- Hemorrhagic infarction
- Venous sinus thrombosis
- Other

Head trauma
- Head trauma with intracranial hemorrhage
- Penetrating head injury
- Closed head injury

Inheritable conditions
- Tuberous sclerosis
- Progressive myoclonic epilepsy
- Metabolic syndrome
- Channelopathy
- Mitochondrial disorder
- Chromosomal aberration
- Presumed genetic cause
- Other

Structural brain abnormality of unknown cause
Other
Unknown—unclear etiology based on the current information

Abbreviation: CNS, central nervous system.

seizure phases by arrows in the order of occurrence (e.g., abdominal aura → automotor seizure → generalized tonic-clonic seizure). To avoid excessive semiologic detail, up to four seizure phases can be separately classified. This restriction is arbitrary but usually sufficient to classify all the important seizure components based on clinical experience with this system in the past decade.

Dimension 3: Etiology
Seizures are caused by the co-occurrence of multiple triggering factors. On the basis of investigational methods used to determine the cause of the epilepsy (e.g., histopathology, metabolic testing, MRI imaging, genetic testing), factors responsible for the generation of seizures can be found simultaneously at different diagnostic levels. To account for multiple coexisting etiologic factors, the etiology dimension permits the classification of several factors in one patient. These factors can be chosen from a list of 12 different categories (Table 22.3). The category "other" permits the free text insertions of rare, not listed causes. Causes defined by histopathologic findings are the most frequently identified etiologies in patients with epilepsies, perhaps because histopathologic causes have been identified for more than a century and are among the best described. Other diagnostic techniques, such as

genetics, have led to the identification of other coexisting causes, and with the results from further research in newer fields, will gain in importance in the future. As a result of this current histopathologic preference, we propose selection of the underlying histopathologic cause first and placement of other coexisting causes in parentheses. Because the classification of etiologies depends greatly on scientific progress, we refrained from listing all possible causes.

Dimension 4: Seizure Frequency
Severity of the epilepsy, as quantified by combined frequency of all seizure types, indicates the acuity of the disease. Categories include "daily," "persistent," "rare or none," "undefined," and "unknown" (Table 22.4). The number of seizures per time unit can be included in parentheses (e.g., 1/day).

Dimension 5: Related Medical Information
This dimension provides additional information in free text on associated medical conditions acquired in the history and examination or in previous diagnostic procedures. Samples include "febrile convulsions at age 1 year," "developmental delay," "right hemianopia," or "generalized slow spike-and-wave complexes on routine EEG 10/2000."

TABLE 22.4
SEIZURE FREQUENCY (FIVE-DIMENSIONAL EPILEPSY CLASSIFICATION)

Daily
    One or more seizures per day.
Rare or none
    Fewer than one seizure per 6 months; these patients are
        required to have had more than two documented seizures,
        with the last seizure occurring more than 6 months ago.
Persistent
    Fewer than one seizure per day but at least one seizure within
        the past 6 months. A persistent pattern must be recognizable
        in the period before the past 6 months. Single seizures, recent
        onset of epilepsy, breakthrough seizures in an otherwise well-
        controlled patient, and patients with fewer than 6 months of
        follow-up are classified as undefined (see below).
Undefined
    Impossible to predict seizure frequency because of unknown
        frequency, recent onset of epilepsy, breakthrough seizures in
        an otherwise well-controlled patient caused by medication
        change/reduction or other provoking factors (sleep
        deprivation, alcohol, hypoxia, chemotherapy, etc.), and
        patients with fewer than 6 months follow-up after epilepsy
        surgery.

The previously described 3-year-old patient with daily myoclonic seizures followed by astatic seizures frequently triggered by light and photic stimulation would be classified by the above methods as:

Epileptogenic zone—generalized (epilepsy with myoclonic astatic seizures/Doose syndrome)
Semiology—myoclonic seizure → astatic seizure
Etiology—unknown
Seizure frequency—daily (20/day)
Related medical information—seizures triggered by photic stimulation

Advantages of the Five-Dimensional Patient-Oriented Classification

Independence of Dimensions
Except for dimension 1 (epileptogenic zone), which summarizes all dimensions, the other four dimensions are independent and separate entities without overlap or duplication of information.

Universal Classification
The five-dimensional classification allows for the categorization of every patient. Independence from epilepsy syndromes permits classification of patients at a less specific level, at different stages in the diagnostic process, and by physicians with different training and background. All patients can be classified, and everyone can use the system. The diagnostic process is independent of the amount of available diagnostic information (medical history, electroencephalography, MRI, PET, single-photon-emission computed tomography). The more information available, the more specific the classification becomes.

Additionally, to preserve clinically important key words and technical terms that can rapidly convey information, epilepsy syndromes can be optionally included in parentheses after the localization in dimension 1.

Essential Characterization of Patients
The five-dimensional classification conveys the information necessary for a brief assessment of each case. A syndromic term can be added on rare occasions when the classified case actually represents a typical syndromic manifestation and use of the syndromic name can convey more information with fewer words than can the five-dimensional epilepsy classification. In addition, important variations in clinical presentation can be encoded and accounted for in the classification.

Timelessness of Classification
Many recent electroclinical syndromes are tightly locked to investigational devices, such as the electroencephalograph or the MRI. Sooner or later, additional techniques for localizing the epileptogenic zone will become available. The five-dimensional patient-oriented classification (12) can be performed solely on the basis of observation and history taking and is flexible enough to incorporate future localizing tools and techniques.

Research Perspectives
The five-dimensional classification (12) allows for reproducible and more objective encoding and decoding of information for research. Whereas a syndrome-based classification of patients encodes a variety of heterogeneous patients into one category (e.g., Lennox-Gastaut syndrome), the five-dimensional classification sorts these patients by well-delineated homogenous criteria. A retrospective study (12) demonstrated the practicability and reproducibility of the five-dimensional classification. Charts of 100 pediatric and 100 adult patients were randomly selected, and each case was classified independently by two investigators according to the patient-oriented classification. Inter-rater reliability was high (kappa 0.8 to 0.9). Therefore, the five-dimensional classification also opens new perspectives for research trials to recognize groups of seizures, etiologies, and epileptogenic zones that may represent clinically or scientifically important entities. Data can be analyzed in a multidimensional fashion by grouping patients according to each dimension.

Close Relationship to General Neurologic Localization Principles
The patient-oriented epilepsy classification follows general neurologic localization principles of symptom description, localization of the brain lesion, and search for etiology. On the basis of a presenting symptom (seizure), a working hypothesis on the localization of the lesion is generated

(epileptogenic zone), and further information is gathered to determine the cause of the lesion (etiology). This process includes a continuous refinement of the seizure semiology, epileptogenic zone, and etiology as more information (e.g., from video-electroencephalography, MRI) becomes available and as the patient is referred and evaluated by a more experienced physician (e.g., from general practitioner to neurologist to epileptologist).

Seizures Listed as Independent Neurologic Symptoms

Repeated epileptic seizures are the presenting symptoms of localized or widespread cortical lesions caused by multiple etiologic factors. There is no one-to-one relationship between seizure semiology and etiologies as frequently suggested by epilepsy syndromes. This multifaceted approach pictures the epileptic seizure as an independent neurologic symptom due to multiple etiologies at various cortical locations occurring at different frequencies and in conjunction with other clinical findings.

Limitations of the Patient-Oriented Classification

Orientation Toward Focal Epilepsy and Epilepsy Surgery Candidates

The five-dimensional classification places more emphasis on focal epilepsies and is designed to provide the epileptologist with a brief outline of important presurgical information. It is therefore more surgically oriented and neglects subtypes of generalized epilepsies at first sight.

Concept of the Epileptogenic Zone

Although the concept of the epileptogenic zone is congenial to the multifactorial approach to epilepsy, it always remains a hypothetical construct, "the best possible guess," and its accuracy may be influenced by the extent of the observers' training and the available tests. However, these arguments apply also to a syndromatic approach and any kind of classification that requires decision making.

Inconsistencies in Etiologic Dimension

Despite attempts to base the etiologic dimension on an isolated modality such as genetics, pathology, pathophysiology, or anatomy, we were not able to describe epilepsy etiology at only one level. This makes the etiologic dimension itself a multifaceted approach with different layers. Frequently, it is difficult to name a single etiology, as in a patient with a malformation of cortical development, a related neurotransmitter imbalance in the region of the malformation, and an underlying genetic mutation accounting for the malformation.

CONCLUSION

The classification of epilepsies is currently controversial, with various proposals under vigorous discussion. The terminology of the 1989 ILAE proposal (1) is in widespread use and is reproduced here as an Appendix. Newer approaches (7,12) are an attempt to improve on its limitations, with the ultimate goal of improving treatment.

REFERENCES

1. Commission on Classification and Terminology of the International League Against Epilepsy. Proposal for revised classification of epilepsies and epileptic syndromes. *Epilepsia* 1989;30:389–399.
2. Commission on Classification and Terminology of the International League Against Epilepsy. Proposal for revised clinical and electroencephalographic classification of epileptic seizures. *Epilepsia* 1981;22:489–501.
3. Merlis JK. Proposal for an international classification of the epilepsies. *Epilepsia* 1970;11:114–119.
4. Commission on Classification and Terminology of the International League Against Epilepsy. Proposal for classification of epilepsies and epileptic syndromes. *Epilepsia* 1985;26:268–278.
5. Gastaut H. Classification of the epilepsies. Proposal for an international classification. *Epilepsia* 1969;10:14–21.
6. Blume WT, Luders HO, Mizrahi E, et al. Glossary of descriptive terminology for ictal semiology: report of the ILAE Task Force on Classification and Terminology. *Epilepsia* 2001;42:1212–1218.
7. Engel J Jr. A proposed diagnostic scheme for people with epileptic seizures and with epilepsy: report of the ILAE Task Force on Classification and Terminology. *Epilepsia* 2001;42:796–803.
8. Gibbs F, Gibbs E, Lennox W. Epilepsy: a paroxysmal cerebral dysrhythmia. *Brain* 1937;60:377–388.
9. Manford M, Hart YM, Sander JW, et al. The National General Practice Study of Epilepsy. The syndromic classification of the International League Against Epilepsy applied to epilepsy in a general population. *Arch Neurol* 1992;49:801–808.
10. Murthy JM, Yangala R, Srinivas M. The syndromic classification of the International League Against Epilepsy: a hospital-based study from South India. *Epilepsia* 1998;39:48–54.
11. Osservatorio Regionale per L'Epilessia (OREp), Lombardy. ILAE classification of epilepsies: its applicability and practical value of different diagnostic categories. *Epilepsia* 1996;37:1051–1059.
12. Kellinghaus C, Loddenkemper T, Najm IM, et al. Specific epileptic syndromes are rare even in tertiary epilepsy centers: a patient-oriented approach to epilepsy classification. *Epilepsia* 2004;45:268–275.
13. Gates JR. Epidemiology and classification of non-epileptic events. In: Gates JR, Rowan AJ, eds. *Epidemiology and classification of non-epileptic events*, 2nd ed. Boston: Butterworth Heinemann, 2000:3–14.
14. Kuzniecky R, Morawetz R, Faught E, et al. Frontal and central lobe focal dysplasia: clinical, EEG and imaging features. *Dev Med Child Neurol* 1995;37:159–166.
15. Benbadis S, Luders H. Classification of epileptic seizures. Comparison of two systems. *Neurophysiol Clin* 1995;25:297–302.
16. Kim KJ, Lee R, Chae JH, et al. Application of semiological seizure classification to epileptic seizures in children. *Seizure* 2002;11:281–284.
17. Luders H, Acharya J, Baumgartner C, et al. Semiological seizure classification. *Epilepsia* 1998;39:1006–1013.
18. Luders H, Acharya J, Baumgartner C, et al. A new epileptic seizure classification based exclusively on ictal semiology. *Acta Neurol Scand* 1999;99:137–141.
19. Luders HO, Burgess R, Noachtar S. Expanding the international classification of seizures to provide localization information. *Neurology* 1993;43:1650–1655.

Proposal for Revised Classification of Epilepsies and Epileptic Syndromes

Commission on Classification and Terminology of the International League Against Epilepsy (1989) *

PART I: INTERNATIONAL CLASSIFICATION OF EPILEPSIES AND EPILEPTIC SYNDROMES

1. Localization-related (focal, local, partial) epilepsies and syndromes
   1.1 Idiopathic (with age-related onset)
   At present, the following syndromes are established, but more may be identified in the future:
   - Benign childhood epilepsy with centrotemporal spike
   - Childhood epilepsy with occipital paroxysms
   - Primary reading epilepsy
   1.2 Symptomatic (Part III)
   - Chronic progressive epilepsia partialis continua of childhood (Kojewnikow's syndrome)
   - Syndromes characterized by seizures with specific modes of precipitation (see Part IV)

Apart from these rare conditions, the symptomatic category comprises syndromes of great individual variability which are based mainly on seizure types and other clinical features, as well as anatomic localization and etiology—as far as these are known.

The seizure types refer to the International Classification of Epileptic Seizures. Inferences regarding anatomic

*Reproduced, with permission, from Raven Press. *Epilepsia* 1989;30: 389–399.

localization must be drawn carefully. The scalp EEG (both interictal and ictal) may be misleading, and even local morphological findings detected by neuroimaging techniques are not necessarily identical with an epileptogenic lesion. Seizure symptomatology and, sometimes, additional clinical features often provide important clues. The first sign or symptom of a seizure is often the most important indicator of the site of origin of seizure discharge, whereas the following sequence of ictal events can reflect its further propagation through the brain. This sequence, however, can still be of high localizing importance. One must bear in mind that a seizure may start in a clinically silent region, so that the first clinical event occurs only after spread to a site more or less distant from the locus of initial discharge. The following tentative descriptions of syndromes related to anatomic localizations are based on data which include findings in studies with depth electrodes.

Temporal Lobe Epilepsies

Temporal lobe syndromes are characterized by simple partial seizures, complex partial seizures, and secondarily generalized seizures, or combinations of these. Frequently, there is a history of febrile seizures, and a family history of seizures is common. Memory deficits may occur. On metabolic imaging studies, hypometabolism is frequently observed [e.g., positron emission tomography (PET)]. Unilateral or bilateral temporal lobe spikes are common on EEG. Onset is frequently in childhood or young adulthood. Seizures occur in clusters at intervals or randomly.

General Characteristics

Features strongly suggestive of the diagnosis when present include:

1. Simple partial seizures typically characterized by autonomic and/or psychic symptoms and certain sensory phenomena such as olfactory and auditory (including illusions). Most common is an epigastric, often rising, sensation.
2. Complex partial seizures often but not always beginning with motor arrest typically followed by oroalimentary automatism. Other automatisms frequently follow. The duration is typically >1 min. Postictal confusion usually occurs. The attacks are followed by amnesia. Recovery is gradual.

Electroencephalographic Characteristics

In temporal lobe epilepsies the interictal scalp EEG may show the following:

1. No abnormality.
2. Slight or marked asymmetry of the background activity.
3. Temporal spikes, sharp waves and/or slow waves, unilateral or bilateral, synchronous but also asynchronous. These findings are not always confined to the temporal region.
4. In addition to scalp EEG findings, intracranial recordings may allow better definition of the intracranial distribution of the interictal abnormalities.

In temporal lobe epilepsies various EEG patterns may accompany the initial clinical ictal symptomatology, including (a) a unilateral or bilateral interruption of background activity; and (b) temporal or multilobar low-amplitude fast activity, rhythmic spikes, or rhythmic slow waves. The onset of the EEG may not correlate with the clinical onset depending on methodology. Intracranial recordings may provide additional information regarding the chronologic and spatial evolution of the discharges.

Amygdalo-Hippocampal (Mesiobasal Limbic or Rhinencephalic) Seizures

Hippocampal seizures are the most common form; the symptoms are those described in the previous paragraphs except that auditory symptoms may not occur. The interictal scalp EEG may be normal, may show interictal unilateral temporal sharp or slow waves, and may show bilateral sharp or slow waves, synchronous or asynchronous. The intracranial interictal EEG may show mesial anterior temporal spikes or sharp waves. Seizures are characterized by rising epigastric discomfort, nausea, marked autonomic signs, and other symptoms, including borborygmi, belching, pallor, fullness of the face, flushing of the face, arrest of respiration, pupillary dilatation, fear, panic, and olfactory-gustatory hallucinations.

Lateral Temporal Seizures

Simple seizures characterized by auditory hallucinations or illusions or dreamy states, visual misperceptions, or language disorders in case of language dominant hemisphere focus. These may progress to complex partial seizures if propagation to mesial temporal or extratemporal structures occurs. The scalp EEG shows unilateral or bilateral midtemporal or posterior temporal spikes which are most prominent in the lateral derivations.

Frontal Lobe Epilepsies

Frontal lobe epilepsies are characterized by simple partial, complex partial, secondarily generalized seizures or combinations of these. Seizures often occur several times a day and frequently occur during sleep. Frontal lobe partial seizures are sometimes mistaken for psychogenic seizures. Status epilepticus is a frequent complication.

General Characteristics

Features strongly suggestive of the diagnosis include:

1. Generally short seizures.
2. Complex partial seizures arising from the frontal lobe, often with minimal or no postictal confusion.
3. Rapid secondary generalization (more common in seizures of frontal than of temporal lobe epilepsy).
4. Prominent motor manifestations which are tonic or postural.
5. Complex gestural automatisms frequent at onset.
6. Frequent falling when the discharge is bilateral.

A number of seizure types are described below; however, multiple frontal areas may be involved rapidly and specific seizure types may not be discernible.

Supplementary Motor Seizures

In supplementary motor seizures, the seizure patterns are postural, focal tonic, with vocalization, speech arrest, and fencing postures.

Cingulate

Cingulate seizure patterns are complex partial with complex motor gestural automatisms at onset. Autonomic signs are common, as are changes in mood and affect.

Anterior Frontopolar Region

Anterior frontopolar seizure patterns include forced thinking or initial loss of contact and adversive movements of head and eyes, with possible evolution including contraversive movements and axial clonic jerks and falls and autonomic signs.

Orbitofrontal

The orbitofrontal seizure pattern is one of complex partial seizures with initial motor and gestural automatisms, olfactory hallucinations and illusions, and autonomic signs.

Dorsolateral

Dorsolateral seizure patterns may be tonic or, less commonly, clonic with versive eye and head movements and speech arrest.

Opercular

Opercular seizure characteristics include mastication, salivation, swallowing, laryngeal symptoms, speech arrest, epigastric aura, fear, and autonomic phenomena. Simple partial seizures, particularly partial clonic facial seizures, are common and may be ipsilateral. If secondary sensory changes occur, numbness may be a symptom, particularly in the hands. Gustatory hallucinations are particularly common in this area.

Motor Cortex

Motor cortex epilepsies are mainly characterized by simple partial seizures, and their localization depends on the side and topography of the area involved. In cases of the lower prerolandic area, there may be speech arrest, vocalization or dysphasia, tonic-clonic movements of the face on the contralateral side, or swallowing. Generalization of the seizure frequently occurs. In the rolandic area, partial motor seizures without march or jacksonian seizures occur, particularly beginning in the contralateral upper extremities. In the case of seizures involving the paracentral lobule, tonic movements of the ipsilateral foot may occur, as well as the expected contralateral leg movements. Postictal or Todd's paralysis is frequent.

Kojewnikow's Syndrome

Two types of Kojewnikow's syndrome are recognized, one of which is also known as Rasmussen's syndrome and is included among the epileptic syndromes of childhood noted under symptomatic seizures. The other type represents a particular form of rolandic partial epilepsy in both adults and children and is related to a variable lesion of the motor cortex. Its principal features are (a) motor partial seizures, always well localized; (b) often late appearance of myoclonus in the same site where somatomotor seizures occur; (c) an EEG with normal background activity and a focal paroxysmal abnormality (spikes and slow waves); (d) occurrence at any age in childhood and adulthood; (e) frequently demonstrable etiology (tumor, vascular); and (f) no progressive evolution of the syndrome (clinical, electroencephalographic or psychological, except in relation to the evolution of the causal lesion). This condition may result from mitochondrial encephalopathy (MELAS). NOTE: Anatomical origins of some epilepsies are difficult to assign to specific lobes. Such epilepsies include those with pre- and postcentral symptomatology (perirolandic seizures). Such overlap to adjacent anatomic regions also occurs in opercular epilepsy.

In frontal lobe epilepsies, the interictal scalp recordings may show (a) no abnormality; (b) sometimes background asymmetry, frontal spikes or sharp waves; or (c) sharp waves or slow waves (either unilateral or frequently bilateral or unilateral multilobar). Intracranial recordings can sometimes distinguish unilateral from bilateral involvement.

In frontal lobe seizures, various EEG patterns can accompany the initial clinical symptomatology. Uncommonly, the EEG abnormality precedes the seizure onset and then provides important localizing information, such as: (a) frontal or multilobar, often bilateral, low-amplitude fast activity, mixed spikes, rhythmic spikes, rhythmic spike waves, or rhythmic slow waves; or (b) bilateral high amplitude single sharp waves followed by diffuse flattening.

Depending on the methodology, intracranial recordings may provide additional information regarding the chronologic and spatial evolution of the discharges; localization may be difficult.

Parietal Lobe Epilepsies

Parietal lobe epilepsy syndromes are usually characterized by simple partial and secondarily generalized seizures. Most seizures arising in the parietal lobe remain as simple partial seizures, but complex partial seizures may arise out of simple partial seizures and occur with spread beyond the parietal lobe. Seizures arising from the parietal lobe have the following features: Seizures are predominantly sensory with many characteristics. Positive phenomena consist of tingling and a feeling of electricity, which may be confined or may spread in a jacksonian manner. There may be a desire to move a body part or a sensation as if a part were being moved. Muscle tone may be lost. The parts most frequently involved are those with the largest cortical representation (e.g., the hand, arm, and face). There may be tongue sensations of crawling, stiffness, or coldness, and facial sensory phenomena may occur bilaterally. Occasionally an intraabdominal sensation of sinking, choking, or nausea may occur, particularly in cases of inferior and lateral parietal lobe involvement. Rarely, there may be pain, which may take the form of a superficial burning dysesthesia or a vague, very severe, painful sensation. Parietal lobe visual phenomena may occur as hallucinations of a formed variety. Metamorphopsia with distortions, foreshortenings, and elongations may occur, and are more frequently observed in cases of nondominant hemisphere discharges. Negative phenomena include numbness, a feeling that a body part is absent, and a loss of awareness of a part or a half of the body, known as asomatognosia. This is particularly the case with nondominant hemisphere involvement. Severe vertigo or disorientation in space may be indicative of inferior parietal lobe seizures. Seizures in the dominant parietal lobe result in a variety of receptive or conductive language disturbances. Some well-lateralized genital sensations may occur with paracentral involvement. Some rotatory or postural motor phenomena may occur. Seizures of the paracentral lobule have a tendency to become secondarily generalized.

Occipital Lobe Epilepsies

Occipital lobe epilepsy syndromes are usually characterized by simple partial and secondarily generalized seizures. Complex partial seizures may occur with spread beyond the occipital lobe. The frequent association of occipital lobe seizures and migraine is complicated and controversial. The clinical seizure manifestations usually, but not always, include visual manifestations. Elementary visual seizures are characterized by fleeting visual manifestations that may be either negative (scotoma, hemianopsia, amaurosis) or, more commonly, positive (sparks or flashes, phosphenes). Such sensations appear in the visual field contralateral to the discharge in the specific visual cortex, but can spread to the entire visual field. Perceptive illusions, in which the objects appear to be distorted, may occur. The following varieties can be distinguished: a change in size (macropsia or micropsia) or a change in distance, an inclination of objects in a given plane of space, and distortion of objects or a sudden change of shape (metamorphopsia). Visual hallucinatory seizures are occasionally characterized by complex visual perceptions (e.g., colorful scenes of varying complexity). In some cases, the scene is distorted or made smaller, and in rare instances, the subject sees his own image (heutoscopy). Such illusional and hallucinatory visual seizures involve epileptic discharge in the temporoparieto-occipital junction. The initial signs may also include tonic and/or clonic contraversion of eyes and head or eyes only (oculoclonic or oculogyric deviation), palpebral jerks, and forced closure of eyelids. Sensation of ocular oscillation or of the whole body may occur. The discharge may spread to the temporal lobe, producing seizure manifestations of either lateral posterior temporal or hippocampoamygdala seizures. When the primary focus is located in the supracalcarine area, the discharge can spread forward to the suprasylvian convexity or the mesial surface, mimicking those of parietal or frontal lobe seizures. Spread to contralateral occipital lobe may be rapid. Occasionally the seizure tends to become secondarily generalized.

1.3 Cryptogenic

Cryptogenic epilepsies are presumed to be symptomatic and the etiology is unknown. Thus, this category differs from the previous one by the lack of etiologic evidence (see definitions).

2. Generalized epilepsies and syndromes
   2.1 Idiopathic (with age-related onset—listed in order of age)
   - Benign neonatal familial convulsions
   - Benign neonatal convulsions
   - Benign myoclonic epilepsy in infancy
   - Childhood absence epilepsy (pyknolepsy)
   - Juvenile absence epilepsy
   - Juvenile myoclonic epilepsy (impulsive petit mal)
   - Epilepsy with grand mal (GTCS) seizures on awakening
   - Other generalized idiopathic epilepsies not defined above
   - Epilepsies with seizures precipitated by specific modes of activation (see Appendix II)
   2.2 Cryptogenic or symptomatic (in order of age)
   - West syndrome (infantile spasms, Blitz-Nick-Salaam Krämpfe)
   - Lennox-Gastaut syndrome
   - Epilepsy with myoclonic-astatic seizures
   - Epilepsy with myoclonic absences
   2.3 Symptomatic
      2.3.1 Nonspecific etiology
      - Early myoclonic encephalopathy
      - Early infantile epileptic encephalopathy with suppression burst
      - Other symptomatic generalized epilepsies not defined above
      2.3.2 Specific syndromes
      - Epileptic seizures may complicate many disease states. Under this heading are included diseases in which seizures are a presenting or predominant feature.
3. Epilepsies and syndromes undetermined whether focal or generalized
   3.1 With both generalized and focal seizures
   - Neonatal seizures
   - Severe myoclonic epilepsy in infancy
   - Epilepsy with continuous spike-waves during slow wave sleep
   - Acquired epileptic aphasia (Landau-Kleffner syndrome)
   - Other undetermined epilepsies not defined above
   3.2 Without unequivocal generalized or focal features. All cases with generalized tonic-clonic seizures in which clinical and EEG findings do not permit classification as clearly generalized or localization related, such as in many cases of sleep-grand mal (GTCS), are considered not to have unequivocal generalized or focal features.
4. Special syndromes
   4.1 Situation-related seizures (Gelegenheitsanfälle)
   - Febrile convulsions
   - Isolated seizures or isolated status epilepticus
   - Seizures occurring only when there is an acute metabolic or toxic event due to factors such as alcohol, drugs, eclampsia, and nonketotic hyperglycemia.

PART II: DEFINITIONS

Localization-Related (Focal, Local, Partial) Epilepsies and Syndromes

Localization-related epilepsies and syndromes are epileptic disorders in which seizure semiology or findings at investigation disclose a localized origin of the seizures. This includes not only patients with small circumscribed constant epileptogenic lesions (anatomic or functional), i.e., true focal epilepsies, but also patients with less well-defined lesions, whose seizures may originate from variable loci. In most symptomatic localization-related epilepsies, the epileptogenic lesions can be traced to one part of one cerebral hemisphere, but in idiopathic age-related epilepsies with focal seizures, corresponding regions of both hemispheres may be functionally involved.

Generalized Epilepsies and Syndromes

According to the International Classification of Epilepsies and Epileptic Syndromes, generalized epilepsies and syndromes are epileptic disorders with generalized seizures, i.e., "seizures in which the first clinical changes indicate initial involvement of both hemispheres.... The ictal encephalographic patterns initially are bilateral."

Epilepsies and Syndromes Undetermined As to Whether They Are Focal or Generalized

There may be two reasons why a determination of whether seizures are focal or generalized cannot be made: (a) The patient has both focal and generalized seizures together or in succession (e.g., partial seizures plus absences), and has both focal and generalized EEG seizure discharges (e.g., temporal spike focus plus independent bilateral spike-wave discharges); and (b) There are no positive signs of either focal or generalized seizure onset. The most common reasons for this are the seizures occur during sleep, the patient recalls no aura, and ancillary investigations, including EEG, are not revealing.

Idiopathic Localization-Related Epilepsies

Idiopathic localization-related epilepsies are childhood epilepsies with partial seizures and focal EEG abnormalities. They are age-related, without demonstrable anatomic lesions, and are subject to spontaneous remission. Clinically, patients have neither neurologic and intellectual deficit nor a history of antecedent illness, but frequently have a family history of benign epilepsy. The seizures are usually brief and rare, but may be frequent early in the course of the disorder. The seizure patterns may vary from case to case, but usually remain constant in the same child. The EEG is characterized by normal background activity and localized high-voltage repetitive spikes, which are sometimes independently multifocal. Brief bursts of generalized spike-waves can occur. Focal abnormalities are increased by sleep and are without change in morphology.

Benign Childhood Epilepsy with Centrotemporal Spikes

Benign childhood epilepsy with centrotemporal spikes is a syndrome of brief, simple, partial, hemifacial motor seizures,

frequently having associated somatosensory symptoms that have a tendency to evolve into GTCS. Both seizure types are often related to sleep. Onset occurs between the ages of 3 and 13 years (peak, 9–10 years), and recovery occurs before the age of 15–16 years. Genetic predisposition is frequent, and there is male predominance. The EEG has blunt high-voltage centrotemporal spikes, often followed by slow waves that are activated by sleep and tend to spread or shift from side to side.

Childhood Epilepsy with Occipital Paroxysms

The syndrome of childhood epilepsy with occipital paroxysms is, in general respects, similar to that of benign childhood epilepsy with centrotemporal spikes. The seizures start with visual symptoms (amaurosis, phosphenes, illusions, or hallucinations) and are often followed by a hemiclonic seizure or automatisms. In 25% of cases, the seizures are immediately followed by migrainous headache. The EEG has paroxysms of high-amplitude spike-waves or sharp waves recurring rhythmically on the occipital and posterior temporal areas of one or both hemispheres, but only when the eyes are closed. During seizures, the occipital discharge may spread to the central or temporal region. At present, no definite statement on prognosis is possible.

Idiopathic Generalized Epilepsies (Age-Related)

Idiopathic generalized epilepsies are forms of generalized epilepsies in which all seizures are initially generalized, with an EEG expression that is a generalized, bilateral, synchronous, symmetrical discharge (such as is described in the seizure classification of the corresponding type). The patient usually has a normal interictal state, without neurologic or neuroradiologic signs. In general, interictal EEGs show normal background activity and generalized discharges, such as spikes, polyspike, spike-wave, and polyspike waves ≥3 Hz. The discharges are increased by slow sleep. The various syndromes of idiopathic generalized epilepsies differ mainly in age of onset.

Benign Neonatal Familial Convulsions

Benign neonatal familial convulsions are rare, dominantly inherited disorders manifesting mostly on the second and third days of life, with clonic or apneic seizures and no specific EEG criteria. History and investigations reveal no etiologic factors. About 14% of these patients later develop epilepsy.

Benign Neonatal Convulsions

Benign neonatal convulsions are very frequently repeated clonic or apneic seizures occurring at about the fifth day of life, without known etiology or concomitant metabolic disturbance. Interictal EEG often shows alternating sharp theta waves. There is no recurrence of seizures, and the psychomotor development is not affected.

Benign Myoclonic Epilepsy in Infancy

Benign myoclonic epilepsy in infancy is characterized by brief bursts of generalized myoclonus that occur during the first or second year of life in otherwise normal children who often have a family history of convulsions or epilepsy. EEG recording shows generalized spike-waves occurring in brief bursts during the early stages of sleep. These attacks are easily controlled by appropriate treatment. They are not accompanied by any other type of seizure, although GTCS may occur during adolescence. The epilepsy may be accompanied by a relative delay of intellectual development and minor personality disorders.

Childhood Absence Epilepsy (Pyknolepsy)

Pyknolepsy occurs in children of school age (peak manifestation, ages 6–7 years), with a strong genetic predisposition in otherwise normal children. It appears more frequently in girls than in boys. It is characterized by very frequent (several to many per day) absences. The EEG reveals bilateral, synchronous symmetrical spike-waves, usually 3 Hz, on a normal background activity. During adolescence, GTCS often develop. Otherwise, absences may remit or, more rarely, persist as the only seizure type.

Juvenile Absence Epilepsy

The absences of juvenile absence epilepsy are the same as in pyknolepsy, but absences with retropulsive movements are less common. Manifestation occurs around puberty. Seizure frequency is lower than in pyknolepsy, with absences occurring less frequently than every day, mostly sporadically. Association with GTCS is frequent, and GTCS precede the absence manifestations more often than in childhood absence epilepsy, often occurring on awakening. Not infrequently, the patients also have myoclonic seizures. Sex distribution is equal. The spike-waves are often >3 Hz. Response to therapy is excellent.

Juvenile Myoclonic Epilepsy (Impulsive Petit Mal)

Impulsive petit mal appears around puberty and is characterized by seizures with bilateral, single or repetitive, arrhythmic, irregular myoclonic jerks, predominantly in the arms. Jerks may cause some patients to fall suddenly. No disturbance of consciousness is noticeable. The disorder may be inherited, and sex distribution is equal. Often, there are GTCS and, less often, infrequent absences. The seizures usually occur shortly after awakening and are often precipitated by sleep deprivation. Interictal and ictal EEG have rapid, generalized, often irregular spike-waves and polyspike-waves; there is no close phase correlation between EEG spikes and jerks. Frequently, the patients are photosensitive. Response to appropriate drugs is good.

Epilepsy with GTCS on Awakening

Epilepsy with GTCS on awakening is a syndrome with onset occurring mostly in the second decade of life. The GTCS occur exclusively or predominantly (>90% of the time) shortly after awakening regardless of the time of day or in a second seizure peak in the evening period of relaxation. If other seizures occur, they are mostly absence or myoclonic, as in juvenile myoclonic epilepsy. Seizures may be precipitated by sleep deprivation and other external factors. Genetic predisposition is relatively frequent. The EEG shows one of the patterns of idiopathic generalized epilepsy. There is a significant correlation with photosensitivity.

Generalized Cryptogenic or Symptomatic Epilepsies (Age-Related)

West Syndrome (Infantile Spasms, Blitz-Nick-Salaam Krämpfe)

Usually, West syndrome consists of a characteristic triad: infantile spasms, arrest of psychomotor development, and hypsarrhythmia, although one element may be missing. Spasms may be flexor, extensor, lightning, or nods, but most commonly they are mixed. Onset peaks between the ages of 4 and 7 months and always occurs before the age of 1 year. Boys are more commonly affected. The prognosis is generally poor. West syndrome may be separated into two groups. The symptomatic group is characterized by previous existence of brain damage signs (psychomotor retardation, neurologic signs, radiologic signs, or other types of seizures) or by a known etiology. The smaller, cryptogenic group is characterized by a lack of previous signs of brain damage and of known etiology. The prognosis appears to be partly based on early therapy with adrenocorticotropic hormone (ACTH) or oral steroids.

Lennox-Gastaut Syndrome

Lennox-Gastaut syndrome manifests itself in children ages 1–8 years, but appears mainly in preschool-age children. The most common seizure types are tonic-axial, atonic, and absence seizures, but other types such as myoclonic, GTCS, or partial are frequently associated with this syndrome. Seizure frequency is high, and status epilepticus is frequent (stuporous states with myoclonias, tonic, and atonic seizures). The EEG usually has abnormal background activity, slow spike-waves <3 Hz and, often, multifocal abnormalities. During sleep, bursts of fast rhythms (~10 Hz) appear. In general, there is mental retardation. Seizures are difficult to control, and the development is mostly unfavorable. In 60% of cases, the syndrome occurs in children suffering from a previous encephalopathy but is primary in other cases.

Epilepsy with Myoclonic-Astatic Seizures

Manifestations of myoclonic-astatic seizures begin between the ages of 7 months and 6 years (mostly between the ages of 2 and 5 years), with (except if seizures begin in the first year) twice as many boys affected. There is frequently hereditary predisposition and usually a normal developmental background. The seizures are myoclonic, astatic, myoclonic-astatic, absence with clonic and tonic components, and tonic-clonic. Status frequently occurs. Tonic seizures develop late in the course of unfavorable cases. The EEG, initially often normal except for 4–7-Hz rhythms, may have irregular fast spike-wave or polyspike wave. Course and outcome are variable.

Epilepsy with Myoclonic Absences

The syndrome of epilepsy with myoclonic absences is clinically characterized by absences accompanied by severe bilateral rhythmical clonic jerks, often associated with a tonic contraction. On the EEG, these clinical features are always accompanied by bilateral, synchronous, and symmetrical discharge of rhythmical spike-waves at 3 Hz, similar to childhood absence. Seizures occur many times a day. Awareness of the jerks may be maintained. Associated seizures are rare. Age of onset is ~7 years, and there is a male preponderance. Prognosis is less favorable than in pyknolepsy owing to resistance to therapy of the seizures, mental deterioration, and possible evolution to other types of epilepsy such as Lennox-Gastaut syndrome.

Symptomatic Generalized Epilepsies and Syndromes

Symptomatic generalized epilepsies, most often occurring in infancy and childhood, are characterized by generalized seizures with clinical and EEG features different from those of idiopathic generalized epilepsies. There may be only one type, but more often there are several types, including myoclonic jerks, tonic seizures, atonic seizures, and atypical absences. EEG expression is bilateral but less rhythmical than in idiopathic generalized epilepsies and is more or less asymmetrical. Interictal EEG abnormalities differ from idiopathic generalized epilepsies, appearing as suppression bursts, hypsarrhythmia, slow spike-waves, or generalized fast rhythms. Focal abnormalities may be associated with any of the above. There are clinical, neuropsychologic, and neuroradiologic signs of a usually diffuse, specific, or nonspecific encephalopathy.

Generalized Symptomatic Epilepsies of Nonspecific Etiology (Age-Related)

Early Myoclonic Encephalopathy

The principal features of early myoclonic encephalopathy are onset occurring before age 3 months, initially fragmentary myoclonus, and then erratic partial seizures, massive myoclonias, or tonic spasms. The EEG is characterized by suppression-burst activity, which may evolve into hypsarrhythmia. The course is severe, psychomotor development is arrested, and death may occur in the first year. Familial cases are frequent and suggest the influence of one or several congenital metabolic errors, but there is no constant genetic pattern.

Early Infantile Epileptic Encephalopathy with Suppression Burst

This syndrome is defined by very early onset, within the first few months of life, frequent tonic spasms, and suppression burst EEG pattern in both waking and sleeping states. Partial seizures may occur. Myoclonic seizures are rare. Etiology and underlying pathology are obscure. The prognosis is serious with severe psychomotor retardation and seizure intractability; often there is evolution to the West syndrome at age 4–6 months.

Epilepsies and Syndromes Undetermined As to Whether They are Focal or Generalized

Neonatal Seizures

Neonatal seizures differ from those of older children and adults. The most frequent neonatal seizures are described as subtle because the clinical manifestations are frequently overlooked. These include tonic, horizontal deviation of the eyes with or without jerking, eyelid blinking or fluttering, sucking, smacking, or other buccal-lingual oral movements, swimming or pedaling movements and, occasionally, apneic spells. Other neonatal seizures occur as tonic extension of the limbs, mimicking decerebrate or decorticate posturing. These occur particularly in premature infants. Multifocal clonic seizures characterized by clonic movements of a limb, which may migrate to other body parts or other limbs, or focal clonic seizures, which are much more localized, may occur. In the latter, the infant is usually not unconscious. Rarely, myoclonic seizures may occur, and the EEG pattern is frequently that of suppression-burst activity. The tonic seizures have a poor prognosis, because they frequently accompany intraventricular hemorrhage. The myoclonic seizures also have a poor prognosis, because they are frequently a part of the early myoclonic encephalopathy syndrome.

Severe Myoclonic Epilepsy in Infancy

Severe myoclonic epilepsy in infancy is a recently defined syndrome. The characteristics include a family history of epilepsy or febrile convulsions, normal development before onset, seizures beginning during the first year of life in the form of generalized or unilateral febrile clonic seizures, secondary appearance of myoclonic jerks, and often partial seizures. EEGs show generalized spike-waves and polyspike-waves, early photosensitivity, and focal abnormalities. Psychomotor development is retarded from the second year of life on, and ataxia, pyramidal signs, and interictal myoclonus appear. This type of epilepsy is very resistant to all forms of treatment.

Epilepsy with Continuous Spike-Waves During Slow-Wave Sleep

Epilepsy with continuous spike-waves during slow-wave sleep results from the association of various seizure types, partial or generalized, occurring during sleep, and atypical absences when awake. Tonic seizures do not occur. The characteristic EEG pattern consists of continuous diffuse spike-waves during slow wave sleep, which is noted after onset of seizures. Duration varies from months to years. Despite the usually benign evolution of seizures, prognosis is guarded because of the appearance of neuropsychologic disorders.

Acquired Epileptic Aphasia (Landau-Kleffner Syndrome)

The Landau-Kleffner syndrome is a childhood disorder in which an acquired aphasia, multifocal spike, and spike and wave discharges are associated. Epileptic seizures and behavioral and psychomotor disturbances occur in two-thirds of the patients. There is verbal auditory agnosia and rapid reduction of spontaneous speech. The seizures, usually GTCS or partial motor, are rare and remit before the age of 15 years, as do the EEG abnormalities.

Special Syndromes

Febrile Convulsions

Febrile convulsions are an age-related disorder almost always characterized by generalized seizures occurring during an acute febrile illness. Most febrile convulsions are brief and uncomplicated, but some may be more prolonged and followed by transient or permanent neurological sequelae, such as the hemiplegia-hemiatrophy-epilepsy (HHE) syndrome. Febrile convulsions tend to recur in about one-third of affected patients. Controversy about the risks of developing epilepsy later have largely been resolved by some recent large studies; the overall risk is probably not more than 4%. The indications for prolonged drug prophylaxis against recurrence of febrile convulsions are now more clearly defined, and most individuals do not require prophylaxis. Essentially, this condition is a relatively benign disorder of early childhood.

PART III: SYMPTOMATIC GENERALIZED EPILEPSIES OF SPECIFIC ETIOLOGIES

Only diseases in which epileptic seizures are the presenting or a prominent feature are classified. These diseases often have epileptic pictures that resemble symptomatic generalized epilepsies without specific etiology, appearing at similar ages.

Malformations

Aicardi syndrome occurs in females and is noted for retinal lacunae and absence of the corpus callosum; infantile spasms with early onset; and often asymmetric, diffuse EEG abnormalities generally asynchronous with suppression burst and/or atypical hypsarrhythmia.

Lissencephaly-pachygyria is characterized by facial abnormalities and specific computed tomography (CT) scan features, axial hypotonia, and infantile spasms. The

EEG shows fast activity of high voltage "alpha-like" patterns without change during wakefulness and sleep.

The individual phacomatoses have no typical electroclinical pattern. We emphasize that West syndrome is frequent in tuberous sclerosis, and that generalized and partial seizures may follow the otherwise typical course of infantile spasms. Sturge-Weber syndrome is a frequent cause of simple partial seizures followed by hemiparesis.

Hypothalamic hamartomas may present with gelastic seizures, precocious puberty, and retardation.

Proven or Suspected Inborn Errors of Metabolism

Neonate

Metabolism errors in the neonate include nonketotic hyperglycinemia and D-glyceric acidemia, showing early myoclonic encephalopathy with erratic myoclonus, partial seizures, and suppression-burst EEG patterns.

Infant

The classical phenylketonuria can express itself as a West syndrome. A variant of phenylketonuria with biopterin deficiency causes seizures starting in the second 6 months of life in infants who have been hypotonic since birth. The seizures are generalized motor seizures associated with erratic myoclonic jerks and oculogyric seizures.

Tay-Sachs and Sandhoff disease present with acoustic startle or myoclonus in the first months of life, without EEG manifestations. In the second year, myoclonic jerks and erratic partial seizures occur, along with marked slowing of the background rhythms.

Another type of metabolic error is early infantile type of ceroid-lipofuscinosis (Santavuori-Haltia-Hagberg disease). Massive myoclonus begins between the ages of 5 and 18 months, with a highly suggestive EEG pattern of vanishing EEG.

Pyridoxine dependency is manifested by seizures that have no suggestive characteristics, but this condition must always be suspected since therapeutic intervention is possible.

Child

Late infantile ceroid-lipofuscinosis (Jansky Bielschowski disease) is characterized by onset between the ages of 2 and 4 years of massive myoclonic jerks, atonic, or astatic seizures. The EEG shows slow background rhythms, multifocal spikes, and a characteristic response to intermittent photic stimulation at a slow rate.

An infantile type of Huntington's disease appears after age 3 years, with a slowing of mental development, followed by dystonia, GTCS, atypical absence seizures, and myoclonic seizures. The EEG shows discharges of generalized spike-waves and polyspike-waves, with the usual photic stimulation rate.

Child and Adolescent

A juvenile form of Gaucher disease is marked by onset at approximately 6–8 years of age, with epileptic seizures of various types, most commonly GTCS or partial motor. The EEG shows progressive deterioration of background activity, abnormal photic response, diffuse paroxysmal abnormalities, and multifocal abnormalities with a clear posterior predominance.

The juvenile form of ceroid-lipofuscinosis (Spielmeyer-Vogt-Sjögren disease) is characterized by onset between the ages of 6 and 8 years, a decrease in visual acuity, slowing of psychomotor development, and appearance of cerebellar and extrapyramidal signs. After 1 to 4 years, GTCS and fragmentary, segmental, and massive myoclonus occur. The EEG shows bursts of slow waves and slow spikes and waves.

Onset of Lafora's disease occurs between the ages of 6 and 19 years (mean 11.5 years) and is characterized by generalized clonic, GTCS, with a frequent association of partial seizures with visual symptomatology, constant myoclonic jerks (fragmentary, segmental, and massive myoclonus), and rapidly progressive mental deterioration. The EEG shows discharges of fast spike-waves and poly-spike-waves, photosensitivity, deterioration of background activity, and the appearance of multifocal abnormalities, particularly posteriorly. On the average, death occurs 5.5 years after onset.

The so-called degenerative progressive myoclonic epilepsy (Lundborg type) also falls into this category. The only significant well-individualized group is the Finnish type, described by Koskiniemi et al. Onset occurs between the ages of 8 and 13 years, with myoclonus (segmental, fragmentary, and massive) and GTCS, associated cerebellar ataxia, and slowly progressive although generally mild mental deterioration. The EEG shows slow abnormalities (theta rhythms and later, delta rhythms), with generalized spike-waves predominantly in the frontal area and photosensitivity. Patients survive ≥15 years.

Dyssynergia cerebellaris myoclonia (DCM) with epilepsy (Ramsay-Hunt syndrome) appears between the ages of 6 and 20 years (mean 11 years) with myoclonias or GTCS. Above all, the myoclonic syndrome is characterized by action and intention myoclonus. The GTCS are rare and sensitive to therapy. Mental deterioration, when present, is slow. Most of the neurologic manifestations are limited to cerebellar signs. In the EEG, the background activity remains normal, with generalized paroxysmal abnormalities (spikes, spike-waves, and polyspike-waves), and photosensitivity. During REM sleep, rapid polyspikes appear, localized in the central and vertex regions.

The clinical picture for the cherry red spot myoclonus syndrome (sialidosis with isolated deficit in neuraminidase) is very similar to that of the Ramsay-Hunt syndrome, with myoclonus, photosensitivity, and cerebellar syndrome. Other characteristics include the nearly constant existence of amblyopia and presence of a cherry red spot on funduscopic examination. The EEG is similar to that of DCM with the following specific features: the poly-spike-wave discharges always correspond to a massive myoclonus and there is no photosensitivity.

A Ramsay-Hunt-like syndrome can also be associated with a mitochondrial myopathy, with abnormalities of lactate and pyruvate metabolism (7).

Adult

Kuf's disease (adult ceroid lipofuscinosis) is a relatively slow, progressive storage disease with frequent generalized seizures that may be very intractable. Unlike juvenile storage disease, the optic fundi may be normal. The main characteristic is an extreme photic sensitivity on slow photic stimulation.

A large number of epilepsy-related diseases in childhood, adulthood, and old age are not enumerated here because the seizures are not distinctively different from other seizure types and are not critical for diagnosis.

PART IV

Precipitated seizures are those in which environmental or internal factors consistently precede the attacks and are differentiated from spontaneous epileptic attacks in which precipitating factors cannot be identified. Certain nonspecific factors (e.g., sleeplessness, alcohol or drug withdrawal, or hyperventilation) are common precipitators and are not *specific* modes of seizure precipitation. In certain epileptic syndromes, the seizures clearly may be somewhat more susceptible to nonspecific factors, but this is only occasionally useful in classifying epileptic syndromes. An epilepsy characterized by specific modes of seizure precipitation, however, is one in which a consistent relationship can be recognized between the occurrence of one or more definable nonictal events and subsequent occurrence of a specific stereotyped seizure. Some epilepsies have seizures precipitated by specific sensation or perception (the reflex epilepsies) in which seizures occur in response to discrete or specific stimuli. These stimuli are usually limited in individual patients to a single specific stimulus or a limited number of closely related stimuli. Although the epilepsies that result are usually generalized and of idiopathic nature, certain partial seizures may also occur following acquired lesions, usually involving tactile or proprioceptive stimuli.

Epileptic seizures may also be precipitated by sudden arousal (startle epilepsy); the stimulus is unexpected in nature. The seizures are usually generalized tonic but may be partial and are usually symptomatic.

Seizures precipitated by integration of higher cerebral function such as memory or pattern recognition are most often associated with complex partial epilepsies but are occasionally observed in generalized epilepsies (such as reading epilepsy). Seizures also occur spontaneously in most such patients.

Primary Reading Epilepsy

All or almost all seizures in this syndrome are precipitated by reading (especially aloud) and are independent of the content of the text. They are simple partial motor-involving masticatory muscles, or visual, and if the stimulus is not interrupted, GTCS may occur. The syndrome may be inherited. Onset is typically in late puberty and the course is benign with little tendency to spontaneous seizures. Physical examination and imaging studies are normal, but EEG shows spikes or spike-waves in the dominant parieto-temporal region. Generalized spike and wave may also occur.

Symptomatic Focal Epilepsies

23

Nancy Foldvary-Schaefer

Certain epileptic disorders are characterized by clusters of signs and symptoms that are considered epileptic syndromes. Because most of these syndromes have numerous etiologic factors, few are defined as specific diseases. The 1989 International League Against Epilepsy (ILAE) classification system subdivides epilepsies and epileptic syndromes into three categories based on clinical history, electroencephalographic manifestations, and etiologic factors (Table 23.1) (1). Localization-related epilepsies and syndromes involve seizures that originate from a localized cortical region. Symptomatic epilepsies have an identifiable cause, such as mesial temporal sclerosis (MTS). Cryptogenic syndromes are presumed to be symptomatic, but they have no known cause and occur with or without accompanying neurologic abnormalities. Idiopathic epilepsies and syndromes are presumed to be inherited.

TEMPORAL LOBE EPILEPSY

Temporal lobe epilepsy (TLE) constitutes nearly two thirds of localization-related epilepsies of adolescence and adulthood (2). Although mesial temporal lobe epilepsy (MTLE) is believed to represent most cases, recent advances in neuroimaging increasingly identify seizures arising from the temporal neocortex. The natural history of TLE is variable, with as many as 30% to 40% of patients continuing to have seizures despite appropriate medical management (2).

Mesial Temporal Lobe Epilepsy

The seizures of MTLE, the most widely recognized symptomatic focal epilepsy, arise from the hippocampus, amygdala, and parahippocampal gyrus. Birth and development are normal, and febrile seizures in infancy or childhood

are the most common risk factor. In one series (3), 45 (67%) of 67 patients had febrile seizures without a recognized central nervous system (CNS) infection prior to onset; seizures were complicated in 33 (73%) of 45 cases. Other risk factors include CNS infection, head trauma, and perinatal injury. Onset ranges from the latter half of the first decade of life to early adulthood, typically after a latency period following the presumed cerebral insult.

Most patients report auras, such as rising abdominal sensations and fearful feelings. Anxiety, olfactory disturbances, psychic phenomena such as déjà vu, and nonspecific cephalic sensations are frequently experienced. Virtually all patients have complex partial seizures with oral or manual automatisms (3–5); unilateral dystonic posturing of a contralateral extremity occurs in approximately 25% of patients (6). Postictal language disturbances are highly predictive of epilepsy arising from the dominant temporal lobe, whereas interpretable speech during the ictus strongly suggests nondominant temporal lobe origin (7), as do the less common ictal vomiting and automatisms with preserved responsiveness (8,9). Motor manifestations, such as facial clonic activity and tonic posturing of one or more extremities, appear 10 or more seconds after clinical onset, once the ictal discharge has spread to extratemporal or neocortical temporal structures (10). Autonomic manifestations include hyperventilation and changes in blood pressure and heart rate. Postictal coughing or nose wiping can occur; both are more common in patients with MTLE than in those with neocortical temporal lobe seizures (11–13). The hand used for nose wiping is usually ipsilateral to the seizure origin. In addition to complex partial seizures, about half of patients with MTLE also experience secondary generalized tonic-clonic seizures (GTCSs), which may be preceded by version of the head or eyes, or focal clonic activity of the

TABLE 23.1
SYMPTOMATIC FOCAL EPILEPSIES

Temporal lobe
  Mesial
  Neocortical
Frontal lobe
  Supplementary motor
  Cingulate
  Anterior frontopolar
  Orbitofrontal
  Dorsolateral
  Opercular
  Motor cortex
Parietal lobe
Occipital lobe

face or upper extremity contralateral to the epileptogenic temporal lobe. Stress, sleep deprivation, alcohol ingestion, and menstruation may all precipitate seizures. Status epilepticus occurs in a minority of patients.

During prolonged electroencephalographic monitoring, more than 90% of patients with MTLE demonstrate epileptic discharges localized to the sphenoidal or anterior temporal electrodes (14,15). Bitemporal independent spikes or sharp waves, maximal on the side of seizure origin, occur in 25% to 50% of cases (14–16). Additional closely spaced electrodes designed to record from the basal or mesial temporal regions facilitate definition of anterior temporal discharges. Surface electrodes placed 1 cm above a point one-third the distance between the external auditory meatus and the external canthus (T1 and T2 placements), FT9 and FT10 in the International 10–10 Electrode Placement System, or sphenoidal electrodes may be used (17). Sphenoidal electrodes are positioned beneath the zygomatic arch approximately 2.5 cm anterior to the incisura intertragica, roughly 10 degrees superiorly from the horizontal plane and posteriorly from the coronal plane (18); they are well tolerated and relatively free of artifacts and complications. Mesial temporal spikes have maximal negativity at anterior temporal or sphenoidal electrodes and widespread positivity over the vertex (8,19,20). Epileptic discharges are absent on serial electroencephalograms (EEGs) in less than 10% of cases (15). One-third of patients have temporal intermittent rhythmic delta activity, consisting of repetitive, rhythmic, saw-toothed or sinusoidal 1- to 4-Hz activity, 50 to 100 μV in amplitude, occurring in the anterior regions (21).

Most temporal lobe seizures involve a gradual buildup of lateralized or localized rhythmic alpha or theta activity, which may be preceded by diffuse or lateralized suppression or arrhythmic activity (11,16,22). The rhythmic activity occurring in the ipsilateral temporal region within 30 seconds of clinical or electrographic seizure onset (8,15,22) correctly predicts an ipsilateral temporal onset in more than 80% of cases, as confirmed by invasive recordings (22). An initial, regular 5- to 9-Hz inferotemporal rhythm is more specific for seizures of hippocampal origin, although this pattern requires the synchronous recruitment of adjacent inferolateral temporal neocortex (23). Seizures confined to the hippocampus, as revealed on intracranial EEG, produce no change on scalp recordings (24). Because of the vertical orientation of dipole sources, seizures of mesiobasal temporal origin may produce rhythmic activity of positive polarity at the vertex coincident with a negative rhythm at the sphenoidal or temporobasal surface electrodes (23,24). Lateralized postictal slowing or background attenuation correctly predicts the side of origin in 96% to 100% of seizures (15,25). False lateralization is observed in 3% to 13% of patients with MTLE (8,11,15) and, like nonlateralized patterns, is more common in patients with bitemporal-independent epileptic discharges (26). In a study of 184 patients with TLE, all patients with unilateral hippocampal atrophy had concordant interictal and ictal EEG lateralization (27).

High-resolution magnetic resonance imaging (MRI) frequently reveals hippocampal atrophy and abnormal signal intensity in the mesial temporal region suggestive of MTS. ^{18}F-fluorodeoxyglucose positron emission tomography (PET) demonstrates temporal lobe hypometabolism that usually extends to the ipsilateral frontoparietal cortices and basal ganglia. Both ictal and interictal single-photon emission computed tomography (SPECT) scans show unilateral abnormalities, although the spatial resolution is inferior to that of PET and time of injection relative to seizure onset dramatically influences results.

MTS is the most common pathologic substrate of MTLE (28), with marked neuronal loss in CA1, CA3, CA4, and the dentate granule cells, and relative sparing of the CA2 pyramidal cells, subiculum, entorhinal cortex, and temporal neocortex. Loss of granule cell innervation leads to reactive synaptogenesis and a subsequent excitatory process capable of initiating and propagating seizures. The coexistence of MTS and extralimbic lesions is observed in approximately 30% of surgical specimens (29). Neoplasms, vascular malformations, and developmental malformations of the mesial temporal structures can also produce epilepsy with clinical and electrophysiologic features similar to those of MTLE caused by MTS.

Neocortical Temporal Lobe Epilepsy

The clinical, neuroradiologic, and electrophysiologic manifestations of neocortical temporal lobe epilepsy (NTLE) are less well defined than in MTLE. Because its pathologic substrates are more diverse than those in MTLE, age of onset is variable, with seizures often beginning in the third decade of life or later (30). Febrile seizures in infancy or early childhood are relatively rare (25,30,31–33), but head trauma, birth injury, and CNS infection are found more frequently in these patients than in those with MTLE (30,33).

Ictal activation of identical structures may render the clinical symptoms of neocortical temporal seizures indistinguishable from those observed with seizures originating from mesial temporal structures. Abdominal auras, psychic phenomena, and nonspecific sensations are frequently reported. In one study (34), abdominal auras were common in patients with MTLE, whereas patients with NTLE described psychic phenomena. However, abdominal auras did occur in patients with NTLE, particularly when the ictal discharge propagated to the mesial temporal structures. Auditory, vestibular, and complex visual phenomena caused by activation of the Heschl gyrus and visual and auditory association cortices are relatively rare, but reliably predict temporal neocortical activation. Complex partial seizures occur in most patients, and GTCSs are also observed. Automatisms and contralateral dystonic posturing occurring early in the attack are less common in patients with NTLE than in those with MTLE; early clonic activity of the contralateral upper extremity or facial grimacing is suggestive of a neocortical temporal origin (30,31,33–36). Autonomic manifestations were notably absent in a small study of NTLE seizures (30).

The electrophysiologic manifestations of NTLE may also be indistinguishable from those of MTLE. The distribution of epileptiform activity in NTLE varies with the location of the epileptogenic zone. Interictal spiking may be maximal at lateral or posterior temporal electrodes; however, sphenoidal and anterior temporal interictal discharges also are observed (24,30,33). Ictal patterns include temporal rhythmic theta or alpha activity, as seen in seizures of mesial temporal origin; irregular, polymorphic 2- to 5-Hz lateralized or localized patterns; and nonlateralized arrhythmic activity (24,30,33). Bilateral ictal patterns are more common and appear earlier in patients with NTLE than in those with MTLE, and rhythmic activity is hemispheric rather than temporal in distribution (11,30,33).

FRONTAL LOBE EPILEPSY

Frontal lobe epilepsies (FLEs) are subclassified according to the presumed location of the epileptogenic zone. Several distinct syndromes have been described, but in some cases, the clinical, electrographic, and neuroimaging features are variable and localization is not possible. After TLE, FLE is the most common type of epilepsy, accounting for 20% to 30% of cases in surgical series (34,37). Frontal lobe seizures take the form of simple partial, complex partial, atonic, tonic, myoclonic, and tonic-clonic attacks. Simple partial seizures involve motor, sensory, autonomic, affective, and cognitive phenomena. Complex partial seizures differ from those originating in the temporal lobe by their abrupt onset, short duration, rapid secondary generalization, and minimal or no postictal state (37). Status epilepticus and seizure clusters are relatively common. Generalized motor activity, version, and focal clonic and tonic activity are frequently observed. Complex motor automatisms, including bicycling and thrashing movements, sexual

automatisms, laughter, and vocalizations, may result in misdiagnosis as psychogenic seizures and, when present early in the attack, distinguish FLE from TLE (5,38). Complex partial status epilepticus occurs in 40% of patients with FLE (37). Prolonged absence seizures with generalized 3-Hz spike-wave complexes and focal motor features or language disturbances also have been observed (39).

Ictal symptomatology may be more helpful than an EEG in localizing frontal lobe seizures. The inaccessibility of a large portion of the frontal lobes to surface electrodes, the rapid spread of seizures within and outside this area, secondary bilateral synchrony and bilateral epileptogenesis as a consequence of bifrontal injury, and variably sized seizure onset zones all contribute to the lack of electroencephalographic localization or mislocalization in patients with FLE (40,41). The interictal EEG may be entirely normal or may reveal generalized or lateralized slowing, focal, hemispheric, multiregional, or generalized spikes or polyspikes, or low-voltage fast activity. In a large study of patients with FLE, interictal epileptiform activity appeared bilaterally synchronous in 37%, lobar in 32%, multilobar in 24%, focal in 12%, and hemispheric or bifrontal and independent each in 9% of cases (42). Epileptiform activity is restricted to the frontal lobes in only 25% of patients and to other areas in 20% to 50%; in 20% to 70% of patients, epileptiform activity is absent (37,43). Supra- and infraorbital, sphenoidal, and additional closely spaced scalp electrodes enhance spike detection in patients with suspected orbitofrontal or mesial frontal seizures. Midline epileptiform activity may be mistaken for vertex sharp transients that appear spike-like in children or may escape detection if viewed on montages not incorporating midline electrodes. Secondary bilateral synchrony, in which a unilateral epileptogenic focus near the midline produces seemingly bilaterally synchronous generalized epileptiform activity, is observed in up to 20% of patients (37). Unilateral discharges that precede and initiate the bilateral epileptiform activity, distinct morphology of focal and bilateral discharges, isolated unilateral discharges, and focal slowing distinguish secondary bilateral synchrony from the generalized epileptiform activity characteristic of idiopathic generalized epilepsies. Bilaterally synchronous bursts of spike-and-wave complexes occurred in 26 of 31 patients whose epilepsy was associated with frontal parasagittal lesions (44).

Frontal lobe complex partial seizures are brief, begin and end abruptly, and frequently involve excessive movement or tonic posturing that obscures the EEG pattern. Approximately one-third of such seizures are not accompanied by any electroencephalographic changes, whereas another one-third feature nonlateralized slowing, rhythmic activity, or repetitive spiking (37,40,43). Lateralized or localized ictal patterns characterize 33% to 50% of these seizures (37,43,45). Seizures arising from the dorsolateral frontal cortex are more likely than mesial frontal seizures to produce localized rhythmic alpha or beta activity, or repetitive spiking (11,46). Occasionally, the ictal onset appears contralateral to the hemisphere of seizure origin (43,47). This phenomena, known as paradoxical lateralization, occurs when a generator located within the interhemispheric fissure produces an obliquely oriented dipole that projects to the opposite hemisphere, as in supplementary sensorimotor area (SSMA) epilepsy.

FLE encompasses several distinct seizure types based on the anatomical site of the presumed ictal generator (Table 23.1) (36,48). However, rapid propagation of the ictal discharge within the frontal lobes and to remote areas limits the localization value of ictal symptomatology alone.

Supplementary Sensorimotor Area Epilepsy

The seizures of SSMA epilepsy typically involve bilateral, asymmetric, tonic, or dystonic posturing of the extremities and facial grimacing, with vocalization or speech arrest and preservation of consciousness (49). One arm is flexed, the other extended; the legs are flexed or extended. Occasionally, posturing is symmetric. The classic fencing posture (elevation of the contralateral arm that is externally rotated and flexed at the elbow, with head turning toward the elevated arm and extension of the opposite arm) is uncommon (49). The tonic phase may culminate in focal clonic activity of one or more extremities that serves as a reliable lateralizing sign. Before tonic posturing, some patients describe nonspecific sensations or sensory disturbances of the extremities—pulling, pulsing, heaviness, or numbness and tingling—that may be ipsilateral or contralateral to the focus (47). Seizures last less than 30 seconds, begin and end abruptly, and tend to cluster. They commonly occur in sleep and, in many cases, are limited to sleep. Postictal manifestations are absent or mild and short-lived. Their shorter duration, stereotypical nature, occurrence in sleep, and the presence of a tonic contraction of the abducted upper extremities distinguish SSMA seizures from nonepileptic attacks.

The interhemispheric location of the ictal generator reduces the yield of ictal and interictal electroencephalographic abnormalities in epilepsy arising from the SSMA compared with that arising from other areas. The interictal record is often entirely normal, particularly if viewed on montages not incorporating midline electrodes. Coronal montages increase the likelihood of detecting abnormalities, as do additional scalp electrodes, which in one study detected midline interictal epileptiform activity in 7 of 11 patients with SSMA epilepsy (47). Sharp waves near the midline may be mistaken for vertex sharp transients that tend to have a spike-like morphology in children. In a pediatric study, midline spikes, sharp waves, positive sharp waves, or delta activity that often spreads unilaterally or bilaterally over the frontal, central, or parietal regions was identified interictally in 11 of 12 cases (50). These abnormalities were observed more often in sleep (exclusively in four cases), and their frequency increased with age.

The identification of ictal patterns is even more challenging. The ictal EEG is often obscured by myogenic and movement artifact or shows no clear change (11). Paroxysmal fast activity in the parasagittal regions and generalized electrodecremental patterns, sometimes preceded by a single, high-amplitude sharp wave or transient, are the most common ictal findings (11,47).

Orbitofrontal Epilepsy

Because of connections with the limbic system, seizures arising from the orbitofrontal cortex resemble those originating from the temporal lobes (34,51–53). Staring, loss of awareness, oral and gestural automatisms, motor agitation, and version of the head or eyes are all characteristic of this form of epilepsy. Autonomic features include epigastric sensations, fear, tachycardia, tachypnea, pallor, sweating, flushing, piloerection, sensation of hunger or thirst, and pupillary dilatation (54). Olfactory hallucinations are not uncommon, and ictal urination occurs rarely. Tharp (38) described three children with seizure clusters characterized by intense autonomic manifestations, loud vocalization, ambulation, oral and manual automatisms, and infrequent urinary incontinence associated with high-amplitude bifrontal spike and slow waves. Screaming, laughing, coughing, sexual automatisms, and pelvic thrusting have been observed with bilaterally synchronous sharp waves or spike-wave complexes maximal in the frontal regions (34,35,53). Ictal onset recorded with depth electrodes may precede the clinical manifestations of disease by as much as 60 seconds, suggesting asymptomatic activation of this area (34).

Anterior Frontopolar Epilepsy

Version, forced thinking, falls, and autonomic signs are all prominent features of frontopolar seizures, along with focal clonic and generalized tonic seizures and GTCSs. Early and complete loss of contact with the environment has been described (55). Penfield and Kristiansen (56) produced version with loss of awareness by stimulating the frontopolar region; stimulation of the premotor area resulted in version alone. Absence seizures associated with seemingly generalized 3-Hz spike-wave activity have been reported (57), but clinical manifestations may be minimal when ictal discharges remain confined to the frontal pole (36).

Dorsolateral Frontal Lobe Epilepsy

Activation of the dorsolateral frontal convexity produces tonic and clonic activity, version of the head or eyes, and arrest of activity sometimes preceded by ill-defined cephalic sensations, epigastric and visual sensations, dizziness, and fear (58). Focal clonic manifestations are seen contralateral to the epileptogenic frontal lobe.

Aphasia and speech arrest occur in seizures arising from the Broca area. Consciousness is often preserved unless the frontopolar regions are involved (59). Quesney and colleagues (58) distinguished seizures arising in the anterior dorsolateral convexity from those of parasagittal origin by automatisms (30% of convexity seizures versus 0% of parasagittal seizures) and somatosensory auras (0% versus 60%, respectively). Version occurred during a period of altered awareness in patients with dorsolateral seizures, whereas those with parasagittal seizures could recall the head turning. In the same series, focal clonic activity contralateral to the epileptogenic focus characterized dorsolateral seizures; bilateral tonic postural changes in the extremities were common in patients with parasagittal seizures.

Cingulate Gyrus Epilepsy

The intimate connections of the cingulate gyrus with the temporal lobe explain why seizures from this region share many features of MTLE. Partial seizures involve loss of awareness and oral, manual, and gestural automatisms (60). Affective manifestations, including aggressive behavior, screaming, and intense fear (61), as well as autonomic changes, such as tachycardia, tachypnea, sweating, and pallor, have been noted. Clonic mouth movements, as well as tonic-clonic and atonic seizures, are also observed (62). Facial grimacing, followed by either laughter or crying, were reported in a woman with a cavernous angioma and seizures arising from the left cingulate gyrus (63). Electrical stimulation of Brodmann area 24 in 83 patients with epilepsy produced arousal; highly integrated movements of the fingers and hands, mouth, legs, and eyes; and hallucinations (61). Mazars (64) described 36 patients with epilepsy who were "cured" after removal of one or both cingulate gyri. Of these, 16 patients experienced generalized seizures (without focal features), and 13 had absence seizures only. In seven patients, absence and generalized seizures were preceded by elevation of one arm, head rotation, clonic facial movements, speech arrest, and staring or nodding. Absence seizures characterized by short periods of blurred consciousness were at times associated with head drops or nodding and blushing. The interictal EEG showed generalized, bilateral spike-and-wave activity in three patients and unilateral frontal arrhythmic slowing in one patient. The remaining patients had no interictal abnormalities.

Opercular Area Epilepsy

Few detailed descriptions of opercular seizures exist, but salivation, mastication, swallowing, speech arrest, laryngeal symptoms, autonomic features, and somatomotor manifestations have been reported. Loss of awareness late in the seizure is often preceded by motor involvement of the face (ipsilateral, contralateral, or bilateral), upper extremities (contralateral), lower extremities (bilateral), or eyes (nonconjugate deviation) (55). Patients have described epigastric and gustatory sensations and fear. Postictal language disturbances may occur with seizures arising from the opercular region of the dominant hemisphere (55).

Motor Area Epilepsy

The clinical manifestations of seizures arising near the motor cortex are a function of the area activated. The lower motor area produces tonic or clonic activity of the contralateral face, speech arrest, dysphasia, and vocalizations. Involvement of the motor strip representing the upper extremity causes clonic activity of the upper extremity, occasionally evolving into a jacksonian march that begins in the distal muscles of the extremity and moves up the arm. Activation of the superior and mesial aspect of the primary motor area gives rise to clonic activity of the contralateral lower extremity. Ipsilateral tonic movements of the leg may also occur as the ictal discharge spreads to the nearby SSMA. Secondary generalized seizures are common. Other features of motor area seizures include postictal hemiparesis or hemiplegia (Todd paralysis) and a tendency for focal motor status epilepticus, or epilepsia partialis continua. Kojewnikow syndrome, characterized by repetitive focal motor seizures, myoclonus, and focal motor status epilepticus, may be associated with perirolandic tumors and vascular malformations (58). This nonprogressive disorder can occur in either childhood or adulthood. Rasmussen syndrome, which also presents with focal motor seizures or epilepsia partialis continua, is discussed elsewhere in this book.

Parietal Lobe Epilepsy

Parietal lobe seizures constitute 5% to 6% of cases of focal epilepsy in medical and surgical series (65–67). Few descriptions are available, because prior to recent advances in neuroimaging, the parietal and occipital lobes were usually considered together. Somatosensory seizures involve the contralateral face or limb(s) and are occasionally bilateral. Numbness, tingling, pain, and thermal sensations of cold or burning have been described, along with nonspecific cephalic sensations, visual hallucinations, vertigo, disturbances in body image, gustatory phenomena, panic, and genital sensations (67–71). Ideomotor apraxia and nystagmus are rare. Psychic auras, epigastric sensations, and ictal amaurosis suggest activation of extraparietal regions (71), and the clinical features of parietal lobe complex partial seizures hint at variable spread patterns. Seizures characterized by asymmetric tonic posturing of the extremities, unilateral clonic activity, contralateral version, and hyperkinetic activity occur with secondary activation of the frontal regions; spread to the temporal lobes produces automatisms and altered consciousness (67,69,71,72). In an ictal SPECT analysis (73), parietal seizures with sensorimotor manifestations were associated with anterior parietal hyperperfusion, whereas seizures with staring and altered awareness produced hyperperfusion involving the posterior parietal region (73).

Not unlike FLE, the surface electroencephalographic characteristics of parietal lobe epilepsy are often poorly localized or mislocalized. The interictal record may be normal, or it may show lateralized or generalized intermittent slowing (66). Interictal epileptiform activity is usually multiregional, suggesting involvement of areas distant from the epileptogenic zone (66,67,69,71,74). Centroparietal epileptiform activity is the sole interictal abnormality in 5% to 20% of cases (67,69,71,74), whereas secondary bilateral synchrony is seen in one-third of patients (69). Ictal patterns depend on the pathway of propagation and may erroneously suggest a temporal or frontal lobe focus (67,69,71). Simple partial seizures of parietal lobe origin frequently have no electroencephalographic correlate (74,75). Compared with TLE, generalized or lateralized ictal patterns are often observed (11,69,71). In a recent study, 62% of parietal seizures had localizing features, although 16% were falsely localized or lateralized (11).

Occipital Lobe Epilepsy

Representing 8% of the symptomatic focal epilepsies (65), seizures of occipital lobe epilepsy involve visual phenomena, sensations of ocular movement, nystagmus, eye flutter, forced eye blinking, and versive head and eye movements (76,77). Visual symptoms may be positive (colored or bright lights) or negative (scotomas, hemianopias, amaurosis). Elementary visual hallucinations that may be limited to the contralateral hemifield occur in 50% to 60% of cases (76,77), but auras suggesting origin outside the occipital lobe, including abdominal, psychic, olfactory, and gustatory sensations, also have been reported. Impairment of consciousness and motor signs, usually version, were observed in nearly 75% of children with symptomatic occipital lobe epilepsy (78). The clinical manifestations of occipital lobe complex partial seizures reflect different patterns of ictal propagation. Infrasylvian spread to the temporal lobe—the most common pathway (48,77)—is associated with automatisms and loss of awareness. Suprasylvian spread to the mesial frontal lobe produces asymmetric tonic posturing, whereas propagation laterally results in focal motor or sensory seizures. Between one-third and one-half of all patients experience multiple seizure types (76,77).

In patients with occipital lobe epilepsy, the interictal EEG reveals widespread epileptiform activity or activity maximal in the posterior temporal regions (76,77). Bitemporal independent, bilateral synchronous frontal complexes, bioccipital and diffuse epileptiform activity are observed in 30% to 50% of cases (76); activity restricted to the occipital lobes occurs in only 8% to 18% of patients (76,77). Ictal recordings show diffuse suppression or rhythmic activity that is usually generalized, but may appear lateralized or maximal over the temporooccipital region (76,77). Salanova and colleagues (76) found localized ictal patterns in half of all patients studied, but only

17% had onset confined to the occipital region. In another surgical series (79), electroencephalographic onset was localized to the occipital or occipitotemporal region in 57% of patients. One study (11) noted correctly localized ictal patterns in 41% of occipital seizures; false localization/lateralization occurred in 28% of seizures. Invasive recordings show ictal propagation to mesial temporal structures, supplementary motor area, or dorsolateral frontal convexity before secondary generalization (74).

ETIOLOGIC FACTORS

With few exceptions, the location of an epileptic focus is not helpful in predicting the etiology of focal seizures. Head trauma often produces contusions of the frontal and temporal polar regions and orbitofrontal cortex. Epilepsy associated with bilateral occipital lobe calcifications, mitochondrial encephalopathy with lactic acidosis and stroke-like episodes, myoclonus epilepsy with ragged red fibers, and Lafora disease preferentially affect the occipital lobes (80). In general, pathologic substrates include malformations of cortical development, neoplasms, head injury, CNS infection, and vascular malformations. In 346 surgical patients from the Montreal Neurological Institute, postnatal trauma (32%) and tumor (28%) were the most common etiologic factors, with inflammatory processes, birth trauma or anoxia, and miscellaneous causes each accounting for fewer than 10% of cases (41); the cause was unknown in 15% of cases. Recent advances in neuroimaging have improved the recognition of MTS and malformations of cortical development—the primary causes of refractory epilepsy at most surgical centers—but the cause remains elusive in approximately 70% of patients with epilepsy and in approximately 25% of surgical patients (81).

MANAGEMENT

Treatment of the focal epilepsies is independent of cause and epileptogenic location. No studies have compared response to antiepileptic drugs (AEDs) and remission rates of epilepsies from different regions. For many years, carbamazepine and phenytoin have been the agents of choice for patients with complex partial seizures with or without secondary GTCSs (82); outcome is poorer and adverse effects more common with phenobarbital or primidone. Carbamazepine and valproic acid have demonstrated similar efficacy against GTCSs, although carbamazepine was superior for complex partial seizures and was associated with fewer adverse effects (83). Over the last decade, however, use of these older agents has diminished with the introduction of newer AEDs. Lamotrigine and oxcarbazepine are approved for use as monotherapy in adults with focal seizures (84,85). In many cases, these agents are better tolerated and have fewer adverse effects. In addition, laboratory monitoring is typically not required. Gabapentin, topiramate, tiagabine, levetiracetam, and zonisamide are also acceptable choices for adjunctive therapy.

Appropriate medical management of focal epilepsies is associated with good control or remission in 60% to 70% of patients (86). Known cause, congenital neurologic deficit, frequent generalized seizures, need for multiple medications, and epileptiform electroencephalographic abnormalities all reduce the likelihood of remission (87). Patients with structural abnormalities on MRI and those with resistant seizures after 1 to 2 years of treatment should be referred for surgical consideration. Surgical outcome depends on the extent of resection, which may be limited by involvement of cortical regions subserving motor or language functions. A seizure-free state is realized in 60% to 70% of patients with TLE after temporal lobectomy, but ranges from 23% to 67% after extratemporal resection (88). The prognosis is less favorable in the absence of a causative lesion on MRI.

REFERENCES

1. Commission on Classification and Terminology of the International League Against Epilepsy. Proposal for revised classification of epilepsies and epileptic syndromes. *Epilepsia* 1989;30: 389–399.
2. Hauser WA. The natural history of temporal lobe epilepsy. In: Lüders H, ed. *Epilepsy surgery.* New York: Raven Press, 1991:133–141.
3. French JA, Williamson PD, Thadani VM, et al. Characteristics of medial temporal lobe epilepsy, I: Results of history and physical examination. *Ann Neurol* 1993;34:774–780.
4. Maldonado HM, Delgado-Escueta AV, Walsh GO, et al. Complex partial seizures of hippocampal and amygdalar origin. *Epilepsia* 1988;29:420–433.
5. Quesney LF. Clinical and EEG features of complex partial seizures of temporal lobe origin. *Epilepsia* 1986;27(Suppl 2):S27–S45.
6. Kotagal P, Lüders H, Morris HH, et al. Dystonic posturing in complex partial seizures of temporal lobe onset: a new lateralizing sign. *Neurology* 1989;39:196–201.
7. Gabr M, Lüders H, Dinner D, et al. Speech manifestations in lateralization of temporal lobe seizures. *Ann Neurol* 1989;25:82–87.
8. Ebner A, Dinner DS, Noachtar S, et al. Automatisms with preserved responsiveness: a lateralizing sign in psychomotor seizures. *Neurology* 1995;45:61–64.
9. Kramer RE, Lüders H, Goldstick LP, et al. Ictus emeticus: an electroclinical analysis. *Neurology* 1988;38:1048–1052.
10. Bossi L, Munari C, Stoffels C, et al. Somatomotor manifestations in temporal lobe seizures. *Epilepsia* 1984;25:70–76.
11. Foldvary N, Klem G, Hammel J, et al. The localizing value of ictal EEG in focal epilepsy. *Neurology* 2001;57:2022–2028.
12. Leutmezer F, Serles W, Lehrner J, et al. Postictal nose wiping: a lateralizing sign in temporal lobe complex partial seizures. *Neurology* 1998;51:1175–1177.
13. Van Ness PC, Marotta J, Kucera A, et al. Postictal cough is a sign of temporal lobe epilepsy. *Neurology* 1993;43:A273.
14. Ebner A, Hoppe M. Noninvasive electroencephalography and mesial temporal sclerosis. *J Clin Neurophysiol* 1995;12:23–31.
15. Williamson PD, French JA, Thadani VM. Characteristics of medial temporal lobe epilepsy, II: Interictal and ictal scalp electroencephalography, neuropsychological testing, neuroimaging, surgical results, and pathology. *Ann Neurol* 1993;34:781–787.
16. Jasper H, Pertuisset B, Flanigin H. EEG and cortical electrograms in patients with temporal lobe seizures. *Arch Neurol* 1951; 65:272–290.
17. Silverman D. The anterior temporal electrode and the ten-twenty system. *Electroencephalogr Clin Neurophysiol* 1960;12:735–737.
18. King DW, So EL, Marcus R, et al. Techniques and applications of sphenoidal recording. *J Clin Neurophysiol* 1986;3:51–65.
19. Baumgartner C, Lindinger G, Ebner A, et al. Propagation of interictal epileptic activity in temporal lobe epilepsy. *Neurology* 1995; 45:118–122.
20. Ebersole JS, Wade PB. Spike voltage topography identifies two types of frontotemporal epileptic foci. *Neurology* 1991;41; 1425–1433.
21. Reiher J, Beaudry M, Leduc CP. Temporal intermittent rhythmic delta activity (TIRDA) in the diagnosis of complex partial epilepsy: sensitivity, specificity and predictive value. *Can J Neurol Sci* 1989;16:398–401.
22. Risinger MW, Engel J Jr, Van Ness PC, et al. Ictal localization of temporal lobe seizures with scalp/sphenoidal recordings. *Neurology* 1989;39:1288–1293.
23. Ebersole JS, Pacia SV. Localization of temporal lobe foci by ictal EEG patterns. *Epilepsia* 1996;37:386–399.
24. Pacia SV, Ebersole JS. Intracranial EEG substrates of scalp ictal patterns from temporal lobe foci. *Epilepsia* 1997;38:642–654.
25. Walczak TS, Radtke RA, Lewis DV. Accuracy and interobserver reliability of scalp ictal EEG. *Neurology* 1992;42:2279–2285.
26. Steinhoff BJ, So NK, Lim S, et al. Ictal scalp EEG in temporal lobe epilepsy with unitemporal versus bitemporal interictal epileptiform discharges. *Neurology* 1995;45:889–896.
27. Cendes F, Li LM, Watson C, et al. Is ictal recording mandatory in temporal lobe epilepsy? Not when the interictal electroencephalogram and hippocampal atrophy coincide. *Arch Neurol* 2000;57:497–500.
28. Wieser HG, Engel J Jr, Williamson PD, et al. Surgically remedial temporal lobe syndromes. In: Engel J Jr, ed. *Surgical treatment of the epilepsies.* New York: Raven Press, 1993:49–63.
29. Lévesque MF, Nakasato N, Vinters HV, et al. Surgical treatment of limbic epilepsy associated with extrahippocampal lesions: the problem of dual pathology. *J Neurosurg* 1991;75:364–370.
30. Foldvary N, Lee N, Thwaites G, et al. Clinical and electrographic manifestations of lesional neocortical temporal lobe epilepsy. *Neurology* 1997;49:757–763.
31. Gil-Nagel A, Risinger MW. Ictal semiology in hippocampal versus extrahippocampal temporal lobe epilepsy. *Brain* 1997;120: 183–192.
32. O'Brien TJ, Kilpatrick C, Murrie V, et al. Temporal lobe epilepsy caused by mesial temporal sclerosis and temporal neocortical lesions. A clinical and electroencephalographic study of 46 pathologically proven cases. *Brain* 1996;119:2133–2141.
33. Pacia SV, Devinsky O, Perrine K, et al. The clinical features of neocortical temporal lobe epilepsy [abstract]. *Epilepsia* 1995;36:113.
34. Mihara T, Inoue Y, Hiyoshi T, et al. Localizing value of seizure manifestations of temporal lobe epilepsies and the consequence of analyzing their sequential appearance. *Jpn J Psychiatry Neurol* 1993;47:175–182.
35. Duchowny M, Jayakar P, Resnick T, et al. Posterior temporal epilepsy: electroclinical features. *Ann Neurol* 1994;35:427–431.
36. Wieser HG, Hajek M. Frontal lobe epilepsy: compartmentalization, surgical evaluation and operative results. In: Jasper HH, Riggio S, Goldman-Rakic PS, eds. *Epilepsy and the functional anatomy of the frontal lobe.* New York: Raven Press, 1995:297–318.
37. Williamson PD, Spencer DD, Spencer SS, et al. Complex partial seizures of frontal lobe origin. *Ann Neurol* 1985;18:497–504.
38. Tharp BR. Orbital frontal seizures. An unique electroencephalographic and clinical syndrome. *Epilepsia* 1972;13:627–642.
39. Niedermeyer E, Fineyre F, Riley T, et al. Absence status (petit mal status) with focal characteristics. *Arch Neurol* 1979;36:417–421.
40. Quesney LF, Constain M, Fish DR, et al. The clinical differentiation of seizures arising in the parasagittal and anterolaterodorsal frontal convexities. *Arch Neurol* 1990;47:677–679.
41. Rasmussen T. Surgery of frontal lobe epilepsy. In: Purpura DP, Penry JK, Walter RD, eds. *Neurosurgical management of the epilepsies.* New York: Raven Press, 1975:197–205.
42. Quesney LF. Preoperative electroencephalographic investigation in frontal lobe epilepsy: electroencephalographic and electrocorticographic recordings. *Can J Neurol Sci* 1991;18(Suppl 4):559–563.
43. Laskowitz DT, Sperling MR, French JA, et al. The syndrome of frontal lobe epilepsy: characteristics and surgical management. *Neurology* 1995;45:780–787.

44. Tükel K, Jasper H. The electroencephalogram in parasagittal lesions. *Electroencephalogr Clin Neurophysiol* 1952;4:481–494.

45. Swartz BE, Walsh GO, Delgado-Escueta AV, et al. Surface ictal electroencephalographic pattern in frontal vs temporal lobe epilepsy. *Can J Neurol Sci* 1991;18:649–662.

46. Baustista RE, Spencer DD, Spencer SS. EEG findings in frontal lobe epilepsies. *Neurology* 1998;50:1765–1771.

47. Morris HH III, Dinner DS, Lüders H, et al. Supplementary motor seizures: clinical and electroencephalographic findings. *Neurology* 1988;38:1075–1082.

48. Blume WT, Whiting SE, Girvin JP. Epilepsy surgery in the posterior cortex. *Ann Neurol* 1991;29:638–645.

49. Bleasel AF, Morris HH. Supplementary sensorimotor area epilepsy in adults. In: Lüders HO, ed. *Supplementary sensorimotor area epilepsy. Advances in neurology*, vol 70. Philadelphia: Lippincott–Raven, 1996:271–284.

50. Connolly MB, Langill L, Wong PK, et al. Seizures involving the supplementary sensorimotor area in children: a video-EEG analysis. *Epilepsia* 1995;36:1025–1032.

51. Chang CN, Ojemann LM, Ojemann GA, et al. Seizures of fronto-orbital origin: a proven case. *Epilepsia* 1991;32:487–491.

52. Ludwig B, Marsan CA, Van Buren J. Cerebral seizures of probable orbitofrontal origin. *Epilepsia* 1975;16:141–158.

53. Rougier A, Loiseau P. Orbitofrontal epilepsy: a case report. *J Neurol Neurosurg Psychiatry* 1988;51:146–147.

54. Munari C, Bancaud J. Electroclinical symptomatology of partial seizures of orbitofrontal origin. In: Chauvel P, Delgado-Escueta AV, Halgren E, et al., eds. *Frontal lobe seizures and epilepsy. Advances in neurology*, vol 57. New York: Raven Press, 1992: 257–265.

55. Bancaud J, Talairach J. Clinical semiology of frontal lobe seizures. In: Chauvel P, Delgado-Escueta AV, Halgren E, et al., eds. *Frontal lobe seizures and epilepsy. Advances in neurology*, vol 57. New York: Raven Press, 1992:3–58.

56. Penfield WG, Kristiansen K. Epileptic seizure patterns. Springfield, IL: Charles C Thomas, 1951.

57. Riggio S, Harner RN. Repetitive motor activity in frontal lobe epilepsy. In: Jasper HH, Riggio S, Goldman-Rakic PS, eds. *Epilepsy and the functional anatomy of the frontal lobe*. New York: Raven Press, 1995:153–164.

58. Quesney LF, Constain M, Rasmussen T. Seizures from the dorsolateral frontal lobe. In: Chauvel P, Delgado-Escueta AV, Halgren E, et al., eds. *Frontal lobe seizures and epilepsy. Advances in neurology*, vol 57. New York: Raven Press, 1992:233–255.

59. Niedermeyer E. Frontal lobe epilepsy: the next frontier. *Clin Electroencephalogr* 1998;29:163–169.

60. Levin B, Duchowny M. Childhood obsessive-compulsive disorder and cingulate epilepsy. *Biol Psychiatry* 1991;30:1049–1055.

61. Bancaud J, Talairach J, Geier S, et al. Behavioral manifestations induced by electric stimulation of the anterior cingulate gyrus in man. *Rev Neurol (Paris)* 1976;132:705–724.

62. Bancaud J. Physiopathogenesis of generalized epilepsies of organic nature (stereoelectroencephalographic study). In: Gastaut H, Jasper H, Bancaud J, et al, eds. *The physiopathogenesis of the epilepsies*. Springfield, IL: Charles C. Thomas, 1969: 158–185.

63. Arroyo S, Lesser RP, Gordon B, et al. Mirth, laughter and gelastic seizures. *Brain* 1993;116:757–780.

64. Mazars G. Cingulate gyrus epileptogenic foci as an origin for generalized seizures. In: Gastaut H, Jasper H, Bancaud J, et al., eds. *The physiopathogenesis of the epilepsies*. Springfield, IL: Charles C Thomas, 1969:186–189.

65. Gibbs FA, Gibbs EL, Lennox WG. Epilepsy: a paroxysmal cerebral dysrhythmia. *Brain* 1937;60:377–388.

66. Mauguiere F, Courjon J. Somatosensory epilepsy: a review of 127 cases. *Brain* 1978;101:307–332.

67. Salanova V, Andermann F, Rasmussen T, et al. Tumoural parietal lobe epilepsy. Clinical manifestations and outcome in 34 patients treated between 1934 and 1988. *Brain* 1995;118:1289–1304.

68. Alemayehu S, Bergey GK, Barry E, et al. Panic attacks as ictal manifestations of parietal lobe seizures. *Epilepsia* 1995;36:824–830.

69. Salanova V, Andermann F, Rasmussen T, et al. Parietal lobe epilepsy. Clinical manifestations and outcome in 82 patients treated surgically between 1929 and 1988. *Brain* 1995;118:607–627.

70. Sveinbjornsdottir S, Duncan JS. Parietal and occipital lobe epilepsy: a review. *Epilepsia* 1993;34:493–521.

71. Williamson PD, Boon PA, Thadani VM, et al. Parietal lobe epilepsy: diagnostic considerations and results of surgery. *Ann Neurol* 1992;31:193–201.

72. Geier S, Bancaud J, Talairach J, et al. Ictal tonic postural changes and automatisms of the upper limb during epileptic parietal lobe discharges. *Epilepsia* 1977;18:517–524.

73. Ho SS, Berkovic SF, Newton MR, et al. Parietal lobe epilepsy: clinical features and seizure localization by ictal SPECT. *Neurology* 1994;44:2277–2284.

74. Cascino GD, Hulihan JF, Sharbrough FW, et al. Parietal lobe lesional epilepsy: electroclinical correlation and operative outcome. *Epilepsia* 1993;34:522–527.

75. Devinsky O, Kelley K, Porter RJ, et al. Clinical and electroencephalographic features of simple partial seizures. *Neurology* 1988;38:1347–1352.

76. Salanova V, Andermann F, Olivier A, et al. Occipital lobe epilepsy: electroclinical manifestations, electrocorticography, cortical stimulation and outcome in 42 patients treated between 1930 and 1991. *Brain* 1992;115:1655–1680.

77. Williamson PD, Thadani VM, Darcey TM, et al. Occipital lobe epilepsy: clinical characteristics, seizure spread patterns, and results of surgery. *Ann Neurol* 1992;31:3–13.

78. Van den Hout BM, Van der Meij W, Wieneke GH, et al. Seizure semiology of occipital lobe epilepsy in children. *Epilepsia* 1997;38:1188–1191.

79. Aykut-Bingol C, Bronen RA, Kim JH, et al. Surgical outcome in occipital lobe epilepsy: implications for pathophysiology. *Ann Neurol* 1998;44:60–69.

80. Kuzniecky R. Symptomatic occipital lobe epilepsy. *Epilepsia* 1998;39(Suppl 4):S24–S31.

81. Annegers JF. The epidemiology of epilepsy. In: Wyllie E, ed. *The treatment of epilepsy: principles & practice*, 2nd ed. Baltimore, MD: Williams & Wilkins, 1997:165–172.

82. Mattson RH, Cramer JA, Collins JF. Comparison of carbamazepine, phenobarbital, phenytoin, and primidone in partial and secondarily generalized tonic-clonic seizures. *N Engl J Med* 1985;313:145–151.

83. Mattson RH, Cramer JA, Collins JF. A comparison of valproate with carbamazepine for the treatment of complex partial seizures and secondarily generalized tonic-clonic seizures in adults. *N Engl J Med* 1992;327:765–771.

84. Gilliam F, Vazquez B, Sackellares JC, et al. An active-control trial of lamotrigine monotherapy for partial seizures. *Neurology* 1998;51:1018–1025.

85. Beydoun A, Sachedo RC, Rosenfeld WE, et al. Oxcarbazepine monotherapy for partial-onset seizures: a multicenter, double-blind, clinical trial. *Neurology* 2000;54:2245–2251.

86. Annegers JF, Hauser WA, Elveback LR. Remission of seizures and relapse in patients with epilepsy. *Epilepsia* 1979;20:729–737.

87. Hauser WA, Hesdorffer DC. The natural history of seizures. In: Wyllie E, ed. *The treatment of epilepsy: principles & practice*, 2nd ed. Baltimore, MD: Williams & Wilkins, 1997:173–178.

88. Benbadis SR, Chelune GJ, Stanford LD, et al. Outcome and complications of epilepsy surgery. In: Wyllie E, ed. *The treatment of epilepsy: principles and practice*, 2nd ed. Baltimore, MD: Williams & Wilkins, 1997:1103–1118.

Idiopathic and Benign Partial Epilepsies of Childhood

24

Elaine C. Wirrell   Carol S. Camfield   Peter R. Camfield

The benign and idiopathic partial epilepsies (IPEs) of childhood account for approximately one-fifth of all epilepsies in children and adolescents. IPEs differ in two ways from most other focal epilepsy syndromes. First, IPEs are genetically determined focal disturbances of cerebral activity without any apparent structural abnormality detectable on magnetic resonance imaging (MRI), whereas most focal epilepsies are "lesional," resulting from a localized area of cortical damage or dysgenesis. Second, most IPEs remit by adolescence, unlike lesional focal epilepsies, which are often refractory.

In a survey of seizure disorders in the southwest of France, the annual incidence of IPEs in children 0 to 15 years of age was estimated to be 8.63 per 100,000 (1), representing one-half of all partial seizures in this age group. The actual incidence of IPE may be higher, however, as many children with partial seizures do not clearly fit into one of the IPE phenotypes and yet have spontaneous remission and no underlying abnormality on neuroimaging. Identification of these epileptic syndromes is paramount to providing these children and their families a favorable prognosis and appropriate management.

Although controversy surrounds their exact clinical boundaries, IPEs of childhood include (2,3):

- Age-dependent occurrence—onset generally after 18 months, with specific peak ages for each subtype
- Absence of significant anatomic lesions on neuroimaging
- Normal neurologic status, with most children intellectually intact and without prior neurologic insult

- Favorable long-term outcome, with remission occurring prior to adolescence in most children, even those whose seizures were initially frequent or difficult to control
- Possible genetic predisposition—other family members with benign forms of epilepsy that resolved in adolescence
- Specific semiology—most seizures are simple partial motor or sensory, although complex partial and secondarily generalized seizures also may be seen; nocturnal occurrence is common and frequency is usually low
- Rapid response to antiepileptic medication in most cases
- Specific electroencephalographic (EEG) features—spikes of distinctive morphology and variable location superimposed on a normal background, with occasional multifocal sharp waves or brief bursts of generalized spike wave; epileptiform discharges are often activated by sleep

The International League Against Epilepsy (ILAE) currently recognizes two types of IPE in childhood (4): benign childhood epilepsy with centrotemporal spikes (BCECTS) and benign occipital epilepsy (BOE). BOE has been further subdivided into early onset (Panayiotopoulos) and late-onset (Gastaut) types. Other proposed but less well-studied syndromes include benign epilepsy in infancy (BPEI) with complex partial or secondarily generalized seizures (5,6), benign partial epilepsy with affective symptoms (BPEAS) (7–10), benign partial epilepsy with extreme somatosensory evoked potentials (BPE-ESEP) (11–13), benign frontal epilepsy (BFE) (14), and benign partial epilepsy of adolescence (BPEA) (15,16). Table 24.1 summarizes the core/classic features of these syndromes.

TABLE 24.1

BENIGN PARTIAL EPILEPSY SYNDROMES

Syndrome	Age of Presentation	Clinical Features	Interictal Electroencephalographic Features	Prognosis
Well-defined syndromes accepted in 1989 ILAE classification				
Benign childhood epilepsy with centrotemporal spikes	Range, 3–13 y Peak, 7–8 y	Diurnal or nocturnal simple partial seizures affecting the lower face with numbness, clonic activity, drooling, and/or dysarthria, nocturnal generalized seizure	High-voltage centrotemporal spikes with horizontal dipole, activated with sleep; normal background	Remission by adolescence
Early onset benign occipital epilepsy (Panayiotopoulos type)	Range, 2–8 y Peak, 5 y	Nocturnal seizure with tonic eye deviation, nausea, and vomiting; often prolonged	High-amplitude, repetitive occipital spike and wave, with fixation-off sensitivity Electroencephalogram may be normal or nonspecific	Remission by 1–2 y after onset
Late-onset benign occipital epilepsy (Gastaut type)	Range, 3–16 y Peak, 8 y	Brief diurnal seizures with elementary visual hallucinations, often with migraine-like, postictal headache	As above	5% suffer recurrent seizures in adulthood
Other rare syndromes				
Benign partial epilepsy in infancy	Range, 3–10 mo Peak, 4–6 mo	Motion arrest, decreased responsiveness, staring, simple automatisms, mild convulsive movements with possible secondary generalization	Normal- or low-voltage rolandic or vertex spikes in sleep	Remission by age 2 y
Benign partial epilepsy in adolescence	Range, adolescence Peak, 13–14 y	Motor or sensory symptoms, often with jacksonian march; auditory, olfactory, or gustatory symptoms never seen	Normal or nonspecific epileptiform discharge	Infrequent seizures that usually abate soon
Benign frontal epilepsy	Range, 4–8 y	Head version ± trunk turning; fencing posture, sometimes followed by truncal, bipedal, or pelvic movements	Unilateral or bilateral frontal or posterior-frontal foci	May persist into adulthood
Benign partial epilepsy with extreme somatosensory-evoked potentials	Range, 4–6 y	Diurnal partial motor seizures with head and body version	High-voltage spikes in parietal and parasagittal regions evoked by tapping of feet	Resolution by adolescence
Benign partial epilepsy with affective symptoms	Range, 2–9 y	Brief episodes with sudden fear, screaming, autonomic disturbance, automatisms, and altered awareness	Rolandic-like spikes in frontotemporal and parietotemporal regions in wakefulness and sleep	Remission within 1–2 y

BENIGN PARTIAL EPILEPSY SYNDROMES RECOGNIZED BY THE ILAE

Benign Childhood Epilepsy with Centrotemporal Spikes

Although Martinus Rulandus described the first case of rolandic epilepsy in 1597 (17), its specific electrographic and clinical features were recognized only during the past 50 years. In 1952, Gastaut (18) noted that these "pre-rolandic" spikes were unrelated to focal pathology, and 2 years later, Gibbs and coworkers (19) observed that the discharges may occur without clinical seizures. In 1958,

Nayrac and Beaussart (20) described the clinical symptoms in 21 patients. The excellent prognosis of this syndrome, compared with the poor outcome in psychomotor epilepsy, was apparent in the early literature (21,22).

Although BCECTS is easily recognized in its "pure" form, atypical features are common and may make a confident diagnosis difficult.

Epidemiology

With an incidence of 6.2 to 21 per 100,000 children age 15 years and younger (23–25), BCECTS accounts for between 13% and 23% of all childhood epilepsies (23,26)

and approximately two-thirds of all IPEs (27–30). Onset is between 3 and 13 years, with a peak at 7 to 8 years; BCECTS always resolves by age 16 years (26). Slightly more boys than girls are affected, with a gender ratio of approximately 6:4 (31–33).

Genetics

The hallmark centrotemporal sharp waves are often found in siblings of children with BCECTS. An autosomal dominant inheritance with an age-specific expression has been suggested (34–36), but most children with these EEG features never experience clinical seizures, which suggests that development of BCECTS depends on other genetic and environmental factors (37–40). The first positive evidence for linkage was found on chromosome 15q14, and either the α_7 acetylcholine receptor subunit gene or another closely linked gene may be implicated in pedigrees with BCECTS, but the disorder is genetically heterogeneous (41).

Scheffer and coworkers (42) described a syndrome of autosomal dominant rolandic epilepsy with speech dyspraxia that may also present an opportunity to identify genes involved in BCECTS. This syndrome begins at a mean age of 5.3 years, and its electroclinical manifestations are identical to those of BCECTS, with nocturnal rolandic seizures and centrotemporal spikes with a horizontal dipole. Oromotor and speech dyspraxia are also present, however, and epilepsy and cognitive impairment worsen in subsequent generations.

Pathophysiology

Seizures in BCECTS involve the lower portion of the perirolandic region in the upper sylvian bank. By stimulating this cortical area, Penfield and Rasmussen, according to Lombroso (21), were able to produce symptoms suggestive of BCECTS.

BCECTS most likely represents a "hereditary impairment in brain maturation" (43–45), and Prince (46) proposed that it may be influenced by out-of-phase developmental timetables for excitation and inhibition. The number of axonal branches and synaptic connections is greater early in development than in the mature animal. Developmental "pruning" of these connections may limit the expression of epilepsy. Younger children may also have hyperexcitable cortical circuits that may be modulated by new or more effective inhibitory connections that appear with maturation. Developmental regulation of voltage-dependent channels may also explain decreased cortical excitability with age.

Clinical Manifestations

Seizures characteristically occur either shortly after falling asleep or before awakening. However, in 15% of patients they happen both in sleep and wakefulness, and in 20% to 30% of patients in the waking state alone (31,32). During wakefulness, simple partial seizures are the rule, with (a) unilateral paresthesias of the tongue, lips, gum, and cheek; (b) unilateral clonic or tonic activity involving the face, lips, and tongue; (c) dysarthria; and (d) drooling (21). Stiffness of the jaw or tongue and a choking sensation are also common. Three types of nocturnal seizures have been described: (a) brief hemifacial seizures with speech arrest and drooling in a conscious state (simple partial seizures); (b) hemifacial seizures, but with loss of consciousness (complex partial seizures), often with gurgling or grunting noises that may terminate with vomiting; and (c) secondarily generalized convulsions (32). Postictal confusion and amnesia are rare (47).

In a small number of cases, Loiseau and Beaussart (48) noted unusual paresthesias or jerking of a single arm or leg, abdominal pain, blindness, or vertigo, which likely reflected seizure foci outside the centrotemporal region, as children with BCECTS may also have interictal sharp waves in other areas. Very young children with BCECTS commonly present with hemiconvulsions instead of the typical facial seizure (32). Rarely, partial motor seizures may change sides without becoming generalized (32).

Seizures are usually infrequent. Loiseau and coworkers (49) reported that 35 (20.8%) of 168 patients suffered a single seizure, and only 10 (5.9%) had very frequent events. Kramer and colleagues (50) described only 13 of 100 patients suffering a single seizure. Very frequent seizures may be more likely in children whose epilepsy begins before 3 years of age (50). Seizures often occur in clusters, followed by long seizure-free intervals. There is no known correlation between severity of the EEG abnormality, seizure frequency, and final outcome (32).

Postictal Todd paresis occurs in 7% to 16% of cases and often suggests a focal onset in patients who present with an apparently primarily generalized seizure (48,51,52).

In most children, seizures last from seconds to several minutes; however, status epilepticus has been described in some children with atypical features (51,52). Temporary oromotor and speech disturbances may be associated with intermittent facial twitching, a disorder that resembles anterior opercular syndrome and correlates with very frequent or continuous spike discharge in the perisylvian region (53–57). This problem does not always respond to intravenous antiepileptic medication, and long-term use of steroids has sometimes seemed beneficial (53). Eventually, all children recover over 6 months to 8 years. Some are left with mild speech disfluency or minor slowing of tongue or jaw movements, while others are completely normal. Positron emission tomography demonstrated a bilateral increase of glucose metabolism in the opercular regions in one patient with this type of nonconvulsive status (58). Recognition of this unusual presentation as a benign focal epilepsy is important to avoid epilepsy surgery before spontaneous resolution occurs at a later age.

A few children whose initial presentation is typical for BCECTS evolve to "atypical benign partial epilepsy" or "pseudo-Lennox" syndrome (59–63). In addition to partial motor seizures, they develop frequent atonic, atypical absence and myoclonic seizures, often with nonconvulsive status epilepticus, as well as cognitive and behavioral disturbances. The sleep electroencephalograms show nearly continuous, bilaterally synchronous spike-and-wave activity. Although these children ultimately have remission of their epilepsy, many are left with varying degrees of mental handicap.

Children with BCECTS usually have an uneventful medical history, although 6% to 10% experience neonatal difficulties (including 3% with neonatal seizures) and 4% to 5% have preceding mild head injuries (32,40). Up to 16% have antecedent febrile seizures, which are likely to be focal or prolonged (40).

The incidence of migraine may be increased in children with BCECTS, although studies have lacked uniformity in migraine diagnosis (64,65). Giroud and colleagues (64) compared four groups of children and found migraine in 62% of 42 children with BCECTS, 34% of 28 children with absence epilepsy, 8% of 38 children with partial epilepsy,

and 6% of 30 children with head trauma. Bladin (65) followed up 30 cases of BCECTS, noting that 20 (67%) patients had recurrent headaches during the evolution of seizures and 24 (80%) developed typical migraine after remission of BCECTS. The pathophysiologic link between BCECTS and migraine is unknown.

Electroencephalographic Manifestations

The electroencephalogram shows high-amplitude diphasic spikes or sharp waves with a prominent aftercoming slow wave (Fig. 24.1). Spikes have a characteristic horizontal dipole, with maximal negativity in centrotemporal (inferior rolandic) and positivity in frontal regions (66,67). They frequently cluster and are markedly activated in drowsiness and nonrapid eye movement sleep (Fig. 24.2); approximately 30% of patients show spikes only during sleep (68). The focus is unilateral in 60% of cases and bilateral in 40%, and may be synchronous or asynchronous (32). The location is usually centrotemporal. Legarda and coworkers (69) described two electroclinical subgroups of BCECTS: a

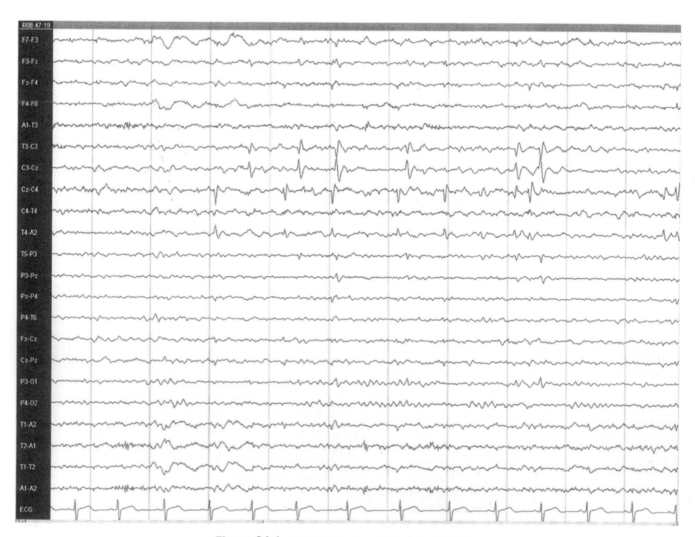

Figure 24.1 Typical rolandic spikes at C_3 and C_4-T_4.

high-central group, with maximum electronegativity at C_3/C_4 and seizures with frequent hand involvement, and a low-central group, with maximum electronegativity at C_5/C_6, ictal drooling, and oromotor involvement.

Atypical locations are frequent, and spikes may shift location on subsequent EEG recordings. On 24-hour electroencephalograms in children with typical BCECTS, Drury and Beydoun (70) found 21% of the patients to have a single focus outside the centrotemporal area. Follow-up recordings showed shifts in foci both toward and away from the centrotemporal area; no clinical differences were found between patients with foci in or outside the centrotemporal zone. Only half of their patients had a horizontal dipole. Wirrell and coworkers (51) also noted atypical spike location in 17% of their patients. Mild background slowing has been observed (47,51), and while generalized spike-and-wave discharge may be present, coexistent absence seizures are rare. With remission, spikes disappear first from the waking record and later from the sleep recording (32).

Few reports of recorded rolandic seizures (Fig. 24.3) exist, but two unique features are noted (32,71–75). Ictal

spike-and-wave discharges may show dipole reversal, with electropositivity in the centrotemporal region and negativity in the frontal area; postictal slowing is not seen.

BCECTS develops in only a small minority of children with typical rolandic spikes or sharp waves on their electroencephalograms. Rolandic discharge was found in 27 of 3726 (0.7%) waking EEG recordings of normal children without a history of seizures (37); if recordings had included sleep, the actual number might have been higher. The percentage of children with rolandic sharp waves who develop clinically apparent seizures is unclear. On the basis of reported incidences of BCECTS and of rolandic EEG discharge in normal children, the risk is probably less than 10%. Therefore, rolandic discharges should be considered most likely an incidental finding in children with other potentially nonepileptic presentations such as staring spells.

Neuropsychological Aspects

A variety of neuropsychological problems have been identified in children with active epilepsy and EEG discharge.

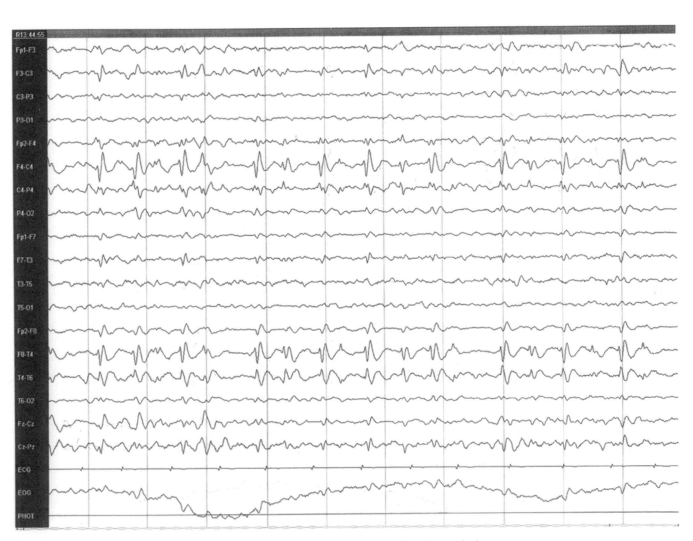

Figure 24.2 Marked activation of rolandic spikes with sleep.

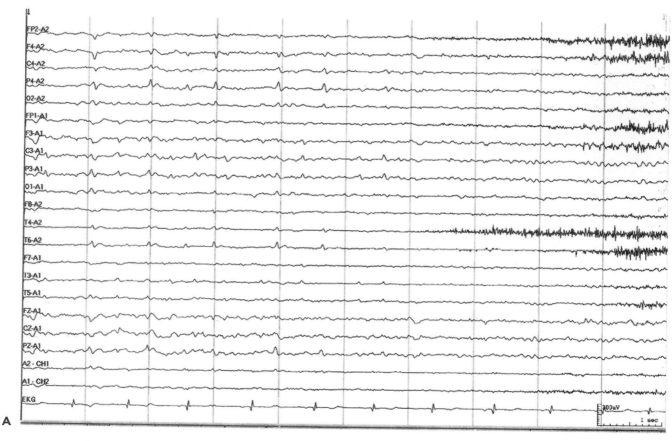

Figure 24.3 **A-C:** Recorded rolandic seizure. **A:** Start of seizure. **B:** Ten seconds later. **C:** End of seizure. (Courtesy of Dr. Mary Connolly, British Columbia Children's Hospital and University of British Columbia.)

Several early studies noted frequent behavior problems, hyperactivity, inattention, and learning disorders in children with BCECTS, but attributed these difficulties to the social stigma of epilepsy or to side effects of antiepileptic medication (33,49,76). More recent comparisons with normal controls yielded interesting results. On neuropsychological assessments, Croona and colleagues (77) found that children with BCECTS had more problems than matched controls with auditory-verbal memory, learning, and some executive functions, as evidenced by poorer performance on the trailmaking, verbal fluency, and Tower of London tests. No deficits were documented in immediate memory or visuospatial memory and learning. Teachers noted greater difficulty with reading comprehension in the BCECTS group, but not to the degree predicted by the neuropsychological data. In other comparisons with controls, Gunduz and coworkers (78) described more problems in go-no-go testing and language and minor motor deficits, and Baglietto and colleagues (79) documented poorer performance on tests of visuospatial short-term memory, attention, cognitive flexibility, picture naming, verbal fluency, and visuoperceptual and visuomotor coordination. Other uncontrolled studies (80,81) have reported high rates of learning disorders and difficulties with impulsiveness and temperament in children with BCECTS.

Neurocognitive deficits appear to correlate with the amount and location of interictal spike discharge. Binnie and Marston (82) tested 10 children to determine whether their interictal rolandic discharge caused any cognitive impairment. In a video-game test of short-term memory, rectangles would appear on the screen, disappear one by one, and reappear again in sequence. Subjects were asked to reproduce the sequence and were monitored by continuous EEG recording; multiple trials of stimulus presentation and response were performed. Trials with epileptiform discharge during the stimulus period were compared to trials without discharge; each subject acted as his own control. Four (57%) of the seven patients with BCECTS showed a significantly increased error rate during trials with discharges, and all of these children had behavioral or learning problems. The effect of epileptiform discharge in the three patients without seizures was much less convincing. Those with right-sided spikes did not have greater difficulty, even though the test emphasized visuospatial tasks.

Several studies suggested that the laterality of the EEG discharge predicts the nature of the neurocognitive deficit and that patients with bilateral discharges have the greatest difficulties. D'Alessandro and coworkers (83) subjected 44 children with BCECTS and normal controls to an extended battery of neuropsychological tests. All patients

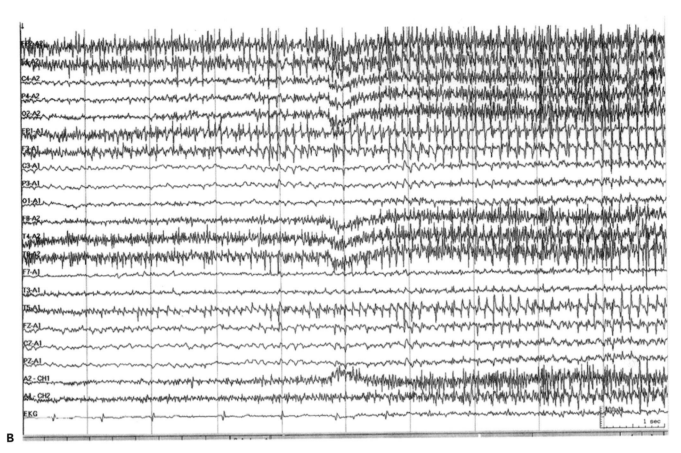

Figure 24.3 Continued.

were right-handed and seizure-free for a minimum of 6 months prior to testing without medication. Despite similar intelligence quotient (IQ) scores, the BCECTS group performed significantly less well on tests of attention and visuomotor skills. Children with BCECTS were then subdivided into three groups on the basis of side of epileptiform discharge on at least three electroencephalograms in the previous year. Eleven children had exclusively right-sided, 18 had exclusively left-sided, and 15 had bilateral centrotemporal discharges. Those with bilateral discharge scored the lowest overall; those with only right-sided discharge performed best. After at least 4 years without seizures and electroencephalogram abnormalities, a follow-up assessment of 13 patients showed resolution of the neuropsychological abnormalities, indicating that they are also "benign" and resolve around the time of puberty.

Piccirilli and colleagues (84) used a dual-task procedure to study language lateralization in 22 right-handed children with BCECTS and unilateral EEG discharge (14 left, 8 right centrotemporal discharges) and a group of normal right-handed controls. The theory is that when a subject is asked to perform two tasks simultaneously, the activities interfere with each other and reduce performance. If the two activities require the same cerebral hemisphere for processing, the interference will be even more marked. As the left hemisphere is dominant for speech and right-sided

movements in a right-handed person, a verbal task should decrease right finger tapping more than left finger tapping. As expected, all controls and patients with right centrotemporal discharge showed left lateralization of language. BCECTS patients with left centrotemporal discharge demonstrated bihemispheric representation of language, raising the possibility that focal epileptic activity may alter cerebral mechanisms that underlie cognitive functioning.

In another study of laterality, Piccirilli and coworkers (85) enrolled 43 right-handed children with BCECTS who were seizure-free for at least 6 months at testing and without daily antiepileptic treatment. Assignment into one of three groups was based on the side of epileptiform discharge on a minimum of three EEGs during the previous year. A figure cancellation test assessed attention and processing of visuomotor information, which is controlled by the right hemisphere in right-handed persons. Children with bilateral or right centrotemporal discharge scored significantly lower than either controls or those with left centrotemporal discharge, suggesting that focal epileptic discharge in the right hemisphere may interfere with visuomotor processing.

By contrast, Laub and coworkers (86) found no correlation between neuropsychological test results, EEG focus, and single-photon-emission computed tomography findings in nine children with BCECTS.

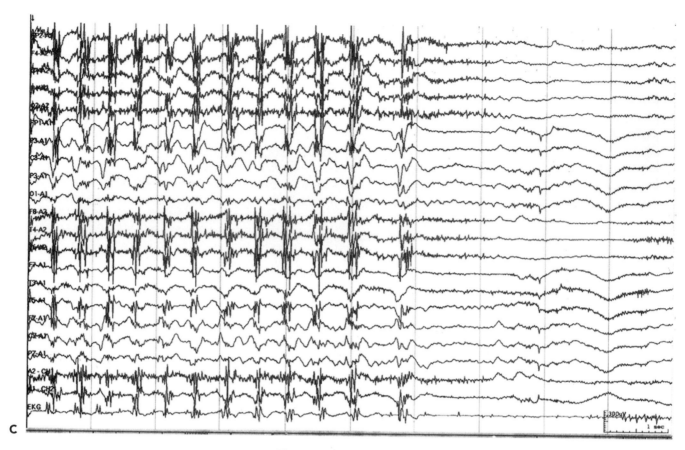

Figure 24.3   Continued.

Higher spike frequency on EEG appears to correlate with poorer neuropsychological outcome. Weglage and colleagues (87) compared 40 right-handed children with rolandic spikes (20 with and 20 without seizures) and 40 healthy controls. Those with rolandic spikes had significantly lower full-scale and performance IQ, as well as poorer outcomes in visual perception, fine motor performance, short-term memory, and behavioral status. Interestingly, in these children, no significant differences were seen in those with and without seizures. Neuropsychological deficits were not related to seizure frequency, lateralization of the rolandic focus, or time since diagnosis. Higher spike frequency was associated with the greatest deficits, however.

Three prospective studies (79,88,89) show that, like the seizures and epileptiform discharges, the cognitive difficulties that occur in many children with BCECTS also appear to resolve with time. Deonna and coworkers (88) observed 22 children with benign focal epilepsy; 4 had delayed language development, and 8 had transient weak scores in one isolated domain (verbal, visuospatial, memory). Cognitive difficulties improved or normalized over 1 to 3 years, with concomitant EEG improvement or normalization. Two of three children whose EEG discharge increased showed greater cognitive problems. In 22 children with BCECTS, Metz-Lutz and coworkers (89) noted that nonverbal cognitive difficulties were correlated with frequency of

seizures and spike-wave discharges and to lateralization of the epileptic focus in the right hemisphere. Frontal functions such as attention, response organization, and fine motor speed were impaired in the presence of active epilepsy, independent of the lateralization of the epileptic focus. After 18 months of follow-up, children who had remission of seizures and EEG abnormalities scored significantly higher on neuropsychological assessment than did those with ongoing epilepsy. Similarly, Baglietto and coworkers (79) reported significant improvements occurring over time in nine children with BCECTS and marked activation of epileptiform discharge during sleep.

In summary, neurocognitive deficits are seen in a significant proportion of children with BCECTS. Because they appear to correlate with the amount and side of interictal spike discharge, these discharges may cause "transient cognitive impairment." The neurocognitive deficits also resolve as seizures and epileptiform discharges abate with age.

Investigations

If the clinical history and electroencephalogram suggest BCECTS, and if the child is neurologically and developmentally intact, no further investigations are required. An MRI scan should be considered if atypical clinical or EEG features are present. EEG recordings of siblings may help to support the diagnosis of highly atypical cases. BCECTS has been reported in children with other central nervous system pathologic findings, yet the prognosis appears to be as favorable in brain-injured patients as in normal children (33,70,90).

One study (91) reporting MRI findings in 18 children with typical BCECTS found hippocampal asymmetries in 28% and white-matter abnormalities in 17% of the children. The latter finding may indicate maturational delay with defective myelination, but the hippocampal changes were unexplained. Gelisse and coworkers (92) reported neuroimaging abnormalities in 10 (14%) of 71 children with BCECTS, including ventricular enlargement, white-matter hyperintensities, hippocampal atrophy, cortical dysplasia, and agenesis of the corpus callosum and cavum septum pellucidum. They propose that these brain lesions may lower the epileptogenic threshold and transform a "genetic predisposition" into a clinical condition; however, the presence of these lesions did not alter the benign course of BCECTS.

Treatment

Children with BCECTS achieve remission regardless of antiepileptic drug therapy. Although treatment decreases generalized seizures (93), it may not reduce partial seizures, seizure recurrence, or duration of active epilepsy or improve social adjustment (94). We are unaware of any peer-reviewed reports of children with BCECTS dying of sudden unexpected death in epilepsy or sustaining brain injury from a seizure. A no-medication strategy is reasonable for the majority of children who have infrequent, nocturnal, partial seizures. If recurrent generalized or diurnal seizures occur, or if the seizures are sufficiently disturbing to the child or the family, treatment is generally started. Short intervals between the first three seizures and younger age at onset predict high seizure frequency.

Only sulthiame and gabapentin have been studied in randomized trials of children with BCECTS. On the basis of case series and a recent meta-analysis of 794 children (95), the usual antiepileptic drugs prescribed for partial seizures—phenytoin, phenobarbital, valproate, carbamazepine, clobazam, and clonazepam—have equivalent efficacy, and 50% to 65% of patients will have no further seizures once medication is started (26,31,33).

An American study (96) of 220 children showed that gabapentin was probably more effective than placebo. The study only considered time to first recurrence over 36 weeks, however, and the results did not reach statistical significance ($P = .06$).

Sulthiame, available outside the United States, is effective and appears additionally to significantly improve the electroencephalogram findings as well as decrease clinical seizures (97–101). In a randomized, double-blind trial, Rating and coworkers (101) compared sulthiame with placebo in 66 children with BCECTS. Twenty-five (81%) of 31 patients taking sulthiame completed 6 months of therapy with no further seizures or adverse events, compared with only 10 (29%) of 35 children taking placebo ($P < .00002$). Of 25 patients remaining on sulthiame at 6 months, 10 (40%) had a normal electroencephalogram, compared with only 1 (10%) of 10 in the placebo group.

Two other retrospective reports suggest the efficacy of sulthiame. Doose and coworkers (97) used low doses (4 to 6 mg/kg per day) to treat 56 children with benign partial epilepsy and reported that 96% became seizure-free, although 11% later had relapses. EEG recordings became initially normal in 88%, but sharp waves later reappeared in 37%. In a nonrandomized study, Gross-Selbeck (98) compared 35 children with BCECTS who received first-line therapy with either sulthiame (n=17) or carbamazepine, phenytoin, or primidone (n=18). Eighty-eight percent of the sulthiame group and only 56% of the group receiving other antiepileptic medications achieved complete remission ($P < .04$). The electroencephalogram became normal in 44% of the sulthiame group and improved in another 44%; the tracing remained unchanged in all children receiving the other medications.

The ideal treatment for BCECTS should relieve both seizures and interictal discharges, especially in patients with neuropsychological deficits. The literature is largely silent as regards the child with cognitive problems and frequent interictal spikes. Sulthiame does decrease interictal discharge, and while it is tempting to think that it may improve neuropsychological dysfunction, no study has yet examined this possibility.

Rarely, antiepileptic drugs may aggravate BCECTS, markedly increasing EEG discharge, often with continuous spike and wave during slow sleep, and causing neuropsychological deterioration. This deterioration has been reported with carbamazepine (102–104), phenobarbital (102), and lamotrigine (105).

Seizures may initially appear refractory in a small number of children (106). Deonna and coworkers (52) reported that one-third of 38 children with BCECTS had persistent seizures despite treatment, and 24% had severe seizures. Beaussart (31) noted that 14% of 221 children had occurrence of seizures that lasted longer than 1 year despite medication or that recurred after 1 to many years.

Prognosis

The long-term prognosis of BCECTS is excellent, even in those with initially frequent, troublesome seizures, and nearly all patients achieve remission by mid-adolescence (31,49,106,107). In a meta-analysis (95), Bouma and coworkers found that 50% of patients were in remission at age 6 years, 92% at age 12 years, and 99.8% at age 18 years. Kurtzke survival analysis was used to calculate a life table that showed the proportion of seizure-free patients as a function of age (Fig. 24.4). Remission occurs sooner in children older at onset and in those with sporadic seizures or seizure clusters (49).

Proportion remission

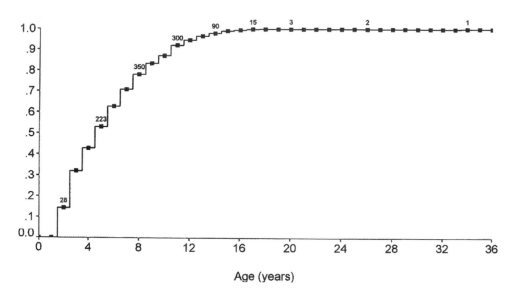

Figure 24.4 Remission of benign childhood epilepsy with centrotemporal spikes (BCECTS) by age. Numbers in the figure represent the number of patients in the analysis. (From Bouma PAD, Bovenkerk AC, Westendorp RGJ, et al. The course of benign partial epilepsy of childhood with centrotemporal spikes: a meta-analysis. *Neurology* 1997;48:430–437, with permission.)

Although learning and behavior problems may be seen in the acute phase, long-term psychosocial outcome is excellent. Following up 79 patients for a mean of 15.8 years, Loiseau and associates (108) found no increase in psychiatric problems and generally normal adult personalities. With respect to occupational status, patients had a better outcome than normal controls. A follow-up of 79 patients at a mean age of 16 years also revealed favorable social and educational outcome (93).

BENIGN OCCIPITAL EPILEPSY OF CHILDHOOD

Gibbs and Gibbs were the first to recognize that some children with occipital epilepsy had a benign course (109). BOE is now divided into two syndromes: the more common, early onset (Panayiotopoulos) type and the later-onset (Gastaut) type.

Epidemiology

Early onset BOE, the second most common type of IPE, occurs much less frequently than BCECTS (110,111). The peak age of onset is 5 years (range, 2 to 8 years) with a female preponderance.

Late-onset BOE begins in mid- to late childhood, with a peak age of 8 years (range, 3 to 16 years); both sexes are equally affected (111).

Genetics

Reporting a large kindred with BOE, Kuzniecky and Rosenblatt (112) suggested that, as in BCECTS, the EEG abnormality was inherited in an autosomal dominant pat-

tern, with age-dependent expression and variable penetrance of the disorder. Other investigators (113,114) found that most affected children lack a family history of similar disorders.

Clinical

Early Onset Benign Occipital Epilepsy

Tonic eye deviation, nausea, and vomiting are nearly always involved (110,111), although other autonomic manifestations may be seen as the seizure evolves (115). Ictal syncope, with loss of tone and unresponsiveness, may precede convulsions or occur without them. Rarely, autonomic symptoms may be extreme, with cardiopulmonary arrest and fixed, dilated pupils (115). According to Panayiotopoulos, ictal visual symptoms occur in only 10% of patients and consist of elementary or complex visual hallucinations, visual illusions, blindness, or blurring. Unlike in the late-onset form, the visual symptoms are never the predominant ictal manifestation, always accompany more typical semiology such as vomiting and eye deviation, and usually follow other seizure manifestations (115). Other authors (116), however, have noted ictal visual phenomena more often. Scarcity of complex ictal visual symptoms may also be due to age-related difficulty in describing symptoms.

Consciousness may be impaired, and seizures can evolve to hemiconvulsions or become secondarily generalized. One-third of children have only single events (113,115,117,118). In one-third to one-half of patients, however, attacks may last longer than 30 minutes (115,118). Whereas all subjects have seizures during sleep, one-third may also have awake events (113,118). A history of febrile seizures is found in approximately 17% of children (115). Rarely, early onset BOE may evolve atypically,

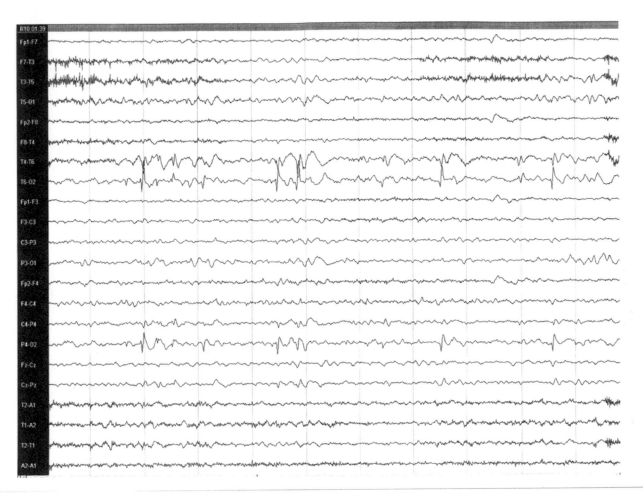

Figure 24.5 Posterior temporal-occipital spikes in a 4-year-old girl who presented with a 65-minute seizure consisting of focal eye deviation and retching.

with appearance of many seizure types, including absences and atonic seizures, and intellectual deterioration (119).

Late-Onset Benign Occipital Epilepsy

Late-onset syndrome manifests as diurnal, brief, visual seizures consisting of elementary visual hallucinations such as multicolored, spherical phenomena (111,120). Other occipital symptoms, such as sensory illusions of ocular movements or pain, tonic eye deviation, or eyelid closures, may coexist. Ictal blindness is usually brief. Consciousness is typically intact, but may be impaired or lost if the seizure progresses or becomes secondarily generalized. Seizures often occur daily. Postictal headache, indistinguishable from migraine, is seen in more than 50% of cases.

Rarely, late-onset BOE may have a stormy onset. Verrotti and coworkers (121) described six children presenting with loss of consciousness lasting 6 to 14 hours that was preceded by visual symptoms. Only two of these patients had further seizures, and all did well at follow-up.

The diagnosis of late-onset BOE should be made cautiously, as the semiology may also be seen with symptomatic occipital epilepsy. In Gastaut's series, prognosis was not always benign, and many patients had ongoing seizures (27).

Electroencephalography Manifestations

The EEG changes are not always stereotypical and may not confirm the diagnosis. Most often, in both early and late-onset forms of BOE, high-amplitude, often bilateral, runs of repetitive occipital spikes and sharp waves are seen (Fig. 24.5). In approximately 25% to 33% of cases of early onset BOE, the electroencephalogram may be normal, but spikes can appear several months later (110,111,113,115,122,123). Extraoccipital spikes are common in Panayiotopoulos syndrome, being the sole EEG abnormality in 21% of cases and occurring with occipital spikes in 40% of cases (115). On follow-up, the EEG foci frequently shift to frontopolar and centroparietotemporal regions and may become generalized (124). Extraoccipital spikes are much less common in Gastaut-type BOE (27). Epileptiform discharge is morphologically similar to that in BCECTS and is also activated with sleep. The spikes are said to show "fixation-off sensitivity," that is, they attenuate with eye opening and are induced by elimination of central vision such as eye closure, darkness, or vision through +10 spherical lenses (Fig. 25.6) (111). Suppression of epileptiform discharges with eye opening is not specific for BOE, however, and may be

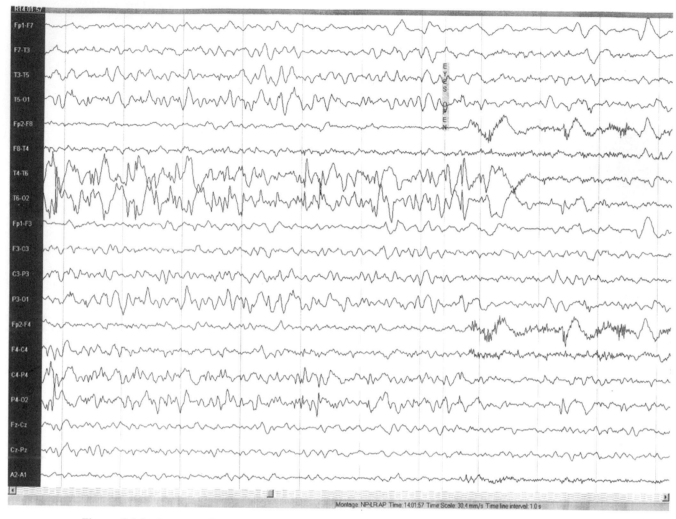

Figure 24.6   Prominent fixation-off sensitivity in the same 4-year-old girl as in Figure 24.5.

seen in symptomatic epilepsies with poorer prognoses (125,126). A superficial rather than a deep dipole source location of the occipital spikes suggests a benign disorder rather than symptomatic occipital epilepsy (127).

The ictal electroencephalogram in early onset BOE shows rhythmic theta or delta activity with intermixed spikes that usually starts posteriorly, although anterior onset has been reported (28,128–130). In late-onset BOE, the discharge is more localized, with fast rhythms appearing in the occipital lobe at the onset of visual symptoms (128).

Neuropsychology

One study (131) examined neuropsychological functioning in 21 children with BOE and in normal controls, matched for age, sex, and socioeconomic status. Compared to controls, the patients had lower scores in attention, memory, and intellectual functioning, and performed significantly more poorly on all verbal and visual tests combined. This study, however, recruited the entire control group from a single private school that may have represented a higher-than-usual educational standard. In addition, neuroimaging was not performed to rule out symptomatic occipital epilepsies. No comment was made about whether the observed differences resolved with remission of epilepsy. Some studies suggest that in rare cases BOE may evolve to continuous spike wave in slow-wave sleep (132,133).

Investigations

Imaging is probably not required in a neurologically and developmentally normal child with a typical clinical history of early onset BOE and an electroencephalogram showing occipital paroxysms with fixation-off sensitivity. Nevertheless, MRI is usually performed to rule out a symptomatic etiology, particularly if the typical electroencephalogram is not present or the clinical picture is atypical. Because lesional occipital lobe epilepsy may mimic the semiologic and EEG features of Gastaut-type BOE, MRI should always be obtained.

Treatment

Most children with early onset BOE have infrequent seizures and do not need antiepileptic drug treatment. Intermittent use of benzodiazepines could be considered for the child with rare but prolonged events. No particular antiepileptic drug has been shown to be superior (113), although carbamazepine is most frequently prescribed.

In contrast, most cases of late-onset BOE require treatment, as seizures are more frequent. Although Panayiotopoulos reported a favorable response to carbamazepine (27,134), only 60% of 63 patients reported by Gastaut achieved complete seizure control (135).

Prognosis

In Panayiotopoulos syndrome, remission of active epilepsy occurs 1 to 2 years from onset, although up to 15% of patients have concurrent symptoms of rolandic epilepsy or later develop BCECTS (118). As in BCECTS, even those with many seizures usually achieve long-term remission.

The prognosis is less clear in Gastaut syndrome, although Gastaut reported that 5% of his 63 cases had recurrent seizures into adulthood (135).

PROPOSED BENIGN PARTIAL EPILEPSY SYNDROMES NOT YET RECOGNIZED BY THE ILAE

Five syndromes have been proposed as possible subtypes of idiopathic and benign focal epilepsy, but not all may be confirmed as diagnostically discrete. The diagnosis is usually made after initiation of treatment and observation of the clinical course.

Benign Partial Epilepsy in Infancy

Watanabe proposed this disorder in 1987, and described two forms: one with partial complex seizures alone (5) and another with partial complex and secondarily generalized seizures (6).

BPEI represents approximately 6.6% to 29% of all epilepsies in the first 2 years of life and may be somewhat more common in Japan. Okumura and colleagues (136) noted that 22 (29%) of 75 infants younger than 2 years of age presenting with epilepsy met the criteria for BPEI, whereas Nelson and coworkers (137) made this diagnosis in only 22 (6.6%) of 331 in their population. Both reports noted that the form with secondarily generalized seizures was slightly more common, accounting for 64% to 73% of all BPEI cases. Peak age at onset is 4 to 6 months, with a range of 3 to 10 months.

Seizures occur in 50% of developmentally normal infants whose family histories reveal benign forms of infantile seizures in 50% of cases (5,6). Motion arrest, decreased responsiveness, staring, simple automatisms,

and mild convulsive movements are usual, with possible secondary generalization. Seizures frequently cluster. Neuroimaging is normal, and seizures are easily controlled with antiepileptic drugs. Remission occurs in 91% within 4 months (137) and in all children by age 2 years.

To determine how well BPEI was recognized, Okumura and coworkers followed up 25 children who were believed to have the syndrome (138). At 5 years, 19 had achieved remission, no longer received antiepileptic drugs, and were developmentally normal. In retrospect, six were thought to not have BPEI, as they had recurrent seizures after 2 years or showed developmental delay. Clearly, this diagnosis is not always easy to make prospectively, with experts being incorrect nearly 25% of the time.

The interictal electroencephalogram is said to be normal, but some infants show low-voltage rolandic and vertex spikes in sleep (139). Ictal recordings demonstrate spikes that are maximal in the temporal regions, in infants with partial complex seizures alone, or in the central, parietal, or occipital regions, in those with secondarily generalized seizures.

Benign Partial Epilepsy of Adolescence

Difficult to recognize with any certainty at presentation, BPEA was initially described by Loiseau and Orgogozo in 1978 (15). Definitive diagnosis usually requires neuroimaging and long-term follow-up to confirm the benign course.

Loiseau's 108 cases accounted for 25% of all partial seizures with onset in the teenage years (16). King and colleagues (140) noted that 8 (22%) of 37 adolescents with new-onset partial seizures met criteria for BPEA. Peak age at onset is 13 to 14 years and boys are more commonly affected (16,141).

Most seizures come on diurnally in neurologically normal adolescents. Family history of epilepsy is exceptional (only 3% of Loiseau's cohort) (16). Either motor or sensory manifestations may be present, and a jacksonian-type march is frequently described. Auditory, olfactory, or gustatory symptoms are never reported. Seizures may be partial simple, partial complex, or secondarily generalized. In Loiseau's series, approximately 80% had an isolated seizure only, while most of the remainder had a cluster of two to five attacks within 36 hours with no recurrences (16). Of King's eight patients, 38% had ongoing, infrequent, simple partial seizures after 2 years of follow-up (140).

Imaging is normal, and the interictal electroencephalogram is either normal or may show bilateral posterior slowing; diffuse slow waves may be seen if electroencephalography is done within the first few days after a seizure. Although no interictal epileptiform discharges were noted in the Loiseau cohort (15), 63% of the King group showed epileptiform abnormalities, even though these lacked distinctive morphology or distribution (140).

Benign Frontal Epilepsy

In 1983, Beaumanoir and Nahory (14) described 11 cases of frontal lobe epilepsy with normal neurologic status and benign course that involved head deviation, sometimes with trunk turning. All the patients had a frontal spike focus on electroencephalography and resolution of both the seizures and the EEG focus within 5 years of follow-up. Four, however, had rare generalized or partial seizures that reappeared years after therapy ended and the EEG focus resolved. Vigevano and Fusco (142) described 10 children with tonic partial seizures in sleep, all of whom had a benign course, many with a positive family history. These cases may represent the early presentation of autosomal dominant frontal lobe epilepsy (143).

Benign Partial Epilepsy with Extreme Somatosensory Evoked Potentials

In 1981, De Marco and Tassinari (12) described 16 children with BPE-ESEP. De Marco (11) had previously noted that approximately 0.01% (155 of 15,000) of children undergoing routine EEG studies showed high-voltage spikes in parietal and parasagittal regions (extreme somatosensory evoked potentials [SSEPs]) evoked by tapping of their feet (11). This pattern was seen at a peak age of 4 to 6 years, occurred in neurologically normal children without any lesions on neuroimaging, and was much more common in males. An increased risk of febrile seizures was noted.

Of the 155 patients in De Marco's group, 46 (30%) either had (n=30) or went on to develop (n=16) epilepsy (13). In another report (144), 91 (24%) of 385 children with this pattern had afebrile seizures. Diurnal partial motor seizures with head and body version were most frequent; however, other IPEs including BCECTS and BOE have also been reported with this EEG picture. Seizure frequency is usually low, but more frequent events are possible, and focal motor status epilepticus has also been reported. In all cases, seizures resolved by age 9 years, with slower resolution of EEG changes and extreme SSEPs.

Benign Partial Epilepsy with Affective Symptoms

BPEAS, or benign psychomotor epilepsy, was proposed as a distinct entity in 1980 (7–9), and 26 cases have been documented (10). Nineteen percent of patients had febrile seizures, and 38% had a family history of epilepsy. Onset is between 2 and 9 years of age, and seizures can occur in either wakefulness or sleep. The hallmark symptom is sudden fear, often with screaming, autonomic disturbance (pallor, sweating, abdominal pain), automatisms such as chewing or swallowing, and altered awareness. Mostly short-lived, seizures may be followed by brief postictal confusion and fatigue, but not unilateral deficits. Secondary generalization does not occur. Although seizures may occur up to several times per day shortly after onset, they respond promptly to antiepileptic drugs.

The EEG background is normal, but rolandic-like spikes are seen in frontotemporal and parietotemporal regions both in wakefulness and sleep. Remission occurs within 1 to 2 years, and long-term intellectual and social outcome is excellent.

SUMMARY

The IPEs of childhood account for a significant proportion of seizure disorders in the pediatric group. In its classic form, BCECTS is easily recognizable, occurring in neurologically normal children and having a distinct semiology and EEG pattern. Early onset BOE, with characteristic ictal semiology and clear occipital discharge on the electroencephalogram, also lends itself to a confident diagnosis. Such is not the case for the other IPEs or for BCECTS or early onset BOE with atypical clinical or EEG features. These diagnoses may be made definitively only in retrospect.

Minor cognitive changes during the active period of epilepsy occur in some children with IPE, but also appear to remit with time. In these cases, treatment to ameliorate the EEG changes as well as the clinical seizures may be beneficial. Many children with IPEs, however, will not require antiepileptic drugs, as most have infrequent seizures. Recognition of these benign epilepsy syndromes is important for appropriate counseling of the child and family.

REFERENCES

1. Loiseau J, Loiseau P, Guyot M, et al. Survey of seizure disorders in the French Southwest, I: incidence of epileptic syndromes. *Epilepsia* 1990;31:391–396.
2. Dalla Bernardina B, Sgrò V, Fontana E, et al. Idiopathic partial epilepsies in children. In: Roger J, Dravet C, Bureau M, et al., eds. *Epileptic syndromes in infancy, childhood and adolescence*, 2nd ed. London: John Libbey, 1992:173–188.
3. Holmes G. Benign focal epilepsies of childhood. *Epilepsia* 1993(Suppl 3):S49–S61.
4. Commission on Classification and Terminology of the International League Against Epilepsy. Proposal for revised classification of epilepsies and epileptic syndromes. *Epilepsia* 1989;30:389–399.
5. Watanabe K, Yamamoto N, Negoro T, et al. Benign complex partial epilepsies in infancy. *Pediatr Neurol* 1987;3:208–211.
6. Watanabe K, Negoro T, Aso K. Benign partial epilepsy with secondarily generalized seizures in infancy. *Epilepsia* 1993;34:635–638.
7. Dalla Bernardina B, Bureau M, Dravet C, et al. Affective symptoms during attacks of epilepsy in children [French]. *Rev Electroencephalogr Neurophysio Clin* 1980;10:8–18.
8. Plouin P, Lerique A, Dulac O. Etude électroclinique et évolution dans 7 observations de crises partielles complexes dominées par un comportement de terreur chez l'enfant. *Boll Lega Ital Epil* 1980;29/30:139–143.
9. Dulac O, Arthuis M. Epilepsie psychomotrice bénigne de l'enfant. In: Flammanon Medecine Science eds. *Journées Parisiennes de pédiatrie*. Paris: Flammarion, 1980: 211–220.

10. Dalla Bernardina B, Colamaria V, Chiamenti C, et al. Benign partial epilepsy with affective symptoms (benign psychomotor epilepsy). In: Roger J, Dravet C, Bureau M, et al., eds. *Epileptic syndromes in infancy, childhood and adolescence*, 2nd ed. London: John Libbey, 1992:219–223.

11. De Marco P. Possibilities of a temporal relationship between the morphology and frequency of a parietal somatosensory evoked spike and the occurrence of epileptic manifestations. *Clin Electroencephalogr* 1980;11:132–135.

12. De Marco P, Tassinari CA. Extreme somatosensory evoked potentials (ESEP): an EEG sign forecasting the possible occurrence of seizures in children. *Epilepsia* 1981;22:569–585.

13. Tassinari CA, De Marco P. Benign partial epilepsy with extreme somatosensory evoked potentials. In: Roger J, Dravet C, Bureau M, et al., eds. *Epileptic syndromes in infancy, childhood and adolescence*, 2nd ed. London: John Libbey, 1992:225–229.

14. Beaumanoir A, Nahory A. Benign partial epilepsies: 11 cases of frontal partial epilepsy with favorable prognosis [French]. *Rev Electroencephalogr Neurophysiol Clin* 1983;13:207–211.

15. Loiseau P, Orgogozo JM. An unrecognized syndrome of benign focal epileptic seizures in teenagers. *Lancet* 1978;2:1070–1071.

16. Loiseau P, Louiset P. Benign partial seizures of adolescence. In: Roger J, Dravet C, Bureau M, et al., eds. *Epileptic syndromes in infancy, childhood and adolescence*, 2nd ed. London: John Libbey, 1992: 343–345.

17. van Huffelen AC. A tribute to Martinus Rulandus: a 16th-century description of benign focal epilepsy of childhood. *Arch Neurol* 1989;46:445–447.

18. Gastaut Y. Un element deroutant de la sémeiologie electroencephalographique: les pointes prerolandiques sans signification focale. *Rev Neurol (Paris)* 1952;87:488–490.

19. Gibbs EL, Gillen HW, Gibbs PA. Disappearance and migration of epileptic foci in children. *Am J Dis Child* 1954;88:596–603.

20. Nayrac P, Beaussart M. Pre-rolandic spike-waves: a very peculiar EEG reading; electroclinical study of 21 cases [French]. *Rev Neurol (Paris)* 1958;99:201–206.

21. Lombroso CT. Sylvian seizures and midtemporal spike foci in children. *Arch Neurol* 1967;17:52–59.

22. Gibbs FA, Gibbs EL. Good prognosis of midtemporal epilepsy. *Epilepsia* 1960;1:448–453.

23. Cavazzuti GB. Epidemiology of different types of epilepsy in school age children of Modena, Italy. *Epilepsia* 1980;21:57–62.

24. Astradsson A, Olafsson E, Ludvigsson P, et al. Rolandic epilepsy: an incidence study in Iceland. *Epilepsia* 1998;39:884–886.

25. Heijbel J, Blom S, Bergfors PG. Benign epilepsy of children with centrotemporal EEG foci: a study of incidence rate in outpatient care. *Epilepsia* 1975;16:657–664.

26. Kriz M, Gadzik M. Epilepsy with centrotemporal (rolandic) spikes. A peculiar seizure disorder of childhood. *Neurol Neurochir Pol* 1978;12:413–419.

27. Panayiotopoulos CP. Benign childhood partial seizures and related epileptic syndromes. London: John Libbey, 1999.

28. Oguni H, Hayashi K, Imai K, et al. Study on the early-onset variant of benign childhood epilepsy with occipital paroxysms, otherwise described as early-onset benign occipital seizure susceptibility syndrome. *Epilepsia* 1999;40:1020–1030.

29. Carabello R, Cersósimo R, Fejerman N. Idiopathic partial epilepsies with rolandic and occipital spikes appearing in the same children. *J Epilepsy* 1998;11:261–264.

30. Guerrini R, Belmonte A, Veggiotti P, et al. Delayed appearance of interictal EEG abnormalities in early onset childhood epilepsy with occipital paroxysms. *Brain Dev* 1997;19:343–346.

31. Beaussart M. Benign epilepsy of children with rolandic (centrotemporal) paroxysmal foci: a clinical entity. Study of 221 cases. *Epilepsia* 1972;13:795–811.

32. Lerman P. Benign partial epilepsy with centrotemporal spikes. In: Roger J, Bureau M, Dravet C, et al., eds. *Epileptic syndromes in infancy, childhood and adolescence*. London: John Libbey, 1992: 189–200.

33. Lerman P, Kivity S. Benign focal epilepsy of childhood: a follow-up study of 100 recovered patients. *Arch Neurol* 1975;32:261–264.

34. Bray PF, Wiser WC. Evidence for a genetic etiology of temporal-central abnormalities in focal epilepsy. *N Engl J Med* 1964;271: 926–933.

35. Heijbel J, Blom S, Rasmuson M. Benign epilepsy of children with centrotemporal EEG foci: a genetic study. *Epilepsia* 1975;16: 285–293.

36. Degen R, Degen HE. Contribution to the genetics of rolandic epilepsy: waking and sleep EEGs in siblings. *Epilepsy Res Suppl* 1992;6:49–52.

37. Cavazzuti GB, Cappella L, Nalin A. Longitudinal study of epileptiform EEG patterns in normal children. *Epilepsia* 1980;21: 43–55.

38. Doose H, Baier WK. A genetically determined basic mechanism in benign partial epilepsies and related non-convulsive conditions. *Epilepsy Res Suppl* 1991;4:113–117.

39. Doose H. Symptomatology in children with focal sharp waves of genetic origin. *Eur J Pediatr* 1989;149:210–215.

40. Doose H, Brigger-Heuer B, Neubauer B. Children with focal sharp waves: clinical and genetic aspects. *Epilepsia* 1997;38: 788–796.

41. Neubauer BA, Fiedler B, Himmelein B, et al. Centrotemporal spikes in families with rolandic epilepsy: linkage to chromosome 15q14. *Neurology* 1998;51:1608–1612.

42. Scheffer IE, Jones L, Pozzebon M, et al. Autosomal dominant rolandic epilepsy and speech dyspraxia: a new syndrome with anticipation. *Ann Neurol* 1995;38:633–642.

43. Doose H, Baier WK. Benign partial epilepsy and related conditions: multifactorial pathogenesis with hereditary impairment of brain maturation. *Eur J Pediatr* 1989;149:152–158.

44. Doose H, Neubauer B, Carlsson G. Children with benign focal sharp waves in the EEG—developmental disorders and epilepsy. *Neuropediatrics* 1996;27:227–241.

45. Doose H, Neubauer BA, Peterson B. The concept of hereditary impairment of brain maturation. *Epileptic Disord* 2000;2 (Suppl 1):S45–S46.

46. Prince DA. Benign focal epilepsies of childhood: genetically determined pathophysiology—epilepsy that comes and goes. *Epilepsia* 2000;41:1085–1087.

47. Holmes GL. Rolandic epilepsy: clinical and electroencephalographic features. *Epilepsy Res Suppl* 1992;6:29–43.

48. Loiseau P, Beaussart M. The seizures of benign childhood epilepsy with rolandic paroxysmal discharges. *Epilepsia* 1973; 14:381–389.

49. Loiseau P, Duche B, Cordova S, et al. Prognosis of benign childhood epilepsy with centrotemporal spikes: a follow-up study of 168 patients. *Epilepsia* 1988;29:229–235.

50. Kramer U, Zelnick N, Lerman-Sagie T, et al. Benign childhood epilepsy with centrotemporal spikes: clinical characteristics and identification of patients at risk for multiple seizures. *J Child Neurol* 2002;17:17–19.

51. Wirrell EC, Camfield PR, Gordon KE, et al. Benign rolandic epilepsy: atypical features are very common. *J Child Neurol* 1995;10:455–458.

52. Deonna T, Ziegler AL, Despland PA, et al. Partial epilepsy in neurologically normal children: clinical syndromes and prognosis. *Epilepsia* 1986;27:241–247.

53. Fejerman N, Di Blasi AM. Status epilepticus of benign partial epilepsies in children: report of two cases. *Epilepsia* 1987;28: 351–355.

54. Colamaria V, Sgro V, Caraballo R, et al. Status epilepticus in benign rolandic epilepsy manifesting as anterior operculum syndrome. *Epilepsia* 1991;32:329–334.

55. Boulloche J, Le Luyer B, Husson A, et al. Dysphagie et troubles du langage: manifestations d'un état de mal épileptique à pointes temporales. In: *Proceedings IVeme Congres de la Société Européenne de Neurologie Pédiatrique*. Barcelona, November 1989:131.

56. Deonna TW, Roulet E, Fontan D, et al. Speech and oromotor deficits of epileptic origin in benign partial epilepsy of childhood with rolandic spikes (BPERS): relationship to the acquired aphasia-epilepsy syndrome. *Neuropediatrics* 1993;24:83–87.

57. Roulet E, Deonna T, Despland PA. Prolonged intermittent drooling and oromotor dyspraxia in benign childhood epilepsy with centrotemporal spikes. *Epilepsia* 1989;30:564–568.

58. de Saint-Martin A, Petiau C, Massa R, et al. Idiopathic rolandic epilepsy with "interictal" facial myoclonia and oromotor deficit: a longitudinal EEG and PET study. *Epilepsia* 1999;40:614–620.

59. Aicardi J, Chevrie JJ. Atypical benign partial epilepsy of childhood. *Dev Med Child Neurol* 1982;24:281–292.

60. Fejerman N, Caraballo R, Tenembaum SN. Atypical evolutions of benign partial epilepsy of infancy with centro-temporal spikes [Spanish]. *Rev Neurol* 2000;31:389–396.

61. Hahn A, Pistohl J, Neubauer BA, et al. Atypical "benign" partial epilepsy or pseudo-Lennox syndrome. Part 1: symptomatology and long-term prognosis. *Neuropediatrics* 2001;32:1–8.

62. Dalla Bernardina B, Tassinari CA, et al. Benign focal epilepsy and "electrical status epilepticus" during sleep. *Rev Electroencephalogr Neurophysiol Clin* 1978;8:350–353.

63. Deonna T, Ziegler AL, Despland PA. Combined myoclonic-astatic and "benign" focal epilepsy of childhood ("atypical benign partial epilepsy of childhood"). A separate syndrome? *Neuropediatrics* 1986;17:144–151.

64. Giroud M, Couillault G, Arnould S, et al. Centro-temporal epilepsy and migraine. A controlled study. Evidence for a non-fortuitous association. *Pediatrie* 1989;44:659–664.

65. Bladin PF. The association of benign rolandic epilepsy with migraine. In: Andermann F, Lugaresi E, eds. *Migraine and epilepsy.* Boston: Butterworths, 1987:145–152.

66. Gregory DL, Wong PK. Topographic analysis of the centrotemporal discharges in benign rolandic epilepsy of childhood. *Epilepsia* 1984;25:705–711.

67. Gregory DL, Wong PK. Clinical relevance of a dipole field in rolandic spikes. *Epilepsia* 1992;33:36–44.

68. Blom S, Heijbel J. Benign epilepsy of children with centro-temporal EEG foci. Discharge rate during sleep. *Epilepsia* 1975;16:133–140.

69. Legarda S, Jayakar P, Duchowny M, et al. Benign rolandic epilepsy: high central and low central subgroups. *Epilepsia* 1994;35:1125–1129.

70. Drury I, Beydoun A. Benign partial epilepsy of childhood with monomorphic sharp waves in centrotemporal and other locations. *Epilepsia* 1991;32:662–667.

71. Dalla Bernardina BD, Tassinari CA. EEG of a nocturnal seizure in a patient with "benign epilepsy of childhood with rolandic spikes." *Epilepsia* 1975;16:497–501.

72. Wirrell EC. Benign epilepsy of childhood with centrotemporal spikes. *Epilepsia* 1998;39(Suppl 4):S32–S41.

73. Gutierrez AR, Brick JF, Bodensteiner J. Dipole reversal: an ictal feature of benign partial epilepsy with centrotemporal spikes. *Epilepsia* 1990;31:544–548.

74. Silva DF, Lima MM, Anghinah R, et al. Dipole reversal: an ictal feature in a patient with benign partial epilepsy of childhood with centro-temporal spike. *Arq Neuropsiquiatr* 1995;53:270–273.

75. Clemens B. Ictal electroencephalography in a case of benign centrotemporal epilepsy. *J Child Neurol* 2002;17:297–300.

76. Heijbel J, Bohman M. Benign epilepsy of children with centrotemporal EEG foci: intelligence, behavior and school adjustment. *Epilepsia* 1975;16:679–687.

77. Croona C, Kihlgren M, Lundberg S, et al. Neuropsychological findings in children with benign childhood epilepsy with centrotemporal spikes. *Dev Med Child Neurol* 1999;41:813–818.

78. Gunduz E, Demirbilek V, Korkmaz B. Benign rolandic epilepsy: neuropsychological findings. *Seizure* 1999;8:246–249.

79. Baglietto MG, Battaglia FM, Nobili L, et al. Neuropsychological disorders related to interictal epileptic discharges during sleep in benign epilepsy of childhood with centrotemporal or rolandic spikes. *Dev Med Child Neurol* 2001;43:407–412.

80. Staden U, Isaacs E, Boyd SG, et al. Language dysfunction in children with rolandic epilepsy. *Neuropediatrics* 1998;29:242–248.

81. Yung AW, Park YD, Cohen MJ, et al. Cognitive and behavioral problems in children with centrotemporal spikes. *Pediatr Neurol* 2000;23:391–395.

82. Binnie CD, Marston D. Cognitive correlates of interictal discharges. *Epilepsia* 1992;33(Suppl 6):S11–S17.

83. D'Alessandro P, Piccirilli M, Tiacci C, et al. Neuropsychological features of benign partial epilepsy in children. *Ital J Neurol Sci* 1990;11:265–269.

84. Piccirilli M, D'Alessandro P, Tiacci C, et al. Language lateralization in children with benign partial epilepsy. *Epilepsia* 1988;29:19–25.

85. Piccirilli M, D'Alessandro P, Sciarma T, et al. Attention problems in epilepsy: possible significance of the epileptogenic focus. *Epilepsia* 1994;35:1091–1096.

86. Laub MC, Funke R, Kirsch CM, et al. BECTS: comparison of cerebral blood flow imaging, neuropsychological testing and long-term EEG findings. *Epilepsy Res Suppl* 1992;6:95–98.

87. Weglage J, Demsky A, Pietsch M, et al. Neuropsychological, intellectual, and behavioral findings in patients with centrotemporal spikes with and without seizures. *Dev Med Child Neurol* 1997;39:646–651.

88. Deonna T, Zesiger P, Davidoff V, et al. Benign partial epilepsy of childhood: a longitudinal neuropsychological and EEG study of cognitive function. *Dev Med Child Neurol* 2000;42:595–603.

89. Metz-Lutz MN, Kleitz C, de Saint Martin A, et al. Cognitive development in benign focal epilepsies of childhood. *Dev Neurosci* 1999;21:182–190.

90. Santanelli P, Bureau M, Magaudda A et al. Benign partial epilepsy with centrotemporal (or rolandic) spikes and brain lesion. *Epilepsia* 1989;30:182–188.

91. Lundberg S, Eeg-Olofsson O, Raininko R, et al. Hippocampal asymmetries and white matter abnormalities on MRI in benign childhood epilepsy with centrotemporal spikes. *Epilepsia* 1999;40:1808–1815.

92. Gelisse P, Corda D, Raybaud C, et al. Abnormal neuroimaging in patients with benign epilepsy with centrotemporal spikes. *Epilepsia* 2003;44:372–378.

93. Peters JM, Camfield CS, Camfield PR. Population study of benign rolandic epilepsy: is treatment needed? *Neurology* 2001;57:537–539.

94. Ambrosetto G, Tassinari CA. Antiepileptic drug treatment of benign childhood epilepsy with rolandic spikes: is it necessary? *Epilepsia* 1990;31:802–805.

95. Bouma PAD, Bovenkerk AC, Westendorp RGJ, et al. The course of benign partial epilepsy of childhood with centrotemporal spikes: a meta-analysis. *Neurology* 1997;48:430–437.

96. Bourgeois BF, Brown LW, Pellock JM, et al. Gabapentin (Neurontin) monotherapy in children with benign childhood epilepsy with centrotemporal spikes (BECTS): a 36-week, double-blind, placebo-controlled study. *Epilepsia* 1998;39(Suppl 6):163.

97. Doose H, Baier WK, Ernst JP, et al. Benign partial epilepsy—treatment with sulthiame. *Dev Med Child Neurol* 1988;30:683–691.

98. Gross-Selbeck G. Treatment of "benign" partial epilepsies of childhood, including atypical forms. *Neuropediatrics* 1995;26:45–50.

99. Lerman P, Lerman-Sagie T. Sulthiame revisited. *J Child Neurol* 1995;10:241–242.

100. Rating D. Treatment in typical and atypical rolandic epilepsy. *Epileptic Disord* 2000;2(Suppl 1):S69–S72.

101. Rating D, Wolf C, Bast T. Sulthiame as monotherapy in children with benign childhood epilepsy with centrotemporal spikes: a 6-month randomized, double-blind, placebo-controlled study. *Epilepsia* 2000;41:1284–1288.

102. Corda D, Gelisse P, Genton P, et al. Incidence of drug-induced aggravation in benign epilepsy with centrotemporal spikes. *Epilepsia* 2001;42:754–759.

103. Prats JM, Garaizar C, Garcia-Nieto ML, et al. Antiepileptic drugs and atypical evolution of idiopathic partial epilepsy. *Pediatr Neurol* 1998;18:402–406.

104. Nanba Y, Maegaki Y. Epileptic negative myoclonus induced by carbamazepine in a child with BECTS. Benign childhood epilepsy with centrotemporal spikes. *Pediatr Neurol* 1999;21:664–667.

105. Catania S, Cross H, de Sousa C, et al. Paradoxic reaction to lamotrigine in a child with benign focal epilepsy of childhood with centrotemporal spikes. *Epilepsia* 1999;40:1657–1660.

106. Blom S, Heijbel J. Benign epilepsy of children with centrotemporal EEG foci: a follow-up in adulthood of patients initially studied as children. *Epilepsia* 1982;23:629–631.

107. De Romanis F, Feliciani M, Ruggieri S. Rolandic paroxysmal epilepsy: a long term study in 150 children. *Ital J Neurol Sci* 1986;7:77–80.

108. Loiseau P, Pestre M, Dartigues JF, et al. Long-term prognosis in two forms of childhood epilepsy: typical absence seizures and epilepsy with rolandic (centrotemporal) EEG foci. *Ann Neurol* 1983;13:642–648.

109. Gibbs F, Gibbs E. *Atlas of electroencephalography, epilepsy, II.* Cambridge: Addison[FES5]-Wesley, 1952:222–224.
110. Panayiotopoulos CP. Benign childhood epilepsy with occipital paroxysms. A 15-year prospective study. *Ann Neurol* 1989;26: 51–56.
111. Panayiotopoulos CP. Benign childhood epileptic syndromes with occipital spikes: new classification proposed by the International League Against Epilepsy. *J Child Neurol* 2000;15:548–552.
112. Kuzniecky R, Rosenblatt B. Benign occipital epilepsy: a family study. *Epilepsia* 1987;28:346–350.
113. Ferrie CD, Beaumanoir A, Guerrini R, et al. Early onset benign occipital seizure susceptibility syndrome. *Epilepsia* 1997;38: 285–932.
114. Lada C, Skiadas K, Theodorou V, et al. A study of 43 patients with Panayiotopoulos syndrome, a common and benign childhood seizure susceptibility. *Epilepsia* 2003;44:81–88.
115. Panayiotopoulos CP. *Panayiotopoulos syndrome: a common and benign childhood epileptic syndrome.* London: John Libbey, 2002.
116. Guerrini R, Battaglia A, Dravet C, et al. Outcome of idiopathic childhood epilepsy with occipital paroxysms. In: Andermann F, Beaumanoir A, Mira L, et al., eds. *Occipital seizures and epilepsies in children.* London: John Libbey, 1993:71–86.
117. Panayiotopoulos CP. Early onset benign childhood occipital seizure susceptibility syndrome: a syndrome to recognize. *Epilepsia* 1999;40:621–630.
118. Caraballo R, Cersosimo R, Medina C, et al. Panayiotopoulos-type benign childhood occipital epilepsy: a prospective study. *Neurology* 2000;55:1096–1100.
119. Ferrie CD, Koutroumanidis M, Rowlinson S, et al. Atypical evolution of Panayiotopoulos syndrome: a case report. *Epileptic Disord* 2002;4:35–42.
120. Gastaut H. Benign spike-wave occipital epilepsy in children. *Rev Electroencephalogr Neurophysiol Clin* 1982;12:179–201.
121. Verrotti A, Domizio S, Melchionda D, et al. Stormy onset of benign childhood epilepsy with occipital paroxysmal discharges. *Childs Nerv Syst* 2000;16:35–39.
122. Guerrini R, Belmonte A, Veggiotti P, et al. Delayed appearance of interictal EEG abnormalities in early onset childhood epilepsy with occipital paroxysms. *Brain Dev* 1997;19:343–346.
123. Oguni H, Hayashi K, Funatsuka M, et al. Study on early-onset benign occipital seizure susceptibility syndrome. *Pediatr Neurol* 2001;25:312–318.
124. Ohtsu M, Oguni H, Hayashi K, et al. EEG in children with early-onset benign occipital seizure susceptibility syndrome: Panayiotopoulos syndrome. *Epilepsia* 2003;44:435–442.
125. Maher J, Ronen GM, Ogunyemi AO, et al. Occipital paroxysmal discharges suppressed by eye opening: variability in clinical and seizure manifestations in childhood. *Epilepsia* 1995;36:52–57.
126. Cooper GW, Lee SI. Reactive occipital epileptiform activity: is it benign? *Epilepsia* 1991;32:63–68.
127. Van der Meij W, Van der Dussen D, Van Huffelen AC, et al. Dipole source analysis may differentiate benign focal epilepsy of childhood with occipital paroxysms from symptomatic occipital lobe epilepsy. *Brain Topogr* 1997;10:115–120.
128. Beaumanoir A. Semiology of occipital seizures in infants and children. In: Andermann F, Beaumanoir A, Mira L, et al., eds. *Occipital seizures and epilepsies in children.* London: John Libbey, 1993:71–86.
129. Vigevano F, Lispi ML, Ricci S. Early onset benign occipital susceptibility syndrome: video-EEG documentation of an illustrative case. *Clin Neurophysiol* 2000;111(Suppl 2):S81–S86.
130. Vigevano F, Ricci S. Benign occipital epilepsy of childhood with prolonged seizures and autonomic symptoms. In: Andermann F, Beaumanoir A, Mira L, et al., eds. *Occipital seizures and epilepsies in children.* London: John Libbey, 1993:133–140.
131. Gulgonen S, Demirbilik V, Korkmaz B, et al. Neuropsychological functions in idiopathic occipital lobe epilepsy. *Epilepsia* 2000;41:405–411.
132. Tenembaum SN, Deonna TW, Fejerman N, et al. Continuous spike-waves and dementia in childhood epilepsy with occipital paroxysms. *J Epilepsy* 1997;10:139–145.
133. Nass R, Gross A, Devinsky O. Autism and autistic epileptiform regression with occipital spikes. *Dev Med Child Neurol* 1998;40: 453–458.
134. Panayiotopoulos CP. Elementary visual hallucinations, blindness and headache in idiopathic occipital epilepsy: differentiation from migraine. *J Neurol Neurosurg Psychiatry* 1999;66: 536–540.
135. Gastaut H. Benign epilepsy of childhood with occipital paroxysms. In: Roger J, Dravet C, Bureau M, et al., eds. *Epilepsy syndromes in infancy, childhood and adolescence.* London: John Libbey, 1985:159–170.
136. Okumura A, Hayakawa F, Kuno K, et al. Benign partial epilepsy in infancy. *Arch Dis Child* 1996;74:19–21.
137. Nelson GB, Olson DM, Hahn JS. Short duration of benign partial epilepsy in infancy. *J Child Neurol* 2002;17:440–445.
138. Okumura A, Hayakawa F, Kato T, et al. Early recognition of benign partial epilepsy in infancy. *Epilepsia* 2000;41:714–717.
139. Bureau M, Cokar O, Maton B, et al. Sleep-related, low voltage rolandic and vertex spikes: an EEG marker of benignity in infancy-onset focal epilepsies. *Epileptic Disord* 2002;4:15–22.
140. King MA, Newton MR, Berkovic SF. Benign partial seizures of adolescence. *Epilepsia* 1999;40:1244–1247.
141. Capovilla G, Gambardella A, Romeo A, et al. Benign partial epilepsies of adolescence: a report of 37 new cases. *Epilepsia* 2001;42:1549–1552.
142. Vigevano F, Fusco L. Hypnic tonic postural seizures in healthy children provide evidence for a partial epileptic syndrome of frontal lobe origin. *Epilepsia* 1993;34:110–119.
143. Scheffer IE, Bhatia KP, Lopes-Cendes I, et al. Autosomal dominant nocturnal frontal lobe epilepsy. A distinctive clinical disorder. *Brain* 1995;118(Pt 1):61–73.
144. Fonseca LC, Tedrus GM. Somatosensory evoked spikes and epileptic seizures: a study of 385 cases. *Clin Electroencephalogr* 2000;31:71–75.

Idiopathic Generalized Epilepsy Syndromes of Childhood and Adolescence

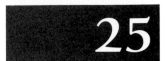

Tobias Loddenkemper   *Selim R. Benbadis*   *Jose M. Serratosa*
Samuel F. Berkovic

TERMINOLOGY

The term *idiopathic generalized epilepsy* (IGE) was defined in the International Classification of Epilepsies and Epileptic Syndromes in 1989 (1). In addition to establishing the difference between partial and generalized, this classification added the terms *idiopathic, cryptogenic,* and *symptomatic*. In the previous version of the classification, IGEs were referred to as "primary" generalized epilepsies and the symptomatic and cryptogenic types as "secondary" generalized epilepsies (2). However, confusion existed, because secondary in the context of a generalized epilepsy meant "secondary to cause," whereas in the context of generalized seizures it referred to seizures with focal electroencephalographic (EEG) features followed by generalization.

In all other areas of medicine idiopathic usually means "of unknown cause"; IGEs, however, actually describe a genetically low threshold for seizures. This unusual meaning was not changed in the most recent multiaxial classification (3), in which an idiopathic epilepsy syndrome is defined as "a syndrome that is only epilepsy, with no underlying structural brain lesion or other neurologic signs or symptoms. These are presumed to be genetic and are usually age dependent." IGE syndromes are characterized by onset in childhood, good response to medical treatment and good prognosis, lack of a structural cerebral abnormality, and a presumed genetic cause (4). The absence of an underlying brain abnormality may be debat-

able, as more evidence for focal structural (5,6), functional (7), and biochemical (8) heterogeneity and abnormalities becomes available.

Specific Idiopathic Generalized Epilepsy Syndromes as a Continuum

Specific syndromes in the current classification of IGEs are childhood absence epilepsy (CAE); juvenile myoclonic epilepsy (JME); juvenile absence epilepsy (JAE); benign myoclonic epilepsy in infancy; epilepsy with generalized tonic-clonic seizures only; epilepsy with myoclonic astatic seizures (Doose syndrome); epilepsy with myoclonic absences; and generalized epilepsies with febrile seizures plus. However, separation of specific IGE syndromes may be difficult, and many patients may be placed in unspecified categories. To determine the frequency of epilepsy syndromes, pediatric patients with IGE were studied as a cohort: 76% received a diagnosis "idiopathic generalized epilepsy, not otherwise specified" (9), a classification that could not be changed even after 2 years of follow-up. Many authors therefore refer to IGE as a spectrum of disorders rather than as multiple separate entities (10–14). A study at a tertiary epilepsy center found 12 of 89 randomly selected patients to have IGE, but only 4 of these 12 could be placed into a specific subcategory of IGEs (15). Further evidence for overlap among the spectrum of IGE derives from genetic studies suggesting that the analysis of seizure types as compared to IGE syndromes may be more helpful in genetic linkage studies (16).

Response to pharmacologic treatment and prognosis is usually good. Benbadis and coworkers reviewed the initial treatment regimen of 58 patients with EEG-confirmed IGE (17). Only 29% were on adequate pharmacologic treatment whereas 48% were treated with ill-advised antiepileptic drugs (AEDs) only and 22% on a combination of ill-advised and adequate AEDs (17). Therefore, improvement in recognition of IGE and appropriate choice of medication is crucial to management and outcome in these patients.

GENERALIZED IDIOPATHIC EPILEPSY SYNDROMES OF CHILDHOOD AND ADOLESCENCE

Juvenile Myoclonic Epilepsy

History

Sudden and brisk muscular contractions during epileptic seizures were first described in the second century by Galen (18). The term *myoclonus* is derived from Friedreich's description of paramyoclonus multiplex to indicate symmetric and multifocal jerks (19). Other 19th century authors, such as Delasiauve (20), Gowers (21), Féré (22), and Reynolds (23), also mentioned the isolated myoclonic jerks that occur in some epilepsy patients, but it was Herpin (24), in 1867, who gave the first detailed description of a patient with JME. He called the myoclonic jerks "secousses," "impulsions," and "commotions épileptiques," that is, compulsions that shake the body as an electric shock would.

In Penfield and Jasper's *Epilepsy and the Functional Anatomy of the Human Brain,* Penfield used the term "myoclonic petit mal" (25). In 1957, Janz and Christian described the characteristics of the syndrome in 47 patients (26). The following year, Castells and Mendilaharsu independently described 70 patients with "bilateral and conscious myoclonic epilepsy" (27). Jeavons, in 1977, was the first to describe the excellent response of patients with JME to valproate (28,29). In 1984, Asconape and Penry (30) and Delgado-Escueta and Enrile-Bacsal (31) reported the clinical and electrophysiologic characteristics of this syndrome.

Epidemiologic Factors

JME is estimated to account for approximately 10% of all epilepsies, with a range from 4% to 11% (12,30,32–35). Underdiagnosed in the past, JME recently became a well-recognized epilepsy syndrome. Previously, myoclonias were frequently recognized only after detailed history taking or after recording myoclonic seizures on video-electroencephalography. The attention given to genetic studies and the widespread use of video-EEG monitoring have made JME an easily recognizable syndrome. Its true prevalence in the general population is difficult to ascertain,

as many patients may misinterpret myoclonic seizures as clumsiness or nervousness (36). There is no male or female predominance in most series.

Clinical Features

Age of Onset

According to Janz, JME begins between 12 and 18 years of age (mean, 14.6 years) (32,37) but can manifest in all age groups (38). Dialeptic (or absence) seizures may occur earlier (mean, 11.5 years; range, 8 to 16 years) than myoclonic seizures (mean, 15.4 years; range, 8 to 30 years) or generalized tonic-clonic seizures (mean, 15.5 years; range, 8 to 30 years) (39).

Precipitating Factors

Myoclonic seizures and generalized tonic-clonic seizures occur mainly on awakening in the morning (40) or after afternoon naps (30) and are triggered by sleep deprivation, fatigue (41), and alcohol (42). In 41% to 42%, menstruation may precipitate myoclonic seizures (30,31). Cocaine and marijuana appear to aggravate seizures in JME (43).

Neurologic Examination

Patients with JME have normal findings on neurologic examination and a normal developmental history. Janz reported no abnormal findings in a series of 181 patients (12). Tsuboi noted abnormal neurologic findings probably not related to JME in 24 of 399 cases (34).

Imaging

Imaging studies do not reveal a cause for the epilepsy. Quantitative magnetic resonance imaging has shown that patients with JME, as well as those with other IGEs, have a significantly larger volume of cortical gray matter than control subjects, with frequent abnormalities in the regional distribution of cerebral gray and white matter (5,6). In JME patients, this cerebral abnormality affects the mesial frontal lobes more severely. Swartz and colleagues (44), using ^{18}F-2-fluoro-2-deoxyglucose positron emission tomography during visual working memory tasks, found differences in regional metabolic patterns between JME patients and control subjects. Their findings support the concept that individuals with JME may suffer from cortical disorganization and abnormal patterns of cortical activation that are associated with subtle cognitive dysfunction.

Seizure Semiology

Myoclonic Seizures

The typical myoclonic seizures of JME consist of mild to moderate jerks of the neck, shoulders, arms, or legs. The jerks are more frequent in the upper than in the lower extremities and are usually bilaterally symmetric but may be unilateral (12,31,45,46). Lancman and associates (45) found asymmetric myoclonic seizures manifested as predominantly unilateral or initially unilateral jerks followed by bilateral jerks in 11 of 85 patients with JME. Myoclonic jerks of the upper extremities can often cause patients to drop objects and can interfere with morning activities such as eating breakfast, brushing the teeth, or applying cosmetics. The jerks can be single or repetitive and frequently involve extensor muscles. If repetitive, they are not rhythmic and usually do not exceed more than a few movements. Falling to the floor is uncommon, but falls may occur when patients are in an awkward position and are "surprised" by a myoclonic seizure. The amplitude of the movement is variable, but the jerk is not forceful or massive. Recovery is immediate, without loss of consciousness. These myoclonias should be distinguished from the massive sudden myoclonic seizures that propel patients to the ground with great force (as seen in Lennox-Gastaut syndrome and in progressive myoclonus epilepsies). A series of repetitive myoclonic jerks may precede a generalized tonic-clonic seizure, producing a clonic-tonic-clonic seizure (47).

Sometimes the myoclonic seizures of JME are perceived only as an electric shock or a "feeling" inside the body, and there is no evidence of movement. Consciousness is either not affected or is so briefly and mildly impaired that the deficit is difficult to perceive. This clearly distinguishes the myoclonic jerks of JME from dialeptic seizures associated with myoclonic jerks ("myoclonic absences") in which shoulder, arm, and leg jerks occur against a background of loss of consciousness, during which patients are unaware of the seizure as jerking continues (48). In contrast, just after a myoclonic seizure, JME patients know that a seizure has occurred. Even successive jerks may not impair consciousness (12).

Generalized Tonic-Clonic Seizures

Generalized tonic-clonic seizures are often preceded by a few minutes of generalized, mild to moderate jerks of increasing frequency and intensity, a seizure pattern known as clonic-tonic-clonic. Because consciousness is preserved during myoclonic jerks, patients may predict a grand mal seizure a few minutes before it occurs and adopt a safe position to prevent major injuries. Consciousness is abruptly lost when the head, face, neck, and trunk extend with a tonic contraction. The tonic phase lasts approximately 10 to 20 seconds and leads to a final phase of clonic trunk and limb jerks. Generalized tonic-clonic seizures are present in 87% to 95% of patients with JME (33,37,49) and are frequently precipitated by lack of sleep, alcohol intake, and stress (41,42).

Dialeptic Seizures (Absences)

Typical dialeptic seizures (or absences) occur in 10% to 33% of JME patients (31,37,49,50). Dialeptic seizures of JME are relatively infrequent, of short duration, and not associated with automatisms (51,52). A prospective study in JME found dialeptic seizures in 16 (31.9%) of 42 patients (53). Clinical changes were subtle and became apparent only with adequate testing. When dialeptic seizures occurred before the age of 10 years, the patient would stop activities, not answer questions, and stare. No postictal symptoms or memory recollections of ictal events were observed. When dialeptic seizures appeared after the age of 10 years, the manifestations were usually less severe and consisted of subjective instant loss of contact and concentration or brief impairment of concentration revealed on questioning (53).

Electroencephalographic Findings

Interictal Electroencephalography

The characteristic EEG pattern of JME consists of discharges of diffuse bilateral, symmetric, and synchronous 4- to 6-Hz polyspike-wave complexes (Fig. 25.1). Discharges may be accentuated over the frontocentral regions. The interictal complexes usually have two or more high-voltage (150 to 300 μV) surface-negative spikes, widespread but of higher voltage in the anterior head region (32). Delgado-Escueta and Enrile-Bascal (31) found 4- to 6-Hz polyspike-wave complexes in all untreated individuals and diffuse 3-Hz spike-wave complexes in 17% of patients. Asymmetric, as well as focal, EEG abnormalities have also been described (45). The resting electroencephalogram background is normal.

Ictal Electroencephalography

The ictal electroencephalogram demonstrates 10- to 16-Hz generalized polyspikes followed by slow waves. Also seen are 4- to 6-Hz diffuse polyspike-wave complexes.

Genetics and Etiology

In 1973, Tsuboi and Christian (54) studied families of patients with "primary generalized epilepsy and sporadic myoclonias of impulsive petit mal." Of 319 probands, 27.3% had at least one near or distant relative affected with epilepsy. Of 390 family members, 15% had diffuse polyspike-wave complexes, and another 39.8% had nonspecific paroxysmal EEG abnormalities. Inheritance was interpreted to follow a polygenic-threshold pattern, with female relatives being more affected than male relatives.

Family studies of JME since then have resulted in conflicting results regarding the mode of inheritance. Polygenic (54), digenic (recessive-dominant or recessive-recessive) (55), single-gene autosomal dominant (56), and recessive models have been proposed. In the families of JME patients, affected family members usually express different idiopathic generalized epilepsy syndromes, such as childhood absence epilepsy, juvenile absence epilepsy, or epilepsy with generalized tonic-clonic seizures on awakening (57–60). Some asymptomatic family members show

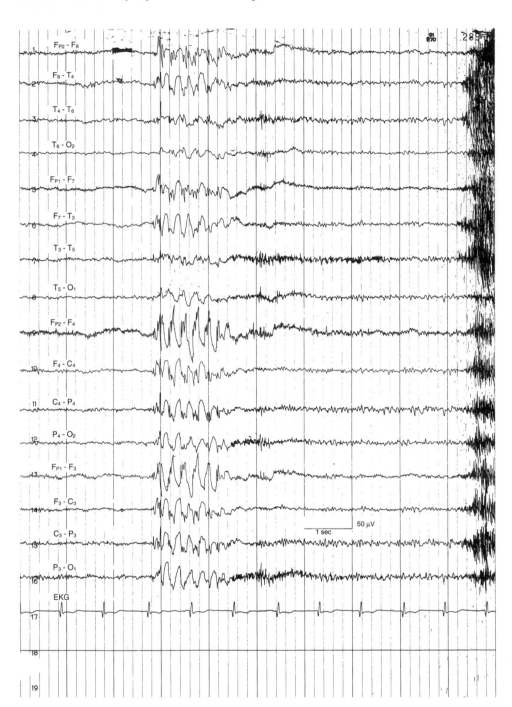

Figure 25.1 Interictal 4- to 6-Hz polyspike-wave discharge of frontocentral predominance in juvenile myoclonic epilepsy. No clinical changes were seen, and the patient could recall a word given during the discharge.

the typical 4- to 6-Hz polyspike-wave complexes on the electroencephalogram (59,61).

Recent studies revealed that JME is a heterogeneous entity related to several mutations. Major genetic susceptibility loci for JME have been termed EJM 1, 2, and 3. Depending on modifying genetic mutations in other loci, phenotypic expression can vary.

In addition, there have been descriptions of individual JME families that appear to be clearly affected by a major autosomal recessive (62) or dominant gene (61). Autosomal dominant inheritance patterns have been described in associ-

ation with mutations in the *GABRA1* gene on chromosome 5q34-q35 (63), the *CACNB4* gene on chromosome 2q22-q23 (64), and the *CLCN2* gene on chromosome 3q26 (65).

The term *EJM 1* is used to characterize the JME phenotype caused by *EFHC1* gene mutations located on 6p12-p11. Families with JME from Mexico, Belize, and Los Angeles had high limit of detection (LOD) scores at the 6p11-p12 locus (66–68). Another study from the Netherlands confirmed the 6p12-p11 marker in conjunction with JME (69). In 2004, Suzuki and colleagues (70), demonstrated mutations in the *EFHC1* gene in six different families, including the ones previously described by Liu and associates (67,68) and Bai and coworkers (66).

EJM 2 is used to characterize the mutation in the α_7 subunit of the neuronal nicotinic acetylcholine receptor on chromosome 15q14. Based on the previous description of autosomal dominant nocturnal frontal lobe epilepsy as a mutation in the α_4 subunit (CHRNA4) of the neuronal nicotinic acetylcholine receptor (71–73), linkage analysis of this region was performed in 34 families with JME and suggested that this region was a major susceptibility locus for JME (74). A maximum multipoint LOD score of 4.42 was obtained at a point 1.7 centimorgans (cM) telomeric to marker D15S144. In this study, 25 of 27 sib pairs had identical haplotypes by descent in one or both chromosomes in the chromosome 15 region. Haplotype sharing analysis allowed placement of the candidate gene in a 15.1-cM region on chromosome 15q. Of interest, a transgenic mouse deficient in this subunit showed generalized hypersynchronous 4- to 7-Hz sharp wave activity on EEG, similar to EEG abnormalities found in JME patients.

EJM 3 is used to characterize a mutation in the *BRD2* gene, a presumed transcription regulator on chromosome 6p21(75). This locus was initially named EJM1 (76), but now mutations in the *EFHC1* gene on 6p12-p11 are called EJM 1 because of phenotype variations. Greenberg and coworkers (55) performed segregation analysis on 28 pedigrees. Including asymptomatic family members with abnormal electroencephalograms as affected or unaffected, these authors rejected the fully penetrant recessive model. Initial linkage studies reported evidence of linkage to chromosome 6p using human leukocyte antigen (HLA) and properdin (Bf) as markers (59). The clinical phenotype for this 6p epilepsy locus consisted of myoclonic seizures, generalized tonic-clonic or clonic-tonic-clonic seizures, absences, and, in asymptomatic individuals, diffuse 4- to 6-Hz polyspike-wave complexes. Maximum LOD scores were obtained using a recessive mode of inheritance with 60% penetrance. Subsequently, other studies reported similar findings (58,77).

A single pedigree, including 10 members showing JME or asymptomatic polyspike-wave complexes on EEG, has supported linkage to chromosome 6p by resulting in LOD scores of 3.4 for several 6p markers (61). Recombinant events defined the *JME* gene region to be a 43-cM interval flanked by marker D6S258 (HLA region) and marker D6S313 (centromere). Results in this large family independently prove linkage of JME and the subclinical polyspike-wave EEG pattern to chromosome 6p markers. Another study by Sander and coworkers (78) has provided further evidence of a JME locus on chromosome 6p. This locus would confer susceptibility to idiopathic generalized seizures in a majority of German families of JME patients. In this study, the *6p* gene was proposed to be in a 10-cM region on chromosome 6p between HLA-DQ and marker D6S1019.

Pal and colleagues noted a linkage disequilibrium between JME and markers in the critical region 6p21, with a peak in the area of the *BRD2* gene (75). DNA-sequencing demonstrated two JME-related single nucleotide polymorphisms in the *BRD2* promotor region, and could not identify any other related mutation (75). Of interest, reported abnormalities of cerebral microanatomy as reported in JME would be compatible with *BRD2* involvement (6).

A mutation in the *GABRA1* gene on 5q34-q35 has been described in 14 members of a French-Canadian family with JME (63). Transmission was autosomal dominant. The authors speculate that seizures are caused by a dysfunction in this ligand-gated channel, because the mutation in the channels produces a reduction in GABA-activated currents *in vitro* (63).

Additionally, a mutation of the *CACNB4* gene on chromosome 2q22-q23 encoding for the β_4 subunit of a voltage-dependent calcium channel has been described in a patient presenting with bilateral myoclonic jerks of the shoulders, rare dialeptic seizures, and generalized tonic-clonic seizures after awakening. This patient was diagnosed with JME. Of note, the proband's daughter presented with generalized 3-Hz spike-and-wave complexes without clinical change (64).

Furthermore, a *CLCN2* gene mutation encoding for a chloride channel 2 on chromosome 3q26 has been identified in a family presenting with serial myoclonic jerks, frequently followed by a generalized tonic-clonic seizure (65). Four family members were diagnosed with autosomal dominant JME and one member had epilepsy with generalized tonic-clonic seizures only (65). The mutation causes functional alteration of the channel function leading to increased chloride concentration within the cell, reduced γ-aminobutyric acid (GABA) response, and neuronal hyperexcitability and seizures (65).

Pharmacologic Treatment

Valproic acid is effective in 86% to 90% of JME patients (29–31,79–81), stopping myoclonias and tonic-clonic, clonic-tonic-clonic, and absence seizures without significant side effects. Newer AEDs, such as lamotrigine or topiramate, may also be useful, but valproic acid enjoys the widest experience. As soon as a diagnosis of JME with grand mal convulsions is entertained, treatment with valproic acid or an alternative drug should be started. Seizures invariably return after drug withdrawal, and lifetime treatment is usually required (31).

Therapeutic doses of valproic acid range from 20 to 30 mg/kg. Patients receiving monotherapy require a lower dose than do those taking valproic acid in combination with other AEDs (29). Most patients are controlled with blood levels of 40 to 100 mg/mL, but in resistant cases, levels of up to 150 mg/mL may be necessary. Penry and colleagues (81) reported that 50% of their patients relapsed at some time between 2 months and 9 years of valproic acid treatment. Relapses were a result of fatigue, drug noncompliance, stress, sleep deprivation, and alcohol consumption.

Lamotrigine is a useful alternative, especially when valproic acid alone is not effective or not well tolerated. In some patients, however, lamotrigine must be combined with valproic acid for seizure control (82). Topiramate is effective in JME, but controlled studies are lacking (83).

Phenytoin, phenobarbital, or primidone may also be added as a second drug to valproic acid in resistant cases. When used as monotherapy, control rates are much lower than those for valproic acid. According to Janz, primidone monotherapy was the treatment of choice before valproic acid became available (37), and 74% of his patients were treated with phenobarbital, phenytoin, or primidone alone. With phenytoin monotherapy, up to 40% of patients experienced an increased frequency of myoclonic jerks (84).

Ethosuximide may be added to valproic acid in JME patients with uncontrolled absences. Clonazepam should be added in patients with uncontrolled jerks. Clonazepam alone is ineffective, controlling only the myoclonic jerks and not the grand mal seizures (33). As adjunctive therapy (with valproic acid or other first-line AEDs), it may be useful in patients with persistent myoclonic jerks. Used alone, clonazepam may suppress the jerks that herald a generalized tonic-clonic seizure and not allow patients to prepare for this type of attack. Some clinicians have favored acetazolamide monotherapy for patients who continue to have generalized tonic-clonic seizures despite trials of first-line AEDs or for patients who have difficulty tolerating valproic acid (85). According to these investigators, acetazolamide does not control myoclonus as well as valproic acid does, but it controls generalized tonic-clonic seizures and is a useful adjunct to valproic acid for resistant cases.

Vigabatrin and gabapentin are not indicated in JME because myoclonic jerks and absence seizures may increase. Carbamazepine, vigabatrin, and tiagabine (86) are associated with absence status epilepticus in patients with IGEs and should not be used in JME.

Levetiracetam has been tested in patients with IGE resistant to medical treatment. Of 10 patients with JME who responded, 2 became seizure free (87). Eight of nine patients responded to zonisamide, with five becoming seizure free (88).

Carbamazepine monotherapy increased the frequency of myoclonic seizures in 19 of 28 patients and decreased seizure frequency in 6 of 28 patients (84). In this study, carbamazepine had a stronger seizure-aggravating effect than did phenytoin in patients with JME (84).

Pregnancy, Juvenile Myoclonic Epilepsy, and Valproic Acid

Female patients receiving valproic acid should be advised of reports that link its use to neural tube defects. These defects occur in 0.5% to 1% of pregnancies in patients receiving valproic acid monotherapy, and in 1% to 2% of pregnancies in patients receiving valproic acid in combination with other AEDs. Supplementation with folic acid may ameliorate the risk. Withdrawal of AEDs in patients who suffer few myoclonic jerks only before pregnancy is planned and rein-

statement after the first trimester may be a treatment option in selected patients after a discussion with the patient of the risks and benefits. All seizure precipitants should be avoided, and when myoclonic seizures on awakening suggest particular vulnerability to convulsive seizures, a fast-acting benzodiazepine should be administered orally or rectally (89). The effects of AEDs on birth control medications should also be discussed with the patient. For women of child-bearing age, lamotrigine or topiramate may be considered.

Outcome and Prognosis

JME carries an excellent prognosis because AED treatment controls seizures in most patients. Nevertheless, any condition that places a patient at risk for a generalized tonic-clonic seizure is not benign. Sudden loss of consciousness can lead to injuries or even death. In swimming or driving, for example, a generalized tonic-clonic seizure can have devastating effects. Recognition of this syndrome is important because of the good response to valproic acid and the high incidence of relapse after medication withdrawal. JME is one form of epilepsy in which discontinuation of pharmacotherapy cannot be recommended, even after long seizure-free periods. Delgado-Escueta and Enrile-Bacsal (31) found a 90% relapse rate after withdrawal of AEDs. In our experience, not a single patient has been seizure free after medication was withdrawn. The patient should be treated as soon as a diagnosis is made and, if possible, before a grand mal seizure occurs. According to Janz (12,32), patients who did not achieve freedom from seizures had their condition untreated 9 years longer than those who responded well to medication. Penry's study showed that 86% of patients with JME are seizure free or well controlled with valproic acid alone or in combination with other AEDs (81).

Childhood Absence Epilepsy

History

CAE, the most widely recognized type of absence epilepsy, was described early in the 20th century as pyknolepsy by Sauer and Adie, who noted its childhood onset, multiple clustered minor attacks (*pyknos*, Greek for "crowded" or "dense"), and usual spontaneous resolution (90,91). Synonyms include petit mal epilepsy, true petit mal, and pyknoleptic petit mal.

Epidemiologic Factors

CAE accounts for 2% to 8% of patients with epilepsy (92–96); the variation depends largely on the mode and source of case collection. In Swedish children 1 to 15 years of age, Olsson found an annual incidence of JAE without diffuse brain damage in 6.3 per 100,000 children (97); the majority had CAE. The cumulative incidence of absence seizures (number of persons who will have absence seizures at some time in their lives) was 98 per 100,000 children in this Swedish study (97), but only 49 per 100,000 children in a Danish study (98). A female bias in affected children is frequently observed (13,99–102), although in some studies boys and girls were equally represented (103,104).

Clinical Features

Age of Onset

CAE characteristically begins between the ages of 4 and 10 years with absence seizures (13,105), but age of onset is not strictly limited and can vary between 2 and 10 years (peak incidence is about 5 years of age). Absences occurring before age 3 years are unusual, although an apparently typical case beginning at 6.5 months has been described (106). Approximately 10% of patients have febrile convulsions before the onset of absences (99,104,105,107). The latest age limit is also difficult to define, and classification of early adolescent cases as CAE or JAE can be somewhat arbitrary. Onset after 11 years of age with the typical pyknoleptic pattern of CAE is unusual (13).

Neurologic Examination

Neurologic findings are usually normal.

Seizure Semiology

By definition, all patients suffer typical absence seizures, which occur several times per day (usually more than 10 times), last on average 9 seconds (range, 5 to 30 seconds), and can be accompanied by mild clonic activity, atonic or tonic components, and automatisms during longer seizures (108–110). Mild myoclonic jerks of the eyelids ("eyelid flutter") can be seen at the beginning of a typical absence seizure. Clinical seizures begin and end abruptly and almost all can be triggered by hyperventilation. Tonic-clonic seizures affect approximately 40% of patients (13,99,105, 107,111,112) but are usually infrequent and easily controlled. They often begin near puberty but can occur in the first decade or, rarely, in early adult life. Afebrile tonic-clonic seizures in early childhood occasionally precede the onset of absences. These patients may represent a separate nosologic group with a male preponderance and a slightly worse prognosis than is seen in typical CAE (113–117). Some authors have suggested that all patients with tonic-clonic seizures, whether of early childhood or adolescent onset, should be excluded from the strict definition of CAE (101,118,119). This would confine CAE to children with absences alone—a view we do not support.

Absence status occurs in 10% to 15% of CAE patients (99,120,121). Although hundreds of absence seizures may occur throughout the day, continuous spike-and-wave discharges are relatively unusual. Absence status seems to be more common in JAE than in CAE.

Myoclonic seizures usually are not seen in CAE. Patients may have some degree of clonic or myoclonic twitching as part of their absences, but distinct myoclonic jerks without impairment of consciousness are uncommon, occurring mainly in teenagers with persisting CAE (122). Some patients also may "evolve" into JME (123), again illustrating

the concept that IGEs represent a spectrum of conditions whose borders are at times blurred (10).

Electroencephalographic Findings

Interictal Electroencephalography

The electroencephalogram demonstrates 3-Hz spike-and-wave complexes as well as generalized spike-and-wave complexes and, rarely, polyspikes between seizures. Occasionally, asymmetries can be observed, but if the complete recording is evaluated, the diagnosis of generalized epilepsy becomes more evident. Background activity is normal. In up to 50% of patients bursts of intermittent rhythmic slowing, lasting 2 to 4 seconds, can be observed in the occipital leads (124).

Ictal Electroencephalography

Ictal patterns initially present with rhythmic 3- to 3.5-Hz sharp waves that slow to 2.5 to 3 Hz. These can be provoked in untreated patients by hyperventilation and in 10% to 15% of patients by photic stimulation.

Etiology and Genetics

Genetic factors predominate in the etiology of CAE. About one-third of patients have a family history of epilepsy, and siblings of affected individuals have an approximately 10% chance of suffering seizures (115,116,125–129). In addition to classical family studies, compelling data from twin studies show a high concordance in identical twins. Lennox and Lennox (130,131) originally described a series of 20 monozygous twins with absence seizures; 75% were concordant for absences and 84% for the spike-and-wave trait. CAE was not isolated from other absence syndromes at the time of the Lennox study, but a review of the original twin files disclosed a number of typical cases of CAE, according to Berkovic and Andermann (unpublished data, 1991).

The Australian Twin Study of Epilepsies (132) used the 1989 classification devised by the International League Against Epilepsy (ILAE) (1). Twenty monozygous pairs of twins with IGEs were identified, of whom 13 had seizures and 16 had the spike-and-wave trait. In all 13 clinically concordant pairs, both twins had the same syndrome, including eight pairs with CAE. In contrast, syndrome heterogeneity was seen among concordant dizygous pairs and other affected family members, strongly suggesting that these syndromes were determined by more than one gene (132). A genetic linkage to chromosome 6p may be present in JME (59); it is not clear whether this genetic locus is relevant in CAE (76).

Because concordance in monozygous twins is less than 100%, nongenetic factors also may play a role. However, a case-controlled study (103) failed to identify any specific prenatal or perinatal risk factors, although the small number of participants limited the study's power.

The data in CAE best fit a multifactorial model of causation (133,134), although typical cases are determined predominantly by genetic factors. Acquired factors may be relatively important in cases with unusual features, including focal neurologic signs, intellectual disability, or atypical spike-and-wave discharges (92,104). To understand the variation of features in absence epilepsies, it is best to regard these disorders as lying on a neurobiologic continuum, with genetically determined, typical CAE at one end and acquired, severe, symptomatic generalized epilepsies at the other (92,135). Community-based practitioners see mainly classic CAE, whereas hospital-based series are weighted to the more complex and less typical cases.

Fong and coworkers suggested three subtypes of CAE and termed these ECA 1, 2, and 3 (136). ECA 1 (40% to 60% of all CAE patients) is characterized by dialeptic seizures that remit in adolescence (136). ECA 2 (40% of all CAE patients) is characterized by seizures that persist into adolescence and development of generalized tonic-clonic seizures. ECA 3 (10% of all CAE patients) presents with features of ECA 2. In addition, patients with ECA 3 also have myoclonic seizures (136). ECA 1 has been linked to chromosome 8q24 (136,137). ECA 2 and 3 are associated with mutations in the *GABRG2* gene on 5q31.1 (138) (see "Etiology and Genetics" under "Generalized Epilepsy with Febrile Seizures PlusGEFS+") and the *CLCN2* gene on 3q26 (12) (see "Genetics and Etiology" under "Juvenile Myoclonic Epilepsy").

Treatment

Both ethosuximide and valproate suppress absence seizures in more than 80% of patients (13,28,91,99,120, 139–141). Because valproate is associated with rare hepatotoxic reactions and other adverse effects, ethosuximide is recommended as the first choice for younger children. However, valproate is at least as effective as ethosuximide and produces fewer neurotoxic side effects. Hepatotoxicity is not an issue in children with CAE.

Ethosuximide does not suppress tonic-clonic seizures, whereas valproate is highly effective. In patients with both absence and tonic-clonic attacks, valproate is clearly preferred. In the past, patients with both seizure types required combination therapy with ethosuximide and phenytoin, carbamazepine, or a barbiturate; this strategy is no longer appropriate.

Patients with refractory absences comprise a small but important minority. Penry (120) and Dieterich and colleagues (99) estimated that in fewer than 5% of cases is the disease truly refractory to modern treatment, although the generally quoted figure is 20% (91,139). Valproate and ethosuximide should be tried sequentially and then in combination. Side effects may limit the use of benzodiazepines (clonazepam, nitrazepam, clobazam). Acetazolamide occasionally is effective. The diones (trimethadione and paramethadione) were the first efficacious antiabsence drugs, but toxic side effects resulted in discontinuation of their use in this application.

Among the newer AEDs, lamotrigine appears effective (142–145). Gabapentin is ineffective (146), as is topiramate. Tiagabine and vigabatrin are contraindicated in the treatment of absence seizures (86,147).

The decision to stop therapy is often difficult. A minimum seizure-free interval of 2 years is usually recommended before withdrawal of medication, but each case must be evaluated individually in terms of attitude of patient and family, participation in sports activities, occupation, and, in adolescents, driving an automobile. The EEG findings may help guide the decision (148), but occasional brief epileptiform discharges should not preclude drug withdrawal in the seizure-free patient.

Outcome and Prognosis

CAE is one of the relatively benign childhood epilepsies, but not all patients become seizure free. The prognosis of absence epilepsies has generated considerable debate in the literature, probably because some series included a high proportion of children with intellectual retardation, focal signs, atypical spike-and-wave discharges, or abnormal EEG background activity. Such patients do not have true CAE but lie toward the middle of the neurobiologic continuum of generalized epilepsies (10). Completeness of follow-up is also a problem; patients with persisting seizures are more likely to continue with clinic visits, whereas those in remission may be hard to trace. Remission occurs usually between 10 and 12 years of age.

The response rate of absence seizures in CAE ranges from 80% to as high as 95% (13,99,120). Before the discovery of effective drugs, absences were known to remit usually by mid-adolescence (90). Absence seizures persisting into adult life are rare, but occasional cases have continued into old age (149,150) or presented *de novo* in adulthood (151). Adults with persisting absence seizures did not appear to have any specific distinguishing features and, in particular, did not demonstrate intellectual impairment or progressive dementia, despite having experienced millions of seizures during their life (149). Remission rates range from 21% to 89%, averaging about 50% (152).

Tonic-clonic seizures are the most likely to persist but are nearly always easy to control. Their occurrence or recurrence when medication is discontinued accounts for most adult patients with CAE who are not in remission (105). Remission rates are probably higher for patients who have only absence seizures than for those who also have tonic-clonic seizures (152). Polyspikes on the EEG are also a negative prognostic factor (153).

Early institution of effective therapy is believed to improve prognosis in terms of the later development of tonic-clonic seizures and relapse of absences (99,112,120, 150,154,155). Although no controlled data support this claim—nor could such studies be ethically countenanced—absences should be treated promptly with the aim of completely suppressing clinical attacks.

Despite normal intelligence and good response to treatment, up to one-third of patients (105,112,155,156) have poor social adaptation as a result of toxic drug reactions, attitude about the condition, or social prejudice, among other factors. Proper education and counseling of patient, family, and teachers, together with optimal medical management, should alleviate many of these problems (91).

Juvenile Absence Epilepsy

History

JAE has only recently been brought to general attention (1,122,157,158), although Doose and Janz and associates in Germany recognized it some years ago (26,37,114,117). Credit for distinguishing JAE as a separate syndrome belongs to the German authors. Many studies of absence epilepsy show the peak age of onset at 6 to 7 years (corresponding to CAE), with a second peak near 12 years (99,100,102,107,121,150) (corresponding to JAE).

Epidemiologic Factors

Because of the relatively recent differentiation of JAE and other absence epilepsies, little is known about specific etiologic factors, although those that determine CAE are probably operative in JAE. Studies in twins confirm the importance of genetic factors, with concordant clinical or EEG features seen in monozygous pairs (132). Contemporary review of Lennox's original material reveals similar findings. The frequency of a family history of seizures has not been extensively investigated but appears to resemble that in CAE (37,116,122,157).

Clinical Features

Age of Onset

Most cases begin near or after puberty, between 10 and 17 years of age (13,122). At the lower age limit, an overlap with CAE clearly occurs, and the neurobiologic relationship of these two disorders is undefined. In patients 10 to 12 years of age, it is unclear whether the presence of pyknoleptic absences, the onset of puberty, or the actual age of onset should be used to distinguish JAE from CAE (13,14). Onset in early adult life is unusual.

Neurologic Examination

Findings on neurologic examination are normal.

Seizures

Absences occur in all cases. Unlike the multiple clustered (pyknoleptic) pattern in CAE, which may involve dozens or hundreds of seizures per day, absences in JAE are relatively uncommon, with only one episode or a few episodes daily. According to Janz (37) and Wolf (122), the absences often have a retropulsive component, although this feature was not observed in a video-EEG study (53). Panayiotopoulos and colleagues (53) found that the absences of JAE were similar to those of CAE, except that consciousness was not as severely impaired as in the latter, even though the paroxysmal discharges were slightly

longer in JAE. Absences may sometimes be activated by calculation or spatial tasks (159).

Tonic-clonic seizures are considerably more common in JAE than in CAE, occurring in approximately 80% of patients (13,122,158). Usually the presenting feature and often appearing shortly after waking, they also may occur randomly throughout the day (14,122).

Absence status is relatively common, although it can be overlooked if not specifically sought in the history (92). In one series of 229 adolescents and adults with absence (158), 87 (38%) had absence status; however, those with JAE were not distinguished from patients with persisting CAE.

Myoclonic seizures occur in approximately 15% of patients, raising the issue of differential diagnosis of JME (14,37,122). In that syndrome, the myoclonic seizures are prominent and characteristic, whereas absences occur in only a minority of cases and are fleeting and subtle (52,160). In JAE the reverse is true: myoclonic seizures should be infrequent and inconspicuous. The clinical overlap suggests that JAE and JME share some underlying genetic determinants (14,52,122).

Electroencephalographic Findings

Interictal Electroencephalography

The electroencephalogram, the key investigation tool, shows generalized spike-and-wave discharges. Although generally similar to those in CAE, the discharges in JAE are slightly less regular and rhythmic and may be faster, with multiple spike-and-wave formations. The discharges are induced by hyperventilation, but photosensitivity is unusual. Background activity is normal (14,122,160).

Ictal Electroencephalography

The ictal electroencephalogram presents with 3-Hz spike-and-wave complexes (slightly less regular and faster) and polyspikes.

Etiology and Genetics

Because of the relatively recent differentiation of JAE and other absence epilepsies, little is known about specific etiologic factors, although the factors that determine CAE are probably operative in JAE. Studies in twins confirm the importance of genetic factors, with concordant clinical or EEG features seen in monozygous pairs (132). Contemporary review of Lennox's original material reveals similar findings. The frequency of a family history of seizures has not been extensively investigated but appears to resemble that in CAE (37,116,122,157).

Sander and colleagues identified a new IGE susceptibility (including JAE) locus at 3q26 via linkage analysis (161). The *CLCN2* gene at 3q26 causing increased intracellular chloride concentration and hyperexcitability was described by Haug and associates in 2003 (65) (see also sections "Juvenile Myoclonic Epilepsy," "Childhood Absence Epilepsy," and "Epilepsy with Generalized Tonic-Clonic Seizures Only").

Treatment

Valproate is an effective choice, satisfactorily controlling absences, absence status, and tonic-clonic seizures (14, 92,122). Lamotrigine, either in combination with valproate or as monotherapy, can be effective for both absences and tonic-clonic seizures (142). If these strategies fail, a therapeutic response is somewhat remote, but ethosuximide or acetazolamide in combination with valproate can be tried. Carbamazepine may be considered for refractory tonic-clonic seizures, but may worsen absences (162–164). Education about the disorder, attention to drug compliance, avoidance of sleep deprivation, and moderation in, if not abstinence from, alcohol consumption are essential components of management in the adolescent patient.

Outcome and Prognosis

At least 80% of patients can be treated with valproate alone (158). Absences usually respond well to therapy, as do tonic-clonic seizures, but unlike CAE, in which most patients eventually become seizure free, the long-term evolution of JAE has not yet been properly characterized.

Epilepsy with Generalized Tonic-Clonic Seizures Only

History

"Epilepsy with generalized tonic-clonic seizures only" was first described as a separate syndrome by the ILAE in its most recent proposed diagnostic scheme for people with epileptic seizures and epilepsy (165). It includes "Epilepsy with generalized tonic clonic seizures on awakening," which was previously described as a separate syndrome.

Frequent seizures after awakening were first described by Gowers in 1885 (166). Epilepsy with generalized tonic-clonic seizures on awakening or "Aufwach-Epilepsie" was first described as a syndrome by Janz in 1953 (167). At this point it remains unclear whether the ILAE meant to include solely patients with generalized tonic-clonic seizures (GTCSs), or intends also to include patients with less frequent dialeptic and myoclonic seizures.

Epidemiology

The prevalence of this syndrome depends on the interpretation of the syndrome. Patients with GTCSs as the sole clinical manifestation comprise approximately 1% of all patients with generalized epilepsy, whereas patients with predominantly GTCSs and also dialeptic and myoclonic seizures represent up to 15% of all patients with generalized epilepsies (168). Males are more frequently affected than females and this may be related to seizure provocation by increased alcohol intake.

Clinical Features

Age of Onset

The peak age of onset is at the end of the second decade, with an age range between 5 and 50 years.

Exam

Neurologic examination and imaging are normal and other tests, except for electroencephalography, do not reveal any other neurologic abnormalities.

Seizures

The predominant seizure type is generalized tonic-clonic. Dialeptic seizures and myoclonic seizures are seen less frequently. Seizures are mainly provoked by alcohol and sleep deprivation, and can also be brought out by photic stimulation. Seizures tend to worsen with age. Wolf reported generalized tonic-clonic seizures on awakening in 17% to 53%, during wakefulness in 23% to 36%, during sleep in 27% to 44%, and not related to pattern in 13% to 26% of patients (169). In the subcategory of generalized tonic-clonic seizures on awakening, GTCSs occur in more than 90% within 1 to 2 hours after awakening or at the end of the day (during relaxation, "Feierabend"), with only rare myoclonic or dialeptic seizures (170). Unterberger and coworkers compared epilepsy with generalized tonic-clonic seizures on awakening and randomly occurring GTCSs and found that patients with early morning seizures had a longer duration of epilepsy, a higher relapse rate, and a stronger relationship to seizure-provoking factors (171).

Electroencephalography

Interictal features on electroencephalography consist of generalized epileptiform discharges presenting either as generalized 4- to 5-Hz spike-and-waves and spike-and-wave complexes or as generalized polyspikes. Discharges can be seen bilaterally with occasional asynchrony or asymmetry of bursts.

Ictal electroencephalography is characterized by generalized fast rhythmic spiking with a bifrontal maximum during the tonic phase of a GTCS. EEG activity is frequently obscured by tonic or clonic muscle artifact. Spiking can be asymmetric and asynchronous. This activity slows down and evolves into discontinuous repetitive generalized bursts of generalized (poly)spikes and waves intermingled with rhythmic slow waves. Clonic jerks start approximately at a spike frequency of 4 Hz. Postictally, electrical activity is reduced and can occasionally appear silent (less than 10 μV) for a brief period and is usually followed by irregular diffuse slowing.

Etiology and Genetics

Patients with epilepsy with GTCSs only frequently have a positive family history of epilepsy. Different mutations in unrelated families of the chloride channel-2 gene (*CLCN2*) on chromosome 3q26-qter are associated with generalized tonic-clonic seizures on awakening (65). Of note, CAE, JAE, and JME are also found in families with this mutation (65) (OMIM 607628).

Treatment

Monotherapy with lamotrigine or valproate is recommended, with valproate having higher efficacy and lamotrigine fewer side effects. Other options include topiramate, levetiracetam, and zonisamide. If the maximum tolerated dose does not reduce seizure frequency, an alternative medication should be tried. In case of monotherapy failure, combination therapy of lamotrigine and valproate may be effective (172). Gabapentin is not helpful (173). Tiagabine (174) and vigabatrin (175) may exacerbate dialeptic seizures. Moreover, the prevention of precipitating factors of seizures, such as sleep deprivation and alcohol intake, and drug treatment are beneficial.

Outcome and Prognosis

The prognosis of patients with GTCSs of unknown cause is very good and usually better than in patients with focal epilepsy and secondary generalized seizures (176). Up to 95% of patients with GTCSs of unknown cause will have a continuous 5-year seizure-free period within 20 years after epilepsy onset (176). Of patients who have been seizure free for 5 years or longer, 21% relapse within a 20-year observation period (176). Frequency of GTCS at the time of diagnosis predicts outcome and remission (177). Failure to remit within 2 years of diagnosis reduces the chance of remission in the following years (178).

Generalized Epilepsy with Febrile Seizures Plus (GEFS+)

History

Approximately 2% to 5% of children younger than age 6 years are affected by febrile seizures (179). Few children with febrile seizures actually continue to have afebrile seizures later in life. Although febrile seizures usually are related to multigenetic inheritance, an autosomal dominant form was described by Scheffer and Berkovic in 1997 in a large Australian family with variable seizure phenotype on a background of febrile seizures (180). In 1998, Wallace and coworkers reported linkage in a region on chromosome 19q13.1 encoding for a subunit of a voltage-gated sodium channel (SCN1B) (181). This has been identified as generalized epilepsy with febrile seizures plus (GEFS+) type 1.

In 1999, Baulac and colleagues investigated a family with clinical presentation of GEFS+ in three generations and excluded linkage to the previously described SCN1B as well as to FEB1 and FEB2 in a French family. They found a new locus on chromosome 2q21-33 in the region of alpha subunits of a sodium channel (SCN1A) (182). In the same year, Moulard and associates identified another family with GEFS+ and linkage to 2q24-q33 in a different French family (183). Escayg and coworkers showed that both French families had mutations in the SCN1A gene, but presented with different amino acid substitutions (64). This mutation has been identified as GEFS+ type 2.

In 2001, Baulac and colleagues (184) and Wallace and associates (138) found a GABA-A (gamma-subunit) mutation (GABRG2) located on chromosome 5q34. This type has been termed GEFS+ type 3.

GEFS+ is associated with an extremely variable phenotype and may clinically overlap with other IGEs. Differences in phenotypic presentation may be related to additional modifying genes, additional susceptibility, and environmental factors.

Epidemiology

According to the most recently proposed diagnostic scheme "generalized epilepsies with febrile seizure plus" (GEFS+) is considered a "syndrome in development." It is a rare syndrome that has been described in at least 21 family pedigrees (185).

Clinical Features

GEFS+ mutations have been described to overlap with myoclonic-astatic epilepsy, JME, CAE, generalized epilepsy with generalized tonic-clonic seizures only (186), and focal epilepsies such as frontal and temporal lobe epilepsy (182,183,187,188). Therefore, the phenotypic spectrum is extremely variable and clinical features may overlap with other IGEs and even with focal epilepsies.

Most patients with GEFS+ present with multiple febrile seizures in early childhood. Febrile seizures persisting beyond the age of 6 years may be associated with afebrile, usually generalized, and in rare instances focal, seizures. Seizures can persist into late adolescence or longer, but usually remit in the early teenage years. A history of febrile seizures in other family members is crucial to the diagnosis.

Age of Onset

Febrile seizures begin approximately at the age of 1 year, slightly earlier than in the average infant with febrile seizures. Onset of afebrile seizures may overlap with febrile seizures or may occur after a seizure-free interval between febrile and afebrile seizures.

Exam

Neurologic examination is usually normal. Among 53 patients with GEFS+ type 2, only one patient presented with mild learning difficulties (188). Mild developmental (187) and intellectual (188) impairment have been described.

Seizures

Clinical seizures consist of febrile seizures in association with afebrile seizures presenting as GTCSs, dialeptic seizures (absences), occasionally associated with automatisms (187), myoclonic, atonic, and tonic seizures (185). Unilateral clonic seizures (182,180) and unilateral face motor seizures (189), as well as visual and psychic auras (187), have also been described in affected family members. Seizures usually persist beyond 6 years of age, until adolescence or longer.

Electroencephalography

The syndrome lacks a clear electroclinical pattern and interictal electroencephalography can be normal. However, interictal epileptiform discharges frequently consist of irregular generalized spike and waves or polyspikes with infrequent 2- to 3-Hz generalized spike-and-wave complexes (180). As a consequence of variable clinical presentations, interictal electroencephalography may also present with focal epileptiform discharges, for example, in the frontal, temporal, and occipital regions (186,187).

Etiology and Genetics

The mode of inheritance is autosomal dominant (OMIM 604233). Incomplete penetrance of genes leads to a large variability in phenotypic presentation. The following subtypes have been described:

> GEFS+ type 1 consists of a mutation in the SCN1B gene and maps to the chromosomal region 19q13.1. This gene encodes the μ_1 subunit of a sodium channel and interferes with modulation of channel gating (181,190,191).

> GEFS+ type 2 is defined by a mutation in the SCN1A gene located at 2q21-33. This gene encodes the α_1 subunit which forms the opening of a sodium channel. Changes result in hyperexcitability of the neuron, predominantly by altered inactivation of the channel (63,64,182,183,187,192–196).

> GEFS+ type 3 has a mutation in the GABRG2 gene which maps to 5q31-33. This gene encodes the γ_2 subunit at the benzodiazepine binding site of the GABA$_A$ receptor (138,184,186,197,198).

SCN2A

A mutation of the SCN2A gene encoding the α_2 subunit of a sodium channel has been identified as the underlying mutation in a patient with GEFS+ and may constitute a new GEFS+ gene at location 2q21-33 (196).

In 2002, Gerard and coworkers were able to exclude all known genes for febrile seizures and GEFS+ by linkage analysis in a newly discovered multigenerational family in France (189). These findings may suggest an additional GEFS+ genetic locus for this phenotype of febrile seizures that persist beyond the age of 6 years and for afebrile seizures (189).

Treatment

The decision to treat pharmacologically should be based on seizure frequency and severity of afebrile seizures. Clinical presentation and individual seizure types should determine the treatment approach and selection of AED if applicable. Because of the paucity of reported cases (approximately 160 reported individuals to date [185]), little information on the efficacy of specific pharmacologic treatments is available. Gerard and coworkers report pharmacologic treatment in 6 of 15 affected individuals "with success and seizure control in most" (189). Interestingly, in one family with a mutation in the GABRG2 gene (GEFS+ type 3), decreased benzodiazepine sensitivity was reported (188).

Prognosis

The prognosis is usually very good. Spontaneous remission occurs frequently in the early teenage years (age 10 to 12 years) (185). However, seizures can persist, and several other epilepsy syndromes can develop (CAE, JME, myoclonic astatic epilepsy, focal epilepsy) (186).

Idiopathic Generalized Epilepsy Syndromes as Part of the Generalized Epilepsy Spectrum

Overall, the types of IGE syndromes just described share many similarities. According to Janz (37), 4.6% of CAE cases evolve into JME when patients reach the usual age of JME onset. A population-based study of 81 children with CAE found that 15% had progressed to JME 9 to 25 years after seizure onset (123). In this study, the development of generalized tonic-clonic or myoclonic seizures in a patient with CAE receiving AEDs made the progression to JME highly likely (123). Syndromes manifest with the same seizure types, have similar EEG changes, may evolve into one another, and have overlapping genetic origins. Findings of neurologic examination as well as imaging studies are normal. Therefore, IGEs may be viewed as a continuous spectrum of conditions, representing a single entity with slightly different phenotypes (11–14,135).

REFERENCES

1. Commission on Classification and Terminology of the International League Against Epilepsy. Proposal for revised classification of epilepsies and epileptic syndromes. *Epilepsia* 1989;30:389–399.
2. Commission on Classification and Terminology of the International League Against Epilepsy. Proposal for revised clinical and electroencephalographic classification of epileptic seizures. *Epilepsia* 1981;22:489–501.
3. Engel J Jr. A proposed diagnostic scheme for people with epileptic seizures and with epilepsy: report of the ILAE Task Force on Classification and Terminology. *Epilepsia* 2001;42:796–803.
4. Mattson RH. Overview: idiopathic generalized epilepsies. *Epilepsia* 2003;44(Suppl 2):2–6.
5. Woermann FG, Sisodiya SM, Free SL, et al. Quantitative MRI in patients with idiopathic generalized epilepsy. Evidence of widespread cerebral structural changes. *Brain* 1998;121(Pt 9):1661–1667.
6. Woermann FG, Free SL, Koepp MJ, et al. Abnormal cerebral structure in juvenile myoclonic epilepsy demonstrated with voxel-based analysis of MRI. *Brain* 1999;122(Pt 11):2101–2108.
7. Nersesyan H, Hyder F, Rothman D, et al. BOLD fMRI and electrophysiological recordings of spike-wave seizures in WAG/Rij rats. *Epilepsia* 2002;43(Suppl 7):272.
8. Meeren HK, Pijn JP, Van Luijtelaar EL, et al. Cortical focus drives widespread corticothalamic networks during spontaneous absence seizures in rats. *J Neurosci* 2002;22:1480–1495.
9. Middeldorp CM, Geerts AT, Brouwer OF, et al. Nonsymptomatic generalized epilepsy in children younger than six years: excellent prognosis, but classification should be reconsidered after follow-up: the Dutch Study of Epilepsy in Childhood. *Epilepsia* 2002;43:734–739.
10. Berkovic SF, Andermann F, Andermann E, et al. Concepts of absence epilepsies: discrete syndromes or biological continuum? *Neurology* 1987;37:993–1000.
11. Briellmann RS, Torn-Broers Y, Berkovic SF. Idiopathic generalized epilepsies: do sporadic and familial cases differ? *Epilepsia* 2001;42:1399–1402.

12. Janz D. Juvenile myoclonic epilepsy. Epilepsy with impulsive petit mal. *Cleve Clin J Med* 1989;56(Suppl Pt 1):S23–S33.

13. Loiseau P, Duche B, Pedespan JM. Absence epilepsies. *Epilepsia* 1995;36:1182–1186.

14. Reutens DC, Berkovic SF. Idiopathic generalized epilepsy of adolescence: are the syndromes clinically distinct? *Neurology* 1995;45:1469–1476.

15. Kellinghaus C, Loddenkemper T, Najm IM, et al. Specific epileptic syndromes are rare even in tertiary epilepsy centers: a patient-oriented approach to epilepsy classification. *Epilepsia* 2004;45: 268–275.

16. Winawer MR, Rabinowitz D, Pedley TA, et al. Genetic influences on myoclonic and absence seizures. *Neurology* 2003;61: 1576–1581.

17. Benbadis SR, Tatum WO, Gieron M. Idiopathic generalized epilepsy and choice of antiepileptic drugs. *Neurology* 2003;61: 1793–1795.

18. Temkin O. *The falling sickness: a history of epilepsy from the Greeks to the beginning of modern neurology.* Baltimore, MD: Johns Hopkins Press, 1971.

19. Friedreich N. Neuropathologische Beobbachtung beim Paramyoklonus Multiplex. *Virchows Arch Pathol Anat Physiol* 1881;86: 421–434.

20. Delasiauve LJF. *Traité de l'épilepsie.* Paris: Masson, 1854.

21. Gowers WR. *Epilepsy and other chronic diseases.* London: John Churchill, 1881.

22. Féré C. *Les épilepsies et les épileptiques.* Paris: Alcan, 1890.

23. Reynolds JR. *Epilepsy: its symptoms, treatment and relation to other chronic convulsive diseases. London:* John Churchill, 1861.

24. Herpin TH. *Des accès incomplets de l'épilepsie.* Paris: J Balliere et Fils, 1867.

25. Penfield W, Jasper H. *Epilepsy and the functional anatomy of the human brain.* Boston: Little, Brown, 1954.

26. Janz D, Christian W. Impulsive petit mal. *Dtsch Z Nervenheilk* 1957;176:346–386.

27. Castells C, Medilaharsu C. La epilepsia mioclonica bilateral y consciente. *Acta Neurol Latinoam* 1958;4:23–48.

28. Jeavons PM, Clark JE, Maheshwari MC. Treatment of generalized epilepsies of childhood and adolescence with sodium valproate ("epilim"). *Dev Med Child Neurol* 1977;19:9–25.

29. Jeavons PM. Nosological problems of myoclonic epilepsies in childhood and adolescence. *Dev Med Child Neurol* 1977;19:3–8.

30. Asconape J, Penry JK. Some clinical and EEG aspects of benign juvenile myoclonic epilepsy. *Epilepsia* 1984;25:108–114.

31. Delgado-Escueta AV, Enrile-Bacsal F. Juvenile myoclonic epilepsy of Janz. *Neurology* 1984;34:285–294.

32. Janz D. Juvenile myoclonic epilepsy. In: Dam M, Gram L, eds. *Comprehensive epileptology.* New York: Raven Press, 1990:171–185.

33. Obeid T, Panayiotopoulos CP. Clonazepam in juvenile myoclonic epilepsy. *Epilepsia* 1989;30:603–606.

34. Tsuboi T. Primary generalized epilepsy with sporadic myoclonias of myoclonic petit mal type. Stuttgart: Thieme, 1977.

35. Wolf P, Goosses R. Relation of photosensitivity to epileptic syndromes. *J Neurol Neurosurg Psychiatry* 1986;49:1386–1391.

36. Lee AG, Delgado-Escueta AV, Maldonado HM, et al. Closed-circuit television videotaping and electroencephalography biotelemetry (video/EEG) in primary generalized epilepsies. In: Gumnit R, ed. *Intensive neurodiagnostic monitoring.* New York: Raven Press, 1986:27–68.

37. Janz D. *Die Epilepsien.* Stuttgart: Thieme, 1969.

38. Gram L, Alving J, Sagild JC, et al. Juvenile myoclonic epilepsy in unexpected age groups. *Epilepsy Res* 1988;2:137–140.

39. Serratosa JM. Juvenile myoclonic epilepsy. In: Wyllie E, ed. *The treatment of epilepsy: principles & practice,* 3rd ed. Philadelphia: Lippincott Williams & Wilkins, 2001:491–507.

40. Touchon J. Effect of awakening on epileptic activity in primary generalized myoclonic epilepsy. In: Sterman MB, Shouse MN, Passouant P, eds. *Sleep and epilepsy.* New York: Academic Press, 1982:239–248.

41. Janz D. Epilepsy and the sleep-waking cycle. In: Vinken PJ, Bruym GW, eds. *Handbook of clinical neurology,* vol 15. New York: Elsevier Science, 1974:15.

42. Mattson R, Linda Fay M, Sturman J, et al. The effect of various patterns of alcohol use on seizures in patients with epilepsy. In: Porter

R, Mattson R, Cramer J, et al., eds. *Alcohol and seizures: basic mechanisms and clinical concepts.* Philadelphia: FA Davis, 1990:233–240.

43. Ferrendelli J, Delgado-Escueta A, Dreifuss F, et al. Panel discussion. *Epilepsia* 1989;40:S24–S27.

44. Swartz BE, Simpkins F, Halgren E, et al. Visual working memory in primary generalized epilepsy: an ^{18}FDG-PET study. *Neurology* 1996;47:1203–1212.

45. Lancman ME, Asconape JJ, Penry JK. Clinical and EEG asymmetries in juvenile myoclonic epilepsy. *Epilepsia* 1994;35:302–306.

46. Oguni H, Mukahira K, Oguni M, et al. Video-polygraphic analysis of myoclonic seizures in juvenile myoclonic epilepsy. *Epilepsia* 1994;35:307–316.

47. Delgado-Escueta AV, Treiman DM, Enrile-Bascal F. Phenotypic variations of seizures in adolescents and adults. In: Andersen V, Hauser W, Penry J, et al., eds. *Genetic basis of the epilepsies.* New York: Raven Press, 1982:49–81.

48. Tassinari C, Bureau M. Epilepsy with myoclonic absences. In: Roger J, Bureau M, Dravet C, et al., eds. *Epileptic syndromes in infancy, childhood and adolescence,* 2nd ed. London: John Libbey, 1992:151–160.

49. Salas Puig J, Tunon A, Vidal JA, et al. Janz's juvenile myoclonic epilepsy: a little-known frequent syndrome [Spanish]. A study of 85 patients. *Med Clin (Barc)* 1994;103:684–689.

50. Obeid T, Panayiotopoulos CP. Juvenile myoclonic epilepsy: a study in Saudi Arabia. *Epilepsia* 1988;29:280–282.

51. Janz D. The natural history of primary generalized epilepsies with sporadic myoclonias of the "impulsive petit mal" type. In: Lugaresi E, Pazzaglia P, Tassinari C, eds. *Evolution and prognosis of epilepsies.* Bologna: Aulo Gaggi, 1973:55–61.

52. Janz D. Epilepsy with impulsive petit mal (juvenile myoclonic epilepsy). *Acta Neurol Scand* 1985;72:449–459.

53. Panayiotopoulos CP, Obeid T, Waheed G. Absences in juvenile myoclonic epilepsy: a clinical and video-electroencephalographic study. *Ann Neurol* 1989;25:391–397.

54. Tsuboi T, Christian W. On the genetics of the primary generalized epilepsy with sporadic myoclonias of impulsive petit mal type. A clinical and electroencephalographic study of 399 probands. *Humangenetik* 1973;19:155–182.

55. Greenberg DA, Delgado-Escueta AV, Maldonado HM, et al. Segregation analysis of juvenile myoclonic epilepsy. *Genet Epidemiol* 1988;5:81–94.

56. Greenberg DA, Delgado-Escueta AV. The chromosome 6p epilepsy locus: exploring mode of inheritance and heterogeneity through linkage analysis. *Epilepsia* 1993;34(Suppl 3):S12–S18.

57. Delgado-Escueta AV, Greenberg D, Weissbecker K, et al. Gene mapping in the idiopathic generalized epilepsies: juvenile myoclonic epilepsy, childhood absence epilepsy, epilepsy with grand mal seizures, and early childhood myoclonic epilepsy. *Epilepsia* 1990;31(Suppl 3):S19–S29.

58. Durner M, Sander T, Greenberg DA, et al. Localization of idiopathic generalized epilepsy on chromosome 6p in families of juvenile myoclonic epilepsy patients. *Neurology* 1991;41:1651–1655.

59. Greenberg DA, Delgado-Escueta AV, Widelitz H, et al. Juvenile myoclonic epilepsy (JME) may be linked to the BF and HLA loci on human chromosome 6. *Am J Med Genet* 1988;31:185–192.

60. Whitehouse WP, Rees M, Curtis D, et al. Linkage analysis of idiopathic generalized epilepsy (IGE) and marker loci on chromosome 6p in families of patients with juvenile myoclonic epilepsy: no evidence for an epilepsy locus in the HLA region. *Am J Hum Genet* 1993;53:652–662.

61. Serratosa JM, Delgado-Escueta AV, Medina MT, et al. Clinical and genetic analysis of a large pedigree with juvenile myoclonic epilepsy. *Ann Neurol* 1996;39:187–195.

62. Panayiotopoulos CP, Obeid T. Juvenile myoclonic epilepsy: an autosomal recessive disease. *Ann Neurol* 1989;25:440–443.

63. Cossette P, Loukas A, Lafreniere RG, et al. Functional characterization of the D188V mutation in neuronal voltage-gated sodium channel causing generalized epilepsy with febrile seizures plus (GEFS+). *Epilepsy Res* 2003;53:107–117.

64. Escayg A, MacDonald BT, Meisler MH, et al. Mutations of SCN1A, encoding a neuronal sodium channel, in two families with GEFS+2. *Nat Genet* 2000;24:343–345.

65. Haug K, Warnstedt M, Alekov AK, et al. Mutations in CLCN2 encoding a voltage-gated chloride channel are associated with idiopathic generalized epilepsies. *Nat Genet* 2003;33:527–532.

66. Bai D, Alonso ME, Medina MT, et al. Juvenile myoclonic epilepsy: linkage to chromosome 6p12 in Mexico families. *Am J Med Genet* 2002;113:268–274.

67. Liu AW, Delgado-Escueta AV, Serratosa JM, et al. Juvenile myoclonic epilepsy locus in chromosome 6p21.2-p11: linkage to convulsions and electroencephalography trait. *Am J Hum Genet* 1995;57:368–381.

68. Liu AW, Delgado-Escueta AV, Gee MN, et al. Juvenile myoclonic epilepsy in chromosome 6p12-p11: locus heterogeneity and recombinations. *Am J Med Genet* 1996;63:438–446.

69. Pinto D, de Haan GJ, Janssen GA, et al. Evidence for linkage between juvenile myoclonic epilepsy-related idiopathic generalized epilepsy and 6p11-12 in Dutch families. *Epilepsia* 2004;45:211–217.

70. Suzuki T, Delgado-Escueta AV, Aguan K, et al. Mutations in EFHC1 cause juvenile myoclonic epilepsy. *Nat Genet* 2004;36:842–849.

71. Phillips HA, Scheffer IE, Berkovic SF, et al. Localization of a gene for autosomal dominant nocturnal frontal lobe epilepsy to chromosome 20q 13.2. *Nat Genet* 1995;10:117–118.

72. Scheffer IE, Bhatia KP, Lopes-Cendes I, et al. Autosomal dominant nocturnal frontal lobe epilepsy. A distinctive clinical disorder. *Brain* 1995;118(Pt 1):61–73.

73. Steinlein OK, Mulley JC, Propping P, et al. A missense mutation in the neuronal nicotinic acetylcholine receptor alpha 4 subunit is associated with autosomal dominant nocturnal frontal lobe epilepsy. *Nat Genet* 1995;11:201–203.

74. Elmslie FV, Rees M, Williamson MP, et al. Genetic mapping of a major susceptibility locus for juvenile myoclonic epilepsy on chromosome 15q. *Hum Mol Genet* 1997;6:1329–1334.

75. Pal DK, Evgrafov OV, Tabares P, et al. BRD2 (RING3) is a probable major susceptibility gene for common juvenile myoclonic epilepsy. *Am J Hum Genet* 2003;73:261–270.

76. Sander T, Hildmann T, Janz D, et al. The phenotypic spectrum related to the human epilepsy susceptibility gene "EJM1." *Ann Neurol* 1995;38:210–217.

77. Weissbecker KA, Durner M, Janz D, et al. Confirmation of linkage between juvenile myoclonic epilepsy locus and the HLA region of chromosome 6. *Am J Med Genet* 1991;38:32–36.

78. Sander T, Bockenkamp B, Hildmann T, et al. Refined mapping of the epilepsy susceptibility locus EJM1 on chromosome 6. *Neurology* 1997;49:842–847.

79. Covanis A, Gupta AK, Jeavons PM. Sodium valproate: monotherapy and polytherapy. *Epilepsia* 1982;23:693–720.

80. Delgado-Escueta AV, Treiman DM, Walsh GO. The treatable epilepsies. *N Engl J Med* 1983;308:1508–1514.

81. Penry JK, Dean JC, Riela AR. Juvenile myoclonic epilepsy: long-term response to therapy. *Epilepsia* 1989;30(Suppl 4):S19–S23.

82. Buchanan N. The use of lamotrigine in juvenile myoclonic epilepsy. *Seizure* 1996;5:149–151.

83. Kellett MW, Smith DF, Stockton PA, et al. Topiramate in clinical practice: first year's postlicensing experience in a specialist epilepsy clinic. *J Neurol Neurosurg Psychiatry* 1999;66:759–763.

84. Genton P, Gelisse P, Thomas P, et al. Do carbamazepine and phenytoin aggravate juvenile myoclonic epilepsy? *Neurology* 2000;55:1106–1109.

85. Resor SR Jr, Resor LD. Chronic acetazolamide monotherapy in the treatment of juvenile myoclonic epilepsy. *Neurology* 1990;40:1677–1681.

86. Knake S, Hamer HM, Schomburg U, et al. Tiagabine-induced absence status in idiopathic generalized epilepsy. *Seizure* 1999;8:314–317.

87. Krauss GL, Betts T, Abou-Khalil B, et al. Levetiracetam treatment of idiopathic generalised epilepsy. *Seizure* 2003;12:617–620.

88. Mullin P, Stern J, Delgado-Escueta AV, et al. Effectiveness of open-label zonisamide in juvenile myoclonic epilepsy. *Epilepsia* 2001;42(Suppl 7):184.

89. Resor SR Jr, Resor LD. The neuropharmacology of juvenile myoclonic epilepsy. *Clin Neuropharmacol* 1990;13:465–491.

90. Adie WJ. Pyknolepsy: a form of epilepsy occurring in children with a good prognosis. *Brain* 1924;47:96–102.

91. Drury I, Dreifuss FE. Pyknoleptic petit mal. *Acta Neurol Scand* 1985;72:353–362.

92. Berkovic SF, Andermann F, Guberman A, et al. Valproate prevents the recurrence of absence status. *Neurology* 1989;39:1294–1297.

93. Chadwick D. Gabapentin and felbamate. In: Duncan JS, Panayiotopoulos CP, eds. *Typical absences and related epileptic syndromes*. London: Elsevier, 1995:376–380.

94. Duncan JS, Panayiotopoulos CP. Juvenile absence epilepsy: an alternative view. In: Duncan JS, Panayiotopoulos CP, eds. *Typical absences and related epileptic syndromes*. London: Elsevier, 1995:167–173.

95. Genton P. Epilepsy with 3 Hz spike-and-waves without clinically evident absences. In: Duncan JS, Panayiotopoulos CP, eds. *Typical absences and related epileptic syndromes*. London: Elsevier, 1995:231–238.

96. Gumnit RJ, Niedermeyer E, Spreen O. Seizure activity uniquely inhibited by patterned vision. *Arch Neurol* 1965;13:363–368.

97. Olsson I. Epidemiology of absence epilepsy, I: concept and incidence. *Acta Paediatr Scand* 1988;77:860–866.

98. Juul-Jensen P, Foldspang A. Natural history of epileptic seizures. *Epilepsia* 1983;24:297–312.

99. Dieterich E, Baier WK, Doose H, et al. Long-term follow-up of childhood epilepsy with absences, I: epilepsy with absences at onset. *Neuropediatrics* 1985;16:149–154.

100. Gibberd FB. The prognosis of petit mal. *Brain* 1966;89:531–538.

101. Hirsch E, Blanc-Platier A, Marescaux C. What are the relevant criteria for a better classification of epileptic syndromes with typical absences? In: Malafosse A, Genton P, Hirsch E, et al., eds. *Idiopathic generalized epilepsies: clinical, experimental and genetic aspects*. London: John Libbey, 1995:87–93.

102. Sato S, Dreifuss FE, Penry JK. Prognostic factors in absence seizures. *Neurology* 1976;26:788–796.

103. Rocca WA, Sharbrough FW, Hauser WA, et al. Risk factors for absence seizures: a population-based case-control study in Rochester, Minnesota. *Neurology* 1987;37:1309–1314.

104. Holowach J, Thurston D, O'Leary JL. Petit mal epilepsy. *Pediatrics* 1962;60:893–901.

105. Loiseau P. Childhood absence epilepsy. In: Roger J, Bureau M, Dravet C, et al., eds. *Epileptic syndromes in infancy, childhood and adolescence*, 2nd ed. London: John Libbey, 1992:135–150.

106. Cavazzuti GB, Ferrari F, Galli V, et al. Epilepsy with typical absence seizures with onset during the first year of life. *Epilepsia* 1989;30:802–806.

107. Livingston S, Torres I, Pauli LL, et al. Petit mal epilepsy. Results of a prolonged follow-up study of 117 patients. *JAMA* 1965;194:227–232.

108. Penry JK, Dreifuss FE. A study of automatisms associated with the absence of petit mal. *Epilepsia* 1969;10:417–418.

109. Penry JK, Dreifuss FE. Automatisms associated with the absence of petit mal epilepsy. *Arch Neurol* 1969;21:142–149.

110. Yoshinaga H, Ohtsuka Y, Tamai K, et al. EEG in childhood absence epilepsy. *Seizure* 2004;13:296–302.

111. Charlton MH, Yahr MD. Long-term follow-up of patients with petit mal. *Arch Neurol* 1967;16:595–598.

112. Loiseau P, Pestre M, Dartigues JF, et al. Long-term prognosis in two forms of childhood epilepsy: typical absence seizures and epilepsy with rolandic (centrotemporal) EEG foci. *Ann Neurol* 1983;13:642–648.

113. Dalby MA. Epilepsy and 3 per second spike and wave rhythms. A clinical, electroencephalographic and prognostic analysis of 346 patients. *Acta Neurol Scand* 1969;45(Suppl):1–183.

114. Dieterich E, Doose H, Baier WK, et al. Long-term follow-up of childhood epilepsy with absences, II: absence-epilepsy with initial grand mal. *Neuropediatrics* 1985;16:155–158.

115. Doose H. Absence epilepsy of early childhood—genetic aspects. *Eur J Pediatr* 1994;153:372–377.

116. Doose H, Baier WK. Genetic factors in epilepsies with primary generalized minor seizures. *Neuropediatrics* 1987;18(Suppl 1):1–64.

117. Doose H, Volzke E, Scheffner D. Course forms of infantile epilepsies with spike waves absences [German]. *Arch Psychiatr Nervenkr* 1965;207:394–415.

118. Hedstrom A, Olsson I. Epidemiology of absence epilepsy: EEG findings and their predictive value. *Pediatr Neurol* 1991;7:100–104.

119. Panayiotopoulos CP. The clinical spectrum of typical absence seizures and absence epilepsies. In: Malafosse A, Genton P,

Hirsch E, et al., eds. *Idiopathic generalized epilepsies: clinical experimental and genetic aspects.* London: John Libbey, 1994:75–85.

120. Penry JK. Diagnosis and treatment of absence seizures. *Cleve Clin Q* 1984;51:283–286.

121. Sato S, Dreifuss FE, Penry JK, et al. Long-term follow-up of absence seizures. *Neurology* 1983;33:1590–1595.

122. Wolf P. Juvenile absence epilepsy. In: Roger J, Bureau M, Dravet C, eds. *Epileptic syndromes in infancy, childhood and adolescence,* 2nd ed. London: John Libbey, 1992:307–312.

123. Wirrell EC, Camfield CS, Camfield PR, et al. Long-term prognosis of typical childhood absence epilepsy: remission or progression to juvenile myoclonic epilepsy. *Neurology* 1996;47:912–918.

124. Aird RB, Gastaut Y. Occipital and posterior electroencephalographic rhythms. *Electroencephalogr Clin Neurophysiol* 1959;11:637–656.

125. Gerken H, Doose H. On the genetics of EEG-anomalies in childhood, 3: spikes and waves. *Neuropadiatrie* 1973;4:88–97.

126. Matthes A, Weber H. Clinical and electroencephalographic family studies on pyknolepsy [German]. *Dtsch Med Wochenschr* 1968;93:429–435.

127. Metrakos JD, Metrakos K. Childhood epilepsy of subcortical ("centrencephalic") origin. Some questions and answers for the pediatrician. *Clin Pediatr (Phila)* 1966;5:537–542.

128. Metrakos K, Metrakos JD. Genetics of convulsive disorders, II: genetic and electroencephalographic studies in centrencephalic epilepsy. *Neurology* 1961;11:474–483.

129. Metrakos K, Metrakos JD. Genetics of epilepsy. In: Vinken PJ, Bruyn GW, eds. *Handbook of clinical neurology,* vol 15. Amsterdam: North Holland, 1974:429–439.

130. Lennox W. The heredity of epilepsy as told by relatives and twins. *JAMA* 1951;146:529–536.

131. Lennox W, Lennox M. The genetics of epilepsy. *Epilepsy and related disorders.* Boston: Little, Brown, 1960:548–574.

132. Berkovic SF, Howell R, Hay D, et al. Epilepsies in twins. In: Wolf P, ed. *Epileptic seizures and syndromes.* London: John Libbey, 1994:157–164.

133. Andermann E. Multifactorial inheritance of generalized and focal epilepsy. In: Andersen V, Hauser WA, Penry JK, et al., eds. *Genetic basis of the epilepsies.* New York: Raven Press, 1982:355–374.

134. Andermann E. Genetic aspects of the epilepsies. In Sakai T, Tsuboi T, eds. *Genetic aspects of human behaviour.* Tokyo: Igaku-Shoin, 1985:129–145.

135. Berkovic SF, Reutens DC, Andermann E, et al. The epilepsies: specific syndromes or a neurobiological continuum? In: Wolf P, ed. *Epileptic seizures and syndromes.* London: John Libbey, 1994:25–37.

136. Fong GC, Shah PU, Gee MN, et al. Childhood absence epilepsy with tonic-clonic seizures and electroencephalogram 3–4-Hz spike and multispike-slow wave complexes: linkage to chromosome 8q24. *Am J Hum Genet* 1998;63:1117–1129.

137. Sugimoto Y, Morita R, Amano K, et al. Childhood absence epilepsy in 8q24: refinement of candidate region and construction of physical map. *Genomics* 2000;68:264–272.

138. Wallace RH, Marini C, Petrou S, et al. Mutant GABA(A) receptor gamma2-subunit in childhood absence epilepsy and febrile seizures. *Nat Genet* 2001;28:49–52.

139. Aicardi J. *Epilepsy in children.* New York: Raven Press, 1994.

140. Bourgeois B, Beaumanoir A, Blajev B, et al. Monotherapy with valproate in primary generalized epilepsies. *Epilepsia* 1987;28 (Supp 2):S8–S11.

141. Sato S, White BG, Penry JK, et al. Valproic acid versus ethosuximide in the treatment of absence seizures. *Neurology* 1982;32:157–163.

142. Brodie MJ. The treatment of typical absences in related epileptic syndromes. In: Duncan JS, Panayiotopoulos CP, eds. *Typical absences and related epileptic syndromes.* London: Churchill Communications, 1995:381–383.

143. Buoni S, Grosso S, Fois A. Lamotrigine in typical absence epilepsy. *Brain Dev* 1999;21:303–306.

144. Frank LM, Enlow T, Holmes GL, et al. Lamictal (lamotrigine) monotherapy for typical absence seizures in children. *Epilepsia* 1999;40:973–979.

145. Schlumberger E, Chavez F, Palacios L, et al. Lamotrigine in treatment of 120 children with epilepsy. *Epilepsia* 1994;35:359–367.

146. Trudeau V, Myers S, LaMoreaux L, et al. Gabapentin in naive childhood absence epilepsy: results from two double-blind, placebo-controlled, multicenter studies. *J Child Neurol* 1996;11:470–475.

147. Parker AP, Agathonikou A, Robinson RO, et al. Inappropriate use of carbamazepine and vigabatrin in typical absence seizures. *Dev Med Child Neurol* 1998;40:517–519.

148. Appleton RE, Beirne M. Absence epilepsy in children: the role of EEG in monitoring response to treatment. *Seizure* 1996;5:147–148.

149. Gastaut H, Zifkin BG, Mariani E, et al. The long-term course of primary generalized epilepsy with persisting absences. *Neurology* 1986;36:1021–1028.

150. Oller-Daurella L, Sanchez ME. Evolucion de las aussencias typicas. *Rev Neurol* 1981;9:81–102.

151. Thomas P, Beaumanoir A, Genton P, et al. 'De novo' absence status of late onset: report of 11 cases. *Neurology* 1992;42:104–110.

152. Bouma PA, Westendorp RG, van Dijk JG, et al. The outcome of absence epilepsy: a meta-analysis. *Neurology* 1996;47:802–808.

153. Bartolomei F, Roger J, Bureau M, et al. Prognostic factors for childhood and juvenile absence epilepsies. *Eur Neurol* 1997;37:169–175.

154. Dreifuss FE. Absence epilepsies. In: Dam M, Gram L, eds. *Comprehensive epileptology.* New York: Raven Press, 1991:145–153.

155. Hertoft P. The clinical, electroencephalographic and social prognosis in petit mal epilepsy. *Epilepsia* 1963;74:298–314.

156. Olsson I, Campenhausen G. Social adjustment in young adults with absence epilepsies. *Epilepsia* 1993;34:846–851.

157. Obeid T. Clinical and genetic aspects of juvenile absence epilepsy. *J Neurol* 1994;241:487–491.

158. Wolf P, Inoue Y. Therapeutic response of absence seizures in patients of an epilepsy clinic for adolescents and adults. *J Neurol* 1984;231:225–229.

159. Goossens LA, Andermann F, Andermann E, et al. Reflex seizures induced by calculation, card or board games, and spatial tasks: a review of 25 patients and delineation of the epileptic syndrome. *Neurology* 1990;40:1171–1176.

160. Panayiotopoulos CP, Obeid T, Waheed G. Differentiation of typical absence seizures in epileptic syndromes. A video EEG study of 224 seizures in 20 patients. *Brain* 1989;112(Pt 4):1039–1056.

161. Sander T, Schulz H, Saar K, et al. Genome search for susceptibility loci of common idiopathic generalised epilepsies. *Hum Mol Genet* 2000;9:1465–1472.

162. Callahan DJ, Noetzel MJ. Prolonged absence status epilepticus associated with carbamazepine therapy, increased intracranial pressure, and transient MRI abnormalities. *Neurology* 1992;42:2198–2201.

163. Liporace JD, Sperling MR, Dichter MA. Absence seizures and carbamazepine in adults. *Epilepsia* 1994;35:1026–1028.

164. Shields WD, Saslow E. Myoclonic, atonic, and absence seizures following institution of carbamazepine therapy in children. *Neurology* 1983;33:1487–1489.

165. Engel J Jr. A proposed diagnostic scheme for people with epileptic seizures and with epilepsy: report of the ILAE Task Force on Classification and Terminology. *Epilepsia* 2001;42:796–803.

166. Gowers WR. Epilepsy and other chronic convulsive diseases: their causes, symptoms and treatment. London: Churchill, 1885.

167. Janz D. "Aufwach"-Epilepsien (als Ausdruck einer den "Nacht"-oder "Schlaf"-Epilepsien gegenüberstehenden Verlaufsform epileptischer Erkrankungen). *Arch Psychiatr Nervenkr* 1953;191:73–98.

168. Roger J, Bureau M, Oller Ferrer-Vidal L, et al. Clinical and electroencephalographic characteristics of idiopathic generalised epilepsies. In: Malafosse A, Genton P, Hirsch E, et al., eds. *Clinical and electroencephalographic characteristics of idiopathic generalised epilepsies.* London: John Libbey, 1994:7–18.

169. Wolf P. Epilepsy with grand mal on awakening. In: Roger J, Bureau M, Dravet C, et al., eds. *Epileptic syndromes in infancy, childhood and adolescence.* London: John Libbey, 1992:329–341.

170. Loiseau P. Crises epileptiques survenant au reveil et epilepsie du reveil. *Sud Med Chirurgical* 1964;99:11492–11502.

171. Unterberger I, Trinka E, Luef G, et al. Idiopathic generalized epilepsies with pure grand mal: clinical data and genetics. *Epilepsy Res* 2001;44:19–25.

172. Panayiotopoulos CP. Treatment of typical absence seizures and related epileptic syndromes. *Paediatr Drugs* 2001;3:379–403.

173. Chadwick D, Leiderman DB, Sauermann W, et al. Gabapentin in generalized seizures. *Epilepsy Res* 1996;25:191–197.

174. Kellinghaus C, Dziewas R, Ludemann P. Tiagabine-related non-convulsive status epilepticus in partial epilepsy: three case reports and a review of the literature. *Seizure* 2002;11:243–249.

175. Panayiotopoulos CP, Agathonikou A, Sharoqi IA, et al. Vigabatrin aggravates absences and absence status. *Neurology* 1997;49: 1467.

176. Annegers JF, Hauser WA, Elveback LR. Remission of seizures and relapse in patients with epilepsy. *Epilepsia* 1979;20: 729–737.

177. Emerson R, D'Souza BJ, Vining EP, et al. Stopping medication in children with epilepsy: predictors of outcome. *N Engl J Med* 1981;304:1125–1129.

178. Elwes RD, Johnson AL, Shorvon SD, et al. The prognosis for seizure control in newly diagnosed epilepsy. *N Engl J Med* 1984; 311:944–947.

179. Shinnar S, Glauser TA. Febrile seizures. *J Child Neurol* 2002;17 (Suppl 1):S44–S52.

180. Scheffer IE, Berkovic SF. Generalized epilepsy with febrile seizures plus. A genetic disorder with heterogeneous clinical phenotypes. *Brain* 1997;120(Pt 3):479–490.

181. Wallace RH, Wang DW, Singh R, et al. Febrile seizures and generalized epilepsy associated with a mutation in the Na+-channel beta1 subunit gene SCN1B. *Nat Genet* 1998;19:366–370.

182. Baulac S, Gourfinkel-An I, Picard F, et al. A second locus for familial generalized epilepsy with febrile seizures plus maps to chromosome 2q21-q33. *Am J Hum Genet* 1999;65: 1078–1085.

183. Moulard B, Guipponi M, Chaigne D, et al. Identification of a new locus for generalized epilepsy with febrile seizures plus (GEFS+) on chromosome 2q24-q33. *Am J Hum Genet* 1999;65:1396–1400.

184. Baulac S, Huberfeld G, Gourfinkel-An I, et al. First genetic evidence of GABA(A) receptor dysfunction in epilepsy: a mutation in the gamma2-subunit gene. *Nat Genet* 2001;28:46–48.

185. Baulac S, Gourfinkel-An I, Nabbout R, et al. Fever, genes, and epilepsy. *Lancet Neurol* 2004;3:421–430.

186. Marini C, Harkin LA, Wallace RH, et al. Childhood absence epilepsy and febrile seizures: a family with a GABA(A) receptor mutation. *Brain* 2003;126:230–240.

187. Ito M, Nagafuji H, Okazawa H, et al. Autosomal dominant epilepsy with febrile seizures plus with missense mutations of the (Na+)-channel alpha 1 subunit gene, SCN1A. *Epilepsy Res* 2002;48:15–23.

188. Wallace RH, Scheffer IE, Barnett S, et al. Neuronal sodium-channel alpha1-subunit mutations in generalized epilepsy with febrile seizures plus. *Am J Hum Genet* 2001;68:859–865.

189. Gerard F, Pereira S, Robaglia-Schlupp A, et al. Clinical and genetic analysis of a new multigenerational pedigree with GEFS+ (generalized epilepsy with febrile seizures plus). *Epilepsia* 2002;43: 581–586.

190. Audenaert D, Claes L, Ceulemans B, et al. A deletion in SCN1B is associated with febrile seizures and early-onset absence epilepsy. *Neurology* 2003;61:854–856.

191. Wallace RH, Scheffer IE, Parasivam G, et al. Generalized epilepsy with febrile seizures plus: mutation of the sodium channel subunit SCN1B. *Neurology* 2002;58:1426–1429.

192. Abou-Khalil B, Ge Q, Desai R, et al. Partial and generalized epilepsy with febrile seizures plus and a novel SCN1A mutation. *Neurology* 2001;57:2265–2272.

193. Annesi G, Gambardella A, Carrideo S, et al. Two novel SCN1A missense mutations in generalized epilepsy with febrile seizures plus. *Epilepsia* 2003;44:1257–1258.

194. Fujiwara T, Sugawara T, Mazaki-Miyazaki E, et al. Mutations of sodium channel alpha subunit type 1 (SCN1A) in intractable childhood epilepsies with frequent generalized tonic-clonic seizures. *Brain* 2003;126:531–546.

195. Nabbout R, Gennaro E, Dalla BB, et al. Spectrum of SCN1A mutations in severe myoclonic epilepsy of infancy. *Neurology* 2003;60:1961–1967.

196. Sugawara T, Tsurubuchi Y, Agarwala KL, et al. A missense mutation of the Na+ channel alpha II subunit gene Na(v)1.2 in a patient with febrile and afebrile seizures causes channel dysfunction. *Proc Natl Acad Sci U S A* 2001;98:6384–6389.

197. Harkin LA, Bowser DN, Dibbens LM, et al. Truncation of the GABA(A)-receptor gamma2 subunit in a family with generalized epilepsy with febrile seizures plus. *Am J Hum Genet* 2002;70: 530–536.

198. Kananura C, Haug K, Sander T, et al. A splice-site mutation in GABRG2 associated with childhood absence epilepsy and febrile convulsions. *Arch Neurol* 2002;59:1137–1141.

The Myoclonic Epilepsies

26

Renzo Guerrini   Paolo Bonanni   Carla Marini   Lucio Parmeggiani

The term *myoclonic* has traditionally designated a large group of epilepsies characterized by repeated brief jerks, often responsible for multiple falls, by severe seizures resistant to antiepileptic drugs, and by an association with cognitive impairment (1,2). However, not all the ictal manifestations that cause falls are myoclonic, and not all myoclonic epilepsies predict a poor outcome. Myoclonic jerks are the only seizure type in but a minority of patients with myoclonic epilepsy (1,2), which is commonly associated with generalized tonic-clonic seizures (2,3), as well as generalized clonic, atypical absence, and atonic seizures (4,5). Tonic seizures are uncommon in myoclonic epilepsies, but isolated tonic attacks during sleep are not rare in children with myoclonic-astatic epilepsy (MAE) (1,6). As a result, confusion arose in classifying myoclonic epilepsies, because they represent a broad group of diseases and epilepsy syndromes that differ in evolution and prognosis. This chapter defines clinical and electroencephalographic (EEG) features of myoclonic seizures, distinguishes them from other seizure types, and describes diagnosis and treatment of various syndromes with prominent myoclonic seizures, including progressive disorders.

DEFINITION

Myoclonus, which is used to describe involuntary, jerky movements frequently involving antagonist muscles (7), can be classified physiologically as epileptic and nonepileptic. Epileptic myoclonus is an elementary electroclinical manifestation of epilepsy involving descending neurons, whose spatial (spread) or temporal (self-sustained repetition) amplification can trigger overt epileptic activity (1). Myoclonus can have a focal, multifocal, or generalized distribution (8). Epileptic myoclonus is characterized neurophysiologically by a myoclonic electromyographic (EMG)

burst ranging between 10 and 100 milliseconds, synchronous EMG bursts or silent periods on antagonist muscles, and an EEG correlate detectable by routine surface electroencephalography or burst-locked EEG averaging (1).

CLINICAL AND ELECTROENCEPHALOGRAPHIC FEATURES

Myoclonic seizures can produce only slight head nodding or abduction of the arms (or both) or be responsible for falls when the lower limbs are also involved or when the atonic phenomenon immediately after the jerk is prominent (3,9). Myoclonic seizures are short and usually cluster, with a repetition rate of 2 to 3 Hz, and most commonly affect axial muscles, but in 57% of patients, may also involve the extraocular muscles, eyelids, and face, especially perioral muscles (10). Most occur spontaneously on awakening, as in juvenile myoclonic epilepsy (JME), or during drowsiness, as in benign myoclonic epilepsy. Jerks may sometimes be precipitated by photic stimulation in the electroencephalography laboratory or induced by natural photic stimuli. Tapping or sudden acoustic stimuli may also cause generalized myoclonic jerks of epileptic origin (11). Usually isolated events, myoclonic seizures at times are repeated in prolonged series and, in some cases, can progress to a myoclonic status with partial preservation of consciousness (5,12).

The electromyographic (EMG) recording shows a biphasic or polyphasic potential lasting from 20 to 150 milliseconds. Generalized bursts of polyspike and waves are evident on ictal electroencephalography. The interictal recording may be entirely normal or show slow background activity, depending on whether the myoclonic attacks are part of an idiopathic or a symptomatic epilepsy. Focal abnormalities are rare. Interictal bursts of irregular polyspike waves lasting

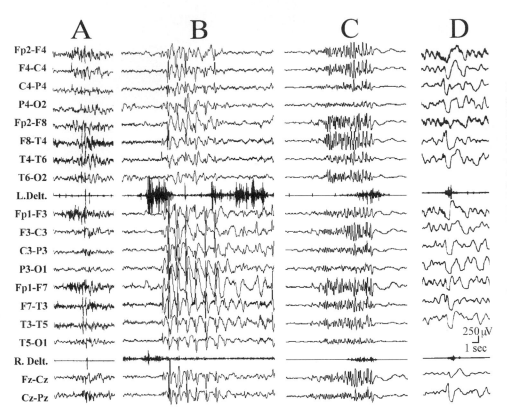

Figure 26.1 Types of brief seizures that clinically manifest as body jerks, shown by their neurophysiologic correlates. **A:** Myoclonic seizure; electromyographic (EMG) burst lasts less than 100 milliseconds and is time-locked to a polyspike-and-wave discharge. **B:** Atonic seizure; a spike-and-wave discharge is accompanied by an EMG silent period lasting as long as the discharge on scalp electroencephalography. Note the progressive onset of the silent period and the transient resumption of muscle tone, resembling a myoclonic jerk, interrupting the EMG silence. **C:** Brief tonic seizure; a polyspike discharge is associated with a bilateral tonic contraction of both deltoid muscles lasting about 5 seconds, that begins with a crescendo pattern. **D:** Epileptic spasm; a brief (approximately 500 milliseconds), diamond-shaped EMG burst correlated with a high-amplitude, diffuse, polyphasic slow transient on EEG channels.

less than 3 seconds can be spontaneous or induced by photic stimulation (2,5). Discharges featuring multiple generalized spikes and waves often increase in frequency during nonrapid eye movement (NREM) sleep (2,5).

DIFFERENTIAL DIAGNOSIS

The recognition and classification of seizures described as a "sudden and brief jerk" are not always easy; misdiagnosis is possible if not frequent. When the description of ictal manifestations is combined with data from electroencephalography, electromyography, and video monitoring, three seizure types that may mimic myoclonic seizure—atonic and tonic seizures and epileptic spasms—can be recognized (Fig. 26.1). During *atonic seizures*, loss of muscle tone causes the patient to fall to the ground suddenly or slump in a rhythmic, step-by-step fashion (3). However, if only the neck muscles are involved, brief head nodding is the sole manifestation. Atonic seizures are also accompanied by loss of consciousness, with the patient unaware of falling, and the drop is followed by immediate recovery. EEG recordings show slow spike waves (13), 3-Hz spike waves (2), polyspike waves (Fig. 26.1B), or fast recruiting rhythms (14,15). EMG channels show suppression of muscle activity (13). *Tonic seizures* involve the tonic contraction of certain muscle groups without progression to a clonic phase (3,16). They also can cause a fall when the lower extremities are forcibly flexed or if the patient is thrown off

balance. The electromyogram shows an interferential muscle discharge similar to that in voluntary contraction (Fig. 26.1C). The electroencephalogram may show flattening of the background activity, very fast activity (20 Hz) increasing in amplitude, or a 10-Hz rhythmic, high-amplitude activity similar to the "epileptic recruiting rhythm" (Fig. 26.1C) (15,17,18). Symmetric or asymmetric spasms are similar to brief tonic seizures and are an important cause of sudden falls (19). They generally occur in prolonged clusters. The EEG-EMG recordings are unequivocally diagnostic, showing a brief (0.5 to 3 seconds), electromyographically diamond-shaped burst accompanied by a high-amplitude, diffuse slow wave with superimposed fast rhythms (Fig. 26.1D).

ETIOLOGY

The vast majority of myoclonic epilepsies are idiopathic or cryptogenic, and genetic factors are important, as indicated by the frequency of epilepsy in family members. Mutations in the β_1 and α_2 subunits of the sodium-channel receptor (*SCN1B* and *SCN2A*) genes have been reported in a few patients with the MAE phenotype within generalized epilepsy with febrile seizures plus (GEFS+) families, as well as in patients with severe myoclonic epilepsy of infancy (Dravet syndrome) (20,21). A family with JME was found to harbor a mutation in the α_1 γ-aminobutyric acid A (GABA$_A$) receptor subunit (*GABRA1*) gene (22). These findings suggest that functional impairment of the ion

TABLE 26.1

CLASSIFICATION OF MYOCLONIC EPILEPSIES BY AGE OF ONSET

Neonatal period
Early myoclonic encephalopathy

Infancy and early childhood
Benign myoclonic epilepsy of infancy (5 months to 5 years)
Severe myoclonic epilepsy of infants or Dravet syndrome (2 months to 1 year)
Myoclonic-astatic epilepsy (7 months to 6 years, usually after 2 years)

Late childhood and adolescence
Myoclonic (or clonic) absence epilepsy (1 to 12 years)
Juvenile myoclonic epilepsy (6 to 22 years)
Photosensitive myoclonic epilepsy (including eyelid myoclonia)

Variable age
Epilepsies with prominent rhythmic distal myoclonus
Angelman syndrome (3 months to 20 years)
Autosomal dominant cortical reflex myoclonus and epilepsy (12 to 59 years)
Familial adult myoclonic epilepsy (19 to 73 years)
  Progressive myoclonus epilepsies[a]

[a]See Table 26.2 for clinical classification and range of age of onset.

channel may represent the pathophysiologic substrate for at least some of the nonprogressive myoclonic epilepsies. On the other hand, the progressive myoclonic epilepsies (PMEs), which are also genetically determined, follow an autosomal recessive inheritance and have been related to gene defects causing abnormal deposit material to accumulate in various organs including the brain.

Cases that are symptomatic of an acquired, fixed brain lesion are uncommon and most often the result of prenatal or perinatal hypoxic-ischemic encephalopathies. Patients with brain damage start having myoclonic seizures between a few months and the third year of life (1,23,24). Other seizure types usually are also present. Myoclonic status may be prominent (23).

Table 26.1 lists the myoclonic epilepsies, by age of onset, that are discussed in this chapter.

MYOCLONIC EPILEPSIES IN THE NEWBORN

The only syndrome in which myoclonic seizures begin in the neonatal period is early myoclonic encephalopathy (EME). Myoclonic seizures at this early age have peculiar features that do not quite overlap with the general characteristics of myoclonic epilepsies.

Early Myoclonic Encephalopathy

This rare syndrome is classified among the generalized symptomatic epilepsies of nonspecific etiology (25).

Among its multiple, prenatal causes are inborn errors of metabolism, such as methylmalonic acidemia and nonketotic hyperglycinemia. Fragmentary, erratic, and severe myoclonus begins neonatally or during the first month of life and is followed by partial seizures and tonic spasms. Fragmentary myoclonus involves the muscles of the face and extremities, with a multifocal distribution. Frequency varies from occasional to almost continuous. Neurologic development is severely delayed, with marked hypotonia, impaired alertness, and, often, a vegetative state (26).

Bursts of spikes, sharp waves, and slow waves are irregularly intermingled and separated by periods of electrical silence (suppression bursts). Erratic myoclonus generally does not have an EEG correlate (26). In patients with nonketotic hyperglycinemia, whole-body myoclonus can be either spontaneous or triggered by tactile-proprioceptive stimuli and is often associated with generalized EEG discharges (27). Spongy leukodystrophy of all myelinated tracts, especially of the reticular activating system, confirms the role of the nonspecific diffuse somatosensory projection system in the generation of generalized myoclonus (27).

MYOCLONIC EPILEPSIES IN INFANCY AND EARLY CHILDHOOD

Benign Myoclonic Epilepsy of Infancy

Characterized by symmetric, frequent, axial or generalized myoclonic seizures, benign myoclonic epilepsy of infancy (BMEI), especially if of late onset, may be difficult to distinguish from milder cases of MAE. A complete differentiation may even be improper, as these conditions might represent two extreme phenotypes of one epilepsy syndrome.

Nosologic Aspects

Because the original descriptions (28,29) involved only children younger than age 2 years at onset and without other seizure types (except febrile seizures), benign myoclonic epilepsy was understood to be an early and minor expression of idiopathic generalized epilepsy. Similar cases were subsequently recognized (30), as was a special subgroup represented by cases of "touch" myoclonic epilepsy in infants whose myoclonic jerks were triggered by tactile or sudden acoustic stimuli, with or without spontaneous jerking (11,31,32). The total number of cases initially remained low, and about half of the patients (29) were mildly retarded or behaviorally disturbed at follow-up, casting some doubts on the syndrome's benign outcome. A series of infants and young children with only myoclonic seizures and occasional generalized tonic-clonic seizures did have a relatively favorable outcome, although about half exhibited behavioral or learning problems (or both) at school age (33). It appeared that patients with only early onset myoclonic seizures could have a variable prognosis.

A review of the 103 cases of benign myoclonic epilepsy reported so far (34) acknowledged that age at onset may be as late as 5 years (35,36), that the term *benign* is questionable according to the most recent International League Against Epilepsy (ILAE) definitions (37), and that the difference from milder cases of MAE may not be entirely clear.

Etiology and Epidemiology

Affecting less than 1% of the epilepsy population in specialized centers, BMEI represents approximately 2% of all idiopathic generalized epilepsies (34). Diagnosis is possible in approximately 1.3% to 1.7% of all children with seizure onset in the first year of life and in 2% of those with onset within 3 years. Boys are affected almost twice as frequently as girls (34,38). There are no familial cases of BMEI; however, a family history of epilepsy or febrile seizures is seen in 39% of cases (39). A single individual with reflex BMEI was described in a family whose other relatives had GEFS + phenotypes and idiopathic generalized epilepsy (40). These data support the role of genetic factors in the etiology of BMEI and raise the likely possibility of etiologic heterogeneity.

Clinical and Electroencephalographic Features

Seizure onset ranges from 5 months to 5 years in otherwise normal children. Mild and rare at onset, myoclonic jerks increase gradually in frequency, becoming multiple daily events presenting in brief clusters of a few jerks. In 30% of children, myoclonic seizures are preceded by infrequent, simple febrile seizures (34). Parents describe head nodding or upward rolling of the eyes, accompanied by brisk abduction of the upper limbs. Jerks might vary in intensity; however, jerking with projection of objects or falling is rare and may appear later in the disease. Falling is followed by immediate recovery, usually without injury. This is an important feature in the differentiation with drop attacks associated with epileptic spasms, atonic seizures, or major myoclonic-astatic disorders, after which children appear confused and often cry because of fear or injuries. Myoclonic seizures may be asymmetric or even unilateral. Drowsiness facilitates the jerks. Impairment of consciousness is difficult to appreciate as jerks are too brief but when repeated may be accompanied by reduced awareness.

In some patients, generalized myoclonic jerks are triggered only by tapping or acoustic stimuli (11,31,32). Reflex jerks, which may begin as early as 4 months (11), can be provoked while awake or during sleep. This "benign reflex myoclonic epilepsy of infancy" may have an even more benign evolution than do other forms of BMEI (34).

The electroencephalogram shows normal background activity (34,35). Spike-and-wave discharges are usually concomitant to myoclonic jerks. Focal abnormalities are not a consistent feature (34,36,41). Ictal discharges, often observed during sleep, consist of 1- to 3-second bursts of generalized fast spike and waves or polyspike and waves. Most jerks are isolated and time-locked with the spike component (42). In the reflex form of BMEI, a refractory period lasting up to 2 minutes may follow a reflex-induced jerk (11). Jerks can be triggered by intermittent photic stimulation in approximately 10% of all affected children (34,35).

Course and Outcome

The benign course is an opinion based largely on retrospective studies. Among the proposed criteria for diagnosis was a rapid response to valproate monotherapy, which is also a feature of benign epilepsy syndromes. Moreover, some children had cognitive or behavioral sequelae, indicating that, even with these strict criteria, a benign outcome could not be guaranteed.

In general, the epilepsy outcome is favorable, and myoclonic jerks reportedly disappeared in all children followed up long-term (34). Myoclonic seizures were estimated to have been present for less than 1 year in most of the 52 published cases with this information (34), although the mean delay in initiating effective treatment was not known. Treatment had been withdrawn in most patients older than age 6 years at follow-up. A minority had rare generalized tonic-clonic seizures between 9 and 16 years of age (34,36), some during valproate withdrawal, which were subsequently controlled by reinstitution of treatment (34). No detailed information is available for the remaining patients. The main reason for continued treatment after age 16 years was photosensitivity, either persisting or emerging after spontaneous myoclonic jerks had disappeared (34,36,41).

Myoclonic jerks persisted in some children who did not receive any drug treatment (34), although no additional seizure types were seen. Such patients were thought to be at increased risk of impaired psychomotor development and behavioral disturbances, but the evidence is unconvincing.

The cognitive and behavioral outcome is favorable (34), and only 17% of affected children experienced mild cognitive difficulties. Clearly, the good outcome fulfilling the early criteria (34) also might be a result of the additional requirements for benignity, such as rapid response to therapy, rather than to an intrinsic difference in severity. Similar remarks could apply to cases classified as MAE with a favorable outcome (6,43). Thus BMEI is neither always benign nor is it the only relatively benign syndrome among the myoclonic epilepsies. Further advances in the genetics of idiopathic generalized epilepsies will likely reveal that the clinical syndrome of BMEI is etiologically (genetically) heterogeneous.

Treatment

See "Myoclonic-Astatic Epilepsy" below.

Differential Diagnosis

Early onset BMEI can be mistaken for cryptogenic infantile spasms, although the latter involve a more sustained muscle contraction and occur in clusters. Polygraphic EEG-EMG recordings easily clarify the clinical picture. Benign nonepileptic myoclonus of early infancy should be considered in the differential diagnosis of developmentally normal children who present with clusters of jerky movements of the limbs, nodding, or axial shudder but have normal interictal and ictal EEG findings (44,45). In such cases, polygraphic recordings show a tonic, rather than a myoclonic, contraction lasting 0.5 to 3 seconds (44).

Myoclonic-Astatic Epilepsy

A form of generalized epilepsy, MAE includes myoclonic-astatic, absence, and tonic seizures and begins between 7 months and 6 years of age (25).

Nosologic Aspects

MAE is used to designate the primary generalized epilepsies of childhood whose main clinical manifestations include myoclonic or astatic seizures (or both) (12). However, major myoclonic attacks and astatic falls attributed to lapses of muscle tone may be impossible to distinguish without extensive polygraphic EEG-EMG recordings. Additional features include genetic factors, the idiopathic and generalized nature of the disorder, and EEG findings of biparietal θ activity and prominent generalized spike-wave or polyspike-wave complexes. Forgoing a "rigidly defined syndrome," Doose and coworkers (12) identified a large subgroup of idiopathic epilepsies characterized by myoclonic and atonic seizures whose recognized variability was attributed to a multifactorial background. Such defining features, based mainly on etiology, apparently included all forms of idiopathic myoclonic epilepsies, as well as cases that would now be classified as benign myoclonic epilepsy, severe myoclonic epilepsy, and other difficult-to-classify forms. The ILAE classification (25) included "Doose's syndrome" among types of myoclonic epilepsy (in addition to severe and benign forms) on the basis of clinical and EEG characteristics, and listed it with other "cryptogenic and symptomatic epilepsy syndromes" involving developmental delay. This practice, however, contrasts with Doose's criteria that were based mainly on a primary or idiopathic etiologic background. Such inconsistencies have contributed to the different ways MAE is defined. For example, it is not clear whether some series considered falls necessary for inclusion (43,46). Because of these discrepancies, prognostic indicators are unclear, and the prognosis may vary in different series. It seems likely that epilepsies with prominent myoclonic activity, including BMEI, MAE, and other unclassifiable cases (but excluding severe myoclonic epilepsy of infants [SMEI] and Lennox-Gastaut syndrome that clearly belong to separate categories) are part of a continuum in which, despite differing severity and outcome, the clinical presentation and etiologic (e.g., genetic) factors may be closely related.

Etiology and Epidemiology

MAE represents 1% to 2.2% of all childhood epilepsies with onset up to age 10 years (12,43) and has a male preponderance (12,43). A family history of epilepsy is present in 14% to 32% of children (12,43), some of whom belonged to large families with GEFS+, carrying missense mutations of the SCN1A gene (21). Consequently, MAE has been considered part of the GEFS+ spectrum.

Clinical and Electroencephalographic Features

Seizures begin between 7 months and 6 years, with a peak incidence between 2 and 6 years, in previously normal children (12,47). Brief, massive or axial, symmetric jerks involving the neck, shoulders, arms, and legs often result in head nodding, abduction of arms, and flexion of the legs at the knees. Each jerk is immediately followed by an abrupt loss of muscle tone that causes a drop to the floor (48), although falls can also result from purely myoclonic seizures (49). Violent myoclonus, followed by an abrupt fall to the ground or on the table, may severely injure the nose, teeth, and face. Such episodes last less than 2 to 3 seconds. The jerks may be isolated or occur in short series at an approximately 3-Hz rhythm and lead to saccadic flexion of the head or abduction of the arms (or both).

The electroencephalogram shows bursts of spike/polyspike-and-wave complexes at 2 to 4 Hz. The muscle contraction responsible for the myoclonic jerk is usually followed by an EMG silence lasting up to 500 milliseconds (Fig. 26.2). The silent period is sometimes without a clear preceding jerk, although a mild contraction in nonsampled muscles is difficult to exclude. Bilateral synchronous EEG discharges and synchronous jerks in muscles from both sides of the body indicate a primary generalized myoclonus (50). Some patients can present with pure atonic seizures (46). Generalized tonic-clonic attacks and atypical absences usually occur as well.

Nonconvulsive status manifests as episodes of somnolence, stupor, apathy, or mild obtundation with drooling, associated with erratic muscle twitching and head nods. Beginning insidiously and progressing, such episodes may last from hours to days or even weeks, often with fluctuations, and have been considered indicative of a poor prognosis (43). In our experience, however, this is not necessarily the case. Nonconvulsive status is often accompanied by long runs of slow waves or spike-wave complexes so severely disorganized as to simulate a hypsarrhythmic pattern (35).

Tonic seizures, considered absent by some authors (6,51), have been found in up to 38% of cases in some series (43). Their presence does not necessarily predict an unfavorable outcome. "Vibratory" tonic seizures have also been mentioned (6,43).

The interictal electroencephalogram may be normal at onset (52). Bursts of 3-Hz spike waves may occur without apparent clinical manifestations and could be activated by sleep. The most suggestive findings are 4- to 7-Hz θ rhythms

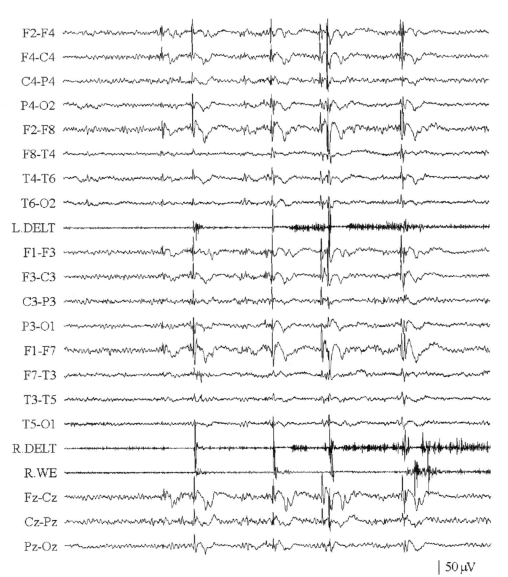

Figure 26.2 Surface electroencephalographic (EEG)-electromyographic (EMG) polygraphic recording of a 13-year-old boy with myoclonicastatic epilepsy. Generalized myoclonic jerks are visible as high-amplitude myoclonic potentials on the EMG channels accompanied by a diffuse discharge of spike-wave complexes. A clear time-locked correlation is observed between the EEG spikes and the myoclonic EMG potentials. L.DELT = left deltoid muscle; R.DELT = right deltoid muscle; R.WE = right wrist extensor.

| 50 µV

with parietal accentuation and occipital 4-Hz rhythms, constantly blocked by eye opening (6). Variable lateralization of paroxysmal bursts is possible, although a consistently localized focus is unusual (50). A subset of patients are photosensitive.

Course and Outcome

Despite the frequent seizure types, MAE is often self-limited and the seizures abate within 3 years in 50% to 89% of patients (6,43). Up to 58% of patients had normal intelligence quotients, while 20% had mild and 22% had severe mental retardation (6). Some children have mild behavioral problems, especially hyperactivity (43); others have intractable epilepsy. Pathophysiologic predictors of the outcome are poorly understood. The association between a poor mental outcome and frequent, especially prolonged, episodes of nonconvulsive status has been emphasized (12). Atypical absences, repeated generalized tonic-clonic seizures, and frequent falls have also been variably linked to a less favorable outcome. Nocturnal tonic seizures have been considered a bad prognostic indicator in some, but not all, reported series (43,52).

Differential Diagnosis

The progressive myoclonic epilepsies such as myoclonus epilepsy with ragged-red fibers (MERRF), Unverricht-Lundborg disease, and late-infantile neuronal ceroid lipofuscinoses (NCL) can be confused with MAE at onset, but later appearance of neurologic signs and continuous, multifocal myoclonus is usually sufficient for diagnosis. Late-onset cryptogenic epileptic spasms (53) can mimic myoclonic-astatic seizures, presenting as multiple daily episodes of violent falls; however, spasms tend to cluster in series with a typical periodicity, and the EEG recording shows different ictal, and usually interictal, features. Differentiation of MAE and Lennox-Gastaut syndrome is usually straightforward. The tonic and atonic attacks with slow spike-wave complexes is more consistent with the latter but not incompatible with MAE. Other childhood epilepsies with predominant myoclonic attacks remain difficult to classify and in some cases may belong to the spectrum of MAE. It is difficult to subsume all myoclonic patients into single, well-defined syndromic entities (51). Of more use is to consider idiopathic epilepsies with prominent myoclonic seizures, such as BMEI, MAE, and other unclassifiable cases, as part of a continuum with different degrees of severity.

Treatment of Benign Myoclonic Epilepsy of Infancy and Myoclonic-Astatic Epilepsy

Treatment of myoclonic seizures is primarily with sodium valproate, ethosuximide, and the benzodiazepines. Lamotrigine does not seem to be effective but may be useful against generalized seizures, especially in MAE (54).

Patients with only myoclonic seizures often respond dramatically to regular doses of either valproate or ethosuximide. Ethosuximide produced a "good response rate" in 64% of patients (6); others may require higher doses of valproate (41). The combination is worth trying even when monotherapy with either drug has failed. Clonazepam may be effective but limited by behavioral side effects. Anecdotal reports (55,56) have championed topiramate, levetiracetam, acetazolamide, methsuximide, and sulthiame.

Resistant myoclonic-astatic seizures that cause disabling falls pose a therapeutic challenge. Uncontrolled trials of steroids or corticotropin have had limited success. Management should include practical measures, such as wearing a helmet, and considerable psychosocial support. The ketogenic diet may be effective but is difficult to maintain for long periods (6). Surgery, including callosotomy, is not generally indicated.

Severe Myoclonic Epilepsy of Infancy or Dravet Syndrome

Including SMEI with the myoclonic epilepsies is controversial, as myoclonus, although present in most children, can be transient and is not this syndrome's main characteristic. Moreover, a subgroup of patients with SMEI do not present with myoclonic seizures at all (5,57). SMEI is characterized by multiple seizure types, including myoclonus, intractability despite treatment, and unfavorable evolution. It represents the prototype of an epileptic encephalopathy in which seizures are thought to be responsible for the deterioration of cerebral functions (58). Prolonged, often lateralized febrile seizures at onset are the most distinctive feature.

Etiology and Epidemiology

Although SMEI has a calculated incidence of 0.5 to 1 per 40,000 children (59,60), it represents 3% to 5% of all epilepsies starting in the first year of life (60) and 6.1% to 8.2% of those starting in the first 3 years of life (5,29). A 2:1 male preponderance is reported (60).

Genetic factors play a major pathogenetic role. A family history of febrile seizures or epilepsy is reported in 25% to 71% of patients (59,61), and affected monozygotic twins are on record (61,62). A link between SMEI and GEFS+ had been identified in several families (63). GEFS+ is associated with mutations of the SCN1A gene in approximately 10% of families (64); a study of seven children with SMEI found *de novo* truncating mutations of SCN1A in all of them (20). Similar results were subsequently confirmed (65). According to a genetic study of 93 patients with SMEI, SCN1A mutations are observed in approximately 35% of patients; in 10% of cases, mutations are inherited from asymptomatic or mildly affected parents (66). These data suggest a genetic heterogeneity with the possible involvement of a second gene, yet to be identified.

Clinical and Electroencephalographic Features

Frequent, usually (70%) febrile seizures, lasting several minutes to more than 1 hour, begin between age 2 months and the end of the first year of life in a normal child (5,67). Triggering factors are fever, infectious episodes without overt fever, and hot water immersion (5). Febrile seizures recur with a mean latency of 6 weeks between the first and second events, while afebrile seizures occur later (5-month mean latency from the first febrile seizure) (61). In the second and third years of life, myoclonic and atypical absences appear, but convulsive seizures remain a constant feature.

According to a detailed video-EEG description (5), generalized seizures are clinically and electrographically similar to those of idiopathic epilepsies, but the initial tonic phase can acquire a vibratory appearance, with high-frequency clonic activity. Unilateral clonic seizures, switching from side to side in different events or occasionally during the same seizure, are frequent at onset but rare after age 3 years. Postictal paresis is common, and EEG ictal activity is highly asymmetric. The so-called falsely generalized seizures are bilateral, tonic, and asymmetric followed by a clonic phase that is highly asymmetric in distribution of involved body segments and frequency of muscle activity. Ictally, electrodecremental activity is followed by slow spike-and-wave discharges, bilateral from onset, with variable asymmetry. In the classically similar "unstable" seizures, however, EEG ictal activity seems to migrate from one area of the brain to another during a single event.

Myoclonic seizures may appear between 1 and 5 years of age as massive, generalized myoclonic jerks, involving the axial muscles and causing falls to the ground. Highly variable in intensity, the jerks can present as nodding of the head, shrugging of shoulders, or abduction of the arms. Jerks can be isolated or grouped in brief clusters and can occur frequently during the entire day or concentrate on awakening, but tend to disappear during sleep (5). Polygraphic recordings show a generalized polyspike-and-wave discharge, time-locked to a brief EMG burst. These seizures appear to be generalized events; however, on EEG-EMG latency analysis, they are seen to spread contralaterally from a focal cortical activity in the motor cortex of one hemisphere and either hemisphere can be activated in subsequent discharges (1). Multifocal erratic myoclonic jerks can involve the hands and face (5). Their origin remains speculative, as back-averaging studies did not produce any cortical transient time-locked to the jerks (1).

Atypical absences accompanied by head nodding or loss of postural control occur in 60% of patients (5) either between ages 1 and 3 years, concomitantly with myoclonic seizures, or between ages 5 and 12 years. EEG recordings show generalized, irregular 2- to 3.5-Hz spike-wave discharges lasting 3 to 10 seconds.

Nonconvulsive status epilepticus has been reported as fluctuating episodes of obtundation, with distal jerks, unsteadiness, and dribbling lasting from hours to several days (5).

Approximately 45% to 80% of patients experience focal seizures, either simple partial motor or complex partial, as early as 4 months or until 4 years of age (61). Prominent autonomic phenomena accompany complex partial seizures (5,67). Focal seizures may evolve to generalized or unilateral seizures.

Rare in SMEI (5,57), tonic seizures tend to present at night as brief, infrequent events.

Interictal EEG deteriorates progressively but lacks specific features. Background activity often remains normal for several years but becomes slower over time. A rhythmic activity at 5 to 6 Hz, involving the central and vertex leads, is sometimes seen (68). Generalized or asymmetric spike/polyspike-and-wave complexes appear later in the disease and are prominent in patients with myoclonic seizures (5). Focal or multifocal spikes predominate in the central or posterior regions. Paroxysmal EEG abnormalities are enhanced during slow-wave sleep. Early photosensitivity occurs in 40% of patients.

Evolution and Outcome

Development is initially normal despite the frequent and prolonged febrile seizures, but cognition becomes progressively impaired during the second and third years of life (58,69). Longitudinal assessment showed values within the normal range before ages 1 to 2 years and a dramatic decrease between ages 2 and 4, followed by a plateau on severely low levels (58). Prolonged convulsive seizures seem to play a major role in cognitive deficits. Most children usually are severely or moderately retarded (2), with frequent attention deficit and hyperactivity.

Myoclonic seizures tend to disappear with age but the other types persist, although becoming shorter (2,34). Fever and afebrile infections maintain a strong triggering potential in late infancy and adolescence.

Accidents or sudden death account for the substantial mortality rate (67). Physicians and parents should be aware that repeated prolonged seizures carry a risk of death higher than in the epilepsy population at large and that the child with SMEI requires close attention.

Treatment

SMEI is highly refractory to all medications but may be slightly improved by valproate and benzodiazepines (5). The combination of clobazam and the cytochrome P450 inhibitor stiripentol, with or without the noninducer valproate, has proved effective (70), possibly because of the enhanced antiepileptic action of the active metabolite norclobazam.

Differential Diagnosis

Early recognition may be difficult; at onset, the main differential diagnosis is febrile seizures. The diagnosis can be established only when other seizure types emerge or if a photoparoxysmal response is observed at an unusually early age. Early onset myoclonic seizures as the only seizure type are the cardinal feature of BMEI, distinguishing it from SMEI.

MAE has a different course, and myoclonic seizures accompanied by falls to the ground represent the main seizure types. Febrile convulsions can be observed at onset, but are usually rare. The electroencephalogram shows generalized polyspike-and-wave discharges but never focal abnormalities, as focal seizures are not a part of MAE.

Lennox-Gastaut syndrome does not confound the differential diagnosis when the clinical history is collected and polygraphic EEG (including sleep) recordings are performed. Epilepsy onset is variable, and affected children often have a pre-existing cerebral lesion. The EEG shows typical slow spike-and-wave discharges and polyspike discharges during sleep, often accompanied by tonic seizures. Myoclonus affects only 18% of patients (71).

PME can sometimes be suspected in children with SMEI because of the clinical course. In children aged less than 4–5 years ceroid lipofuscinoses represent the main clinical entity to rule out. However, lack of progressive visual disturbances, absence of low-frequency intermittent photic stimulation (IPS) giant responses, and negativity of biologic investigations can prompt the correct diagnosis.

MYOCLONIC EPILEPSIES OF LATE CHILDHOOD AND ADOLESCENCE

Myoclonic (or Clonic) Absence Epilepsy

Patients with myoclonic absences differ from those just described in that the jerks are an integral part of the absences. Age at onset ranges from 1 to 12 years (72), with a peak near age 7 years. The 70% male preponderance is opposite that usually seen in absence epilepsies. Approximately 20% of affected children have a family history of epilepsy. The 3-Hz jerks are temporally correlated with the spike component of the spike-wave complex (72). The EEG discharge during myoclonic absences is indistinguishable from the discharges that accompany typical absences (9). Approximately 66% of cases present additional seizure types, especially generalized tonic-clonic, of variable severity (72). Myoclonic absences are resistant to drug therapy or evolve to other seizure types approximately 60% of the time. Cognitive impairment, already obvious before the onset of myoclonic absences in approximately 50% of children, becomes more severe, especially in children who also experience frequent generalized tonic-clonic seizures (72).

Juvenile Myoclonic Epilepsy

Once called "impulsive petit mal" (73), JME belongs to the idiopathic generalized epilepsies (25).

Etiology and Epidemiology

The frequency of JME varies from 3.1% (74) to 11.9% (75,76). Among idiopathic generalized epilepsies, JME is diagnosed in 20% to 27% of cases (77,78). Approximately 17% to 50% of patients have a family history of epilepsy (73). The risk of recurrent epilepsy in family members of JME patients is between 3% and 7% (79,80), and is higher in girls.

Autosomal dominant and recessive, complex, and a two-locus model of inheritance have been proposed (22,81,82). The greater heritability and lower threshold for females (79) accounts for the 2:1 female-to-male ratio reported in some series (79,83,84). Linkage studies have yielded discordant results. A linkage between a major gene for JME and the HLA-BF locus on the short arm of chromosome 6 was initially reported (85–87). Subsequently, the initial candidate region (EMJ1) was refined and an additional locus identified on the short arm of chromosome 6 (88,89). The locus, however, was not confirmed in other studies (90,91), and a second susceptibility locus on chromosome 15q was identified but not replicated (92). A Mexican family with JME with absence has been linked to chromosome 1p (93). A large French Canadian family in which JME followed an autosomal dominant inheritance (22) was found to harbor a mutation of the GABRA1 gene. The uncertain mode of inheritance and the heterogeneous phenotypes in relatives may explain the difficulty in finding common genes for JME.

Clinical and Electroencephalographic Features

Except for febrile seizures, no history of neurologic disorders is present. Females (61%) are more commonly affected than males (57%) (77). Onset is between 6 and 22 years of age; more than 75% of patients have their initial seizures between their 12th and 18th year (94). Myoclonic jerks usually appear between the ages of 12 and 16 years. Generalized tonic-clonic seizures peak at about 16 years (77) and often prompt medical attention.

The myoclonic jerks are sudden and spontaneous, affecting mainly the shoulders and arms symmetrically, occasionally the lower extremities or the entire body; falls are rare. In exceptional cases, asymmetric or even unilateral jerks may cause a misdiagnosis of focal epilepsy (77). Jerks

may occur singularly at irregular intervals or in brief arrhythmic series, with no apparent alteration of consciousness. While massive jerks are visible, mild ones may mimic postawakening clumsiness with throwing of objects and are described by patients as a "sort of internal electrical shock." Most jerks occur within 20 to 30 minutes after awakening in the morning; some may also supervene with tiredness at the end of the day or in relaxing situations (84), but not on falling asleep. Sleep deprivation is the most effective trigger. A sharp increase in frequency of jerks may herald episodes of myoclonic status epilepticus; relatively common in the past (95), these have become rarer (96) with improved recognition. Indeed, drug withdrawal or inappropriate drug choice may precipitate myoclonic status (77) lasting from a few minutes to several hours and characterized by jerks that recur every few seconds. Often, the jerks may be so mild that only the patient can perceive them. Isolated facial or lingual and perioral jerks may be precipitated by talking (97), a phenomenon analogous to the jerking in primary reading epilepsy.

Infrequent generalized tonic-clonic seizures occur in approximately 85% of patients (84,98), many preceded by a crescendo of myoclonic jerks. Like jerks, these seizures are often precipitated by sleep deprivation (84%), stress (70%), and alcohol intake (51%) (99), and patients with irregular lifestyles or noncompliance may have several episodes. A triggering role of mental activities implying planning of manual praxis or decision making has been reported (100) in up to one-third of patients who are specifically questioned (97).

Short absence attacks sometimes occur independently of the jerks and although not evident to the patient or witnesses, may be uncovered during electroencephalography (77). Intensive video-EEG monitoring suggests that from 33% to 38% of patients may suffer brief absence seizures (78). Typical "pyknoleptic" absences are rare (6% in Janz's series) (98). Approximately 5% of patients have clinical photosensitivity (101).

The ictal electroencephalogram of myoclonic jerks consists of generalized symmetric discharges of high-frequency spikes (10 to 16 per second), followed by several slow waves; amplitude is maximum in the frontocentral areas. Such tracings were found in 85% to 95% of patients by some authors (84,98), but much less frequently by others (83,95). Focal slow waves or asymmetric interictal discharges with inconsistent lateralization are reported in 15% to 55% of patients (77,101,102). Background activity is consistently normal. Approximately 30% to 40% of patients have a photoparoxysmal response often accompanied by myoclonic jerks (98,103) that does not, however, translate into clinical photosensitivity in everyday life. The risk of a photoparoxysmal response is twice as high in girls. Discharges of polyspike-wave complexes occur on eye closure in up to 21% of patients (84). Sleep does not induce jerks, but the rate of discharges may be increased during stage 1 sleep and is particularly high on awakening (104).

Course and Outcome

Response to treatment is excellent or good, with complete control in 80% to 90% of cases (77,106), but spontaneous remission is very rare. After discontinuation of medication, relapses are frequent, even after many years of control (107), but can sometimes be delayed for several years (108). Approximately 15% of patients have treatment-resistant disease; the risk of continued seizures is higher if all three seizures types are present (77). Sudden unexplained death is not a negligible risk in patients who continue to have generalized tonic-clonic seizures (109).

Differential Diagnosis

The myoclonic attacks of JME should be separated from the myoclonic or clonic absences, which have a more adverse prognosis. In JME, consciousness is preserved, and the clonic jerks are arrhythmic. The differentiation of JME and the PMEs is based on the presence of mental deterioration, occurrence of other types of myoclonus in addition to massive myoclonic jerks (particularly erratic and/or intention myoclonus), and other clinical and EEG characteristics in PMEs. Lafora disease and some cases of Unverricht-Lundborg disease may initially be mistaken for JME. Subsequent worsening of the myoclonic syndrome, appearance of slow background EEG activity, and cognitive deterioration suggest the possibility of a progressive disorder.

There is no indication that any of the myoclonic epilepsies of infancy and childhood (i.e., benign myoclonic epilepsy and MAE) may evolve into JME. Confusion may arise from cases of late-onset MAE (ages 5 to 7 years), but the association of myoclonic-astatic seizures, nocturnal brief generalized tonic-clonic seizures, or tonic seizures and episodes of absence status is clearly different from JME. Approximately 5% of childhood absence epilepsy may evolve into JME during adolescence.

Treatment

Monotherapy with sodium valproate controls the jerks and other types of attacks in approximately 85% of patients (78,108). Methsuximide is an alternative monotherapy (110). Phenobarbital and primidone, originally recommended by Janz, are more useful against grand mal seizures than myoclonic jerks. In resistant cases, the addition of small doses of clonazepam or clobazam may be effective (94). Lamotrigine has been used either as an alternative to or in association with valproic acid (111–113); however, withdrawal of valproic acid led to a recrudescence of both myoclonic and generalized tonic-clonic seizures, suggesting that a specific pharmacodynamic action of lamotrigine caused the clinical worsening. Preliminary data suggest that topiramate might be an interesting alternative in some patients with difficult-to-treat JME (114). Long-term acetazolamide monotherapy may help about half of patients who respond poorly to conventional antiepileptic drugs or suffer valproate-associated adverse effects (115).

Undefined Epilepsies with Myoclonic Seizures

Epilepsy with myoclonic seizures that manifests in childhood or adolescence may have atypical features. Whether these entities represent distinct syndromes with prominent myoclonic seizures is still uncertain.

Eyelid Myoclonia with and without Absences

Eyelid myoclonia with absences is characterized by prominent jerking of the eyelids with upward deviation of the eyes. The severity of eyelid jerking contrasts with the slight eyelid flicker seen in typical absences (116,117). The brevity of the phenomenon (1 to 2 seconds) may make it impossible to establish whether there is concomitant lapse of consciousness. The intensity of the jerking justifies the inclusion among myoclonic epilepsies, as the myoclonic phenomena are usually difficult to control and persist into adulthood, whereas the absences are relatively easily controlled. Marked photosensitivity and frequent autostimulation are also features that eyelid myoclonia, with and without absences, shares with other myoclonic epilepsies of infancy and childhood.

Myoclonic Seizures Induced by Photic Stimuli

Myoclonic attacks can be induced by photic stimuli. Jeavons and Harding (117) found that only 1.5% of pure photosensitive epilepsies (i.e., epilepsies induced exclusively by exposure to visual stimuli without any spontaneous attacks) were myoclonic. Visually induced generalized myoclonic jerks are usually symmetric and predominate in the upper extremities. Usually they produce only head nodding and slight arm abduction. More generalized jerks involving the face, trunk, and legs may occasionally cause falls. The relationship of myoclonic jerks to the stimulus is complex. Sometimes there is no definite time association; on other occasions the jerks may be repeated rhythmically with the same frequency as the stimulus or at one of its subharmonics (118). On the electroencephalogram, the jerks are associated with the photoparoxysmal response, consisting of a bilateral polyspike or polyspike-and-wave discharge (16,118).

Spontaneous seizures are said to occur mainly, but not exclusively, when the polyspike-wave discharge persists after the stimulation is discontinued (118); this is sometimes called a "prolonged photoconvulsive response" (119). Myoclonic attacks can be provoked by television watching, especially when patients are close to the screen, and by playing video games. Mentally retarded patients especially induce the myoclonic attacks by waving a hand between their eyes and a source of light, flickering their eyelids in front of a light source, staring at patterned surfaces, or by similar maneuvers (117,120,121). Reporting on 27 patients who had a combination of myoclonic absence, myoclonic jerks, and generalized tonic-clonic seizures (122), Seino and Fujihara (cited by Dreifuss [122]) considered photosensitive myoclonic epilepsy a new epileptic syndrome, always associated with mental retardation and an obvious tendency toward resistance to drug therapy.

MYOCLONIC EPILEPSIES WITH VARIABLE AGE OF ONSET

Epilepsies with Prominent Rhythmic Distal Myoclonus

Angelman Syndrome

This neurogenetic disorder is caused by a defect on maternal chromosome 15q11-q13. A cytogenetic deletion including three genes coding for the α_5, β_3, and γ_3 subunits of the GABA$_A$ (*GABRB3*, *GABRA5*, and *GABRG3*) and the *UBE3A* gene is present in 70% of patients (123). A less-frequent cause is uniparental paternal disomy or mutations in the imprinting center or in the *UBE3A* gene (124). Patients present with moderate to severe mental retardation, absence of language, microbrachycephaly, inappropriate paroxysmal laughter, epilepsy, EEG abnormalities, ataxic gait, tremor, and jerky movements. Neurophysiologic investigations reveal a spectrum of myoclonic manifestations (125). Rapid distal jerking of fluctuating amplitude causes a coarse tremor combined with dystonic limb posturing. Jerks occur at rest in prolonged runs. Myoclonic and absence seizures, as well as episodes of myoclonic status are also present. Bilateral jerks of myoclonic absences show rhythmic repetition at approximately 2.5 Hz (Fig. 26.3) and are time-locked with a cortical spike. Interside latency of both spikes and jerks is consistent with transcallosal spread, and spike-to-jerk latency indicates propagation through rapid conduction through corticospinal pathways. Because epilepsy tends to be more severe in patients with a cytogenetic deletion, in addition to *UBE3A*, other genes in 15q11-13 (especially *GABRB3*) could play a major role in epileptogenesis (126).

Treatment

Episodes of myoclonic or nonconvulsive status are usually controlled with intravenous benzodiazepines (125,127). For the long-term treatment of epilepsy, the combination of benzodiazepines and valproic acid is particularly effective (125–128). Ethosuximide, in addition to valproic acid, controls refractory atypical absences.

Familial Autosomal Dominant Myoclonic Epilepsy and Autosomal Dominant Cortical Reflex Myoclonus and Epilepsy

Benign familial autosomal dominant myoclonic epilepsy (BFAME or FAME) has been described in several families of mostly Japanese origin (129,130). Patients present with homogeneous characteristics: autosomal dominant inheritance; adult onset (mean age, 38 years; range, 19–73 years); nonprogressive course; distal, rhythmic myoclonus enhanced during posture maintenance (cortical tremor);

rare, apparently generalized seizures often preceded by worsening myoclonus; absence of other neurologic signs; generalized interictal spike-and-wave discharges; photoparoxysmal response; giant somatosensory evoked potentials; hyperexcitability of the C-reflex; and cortical EEG potential time-locked to the jerks. Analysis in the original Japanese families indicated a linkage to chromosome 8q23.3-q24 locus (131); however, European families with a similar phenotype did not link to the same locus (130, 132–134).

Autosomal dominant cortical reflex myoclonus and epilepsy (ADCME) (135) has been described in patients who present with a homogeneous syndromic core that includes nonprogressive cortical reflex myoclonus, expressed with semicontinuous rhythmic distal jerking (cortical tremor); generalized tonic-clonic seizures sometimes preceded by generalized myoclonic jerks; and generalized EEG abnormalities. Ages at onset of cortical tremor and of generalized tonic-clonic seizures overlap in a given individual but vary between individuals, ranging from 12 to 50 years. This clinical picture shares some features with FAME (131), but all ADCME patients also have focal frontotemporal EEG abnormalities and some have focal seizures that start about the same age as the other manifestations and are either intractable or remit after several years.

Inheritance is autosomal dominant with high penetrance. Linkage analysis has identified a critical region on chromosome 2p11.1-q12.2. The exclusion of the locus for FAME on chromosome 8q23.3-q24 from linkage to an ADCME family and the new localization of the responsible gene to chromosome 2, together with the different phenotype, define a new epilepsy syndrome (135). Three Italian families with familial adult myoclonic epilepsy are possibly linked to 2p11.1-q12.2, suggesting a possible allelism with ADCME (133,134).

Progressive Myoclonus Epilepsies

This group of rare heterogeneous genetic disorders shares clinical features including myoclonic jerks that are segmental, arrhythmic, usually asynchronous (Fig. 26.4), and often stimulus sensitive; epileptic seizures, predominantly generalized tonic-clonic, but also clonic, absence, and focal seizures; progressive mental deterioration; and variable neurologic signs and symptoms, including cerebellar, extrapyramidal, and action myoclonus (136). Table 26.2 lists the clinical classification (136–139).

Epidemiology

PMEs represent less than 1% of all epilepsy cases and have a variable geographic and ethnic distribution. Between 1960 and 2002, 128 patients were seen in the Saint Paul Centre (Marseille), most with Unverricht-Lundborg and Lafora diseases (139). The NCLs have the highest incidence (1 in about 10,000 children) in northern European populations,

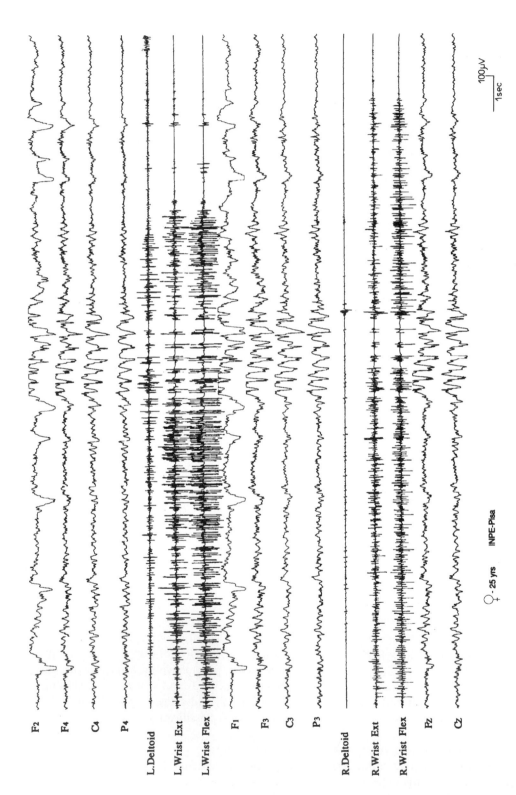

F2
F4
C4
P4
L.Deltoid
L.Wrist Ext
L.Wrist Flex
F1
F3
C3
P3
R.Deltoid
R.Wrist Ext
R.Wrist Flex
Pz
Cz

100μV

1sec

♀ - 25 yrs   INPE-Pisa

Figure 26.3 Surface electroencephalographic (EEG)-electromyographic (EMG) polygraphic recording of a 16-year-old girl with Angelman syndrome. Rhythmic 12- to 15-Hz myoclonus, involving all muscles recorded, is accompanied by diffuse, rhythmic, 5- to 8-Hz sharp EEG activity. During a short myoclonic absence, a discharge of generalized spike-and-wave complexes is associated with rhythmic EMG bursts of 2 to 4 myoclonic potentials, each time-locked with the spikes. After the absence, recordings resume the rhythmic pattern of myoclonus that disappears 3 seconds later in the right hemisphere and left muscles, but it persists for 3 more seconds contralaterally.

Awake at rest

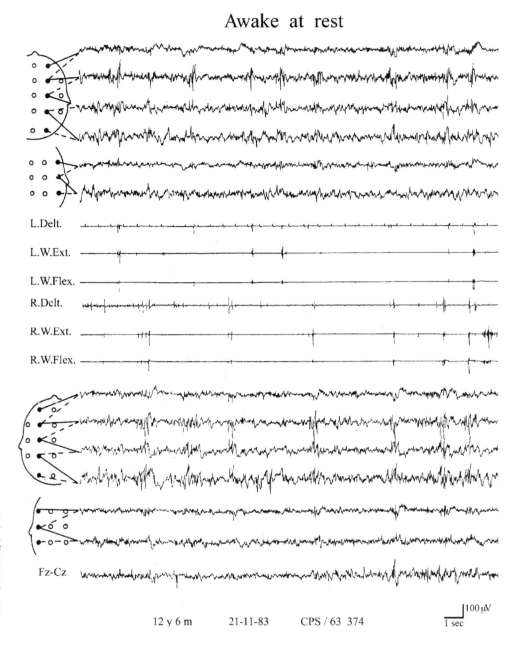

L.Delt.

L.W.Ext.

L.W.Flex.

R.Delt.

R.W.Ext.

R.W.Flex.

Fz-Cz

Figure 26.4 Gaucher disease type III. Waking electroencephalographic (EEG) polygraphic recording including electromyography of left and right deltoids, flexor, and extensor wrists muscles, showing myoclonic jerks on the electromyographic channels correlated with bilateral polyspike discharges on the EEG channels.

12 y 6 m   21-11-83   CPS / 63 374

$100 \mu V$

1 sec

although a focus was identified in Newfoundland (Canada) (140). Dentatorubral-pallidoluysian atrophy (DRPLA) and galactosialidosis occur frequently in Japan, sialidosis occurs frequently in Italy, and Gaucher disease is prevalent among Ashkenazic Jews.

Molecular Genetics

Excluding DRPLA and adult NCL with autosomal dominant inheritance and MERRF with mitochondrial inheritance, the other PMEs follow a recessive inheritance. The underlying gene defects have been identified (Table 26.3) (141–155).

Most PMEs result from the accumulation of abnormal deposit material but the pathogenetic pathway leading to the phenotype from the gene defect is not yet known.

Diagnostic methods are available for the great majority of patients (Table 26.4).

This section describes the four major conditions responsible for PMEs in infancy, childhood, and adolescence.

Unverricht-Lundborg Disease

This classic form of PME with stimulus-sensitive myoclonus begins between the ages of 6 and 18 years (139,156). Incidence is high around the Baltic sea (157) and in the Mediterranean region (158). Usually precipitated by passive joint movements, as well as auditory and light stimuli, myoclonic jerks of the arms and legs ultimately interfere with speech, gait, swallowing, and ambulation, until all voluntary actions become almost impossible. Later, generalized tonic-clonic seizures are often preceded by a

TABLE 26.2
CLINICAL CLASSIFICATION OF THE PROGRESSIVE MYOCLONUS EPILEPSIES

Type	Age of Onset (years)
Unverricht-Lundborg disease	7–16
Lafora disease	6–19
Neuronal ceroid-lipofuscinoses	
Infantile (Haltia-Santavuori)	6 months–2 years
Late infantile (Jansky-Bielschowsky)	1–4
Intermediate (Lake or Cavanagh)	5–8
Juvenile (Spielmeyer-Vogt)	4–14
Adult (Kufs)	15–50
Myoclonic epilepsy with ragged-red fibers	3–65
Sialidosis	8–15
Type 1	
Galactosialidosis (type 2)	
Dentatorubral-pallidoluysian atrophy	Childhood
Gaucher disease (type III)	Variable

crescendo of massive myoclonic jerks. Both seizures and myoclonias appear on awakening and are distinguished from those of JME by their sensitivity to stimuli. Generally, the disease progresses slowly: patients maintain normal cognitive functions until moderate deterioration develops in 10 to 20 years. Symptoms often fluctuate sharply between "good periods" of slightly impaired function and "bad periods" of frequent and severe myoclonic jerks culminating in tonic-clonic seizures. The disease stabi-

lizes in adulthood, when the debilitating effects of myoclonic jerks subside, and patients survive to old age (139,159).

The electroencephalogram shows normal or slightly slow background activity, generalized polyspike and 3- to 5-Hz spike-wave discharges resembling those of JME (160). Unlike in JME, however, epileptiform activity decreases during NREM sleep, and discharges are often seen during REM sleep (160). Photosensitivity is present in more than 90% of cases. Giant somatosensory evoked potentials have abnormally high amplitude.

This recessively inherited disease was the first PME in which the gene defect—mutations of the cystatin B (*CSTB* or *EPM1*) gene on chromosome 21q22.3—was discovered. (141,161). The most common mutation consists of a dodecamer repeat in the promoter region (162); only a minority of patients harbor mutations within the transcriptional unit of *CSTB* (163). All patients carry *CSTB* gene mutations, but how this defect can cause the phenotype is not yet understood. Neuropathologic studies have shown widespread degenerative changes in the central nervous system including loss of Purkinje cells but no storage material in the brain (138). Mice that are deficient in cystatin B do not manifest epileptic seizures and myoclonus; however, *CSTB* knockout mice and kindling studies in rats support evidence favoring a neuroprotective role for cystatin B (141,164).

Lafora Body Disease

This autosomal recessive condition begins between the ages of 10 and 18 years (137,165) with generalized tonic-clonic

TABLE 26.3
MOLECULAR GENETICS OF PROGRESSIVE MYOCLONUS EPILEPSIES

PME Type	Inheritance	Locus	Gene
Unverricht-Lundborg disease (141)	AR	21q22.3	EPM1
Lafora disease (142,143)	AR	6q 24	EPMA
		6p22.3	EPM2B
NCL	AR		
Infantile (144)		1p32	CLN1
Late-infantile (145)		11p15.5	CLN2
Finnish variant (146)		13q21	CLN5
Gipsy variant (147)		15q21-23	CLN6
Turkish variant (148)		?	CLN7
Juvenile (149)		16p12.1	CLN3
Juvenile variant (150)		8p22	CLN8
Adult	AR and AD	?	CLN4
MERRF (154)	Mitochondrial	Mt DNA	tRNA^{Lys}
Sialidosis (152)	AR	6p21.3	NEU
Galactosialidosis (153)		20q13	PPCA
Gaucher type III (154)	AR	1q21	GBA
DRPLA (155)	AD	12p.13.31	CAG repeats

AD, autosomal dominant; AR, autosomal recessive; DRPLA, dentatorubral-pallidoluysian atrophy; MERRF, myoclonus epilepsy with ragged-red fibers; Mt DNA, mitochondrial DNA; NCL, neuronal ceroid lipofuscinosis; PME, progressive myoclonus epilepsy.

TABLE 26.4

DIAGNOSTIC TOOLS FOR THE PROGRESSIVE MYOCLONUS EPILEPSIES

PME Type	Methods	Marker
Unverricht-Lundborg disease	Molecular biology	*EPM1*
Lafora disease	Biopsy	Lafora bodies
	Molecular biology	*EPM2A* and *EPM2B*
NCL	Biopsy	Storage lipopigment in lysosomes
	Molecular biology	*CLN1, 2, 3, 5, 6, 8*
MERRF	Muscle biopsy	Ragged-red fibers
	Molecular biology	A8344G substitution (90%)
Sialidosis	Urine	*Urinary oligosaccharides
	Lymphocytes, fibroblasts	α-N-acetyl neuroaminidase deficit
	Molecular biology	*NEU*
Galactosialidosis	Urine, leukocytes, fibroblasts	β-Galactosidase deficit
	Molecular biology	*PPCA*
Gaucher	Lymphocytes, fibroblast	β-Glucocerebrosidase deficit
	Molecular biology	*GBA*
DRPLA	Molecular biology	GAC expansion

DRPLA, dentatorubral-pallidoluysian atrophy; MERRF, myoclonus epilepsy with ragged-red fibers; NCL, neuronal ceroid lipofuscinosis; PME, progressive myoclonus epilepsy.

and focal-visual seizures (137,166). Later, low-amplitude myoclonic jerks produce muscle twitches that may be visible but do not induce any movement. Subsequent spontaneous jerks are increased by sudden noises, flashing lights, touch, or movement. Myoclonus eventually becomes almost constant and is often accompanied by massive myoclonic seizures. Mental deterioration is rapid. Patients become totally disabled and die within 5 to 10 years from the first symptoms (139).

When the disease begins, the electroencephalogram shows relatively normal background activity, spontaneous polyspike-wave discharges, and a photoconvulsive response (167) that could lead to a misdiagnosis of JME. The background activity eventually becomes slow and disorganized, with almost continuous generalized and multifocal epileptiform discharges (167).

The hallmark Lafora bodies are para-aminosalicylic acid–positive cytoplasmic inclusions containing polyglucosans. Found in the brain, spinal cord, heart, skeletal muscle, liver, and skin, Lafora bodies can also be seen in the myoepithelial cells of the apocrine sweat glands and in the apocrine and eccrine sweat duct cells. The axillary skin biopsy is the diagnostic procedure of choice (168).

Mutations of the *EPM2A* gene on chromosome 6q23-25, which codes for laforin, cause 80% of cases (142,169). Laforin is a dual-specificity protein tyrosine phosphatase, which is active in the growth, development, and survival of neurons, dendrites, and synapses. Not surprisingly, therefore, mutations of *EPM2A* cause a disease with rapid cognitive decline and epilepsy but the exact pathogenetic mechanism is not understood. A second gene has been identified (143): *EPM2B*, on chromosome 6p22.3, encoding for a protein named "malin" with an as-yet unknown function.

Neuronal Ceroid Lipofuscinoses

The most frequent neurodegenerative disorders in childhood (167), NCLs are divided into four main subtypes based on age of onset and anatomopathologic findings: infantile (Santavuori-Haltia disease; *CLN1*), late infantile (Jansky-Bielschowsky disease; *CLN2*), juvenile (Spielmeyer-Vogt-Sjögren or Batten disease; *CLN3*), and adult (Kufs disease; *CLN4*). In addition to the classic PME symptoms, NCLs involve impaired vision. All are characterized by the storage in multiple tissues of lipopigments, but the ultrastructure of inclusion bodies differs in each NCL subtype.

Because of its very early onset and rapid progression, the infantile type is not considered a PME and is not discussed further.

In late-infantile NCL, myoclonic, generalized tonic-clonic, and atypical absence seizures begin between the ages of 2 and 4 years (137), followed soon after by mental deterioration, ataxia, and spasticity; visual impairment usually develops between 4 and 6 years. Death occurs before age 10 years. The EEG shows slow background activity with generalized epileptiform discharges and spikes in the occipital regions in response to photic stimulation, corresponding to giant visual evoked potentials; somatosensory evoked potentials are also abnormal. Biopsy specimens of the skin, conjunctiva, or rectum show the pathognomonic curvilinear bodies; however, mixed lysosomal inclusions featuring curvilinear profiles and rectilinear complexes are also seen and could be misleading (170). Ultrastructural studies of amniotic fluid cells, choroid villi, fetal skin, or lymphocytes have been used for prenatal diagnosis (171). Late-infantile NCL was initially mapped to chromosome 11p15, and the causative gene, *CLN2*, encoding for a lysosomal enzyme (TTP1) was subsequently identified (145,147). Although more than 30 mutations have been reported, two (T523-1G>C and 636 C>T) account for approximately 60% to 78% of patients (172,173). Molecular biology diagnosis can be made using specific polyclonal antibodies against *CLN2* product or by testing the decreased activity of TTP1.

Three genetic variants have been described: Finnish and early juvenile, whose mutated *CLN5* and *CLN6* genes have been mapped to the chromosomal regions 13q21 and 15q21 (147,149,174), and a Turkish variant (*CLN7*), not yet chromosomally linked (148).

The juvenile subtype, the most common form of NCL, manifests as rapidly progressing visual impairment between 4 and 7 years of age, followed by myoclonus, generalized tonic-clonic and absence seizures, and neurologic deterioration. Speech disturbances, behavioral problems, extrapyramidal signs, and sleep disturbances complete the clinical picture. Death usually occurs in the late teens or early twenties. The EEG resembles the late-infantile form but without photosensitivity. The diagnosis is confirmed by fingerprints in the skin biopsy material. Juvenile NCL was mapped to chromosome 16, and the *CLN3* gene was subsequently cloned (175,176). Although several mutations (deletions, insertions, missense, non-sense, or splice-site) have been identified, approximately 80% of patients carry a deletion that removes exons 7 and 8 (177). *CLN3* encodes for a protein whose function is not known.

Some patients show inclusion bodies with the ultrastructure profile of the granular osmiophilic deposits typical of the infantile form; these patients carry mutations in the *CLN1* gene (178). A progressive epilepsy with mental retardation, known as northern epilepsy, has been included in the NCLs and is considered a variant of the juvenile form (179). *CLN8*, the disease-causing mutated gene, maps to chromosome 8p (150).

The rare adult subtype is characterized by myoclonus, ataxia, and dementia (167). A distinct clinical phenotype involves presenile onset of behavioral abnormalities, dementia, motor dysfunction, ataxia, and extrapyramidal and suprabulbar signs (180). The electroencephalogram shows generalized spike-wave discharges, with photosensitivity to low frequencies; somatosensory evoked potentials are usually enlarged. Electron microscopic study of skin biopsy material shows either fingerprints, curvilinear bodies, or granular osmiophilic deposits. Adult NCL can have a recessive or autosomal dominant inheritance, but a locus for *CLN4* has not been identified.

MERRF has a highly variable age of onset, from childhood to late adulthood (181,182), and is clinically characterized by myoclonus, generalized tonic-clonic seizures, and, sometimes, atypical absences. Other features include deafness, short stature, optic atrophy, neuropathy, migraine, fatigue, and diabetes. The electroencephalogram shows generalized atypical spike- and polyspike-wave discharges; rare focal epileptiform abnormalities can also be seen with photosensitivity. Somatosensory evoked potentials are usually giant. Muscle biopsy specimens reveal subsar-

colemmal aggregates of mitochondria, the so-called ragged-red fibers. Inheritance is consistent with mitochondrial transmission: the disorder is associated with an A-to-G substitution at nucleotide 8344 in the transfer RNA (tRNA) Lys in the mitochondrial DNA (151). At least two other mutations (T8356C and G8363A) in the same gene can cause a similar picture (183,184). MERRF may also involve the A-to-G transition at nucleotide 3243 of the tRNA^{Leu} (UUR), which is usually associated with other mitochondrial disorders (185,186). These mutations lead to functionally incompetent mitochondria that result in energy-deficient cells.

Treatment

Absent an etiologic therapy, the treatment of PMEs focuses on controlling seizures and myoclonus. Valproic acid, as monotherapy or combined with clonazepam or clobazam and phenobarbital, is the drug of choice for seizures. Phenytoin had been used in the past but caused rapid progression of symptoms with very severe myoclonus and ataxia, especially in patients with Unverricht-Lundborg disease, in whom it is contraindicated (187). High doses of piracetam (24 to 36 g/day; available outside the United States) are tolerated relatively well, with few adverse effects and with clinically relevant and sustained improvement of the myoclonus and the motor impairment (188,189). Levetiracetam is also used for myoclonus (190).

The antioxidant *N*-acetylcysteine, zonisamide, and oral 5-hydroxy-L-tryptophan prevent further deterioration and control seizures and the disabling stimulus-sensitivity myoclonus (191–194); long-term efficacy trials have not been performed, however. Coenzyme Q10, vitamin K$_3$, vitamin C, riboflavin, thiamine, and dichloroacetate may be effective in MERRF (195). In one patient with progressive myoclonus epilepsy, vagus nerve stimulation reduced seizures more than 90% and significantly improved cerebellar function (196). Gene therapy for PMEs remains only theoretical and speculative.

Drug-Induced Myoclonic Seizures

Either because of a paradoxical reaction or inappropriate choice, antiepileptic drugs can aggravate or induce myoclonic seizures, priming a vicious circle of intensive treatment in which the original disorder is no longer recognizable and is transformed into an epileptic encephalopathy.

Anecdotal reports suggest the use of lamotrigine in some myoclonic epilepsies, but convincing data are lacking. Conversely, lamotrigine as add-on treatment may worsen seizures in patients with SMEI (197). Carbamazepine and vigabatrin should be avoided in MAE, because they can trigger episodes of myoclonic status (43,52). JME, like other idiopathic generalized epilepsies, can be aggravated by phenytoin and especially carbamazepine, which may even precipitate myoclonic status (109). Lamotrigine reportedly aggravates seizures in JME (198). Carbamazepine

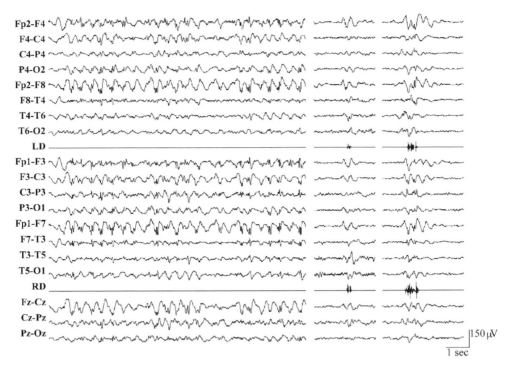

Figure 26.5 A   14-year-old girl presented with a "confusional state," described by her parents as day-long episodes of confusion and awkward behavior, starting at age 9 years and recurring once a month until age 12 years. At age 12 years, carbamazepine treatment was begun for a generalized tonic-clonic seizure, which did not recur, although the confusional episodes became weekly events.

The electroencephalogram shows almost continuous 3- to 4-Hz generalized polyspike-and-wave discharges (*left panel*). Although confused, the girl could perform simple motor tasks when encouraged. Administration of clobazam was followed by gradual abatement of spike-and-wave discharges and recovery of a normal background activity. During this phase (*right panel*), occasional whole-body myoclonic jerks accompanied by a generalized polyspike-and-wave discharge were recorded. On substitution with valproic acid, the confusional states disappeared during the past few months. Carbamazepine seems to have increased seizure frequency in this patient and induced *de novo* myoclonic seizures previously unreported.

or oxcarbazepine (126–128), phenytoin (126), or vigabatrin (199) may worsen myoclonic and absence seizures in Angelman syndrome.

De novo appearance of myoclonic jerks was described in children and adults with cryptogenic or partial epilepsy treated with add-on vigabatrin (197,200), and in children with childhood absence epilepsy treated with vigabatrin and carbamazepine (201) (Fig. 26.5). *De novo* myoclonic status epilepticus has been reported following high doses of lamotrigine in Lennox-Gastaut syndrome (202).

REFERENCES

1. Guerrini R, Bonanni P, Rothwell J, et al. Myoclonus and epilepsy. In: Guerrini R, Aicardi J, Andermann F, et al., eds. *Epilepsy and movement disorders.* Cambridge, UK: Cambridge University Press, 2002:165–210.
2. Aicardi J, Levy Gomes A. Myoclonic epilepsies in childhood. *Int Pediatr* 1991;6:195–200.
3. Erba G, Browne TR. Atypical absence, myoclonic, atonic, and tonic seizures, and the "Lennox-Gastaut syndrome." In: Browne T, Feldman RG, eds. *Epilepsy: diagnosis and management.* Boston: Little Brown, 1983:75–94.
4. Dalla Bernardina B, Capovilla G, Chiamenti C, et al. Cryptogenic myoclonic epilepsies of infancy and early childhood: nosological and prognostic approach. In: Wolf P, Janz D, Dreifuss FE, eds. *Advances in epileptology.* New York: Raven Press, 1987:175–179.
5. Dravet C, Bureau M, Oguni H, et al. Severe myoclonic epilepsy in infancy (Dravet syndrome). In: Roger J, Bureau M, Dravet C, et al., eds. *Epileptic syndromes in infancy, childhood and adolescence,* 3rd ed. London: John Libbey, 2002:81–103.
6. Oguni H, Tanaka T, Hayashi K, et al. Treatment and long-term prognosis of myoclonic-astatic epilepsy of early childhood. *Neuropediatrics* 2002;33:122–132.
7. Patel V, Jankovic J. Myoclonus. *Curr Neurol* 1988;8:109–156.
8. Hallett M. Myoclonus: relation to epilepsy. *Epilepsia* 1985;26:S67–S77.
9. Tassinari C, Bureau M, Thomas P. Epilepsy with myoclonic absences. In: Roger J, Bureau M, Dravet C, et al., eds. *Epileptic syndromes in infancy, childhood and adolescence,* 2nd ed. London: John Libbey, 1992:151–160.
10. Aicardi J, Chevrie JJ. Myoclonic epilepsies of childhood. *Neuropadiatrie* 1971;3:177–190.
11. Ricci S, Cusmai R, Fusco L, et al. Reflex myoclonic epilepsy in infancy: a new age-dependent idiopathic epileptic syndrome related to startle reaction. *Epilepsia* 1995;36:342–348.
12. Doose H. Myoclonic-astatic epilepsy. *Epilepsy Res Suppl* 1992;6:163–168.
13. Gastaut H, Broughton R, Roger J, et al. Generalized convulsive seizures without local onset. In: Vinken P, Bruyn GW, eds. *The epilepsies. Handbook of clinical neurology.* Amsterdam: Elsevier, 1974:107–129.
14. Chayasirisobhon S, Rodin EA. Atonic-akinetic seizures. *Electroencephalogr Clin Neurophysiol* 1981;50:225.

15. Fariello RG, Doro JM, Forster FM. Generalized cortical electrodecremental event. Clinical and neurophysiological observations in patients with dystonic seizures. *Arch Neurol* 1979;36: 285–291.

16. Gastaut H, Broughton R. *Epileptic seizures.* Springfield, IL: Charles C Thomas, 1972.

17. Brenner RP, Atkinson R. Generalized paroxysmal fast activity: electroencephalographic and clinical features. *Ann Neurol* 1982;11:386–390.

18. Gastaut H, Roger J, Ouahchi S, et al. An electro-clinical study of generalized epileptic seizures of tonic expression. *Epilepsia* 1963;4:15–44.

19. Egli M, Mothersill I, O'Kane M, et al. The axial spasm—the predominant type of drop seizure in patients with secondary generalized epilepsy. *Epilepsia* 1985;26:401–415.

20. Claes L, Del-Favero J, Ceulemans B, et al. De novo mutations in the sodium-channel gene *SCN1A* cause severe myoclonic epilepsy of infancy. *Am J Hum Genet* 2001;68:1327–1332.

21. Wallace RH, Wang DW, Singh R, et al. Febrile seizures and generalized epilepsy associated with a mutation in the Na$^+$-channel β$_1$ subunit gene *SCN1B. Nat Genet* 1998;19:366–370.

22. Cossette P, Liu L, Brisebois K, et al. Mutation of *GABRA1* in an autosomal dominant form of juvenile myoclonic epilepsy. *Nat Genet* 2002;31:184–189.

23. Dalla Bernardina B, Fontana E, Darra F. Myoclonic status in nonprogressive encephalopathies. In: Roger J, Bureau M, Dravet C, et al., eds. *Epileptic syndromes in infancy, childhood and adolescence.* London: John Libbey, 2002:137–144.

24. Elia M, Musumeci SA, Ferri R, et al. Trisomy 12p and epilepsy with myoclonic absences. *Brain Dev* 1998;20:127–130.

25. Commission on Classification and Terminology of the International League Against Epilepsy. Proposal for revised classification of epilepsies and epileptic syndromes. *Epilepsia* 1989;30: 389–399.

26. Aicardi J. Early myoclonic encephalopathy (neonatal myoclonic encephalopathy). In: Roger J, Bureau M, Dravet C, et al., eds. *Epileptic syndromes in infancy, childhood and adolescence,* 2nd ed. London: John Libbey, 1992:13–23.

27. Scher MS, Bergman I, Ahdab-Barmada M, et al. Neurophysiological and anatomical correlations in neonatal nonketotic hyperglycinemia. *Neuropediatrics* 1986;17:137–143.

28. Dravet C, Bureau M. The benign myoclonic epilepsy of infancy [author's translation]. *Rev Electroencephalogr Neurophysiol Clin* 1981;11:438–444.

29. Dravet C, Bureau M, Genton P. Benign myoclonic epilepsy of infancy: electroclinical symptomatology and differential diagnosis from the other types of generalized epilepsy of infancy. *Epilepsy Res Suppl* 1992;6:131–135.

30. Ohtsuka Y, Ohno S, Oka E, et al. Classification of epilepsies and epileptic syndromes of childhood according to the 1989 ILAE classification. *J Epilepsy* 1993;6:272–276.

31. Revol M, Isnard H, Beaumanoir A, et al. Touch evoked myoclonic seizures in infancy. In: Beaumanoir A, Naquet R, Gastaut H, eds. *Reflex seizures and reflex epilepsies.* Geneva: Médicine et Hygiène, 1989:103–105.

32. Deonna T, Despland PA. Sensory-evoked (touch) idiopathic myoclonic epilepsy of infancy. In: Beaumanoir A, Naquet R, Gastaut H, eds. *Reflex seizures and reflex epilepsies.* Geneva: Médicine et Hygiène, 1989:99–102.

33. Aicardi J, Levy Gomes A. The Lennox-Gastaut syndrome: clinical and electroencephalographic features. In: Niedermeyer E, Degen R, eds. *The Lennox-Gastaut syndrome.* New York: Allan R. Liss, 1988:25–46.

34. Dravet C, Bureau M. Benign myoclonic epilepsy in infancy. In: Roger J, Bureau M, Dravet C, et al., eds. *Epileptic syndromes in infancy, childhood and adolescence,* 3rd ed. London: John Libbey, 2002:69–79.

35. Guerrini R, Dravet C, Gobbi G, et al. Idiopathic generalized epilepsies with myoclonus in infancy and childhood. In: Malafosse A, Genton P, Hirsch E, et al., eds. *Idiopathic generalized epilepsies: clinical, experimental and genetics aspects.* London: John Libbey, 1994:267–280.

36. Giovanardi Rossi P, Parmeggiani A, Posar A, et al. Benign myoclonic epilepsy: long-term follow-up of 11 new cases. *Brain Dev* 1997;19:473–479.

37. Engel J Jr. A proposed diagnostic scheme for people with epileptic seizures and with epilepsy: report of the ILAE Task Force on Classification and Terminology. *Epilepsia* 2001;42: 796–803.

38. Sarisjulis N, Gamboni B, Plouin P, et al. Diagnosing idiopathic/cryptogenic epilepsy syndromes in infancy. *Arch Dis Child* 2000;82:226–230.

39. Arzimanoglou A, Prudent M, Salefanque F. Epilepsie myoclonoastatique et épilepsie myoclonique bénigne du nourrisson dans une même famille: quelques réflexions sur la classification des épilepsies. *Epilepsies* 1996;8:307–315.

40. Bonanni P, Malcarne M, Moro F, et al. Generalized epilepsy with febrile seizures plus (GEFS+): clinical spectrum in seven Italian families unrelated to *SCN1A, SCN1B,* and *GABRG2* gene mutations. *Epilepsia* 2004;45:149–158.

41. Lin Y, Itomi K, Takada H, et al. Benign myoclonic epilepsy in infants: video-EEG features and long-term follow-up. *Neuropediatrics* 1998;29:268–271.

42. Guerrini R, Bonanni P, Parmeggiani L, et al. Cortical reflex myoclonus in Rett syndrome. *Ann Neurol* 1998;43:472–479.

43. Kaminska A, Ickowicz A, Plouin P, et al. Delineation of cryptogenic Lennox-Gastaut syndrome and myoclonic astatic epilepsy using multiple correspondence analysis. *Epilepsy Res* 1999;36:15–29.

44. Pachatz C, Fusco L, Vigevano F. Benign myoclonus of early infancy. *Epileptic Disord* 1999;1:57–61.

45. Dravet C, Giraud N, Bureau M, et al. Benign myoclonus of early infancy or benign non-epileptic infantile spasms. *Neuropediatrics* 1986;17:33–38.

46. Oguni H, Fukuyama Y, Tanaka T, et al. Myoclonic-astatic epilepsy of early childhood—clinical and EEG analysis of myoclonic-astatic seizures, and discussions on the nosology of the syndrome. *Brain Dev* 2001;23:757–764.

47. Doose H, Gerken H, Leonhardt R, et al. Centrencephalic myoclonic-astatic petit mal. Clinical and genetic investigation. *Neuropadiatrie* 1970;2:59–78.

48. Tassinari CA, Rubboli G, Shibasaki H. Neurophysiology of positive and negative myoclonus. *Electroencephalogr Clin Neurophysiol* 1998;107:181–195.

49. Dravet C, Guerrini R, Bureau M. Epileptic syndromes with drop seizures in children. In: Beaumanoir A, Andermann F, Avanzini G, et al., eds. *Falls in epileptic and non-epileptic seizures during childhood.* London: John Libbey, 1997:95–111.

50. Bonanni P, Parmeggiani L, Guerrini R. Different neurophysiologic patterns of myoclonus characterize Lennox-Gastaut syndrome and myoclonic astatic epilepsy. *Epilepsia* 2002;43: 609–615.

51. Giovanardi Rossi P, Gobbi G, Melideo G, et al. Myoclonic manifestations in Lennox-Gastaut syndrome and other childhood epilepsies. In: Niedermeyer E, Degen R, eds. *The Lennox-Gastaut syndrome.* New York: Alan R. Liss, 1988:137–158.

52. Guerrini R, Parmeggiani L, Kaminska A, et al. Myoclonic astatic epilepsy. In: Roger J, Bureau M, Dravet C, et al., eds. *Epileptic syndromes in infancy, childhood and adolescence,* 3rd ed. London: John Libbey, 2002:105–112.

53. Bednarek N, Motte J, Soufflet C, et al. Evidence of late-onset infantile spasms. *Epilepsia* 1998;39:55–60.

54. Dulac O, Kaminska A. Use of lamotrigine in Lennox-Gastaut and related epilepsy syndromes. *J Child Neurol* 1997;12:S23–S28.

55. Tennison MB, Greenwood RS, Miles MV. Methsuximide for intractable childhood seizures. *Pediatrics* 1991;87:186–189.

56. Mikaeloff Y, de Saint-Martin A, Mancini J, et al. Topiramate: efficacy and tolerability in children according to epilepsy syndromes. *Epilepsy Res* 2003;53:225–232.

57. Oguni H, Hayashi K, Awaya Y, et al. Severe myoclonic epilepsy in infants—a review based on the Tokyo Women's Medical University series of 84 cases. *Brain Dev* 2001;23:736–748.

58. Chiron C. Prognosis of severe myoclonic epilepsy in infancy (Dravet syndrome). In: Jallon P, Berg A, Dulac O, et al., eds. *Prognosis of epilepsies.* Paris: John Libbey, 2003:239–248.

59. Hurst DL. Epidemiology of severe myoclonic epilepsy of infancy. *Epilepsia* 1990;31:397–400.

60. Yakoub M, Dulac O, Jambaque I, et al. Early diagnosis of severe myoclonic epilepsy in infancy. *Brain Dev* 1992;14:299–303.

61. Ohki T, Watanabe K, Negoro T, et al. Severe myoclonic epilepsy in infancy: evolution of seizures. *Seizure* 1997;6:219–224.

62. Fujiwara T, Nakamura H, Watanabe M, et al. Clinicoelectrographic concordance between monozygotic twins with severe myoclonic epilepsy in infancy. *Epilepsia* 1990;31:281–286.
63. Singh R, Scheffer IE, Whitehouse W, et al. Severe myoclonic epilepsy of infancy is part of the spectrum of generalized epilepsy with febrile seizures plus (GEFS+). *Epilepsia* 1999;40:175.
64. Escayg A, Heils A, MacDonald BT, et al. A novel SCN1A mutation associated with generalized epilepsy with febrile seizures plus—and prevalence of variants in patients with epilepsy. *Am J Hum Genet* 2001;68:866–873.
65. Sugawara T, Mazaki-Miyazaki E, Fukushima K, et al. Frequent mutations of SCN1A in severe myoclonic epilepsy in infancy. *Neurology* 2002;58:1122–1124.
66. Nabbout R, Gennaro E, Dalla Bernardina B, et al. Spectrum of SCN1A mutations in severe myoclonic epilepsy of infancy. *Neurology* 2003;60:1961–1967.
67. Doose H, Lunau H, Castiglione E, et al. Severe idiopathic generalized epilepsy of infancy with generalized tonic-clonic seizures. *Neuropediatrics* 1998;29:229–238.
68. Hurst DL. Severe myoclonic epilepsy of infants. *Pediatr Neurol* 1987;3:269–272.
69. Cassé-Perrot C, Wolff M, Dravet C. Neuropsychological aspects of severe myoclonic epilepsy in infancy. In: Jambaqué I, Lassonde M, Dulac O, eds. *The neuropsychology of childhood epilepsy*. New York: Plenum Press, 2001:131–140.
70. Chiron C, Marchand MC, Tran A, et al. Stiripentol in severe myoclonic epilepsy in infancy: a randomised placebo-controlled syndrome-dedicated trial. *Lancet* 2000;356:1638–1642.
71. Chevrie JJ, Aicardi J. Childhood epileptic encephalopathy with slow spike-wave. A statistical study of 80 cases. *Epilepsia* 1972;13:259–271.
72. Bureau M, Tassinari CA. Epileptic syndromes in infancy, childhood and adolescence. In: Roger J, Bureau M, Dravet C, et al., eds. *The syndrome of myoclonic absences*, 3rd ed. London: John Libbey, 2002:305–309.
73. Janz D. Epilepsy with impulsive petit mal (juvenile myoclonic epilepsy). *Acta Neurol Scand* 1985;72:449–459.
74. Bamberger P, Matthes, A. *Anfälle in kindesalter*. Basel: Karger, 1959.
75. Janz D. Juvenile myoclonic epilepsy. *Cleve Clin J Med* 1989;56:23–33.
76. Delgado-Escueta AV, Serratosa JM, Medina MT. Juvenile myoclonic epilepsy. In: Wyllie E, ed. *The treatment of epilepsy: principles and practice*, 2nd ed. Baltimore, MD: Williams & Wilkins, 1996: 484–501.
77. Thomas P, Genton P, Gelisse P, et al. Juvenile myoclonic epilepsy. In: Roger J, Bureau M, Dravet C, et al., eds. *Epileptic syndromes in infancy, childhood and adolescence*, 3rd ed. London: John Libbey, 2002:335–356.
78. Genton P, Gelisse P, Thomas P. Juvenile myoclonic epilepsy today: current definitions and limits. In: Schmitz B, Sander T, eds. *Juvenile myoclonic epilepsy: the Janz syndrome*. Petersfield, UK and Philadelphia, USA: Wrightson Biomedical, 2000:11–32.
79. Tsuboi T, Christian W. On the genetics of the primary generalized epilepsy with sporadic myoclonias of impulsive petit mal type. *Humangenetik* 1973;19:155–182.
80. Beck-Mannagetta G, Janz D. Syndrome-related genetics in generalized epilepsy. In: Anderson VE, Hauser WA, Leppik IE, et al., eds. *Genetic strategies in epilepsy research*. Amsterdam: Elsevier, 1991:105–111.
81. Panayiotopoulos CP, Obeid T. Juvenile myoclonic epilepsy: an autosomal recessive disease. *Ann Neurol* 1989;25:440–443.
82. Greenberg DA, Durner M, Delgado-Escueta AV. Evidence for multiple gene loci in the expression of the common generalized epilepsies. *Neurology* 1992;42:56–62.
83. Tsuboi T, Endo S. Incidence of seizures and EEG abnormalities among offspring of epileptic patients. *Hum Genet* 1977;36:173–189.
84. Wolf P. Juvenile myoclonic epilepsy. In: Roger J, Dravet C, Bureau M, et al., eds. *Epileptic syndromes in infancy, childhood and adolescence*. London: John Libbey, 1992:313–327.
85. Greenberg DA, Delgado-Escueta AV, Widelitz H, et al. Juvenile myoclonic epilepsy (JME) may be linked to the BF and HLA loci on human chromosome 6. *Am J Med Genet* 1988;31:185–192.
86. Durner M, Sander T, Greenberg DA, et al. Localization of idiopathic generalized epilepsy on chromosome 6p in families of juvenile myoclonic epilepsy patients. *Neurology* 1991;41:1651–1655.
87. Weissbecker KA, Durner M, Janz D, et al. Confirmation of linkage between juvenile myoclonic epilepsy locus and the HLA region of chromosome 6. *Am J Med Genet* 1991;38:32–36.
88. Liu AW, Delgado-Escueta AV, Serratosa JM, et al. Juvenile myoclonic epilepsy locus in chromosome 6p21.2-p11: linkage to convulsions and electroencephalography trait. *Am J Hum Genet* 1995;57:368–381.
89. Serratosa JM, Delgado-Escueta AV, Medina MT, et al. Clinical and genetic analysis of a large pedigree with juvenile myoclonic epilepsy. *Ann Neurol* 1996;39:187–195.
90. Elmslie FV, Williamson MP, Rees M, et al. Linkage analysis of juvenile myoclonic epilepsy and microsatellite loci spanning 61cM of human chromosome 6p in 19 nuclear pedigrees provides no evidence for a susceptibility locus in this region. *Am J Hum Genet* 1996;59:653–663.
91. Whitehouse WP, Rees M, Curtis D, et al. Linkage analysis of idiopathic generalized epilepsy (IGE) and marker loci on chromosome 6p in families of patients with juvenile myoclonic epilepsy: no evidence for an epilepsy locus in the HLA region. *Am J Hum Genet* 1993;53:652–662.
92. Elmslie FV, Rees M, Williamson MP, et al. Genetic mapping of a major susceptibility locus for juvenile myoclonic epilepsy on chromosome 15q. *Hum Mol Genet* 1997;6:1329–1334.
93. Westling B, Weissbecker K, Serratosa JM, et al. Evidence for linkage of juvenile myoclonic epilepsy with absence to chromosome 1p. *Am J Hum Genet* 1996;59:241.
94. Obeid T, Panayiotopoulos CP. Juvenile myoclonic epilepsy: a study in Saudi Arabia. *Epilepsia* 1988;29:280–282.
95. Asconape J, Penry JK. Some clinical and EEG aspects of benign juvenile myoclonic epilepsy. *Epilepsia* 1984;25:108–114.
96. Salas-Puig X, Camara da Silva AM, Dravet C, et al. L'épilepsie myoclonique juvénile dans la population du Centre Saint Paul. *Epilepsies* 1990;2:108–113.
97. Wolf P, Mayer T. Juvenile myoclonic epilepsy: a syndrome challenging syndromic concepts? In: Schmitz B, Sander, T, eds. *Juvenile myoclonic epilepsy: the Janz syndrome*. Petersfield, UK and Philadelphia, USA: Wrightson Biomedical, 2000:33–39.
98. Janz D. Juvenile myoclonic epilepsy. In: Dam M, Gram L, eds. *Comprehensive epileptology*. New York: Raven Press, 1991:71–185.
99. Pedersen SB, Petersen KA. Juvenile myoclonic epilepsy: clinical and EEG features. *Acta Neurol Scand* 1998;97:160–163.
100. Matsuoka H, Takahashi T, Sasaki M, et al. Neuropsychological EEG activation in patients with epilepsy. *Brain* 2000;123:318–330.
101. Genton P, Salas Puig J, Tunon A, et al. Juvenile myoclonic epilepsy and related syndromes: clinical and neurophysiological aspects. In: Malafosse A, Genton P, Hirsch E, et al., eds. *Idiopathic generalized epilepsies: clinical, experimental and genetic aspects*. London: John Libbey, 1994:253–265.
102. Aliberti V, Grunewald RA, Panayiotopoulos CP, et al. Focal electroencephalographic abnormalities in juvenile myoclonic epilepsy. *Epilepsia* 1994;35:297–301.
103. Wolf P, Goosses R. Relation of photosensitivity to epileptic syndromes. *J Neurol Neurosurg Psychiatry* 1986;49:1386–1391.
104. Touchon J. Effect of awakening on epileptic activity in primary generalized myoclonic epilepsy. In: Sterman MB, Shouse MN, Passouant P, eds. *Sleep and epilepsy*. New York: Academic Press, 1982:239–248.
105. Lennox-Buchthal MA. Febrile convulsions. A reappraisal. *Electroencephalogr Clin Neurophysiol* 1973;32(Suppl):1–138.
106. Jeavons PM, Clark JE, Maheshwari MC. Treatment of generalized epilepsies of childhood and adolescence with sodium valproate ("epilim"). *Dev Med Child Neurol* 1977;19:9–25.
107. Baruzzi A, Procaccianti G, Tinuper P, et al. Antiepileptic drug withdrawal in childhood epilepsies: preliminary results of a prospective study. In: Faienza C, Prati G, eds. *Diagnostic and therapeutic problems in paediatric epileptology*. Amsterdam: Elsevier, 1988:117–123.
108. Penry JK, Dean JC, Riela AR. Juvenile myoclonic epilepsy: long-term response to therapy. *Epilepsia* 1989;30:S19–S23.
109. Genton P, Gelisse P, Thomas P, et al. Do carbamazepine and phenytoin aggravate juvenile myoclonic epilepsy? *Neurology* 2000;55:1106–1109.

110. Hurst DL. Methsuximide therapy of juvenile myoclonic epilepsy. *Seizure* 1996;5:47–50.

111. Buchanan N. The use of lamotrigine in juvenile myoclonic epilepsy. *Seizure* 1996;5:149–151.

112. Wallace SJ. Myoclonus and epilepsy in childhood: a review of treatment with valproate, ethosuximide, lamotrigine and zonisamide. *Epilepsy Res* 1998;29:147–154.

113. Biraben A, Allain H, Scarabin JM, et al. Exacerbation of juvenile myoclonic epilepsy with lamotrigine. *Neurology* 2000;55:1758.

114. Kellett MW, Smith DF, Stockton PA, et al. Topiramate in clinical practice: first year's postlicensing experience in a specialist epilepsy clinic. *J Neurol Neurosurg Psychiatry* 1999;66:759–763.

115. Resor SR Jr, Resor LD. Chronic acetazolamide monotherapy in the treatment of juvenile myoclonic epilepsy. *Neurology* 1990;40:1677–1681.

116. Jeavons P. Myoclonic epilepsies: therapy and prognosis. In: Akimoto H, Kazamatsuri H, Seino M, et al., ed. *Advances in epileptology: XIIIth epilepsy international symposium*. New York: Raven Press, 1982:141–144.

117. Jeavons PM, Harding GFA. *Photosensitive epilepsy*. London: Heinemann, 1975.

118. Kasteleijn-Nolst Trenite DG, Guerrini R, Binnie CD, et al. Visual sensitivity and epilepsy: a proposed terminology and classification for clinical and EEG phenomenology. *Epilepsia* 2001;42:692–701.

119. Reilly EL, Peters JF. Relationship of some varieties of electroencephalographic photosensitivity to clinical convulsive disorders. *Neurology* 1973;23:1050–1057.

120. Binnie CD, Darby CE, De Korte RA, et al. Self-induction of epileptic seizures by eye closure: incidence and recognition. *J Neurol Neurosurg Psychiatry* 1980;43:386–389.

121. Tassinari CA, Rubboli G, Michelucci R. Reflex epilepsy. In: Dam M, Gram L, eds. *Comprehensive epileptology*. New York: Raven Press, 1990:233–243.

122. Dreifuss FE. Discussion of absence and photosensitive epilepsy. In: Roger J, Dravet C, Bureau M, et al., eds. *Epileptic syndromes in infancy, childhood and adolescence*. London: John Libbey, 1985:237–241.

123. Guerrini R, Carrozzo R, Rinaldi R, et al. Angelman syndrome: etiology, clinical features, diagnosis, and management of symptoms. *Paediatr Drugs* 2003;5:647–661.

124. Matsuura T, Sutcliffe JS, Fang P, et al. De novo truncating mutations in E6-AP ubiquitin-protein ligase gene (UBE3A) in Angelman syndrome. *Nat Genet* 1997;15:74–77.

125. Guerrini R, De Lorey TM, Bonanni P, et al. Cortical myoclonus in Angelman syndrome. *Ann Neurol* 1996;40:39–48.

126. Minassian BA, DeLorey TM, Olsen RW, et al. Angelman syndrome: correlations between epilepsy phenotypes and genotypes. *Ann Neurol* 1998;43:485–493.

127. Viani F, Romeo A, Viri M, et al. Seizure and EEG patterns in Angelman's syndrome. *J Child Neurol* 1995;10:467–471.

128. Laan LA, Renier WO, Arts WF, et al. Evolution of epilepsy and EEG findings in Angelman syndrome. *Epilepsia* 1997;38:195–199.

129. Okuma Y, Shimo Y, Shimura H, et al. Familial cortical tremor with epilepsy: an under-recognized familial tremor. *Clin Neurol Neurosurg* 1998;100:75–78.

130. Labauge P, Amer LO, Simonetta-Moreau M, et al. Absence of linkage to 8q24 in a European family with familial adult myoclonic epilepsy (FAME). *Neurology* 2002;58:941–944.

131. Mikami M, Yasuda T, Terao A, et al. Localization of a gene for benign adult familial myoclonic epilepsy to chromosome 8q23.3-q24.1. *Am J Hum Genet* 1999;65:745–751.

132. van Rootselaar F, Callenbach PM, Hottenga JJ, et al. A Dutch family with "familial cortical tremor with epilepsy." Clinical characteristics and exclusion of linkage to chromosome 8q23.3-q24.1. *J Neurol* 2002;249:829–834.

133. De Falco FA, Striano P, De Falco A, et al. Benign adult familial myoclonic epilepsy: genetic heterogeneity and allelism with ADCME. *Neurology* 2003;60:1381–1385.

134. Striano P, Chifari R, Striano S, et al. A new benign adult familial myoclonic epilepsy (BAFME) pedigree suggesting linkage to chromosome 2p11.1-q12.2. *Epilepsia* 2004;45:190–192.

135. Guerrini R, Bonanni P, Patrignani A, et al. Autosomal dominant cortical myoclonus and epilepsy (ADCME) with complex partial and generalized seizures: a newly recognized epilepsy syndrome

with linkage to chromosome 2p11.1-q12.2. *Brain* 2001;124:2459–2475.

136. Marseille Consensus Group Classification of progressive myoclonus epilepsies and related disorders. *Ann Neurol* 1990;28:113–116.

137. Berkovic SF, Andermann F, Carpenter S, et al. Progressive myoclonus epilepsies: specific causes and diagnosis. *N Engl J Med* 1986;315:296–305.

138. Delgado-Escueta AV, Ganesh S, Yamakawa K. Advances in the genetics of progressive myoclonus epilepsy. *Am J Med Genet* 2001;106:129–138.

139. Genton P, Malafosse A, Moulard B, et al. Progressive myoclonus epilepsies. In: Roger J, Bureau M, Dravet C, et al., eds. *Epileptic syndromes in infancy, childhood and adolescence*, 3rd ed. London: John Libbey, 2002:407–430.

140. Andermann E, Jacob JC, Andermann F, et al. The Newfoundland aggregate of neuronal ceroid-lipofuscinosis. *Am J Med Genet Suppl* 1988;5:111–116.

141. Pennacchio LA, Lehesjoki A-E, Stone NE, et al. Mutations in the gene encoding cystatin B in progressive myoclonus epilepsy (*EPM1*). *Science* 1996;271:1731–1734.

142. Minassian B, Lee J, Herbrick J, et al. Mutations in a gene encoding a novel protein tyrosine phosphatase cause progressive myoclonus epilepsy. *Nat Genet* 1998;20:171–174.

143. Chan EM, Young EJ, Ianzano L, et al. Mutations in NHLRC1 cause progressive myoclonus epilepsy. *Nat Genet* 2003;35:125–127.

144. Vesa J, Hellsten E, Verkruyse LA, et al. Mutations in the palmitoyl protein thioesterase gene causing infantile neuronal ceroid lipofuscinosis. *Nature* 1995;376:584–587.

145. Sleat D, Donnelly R, Lackland H, et al. Association of mutations in a lysosomal protein with classical late-infantile neuronal ceroid lipofuscinosis. *Science* 1997;277:1802–1805.

146. Savukoski M, Kestila M, Williams R, et al. Defined chromosomal assignment of CLN5 demonstrates that at least four genetic loci are involved in the pathogenesis of human ceroid lipofuscinoses. *Am J Hum Genet* 1994;55:695–701.

147. Sharp JD, Wheeler RB, Lake BD, et al. Loci for classical and a variant late infantile neuronal ceroid lipofuscinosis map to chromosomes 11p15 and 15q21-23. *Hum Mol Genet* 1997;6:591–595.

148. Wheeler RB, Sharp JD, Mitchell WA, et al. A new locus for variant late infantile neuronal ceroid lipofuscinosis-CLN7. *Mol Genet Metab* 1999;66:337–338.

149. Sharp JD, Wheeler RB, Lake BD, et al. Genetic and physical mapping of the CLN6 gene on chromosome 15q21-23. *Mol Genet Metab* 1999;66:329–331.

150. Ranta S, Zhang Y, Ross B, et al. The neuronal ceroid lipofuscinoses in human EPMR and mnd mice are associated with mutations in CLN8. *Nat Genet* 1999;23:233–236.

151. Shoffner JM, Lott MT, Lezza AM, et al. Myoclonic epilepsy and ragged-red fiber disease (MERRF) is associated with a mitochondrial DNA tRNA(Lys) mutation. *Cell* 1990;61:931–937.

152. Bonten EJ, Arts WF, Beck M, et al. Novel mutations in lysosomal neuraminidase identify functional domains and determine clinical severity in sialidosis. *Hum Mol Genet* 2000;9:2715–2725.

153. D'Azzo A, Hoogeveen A, Reuser AJ, et al. Molecular defect in combined beta-galactosidase and neuraminidase deficiency in man. *Proc Natl Acad Sci U S A* 1982;79:4535–4539.

154. Grabowski GA, Dinur T, Osiecki KM, et al. Gaucher disease types 1, 2, and 3: differential mutations of the acid beta-glucosidase active site identified with conduritol B epoxide derivatives and sphingosine. *Am J Hum Genet* 1985;37:499–510.

155. Koide R, Ikeuchi T, Onodera O, et al. Unstable expansion of CAG repeat in hereditary dentatorubral-pallidoluysian atrophy (DRPLA). *Nat Genet* 1994;6:9–13.

156. Berkovic SF, So NK, Andermann F. Progressive myoclonus epilepsies: clinical and neurophysiological diagnosis. *J Clin Neurophysiol* 1991;8:261–274.

157. Norio R, Koskiniemi M. Progressive myoclonus epilepsy: genetic and nosological aspects with special reference to 107 Finnish patients. *Clin Genet* 1979;15:382–398.

158. Roger J, Genton P, Bureau M, et al. Progressive myoclonus epilepsies in childhood and adolescence. In: Roger J, Bureau M, Dravet C, et al., eds. *Epilepsy syndromes in infancy, childhood and adolescence*. London: John Libbey, 1992:381–400.

159. Berkovic SF, Cochius J, Andermann E, et al. Progressive myoclonus epilepsies: clinical and genetic aspects. *Epilepsia* 1993;34:S19–S30.

160. Tassinari CA, Bureau-Paillas M, Grasso E, et al. Electroencephalographic study of myoclonic cerebellar dyssynergia with epilepsy (Ramsay-Hunt syndrome). *Rev Electroencephalogr Neurophysiol Clin* 1974;4:407–428.

161. Lehesjoki A-E, Koskiniemi M, Sistonen P, et al. Localization of a gene for progressive myoclonus epilepsy to chromosome 21q22. *Proc Natl Acad Sci U S A* 1991;88:3696–3699.

162. Lalioti MD, Scott HS, Buresi C, et al. Dodecamer repeat expansion in cystatin B gene in progressive myoclonus epilepsy. *Nature* 1997;386:847–851.

163. Virtaneva K, D'Amato E, Miao J, et al. Unstable minisatellite expansion causing recessively inherited myoclonus epilepsy, EPM1. *Nat Genet* 1997;15:393–396.

164. D'Amato E, Kokaia Z, Nanobashvili A, et al. Seizures induce widespread upregulation of cystatin B, the gene mutated in progressive myoclonus epilepsy, in rat forebrain neurons. *Eur J Neurosci* 2000;12:1687–1695.

165. Lafora GR. Beitrag zur Histopathologie der myoklonischen Epilepsie. *Z Gesamte Neurol Psychiatrie* 1911;6:1–14.

166. Tinuper P, Aguglia U, Pellissier JF, et al. Visual ictal phenomena in a case of Lafora disease proven by skin biopsy. *Epilepsia* 1983; 24:214–218.

167. Serratosa JM. The progressive *myoclonus epilepsies*. In: Wyllie E, ed. *The treatment of epilepsy: principles and practice*, 3rd ed. Philadelphia: Lippincott Williams & Wilkins, 2001:509–524.

168. Carpenter S, Karpati G. Sweat gland duct cells in Lafora disease: diagnosis by skin biopsy. *Neurology* 1981;31:1564–1568.

169. Serratosa JM, Delgado-Escueta AV, Posada I, et al. The gene for progressive myoclonus epilepsy of Lafora type maps to chromosome 6q. *Hum Mol Genet* 1995;4:1657–1663.

170. Wisniewski KE, Kida E, Patxot OF, et al. Variability in the clinical and pathological findings in the neuronal ceroid lipofuscinoses: review of data and observations. *Am J Med Genet* 1992;42:525–532.

171. Chow CW, Borg J, Billson VR, et al. Fetal tissue involvement in the late infantile type of neuronal ceroid lipofuscinosis. *Prenat Diagn* 1993;13:833–841.

172. Zhong NA, Wisniewski KE, Ju W, et al. Molecular diagnosis of and carrier screening for the neuronal ceroid lipofuscinoses. *Genet Test* 2000;4:243–248.

173. Sleat DE, Gin RM, Sohar I, et al. Mutational analysis of the defective protease in classic late-infantile neuronal ceroid lipofuscinosis, a neurodegenerative lysosomal storage disorder. *Am J Hum Genet* 1999;64:1511–1523.

174. Savukoski M, Klockars T, Holmberg V, et al. CLN5, a novel gene encoding a putative transmembrane protein mutated in Finnish variant late infantile neuronal ceroid lipofuscinosis. *Nat Genet* 1998;19:286–288.

175. Eiberg H, Gardiner RM, Mohr J. Batten disease (Spielmeyer-Sjögren disease) and haptoglobins (HP): indication of linkage and assignment to chr. 16. *Clin Genet* 1989;36:217–218.

176. The International Batten Disease Consortium. Isolation of a novel gene underlying Batten disease, CLN3. *Cell* 1995;82:949–957.

177. Munroe PB, Mitchison HM, O'Rawe AM, et al. Spectrum of mutations in the Batten disease gene, CLN3. *Am J Hum Genet* 1997;61:310–316.

178. Mitchison HM, Hofmann SL, Becerra CH, et al. Mutations in the palmitoyl-protein thioesterase gene (PPT; CLN1) causing juvenile neuronal ceroid lipofuscinosis with granular osmiophilic deposits. *Hum Mol Genet* 1998;7:291–297.

179. Herva R, Tyynela J, Hirvasniemi A, et al. Northern epilepsy: a novel form of neuronal ceroid-lipofuscinosis. *Brain Pathol* 2000; 10:215–222.

180. Wisniewski KE, Zhong N, Philippart M. Pheno/genotypic correlations of neuronal ceroid lipofuscinoses. *Neurology* 2001;57: 576–581.

181. Garcia Silva MT, Aicardi J, Goutieres F, et al. The syndrome of myoclonic epilepsy with ragged-red fibers. Report of a case and review of the literature. *Neuropediatrics* 1987;18:200–204.

182. Berkovic SF, Carpenter S, Evans A, et al. Myoclonus epilepsy and ragged-red fibres (MERRF). 1. A clinical, pathological, biochemical, magnetic resonance spectrographic and positron emission tomographic study. *Brain* 1989;112:1231–1260.

183. Ozawa M, Nishino I, Horai S, et al. Myoclonus epilepsy associated with ragged-red fibers: a G-to-A mutation at nucleotide pair 8363 in mitochondrial tRNA(Lys) in two families. *Muscle Nerve* 1997;20:271–278.

184. Silvestri G, Moraes CT, Shanske S, et al. A new mtDNA mutation in the tRNA(Lys) gene associated with myoclonic epilepsy and ragged-red fibers (MERRF). *Am J Hum Genet* 1992;51: 1213–1217.

185. Campos Y, Martin MA, Lorenzo G, et al. Sporadic MERRF/MELAS overlap syndrome associated with the 3243 tRNA(Leu(UUR)) mutation of mitochondrial DNA. *Muscle Nerve* 1996;19: 187–190.

186. Fabrizi GM, Cardaioli E, Grieco GS, et al. The A to G transition at nt 3243 of the mitochondrial tRNALeu(UUR) may cause an MERRF syndrome. *J Neurol Neurosurg Psychiatry* 1996;61: 47–51.

187. Eldridge R, Iivanainen M, Stern R, et al. "Baltic" myoclonus epilepsy: hereditary disorder of childhood made worse by phenytoin. *Lancet* 1983;2:838–842.

188. Koskiniemi M, Van Vleymen B, Hakamies L, et al. Piracetam relieves symptoms in progressive myoclonus epilepsy: a multicentre, randomised, double blind, crossover study comparing the efficacy and safety of three dosages of oral piracetam with placebo. *J Neurol Neurosurg Psychiatry* 1998;64:344–348.

189. Fedi M, Reutens D, Dubeau F, et al. Long-term efficacy and safety of piracetam in the treatment of progressive myoclonus epilepsy. *Arch Neurol* 2001;58:781–786.

190. Genton P, Gelisse P. Antimyoclonic effect of levetiracetam. *Epileptic Disord* 2000;2:209–212.

191. Henry TR, Leppik IE, Gumnit RJ, et al. Progressive myoclonus epilepsy treated with zonisamide. *Neurology* 1988;38:928–931.

192. Hurd RW, Wilder BJ, Helveston WR, et al. Treatment of four siblings with progressive myoclonus epilepsy of the Unverricht-Lundborg type with N-acetylcysteine. *Neurology* 1996;47:1264–1268.

193. Kyllerman M, Ben-Menachem E. Zonisamide for progressive myoclonus epilepsy: long-term observations in seven patients. *Epilepsy Res* 1998;29:109–114.

194. Pranzatelli MR, Tate E, Huang Y, et al. Neuropharmacology of progressive myoclonus epilepsy: response to 5-hydroxy-L-tryptophan. *Epilepsia* 1995;36:783–791.

195. Sperl W. Diagnosis and therapy of mitochondriopathies. *Wien Klin Wochenschr* 1997;109:93–99.

196. Smith B, Shatz R, Elisevich K, et al. Effects of vagus nerve stimulation on progressive myoclonus epilepsy of Unverricht-Lundborg type. *Epilepsia* 2000;41:1046–1048.

197. Guerrini R, Belmonte A, Genton P. Antiepileptic drug-induced worsening of seizures in children. *Epilepsia* 1998;39:S2–S10.

198. Biraben A, Allain H, Scarabin JM, et al. Exacerbation of juvenile myoclonic epilepsy with lamotrigine. *Neurology* 2000;55: 1758.

199. Kuenzle C, Steinlin M, Wohlrab G, et al. Adverse effects of vigabatrin in Angelman syndrome. *Epilepsia* 1998;39:1213–1215.

200. Marciani MG, Maschio M, Spanedda F, et al. Development of myoclonus in patients with partial epilepsy during treatment with vigabatrin: an electroencephalographic study. *Acta Neurol Scand* 1995;91:1–5.

201. Snead OC 3rd, Hosey LC. Exacerbation of seizures in children by carbamazepine. *N Engl J Med* 1985;313:916–921.

202. Guerrini R, Belmonte A, Parmeggiani L, et al. Myoclonic status epilepticus following high-dosage lamotrigine therapy. *Brain Dev* 1999;21:420–424.

Encephalopathic Generalized Epilepsy and Lennox-Gastaut Syndrome

27

Kevin Farrell   *William O. Tatum IV*

Some generalized epilepsies are associated with cognitive dysfunction and encephalopathy. The clinical features of the seizures commonly observed in the encephalopathic generalized epilepsies were described in the 18th and 19th centuries (1). The development of electroencephalography demonstrated that patients with encephalopathic generalized epilepsy often had characteristic electroencephalographic (EEG) abnormalities. For instance, slow spike-and-wave discharges were observed in patients who often displayed brief motor seizures resistant to antiepileptic medications (2). As it became apparent that the natural history and response to treatment were often influenced by factors other than seizure type—for example, age of onset, intellectual function—the concept of epileptic syndromes became accepted and was embodied in the Classification of Epileptic Syndromes of the International League Against Epilepsy (3). In this classification, the term *symptomatic generalized epilepsies* was used for generalized epilepsies with encephalopathy and mental retardation. In 2001, a revision of the classification of both seizures and epileptic syndromes was proposed, suggesting that the term *cryptogenic* be replaced by *probably symptomatic* (4). Despite these proposals, many patients with encephalopathic generalized epilepsy do not fit clearly into a recognized syndrome. This chapter describes the clinical features, EEG abnormalities, response to treatment, and natural history of these epilepsies, including the Lennox-Gastaut syndrome, which is perhaps the best documented of these epilepsies.

SYNDROMES

Lennox-Gastaut Syndrome

The term *Lennox-Gastaut syndrome* (LGS) (5) has been used to describe a broad group of patients with (a) multiple generalized seizure types, typically tonic, atonic, myoclonic, and atypical absence; (b) an interictal EEG pattern characterized by diffuse slow spike-and-wave complexes; and (c) cognitive dysfunction, which develops in most but not all patients (5,6). Although cognitive dysfunction is common in patients with LGS (5,6), this often does not become apparent until later in the course of the disorder (5,7,8). Some authors have suggested that tonic seizures and paroxysmal fast rhythms at approximately 10 to 12 Hz during nonrapid eye movement (NREM) sleep are virtually never absent in LGS (7). Nonconvulsive status epilepticus is a common feature. The seizures are usually refractory to medical treatment.

The first seizure usually occurs between 1 and 8 years of age, with a peak between 3 and 5 years of age (8). The initial seizures may be partial or tonic-clonic, rather than the characteristic mixed motor seizures. Approximately 25% of children are neurologically normal prior to the onset of the epilepsy and have normal neuroimaging. In an additional 30% to 41% of patients, LGS is preceded by West syndrome (9,10). LGS occasionally occurs for the first time in the second decade of life (6,11). The onset of LGS in the second decade has also been described in patients who presented initially with features of idiopathic generalized epilepsy, characterized by absence and generalized tonic-clonic seizures and by 3-Hz spike waves (6). In some of these patients, the clinical and EEG features of LGS developed after an episode of status epilepticus that was associated with an unsupervised withdrawal of antiepileptic medication, and treatment could be associated with seizure control and a disappearance of the slow spike-and-wave complexes (12). During adulthood, patients with partial epilepsy may develop drop attacks and slow spike-and-wave discharges that superficially resemble adult-onset LGS. Most of these patients probably have focal or multifocal epilepsy with secondary bilateral synchrony (8).

It is clear that the term LGS is descriptive of a heterogeneous group of patients with differing etiologies and long-term outcomes. Categorizing a subgroup of patients with encephalopathic generalized epilepsy as LGS may add little toward treatment or prognosis and may have an inadvertent negative effect on parents and physicians, especially early in the course, by suggesting a very poor prognosis before long-term outcome is clear. Families who receive a diagnosis of LGS are often devastated when they research the issue independently, and in some cases, this dire interpretation is unwarranted. In other instances, a diagnosis of LGS may discourage physicians from continued aggressive efforts toward better seizure control. Although reference to LGS continues to appear in the remaining text, readers may want to reflect on the prudence of assigning the term LGS sparingly and instead use the broader term *encephalopathic generalized epilepsy* because of its greater phenotypic variability.

Other Encephalopathic Generalized Epilepsies

Many patients with multiple generalized seizure types and cognitive dysfunction do not demonstrate the generalized sharp and slow-wave complexes characteristic of LGS. A few of these patients have one of the syndromes described later in the differential diagnosis section. Most, however, are not amenable to syndromic diagnosis. Some are categorized by the dominant EEG abnormality. Thus, the multiple independent spike foci pattern on electroencephalograms is characterized by generalized motor seizures in most patients, with half of the patients having multiple seizure types, half having daily seizures, and two thirds being intellectually subnormal (13). With the advent of magnetic resonance imaging (MRI) and molecular genetics, many of these patients are now being categorized according to the underlying brain abnormality (e.g., hypothalamic hamartomas) (14) or molecular genetic disorder (e.g., mental retardation and seizures in males associated with mutation in the creatine-transporter gene located in Xq28) (15). The increasing ability to identify the underlying brain disease will clearly facilitate genetic counseling and also may prove very useful in counseling regarding the natural history of the epilepsy.

SEIZURE TYPES

Tonic, atypical absence, myoclonic, and atonic seizures are the characteristic seizure types in LGS and also are common in other encephalopathic generalized epilepsies. Tonic-clonic, clonic, or partial seizures may also be observed in patients with LGS and other encephalopathic generalized epilepsies, and are often the initial seizure type.

Tonic Seizures

Tonic seizures are the most common seizure type in LGS, particularly in patients with seizure onset at an early age (16). The prevalence of tonic seizures in LGS is between 74% and 90% in studies involving sleep EEG recordings (8). Mild episodes may be limited to a minimal upward deviation of the eyes (*sursum vergens*) and a brief respiratory disturbance. These mild seizures are common during sleep (17), and their clinical manifestations are often difficult to recognize without video-EEG recording (18,19). Tonic seizures may be restricted to neck flexors, and to facial and masticatory muscles; may involve the proximal muscles of the extremities, causing elevation and abduction of the arms; or may be associated with tonic involvement of the distal extremity muscles (8). Involvement of the extremities is often associated with a sudden fall, and these seizures may be difficult to distinguish from myoclonic or atonic seizures. Tonic seizures that last for longer than 20 seconds often have a vibratory component, with rapid and discrete clonic jerks. Such seizures are often mischaracterized as generalized tonic-clonic seizures. Altered consciousness may not be apparent for up to 1 second after onset of the EEG discharge, but recovery occurs within seconds of the end of the discharge (7). Gestural and ambulatory automatisms may follow the tonic phase, particularly in patients with late-onset LGS (20). Involvement of respiratory musculature is common and may result in apnea. Facial flushing, tachycardia, and pupillary dilation also have been described (21).

Atypical Absence Seizures

Atypical absence seizures are commonly seen in patients with LGS and other encephalopathic generalized epilepsies (7). They may be associated with eyelid myoclonias, mild tonic stiffening, autonomic features, and mild automatisms. Atypical absence seizures are not precipitated by photic stimulation. Gradual onset and offset, which are characteristic of atypical absence seizures, often make it difficult for caregivers to recognize these seizures (22).

Atonic Seizures

Atonic seizures may be difficult to distinguish clinically from myoclonias, myoclonic atonias, and tonic seizures, which may also cause the patient to fall (7). Studies involving polygraphic recordings of muscle activity have demonstrated that drop seizures most often result from tonic seizures and that atonic seizures are less uncommon (23–25).

Myoclonic Seizures

Myoclonic seizures occur in 30% of patients with LGS (26); the term *myoclonic variant of LGS* has been used to describe such patients (27,28). The prognosis for mental development tends to be better in patients with LGS when myoclonic seizures are prominent (28).

Nonconvulsive Status Epilepticus

Nonconvulsive status epilepticus has been reported in 54% to 97% of patients with LGS, with higher rates observed in studies that included only patients with the classic features of LGS (29). Tonic seizures and confusion are the most common ictal manifestations (29). The confusional state may fluctuate and is often not recognized as a seizure, particularly in mentally retarded individuals. In patients with LGS, status epilepticus may last hours to weeks. In one study (30), the duration was longer than 1 week in 15 of 30 patients. Pure tonic status epilepticus occurs mostly in adults, is more frequent in patients whose initial seizures were tonic or tonic-clonic (30), and may be precipitated by intravenous (IV) administration of benzodiazepines (31–34). Nonconvulsive status epilepticus may be inhibited by active wakefulness and facilitated by drowsiness; consequently, overmedication may compound the problem. The EEG pattern during status epilepticus may be difficult to distinguish from the interictal EEG pattern (29). The abnormalities include an increased amount of generalized slow spike-and-wave or polyspike-and-wave complexes, a hypsarrhythmia-like pattern, and 10-Hz discharges of variable duration (29).

ELECTROENCEPHALOGRAPHIC FEATURES

Interictal Electroencephalography

The interictal EEG background in LGS demonstrates a lower-than-normal frequency of the posterior dominant rhythm (35) and, generally, an increased amount of slow activity. Persistent background slowing is observed in 67% of patients and is associated with a poor prognosis for normal mental development (8). Background slowing is increased when the seizures are poorly controlled. Disturbances in NREM sleep patterns and total duration of REM sleep are observed in most patients with LGS who have severe mental retardation or frequent seizures (36), but these sleep features may be difficult to appreciate without a prolonged EEG recording and may be absent if the seizures are not frequent (37).

The interictal electroencephalogram in LGS is characterized by 2- to 2.5-Hz spike-and-wave and polyspike-and-wave discharges, although this pattern may be seen in other epilepsies as well. The spike-and-wave discharges are usually diffuse and maximal bifrontally, but are sometimes confined to the anterior or posterior head regions (38) (Fig. 27.1). The complexes are most often symmetrical, but focal or multifocal spikes and sharp waves are observed in 75% of patients, usually in the frontal or temporal regions (8). The slow spike waves are not induced by photic stimulation and are only rarely enhanced by hyperventilation (38). During slow-wave sleep, the discharges are more obviously bisynchronous and are often associated with polyspikes. Slow spike-wave complexes are often not present when the seizures initially occur, and in one series (16) they were first observed at a mean age of 44 months, in contrast to the mean age of seizure onset of 26 months. In later childhood, the slow spike-wave discharges gradually decrease in frequency or may disappear altogether.

Generalized paroxysmal fast activity manifesting as bursts of greater than 10-Hz rhythms, particularly during slow-wave sleep, are considered by some to be an integral feature of LGS (7,8) (Fig. 27.2). Nevertheless, this activity may not be present in all sleep recordings, and its prevalence depends on the duration of sleep recorded (39). The discharges are distributed diffusely, but are usually more prominent anteriorly and may be accompanied by tonic seizures. Polygraphic or video-EEG recordings may demonstrate subtle clinical signs that can be very brief and difficult to detect by observation alone.

The interictal EEG pattern in the other encephalopathic generalized epilepsies is variable. There is usually a poorly organized posterior dominant rhythm, and focal or multifocal abnormalities are common. Blume has described the clinical and EEG features in patients with multiple independent spike foci (13).

Ictal Electroencephalography

The ictal electroencephalogram during tonic seizures demonstrates bilaterally synchronous (10- to 25-Hz) activity maximal in the anterior and vertex regions, or attenuation of the background rhythm, which may be preceded by polyspikes, which may, in turn, be preceded or followed by generalized slow spike-and-wave activity. In contrast to generalized tonic-clonic seizures, postictal depression of EEG activity is uncommon. Tonic-automatic seizures are characterized by bilateral rapid discharges during the tonic phase and by diffuse slow spike-wave activity during automatism (7). The clinical features of a tonic seizure may not be apparent for up to 1 second after onset of the EEG discharge and may persist for several seconds after the discharge ends (40).

Atypical absence seizures are characterized by irregular, diffuse slow spike-and-wave discharges at approximately 2 to 2.5 Hz, which may be difficult to distinguish from the

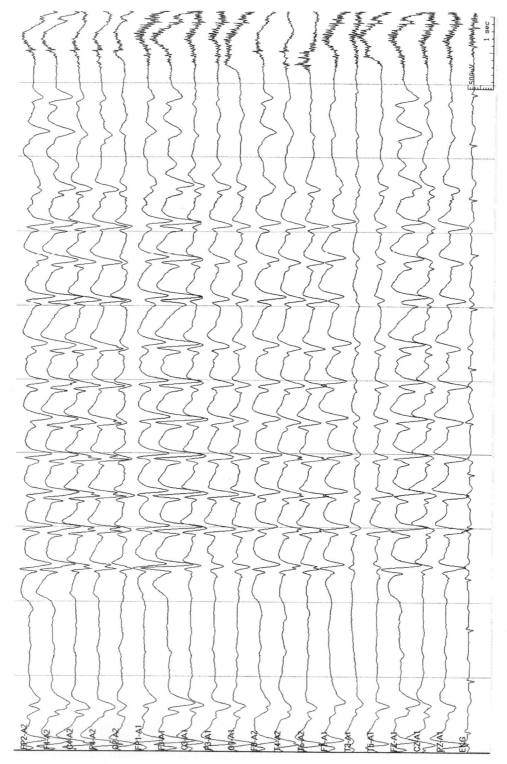

Figure 27.1 Interictal electroencephalogram demonstrates generalized sharp and slow-wave complexes.

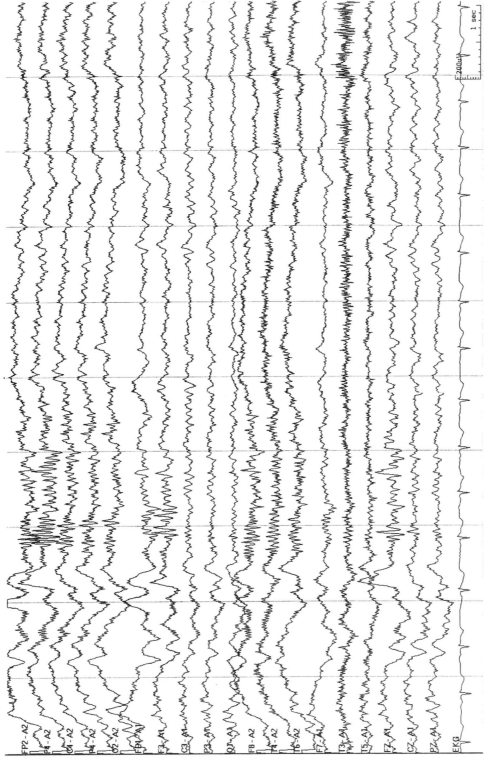

Figure 27.2 Paroxysmal fast activity occurs during nonrapid eye movement sleep without recognized clinical accompaniment.

interictal slow spike-wave pattern. Rapid rhythms may be occasionally observed. Atonic and myoclonic seizures usually result in a loss of posture and may be difficult to detect without polygraphic video-EEG recordings. A variety of ictal abnormalities may be seen, including polyspike waves and, less commonly, slow spike waves or diffuse rapid rhythms (8).

ASSOCIATED NEUROLOGIC DYSFUNCTION

In children with LGS, diffuse cognitive dysfunction is often not evident at seizure onset but becomes more apparent with time. In one series, 34% of patients had normal mental development at 4 years of age; however, 78% to 96% eventually developed mental retardation (41). Severe retardation occurs more often in patients with seizure onset before 3 years of age, frequent seizures, repeated episodes of status epilepticus, or symptomatic LGS, particularly in those with previous West syndrome (16,42). The cognitive dysfunction is exacerbated by several factors: the use of multiple medications, the tendency to increase the dose repeatedly because of poor seizure control, the effect of subtle seizures, and postictal confusion. Impaired information processing and prolonged reaction time are particularly prominent, with these patients consequently performing poorly on timed tests (43). Behavioral and personality disturbances, such as short attention span, aggressiveness, and disinhibition, complicate social adjustment and often confound attempts to integrate these individuals into the classroom and the community.

In children with LGS, motor development is affected less than cognitive development. Normal motor milestones were observed at 4 years of age in 79% of children with the disorder (41); however, many patients become ataxic or clumsy with time. Deterioration of gait over several years was a prominent feature in 17% of children in one series and, together with an increase in drop attacks, resulted in many becoming wheelchair-bound (44).

The degree of neurologic dysfunction observed in other encephalopathic epilepsies depends on the etiology and the severity of the underlying brain abnormality. Patients with secondary generalized epilepsy as a consequence of perinatal or postnatal brain injury are more likely to have spasticity.

ETIOLOGY

Congenital abnormalities of brain development are the most common cause of encephalopathic generalized epilepsy. They are demonstrated less often in LGS, and some abnormalities, such as Aicardi syndrome and lissencephaly, are rarely associated with LGS (5). In 20% to 30% of patients with LGS, there is normal psychomotor development at the onset, no history of brain injury, nor-

---

TABLE 27.1

DISORDERS ASSOCIATED WITH THE LENNOX-GASTAUT SYNDROME

More common
- Brain malformations, including focal cortical dysplasia, bilateral perisylvian polymicrogyria, subcortical band heterotopia, and hypothalamic hamartoma
- Neurocutaneous disorders, including tuberous sclerosis, nevus sebaceous, and hypomelanosis of Ito
- Perinatal and postnatal hypoxic-ischemic brain injury
- Meningitis and encephalitis
- Genetic abnormalities, including generalized epilepsy with febrile seizures plus

Rare
- Inborn errors of metabolism, such as mitochondrial cytopathies
- Brain tumor

---

mal brain imaging, and indeterminate cause (8,16,45). Even in patients with LGS who have evidence of neurologic abnormality at presentation, the cause was determined in only 35 of 99 patients in one study (45). The most commonly reported abnormalities in LGS are congenital brain malformations, hypoxic-ischemic brain injury, encephalitis, meningitis, and tuberous sclerosis (5,45) (Table 27.1). Genetic and metabolic diseases are often associated with myoclonic seizures, but such conditions are rarely seen in LGS and are more often observed with other forms of encephalopathic generalized epilepsy. Mitochondrial disorders and neuronal ceroid lipofuscinosis are the most common genetic and metabolic disorders associated with encephalopathic generalized epilepsy. In individuals with encephalopathic epilepsy and absence of a developmental brain abnormality on head MRI scan, it is also important to evaluate the patient for possible aminoacidopathies, organic acidurias, and urea cycle disorders. Genetically determined diseases are increasingly being shown to be the pathologic basis of many cases of encephalopathic epilepsy. Genetic factors also play a role in LGS, with a family history of febrile seizures or epilepsy reported in 48% of patients with cryptogenic LGS (46). In addition, LGS has been reported to be a phenotype of generalized epilepsy with febrile seizures plus (GEFS+) (47).

LGS and other encephalopathic generalized epilepsies may occur in patients with focal brain lesions. Abnormalities of the frontal lobe (48) are more likely to be associated with LGS than are focal lesions in other brain areas, but recovery from the syndrome has been described after removal of a parietotemporal astrocytoma (49). LGS also has been reported following head trauma (17).

NEUROPATHOLOGY

Although neuroimaging rarely demonstrates congenital brain abnormalities in patients with LGS, abnormalities of brain development were observed in 16 of the 30 postmortem samples (50). Cerebellar lesions were found in 20 of these specimens and were the only abnormalities in 4 patients. Diffuse or focal neuronal necrosis was described in at least 23 of the 30 postmortem samples and was limited to the cerebellum in 8 patients. It is not clear, however, whether the cerebellar lesions and neuronal necrosis preceded seizure onset or resulted from the seizures or the treatment. Cortical biopsies from patients with LGS also have revealed neuronal loss, reduction of dendritic spines, dilation of the presynaptic and postsynaptic vesicles, and abnormal mitochondria (50,51).

NEUROIMAGING

Abnormalities of brain development are the most common cause of encephalopathic generalized epilepsy, and MRI is the most sensitive and specific method for imaging these disorders. In other patients, nonspecific changes are the most common abnormality, except in those with a history of a perinatal or postnatal brain insult (e.g., hypoxic-ischemic brain injury, meningitis/encephalitis). Diffuse cerebral atrophy was described in approximately 75% of patients studied with computed tomography (CT) of the head (52). Focal CT abnormalities, although observed less often, have included tuberous sclerosis, brain tumors, and cortical lesions (5).

Positron emission tomography (PET) has not demonstrated consistent abnormalities of cerebral metabolism in this syndrome (53-55), but cortical metabolic activity was diffusely reduced in approximately half of the patients studied by Chugani and associates (53). Unilateral hypometabolism and focal metabolic abnormalities affecting the frontal or temporal lobes (53,54) may be related to the heterogeneous nature of the syndrome and imply different pathophysiologic mechanisms.

DIFFERENTIAL DIAGNOSIS AND OTHER SYNDROMES

Many of the EEG and clinical features of LGS evolve with time and are not present at the onset of the epilepsy. Thus, partial or generalized tonic-clonic seizures may be the initial ictal manifestation, with the more classic seizure types not evident until later. Similarly, slow spike-wave complexes are frequently not observed on an EEG when the seizures first occur. In one study, all the features of LGS were present in only 29% of children when they first developed seizures (56). Similarly, it is often difficult to classify a specific epileptic syndrome in patients with other symptomatic generalized epilepsies. Table 27.2 lists several epileptic syndromes and diseases that share some of the features of LGS and other encephalopathic generalized epilepsies.

TABLE 27.2

EPILEPTIC SYNDROMES AND DISEASES THAT MIMIC LENNOX-GASTAUT SYNDROME

- Myoclonic epilepsies of early childhood
  - Severe myoclonic epilepsy of infancy
  - Epilepsy with myoclonic absences
  - Myoclonic-astatic epilepsy
  - Myoclonic epilepsy of infancy associated with a fixed encephalopathy
- Atypical partial benign epilepsy of childhood
- Epilepsy with electrical status epilepticus during slow-wave sleep
- Neuronal ceroid lipofuscinosis
- Angelman syndrome

Myoclonic-Astatic Epilepsy

Myoclonic-astatic epilepsy is a syndrome characterized by myoclonic, astatic, typical absence, and tonic-clonic seizures. The distinction between LGS associated with myoclonic seizures and myoclonic-astatic epilepsy is not always clear. The absence of tonic seizures is considered a criterion for the diagnosis of myoclonic-astatic epilepsy (27), although tonic seizures can be observed later in the course of the epilepsy (5). In patients with myoclonic-astatic epilepsy, partial seizures are unusual (57). Seizures begin between 1 and 5 years of age, with tonic-clonic attacks the initial type in more than half of the patients (58). Most patients are neurologically normal before seizure onset, but approximately 50% exhibit slowing in mental development. This occurs more often in those with frequent nonconvulsive status epilepticus, which affects approximately one-third of the patients (59). A strong genetic component was suggested by a history of epilepsy in 37% of first- and second-degree relatives (59). Subsequently, myoclonic-astatic epilepsy was demonstrated to be a phenotype of the genetic disorder GEFS+ (60). The electroencephalogram demonstrates generalized spike waves, photosensitivity, and 4- to 7-Hz rhythms with parietal accentuation. The prognosis for seizure control and mental development is better in patients with myoclonic-astatic epilepsy than in most patients with LGS. There have been no controlled studies of treatment in patients with myoclonic-astatic epilepsy. Valproic acid, benzodiazepines, and lamotrigine are often used initially, although in a retrospective study, the most effective treatment was the ketogenic diet, followed by adrenocorticotropic hormone (ACTH) and ethosuximide (61).

Atypical Partial Benign Epilepsy

Myoclonic and atonic seizures occur in clusters that last between 2 and 4 weeks, beginning between 2 and 6 years of age in children with normal development (62). Nocturnal partial seizures are prominent, particularly at the onset of the epilepsy, but tonic seizures do not occur. Diffuse 3-Hz spike waves are observed in the waking record, and very often diffuse slow spike-wave activity is seen during drowsiness and slow-wave sleep. The EEG pattern is frequently less abnormal during seizure-free intervals, and central spikes are common. Seizures remit in most patients before the age of 10 years, and mental and behavioral regression is not significant.

Continuous Spike Waves During Slow-Wave Sleep

Some patients with progressive cognitive dysfunction demonstrate continuous spike-wave activity during slow-wave sleep (63). Atonic seizures may occur, but tonic seizures have not been demonstrated despite prolonged sleep recordings (64).

Angelman Syndrome

Angelman syndrome is characterized by microcephaly, flat occiput, severe mental retardation, ataxia, jerky limb movements, and a cheerful disposition. Most of these children have epilepsy, which usually begins in infancy or early childhood (65). The most common seizure types are atypical absence, myoclonic, tonic, unilateral clonic, and complex partial with eye deviation and vomiting (65,66). Myoclonic status, which may manifest with hypotonia, drowsiness, and mild clonic jerking, occurs in approximately half of the children, but is rare after 6 years of age (66). The electroencephalogram demonstrates diffuse, bifrontally dominant high-amplitude 1- to 3-Hz notched, triphasic, or polyphasic slow waves or slow and sharp waves, particularly during stage 3 and 4 sleep (66). A deletion at 15q11-q13 can be demonstrated in approximately 70% of patients with Angelman syndrome, and these patients tend to have a more severe form of epilepsy. In contrast, the epilepsy is less severe in those rare patients with methylation imprint abnormalities, uniparental disomy, or mutations of the *UBE3A* gene, as well as in the group of patients (25%) in whom the underlying abnormality cannot be demonstrated (66). Several γ-aminobutyric acid A (GABA$_A$) receptor subunit genes are located in the 15q11-q13 region, and it has been suggested that the cortical hyperexcitability associated with Angelman syndrome may be related to reduced GABAergic inhibition (66).

TREATMENT

The treatment of patients with LGS and other encephalopathic generalized epilepsies includes control of the seizures, management of the associated cognitive and behavioral dysfunction, and support for the whole family.

Antiepileptic Drugs

Antiepileptic drugs (AEDs) often are ineffective in the treatment of LGS and other encephalopathic generalized epilepsies. Because of this, patients often receive multiple-drug therapy, with sedation and other neurotoxic effects being common complications. It is important to minimize the sedative side effects of AEDs in these patients because of the much higher incidence of seizures during drowsiness and inactive wakefulness (67). Myoclonic and atonic seizures are controlled more easily than are tonic seizures (5), but tolerance is a particular problem in patients with LGS and other encephalopathic generalized epilepsies.

Both the 1,4-(clonazepam, nitrazepam, diazepam) and 1,5-(clobazam) benzodiazepines have been used extensively (68–70). Their mechanisms of action may differ, and one agent may be effective when another has failed (68). Tolerance has been reported to be a particular problem with benzodiazepines (71,72). Diazepam is less effective than other benzodiazepines, and IV diazepam (31,34) and lorazepam (32) may induce tonic seizures in patients with LGS and other encephalopathic generalized epilepsies. Clonazepam and nitrazepam are often associated with troublesome side effects, particularly drowsiness, drooling, incoordination, and hyperactivity, whereas clobazam is associated with less sedation than the 1,4-benzodiazepines (73).

Valproic acid has been reported to be more effective in cryptogenic than in symptomatic LGS (69), and is most effective in controlling myoclonic, atypical absence, and atonic seizures (69,74). Valproic acid is associated with significantly fewer neurologic side effects than the benzodiazepines, but many of the children being treated with the agent are receiving polytherapy, which increases the risk for serious hepatotoxicity particularly in the very young child.

Lamotrigine has a broad spectrum of antiepileptic action and is effective against partial and generalized seizures (75). In two placebo-controlled studies, lamotrigine was shown to be effective in the treatment of LGS (76,77). The relative infrequency of drowsiness and behavioral side effects adds to the usefulness of lamotrigine, but the slow dosage escalation that is recommended in children, in order to reduce the risk for drug-induced rash, is a problem for those with very frequent seizures.

Topiramate was effective in reducing the number of drop attacks and major motor seizures in a placebo-controlled study of patients with LGS (78). In an open study, topiramate was associated with a 50% or greater reduction in seizure frequency in 11 of 20 adults with developmental disabilities and complete control in 2 adults (79). Anorexia and behavioral dysfunction are the major disadvantages of topiramate use in these patients. The behavioral side effects may be ameliorated by slow dosage escalation.

The older AEDs are often not effective in the treatment of LGS. Phenobarbital and primidone may be useful in controlling some seizure types, but these agents exacerbate the hyperactivity and aggressiveness often seen in children with LGS. In addition, barbiturates often produce sedation, which may increase the frequency of astatic seizures. Some experts consider phenytoin to be the treatment of choice for tonic status epilepticus, and it also may be effective against tonic seizures (80). Although carbamazepine may be effective against partial seizures, it can precipitate or exacerbate generalized seizures (81). Ethosuximide is reported to be the most effective AED in the treatment of myoclonic-astatic epilepsy (61).

Several of the other newer AEDs may play a role in the treatment of LGS and symptomatic generalized epilepsy. Treatment with felbamate reduced atonic and tonic-clonic seizures in a placebo-controlled study of patients with LGS (82), although the risk for aplastic anemia and liver failure limit the use of this agent to those in whom other treatments have failed. In open Japanese studies, zonisamide was reported to be effective in 26% to 50% of patients with LGS (83). There are limited data on the use of levetiracetam in patients with LGS and encephalopathic epilepsy. In open studies, vigabatrin has been reported to improve seizure control in patients with LGS and secondary generalized epilepsy (84,85). Gabapentin is not useful and may exacerbate atypical absence and myoclonic seizures in patients with these epilepsies (86).

Ketogenic Diet

The ketogenic diet may be effective in the treatment of LGS and other encephalopathic generalized epilepsies (87,88). In an open, prospective, multicenter study of 51 children with intractable generalized epilepsy, 10% were seizure free after 1 year on the ketogenic diet and an additional 30% had greater than 90% improvement in seizure control (89). The ketogenic diet is reported to be particularly effective in patients with myoclonic-astatic epilepsy (61). In those who respond, a reduction in the frequency of atonic and myoclonic seizures is usually observed within days of introduction of the diet (90). An experienced dietitian is key to the success of this approach (88). Although treatment with topiramate, zonisamide, and acetazolamide may be complicated by kidney stones, the combination of the ketogenic diet with one of these agents does not appear to increase the risk over that of the diet alone (91). Patients receiving phenobarbital or benzodiazepines may experience increased sedation when on the ketogenic diet.

Hormonal and Other Drug Therapies

Treatment with corticosteroids and ACTH may be effective, particularly if begun shortly after onset of the cryptogenic form of LGS (92). ACTH doses of 30 to 40 IU (9,92) controlled seizures between 1 and 6 weeks after treatment began (92,93), necessitating a prolonged trial of therapy in some patients. Because of the high relapse rate, the use of steroids is usually limited to episodes of nonconvulsive status epilepticus and to periods of frequent seizures (19,94). The intractability of this syndrome has encouraged a variety of antiepileptic treatments, such as IV immunoglobulin (95,96), amantadine (97), imipramine (98,99), and a thyroid-releasing hormone analogue (100). However, most of these studies have been uncontrolled and have enrolled small numbers of patients.

Surgery

Callosotomy may reduce both seizure frequency and seizure severity in patients with LGS and other encephalopathic epilepsies, although complete control is rare. Improvement in behavior and alertness has been observed in patients with decreased seizure frequency (101). Tonic seizures resulting in falls are the seizure type most improved by this procedure (101). A lateralized frontal focus and secondary bilateral synchrony may imply a favorable prognosis (102), but patients with cryptogenic LGS may also be helped significantly (101). In one series (103), anterior callosotomy was most useful against the cryptogenic form of LGS and was ineffective in patients with prior West syndrome, although in another report (19), completion of the callosotomy enhanced seizure control in two-thirds of these patients.

Vagus Nerve Stimulation

Vagus nerve stimulation may be useful for the management of both the seizures and the behavior of patients with LGS (104–107); this technique is also effective in children with other encephalopathic epilepsies and hypothalamic hamartomas (108).

Nonmedical Management

The intractability of the seizures and the associated behavioral and cognitive dysfunction mandate a multidisciplinary approach to the management of patients with LGS. Most children require individualized educational plans. Although the development of life skills is a well-recognized goal, social skills are equally important. Most children with encephalopathic epilepsy and LGS form few friendships with their peers, and their lack of social competence as adults is a major handicap. The needs of parents and siblings must be recognized, and respite care for the family should be encouraged.

PROGNOSIS

LGS has a poor prognosis. Only a few patients achieve seizure control, and cognitive dysfunction and behavioral abnormalities are common. Consequently, very few patients are able to lead independent adult lives.

Seizures occur daily in most patients and persist in 60% to 80% (41,109). Seizure onset before the age of 3 years (16), a history of West syndrome (109), symptomatic LGS, severe cognitive dysfunction (41), and difficulty in achieving control (41) are predictive of refractory seizures. Approximately one-third of patients with cryptogenic and half of those with symptomatic LGS lose the electroclinical characteristics of LGS (44). These patients develop the electroclinical features of other encephalopathic epilepsies or localization-related epilepsy. Electroclinical features in early childhood also may influence the evolution of the seizure type. Patients with tonic seizures, nonconvulsive or tonic status epilepticus, and 10-Hz discharges during sleep are more likely as adults to manifest the same seizure types (110). In contrast, those with atypical absences and slow spike-wave activity who lack one or more of these features tend not to have the characteristic Lennox-Gastaut seizure types as adults, being more likely to have partial seizures, particularly complex partial or multifocal seizures (110). Lennox-Gastaut features in this group may represent an age-related expression of focal epilepsy associated with diffuse brain dysfunction.

The prognosis for normal mental development is poor, with an extremely bleak long-term social outcome. Only 21% of patients observed for at least 12 years were in regular classrooms or nonsheltered occupations (14). The severity of the mental delay becomes more obvious with time (14,16). The age of seizure onset correlates best with mental outcome. Onset before 3 years of age is strongly associated with mental retardation (16), and severe retardation occurs more often in cases of symptomatic LGS (72%) than in the cryptogenic form (22%) (16). Repeated episodes of petit mal status portend a poor outcome (42), and mental ability often regresses after an episode of status epilepticus (7). In contrast, atypical absence or myoclonic seizures carry a more hopeful prognosis (16), as does the coexistence of fast spike-wave activity and the precipitation of spike-wave activity by hyperventilation (39,41).

REFERENCES

1. Karbowski K. Developments in epileptology in the 18th and 19th century prior to the delineation of the Lennox-Gastaut syndrome. In: Niedermeyer E, Degen R, eds. *The Lennox-Gastaut syndrome.* New York: Alan R. Liss, 1988:1–8.
2. Lennox WG, Davis JP. Clinical correlates of the fast and slow spike-wave electroencephalogram. *Pediatrics* 1950;5:626–644.
3. Commission on Classification and Terminology of the International League Against Epilepsy. Proposal for revised classification of epilepsies and epileptic syndromes. *Epilepsia* 1989;30:389–399.
4. Engel J. A proposed diagnostic scheme for people with epileptic seizures and epilepsy. Report of the ILAE Task Force on Classification and Terminology. *Epilepsia* 2001;42: 796–803.
5. Aicardi J. *Diseases of the nervous system in childhood,* 2nd ed. London: MacKeith Press, 1998:585–589.
6. Bauer G, Benke T, Bohr K. The Lennox-Gastaut syndrome in adulthood. In: Niedermeyer E, Degen R, eds. *The Lennox-Gastaut syndrome.* New York: Alan R. Liss, 1988:317–328.
7. Beaumanoir A, Blume W. The Lennox-Gastaut syndrome. In: Roger J, Bureau M, Dravet C, et al., eds. *Epileptic syndromes in infancy, childhood and adolescence,* 3rd Ed. London: John Libbey, 2002:113–136.
8. Roger J, Dravet C, Bureau M. The Lennox-Gastaut syndrome. *Cleve Clin J Med* 1989;56(Suppl Pt 2):S172–S180.
9. O'Donohoe NV. *Epilepsies of childhood,* 2nd ed. London: Butterworths, 1985.
10. Weinmann HM. Lennox-Gastaut syndrome and its relationship to infantile spasms (West syndrome). In: Niedermeyer E, Degen R, eds. *The Lennox-Gastaut syndrome.* New York: Alan R. Liss, 1988:301–316.
11. Roger J, Remy C, Bureau M, et al. Lennox-Gastaut syndrome in the adult. *Rev Neurol (Paris)* 1987;143:401–405.
12. Dravet C. The Lennox-Gastaut syndrome: from baby to adolescent. In: Nehlig A, Motte J, Moshe SL, et al., eds. *Childhood epilepsies and brain development.* London: John Libbey, 1999:103–112.
13. Blume WT. Clinical and electroencephalographic correlates of the multiple independent spike foci pattern in children. *Ann Neurol* 1978;4:541–547.
14. Freeman JL, Harvey AS, Rosenfeld JV, et al. Generalized epilepsy in hypothalamic hamartoma: evolution and postoperative resolution. *Neurology* 2003;60:762–767.
15. Hahn KA, Salomons GS, Tackels-Horne D, et al. X-linked mental retardation with seizures and carrier manifestations is caused by a mutation in the creatine-transporter gene (SLC6A8) located in Xq28. *Am J Hum Genet* 2002;70:1349–1356.
16. Chevrie JJ, Aicardi J. Childhood epileptic encephalopathy with slow spike-wave: a statistical study of 80 cases. *Epilepsia* 1972; 13:259–271.
17. Niedermeyer E. *The generalized epilepsies.* Springfield, IL: Charles C Thomas, 1972.
18. Connolly MB, Farrell K, Karim Y, et al. Video-EEG in paediatric outpatients. *Epilepsia* 1994;35:477–481.
19. Dulac O, N'Guyen T. The Lennox-Gastaut syndrome. *Epilepsia* 1993;34(Suppl 7):S7–S17.
20. Oller-Daurella L. A special type of delayed crisis in Lennox-Gastaut syndrome. *Rev Neurol (Paris)* 1970;122:459–462.
21. Chatrian GE, Lettich E, Wilkus RJ, et al. Polygraphic and clinical observations on tonic-autonomic seizures. In: Broughton RJ, ed. *Henri Gastaut and the Marseilles School's contribution to the neurosciences.* Amsterdam: Elsevier Biomedical, 1982:100–124.
22. Bare MA, Glauser TA, Strawsburg RH. Need for electroencephalogram video confirmation with atypical absence seizures in children with Lennox-Gastaut syndrome. *J Child Neurol* 1998;13:498–500.
23. Egli M, Mothersill I, O'Kane M, et al. The axial spasm: the predominant type of drop seizure in patients with secondary generalized epilepsy. *Epilepsia* 1985;26:401–415.
24. Gastaut H. The Lennox-Gastaut syndrome: comments on the syndrome's terminology and nosological position among the secondary generalized epilepsies of childhood. *Electroencephalogr Clin Neurophysiol* 1982:35(Suppl 1):S71–S84.
25. Ikeno T, Shigematsu H, Miyakoshi M, et al. An analytic study of epileptic falls. *Epilepsia* 1985;26:612–621.
26. Giovanardi Rossi P, Gobbi G, Melideo G, et al. Myoclonic manifestations in the Lennox-Gastaut syndrome and other childhood epilepsies. In: Niedermeyer E, Degen R, eds. *The Lennox-Gastaut syndrome.* New York: Alan R. Liss, 1988:109–124.
27. Aicardi J. Course and prognosis of certain childhood epilepsies with predominantly myoclonic seizures. In: Wada JA, Penry JK, eds. *Advances in epileptology:* Xth Epilepsy International Symposium. New York: Raven Press, 1980:159–163.
28. Aicardi J, Chevrie JJ. Myoclonic epilepsies of childhood. *Neuropadiatrie* 1971;3:177–190.
29. Beaumanoir A, Foletti G, Magistris M, et al. Status epilepticus in the Lennox-Gastaut syndrome. In: Niedermeyer E, Degen R, eds. *The Lennox-Gastaut syndrome.* New York: Alan R. Liss, 1988:283–300.
30. Dravet C, Natale O, Magaudda A, et al. Status epilepticus in the Lennox-Gastaut syndrome. *Rev Electroencephalogr Neurophysiol Clin* 1986;15:361–368.
31. Bittencourt PRM, Richens A. Anticonvulsant-induced status epilepticus in Lennox-Gastaut syndrome. *Epilepsia* 1981;22:129–134.
32. Dimario FJ, Clancy RR. Paradoxical precipitation of tonic seizures by lorazepam in a child with atypical absence seizures. *Pediatr Neurol* 1988;4:249–251.

33. Prior PF, McLaine GN, Scott DF, et al. Tonic status epilepticus precipitated by intravenous diazepam in a child with petit mal status. *Epilepsia* 1972;13:467–472.

34. Tassinari CA, Dravet C, Roger J, et al. Tonic status epilepticus precipitated by intravenous benzodiazepines in five patients with Lennox-Gastaut syndrome. *Epilepsia* 1972;13:421–435.

35. Fitzgerald LF, Stone JL, Hughes JR, et al. The Lennox-Gastaut syndrome: electroencephalographic characteristics, clinical correlates, and follow-up studies. *Clin Electroencephalogr* 1992;23:180–189.

36. Baldy-Moulinier M, Touchon J, Billiard M, et al. Nocturnal sleep studies in the Lennox-Gastaut syndrome. In: Niedermeyer E, Degen R, eds. *The Lennox-Gastaut syndrome.* New York: Alan R. Liss, 1988:243–260.

37. Degen R, Degen HE. Sleep EEG in patients with myoclonic-astatic seizures (Lennox-Gastaut syndrome). *EEG EMG Z Elektroenzephalogr Elektromyogr Verwandte Geb* 1983;14:106–112.

38. Blume WT. Lennox-Gastaut syndrome. In: Lüders H, Lesser RP, eds. *Epilepsy: electroclinical syndromes.* Heidelberg: Springer-Verlag, 1987:73–92.

39. Aicardi J, Levy Gomes A. Clinical and electroencephalographic symptomatology of the "genuine" Lennox-Gastaut syndrome and its differentiation from other forms of epilepsy of early childhood. *Epilepsy Res Suppl* 1992;6:185–193.

40. Tassinari CA, Ambrosetto G. Tonic seizures in the Lennox-Gastaut syndrome: semiology and differential diagnosis. In: Niedermeyer E, Degen R, eds. *The Lennox-Gastaut syndrome.* New York: Alan R. Liss, 1988:109–124.

41. Blume WT, David RB, Gomez MR. Generalized sharp and slow wave complexes: associated clinical features and long-term follow-up. *Brain* 1973;96:289–306.

42. Doose H, Volzke E. Petit mal status in early childhood and dementia. *Neuropadiatrie* 1979;10:10–14.

43. Erba G, Cavazzuti V. Ictal and interictal response latency in Lennox-Gastaut syndrome. *Electroencephalogr Clin Neurophysiol* 1977;42:717.

44. Oguni H, Hayashi K, Osawa M. Long-term prognosis of Lennox-Gastaut syndrome. *Epilepsia* 1996;37(Suppl 3):44–47.

45. Ohtahara S, Ohtsuka Y, Yoshinaga H, et al. Lennox-Gastaut syndrome: etiological considerations. In: Niedermeyer E, Degen R, eds. *The Lennox-Gastaut syndrome.* New York: Alan R. Liss, 1988;45:47–63.

46. Boniver C, Dravet C, Bureau M, et al. Idiopathic Lennox-Gastaut syndrome. In: Wolf P, Dam M, Janz D, et al., eds. *Advances in epileptology:* XVIth Epilepsy International Symposium. New York: Raven Press, 1987:195–200.

47. Singh R, Andermann E, Whitehouse WP, et al. Severe myoclonic epilepsy of infancy: extended spectrum of GEFS+? *Epilepsia* 2001;42:837–844.

48. Bancaud J, Talairach J, Geier S, et al. Behavioral manifestations induced by electric stimulation of the anterior cingulate gyrus in man. *Rev Neurol (Paris)* 1976;132:705–724.

49. Angelini L, Broggi G, Riva D, et al. A case of Lennox-Gastaut syndrome successfully treated by removal of a parietotemporal astrocytoma. *Epilepsia* 1979;20:665–669.

50. Roger J, Gambarelli-Dubois D. Neuropathological studies of the Lennox-Gastaut syndrome. In: Niedermeyer E, Degen R, eds. *The Lennox-Gastaut syndrome.* New York: Alan R. Liss, 1988:73–93.

51. Renier WO. Neuromorphological and biochemical analysis of a brain biopsy in a second case of idiopathic Lennox-Gastaut syndrome. In: Niedermeyer E, Degen R, eds. *The Lennox-Gastaut syndrome.* New York: Alan R. Liss, 1988:427–432.

52. Gastaut H, Gastaut JL. Computerized transverse axial tomography in epilepsy. *Epilepsia* 1976;17:325–336.

53. Chugani HT, Mazziotta JC, Engel J Jr, et al. The Lennox-Gastaut syndrome: metabolic subtypes determined by 2-deoxy-2[^{18}F] fluoro-D-glucose positron emission tomography. *Ann Neurol* 1987;21:4–13.

54. Iinuma K, Yanai K, Yanagisawa T, et al. Cerebral glucose metabolism in five patients with Lennox-Gastaut syndrome. *Pediatr Neurol* 1987;3:12–18.

55. Theodore WH, Rose D, Patronas N, et al. Cerebral glucose metabolism in the Lennox-Gastaut syndrome. *Ann Neurol* 1987;21:14–21.

56. Goldsmith IL, Zupanc ML, Buchhalter JR. Long-term seizure outcome in 74 patients with Lennox-Gastaut syndrome: effects of incorporating MRI head imaging in defining the cryptogenic subgroup. *Epilepsia* 2000;41:395–399.

57. Doose H, Gerken H, Leonhardt R, et al. Centrencephalic myoclonic-astatic petit mal. Clinical and genetic investigation. *Neuropadiatrie* 1970;2:59–78.

58. Doose H. Myoclonic astatic epilepsy of early childhood. In: Roger J, Bureau M, Dravet C, et al., eds. *Epileptic syndromes in infancy, childhood and adolescence,* 2nd ed. London: John Libbey, 1992:103–114.

59. Doose H. Myoclonic astatic epilepsy of early childhood. In: Roger J, Bureau M, Dravet C, et al., eds. *Epileptic syndromes in infancy, childhood and adolescence.* London: John Libbey, 1985:78–88.

60. Singh R, Scheffer IE, Crossland K, et al. Generalized epilepsy with febrile seizures plus: a common childhood-onset genetic epilepsy syndrome. *Ann Neurol* 1999;45:75–81.

61. Oguni H, Tanaka T, Hayashi K, et al. Treatment and long-term prognosis of myoclonic-astatic epilepsy of early childhood. *Neuropediatrics* 2002;33:122–132.

62. Aicardi J, Chevrie JJ. Atypical benign epilepsy of childhood. *Dev Med Child Neurol* 1982;24:281–292.

63. Patry G, Lyagoubi S, Tassinari CA. Subclinical "electrical status epilepticus" induced by sleep. An electroencephalographic study of six cases. *Arch Neurol* 1971;24:242–252.

64. Tassinari CA, Rubboli G, Volpi L, et al. Electrical status epilepticus during slow sleep (ESES or CSWS) including acquired epileptic aphasia (Landau-Kleffner syndrome) In: Roger J, Bureau M, Dravet C, et al., eds. *Epileptic syndromes in infancy, childhood and adolescence,* 3rd ed. London: John Libbey, 2002:265–284.

65. Viani F, Romeo A, Viri M, et al. Seizure and EEG patterns in Angelman's syndrome. *J Child Neurol* 1995;10:467–471.

66. Minassian BA, DeLorey TM, Olsen RW, et al. Angelman syndrome: correlation between epilepsy phenotypes and genotypes. *Ann Neurol* 1998;43:485–493.

67. Papini M, Pasquinelli A, Armellini M, et al. Alertness and incidence of seizures in patients with Lennox-Gastaut syndrome. *Epilepsia* 1984;25:161–167.

68. Munn RI, Farrell K. Open study of clobazam in refractory epilepsy. *Pediatr Neurol* 1993;9:465–469.

69. O'Donohoe NV, Paes BA. A trial of clonazepam in the treatment of severe epilepsy in infancy and childhood. In: Penry JK, ed. *Epilepsy: Eighth International Symposium.* New York: Raven Press, 1977:159–162.

70. Hosain SA, Green NS, Solomon GE, et al. Nitrazepam for the treatment of Lennox-Gastaut syndrome. *Pediatr Neurol* 2003;28:16–19.

71. Farrell K. Benzodiazepines in the treatment of children with epilepsy. *Epilepsia* 1986;27:S45–S51.

72. Frey HH. Experimental evidence for the development of tolerance to anticonvulsant drug effects. In: Frey HH, Fröscher W, Koella WP, et al., eds. *Tolerance to beneficial and adverse effects of antiepileptic drugs.* New York: Raven Press, 1986:7–14.

73. Cull CA, Trimble MR. Anticonvulsant benzodiazepines and performance. *R Soc Med Int Congr Symp Series* 1985;74:121–128.

74. Jeavons PM, Clark JE, Maheshwari MC. Treatment of generalized epilepsies of childhood and adolescence with sodium valproate ("epilim"). *Dev Med Child Neurol* 1977;19:9–25.

75. Schlumberger E, Chavez F, Palacios L, et al. Lamotrigine in treatment of 120 children with epilepsy. *Epilepsia* 1994;35:359–367.

76. Eriksson AS, Nergardh A, Hoppu K. The efficacy of lamotrigine in children and adolescents with refractory generalized epilepsy: a randomized, double-blind, crossover study. *Epilepsia* 1998;39:495–501.

77. Motte J, Trevathan E, Arvidsson JF, et al. Lamotrigine for generalized seizures associated with Lennox-Gastaut syndrome. *N Engl J Med* 1997;337:1807–1812.

78. Sachdeo RC, Glauser TA, Ritter F, et al. A double-blind, randomized trial of topiramate in Lennox-Gastaut syndrome. *Neurology* 1999;52:1882–1887.

79. Singh BK, White-Scott S. Role of topiramate in adults with intractable epilepsy, mental retardation, and developmental disabilities. *Seizure* 2002;11:47–50.

80. Erba G, Browne TR. Atypical absence, myoclonic, atonic, and tonic seizures and the "Lennox-Gastaut syndrome." In: Browne TR, Feldman RG, eds. *Epilepsy, diagnosis and management.* Boston: Little, Brown, 1983:75–94.

81. Snead OC III, Hosey LC. Exacerbation of seizures in children by carbamazepine. *N Engl J Med* 1985;313:916–921.

82. Felbamate Study Group in Lennox-Gastaut Syndrome. Efficacy of felbamate in childhood epileptic encephalopathy (Lennox-Gastaut syndrome). *N Engl J Med* 1993;328:29–33.

83. Glauser TA, Pellock JM. Zonisamide in pediatric epilepsy: review of the Japanese experience. *J Child Neurol* 2002;17:87–96.

84. Livingston JH, Beaumont D, Arzimanoglou A, et al. Vigabatrin in the treatment of epilepsy in children. *Br J Clin Pharmacol* 1989;27:109S–112S.

85. Luna D, Dulac O, Pajot N, et al: Vigabatrin in the treatment of childhood epilepsies: a single-blind placebo-controlled study. *Epilepsia* 1989;30:430–437.

86. Vossler DG. Exacerbation of seizures in Lennox-Gastaut syndrome by gabapentin. *Neurology* 1996;46:852–853.

87. Freeman JM, Vining EPG, Pillas DJ, et al. The efficacy of the ketogenic diet—1998: a prospective evaluation of intervention in 150 children. *Pediatrics* 1998;102:1358–1363.

88. Kinsman SL, Vining EPG, Quaskey SA, et al. Efficacy of the ketogenic diet for intractable seizure disorders: review of 58 cases. *Epilepsia* 1992;33:1132–1136.

89. Vining EPG, Freeman JM, Balaban-Gil K, et al. A multicenter study of the efficacy of the ketogenic diet. *Arch Neurol* 1998;55:1433–1437.

90. Freeman JM, Vining EPG. Seizures decrease rapidly after fasting: preliminary studies of the ketogenic diet. *Arch Pediatr Adolesc Med* 1999;153:946–949.

91. Kossoff EH, Pyzik PL, Furth SL, et al. Kidney stones, carbonic anhydrase inhibitors, and the ketogenic diet. *Epilepsia* 2002;43:1168–1171.

92. Yamatogi Y, Ohtsuka Y, Ishida T, et al. Hydrocortisone therapy of secondary generalized epilepsy in children. *Brain Dev* 1979;1:267–276.

93. Hasaerts D, Dulac O. Hydrocortisone therapy of secondary generalized epilepsy in children. *Arch Fr Pediatr* 1989;46:635–639.

94. Brett EM. The Lennox-Gastaut syndrome: therapeutic aspects. In: Niedermeyer E, Degen R, eds. *The Lennox-Gastaut syndrome.* New York: Alan R. Liss, 1988:329–339.

95. Ariizumi M, Baba K, Shiihara H, et al. High dose gammaglobulin for intractable childhood epilepsy. *Lancet* 1983;2:162–163.

96. Sandstedt P, Kostulas V, Larsson LE. Intravenous gammaglobulin for postencephalitic epilepsy. *Lancet* 1984;2:1154–1155.

97. Shields WD, Lake JL, Chugani HT. Amantadine in the treatment of refractory epilepsy in childhood: an open trial in 10 patients. *Neurology* 1985;35:579–581.

98. Fromm GH, Wessel HB, Glass JD, et al. Imipramine in absence and myoclonic-astatic seizures. Neurology 1978;28:953–957.

99. Hurst DL. The use of imipramine in minor motor seizures. *Pediatr Neurol* 1986;2:13–17.

100. Inanaga K, Inoue Y. Effect of thyrotropin releasing hormone analog in a patient with myoclonus epilepsy. *Kurume Med J* 1981;28:201–210.

101. Andermann F, Olivier A, Gotman J, et al. Callosotomy for the treatment of patients with intractable epilepsy and the Lennox-Gastaut syndrome. In: Niedermeyer E, Degen R, eds. *The Lennox-Gastaut syndrome.* New York: Alan R. Liss, 1988:361–376.

102. Wyllie E. Corpus callosotomy for intractable generalized epilepsy. *J Pediatr* 1988;113:255–261.

103. Pinard JM, Delande OJ, Plouin P, et al. Results of callosotomy in children according to etiology and epileptic syndromes. *Epilepsia* 1992;33(Suppl 3):27.

104. Lundgren J, Åmark P, Blennöw G, et al. Vagus nerve stimulation in 16 children with refractory epilepsy. *Epilepsia* 1998;39:809–813.

105. Hosain S, Nikalov B, Harden C, et al. Vagus nerve stimulation treatment for Lennox-Gastaut syndrome. *J Child Neurol* 2000;15:509–512.

106. Frost M, Gates J, Helmers SL, et al. Vagal nerve stimulation in children with refractory seizures associated with Lennox-Gastaut syndrome. *Epilepsia* 2001;42:1148–1152.

107. Aldenkamp AP, Van de Veerdonk SHA, Majoie HJM, et al. Effects of 6 months of treatment with vagus nerve stimulation on behavior in children with Lennox-Gastaut syndrome in an open clinical and nonrandomized study. *Epilepsy Behav* 2001:2:343–350.

108. Murphy JV, Wheless JW, Schmoll CM. Left vagal nerve stimulation in six patients with hypothalamic hamartomas. *Pediatr Neurol* 2000;23:167–168.

109. Ohtahara S, Yamatogi Y, Ohtsuka Y. Prognosis of the Lennox syndrome–long-term clinical and electroencephalographic follow-up study, especially with special reference to relationship with the West syndrome. *Folia Psychiatr Neurol Jpn* 1976;30:275–287.

110. Beaumanoir A. Nosological limits of the Lennox-Gastaut syndrome [author's translation]. *Rev Electroencephalogr Neurophysiol Clin* 1981;11:468–473.

Rasmussen's Encephalitis (Chronic Focal Encephalitis)

28

François Dubeau

Rasmussen encephalitis is a progressive disorder of childhood, associated with hemispheric atrophy, severe focal epilepsy, intellectual decline, and hemiparesis. Neuropathologic features described in the surgical specimens show characteristics of chronic inflammation such as perivascular and leptomeningeal lymphocytic infiltration, microglial nodules, astrocytosis, and neuronal degeneration. There are variants of this syndrome with regard to age at onset, staging, localization, progression, and outcome. Treatment options are limited. Antiepileptic drugs (AEDs) usually show no significant benefit. Immunotherapy trials (undertaken mostly during the 1990s) showed modest transient improvement in symptoms and disease progression in some patients. Only hemispherectomy seems to produce persistent relief of seizures and functional improvement.

The disorder was first described by Dr. Theodore Rasmussen in 1958, who, together with Jerzy Olszewski and Donald Lloyd-Smith, published the clinical and histopathologic features of three patients with focal seizures caused by chronic focal encephalitis (1). The original proband, FS, a 10-year-old boy, was referred in 1945 to Dr. Wilder Penfield by Dr. Edgar Fincher, chief of neurosurgery at Emory University in Atlanta, Georgia, because of intractable right-sided focal motor seizures starting at 6 years of age (2). FS developed a right hemiparesis and underwent, between 1941 and 1956, three surgical interventions (two at the Montreal Neurological Hospital and Institute [MNHI]) at 7, 10, and 21 years of age in an attempt to control the evolution of the disease. In the first chapter of the monograph on chronic encephalitis published by Dr. Frederick Andermann in 1991, Dr. Rasmussen

reported a letter by Dr. Fincher to Dr. Penfield (dated 1956) urging him to consider a more extensive cortical excision and concluded, "I note in your discussion that you list the cause as unknown, but if this youngster doesn't have a chronic low-grade encephalitic process which has likely, by now, burned itself out, I will buy you a new hat." The last intervention was a left hemispherectomy performed by Dr. Rasmussen, and histology showed sparse perivascular inflammation and glial nodules. FS remained seizure-free until his last follow-up at 51 years of age. He was mildly retarded and had a fixed right hemiplegia. He developed hydrocephalus as a late complication of the surgical procedure and required a shunt. Dr. Penfield, who was consulted in this case, remained skeptical of the postulate that the syndrome was a primary inflammatory disorder, and he raised most of the issues that continue to be debated: if it is an encephalitic process, would it not involve both hemispheres? Is the encephalitic process the result of recurrent seizures caused by a small focal lesion in one hemisphere? Why it is that epileptic seizures are destructive in one case and not in another? Dr. Rasmussen himself recognized that Fincher's 1941 diagnosis of chronic encephalitis in FS's case was made 14 years before case 2 of the original 1958 report (1). The story does not say, however, if Dr. Penfield had to provide his colleague and friend Dr. Fincher with a new hat (3).

This diagnosis, later recognized as "Rasmussen encephalitis (RE) or syndrome," became the subject of extensive discussion in the literature, initially debating the best timing for surgery and best surgical approaches, and, more recently, the etiology and pathogenesis of this unusual and enigmatic disease. A large number of publications can now be found in the literature, and two international symposia were held in Montreal, first in 1988 and again in December 2002. The interest in this disease, which is usually described in children, was initially driven by the severity and inescapability of its course, which rapidly led to its description as a prototype of "catastrophic epilepsy." Physicians and scientists became interested by the unusual pathogenesis and evolution of the syndrome and are now trying to reconcile the apparent focal nature of the disease with the postulated viral and autoimmune etiologies that may or may not be mutually exclusive. This chapter reviews and updates a number of issues regarding RE, particularly the putative mechanisms of the disease, the variability of the clinical presentations, and the indications and rationale of new medical therapies, such as immunomodulation and receptor-directed pharmacotherapy.

CLINICAL PRESENTATIONS

Typical Course

In the early stages of the disease, the major issue is diagnosis. A combination of characteristic clinical, electrophysiologic, and imaging findings aid in the diagnosis. The 48 patients studied at the MNHI were collected over a period of 30 years and consisted mostly of referrals from outside Canada. Although now easier to recognize, this disease remains rare. During the last decade, an additional 10 patients at the MNHI were studied, a small number compared to the 100 to 150 patients with intractable focal epilepsy due to other causes studied each year at the center. Typically, the disease starts in healthy children between 1 and 13 years (mean age, 6.8 years) with 80% developing seizures before the age of 10 years (4). There is no difference in incidence between the sexes. In approximately half the patients, a history of infectious or inflammatory episode was described 6 months prior to the onset of seizures.

The first sign of the disease is the development of seizures. Seizures are usually partial or secondarily generalized tonic-clonic seizures; 20% of patients in the MNHI series presented with status epilepticus as the first manifestation. Early seizures could be polymorphic with variable semiology, but motor seizures are almost always reported. Other variable semiology of seizures with somatosensory, autonomic, visual, and psychic features has been described (4,5). The seizures rapidly become refractory, with little response to AEDs. Epilepsia partialis continua (EPC) and other forms of focal seizures are particularly unresponsive to AEDs (6–9). We reviewed the AED therapy of 25 patients of the MNHI series and found no specific agent or combination therapy that appeared to be more effective or less toxic than other regimens (8). Our experience with newer AEDs in seven other patients with RE did not support improved effectiveness or tolerability for the new agents. The new AEDs levetiracetam and topiramate may theoretically have a role in the treatment of RE, because levetirac-

etam has efficacy in treating cortical myoclonus (10,11) and topiramate has a direct effect on glutamate receptors and release of N-methyl-D-glutamine (NMDA) (12).

A variety of seizure types develop over time. The most common are focal motor and EPC (in 56% of the patients), with scalp electroencephalogram (EEG) patterns suggesting perirolandic onset. Secondarily generalized motor seizures are also common in many patients, but these appear to be easier to control with AEDs. Other, less frequent types of motor seizures include jacksonian march (12%), posturing (25%), or versive movements of the head and eyes (13%), suggesting involvement of the primary motor, premotor, and supplementary motor areas. Drop attacks, however, are rare. Focal seizures with somatosensory (22% of the patients), visual (16%), or auditory (2%) manifestations are less frequent and appear later in the course of the disease, suggesting that the epileptogenic process has migrated from frontocentral regions to more posterior cortical areas.

Oguni and colleagues (4) empirically divided the progression of the disease into three stages: *stage 1*, from the onset of the seizures and before the development of a fixed hemiparesis (3 months to 10 years, mean duration, 2.8 years); *stage 2*, from the development of a fixed hemiparesis (occurring in all 48 patients) to the completion of neurologic deterioration, including intellectual decline (85%), visual (49%) and sensory (29%) cortical deficits, and speech problems (dysarthria 23%, dysphasia 19%) dependent or independent of the burden of seizure activity (2 months to 10 years, mean duration, 3.7 years); and *stage 3*, stabilization of the condition in which further progression no longer occurs, and even the seizures tend to decrease in severity and frequency.

A study by Bien and colleagues (13) presented the clinical natural history of RE in parallel with the time course of brain destruction as measured by serial magnetic resonance imaging (MRI), in a series of 13 patients studied histologically. They separated the progression of the disease into prodromal, acute, and residual stages comparable to the three stages of Oguni and colleagues. However, Bien and colleagues distinguished two patterns of disease: one with an earlier and more severe disorder starting during childhood (mean age at first seizure, 4.4 years; range, 1.6 to 6.4 years) and a second with a more protracted and milder course starting during adolescence or adult life (mean age at first seizure, 21.9 years; range, 6.4 to 40.9 years), the second pattern representing a well-described variant of RE in the last decade (14–18).

Clinical Variants of Rasmussen Encephalitis

RE has been known for more than 50 years. After the initial description, it became clear that the disease is clinically heterogeneous despite the pathologic hallmark of nonspecific chronic inflammation in the affected hemisphere. This heterogeneity may be explained by different etiologies (viral,

viral- and nonviral-mediated autoimmune disease), by different reactions of the host's immune system to exogenous or endogenous insults (age, genetic background, presence of another lesion, or "double pathology"), and by the modulating effect of a variety of antiviral, immunosuppressant, and immunomodulatory agents, or receptor-directed pharmacotherapy used in variable combinations and durations to treat these patients. Atypical or unusual clinical features include early onset (usually younger than 2 years of age) with rapid progression of the disease; bilateral cerebral involvement; relatively late onset during adolescence or adult life with slow progression; atypical anatomic location of the initial brain MRI findings; focal or protracted or subcortical variants of RE; and double pathology.

Bilateral Hemispheric Involvement

Usually the disease affects only one hemisphere, and most autopsy studies available confirmed unilateral cerebral involvement (19). Over time, however, there may be some contralateral ventricular enlargement and cortical atrophy attributed either to the effect of recurrent seizures and secondary epileptogenesis or to Wallerian changes. Patients with definite bilateral inflammatory involvement are exceptional and such involvement has been described so far in no more than a dozen patients (15,20–25). Bilateral disease tends to occur in children with early onset (before age 2 years), but was also described in the late-onset adolescent or adult forms. A small number had received high-dose steroids or an intrathecal antiviral agent, which suggested that early aggressive immunologic therapy may have predisposed them to contralateral spread of the disease.

Late-onset Adolescent and Adult Variants

A number of papers report the development of RE in adolescence or adult life as representing approximately 10% of the total number of patients with RE described in the literature over the last 40 years (13–18,26–34). In the MNHI series, 9 (16%) of 55 patients collected between 1945 and 2000 started to have seizures after the age of 12 years. The largest series, described by Hart and colleagues (18), included 13 adults and adolescents collected from 5 centers. In comparison with the childhood form, late-onset RE has a more variable evolution (13,18), a generally more insidious onset of focal neurologic defects and cognitive impairment, and an increased incidence of occipital involvement (23% in the series described by Hart and coworkers versus 7% in children younger than 12 years old in the MNHI series). Hemiparesis and hemispheric atrophy are often late and may not be as severe when compared with the more typical childhood form (13). Occasionally the outcome in late-onset RE is similar to or worse than in children (15,26,27), but because of the generally more benign and protracted course, early hemispherectomy seems less appropriate in this group of patients in whom

neurologic deficits are usually less pronounced. Moreover, because of a lack of plasticity in adults, the decision for hemispherectomy is complicated because of potential risk of new irreversible postoperative deficits in the form of severe motor, visual, and speech and language (dominant hemisphere) impairment.

Focal and Chronic Protracted Variants

There are rare reports of patients with RE whose seizures were relatively well controlled with AEDs or focal resections, and in whom the neurologic status stabilized spontaneously (18,30,33,35). Rasmussen had already suggested the existence of a "nonprogressive focal form of encephalitis." With Aguilar, he reviewed 512 surgical specimens from 449 patients and found 32 cases with histologic evidence suggesting the presence of active encephalitis (14). Twelve demonstrated progressive neurologic deterioration compatible with RE, and 20 (4.4%) showed no or mild neurologic deterioration. In his review of patients who underwent temporal resections for intractable focal seizures, Laxer (35) found 5 patients (3.8% of a series of 160 patients) with what he thought was a benign, focal, nonprogressive form of RE. These patients (children or adults) with no evidence of progression are indistinguishable clinically from those with refractory seizures due to other causes, including mesial temporal sclerosis (33,35).

Basal Ganglia Involvement

EPC and other types of focal motor seizures are a common finding in patients with RE. Chorea, athetosis, or dystonia were infrequently described and may have been overlooked because of the preponderance of the epileptic disorder and of the hemiparesis. In 27 of the 48 patients of the MNHI series who had EPC, 9 additionally had writhing or choreiform movements, and a diagnosis of Sydenham chorea was made in 3 of the patients early in the disease course (4). Matthews and colleagues (36) described a 10-year-old girl with a 1-year history of progressive right-sided hemiparesis, EPC, and secondary generalized seizures. MRI showed diffuse cortical and subcortical changes maximum in the perisylvian frontotemporoparietal area. At examination, she had choreic movements of the right arm and hand in addition to EPC. Tien and colleagues (37) were the first to describe in an 8.5-year-old girl with intractable focal motor seizures, atrophy of the caudate and putamen with abnormal high signals and severe left hemispheric atrophy. They interpreted these findings as the result of gliosis and chronic brain damage. Topçu and colleagues (9) described a patient who developed hemidystonia as a result of involvement of the contralateral basal ganglia. The movement disorder appeared 3 years after the onset of seizures. A rather typical subsequent evolution suggested RE. The movement disorder started during intravenous immunoglobulin (IVIG) and interferon therapy, and did not respond to anticholinergic drugs nor to a frontal resection. Ben-Zeev and colleagues (38), Koehn and Zupanc (39), Frucht (34) and, finally, Lascelles and colleagues (40) each reported a case of RE whose clinical presentation was dominated by a hemidyskinesia, with EPC in three of those patients, and progressive hemiparesis. Two cases showed selective frontal cortical and caudate atrophy on MRI; one developed progressive left basal ganglia atrophy and later focal frontotemporoparietal atrophy; and one had only pronounced right caudate, globus pallidus, and putamen atrophy. In the case of Frucht, IVIG dramatically improved both the hyperkinetic movements and the EPC, but the effect was transient, suggesting a common neuroanatomic mechanism or humoral autoimmune process. In a series of 21 patients with RE, Bhatjiwale and colleagues (41) looked specifically at the involvement of the basal ganglia. Fifteen (71%) patients showed mild to severe basal ganglia involvement on imaging in three different patterns: predominantly cortical in six cases, predominantly basal ganglia in six cases, and both cortical and basal ganglia involvement in three cases. In five cases, the changes found in the basal ganglia were static, whereas in the others there was steady progression. The caudate nucleus was generally more prominently involved, usually in association with frontal atrophy. Five cases also showed putaminal involvement, always with temporoinsular atrophy. Interestingly, two of the six patients with prominent basal ganglia involvement had dystonia as a presenting feature. The authors postulated that the disease may proceed from different foci, including cases where RE seems to start in deep gray matter. Similar findings were recently described by the Italian Study Group on Rasmussen encephalitis (42), which found basal ganglia atrophy in 9 of 13 patients studied. They suggested that atrophy of the basal ganglia represents only secondary change because of disconnection from the affected overlying frontal and insular cortex.

Brainstem Variant

McDonald and colleagues (43) recently reported a 3-year-old boy with RE manifested by chronic brainstem encephalitis. After a prolonged febrile seizure associated with an acute varicella infection, he developed recurrent partial motor seizures, EPC, and left hemiparesis within a few weeks. After a few more weeks, signs of brainstem involvement appeared, repeated MRI showed increased signal in the pons, but a complete infectious and inflammatory evaluation, including brain biopsy, was negative. He died 14 months after the onset of his illness. Neuropathologic findings in the brainstem were typical of those found in RE. Bilateral mesial temporal sclerosis was also present. The authors proposed that this case represents a rare focal form of RE with primarily involvement of the brainstem, and hemiparesis and mesial temporal sclerosis resulting from seizure activity. However, this is an isolated case report in a complicated patient, and existence of this variant is questionable.

Multifocal Variant

Maeda and colleagues (44) described a 6-year-old girl with typical RE. One year following the onset of seizures, MRI-FLAIR (fluid attenuated inversion recovery) sequences showed multiple high-signal-intensity areas in the right hemisphere, and a methionine-PET (positron emission tomography) performed at the same time exhibited multifocal methionine uptake areas concordant with the MRI lesions, suggesting multiple independent sites of chronic inflammation. The authors proposed that the inflammatory process in RE may spread from multifocal lesions and not necessarily originate from localized temporal, insular, or frontocentral lesions, as usually described, before spreading across adjacent regions to the entire hemisphere.

Double Pathology

A small number of reports have documented coexisting brain pathologies with RE: a tumor (anaplastic astrocytoma, ganglioglioma) in two patients (45,46), dysgenetic tissue in four patients (19,45,47,48), multifocal perivasculitis in seven patients (19), and cavernous angiomas with signs of vasculitis in two patients (19,45). Double pathology in RE supports the theory of focal disruption (trauma, infection, or other pathology) of the blood–brain barrier (BBB), allowing access of antibodies produced by the host to neurons expressing the target receptor and production of focal inflammation (3,49). So far, however, only one case of double pathology provided reasonable support for this hypothesis (48). Strongly positive anti-GluR3 (glutamate receptor 3 subunit) antibodies were measured in one case of RE with concomitant cortical dysplasia in a 2.5-year-old girl with catastrophic epilepsy starting at age 2 years. She underwent a right, partial frontal lobectomy, plasmapheresis, and therapy with IVIG with a transient response, and, finally, a right functional hemispherectomy with good seizure control. GluR3 antibodies were measured serially throughout the course of her treatment and correlated with her clinical status. They were undetectable 1 year after her last surgery.

There are also reports of coexisting autoimmune diseases such as Parry-Romberg syndrome (50,51), linear scleroderma (52,53), and systemic lupus erythematosus (40) with changes suggestive of RE. Such changes have also been described in disorders with impaired immunity such as agammaglobulinemia (54) and multiple endocrinopathies, chronic mucocutaneous candidiasis, and impaired cellular immunity (55). The occurrence of two conditions presumably caused by impaired immunity in the same individual may strengthen the view that immune-mediated mechanisms are responsible for the development of RE.

Finally, the rare association of uveitis (three cases) or choroiditis (one case) with typical features of RE has led to the speculation that a viral infection may have been responsible for both (26,56,57). In all cases, the ocular pathology was ipsilateral to the involved hemisphere that showed chronic encephalitis. In three cases (26,56), the uveitis or choroiditis was detected 2 to 4 months after epilepsy onset. In one case (57), ocular diagnosis preceded the onset of chronic encephalitis. In light of these cases, it was hypothesized that a primary ocular infection, in particular a viral infection with herpes simplex virus (HSV), varicella-zoster virus (VZV), Epstein-Barr virus (EBV), cytomegalovirus (CMV), measles, or rubella, followed by vascular or neurotropic spread to the brain, was a possible mechanism for development of RE.

ELECTROENCEPHALOGRAPHY

Few studies specifically reported the EEG changes associated with RE (58–62), and even fewer tried to correlate the clinical and EEG features of the disease over time (63–65). So and Gloor (62) reported the scalp and perioperative (ECoG, electrocorticogram) EEG findings in the MNHI series of patients with RE. They summarized the EEG features as (a) disturbance of background activity in all except one patient with more severe slowing and relative depression of background rhythms in the diseased hemisphere; polymorphic or rhythmic delta activity was found in all (more commonly bilateral with lateralized preponderance); (b) interictal epileptiform activity in 94% of patients, rarely focal (more commonly multifocal and lateralized to one hemisphere or bilateral independent, but strongly lateralized discharges with or without bilateral synchrony); (c) clinical or subclinical seizure onsets were variable and occasionally focal, but more often poorly localized, lateralized, bilateral, or even generalized; and (d) no clear electroclinical correlation apparent in many of the recorded clinical seizures, in particular in EPC. The electrographic lateralization of these abnormalities (focal slowing, progressive deterioration of unilateral background activity, ictal, and multifocal interictal hemispheric epileptiform activity) was sufficiently concordant with the clinical lateralization to provide essential information about the abnormal hemisphere in 90% of cases. These EEG features, indicative of a widespread destructive and epileptogenic process, in the specific clinical context of catastrophic epilepsy and worsening neurologic deficits involving one hemisphere, suggest the diagnosis of chronic encephalitis.

The evolution of the electroencephalogram was studied longitudinally in a small number of patients (62–65). The studies showed progression of the EEG abnormalities. At the onset of the disease, EEG abnormalities tended to be lateralized and nonspecific, with unilateral slowing of background activity. As the disease progressed, it tended to become bilateral and widespread, multifocal or synchronous, suggesting a more diffuse hemispheric process, but not always confined to one hemisphere. It is not clear if this late bilateralization of the EEG abnormalities represented functional interference, secondary epileptogenesis, or, much less likely, inflammatory process directly involving the contralateral hemisphere.

IMAGING

Anatomic Imaging

Imaging studies, although not specific, are extremely important for the diagnosis of RE. Typically, they show progressive, lateralized atrophy coupled with localized or lateralized functional abnormalities (5,7,13,37,41,42, 47,66–70). Brain magnetic resonance studies early in the course of the illness may be normal, rapidly followed by a combination of characteristic features that parallel the clinical and electrophysiologic deterioration, reflecting the nature of the pathologic process. Recent studies using serial MRIs in a relatively large number of patients with RE provided better insight into the early, progressive, and late gray and white matter changes expected in this disease: cortical swelling, atrophy of cortical and deep gray matter nuclei, particularly the caudate, a hyperintense signal in gray and white matter, and secondary changes (5,13,41,42,70). In the early phase of the disease, when the MRI still appears normal, a few studies demonstrated abnormalities of perfusion or metabolism by single-photon-emission computed tomography (SPECT) or PET, suggesting that these imaging procedures may aid in early identification of the disease and of the abnormal hemisphere (37,69,71). Rapidly on early magnetic resonance scans, however, the cortex shows focal hyperintense signals on T2 or FLAIR sequences (42) and may appear swollen. This can be explained by brain edema at the onset of inflammation (70) or, alternatively, by recurrent focal seizures (72). Very early signal change in the white matter (within 4 months) is also frequent, usually focal, with or without swelling (42). Later, progressive atrophy of the affected hemisphere occurs, reflecting the manner in which the disease spreads, and with most of the hemispheric volume loss occurring during the first 2 years (42,70). The cortical atrophy is initially either temporal, frontoinsular, or frontocentral, and, more rarely, parietooccipital, later spreading across the hemisphere. Basal ganglia involvement, mostly of the putamen and caudate, is also characteristic and may be a result of direct damage by the pathologic process or secondary to changes caused by disconnection of the basal ganglia from the affected overlying frontocentral and insular cortices (41,42). Other secondary changes usually associated with severe hemispheric tissue loss are atrophy of the brainstem, particularly of the cerebral peduncle and pons, thinning of the corpus callosum, and atrophy of the contralateral cerebellar hemisphere (42). Surprisingly, gadolinium enhancement on MRI is rarely observed (31,42,47,69,70,73,74).

Functional Imaging

Several studies, often case reports, have emphasized the utility of functional imaging such as PET, SPECT, and proton magnetic resonance spectroscopy (MRS) in the diagnosis and follow up. Functional abnormalities may be useful in cases in which MRI is normal, usually at the onset of the disease, or when structural imaging fails to provide satisfactory localizing information. Combined anatomic and functional neuroimaging may serve to focus the diagnostic work-up, hasten brain biopsy for definitive diagnosis, or define the appropriate surgical approach. It may be useful to follow the evolution of the disease or the result of treatment. Finally, functional studies may provide insight in the cortical reorganization of speech areas and of motor and somatosensory cortices.

Fiorella and colleagues (69) reviewed 2-deoxy-2-[^{18}F]-fluoro-D-glucose PET (FDG-PET) and MRI studies of 11 patients with surgically proven RE. All had diffuse, unilateral cerebral hypometabolism on PET images, closely correlated with the distribution of cerebral atrophy on MRI. Even subtle diffuse atrophic changes were accompanied by marked decreases in cerebral glucose use that, according to the authors, increased diagnostic confidence and aided in the identification of the abnormal hemisphere. During ictal studies, patients had multiple foci of hypermetabolism, indicative of multifocal seizure activity within the affected hemisphere, and never showed such changes in the contralateral one. Similar findings had been reported previously but in smaller series (37,42,73,75–78). Although MRI alone is generally sufficient to identify the affected hemisphere, FDG-PET unequivocally confirms the findings in each case. Blood flow or perfusion studies using Oxygen-15 PET showed a similar correlation, with regions of perfusion change corresponding with structural MRI changes (78). Using a specific radioligand ([^{11}C](R)-PK11195) for peripheral benzodiazepine-binding sites on cells of mononuclear phagocyte lineage, Banati and colleagues (79) demonstrated *in vivo* the widespread activation of microglia in three patients which is usually found by neuropathologic study.

SPECT was used to study regional blood flow in a number of patients (7,9,42,66,71,75,77,80–86). The findings may be of some help and more sensitive than anatomic neuroimaging early in the disease, but are nonspecific. As with FDG-PET, the regions of functional change usually correlate with anatomic abnormalities. Interictal SPECT scans reveal diminished perfusion in a large zone surrounding the epileptic area shown on electroencephalography. This hypoperfusion may show some variability depending on fluctuation of the epileptic activity. Ictal studies often show zones of hyperperfusion representing likely areas of more intense seizure activity. Sequential scans may be helpful to follow the progression of the disease (66) or the effect of a treatment (84).

MRS has been used in a number of patients with RE (36,42,84,87–92). Localized proton MRS was described for the first time in two patients by Matthews and colleagues (36). They showed reduced *N*-acetylaspartate (NAA) concentrations—a compound exclusively found in neurons and their processes—in diseased areas in both patients, suggesting neuronal loss. In addition, MRS

showed increased lactate in a patient with EPC, probably the result of excessive and repetitive seizure activity. These findings were confirmed by Peeling and Sutherland (87) and by Cendes and colleagues (88). Peeling and Sutherland also showed that the concentration of NAA *in vitro* (MRS on tissue obtained from surgical patients) was reduced in proportion to the severity and extent of the encephalitis. Cendes and colleagues did sequential studies at 1 year in three patients and demonstrated progression of the MRS changes. They noted that those changes were more widespread than the structural changes seen on anatomic MRI. Overall, the studies using NAA indicate that MRS can identify and quantify neuronal damage and loss throughout the affected hemisphere, including areas that appear anatomically normal. In addition to NAA and lactate, other compounds measured included choline, creatine, *myo*-inositol, glutamine, and glutamate. Choline is usually elevated, which probably indicates demyelination and increased membrane turnover (83,88,89,92). *Myo*-inositol, a glial cell marker, was found to be elevated in a small number of patients (83,90,92), indicating glial proliferation or prominent gliotic activity. Hypothetically, *myo*-inositol signal should increase with the progression of the disease. Lactate was almost always elevated, and this increase probably results from ongoing or repetitive focal epileptic activity rather than being a marker of the inflammatory process itself (87–89,91). The largest peaks in lactate were usually detected in patients with EPC. Glutamine and glutamate levels were also elevated in two patients so far, a finding of interest considering the potential role of excitatory neurotransmitters in the disease (83).

ETIOLOGY AND PATHOGENESIS

The etiology and pathogenesis of RE remain unknown. Typical histologic findings reported in surgical or autopsy specimens are perivascular lymphocytic cuffing, proliferation of microglial nodules, neuronal loss, and gliosis in the affected hemisphere. The microglial nodules are associated with frequent nonspecific neuronophagia and occur particularly near perivascular cuffs of lymphocytes and monocytes. There is some evidence of spongiosis, but this is not as widespread as in the true spongiform encephalopathies. Lesions tend to extend in a confluent rather than a multifocal manner. Finally, the main inflammatory changes are found in the cortex and their intensity is inversely correlated with disease duration with slow progress toward a "burnt-out" stage (13,19). Three mechanisms or processes, not mutually exclusive, have been proposed to explain the initiation and unusual evolution of this rare clinical syndrome: first, *viral infections directly inducing central nervous system (CNS) injury*; second, *a viral-triggered autoimmune CNS process*; and third, *a primary autoimmune CNS process*. It is also possible that RE has a noninflammatory origin, and that the observed inflammation merely represents a response to injury.

The observation of the type of inflammatory process found within the lesions has led over the last few years to multifaceted approaches to uncover a possible infectious or immune-mediated (humoral or cellular) etiology. Epidemiologic studies have not identified a genetic, environmental (geographical or seasonal), or clustering effect, and failed to demonstrate any association between exposure to various factors, including viruses, and the subsequent development of RE. In many cases, there is no apparent increase in preexistent febrile convulsions, or immediately preceding or associated infectious illness. Serologic studies to detect antecedent viral infection have been contradictory or inconclusive (15,93–102), the search for a pathogenic virus has so far mostly focused on the herpesvirus family, and direct brain tissue analysis has also yielded inconsistent results (15,97,98,101–103). The role of an infectious agent, and the *viral hypothesis*, in the causation of RE remains, at best, uncertain. It should be noted, however, that a few patients were reported to improve with antiviral therapy (22,104–106).

Systemic (40,50–55) and cerebrospinal fluid (CSF) compartment immune responses still fail to indicate clear evidence of either ongoing or deficient immune reactivity (107). A primary role for pathogenic antibodies in the etiology of RE was proposed after Rogers and colleagues (108) described rabbits immunized with fusion proteins containing a portion of the GluR3. Those animals developed intractable seizures, and, on histopathologic examination, their brains showed changes characteristic of RE with perivascular lymphocytic infiltrate and microglial nodules. The subsequent finding of autoantibodies to GluR3 in the sera of some affected patients with RE led to the definition of a *GluR3 autoantibody hypothesis* and allowed new speculation into its pathogenesis. GluR3 autoantibodies may cause damage to the brain, and eventually epilepsy, by excitotoxic mechanisms. In the animal model, GluR3 autoantibodies appear to activate the excitatory receptor that leads to massive influx of ions, neuronal cell death, local inflammation, and further disruption of the BBB, allowing entrance of more autoantibodies (49,109). Another proposed mechanism suggests that GluR3 autoantibodies can cause damage by activating complement cascades that lead to neuronal cell death and inflammation (110,111). These hypotheses prompted a number of open-labeled therapeutic attempts to modulate the immune system of patients, especially by removing or annihilating the circulating pathogenic factors presumably responsible for the disease (49,108,110–114). Among cases with no detectable anti-GluR3 antibodies, several were also described to respond well to immunosuppressive treatments (3,17). Other reports in several patients showed no response to plasma exchange (17,112). Finally, more recent work shows that anti-GluR3 antibodies are not specific for RE but can be detected in other neurologic disorders, particularly in non-RE patients with catastrophic epilepsy. Since the sensitivity of detection is low for the RE population

and the presence of GluR3 antibodies does not distinguish RE from other forms of epilepsy, the anti-GluR3 antibody test is not useful for a diagnosis of RE (115–117). Whether GluR3 autoantibodies in severe forms of epilepsy are responsible for the seizures or whether they result from an underlying degenerative or inflammatory process is still unclear. Passive transfer of the disease into naïve animals remains unsuccessful so far, and additional animal models of this illness are lacking.

Various other autoantibodies against neural molecules were described in RE: autoantibodies against munc-18 (118), neuronal acetylcholine receptor α_7 subunit (119), and NMDAAR2A to 2D, specifically GluR epsilon$_2$ (120), have been reported in some patients. Again, however, these autoantibodies could be detected in neurologic diseases other than RE, confirming that none of the described autoantibodies is specifically associated with this disease, and that a variety of autoantibodies to neuronal and synaptic structures can be found that may contribute to the inflammatory process, or represent an epiphenomenon of an activated immune system. Takahashi and colleagues (120) showed that GluR epsilon$_2$ were present only in patients with EPC (15 patients, including 10 with histologically proven or clinical RE, 3 with acute encephalitis/encephalopathy, and 2 with nonprogressive EPC), and antibodies were directed primarily against cytoplasmic epitopes, suggesting the involvement of T-cell–mediated autoimmunity.

Recent reports indeed suggested that a T-cell–mediated inflammatory response may be another initiating or perpetuating mechanism in RE. Active inflammatory brain lesions contain large numbers of T lymphocytes (121). These are recruited early within the lesions, suggesting that a T-cell–dependent immune response contributes to the onset and evolution of the disease. Li and colleagues (122) analyzed T-cell receptor expression in the lesions of patients with RE and found that the local immune response includes restricted T-cell populations that are likely to have expanded from a small number of precursor T cells, responding themselves to discrete antigenic epitopes. However, the nature of the antigen that triggers such a response is unknown. Nevertheless, recent work provides further credence to the hypothesis that a T-cell–mediated cytotoxic reaction (CD8$^+$ T-cell cytotoxicity) induces damage and apoptotic death of cortical neurons in RE (123,124). In an attempt to combine existing knowledge, these investigators (123) proposed a new scheme of pathogenesis. First, a focal event initiates the process (e.g., infection, trauma, immune-mediated brain damage, even focal seizure activity) and an immune reaction with antigen presentation in the CNS and entry of cytotoxic T lymphocytes into the CNS across the disrupted BBB. Second, activated cytotoxic T lymphocytes attack CNS neurons while the inflammatory process, together with the release of cytokines, causes a spread of the inflammatory reaction and recruitment of more activated cytotoxic T lymphocytes.

Third, the generation of potentially antigenic fragments, including GluR3, gives rise to autoantibodies (125), and may lead to an antibody-mediated "second wave of attack."

CRITERIA FOR (EARLY) DIAGNOSIS

The clinical changes of RE are nonspecific, particularly at the beginning of the disease, and clearly at this stage the major issue is diagnosis. We now have better diagnostic criteria that can lead to early diagnosis (Table 28.1). The onset in a previously healthy child is of rapidly increasing frequency and severity of simple focal, usually motor, seizures often followed by postictal deficit. This, and a lack of evidence of anatomic abnormalities on early brain MRI, should raise suspicion regarding the diagnosis of RE. Further course and evaluation with scalp EEG showing unilateral findings with focal or regional slowing, deterioration of background activity, multifocal interictal epileptiform discharges, and seizure onset or EPC, particularly corresponding to the cortical motor area, are major neurophysiologic features in favor of RE. Early MRI characteristics include the association of focal white matter hyperintensity and cortical swelling with hyperintense signal, particularly in the insular and peri-insular regions. This is later followed by hemispheric atrophy that is usually predominant in the peri-insular and frontal regions, and the head of the caudate nucleus contralateral to the clinical manifestations. Functional imaging studies may reveal abnormalities before any visible structural changes. Typically, FDG-PET shows diffuse hemispheric glucose hypometabolism. SPECT shows unilateral interictal hypoperfusion and ictal multifocal areas of hyperperfusion confirming the lateralized hemispheric nature of the lesion and its extent. MRS may also help in the early detection of brain damage and shows a lateralized decrease in NAA intensity relative to creatine, suggesting neuronal loss or damage in one hemisphere. There is no consistent systemic and CSF response that may contribute to the diagnosis, and, in fact, the most common feature is the lack of cellular or protein response in the CSF of patients with RE. Brain biopsy is often used as a diagnostic tool in many centers for confirming the diagnosis. However, histologic findings in RE are nonspecific chronic inflammatory changes that may be subtle enough to be missed by an inexperienced pathologist. Furthermore, the brain involvement may be patchy, and a normal biopsy does not rule out the diagnosis of RE. In some experienced centers, brain biopsy is not routinely done, and clinical evolution in association with scalp electroencephalography and brain MRI are considered diagnostic of RE.

TABLE 28.1

CRITERIA FOR (EARLY) DIAGNOSIS OF RASMUSSEN ENCEPHALITIS

Clinical	• Refractory focal motor seizures rapidly increasing in frequency and severity, and often polymorphic • Epilepsia partialis continua • Motor, progressive hemiparesis, and cognitive deterioration
Electroencephalography	• Focal or regional slow wave activity contralateral to motor manifestations • Multifocal, usually lateralized, interictal, and ictal epileptiform discharges • Progressive, lateralized impoverishment of background activity
Imaging	• *MRI*: focal cortical swelling with hyperintensity and white matter signal hyperintensity, insular cortical atrophy, atrophy of the head of caudate nucleus, and progressive gray and white matter atrophy, unilateral • *PET*: unilateral, hemispheric, but during early stage may be restricted to frontal and temporal regions, glucose hypometabolism • *SPECT*: unilateral interictal hemispheric hypoperfusion and ictal multifocal hyperperfusion • *MRS*: unilateral reduced NAA, and increased lactate, choline, myoinositol and glutamine/glutamate
Blood	• None, except inconsistent finding of anti-GluR3 antibodies
Cerebrospinal fluid	• None, except sometimes presence of oligoclonal bands and inconsistent elevated levels of anti-GluR3 antibodies
Histopathology	• Microglial nodules, perivascular lymphocytic infiltration, neuron degeneration, and spongy degeneration • Combination of active and remote, multifocal, intracortical and white matter lesions

Abbreviations: GluR3 = glutamate receptor 3 subunit; MRI = magnetic resonance imaging; MRS = magnetic resonance spectroscopy; NAA = *N*-acetylaspartate; PET = positron emission tomography; SPECT = single-photon-emission computed tomography.

The differential diagnosis is from focal cortical dysplasia and tuberous sclerosis, mitochondrial encephalopathy, such as mitochondrial encephalopathy with lactic acidosis and stroke-like episodes (MELAS), brain tumors, cerebral vasculitis, degenerative cortical gray matter diseases, and some forms of meningoencephalitis. Although several diagnostic criteria have been proposed, especially for an early diagnosis of RE, the correct identification of patients with this disease remains a matter of experience, particularly if specific investigative or therapeutic interventions are considered. When a constellation of clinical and laboratory findings highlights the possibility of RE, close follow-up is necessary to assess progression of the disease and eventually confirm its diagnosis.

MEDICAL AND SURGICAL TREATMENTS

The typical evolution of RE is characterized by the development of intractable seizures, progressive neurologic deficits, and intellectual impairment. AEDs usually fail to provide any significant improvement in seizures. This has led clinicians to try a variety of empiric treatments, including antiviral agents and immunomodulatory or immunosuppressive therapies. Surgery, and specifically hemispherectomy, appears to be successful in arresting the disease process. However, the ensuing neurologic deficits due to surgery usually lead to reluctance to carry out this procedure until significant hemiparesis or other functional deficits have already occurred. Apart from the surgical treatment, there is no established treatment for RE.

Antiepileptic Drug Therapy

Guidelines for AED treatment in RE are difficult to define and have always been empirical. No AED, or any polytherapy regimen, has been proven to be superior (8), and the choice of the ideal AED rests on its clinical efficacy and side-effect profile. Because of the nature of this disease, the danger of overtreatment is high. AED pharmacokinetics, toxicity, and interactions may be better determinants of AED selection and combination therapy. EPC is particularly difficult to treat, but AEDs can reduce the frequency and severity of other focal and secondarily generalized seizures. Since the author's original report on AED efficacy in RE (8), several new agents have been introduced. Drugs such as topiramate, that act on excitatory neurotransmitters, or those that may affect cortically generated myoclonus, like levetiracetam in EPC, may have a more specific role in treatment.

Antiviral Therapy

Most treatments directed at aborting the progression of the disease were based on the assumption that RE is either an infectious, viral, or an autoimmune disorder. Examples of antiviral treatments are scarce, and only two reports (22,105) are published: one on the treatment of four patients with ganciclovir, a potent anticytomegalovirus drug, and another on the treatment of a single patient with zidovudine. Although definite improvement was documented in four of the five patients, no further reports using antiviral agents in RE have been published.

Immune Therapy

Evidence implicating humoral and cellular immune responses in the pathophysiology of RE has led to various therapeutic initiatives. A number of case reports and small series suggesting potential therapeutic roles of immune-directed interventions have now been published. These include interferon, steroids, IVIG, plasmapheresis, selective immunoglobulin (Ig) G immunoadsorption by protein A, and immunosuppression with drugs such as cyclophosphamide. Rarely, such approaches have been associated with sustained cessation of seizure activity and arrest in the progression of the inflammatory process. In the majority of the cases, only transient or partial improvements because of immunomodulator or immunosuppressor use have been noted. Of potential importance is the observation that, to date, the more aggressive immune therapies have been deferred to later stages of the disease, where the burden of the disease is considered to outweigh the toxicity of these interventions. The challenge is to develop safe therapeutic protocols that can be tested in patients soon after the diagnosis, and at a time when less damage has occurred and the process may have a better chance to respond to therapy. Eventually, regimens that strike the proper balance between safety and efficacy in typical RE could be applied to the more unusual variants.

Interferon-alpha

Intraventricular interferon-alpha has been tried in only two children (104,106) with the rationale that interferons have both immunomodulating (enhancement of phagocytic activity of macrophages and augmentation of the cytotoxicity of target-specific lymphocytes) and antiviral activity (inhibition of viral replication in virus-infected cells). In both cases, improvement of the epileptic and neurologic syndrome was observed.

Steroids

Relatively low- and high-dose steroid regimens were used either alone or in association with other agents such as IVIG. Initial reports were somewhat discouraging (7,54), but eventually the use of high-dose intravenous (IV) boluses led to encouraging results. When applied during the first year of the disease, pulse IV steroids were effective in suppressing, at least temporarily, the inflammatory process (17,20,21,84). The proposed modes of action of steroids include an antiepileptic effect, an improvement of BBB function—and hence reduction of entry into the brain of potentially deleterious toxic or immune mediators—

and a direct anti-inflammatory effect. Because of a less favorable response and of the adverse effects of prolonged high-dose steroids, Hart and colleagues (20) suggested the use of IVIG as initial treatment followed by high-dose steroids, or both, to control seizures and improve the end point of the disease. The long-term efficacy of steroids in RE remains unknown, but they may be effective when used in pulses to stop status epilepticus.

Immunoglobulin

The use of IVIG in RE was first described by Walsh (126) in a 9-year-old child who received repeated infusions of IVIG over a period of several months with initial improvement, but later followed by protracted deterioration and cessation of the treatment. Six subsequent studies reported on the effect of IVIG, alone or in combination with other treatment modalities (17,20,29,32,84,127,128). These reports show similar results with initial benefit, but with a much less clear-cut, long-term effect. They indicate variable results, ranging from no benefit to significant improvement, maintained in a single case for a period of close to 4 years (127). IVIG is usually much better tolerated than steroids. The basis for a potential therapeutic effect of immunoglobulin in RE is not known, but may reflect the functions of natural antibodies in maintaining immune homeostasis in healthy people. Leach and colleagues showed a delayed but more persistent response in two adults and suggested that IVIG is more effective in adults than in children. They also proposed that IVIG may have a disease-modifying effect. This phenomenon is probably real but, to date, no one has shown that the early use of immune therapy can modify the long-term course of RE.

Plasmapheresis and Selective IgG Immunoadsorption

Plasma exchange is used with the assumption that circulating factors, likely autoantibodies, are pathogenic in at least some patients (17,108,112–114). The majority of patients treated with apheresis showed repeated, and at times dramatic, but transient responses. Because of the lack of long-term efficacy, the complications, and the expense, plasmapheresis should probably be used as adjunctive therapy and may be especially useful in patients with acute deterioration, such as status epilepticus.

Immunosuppressive Therapy

Only one study reported a single patient treated with intermittent cyclophosphamide (17), suggesting the possibility of steroid-sparing treatment with intermittent IV cyclophosphamide for patients with steroid-responsive RE. The authors proposed that intermittent cyclophosphamide may well replace steroid therapy because it is associated with less risk of systemic complications.

Immunosuppressants are used in other autoimmune disorders and also in the prevention and treatment of transplant rejection. They act against the activation of T cells, which, in view of the recent findings of cytotoxic T-lymphocyte–mediated damage in RE (122), may lead to their acquiring a more prominent role in medical treatment.

Surgery

The only effective surgical procedure seems to be the resection and/or disconnection of the abnormal hemisphere (68,129–131). Alternative procedures such as partial corticectomies, subpial transection, and callosal section have limited results and did not render patients seizure-free (7,132–135). The recent publication by Kossoff and colleagues (131) clearly demonstrated the benefits of hemispherectomy in children with RE. They showed that 91% of 46 children (mean age at surgery, 9.2 years) with severe RE who underwent hemispherectomy (in the majority hemidecortication) between 1975 and 2002 became seizure-free (65%) or had nondisabling seizures (26%) that often did not require medications. Patients were walking independently, and all were talking at the time of their most recent follow-up, with relatively minor or moderate residual speech problems. Twenty-one had left-sided pathology (presumably involving the dominant hemisphere) with a mean age at surgery of 8.8 years.

Hemispherectomy, hemidecortication, functional hemispherectomy, or hemispherotomy have proven efficacy for control of seizures in patients with RE. The decision on how early in the course of the disease surgery should be undertaken depends on the certainty of the diagnosis, the severity and frequency of the seizures, and the impact on the psychosocial development of the patient. The natural evolution of the disease and the severity of the epilepsy often justify early intervention, even prior to maximal neurologic deficit. The decision about such a radical procedure requires considerable time and thought, and the psychological preparation of the patients and their families is essential (68,136). Finally, involvement of the dominant hemisphere by the disease process provides important observations on brain plasticity, especially on the shift of language (137–142). Recent reports looking at language outcomes after long-term RE, serial Amytal tests, functional MRI studies, and hemispherectomy illustrate the great plasticity of the child's brain and the ability of the nondominant hemisphere to take over some language function even at a relatively late age.

CONCLUSION AND FUTURE PERSPECTIVES

RE, although a rare disorder, is now much better delineated and understood by the wider clinical and scientific community. However, recognition of the disease in a naïve patient to make an early diagnosis continues to be a challenge. Although confirmation of the clinical diagnosis of RE rests on pathologic findings, *in vivo* combinations of diagnostic approaches such as clinical course, scalp EEG findings, and high-resolution MRI suggest the diagnosis with a high degree of accuracy. The syndrome, however, appears more clinically heterogeneous than initially thought; localized, protracted, or slowly progressive forms of the disease have now been described suggesting that distinct pathophysiologic mechanisms may be at play. Evidence implicating immune responses in the pathophysiology of RE has accumulated involving both B- and T-cell–mediated processes, but the mechanisms by which the immune system is activated remain to be elucidated. The identification of autoantigens provides evidence that RE can be associated with an immune attack on synaptic antigens, and impaired synaptic function leading to seizures and cell death. In addition, T-cell–mediated cytotoxicity may lead to neuronal damage and apoptotic death. Identification of the initiating event (possibly the antigen that triggered the autoimmune response) and of the sequence of immune reactivities occurring in the course of the disease will hopefully allow timely and specific immunotherapy. Patients with RE, however, usually present with rapid progression, and questions on the type and timing of surgical intervention are still being raised. It seems clear that most will fare better with earlier surgery, and only hemispherectomy techniques can provide definitive and satisfactory results with good seizure, cognitive, and psychosocial outcome.

ACKNOWLEDGMENT

I thank Drs. Frederick Andermann and Amit Bar-Or for thoughtful comments.

REFERENCES

1. Rasmussen T, Olszewski J, Lloyd-Smith D. Focal seizures due to chronic localized encephalitis. *Neurology* 1958;8:435–445.
2. Rasmussen T. Chronic encephalitis and seizures: historical introduction. In: Andermann F, ed. *Encephalitis and epilepsy: Rasmussen's syndrome.* London: Butterworth-Heinemann, 1991:1–4.
3. Antel JP, Rasmussen T. Rasmussen's encephalitis and the new hat. *Neurology* 1996;46:9–11.
4. Oguni H, Andermann F, Rasmussen T. The natural history of the syndrome of chronic encephalitis and epilepsy: A study of the MNHI series of forty-eight cases. In: Andermann F, ed. *Encephalitis and epilepsy: Rasmussen's syndrome.* London: Butterworth-Heinemann, 1991:7–35.
5. Granata T, Gobbi G, Spreafico R, et al. Rasmussen's encephalitis. Early characteristics allow diagnosis. *Neurology* 2003;60:422–425.
6. Gupta PC, Roy S, Tandon PN. Progressive epilepsy due to chronic persistent encephalitis. Report of 4 cases. *J Neurol Sci* 1974; 22:105–120.
7. Piatt JH Jr, Hwang PA, Armstrong DC, et al. Chronic focal encephalitis (Rasmussen syndrome): six cases. *Epilepsia* 1988; 29:268–279.
8. Dubeau F, Sherwin A. Pharmacologic principles in the management of chronic focal encephalitis. In: Andermann F, ed. *Encephalitis and epilepsy: Rasmussen's syndrome.* London: Butterworth-Heineman, 1991:179–192.
9. Topçu M, Turanli G, Aynaci FM, et al. Rasmussen's encephalitis in childhood. *Child Nerv Syst* 1999;15:395–402.
10. Genton P, Gelisse P. Antimyoclonic effect of levetiracetam. *Epileptic Disord* 2000;2:209–212.
11. Frucht SJ, Louis ED, Chuang C, et al. A pilot tolerability and efficacy study of levetiracetam in patients with chronic myoclonus. *Neurology* 2001;57:1112–1114.
12. Moshé SL. Mechanisms of action of anticonvulsant agents. *Neurology* 2000;55(Suppl 1):S32–S40.
13. Bien CG, Widman G, Urbach H, et al. The natural history of Rasmussen's encephalitis. *Brain* 2002;125:1751–1759.
14. Aguilar MJ, Rasmussen T. Role of encephalitis in pathogenesis of epilepsy. *Arch Neurol* 1960;2:663–676.
15. McLachlan RS, Girvin JP, Blume WT, et al. Rasmussen's chronic encephalitis in adults. *Arch Neurol* 1993;50:269–274.
16. Larner AJ, Smith SJ, Duncan JS, et al. Late-onset Rasmussen's syndrome with first seizure during pregnancy. *Eur Neurol* 1995; 35:172.
17. Krauss GL, Campbell ML, Roche KW, et al. Chronic steroid-responsive encephalitis without autoantibodies to glutamate receptor GluR3. *Neurology* 1996;46:247–249.
18. Hart YM, Andermann F, Fish DR, et al. Chronic encephalitis and epilepsy in adults and adolescents: a variant of Rasmussen's syndrome? *Neurology* 1997;48:418–424.
19. Robitaille Y. Neuropathological aspects of chronic encephalitis. In: Andermann F, ed. *Encephalitis and epilepsy: Rasmussen's syndrome.* London: Butterworth-Heinemann, 1991:79–110.
20. Hart YM, Cortez M, Andermann F, et al. Medical treatment of Rasmussen's syndrome (chronic encephalitis and epilepsy): effect of high-dose steroids or immunoglobulins in 19 patients. *Neurology* 1994;44:1030–1036.
21. Chinchilla D, Dulac O, Robain O, et al. Reappraisal of Rasmussen's syndrome with special emphasis on treatment with high dose of steroids. *J Neurol Neurosurg Psychiatry* 1994;57: 1325–1333.
22. De Toledo JC, Smith DB. Partially successful treatment of Rasmussen's encephalitis with zidovudine: symptomatic improvement followed by involvement of the contralateral hemisphere. *Epilepsia* 1994;35:352–355.
23. Takahashi Y, Kubota H, Fujiwara T, et al. Epilepsia partialis continua of childhood involving bilateral brain hemispheres. *Acta Neurol Scand* 1997;96:345–352.
24. Silver K, Andermann F, Meagher-Villemure K. Familial alternating epilepsia partialis continua with chronic encephalitis: another variant of Rasmussen syndrome? *Arch Neurol* 1998; 55:733–736.
25. Tobias SM, Robitaille Y, Hickey WF, et al. Bilateral Rasmussen encephalitis: postmortem documentation in a five-year-old. *Epilepsia* 2003;44:127–130.
26. Gray F, Serdaru M, Baron H, et al. Chronic localised encephalitis (Rasmussen's) in an adult with epilepsia partialis continua. *J Neurol Neurosurg Psychiatry* 1987;50:747–751.
27. Stephen LJ, Brodie MJ. An islander with seizures. *Scott Med J* 1998;43:183–184.
28. Coral LC, Haas LJ. Probable Rasmussen's syndrome. Case report. *Arq Neuropsiquiatr* 1999;57:1032–1035. Portuguese.
29. Leach JP, Chadwick DW, Miles JB, et al. Improvement in adult onset Rasmussen's encephalitis with long-term immunomodulatory therapy. *Neurology* 1999;52:738–742.
30. Yeh PS, Lin CN, Lin HJ, Tsai TC. Chronic focal encephalitis (Rasmussen's syndrome) in an adult. *J Formos Med Assoc* 2000;99:568–571.
31. Vadlamudi L, Galton CJ, Jeavons SJ, et al. Rasmussen's syndrome in a 54-year-old female: more support for an adult variant. *J Clin Neurosci* 2000;7:154–156.
32. Villani F, Spreafico R, Farina L, et al. Immunomodulatory therapy in an adult patient with Rasmussen's encephalitis. *Neurology* 2001;56:248–250.
33. Hennessy MJ, Koutroumanidis M, Dean AF, et al. Chronic encephalitis and temporal lobe epilepsy: a variant of Rasmussen's syndrome? *Neurology* 2001;56:678–681.
34. Frucht S. Dystonia, athetosis, and epilepsia partialis continua in a patient with late-onset Rasmussen's encephalitis. *Mov Disord* 2002;17:609–612.
35. Laxer KD. Temporal lobe epilepsy with inflammatory changes. In: Andermann F, ed. *Encephalitis and epilepsy: Rasmussen's syndrome.* London: Butterworth-Heinemann, 1991:135–140.
36. Matthews PM, Andermann F, Arnold DL. A proton magnetic resonance spectroscopy study of focal epilepsy in humans. *Neurology* 1990;40:985–989.

37. Tien RD, Ashdown BC, Lewis DV Jr, et al. Rasmussen's encephalitis: neuroimaging findings in four patients. *Am J Roentgenol* 1992;158:1329–1332.
38. Ben-Zeev B, Nass D, Polack S, et al. Progressive unilateral basal ganglia atrophy and hemidystonia: a new form of chronic focal encephalitis. *Neurology* 1999;S2:A42.
39. Koehn MA, Zupanc ML. Unusual presentation and MRI findings in Rasmussen's syndrome. *Pediatr Neurol* 1999;21:839–842.
40. Lascelles K, Dean AF, Robinson RO. Rasmussen's encephalitis followed by lupus erythematosus. *Dev Med Child Neurol* 2002; 44:572–574.
41. Bhatjiwale MG, Polkey C, Cox TC, et al. Rasmussen's encephalitis: neuroimaging findings in 21 patients with a closer look at the basal ganglia. *Pediatr Neurosurg* 1998;29:142–148.
42. Chiapparini L, Granata T, Farina L, et al. Diagnostic imaging in 13 cases of Rasmussen's encephalitis: can early MRI suggest the diagnosis? *Neuroradiology* 2003;45:171–183.
43. McDonald D, Farrell MA, McMenamin J. Rasmussen's syndrome associated with chronic brain stem encephalitis. *Eur J Paediatr Neurol* 2001;5:203–206.
44. Maeda Y, Oguni H, Saitou Y, et al. Rasmussen syndrome: multifocal spread of inflammation suggested from MRI and PET findings. *Epilepsia* 2003;44:1118–1121.
45. Hart Y, Andermann F, Robitaille Y, et al. Double pathology in Rasmussen's syndrome: a window on the etiology? *Neurology* 1998;50:731–735.
46. Firlik KS, Adelson PD, Hamilton RL. Coexistence of a ganglioglioma and Rasmussen's encephalitis. *Pediatr Neurosurg* 1999;30:278–282.
47. Yacubian EM, Rosemberg S, Marie SK, et al. Double pathology in Rasmussen's encephalitis: etiological considerations. *Epilepsia* 1996;37:495–500.
48. Palmer CA, Geyer JD, Keating JM, et al. Rasmussen's encephalitis with concomitant cortical dysplasia: the role of GluR3. *Epilepsia* 1999;40:242–247.
49. Twyman RE, Gahring LC, Spiess J, et al. Glutamate receptor antibodies activate a subset of receptors and reveal an agonist binding site. *Neuron* 1995;14:755–762.
50. Straube A, Padovan CS, Seelos K. Parry-Romberg syndrome and Rasmussen syndrome: only an incidental similarity? *Nervenarzt* 2001;72:641–646.
51. Shah JR, Juhasz C, Kupsky WJ, et al. Rasmussen encephalitis associated with Parry-Romberg syndrome. *Neurology* 2003;61: 395–397.
52. Pupillo G, Andermann F, Dubeau F. Linear scleroderma and intractable epilepsy: neuropathologic evidence for a chronic inflammatory process. *Ann Neurol* 1996;39:277–278.
53. Stone J, Franks AJ, Guthrie JA, et al. Scleroderma 'en coup de sabre': pathological evidence of intracerebral inflammation. *J Neurol Neurosurg Psychiatry* 2001;70:382–385.
54. Lyon G, Griscelli C, Fernandez-Alvarez E, et al. Chronic progressive encephalitis in children with X-linked hypogammaglobulinemia. *Neuropaediatrie* 1980;11:57–71.
55. Gupta PC, Rapin I, Houroupian DS, et al. Smoldering encephalitis in children. *Neuropediatrics* 1984;15:191–197.
56. Harvey AS, Andermann F, Hopkins IJ, et al. Chronic encephalitis (Rasmussen's syndrome) and ipsilateral uveitis. *Ann Neurol* 1992;32:826–829.
57. Fukuda T, Oguni H, Yanagaki S, et al. Chronic localized encephalitis (Rasmussen's syndrome) preceded by ipsilateral uveitis: a case report. *Epilepsia* 1994;35:1328–1331.
58. Bancaud J, Bonis A, Trottier S, et al. Continuous partial epilepsy: syndrome and disease [French]. *Rev Neurol* 1982;138:803–814.
59. Bancaud J. Kojewnikow's syndrome (epilepsia partialis continua) in children. In: Roger J, Dravet C, Bureau M, et al, eds. *Epileptic syndromes in infancy, childhood and adolescence*, 2nd ed. London: John Libbey, 1992:363–379.
60. Dulac O, Dravet C, Plouin P, et al. Nosological aspects of epilepsia partialis continua in children [French]. *Arch Fr Pediatr* 1983;40:689–695.
61. Hwang PA, Piatt J, Cyr L, et al. The EEG of Rasmussen's encephalitis. *Electromyogr Clin Neurophysiol* 1988;69:51P–52P.
62. So NK, Gloor P. Electroencephalographic and electrocorticographic findings in chronic encephalitis of the Rasmussen type.

In: Andermann F, ed. *Encephalitis and epilepsy: Rasmussen's syndrome.* London: Butterworth-Heinemann, 1991:37–45.
63. Campovilla G, Paladin F, Dalla Bernardina B. Rasmussen's syndrome: longitudinal EEG study from the first seizure to epilepsia partialis continua. *Epilepsia* 1997;38:483–488.
64. Andrews PI, McNamara JO, Lewis DV. Clinical and electroencephalographic correlates in Rasmussen's encephalitis. *Epilepsia* 1997;38:189–194.
65. Beaumanoir A, Grioni D, Kullman G, et al. EEG anomalies in the prodromic phase of Rasmussen's syndrome. Report of two cases [French]. *Neurophysiol Clin* 1997;27:25–32.
66. English R, Soper N, Shepstone BJ, et al. Five patients with Rasmussen's syndrome investigated by single-photon-emission computed tomography. *Nucl Med Commun* 1989;10:5–14.
67. Tampieri D, Melanson D, Ethier R. Imaging of chronic encephalitis. In: Andermann F, ed. *Encephalitis and epilepsy: Rasmussen's syndrome.* London: Butterworth-Heinemann, 1991: 47–69.
68. Vining EP, Freeman JM, Brandt J, et al. Progressive unilateral encephalopathy of childhood (Rasmussen's syndrome): a reappraisal. *Epilepsia* 1993;34:639–650.
69. Fiorella DJ, Provenzale JM, Coleman RE, et al. 18F-fluorodeoxyglucose positron emission tomography and MR imaging findings in Rasmussen encephalitis. *Am J Neuroradiol* 2001;22: 1291–1299.
70. Bien CG, Urbach H, Deckert M, et al. Diagnosis and staging of Rasmussen's encephalitis by serial MRI and histopathology. *Neurology* 2003;58:250–257.
71. Burke GJ, Fifer SA, Yoder J. Early detection of Rasmussen's syndrome by brain SPECT imaging. *Clin Nucl Med* 1992;17: 730–731.
72. Sammaritano M, Andermann F, Melanson, et al. Prolonged focal cerebral edema associated with partial status epilepticus. *Epilepsia* 1985;26:334–339.
73. Zupanc ML, Handler EG, Levine RL, et al. Rasmussen encephalitis: epilepsia partialis continua secondary to chronic encephalitis. *Pediatr Neurol* 1990;6:397–401.
74. Nakasu S, Isozumi T, Yamamoto A, et al. Serial magnetic resonance imaging findings of Rasmussen's encephalitis. *Neurol Med Chir* 1997;37:924–928.
75. Hwang PA, Gilday DL, Spire JP, et al. Chronic focal encephalitis of Rasmussen: functional neuroimaging studies with positron emission tomography and single-photon emission computed tomography scanning. In: Andermann F, ed. *Encephalitis and epilepsy: Rasmussen's syndrome.* London: Butterworth-Heinemann, 1991:61–72.
76. Hajek M, Antonini A, Leenders KL, et al. Epilepsia partialis continua studied by PET. *Epilepsy Res* 1991;9:44–48.
77. Duprez TPJ, Grandin C, Gadisseux JF, et al. MR-monitored remitting-relapsing pattern of cortical involvement in Rasmussen syndrome: comparative evaluation of serial MR and PET/SPECT features. *J Comput Assist Tomogr* 1997;21:900–904.
78. Kaiboriboon K, Cortese C, Hogan RE. Magnetic resonance and positron emission tomography changes during the clinical progression of Rasmussen encephalitis. *J Neuroimaging* 2000;10: 122–125.
79. Banati RB, Guerra GW, Myers R, et al. [^{11}C](R)-PK11195 positron emission tomography imaging of activated microglia *in vivo* in Rasmussen's encephalitis. *Neurology* 1999;53:2199–2203.
80. Aguilar Rebolledo F, Rojas Bautista J, Villanueva Perez R, et al. SPECT-99mTc-HMPAO in a case of epilepsia partialis continua and focal encephalitis [Spanish]. *Rev Invest Clin* 1996;48: 199–205.
81. Yacubian EMT, Sueli KNM, Valério RMF, et al. Neuroimaging findings in Rasmussen's syndrome. *J Neuroimaging* 1997;7: 16–22.
82. Paladin F, Capovilla G, Bonazza A, et al. Utility of Tc 99m HMPAO SPECT in the early diagnosis of Rasmussen's syndrome. *Ital J Neurol Sci* 1998;19:217–220.
83. Geller E, Faerber EN, Legido A, et al. Rasmussen encephalitis: complementary role of multitechnique neuroimaging. *Am J Neuroradiol* 1998;19:445–449.
84. Vinjamuri S, Leach JP, Hart IK. Serial perfusion brain tomographic scans detect reversible focal ischemia in Rasmussen's encephalitis. *Postgrad Med J* 2000;76:33–40.
85. Ishibashi H, Simos PG, Wheless JW, et al. Multimodality functional imaging evaluation in a patient with Rasmussen's encephalitis. *Brain Dev* 2002;24:239–244.

86. Hartley LM, Harkness W, Harding B, et al. Correlation of SPECT with pathology and seizure outcome in children undergoing epilepsy surgery. *Dev Med Child Neurol* 2002;44:676–680.

87. Peeling J, Sutherland G. 1H magnetic resonance spectroscopy of extracts of human epileptic neocortex and hippocampus. *Neurology* 1993;43:589–594.

88. Cendes F, Andermann F, Silver K, et al. Imaging of axonal damage *in vivo* in Rasmussen's syndrome. *Brain* 1995;118:753–758.

89. Sundgren PC, Burtsher IM, Lundgren J, et al. MRI and proton spectroscopy in a child with Rasmussen's encephalitis. Case report. *Neuroradiology* 1999;41:935–940.

90. Tükdogan-Sözüer D, Özek MM, Sav A, et al. Serial MRI and MRS studies with unusual findings in Rasmussen's encephalitis. *Eur Radiol* 2000;10:962–966.

91. Park YD, Allison JD, Weiss KL, et al. Proton magnetic resonance spectroscopic observations of epilepsia partialis continua in children. *J Child Neurol* 2000;15:729–733.

92. Sener RN. Rasmussen's encephalitis: proton MR spectroscopy and diffusion MR findings. *J Neuroradiol* 2000;27:179–184.

93. Friedman H, Ch'ien L, Parham D. Virus in brain of child with hemiplegia, hemiconvulsions, and epilepsy. *Lancet* 1977;ii:666.

94. Riikonen R. Cytomegalovirus infection and infantile spasms. *Dev Med Child Neurol* 1978;20:570–579.

95. Mizuno Y, Chou SM, Estes ML, et al. Chronic localized encephalitis (Rasmussen's) with focal cerebral seizures revisited. *J Neuropathol Exp Neurol* 1985;44:351.

96. Asher DM, Gadjusek DC. Virologic studies in chronic encephalitis. In: Andermann F, ed. *Encephalitis and epilepsy: Rasmussen's syndrome.* London: Butterworth-Heinemann, 1991: 147–158.

97. Walter GF, Renella RR. Epstein-Barr virus in brain and Rasmussen's encephalitis. *Lancet* 1989;1:279–280.

98. Power C, Poland SD, Blume WT, et al. Cytomegalovirus and Rasmussen's encephalitis. *Lancet* 1990;336:1282–1284.

99. Farrell MA, Cheng L, Cornford ME, et al. Cytomegalovirus and Rasmussen's encephalitis. *Lancet* 1991;337:1551–1552.

100. Vinters HV, Wang R, Wiley CA. Herpesviruses in chronic encephalitis associated with intractable childhood epilepsy. *Hum Pathol* 1993;24:871–879.

101. Atkins MR, Terrell W, Hulette CM. Rasmussen's syndrome: a study of potential viral etiology. *Clin Neuropathol* 1995; 14:7–12.

102. Jay V, Becker LE, Otsubo H, et al. Chronic encephalitis and epilepsy (Rasmussen's encephalitis): detection of cytomegalovirus and herpes simplex virus 1 by the polymerase chain reaction and *in situ* hybridization. *Neurology* 1995;45: 108–117.

103. Prayson RA, Frater JL. Rasmussen encephalitis. A clinicopathologic and immunohistochemical study of seven patients. *Am J Clin Pathol* 2002;117:776–782.

104. Maria BL, Ringdahl DM, Mickle JP, et al. Intraventricular alpha interferon therapy for Rasmussen's syndrome. *Can J Neurol Sci* 1993;20:333–336.

105. McLachlan RS, Levin S, Blume WT. Treatment of Rasmussen's syndrome with ganciclovir. *Neurology* 1996;47:925–928.

106. Dabbagh O, Gascon G, Crowell J, et al. Intraventricular interferon-α stops seizures in Rasmussen's encephalitis: a case report. *Epilepsia* 1997;38:1045–1049.

107. Grenier Y, Antel JP, Osterland CK. Immunologic studies in chronic encephalitis of Rasmussen. In: Andermann F, ed. *Encephalitis and epilepsy: Rasmussen's syndrome.* London: Butterworth-Heinemann, 1991:125–134.

108. Rogers SW, Andrews PI, Garhing LC, et al. Autoantibodies to glutamate receptor GluR3 in Rasmussen's encephalitis. *Science* 1994;265:648–651.

109. Levite M, Fleidervish IA, Schwarz A, et al. Autoantibodies to the glutamate receptor kill neurons via activation of the receptor ion channel. *J Autoimmun* 1999;13:61–72.

110. He XP, Patel M, Whitney KD, et al. Glutamate receptor GluR3 antibodies and death of cortical cells. *Neuron* 1998;20:153–163.

111. Whitney KD, Andrews JM, McNamara JO. Immunoglobulin G and complement immunoreactivity in the cerebral cortex of patients with Rasmussen's encephalitis. *Neurology* 1999;53: 699–708.

112. Andrews PI, Ditcher MA, Berkovic SF, et al. Plasmapheresis in Rasmussen's encephalitis. *Neurology* 1996;46:242–246.

113. Palcoux JB, Carla H, Tardieu M, et al. Plasma exchange in Rasmussen's encephalitis. *Ther Apher* 1997;1:79–82.

114. Antozzi C, Granata T, Aurisano N, et al. Long-term selective IgG immunoadsorption improves Rasmussen's encephalitis. *Neurology* 1998;51:302–305.

115. Wiendl H, Bien CG, Bernasconi P, et al. GluR3 antibodies: prevalence in focal epilepsy but no specificity for Rasmussen's encephalitis. *Neurology* 2001;57:1511–1514.

116. Baranzini SE, Laxer K, Saketkhoo R, et al. Analysis of antibody gene rearrangement, usage, and specificity in chronic focal encephalitis. *Neurology* 2002;58:709–716.

117. Mantegazza R, Bernasconi P, Baggi F, et al. Antibodies against GluR3 peptides are not specific for Rasmussen's encephalitis but are also present in epilepsy patients with severe, early onset disease and intractable seizures. *J Neuroimmunol* 2002;131: 179–185.

118. Yang R, Puranam RS, Butler LS, et al. Autoimmunity to munc-18 in Rasmussen's encephalitis. *Neuron* 2000;28:375–383.

119. Watson R, Lang B, Bermudez I, et al. Autoantibodies in Rasmussen's encephalitis. *J Neuroimmunol* 2001;118:148.

120. Takahashi Y, Mori H, Mishina M, et al. Autoantibodies to NMDA receptor in patients with chronic forms of epilepsia partialis continua. *Neurology* 2003;61:891–896.

121. Farrell MA, Droogan O, Secor DL, et al. Chronic encephalitis associated with epilepsy: immunohistochemical and ultrastructural studies. *Acta Neuropathol* 1995;89:313–321.

122. Li Y, Uccelli A, Laxer KD, et al. Local-clonal expansion of infiltrating T lymphocytes in chronic encephalitis of Rasmussen. *J Immunol* 1997;158:1428–1437.

123. Bauer J, Bien CG, Lassmann H. Rasmussen's encephalitis: a role for autoimmune cytotoxic T lymphocytes. *Curr Opin Neurol* 2002;15:197–200.

124. Gahring LC, Carlson NG, Meyer EL, et al. Cutting edge: granzyme B proteolysis of a neuronal glutamate receptor generates an autoantigen and is modulated by glycosylation. *J Immunol* 2001;166:1433–1438.

125. Bien CG, Elger CE, Wiendl H. Advances in pathogenic concepts and therapeutic agents in Rasmussen's encephalitis. *Expert Opin Investig Drugs* 2002;11:981–989.

126. Walsh PJ. Treatment of Rasmussen's syndrome with intravenous gammaglobulin. In: Andermann F, ed. *Encephalitis and epilepsy: Rasmussen's syndrome.* London: Butterworth-Heinemann, 1991: 201–204.

127. Wise MS, Rutledge SL, Kuzniecky RI. Rasmussen syndrome and long-term response to gamma globulin. *Pediatr Neurol* 1996;14:149–152.

128. Caraballo R, Tenembaum S, Cersosimo R, et al. Rasmussen syndrome [Spanish]. *Rev Neurol* 1998;26:978–983.

129. Villemure JG, Andermann F, Rasmussen TB. Hemispherectomy for the treatment of epilepsy due to chronic encephalitis. In: Andermann F, ed. *Encephalitis and epilepsy: Rasmussen's syndrome.* London: Butterworth-Heinemann; 1991:235–244.

130. DeLalande O, Pinard JM, Jalin O, et al. Surgical results of hemispherotomy. *Epilepsia* 1995;36(Suppl 3):241.

131. Kossoff EH, Vining EPG, Pillas DJ, et al. Hemispherectomy for intractable unihemispheric epilepsy. Etiology and outcome. *Neurology* 2003;61:887–890.

132. Olivier A. Corticectomy for the treatment of seizures due to chronic encephalitis. In: Andermann F, ed. *Encephalitis and epilepsy: Rasmussen's syndrome.* London: Butterworth-Heinemann, 1991:205–212.

133. Spencer SS, Spencer DD. Corpus callosotomy in chronic encephalitis. In: Andermann F, ed. *Encephalitis and epilepsy: Rasmussen's syndrome.* London: Butterworth-Heinemann, 1991; 213–218.

134. Morrell F, Whisler WW, Cremin Smith M. Multiple subpial transection in Rasmussen's encephalitis. In: Andermann F, ed. *Encephalitis and epilepsy: Rasmussen's syndrome.* London: Butterworth-Heinemann, 1991;219–234.

135. Honavar M, Janota I, Polkey CE. Rasmussen's encephalitis in surgery for epilepsy. *Dev Med Child Neurol* 1992;34:3–14.

136. Guimarães CA, Souza EAP, Montenegro MA, et al. Rasmussen's encephalitis. The relevance of neuropsychological assessment in patient's treatment and follow up. *Arq Neuropsiquiatr* 2002; 60:378–381.

137. Taylor LB. Neuropsychological assessment of patients with chronic encephalitis. In: Andermann F, ed. *Encephalitis and epilepsy: Rasmussen's syndrome*. London: Butterworth-Heinemann, 1991:111–124.

138. Boatman D, Freeman J, Vining E, et al. Language recovery after left hemispherectomy in children with late-onset seizures. *Ann Neurol* 1999;46:579–586.

139. Curtiss S, de Bode S. Age and etiology as predictors of language outcome following hemispherectomy. *Dev Neurosci* 1999;21: 174–181.

140. Curtiss S, de Bode S, Mathern GW. Spoken language outcomes after hemispherectomy: factoring in etiology. *Brain Lang* 2001;79:379–396.

141. Telfeian AE, Berqvist C, Danielak C, et al. Recovery of language after left hemispherectomy in a sixteen-year-old girl with late-onset seizures. *Pediatr Neurosurg* 2002;37:19–21.

142. Hertz-Pannier L, Chiron C, Jambaqué I, et al. Late plasticity for language in a child's non-dominant hemisphere. A pre- and post-surgery fMRI study. *Brain* 2002;125:361–372.

Continuous Spike Wave of Slow Sleep and Landau-Kleffner Syndrome

29

Brian Neville   *J. Helen Cross*

Epileptic encephalopathies are disturbances of cognition, behavior and motor control that occur with epileptic seizures and are attributed to epileptiform activity, which may be subclinical. The definition generally excludes impairments caused by brain damage, either pre-existing or disease related, and those caused by drug treatment. Such encephalopathies can have permanent or reversible, mild or severe, and global or selective effects. This chapter discusses two uncommon epileptic encephalopathies, Landau-Kleffner syndrome (LKS) and continuous spike wave of slow sleep (CSWS). A major focus of the discussion is the degree to which these conditions overlap. CSWS manifests clinically in various ways, including LKS, whereas LKS in a similar clinical form may feature less-florid electroencephalographic (EEG) abnormalities not fulfilling the criteria for CSWS.

LKS was not mentioned in the 1969 and 1981 classifications of the International League Against Epilepsy because encephalopathies were not included (1). The 1989 proposal classifies "acquired epileptic aphasia (LKS)" under "epilepsies and the epileptic syndromes undetermined whether associated with focal and/or generalized seizures"; however, this revision used the clinical and electrical phenomenology of the seizures as the handle for definition when encephalopathy is the main issue (2). CSWS is defined as the association of partial or generalized seizures during sleep and atypical absences during wakefulness with a characteristic EEG pattern of continuous, diffuse spike-and-wave complexes during slow-wave sleep, which

is noted after onset of the seizures (2). The relationship between CSWS syndrome, also known as electrical status epilepticus of slow sleep (ESES), and LKS, as well as with the much-less-severe benign epilepsy with centrotemporal spikes (BECTS), has been extensively discussed (3–6). Children with cognitive or language regression, high rates of centrotemporal or wider epileptiform activity, and normal magnetic resonance imaging (MRI) scans can be placed into a single category. Until our understanding of these disorders improves, LKS may best be regarded as a specific subgroup of CSWS, at least for historical and treatment purposes.

CONTINUOUS SPIKE WAVES OF SLOW SLEEP

Definition

CSWS is characterized by neuropsychological and behavioral changes temporally related to the almost continuous spike-wave activity on electroencephalography that is most prominent and pervasive during slow-wave sleep. It was first described in 1971 as "subclinical status epilepticus" induced by sleep in children (7). Subsequently, other terminology has followed on further descriptions of the syndrome. Although CSWS and ESES are used synonymously, some investigators have proposed that ESES designate the

EEG abnormalities and CSWS the combined electroclinical picture (3); this definition is used in this chapter. The prevalence of CSWS among the epilepsies is unknown, although Morikawa and colleagues (8) found an incidence of 0.5% in 12,854 children reviewed at their center over 10 years. Other investigators (9) have reported similar figures.

Diagnosis

The diagnosis is made primarily on the basis of electrical findings in association with clinical manifestations. Tassinari and colleagues proposed the following characteristics (10):

- Neuropsychological impairment seen as global or selective regression of cognitive or expressive functions such as acquired aphasia
- Motor impairment in the form of ataxia, dyspraxia, dystonia, or unilateral deficit
- Epilepsy with focal and or apparently generalized seizures, tonic-clonic seizures, absences, partial motor seizures, complex partial seizures, or epileptic falls (tonic seizures are not typical)
- Electrographic status epilepticus occurring during at least 85% of slow sleep and persisting on three or more records for at least 1 month

The diagnostic continuous spike-wave discharges occur at 1.5 to 2.5 Hz and persist during slow-wave sleep (Fig. 29.1), particularly in the first sleep cycle (11). Although early investigators required spike-wave activity during 85% of slow sleep for diagnosis, several authors now accept a lower proportion with a clear sleep/wake discrepancy. Previously the abnormality was described as "spatially diffuse"; however, more focal abnormalities have been reported.

Initial reports also proposed that the condition be present over more than three records for at least 1 month (7). Subsequent definitions do not consider duration, which may be related to the timing of the diagnosis.

Early investigations suggested that both sexes are equally affected, but larger collections of case studies show a male preponderance (12).

Clinical Presentation

Even with supposedly similar electrical findings, the clinical presentation remains diverse. Moreover because of considerable overlap it is generally difficult to differentiate CSWS and LKS solely on the basis of clinical features. Some children present with classic regression of language after onset of seizures. In others changes in cognitive performance, varying from the severe to subtle, may be seen within the context of normal or abnormal early developmental progress (8,13,14). In 62% to 74% of patients reported, cognitive development prior to onset was normal (8,13,15), necessitating a high degree of clinical vigilance

for diagnosis. Reviewing 209 cases from the literature, Rouselle and Revol (16) classified the neuropsychological presentation into four groups: Group 1 (n=35) had an initially normal neurologic state (except for one child); all children presented with severe epilepsy and little or no neuropsychological deterioration (although cognitive state was often poorly documented). Group 2 (n=33) presented with language deterioration and 28 were classified as having LKS. Group 3 (n=99) included children who were initially neurologically normal and had deterioration of neuropsychological (global or selective) but not language function. Group 4 (n=42) presented with either focal or diffuse brain lesions and unknown clinical manifestations.

The key points of differentiation among the groups were the topographic features of the main electrical focus and the duration of ESES. The neuropsychologically normal children (group 1) had a predominantly rolandic focus and ESES for 6 months. The children with language deterioration (group 2) exhibited a temporal lobe prominence on the electroencephalogram and ESES for 18 months. Children with global deterioration (groups 3 and 4) showed a frontal prominence on the electroencephalogram and ESES for more than 2 years.

Whether the clinical presentation can be correlated with diffuse frontal or temporal predominance of scalp EEG abnormalities during sleep is unclear from the number of cases published. Some researchers propose that acquired aphasia may accompany a temporal prominence of EEG discharges, whereas more global deficits may be linked to diffuse EEG changes with a frontal prominence (16). Analysis of cases involving unilateral pathologic lesions shows that at least some discharges arise focally but propagate rapidly within and between hemispheres, suggesting secondary bilateral synchrony (17,18). Another presentation may involve bilateral pathologic lesions, such as perisylvian polymicrogyria.

Seizures are often not the major feature but often present between 3 and 5 years of age before the diagnosis is made. These are typically focal or generalized motor seizures that tend to occur at night. Drop attacks, such as atonic seizures, occur in approximately 50% of the patients, heralding the appearance of ESES (8). Absence seizures are associated with bursts of spike-wave activity. Some children may have myoclonic absences and generalized nonconvulsive seizures (19,20). Tassinari and associates (10) noted that the severity and frequency of seizures often change when ESES is discovered; to what extent this may be related to the change in EEG pattern that prompts further investigation is unknown. These authors proposed three groups based on seizure patterns: group 1 with rare nocturnal motor seizures (11%); group 2 with unilateral partial motor seizures or generalized tonic-clonic seizures occurring mainly during sleep with absences in wakefulness (44.5%); and group 3 with rare nocturnal seizures but with atypical absences, frequently involving atonic or tonic components, that lead to sudden falls. Negative myoclonus

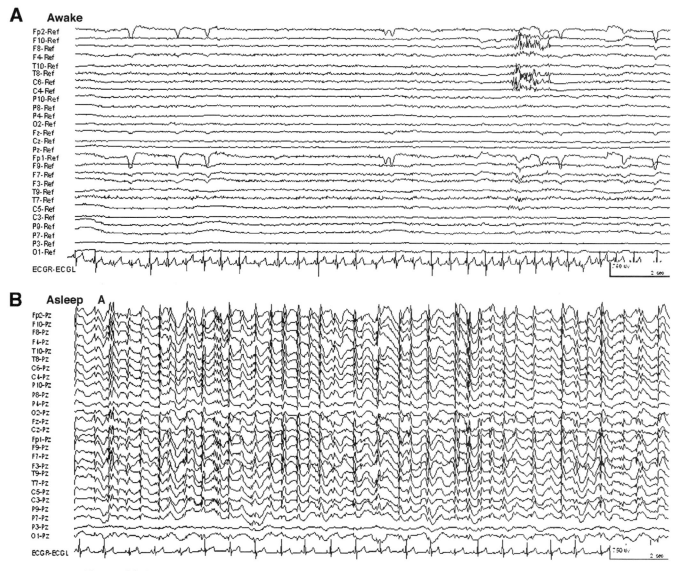

Figure 29.1 Waking (**A**) and sleeping (**B**) electroencephalographic recordings of a 7-year-old boy who presented with impulsive behavior, progressive memory difficulty, and occasional "absence" episodes. The waking record shows no abnormality; continuous spike-wave activity is seen in slow sleep.

is common and contributes to the motor impairment (15,21,22).

Etiologic Factors

Genetic factors are unknown although there is one report of monozygotic twins (23) and of familial seizure disorders, including febrile convulsions in 15% of patients (24). Of 71 cases collected for discussion at a 1995 symposium, MRI or computed tomography scan was performed in 58, and 33% of these were abnormal. Children with CSWS are more likely to have abnormal radiologic findings than are children who present with acquired epileptic aphasia, with or without ESES. The most common abnormality is diffuse or unilateral cerebral atrophy, but developmental disorders also figure in a significant proportion of the cases. A

particular association has been noted between ESES and multilobar polymicrogyria (18). Atonic seizures (negative myoclonus) were notable in these children, as was the lack of apparent cognitive deterioration at diagnosis, although neuropsychological assessment was difficult.

Kobayashi and colleagues (25) hypothesized two mechanisms of secondary bilateral synchrony that may explain ESES. The first mechanism may involve spread through the corpus callosum. In the second mechanism an initial diffusion of discharges through the corpus callosum may be followed by generalization of discharges through the corticothalamic system. Whether ESES activity in all cases is the result of secondary bilateral synchrony is unclear. Recently, neonatal lesions in the thalamus have been found in cases of CSWS (26,27). The underlying mechanisms leading to ESES are probably complex and poorly understood.

Outcome

CSWS is generally believed to be an age-related phenomenon and prognosis for the EEG abnormality and seizures is relatively good. In most children seizures resolve by the teenage years, preceding (30%), coinciding with (30%) or following (40%) the resolution of ESES. One case report described an adult with nearly continuous spike wave of slow sleep that were present over 4 years (28).

The major long-term morbidity relates to neuropsychological outcome, which is difficult to predict and at best remains guarded. In most cases, a significant, though often partial, improvement occurs after resolution of ESES, and 50% of patients have a nearly average neuropsychological outcome and can lead independent lives (13,29). To what extent cognitive recovery is related to early aggressive treatment (and presumed resolution) of ESES is difficult to determine from the literature; however, trials of aggressive treatment under close supervision may be indicated in an attempt to normalize the EEG pattern when cognitive decline is documented.

LANDAU-KLEFFNER SYNDROME

An uncommon condition, LKS is probably the clearest illustration of the acquired epileptic encephalopathies. A "classical" definition has been articulated since the original description in 1957 (30), but several of the first six patients had wider impairments than some authorities might accept. In LKS, normal development including language for at least the first 2 years of life is followed by loss of language, particularly speech comprehension, in association with partial epilepsy of centrotemporal origin. In 20% to 30% of children, no clinical seizures are obvious at presentation but a typical EEG abnormality is enhanced during sleep. MRI scanning shows negative results. Even with these strict criteria, however, children with LKS commonly have additional impairments that are often more amenable to treatment than is the aphasia. Consequently, we prefer a broad definition with acquired aphasia being an early feature and the inclusion of additional attention deficit, hyperactivity, motor organization problems, features of autistic spectrum disorder, and global cognitive regression. Some authorities choose to restrict use of the term LKS to children who retain social responsiveness and regard the development of autism as a different condition (31). We include children with these disorders if they otherwise satisfy the criteria for LKS. We recognize two variant forms: one with mild primary language delay and typical regression after 2 years of age and a second variant with a lesion, usually temporal. Children younger than 2 years of age with regression are excluded despite evidence of concurrent epileptiform activity.

A review of more than 300 published patients reveals that LKS usually presents between 3 and 7 years of age but may occur as early as 2 and as late as 14 years of age. The male-to-female ratio is 2:1. Family history is only occasionally positive (12,32). Although a strict definition requires normal early development, approximately 13% of reported cases had some pre-existing language abnormality. Onset is usually insidious and loss of language abilities, often with fluctuations, may take place over a period of up to 1 year. Rarely parents may report sudden loss of language after a seizure.

Clinical Presentation

Seventy percent of patients present with seizures of various types that are infrequent and usually respond well to medical treatment. Treatment of seizures usually has little impact on the aphasia except in a minority of patients who may show some improvement after seizure control. The predominant seizure types are partial motor, often involving bulbar structures with or without disturbance of consciousness (19,32). Focal myoclonic jerks, complex absences, and generalized tonic-clonic seizures also are seen. Occasionally, generalized motor seizures occur during sleep; prolonged generalized seizures are rare. Postictal hemiparesis (Todd paresis) or postictal aphasia seems to be particularly common. Sometimes, an attempt to understand or produce speech may provoke a seizure (33). Seizures tend to remit in the second decade, but most children are left with significant language and cognitive impairment.

The language impairment varies but is usually progressive (34) and involves severe verbal auditory agnosia with subsequent loss of speech and preserved hearing. The language deficit may lead to mutism and inability to recognize familiar environmental sounds. Written language may be preserved or selectively impaired (35). Any part of the language system may be affected, with the dysfunction including predominantly expressive aphasia (36), as well as fluent and mixed aphasia. The type of aphasia may change over time. No compelling correlation has been observed between types of aphasia and site of main EEG focus. It is often difficult to formally evaluate the cognitive state of children with dense aphasia, but there are suggestions of surviving receptive potential from the speed and extent of later recovery, based on the account given by recovered children (33) and preserved auditory evoked responses (37).

Although the behavioral problems that occur with LKS have been ascribed to the frustration engendered by acquired aphasia, distinct and often severe impairments are present that do not conform to this notion. Probably at least 50% of children with LKS have some behavior problems (38).

Hyperactivity, often with impulsivity and aggressiveness, is common. In a densely aphasic child aggressive behavior can be difficult to manage, especially when associated with violent manic outbursts. When combined with loss of social functioning, repetitive behavior and obsessionality the criteria for an autistic spectrum disorder are satisfied. Sleep is often disturbed and settling at night is a problem. Some global cognitive regression is present in severely affected children. A state of apathy rather than hyperactivity sometimes develops.

Motor problems, including organizational difficulties, ataxia, bulbar symptoms and dystonia (39,40) may be found in up to two-thirds of patients and impair writing, dressing, feeding and walking. Todd paresis is common, and the child may continue to prefer the opposite hand for writing for an extended time despite the seemingly complete recovery of the paretic hand.

The diagnosis of this type of regression in the context of clinical or subclinical epilepsy is usually not difficult. The progressive history of language deterioration is unlike the acute onset of cerebrovascular disease. MRI scan and sleep electroencephalography are the primary investigative techniques. Usually, neurodegenerative diseases have specific physical signs and MRI abnormalities, with distinct EEG findings. Fluctuation in clinical severity and a good response to treatment with antiepileptic medications offer confirmatory evidence, although in atypical cases detailed neurodegenerative investigation may be appropriate.

Electrophysiologic Findings

The EEG abnormalities consist of slow waves, spikes and spike-wave complexes in the centrotemporoparietal regions (19,41,42). A predominant scalp localization to the frontal lobes has been reported in one-third of some series (40). The discharges are bilateral, independent, or synchronous and may have a fluctuating left- or right-sided predominance. The development of surgical treatments has prompted more precise electrophysiologic localization, and most studies have pointed to the temporal lobe (43), particularly the superior temporal gyrus and into the sylvian fissure. Results of methohexital suppression tests (44), intraoperative electrocorticography of limited parts of the cortex, and magnetoencephalography (MEG) (45) also offer evidence for a perisylvian location. MEG has also shown intrasylvian involvement. Dichotic listening studies and auditory evoked responses implicate the primary auditory cortex (46,47), but EEG foci may be multiple and extrasylvian (45). Enhancement of epileptiform activity in slow-wave sleep is variable, occupying 85% of slow-wave sleep in 20% of patients (fulfilling the arbitrary definition of CSWS), 50% to 80% of sleep in 26% of patients, and less than 50% of sleep in the rest of patients (40). The abnormal sleep-related activity also may switch off temporarily so that a single, normal electroencephalogram during sleep does not exclude LKS (34). Prolonged spike-wave discharges in slow sleep may persist for months to years (6), and the extent of natural recovery seems to be inversely related to the length of time the EEG abnormality has been present (48).

Pathogenesis

The frequent subclinical EEG discharges in sleep and wakefulness are presumed to disrupt the central pathways for language processing. This relationship between seizures and language difficulties is also seen in the less severe but similar syndrome of BECTS. Although the seizures of BECTS are usually mild, infrequent and self-limiting at least 50% of the children have problems with language processing (49).

High-resolution brain MRI shows normal results. Two reports of inflammatory disease of the brain (50) and arteries (51) in LKS raise the possibility of an immune-mediated cause. Anecdotal reports describe prompt response to immunoglobulin treatment in patients with a diagnosis of LKS (52,53).

Functional imaging studies using singe-photon-emission computed tomography (SPECT) often show hypoperfusion and hypometabolism in the temporal regions may be evident on positron emission tomography. Some reports also described temporal hypermetabolism identified on SPECT (54–56), compatible with active epileptic discharges arising from this part of the brain.

Outcome

The long-term natural history of LKS is not well known but partial improvements in communication, behavior, and motor competence can extend into the second and third decades.

Late recurrence of severe symptoms after a good recovery is rare, but subtle language and communication deficits have not been investigated in apparently recovered patients.

TREATMENT

A multidisciplinary team consisting of a developmental speech and language therapist, a neuropsychologist, and a pediatric neurologist is necessary to comprehensively assess and monitor the entire cognitive profile in LKS is often required and CSWS. Assessment of the use of gestures, but only a minority find it possible to master a signing system (57). Facial expression and use of gaze are often lacking in LKS (58).

Management of these syndromes entails four aspects.

Treatment of Seizures

Seizures usually respond to appropriate anticonvulsants. Some seizures, refractory to routine medication, may remit when corticosteroid drugs are used for the encephalopathy or after surgical treatment.

Treatment of Encephalopathy

There is no evidence that treatment of subclinical abnormal EEG activity with antiepileptic drugs will alter the course and outcome of encephalopathy in CSWS and LKS. However, some authorities believe that aggressive trials of antiepileptic drugs may be used together with close monitoring of sleep electroencephalography, particularly in CSWS. Neuropsychological progress should be closely monitored with goal-oriented speech and occupational therapy.

Improvement in seizures and encephalopathy has been reported after treatment with corticosteroids (54,59), but no definitive conclusions are possible, as the series were open label, involved small numbers of children, and used variable inclusion criteria, treatment regimens, and outcome measures. In a study of 20 children with LKS (60), prospective treatment with prednisolone 2 mg/kg for 6 weeks followed by a 6-week weaning period produced useful improvement in more than half, as determined by formal developmental assessments. A trial of oral steroids for 6 to 12 weeks is generally suggested in children with CSWS and LKS who have seizures, progressive encephalopathy, cognitive impairment and significant sleep-related abnormal EEG activity. Close monitoring for steroid-related side effects is required. If a good response is followed by a relapse on weaning or withdrawal, a pulsed regimen of prednisolone 4 mg/kg (3 mg/kg in children over 8 years) given weekly may be effective and produce relatively few side effects. Although the mechanism of action of steroids is unknown, corticosteroids are assumed to work as anticonvulsants as in other early onset epileptic encephalopathies.

Individual patients may respond to benzodiazepines, particularly clobazam (54), and there are anecdotal reports of clinical response to immunoglobulin (52,53). Sodium valproate and ethosuximide have been helpful in CSWS (23). Repeated high doses of diazepam have reportedly resolved the electrical abnormality but tolerance can be a problem (61,62). Some medication, particularly carbamazepine, can aggravate CSWS and weaning may lead to clinical and EEG improvement. Such drugs should be avoided in these syndromes despite the presence of focal motor seizures.

A few centers have used multiple subpial transections as therapy for LKS in a small number of patients (44,63–67). One study (64) found the procedure useful in patients with seizures, ESES and pure language regression but without autistic features or global cognitive impairment. Other series have reported variable success in broad categories of patients with ESES and autistic features (68). Although not entirely clear, the major criterion for surgery is believed to be convincing evidence of predominantly one affected cerebral hemisphere provided by use of scalp EEG, methohexital suppression tests, the intracarotid Amytal test, and MEG. A child with ongoing seizures and significant progressive language and cognitive impairment in whom antiepileptic medications and steroids have failed may be considered a surgical candidate. The precise extent of cortex to be transected remains a matter of debate and may be clarified by intraoperative electrocorticography.

Surgery is associated with improvement in more than 50% of cases, with only partial improvement in seizures and cognition. It is not clear whether the extent of improvement ultimately has a positive impact on the child's quality of life and long-term outcome (69). Some reports suggest improvement in autistic features and other behavioral disorders postoperatively (31,67,68), but typically without a return to completely normal functioning. Whether the long-term outcome is significantly influenced by treatment is not yet resolved.

Specific Behavioral Intervention

Behavioral impairments should be identified and managed using parental counselling, therapy and medication. Attention deficit hyperactivity disorder may respond well to methylphenidate; severe impulsivity, hyperactivity, and aggressive behavior to clonidine or risperidone; obsessional behavior and anxiety to serotonin reuptake inhibitors; and difficulty in getting to sleep may be lessened with melatonin and short-acting benzodiazepines. In each situation, drug treatment is preceded by family and school education about management and the provision of structure and support as appropriate. The possibility of enhanced side effects of antiepileptic drugs (e.g., irritability with sodium valproate and sleeping problems with lamotrigine) must be kept in mind. A severe behavioral disorder may pose a formidable challenge in the investigation and treatment of LKS and CSWS.

General Behavioral, Educational and Communication Support

Integrated medical, psychiatric, and psychological care, along with support from educational and social services, is required for the management of LKS. Parent support groups also can be helpful.

REFERENCES

1. Commission on Classification and Terminology of the International League Against Epilepsy. Proposal for revised clinical and electroencephalographic classification of epileptic seizures. *Epilepsia* 1981;22:489–501.
2. Commission on Classification and Terminology of the International League Against Epilepsy. Proposal for revised classification of epilepsies and epileptic syndromes. *Epilepsia* 1989;30:389–399.
3. Galanopolou AS, Bojko A, Lado F, et al. The spectrum of neuropsychiatric abnormalities associated with electrical status epilepticus in sleep. *Brain Dev* 2000;22:279–295.
4. Yung A, Park YD, Cohen M, et al. Cognitive and behavioural problems in children with centrotemporal spikes. *Pediatr Neurol* 2000;23:391–395.
5. Veggiotti P, Beccaria F, Guerrini R, et al. Continuous spike and wave activity during slow wave sleep: syndrome or EEG pattern. *Epilepsia* 1999;40:1593–1601.
6. Tassinari CA, Rubboli G, Michelucci R, et al. Acquired epileptic aphasia or Landau Kleffner syndrome. In: Meinardi H, ed. *The epilepsies, part II,* vol 73. *Handbook of clinical neurology.* New York: Elsevier, 2000:281–292.

7. Patry G, Lyagoubi S, Tassinari CA. Subclinical "electrical status epilepticus" induced by sleep in children. *Arch Neurol* 1971; 24:242–252.

8. Morikawa T, Seino M, Watanabe Y, et al. Clinical relevance of continuous spike waves during slow wave sleep. In: Manelis S, Bental E, Loeber JN, et al., eds. *Advances in epileptology.* New York: Raven Press, 1989:359–363.

9. Kramer U, Nevo M, Neufeld Y, et al. Epidemiology of epilepsy in childhood; a cohort of 440 consecutive patients. *Pediatr Neurol* 1998;18:46–50.

10. Tassinari CA, Rubboli G, Volpi L, et al. Encephalopathy with electrical status epilepticus during slow sleep or ESES syndrome including the acquired aphasia. *Clin Neurophysiol* 2000;111:S94–S102.

11. Genton P, Guerrini R, Bureau M, et al. Continuous focal discharges during REM sleep in a case of Landau Kleffner syndrome: a three year follow up. In: Beaumanoir A, Bureau M, Deonna T, et al., eds. *Continuous spikes and waves during slow sleep. Electrical status epilepticus during slow sleep: acquired epileptic aphasia and related conditions.* London: John Libbey, 1995:155–159.

12. Bureau M. Outstanding cases of CSWS and LKS: analysis of the data sheets provided by the participants. In: Beaumanoir A, Bureau M, Deonna T, et al., eds. *Continuous spikes and waves during slow sleep. Electrical status epilepticus during slow sleep: acquired epileptic aphasia and related conditions.* London: John Libbey, 1995:213–216.

13. Tassinari CA, Bureau M, Dravet C, et al. Epilepsy with continuous spikes and waves during slow sleep—otherwise described as ESES (epilepsy with electrical status epilepticus during slow sleep). In: Roger J, Bureau M, Dravet C, et al., eds. *Epileptic syndromes in infancy, childhood and adolescence.* London: John Libbey, 1992: 245–256.

14. Dalla Bernardina B, Tassinari CA, Dravet C, et al. Benign focal epilepsy and "electrical status epilepticus" during sleep [author's translation; French]. *Rev Electroencephalogr Neurophysiol Clin* 1978;8:350–353.

15. Dalla Bernardina B, Fontana E, Michelizza B, et al. Partial epilepsies of childhood, bilateral synchronization, continuous spike waves during slow sleep. In: Manelis S, Bental E, Loeber JN, eds. *Advances in epileptology.* New York: Raven Press, 1989:295–302.

16. Rouselle C, Revol M. Relations between cognitive functions and CSWS. In: Beaumanoir A, Bureau M, Deonna T, et al., eds. *Continuous spikes and waves during slow sleep. Electrical status epilepticus during slow sleep: acquired epileptic aphasia and related conditions.* London: John Libbey, 1995:123–133.

17. Kobayashi K, Nishibayashi N, Ohtsuka Y, et al. Epilepsy with electrical status epilepticus during slow sleep and secondary bilateral synchrony. *Epilepsia* 1994;35:1097–1103.

18. Guerrini R, Genton P, Bureau M, et al. Multilobar polymicrogyria, intractable drop attack seizures and sleep-related electrical status epilepticus. *Neurology* 1998;51:504–512.

19. Dulac O, Billard C, Arthuis M. Electroclinical and developmental aspects of epilepsy in the aphasia-epilepsy syndrome [French]. *Arch Fr Pediatr* 1983;40:299–308.

20. Gaggero R, Caputo M, Fiorio P, et al. SPECT and epilepsy with continuous spike waves during slow-wave sleep. *Childs Nerv Syst* 1995;11:154–160.

21. Tassinari CA, Rubboli G, Parmeggiani L, et al. Epileptic negative myoclonus. *Adv Neurol* 1995;67:181–197.

22. Tassinari CA, Rubboli G, Shibasaki H. Neurophysiology of positive and negative myoclonus. *Electroencephalogr Clin Neurophysiol* 1998;107:181–195.

23. Case reports. In: Beaumanoir A, Bureau M, Deonna T, et al., eds. *Continuous spike waves during slow sleep. Electrical status epilepticus during slow sleep: acquired epileptic aphasia and related conditions.* London: John Libbey, 1995:169–210.

24. Tassinari CA, Rubboli G, Volpi L, et al. Electrical status epilepticus during slow sleep (ESES or CSWS) including acquired epileptic aphasia (Landau-Kleffner syndrome). In: Roger J, Bureau M, Dravet C, et al., eds. *Epileptic syndromes in infancy, childhood and adolescence.* London: John Libbey, 2002:265–283.

25. Kobayashi K, Ohtsuka Y, Oka E, et al. Primary and secondary bilateral synchrony in epilepsy: differentiation by estimation of interhemispheric small time differences during short spike-wave activity. *Electroencephalogr Clin Neurophysiol* 1992;83:93–103.

26. Monteiro JP, Roulet Perez E, Davidoff V, et al. Primary neonatal thalamic haemorrhage and epilepsy with continuous spike-wave during sleep: a longitudinal followup of a possible significant relation. *Eur J Paediatr Neurol* 2001;5:41–47.

27. Incorpora G, Pavone P, Smilari PG, et al. Late unilateral thalamic hemorrhage in infancy: report of two cases. *Neuropediatrics* 2004; 30:264–267.

28. Mariotti P, Della Marca G, Iuvone L, et al. Is ESES/CSWS a strictly age related disorder? *Clin Neurophysiol* 2000;111:452–456.

29. Mira L, Oxilia B, van Lierde A. Cognitive assessment of children with CSWS syndrome: a critical review of data from 155 cases submitted to the Venice colloquium. In: Beaumanoir A, Bureau M, Deonna T, et al., eds. *Continuous spike waves during slow sleep. Electrical status epilepticus during slow sleep: acquired epileptic aphasia and related conditions.* London: John Libbey, 1995:229–242.

30. Landau WM, Kleffner FR. Syndrome of acquired aphasia with convulsive disorder in children. *Neurology* 1957;7:523–530.

31. Nass R, Heier L, Walker R. Outcome of multiple subpial transections for autistic epileptiform regression. *Pediatr Neurol* 1999;21: 464–470.

32. Beaumanoir A. The Landau Kleffner syndrome. In: Beaumanoir A, Bureau M, Deonna T, et al., eds. *Epileptic syndromes in infancy, childhood and adolescence.* London: John Libbey, 1992:231–244.

33. Neville BG, Boyd SG. Selective epileptic gait disorder. *J Neurol Neurosurg Psychiatry* 1995;58:371–373.

34. Deonna T, Roulet E. Acquired epileptic aphasia (AEA): definition of the syndrome and current problems. In: Beaumanoir A, Bureau M, Deonna T, et al., eds. *Continuous spikes and waves during slow sleep. Electrical status epilepticus during slow sleep; acquired epileptic aphasia and related conditions.* London: John Libbey, 1995:37–45.

35. Maquet P, Hirsch E, Metz-Lutz MN, et al. Regional cerebral glucose metabolism in children with deterioration of one or more cognitive functions and continuous spike and wave discharges in sleep. *Brain* 1995;118:1497–1520.

36. Rapin I, Mattis S, Rowan AJ, et al. Verbal auditory agnosia and seizures in children. *Dev Med Child Neurol* 1977;19:192–207.

37. Boyd SG, River-Gaxiola M, Towell AD, et al. Discrimination of speech sounds in a boy with Landau-Kleffner syndrome: an intraoperative event-related potential study. *Neuropädiatrie* 1996;27:211–215.

38. Neville BG, Burch VM, Cass H, et al. Behavioural aspects of Landau-Kleffner syndrome. In: Gillberg C, O'Brien G, eds. *Developmental disability and behaviour.* London: Cambridge University Press, 2000:56–63.

39. Neville BG, Burch VM, Cass H, et al. Motor disorders in Landau Kleffner syndrome. *Epilepsia* 1998;(Suppl 6):123.

40. Hirsch E, Maquet P, Metz-Lutz MN, et al. The eponym "Landau Kleffner syndrome" should not be restricted to childhood acquired aphasia with epilepsy. In: Beaumanoir A, Bureau M, Deonna T, et al, eds. *Continuous spike and wave during slow sleep. Electrical status epilepticus during slow sleep. Acquired epileptic aphasia and related conditions.* London: John Libbey, 1995:57–62.

41. Hirsch E, Marescaux C, Maquet P, et al. Landau Kleffner syndrome: a clinical and EEG study of five cases. *Epilepsia* 1990;31: 756–767.

42. Mantovani JF. Autistic regression and Landau Kleffner syndrome: prognosis and confusion? *Dev Med Child Neurol* 2000;42: 349–353.

43. Tuchman RF. Acquired epileptiform aphasia. *Semin Pediatr Neurol* 1997;4:93–101.

44. Morrell F, Whisler WW, Smith MC, et al. Landau-Kleffner syndrome: treatment with subpial intracortical transection. *Brain* 1995;118:1529–1546.

45. Paetau R, Granstrom ML, Blomstedt G, et al. Magnetoencephalography in presurgical evaluation of children with Landau Kleffner syndrome. *Epilepsia* 1999;40:326–335.

46. Seri S, Cerquiglini A, Pisani F. Spike-induced interference in auditory sensory processing in Landau Kleffner syndrome. *Electroencephalogr Clin Neurophysiol* 1999;108:506–510.

47. Metz-Lutz MN, Hirsch E, Maquet P, et al. Dichotic listening performances in the follow-up of Landau Kleffner syndrome. *Child Neuropsychol* 1997;3:47–60.

48. Robinson RO, Baird G, Robinson G, et al. Landau Kleffner syndrome: course and correlates with outcome. *Dev Med Child Neurol* 2001;43:243–247.

49. Staden U, Isaacs E, Boyd SG, et al. Language dysfunction in children with rolandic epilepsy. *Neuropediatrics* 1998;29:242–248.

50. Lou HC, Brandt S, Bruhn P. Aphasia and epilepsy in children. *Acta Neurol Scand* 1977;56:46–54.

51. Pascual-Castroviejo I, Lopez Martin L, Martinez Bermejo A, et al. Is cerebral arteritis the cause of the Landau Kleffner syndrome? Four cases in childhood with angiographic study. *Can J Neurol Sci* 1992;19:46–52.

52. Mikati MA, Saab R, Fayad MN, et al. Efficacy of intravenous immunoglobulin in Landau Kleffner syndrome. *Pediatr Neurol* 2002;26:298–300.

53. Lagae LG, Silberstein J, Casaer P. Successful use of intravenous immunoglobulins in Landau Kleffner syndrome. *Pediatr Neurol* 1998;18:165–168.

54. O'Regan ME, Brown JK, Goodwin GM, et al. Epileptic aphasia: a consequence of regional hypometabolic encephalopathy? *Dev Med Child Neurol* 1998;40:508–516.

55. Maquet P, Hirsch E, Dive D, et al. Cerebral glucose utilization during sleep in Landau Kleffner syndrome: a PET study. *Epilepsia* 1990;31:778–783.

56. Cooper JA, Ferry PC. Acquired auditory verbal agnosia and seizures in childhood. *J Speech Hear Disord* 1978;43:176–184.

57. Bishop DV. Comprehension of spoken, written and signed sentences in childhood language disorders. *Child Psychol Psychiatry* 1982;23:1–20.

58. Roulet Perez E, Davidoff V, Prelaz AC, et al. Sign language in childhood epileptic aphasia (Landau Kleffner syndrome). *Dev Med Child Neurol* 2001;43:739–744.

59. Neville BG, Burch VM, Cass H, et al. The Landau Kleffner syndrome. In: Oxbury JM, Polkey C, Duchowny M, eds. *Intractable focal epilepsy: medical and surgical treatment.* London: WB Saunders, 2000:277–284.

60. Lees JA, Cass H, Waring M, et al. Measuring response to pharmacological treatment in children with epilepsy related aphasia (Landau-Kleffner syndrome). *Dev Med Child Neurol* 1998;77:9.

61. De Negri M, Baglietto MG, Biancheri R. Electrical status epilepticus in childhood: treatment with short cycles of high dosage benzodiazepine (preliminary note). *Brain Dev* 1993;15: 311–312.

62. De Negri M, Baglietto MG, Battaglia FM, et al. Treatment of electrical status epilepticus by short diazepam (DZP) cycles after DZP rectal bolus test. *Brain Dev* 1995;17:330–333.

63. Morrell F, Kanner AM, Whisler WW. Multiple subpial transection: application to paediatric epilepsy surgery. In: Tuxhorn I, Holthausen H, Boenigk H, eds. *Paediatric epilepsy syndromes and their surgical treatment.* London: John Libbey, 1997:865–875.

64. Morrell F, Whisler WW, Bleck TP. Multiple subpial transection: a new approach to the surgical treatment of focal epilepsy. *J Neurosurg* 1989;70:231–239.

65. Sawhey IM, Robertson IJ, Polkey CE, et al. Multiple subpial transection: a review of 21 cases. *J Neurol Neurosurg Psychiatry* 1995; 58:344–349.

66. Polkey CE. Surgery for epilepsy. *Arch Dis Child* 2004;64:185–187.

67. Polkey C. Alternative surgical procedures to help drug resistant epilepsy—a review. *Epileptic Disord* 2003;5:63–75.

68. Neville BG, Harkness W, Cross JH, et al. Surgical treatment of severe autistic regression in childhood epilepsy. *Pediatr Neurol* 1997;16:137–140.

69. Grote CL, Van Slyke P, Hoeppner JA. Language outcome following multiple subpial transection for Landau Kleffner syndrome. *Brain* 1999;122:561–566.

Epilepsy with Reflex Seizures

30

Benjamin G. Zifkin   *Frederick Andermann*

DEFINITION AND CLASSIFICATION

The seizures of reflex epilepsy are reliably precipitated by some identifiable factor (1). The International League Against Epilepsy (2) describes reflex epilepsies as "characterized by specific modes of seizure precipitation"; its 2001 classification proposal (3) redefines reflex epilepsy syndromes as those in which "all epileptic seizures are precipitated by sensory stimuli." Reflex seizures that occur in focal and generalized epilepsy syndromes that are also associated with spontaneous seizures are generally listed as seizure types; for example, photosensitive seizures in patients with juvenile myoclonic epilepsy. Reflex seizures also can be classified according to the seizure trigger, and although they may not otherwise differ clinically from seizures in other forms of epilepsy, understanding the seizure trigger is important in treating patients and studying the mechanisms of epileptogenesis. Seizures triggered by factors such as alcohol withdrawal are not included among reflex seizures.

The use of the term *reflex* is controversial. Hall (4) first applied it to epilepsy in 1850. Arguing that no reflex arc is involved in reflex epilepsy, others proposed terms such as *sensory precipitation* (5,6) or *stimulus sensitive epilepsies* (7). Wieser (8) noted that sensory precipitation epilepsy is a misnomer because some reflex seizures are not precipitated by sensory stimuli. We and others retain *reflex epilepsy* to mean that a certain stimulus regularly elicits an observable response in the form of abnormal, paroxysmal, electroencephalographic (EEG) activity with or without a clinical seizure. Although some investigators restrict the term *reflex epilepsy* to cases in which a certain stimulus always induces seizures (9), it can include cases in which spontaneous seizures also occur or instances in which the epileptogenic stimulus does not invariably induce an attack (10), which often occurs in patients taking antiepileptic drugs.

The term *epilepsy with reflex seizures,* although more cumbersome, perhaps better reflects clinical reality and more accurately describes cases with reflex and spontaneous attacks.

Reflex seizures have long fascinated epileptologists. Apart from epileptic photosensitivity to flickering light, cases of reflex epilepsy are relatively rare and permit glimpses into the mechanisms of epileptogenesis and the organization of cognitive function. The identification of a patient with reflex epilepsy depends on the physician's awareness and on the observations of the patient and witnesses. The epileptogenic trigger must occur often enough in everyday life so that the patient suspects its relation to the resulting seizures. If the trigger is ubiquitous, however, the seizures appear to occur by chance or with no obvious antecedent. Many triggers have been recognized and studied. This chapter reviews the neurophysiology of reflex epilepsy from available human and animal studies. It also discusses the clinical syndrome of reflex epilepsy classified by the triggering stimulus.

BASIC MECHANISMS OF REFLEX EPILEPSY

There are two types of animal model of reflex epilepsy. In the first, irritative cortical lesions are created, and their activation by specific stimuli is studied. The second involves naturally occurring reflex epilepsies or seizures induced by specific sensory stimulation in genetically predisposed animals.

The first approach has been used since 1929, when Clementi (11) induced convulsions with intermittent photic stimulation after applying strychnine to the visual cortex. This technique also demonstrated that strychninization of auditory (12), gustatory (13), and olfactory cortex (14) produced focal irritative lesions that may produce seizures with the appropriate afferent stimulus. EEG studies showed that the clinical seizures (chewing movements), which were induced by photic stimulation in rabbits with strychnine lesions of the visual cortex, resulted from rapid transmission of the epileptic discharge from the visual cortex to masticatory areas (15). The spread of paroxysmal discharge from the visual cortex may also extend to frontorolandic areas during seizures (16,17). The ictal EEG spread was thought to represent corticocortical conduction (11,16), although later work with pentylenetetrazol also implicated thalamic relays (17) and demonstrated spread of the visual evoked potential to the brainstem reticular formation (18). Hunter and Ingvar (19) identified a subcortical pathway involving the thalamus and reticular system and an independent corticocortical system for radiation of visual evoked responses to the frontal lobe. In cats and monkeys, the frontorolandic region was also shown to receive spreading evoked paroxysmal activity from auditory and other stimuli (20,21).

The second approach, the study of naturally occurring or induced reflex seizures in genetically susceptible animals, has been pursued in photosensitive chickens (22,23); rodents susceptible to sound-induced convulsions (24); the E1 mouse, sensitive to vestibular stimulation (25); and the Mongolian gerbil, sensitive to a variety of stimuli (26,27). The only species in which the reflex seizures and EEG findings are similar to those in humans is the baboon *Papio papio* (28), except that the light-induced epileptic discharges in baboons occur in the frontorolandic area rather than in the occipital lobe (29). EEG, visual evoked potentials, intracerebral recording, and lesion and pharmacologic studies show that visual afferents are necessary to trigger frontorolandic light-induced epileptic discharges. The occipital lobe does not generate this abnormal activity, but sends corticocortical visual afferents to hyperexcitable frontal cortex, which is responsible for the epileptiform activity (30). The interhemispheric synchronization of the light-induced paroxysmal EEG activity and seizures depends mainly on the corpus callosum and not on the brainstem. Brainstem reticular activation depends initially on frontal cortical mechanisms until a seizure is about to begin, at which point the cortex can no longer control reticular activation. The genetically determined hyperexcitability may be related to cortical biochemical abnormalities, involving regulation of extracellular calcium concentration (31,32), or to an imbalance between excitatory and inhibitory neurotransmitter amino acids (33) similar to those described in feline generalized penicillin epilepsy and in human epilepsy (34). This model, however, more closely resembles photic-induced cortical myoclonus than typical human photosensitive epilepsy.

In human epileptic photosensitivity, generalized epileptiform activity and clinical seizures can be activated by the localized occipital trigger. Studies in photosensitive patients who are also pattern sensitive suggest that generalized seizures and EEG paroxysmal activity can occur in these

subjects if normal excitation of visual cortex involves a certain "critical mass" of cortical area with synchronization and subsequent spreading of excitation (35–38). We (39) suggested that a similar mechanism involving recruitment of a critical mass of parietal rather than visual cortex is responsible for generalized seizures induced by thinking or by spatial tasks. Studies of reading epilepsy also suggest that increased task difficulty, complexity, or duration increases the chance of EEG or clinical activation (40,41).

Wieser (8) proposed a neurophysiologic model for critical mass, referring to the group 1 and group 2 epileptic neurons of the chronic experimental epileptic focus described by Wyler and Ward (42). Group 1 neurons produce abundant, spontaneous, high-frequency bursts of action potentials. Group 2 neurons have a variable interspike interval, and their spontaneous epileptic activity is less marked. Moreover, these properties are influenced by external stimuli that can promote or inhibit the incorporation of group 2 neurons into the effective quantity of epileptic tissue and thus trigger or inhibit a seizure. The stimuli effective in eliciting reflex seizures would act on this population of neurons, recruiting them into the highly epileptic group 1 neuron pool to form the critical mass needed to produce epileptogenic EEG activity or clinical seizures. This mechanism also can explain conditioning (43) and deconditioning (44) of reflex epileptic responses. A further generalizing system also must be postulated to account for the seizures observed with photic or cognitive stimulation, analogous to the corticocortical pathways linking occipital cortex with frontorolandic cortex in *Papio papio*. A role for reticulothalamic structures has been suggested but seems unnecessary, at least in certain animal models in which corticocortical spread of evoked epileptic activity persists after mesencephalic and diencephalic ablation (19).

Patients with reflex seizures may report that emotion plays a role in seizure induction and, sometimes, in seizure inhibition. Gras and coworkers (45) emphasized the influence of emotional content in activating EEG spikes in a patient with reading epilepsy. An emotional component was also obvious in several cases of musicogenic and eating epilepsy. Fenwick (46) described psychogenic seizures as epileptic seizures generated by an action of mind, self-induced attacks (e.g., by thinking sad thoughts) and those unintentionally triggered by specific mental activity such as thinking. This use of the term *psychogenic seizures*, common in European epileptology, does not refer to nonepileptic events. Fenwick (46) related seizure induction and inhibition in some individuals with or without typical reflex seizures to the neuronal excitation and inhibition accompanying mental activity. He also referred to the alumina cream model, with recruitment of group 2 neurons and evoked change in neuronal activity surrounding the seizure focus as factors in seizure occurrence, spread, and inhibition.

Wolf (47) believed that two pathophysiologic theories arose in the discussion of reflex epilepsies. Arguing that primary reading epilepsy is an age-related idiopathic epilepsy syndrome (48), he observed that seizure evocation would depend on involvement of the multiple processes used for reading, an activity involving both hemispheres, with a functional rather than a topographic anatomy. "Maximal interactive neuronal performance is at least a facilitating factor," he wrote (47), and suggested that the functional complexity of the epileptogenic tasks leads to seizure precipitation. He contrasted this with the suggestion described previously that the latency, dependence on task duration and complexity, and influence of nonspecific factors such as attention and arousal often observed in these seizures depend on the ad hoc recruitment of a critical mass of epileptogenic tissue to produce a clinical seizure or paroxysmal EEG activity in response to the different characteristics of an effective triggering stimulus. In seizures induced by reading, thinking, photic response, and pattern sensitivity, the relatively localized trigger induces generalized or bilateral EEG abnormalities and seizures. The recruitment that produces these seizures, however, need not be confined to physically contiguous brain tissue or fixed neuronal links. Instead, it may depend on the activity of a function-related network of both established and plastic links between brain regions, modified by the effects of factors such as arousal. These two approaches share much common ground.

Disorders of cortical development may be present in some patients with reflex seizures. Especially in early work, reportedly normal imaging results may be misleading. Subtle changes or dysplastic lesions may be missed without special magnetic resonance imaging (MRI) techniques or may be found only in a surgical specimen (49,50).

REFLEX EPILEPSY WITH VISUAL TRIGGERS

Epilepsy with reflex seizures evoked by visual stimuli is the most common reflex epilepsy. Of the several abnormal EEG responses to laboratory intermittent photic stimulation (IPS) described, only generalized paroxysmal epileptiform discharges (e.g., spikes, polyspikes, spike-and-wave complexes) are clearly linked to epilepsy in humans. Approximately 5% of patients with epilepsy show this response to IPS (51,52). Photosensitivity is genetically determined (53,54), but studies of the epileptic response to IPS are complicated by the age and sex dependence of the phenomenon, which occurs most frequently in adolescents and women, and by differences in how IPS is performed. An expert panel has published a protocol for performing IPS and guidelines for interpreting the EEG responses (55).

Sensitivity to IPS is customarily divided into three groups: patients with light-induced seizures only, patients with photosensitivity and other seizure types, and asymptomatic individuals with isolated photosensitivity. Kasteleijn-Nolst Trenité (56) showed that more than half

of known photosensitive patients questioned immediately after stimulation denied having had brief but clear-cut seizures induced by IPS and documented by video-EEG monitoring. Photosensitive epilepsy may be classified into two major groups, depending on whether the seizures are induced by flickering light. Further classification into subgroups is as follows:

> Seizures induced by flicker
>> Pure photosensitive epilepsy including idiopathic photosensitive occipital epilepsy
>> Photosensitive epilepsy with spontaneous seizures
>> Self-induced seizures
> Visually evoked seizures not induced by flicker
>> Pattern-sensitive seizures
>> Seizures induced by eye closure
>> Self-induced seizures

Pure Photosensitive Epilepsy

Pure photosensitive epilepsy is characterized by generalized seizures provoked exclusively by flickering light. According to Jeavons (57), 40% of photosensitive patients have this variety of epilepsy, and television is the most common precipitating factor. Video games may trigger these seizures, although not all such events represent pure photosensitive epilepsy (58,59). Other typical environmental stimuli include discothèque lights and sunlight reflected from snow or the sea or interrupted by roadside structures or trees.

Pure photosensitive epilepsy is typically a disorder of adolescence, with a female predominance. Reviews of the topic have been provided by several authors (51,52,55,56,60). The seizures are generalized tonic-clonic in 84% of patients (61), absences in 6% of patients, partial motor seizures (possibly asymmetric myoclonus in some cases) in 2.5% of patients, and myoclonic seizures in 1.5% of patients. Subtle myoclonic seizures may go unnoticed until an obvious seizure occurs. The developmental and neurologic examinations are normal. The resting electroencephalogram may be normal in approximately 50% of patients, but spike-and-wave complexes may be seen with eye closure. Intermittent photic stimulation evokes a photoparoxysmal response in virtually all patients. Depending on the photic stimulus and on the patient's degree of photosensitivity, the clinical response ranges from subtle eyelid myoclonus to a generalized tonic-clonic convulsion.

Pure photosensitive epilepsy is typically conceptualized as a variety of idiopathic generalized epilepsy, but cases occur in which electroencephalography and clinical evidence favors the occipital lobe origin, as predicted by theoretical and animal models (62,63). Recently, there has been increased recognition that IPS can induce clear-cut partial seizures originating in the occipital lobe (64,65). As in more typical photosensitive subjects, environmental triggers include television and video games. Many of these patients have idiopathic photosensitive occipital lobe epilepsy, a relatively benign, age-related syndrome without spontaneous seizures, although cases with occipital lesions have been reported, including patients with celiac disease. The clinical seizure pattern depends on the pattern of spread. The visual stimulus triggers initial visual symptoms that may be followed by versive movements and motor seizures; however, migraine-like symptoms of throbbing headache, nausea, and, sometimes, vomiting are common and can lead to delayed or incorrect diagnosis.

Photosensitivity with Spontaneous Seizures

Jeavons and Harding (61) found that about one-third of their photosensitive patients with environmentally precipitated attacks also had spontaneous seizures similar to those of pure photosensitive epilepsy. Spike-and-wave activity was common in the resting EEG patterns of patients with spontaneous seizures, and only 39% of patients had normal resting electroencephalograms. Photosensitivity may accompany idiopathic generalized epilepsies, especially juvenile myoclonic epilepsy (JME), and is associated with onset in childhood and adolescence, normal intellectual development and neurologic examination, normal EEG background rhythm, and generally good response to treatment with valproate. It also may occur with severe myoclonic epilepsy of infancy (Dravet syndrome) or with disorders associated with progressive myoclonic epilepsy like Lafora disease, Unverricht-Lundborg disease, Kufs disease, and the neuronal ceroid lipofuscinoses (66). Photosensitivity is usual in eyelid myoclonia with absences (EMA) but not in benign occipital epilepsies of childhood of the Gastaut or Panayiotopoulos types (67).

Pure photosensitive epilepsy may be treated by avoiding or modifying environmental light stimuli. Increasing the distance from the television set, watching a small screen in a well-lighted room, using a remote control so that the set need not be approached, and monocular viewing or the use of polarized spectacles to block one eye should provide protection (57,68). Colored spectacles may be useful in selected patients (69,70). Drug treatment is needed if these measures are impractical or unsuccessful, if photosensitivity is severe, or if spontaneous attacks occur. The drug of choice is valproate, which in one study (71) abolished photosensitivity in 54% of patients and markedly reduced it in a further 24%. Lamotrigine, topiramate, ethosuximide, benzodiazepines such as clobazam (72), and levetiracetam (56) also may be useful. Quesney and associates (73) proposed a dopaminergic mechanism in human epileptic photosensitivity based on the transient abolition of photosensitivity with apomorphine, and bromocriptine and parenteral L-dopa are reported to alleviate photosensitivity (74,75). About one-fourth of patients with pure photosensitive epilepsy lose their photosensitivity by 25 years of age (76). Because this resolution usually occurs only in the third decade, withdrawal of treatment too early may lead to

seizure recurrence; serial EEG recordings to determine the photosensitivity range may be helpful in assessment and follow-up (56).

Seizures with Self-Induced Flicker

Reports of self-induced epileptic attacks using visual sensitivity antedated the discovery of the photoparoxysmal EEG response (77). Regarded as rare, self-induction was reported particularly in mentally retarded children and adolescents, with a female preponderance (51,52,78,79). More recent information, however, shows that although some affected patients are retarded, most are not (80–82). When carefully sought, the syndrome is not rare; it was found in approximately 40% of photosensitive patients studied by Kasteleijn-Nolst Trenité and coworkers (80). The electroencephalogram usually shows spontaneous generalized spikes or spike-and-wave complexes, and approximately 75% of patients are sensitive to IPS. The self-induced seizures are usually myoclonic, especially with palpebral myoclonus, or absences, and some patients have EMA. Patients induce seizures with maneuvers that cause flicker, such as waving a hand with fingers spread apart in front of their eyes or gazing at a vertically rolling television image. Monitoring (82,83) shows that these behaviors, once thought to be part of the seizure, precede the attacks and are responsible for inducing them. The compulsive nature of this behavior has been observed often and has been likened to self-stimulation (84) in experimental animals. Patients have reported intensely pleasant sensations and relief of stress with self-induced photosensitive absence seizures (81,82). Frank sexual arousal has been described (85,86). Patients are often unwilling to give up their seizures, and noncompliance with standard, well-tolerated antiepileptic drugs is common (80,81). Treatment is difficult, however, even in compliant patients (79). Drugs that suppress self-stimulation in animals, such as chlorpromazine and pimozide, may block the pleasurable response without affecting the response to IPS and have partially reduced or completely terminated self-induction (79,87). The effectiveness of valproate in reducing or abolishing photosensitivity has resulted in virtual disappearance of this form of self-induction, which is now encountered in patients for whom the drug has not been prescribed and in those with inadequate drug levels for any reason. Many patients appear not to want treatment for their self-induced attacks.

VISUALLY EVOKED SEIZURES NOT INDUCED BY FLICKER

Pattern-Sensitive Seizures

Absences, myoclonus, or, more rarely, tonic-clonic seizures may occur in response to epileptogenic patterns. These are striped and include common objects such as the television screen at short distances, curtains or wallpaper, escalator steps, and striped clothing. Pattern sensitivity is seen in approximately 70% of photosensitive patients tested with patterned IPS in the EEG laboratory, but sensitivity to stationary striped patterns affects only about 30% of photosensitive patients (37). Clinical pattern sensitivity is, however, rare, and patients often may not make the association, the family may be unaware of it, and physicians may not inquire about it.

Wilkins and coworkers (36,38,88–90) studied the properties of epileptogenic patterns, isolating visual arc size, brightness, contrast, orientation, duty cycle, and sensitivity to movement and binocularity. They concluded that the seizures involve excitation and synchronization of a sufficiently large number of cells in the primary visual cortex with subsequent generalization. We can compare this with the previously described animal experiments and Wieser's theory. Pattern sensitivity optimally requires binocular viewing, and treatment may be aided by avoidance of environmental stimuli (admittedly often impractical) as well as by alternating occlusion of one eye with polarizing spectacles and increased distance from the television set. Spontaneous attacks or a high degree of pattern sensitivity requires antiepileptic drug treatment, as described earlier.

Seizures Induced by Eye Closure

Although eye closure may evoke paroxysmal activity in photosensitive patients, especially those with EMA, seizures induced by eye closure are unusual. They are rare in patients not sensitive to simple flash IPS. Seizures with eye closure are typically absences or myoclonic attacks and are not specific for any one cause. They must be distinguished from rare seizures occurring with eyes closed or with loss of central fixation. Panayiotopoulos and colleagues (67,91) studied these extensively and described syndromes in which they occur.

Self-Induced Seizures

Photosensitive patients may induce seizures with maneuvers that do not produce flicker. These attacks are similar to flicker-induced seizures, but the inducing behaviors are not. Pattern-sensitive patients may be irresistibly drawn to television screens, which they must approach closely to resolve the epileptogenic pattern of vibrating lines, or they may spend hours gazing through venetian blinds or at other sources of pattern stimulation. Those sensitive to eye closure have been observed to use forceful slow upward gaze with eyelid flutter (92,93) to induce paroxysmal EEG discharge and, at times, frank seizures. These patients are often children, who describe the responses as pleasant: "as nice as being hugged, but not as nice as eating pudding," (C.D. Binnie, personal communication). We have observed that these tonic eyeball movements are always associated with spike-and-wave activity in children.

As they mature, their eyeball movements may persist but no longer elicit epileptiform activity and can be likened to a tic learned in response to positive reinforcement. These observations and the compulsive seizure-inducing behavior of many such patients suggest that, as in flicker-induced seizures, the self-induced attacks give pleasure or relieve stress. Experience suggests that treatment is similarly difficult (79).

SEIZURES INDUCED BY TELEVISION AND OTHER ELECTRONIC SCREENS

Television is probably the most common environmental trigger of photosensitive seizures. A television screen produces flicker at the mains frequency, generating IPS at 60 Hz in North America and 50 Hz in Europe. Jeavons and Harding (61) found that photosensitivity was more common at the lower frequency, which partly explained the higher incidence of television-induced seizures in Europe than in North America. Television-induced seizures, however, are not related to alternating current (AC) frequency flicker alone. Wilkins and coworkers (89,90) described two types of television-sensitive patients: those sensitive to IPS at 50 Hz, who apparently were sensitive to whole-screen flicker even at distances greater than 1 m from the screen, and patients not sensitive to the "mains" or "AC" frequency flicker but who responded to the vibrating pattern of interleaved lines at half the AC frequency, which can be discerned only near the screen. They emphasized that increased distance from the screen decreased the ability to resolve the line pattern and that a small screen evoked less epileptiform activity than a large one. Binocular viewing was also needed to trigger attacks.

Domestic video games using the home television screen, viewed at close distances for long periods and sometimes under conditions of sleep deprivation and possible alcohol or nonmedical drug use, can thus not surprisingly trigger seizures in predisposed individuals, some of whom were not known to be photosensitive. Some individuals are not photosensitive and may have seizures by chance or induced by thinking or other factors. These events, however, have caused many patients with epilepsy to believe erroneously that they are at risk from video games, and they need accurate information about their personal risk (94).

Not all seizures triggered by television and similar screens fit this pattern. Seizures can be triggered even at greater distances and by noninterlaced screens without inherent flicker; flashing or patterned screen content has been implicated in such episodes. Nevertheless, the 50/25-Hz frequency appears to be a powerful determinant of screen sensitivity, and in countries with 50-Hz AC, special 100-Hz television sets have been shown to greatly reduce the risk of attacks (95). Other preventive measures include watching a small screen from afar in a well-lighted room, using a remote control to avoid approaching the set, and covering one eye and looking away if the picture flickers or if myoclonia occurs (96).

Broadcasting of certain forms of flashing or patterned screen content has been responsible for outbreaks of photosensitive seizures, most notably in Japan, where 685 people, mostly children and young adults with no history of epilepsy, were hospitalized after viewing a cartoon (97). Broadcast standards in the United Kingdom and Japan now reduce this risk. Electronic filters have also been proposed (98). Further outbreaks are to be expected if viewers, especially mass audiences of adolescents, are exposed to such screen content when guidelines do not exist or are violated (99).

SEIZURES INDUCED BY COMPLEX NONVISUAL ACTIVITY

Reflex epilepsy with nonvisual stimuli is rare. Seizures may be classified as those with relatively simple somatosensory triggers and those triggered by complex activity, such as thinking, eating, or listening to music.

Seizures Induced by Thinking

Wilkins and colleagues (39) introduced the term *seizures induced by thinking* to describe a patient who reported seizures induced by mental arithmetic but who proved also to be sensitive to tasks involving manipulation of spatial information with or without any motor activity. Other complex mental activities have been reported to trigger seizures, such as card games and board games such as checkers (British, draughts) or making complex decisions. A rather consistent electroclinical syndrome emerges, most succinctly called seizures induced by thinking, reviewed in Andermann and coworkers (100).

Approximately 80% of patients have more than one trigger, but because EEG monitoring of detailed neuropsychological testing was not always performed, this may be an underestimate. Reading is not usually an effective trigger, and unlike reading epilepsy, most patients also have apparently spontaneous attacks. The seizures are typically generalized myoclonus, absences, or tonic-clonic attacks, and the induced EEG abnormalities are almost always generalized spike-and-wave or polyspike-and-wave activity. Focal spiking is found in approximately 10% of patients, and photosensitivity is seen in approximately 25%. Although numbers are small, most subjects are male. The mean age of onset is 15 years. Family histories of epilepsy are neither typical nor helpful in the diagnosis. Avoidance of triggering stimuli is practical only when activation is related to cards or other games, but drugs effective in idiopathic generalized epilepsies have been most useful. Epileptogenic tasks in these patients involve the processing of spatial information and possibly sequential decisions.

The generalized seizures and EEG discharges may depend on initial involvement of parietal or, possibly, frontal cortex and subsequent generalization, much as pattern-sensitive seizures depend on initial activation of primary visual cortex (39). Recent studies provide more detail on the cerebral representation of calculation and spatial thought and document a bilateral functional network activated by such tasks (101).

Praxis-Induced Seizures

Japanese investigators (102) have described praxis-induced seizures as myoclonic seizures, absences, or generalized convulsions triggered by activities as in seizures induced by thinking, but with the difference that precipitation depends on using a part of the body to perform the task (e.g., typing). Hand or finger movements without "action-programming activity" (defined as "higher mental activity requiring hand movement" and apparently synonymous with praxis) are not effective triggers (103). The EEG responses consist of bisynchronous spike or polyspike-and-wave bursts at times predominant over centroparietal regions. Most subjects have JME; some have another idiopathic generalized epilepsy syndrome. None have clear-cut localization-related epilepsy. In its milder forms, such as the morning myoclonic jerk of the arm manipulating a utensil (M. Seino, personal communication, 1999), this phenomenon resembles cortical reflex myoclonus as part of a "continuum of epileptic activity centered on the sensorimotor cortex" (104). It also appears to be another manifestation of triggering of a generalized or bilateral epileptiform response by a local or functional trigger, in this case requiring participation of the rolandic region of one or both hemispheres, which may be regionally hyperexcitable in JME (105). The seizures of idiopathic generalized epilepsy may involve only selected thalamocortical networks (106).

Reading Epilepsy

Bickford and colleagues (107) first identified primary and secondary forms of reading epilepsy. The primary form consists of attacks triggered exclusively by reading, without spontaneous seizures. Age at onset is typically between 12 and 25 years. Patients report characteristic jaw jerks or clicks. If reading continues, a generalized convulsion may occur. Prolonged reading-induced partial seizures with ictal dyslexia or speech arrest, bilateral myoclonic seizures, and absences are reported. The resting electroencephalogram is normal, but during reading, abnormal paroxysmal activity is recorded, often consisting of sharp theta activity that may be generalized (92,107–110) or localized to either temporoparietal region, especially on the dominant side (111–113) These abnormalities frequently correlate with the jaw jerks. Bilateral or asymmetric myoclonic attacks may also occur with bilaterally synchronous spike-and-wave activity.

Patients with primary reading epilepsy are typically developmentally normal, with normal neurologic examinations. No structural lesions have been demonstrated. A family history of epilepsy is common, and familial reading epilepsy has been reported (112–114). Patients with secondary reading epilepsy also have spontaneous seizures without jaw jerking and often have an abnormal baseline electroencephalogram. Primary reading epilepsy is classified as an idiopathic, age-related, localization-related epilepsy. This definition is being revised, and some investigators believe that it does not fully reflect the variety of associated electroclinical patterns.

The triggering stimulus in reading epilepsy is unknown. Bickford and coworkers (107) proposed that normal sensory stimuli influenced some hyperexcitable cortical focus, and Wolf (48) suggested that this "locus-relation" involved maturational change in the region of the angular gyrus of the dominant hemisphere. Critchley and colleagues (111) emphasized several factors: the visual pattern of printed words; attention; proprioceptive input from jaw and extraocular muscles; and conditioning. Forster (44) theorized that the seizures were evoked by higher cognitive functions; however, patients with primary reading epilepsy are not photosensitive, deny other precipitating cognitive stimuli, and do not appear to have thinking-induced seizures. Patients with the latter almost always deny activation by reading. A single patient with otherwise clear-cut primary reading epilepsy reported induction by card playing while drinking beer (115). Comprehension of the material being read is essential in some cases and irrelevant in others, suggesting that attention is not sufficient to precipitate seizures. Studies suggest that increased difficulty, complexity, or duration of a task increases the chance of EEG or clinical activation (40,41). Functional imaging shows that these seizures result from activation of parts of a speech and language network in both hemispheres (116), confirming that the hyperexcitable neuronal tissue forming the critical mass is not necessarily contiguous but is functionally linked, as discussed by Wolf (41) and by Rémillard and coworkers (117). A mechanism similar to that in pattern-sensitive epilepsy, in which generalized activity is activated by the occipital cortical stimuli, may operate in some cases of primary reading epilepsy in which bilateral myoclonic attacks or bilaterally synchronous epileptiform activity is triggered. Primary reading epilepsy generally responds well to valproate, and benzodiazepines or lamotrigine are expected to be useful as well; however, patients often decline treatment, especially if they only have jaw jerks.

Language-Induced Epilepsy

Geschwind and Sherwin (118) described a patient whose seizures were induced by three components of language: speaking, reading, and writing. Other cases have been reported since. Similar to those in primary reading epilepsy,

the seizures consist of jaw jerks, with focal (108,119–121) or generalized (118) abnormal paroxysmal EEG activity during language tasks. In some patients, isolated components of language were the only effective seizure triggers. Writing (122,123), typing (124), listening to spoken language (125), and singing or recitation (126) have been reported as isolated triggers. Writing or speaking may activate patients with reading epilepsy (121,127); exceptionally, reading epilepsy activated by card games occurred in one patient (115). We consider activation by drawing (128) to be part of seizures induced by thinking, and other patients believed to have language-induced epilepsy may have thinking-induced seizures. This heterogeneity suggests that the definition of a language-induced epilepsy is not clear-cut. Cases may form part of relatively more stereotyped syndromes of reading epilepsy, whose definition should be broadened. Alternatively, Koutroumanidis and colleagues (116) suggested that primary reading epilepsy might be classified as a variant of a more broadly defined language-induced epilepsy.

Musicogenic Epilepsy

The rare musicogenic epilepsy consists of seizures provoked by hearing music. The music that triggers seizures often is remarkably patient-specific and no consistently epileptogenic features of musical sound can be identified. A startle effect is not required. Many patients have spontaneous attacks as well. Some attacks can be provoked by music and by nonmusical sounds, such as ringing or whirring noises. In some patients, an effective musical stimulus often induces emotional and autonomic manifestations before the clinical seizure begins. Patients may report triggers with personal emotional significance. However, in some patients, the triggers have no particular connotations (129), whereas in others they may (130). Triggers without particular emotional significance can induce the typical autonomic features before the clinical attack (131,132). Establishment of the seizure as a conditioned response has also been suggested (92,130,132, 133), but this view is not generally accepted (134). A case with self-induction possibly motivated by emotional factors has been described (135). Musicogenic attacks may appear only in adulthood, often in the context of a preexisting symptomatic localization-related epilepsy. Many case reports antedate intensive monitoring and modern imaging, but the seizures appear to be simple or complex partial, and epileptiform EEG abnormalities are recorded focally from either temporal lobe.

The pathophysiology of musicogenic epilepsy is obscure. Studies in epileptic subjects not sensitive to music show that musical stimuli may have widespread effects on neuronal activity in human temporal lobes, extending well beyond the rather restricted primary auditory area (136); that different components of music have different effects, possibly with specialized lateralization and localization;

and that the effects of music differ from those of speech (137,138). Components of musical stimuli such as melodic contour and perception of unfamiliar pitch patterns are processed by cortical subsystems rather than by a nonspecific music area of the brain (139–141). Functional imaging of musical perception has been reviewed (142). Wieser and coworkers (143) suggested a right temporal predominance for musicogenic seizures. Right anterior and mesial hyperperfusion during ictal single-photon-emission computed tomography has been documented (143,144). Zifkin and Zatorre (145) note that more complex musical processing tasks activate more cortical and subcortical territory bilaterally, although with right hemisphere predominance. Hyperexcitable cortical areas could be stimulated to different degrees and extents by different musical stimuli in patients sensitive to these triggers. Gloor (146) suggested that responses to limbic stimulation in epileptic subjects depend on widespread neuronal matrices linked through connections that have become strengthened through repeated use. This view is of interest in a consideration of the delay from seizure onset to the development of sensitivity to music and the extent of the networks involved in musical perception.

The extreme specificity of the stimulus in some patients and the delay from stimulus to seizure onset can be useful in preventing attacks but these seizures usually occur in patients with partial seizures, and appropriate antiepileptic drugs are generally required. Intractable seizures should prompt evaluation for surgical treatment.

Seizures Induced by Eating (Eating Epilepsy)

Boudouresques and Gastaut (147) first described eating epilepsy in four patients who experienced seizures after a heavy meal. Gastric distention may have been at least partly responsible for these attacks (148), but most such seizures occur early in a meal and are unrelated to gastric distention (149,150). The clinical characteristics are usually stereotyped in individual patients but there are few common features among patients. Some patients have seizures at the very sight or smell of food, whereas others have them only in the middle of a meal or shortly afterward. In some patients, the seizures may be associated with the emotional or autonomic components of eating; in others, they are associated with sensory afferents from tongue or pharynx. These seizures have also been documented in children, in whom they can be mistaken for gastroesophageal reflux (151).

Seizures with eating are almost always related to a symptomatic partial epilepsy. Cases in whom the seizures were generalized from onset are exceptional (152). Rémillard and colleagues (117) suggest that patients with these seizures and temporolimbic epilepsy are activated by eating from the beginning of their seizure disorder and continue to have most seizures with meals. In contrast, patients with localized extralimbic, usually postcentral,

seizure onset develop reflex activation of seizures later in their course, with less constant triggering by eating and more prominent spontaneous seizures. These patients typically have more obvious lesions and findings on neurologic examination.

The mechanism of eating epilepsy is unclear. Several investigators suggest that interaction of limbic and extralimbic cortices (153) and contributions from subcortical structures, such as hypothalamus (148,154,155), are particularly important. Other proposed triggering mechanisms include a conditioned response, mastication (155), stimulation of the esophagus (156), and satisfaction of a basic drive (152). Rémillard and coworkers (117) suggested that seizures with extralimbic, suprasylvian onset, often involving obvious structural lesions, may be activated by specific thalamocortical afferents. That obvious combinations of several stimuli are required in some cases (157,158) enhances the circumstantial evidence favoring an interaction among cortical areas and diencephalic structures, which in other cases could involve less obvious combinations of stimuli. When the abnormal cortex is located in regions responding to proprioceptive and other sensory afferents (especially lingual, buccal, or pharyngeal) activated by the extensive sensory input generated by a complex behavior such as eating, patients may be more sensitive to the physical manipulation of food, texture, temperature, and chewing. They may also have seizures induced by activities such as brushing teeth. These patients have extralimbic seizure onset. This mechanism may be similar to that described for other proprioceptive or somatosensory-induced seizures (104). A similar mechanism, but with afferents recruiting hyperexcitable temporolimbic structures, may also operate in subjects with temporolimbic seizure onset, who may be more sensitive to gustatory, olfactory, affective, or emotional stimuli or to stimuli arising from more distal parts of the gut. Alerting stimuli have been reported to abolish attacks (159), providing further circumstantial evidence for the participation of an increasing cortical mass and of subcortical influences in some cases of reflex epilepsy.

The extraordinarily high frequency of seizures associated with meals in Sri Lanka (160) may be ascribed to the inclusion of all attacks occurring from 30 minutes before to 30 minutes after eating. This does not correspond to eating epilepsy as defined here.

Proprioceptive-Induced Seizures and Startle Epilepsy

Proprioceptive-induced seizures include those that appear to be evoked by active or passive movements. Gowers (161) first described seizures induced by movement in humans, and they have been characterized as movement-induced seizures. Studies in the monkey by Chauvel and Lamarche (162) suggest that proprioception is the most important trigger and that the term *movement-induced seizures* is incorrect. With a chronic alumina focus in the cortical foot area, spontaneous and reflex seizures have been observed. Reflex motor attacks were triggered by active or passive movement of the contralateral limb and by tapping the hind limb tendons. The stimuli activating proprioceptive afferents to a hyperexcitable cortical area triggered seizures. Seizures could not be elicited in the curarized animal. In humans, focal reflex or posture-induced seizures can be transiently observed in patients with nonketotic hyperglycemia, resolving only with metabolic correction. Interictal focal neurologic deficits are seen as evidence of underlying cortical dysfunction (104,163). Proprioceptive afferents, rather than the observed movements, are implicated in seizure precipitation in animal studies and probably in humans (164), although the case reported by Gabor (165) is a possible exception. Arseni and colleagues (166) and Oller-Daurella and Dini (167) have confirmed the epileptic nature of these attacks.

Startle epilepsy involves seizures induced by sudden and unexpected stimuli (168,169). Typically lateralized and tonic, the seizures are often associated with developmental delay, gross neurologic signs such as hemiplegia, and cerebral lesions (170–172). Computed tomography scans often show unilateral or bilateral mesial frontal lesions (168); patients with normal scans have had dysplastic lesions identified on MRI (173). Electroencephalograms with depth electrodes show initial ictal discharge in the supplementary motor area (174) and mesial frontal cortex (175). These represent a symptomatic localization-related epilepsy and are often medically intractable. Most patients have other spontaneous seizures.

Proprioceptive-induced seizures can be confused with nonepileptic conditions. Clinical and EEG findings should permit differentiation of startle epilepsy from startle disease or hyperekplexia and from other excessive startle disorders (176–178), and should exclude cataplexy and myoclonic epilepsy syndromes. Apparent movement-induced seizures without startle must be distinguished from paroxysmal kinesigenic choreoathetosis, in which movements are clearly tonic and choreoathetoid, consciousness is preserved, and the EEG pattern remains normal during attacks (179).

Seizures Triggered by Somatosensory Stimulation

Seizures may be induced by tapping or rubbing individual regions of the body (104). These are partial seizures, often with initial localized sensory symptoms and tonic features, and typically occur in patients with lesions involving postrolandic cortex. A well-defined trigger zone may be found. Drugs for partial seizures are needed, but the seizures may be intractable and require evaluation for surgery.

Reflex drop attacks elicited by walking (180) are seen rarely in patients with reflex interictal spikes evoked by percussion of the foot (181). We consider these to be a variety of seizures induced by proprioceptive stimulation. They are interesting because, unexpectedly, individuals with the interictal evoked spikes do not usually have such attacks. This disorder probably represents a form of idiopathic localization-related epilepsy of childhood, distinct because of the parietal lobe involvement, though underlying dysplastic lesions cannot be excluded. Participation of a more elaborate network for motor programming cannot be excluded in some cases, especially if the effective stimulus seems restricted to activities such as walking (182).

Touch-Evoked Seizures

Seizures can be evoked by simple touch (i.e., "tap" seizures), apparently unrelated to proprioceptive afferents (183,184), although startle may be important. These reflex generalized myoclonic attacks and associated bilateral spike-and-wave EEG discharges occur without evidence of lateralized lesions; the family history may also be positive (185). These typically occur in normal infants and toddlers and can represent an idiopathic and relatively benign generalized myoclonic epilepsy syndrome rather than a progressive myoclonic encephalopathy (186,187). They usually respond to valproate, but prolonged treatment may not be needed.

Hot Water Epilepsy

Seizures triggered by immersion in hot water were first described in 1945 (188). The condition is rare in Japan, the Americas, and Europe, but seems more common in India (189,190). Little EEG documentation is available, but the epileptic nature of these attacks has been confirmed in some patients (191,192). Indian patients are typically male, with a mean age at onset of 13.4 years, who are reported to have complex partial or generalized tonic-clonic seizures during ritual bathing when jugs of hot water are poured over the head. Startle and vasovagal events cannot be excluded in many cases, nor can they be discounted in some North American, European, and Japanese reports. These cases typically involve younger children than in India, with complex partial seizures occurring as soon as the child is immersed in hot water; sensitivity often diminishes with time (193). A mechanism involving defective thermoregulation has been proposed, and some of the attacks may be a form of situation-related seizure with age-dependent occurrence similar to febrile convulsions (190). However, spontaneous seizures have been reported in subjects in a study performed in Turkey, if the reflex attacks begin after early childhood (194).

Miscellaneous Reflex Seizures

Other unusual reflex stimuli have been described, usually as occasional case reports, but more recently with improved EEG and radiologic documentation. Vestibular stimuli are reported to induce seizures. It is important to exclude startle effects with caloric stimulation, for example, and to take into account the time required for caloric stimulation to be effective (195).

Klass and Daly (196) reported the extraordinary case of a child with generalized seizures self-induced by looking at his own hand. By 4 years of age, medications were withdrawn, and no further seizures, reflex or otherwise, occurred in 26 years of follow-up (196). The electroencephalogram was said to be normal. A similar case has been reported (44).

CONCLUSIONS

Reflex seizures and reflex epilepsy continue to challenge and puzzle neurologists and neurophysiologists. Intensive monitoring and advances in imaging have helped to clarify some of the mechanisms involved in these cases, which must represent some of nature's more complex experiments. Continued progress depends on the skill and imagination of neurologists and on their patients, to whom these studies are really dedicated.

REFERENCES

1. Wilkins AJ. http://www.essex.ac.uk/psychology/overlays/ epilepsy%20POT2.htm
2. Commission on classification and terminology of the international league against epilepsy. Proposal for revised classification of epilepsies and epileptic syndromes. *Epilepsia* 1989;30:389–399.
3. Engel J Jr. A proposed diagnostic scheme for people with epileptic seizures and with epilepsy: report of the ILAE Task Force on Classification and Terminology. *Epilepsia* 2001;42:796–803.
4. Hall M. *Synopsis of the diastaltic nervous system.* London: Joseph Mallet, 1850:112.
5. Gastaut H. Reflex mechanisms in the genesis of epilepsy. *Epilepsia* 1962;3:457–460.
6. Penfield W, Erickson T. *Epilepsy and cerebral localization.* Springfield, IL: Charles C Thomas, 1941:28.
7. Commission on Classification and Terminology of the International League Against Epilepsy. Proposal for classification of epilepsies and epileptic syndromes. *Epilepsia* 1985;26:268–278.
8. Wieser HG. Seizure-inducing and preventing mechanisms. In: Beaumanoir A, Gastaut H, Naquet R, eds. *Reflex seizures and reflex epilepsies.* Geneva: Editions Médecine et Hygiène, 1989:49–60.
9. Henner K. Reflex epileptic mechanisms: conceptions and experiences of a clinical neurologist. *Epilepsia* 1962;3:236–250.
10. Beaumanoir A, Gastaut H, Naquet R, eds. *Reflex seizures and reflex epilepsies.* Geneva: Editions Médecine et Hygiène, 1989:554.
11. Clementi A. Stricninizzazione della sfera corticale visiva ed epilessia sperimentale da stimoli luminosi. *Arch Fisiol* 1929;27:356–387.
12. Clementi A. Stricninizzazione della sfera corticale visiva ed epilessia sperimentale da stimoli acustici. *Arch Fisiol* 1929;27:388–414.
13. Clementi A. Sfera gustativa della corteccia cerebrale del cane ed epilessia sperimentale riflessa a tipo sensoriale gustativo. *Boll Soc Ital Biol* 1935;10:902–904.
14. Moruzzi G. *L'Epilessia sperimentale.* Bologna, Italy: Nicolo Zanichelli, 1946:128.
15. Terzian H, Terzuolo C. Richerche electrofisiologiche sull'epilessia fotica di Clementi. *Arch Fisiol* 1951;5:301–320.
16. Fulchignoni S. Contributo alla conoscenza dell'epilessia sperimentale riflessa per stimoli luminosi. *Riv Pat Nerv Ment* 1938;51:154.
17. Gastaut H, Hunter J. An experimental study of the mechanism of photic activation in idiopathic epilepsy. *Electroencephalogr Clin Neurophysiol* 1950;2:263–287.
18. Gastaut H. L'épilepsie photogénique. *Rev Prat* 1951;1:105–109.
19. Hunter J, Ingvar D. Pathways mediating Metrazol-induced irradiation of visual impulses. *Electroencephalogr Clin Neurophysiol* 1955;7:39–60.
20. Bignall KE, Imbert M. Polysensory and corticocortical projections to the frontal lobe of squirrel and rhesus monkey. *Electroencephalogr Clin Neurophysiol* 1969;26:206–215.
21. Buser P, Ascher P, Bruner J, et al. Aspects of sensory motor reverberations to acoustic and visual stimuli: the role of primary specific cortical areas. In: Moruzzi G, Fessard A, Jasper HH, eds. *Brain mechanisms. Progress in brain research.* Amsterdam: Elsevier, 1963;1:294–322.
22. Crichlow EC, Crawford RD. Epileptiform seizures in domestic fowl, II: intermittent light stimulation and the electroencephalogram. *Can J Physiol Pharmacol* 1974;52:424–429.
23. Johnson DD, Davis HL. Drug responses and brain biochemistry of the Epi mutant chicken. In: Ookawa T, ed. *The brain and behavior of the fowl.* Tokyo: Japan Scientific Society Press, 1983:281–296.
24. Chapman AG, Meldrum BS. Epilepsy-prone mice: genetically determined sound-induced seizures. In: Jobe PC, Laird HE II, eds. *Neurotransmitters and epilepsy.* Clifton, NJ: Humana Press, 1987.
25. Seyfried TN, Glaser GH. A review of mouse mutants as genetic models of epilepsy. *Epilepsia* 1985;26:143–150.
26. Löscher W, Schmidt D. Which animal models should be used in the search for new antiepileptic drugs: a proposal based on experimental and clinical considerations. *Epilepsy Res* 1988;2:145–181.
27. Loskota WJ, Lomax P, Rich ST. The gerbil as a model for the study of the epilepsies: seizure patterns and ontogenesis. *Epilepsia* 1974;15:109–119.
28. Killam KF, Killam EK, Naquet R. An animal model of light sensitive epilepsy. *Electroencephalogr Clin Neurophysiol* 1967;22 (Suppl):497–513.
29. Killam KF, Killam EK, Naquet R. Mise en évidence chez certains singes d'un syndrome myoclonique. *C R Acad Sci (Paris)* 1966;262:1010–1012.
30. Menini C, Silva-Barrat C. The photosensitive epilepsy of the baboon. A model of generalized reflex epilepsy. In: Zifkin BG, Andermann F, Beaumanoir A, Rowan AJ, eds. *Reflex epilepsies and reflex seizures. Advances in neurology,* vol 75. Philadelphia: Lippincott-Raven Press, 1998:29–47.
31. DeSarro GB Nistico G, Meldrum BS. Anticonvulsant properties of flunarizine on reflex and generalized models of epilepsy. *Neuropharmacology* 1986;25:695–701.
32. Pumain R, Menini C, Heinemann U, et al. Chemical synaptic transmission is not necessary for epileptic seizures to persist in the baboon *Papio papio. Exp Neurol* 1985;89:250–258.
33. Lloyd KG, Scatton B, Voltz C, et al. Cerebrospinal fluid amino acid and monoamine metabolite levels of *Papio papio*: correlation with photosensitivity. *Brain Res* 1986;363:390–394.
34. Gloor P, Metrakos J, Metrakos K, et al. Neurophysiological, genetic and biochemical nature of the epileptic diathesis. In: Broughton RJ, ed. *Henri Gastaut and the Marseilles School's contribution to the neurosciences.* Amsterdam: Elsevier, 1982:45–56.
35. Binnie CD, Findlay J, Wilkins AJ. Mechanisms of epileptogenesis in photosensitive epilepsy implied by the effects of moving patterns. *Electroencephalogr Clin Neurophysiol* 1985;61:1–6.
36. Wilkins AJ, Andermann F, Ives J. Stripes, complex cells and seizures: an attempt to determine the locus and nature of the trigger mechanism in pattern-sensitive epilepsy. *Brain* 1975;98:365–380.
37. Wilkins AJ, Binnie CD, Darby CE. Visually induced seizures. *Prog Neurobiol* 1980;15:85–117.
38. Wilkins AJ, Binnie CD, Darby CE. Interhemispheric differences in photosensitive epilepsy, I: pattern sensitivity threshold. *Electroencephalogr Clin Neurophysiol* 1981;52:461–468.
39. Wilkins AJ, Zifkin B, Andermann F, et al. Seizures induced by thinking. *Ann Neurol* 1982;11:608–612.
40. Christie S, Guberman A, Tansley BW, et al. Primary reading epilepsy: investigation of critical seizure-provoking stimuli. *Epilepsia* 1988;29:288–293.

41. Wolf P, Mayer T, Reker M. Reading epilepsy: report of five new cases and further considerations on the pathophysiology. *Seizure* 1998;7:271–279.

42. Wyler AR, Ward AA Jr. Epileptic neurons. In: Lockard JS, Ward AA Jr, eds. *Epilepsy: a window to brain mechanisms.* New York: Raven Press, 1980:51–68.

43. Gastaut H, Régis H, Dongier S, et al. Conditionnement électroencéphalographique des décharges épileptiques et notion d'épilepsie réflexo-conditionnée. *Rev Neurol* 1956;94:829–835.

44. Forster FM. Reflex epilepsy, behavioral therapy and conditional reflexes. Springfield, IL: Charles C Thomas, 1977:318.

45. Gras P, Grosmaire N, Giroud M, et al. Exploration d'un cas d'épilepsie à la lecture par EEG avec électrodes sphénoïdales: rôle des régions temporales dans le déclenchement émotionnel des crises. *Neurophysiol Clin* 1992;22:313–320.

46. Fenwick P. Self-generation of seizures by an action of mind. In: Zifkin BG, Andermann F, Beaumanoir A, Rowan AJ, eds. *Reflex epilepsies and reflex seizures. Advances in neurology,* vol 75. Philadelphia: Lippincott-Raven Press, 1998:87–92.

47. Wolf P. From seizures to syndromes. In: Wolf P, ed. *Epileptic seizures and syndromes.* London: John Libbey, 1994:39–40.

48. Wolf P. Reflex epilepsies and syndrome classification: an argument for considering primary reading epilepsy as an idiopathic localization-related epilepsy. In: Beaumanoir A, Gastaut H, Naquet R, eds. *Reflex seizures and reflex epilepsies.* Geneva: Editions Médecine et Hygiène, 1989:283–288.

49. Woermann FG, Free SL, Koepp MJ, Sisodiya SM, Duncan JS. Abnormal cerebral structure in juvenile myoclonic epilepsy demonstrated with voxel-based analysis of MRI. *Brain* 1999;122:2111–2118.

50. Martinez O, Reisin R, Zifkin BG, Andermann F, Sevlever G. Evidence for reflex activation of experiential complex partial seizures. *Neurology* 2000;56:121–123.

51. Kasteleijn-Nolst Trenité DG. Photosensitivity in epilepsy: electrophysiological and clinical correlates. *Acta Neurol Scand* 1989;125(Suppl):31–49.

52. Newmark ME, Penry JK. *Photosensitivity and epilepsy: a review.* New York: Raven Press, 1979:220.

53. Doose H, Gerken H. On the genetics of EEG anomalies in childhood, IV: photoconvulsive reaction. *Neuropaediatrie* 1973;4:162–171.

54. Waltz S, Stephani U. Inheritance of photosensitivity. *Neuropediatrics* 2000; 31:82–85.

55. Zifkin BG, Kasteleijn-Nolst Trenité D. Reflex epilepsy and reflex seizures of the visual system: a clinical review. *Epileptic Disord* 2000;2:129–136.

56. Kasteleijn-Nolst Trenité DGA. Reflex seizures induced by intermittent light stimulation. In: Zifkin BG, Andermann F, Beaumanoir A, Rowan AJ, eds. *Reflex epilepsies and reflex seizures. Advances in neurology,* vol 75. Philadelphia: Lippincott-Raven Press, 1998:99–121.

57. Jeavons PM. Photosensitive epilepsy. In: Laidlaw J, Richens A, eds. *A textbook of epilepsy,* 2nd ed. Edinburgh: Churchill Livingstone, 1982:195–210.

58. DeMarco P, Ghersini L. Videogames and epilepsy. *Dev Med Child Neurol* 1985;27:519–521.

59. Kasteleijn-Nolst Trenité DGA, Dekker E, Spekreijse S, et al. Role of television, video games and computers in epileptic photosensitive patients: preliminary results. *Epilepsia* 1994;35(Suppl 7):37.

60. Harding GFA, Jeavons PM. *Photosensitive epilepsy.* London: MacKeith Press, 1994.

61. Jeavons PM, Harding GFA. Photosensitive epilepsy. In: *Clinics in developmental medicine.* London: Heinemann Medical, 1975:56–121.

62. Aso K, Watanabe K, Negoro T, et al. Photosensitive partial seizure: the origin of abnormal discharges. *J Epilepsy* 1988;1:87–93.

63. Rubboli G, Michelucci R, Ambrosetto G, et al. Le crisi indotte dalla televisione: epilessia generalizzata od occipitale? *Boll Lega Ital Epil* 1988;6263:207–208.

64. Guerrini R, Bonanni P, Parmeggiani L, et al. Induction of partial seizures by visual stimulation. In: Zifkin BG, Andermann F, Beaumanoir A, Rowan AJ, eds. *Reflex epilepsies and reflex seizures. Advances in neurology,* vol 75. Philadelphia: Lippincott-Raven Press, 1998:159–178.

65. Hennessy M, Binnie CD. Photogenic partial seizures. *Epilepsia* 2000;41:59–64.

66. Berkovic SF, Andermann F, Carpenter S, et al. Progressive myoclonus epilepsies: specific causes and diagnosis. *N Engl J Med* 1986;315:296–305.

67. Panayiotopoulos CP. Fixation-off, scotosensitive, and other visual-related epilepsies. In: Zifkin BG, Andermann F, Beaumanoir A, Rowan AJ, eds. *Reflex epilepsies and reflex seizures. Advances in neurology,* vol 75. Philadelphia: Lippincott-Raven Press, 1998:139–157.

68. Wilkins AJ, Darby CE, Binnie CD. Optical treatment of photosensitive epilepsy. *Electroencephalogr Clin Neurophysiol* 1977;43:577.

69. Capovilla G, Beccaria F, Romeo A, Veggiotti P, Canger R, Paladin F. Effectiveness of a particular blue lens on photoparoxysmal response in photosensitive epileptic patients. *Ital J Neurol Sci.* 1999;20:161–166.

70. Wilkins AJ, Baker A, Amin D, et al. Treatment of photosensitive epilepsy using coloured glasses. *Seizure* 1999;8:444–449.

71. Harding GFA, Herrick CE, Jeavons PM. A controlled study of the effect of sodium valproate on photosensitive epilepsy and its prognosis. *Epilepsia* 1979;19:555–565.

72. Chapman AG, Horton RW, Meldrum BS. Anticonvulsant action of a 1,5 benzodiazepine, clobazam, in reflex epilepsy. *Epilepsia* 1978;19:293–299.

73. Quesney LF, Andermann F, Gloor P. Dopaminergic mechanism in generalized photosensitive epilepsy. *Neurology* 1981;31:1542–1544.

74. Clemens B. Dopamine agonist treatment of self-induced pattern-sensitive epilepsy: a case report. *Epilepsy Res* 1988;2:340–343.

75. Morimoto T, Hayakawa T, Sugie H, et al. Epileptic seizures precipitated by constant light, movement in daily life, and hot water immersion. *Epilepsia* 1985;26:237–242.

76. Harding GF, Edson A, Jeavons PM. Persistence of photosensitivity. *Epilepsia* 1997;38:663–669.

77. Radovici A, Misirliou V, Gluckman M. Épilepsie réflexe provoquée par éxcitations optiques des rayons solaires. *Rev Neurol* 1932;1:1305–1308.

78. Andermann K, Berman S, Cooke PM, et al. Self-induced epilepsy. A collection of self-induced epilepsy cases compared with some other photoconvulsive cases. *Arch Neurol* 1962;6:49–65.

79. Binnie CD. Self-induction of seizures: the ultimate noncompliance. *Epilepsy Res* 1988;1(Suppl):153–158.

80. Kasteleijn-Nolst Trenité DG, Binnie CD, Overweg J, et al. Treatment of self-induction in epileptic patients: who wants it? In: Beaumanoir A, Gastaut H, Naquet R, eds. *Reflex seizures and reflex epilepsies.* Geneva: Editions Médecine et Hygiène, 1989:439–446.

81. Lerman P, Kivity S. Self-induced photogenic epilepsy: a report of 14 cases. In: Beaumanoir A, Gastaut H, Naquet R, eds. *Reflex seizures and reflex epilepsies.* Geneva: Editions Médecine et Hygiène, 1989:379–384.

82. Tassinari CA, Rubboli G, Rizzi R, et al. Self-induction of visually induced seizures. In: Zifkin BG, Andermann F, Beaumanoir A, Rowan AJ, eds. *Reflex epilepsies and reflex seizures. Advances in neurology,* vol 75. Philadelphia: Lippincott-Raven Press, 1998:179–192.

83. Watanabe K, Negoro T, Matsumoto A, et al. Self-induced photogenic epilepsy in infants. *Arch Neurol* 1985;42:406–407.

84. Olds J, Milner P. Positive reinforcement produced by electrical stimulation of septal area and other areas of rat brain. *J Comp Physiol Psychol* 1954;47:419–427.

85. Ehret R, Schneider E. Photogene Epilepsie mit suchtartiger Selbstauslosung kleiner Anfälle und wiederholten Sexualdelikten. *Arch Psychiatr Nervenkr* 1961;202:75–94.

86. Faught E, Falgout J, Nidiffer FD. Self-induced photosensitive absence seizures with ictal pleasure. *Arch Neurol* 1986;43:408–410.

87. Overweg J, Binnie CD. Pharmacotherapy of self-induced seizures [abstract]. In: *The 12th Epilepsy International Symposium.* Copenhagen, Denmark, 1980.

88. Wilkins AJ, Binnie CD, Darby CE, et al. Epileptic and nonepileptic sensitivity to light. In: Beaumanoir A, Gastaut H, Naquet R, eds. *Reflex seizures and reflex epilepsies.* Geneva: Editions Médecine et Hygiène, 1989:153–162.

89. Wilkins AJ, Darby CE, Binnie CD. Neurophysiological aspects of pattern-sensitive epilepsy. *Brain* 1979;102:125.

90. Wilkins AJ, Darby CE, Binnie CD, et al. Television epilepsy: the role of pattern. *Electroencephalogr Clin Neurophysiol* 1979;47:163–171.

91. Giannakodimos S, Panayiotopoulos CP. Eyelid myoclonia with absences in adults: a clinical and video-EEG study. *Epilepsia* 1996;37:36–44.

92. Gastaut H, Tassinari CA. Triggering mechanisms in epilepsy: the electroclinical point of view. *Epilepsia* 1966;7:85–138.

93. Green JB. Self-induced seizures: clinical and electroencephalographic studies. *Arch Neurol* 1966;15:579–586.

94. Millett CJ, Fish DR, Thompson PJ. A survey of epilepsy-patient perceptions of video-game material/electronic screens and other factors as seizure precipitants. *Seizure* 1997;6:457–459.

95. Ricci S, Vigevano F, Manfredi M, et al. Epilepsy provoked by television and video games: safety of 100-Hz screens. *Neurology* 1998;50:790–793.

96. Binnie CD, Wilkins AJ. Visually induced seizures not caused by flicker (intermittent light stimulation). In: Zifkin BG, Andermann F, Beaumanoir A, Rowan AJ, eds. *Reflex epilepsies and reflex seizures. Advances in neurology,* vol 75. Philadelphia: Lippincott-Raven Press, 1998:123–138.

97. Ishida S, Yamashita Y, Matsuishi T, et al. Photosensitive seizures provoked while viewing "Pocket Monsters," a made-for-television animation program in Japan. *Epilepsia* 1998;39:1340–1344.

98. Takahashi T, Kamijo K, Takaki Y, Yamazaki T. Suppressive efficacies by adaptive temporal filtering system on photoparoxysmal response elicited by flickering pattern stimulation. *Epilepsia* 2002;43:530–534.

99. Harding GFA. TV can be bad for your health. *Nat Med* 1998;4:265–267.

100. Andermann F, Zifkin BG, Andermann E. Epilepsy induced by thinking and spatial tasks. In: Zifkin BG, Andermann F, Beaumanoir A, Rowan AJ, eds. *Reflex epilepsies and reflex seizures. Advances in neurology,* vol 75. Philadelphia: Lippincott-Raven Press, 1998:263–272.

101. Stanescu-Cosson R, Pinel P, van De Moortele PF, Le Bihan D, Cohen L, Dehaene S. Understanding dissociations in dyscalculia: a brain imaging study of the impact of number size on the cerebral networks for exact and approximate calculation. *Brain* 2000;123:2240–2255.

102. Inoue Y, Seino M, Tanaka M, et al. Praxis-induced epilepsy. In: Wolf P, ed. *Epileptic seizures and syndromes.* London: John Libbey, 1994:81–91.

103. Matsuoka H, Takahashi T, Sasaki M, et al. Neuropsychological EEG activation in patients with epilepsy. *Brain* 2000;123:318–330.

104. Vignal J-P, Biraben A, Chauvel PY, et al. Reflex partial seizures of sensorimotor cortex (including cortical reflex myoclonus and startle epilepsy). In: Zifkin BG, Andermann F, Beaumanoir A, Rowan AJ, eds. *Reflex epilepsies and reflex seizures. Advances in neurology,* vol 75. Philadelphia:Lippincott-Raven Press, 1998:207–226.

105. Wolf P. Regional manifestation of idiopathic epilepsy. Introduction. In: Wolf P, ed. *Epileptic seizures and syndromes.* London: John Libbey, 1994:265–267.

106. Blumenfeld H. From molecules to networks: cortical/subcortical interactions in the pathophysiology of idiopathic generalized epilepsy. *Epilepsia* 2003;44(Suppl 2):7–15.

107. Bickford RG, Whelan JL, Klass DW, et al. Reading epilepsy: clinical and electroencephalographic studies of a new syndrome. *Trans Am Neurol Assoc* 1956;81:100–102.

108. Stoupel N. On the reflex epilepsies: epilepsy caused by reading. *Electroencephalogr Clin Neurophysiol* 1968;25:416–417.

109. Kartsounis LD. Comprehension as the effective trigger in a case of primary reading epilepsy. *J Neurol Neurosurg Psychiatry* 1988;51:128–130.

110. Newman PK, Longley BP. Reading epilepsy. *Arch Neurol* 1984;41:13–14.

111. Critchley M, Cobb W, Sears TA. On reading epilepsy. *Epilepsia* 1959;1:403–417.

112. Daly RF, Forster FM. Inheritance of reading epilepsy. *Neurology* 1975;25:1051–1054.

113. Ramani V. Reading epilepsy. In: Zifkin BG, Andermann F, Beaumanoir A, Rowan AJ, eds. *Reflex epilepsies and reflex seizures.*

Advances in neurology, vol 75. Philadelphia: Lippincott-Raven Press, 1998:241–262.

114. Matthews WB, Wright FK. Hereditary primary reading epilepsy. *Neurology* 1967;17:919–921.

115. Bingel A. Reading epilepsy. *Neurology* 1957;7:752–756.

116. Koutroumanidis M, Koepp MJ, Richardson MP, et al. The variants of reading epilepsy. A clinical and video-EEG study of 17 patients with reading-induced seizures. *Brain* 1998;121:1409–1427.

117. Rémillard GM, Zifkin BG, Andermann F. Seizures induced by eating. In: Zifkin BG, Andermann F, Beaumanoir A, Rowan AJ, eds. *Reflex epilepsies and reflex seizures. Advances in neurology,* vol 75. Philadelphia: Lippincott-Raven Press, 1998:227–240.

118. Geschwind N, Sherwin I. Language-induced epilepsy. *Arch Neurol* 1967;16:25–31.

119. Bennett DR, Mavor H, Jarcho LW. Language-induced epilepsy: report of a case. *Electroencephalogr Clin Neurophysiol* 1971;30:159.

120. Brooks JE, Jirauch PM. Primary reading epilepsy: a misnomer. *Arch Neurol* 1971;25:97–104.

121. Lee SI, Sutherling WW, Persing JA, et al. Language-induced seizures. A case of cortical origin. *Arch Neurol* 1980;37:433–436.

122. Asbury AK, Prensky AL. Graphogenic epilepsy. *Trans Am Neurol Assoc* 1963;88:193–194.

123. Sharbrough FW, Westmoreland B. Writing epilepsy. *Electroencephalogr Clin Neurophysiol* 1977;43:506.

124. Cirignotta F, Zucconi M, Mondini S, et al. Writing epilepsy. *Clin Electroencephalogr* 1986;17:21–23.

125. Tsuzuki H, Kasuga I. Paroxysmal discharges triggered by hearing spoken language. *Epilepsia* 1978;19:147–154.

126. Herskowitz J, Rosman NP, Geschwind N. Seizures induced by singing and recitation: a unique form of reflex epilepsy in childhood. *Arch Neurol* 1984;41:1102–1103.

127. Saenz-Lope E, Herranz-Tanarro FJ, Masdeu JC. Primary reading epilepsy. *Epilepsia* 1985;26:649–656.

128. Brenner RP, Seelinger DF. Drawing-induced seizures. *Arch Neurol* 1979;36:515–516.

129. Brien SE, Murray TJ. Musicogenic epilepsy. *Can Med Assoc J* 1984;131:1255–1258.

130. Jallon P, Heraut LA, Vanelle JM. Musicogenic epilepsy. In: Beaumanoir A, Gastaut H, Naquet R, eds. *Reflex seizures and reflex epilepsies.* Geneva: Editions Médecine et Hygiène, 1989:269–274.

131. Critchley M. Musicogenic epilepsy. *Brain* 1937;60:13–27.

132. Scott D. Musicogenic epilepsy. In: Critchley M, Henson RA, eds. *Music and the brain.* London: Heinemann Medical, 1977:354–364.

133. Forster FM, Booker HE, Gascon G. Conditioning in musicogenic epilepsy. *Trans Am Neurol Assoc* 1967;92:236–237.

134. Forster FM. The classification and conditioning treatment of the reflex epilepsies. *Int J Neurol* 1972;9:73–86.

135. Daly DD, Barry MJ Jr. Musicogenic epilepsy. Report of three cases. *Psychosom Med* 1957;19:399–408.

136. Liegeois-Chauvel C, Musolino A, Chauvel P. Localization of the primary auditory area in man. *Brain* 1991;114:139–151.

137. Creutzfeldt O, Ojemann G. Neuronal activity in the human lateral temporal lobe, III: activity changes during music. *Exp Brain Res* 1989;77:490–498.

138. Wieser HG, Mazzola G. Musical consonances and dissonances: are they distinguished independently by the right and left hippocampi? *Neuropsychologia* 1986;24:805–812.

139. Peretz I, Kolinsky R, Tramo R, et al. Functional dissociations following bilateral lesions of auditory cortex. *Brain* 1994;117:1283–1301.

140. Zatorre RJ. Discrimination and recognition of tonal melodies after unilateral cerebral excisions. *Neuropsychologia* 1985;23:31–41.

141. Zatorre RJ, Evans AC, Meyer E. Neural mechanisms underlying melodic perception and memory for pitch. *J Neurosci* 1994;14:1908–1919.

142. Johnsrude IS, Giraud AL, Frackowiak RSJ. Functional imaging of the auditory system: the use of positron emission tomography. *Audiol Neurootol* 2002;7:251–276.

143. Wieser HG, Hungerbühler H, Siegel AM, et al. Musicogenic epilepsy: review of the literature and case report with ictal single photon emission computed tomography. *Epilepsia* 1997;38:200–207.

144. Genc BO, Genc E, Tastekin G, Iihan N. Musicogenic epilepsy with ictal single photon emission computed tomography

(SPECT): could these cases contribute to our knowledge of music processing? *Eur J Neurol* 2001;8:191–194.

145. Zifkin BG, Zatorre R. Musicogenic epilepsy. In: Zifkin BG, Andermann F, Beaumanoir A, Rowan AJ, eds. *Reflex epilepsies and reflex seizures. Advances in neurology*, vol 75. Philadelphia: Lippincott-Raven Press, 1998:273–281.

146. Gloor P. Experiential phenomena of temporal lobe epilepsy. Facts and hypotheses. *Brain* 1990;113:1673–1694.

147. Boudouresques J, Gastaut H. Le mécanisme réflexe de certaines épilepsies temporales. *Rev Neurol* 1954;90:157–158.

148. Gastaut H, Poirier F. Experimental, or "reflex," induction of seizures: report of a case of abdominal (enteric) epilepsy. *Epilepsia* 1964;5:256–270.

149. Hernandez-Cossio O, Diaz G, Hernandez-Fustes O. A case of eating epilepsy. In: Beaumanoir A, Gastaut H, Naquet R, eds. *Reflex seizures and reflex epilepsies*. Geneva: Editions Médecine et Hygiène, 1989:301–304.

150. Loiseau P, Guyot M, Loiseau H, et al. Eating seizures. *Epilepsia* 1986;27:161–163.

151. Plouin P, Ponsot C, Jalin C. Eating seizures in a three year old child. In: Beaumanoir A, Gastaut H, Naquet R, eds. *Reflex seizures and reflex epilepsies*. Geneva: Editions Médecine et Hygiène, 1989:309–313.

152. Cirignotta F, Marcacci G, Lugaresi E. Epileptic seizures precipitated by eating. *Epilepsia* 1977;18:445–449.

153. Fiol ME, Leppik IE, Pretzel K. Eating epilepsy: EEG and clinical study. *Epilepsia* 1986;27:441–445.

154. Robertson WC, Fariello RG. Eating epilepsy with a deep forebrain glioma. *Ann Neurol* 1979;6:271–273.

155. Scollo-Lavizzari G, Hess R. Sensory precipitation of epileptic seizures: report on two unusual cases. *Epilepsia* 1967;8:157–161.

156. Forster FM. Epilepsy associated with eating. *Trans Am Neurol Assoc* 1971;96:106–107.

157. Aguglia U, Tinuper P. Eating seizures. *Eur Neurol* 1983;22: 227–231.

158. Reder AT, Wright FS. Epilepsy evoked by eating: the role of peripheral input. *Neurology* 1982;32:1065–1069.

159. Ganga A, Sechi GP, Porcella V, et al. Eating seizures and distraction-arousal functions. *Eur Neurol* 1988;28:167–170.

160. Senanayake N. Eating epilepsy—a reappraisal. *Epilepsy Res* 1990;5:74–79.

161. Gowers WR. *Epilepsy and other chronic convulsive diseases: their causes, symptoms and treatment.* London: JA Churchill, 1901:320.

162. Chauvel P, Lamarche M. Analyse d'une 'épilepsie du mouvement' chez un singe porteur d'un foyer rolandique. *Neurochirurgie* 1975;21:121–137.

163. Singh BM, Gupta DR, Strobos RJ. Nonketotic hyperglycemia and epilepsia partialis continua. *Arch Neurol* 1973;29:187–190.

164. Rosen I, Fehling C, Sedgwick M, et al. Focal reflex epilepsy with myoclonus: electrophysiological investigation and therapeutic implications. *Electroencephalogr Clin Neurophysiol* 1977;42:95–106.

165. Gabor AJ. Focal seizures induced by movement without sensory feedback mechanisms. *Electroencephalogr Clin Neurophysiol* 1974; 36:403–408.

166. Arseni C, Stoica I, Serbanescu T. Electroclinical investigations on the role of proprioceptive stimuli in the onset and arrest of convulsive epileptic paroxysms. *Epilepsia* 1967;8:162–170.

167. Oller-Daurella L, Dini J. Las crisis epilepticas desencadenadas por movimientos voluntarios. *Med Clin* 1970;54:189–196.

168. Aguglia U, Tinuper P, Gastaut H. Startle-induced epileptic seizures. *Epilepsia* 1984;25:712–720.

169. Alajouanine T, Gastaut H. La syncinésie-sursaut et l'épilepsie-sursaut à déclenchement sensoriel ou sensitif inopiné. *Rev Neurol* 1955;93:29–41.

170. Falconer MA, Driver MV, Serafetinides EA. Seizures induced by movement: report of a case relieved by operation. *J Neurol Neurosurg Psychiatry* 1963;26:300–307.

171. Lishman WA, Symonds CP, Whitty CWM, et al. Seizures induced by movement. *Brain* 1962;85:93–108.

172. Whitty CWM, Lishman WA, Fitzgibbon JP. Seizures induced by movement: a form of reflex epilepsy. *Lancet* 1964;1:1403–1405.

173. Manford MR, Fish DR, Shorvon SD. Startle provoked epileptic seizures: features in 19 patients. *J Neurol Neurosurg Psychiatry* 1996;61:151–156.

174. Bancaud J, Talairach J, Lamarche M, et al. Hypothèses neurophysiopathologiques sur l'épilepsie-sursaut chez l'homme. *Rev Neurol* 1975;131:559–571.

175. Bancaud J, Talairach J, Bonis A. Physiopathogénie des épilepsies-sursaut (à propos d'une épilepsie de l'aire motrice supplémentaire). *Rev Neurol* 1967;117:441–453.

176. Andermann F, Andermann E. Excessive startle syndromes: startle disease, jumping, and startle epilepsy. *Adv Neurol* 1986;43: 321–338.

177. Gastaut H, Villeneuve A. The startle disease or hyperekplexia: pathological surprise reaction. *J Neurol Sci* 1967;5:523–542.

178. Saenz-Lope E, Herranz-Tanarro FJ, Masdeu JC, et al. Hyperekplexia: a syndrome of pathological startle responses. *Ann Neurol* 1984; 15:36–41.

179. Bhatia KP. The paroxysmal dyskinesias. *J Neurol* 1999;246: 149–155.

180. Di Capua M, Vigevano F, Tassinari CA. Drop seizures reflex to walking. In: Beaumanoir A, Gastaut H, Naquet R, eds. *Reflex seizures and reflex epilepsies*. Geneva: Editions Médecine et Hygiène, 1989:83–88.

181. DeMarco P, Tassinari CA. Extreme somatosensory evoked potential (ESEP): an EEG sign forecasting a possible occurrence of seizures in children. *Epilepsia* 1981;22:569–575.

182. Iriarte J, Sanchez-Carpintero R, Schlumberger E, Narbona J, Viteri C, Artieda J. Gait epilepsy. A case report of gait-induced seizures. *Epilepsia* 2001;42:1087–1090.

183. Ravindran M. Single case study. Contact epilepsy: a rare form of reflex epilepsy. *J Nerv Ment Dis* 1978;166:219–221.

184. Schmidt G, Todt H. Durch taktile und viscerale Reize ausgeloste Reflexepilepsie beim Kind. *Kinderartzl Praxis* 1979;47:482–487.

185. Ricci S, Cusmai R, Fusco L, et al. Reflex myoclonic epilepsy of the first year of life (abstract). *Epilepsia* 1993;34(Suppl 6):47.

186. Deonna T. Reflex seizures with somatosensory precipitation. Clinical and electroencephalographic patterns and differential diagnosis, with emphasis on reflex myoclonic epilepsy of infancy. In: Zifkin BG, Andermann F, Beaumanoir A, Rowan AJ, eds. *Reflex epilepsies and reflex seizures. Advances in neurology*, vol 75. Philadelphia: Lippincott-Raven Press, 1998:193–206.

187. Revol M, Isnard H, Beaumanoir A, et al. Touch evoked myoclonic seizures in infancy. In: Beaumanoir A, Gastaut H, Naquet R, eds. *Reflex seizures and reflex epilepsies*. Geneva: Editions Médecine et Hygiène, 1989:103–108.

188. Allen IM. Observations on cases of reflex epilepsy. *N Z Med J* 1945;44:135–142.

189. Satishchandra P, Ullal GR, Shankar SK. Hot water epilepsy. In: Zifkin BG, Andermann F, Beaumanoir A, Rowan AJ, eds. *Reflex epilepsies and reflex seizures. Advances in neurology*, vol 75. Philadelphia: Lippincott-Raven Press, 1998:283–293.

190. Szymonowicz W, Meloff KL. Hot water epilepsy. *Can J Neurol Sci* 1978;5:247–251.

191. Roos RAC, van Dijk JG. Reflex epilepsy induced by immersion in hot water. *Eur Neurol* 1988;28:6–10.

192. Shaw NJ, Livingston JH, Minus RA, et al. Epilepsy precipitated by bathing. *Dev Med Child Neurol* 1988;30:108–114.

193. Ioos C, Fohlen M, Villeneuve N, et al. Hot water epilepsy: a benign and unrecognized form. *J Child Neurol* 2000;15:125–128.

194. Bebek N, Gurses C, Gokyigit A, Baykan B, Ozkara C, Dervent A. Hot water epilepsy: clinical and electrophysiologic findings based on 21 cases. *Epilepsia* 2001;42:1180–1184.

195. Karbowski K. Epileptic seizures induced by vestibular and auditory stimuli. In: Beaumanoir A, Gastaut H, Naquet R, eds. *Reflex seizures and reflex epilepsies*. Geneva: Editions Médecine et Hygiène, 1989: 255–260.

196. Klass DW. Self-induced seizures: long-term follow-up of two unusual cases. In: Beaumanoir A, Gastaut H, Naquet R, eds. *Reflex seizures and reflex epilepsies*. Geneva: Editions Médecine et Hygiène, 1989:369–378.

Less Common Epilepsy Syndromes and Epilepsy Associated with Chromosomal Abnormalities

31

Sophia Varadkar   *J. Helen Cross*

The past 10 years have seen a dramatic increase in the number of described epilepsy syndromes, as evidenced by the proposed revisiting of the International League Against Epilepsy (ILAE) classification (2001). Debate over the revised classification continues, centering, in particular, on when a new syndrome should be "accepted" as opposed to "proposed." Several epilepsy syndromes are described on the basis of specific clinical, neurophysiologic, and neuroimaging findings, and some are not included in the ILAE classification (2001). This chapter discusses rare but well-defined epilepsy syndromes, mainly those of early infancy, but also those associated with chromosomal abnormalities and hemiconvulsion-hemiplegia-epilepsy (HHE).

EPILEPSIES IN INFANCY

Epilepsy in infancy remains a challenge, both in diagnosis (symptomatic as opposed to idiopathic syndromes) and in treatment. In general, epilepsy during the first year of life is widely believed to carry a poor prognosis for seizure control and developmental outcome. However, a group of more benign epilepsies probably are underdiagnosed in view of their prompt response to medication and good developmental outcome.

Migrating partial seizures of infancy, early infantile epileptic encephalopathy (EIEE), and early myoclonic encephalopathy (EME) are aggressive, resistant syndromes that have a devastating impact on neurodevelopment. EIEE and EME are characterized by burst suppression on the electroencephalogram (EEG). Differentiating them from infantile spasms and other malignant epilepsies has therapeutic and prognostic implications. EIEE, in particular, has led to the concept of "age-dependent epileptic encephalopathy," a disorder that evolves to infantile spasms and later to Lennox-Gastaut syndrome (1,2).

Benign myoclonic epilepsy of infancy (BMEI) and benign partial epilepsy of infancy share features with these aggressive syndromes but have a more favorable neurodevelopmental outcome and respond better to treatment. Both BMEI and severe myoclonic epilepsy of infancy (SMEI) may follow febrile convulsions but have a very different course. Distinguishing between them, however, may require initiation of treatment and observation over time.

Symptomatic Generalized Epilepsies

Early Myoclonic Encephalopathy

EME, like EIEE, begins neonatally and carries a poor prognosis (3). It affects both sexes equally, and familial cases have been reported. Because EME is associated with inherited metabolic disorders, such as (most commonly) nonketotic hyperglycinemia, propionic aciduria, methyl-malonic acidemia, D-glycine acidemia, and pyridoxine dependence (4,5), careful metabolic investigation of all cases is required.

Seizures always begin before age 3 months, although overall onset is later than that in EIEE. Whereas the main seizure type in EIEE is tonic spasms, often erratic myoclonus (Fig. 31.1) and frequent partial seizures predominate in EME (6). Massive myoclonias and tonic spasms are sometimes seen, but erratic myoclonus is not a feature of EIEE. Evolution to infantile spasms has been reported with nonketotic hyperglycinemia (7).

The EEG shows burst suppression that is enhanced by sleep (6,8) and may not always be apparent in wakefulness. This pattern may persist but does not evolve with age.

Response to anticonvulsant medication is poor. Sodium valproate remains the first choice, and lamotrigine in combination may be helpful (9). Many children die by 2 years of age, and neurodevelopmental outcome in survivors is dismal. Continued deterioration to death is expected.

Early Infantile Epileptic Encephalopathy (Ohtahara Syndrome)

Still best known by its eponymous title, EIEE was first reported by Ohtahara in 1976 and is the earliest of the age-dependent epileptic encephalopathies. EIEE is characterized by early tonic seizures, a burst-suppression electroencephalographic pattern, poor response to treatment, and poor neurodevelopmental outcome, with evolution to infantile spasms and Lennox-Gastaut syndrome (1,10,11).

No cause is found in most cases, but many associations have been noted, most frequently structural brain anomalies. Aicardi syndrome, migrational disorders, porencephaly, and hemimegalencephaly are other accompanying conditions. Detailed neuroimaging is always warranted. There is no difference between male and female occurrence, and no familial cases have been reported.

Although seizures may begin on the first day of life, most start in the first month and nearly all by 3 months of age. Mainly tonic, the seizures occur in wakefulness and in sleep, singly or in clusters. Partial, focal motor, hemiconvulsion, and, rarely, myoclonic are other types. The typical burst-suppression pattern is seen during both waking and sleeping states and is periodic and consistent. Bursts of high-voltage slow waves and spikes last 1 to 3 seconds, followed by flattening for 3 to 4 seconds. Both the electroencephalographic pattern and the seizures show an age-dependent evolution: infantile spasms emerge clinically and hypsarrhythmia electrographically, either between 3 and 6 months or between 1 and 3 years of age, with later appearance of Lennox-Gastaut syndrome (12). Seizures are highly resistant to anticonvulsant therapy; corticotropin may produce a partial response and zonisamide is useful (13,14). Structural anomalies may be amenable to epilepsy surgery (15,16). Very poor developmental outcome and death in infancy or severe handicap are expected.

Migrating Partial Seizures of Infancy

This rare syndrome, beginning in the first 6 months of life, was first described by Coppola and coworkers in 1995, and

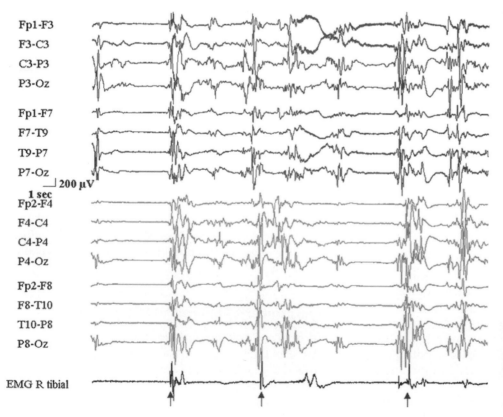

Figure 31.1 Early myoclonic encephalopathy. Electroencephalogram from a 3-month-old child with myoclonic jerking since before birth. *Arrows* indicate clinical jerks of the right leg. Note the markedly abnormal, high-amplitude, discontinuous electroencephalographic activities and the isolated myoclonias on the surface electromyographic recording.

there are now more than 40 cases in the literature. The characteristic multifocal seizures show migration of the focus during the seizure. Cognitive regression, developmental devastation, and high mortality are expected outcomes (17,18).

Males and females are equally affected and present at a mean age of 3 months with frequent partial seizures, initially with particular motor features (17,19). Autonomic manifestations may be striking; secondary generalization may be seen; and status epilepticus may occur (17,19). This initial period lasts an average of 6 to 7 weeks and is followed by months during which seizures increase in frequency, may occur in clusters, and vary in clinical expression. Developmental regression is dramatic (20); infants usually become progressively hypotonic and microcephalic and may demonstrate a movement disorder. The EEG shows nearly continuous seizures involving multiple independent areas. The focus may originate in either hemisphere and migrate from one area of the cortex to another during a single seizure and between consecutive seizures. This characteristic bilateral involvement is usually apparent from early in the disease. Its appearance up to 2 months into the illness may delay diagnosis (21). Interictally, multifocal epileptiform activity continues.

No risk factors have been recognized; a familial tendency seems lacking; extensive investigation has not identified a cause (18). In some cases, postmortem examination has shown hippocampal neuronal loss and gliosis (17).

Response to conventional antiepileptic drugs, steroids, a ketogenic diet, human immunoglobulin, and flunarizine has been disappointing (22). Therapy with oral potassium bromide achieved complete control in one infant and almost complete control in another; both infants evinced some developmental gains on short-term follow-up (23). Response to stiripentol and high doses of clonazepam has been inconsistent (24).

Benign Infantile Epilepsies

Benign partial epilepsy of infancy and BMEI are rare idiopathic syndromes whose diagnosis can be established only after treatment has begun and the benign course has been confirmed. Benign idiopathic and familial neonatal convulsions also have good prognoses but are not discussed here.

Benign Partial Epilepsy of Infancy

Partial epilepsies in infancy differ in etiology, therapy, and prognosis from the generalized epilepsies in this age group that may be manifested by focal seizures. The majority of focal epilepsies in infancy are symptomatic and are caused by neurocutaneous syndromes, brain malformations, focal dysplasias, and tumors. Described by Watanabe and colleagues in 1987 (25), benign partial epilepsy of infancy appears between 3 and 20 months of age. Radiologic and metabolic investigations are negative, although an increased

family history of febrile and infantile convulsions may be present (25). Often occurring in clusters, the seizures are characterized by behavioral arrest and staring, with limb or facial automatisms and prompt secondary generalization in many (26). The EEG is focal at onset with recruiting rhythms. During the seizure, slow waves emerge and dissipate, and, finally, spikes, polyspikes, and sharp-wave complexes are evident in centrotemporal, occipital, and parietal regions bilaterally. The interictal EEG is unremarkable (27). Seizures are easily controlled with carbamazepine or phenobarbital but if untreated may infrequently occur in brief isolated clusters. In retrospect, treatment may not be necessary but is usually undertaken before the diagnosis becomes apparent. Development is normal prior to seizure onset and remains so (26). No association with later epilepsy has been identified. A familial syndrome has been described, with mean seizure onset at a slightly younger age, similar seizure semiology, excellent response to treatment, and normal development (28).

Benign Myoclonic Epilepsy of Infancy

In 1981, Dravet and Bureau described BMEI in infants and children between 4 months and 3 years of age. In contrast to early infantile myoclonic encephalopathy, BMEI involves a favorable neurodevelopmental outcome and usually easy seizure control (29–31). It accounts for approximately 1% to 2% of epilepsies beginning in infancy and early childhood. Development is normal; febrile convulsions may have occurred; 30% of infants have a family history of febrile convulsions or epilepsy (32). Clinical examination and neuroimaging are normal. More males than females are affected.

The myoclonic jerks—brief tonic contractions of the trunk and upper limbs and head drop—may be subtle and unrecognized at first; later they become more obvious and more intense, occurring in short series at any time of the day but more likely when the child is drowsy. Some seizures have an acoustic or tactile "reflex" trigger (33). Other seizure types are not expected.

The EEG shows normal background activity. Generalized spike-wave or polyspike-wave discharges, associated with the myoclonic jerks (32), are activated by drowsiness and during the first stages of sleep. Clinical and electroencephalographic photosensitivity are present in one-third of patients. The interictal EEG is normal for age.

Other conditions considered in the differential diagnoses must be ruled out. Infantile spasms and EME are distinguished by their terrible impact on development. SMEI and BMEI both demonstrate photosensitivity, but there is usually a history of status epilepticus and the later emergence of jerks in SMEI. The runs of myoclonic jerks in BMEI are short compared with those in infantile spasms; they appear early in BMEI. Other than febrile convulsions, no other seizure type is seen in BMEI, whereas multiple seizure types characterize SMEI,

Lennox-Gastaut syndrome, and myoclonic-astatic epilepsy. Development in BMEI continues normally despite the seizures; this is not the case in any of the other epilepsies just described.

Monotherapy with sodium valproate, the drug of choice, is generally efficacious. A good response to add-on therapy with phenobarbital and benzodiazepines has been reported, but ethosuximide and primidone have produced disappointing results. Therapy can usually be withdrawn by 6 years. Generalized tonic-clonic seizures have been observed between 9 and 12 years of age and on drug withdrawal (29,34,35). If withdrawal seizures occur or if photosensitivity persists, treatment continues.

With early diagnosis and institution of treatment, most infants will be seizure free and incur no educational or psychological problems. Despite this optimistic prognosis, however, and the "benign" designation, as many as 25% of patients in some series (35) experience mild learning difficulties.

EPILEPSIES ASSOCIATED WITH CHROMOSOMAL ANOMALIES

Epilepsy is increasingly recognized as a frequent and significant part of the clinical problems associated with chromosomal anomalies. As ongoing investigation documents the involvement of the central nervous system in many chromosomal abnormalities, more patients with epilepsy are noted to have chromosomal anomalies and more chromosomal anomalies are recognized to include epilepsy. Loss or abnormal function of genetic loci on involved chromosomes may lead to increased seizure susceptibility, cortical excitability, or changes in neurotransmitters. Alternatively, epilepsy may originate from structural brain abnormalities occurring with the chromosomal abnormality.

Although epilepsies in the setting of chromosomal anomalies range from very mild to severe, they are generally difficult to treat. In a few, such as Angelman syndrome, the epilepsy or the electroencephalographic pattern is characteristic or highly suggestive of the chromosomal anomaly; in the majority, this is not the case. A deepening knowledge of these epilepsies and their electroencephalographic patterns may contribute to their diagnosis, or, conversely, the chromosomal anomalies may suggest target genes for the investigation of seizure pathogenesis (36).

Ring Chromosomes

Epilepsy associated with ring chromosomes 14 and 20 is well recognized. Infantile spasms and hypoplasia of the corpus callosum have been reported with ring chromosome 9 (37). Epilepsy also has been noted with ring chromosomes 15, 17, and 21 (38–40).

Ring Chromosome 20

The incidence of ring chromosome 20 is unclear, and the syndrome is probably underdiagnosed, as the phenotype does not immediately suggest a chromosomal anomaly. The clinical features are mild to moderate learning difficulties, behavioral problems (usually restlessness and aggression), and epilepsy, often without significant dysmorphism. Usually present are atypical absences and nonconvulsive status with diffuse, slow, rhythmic electroencephalographic and less frequently perioral and eyelid myoclonia (41,42). Bifrontal slow waves can be a striking interictal feature (Fig. 31.2). Subtle nocturnal frontal lobe seizures also have been described (43). Adverse psychological events triggering episodes of status (44) may contribute to misdiagnosis of nonepileptic seizures.

Seizures often resist treatment, and no medication has been found either to be useful or to aggravate seizures. Excision of a cortical dysplasia in one patient did not resolve seizures (22). Vagus nerve stimulation succeeded in one patient (45). Interestingly, the chromosomal telomeric regions p13 and q13 lost in formation of the ring have been implicated in benign neonatal familial convulsions and in autosomal dominant nocturnal frontal lobe epilepsy, yet the actual candidate genes do not seem to have been lost in the cases examined.

Ring Chromosome 14

Ring chromosome 14 presents with a more severe phenotype of early-onset epilepsy, severe to profound learning difficulties, speech impairment, microcephaly, and dysmorphism, particularly with ocular anomalies (46). One

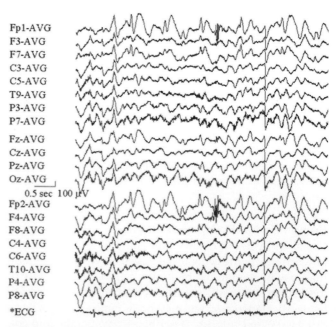

Figure 31.2 Ring chromosome 20. Electroencephalogram from a 7-year-old child with increasingly frequent seizures from the age of 12 months. Note the persistent bilateral frontal sharp waves and slow activity.

case has been reported in association with hypoplasia of the corpus callosum (47). While most are karyotypically mosaic, homogeneous cases are phenotypically identical. Epilepsy usually begins in the first year of life and is generalized and drug resistant. Complex partial seizures that may occur in clusters and seizures of frontocentral origin have been reported (47).

Angelman Syndrome and Rett Syndrome

Before their classic features emerge, these severely disabling, genetically based disorders can be difficult to differentiate, as they have similar clinical presentations and epilepsy and electroencephalographic characteristics.

Angelman Syndrome

Angelman syndrome has an estimated prevalence of 1 in 20,000 (48). The genetic abnormality in the majority of cases is a large deletion of the maternally inherited chromosome 15q11-13. Deletion of this same region of the paternally inherited chromosome results in Prader-Willi syndrome, in which seizures are uncommon (49). Severity of phenotype and risk of recurrence differ according to the genetic etiology (50). Diagnosis can be made by genetic testing and clinical criteria; electroencephalographic features may provide significant contributory evidence. Children present with severe developmental delay, lack of verbal skills, ataxia, tremulous movements, and distinctive behavior previously termed the "happy puppet" syndrome

that includes hand flapping, inappropriate laughter, and hyperactivity (51).

Reported in up to 90% of cases, epilepsy usually begins between 18 and 24 months of age, often with convulsions accompanying fever (52). Tonic-clonic, atypical absence, complex partial, myoclonic, tonic, and atonic seizures, often in clusters, may be quiescent in later childhood, only to emerge again in adulthood (53). Generalized tonic-clonic, absence, and myoclonic status occur (52). The EEG demonstrates three characteristic features, all of which are unusually and often strikingly rhythmic and of high amplitude (Fig. 31.3):

1. Symmetric, persistent, rhythmic activity, 4 to 6 per second, not associated with drowsiness is less frequent. It was not reported after the age of 5 to 6 years in one series or after age 12 years in another (53,54).
2. Posterior sharp theta activity with small spikes often survives until adulthood and may appear spontaneously or be brought about by eye closure (54,55).
3. Anterior rhythmic delta activity is the most common. Variants of this "delta pattern" have been characterized as hypsarrhythmic-like, ill-defined slow spike-and-wave, triphasic-like, and slow (55). Anterior rhythmic, slow triphasic waves persist into adulthood (53).

These features may be present at different times in the same patient, and suggestive features may precede the clinical phenotype or epileptic seizures. If all three electroencephalographic features coexist with developmental delay, the diagnosis is probable. The presence of only one or two

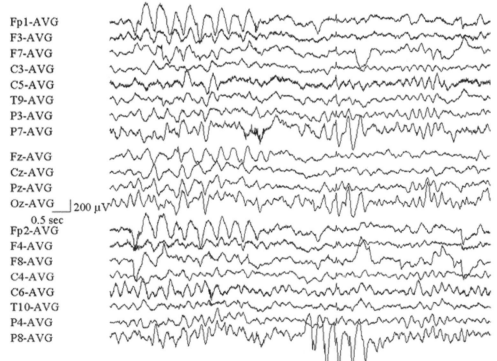

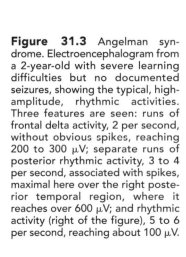

Figure 31.3 Angelman syndrome. Electroencephalogram from a 2-year-old with severe learning difficulties but no documented seizures, showing the typical, high-amplitude, rhythmic activities. Three features are seen: runs of frontal delta activity, 2 per second, without obvious spikes, reaching 200 to 300 μV; separate runs of posterior rhythmic activity, 3 to 4 per second, associated with spikes, maximal here over the right posterior temporal region, where it reaches over 600 μV; and rhythmic activity (right of the figure), 5 to 6 per second, reaching about 100 μV.

features reduces certainty, but the diagnostic possibility is strengthened in the context of the clinical syndrome.

Cortical myoclonus is well described and may respond to piracetam (56). Initially seizures are particularly resistant to treatment, but this lessens in later childhood. Sodium valproate with or without a benzodiazepine has been useful (52), as have topiramate and phenobarbitone (57). Carbamazepine may exacerbate seizures (52).

Rett Syndrome

With an estimated prevalence of 1 in 10,000 females, Rett syndrome predominantly affects females and in most cases arises *de novo*. It is now known to be associated with mutations in the *MECP2* gene in at least 85% of sporadic cases (58), but previously the diagnosis was based on clinical criteria. Apparently normal birth history and development until ages 6 to 18 months are followed by regression of speech, loss of bilateral hand function, sleep disturbance, and agitation. The typical features of severe cognitive impairment, acquired microcephaly, stereotypical hand movements, spasticity, and scoliosis then emerge (59).

Seizures have been reported in up to 66% of patients and in more than 50% were generalized tonic-clonic, although difficulties in distinguishing true seizures from "vacant spells" without the aid of video-electroencephalography may lead to overestimation (60,61).

Electroencephalographic changes are nonspecific, often described as multifocal central and centrotemporal discharges in combination with slow background activity (62). Electroencephalographic patterns more typical of Angelman syndrome have been reported in children with proven *MECP2* mutations (63). Thus, the phenotypic overlap of the two syndromes and reports of patients with the Angelman phenotype and *MECP2* mutations (64) raise the possibility of a common pathogenesis. The phenotypic variability of conditions associated with *MECP2* deletions remains wide (65). Genetic studies for Rett syndrome should be performed in patients with the Angelman phenotype but normal results of 15q DNA methylation studies, as well as in patients who have some but not all the typical features.

Down Syndrome (Trisomy 21)

Down syndrome, the most common genetic cause of learning difficulties, has an estimated incidence of 1 in 800 live births. The extra chromosome 21 results from nondisjunction (in more than 95% of cases), translocation (4%), or mosaicism (1%). The diagnosis is now often made antenatally and confirmed on karyotyping. The characteristic clinical features are well known and usually recognized at birth (66).

The overall incidence of epilepsy in Down syndrome is probably not higher than in the general population, but epileptic syndromes show a bimodal distribution with a particularly increased incidence and later onset of certain age-related epilepsies. Additionally, in as many as 50% of patients, the epilepsy is related to associated medical conditions. The epileptic syndrome determines the treatment and the prognosis. Epilepsy peaks in early childhood and late adulthood and does occur between these extremes, but without peculiarity to Down syndrome.

Epilepsy in Children with Down Syndrome

Infantile spasms, which occur with an increased incidence in children with Down syndrome (2% to 5%), are relatively easy to control, particularly with vigabatrin (67,68). After treatment, some studies report remarkable improvement; others note poor neurodevelopmental outcome (69–72).

Reflex epilepsies affect as many as 20% of children with seizures (73,74). Lennox-Gastaut syndrome, although uncommon, begins later in these children (mean age, 10 years) and may occur in those with reflex seizures (71).

Compared with that in the general population, the incidence of febrile convulsions seems lower (70,71).

Epilepsy in Adults with Down Syndrome

Strongly associated with Alzheimer disease, late-onset epilepsy usually begins after age 40 years and affects nearly half of all adults in the over-50-years age group (75). Seizure types vary, and in this setting, late-onset myoclonic epilepsy in Down syndrome (LOMEDS) has been proposed as a specific myoclonic epilepsy syndrome (76). Myoclonic epilepsy reportedly responds to sodium valproate and topiramate.

Phenytoin should be used with caution, as these adults with late-onset seizures show increased sensitivity to its adverse effects, even without elevated plasma levels (77).

Fragile X

Fragile X is the second most frequent chromosomal abnormality causing mental retardation. Inheritance is X-linked recessive; the phenotype is most severe in males, but obligate female carriers are also mildly affected. The fragile X mental retardation gene (*FMR1*), identified in 1991, contains an unstable nucleotide triplet repeat, whose expansion silences the gene and leads to the syndrome (78). DNA analysis can reliably determine the extent of expansion and detect full mutations.

Prevalence is estimated at 1 in 4000 to 6000 males, possibly as high as 1 in 1250 in some populations (79–81). Moderate learning difficulties, a long face, macrognathism, prominent ears, and macroorchidism comprise the clinical phenotype. The behavioral phenotype includes autistic-like features and hyperactivity.

The reported prevalence of epilepsy in large studies varies from 10% to 20% (82,83). Most seizures begin between 2 and 12 years of age, and the incidence of epilepsy does not seem to correlate with the degree of learning difficulties (71). Generalized tonic-clonic and complex partial seizures are most frequent (71,82,83), and infantile spasms evolving to Lennox-Gastaut have been reported (84). The most consistently noted electroencephalographic abnormalities are medium- to high-voltage unilateral or bilateral spikes in the temporal area, activated by sleep, and similar to the pattern in benign partial epilepsy with centrotemporal spikes (84). These epileptiform changes are also seen in children with fragile X syndrome who have no seizure history (82,83). Focal seizures and focal electroencephalographic patterns have been reported in female carriers (82,85). The epilepsy generally responds to monotherapy with sodium valproate or carbamazepine. Seizures are infrequent, and many remit in childhood. Centrotemporal spikes may be a good prognostic factor for such early remission. In up to 25% of patients, however, seizures persist into adulthood and frontal slowing on the EEG may be a poor prognostic indicator (82).

Klinefelter Syndrome (47, XXY)

The most common sex chromosome abnormality, Klinefelter syndrome, occurs in 1 to 2 per 1000 males and results from one or more extra X chromosomes. It most commonly presents with infertility and is diagnosed on the basis of chromosomal karyotyping. Clinical features include tallness, hypogonadism with small testes, androgen deficiency, and female body habitus with gynecomastia. Intelligence is usually normal, although language-based learning difficulties, frontal-executive dysfunction, and difficulties with social relationships are among the recognized educational and psychological problems (86–88). Reduced gray matter volume in the temporal lobe has been suggested as a structural basis for the observed deficits (89). The neuropsychological phenotype, while mild compared with that of other chromosomal disorders, can cause significant morbidity in affected men, and for this reason, educational and psychological support should be a key aspect of treatment (90).

Epilepsy is more prevalent than in the general population, but the seizures—most commonly febrile convulsions, generalized tonic-clonic seizures, and complex partial seizures—are usually mild and easily controlled with medication (91–93). Electroencephalographic changes are heterogenous and have been noted in patients with and without a history of seizures.

THE HEMICONVULSION-HEMIPLEGIA-EPILEPSY SYNDROME

Recognized in the 1800s and described by Gastaut in 1957, this syndrome is rare (94). Its cause is unknown, although hypoxia, venous thrombosis, trauma, intracranial hemorrhage, and infections have been implicated as possible pathogenetic mechanisms. Recently, a factor V Leiden

mutation has been suggested as causative in two children (95). HHE could also be the severe end along a spectrum of sequelae of complex febrile convulsions, with mesial temporal sclerosis now regarded as a lesser structural consequence (96). Whether an underlying abnormality has gone unrecognized prior to the hemiconvulsion-hemiplegia in many cases is, however, open to debate. The morbidity and mortality from status epilepticus have decreased dramatically (97,98) as the syndrome's incidence has declined in the developed world, whether as a result of prevention of febrile convulsions, earlier intervention to abort status epilepticus and thus prevent HHE, or advances in investigative modalities (particularly neuroimaging) that demonstrate an underlying cause (99).

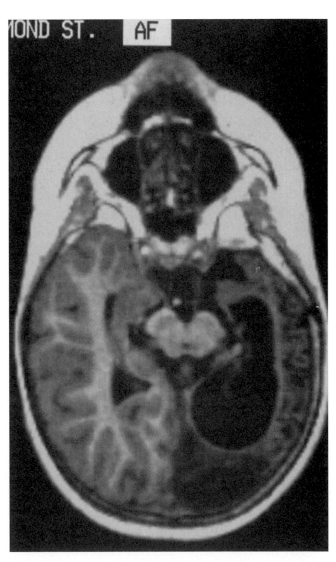

Figure 31.4 Hemiconvulsion-hemiplegia-epilepsy syndrome. Axial T1-weighted magnetic resonance imaging brain scan showing extensive atrophy of the left cerebral hemisphere and multicystic change, predominantly posteriorly. The right hemisphere is normal. This child had prolonged, right-sided febrile status epilepticus at 26 months of age. Right-sided hemiplegia was apparent on recovery, and intractable focal seizures began shortly afterward. She underwent a left functional hemispherectomy at age 5 years, 3 months and remains seizure free at 14 years of age.

The syndrome's hemiconvulsion usually occurs before 4 years of age in the setting of an intercurrent febrile illness. Initially generalized, the convulsion continues as prolonged clonic status epilepticus with a unilateral predominance. Hemifacial twitching or head and eye deviation is a particular feature. Ictal EEGs show predominantly rhythmic slow activity on the contralateral side to the clinical seizure. At this acute stage, unilateral swelling is evident on neuroimaging. Convulsive status epilepticus reportedly ranges from 30 minutes to more than 24 hours. The seizure responds clinically and electrographically to intravenous diazepam. Asymmetry persists on the postictal EEG.

Ipsilateral hemiplegia immediately follows the hemiconvulsion and resolves over days to weeks but can also become persistent and spastic. Neuroimaging evolves to show global cerebral hemiatrophy (Fig. 31.4); hypoperfusion has been reported on interictal single-photon-emission computed tomography studies (100–102). Movement disorder, learning difficulties, and transient aphasia also have been observed as sequelae (103).

Although it may not emerge for several years, the subsequent epilepsy is ipsilateral to the hemiplegia and focal, usually has complex partial semiologic features, and originates in the temporal lobe. Satisfactory control has been described with carbamazepine or phenobarbitone, or both (102). Although only a small number of suitable adults with drug-resistant epilepsy proceeded to surgery, outcomes were better with large resections (99). Improved seizure control followed corpus callosotomy in three atypical cases (104).

ACKNOWLEDGMENTS

The authors thank Dr. Stewart Boyd, consultant clinical neurophysiologist at Great Ormond Street Hospital for Children, NHS Trust, London, who provided the EEG figures and legends.

REFERENCES

1. Yamatogi Y, Ohtahara S. Age-dependent epileptic encephalopathy: a longitudinal study. *Folia Psychiatr Neurol Japon* 1981;35:321–332.
2. Ohtsuka Y, Ogino T, Murakami N, et al. Developmental aspects of epilepsy with special reference to age-dependent epileptic encephalopathy. *Jpn J Psychiatry Neurol* 1986;40:307–313.
3. Aicardi J, Goutieres F. Neonatal myoclonic encephalopathy. *Rev Electroencephalogr Neurophysiol Clin* 1978;8:99–101.
4. Dalla BB, Aicardi J, Goutieres F, et al. Glycine encephalopathy. *Neuropadiatrie* 1979;10:209–225.
5. Chen PT, Young C, Lee WT, et al. Early epileptic encephalopathy with suppression burst electroencephalographic pattern—an analysis of eight Taiwanese patients. *Brain Dev* 2001;23:15–720.
6. Dalla BB, Dulac O, Fejerman N, et al. Early myoclonic epileptic encephalopathy (E.M.E.E.). *Eur J Pediatr* 1983;140:248–252.
7. Wang PJ, Lee WT, Hwu WL, et al. The controversy regarding diagnostic criteria for early myoclonic encephalopathy. *Brain Dev* 1998;20:530–535.
8. Murakami N, Ohtsuka Y, Ohtahara S. Early infantile epileptic syndromes with suppression-bursts: early myoclonic encephalopathy vs. Ohtahara syndrome. *Jpn J Psychiatry Neurol* 1993;47:197–200.
9. Wallace SJ. Myoclonus and epilepsy in childhood: a review of treatment with valproate, ethosuximide, lamotrigine and zonisamide. *Epilepsy Res* 1998;29:147–154.
10. Ohtahara S, Ishida T, Oka E. On the specific age dependent epileptic syndrome: the early-infantile epileptic encephalopathy with suppression-burst. *No To Hattatsu* 1976;8:270–280.
11. Ohtahara S. A study on the age-dependent epileptic encephalopathy. *No To Hattatsu* 1977;9:2–21.
12. Ohtahara S, Ohtsuka Y, Yamatogi Y, et al. The early-infantile epileptic encephalopathy with suppression-burst: developmental aspects. *Brain Dev* 1987;9:371–376.
13. Ohno M, Shimotsuji Y, Abe J, et al. Zonisamide treatment of early infantile epileptic encephalopathy. *Pediatr Neurol* 2000;23:341–344.
14. Sofue A, Hayakawa F, Okumura A. A case of infantile epileptic encephalopathy with frequent focal motor status convulsivus: successful treatment with zonisamide. *No To Hattatsu* 2002;34:43–48.
15. Martinez BA, Roche C, Lopez M, et al. Early infantile epileptic encephalopathy. *Rev Neurol* 1995; 23:297–300.
16. Komaki H, Sugai K, Maehara T, et al. Surgical treatment of early-infantile epileptic encephalopathy with suppression-bursts associated with focal cortical dysplasia. *Brain Dev* 2001;23:727–731.
17. Coppola G, Plouin P, Chiron C, et al. Migrating partial seizures in infancy: a malignant disorder with developmental arrest. *Epilepsia* 1995;36:1017–1024.
18. Wilmshurst JM, Appleton DB, Grattan-Smith PJ. Migrating partial seizures in infancy: two new cases. *J Child Neurol* 2000;15:717–722.
19. Dulac O. Malignant migrating partial seizures in infancy. In: Roger J, Bureau M, Dravet C, et al., eds. *Epileptic syndromes in infancy, childhood and adolescence,* 3rd ed. Eastleigh, UK: John Libbey, 2002:65–68.
20. Veneselli E, Perrone MV, Di Rocco M, et al. Malignant migrating partial seizures in infancy. *Epilepsy Res* 2001;46:27–32.
21. Gerard F, Kaminska A, Plouin P, et al. Focal seizures versus focal epilepsy in infancy: a challenging distinction. *Epileptic Disord* 1999;1:135–139.
22. McLellan A, Kirkpatrick M. Intractable partial seizures in infancy. *Dev Med Child Neurol Suppl* 1997;77:27–28.
23. Okuda K, Yasuhara A, Kamei A, et al. Successful control with bromide of two patients with malignant migrating partial seizures in infancy. *Brain Dev* 2000;22:56–59.
24. Perez J, Chiron C, Musial C, et al. Stiripentol: efficacy and tolerability in children with epilepsy. *Epilepsia* 1999;40:1618–1626.
25. Watanabe K, Yamamoto N, Negoro T, et al. Benign complex partial epilepsies in infancy. *Pediatr Neurol* 1987;3:208–211.
26. Watanabe K, Negoro T, Aso K. Benign partial epilepsy with secondarily generalized seizures in infancy. *Epilepsia* 1993;34:635–638.
27. Watanabe K, Yamamoto N, Negoro T, et al. Benign infantile epilepsy with complex partial seizures. *J Clin Neurophysiol* 1990;7:409–416.
28. Vigevano F, Fusco L, Di Capua M, et al. Benign infantile familial convulsions. *Eur J Pediatr* 1992;151:608–612.
29. Dravet C, Bureau M. The benign myoclonic epilepsy of infancy [French]. *Rev Electroencephalogr Neurophysiol Clin* 1981;11:438–444.
30. Dravet C, Giraud N, Bureau M, et al. Benign myoclonus of early infancy or benign non-epileptic infantile spasms. *Neuropediatrics* 1986;17:33–38.
31. Lombroso CT, Fejerman N. Benign myoclonus of early infancy. *Ann Neurol* 1977;1:138–143.
32. Dravet C, Bureau M, Genton P. Benign myoclonic epilepsy of infancy: electroclinical symptomatology and differential diagnosis from the other types of generalized epilepsy of infancy. *Epilepsy Res Suppl* 1992;6:131–135.
33. Ricci S, Cusmai R, Fusco L, et al. Reflex myoclonic epilepsy in infancy: a new age-dependent idiopathic epileptic syndrome related to startle reaction. *Epilepsia* 1995;36:342–348.
34. Lin Y, Itomi K, Takada H, et al. Benign myoclonic epilepsy in infants: video-EEG features and long-term follow-up. *Neuropediatrics* 1998;29:268–271.
35. Todt H, Muller D. The therapy of benign myoclonic epilepsy in infants. *Epilepsy Res Suppl* 1992;6:137–139.
36. Singh R, Gardner RJ, Crossland KM, et al. Chromosomal abnormalities and epilepsy: a review for clinicians and gene hunters. *Epilepsia* 2002;43:127–140.

37. Lanzi G, Fazzi E, Veggiotti P, et al. Ring chromosome 9: an atypical case. *Brain Dev* 1996;18:216–219.
38. Schinzel A, Niedrist D. Chromosome imbalances associated with epilepsy. *Am J Med Genet* 2001;106:119–124.
39. Gass JD, Taney BS. Flecked retina associated with cafe au lait spots, microcephaly, epilepsy, short stature, and ring 17 chromosome. *Arch Ophthalmol* 1994;112:738–739.
40. Schmid W, Tenconi R, Baccichetti C, et al. Ring chromosome 21 in phenotypically apparently normal persons: report of two families from Switzerland and Italy. *Am J Med Genet* 1983;16: 323–329.
41. Canevini MP, Sgro V, Zuffardi O, et al. Chromosome 20 ring: a chromosomal disorder associated with a particular electroclinical pattern. *Epilepsia* 1998;39:942–951.
42. Inoue Y, Fujiwara T, Matsuda K, et al. Ring chromosome 20 and nonconvulsive status epilepticus. A new epileptic syndrome. *Brain* 1997;120:939–953.
43. Augustijn PB, Parra J, Wouters CH, et al. Ring chromosome 20 epilepsy syndrome in children: electroclinical features. *Neurology* 2001;57:1108–1111.
44. Petit J, Roubertie A, Inoue Y, et al. Non-convulsive status in the ring chromosome 20 syndrome: a video illustration of 3 cases. *Epileptic Disord* 1999;1:237–241.
45. Chawla J, Sucholeiki R, Jones C, et al. Intractable epilepsy with ring chromosome 20 syndrome treated with vagal nerve stimulation: case report and review of the literature. *J Child Neurol* 2002; 17:778–780.
46. Schmidt R, Eviatar L, Nitowsky HM, et al. Ring chromosome 14: a distinct clinical entity. *J Med Genet* 1981;18:304–307.
47. Ono J, Nishiike K, Imai K, et al. Ring chromosome 14 complicated with complex partial seizures and hypoplastic corpus callosum. *Pediatr Neurol* 1999;20:70–72.
48. Clayton-Smith J, Pembrey ME. Angelman syndrome. *J Med Genet* 1992;29:412–415.
49. Magenis RE, Toth-Fejel S, Allen LJ, et al. Comparison of the 15q deletions in Prader-Willi and Angelman syndromes: specific regions, extent of deletions, parental origin, and clinical consequences. *Am J Med Genet* 1990;35:333–349.
50. Clayton-Smith J, Laan L. Angelman syndrome: a review of the clinical and genetic aspects. *J Med Genet* 2003;40:87–95.
51. Williams CA, Angelman H, Clayton-Smith J, et al. Angelman syndrome: consensus for diagnostic criteria. Angelman Syndrome Foundation. *Am J Med Genet* 1995;56:237–238.
52. Viani F, Romeo A, Viri M, et al. Seizure and EEG patterns in Angelman's syndrome. *J Child Neurol* 1995; 10:467–471.
53. Laan LA, den Boer AT, Hennekam RC, et al. Angelman syndrome in adulthood. *Am J Med Genet* 1996;66:356–360.
54. Boyd SG, Harden A, Patton MA. The EEG in early diagnosis of the Angelman (happy puppet) syndrome. *Eur J Pediatr* 1988;147: 508–513.
55. Valente KD, Andrade JQ, Grossmann RM, et al. Angelman syndrome: difficulties in EEG pattern recognition and possible misinterpretations. *Epilepsia* 2003;44:1051–1063.
56. Guerrini R, De Lorey TM, Bonanni P, et al. Cortical myoclonus in Angelman syndrome. *Ann Neurol* 1996;40:39–48.
57. Franz DN, Glauser TA, Tudor C, Williams S. Topiramate therapy of epilepsy associated with Angelman's syndrome. *Neurology* 2000; 54:1185–1188.
58. Amir RE, Van der Veyver IB, Wan M, et al. Rett syndrome is caused by mutations in X-linked MECP2, encoding methyl-CpG-binding protein 2. *Nat Genet* 1999;23:185–188.
59. Hagberg B, Aicardi J, Dias K, et al. A progressive syndrome of autism, dementia, ataxia, and loss of purposeful hand use in girls: Rett's syndrome: report of 35 cases. *Ann Neurol* 1983;14: 471–479.
60. Cass H, Reilly S, Owen L, et al. Findings from a multidisciplinary clinical case series of females with Rett syndrome. *Dev Med Child Neurol* 2003;45:325–337.
61. Glaze DG, Schultz RJ, Frost JD. Rett syndrome: characterization of seizures versus non-seizures. *Electroencephalogr Clin Neurophysiol* 1998;106:79–83.
62. Robb SA, Harden A, Boyd SG. Rett syndrome: an EEG study in 52 girls. *Neuropediatrics* 1989;20:192–195.
63. Laan M, Vein A. A Rett patient with a typical Angelman EEG. *Epilepsia* 2002;43:1590–1592.
64. Watson P, Black G, Ramsden S, et al. Angelman syndrome phenotype associated with mutations in MECP2, a gene encoding a methyl CpG binding protein. *J Med Genet* 2001;38: 224–228.
65. Hammer S, Dorrani N, Dragich J, et al. The phenotypic consequences of MECP2 mutations extend beyond Rett syndrome. *Ment Retard Dev Disabil Res Rev* 2002;8:94–98.
66. Jones KL. *Smith's recognizable patterns of human malformation*, 4th ed. Philadelphia: WB Saunders, 1988.
67. Nabbout R, Melki I, Gerbaka B, et al. Infantile spasms in Down syndrome: good response to a short course of vigabatrin. *Epilepsia* 2001;42:1580–1583.
68. Pollack MA, Golden GS, Schmidt R, et al. Infantile spasms in Down syndrome: a report of 5 cases and review of the literature. *Ann Neurol* 1978;3:406–408.
69. Goldberg-Stern H, Strawsburg RH, Patterson B, et al. Seizure frequency and characteristics in children with Down syndrome. *Brain Dev* 2001;23:375–378.
70. Stafstrom CE, Patxot OF, Gilmore HE, et al. Seizures in children with Down syndrome: etiology, characteristics and outcome. *Dev Med Child Neurol* 1991;33:191–200.
71. Guerrini R, Dravet C, Ferrari AR, et al. The evolution of epilepsy in the most common genetic forms with mental retardation (Down's syndrome and the fragile X syndrome) [Italian]. *Pediatr Med Chir* 1993;15(Suppl 1):19–22.
72. Stafstrom CE, Konkol RJ. Infantile spasms in children with Down syndrome. *Dev Med Child Neurol* 1994;36: 576–585.
73. Guerrini R, Genton P, Bureau M, et al. Reflex seizures are frequent in patients with Down syndrome and epilepsy. *Epilepsia* 1990;31: 406–417.
74. Pueschel SM, Louis S. Reflex seizures in Down syndrome. *Childs Nerv Syst* 1993;9:23–24.
75. McVicker RW, Shanks OE, McClelland RJ. Prevalence and associated features of epilepsy in adults with Down's syndrome. *Br J Psychiatry* 1994;164:528–532.
76. Moller JC, Hamer HM, Oertel WH, et al. Late-onset myoclonic epilepsy in Down's syndrome (LOMEDS). *Seizure* 2001;10: 303–306.
77. Tsiouris JA, Patti PJ, Tipu O, et al. Adverse effects of phenytoin given for late-onset seizures in adults with Down syndrome. *Neurology* 2002;59:779–780.
78. Verkerk AJ, Pieretti M, Sutcliffe JS, et al. Identification of a gene (FMR-1) containing a CGG repeat coincident with a breakpoint cluster region exhibiting length variation in fragile X syndrome. *Cell* 1991;65:905–914.
79. Crawford DC, Meadows KL, Newman JL, et al. Prevalence of the fragile X syndrome in African-Americans. *Am J Med Genet* 2002; 110:226–233.
80. de Vries BB, van den Ouweland AM, Mohkamsing S, et al. Screening and diagnosis for the fragile X syndrome among the mentally retarded: an epidemiological and psychological survey. Collaborative Fragile X Study Group. *Am J Hum Genet* 1997;61: 660–667.
81. Turner G, Webb T, Wake S, et al. Prevalence of fragile X syndrome. *Am J Med Genet* 1996;64:196–197.
82. Berry-Kravis E. Epilepsy in fragile X syndrome. *Dev Med Child Neurol* 2002;44:724–728.
83. Musumeci SA, Hagerman RJ, Ferri R, et al. Epilepsy and EEG findings in males with fragile X syndrome. *Epilepsia* 1999;40: 1092–1099.
84. Musumeci SA, Colognola RM, Ferri R, et al. Fragile-X syndrome: a particular epileptogenic EEG pattern. *Epilepsia* 1988;29: 41–47.
85. Singh R, Sutherland GR, Manson J. Partial seizures with focal epileptogenic electroencephalographic patterns in three related female patients with fragile-X syndrome. *J Child Neurol* 1999;14: 108–112.
86. Boone KB, Swerdloff RS, Miller BL, et al. Neuropsychological profiles of adults with Klinefelter syndrome. *J Int Neuropsychol Soc* 2001;7:446–456.
87. Geschwind DH, Boone KB, Miller BL, et al. Neurobehavioral phenotype of Klinefelter syndrome. *Ment Retard Dev Disabil Res Rev* 2000;6:107–116.

88. Rovet J, Netley C, Keenan M, et al. The psychoeducational profile of boys with Klinefelter syndrome. *J Learn Disabil* 1996;29:180–196.

89. Patwardhan AJ, Eliez S, Bender B, et al. Brain morphology in Klinefelter syndrome: extra X chromosome and testosterone supplementation. *Neurology* 2000;54:2218–2223.

90. Ratcliffe S. Long-term outcome in children of sex chromosome abnormalities. *Arch Dis Child* 1999;80:192–195.

91. Boltshauser E, Meyer M, Deonna T. Klinefelter syndrome and neurological disease. *J Neurol* 1978;219:253–259.

92. Tatum WO, Passaro EA, Elia M, et al. Seizures in Klinefelter's syndrome. *Pediatr Neurol* 1998;19:275–278.

93. Elia M, Musumeci SA, Ferri R, et al. Seizures in Klinefelter's syndrome: a clinical and EEG study of five patients. *Ital J Neurol Sci* 1995;16:231–238.

94. Gastaut H, Vigouroux M, Trevisan C, et al. Le syndrome "hemi-convulsion-hemiplegie-epilepsie" (syndrome HHE). *Rev Neurol* 1957;97:37–52.

95. Scantlebury MH, David M, Carmant L. Association between factor V Leiden mutation and the hemiconvulsion, hemiplegia, and epilepsy syndrome: report of two cases. *J Child Neurol* 2002;17: 713–717.

96. Guerrini R, Bureau M, Dravet C, Genton P. A propos du syndrome hemiconvulsion-hemiplegie-epilepsie (HHE). *Epilepsie* 1996;8:159–166.

97. Chevrie JJ, Aicardi J. Convulsive disorders in the first year of life: neurological and mental outcome and mortality. *Epilepsia* 1978; 19:7–74.

98. Maytal J, Shinnar S, Moshe SL, et al. Low morbidity and mortality of status epilepticus in children. *Pediatrics* 1989;83: 323–331.

99. Chauvel P, Dravet C. The HHE syndrome. In: Roger J, Bureau M, Dravet C, et al., eds. *Epileptic syndromes in infancy, childhood and adolescence.* Eastleigh, UK: John Libbey, 2002:247–263.

100. Kataoka K, Okuno T, Mikawa H, et al. Cranial computed tomographic and electroencephalographic abnormalities in children with post-hemiconvulsive hemiplegia. *Eur Neurol* 1988;28: 279–284.

101. Oe H, Yuasa R, Tsuchiyama M, et al. Neuroimaging findings of hemiconvulsions, hemiplegia, epilepsy (HHE) syndrome. *Rinsho Shinkeigaku* 1999;39:485–488.

102. Salih MA, Kabiraj M, Al Jarallah AS, et al. Hemiconvulsion-hemiplegia-epilepsy syndrome. A clinical, electroencephalographic and neuroradiological study. *Childs Nerv Syst* 1997;13:257–263.

103. Aicardi J, Amsili J, Chevrie JJ. Acute hemiplegia in infancy and childhood. *Dev Med Child Neurol* 1969;11:162–173.

104. Kwan SY, Wong TT, Chang KP, et al. Postcallosotomy seizure outcome in hemiconvulsion-hemiatrophy-epilepsy syndrome. *Zhonghua Yi Xue Za Zhi (Taipei)* 2000;63:503–511.

Neonatal Seizures

32

Robert R. Clancy   *Eli M. Mizrahi*

Neonatal seizures are a classic and ominous neurologic sign that can arise in any newborn infant. Their significance lies in their high incidence, association with acute neonatal encephalopathies, substantial mortality and neurologic morbidity, and the concern that seizures *per se* could extend the acute brain injury. Seizures in the neonate differ clinically and electrographically from those in mature infants and children. Diagnostic and treatment decisions remain limited by a paucity of rigorous scientific data for this population. This chapter reviews the significance of neonatal seizures, the pathophysiologic basis of clinical, electroclinical, and electrographic seizures, prognostic expectations, and etiologies, and surveys current treatment options that might themselves pose a risk to the developing brain.

HISTORICAL BACKGROUND

The appearance of "seizures," "fits," or "convulsions" in newborn infants has been known since antiquity. *Seizure* is derived from a Greek word implying a sudden "attack of disease." The invention of the electroencephalograph by Hans Berger allowed investigators to discover the epileptic mechanisms that underlie seizure expressions in mature individuals. It was naturally assumed that clinical seizures in neonates were always associated with abnormal, excessive, paroxysmal electrical discharges arising from repetitive neuronal firing in the cerebral cortex. Despite the identification of electroclinical correlations of seizures in mature individuals, progress in understanding the nosology of neonatal seizures was only recently notable. Although some neonatal seizures were accompanied by simultaneous epileptic discharges demonstrated by electroencephalography, not every clinical event in a neonate that appears as an abrupt "attack" is truly epileptic, and the relationship between neonatal seizures and the conventional connotations of the term *epilepsy* demands careful scrutiny. Thus, seizures in the neonate are now distributed into three classes (Fig. 32.1). "Electroclinical" seizures are abnormal, clinically observable events that are consistently founded on a specific epileptic mechanism and coincide with an obvious electrographic seizure during simultaneous electroencephalographic (EEG) monitoring. "Clinical-only" seizures refer to other abnormal-appearing abrupt clinical events that are not associated with simultaneous electrographic seizure activity during EEG monitoring; they may be considered a type of *nonepileptic* seizure; "EEG-only" seizures lack definite clinical seizure activity; they are also called "subclinical" or "occult."

SIGNIFICANCE OF NEONATAL SEIZURES

Incidence

The incidence of seizures in the first 28 days of life, one of the highest risk periods for seizures in humans, ranges between 1% and 5%. Depending on the methodology used, seizures occur at a rate of 1.5 to 5.5 per 1000 neonates (1–7), most within the first week of life (4). Incidence varies with specific risk factors. Lanska and colleagues (4) reported the incidence of seizures in all neonates to be 3.5 per 1000, but 57.5 per 1000 in very-low-birth-weight (<1500 g) infants, 4.4 per 1000 in low-birth-weight (1500–2499 g) infants, and 2.8 per 1000 in normal-birth-weight (2500–3999 g) infants. Scher and colleagues (8,9) described seizures in 3.9% of neonates younger than 30 weeks conceptional age and in 1.5% of those older than 30 conceptional weeks.

The human newborn is especially vulnerable to a wide range of toxic or metabolic conditions. Sepsis, meningitis, hypoxic-ischemic encephalopathy (HIE), hypoglycemia, and hyperbilirubinemia are capable of eliciting seizures. This may explain, in part, the frequent occurrence of brain-damaging events in the first 30 days of life. However, the neonatal brain itself may be especially prone to seizures when injured.

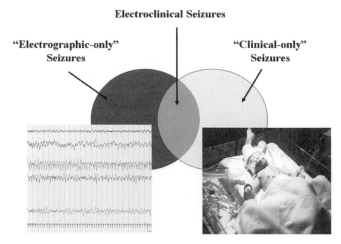

Figure 32.1 Three types of "seizures" in the newborn: "electrographic only," "electroclinical," and "clinical only."

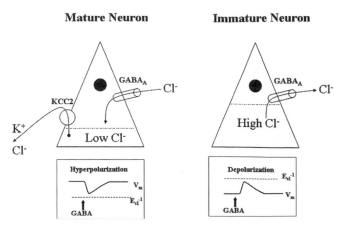

Figure 32.2 The effects of γ-aminobutyric acid may be paradoxically excitatory in early central nervous system development.

One suspected mechanism of enhanced seizure susceptibility in the newborn is the relative imbalance between inhibition and excitation. Compared with more mature brains, the neonatal brain has delayed maturation of inhibitory circuits and precocious maturation of excitatory circuits (10). This "imbalance" reflects a desirable and natural aspect of early central nervous system (CNS) development characterized by exuberant growth of excitatory synapses (10) coupled with activity-dependent pruning necessary for the prodigious rate of novel learning that faces all neonates. Moreover, according to studies in the neonatal rat, γ-aminobutyric acid (GABA) (the chief inhibitory neurotransmitter of the mature brain) may exert paradoxically *excitatory* effects in early CNS development (11,12). A developmentally dependent potassium chloride channel (KCC2) does not reach mature proportions in the rat hippocampus until the 15th postnatal day (Fig. 32.2). This age-dependent channel pumps potassium chloride from the interior of the neuron, reducing intracellular chloride levels. Thus, when the ligand-dependent GABA receptor is opened, extracellular chloride follows its electrochemical gradient into the neuron and hyperpolarizes it as expected. However, before the appearance of KCC2, the intracellular concentration of chloride is high, exceeding that of the extracellular space. In the immature rat, activation of the GABA receptor allows chloride to run along its electrochemical gradient out of the neuron, paradoxically depolarizing it (13).

Although neonatal seizures most commonly result from an underlying acute illness, some are reversible, the outward sign of a *treatable* condition. For example, the presence of hypocalcemia, hypomagnesemia, hypoglycemia, pyridoxine deficiency, or sepsis-meningitis may be heralded by neonatal seizures.

Prognostic Significance

Neonatal seizures are a powerful prognostic indicator of mortality and neurologic morbidity. The summary report from Bergman and associates (2) of 1667 patients noted an overall mortality of 24.7% before 1969 and 18% after 1970. Volpe (14) cited a mortality rate of 40% before 1969 and 20% after 1969. According to Lombroso (15), mortality decreased modestly from about 20% previously to 16% in the early 1980s. These improvements probably reflect better obstetrical management and modern neonatal intensive care. All of these studies relied on seizure diagnosis by clinical criteria and did not require EEG confirmation.

Survivors of neonatal seizures face an exceptionally high risk for cerebral palsy, often with mental retardation and chronic postnatal epilepsy. The National Collaborative Perinatal Population (NCPP) study (16,17) examined numerous clinical perinatal factors for their association with severe mental retardation, cerebral palsy, and microcephaly (Fig. 32.3). The clinical diagnosis of "neonatal seizures" was independently and significantly associated with these adverse outcomes and eclipsed only by "intracranial hemorrhage" in forecasting them. Neurologic functioning may even be impaired in those who appear "normal" after neonatal seizures (18).

Contemporary studies of the prognosis after neonatal seizures have emphasized the inclusion of infants whose seizure type was confirmed by EEG monitoring. Outcome has been assessed in terms of survival, neurologic disability, developmental delay, and postnatal epilepsy. Ortibus and colleagues (19) reported that 28% died; 22% of survivors were neurologically normal at an average of 17 months of age; 14% had mild abnormalities; and 36% were severely abnormal. Six years later, Brunquell and colleagues (20) put the mortality rate at 30%. Neurologic examinations showed abnormalities in 59% of survivors; 40% were mentally retarded; 43% had cerebral palsy; and 21% had postnatal epilepsy when followed up for a mean of 3.5 years.

Preliminary results of the Neonatal Seizures Clinical Research Centers from 1992 to 1997 have been reported (21). Of the 207 full-term infants with video-

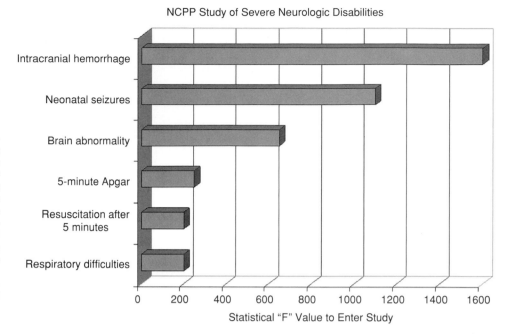

NCPP Study of Severe Neurologic Disabilities

Figure 32.3 The National Collaborative Perinatal Population (NCPP) study prospectively followed more than 34,000 mothers to identify perinatal events associated with adverse outcomes. Fifty neonates were found with subsequent severe neurologic handicaps. Six independent variables, including neonatal seizures, were associated with such neurologically devastating outcomes. (Adapted from Nelson KB, Broman SH. Perinatal risk factors in children with serious motor and mental handicaps. *Ann Neurol* 1977; 2:371–377, with permission.)

electroencephalography–confirmed seizures who were prospectively enrolled, 28% died. Two-year follow-up data were available for 122 patients, or 86% of the survivors. Abnormal neurologic findings were noted in 42%. A Mental Developmental Index (MDI) score below 80 was present in 55%, a Psychomotor Developmental Index (PDI) score less than 80 in 50%, and chronic postnatal epilepsy in 26%.

Whether seizures themselves adversely affect the developing brain is difficult to determine from clinical studies. Seizure *burden* may appear to influence outcome because some infants who experience brief, infrequent seizures may have relatively good long-term outcomes, whereas those with prolonged seizures often do not fare as well. However, easily controlled or self-limited seizures may be the result of transient, successfully treated, or benign CNS disorders of neonates, while medically refractory neonatal seizures may stem from more sustained, less treatable, or more severe brain disorders. Legido and associates (22) studied 40 neonates with electrographic seizures detected on randomly timed routine electroencephalogram examinations, and monitored them for cerebral palsy, mental retardation, and epilepsy. Overall neurologic outcome was more favorable in those with two or fewer seizures per hour than in those with more than that number. In the subgroup with seizures caused by asphyxia, cerebral palsy was more frequent when more than five seizures occurred per hour. However, these results might equally reflect more severe underlying injuries that triggered both the additional short-term seizures and greater morbidity on long-term follow-up. Attempting a balanced approach, McBride and coworkers (23) followed up 68 high-risk neonates with birth asphyxia, meningitis, and other stressors linked to neonatal seizures. All infants underwent long-term EEG

monitoring. Forty developed electrographic seizures, and 28 did not. By logistic regression, electrographic neonatal seizures were significantly correlated with death and cerebral palsy. Other investigators (24), using proton magnetic resonance spectroscopy (^{1}H-MRS) found an association of seizure severity with impaired cerebral metabolism measured by lactate/choline and compromised neuronal integrity measured by *N*-acetylaspartate/choline, and suggested this as evidence of brain injury not limited to structural damage detected by magnetic resonance imaging (MRI).

Neonatal Seizures May Be Inherently Harmful

Neonatal seizures may be intrinsically harmful to the brain (25). Most seizures were long assumed to be the innocuous, albeit conspicuous, result of an acute injury, and the subsequent long-term neurodevelopmental abnormalities, the result of their underlying causes, not the seizures themselves. Basic animal research into how extensively seizure activity may affect the developing brain has not resolved the controversy (26–30). Immature animals are more resistant than older animals to some seizure-induced injury (31). The immature brain may be resistant to acute seizure-induced cell loss (28); however, functional abnormalities such as impairment of visual-spatial memory and reduced seizure threshold (32) occur after seizures, and seizures induce changes in brain development, including altered neurogenesis (33), synaptogenesis, synaptic pruning, neuronal migration, and the sequential expression of genes including neurotransmitter receptors and transporters (34,35).

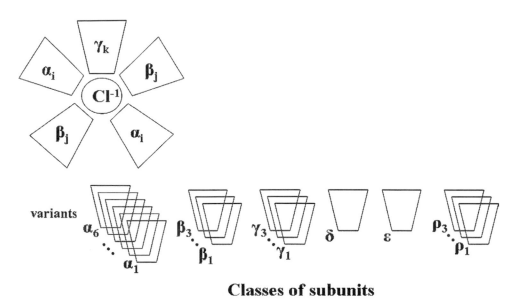

Figure 32.4 γ-Aminobutyric acid is a pentamer structure composed of six possible classes of subunits. The subunits themselves may have multiple variants that are expressed at different developmental ages.

Research by Holmes and colleagues (36) provides a newborn animal model for investigating whether recurrent seizures, induced by proconvulsant drugs that do not otherwise injure the brain, leave long-term undesirable effects on brain structure, learning, and susceptibility to spontaneous seizures. Starting on the first day of life, a series of about 25 seizures was induced by the administration of fluorothyl to neonatal rats. Behavioral testing in these animals as adults showed impaired spatial learning and memory, decreased activity levels, significantly lower threshold to pentylenetetrazol-induced seizures, and sprouting of CA3 mossy fibers, relative to controls that did not have neonatal seizures.

Neonatal seizures induce persistent changes in the inherent electrophysiologic properties of CA1 hippocampal cells in the rat (37). Although the resting membrane potentials in CA1 pyramidal neurons did not differ in controls and neonatal-seizure animals, reductions were noted in CA1 spike frequency adaptation and afterpolarization potentials after a spike train.

Seizures also accelerate neuronal death in the neonatal rat hippocampus in the setting of hypoxia (38). In the presence of hypoxia, the brain usually saves energy by blocking synaptic activity and electrically silencing the neuron; this effectively "turns off" the electroencephalogram. Seizures aggravate the hypoxic state by accelerating rapid anoxic depolarizations in the intact rat hippocampus. In effect, the generation of seizures "breaks the law of neuronal silence."

Finally, neonatal seizures in rats alter the subsequent composition of the GABA$_A$ receptor. GABA$_A$ is a pentamer in which five subunits assemble into a receptor structure (Fig. 32.4). Six subunit classes may comprise the pentamer: six variants of alpha, three of beta, three of gamma, one of delta, one of epsilon, and three of rho. The specific composition of an individual GABA$_A$ receptor depends on developmental age. In the studies of Zhang and associates (12,39), rats with neonatal seizures had a substantially higher proportion of beta-actin in the α_1 GABA$_A$ subunit component than did control animals (Fig. 32.5) (40).

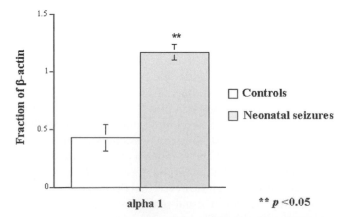

Figure 32.5 Rat pups subjected to seizures had significant differences in γ-aminobutyric acid subunit composition in later life compared with control animals. (Adapted from Brooks-Kayal AR, Shumate MD, Jim H, et al. Gamma-aminobutyric acid (A) receptor subunit expression predicts functional changes in hippocampal dentate granule cells during postnatal development. *J Neurochem* 2001;77:1266–1278, with permission.)

CLASSIFICATION AND CLINICAL FEATURES OF NEONATAL SEIZURES

Application of a syndromic classification to neonatal seizures is limited when considered in light of the classification of the International League Against Epilepsy (ILAE) (41,42). Almost all neonatal seizures are thought to be symptomatic, an acute reaction or consequence of a specific etiology. The ILAE addresses only five neonatal syndromes: benign neonatal convulsions, benign familial neonatal convulsions (BFNC), early myoclonic encephalopathy (EME), early infantile epileptic encephalopathy (EIEE), and migrating partial seizures of infancy. These are discussed later.

Seizures in the neonate are uniquely different from those in older infants and children. These differences are based on mechanisms of epileptogenesis and the developmental state of the immature brain and the relatively greater importance of nonepileptic mechanisms of seizure generation in this age group. Neonatal seizures may be classified by (a) clinical manifestations; (b) the relationship between clinical seizures and electrical activity on the electroencephalogram; and (c) seizure pathophysiology.

Clinical Classifications

A number of clinical classifications of neonatal seizures have been published (43–49). Early classifications focused on the *clinical* differences between seizures in neonates and those in older children: neonatal seizures were reported to be clonic or tonic, not tonic-clonic; when focal, they were either unifocal or multifocal. Later classifications included the term *myoclonus*. Another distinguishing feature of neonatal seizures is the occurrence of events described initially as "anarchic" (43) and thereafter "minimal" (45) or "subtle" (46). These events included oral-buccal-lingual movements such as sucking and chewing; movements of progression, such as bicycling of the legs and swimming movements of the arms; and random eye movements. First considered epileptic in origin, they were later deemed to be exaggerated reflex behaviors and thus were called "brainstem release phenomena" or "motor automatisms" (48). Table 32.1 lists the clinical characteristics of neonatal seizures according to a current classification scheme (50) that can be applied through observation.

Electroclinical Associations

Neonatal seizures may also be classified by the temporal relationship of clinical events to electrical seizure activity recorded on scalp electroencephalogram. In an electroclinical seizure, the clinical event overlaps with electrographic seizure activity. Some clinical-only events characterized as neonatal seizures may occur without any EEG seizure activity. Electrical-only seizures (also called subclinical or occult) occur in the absence of any clinical events.

Seizure Pathophysiology

Seizures may be classified as epileptic or nonepileptic (Table 32.2). Some clinical neonatal seizures are clearly epileptic, occurring in close association with EEG seizure activity, involving clinical events that can neither be provoked by stimulation nor suppressed by restraint, and

directly triggered by hypersynchronous cortical neuronal discharges. The following properties of the developing brain intensify seizure initiation, maintenance, and propagation: increases in cellular and synaptic excitation and a tendency to enhance propagation of an epileptic discharge (29,31,51–53). The clinical events that are most clearly epileptic in origin are focal clonic, focal tonic, some types of myoclonic, and rarely spasms (Tables 32.1 and 32.2). Electrical-only seizures are, by definition, epileptic.

Best considered nonepileptic in origin (48,54) are events that occur in the absence of electrical seizure activity but that have clinical characteristics resembling reflex behaviors. Such clinical events, whether provoked by stimulation or arising spontaneously, can be suppressed or altered by restraining or repositioning the infant. The clinical events may grow in intensity with increases in the repetition rate of stimulation (temporal summation) or the sites of simultaneous stimulation (spatial summation). Some types of myoclonic events, generalized tonic posturing, and motor automatisms can be classified as "nonepileptic" (Tables 32.1 and 32.2).

Paroxysmal clinical changes related to the autonomic nervous system have been proposed as manifestations of seizures. These include stereotyped, episodic alterations in heart rate, respiration, and blood pressure (47,55,56). Skin flushing, salivation, apnea (57,58), and pupillary dilation may also be autonomic signs of seizures, but they are usually associated with other clinical manifestations, except in the therapeutically paralyzed infant (48).

Electrographic Seizures

Although clinical observation is critical to the detection of neonatal seizures, the electroencephalogram offers the most important means of confirmation and characterization. Infants with normal background activity are much less likely to develop seizures than are those with significant background abnormalities (59).

Interictal Background and Prediction Value

The ongoing cerebral electrical activity is the stage on which the drama of the episodic electrographic seizure unfolds. In many ways, the integrity of the EEG background is more critical than the mere presence or absence of the seizures themselves. For example, with or without electrographic seizures, an extremely abnormal EEG background (burst suppression [60] or isoelectric recording) inherently conveys a sense of profound electrophysiologic disruption and forecasts an exceedingly high risk for death or adverse neurologic outcome. Conversely, a nearly normal interictal EEG background suggests relatively preserved neurologic health despite the intrusion of the seizures.

The interictal background also occasionally can offer clues to seizure etiology. Persistently focal sharp waves may

TABLE 32.1

CLINICAL CHARACTERISTICS, CLASSIFICATION, AND PRESUMED PATHOPHYSIOLOGY OF NEONATAL SEIZURES

Classification	Characteristics	Pathophysiologic Basis
Focal clonic	Repetitive, rhythmic contraction of muscle groups of the limbs, face, or trunk May be unifocal or multifocal May occur synchronously or asynchronously in muscle groups on one side of the body May occur simultaneously but asynchronously on both sides Cannot be suppressed by restraint	Epileptic
Focal tonic	Sustained posturing of single limbs Sustained asymmetric posturing of the trunk Sustained eye deviation Cannot be provoked by stimulation or suppressed by restraint	Epileptic
Generalized tonic	Sustained symmetric posturing of limbs, trunk, and neck May be flexor, extensor, or mixed extensor/flexor May be provoked or intensified by stimulation May be suppressed by restraint or repositioning	Presumed nonepileptic
Myoclonic	Random, single, rapid contractions of muscle groups of the limbs, face, or trunk Typically not repetitive or may recur at a slow rate May be generalized, focal, or fragmentary May be provoked by stimulation	Epileptic or nonepileptic
Spasms	May be flexor, extensor, or mixed extensor/flexor May occur in clusters Cannot be provoked by stimulation or suppressed by restraint	Epileptic
Motor Automatisms Ocular signs	Random, roving eye movements or nystagmus (distinct from tonic eye deviation) May be provoked or intensified by tactile stimulation	Nonepileptic
Oral-buccal-lingual movements	Sucking, chewing, tongue protrusions May be provoked or intensified by stimulation	Nonepileptic
Progression movements	Rowing or swimming movements Pedaling or bicycling movements of the legs May be provoked or intensified by stimulation May be suppressed by restraint or repositioning	Nonepileptic
Complex purposeless movements	Sudden arousal with transient increased random activity of limbs May be provoked or intensified by stimulation	Nonepileptic

suggest a restricted injury such as localized subarachnoid hemorrhage, contusion, or stroke, whereas multifocal sharp waves suggest diffuse dysfunction. Hypocalcemia is a consideration if a well-maintained background features excessive bilateral rolandic spikes. Inborn errors of metabolism, such as maple-syrup urine disease, are sometimes associated with distinctive vertex wicket spikes. Pseudoperiodic discharges raise the suspicion of herpes simplex virus encephalitis. A grossly abnormal electroencephalogram in the absence of any obviously acquired disease suggests cerebral dysgenesis.

Interictal EEG spikes *per se* have uncertain diagnostic significance (61). Interictal focal sharp waves and spikes are not typically considered indicators of epileptogenesis in the same way as they are in older children and adults. Compared with those of age-matched neonates without seizures (62,63), the interictal records of infants with electroencephalogram-confirmed seizures have background abnormalities, excessive numbers of "spikes" (lasting <200 milliseconds) compared with sharp waves (lasting >200 milliseconds), excessive occurrence of spikes or sharp waves per minute, and a tendency for "runs," "bursts," or "trains" of repetitive sharp waves. However, only a few infants with confirmed seizures exhibit all of these interictal characteristics, and many show no excessive spikes or sharp waves.

TABLE 32.2

CLASSIFICATION OF NEONATAL SEIZURES BY ELECTROCLINICAL FINDINGS

Clinical seizures with a consistent electrocortical signature (epileptic)
Focal clonic
    Unifocal
    Multifocal
    Hemiconvulsive
    Axial
Focal tonic
    Asymmetric truncal posturing
    Limb posturing
    Sustained eye deviation
Myoclonic
    Generalized
    Focal
Spasms
    Flexor
    Extensor
    Mixed extensor/flexor
Clinical seizures without a consistent electrocortical signature
    (presumed nonepileptic)
Myoclonic
    Generalized
    Focal
    Fragmentary
Generalized tonic
    Flexor
    Extensor
    Mixed extensor/flexor
Motor automatisms
    Oral-buccal-lingual movements
    Ocular signs
    Progression movements
    Complex purposeless movements
Electrical seizures without clinical seizure activity

Characteristics

At the heart of the epileptic process is the abnormal, excessive, repetitive electrical firing of neurons. Affected neurons lose their autonomy and are engulfed by the synchronized bursts of repeated electrical discharges. Sustained trains of action potentials arise in the affected neurons, which repeatedly fire and eventually propagate beyond their site of origin. At the conclusion of the ictus, inhibitory influences terminate the electrophysiologic cascade and end the seizure. Electrographic seizures in the neonate have varied appearances and are relatively rare before 34 to 35 weeks conceptional age. The morphology, spatial distribution, and temporal behavior of the seizure discharges may differ within and between individuals.

Morphology

An electrographic seizure is a discrete abnormal event lasting at least 10 seconds, with a definite beginning, middle, and end (64). No single morphologic pattern characterizes a seizure (Fig. 32.6). Even in the same patient, the ictal EEG activity may appear pleomorphic. The "typical"

neonatal seizure begins as low-amplitude, rhythmic, or sinusoidal waveforms or spike or sharp waves. As the seizure evolves, the amplitude of the ictal activity increases, while its frequency slows. Spikes or sharp waves are not necessarily present. Instead, rhythmic activity of any frequency (delta, theta, alpha, or beta) can make up the ictal patterns at the scalp surface.

Spatial Distribution

In older children generalized seizures may appear simultaneously, synchronously, and symmetrically in both hemispheres. In the neonatal brain, which lacks the physiologic organization necessary for such exquisite orchestration, individual seizures always arise focally, for example, first appearing in the left temporal region (T_3), migrating to adjacent electrode sites FP_3, C_3, or O_1, and finally engaging the entire hemisphere (so-called hemiconvulsive seizure); seizures may also migrate from one hemisphere to another (50). Occasionally, simultaneous focal seizures may appear to behave independently, spreading to all brain regions, and superficially masquerading as a "generalized seizure." However, the ictal patterns are not those of the truly generalized seizures, which usually are composed of spike or polyspike slowwave discharges.

Although diffuse causes of encephalopathy such as meningitis, hypoglycemia, or hypoxia/ischemia may be expected to produce generalized seizures, each seizure instead arises from a restricted area of cortex. Multiple seizures that each originate from different scalp regions are called "multifocal-onset seizures"; those that arise from the same scalp location are unifocal onset and raise the possibility of a localized structural abnormality such as a stroke (65), reflecting the restricted functional disturbance.

Temporal Profile

An electrographic neonatal seizure lasts about 2 minutes and is followed by a variable interictal period (Fig. 32.7). These temporal characteristics were obtained from relatively brief tracings randomly selected during a variety of acute encephalopathies (9). Few studies comprehensively describe the natural history of electrographic seizures during continuous monitoring from the onset of acute neurologic illness. Solitary, prolonged electrographic seizures are rare in newborn infants; more than 90% of those seizures recorded in one study lasted less than 30 minutes (64). Repetitive brief serial seizures are much more characteristic than prolonged seizures lasting many hours.

Special Ictal Electroencephalographic Morphologies

Some ictal patterns unique to the neonatal period are associated with severe encephalopathies. Electrical seizures of the depressed brain are long, low in voltage, and highly localized. They may be unifocal or multifocal and show little tendency to spread or modulate. Not associated with

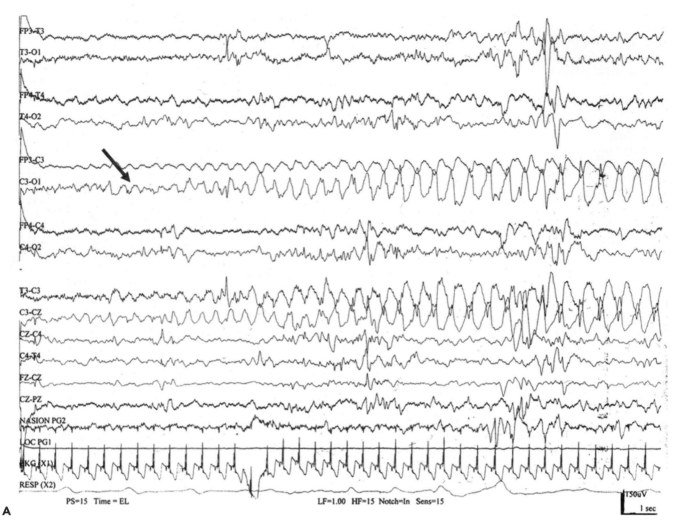

Figure 32.6 No single morphologic pattern characterizes electrographic neonatal seizures; rather, their distinctive behavior as a discrete, evolving electrographic event identifies them as ictal. **A:** A focal seizure arises from C₃ (*arrow*) as low-amplitude, rhythmic theta activity that gradually changes to higher-amplitude delta activity. **B:** An electrographic seizure is in progress as repetitive spikes in the right frontopolar, central, and midline vertex regions (*arrows*).

clinical seizures, they occur when the EEG background is depressed and undifferentiated, and suggest a poor prognosis. Alpha seizure activity (66–68) is characterized by sudden, transient, rhythmic activity of the α frequency (8 to 12 Hz) in the temporal or central region, unaccompanied by clinical events. An α discharge usually indicates a severe encephalopathy and poor prognosis.

Video-EEG monitoring has been the basis of clinical investigations into the classification, therapy, and prognosis of neonatal seizures (69–72), but is not widely available for routine use. Attended electroencephalography with simultaneous observation by trained electroneurodiagnostic technologists remains the conventional method of monitoring newborns with seizures.

Measures of Electrographic Seizure "Burden"

Most electrographic neonatal seizures do not provoke distinctive clinical signs (73) (Fig. 32.8), and, in infants iatro-

genically paralyzed by vecuronium or pancuronium, clinical recognition is useless.

Individual electrographic seizures may remain confined to their area of origin or may spread substantially to other regions (74). Counting the number of seizures or determining the percentage of the record with seizures does not provide information on their *spatial* distribution. An anatomic approach simplifies the entire neonatal electroencephalogram by considering five nonoverlapping areas of interest (75): left and right frontotemporal areas; the two left and right centro-occipital areas; and one midline region (Fig. 32.9). The spatial distribution of electrographic seizures varies considerably among individual neonates (Fig. 32.10) (71).

The simplest way to measure the burden of seizures is to consider them "present" or "absent" (Fig. 32.11). Counting the number of attacks that occur per hour can overstate or understate the seizure burden because the

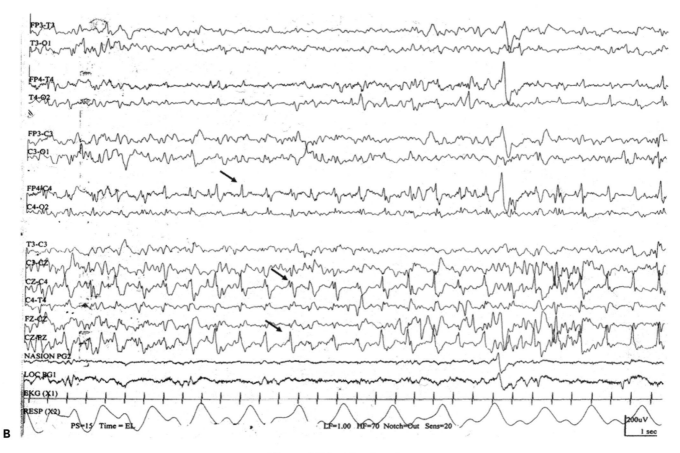

Figure 32.6 (*Continued*)

Etiologic Factors

number of electrographic seizures recorded even in a similar context varies widely. For example, during 48 hours of video-EEG monitoring after heart surgery, 11.5% of 183 newborns had one or more electrographic seizures, but total seizure *counts* varied from 1 to 217 (Fig. 32.12) (71). Because individual seizures also vary in length, a third way to measure seizure burden is to describe the percentage of time in which EEG seizure activity is present in any brain region. This can range from a 0% if no seizures are captured to 100% if the entire record demonstrates seizure activity anywhere in the brain. In the most precise, although time-consuming, *temporal-spatial* analysis, seizure burden is the total amount of time that EEG seizures are detected in each of the five regions of interest. Future investigations may determine whether a "dose– response" curve exists between this fuller measure of seizure burden and eventual long-term neurodevelopmental follow-up.

Etiologic Factors

Acute or chronic conditions can give rise to seizures. In most cases, specific causes can be determined after analysis of clinical and laboratory information (Table 32.3). Table 32.4 lists potential causes of neonatal seizures, but only a few are discussed in detail.

Acute Causes

Hypoxic-Ischemic Etiologies

Probably the most common cause of neonatal seizures, "acute neonatal encephalopathy" (76) is characterized by depressed mental status (lethargy or coma); seizures; axial and appendicular hypotonia with an overall reduction in spontaneous motor activity; and clear evidence of bulbar dysfunction with poor sucking, and swallowing, and an inexpressive face (77). Care should be taken to separate this generic designation from neonatal HIE. Not every infant who is acutely encephalopathic has suffered hypoxia-ischemia (78). The American College of Obstetricians and Gynecologists Task Force on Neonatal Encephalopathy and Cerebral Palsy suggests four diagnostic criteria for HIE: (a) evidence of metabolic acidosis in fetal umbilical cord arterial blood obtained at delivery (pH value less than 7 and base deficit greater than 12 mmol/L); (b) early onset of severe or moderate neonatal encephalopathy in infants born at 34 or more weeks of gestation; (c) subsequent cerebral palsy of the spastic quadriplegic or dyskinetic type; and (d) exclusion of other identifiable etiologies such as trauma, coagulation disorders, infectious conditions, or genetic disorders (79). These four conditions should occur in the context of a "sentinel" hypoxic event immediately

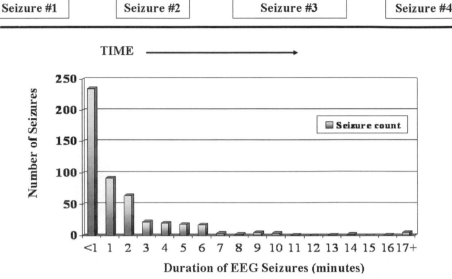

Figure 32.7 In most neonates with electrographic seizures, the electroencephalogram shows a series of brief ictal events, typically lasting about 2 minutes, followed by varying length interictal periods. The histogram shows the distribution of durations (minutes) of 487 electroencephalographic seizures recorded from 42 neonates. (Adapted from Clancy RR, Legido A. The exact ictal and interictal duration of electroencephalographic neonatal seizures. *Epilepsia* 1978; 28:537–541.)

before or during labor, such as uterine rupture, abruption of the placenta, or prolapse of the umbilical cord. There should also be a sudden and sustained fetal bradycardia or the absence of fetal heart rate variability; persistent, late, or variable decelerations; Apgar scores of 0 to 3 after 5 minutes; and multisystem involvement within 72 hours of birth. Examples of multisystem malfunction (80) include acute renal tubular necrosis, elevated values of liver function tests, necrotizing enterocolitis from bowel ischemia, and depressed blood-cell lines (e.g., thrombocytopenia) because of ischemic injury of the bone marrow (81). Early imaging studies should show acute diffuse cerebral abnormalities consistent with hypoxia/ischemia.

Other conditions that can clinically mimic acute neonatal HIE are some inborn errors of metabolism, pyridoxine dependence, stroke, coagulopathies, sinovenous thrombosis, and "fetal sepsis syndrome" (82–85), which can occur with sepsis or chorioamnionitis (86). The latter is suspected in a mother with abdominal pain and tenderness, fever, leukocytosis, and foul-smelling amniotic fluid, and can be confirmed by pathologic examination of the placenta and umbilical cord (87).

Perinatal stroke is defined as a cerebrovascular event occurring between 28 weeks of gestation and 7 days of age. The incidence is 1 in 4000 livebirths (88). There are two main clinical presentations: (a) acute appearance of neonatal seizures, hypotonia, feeding difficulties, and, rarely, hemiparesis (65,89–91) (Fig. 32.13); and (b) later discovery of stroke through the gradual appreciation of a congenital hemiparesis or the onset of a partial seizure disorder in an infant apparently healthy at birth. Risk factors include congenital heart defects (CHDs), blood and lipid

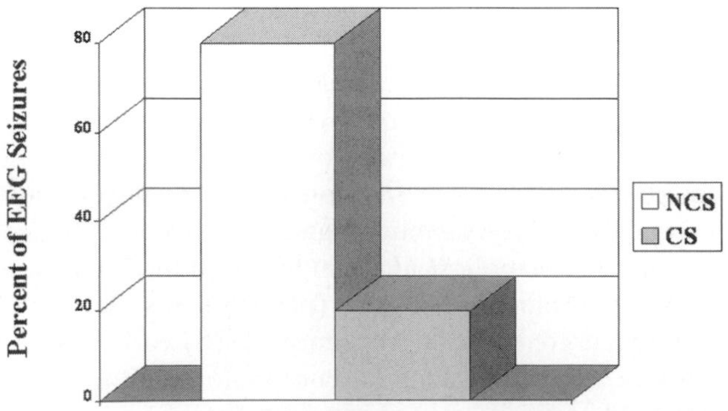

NCS = no clinical signs; CS = definite clinical signs.

Figure 32.8 In one study, only 20% of electrographic neonatal seizures produce definite clinical signs. (Adapted from Clancy RR, Legido A, Lewis D. Occult neonatal seizures. *Epilepsia* 1988; 29:256–261.)

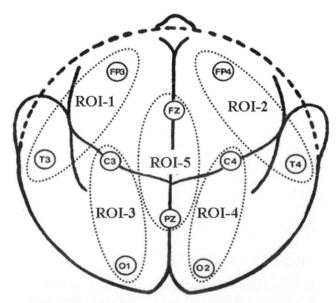

Figure 32.9 The entire array of the standard neonatal electroencephalogram can be reduced to five nonoverlapping regions of interest that identify the spatial characteristics of electroencephalographic seizures.

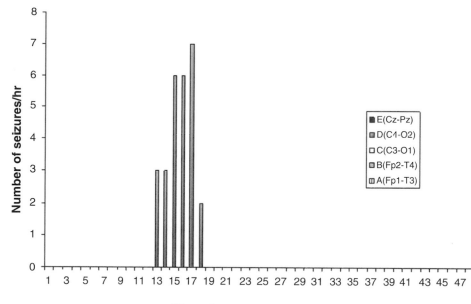

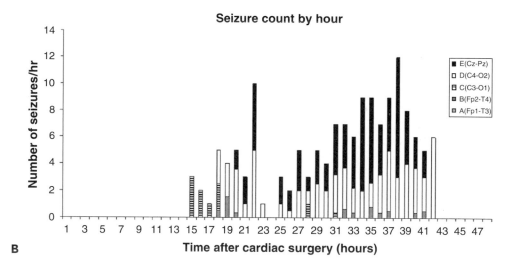

Figure 32.10 The spatial distribution of electroencephalographic (EEG) seizures varies among neonates. **A:** All EEG seizures begin in a single brain region (C_4-O_2). **B:** EEG seizures begin in four locations (C_z-P_z, C_4-O_2, C_3-O_1, and Fp_2-T_4). (Adapted from Sharif U, Ichord R, Saymor JW, et al. Electrographic neonatal seizures after newborn heart surgery. *Epilepsia* 2003;44:164.)

disorders, infection, placental disorders, vasculopathy, trauma, dehydration, and extracorporeal membrane oxygenation (ECMO).

Cerebral sinovenous thrombosis is estimated to occur at a rate of 0.67 cases per 100,000 children per year (92–94) in neonates and older children. The Canadian Stroke Registry includes reports of 160 consecutive children, of whom 43% were neonates. The neonatal presentation included seizures (71%) and nonspecific CNS signs such as lethargy (58%), but only infrequently frank hemiparesis (Fig. 32.14). Among risk factors are perinatal conditions (51%), dehydration (30%), infection (10%), and prothrombotic states (20%). The overall outcome reported in children and neonates included an 8% mortality rate; 54%

developed normally and 38% had long-term neurologic disabilities.

ECMO is an effective therapy for newborn infants with life-threatening respiratory failure unresponsive to maximum conventional medical support. However, the procedure requires ligations of the right common carotid artery and right jugular vein at a time when the infants' underlying lung disease may render them particularly vulnerable to the effects of diffuse CNS hypoxia-ischemia. The high rate of subsequent neurologic morbidity among survivors raises the possibility that ECMO itself may contribute to ischemic-reperfusion brain injuries (95). A high proportion of survivors have MRI-identified focal parenchymal brain lesions, often announced by seizures during ECMO.

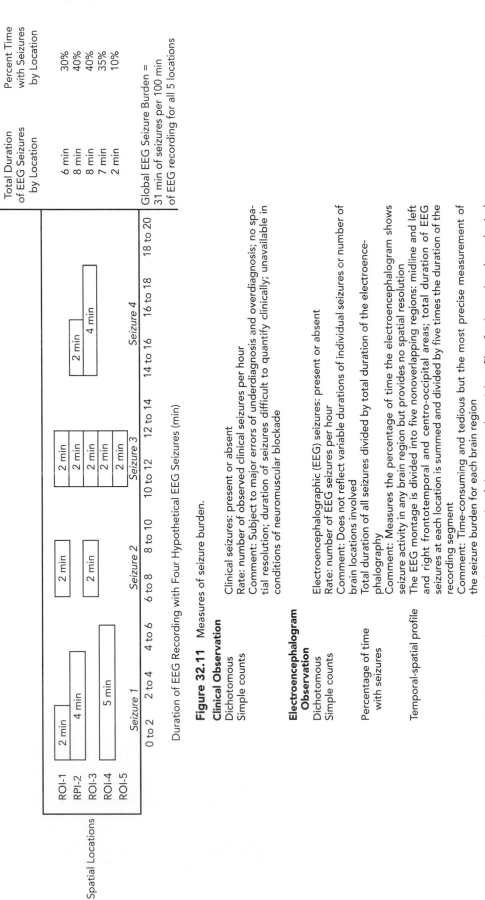

Figure 32.11 Measures of seizure burden.

Clinical Observation

Dichotomous   Clinical seizures: present or absent

Simple counts   Rate: number of observed clinical seizures per hour

Comment: Subject to major errors of underdiagnosis and overdiagnosis; no spatial resolution; duration of seizures difficult to quantify clinically; unavailable in conditions of neuromuscular blockade

Electroencephalogram Observation

Dichotomous   Electroencephalographic (EEG) seizures: present or absent

Simple counts   Rate: number of EEG seizures per hour

Comment: Does not reflect variable durations of individual seizures or number of brain locations involved

Percentage of time with seizures   Total duration of all seizures divided by total duration of the electroencephalography

Comment: Measures the percentage of time the electroencephalogram shows seizure activity in any brain region but provides no spatial resolution

Temporal-spatial profile   The EEG montage is divided into five nonoverlapping regions: midline and left and right frontotemporal and centro-occipital areas; total duration of EEG seizures at each location is summed and divided by five times the duration of the recording segment

Comment: Time-consuming and tedious but the most precise measurement of the seizure burden for each brain region

The illustration above provides an example of the temporal-spatial profile of seizures in a hypothetical neonate. In this case, the burden of seizures can be quantitated in several ways:
Comparison of different measures of seizure burden

1. Dichotomous: EEG seizures present
2. Simple count and rate: 12 seizures per hour
3. Percentage of time with seizures in any location: 65%
4. Spatial-temporal measurement: 31 minutes of seizures in all locations per "5 times duration of record" (100 minutes)

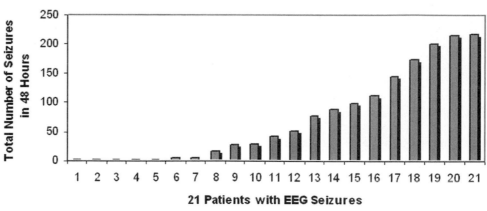

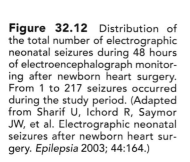

Figure 32.12 Distribution of the total number of electrographic neonatal seizures during 48 hours of electroencephalograph monitoring after newborn heart surgery. From 1 to 217 seizures occurred during the study period. (Adapted from Sharif U, Ichord R, Saymor JW, et al. Electrographic neonatal seizures after newborn heart surgery. *Epilepsia* 2003; 44:164.)

Cerebral hemorrhage and infarction have been reported in 28% to 52% of ECMO-treated infants (96).

CHDs enhance the risk for neonatal seizures (97), which can arise preoperatively or postoperatively. Some of these infants find it difficult to make the transition from intrauterine to extrauterine life, exhibiting depressed Apgar scores and persistent hypoxia leading to hypotension, acidosis, and multisystem failure including encephalopathy with seizures. CHDs also may be associated with the presence of other midline somatic defects including CNS anomalies. Seizures can arise from concurrent cerebral dysgenesis as well (98). Strokes may occur from embolization during cardiac catheterization. Hypocalcemia may trigger seizures in the setting of DiGeorge syndrome. However, seizures usually arise *after* newborn heart surgery; they do not occur at random, but, rather, are influenced by suspected or confirmed genetic disorders, aortic arch obstruction, or the need

for prolonged deep hypothermic circulatory arrest (99). This population is especially valuable for neuroprotection trials, because the child's status can be determined before surgery (100). The hypothesis is that if a neuroprotective agent administered preoperatively prevents seizures, the child has enjoyed neuroprotection from the intervention.

Metabolic Etiologies

Hypoglycemia, hyponatremia, hypernatremia, hypocalcemia, hypomagnesemia, and acute hyperbilirubinemia (acute kernicterus) can be associated with neonatal seizures. These conditions are detectable by simple screening tests (Table 32.3).

Hypoglycemia may itself cause brain damage independent of the seizures. Causes of hypoglycemia that should be evaluated in children include simple prematurity, maternal diabetes, nesidioblastosis, galactosemia, defects of gluconeogenesis, glycogen storage diseases, and respiratory chain defects. Glucose transporter type I syndrome (Glu I deficiency) is characterized by infantile seizures that usually begin between 6 and 12 weeks of life, developmental delay, ataxia, and progressive microcephaly (101–103). Affected newborns appear normal at birth. Neonatal seizures, initially rare, increase in frequency as the developmental delay becomes evident. The resultant diminution in transported glucose at the blood-brain barrier markedly reduces brain and cerebrospinal fluid values. Genetic studies implicate numerous mutations. The ketogenic diet provides an alternate form of fuel for the CNS.

Inborn Errors of Metabolism

For a detailed discussion, see Chapter 37. The discussion below is limited to the diagnosis of common neonatal conditions amenable to treatment with a specific intervention.

Maple syrup urine disease, ketotic and nonketotic hyperglycinemia, and urea cycle disorders may all induce a severe acute encephalopathy with seizures. Maple syrup urine disease produces an inability to decarboxylate branched-chain amino acids such as leucine, isoleucine,

---

TABLE 32.3

DATA TO DETERMINE THE ETIOLOGY OF NEONATAL SEIZURES

Clinical	Complete history, general physical and neurologic examinations, eye examination
Neuroimaging	Computerized tomographic or magnetic resonance imaging
Blood Tests	Arterial blood gases and pH
	Sodium, glucose, calcium, magnesium, ammonia, lactate and pyruvate, serum amino acids
	Comprehensive "neogen" panel[a]
	TORCH (toxoplasmosis, other infections, rubella, cytomegalovirus, and herpes simplex) titers
	Biotin
Urine tests	Reducing substances, sulfites, organic acids
	Toxicologic screen
Cerebrospinal fluid tests	Red and white blood cell counts
	Glucose and protein
	Culture
	Neurotransmitter profile[b]

[a] Varies by U.S. states.
[b] In the proper clinical context.

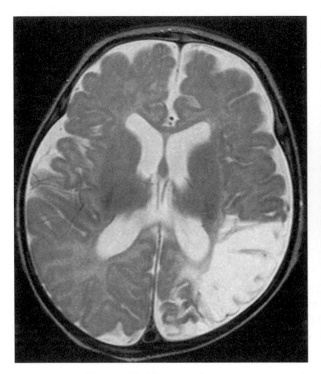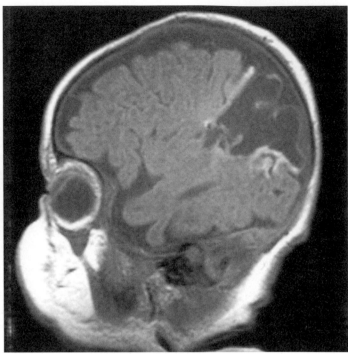

Figure 32.13   Arterial ischemic stroke in the distribution of the left middle cerebral artery in a 41-week estimated-gestational-age infant with a prothrombotic disorder.

and valine. After receiving a protein load from feeding milk, the neonate develops a shrill cry, progressive obtundation, hypotonia punctuated with episodic posturing, and seizures. Urine testing for 2,4-dinitrophenylhydrazine (DNPH) shows positive results, and hypoglycemia may appear from the elevated leucine.

Nonketotic hyperglycinemia has a catastrophic clinical presentation (aptly named glycine encephalopathy) with intractable seizures, coma, hiccups, apnea, pupil-sparing ophthalmoparesis, spontaneous and stimulus-provoked myoclonus, and a burst-suppression pattern on electroencephalography. Glycine levels are elevated in the blood and cerebrospinal fluid. The disorder represents an inability to cleave glycine, which is both an excitatory and inhibitory neurotransmitter. Treatment involves an *N*-methyl-D-aspartate antagonist, as well as magnesium, sodium benzoate, and dextromethorphan.

The ketotic hyperglycinemias, propionic and methylmalonic acidemias, present with overwhelming multisystem failure and dehydration, ketoacidosis, and fulminant CNS signs such as seizures, vomiting, and coma. Diagnosis is made by serum amino acid surveys and measurement of specific enzyme activity.

Carbamoylphosphate synthetase deficiency, ornithine carbamyl transferase deficiency, citrullinemia, and arginosuccinic acidemia, among the large number of urea-cycle abnormalities, each cause neonatal seizures in the first days or weeks of life. Coma and prominent bulbar dysfunction are noted with ophthalmoparesis, fixed pupils, absent gag reflex, poor sucking, and apnea. The degree of serum ammonia elevation may correlate with the discontinuity in the abnormal electroencephalogram backgrounds (104).

Biotinidase deficiency may produce alopecia, seborrheic dermatitis, developmental delay, hypotonia, and ataxia. Seizures may begin as early as the first week of life. The diagnosis is made by measurement of blood levels of biotinidase activity. Oral administration of free biotin daily is the treatment.

Pyridoxine-dependent seizures (105,106) usually arise between birth and 3 months of age, although atypical cases have been reported at 3 years. Some seizures can be appreciated *in utero* (107), especially if a previous pregnancy had been similarly affected with this autosomal recessive disorder. Parental consanguinity is not uncommon. The neonate presents with agitation, irritability, jitteriness, diminished sleep, and intractable clonic seizures. The EEG patterns are entirely nonspecific and include abnormal backgrounds, excessive multifocal sharp waves, and focal electrographic seizures evolving to hypsarrhythmia later in the first year. The diagnosis is made when seizures immediately cease and epileptiform EEG activity disappears within a few hours of the intravenous administration of 50 to 100 mg of pyridoxine. Lifelong therapy with pyridoxine 50 to 100 mg per day is necessary. Despite early treatment, some neonates are eventually retarded and show MRI evidence of a leukodystrophy. The biochemical cause of these seizures is unknown, and the only reliable diagnostic test is an unequivocal response to a trial of pyridoxine.

Folinic acid-responsive neonatal seizures were first described by Hyland as the unexpected appearance of

TABLE 32.4

ETIOLOGIES OF NEONATAL SEIZURES

Acute	Chronic
Acute neonatal encephalopathy (includes classic hypoxic-ischemic encephalopathy, both ante- and intrapartum)	Isolated cerebral dysgenesis, e.g., lissencephaly, hemimegalencephaly
Arterial ischemic stroke	Cerebral dysgenesis associated with inborn errors of metabolism
Sinovenous thrombosis	Chronic infection (TORCH [toxoplasmosis, other infections, rubella, cytomegalovirus, and herpes simplex] syndromes)
Extracorporeal membrane oxygenation	Neurocutaneous syndromes
Congenital heart disease	• Incontinentia pigmenti (Bloch Sulzberger syndrome)
Vein of Galen malformation	• Hypomelanosis of Ito
Giant arteriovenous malformation	• Sturge-Weber syndrome
Hypertensive encephalopathy	• Tuberous sclerosis
Intracranial hemorrhage (subdural subarachnoid, intraventricular, intraparenchymal)	• Linear sebaceous nevus (epidermal nevus syndrome)
Trauma (intrapartum and nonaccidental)	Genetic conditions
Infections (sepsis, meningitis, encephalitis)	• 22Q11 microdeletion
Transient, simple metabolic disorders	• ARX (Aristaless-related homeobox) mutations
Inborn errors of metabolism (including pyridoxine dependent seizures)	Specific very early onset epilepsy syndromes
Intoxication	
	• Fifth day fits (benign neonatal convulsions)
	• Benign familial neonatal seizures
	• Early myoclonic encephalopathy
	• Early infantile epileptic encephalopathy
	• Migrating partial seizures of infancy

seizures in term infants during the first few hours or days of life (108). Subsequently intractable, the seizures were associated with severe developmental delay, progressive atrophy on MRI examination, and frequent bouts of status epilepticus. The patients did not respond to intravenous pyridoxine. Analysis of cerebrospinal fluid by means of high-performance liquid chromatography with electrochemical detection consistently revealed an as yet unidentified compound, now used as the marker for this condition. Seizures ceased and the EEG pattern improved after the administration of 2.5 mg of folinic acid twice daily.

The molybdenum cofactor is essential for the proper functioning of the enzymes sulfite oxidase and xanthine dehydrogenase. Deficiency of the cofactor and isolated sulfite oxidase deficiency are autosomal recessive errors that produce severe neurologic symptoms resulting from a lack of sulfite oxidase activity (109–111). The presentation includes poor feeding, an abnormally pitched cry, jitteriness, and intractable seizures. A fresh urine sample shows positive results of a sulfite test and elevated levels of xanthine and hypoxanthine, coupled with depressed concentrations of uric acid. This array of chemical malfunction can arise from mutations in three molybdenum cofactors or in gephyrin. Synthesis of molybdenum cofactor requires the activities of at least six gene products including gephyrin (112), a polypeptide responsible for the cluster-

ing of inhibitory glycine receptors and postsynaptic membranes in the rat CNS. Mutations in sulfite oxidase are found in patients with isolated sulfite oxidase deficiency. There is no effective treatment, and prognosis for neurologic recovery and survival is poor.

Neonatal Intoxications

Lidocaine or mepivacaine inadvertently injected into the fetal scalp during local pudendal analgesia for the mother, cocaine, heroin (113), amphetamines, propoxyphene, and theophylline also may cause seizures.

Chronic Causes

Cerebral Dysgenesis

Some neonatal seizures result from long-standing disorders, such as cerebral dysgenesis, neurocutaneous syndromes, genetic disorders, or very early onset epilepsy. An MRI scan should be performed early to uncover cerebral dysgenesis (114). In lissencephaly or hemimegalencephaly (Fig. 32.15), no acute cause for seizures such as neonatal depression or birth trauma is present, and the infant appears outwardly well yet experiences seizures. The identification of cerebral dysgenesis on neuroimaging should not dissuade the clinician from seeking evidence of inborn errors of metabolism, as both may coexist (e.g., cytochrome

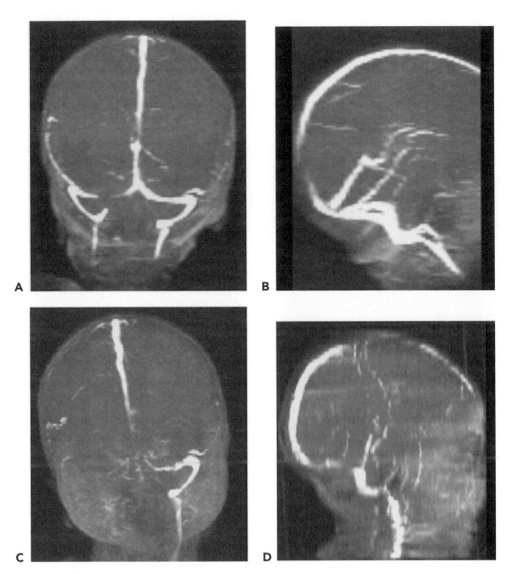

Figure 32.14 Magnetic resonance venogram of a 2-week-old term infant admitted for seizures, lethargy, and dehydration. **A** and **B:** Thrombosis of the right transverse sinus was noted on the first day of hospitalization. **C** and **D:** By day 10, the thromboses had extended to the sigmoid, jugular, and straight sinuses.

oxidase deficiency; glutaric aciduria types I and II; 3-hydroxyisobutaric aciduria; 3-methylglutaconic aciduria; 3-ketothiolase deficiency; sulfite oxidase deficiency; pyruvate dehydrogenase deficiency; neonatal adrenoleukodystrophy; fumaric aciduria; long ketotic hyperglycinemia; and Zellweger syndrome) (115).

TORCH Infections

Chronic TORCH (toxoplasmosis, other infections, rubella, cytomegalovirus, and herpes virus) infections can be identified by ophthalmologic changes, microcephaly, periventricular calcifications on neuroimaging, and blood tests. Congenital infections acquired before the fourth month of gestation may cause an acquired form of migration defect and give rise to dysgenetic patterns on computed tomography (CT) or MRI scanning (116).

Neurocutaneous Syndromes

Among the neurocutaneous syndromes that may give rise to neonatal seizures is familial incontinentia pigmenti, a mixed syndrome of different mosaicisms (117). This X-linked dominant state is presumably lethal in males. Perinatal inflammatory vesicles are followed by verrucous patches that produce a distinctive pattern of hyperpigmentation and finally dermal scarring. The cause is a mutation in the I-κB kinase (IKK)-γ gene located on XQ28. Bloch-Sulzberger syndrome is an earlier described synonym. In contrast to the familial form, sporadic incontinentia pigmenti maps to XP11 and is considered the "negative" pattern. Better known as hypomelanosis of Ito, its cutaneous lesions appear as areas of hypopigmentation.

Tuberous sclerosis may create neonatal seizures in two basic ways (118): first, through cortical tubers, which in the neonate may be easier to appreciate on CT scan than on MRI, and second, embolic stroke from intracardiac tumors. In the neonate, the classic neurocutaneous signs are often not apparent, except for hypomelanotic macules noted at or soon after birth; however, these may be evident only on skin examination under a Wood lamp.

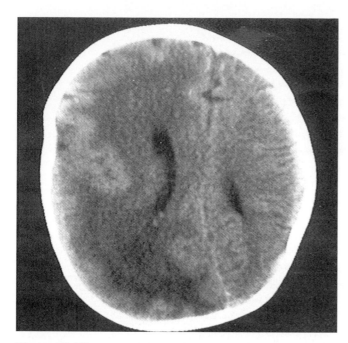

Figure 32.15 Computed tomography scan of the head showing right hemimegalencephaly with dysplastic and enlarged right cerebral hemisphere. Brain magnetic resonance imaging provides better resolution and definition of the abnormality and reveals subtle involvement of the contralateral hemisphere.

Linear sebaceous nevi are a family of disorders with distinctive raised, waxy, sometimes verrucous nevi on the scalp or face, associated with hemihypertrophy, hemimegalencephaly, and neonatal seizures (119).

Sturge-Weber syndrome is a sporadic syndrome featuring the distinctive port wine stain and associated vascular anomaly over the cortical surface. It may manifest with neonatal seizures.

Genetic Conditions

DiGeorge syndrome, caused by a microdeletion in the 22Q11 area, is a risk factor for seizures in infants undergoing newborn heart surgery, with or without hypocalcemia, and also increases risk for seizures in later life.

Recently, mutations in the Aristaless-related homeobox (ARX) gene have been found in patients with early onset infantile spasms, ambiguous genitalia, variable degrees of mental retardation, autism, and cerebral malformations (120). Homeobox genes code for transcription factors that orchestrate the developmental plan of embryos. Mutations in these genes cause holoprosencephaly, schizencephaly, septo-optic dysplasia, and other brain malformations. The ARX gene mutation is now recognized to be responsible for some cases of lissencephaly, agenesis of the corpus callosum, and dysplasia of the thalamus and midbrain.

Epilepsy Syndromes of Early Infantile Onset

In the 1970s, French neurologists coined the "fifth-day fits" (benign neonatal convulsions) to describe an electroclinical syndrome in which seizures unexpectedly arose between the fourth and sixth days of life (121). The seizures were usually partial clonic, often with apnea and status epilepticus. More than half had a distinctive "theta pointu alternant" pattern in which the bursts of cerebral electrical activity in the discontinuous parts of the record showed sharply contoured theta waves, especially in the central regions. This EEG pattern has also been recognized in patients with unmistakable HIE.

Benign *familial* neonatal convulsions (BFNC) was the first idiopathic epilepsy syndrome discovered to be caused by a single gene mutation (122,123). Partial seizures unexpectedly begin by the third day of life in neurologically normal-appearing patients, 10% to 15% of whom progress to epilepsy. Three known genetic defects are responsible for this disorder (122). BFNC type I has a defective gene KCNQ2 at chromosomal locus 20Q13.2 with an aberrant α subunit of a voltage-gated potassium channel. Type II has an abnormal KCNQ3 gene, located on 8Q24, and also codes for an aberrant α subunit of a voltage-gated potassium channel. BFNC with myokymia (124) has been reported as a separate mutation of KCNQ2, also on 20Q13.2. Some so-called benign familial *infantile* seizures (125), which typically appear in the first year of life, present with neonatal seizures. These are associated with the aberrant gene SCN2A, located on 2Q24, that represents a defective α subunit of a voltage-gated sodium channel (122).

Migrating partial seizures in infancy constitute a constellation of unprovoked, alternating electroclinical seizures and subsequent neurodevelopmental devastation that was described in 1995 by Coppola and associates (126). Although multifocal neonatal seizures are not uncommon after infections, metabolic disorders, and hypoxia/ischemia, they can also accompany cerebral dysgenesis and some other neonatal seizure syndromes. In migrating partial seizures in infancy, healthy infants without cerebral dysy display. Multifocal partial seizures that arise independently and sequentially from both hemispheres (Fig. 32.16) within the first 6 months of life and progress through a period of intractability, ultimately leading to severe psychomotor retardation. As described in the original paper and later case reports, prognosis was very poor, with 28% mortality and the majority of survivors profoundly retarded and nonambulatory; however, later patients have fared somewhat better (127).

First described by Aicardi and Goutieres (128), EME is characterized by maternal reports of sustained, rhythmic fetal kicking, oligohydramnios or polyhydramnios, normal Apgar scores, and seizure onset from the first day of life to several months (typical age, 16 days). Clinical seizures include erratic fragments of myoclonic activity, massive myoclonia, stimulus-sensitive myoclonia, and partial seizures. Electroencephalograms are eventually markedly abnormal, frequently with a burst-suppression background. The myoclonic limb movements tend to occur during the burst periods of the burst suppression (Fig. 32.17). All patients are completely resistant to antiepileptic drugs (AEDs). Other clinical features are progressive

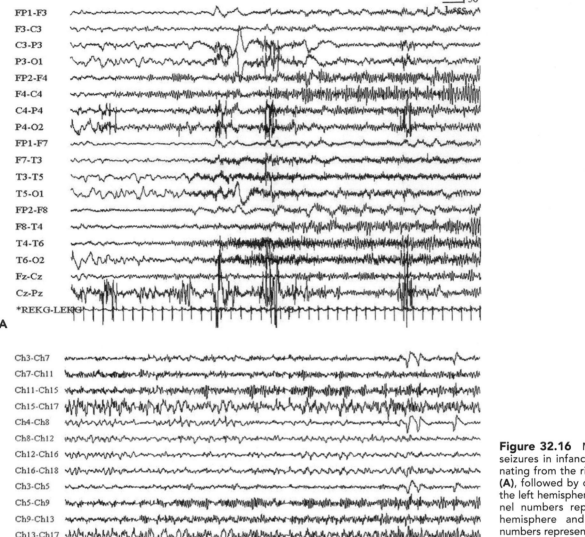

Figure 32.16 Migrating partial seizures in infancy. Seizure originating from the right hemisphere **(A)**, followed by one arising from the left hemisphere **(B)** (odd channel numbers represent the left hemisphere and even channel numbers represent the right hemisphere). Note that the time axis of the electroencephalogram rhythm strip is slightly compressed. The time and amplitude calibration bar appears at the top of the figure: 1 second and 50 μV. (Adapted from Marsh E, Melamed S, Clancy R. Migrating partial seizures in early infancy: expanding the phenotype of a rare neonatal seizure type. *Epilepsia* 2003;44:305.)

decline in head circumference percentiles, bulbar signs (especially apnea), feeding difficulties, cleft or high-arched palate, and severe psychomotor delay. Progressive cerebral atrophy is evident on neuroimaging scans (129). The cause is unknown.

Early infantile epileptic encephalopathy (EIEE), also known as Ohtahara syndrome, is characterized by intractable tonic seizures in the setting of a severe encephalopathy and a burst-suppression background pattern (130). In fact, the EEG findings alone appear similar to those of EME. Many infants with EIEE harbor overt cerebral dysgenesis or cortical dys-

plasias. Survivors often develop typical infantile spasms with hypsarrhythmia and Lennox-Gastaut syndrome accompanied by multifocal spikes on the electroencephalogram.

TREATMENT

Despite the decades-long recognition of neonatal seizures, treatment recommendations rest almost entirely on conventional wisdom and traditional practices. Because AEDs are used to treat neonatal seizures of *epileptic* origin, initial

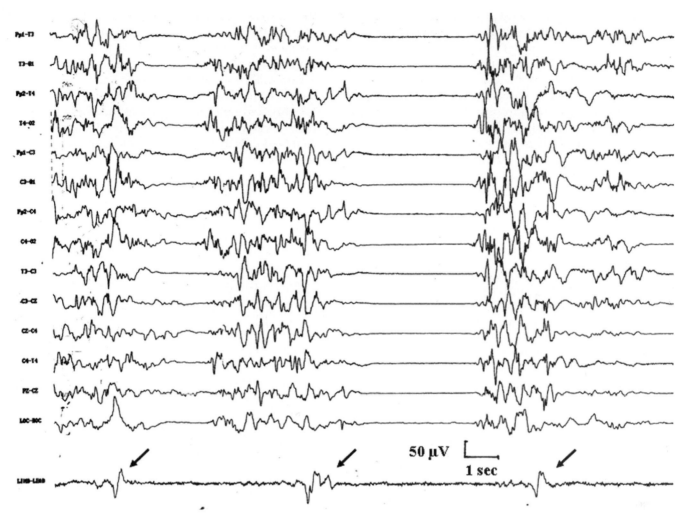

Figure 32.17 Burst-suppression electroencephalographic pattern of early myoclonic epilepsy. The abnormal myoclonic movements, detected by the bottom electromyographic channel (*arrows*), occur during the "burst" periods of the tracing.

consideration is given to the clinical and EEG features of the events. Discussion has also centered on the advisability of treating all epileptic neonatal seizures, as some are brief, infrequent, and self-limited. If the burden of seizures will be minimal, the infant need not be exposed to acute and long-term drug therapy. On the other hand, epileptic neonatal seizures that are long, frequent, and not self-limited are treated acutely and vigorously with AEDs.

No studies unequivocally demonstrate the efficacy of barbiturates in the treatment of neonatal seizures. In a randomized, controlled study (131), thiopental was administered soon after perinatal asphyxia. Seizures were diagnosed by clinical signs and occurred in 76% of treated infants and in 73% of a control (placebo) group. High doses of phenobarbital given after perinatal asphyxia resulted in a lower rate of recurrent seizures compared to placebo, although the difference was not statistically significant (132). Of 31 acutely ill neonates with electrographic seizures detected during continuous electroencephalograph monitoring,

only 2 had a complete cessation of both clinical and EEG seizures with AEDs (133). Six had an equivocal electroclinical response. Clinical seizures stopped in 13, although the electrographic seizures persisted. The remaining 10 had persistent electroclinical seizures. Two studies (70,74) reported a mixed response of electroclinical seizures to phenobarbital. In a comparison study (134), electrographic seizures ceased in 43% of the group treated with phenobarbital and in 45% of the group given phenytoin; however, the lack of a placebo control precluded determination of absolute efficacy. Video-EEG monitoring demonstrated cessation of seizures in 11 of 22 infants after administration of phenobarbital 40 mg/kg (70). The choice of a second-line drug for nonresponders was limited to lignocaine or benzodiazepines. According to a recent Cochrane review (135), "at the present time, anticonvulsant therapy determined in the immediate period following perinatal asphyxia cannot be recommended for routine clinical practice, other than in the treatment of prolonged or frequent clinical seizures."

In summary, despite the frequent empiric selection of phenobarbital in clinical practice for the treatment of neonatal seizures, evidence of its efficacy is limited, and animal studies raise concern that phenobarbital itself may have deleterious effects on the young nervous system (see below). A joint venture by the National Institutes of Health and the Food and Drug Administration, the "newborn drug development initiative," fosters the performance of ethical, well-controlled trials of pharmaceutical agents used in neonatal neurology, cardiology, anesthesia, pain management, and related disorders. Few drugs for use in the newborn have been subjected to adequately powered, randomized, placebo-controlled investigations to demonstrate real safety and efficacy. Drugs with potential for the treatment of neonatal seizures are no exception.

Nevertheless, in ordinary clinical practice, it is common to administer AEDs in an effort to reduce or eliminate seizures in the newborn. Early studies of neonatal seizures recommended loading doses of phenobarbital 15 to 20 mg/kg, with the intention of generating serum levels between 15 and 20 μg/mL, followed by maintenance doses of 3 to 4 mg/kg per day. In the comparative study with phenytoin (134,136), phenobarbital doses were chosen to achieve *free* (unbound) concentrations of 25 μg/mL. This was accomplished by incubating the infant's blood with phenobarbital to determine drug binding. Plasma binding of phenobarbital in neonates varies from 0% to 45%. The "mg/kg" dose needed to provide a free plasma-bound level of 25 μg/mL is calculated by the formula

$$\text{plasma-bound dose} = (25 \text{ mg/kg}) \times \text{Vd (L/kg)}/ \\ (\% \text{ free binding})$$

For phenobarbital, the volume of distribution is assumed to be 1 L/kg.

The "mg/kg" dose of phenytoin should be calculated to achieve, but not exceed, free concentrations of 3 μg/mL (134,136). The formula (3 μg/kg) × Vd (L/kg)/(% free binding) assumes a volume of distribution of 1 L/kg. Phenytoin has nonlinear pharmacokinetics: steady-state plasma concentrations at one dosing schedule do not predict those at another schedule (137,138). There are also variable rates of hepatic metabolism, decreases in elimination rates during the first weeks of life, and variable bioavailability with different generic preparations. A redistribution of the AED after the initial dose decreases brain concentrations thereafter; thus, dosage must be tailored to the individual patient after therapy begins.

Phenytoin should be given by direct intravenous infusion at a rate no faster than 1 mg/kg per minute. Serum binding of the drug is unpredictable in critically ill neonates, and excessively rapid administration or high concentrations can result in serious or lethal cardiac arrhythmias. Furthermore, phenytoin is strongly alkalotic and may lead to local venous thrombosis or tissue irritation. The use of fosphenytoin may reduce these risks.

Benzodiazepines, typically lorazepam (0.15 mg/kg) and diazepam (0.3 mg/kg), are third-line treatments of neonatal seizures. Side effects of acute administration include hypotension and respiratory depression. Alternative or adjuvant AEDs have also been empirically prescribed for refractory neonatal seizures. Clonazepam, lidocaine (139,140), and midazolam (141) are administered intravenously; carbamazepine (142), primidone (143), valproate (144), vigabatrin (145), and lamotrigine (146) are given orally.

Chronic Postnatal Epilepsy and the Need for Long-Term Treatment

Chronic postnatal epilepsy is relatively common in the wake of neonatal seizures (Fig. 32.18). For many patients, permanent, fixed brain injuries, such as resolving stroke, ischemia, or traumatic lesions, serve as the nidus for future epilepsy. As mentioned, repeated neonatal seizures may have "instructed" the brain how to have seizures, resulting in a persistent lowering of the seizure threshold (32). In infants with EME or EIEE, neonatal seizures represent the beginning of very early onset epilepsy, which persists by its nature. The most common occurrence, however, is epilepsy after neonatal seizures triggered by acute neonatal conditions.

Ellenberg and colleagues (147) found that approximately 20% of survivors of neonatal seizures experienced one or more seizures up to 7 years of age; nearly two thirds of the seizures occur within the first 6 months of life. Other researchers (8,19–21,72) reported rates ranging from 17% to 30%. The 56% noted by Clancy and colleagues (22,148) may be explained by the population's relatively serious risk factors for CNS dysfunction. Partial and generalized seizures characterize postneonatal epilepsy and do not seem to be preventable by the long-term administration of AEDs after neonatal seizures.

Not all neonates require extended therapy after acute seizures have been controlled, although no criteria for maintenance AED use have been sufficiently studied. For chronic therapy, either phenobarbital or phenytoin 3 to

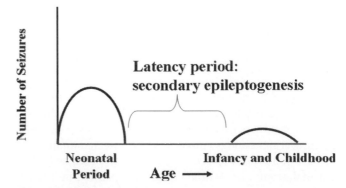

Figure 32.18 Acute neonatal seizures are often followed by chronic postnatal epilepsy. A latent period, during which secondary epileptogenesis develops, gives rise to spontaneous, unprovoked seizures.

4 mg/kg per day is given, and serum levels are monitored. Reported schedules for discontinuation of maintenance therapy range from 1 week to 12 months after the last seizure (149); one currently used schedule withdraws AEDs 2 weeks after the last seizure (150).

Potential Deleterious Effects of Antiepileptic Drug Administration on the Immature Central Nervous System

AEDs prevent or interrupt electrographic seizures by the blockade of voltage-dependent sodium channels and glutamatergic excitatory neurotransmission and enhancing of GABA-mediated inhibition. However, in this critical time of early brain development, suppression of synaptic transmission may have undesirable consequences, because neuronal and synaptic pruning are activity dependent. Since the 1970s, it has been known that rat pups fed phenobarbital later have reductions in brain weight and in total brain cell count (151). How AEDs may harm the developing rat brain remains under investigation, but evidence suggests that these drugs may trigger apoptotic neurodegeneration in the rodent forebrain and suppress an endogenous neuroprotective system already in place (152). The clinical impact of these findings is less certain. Most neonates are given phenobarbital because of seizures, and it is difficult to determine how much of any long-term aftermath is the result of the seizures' underlying etiology, the attacks themselves, or the medications administered to suppress them. Some neonates receive phenobarbital for other reasons, such as to provide sedation or to accelerate hepatic maturity in neonatal hyperbilirubinemia and appear to experience no ill effects. Likewise, benzodiazepines are commonly administered for sedation or to reduce agitation, and no obvious adverse effects are associated with their use, although careful studies are lacking.

REFERENCES

1. Eriksson M, Zetterstrom R. Neonatal convulsions: incidence and causes in the Stockholm area. *Acta Paediatr Scand* 1979;68: 807–811.
2. Bergman I, Painter MJ, Hirsch RP. Outcomes in neonates with convulsions treated in an intensive care unit. *Ann Neurol* 1983;14:642.
3. Spellacy W, Peterson P, Winegar A. Neonatal seizures after cesarean section: higher risk with labor. *Am J Obstet Gynecol* 1987;157:377–379.
4. Lanska MJ, Lanska DJ, Baumann RJ, et al. A population-based study of neonatal seizures in Fayette County, Kentucky. *Neurology* 1995;45:724–732.
5. Ronen G, Penney S. The epidemiology of clinical neonatal seizures in Newfoundland, Canada. *Ann Neurol* 1995;38:518–519.
6. Ronen GM, Penney S, Andrews W. The epidemiology of clinical neonatal seizures in Newfoundland: a population-based study. *J Pediatr* 1999;134:71–75.
7. Saliba RM, Annegers JF, Waller DK, et al. Incidence of neonatal seizures in Harris County, Texas, 1992–1994. *Am J Epidemiol* 1996;150:763–769.
8. Scher M, Aso K, Beggarly M, et al. Electrographic seizures in preterm and full-term neonates: clinical correlates, associated brain lesions and risk for neurologic sequelae. *Pediatrics* 1993; 34:128–134.
9. Scher M, Hamid M, Steppe D, et al. Ictal and interictal electrographic seizure durations in preterm and term neonates. *Epilepsia* 1993;34:284–288.
10. Johnston MV. Selective vulnerability in the neonatal brain. *Ann Neurol* 1998;44:155–156.
11. Zhang G, Hsu FC, Raol YH, et al. Selective alterations of GABA A receptor subunit expression and function in hippocampal dentate granule cells after seizures in the developing brain. *Epilepsia* 2001;42:224.
12. Zhang G, Raol YH, Brooks-Kayal AR. Selective alteration of excitatory and inhibitory receptors and transporters in hippocampal dentate granule cells after seizures in the developing brain. *Epilepsia* 2002;43:27.
13. Staley K. Enhancement of the excitatory actions of GABA by barbiturates and benzodiazepines. *Neurosci Lett* 1992;146:105–107.
14. Volpe J. Neonatal seizures. In: *Neurology of the newborn*, 4th ed. Philadelphia: WB Saunders, 2001:178–214.
15. Lombroso CT. Prognosis in neonatal seizures. *Adv Neurol* 1983; 34:101.
16. Ellenberg JH, Nelson KB. Cluster of perinatal events identifying infants at high risk for death or disability. *J Pediatr* 1988;113: 546–552.
17. Nelson KB, Broman SH. Perinatal risk factors in children with serious motor and mental handicaps. *Ann Neurol* 1977;2:371–377.
18. Temple CM, Dennis J, Carney R, et al. Neonatal seizures: long-term outcome and cognitive development among "normal" survivors. *Dev Med Child Neurol* 1995;37:109–118.
19. Ortibus EL, Sum JM, Hahn JS. Predictive value of EEG for outcome and epilepsy following neonatal seizures. *Electroencephalogr Clin Neurophysiol* 1996;98:175–185.
20. Brunquell PJ, Glennon CM, DiMario FJ Jr, et al. Prediction of outcome based on clinical seizure type in newborn infants. *J Pediatr* 2002;140:707–712.
21. Mizrahi EM, Clancy R, Dunn JK, et al. Neurologic impairment, developmental delay and post-natal seizures two years after video-EEG documented seizures in near-term and full-term neonates: report of the Clinical Research Centers for Neonatal Seizures. *Epilepsia* 2001;102:47.
22. Legido A, Clancy RR, Berman PH. Neurologic outcome after electroencephalographically proven neonatal seizures. *Pediatrics* 1991;88:583–596.
23. McBride MC, Laroia N, Guillet R. Electrographic seizures in neonates correlate with poor neurodevelopmental outcome. *Neurology* 2000;55:506–513.
24. Miller SP, Weiss J, Barnwell A, et al. Seizure-associated brain injury in term newborns with perinatal asphyxia. *Neurology* 2002;58:542–548.
25. Schmid R, Tandon P, Stafstrom CE, et al. Effects of neonatal seizures on subsequent seizure-induced brain injury. *Neurology* 1999;53:1754–1761.
26. Wasterlain CG, Plum F. Retardation of behavioral landmarks after neonatal seizures in rats. *Trans Am Neurol Assoc* 1973;98:320–321.
27. Wasterlain CG. Neonatal seizures and brain growth. *Neuropadiatrie* 1978;9:213–228.
28. Wasterlain C, Niquet J, Thompson K, et al. Seizure-induced neuronal death in the immature brain. *Prog Brain Res* 2002;135: 335–353.
29. Holmes G. Epilepsy in the developing brain. *Epilepsia* 1997;38: 12–30.
30. Yager JY, Armstrong EA, Miyashita H, et al. Prolonged neonatal seizures exacerbate hypoxic-ischemic brain damage: correlation with cerebral energy metabolism and excitatory amino acid release. *Dev Neurosci* 2002;24:367–381.
31. Swann J. Synaptogenesis and epileptogenesis in developing neural networks. In: Schwartzkroin P, Moshe SL, Noebels JL, et al., eds. *Brain development and epilepsy.* New York: Oxford University Press, 1995:195–233.
32. Mazarati A, Bragin A, Baldwin R, et al. Epileptogenesis after self-sustaining status epilepticus. *Epilepsia* 2002;43:74–80.
33. Sankar R, Shin D, Liu H, et al. Granule cell neurogenesis after status epilepticus in the immature rat brain. *Epilepsia* 2000;41: S53–S56.

34. McCabe BK, Silveira DC, Cilio MR, et al. Reduced neurogenesis after neonatal seizures. *J Neurosci* 2001;21:2094–2103.

35. Fando JL, Conn M, Wasterlain CG. Brain protein synthesis during neonatal seizures: an experimental study. *Exp Neurol* 1979; 63:220–228.

36. Holmes GL, Gairsa JL, Chevassus-Au-Louis N, et al. Consequences of neonatal seizures in the rat: morphological and behavioral effects. *Ann Neurol* 1998;44:845–857.

37. Villeneuve N, Ben-Ari Y, Holmes GL, et al. Neonatal seizures induced persistent changes in intrinsic properties of CA1 rat hippocampal cells. *Ann Neurol* 2000;47:729–738.

38. Dzhala V, Ben-Ari Y, Khazipov R. Seizures accelerate anoxia-induced neuronal death in the neonatal rat hippocampus. *Ann Neurol* 2000;48:632–640.

39. Zupan V, Gonzalez P, Lacaze-Masmonteil T, et al. Periventricular leukomalacia: risk factors revisited. *Dev Med Child Neurol* 1996;38:1061–1067.

40. Brooks-Kayal AR, Shumate MD, Jin H, et al. Gamma-aminobutyric acid(A) receptor subunit expression predicts functional changes in hippocampal dentate granule cells during postnatal development. *J Neurochem* 2001;77:1266–1278.

41. Commission on Classification and Terminology of the International League Against Epilepsy. Proposal for revised classification of epilepsies and epileptic syndromes. *Epilepsia* 1989;30:389–399.

42. ILAE Commission Report. A proposed diagnostic scheme for people with epileptic seizures and with epilepsy: report of the ILAE Task Force on Classification and Terminology. *Epilepsia* 2001;42:796–803.

43. Dreyfus-Brisac C, Monod N. Electroclinical studies of status epilepticus and convulsions in the newborn. In: Kellaway P, Petersen I, eds. *Neurological and electroencephalographic correlative studies in infancy.* New York: Grune and Stratton, 1964: 250–272.

44. Rose A, Lombroso C. A study of clinical, pathological and electroencephalographic features in 137 full-term babies with a long-term follow up. *Pediatrics* 1970;45:404–425.

45. Lombroso C. Seizures in the newborn. In: Vinken P, Bruyn G, eds. *The epilepsies. Handbook of clinical neurophysiology,* vol 15. Amsterdam: North Holland, 1974:189–218.

46. Volpe J. Neonatal seizures. *N Engl J Med* 1973;289:413–416.

47. Watanabe K, Hara K, Miyazaki S. Electroclinical studies of seizures in the newborn. *Folia Psychiatr Neurol Jpn* 1977;31: 383–392.

48. Mizrahi EM, Kellaway P. Characterization and classification of neonatal seizures. *Neurology* 1987;37:1837–1844.

49. Volpe J. Neonatal seizures: current concepts and revised classification. *Pediatrics* 1989;84:422–428.

50. Mizrahi EM, Kellaway P. *Diagnosis and management of neonatal seizures.* Philadelphia: Lippincott-Raven, 1998.

51. Hablitz J, Lee W, Prince D. NMDA receptor involvement in epileptogenesis in the immature neocortex. *Epilepsy Res Suppl* 1992;8:139–145.

52. Prince D. Basic mechanisms of focal epileptogenesis. In: Avanzini G, Fariello R, Heinemann U, et al., eds. *Epileptogenic and excitotoxic mechanisms.* London: John Libbey, 1993:17–27.

53. Schwartzkroin P. Plasticity and repair in the immature central nervous system. In: Schwartzkroin P, Moshe SL, Nobels JL, eds. *Brain development and epilepsy.* New York: Oxford University Press, 1995:234–267.

54. Kellaway P, Hrachovy R. Status epilepticus in newborns: a perspective on neonatal seizures. In: Delgado-Escueta A, Wasterlain C, Treiman D, et al., eds. *Advances in neurology.* New York: Raven Press, 1983:93–99.

55. Lou H, Friis-Hansen B. Arterial blood pressure elevations during motor activity and epileptic seizures in the newborn. *Acta Paediatr Scand* 1979;68:803–806.

56. Goldberg R, Goldman S, Ramsay R. Detection of seizure activity in the paralyzed neonate using continuous monitoring. *Pediatrics* 1982;69:583–586.

57. Donati F, Schaffler L, Vassella F. Prolonged epileptic apneas in a newborn: a case report with ictal EEG recording. *Neuropediatrics* 1995;26:223–225.

58. Watanabe K, Hara K, Miyazaki S, et al. Apneic seizures in the newborn. *Am J Dis Child* 1982;136:980–984.

59. Laroia N, Guillet R, Burchfiel J, et al. EEG background as predictor of electrographic seizures in high-risk neonates. *Epilepsia* 1998;39:545–551.

60. Menache C, Bourgeois B, Volpe J. Prognostic value of neonatal discontinuous EEG. *Pediatr Neurol* 2002;27:93–101.

61. Hrachovy R, Mizrahi EM, Kellaway P. Electroencephalography of the newborn. In: Daly D, Pedley T, eds. *Current practice of clinical electroencephalography,* 2nd ed. New York: Raven Press, 1990: 201–242.

62. Clancy R. Interictal sharp EEG transients in neonatal seizures. *J Child Neurol* 1989;4:30–38.

63. Clancy R. Bergqvist AC, Dlugos D. Neonatal electroencephalography. In: Ebersole JS, Pedley T, eds. *Current practice of clinical electroencephalography,* 3rd ed. Philadelphia: Lippincott-Raven, 2003:160–234.

64. Clancy RR, Legido A. The exact ictal and interictal duration of electroencephalographic neonatal seizures. *Epilepsia* 1987;28: 537–541.

65. Clancy R, Malin S, Laraque D, et al. Focal motor seizures heralding stroke in full-term neonates. *Am J Dis Child* 1985;139: 601–606.

66. Knauss T, Carlson C. Neonatal paroxysmal monorhythmic alpha activity. *Arch Neurol* 1978;35:104–107.

67. Willis J, Gould JB. Periodic alpha seizures with apnea in a newborn. *Dev Med Child Neurol* 1980;22:214–222.

68. Watanabe K, Kuroyanagi M, Hara K, et al. Neonatal seizures and subsequent epilepsy. *Brain Dev* 1982;4:341–346.

69. Mizrahi EM. Neonatal seizures: problems in diagnosis and classification. *Epilepsia* 1987;28:S46–S55.

70. Boylan GB, Rennie JM, Pressler RM, et al. Phenobarbitone, neonatal seizures, and video-EEG. *Arch Dis Child Fetal Neonat Ed* 2002;86:F165–F170.

71. Sharif U, Ichord R, Gaynor JW, et al. Electrographic neonatal seizures after newborn heart surgery. *Epilepsia* 2003;44:164.

72. Bye AM, Cunningham CA, Chee KY, et al. Outcome of neonates with electrographically identified seizures, or at risk of seizures. *Pediatr Neurol* 1997;16:225–231.

73. Clancy R, Legido A, Lewis D. Occult neonatal seizures. *Epilepsia* 1988;29:256–261.

74. Bye AM, Flanagan D. Spatial and temporal characteristics of neonatal seizures. *Epilepsia* 1995;36:1009–1016.

75. Clancy RR. The contribution of EEG to the understanding of neonatal seizures. *Epilepsia* 1996;37:S52–S59.

76. Leviton A, Nelson KB. Problems with definitions and classifications of newborn encephalopathy. *Pediatr Neurol* 1992;8:85–90.

77. Durham SR, Clancy R, Leuthardt E, et al. CHOP Infant Coma Scale ("infant face scale"): a novel coma scale for children less than two years of age. *J Neurotrauma* 2000;17:729–737.

78. Graham EM, Holcroft CJ, Blakemore KJ. Evidence of intrapartum hypoxia-ischemia is not present in the majority of cases of neonatal seizures. *J Matern Fetal Neonat Med* 2002;12:123–126.

79. ACOG Task Force on Neonatal Encephalopathy and Cerebral Palsy. *Neonatal encephalopathy and cerebral palsy: defining the pathogenesis and pathophysiology.* Washington, DC: American College of Obstetricians and Gynecologists, 2002:73–80.

80. Martin-Ancel A, Garcia-Alix A, Gaya F, Cabanas F, Burgueros M, Quero J. Multiple organ involvement in perinatal asphyxia. *J Pediatr* 1995;127:786–793.

81. Phelan JP, Korst LM, Ahn MO, Martin GL. Neonatal nucleated red blood cell and lymphocyte counts in fetal brain injury. *Obstet Gynecol* 1998;91:485–489.

82. Dammann O, Leviton A. Maternal intrauterine infection, cytokines, and brain damage in the preterm newborn. *Pediatr Res* 1997;42:1–8.

83. Grether J, Nelson KB. Maternal infection and cerebral palsy in infants of normal birth weight. *JAMA* 1997;278:207–211.

84. Kadhim H, Tabarki B, Verellen G, et al. Inflammatory cytokines in the pathogenesis of periventricular leukomalacia. *Neurology* 2001;56:1278–1284.

85. Svigos JM. The fetal inflammatory response syndrome and cerebral palsy: yet another challenge and dilemma for the obstetrician. *Aust N Z Obstet Gynaecol* 2001;41:170–176.

86. Baud O, Emilie D, Pelletier E, et al. Amniotic fluid concentrations of interleukin-1beta, interleukin-6 and TNF-alpha in

chorioamnionitis before 32 weeks of gestation: histological associations and neonatal outcome. *Br J Obstet Gynaecol* 1999;106: 72–77.

87. Wu YW, Colford JM Jr. Chorioamnionitis as a risk factor for cerebral palsy: a meta-analysis. *JAMA* 2000;284:1417–1424.

88. deVeber G, Monagle P, Chan A, et al. Prothrombotic disorders in infants and children with cerebral thromboembolism. *Arch Neurol* 1998;55:1539–1543.

89. Ment LR, Duncan CC, Ehrenkranz RA. Perinatal cerebral infarction. *Ann Neurol* 1984;16:559–568.

90. Perlman JM, Rollins NK, Evans D. Neonatal stroke: clinical characteristics and cerebral blood flow velocity measurements. *Pediatr Neurol* 1994;11:281–284.

91. Sreenan C, Bhargava R, Robertson CM. Cerebral infarction in the term newborn: clinical presentation and long-term outcome. *J Pediatr* 2000;137:351–355.

92. deVeber G, Andrew M, Canadian Pediatric Ischemic Stroke Study Group. Cerebral sinovenous thrombosis in children. *N Engl J Med* 2001;345:417–423.

93. Barron TF, Gusnard DA, Zimmerman R, et al. Cerebral venous thrombosis in neonates and children. *Pediatr Neurol* 1992; 8:112–116.

94. Rivkin MJ, Anderson ML, Kaye EM. Neonatal idiopathic cerebral venous thrombosis: an unrecognized cause of transient seizures or lethargy. *Ann Neurol* 1992;32:51–56.

95. Korinthenberg R, Kachel W, Koelfen W, et al. Neurological findings in newborn infants after extracorporeal membrane oxygenation, with special reference to the EEG. *Dev Med Child Neurol* 1993;35:249–257.

96. Lago P, Rebsamen S, Clancy R, et al. MRI, MRA and neurodevelopmental outcome following neonatal ECMO. *Pediatr Neurol* 1995;12:294–304.

97. Clancy R. The neurology of hypoplastic left heart syndrome. In: Rychik J, Wenovsky G, eds. *The hypoplastic left heart syndrome.* Boston: Kluwer Academic, 2003:251–273.

98. Natowicz M, Chatten J, Clancy R. Genetic disorders and major extracardiac anomalies associated with the hypoplastic left heart syndrome. *Pediatrics* 1988;82:698–706.

99. Clancy RR, McGaurn S, Wernovsky G, et al. Risk of seizures in survivors of newborn heart surgery using deep hypothermic circulatory arrest. *Pediatrics* 2001;111:592–601.

100. Clancy RR, McGaurn SA, Goin JE, et al. Allopurinol neurocardiac protection trial in infants undergoing heart surgery utilizing deep hypothermic circulatory arrest. *Pediatrics* 2001;107: 61–70.

101. De Vivo DC, Trifiletti RR, Jacobson RI, et al. Defective glucose transport across the blood-brain barrier as a cause of persistent hypoglycorrhachia, seizures and developmental delay. *N Engl J Med* 1991;325:703–709.

102. Fishman RA. The glucose-transporter protein and glucopenic brain injury. *N Engl J Med* 1991;325:731–732.

103. Maher F, Vannucci S, Simpson I. Glucose transporter proteins in the brain. *FASEB J* 1994;8:1003–1011.

104. Clancy R, Chung HJ. EEG changes during recovery from acute severe neonatal citrullinemia. *Electroencephalogr Clin Neurophysiol* 1991;78:222–227.

105. Pettit RE. Pyridoxine dependency seizures: report of a case with unusual features. *J Child Neurol* 1987;2:38–41.

106. Coker SB. Post-neonatal vitamin B6–dependent epilepsy. *Pediatrics* 1992;90:221–223.

107. Osiovich H, Barrington K. Prenatal ultrasound diagnosis of seizures. *Am J Perinatol* 1996;13:499–501.

108. Torres OA, Miller VS, Buist NM, et al. Folinic acid-responsive neonatal seizures. *J Child Neurol* 1999;14:529–532.

109. Slot HMJ, Overweg-Plandsoen WCG, Bakker HD, et al. Molybdenum-cofactor deficiency: an easily missed cause of neonatal convulsions. *Neuropediatrics* 1993;24:139–142.

110. Arnold GL, Greene CL, Stout JP, et al. Molybdenum cofactor deficiency. *J Pediatr* 1993;123:595–598.

111. Johnson JL. Prenatal diagnosis of molybdenum cofactor deficiency and isolated sulfite oxidase deficiency. *Proc Natl Acad Sci U S A* 2002;23:6–8.

112. Stallmeyer B, Schwarz G, Sculze J, et al. The neurotransmitter receptor-anchoring protein gephyrin reconstitutes molybdenum

113. cofactor biosynthesis in bacteria, plants and mammalian cells. *Proc Natl Acad Sci U S A* 1998;96:1333–1338.

113. Herzlinger RA, Kandall SR, Vaughan HG Jr. Neonatal seizures associated with narcotic withdrawal. *J Pediatr* 1977;91: 638–641.

114. Porter BE, Brooks-Kayal AR, Golden JA. Disorders of cortical development and epilepsy. *Arch Neurol* 2002;59:361–365.

115. Tharp BR. Neonatal seizures and syndromes. *Epilepsia* 2002; 43:2–10.

116. Hayward JC, Titelbaum D, Clancy R, et al. Lissencephaly-pachygyria associated with congenital cytomegalovirus infection. *J Child Neurol* 1991;6:109.

117. Bachevalier F, Marchal C, Di Cesare MP, et al. Lethal neurological involvement during incontinentia pigmenti. *Ann Dermatol Venereol* 2003;130:1139–1142.

118. Miller SP, Tasch T, Sylvain M, et al. Tuberous sclerosis complex and neonatal seizures. *J Child Neurol* 1998;13:619–623.

119. Clancy R, Kurtz M, Baker D. Neurological manifestations of the organoid nevus syndrome. *Arch Neurol* 1985;42:236–240.

120. Sherr EH. The ARX story (epilepsy, mental retardation, autism, and cerebral malformations): one gene leads to many phenotypes. *Curr Opin Pediatr* 2003;15:567–571.

121. Dehan M, Navelet Y, d'Allest AM, et al. Quelques precisions sur le syndrome des convulsions du cinquième jour de vie. *Arch Fr Pediatr* 1982;39:405–407.

122. George AJ. Molecular basis of inherited epilepsy. *Arch Neurol* 2004;61:473–478.

123. Cooper EC, Jan LY. Ion channel genes and human neurological disease: recent progress, prospects and challenges. *Proc Natl Acad Sci U S A* 1998;96:4759–4766.

124. Dedek K, Kunath B, Kananura C, et al. Myokymia and neonatal epilepsy caused by a mutation in the voltage sensor of the KCNQ2 K+ channel. *Proc Natl Acad Sci U S A* 2001;98: 12272–12277.

125. Watanabe K, Yamoto N, Negoro T. Benign complex partial epilepsies in infancy. *Pediatr Neurol* 1987;3:208–211.

126. Coppola G, Plouin P, Chiron C, et al. Migrating partial seizures in infancy: a malignant disorder with developmental arrest. *Epilepsia* 1995;36:1017–1024.

127. Marsh E, Melamed S, Clancy R. Migrating partial seizures in early infancy: expanding the phenotype of a rare neonatal seizure type. *Epilepsia* 2003;44:305.

128. Aicardi J, Goutieres F. Encephalopathie myoclonique neonatale. *Rev Electroencephalogr Neurophysiol Clin* 1978;8:99–101.

129. Clancy R, Chung HJ, Hayward JC, et al. Early myoclonic epileptic encephalopathy. *Ann Neurol* 1990;28:472–473.

130. Ohtahara S, Ishida T, Oka E, et al. On the specific age-dependent epileptic syndrome. The early-infantile epileptic encephalopathy with suppression-burst. *No To Hattatsu* 1976;8: 270–280.

131. Goldberg RN, Moscoso P, Bauer CR, et al. Use of barbiturate therapy in severe perinatal asphyxia: a randomized controlled trial. *J Pediatr* 1986;109:851–856.

132. Hall RT, Hall FK, Daily DK. High-dose phenobarbital therapy in term newborn infants with severe perinatal asphyxia: a randomized, prospective study with three-year follow-up. *J Pediatr* 1998;132:345–348.

133. Connell J, Oozeer R, de Vries L, et al. Clinical and EEG response to anticonvulsants in neonatal seizures. *Arch Dis Child* 1989; 64:459–464.

134. Painter MJ, Scher MS, Stein AD, et al. Phenobarbital compared with phenytoin for the treatment of neonatal seizures. *N Engl J Med* 1999;341:485–489.

135. Evans DJ, Levene MI. Anticonvulsants for preventing mortality and morbidity in full term newborns with perinatal asphyxia. *Cochrane Database System Rev* 2001;CD001240.

136. Painter MJ, Alvin J. Neonatal seizures. *Curr Treat Options Neurol* 2001;3:237–248.

137. Bourgeois B, Dodson W. Phenytoin elimination in newborns. *Neurology* 1983;33:173–178.

138. Dodson W. Antiepileptic drug utilization in pediatric patients. *Epilepsia* 1984;25:S132–S139.

139. Hellstrom-Westas L, Westgren U, Rosen I, et al. Lidocaine for treatment of severe seizures in newborn infants, I: clinical effects and cerebral electrical activity monitoring. *Acta Paediatr Scand* 1988;77:79–84.

140. Norell E, Gamstorp I. Neonatal seizures: effect of lidocaine. *Acta Paediatr Scand Suppl* 1970;206:(Suppl):97+.
141. Sheth RD, Buckley DJ, Gutierrez AR, et al. Midazolam in the treatment of refractory neonatal seizures. *Clin Neuropharmacol* 1996;19:165–170.
142. Macintosh D, Baird-Lampert J. Is carbamazepine an alternative maintenance therapy for neonatal seizures? *Dev Pharmacol Ther* 1987;10:100–106.
143. Sapin J, Riviello JJ, Grover W. Efficacy of primidone for seizure control in neonates and young infants. *Pediatr Neurol* 1988;4:292–295.
144. Gal P, Otis K, Gilman J, et al. Valproic acid efficacy, toxicity and pharmacokinetics in neonates with intractable seizures. *Neurology* 1988;38:467–471.
145. Aicardi J, Mumford J, Dumas C. Vigabatrin as initial therapy for infantile spasms: a European retrospective survey. *Epilepsia* 1996;37:638–642.
146. Barr P, Buettiker V, Anthony J. Efficacy of lamotrigine in refractory neonatal seizures. *Pediatr Neurol* 1999;20:161–163.
147. Ellenberg JH, Hirtz D, Nelson KB. Age at onset of seizures in young children. *Ann Neurol* 1984;15:127–134.
148. Clancy RR, Legido A. Postnatal epilepsy after EEG-confirmed neonatal seizures. *Epilepsia* 1991;32:69–76.
149. Boer H, Gal P. Neonatal seizures: a survey of current practice. *Clin Pediatr* 1982;21:453–457.
150. Fenichel G. Paroxysmal disorders. In: *Clinical pediatric neurology*, 3rd ed. Philadelphia: WB Saunders, 2001:1–45.
151. Daval J-L, Pereira de Vasconcelos A, Lartaud I. Development of mammalian cultured neurons following exposure to anticonvulsant drugs. In: Wasterlain CG, Vert P, eds. *Neonatal seizures*. New York: Raven Press, 1990:295–301.
152. Bittigau P, Sifringer M, Genz K. Antiepileptic drugs and apoptotic neurodegeneration in the developing brain. *Proc Natl Acad Sci USA* 2002;99:15089–15094.

Febrile Seizures

33

Michael Duchowny

Almost three decades ago, Livingston (1) observed that children with febrile seizures fared considerably better than those with epileptic convulsions not activated by fever; their prognosis with respect to epilepsy was uniformly more favorable, and they were more likely to be neurologically normal. Febrile seizures are now recognized to be a relatively benign, age-dependent epilepsy syndrome and the most prevalent form of seizure in early life.

The National Institutes of Health (NIH) Consensus Development Conference on the Management of Febrile Seizures defined a febrile seizure as "an event in infancy or childhood, usually occurring between 3 months and 5 years of age, associated with fever but without evidence of intracranial infection or defined cause" (2). This definition is useful because it emphasizes age specificity and the absence of underlying brain abnormalities. It also implies that febrile seizures are not true epilepsy, because affected individuals are not predisposed to recurrent afebrile episodes.

In clinical practice, however, the NIH definition must be interpreted with caution. Intracranial infection may not be readily apparent, especially in very young infants. Although few medical practitioners advocate extensive testing in a healthy child with a brief nonfocal febrile seizure, an infant or child in febrile hemiconvulsive status epilepticus requires immediate medical attention.

Familiarity with the clinical manifestations and long-term prognosis of febrile seizures is essential in caring for affected individuals. Epidemiologic studies have been especially useful in identifying features of the seizure or the patient that involve adverse consequences. Understanding these factors forms the basis of proper seizure management and family counseling.

PREDISPOSING FACTORS

Genetics

There is no consensus regarding the mode of inheritance of febrile seizures or their clinical expression. Autosomal dominant (3), autosomal recessive (4), and polygenic theories (5,6) have all been formulated.

Febrile seizures are approximately two to three times more common among family members of affected children than in the general population (3,7). Affected parents increase the risk for the occurrence of febrile seizures in siblings. The risk increases when both parents are affected and is increased further in proportion to the number of febrile seizures experienced by the proband (8). A higher incidence of afebrile epilepsy has been found in first-degree relatives of patients with febrile seizures (8,9). Conversely, the occurrence of febrile seizures in first-degree relatives is itself a risk factor for febrile seizure recurrence (10). Siblings have the greatest risk, followed by offspring, nieces, and nephews (8). Coexistence of febrile seizures and epilepsy increases the risk for both disorders in siblings (8).

The incidence of febrile seizures also varies according to geographic region and race. Parents and siblings of Asian children are at considerably higher risk for febrile seizures than are Western families. Sibling risk approaches 30% if one parent has had a febrile seizure. The difference in frequency of febrile seizures in Asian compared with European or North American families suggests a strong, genetically determined population effect (11).

Linkage studies in a number of large pedigrees have identified several mutations in sodium channel subunit genes (12). Putative febrile seizure loci include FEB 1 (chromosome 8q13-q21), FEB 2 (chromosome 19p), FEB 3 (chromosome 2q23-24), and FEB 4 (chromosome 5q14-q15) (13,14). All affected individuals present with recurrent febrile seizures by 3 years of age, with no evidence of structural brain pathology or intracranial infection. Although most individuals are predisposed to later afebrile seizures, families mapping to the FEB 3 locus have significantly higher rates of later epilepsy compared with that reported in general population studies or in families with febrile seizures (15).

Despite the identification of multiple febrile seizure loci and mutated genes, little evidence points to their direct contribution toward the majority of febrile seizures reported in most affected individuals. This probably reflects the marked heterogeneous clinical manifestations of febrile seizures and their lack of association with known genetic loci (16). Furthermore, family pedigrees of most known febrile seizure phenotypes are atypical of "common" febrile seizures, in that mutation-specific febrile seizures often have an extended age of onset and offset, and predispose individuals to later afebrile seizures. Pal and associates (17) used a case-control study design to identify specific phenotypic subgroups of febrile seizures and reduce clinical heterogeneity. In a comparison of 83 patients with febrile seizures who had a first-degree family history and 101 control patients with febrile seizures who lacked affected family members, the investigators found that a first-degree family history of febrile seizures and the later occurrence of afebrile seizures were specifically and independently associated with an increased risk for febrile seizure recurrence.

Age

The onset of febrile seizures generally follows a bell-shaped pattern. Ninety percent of these seizures occur within the first 3 years of life (18), 4% before 6 months, and 6% after 3 years of age. Approximately 50% appear during the second year of life, with a peak incidence between 18 and 24 months (18).

Febrile seizures occurring before 6 months of age should always raise the level of suspicion of infectious causes; bacterial meningitis must be excluded by examination of the cerebrospinal fluid (CSF) in patients of this age group. Febrile seizures after 5 years of age also should be managed cautiously, because benign causes are less common in older children.

The limited age range in febrile seizures has never been satisfactorily explained. Immaturity of central neurotransmission may play a role but should affect other childhood seizure types equally. Prostaglandin E_2, but not homovanillic or 5-hydroxyindoleacetic acid, is increased in lumbar CSF following febrile seizures in humans (19,20). Hyperthermia-induced convulsions in the developing rat can alter nicotinic and muscarinic cholinergic function (21). The maximum changes occur 55 days after the last convulsion, suggesting the importance of secondary factors.

Fever

Febrile seizures typically occur relatively early in an infectious illness, usually during the rising phase of the temperature curve. Rectal temperatures at this time may exceed 39.2°C (102.6°F), and approximately one-fourth of seizures occur at temperatures above 40.2°C (104.4°F). Despite the implicit relationship between fever and seizure activation, temperature itself probably does not lower the seizure threshold. The incidence of febrile seizures does not increase in proportion to temperature elevation, and

febrile seizures are generally uncommon in the later stages of a persistent illness. Moreover, children between the ages of 6 and 18 months who experience a fever higher than 40°C (104°F) have a sevenfold reduction in seizure recurrence compared with children with a fever below 40°C (104°F) (22). A brief duration of fever before the initial febrile seizure has been linked to an increased risk for seizure recurrence (23).

Febrile seizures typically are associated with common childhood illnesses, most frequently viral upper respiratory tract, middle ear, and gastrointestinal infections. Bacterial infections, including bacteremia, pneumonia, sepsis, and meningitis, are rare concomitants of febrile seizures. None of the common viral or bacterial childhood infectious illnesses appears to be uniquely capable of activating febrile seizures.

Febrile seizures in conjunction with shigellosis constitute the most frequent extraintestinal manifestation of this infection (24). A direct neurotoxic effect of the *Shigella* bacterium on seizure threshold has been proposed.

Immunization-related seizures also manifest with fever, usually within 48 hours of inoculation (25). Approximately one-fourth of immunization-related seizures are related to administration of diphtheria-pertussis-tetanus (DPT) vaccine, and one-fourth follow measles immunization. Data from the National Collaborative Perinatal Project indicate that age of onset, personal and family history, and clinical presentation of postimmunization seizures resemble those of febrile seizures from infectious causes (26). The risk of DPT-induced febrile seizures increases if a family member has had an afebrile seizure (27,28). These shared features suggest that infectious and immunization-related febrile seizures are expressions of a unitary condition.

Associated Factors

Ancillary factors related to underlying illness or fever may be implicated in the pathogenesis of febrile convulsions, usually with little supportive evidence. Direct viral invasion of brain tissue has been proposed (29), but children with proven viral infections appear no more likely to experience seizure recurrence than do uninfected children (30). Electrolyte disturbances are said to lower seizure threshold, but this mechanism remains relatively unsupported (31). Transient pyridoxine deficiency seems unlikely, and the association of *Shigella* infection and febrile seizures has prompted a search for an epileptogenic neurotoxin.

Proinflammatory cytokines have recently been implicated in the pathogenesis of febrile seizures. Interleukin (IL)-1β, tumor necrosis factor-α, and nitrite levels are all increased in the CSF of children with a febrile seizure (32). Increased secretion of IL-6 and IL-10 by liposaccharide-stimulated mononuclear cells is higher in patients with a history of previous febrile seizures (33).

Girls younger than 18 months of age have a slightly higher risk than boys of experiencing more frequent and severe febrile seizures (34,35). Ounsted (36) proposed that an excess of boys from one-sex sibships may explain the male predominance.

TYPES OF FEBRILE SEIZURES

Simple Febrile Convulsions

Simple febrile convulsions are solitary events, lasting less than 15 minutes and lacking focality. They occur in neurologically normal children and are not associated with persistent deficits. The source of the fever is always outside the central nervous system (CNS).

Between 80% and 90% of all febrile seizures are simple episodes (18,37,38). This figure is probably an underestimate, because most published series are hospital based and thus weighted toward children with complex risk factors (39).

Despite their common occurrence, the sporadic nature and brief duration of febrile seizures make analysis difficult. Descriptions provided by parents and emergency department personnel are retrospective and probably not entirely accurate. Video-electroencephalographic studies of afebrile generalized seizures, for example, often reveal subtle atonic or myoclonic components that were omitted in the witnessed accounts. Lack of objectivity notwithstanding, febrile seizures are described as tonic, clonic, or tonic-clonic events that usually begin without warning and display upward eye deviation as consciousness is lost. Atonic forms are rare, and postictal depression is generally brief.

Electroencephalography has not been particularly useful in the evaluation of simple febrile seizures. Although paroxysmal and nonspecific electroencephalographic (EEG) abnormalities are often evident within 24 hours of seizure onset, they have little prognostic significance. Slow-wave activity occurs in up to one-third of patients (40), and is often bilateral and prominent in the posterior regions (41). Twenty percent of patients, usually older than 2.5 years of age, have generalized spike-and-wave discharges on the electroencephalogram.

In a longitudinal study of 89 patients with febrile seizures followed until puberty, Doose and associates (42) identified three patterns of EEG abnormality: rhythms of 4 to 7 Hz, generalized spike-and-wave discharges, and photosensitivity. None were specific for febrile seizures because all had been described in generalized epilepsies as well. Genetic factors probably account for the age-related expression of these EEG patterns in benign, simple febrile seizures.

Because simple febrile seizures may result from CNS infection, trauma, or electrolyte disturbance, laboratory investigation is usually warranted even when findings on the physical examination are normal. The diagnostic yield of such studies is usually well below 2%, however, and difficult to justify (43). The skull roentgenogram and lumbar puncture are even less likely to contribute useful information in healthy children (44), and the rare febrile seizure caused by electrolyte disturbance usually can be diagnosed from the patient's history. The confirmation of viral meningitis by lumbar puncture does not alter long-term management.

The evaluation of simple febrile seizures should therefore rely primarily on careful history taking, and judicious laboratory and radiologic testing. This approach, which is particularly important in children who are normal, has been underscored in an editorial (45) stating that "children who have their first febrile convulsion need no more tests than the clinical findings dictate." An exception is the requirement for CSF examination in all patients younger than 6 months of age who lack any of the classic signs of bacterial meningitis. The rule that all children younger than 18 months of age with a first febrile seizure should always undergo CSF examination is probably excessive, and each child should be evaluated individually. When meningitis is suspected clinically, lumbar puncture should be performed promptly in the physician's office or emergency department.

Hospitalization is rarely necessary following a simple febrile seizure. Testing can usually be performed in an outpatient setting because risk of seizure recurrence is low. Even so, pediatricians may hospitalize patients who can be sent home safely. In 1975, 24% of practicing pediatricians routinely admitted children after a first febrile seizure; a decade later, 20% still followed this practice (46).

Complex Febrile Seizures

The concept of a "complex" febrile seizure originated with epidemiologic studies indicating that several patient- and seizure-related variables predicted higher rates of subsequent epilepsy: seizure duration longer than 15 minutes, focal seizure manifestations, seizure recurrence within 24 hours, abnormal neurologic status, and afebrile seizures in a parent or sibling (47). Six percent of patients with two or more risk factors developed afebrile epilepsy by the age of 7 years, compared with only 0.9% if risk factors were absent (47).

Studies conducted at the Mayo Clinic also reveal a less favorable prognosis for patients with complex febrile seizures (38). Seventeen percent of neurologically impaired children with complex febrile seizure manifestations developed epilepsy by the third decade, compared with 2.5% of children who lacked risk factors. The occurrence of focal, recurrent, and prolonged seizures raised the risk for afebrile episodes to nearly 50%.

Children with complex febrile convulsions may subsequently exhibit a variety of afebrile seizure patterns. The National Collaborative Perinatal Project (37) found generalized tonic-clonic seizures to be the most frequent and absence or myoclonic seizures less common. In the Mayo Clinic experience (48), 29 cases of afebrile epilepsy developed in a cohort of 666 patients with febrile seizures. Seizures were classified as focal in 16 patients and of temporal origin in 10 patients. Generalized tonic-clonic seizures were reported in 12 patients, 3 of whom also had absence seizures. One patient had unclassifiable seizures. In a retrospective analysis of 504 children with epilepsy, Camfield and colleagues (49) found a 14.9% incidence of prior febrile seizures. Febrile seizures most often preceded generalized tonic-clonic afebrile seizures and were regarded as fundamentally indicative of reduced seizure threshold.

Complex febrile seizures must be managed more aggressively than simple episodes. Meningitis must be excluded by timely performance of CSF examination, and neuroimaging studies are indicated to detect structural lesions. In acute bacterial meningitis, focal febrile seizures may accompany cortical vein or sagittal sinus thrombosis. In North America, parasitic disease and brain abscess are uncommon causes of complex febrile seizures.

Although children with complex febrile seizures may be expected to show a higher rate of abnormal EEG recordings than normal, confirmatory data are sparse. Studies of febrile seizures rarely include EEG findings, although this type of information would enhance the value of electroencephalography in the management of patients with febrile seizures.

Febrile Status Epilepticus

Although most febrile seizures are self-limited, prolonged episodes and febrile status epilepticus are not rare. The reported occurrence of epilepsy, brain damage, or death following febrile status epilepticus further underscores its serious nature. Of 1706 children with febrile seizures followed in the National Collaborative Perinatal Project, 8% experienced seizures for longer than 15 minutes, and 4% had seizures for longer than 30 minutes (37). Febrile status epilepticus accounted for approximately 25% of all cases of status epilepticus in children (27,50), and is often the initial presentation of chronic epilepsy (37).

Children with febrile status epilepticus are usually mentally and physically normal. As with simple febrile seizures, common childhood infectious diseases and immunizations are the primary cause of the fever. An association between female sex and febrile status epilepticus has been observed (51), with younger age strongly predisposing patients toward prolonged unilateral febrile seizures (52).

Postmortem studies of patients dying of febrile status epilepticus reveal widespread neuronal necrosis of the cortex, basal ganglia, thalamus, cerebellum, and temporolimbic structures (53). Rare inflammatory changes suggest that seizures and anoxia, rather than infection, are the primary causes of mortality (41,53,54).

Prospective studies reveal that the risk for death or permanent neurologic impairment following febrile status epilepticus is negligible (37,55). The tendency for febrile status epilepticus to recur is especially low in neurologically normal children (56), and mortality in this group

has markedly declined. None of the 1706 patients followed in the National Collaborative Perinatal Project died as a consequence of febrile seizures, a finding confirmed by others (56).

A few infants present with severe febrile hemiconvulsive status that is followed by permanent hemiplegia. After a variable seizure-free interval, they develop chronic focal epilepsy that can persist for many years. This presentation, called the hemiconvulsion-hemiplegia-epilepsy (HHE) syndrome, was described by Gastaut and associates (57), who regarded it as distinct from other prenatal or perinatal causes of infantile hemiplegia and epilepsy.

The HHE syndrome usually manifests before the age of 2 years as status epilepticus lasting from hours to days. Seizures may be triggered by any of the benign childhood infections or they may be idiopathic in nature. Hemiconvulsions are typical at onset, but generalized patterns usually predominate as the seizure progresses. Postictal unresponsiveness may be prolonged.

After the ictus, the child has a variable degree of residual spastic hemiparesis. Recovery of motor function depends on the severity and topography of the damage and the age at which it is acquired. The later emergence of afebrile seizures changes the designation of the hemiconvulsion-hemiplegia syndrome into the HHE syndrome. Recurrent and often medically resistant seizures may persist for years thereafter. Complex partial seizures are the most prevalent form of later epilepsy. Some patients with the HHE syndrome and intractable disabling partial seizures may achieve freedom from seizures after cortical resection or hemispherectomy. Histopathologic analysis reveals atrophy and gliosis throughout the involved hemisphere, with prominent sclerosis of mesial temporal structures. Improvements in the acute treatment of patients with status epilepticus have made the HHE syndrome rare.

RISK ASSESSMENT IN FEBRILE SEIZURES

Recurrence Risk for Febrile Seizures

Approximately one-third of patients with febrile seizures experience additional attacks; of this group, one-half will have a third seizure (58,59). Only 9% experience three or more attacks (47).

Age of onset is the most important predictor of febrile seizure recurrence. One-half of all infants younger than 1 year of age at the time of their first febrile seizure will have a recurrence, compared with 20% of children older than 3 years of age. Young age at onset, a history of febrile seizures in first-degree relatives, low-grade fever in the emergency department, and brief interval between fever onset and seizure presentation are strong independent predictors of febrile seizure recurrence (60). Recurrences generally occur within 1 year but are no more likely in children who had a complex febrile seizure than in those who experienced a simple febrile seizure.

In those with a subsequent febrile episode (61), approximately one-half of all recurrent febrile seizures occur within the 2 hours following onset of fever. Young age at onset and high temperature favor recurrence.

Children with multiple risk factors experience the highest rates of febrile seizure recurrence. The presence of two or more risk factors is associated with a 30% or greater recurrence risk, whereas three risk factors are associated with a 60% or greater recurrence risk (62). Subsequent febrile seizures are more likely to be prolonged when the initial febrile seizure is prolonged (63). Febrile seizure recurrence is not more likely in children with abnormal neurodevelopmental status (63).

Risk for Epilepsy and Association with Hippocampal Sclerosis

Between 1.5% and 4.6% of children with febrile seizures go on to develop afebrile seizures (64–67). Although this rate is significantly higher than in the general population, it reflects primarily infants and children with one or more complex febrile seizures (47,68). The presence of a neurodevelopmental abnormality, a family history of epilepsy, and prolonged duration of fever are also definite risk factors (69). The forms of later epilepsy are varied and similar to the seizure pattern encountered in children without a history of febrile seizures.

The mechanism by which individuals with febrile seizures are predisposed to later epilepsy is much less clear. Prolonged febrile convulsions in early infancy may precede a variety of seizures but are particularly common in children who develop intractable seizures of temporal lobe origin (70). Histopathologic studies of temporal lobectomy specimens demonstrate hippocampal sclerosis (HS) in approximately half of all surgical cases. HS is hypothesized to result from asphyxia during prolonged febrile seizures, especially febrile status epilepticus (71,72). Prolonged childhood febrile seizures are known to increase cerebral metabolic demand and to induce systemic changes, including hypoxia, hypoglycemia, and arterial hypotension (73). Hyperpyrexia may increase cerebral metabolic rate by as much as 25% (74). Neuronal changes are observed in the neocortex, thalamus, and hippocampus in paralyzed and ventilated seizing animals with controlled systemic factors (73). For reasons that are unclear, there is a significant predominance of right-sided HS in patients with a history of febrile seizures (75).

The association between prolonged febrile seizures and later HS continues to be controversial. In a long-term follow-up study of 24 patients with a prolonged first febrile seizure, Tarkka and colleagues (76) found no reduction in mean hippocampal volumes compared with a control group with a simple febrile seizure and no later epilepsy. Bower and coworkers (77) investigated patients with proven HS and febrile seizures, and found no relationship between hippocampal volume reduction and history of febrile seizures. These larger series contrast with well-documented, individual prospective case studies linking prolonged febrile seizures to subsequent hippocampal swelling, atrophy, and sclerosis (78,79). Prolonged febrile seizures that predispose individuals to HS occur in clusters of unilateral or generalized febrile status, with unilateral ictal EEG discharges and prolonged postictal unresponsiveness.

Alternatively, it is possible that prolonged febrile seizures act in combination with later afebrile seizures to influence the development of HS. Theodore and associates (80) investigated hippocampal volumes in patients with medically uncontrolled temporal lobe epilepsy and found that individuals with a history of complex or prolonged febrile seizures had smaller ipsilateral hippocampal volumes than did those without a history of HS. Epilepsy duration had a significant effect on ipsilateral hippocampal volume, suggesting that damage to the hippocampus after a first prolonged febrile seizure may be progressive. Experimental studies of febrile seizures suggest that progressive hippocampal changes could be modulated through alteration of activity-dependent regulation of cyclic nucleotide-gated channels (81).

The clinical and experimental sequelae of prolonged febrile seizures are difficult to reconcile with epidemiologic data indicating that most severe attacks do not produce long-lasting consequences. Febrile seizures should therefore be considered to represent a continuum of brain dysfunction ranging from very mild local cellular changes to severe generalized damage or hemiatrophy.

Neuroimaging studies further support the concept of selective hippocampal vulnerability to prolonged or recurrent febrile seizures in susceptible individuals (82). Confirmed magnetic resonance imaging evidence of hippocampal damage was identified in 6 of 15 infants with focal or lateralized complex febrile seizures and in none of 12 infants with generalized febrile seizures (83). Signs of pre-existing hippocampal abnormalities and electrographic seizure discharges in the temporal lobe in several infants suggest primary febrile seizure onset in the temporal lobe. Hippocampal volumetry reveals smaller total volumes and a larger right-to-left ratio in children with complex febrile seizures than in controls (84). Increasing duration of the seizure is inversely associated with ipsilateral, but not contralateral, hippocampal volume, suggesting that the deleterious effects of persistent seizures remain localized to the epileptogenic zone (85).

A complex relationship exists among age, sex, and hemispheric vulnerability in children who develop temporal lobe seizures after prolonged febrile convulsions. Left-sided hippocampal sclerosis is more common following prolonged febrile seizures in the first year of life but is rare after 2 years of age, whereas right-sided hippocampal sclerosis is equally prevalent throughout the first 4 years of life (86,87). The risk for hippocampal sclerosis in both sexes is highest in the first year of life, but declines gradually in boys and precipitously in girls. These observations suggest differential rates of vulnerability for each cerebral hemisphere in both sexes.

Genetic factors may contribute to the development of epilepsy in some individuals with febrile seizures. Temporal lobe seizures are more likely to begin early but to remit permanently if a first-degree relative has experienced a febrile seizure (88). A single gene is held responsible, because the siblings of patients with temporal lobe and febrile seizures have a similar incidence of febrile seizures alone.

The autosomal dominantly inherited syndrome of generalized epilepsy with febrile seizures plus (GEFS+) was first described in a large kindred from rural Victoria, Australia (89). The clinical phenotype includes those with febrile seizures in early childhood who develop persistent febrile seizures beyond age 6 years and individuals with a variety of heterogeneous afebrile generalized seizure phenotypes. Seizures typically cease by midadolescence.

GEFS+ demonstrates an autosomal dominant mode of inheritance. In GEFS+ families, a mutation in the voltage-gated sodium channel β_1 subunit (SCN1B) gene at chromosome 19q13.1 and two mutations of the same α_1 subunit (SCN1A) gene at chromosome 2q24 have been identified (90–94). Rather than being a rare disorder, the GEFS+ phenotype has now been identified in multiple families with generalized epilepsy and febrile seizures (95). The phenotypically heterogeneous nature of the later epilepsy is attested to by the recently recognized association of the SCN1A mutation to partial as well as generalized seizures (96). Several large kindreds with autosomal dominant temporal lobe epilepsy and febrile seizures that do not show linkage to candidate regions for familial partial epilepsy and febrile seizures have also been described (97,98).

The spectrum of genetic epilepsies associated with febrile seizures is expanding. Severe myoclonic epilepsy of infancy, also known as Dravet syndrome, is a malignant epileptic encephalopathy that typically presents in the first year of life with prolonged febrile seizures (99). Febrile seizures may be generalized or focal and typically first occur between 5 and 7 months. Initial development and EEG studies are normal, making early diagnosis extremely challenging. Other seizure types and developmental regression subsequently intervene between the ages of 1 and 4 years. Myoclonic seizures are often mild or absent, or disappear after a relatively brief period. Ataxia and pyramidal signs evolve later in some patients and can progressively restrict ambulation. Intellectual functioning is almost always severely impaired.

A high proportion of family members of individuals with Dravet syndrome exhibit various seizure types. It has been suggested that Dravet syndrome should be included within the phenotypic continuum of GEFS+, but at the severe end of the spectrum (100). Missense mutations in the gene that encodes the neuronal voltage-gated SCN1A in families of GEFS+ patients has been identified in

approximately one-third of patients with Dravet syndrome (101,102). A greater frequency of unilateral motor seizures occurs in patients carrying this mutation (102).

FEBRILE SEIZURES AND LATER NEUROPSYCHOLOGICAL STATUS

The consequences of febrile seizures on later intellectual functioning and behavior have been extensively studied. Although some children with febrile seizures can manifest cognitive sequelae, virtually all had neurologic deficits that predated their convulsions (103). A cohort of 381 children with simple and complex febrile seizures was compared with a control group with respect to academic progress, intelligence, and behavior; no differences were observed between the groups in any of the measures (104).

Two large, longitudinal, population-based studies provide strong evidence that febrile seizures do not adversely affect neuropsychological status. Ellenberg and Nelson (55) studied intellectual and academic function following febrile seizures in 431 sibling pairs 7 years of age who were part of the National Collaborative Perinatal Project. Children with febrile seizures and normal intelligence achieved reading and spelling milestones at rates similar to those of their seizure-free siblings. Poor academic performance on the Wide Range Achievement Test was equally common in patients with febrile seizures and sibling controls. The National Child Development Study, completed in the United Kingdom, also found that children with febrile seizures did not differ from controls in behavior, height, head circumference, or academic achievement (65,105).

THERAPY

The American Academy of Pediatrics, through its Committee on Quality Improvement, published two practice parameters dealing with the evaluation of the child with a first febrile seizure and the long-term treatment of the child with simple febrile seizures (106,107). These publications provided an analytic framework for the evaluation and treatment of patients with febrile seizures. Pertinent evidence on individual therapeutic agents, including study results and dosing guidelines, is supplied. These practice parameters were further reviewed and expanded in 2000 (108).

Parents should be taught the importance of prompt use of antipyretics and tepid sponge bathing to control fever. Unfortunately, fever may be recognized only after the onset of convulsion; therefore, attention must be directed to other signs of infection, such as anorexia, diarrhea, or rash (18). Bacterial infections should be treated with the appropriate antibiotic agents.

Prophylactic antiepileptic drug (AED) therapy should be withheld, as the benefits of treatment do not outweigh the risks. Recurrent febrile seizures and later afebrile epilepsy, the major sequelae of a febrile seizure, are both rare. Despite their anxiety, family members should be counseled about the merits of withholding prophylactic treatment. Parents must come to regard simple febrile seizures as a benign disorder that remits with time.

The use of AEDs can sometimes be considered following the occurrence of complex febrile seizures that carry an increased risk for later epilepsy. However, even seemingly life-threatening seizures must be evaluated cautiously. As neurologic impairment and death are extremely unlikely, even after febrile status epilepticus, most children do not require the use of long-term medication. The NIH consensus panel found that high-risk patients with two risk factors (e.g., abnormalities on neurologic examination, prolonged focal seizure, family history of epilepsy) still had only a 13% chance of developing epilepsy. Moreover, even though phenobarbital reduced febrile seizure recurrence, there is no firm evidence that the prevention of recurrent febrile seizures diminishes the risk for later epilepsy.

Febrile seizures often cease by the time a child is examined; prolonged episodes can be terminated with the use of parenteral diazepam, lorazepam, or phenobarbital. Phenobarbital, valproic acid, and diazepam all prevent febrile seizure recurrence (109–114), but slow oral absorption necessitates long-term administration and renders these agents ineffective in short attacks. Therapeutic levels of phenytoin and carbamazepine do not prevent recurrent febrile seizures, although phenytoin may decrease seizure severity (115).

Phenobarbital administration has been associated with rash, sedation, and dysarthria. Hyperactivity, behavioral disorders, irritability, and sleep abnormalities occur in up to 40% of patients, and may provoke parental resistance to medication and noncompliance. Most behavior problems appear shortly after therapy is initiated, are idiosyncratic, and resolve with discontinuation of barbiturates (116).

The long-term effects on cognitive functioning of prolonged barbiturate therapy remain controversial. Prolonged administration was reported not to impair cognitive function (117–119), but serum levels were rarely recorded in these studies, and the populations were highly variable with respect to seizure type, degree of control, and administration of other AEDs. In one study (120), children with febrile seizures receiving daily doses of phenobarbital were compared with carefully matched controls. No differences in performance were apparent on the Wechsler Preschool and Primary Scales of Intelligence, Matching Familiar Figures Test, or Children's Embedded Figures Test (120).

Farwell and colleagues (121) performed the most comprehensive evaluation of phenobarbital administration on intelligence and found an 8-point discrepancy between patients and controls on the Stanford-Binet Scales of Intelligence administered up to 2.5 years after treatment. Barbiturate levels were unrelated to intelligence quotient (IQ) scores, and no difference was detected in the incidence of behavioral problems. Phenobarbital also had no effect on febrile seizure recurrence. Only 25% of the eligible study children completed IQ testing, however, and long-term compliance with medication could not be enforced.

Rectally administered diazepam gel is currently the agent of choice for short-term prophylaxis of febrile seizures (122). Parents are easily instructed on its safe administration. Used intermittently, rectal diazepam gel is equally effective as continuous phenobarbital and terminates most febrile seizures immediately (43,120,123–125). Respiratory depression is a potential concern but is rarely encountered in clinical practice, and tolerance is not associated with infrequent use. Buccal midazolam is as effective as rectal diazepam (126) and intravenous midazolam is as effective as diazepam for controlling seizures in a prehospital setting (127). Nasal midazolam offers rapid seizure termination and can be administered by parents or caretakers of children with recurrent febrile seizures (128).

Intermittent diazepam has rekindled interest in simple febrile seizure prevention. In one study (129), the number of recurrent seizures was reduced in nearly 50% of all children receiving diazepam at fever onset, compared with those receiving placebo. Intermittent therapy for acute seizures is particularly well received by family members because of the considerable anxiety that is provoked. Preventive agents are thus chosen by most parents (130). Rectal diazepam affords primary control over a stressful emergency, thereby improving the quality of life in more than half of affected families (125).

CONCLUSIONS

The syndrome of febrile seizures is the most common seizure presentation in infancy and early childhood. Most events are self-limited and carry only a modest risk for febrile seizure recurrence. Febrile seizures are thus a genetically predetermined, age-dependent response to fever and not an epilepsy. Treatment with prophylactic AEDs is not indicated.

Fewer than 10% of patients with febrile seizures experience severe or recurrent attacks. Risk factors for complex episodes are known, and the likelihood of developing epilepsy remains at less than 5%. Diagnostic procedures or treatment should be considered only on an individual basis; febrile status epilepticus must be treated as a medical emergency. Underlying neurologic disorders require investigation, and "epileptic seizures exacerbated by fever" should be distinguished from febrile seizures per se. Rectal diazepam gel is now considered the agent of choice for acute febrile seizure termination. It is important to counsel families about the benign and genetic nature of febrile seizures and to provide reassurance about the excellent long-term prognosis. There is no evidence that prophylactic administration of AEDs prevents the occurrence of later epilepsy.

REFERENCES

1. Livingston S. *Comprehensive management of epilepsy in infancy, childhood and adolescence.* Springfield, IL: Charles C Thomas, 1972.
2. Consensus Development Conference on Febrile Seizures. Proceedings. *Epilepsia* 1981;22:377–381.
3. Frantzen E, Lennox-Buchthal M, Nygaard A, et al. A genetic study of febrile convulsions. *Neurology* 1970;20:909–917.
4. Gastaut H. On genetic transmission of epilepsies. *Epilepsia* 1969; 10:3–6.
5. Tsuboi T. Polygenic inheritance of epilepsy and febrile convulsions: analysis based on a computational model. *Br J Psychiatry* 1976;129:239–242.
6. Tsuboi T, Endo S. Febrile convulsions followed by nonfebrile convulsions: a clinical, electroencephalographic and follow-up study. *Neuropadiatrie* 1977;8:209–223.
7. Nelson KB, Ellenberg JH. Prenatal and perinatal antecedents of febrile seizures. *Ann Neurol* 1990;27:127–131.
8. Hauser WA, Annegers JF, Anderson VE, et al. The risk of seizure disorders among relatives of children with febrile convulsions. *Neurology* 1985;35:1268–1273.
9. Metrakos JD, Metrakos K. Genetic factors in epilepsy. *Mod Probl Pharmacopsychiatry* 1970;44:77–86.
10. Rantala H, Uhari M. Risk factors for recurrences of febrile convulsions. *Acta Neurol Scand* 1994;90:207–210.
11. Fukuyama YK, Kagawa K, Tanaka KA. A genetic study of febrile convulsions. *Eur Neurol* 1979;18:166–182.
12. Iwasaki N, Nakayama J, Hamano K, et al. Molecular genetics of febrile seizures. *Epilepsia* 2002;43(Suppl 9):32–35.
13. Nakayama J, Hamano K, Iwasaki N, et al. Significant evidence for linkage of febrile seizures to chromosome 5q14-q15. *Hum Mol Genet* 2000;9:87–91.
14. Lopes-Cendes I, Scheffer IE, Berkovic SF, et al. A new locus for generalized epilepsy with febrile seizures plus maps to chromosome 2. *Am J Hum Genet* 2000;66:698–701.
15. Peiffer A, Thompson J, Charlier C, et al. A locus for febrile seizures (FEB3) maps to chromosome 2q23-24. *Ann Neurol* 1999;46:671–678.
16. Racacho LJ, McLachlan RS, Ebers GC, et al. Evidence favoring genetic heterogeneity for febrile convulsions. *Epilepsia* 2000;41: 132–139.
17. Pal DK, Kugler SL, Mandelbaum DE, et al. Phenotypic features of familial febrile seizures: case-control study. *Neurology* 2003; 60:410–414.
18. Verity CM, Butler NR, Golding J. Febrile convulsions in a national cohort followed up from birth. I. Prevalence and recurrence in the first five years of life. *Br Med J* 1985;290:1307–1310.
19. Habel A, Yates CM, McQueen JK, et al. Homovanillic acid and 5-hydroxyindoleacetic acid in lumbar cerebrospinal fluid in children with afebrile and febrile convulsions. *Neurology* 1981;31:488–491.
20. Loscher W, Siemes H. Increased concentration of prostaglandin E-2 in cerebrospinal fluid of children with febrile convulsions. *Epilepsia* 1988;29:307–310.
21. McCaughran JA Jr, Edwards E, Schechter N. Experimental febrile convulsions in the developing rat: effects on the cholinergic system. *Epilepsia* 1984;25:250–258.
22. El-Radhi AS, Withana K, Banajeh S. Recurrence rate of febrile convulsion related to the degree of pyrexia during the first attack. *Clin Pediatr (Phila)* 1986;25:311–313.
23. Berg AT, Shinnar S, Hauser WA, et al. A prospective study of recurrent febrile seizures. *N Engl J Med* 1992;327:1122–1127.
24. Lahat E, Katz Y, Bistritzer T, et al. Recurrent seizures in children with *Shigella*-associated convulsions. *Ann Neurol* 1990;28:393–395.
25. Cody CL, Baraff LJ, Cherry JD, et al. Nature and rates of adverse reactions associated with DTP and DT immunizations in infants and children. *Pediatrics* 1981;68:650–660.
26. Hirtz DG, Nelson KB, Ellenberg JH. Seizures following childhood immunizations. *J Pediatr* 1983;102:14–18.
27. Maytal J, Shinnar S, Moshe SL, et al. Low morbidity and mortality of status epilepticus in children. *Pediatrics* 1989;83:323–331.
28. Livengood JR, Mullen JR, White JW, et al. Family history of convulsions and use of pertussis vaccine. *J Pediatr* 1989;115:527–531.
29. Lewis HM, Parry JV, Parry RP, et al. Role of viruses in febrile convulsions. *Arch Dis Child* 1979;54:869–876.
30. Rantala H, Uhari M, Tuokko H. Viral infections and recurrences of febrile convulsions. *J Pediatr* 1990;116:195–199.
31. Wallace SJ. Factors predisposing to a complicated initial febrile convulsion. *Arch Dis Child* 1975;50:943–947.
32. Haspolat S. Mihci E, Coskun M, et al. Interleukin-1beta, tumor necrosis factor-alpha, and nitrite levels in febrile seizures. *J Child Neurol* 2002;17:749–751.
33. Straussberg R. Amir J. Harel L, et al. Pro- and anti-inflammatory cytokines in children with febrile convulsions. *Pediatr Neurol* 2001;24:49–53.
34. Millichap JG. *Febrile convulsions.* New York: Macmillan, 1968.
35. Taylor DC, Ounsted C. Age, sex, and hemispheric vulnerability in the outcome of seizures in response to fever. In: Brierley JB, Meldrum BS, eds. *Brain hypoxia. Clinics in developmental medicine,* vol 39/40. London: Heinemann, 1971:266–273.
36. Ounsted C. The sex ratio in convulsive disorders with a note on single-sex sib-ships. *J Neurochem* 1953;16:267–274.
37. Nelson KB, Ellenberg JH. Prognosis in children with febrile seizures. *Pediatrics* 1978;61:720–727.
38. Annegers JF, Hauser WA, Shirts SB, et al. Factors prognostic of unprovoked seizures after febrile convulsions. *N Engl J Med* 1987;316:493–498.
39. Ellenberg JH, Nelson KB. Sample selection and the natural history of disease. Studies of febrile seizures. *JAMA* 1980;243:1337–1340.
40. Frantzen E, Lennox-Buchthal M, Nygaard A. Longitudinal EEG and clinical study of children with febrile convulsions. *Electroencephalogr Clin Neurophysiol* 1968;24:197–212.
41. Lennox-Buchthal MA. Febrile convulsions. A reappraisal. *Electroencephalogr Clin Neurophysiol* 1973;32(Suppl):1–138.
42. Doose H, Ritter K, Volzke E. EEG longitudinal studies in febrile convulsions. Genetic aspects. *Neuropediatrics* 1983;14:81–87.
43. Jaffe M, Bar-Joseph G, Tirosh E. Fever and convulsions—indications for laboratory investigations. *Pediatrics* 1981;67:729–731.
44. Kudrajavcev T. Skull x-rays and lumbar puncture in a young child presenting with a seizure and fever. In: Nelson KB, Ellenberg JH, eds. *Febrile seizures.* New York: Raven Press, 1981:221–229.
45. Febrile convulsions: a suitable case for treatment [editorial]? *Lancet* 1980;2:680–681.
46. Hirtz DG, Lee YJ, Ellenberg JH, et al. Survey on the management of febrile seizures. *Am J Dis Child* 1986;140:909–914.
47. Nelson KB, Ellenberg JH. Predictors of epilepsy in children who have experienced febrile seizures. *N Engl J Med* 1976;295: 1029–1033.
48. Annegers JF, Hauser WA, Elveback LR, et al. The risk of epilepsy following febrile convulsions. *Neurology* 1979;29:297–303.
49. Camfield P, Camfield C, Gordon K, et al. What types of epilepsy are preceded by febrile seizures? A population-based study of children. *Dev Med Child Neurol* 1994;36:887–892.
50. Aicardi J, Chevrie JJ. Convulsive status epilepticus in infants and children. A study of 239 cases. *Epilepsia* 1970;11:187–197.
51. Chevrie JJ, Aicardi J. Duration and lateralization of febrile convulsions. Etiological factors. *Epilepsia* 1975;16:781–789.
52. Herlitz GP. Studien über die Sogenannten initalen Fieber-krampfe bei Kindern. *Acta Paediatr Scand* 1941;29(Suppl 1):1–142.
53. Fowler M. Brain damage after febrile convulsions. *Arch Dis Child* 1957;32:67–76.
54. Zimmerman HM. The histopathology of convulsive disorders in children. *J Pediatr* 1938;13:859–890.
55. Ellenberg JH, Nelson KB. Febrile seizures and later intellectual performance. *Arch Neurol* 1978;35:17–21.
56. Maytal J, Shinnar S. Febrile status epilepticus. *Pediatrics* 1990;86: 611–616.
57. Gastaut H, Poirier F, Payan H, et al. HHE syndrome, hemiconvulsions, hemiplegia, epilepsy. *Epilepsia* 1959;1:418–447.
58. Berg AT, Shinnar S, Hauser WA, et al. Predictors of recurrent febrile seizures: a meta-analytic review. *J Pediatr* 1990;116:329–337.
59. Van den Berg BJ. Studies on convulsive disorders in young children. 3. Recurrence of febrile convulsions. *Epilepsia* 1974;15:177–190.
60. Berg AT, Shinnar S, Darefsky AS, et al. Predictors of recurrent febrile seizures. A prospective cohort study. *Arch Pediatr Adolesc Med* 1997;151:371–378.
61. Van Stuijvenberg M, Steyerberg EW, Derksen-Lubsen G, et al. Temperature, age, and recurrence of febrile seizures. *Arch Pediatr Adolesc Med* 1998;152:1170–1175.

62. Berg AT, Shinnar S, Darefsky AS, et al. Predictors of recurrent febrile seizures. A prospective cohort study. *Arch Pediatr Adolesc Med* 1997;151:371–378.
63. Berg AT, Shinnar S. Complex febrile seizures. *Epilepsia* 1996; 37:126–133.
64. Hauser WA, Kurland LT. The epidemiology of epilepsy in Rochester, Minnesota, 1935 through 1967. *Epilepsia* 1975;16:1–66.
65. Ross EM, Peckham CS, West PB, et al. Epilepsy in childhood: findings from the National Child Development Study. *Br Med J* 1980;280:207–210.
66. Ueoka K, Nagano H, Kumanomidou U, et al. Clinical and electroencephalographic study in febrile convulsions with special reference to follow-up study. *Brain Dev* 1979;1:196.
67. Van der Berg BJ, Yerushalmy J. Studies on convulsive disorders in young children. I. Incidence of febrile and nonfebrile convulsions by age and other factors. *Pediatr Res* 1969;3:298–304.
68. Wallace SJ. Recurrence of febrile convulsions. *Arch Dis Child* 1974;49:763–765.
69. Shinnar S, Glauser TA, Febrile seizures. *J Child Neurol* 2002; 17 Suppl 1:S44–S52.
70. Wallace SJ. Spontaneous fits after convulsions with fever. *Arch Dis Child* 1977;52:192–196.
71. Falconer MA. Genetic and related aetological factors in temporal lobe epilepsy. *Epilepsia* 1971;12:13–31.
72. Rasmussen T. Relative significance of isolated infantile convulsions as a primary cause of focal epilepsy. *Epilepsia* 1979;20:395–401.
73. Meldrum BS. Secondary pathology of febrile and experimental convulsions. In: Brazier MAB, Coceani F, eds. *Brain dysfunction in infantile febrile convulsions.* New York: Raven Press, 1976.
74. Nemoto EM, Frankel HM. Cerebral oxygenation and metabolism during progressive hyperthermia. *Am J Physiol* 1970;219: 1784–1788.
75. Janszky J, Woermann FG, Barsi P, et al. Right hippocampal sclerosis is more common than left after febrile seizures. *Neurology* 2003;60:1209–1210.
76. Tarkka R. Paakko E, Pyhtinen J, et al. Febrile seizures and mesial temporal sclerosis: No association in a long-term follow-up study. *Neurology* 2003;60:215–218.
77. Bower SP, Kilpatrick CJ, Vogrin SJ. Degree of hippocampal atrophy is not related to a history of febrile seizures in patients with proved hippocampal sclerosis. *J Neurol Neurosurg Psychiatry* 2000;69:733–738.
78. Schulz R, Ebner A. Prolonged febrile convulsions and mesial temporal lobe epilepsy in an identical twin. *Neurology* 2001;57: 318–320.
79. Sokol DK, Demyer WE, Edwards-Brown M, et al. From swelling to sclerosis: acute change in mesial hippocampus after prolonged febrile seizure. *Seizure* 2003;12:237–240.
80. Theodore WH, Bhatia S, Hatta J, Fazilat S. Hippocampal atrophy, epilepsy duration, and febrile seizures in patients with partial seizures. *Neurology* 1999;52:132–136.
81. Brewster A, Bender RA, Chen Y, et al. Developmental febrile seizures modulate hippocampal gene expression of hyperpolarization-activated channels in an isoform- and cell-specific manner. *J Neurosci* 2002;22:4591–4599.
82. Salanova V, Markand O, Worth R, et al. FDG-PET and MRI in temporal lobe epilepsy: relationship to febrile seizures, hippocampal sclerosis and outcome. *Acta Neurol Scand* 1998;97: 146–153.
83. VanLandingham KE, Heinz ER, Cavazos JE, et al. Magnetic resonance imaging evidence of hippocampal injury after prolonged focal febrile convulsions. *Ann Neurol* 1998;43:413–426.
84. Szabó CA, Wyllie E, Siavalas EL, et al. Hippocampal volumetry in children 6 years or younger: assessment of children with and without complex febrile seizures. *Epilepsy Res* 1999;33:1–9.
85. Theodore WH, Bhatia S, Hatta J, et al. Hippocampal atrophy, epilepsy duration, and febrile seizures in patients with partial seizures. *Neurology* 1999;52:132–136.
86. Taylor DC. Differential rates of cerebral maturation between sexes and between hemispheres. Evidence from epilepsy. *Lancet* 1969;2:140–142.
87. Taylor DC, Ounsted C. Biological mechanisms influencing the outcome of seizures in response to fever. *Epilepsia* 1971;12:33–45.
88. Lindsay J, Ounsted C, Richards P. Long-term outcome in children with temporal lobe seizures. IV. Genetic factors, febrile convulsions and the remission of seizures. *Dev Med Child Neurol* 1980;22:429–439.
89. Scheffer IE, Berkovic SF. Generalized epilepsy with febrile seizures plus. A genetic disorder with heterogeneous clinical phenotypes. *Brain* 1997;120:479–490.
90. Wallace RH, Wang DW, Singh R, et al. Febrile seizures and generalized epilepsy associated with a mutation in the Na+−channel beta 1 subunit gene SCN1B. *Nat Genet* 1998;19:366–370.
91. Wallace RH, Scheffer JE, Parasivam G. Generalized epilepsy with febrile seizures plus: mutation of the sodium channel subunit SCN1B. *Neurology* 2002;58:1426–1429.
92. Sugawara T, Mazaki-Miyazaki E, Ito M, et al. Nav1.1 mutations cause febrile seizures associated with afebrile partial seizures. *Neurology* 2001;57:703–705.
93. Lerche H, Jurkat-Rott K, Lehmann-Horn F. Ion channels and epilepsy. *Am J Med Genet* 2001; 106:146–159.
94. Ito M, Nagafuji H, Okazawa H, et al. Autosomal dominant epilepsy with febrile seizures plus with missense mutations of the (Na+)-channel alpha 1 subunit gene, SCN1A. *Epilepsy Res* 2002;48:15–23.
95. Singh R, Scheffer IE, Crossland K, et al. Generalized epilepsy with febrile seizures plus: a common childhood-onset genetic epilepsy syndrome. *Ann Neurol* 1999;45:75–81.
96. Abou-Khalil B, Ge O, Desai R, et al. Partial and generalized epilepsy with febrile seizures plus and a novel SCN1A mutation. *Neurology* 2001;57:2265–2272.
97. Ward N, Evanson J, Cockerell OC. Idiopathic familial temporal lobe epilepsy with febrile convulsions. *Seizure* 2002;11:16–19.
98. Depondt C, Van Paesschen W, Matthijs G, et al. Familial temporal lobe epilepsy with febrile seizures. *Neurology* 2002;58: 1429–1433.
99. Dravet C, Bureau M, Oguni H, et al. Severe myoclonic epilepsy in infancy: Dravet syndrome. *Adv Neurol* 2005;95:71–102.
100. Singh R, Andermann E, Whitehouse WP, et al. Severe myoclonic epilepsy of infancy: extended spectrum of GEFS+? *Epilepsia* 2001;42:837–844.
101. Claes L, Del Favero J, Ceulemans B, et al. De novo mutations in the sodium-channel gene SCN1A cause severe myoclonic epilepsy of infancy. *Am J Hum Genet* 2001; 68:1327–1332.
102. Nabbout R, Kozlovski A, Gennaro E, et al. Absence of mutations in major GEFS+ genes in myoclonic astatic epilepsy. *Epilepsy Res* 2003;56:127–133.
103. Wallace SJ. Neurological and intellectual deficits: convulsions with fever viewed as acute indications of life-long developmental defects. In: Brazier MAB, Coceani F, eds. *Brain dysfunction in infantile febrile convulsions.* New York: Raven Press, 1976:259–277.
104. Verity CM, Greenwood R, Golding J, Long-term intellectual and behavioral outcomes of children with febrile convulsions. *N Engl J Med* 1998;338:1723–1728.
105. Wolf SM. Controversies in the treatment of febrile convulsions. *Neurology* 1979;29:287–290.
106. Practice parameter: the neurodiagnostic evaluation of the child with a first simple febrile seizure. American Academy of Pediatrics. Provisional Committee on Quality Improvement, Subcommittee on Febrile Seizures. *Pediatrics* 1996;97:769–772.
107. Practice parameter: long-term treatment of the child with simple febrile seizures. American Academy of Pediatrics. Committee on Quality Improvement, Subcommittee on Febrile Seizures. *Pediatrics* 1999; 103:1307–1309.
108. Baumann RJ, Duffner PK. Treatment of children with simple febrile seizures: the AAP practice parameter. American Academy of Pediatrics. *Pediatr Neurol* 2000;23:11–17.
109. Faero O, Kastrup KW, Lykkegaard Nielsen E, et al. Successful prophylaxis of febrile convulsions with phenobarbital. *Epilepsia* 1972;13:279–285.
110. Lee K, Taudorf K, Hvorslev V. Prophylactic treatment with valproic acid or diazepam in children with febrile convulsions. *Acta Paediatr Scand* 1986;75:593–597.
111. Mamelle N, Mamelle JC, Plasse JC, et al. Prevention of recurrent febrile convulsions—a randomized therapeutic assay: sodium valproate, phenobarbital and placebo. *Neuropediatrics* 1984;15:37–42.
112. Ngwane E, Bower B. Continuous sodium valproate or phenobarbitone in the prevention of "simple" febrile convulsions. Comparison by a double-blind trial. *Arch Dis Child* 1980;55:171–174.

113. Wallace SJ, Smith JA. Successful prophylaxis against febrile convulsions with valproic acid or phenobarbitone. *Br Med J* 1980; 280:353–354.
114. Wallace SJ, Smith JA. Prophylaxis against febrile convulsions. *Br Med J* 1980;280:863–864.
115. Melchior JC, Buchthal F, Lennox-Buchthal M. The ineffectiveness of diphenylhydantoin in preventing febrile convulsions in the age of greatest risk, under three years. *Epilepsia* 1971;12:55–62.
116. Wolf SM, Forsythe A. Behavior disturbance, phenobarbital, and febrile seizures. *Pediatrics* 1978;61:728–731.
117. Chaudhry M, Pond DA. Mental deterioration in epileptic children. *J Neurol Neurosurg Psychiatry* 1961;24:213–219.
118. Holdsworth L, Whitmore K. A study of children with epilepsy attending ordinary schools. I. Their seizure patterns, progress and behaviour in school. *Dev Med Child Neurol* 1974;16:746–758.
119. Wapner I, Thurston DL, Holowach J. Phenobarbital. Its effect on learning in epileptic children. *JAMA* 1962;182:937.
120. Wolf SM, Forsythe A, Stunden AA, et al. Long-term effect of phenobarbital on cognitive function in children with febrile convulsions. *Pediatrics* 1981;68:820–823.
121. Farwell JR, Lee YJ, Hirtz DG, et al. Phenobarbital for febrile seizures—effects on intelligence and on seizure recurrence. *N Engl J Med* 1990;322:364–369.
122. Dreifuss FE, Rosman NP, Cloyd JC, et al. A comparison of rectal diazepam gel and placebo for acute repetitive seizures. N Engl J Med. 1998;338:1869–1875.
123. Knudsen FU. Effective short-term diazepam prophylaxis in febrile convulsions. *J Pediatr* 1985;106:487–490.
124. Knudsen FU, Vestermark S. Prophylactic diazepam or phenobarbitone in febrile convulsions: a prospective, controlled study. *Arch Dis Child* 1978;53:660–663.
125. Kriel RL, Cloyd JC, Hadsall RS, et al. Home use of rectal diazepam for cluster and prolonged seizures: efficacy, adverse reactions, quality of life, and cost analysis. *Pediatr Neurol* 1991;7:13–17.
126. Scott RC, Besag FM, Neville BG. Buccal midazolam and rectal diazepam for treatment of prolonged seizures in childhood and adolescence: a randomised trial. *Lancet* 1999;353: 623–626.
127. Rainbow J, Browne GJ, Lam LT. Controlling seizures in the prehospital setting: diazepam or midazolam? *J Paediatr Child Health* 2002;38:582–586.
128. Lehat E, Goldman M, Barr J, Bistritzer T, Berkovitch M. Comparison of intranasal midazolam with intravenous diazepam for treating febrile seizures in children: prospective randomised study. *BMJ* 2000;321:83–86.
129. Rosman NP, Colton T, Labazzo J, et al. A controlled trial of diazepam administered during febrile illnesses to prevent recurrence of febrile seizures. *N Engl J Med* 1993;329:79–84.
130. Millichap JG, Colliver JA. Management of febrile seizures: survey of current practice and phenobarbital usage. *Pediatr Neurol* 1991;7:243–248.

Posttraumatic Epilepsy

34

Jayanthi Mani   Elizabeth Barry

With an estimated annual incidence between 180–220 cases per 100,000 members of the population (1,2), head injury causes significant morbidity and mortality (3). A recognized and preventable cause of seizures (4,5), head trauma is responsible for more than 20% of symptomatic cases of epilepsy and for 5% of all epilepsy (6). Approximately 70% of seizures after head injury occur in the first 2 years, but may begin anytime after the injury, even years after apparent recovery (7,8). Although the annual incidence of head injury has not changed much in the past 30 years, the number of survivors of serious head injuries has risen (9), and more head trauma is occurring among the elderly (10). Both trends may result in an increased incidence of posttraumatic epilepsy.

TERMINOLOGY

Posttraumatic seizures are single or recurrent seizures after penetrating or nonpenetrating traumatic brain injury that cannot be attributed to another obvious cause.

Posttraumatic epilepsy describes late-onset, recurrent, unprovoked seizures that are not attributable to another obvious cause.

TIMING OF SEIZURES

Posttraumatic seizures are classified as early or late, depending on when they appear after head injury (7,11–15), because they represent different pathophysiologic processes.

Early seizures are acute provoked attacks that occur within a week of the injury, when the patient is still suffering from the direct neurologic or systemic effects of the head trauma (16–20). Although not considered epilepsy, these seizures increase the risk for posttraumatic epilepsy (21,22). Approximately 50% of early seizures occur within the first 24 hours (5). Sometimes referred to as immediate seizures, their occurrence between 1 and 24 hours after injury repre-

sents the initial effect of the acute trauma on the brain (11,14,18). These may be confused with impact or concussive convulsions, which occur within seconds of the impact. Concussive convulsions are believed to be nonepileptic, and do not require antiepileptic treatment (23).

Developing more than a week after head injury (12,13, 24,25), late seizures reflect permanent changes in the brain and therefore signal the onset of posttraumatic epilepsy. Nearly 40% of late seizures appear within the first 6 months after injury; more than 50% appear by 1 year and 70% to 80% appear by 2 years after the injury (26,27). Although the risk of posttraumatic epilepsy continues to decline as the postinjury seizure-free interval lengthens, late seizures may begin more than 15 years after the acute damage has resolved (8,28,29). Such a delayed manifestation is established when recurrent focal seizures arise from the area of severe penetrating brain injury.

RISK FACTORS

Severity of Head Injury

The overall risk of early seizures varies from 2% to 15% (16,30,31); that of posttraumatic epilepsy (late seizures) is approximately 5% to 7% (24,26,28). The most important risk factor for either is the severity of the injury (7,13,32), and the greater the severity, the higher the risk of posttraumatic seizures. Stratifying seizure frequency by severity of head injury has been difficult, because definitions of mild, moderate, and severe vary in the published literature. The duration of posttraumatic amnesia, the nature of the brain injury, and the Glasgow Coma Scale have been used to grade severity of injury. Correlating with severity and increasing the seizure risk are prolonged coma or posttraumatic amnesia (longer than 24 hours), brain contusion, intracranial hematoma, depressed skull fracture, dural penetration, and, to a lesser extent, linear skull fractures (12,33,34). Risk also increases when more than one factor is present (35).

Early seizures accompany fewer than 5% of mild or moderate head injuries (16,18,26,30) and often indicate other neurologic or systemic abnormalities, especially in an otherwise mild injury (18,36). The incidence increases to 30% with subdural or intracerebral hematoma, depressed skull fracture, penetrating brain injury, or cortical contusion (19,37). Seizures after the first hour usually imply severe head injury and focal intracranial pathologic lesions, such as hemorrhage or skull fracture.

Late posttraumatic seizures are common with more severe head injury. In the series reported by Annegers and Coan (38), the risk of posttraumatic epilepsy 5 years after closed head injury was 1.5% after mild trauma, similar to the risk for the general population without such injury; 2.9% after moderate damage; and 17.2% after severe insult (mild trauma was defined as coma or amnesia lasting less than 30 minutes, no skull fracture; moderate as coma or amnesia lasting between 30 minutes and 24 hours, skull fracture, but no contusion or intracranial hemorrhage; and severe trauma as coma or amnesia lasting more than 24 hours, and/or brain contusion or intracranial hemorrhage). Temkin (37) reported that the risk of late seizures increases by 400 times of that expected in a general population in the presence of early seizures, coma for more than a week, nonelevated depressed skull fracture, dural penetration injury, one nonreactive pupil, and subdural or intracerebral hematoma. In military personnel who survive high-velocity penetrating head injuries during warfare, the nearly 50% risk of posttraumatic epilepsy (7,27,29,39) is increased by the presence of a brain abscess.

Age

The influence of age on the development of posttraumatic seizures is well documented (12,24,40,41). Children younger than age 5 years are more likely than adults to have seizures within the first hour after mild head injury (16,30,42,43), although early seizures are less predictive of late seizures than in adults (24,26). Adults older than age 65 years are highly vulnerable to severe brain damage and late posttraumatic epilepsy from any type of head injury (28,44).

Early Seizures

Regardless of other risk factors, even a single early seizure increases the risk of late epilepsy to more than 25% in most series (12,24,34,37,45). Late seizures are more likely to begin within the first year if there has been an early seizure.

Immediate Seizures

Jennett (12) defined an immediate, or impact, seizure as "a single generalized seizure . . . occurring within seconds of . . . a mild injury in an adult" and hypothesized that it did not necessarily indicate brain injury or predict later seizures.

Although later investigators (46) adopted this position, universal agreement was lacking. Kollevold (21) found no difference in the risk of late epilepsy between a first seizure occurring within minutes of a head injury or during the ensuing 6 hours. McCrory and colleagues (23) report that convulsions within seconds of impact after concussive brain injury in sport do not increase the risk of long-term epilepsy. Contrary to these observations, Barry and coworkers (47) report that impact seizures may precede late epilepsy. Temkin (37) noted an increased risk for delayed early seizures (from days 1 to 7) in patients whose seizures occurred in the first hour after head trauma. Most researchers do not distinguish between immediate and early seizures as risk factors for late epilepsy.

Genetic Factors

The evidence for genetic influences on posttraumatic seizures is conflicting. Some studies (48) have reported a higher incidence of seizures in family members of patients with posttraumatic seizures; other research has failed to demonstrate a similar relationship (29,49).

Persistence of Posttraumatic Seizures

The ease with which posttraumatic seizures are controlled reflects the factors that determine their development. More than half remit after 2 years (7,8). Seizures that occur after severe head injury or that resist early control tend to persist (25). Seizures that develop within the first year are more likely to remit than those that appear later (33).

PATHOLOGY AND PATHOPHYSIOLOGY

Early Seizures

The immediate or primary insult after a head injury consists of diffuse axonal injury due to shearing forces and focal brain damage from the direct impact to the skull, movement of the brain in the skull, or penetration (50–52). Secondary axonal injury is caused by retraction and swelling of the injured axons with distal wallerian degeneration (53). Subsequent brain necrosis may result from cytotoxic processes such as the release of free oxygen radicals and cytokines and the influx of calcium into open ion channels (51,54). All of these processes contribute to the development of early seizures, as do complications such as hypoxia, increased intracranial pressure, hypotension, brain edema, intracranial bleeding, ischemia, electrolyte imbalances, and secondary infection (36,55).

Late Seizures

The development of late epilepsy is less well understood. Late seizures may be caused by irritating effects of intracerebral hemorrhage or by cortical damage to vulnerable brain regions like the hippocampus. In experimental models, iron deposition on the brain is strongly epileptogenic (56), and the presence of hemosiderin in the brain is a well-recognized cause of seizures (33,45,52,57). Even mild closed head injury can cause intracranial hemorrhage, with subsequent deposition of iron, which affects intracellular calcium concentration and the formation of free radicals (58). Early seizures may cause progressive changes in neural networks and lead to spontaneous recurrent late seizures (59).

Late posttraumatic epilepsy may also be caused by the death of inhibitory neurons and the reorganization of networks, with loss of inhibition and enhancement of intrinsic cellular bursting. In experimental studies of head trauma, selective cell loss in the hippocampus produced abnormal hyperexcitability and enhanced kindling (60–62). Similar changes have been seen in humans after head injury (61).

CLINICAL FEATURES

The full spectrum of seizure semiology can be seen after head trauma with the exception of true absence seizures. The site of injury and the underlying structural damage determine the type of focal manifestations (8,29,39,63, 64). An interaction also exists between the site of injury and the time of seizure onset. Epilepsy appears earliest after lesions of the motor area, followed by temporal lobe lesions and those in the frontal or occipital areas (15). Early posttraumatic seizures are likely to be generalized tonic-clonic (18,30,65) even in the presence of focal brain damage. Late seizures usually have a focal onset (8,63,64). Complex partial seizures, the most common partial type, may develop subsequent to early generalized seizures (29).

Status Epilepticus

Approximately 10% to 20% of early seizures develop into status epilepticus, usually in children (5,16). Continuous electroencephalographic (EEG) monitoring identifies patients with nonconvulsive status after head injury. Mortality is high, even with a mild head injury, although status is most often a sequela of severe trauma (66). Generalized status epilepticus frequently accompanies underlying complications, such as ischemia or metabolic imbalance. Focal motor status is most common with subdural hematomas or depressed skull fractures and can be refractory to treatment. Early status epilepticus after brain injury may increase the risk of later unprovoked seizures (67).

DIAGNOSTIC STUDIES

Imaging Studies

As the preferred diagnostic test for assessing intracranial damage after head injury (64), computed tomography (CT)

has largely confirmed that a focal brain lesion with intracerebral hemorrhage predicts an increased risk of posttraumatic early and late seizures (24,68). Magnetic resonance imaging (MRI) scans detect traumatic white-matter abnormalities with greater sensitivity than does CT (69). Several new magnetic resonance techniques demonstrate increased sensitivity for detecting traumatic brain lesions (70), but the implications of these abnormalities for the subsequent development of seizures are unclear. Seizure occurrence does not correlate with severity and localization of traumatic brain lesions on MRI; patients may have what appears to be extensive damage yet achieve complete neurologic recovery (71). Functional imaging techniques may predict increased susceptibility for seizures after brain injury (72,73).

Electroencephalography

Altered EEG patterns during the acute phase of head injury are usually nonspecific and reflect systemic factors as well as direct brain damage (74,75). Recordings obtained soon after the injury are useful for predicting recovery from coma (76) or detecting ongoing seizure activity in patients whose clinical signs are suppressed by the trauma or iatrogenic intervention. Continuous video-EEG monitoring in the intensive care unit increasingly serves this purpose (66,77).

Electroencephalograms are less useful for predicting the risk of posttraumatic epilepsy (65,78,79). Epileptiform abnormalities may appear as early as a week after injury (80). Early EEG abnormalities only poorly predict late seizures (78), although focal EEG activity seen 1 month after head trauma predicts an increased risk of seizures at 1 year after head injury (45). The conflicting, and therefore inadequate, evidence precludes conclusions on the predictive value of early EEG changes for long-term seizure risk (81).

Patients with severe head injuries, especially with posttraumatic epilepsy, have abnormal EEG findings long after recovery from the trauma (31,82). Central and temporal spikes are associated with a high risk of epilepsy. Prominent epileptiform activity is seen with longer duration and intractable epilepsy (31).

TREATMENT

Early Seizures

Although early seizures may not recur, treatment may minimize the secondary effects of increased intracranial pressure and prevent status epilepticus. Antiepileptic medication, usually a drug that does not cause significant sedation such as phenytoin, should be loaded intravenously and maintained throughout the acute phase in these critically ill patients.

Late Seizures

Carrying an increased risk for injury, continued psychosocial disability, and death (83,84), late posttraumatic seizures, like any other type of focal, symptomatic epilepsy, require long-term maintenance of antiepileptic drug therapy. Medication should not be withdrawn until seizures have been controlled for at least 2 years. The later seizures begin (especially more than a year after trauma), the less likely they are to remit (33). The diagnosis of posttraumatic epilepsy may be difficult to establish, particularly after severe head injury, because accompanying profound cognitive and behavioral disturbances may resemble complex partial seizures (36). Nonepileptic seizures also may occur, usually after minor head injury (85). Long-term video-EEG monitoring should clarify the diagnosis, because the medications themselves may interfere with total recovery.

Patients with intractable epilepsy secondary to head trauma without MRI-detected focal lesions often have seizure foci that are difficult to localize, and this may deter surgical intervention (86). One-third of cases of intractable posttraumatic epilepsy involve mesial temporal sclerosis, and these patients have a good postsurgical outcome (86,87). The causal relationship and mechanisms of mesial temporal sclerosis and hippocampal sclerosis after brain injury are not clear but probably reflect diffuse secondary effects of brain trauma.

PREVENTION

Medical prophylaxis of posttraumatic seizures is controversial. As posttraumatic seizures impede recovery from brain injury (88), so, too, may the medications. A survey of neurosurgeons (89) revealed that most of them routinely prescribe prophylactic medications only for the most severely injured patients or those experiencing early posttraumatic seizures. The duration of treatment varied but usually continued for 6 months.

Late Seizures

In kindling models of epileptogenesis, pretreatment with some antiepileptics prevented clinical seizures (90,91), but clinical studies have yielded contradictory results, even in patients at greatest risk for posttraumatic seizures. Observational studies published in the past two decades demonstrated significant benefit of phenytoin and phenobarbital in the prevention of late seizures (92,93); however, randomized, double-blind, prospective evaluations of antiseizure drug prophylaxis with phenytoin, phenobarbital, carbamazepine, and valproic acid consistently found no benefit (94–97), irrespective of the choice of antiepileptic drug.

Recent preliminary evidence from animal models indicates that the window for intervention against epileptogenesis may be restricted to the period soon after the insult (98). This has to be confirmed in clinical studies.

Early Seizures

A meta-analysis (99) demonstrated a role for phenytoin (relative risk [RR], 0.33; confidence interval [CI], 0.19–0.59) and carbamazepine (RR 0.39; CI 0.17–0.92) in the prevention of early seizures after head trauma, although phenytoin does not have a detectable impact on mortality from brain trauma (100,101). A Cochrane Database Review of six trials also demonstrated a beneficial effect of antiepileptic drugs (RR 0.34; CI 0.21–0.54) (101).

On the basis of an analysis of prospective studies (81), the American Academy of Neurology has published recommendations on the use of antiepileptic drug prophylaxis in adults with severe traumatic brain injury. Their current recommendation is to use phenytoin prophylaxis in adults with severe brain injury to prevent early posttraumatic seizures. Phenytoin may be initiated as an intravenous loading dose as soon as possible after the injury. Current evidence does not support the routine use of antiepileptic drugs beyond the first 7 days after the injury.

Data on the use of antiepileptic drugs to prevent seizures in children are insufficient for treatment recommendations (102–105). Administration of glucocorticoids after brain injury does not decrease late posttraumatic seizures, and early treatment has increased seizure activity (106).

FUTURE DIRECTIONS

The study of posttraumatic epilepsy may yield valuable insights into epileptogenesis after brain injury. Studies are evaluating the role of neuroprotective agents in traumatic brain injury, and prospective trials with some new antiepilepsy medications may offer clues to reducing the incidence of posttraumatic epilepsy. A better understanding of the epileptogenetic processes may assist in the selection of agents relevant to the specific mechanisms of brain injury.

REFERENCES

1. Annegers JF, Grabow JD, Kurland LT, et al. The incidence, causes, and secular trends of head trauma in Olmsted County, Minnesota, 1935–1974. *Neurology* 1980;30:912–919.
2. Bruns J Jr, Hauser WA. The epidemiology of traumatic brain injury: a review. *Epilepsia* 2003;44(Suppl):2–10.
3. Jennett B. Epidemiology of head injury. *J Neurol Neurosurg Psychiatry* 1996;60:362–369.
4. Elvidge AR. Remarks on post-traumatic convulsive state. *Trans Am Neurol Assoc* 1939;65:125–129.
5. Pagni CA. Posttraumatic epilepsy: incidence and prophylaxis. *Acta Neurochir Suppl* 1990;50:38–47.
6. Hauser WA, Annegers JF, Kurland LT. Prevalence of epilepsy in Rochester, Minnesota: 1940–1980. *Epilepsia* 1991;32:429–445.
7. Caveness WF, Meirowsky AM, Rish BL, et al. The nature of posttraumatic epilepsy. *J Neurosurg* 1979;50:545–553.

8. Walker AE, Erculei F. Post-traumatic epilepsy 15 years later. *Epilepsia* 1970;11:17–26.

9. Thurman D, Guerrero J. Trends in hospitalization associated with traumatic brain. *JAMA* 1999;282(10):989–991.

10. Tieves KS, Yang H, Layde PM. The epidemiology of traumatic brain injury in Wisconsin. *WMJ* 2005;104(2):22–5, 54.

11. Dalmady-Israel C, Zasler ND. Post-traumatic seizures: a critical review. *Brain Inj* 1993;7:263–273.

12. Jennett WB. *Epilepsy after blunt head injuries.* Springfield, IL: Charles C Thomas, 1962.

13. Jennett WB, Lewin W. Traumatic epilepsy after closed head injuries. *J Neurol Neurosurg Psychiatry* 1960;23:295–301.

14. Kollevold T. Immediate and early cerebral seizures after head injuries, part I. *J Oslo City Hosp* 1976;26:99–114.

15. Paillas JE, Paillas N, Bureau M. Post-traumatic epilepsy. Introduction and clinical observations. *Epilepsia* 1970;11:5–15.

16. Jennett B. Early traumatic epilepsy. *Arch Neurol* 1974;30:394–398.

17. Kollevold T. Immediate and early cerebral seizures after head injuries, part II. *J Oslo City Hosp* 1977;27:89–99.

18. Lee S-T, Lui T-N. Early seizures after mild closed head injury. *J Neurosurg* 1992;76:435–439.

19. Lee S-T, Lui T-N, Wong C-W, et al. Early seizures after moderate closed head injury. *Acta Neurochir* 1995;137:151–154.

20. Lee S-T, Lui T-N, Wong C-W, et al. Early seizures after severe closed head injury. *Can J Neurol Sci* 1997;24:40–43.

21. Kollevold T. Immediate and early seizures after head injuries, part III. *J Oslo City Hosp* 1978;28:77–86.

22. Walker AE. Pathogenesis and pathophysiology of posttraumatic epilepsy. In: Walker AE, Caveness WF, Critchley M, eds. *The late effects of head injury.* Springfield, IL: Charles C Thomas, 1969: 306–314.

23. McCrory PR, Berkovic SF. Concussive convulsions. Incidence in sport and treatment recommendations. *Sports Med* 1998;25: 131–136.

24. De Santis A, Sganzerla E, Spagnoli D, et al. Risk factors for late posttraumatic epilepsy. *Acta Neurochir Suppl* 1992;55:64–67.

25. Haltiner AM, Temkin NR, Dikmen AA. Risk of seizure recurrence after the first late posttraumatic seizure. *Arch Phys Med Rehabil* 1997;78:835–840.

26. Annegers JF, Grabow JD, Groover RV, et al. Seizures after head trauma: a population study. *Neurology* 1980;30:683–689.

27. Hughes JR. Post-traumatic epilepsy in the military. *Mil Med* 1986;151:416–419.

28. Annegers JF, Hauser WA, Coan SP, et al. A population-based study of seizures after traumatic brain injuries. *N Engl J Med* 1998;338:20–24.

29. Salazar AM, Jabbari B, Vance SC, et al. Epilepsy after penetrating head injury, I: clinical correlates: a report of the Vietnam Head Injury Study. *Neurology* 1985;35:1406–1414.

30. Desai BT, Whitman S, Coonley-Hoganson R, et al. Seizures and civilian head injuries. *Epilepsia* 1983;24:289–296.

31. Martins da Silva A, Rocha Vaz A, Ribeiro I, et al. Controversies in posttraumatic epilepsy. *Acta Neurochir Suppl* 1990;50:48–51.

32. Weiss GH, Caveness WF. Prognostic factors in the persistence of posttraumatic epilepsy. *J Neurosurg* 1972;37:164–169.

33. Jennett B. Epilepsy and acute traumatic intracranial hematoma. *J Neurol Neurosurg Psychiatry* 1975;38:378–381.

34. Weiss GH, Feeney DM, Caveness WF, et al. Prognostic factors for the occurrence of posttraumatic epilepsy. *Arch Neurol* 1983;40:7–10.

35. Jennett B, Teasdale G. *Management of head injuries.* Philadelphia: FA Davis, 1981.

36. Yablon SA. Posttraumatic seizures. *Arch Phys Med Rehabil* 1993; 74:983–1001.

37. Temkin NR. Risk factors for posttraumatic seizures in adults. *Epilepsia* 2003;44(Suppl 10):18–20.

38. Annegers JF, Coan SP. The risks of epilepsy after traumatic brain injury. *Seizure* 2000;9:453–457.

39. Russell WR, Whitty CWM. Studies in traumatic epilepsy, I: factors influencing the incidence of epilepsy after brain wounds. *J Neurol Neurosurg Psychiatry* 1952;15:93–98.

40. Asikainen I, Kaste M, Sarna S. Early and late posttraumatic seizures in traumatic brain injury rehabilitation patients: brain injury factors causing late seizures and influence of seizures on long-term outcome. *Epilepssia* 1999;40:584–589.

41. Bruns J Jr, Hauser WA. The epidemiology of traumatic brain injury: a review. *Epilepsia* 2003;44(Suppl 10):2–10.

42. Hahn YS, Fuchs S, Flannery AM, et al. Factors influencing post-traumatic seizures in children. *Neurosurgery* 1988;22:864–867.

43. Hendrick EB, Harris L. Post-traumatic epilepsy in children. *J Trauma* 1968;8:547–555.

44. Hernesniemi J. Outcome following head injuries in the aged. *Acta Neurochir* 1979;49:67–79.

45. Angeleri F, Majkowski J, Cacchio G, et al. Posttraumatic epilepsy risk factors: one-year prospective study after head injury. *Epilepsia* 1999;40:1222–1230.

46. McCrory PR, Bladin PF, Berkovic SF. Retrospective study of concussive convulsions in elite Australian rules and rugby league footballers: phenomenology, aetiology, and outcome. *BMJ* 1997; 314:171–174.

47. Barry E, Bergey GK, Krumholz A, et al. Posttraumatic seizure types vary with the interval after head injury. *Epilepsia* 1997;38 (Suppl 8):49–50.

48. Evans JH. Post-traumatic epilepsy. *Neurology* 1962;12:665–674.

49. Schaumann BA, Annegers JF, Johnson SB, et al. Family history of seizures in posttraumatic and alcohol-associated seizure disorders. *Epilepsia* 1994;35:48–52.

50. Adams JH, Mitchell DE, Graham DI, et al. Diffuse brain damage of immediate impact type. *Brain* 1977;100:489–502.

51. Miller JD. Head injury. *J Neurol Neurosurg Psychiatry* 1993;56: 440–447.

52. Payan H, Toga M, Bernard-Badier M. The pathology of post-traumatic epilepsy. *Epilepsia* 1970;11:81–94.

53. Povlishock JT. Traumatically induced axonal injury: pathogenesis and pathobiological implications. *Brain Pathol* 1992;2:1–12.

54. Ikeda Y, Long DM. The molecular basis of brain injury and brain edema: the role of oxygen free radicals. *Neurosurgery* 1990;27: 1–11.

55. Miller JD, Becker DP. Secondary insults to the injured brain. *J R Coll Surg Edinb* 1982;27:292–298.

56. Willmore LJ. Recurrent seizures induced by cortical iron injection: a model of posttraumatic epilepsy. *Ann Neurol* 1978;4:329–336.

57. Weisberg LA, Shamsnia M, Elliott D. Seizures caused by nontraumatic parenchymal brain hemorrhages. *Neurology* 1991;41: 1197–1199.

58. Willmore LJ, Hiramatsu M, Kochi H, et al. Formation of superoxide radicals, lipid peroxides and edema after $FeCl_{13}$ injection into rat isocortex. *Brain Res* 1983;277:393–396.

59. Lowenstein DH. Recent advances related to basic mechanisms of epileptogenesis. *Epilepsy Res Suppl* 1996;11:45–60.

60. Coulter DA, Rafiq A, Shumate M, et al. Brain injury-induced enhanced limbic epileptogenesis: anatomical and physiological parallels to an animal model of temporal lobe epilepsy. *Epilepsy Res* 1996;26:81–91.

61. Kotapka MJ, Graham DI, Adams JH, et al. Hippocampal pathology in fatal non-missile human head injury. *Acta Neuropathol* 1992;83:530–534.

62. Lowenstein DH, Thomas MJ, Smith DH, et al. Selective vulnerability of dentate hilar neurons following traumatic brain injury: a potential mechanistic link between head trauma and disorders of the hippocampus. *J Neurosci* 1992;12:4846–4853.

63. Russell WR, Whitty CWM. Studies in traumatic epilepsy, 2: focal motor and somatic sensory fits: a study of 85 cases. *J Neurol Neurosurg Psychiatry* 1953;16:73–97.

64. Russell WR, Whitty CWM. Studies in traumatic epilepsy, 3: visual fits. *J Neurol Neurosurg Psychiatry* 1955;18:79–96.

65. Martins da Silva A, Nunes B, Vaz AR, et al. Posttraumatic epilepsy in civilians: clinical and electroencephalographic studies. *Acta Neurochir Suppl* 1992;55:56–63.

66. Vespa PM, Nuwer MR, Nenov V, et al. Increased incidence and impact of nonconvulsive and convulsive seizures after traumatic brain injury as detected by continuous electroencephalographic monitoring. *J Neurosurg* 1999;91:750–760.

67. Hesdorffer DC, Logroscino G, Cascino G, et al. Risk of unprovoked seizure after acute symptomatic seizure: effect of status epilepticus. *Ann Neurol* 1998;44:908–912.

68. D'Alessandro R, Tinuper P, Ferrara R, et al. CT scan prediction of late post-traumatic epilepsy. *J Neurol Neurosurg Psychiatry* 1982;45: 1153–1155.

69. Mittl RL, Grossman RI, Hiehle JF, et al. Prevalence of MR evidence of diffuse axonal injury in patients with mild head injury and normal head CT findings. *Am J Neuroradiol* 1994;15: 1583–1589.

70. Garnett MR, Cadoux-Hudson TA, Styles P. How useful is magnetic resonance imaging in predicting severity and outcome in traumatic brain injury? *Curr Opin Neurol* 2001;14:753–757.

71. Levin HS, Williams DH, Eisenberg HM, et al. Serial MRI and neurobehavioural findings after mild to moderate closed head injury. *J Neurol Neurosurg Psychiatry* 1992;55:255–262.

72. Kumar R, Gupta RK, Husain M, et al. Magnetization transfer MR imaging in patients with posttraumatic epilepsy. *Am J Neuroradiol* 2003;24:218–224.

73. Mazzini L, Cossa FM, Angelino E, et al. Posttraumatic epilepsy: neuroradiologic and neuropsychological assessment of long-term outcome. *Epilepsia* 2003;44:569–574.

74. Bricolo A. Electroencephalography in neurotraumatology. *Clin Electroencephalogr* 1976;7:184–197.

75. Gutling E, Gonser A, Imhof H-G, et al. EEG reactivity in the prognosis of severe head injury. *Neurology* 1995;45:915–918.

76. Facco E. Current topics. The role of EEG in brain injury. *Intensive Care Med* 1999;25:872–877.

77. Scheuer ML. Continuous EEG monitoring in the intensive care unit. *Epilepsia* 2002;43(Suppl 3):114–127.

78. Jennett B, van de Sande J. EEG prediction of post-traumatic epilepsy. *Epilepsia* 1975;16:251–256.

79. Reisner T, Zeiler K, Wessely P. The value of CT and EEG in cases of posttraumatic epilepsy. *J Neurol* 1979;221:93–100.

80. Courjon JA. Posttraumatic epilepsy in electroclinical practice. In: Walker AE, Caveness WF, Critchley M, eds. *The late effects of head injury*. Springfield, IL: Charles C Thomas, 1969:215–227.

81. Chang BS, Lowenstein DH. Practice parameter: antiepileptic drug prophylaxis in severe traumatic brain injury: report of the Quality Standards Subcommittee of the American Academy of Neurology. *Neurology* 2003;60:10–16.

82. Jabbari B, Vengrow MI, Salazar AM, et al. Clinical and radiological correlates of EEG in the late phase of head injury: a study of 515 Vietnam veterans. *Electroencephalogr Clin Neurophysiol* 1986; 64:285–293.

83. Armstrong KK, Sahgal V, Bloch R, et al. Rehabilitation outcomes in patients with posttraumatic epilepsy. *Arch Phys Med Rehabil* 1990;71:156–160.

84. Walker AE, Blumer D. The fate of World War II veterans with posttraumatic seizures. *Arch Neurol* 1989;46:23–26.

85. Barry E, Krumholz A, Bergey GK, et al. Nonepileptic posttraumatic seizures. *Epilepsia* 1998;39:427–431.

86. Marks DA, Kim J, Spencer DD, et al. Seizure localization and pathology following head injury in patients with uncontrolled epilepsy. *Neurology* 1995;45:2051–2057.

87. Diaz-Arrastia R, Agostini MA, Frol AB, et al. Neurophysiologic and neuroradiologic features of intractable epilepsy after traumatic brain injury in adults. *Arch Neurol* 2000;57:1611–1616.

88. Dikmen SS, Temkin NR, Miller B, et al. Neurobehavioral effects of phenytoin prophylaxis of posttraumatic seizures. *JAMA* 1991;265:1271–1277.

89. Rapport RL, Penry JK. A survey of attitudes toward the pharmacological prophylaxis of posttraumatic epilepsy. *J Neurosurg* 1973; 38:159–166.

90. Turner IM, Newman SM, Louis S, et al. Pharmacological prophylaxis against the development of kindled amygdaloid seizures. *Ann Neurol* 1977;2:221–224.

91. Wada JA, Sato M, Wake A, et al. Prophylactic effects of phenytoin, phenobarbital, and carbamazepine examined in kindling cat preparations. *Arch Neurol* 1976;33;426–434.

92. Rish BL, Caveness WF. Relation of prophylactic medication to the occurrence of early seizures following craniocerebral trauma. *J Neurosurg* 1973;38:155–158.

93. Servit Z, Musil F. Prophylactic treatment of posttraumatic epilepsy: results of a long-term follow-up in Czechoslovakia. *Epilepsia* 1981;22:315–320.

94. McQueen JK, Blackwood DHR, Harris P, et al. Low risk of late post-traumatic seizures following severe head injury: implications for clinical trials of prophylaxis. *J Neurol Neurosurg Psychiatry* 1983;46:899–904.

95. Young B, Rapp RP, Norton JA, et al. Failure of prophylactically administered phenytoin to prevent late posttraumatic seizures. *J Neurosurg* 1983;58.236–241.

96. Glotzner FL, Haubitz I, Miltner F, et al. Seizure prevention using carbamazepine following severe brain injuries [German]. *Neurochirurgia (Stuttg)* 1983;26:66–79.

97. Temkin NR, Dikmen SS, Anderson GD, et al. Valproate therapy for prevention of posttraumatic seizures: a randomized trial. *J Neurosurg* 1999;91:593–600.

98. Benardo LS. Prevention of epilepsy after head trauma: do we need new drugs or a new approach? *Epilepsia* 2003;44(Suppl 10):27–33.

99. Temkin NR. Antiepileptogenesis and seizure prevention trials with antiepileptic drugs: meta-analysis of controlled trials. *Epilepsia* 2001;42:515–524.

100. Schierhout G, Roberts I. Anti-epileptic drugs for preventing seizures following acute traumatic brain injury. *Cochrane Database Syst Rev* 2001;4:CD000173.

101. Haltiner AM, Newell DW, Temkin NR, et al. Side effects and mortality associated with use of phenytoin for early posttraumatic seizure prophylaxis. *J Neurosurg* 1999;91:588–592.

102. Young B, Rapp RP, Norton JA, et al. Failure of prophylactically administered phenytoin to prevent post-traumatic seizures in children. *Childs Brain* 1983;10:185–192.

103. Lewis RJ, Yee L, Inkelis SH, et al. Clinical predictors of post-traumatic seizures in children with head trauma. *Ann Emerg Med* 1993;22:1114–1118.

104. Tilford JM, Simpson PM, Yeh TS, et al. Variation in therapy and outcome for pediatric head trauma patients. *Crit Care Med* 2001; 29:1056–1061.

105. Adelson PD, Bratton SL, Carney NA, et al. Guidelines for the acute medical management of severe traumatic brain injury in infants, children, and adolescents. Chapter 19. The role of antiseizure prophylaxis following severe pediatric traumatic brain injury. *Pediatr Crit Care Med* 2003;4(3 Suppl):S72–S75.

106. Watson NF, Barber JK, Doherty MJ, et al. Does glucocorticoid administration prevent late seizures after head injury? *Epilepsia* 2004;45:690–694.

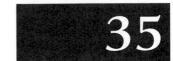

Epilepsy in the Setting of Cerebrovascular Disease

Bernd Pohlmann-Eden   *Martin Del Campo*   *Neil R. Friedman*

Deepak K. Lachhwani

Cerebrovascular disease (CVD) is a leading cause of neurologic morbidity across all age groups. Since the original description by Hughlings Jackson in 1864 of stroke associated with focal epilepsy, it has been known that seizures comprise a significant portion of the morbid manifestations in both the early and the late stages of affliction with ischemic or hemorrhagic stroke, either directly caused by the cortical insult or as a result of the underlying etiology leading up to stroke (e.g., malformations of cerebral vasculature). Whereas seizures may occur in up to 10% to 40% of patients with stroke (1–3), recurrent seizures (i.e., epilepsy) develop in 2% to 4% (4–7). These figures are based on small retrospective studies with heterogeneous patient groups and a variable follow-up, or prospective studies with limited follow-up of 1 to 2 years (5,6). Although only limited long-term follow-up data are available from prospective studies, it seems apparent that epilepsy is infrequent after cerebrovascular insult, and in most patients it is responsive to medical therapy. However, there is a subgroup of patients who present with congenital hemiparesis as a consequence of an antenatal or perinatal stroke. This subgroup has a higher risk of developing epilepsy (up to 60% of the patients) that may be medically refractory (in up to 10%) (8). This chapter discusses aspects of poststroke epilepsy in different age groups as well as the role of epilepsy surgery in patients with medically refractory disease.

ISSUES IN PEDIATRIC PATIENTS

Pediatric stroke has become an increasingly recognized entity over the past decade. Although still relatively uncommon, the reported incidence and prevalence of pediatric stroke have increased with better data collection, improved imaging modalities, and better recognition and awareness among physicians. The incidence of ischemic stroke in childhood, for example, has increased from 0.63 per 100,000 per year (9) to 3.3 per 100,000 per year (10). This may be an underestimate, with reported incidence in some cases as high as 13 per 100,000 per year (11). If one includes the incidence of hemorrhagic stroke, the overall incidence of pediatric stroke is likely to exceed 6 per 100,000 per year (12). Stroke remains one of the top 10 causes of death in children, with a mortality rate of approximately 10% (11). Outcome, in general, is better than that seen in adults, mostly because of brain plasticity and the absence of ubiquitous underlying degenerative vascular disease such as atherosclerosis. Morbidity, however, is now recognized as a serious complication of pediatric stroke, and a majority of survivors will have residual and persistent neurologic and/or cognitive impairment. Neurologic impairment includes residual hemiparesis in about 66% of children, visual field deficits, and/or epilepsy. The recurrence risk for stroke is variable and depends on the underlying etiology and has been estimated to be 20% to 40% (13,14). The etiologies of stroke in childhood are multitudinous, and vary considerably from those seen in adults, with approximately 20% to 30% of cases remaining unresolved.

Seizures are more commonly seen as a heralding symptom in childhood stroke than in adult stroke. In childhood stroke, as compared with neonatal stroke, motor deficits are more commonly the presenting neurologic symptom than are seizures. The reported incidence of poststroke seizures and subsequent epilepsy in children has been highly variable, based partly on population selection and small sample size. In the largest pediatric series to date (15), seizure incidence at presentation was 49% for arterial ischemic stroke and 64% for sinovenous thrombosis. Of these, 13% of the former and 23% of the latter had had seizure recurrence at follow-up. In another series (16), early seizures (within 2 weeks of presentation) were observed in 35% and 39% of ischemic and hemorrhagic stroke, respectively. A smaller study (17) found acute seizures to be the sole presenting feature of the stroke in 11% of their patients, with a further 11% presenting with hemiparesis accompanying the seizure at presentation. Nine (25%) of 35 children subsequently went on to develop epilepsy. In a series of 73 patients (18), acute seizures occurred in 49% of patients, with a further 7% presenting with early seizures (i.e., within 2 weeks of presentation). Eight percent of the cohort presented with late-onset seizures (more than 2 weeks after stroke presentation). Of those patients with seizures, two thirds had cortically based strokes. Epilepsy occurred in 28% of the patients: all with late-onset initial seizures and 50% with acute or early initial seizures. Subcortical (basal ganglia, thalamus) infarcts are also associated with seizures either as an isolated presenting feature or in combination with a hemiplegia (19). The semiology of the seizures is variable, and patients often have more than one seizure type, including focal motor, complex partial seizures, with or without secondary generalization, and, occasionally, primary generalized seizures. Status epilepticus has rarely been reported (20). The occurrence of seizure at the initial presentation of the stroke is associated with an unfavorable neurologic outcome (11,15,21).

Neonatal stroke differs from childhood stroke in a number of ways. It occurs in approximately 1 in 4000 term livebirths per year (22,23), and comprises 25% of all pediatric stroke. Two thirds of neonatal strokes have large-vessel infarcts (24), compared with childhood stroke in which more than 50% of strokes involve small-vessel territory. The anterior circulation is five times more commonly involved than the posterior circulation. The majority of neonatal strokes are ischemic (80%) rather than hemorrhagic (20%), and 60% to 65% involve the left middle cerebral artery territory (24–27). Multiple infarcts are seen in 15% to 20% of cases. Approximately 12% to 14% of all newborn seizures are associated with cerebral infarction, with 80% to 90% occurring within 24 to 48 hours of the infarct (22,25,27–30). Seizures are the most frequent presenting neurologic symptom. They may be obvious (generalized or focal tonic or clonic seizures) or subtle and nondescript (such as orofacial automatisms, episodes of decreased alertness).

In a large prospective series (31), 62 (69%) of 90 term infants who presented only with seizures (and without evidence of a more diffuse neonatal encephalopathy) showed magnetic resonance imaging (MRI) evidence of acute focal ischemia (35 of 62) or hemorrhagic brain injury (27 of 62). Only two of these children showed additional brain

MRI evidence of an antenatal injury. Of the 245 term infants presenting with a neonatal encephalopathy, with or without seizures, only 8 (3.3%) had evidence on brain MRI scan of a focal infarction.

Neonatal seizures have been reported in more than 70% of cases of sinovenous thrombosis (32). In the Canadian Pediatric Ischemic Stroke Registry, the risk of epilepsy was 20% following an infarct caused by sinovenous thrombosis versus 15% when the stroke was caused by arterial ischemia. Interestingly, another series (24) showed no seizure recurrence in a cohort of 24 acute newborn strokes.

The electroencephalogram in neonatal stroke is highly variable and frequently normal. Abnormalities include focal or generalized slowing; focal, multifocal, or bilateral spike or spike-and-wave discharges; low-voltage rhythms; and burst suppression. Periodic lateralized epileptiform discharges (PLEDs) have also been reported in neonatal stroke in the term infant (33). The presence of an abnormal background on the electroencephalogram (24) and seizures are predictors of disability at outcome (30).

The etiology of neonatal stroke remains unknown in many instances; however, there is a growing body of evidence implicating thrombophilic abnormalities as a contributing factor to focal cerebral ischemic lesions. These abnormalities are noted in 30% to 68% of infants in some series (27,31). Some of these include genetic prothrombotic risk factors, while others are transient or acquired (acute-phase reactants) as a result of hypoxia or sepsis. Other factors predisposing to stroke include sinovenous thrombosis, possible thromboembolus from the placenta through a patent foramen ovale, sepsis, and neonatal asphyxia.

ISSUES IN ADULT PATIENTS

CVD is the most frequent underlying etiology of both single seizures and epilepsy in the elderly. In studies looking at both first seizure and new-onset epilepsy, in which sophisticated neuroimaging or high-resolution MRI was available (34–37), the percentage of CVD patients was in the range of 25% to 39% (Fig. 35.1). It is very likely that discrete CVD lesions are often missed. Eighteen percent of patients older than 60 years of age with an unknown cause for new-onset seizures had previously undetected cerebral infarction (38). According to a recent evaluation of the large UK General Practice Research Database, 4709 patients older than age 60 years presenting with their focal seizures "of unknown etiology" were at significantly higher risk to develop stroke ($p < 0.0001$) than was a random control group of 4709 individuals without seizures (39). This suggests that a first seizure in an elderly patient may actually be the tip of an iceberg of a subtle and otherwise undetected CVD and emphasizes the need for a rigorous standardized diagnostic protocol.

The incidence of stroke-associated seizures might be highly underestimated, as they often present as altered

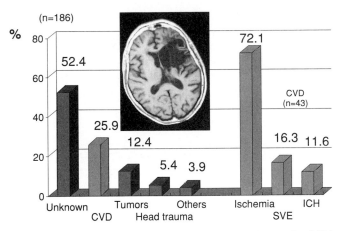

Figure 35.1 Morphologic patterns in a prospective study of 186 patients presenting with their first "unprovoked" seizure, with an example of a patient with a combined cortical-subcortical lesion. CVD, cerebrovascular disease; ICH, intracranial hemorrhage; SVE, subcortical vascular encephalopathy.

mental status, sudden slowing, episodes of confusion, and unexplained episodes of loss of consciousness or memory loss. This variation of presentation is linked to their often extratemporal origin involving frontal areas, which are frequently affected by stroke (37). Within the same study, the Veterans Affair Cooperative Study, a prospective, currently ongoing, randomized, double-blind treatment study in patients older than age 60 years (37), 38.3% of patients presented with complex partial seizures, 14.3% with simple partial, 7.5% with mixed partial, and 39.9% with generalized tonic-clonic seizures, a third of which had focal onset (12.8%). In general, the leading seizure type is focal, and nearly half show secondary generalization (40). Status epilepticus was observed in 31 (19%) of 159 individuals with poststroke seizures in a cohort of 3205 patients, 4 of them presenting during the acute phase of stroke (41). A stroke-associated seizure with subsequent Todd paresis mimicking recurrent stroke is considered to be the most frequent misdiagnosis in referrals to stroke units. Experimental and clinical evidence suggests that *poststroke* seizures induce additional harm to the infarcted area, leading to an irreversible functional deterioration (42). The reported incidence of poststroke seizures varies from 4.4% to 42.8%, and the incidence of poststroke epilepsy ranges from 2.7% to 17%; this variation is a consequence of the confusion of terms and highly variable study designs (40).

It is important to differentiate early seizures (within 14 days) and late seizures, as they seem to have a significantly different pathophysiologic background: acute metabolic disturbances including excessive glutamate release in early seizures versus development of complex epileptogenic scar formation in late seizures (43). In a recent, prospective, hospital-based, multicenter study of 1897 consecutive stroke patients (6), seizures occurred within a mean follow-up of 9 months in 10.6% of the hemorrhagic and 8.6% of the ischemic strokes; half of them manifested within 24 hours

from onset, which is confirmed by other studies. Early seizures presented in 90 of 1640 stroke patients in a large, prospective, community-based study (44); in 89%, the seizures were the initial presentation. In another population-based study (7), 6% of 535 patients followed after stroke developed seizures within the first week, 78% of which occurred within 24 hours. The cumulative probability of developing a late seizure was 7.4% by 5 years and 8.9% by 10 years. The 5-year actuarial risk of poststroke seizures was calculated to be 11.5% in the Oxfordshire Community Stroke Project (5), in which 675 patients were followed for up to 6.3 years; the relative risk of seizures in comparison with the general population was 35-fold in the first year and 19-fold in the second year. The risk of both early and late seizures was reported to be significantly lower in young adults with cryptogenic ischemic stroke (risk for early seizures occurring in less than 1 week in 2.4%; of which 71.0% occurred within 24 hours; risk at 5 years of 5.5%), obviously reflecting more subtle cerebrovascular lesions and lack of other risk factors found in the elderly (45).

Very few data are available about electroencephalograph-monitored functional brain disturbances in the acute setting of stroke. In a prospective series of 30 consecutive stroke patients (46), almost one-third presented with subclinical epileptiform activity such as PLEDs, spikes, or sharp waves, most within the very first hours after the stroke, and significantly more observed in combined cortical-subcortical lesions. This was reconfirmed in an extended series (47), in which 6 of 26 poststroke patients developed subclinical and clinical seizures and in which embolic stroke was found in single cases to induce simultaneous epileptogenic zones in topographically distant areas. PLEDs in particular may hold significant clues to the understanding of focal hyperexcitability after stroke, as stroke was found to be the underlying etiology in 30% to 50% of patients showing this electrographic pattern (48–51). The lack of systematic studies using both a standardized electroencephalography and MRI protocol prohibits further speculation on the predictive value of specific electroencephalographic (EEG) patterns for risk of seizures after stroke (43).

With regard to other predictors for seizures after stroke (40), there is increasing evidence for a higher risk in hemorrhagic conditions. The risk is highest in subarachnoid hemorrhage, followed by intracranial hemorrhage and hemorrhagic stroke as compared with ischemic stroke (6,43,52,53). This finding may refer to the observation that seizures, in particular early seizures, seem to occur more frequently in severe, large, and disabling strokes (54,55). The role of the precise topography and distribution of the cerebrovascular lesion for seizure recurrence is still part of an ongoing debate (43). While it has been repeatedly emphasized that cortical involvement is a strong predictor of seizure recurrence (6,52,53), more sophisticated studies using both computed tomography (CT) and high-resolution MRI favor a concept according to which a critically disturbed interaction (or lesion) of both cortical and subcortical regions leads to an increased risk of seizure recurrence. Support for this hypothesis was found both in a series of first-seizure patients (36) and in an MRI-proven study in subcortical vascular encephalopathy (56). Seizures were reported to occur more frequently if the infarct had an anterior hemispheric location (5,7), or if the parietal or temporal lobe (52) or the posterior area around the lateral sulcus was involved (57). Patients with a preserved cortical island sign (Fig. 35.1) in an extended stroke lesion are considered to represent a high-risk population for seizures (58). According to a CT-based study, late seizures themselves seem to carry a higher risk for poststroke epilepsy than do early seizures (34).

PHARMACOTHERAPY IN POSTSTROKE PATIENTS WITH SEIZURES

Any decision for treatment should weigh the actual risk for seizures in the individual patient against potential side effects such as somnolence, confusion, gait disturbances, memory decline, and long-term sequelae like osteoporosis and weight changes. There is no evidence to date that antiepileptic drugs (AEDs) have a prophylactic effect on seizure occurrence (59) or change the course of epilepsy after withdrawal (60). However, it would be intriguing to systematically study the use of AEDs in the early stage of stroke in patients considered at risk for seizure recurrence.

Acute treatment may be guided by the need for rapid therapeutic effect. Intravenous agents such as benzodiazepines, phenobarbital, or fosphenytoin may be implemented (in that order) in pediatric patients; in patients older than 2 years of age, intravenous valproate may also be included in the list of parenteral choices.

Long-term treatment after a single seizure should be an exception (high-risk patients, safety issues). As a principle, treatment should be started after the second proven seizure. New AEDs, such as oxcarbazepine, lamotrigine, levetiracetam, and topiramate, offer more favorable adverse-effect profiles over older agents. In particular, gabapentin, topiramate, lamotrigine, and levetiracetam should be the first-line therapeutics in the elderly and in patients suffering from stroke-associated seizures. Except that they are more expensive and dependent on renal excretion, they seem to provide a wide range of advantages compared with conventional AEDs with the same efficacy. Two double-blind prospective trials (37,61) proved the superiority of both lamotrigine and gabapentin as compared with carbamazepine, as both new AEDs had fewer side effects, were better tolerated (higher retention rate), and showed the same rate of seizure freedom. New AEDs that are non–liver-enzyme-inducing have significantly fewer interactions, which is crucial for the elderly patient who is taking, on average, six to seven different medications (37), often including warfarin. In addition, endogenous processes such as calcium (and testosterone) metabolism will not be affected, leading to a lower risk for osteoporosis and fracture. "Start low and go slow" is a rule of thumb for the recommended daily average dosages of lamotrigine, topiramate, gabapentin, and levetiracetam. Monotherapy is desired and often sufficient. Long-term prognosis is considered to be good, with seizure-free rates of more than 70%; however, convincing data are lacking.

EPILEPSY SURGERY IN POSTSTROKE PATIENTS WITH REFRACTORY SEIZURES

Fortunately, recurrent seizures occur in fewer than 5% of all patients who suffer a cerebrovascular insult beyond early childhood. Most of these patients have rare seizures and are successfully managed with medical therapy. Patients with congenital hemiparesis caused by antenatal or perinatal cerebrovascular insult comprise a subgroup with greater risk of developing epilepsy, and a significant number of them will progress to medically refractory epilepsy (8). As with other symptomatic etiologies, epilepsy surgery may play a vitally important role in patients with medically refractory seizures and warrants careful consideration after at least two appropriate medical agents have failed.

Most of the outcome data in older poststroke epilepsy patients undergoing resective surgery for control of seizures needs to be extracted from a larger group of symptomatic epilepsy patients in whom seizures were refractory and who needed epilepsy surgery. This is in keeping with the fact that poststroke medically refractory epilepsy patients do not form a large cohort presenting to any given epilepsy center. The guiding principles for presurgical planning in this group include ascertainment of convergent features of seizure semiology and EEG and imaging data, with subsequent surgical resection of the epileptogenic zone. However, because of limited systematic data available for surgery in older poststroke patients, this discussion focuses on the younger poststroke epilepsy patients in whom there is growing experience with epilepsy surgery.

Epilepsy surgery plays an important therapeutic role in selected children with refractory epilepsy and congenital hemiparesis caused by an antenatal or perinatal vascular insult. In a series of 50 patients with infantile hemiplegia who underwent cerebral hemispherectomy for epilepsy (62), seizures were completely or substantially relieved in 82% at a median follow-up of 13 years. A surgical series from our center included 41 patients with vascular hemiplegia of congenital origin (63). Of the 22 patients who underwent surgery and who had adequate follow-up (median, 2.8 years), 55% were seizure free and an additional 30% had significant reduction in seizures. In another pediatric epilepsy surgical series that included 135 patients (64), 37% of the patients had infarct/ischemia as their underlying etiology, and after 5 years of follow-up more than 60% were seizure free.

As a subgroup of poststroke epilepsy patients, these younger patients with antenatal/perinatal infarction share some unique clinical, electrophysiologic, and neuroimaging features. Awareness of these features may be of immense help in the surgical planning.

Clinical Features and Seizure Semiology

Clinically noticeable neurologic deficit may vary from a mild hemiparesis to a complete hemiplegia, with or without a homonymous visual field cut and is not always reflective of the extent of damage evident on MRI films. Twenty-eight percent of the patients in our series were noted to have only a mild hemiparesis although their MRIs showed extensive porencephalic lesions (63).

Seizure burden is significant, and most patients have daily seizures. Multiple seizure types are often encountered, with two-thirds of the patients having at least two seizure types (63). Focal motor seizures are commonly seen, and this is in keeping with an inherently low seizure threshold of a damaged motor cortex; however, exclusively focal or unilateral seizures are uncommon (6). Infantile spasms may be the only seizure type in some patients seen early in the course, and a significant proportion of older patients may carry a history of such a seizure type. Other seizure manifestations are consistent with the topography of the underlying damaged cortex.

Interictal and Ictal Epileptiform Abnormalities

Surface EEG findings typically show a combination of focal slowing, reduced background rhythms, and epileptiform abnormalities overlying the region of damaged cortex, as illustrated in Figure 35.2. However, a wide range of electrical findings, from near normal to diffuse bilateral abnormalities, may be seen (62). Younger patients tend to have more diffuse EEG abnormalities than do older patients. In some cases, the more impressive abnormalities are ipsilateral to the side of hemiplegia, that is, over the "preserved" hemisphere (62). An obvious reason for this finding may be the dysfunction of the structurally preserved hemisphere. However, rapid interhemispheric conduction reflected in the contralateral hemisphere, poor conduction of rhythms through a porencephalic cyst, and evolution of normal and abnormal EEG rhythms in a maturing brain are other factors that may have a bearing on the manifested EEG phenotype in a given patient. These should be considered during interpretation of video-electroencephalograph recordings. Careful attention to semiology and structural abnormality is crucial in hypothesizing the location of the epileptogenic zone in such cases. EEG recordings in our series (63) showed interictal sharp waves to be bilateral or generalized in more than 50% of the patients. Within the damaged hemisphere, EEG seizures were seen to arise from two independent regions in more than one-third of patients. In two patients, EEG seizures evolved unequivocally from the structurally preserved hemisphere, and these patients did not proceed to surgery.

Neuroimaging

MRI findings may be divided in two broad categories. In the first category, a large porencephalic cyst or areas of cystic encephalomalacia are seen (Fig. 35.3). Strokes involving the carotid artery territory are more frequently associated with seizures; hence, epilepsy surgery candidates are likely to show lesions with encephalomalacia in the distribution of the anterior and/or middle cerebral arteries (65). A smaller proportion of patients will have such findings in the posterior head regions. Unilateral periventricular

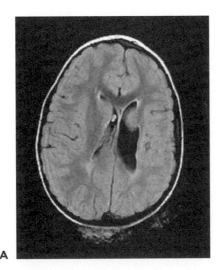
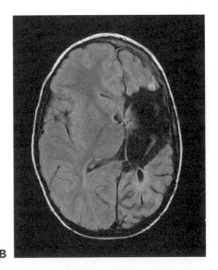

A **B**

Figure 35.2 A 5-year-old girl with refractory automotor seizures (with or without right-hand tonic stiffening) since 11 months of age. Axial magnetic resonance imaging (fluid-attenuated inversion recovery) image (**A**) showing left periventricular leukomalacia with volume loss of overlying cortex and (**B**) postoperative appearance after left functional hemispherectomy. Interictal epileptiform (**C**) and ictal electroencephalographic abnormalities (**D**) were localized to the left posterior quadrant. The child is seizure free 1 year after the surgery.

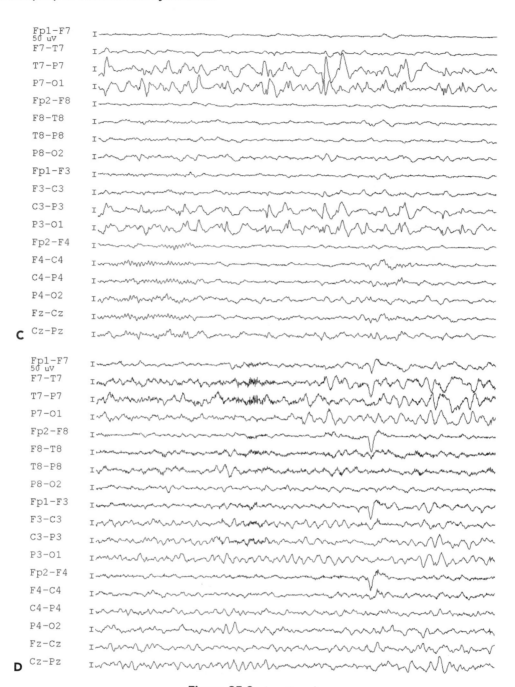

Figure 35.2 *(continued)*

leukomalacia with compensatory ventricular dilatation and somewhat preserved or mild to moderate diffuse atrophy of the overlying cortex may be seen in the second category of MRI findings. Four patients in our surgical series demonstrated such findings (Fig. 35.2). All had moderate to severe hemiparesis as a consequence of the more obvious subcortical damage.

Surgery

In patients with small-vessel stroke with focal encephalomalacia, identification of the epileptogenic zone based on concordant seizure semiology, surface ictal and interictal electroencephalography, and neuroimaging findings may enable a focal resection without further tests. If the epileptogenic zone and eloquent cortex are thought to be in close proximity, functional localization studies with subdural electrodes might be helpful in delineating the surgical roadmap for resection.

In patients with congenital hemiparesis and refractory seizures, the most common surgical procedure is functional hemispherectomy. More than 50% of patients in our (63) and in another (64) surgical series underwent this procedure. Candidates include patients with seizures arising from extensive or multiple areas of epileptogenicity within one hemisphere and preexisting motor deficit on the contralateral side. With no worsening of the preoperative neurologic functional status, this method offers seizure-free outcome in 70% to 80% of patients and is vastly better compared with callosotomy or partial hemispherectomy (62,66). In patients with intact visual fields prior to surgery, homonymous hemianopia is an inevitable but usually acceptable new postoperative deficit.

In patients with a more restricted structural lesion with concordant EEG data, surgical options may include a large resection sparing areas of eloquent cortex. Lobar or multilobar resection was carried out in 25% of our patients (63). Eighty percent of patients in our series (63) and 53% of patients in another series (64) were either seizure free or had auras only after undergoing a lobar or multilobar resection.

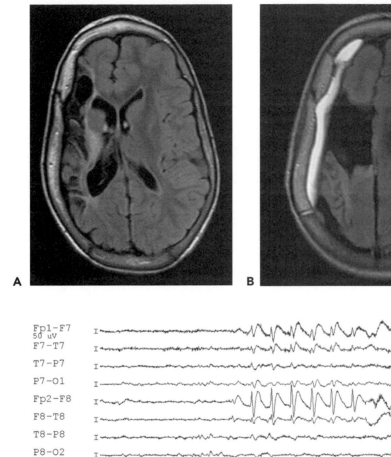

Figure 35.3 A 14-year-old boy with refractory axial tonic seizures since 2 months of age. Early in the course of epilepsy, he had some left-sided motor seizures. Axial magnetic resonance imaging (MRI) (fluid-attenuated inversion recovery) image (**A**) showing areas of encephalomalacia in the distribution of the right middle cerebral artery and (**B**) postoperative appearance. More than 75% of the interictal epileptiform discharges (**C**) were in the form of generalized slow spike-and-wave complexes, and ictal electroencephalography (**D**) was nonlocalizable. The decision to proceed with surgery was based on a unilateral MRI lesion, devastating epilepsy, and coexisting dense contralateral hemiparesis. This decision was arrived at only after careful deliberation at a patient management conference, bioethics consultation, and fully informed parental consent. The child is seizure free 6 months after the surgery.

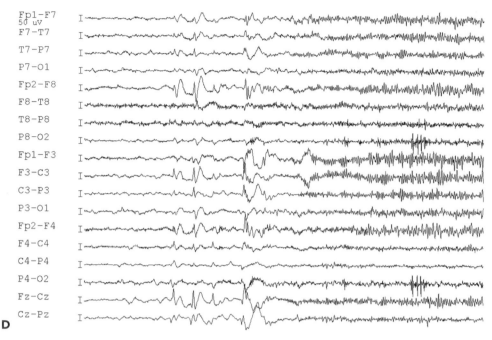

Fp1-F7
50 uv
F7-T7
T7-P7
P7-O1
Fp2-F8
F8-T8
T8-P8
P8-O2
Fp1-F3
F3-C3
C3-P3
P3-O1
Fp2-F4
F4-C4
C4-P4
P4-O2
Fz-Cz
Cz-Pz

D

Figure 35.3   (continued)

Poststroke epilepsy, especially in younger patients presenting with congenital hemiparesis, includes unique clinical, EEG, and imaging features. Seizure semiology consistent with a restricted cortical lesion and concordant localized epileptiform abnormalities lead to presurgical planning similar to that in other focal symptomatic refractory epilepsies. The case in Figure 35.3 illustrates this typical confluence of clinical, EEG, and MRI findings. However, generalized, multiregional, or bihemispheric EEG abnormalities may be seen in younger poststroke patients and may not necessarily portend a contraindication to surgical candidacy, as illustrated in Figure 35.2. Given the nature of medically refractory poststroke epilepsy and its potential for lifelong morbidity, careful consideration of all surgical options is warranted, even in complicated cases.

REFERENCES

1. Lancman ME, Golimstok A, Norscini J, et al. Risk factors for developing seizures after a stroke. *Epilepsia* 1993;34:141–143.
2. Dodge PR, Richardson EP Jr, Victor M. Epilepsy as sequel to cerebral vascular disease; a clinico-pathological study. *Trans Am Neurol Assoc* 1954;13:184–186.
3. Kilpatrick CJ, Davis SM, Tress BM, et al. Epileptic seizures in acute stroke. *Arch Neurol* 1990;47:157–160.
4. Camilo O, Goldstein LB. Seizures and epilepsy after ischemic stroke. *Stroke* 2004;35:1769–1775.
5. Burn J, Dennis M, Bamford J, et al. Epileptic seizures after a first stroke: the Oxfordshire Community Stroke Project. *BMJ* 1997;315:1582–1587.
6. Bladin CF, Alexandrov AV, Bellavance A, et al. Seizures after stroke: a prospective multicenter study. *Arch Neurol* 2000;57:1617–1622.
7. So EL, Annegers JF, Hauser WA, et al. Population-based study of seizure disorders after cerebral infarction. *Neurology* 1996;46:350–355.
8. Uvebrant P. Hemiplegic cerebral palsy. Aetiology and outcome. *Acta Paediatr Scand Suppl* 1988;345:1–100.
9. Schoenberg BS, Mellinger JF, Schoenberg DG. Cerebrovascular disease in infants and children: a study of incidence, clinical features, and survival. *Neurology* 1978;28:763–768.
10. deVeber G, the Canadian Pediatric Stroke Ischemic Stroke Study Group. Canadian Pediatric Ischemic Stroke Registry: analysis of children with arterial ischemic stroke [abstract]. *Ann Neurol* 2000;48:526.
11. Lynch JK, Hirtz DG, deVeber G, et al. Report of the National Institute of Neurological Disorders and Stroke Workshop on Perinatal and Childhood Stroke. *Pediatrics* 2002;109:116–123.
12. deVeber G, Roach S, Riela AR, et al. Stroke in children: recognition, treatment, and future directions. *Semin Pediatr Neurol* 2000;7:309–317.
13. Chabrier S, Husson B, Lasjaunias P, et al. Stroke in childhood: outcome and recurrence by mechanism in 59 patients. *J Child Neurol* 2000;15:290–294.
14. Lanthier S, Carmant L, David M, et al. Stroke in children. The coexistence of multiple risk factors predicts poor outcome. *Neurology* 2000;54:371–378.
15. deVeber GA, MacGregor D, Curtis R, et al. Neurologic outcome in survivors of childhood arterial ischemic stroke and sinovenous thrombosis. *J Child Neurol* 2000;15:316–324.
16. Giroud M, Lemesle M, Madinier G, et al. Stroke in children under 16 years of age. Clinical and etiological differences with adults. *Acta Neurol Scand* 1997;96:401–406.
17. De Schryver ELL, Kappelle LJ, Jennekens-Schinkel A, et al. Prognosis of ischemic stroke in childhood: a long-term follow-up study. *Dev Med Child Neurol* 2000;42:313–318.
18. Yang JS, Park YD, Hartlage PL. Seizures associated with stroke in childhood. *Pediatr Neurol* 1995;12:136–138.
19. Browner MC, Rollins N, Roach ES. Basal ganglia and thalamic infarction in children: causes and clinical features. *Arch Neurol* 1996;53:1252–1256.
20. Mancini J, Girard N, Chabrol B, et al. Ischemic cerebrovascular disease in children: retrospective study of 35 patients. *J Child Neurol* 1997;12:193–199.
21. Delsing BJ, Catsman-Berrevoets CE, Appel IM. Early prognostic indicators of outcome in ischemic childhood stroke. *Pediatr Neurol* 2001;24:283–289.
22. Estan J, Hope P. Unilateral neonatal cerebral infarction in full-term infants. *Arch Dis Child* 1997;76:F88–F93.

23. De Vries L, Groenendal F, Eken P, et al. Infarcts in the vascular distribution of the middle cerebral artery in preterm and full-term infants. *Neuropediatrics* 1997;28:88–96.
24. Mercuri E, Rutherford M, Cowan F, et al. Early prognostic indicators of outcome in infants with neonatal cerebral infarction: a clinical, electroencephalogram, and magnetic resonance imaging study. *Pediatrics* 1999;103:39–46.
25. Pearlman JM, Rollins NK, Evans D. Neonatal stroke: clinical characteristics and cerebral blood flow velocity measurements. *Pediatr Neurol* 1994;11:281–284.
26. Filipek PA, Krishnamorthy KS, Davis KR, et al. Focal cerebral infarction in the neonate: a distinct entity. *Pediatr Neurol* 1987;3: 141–147.
27. Günther G, Junker R, Sträter R, et al. Symptomatic ischemic stroke in full-term neonates: role of acquired and genetic prothrombotic risk factors. *Stroke* 2000;31:2437–2441.
28. Koelfen W, Freund M, Varnholt V. Neonatal stroke involving the middle cerebral artery in term infants: clinical presentation, EEG and imaging study and outcome. *Dev Med Child Neurol* 1995;37: 204–212.
29. Mercuri E, Cowan F, Rutherford M, et al. Ischemic and hemorrhagic brain lesions in newborns with seizures and normal Apgar scores. *Arch Dis Child* 1995;73:F67–F74.
30. Sreenan C, Bhargava R, Robertson CMT. Cerebral infarction in the newborn: clinical presentation and long-term outcome. *J Pediatr* 2000;137:351–355.
31. Cowans F, Rutherford M, Groenendall F, et al. Origin and timing of brain lesions in term infants with neonatal encephalopathy. *Lancet* 2003;361:736–742.
32. deVeber G, Andrew M, Adams C, et al. Cerebral venous thrombosis in children. *N Engl J Med* 2001;345:417–423.
33. Randò T, Ricci D, Mercuir E, et al. Periodic lateralized epileptiform discharges (PLEDs) as early indicator of stroke in full-term newborns. *Neuropediatrics* 2000;31:202–205.
34. Sung CY, Chu NS. Epileptic seizures in elderly people: aetiology and seizure type. *Age Ageing* 1990;19:25–30.
35. Sanders KM, Murray GB. Geriatric epilepsy: a review. *J Geriatr Psychiatr Neurol* 1991;4:98–105.
36. Pohlmann-Eden B, Schreiner A, Hornung T. Predictive value and morphological pattern of cerebrovascular disease lesions in patients presenting with a first "unprovoked" seizure. *Ann Neurol* 1998;44:468.
37. Ramsay RE, Rowan JA, Pryor FM. Special considerations in treating the elderly with epilepsy. *Neurology* 2004;62:S24–S29.
38. Roberts RC, Shorvon SD, Cox TCS, et al. Clinically unsuspected cerebral infarction revealed by computed tomography scanning in late onset epilepsy. *Epilepsia* 1988;29:190–194.
39. Cleary P, Shorvon S, Tallis R. Late-onset seizures as a predictor of subsequent stroke. *Lancet* 2004;363:1184–1186.
40. Pohlmann-Eden B, Hoch DB, Cochius JI, et al. Stroke and epilepsy: critical review of the literature. Part I: epidemiology and risk factors. *Cerebrovasc Dis* 1996;6:332–338.
41. Rumbach L, Sablot D, Berger E, et al. Status epilepticus in stroke. Report on a hospital-based stroke cohort. *Neurology* 2000;54: 350–354.
42. Bogousslavsky J, Martin R, Regli F, et al. Persistent worsening of stroke sequelae after delayed seizures. *Arch Neurol* 1992;49: 385–388.
43. Pohlmann-Eden B, Cochius JI, Hoch DB, et al. Stroke and epilepsy: critical review of the literature, part II: risk factors, pathophysiology and overlap syndromes. *Cerebrovasc Dis* 1997;7: 2–9.
44. Giroud M, Gras P, Fayolle H, et al. Early seizures after acute stroke: a study of 1640 cases. *Epilepsia* 1994;35:959–964.
45. Lamy C, Domingo V, Semah F, et al. Early and late seizures after cryptogenic ischaemic stroke in young adults. *Neurology* 2003;60: 400–404.
46. Pohlmann-Eden B, Mager RD, Hoch DB, et al. The significance of subclinical epileptiform activity after stroke. In: Stalberg E, Deweerd AW, Zidar J, eds. *9th European Congress of Clinical Neurophysiology*. Bologna, Italy: Monduzzi Editore, 1998:523–532.
47. Strittmatter E, Scheuler W, Behrens S, et al. The relevance of early long-term electroencephalography in acute ischemic stroke. *Klin Neurophysiol* 2002;33:34–41.
48. Chatrian GE, Shaw CM, Leffman H. The significance of periodic lateralized epileptiform discharges in EEG: an electrographic, clinical and pathological study. *Electroencephalogr Clin Neurophysiol* 1964;17:177–193.
49. Schwartz MS, Prior PF, Scott DF. The occurrence and evolution in the EEG of a lateralized periodic phenomenon. *Brain* 1973;96: 613–622.
50. Young GB, Goodenough P, Jacono V, et al. Periodic lateralized epileptiform discharges (PLEDs): electrographic and clinical features. *Am J EEG Technol* 1988;28:1–13.
51. Pohlmann-Eden B, Cochius J, Hoch DB, et al. Periodic lateralized epileptiform discharges—an overview. *J Clin Neurophysiol* 1996;13:519–530.
52. Arboix A, García-Eroles L, Massons JB, et al. Predictive factors of early seizures after acute cerebrovascular disease. *Stroke* 1997;28: 1590–1594.
53. Silverman IE, Restrepo L, Mathews GC. Poststroke seizures. *Arch Neurol* 2002;59:195–199.
54. Reith J, Jørgensen HS, Nakayama H, et al. Seizures in acute stroke: predictors and prognostic significance. The Copenhagen Stroke Study. *Stroke* 1997;28:1585–1589.
55. Lossius MI, Ronning OM, Mowinckel P, et al. Incidence and predictors for poststroke epilepsy. *Eur J Neurol* 2002;9:365–368.
56. Schreiner A, Pohlmann-Eden B, Schwartz A, et al. Epileptic seizures in subcortical vascular encephalopathy. *J Neurol Sci* 1995;130:171–173
57. Heuts-van Raak L, Lodder J, Kessels F. Late seizures following a first symptomatic brain infarct are related to large infarcts involving the posterior area around the lateral sulcus. *Seizure* 1996;5: 185–194.
58. Pohlmann-Eden B, Fatar M, Hennerici M. The preserved cortical island sign is highly predictive of postischemic seizures. *Cerebrovasc Dis* 2001;12:282.
59. Schierhout G, Roberts I. Anti-epileptic drugs for preventing seizures following acute traumatic brain injury. *Cochrane Rev* 2003;3.
60. Gilad R, Lampl Y, Eschel M, et al. Antiepileptic treatment in patients with early postischemic stroke seizures: a retrospective study. *Cerebrovasc Dis* 2001;12:39–43.
61. Brodie MJ, Owerstall PW, Giorgio L. Multicentre, double-blind, randomised comparison between lamotrigine and carbamazepine in elderly patients with newly diagnosed epilepsy. The UK Lamotrigine Elderly Study Group. *Epilepsy Res* 1999;37:81–87.
62. Wilson PJ. Cerebral hemispherectomy for infantile hemiplegia. A report of 50 cases. *Brain* 1970;93:147–180.
63. Carreno M, Kotagal P, Perez JA, et al. Intractable epilepsy in vascular congenital hemiparesis: clinical features and surgical options. *Neurology* 2002;59:129–131.
64. Mathern GW, Giza CC, Yudovin S, et al. Postoperative seizure control and antiepileptic drug use in pediatric epilepsy surgery patients: the UCLA experience, 1986–1997. *Epilepsia* 1999;40: 1740–1749.
65. Richardson EP Jr, Dodge PR. Epilepsy in cerebral vascular disease; a study of the incidence and nature of seizures in 104 consecutive autopsy-proven cases of cerebral infarction and hemorrhage. *Epilepsia* 1954;3:49–74.
66. Tinuper P, Andermann F, Villemure JG, et al. Functional hemispherectomy for treatment of epilepsy associated with hemiplegia: rationale, indications, results, and comparison with callosotomy. *Ann Neurol* 1988;24:27–34.

Epilepsy in the Setting of Neurocutaneous Syndromes

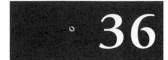

Prakash Kotagal   *Deepak K. Lachhwani*

The neurocutaneous syndromes are a group of unrelated disorders characterized by congenital dysplastic abnormalities involving the skin and nervous system. Epileptic seizures are encountered most frequently in tuberous sclerosis and the Sturge-Weber syndrome. Neurofibromatosis and other lesser-known entities, such as epidermal nevus syndrome, are also known to be accompanied by epilepsy.

TUBEROUS SCLEROSIS

Genetics

Tuberous sclerosis, also known as Bourneville disease, is a congenital hamartomatosis that affects multiple organ systems, especially the central nervous system (CNS). A genetic disorder with high penetrance and variability in expression, it is inherited as an autosomal dominant condition; the prevalence of the gene is estimated at 1 in 9700 persons (1). The gene locus in one-third of tuberous sclerosis families has been mapped to chromosome 9q34 (also known as *TSC1*, or tuberous sclerosis complex-1) (2); in other families, the gene locus is on 16p13 (*TSC2*) (3). Linkage studies initially indicated that there was a high incidence of apparently sporadic cases caused by new mutations; these appeared to account for 60% of all new cases (4–6). However, data using single-strand conformational polymorphism and heteroduplex analysis showed spontaneous mutations to account for only 22% of all cases (7). Hamartin, the product of the *TSC1* gene, appears to be localized to cytoplasmic vesicles. Tuberin, another protein encoded by the *TSC2* gene, functions as a guanosine triphosphatase (GTPase)-accelerating protein for the small-

molecular-weight GTPases Rap1a and Rab5. Tuberin has been colocalized to the perinuclear region of cultured cells and has been shown to colocalize with Rap1 in the stacks of the Golgi apparatus. A coiled-coil domain near the COOH terminus of hamartin was shown to bind specifically to a coiled-coil domain near the NH_2 terminus of tuberin, indicating that the two proteins work together in the same cellular pathway (8). It has been hypothesized that tumorigenesis in tuberous sclerosis could be the result of aberrant vesicular trafficking (9). Lack of tuberin has been shown to trigger inappropriate proliferation and differentiation in the neuroepithelium of the telencephalic vesicles during midgestation (10). Evidence suggests that *TSC* genes participate in multiple signaling cascades, one of which is binding to mTOR (mammalian target of rapamycin), an enzyme that is critical to normal cell growth and proliferation. Disruption a result of loss of *TSC1* and *TSC2* function activates the mTOR cascade, resulting in abnormal growth and proliferation. An understanding of this mechanism provides a unique opportunity to test rapamycin (a highly specific inhibitor and previously approved by the Food and Drug Administration as therapy for some renal neoplasms) as a potential therapeutic agent (11).

Tuberin has also been identified in cortical dysplasia tissue, suggesting that, in addition to its role as a growth suppressor, it may also contribute to cortical maturation and cellular differentiation (12,13).

Both parents of a child who has tuberous sclerosis should be examined for evidence of the disease by means of a complete physical examination, examination under a Wood lamp, dilated eye examination, magnetic resonance imaging (MRI) of the head, and renal ultrasonography. If the parents have no evidence of tuberous sclerosis, the recurrence risk for their next child is approximately 1:10,000 (the same as in the general population); if either parent has the disease, the risk for another affected child is 50%.

Clinical Features

The classic Vogt triad of seizures, mental retardation, and facial angiofibroma is seen in only 29% of patients with tuberous sclerosis (14,15). Gomez (14,15) found that 6% of tuberous sclerosis patients had none of the symptoms of the triad. One of the following major criteria must be present to establish a diagnosis of tuberous sclerosis: facial angiofibroma or periungual fibroma; cortical tuber, subependymal nodule, or giant cell astrocytoma; multiple retinal hamartomas; or multiple renal angiomyolipomas. The diagnosis can also be made if the patient has two of the following minor criteria: infantile spasms; hypomelanotic macules (ash leaf spots); single retinal hamartoma; subependymal or cortical calcification on a computed tomography (CT) scan; bilateral renal angiomyolipomas or cysts; cardiac rhabdomyoma; or history of tuberous sclerosis in a first-degree relative (14,15). More than 90% of patients have calcifications in the subependymal region of the lateral ventricle or cortical tubers. In Gomez's series of 300 tuberous sclerosis patients, skin lesions were seen in 96%, seizures in 84%, retinal hamartomas in 47%, and mental impairment in 45% (15).

Cortical and subcortical tubers are hamartias and constitute a hallmark of the disease. Cortical tuber count and distribution account for the phenotypic variability, with a higher tuber burden being associated with more severe clinical manifestations (16). Tubers also occur in the cerebellum in 15% of patients (17). Ventricular dilation is a common but nonspecific finding. Subependymal nodules are hamartomas, typically located in the lateral ventricles near the foramina of Monro. They are found in a majority of patients and are usually asymptomatic unless their growth results in blocking of the cerebrospinal fluid circulation. The development of brain tumors in these patients is uncommon; however, subependymal giant cell astrocytomas may occur in up to 8% of patients, typically near the foramen of Monro. They are believed to originate from a subependymal nodule (18). Patients may also have heterotopic masses of gray matter, consistent with the concept that tuberous sclerosis is a dysplastic process. Roach and colleagues (16) found that patients with five or more cortical lesions were more likely to have intractable seizures and developmental delay.

MRI has become the imaging tool of choice in the past two decades. Although CT scanning is more fruitful in demonstrating calcified lesions, MRI is superior in detecting these and other smaller lesions, which are likely to be missed on CT scans. In the myelinated brain, tubers appear as regions of low T1 and high T2 signal, and may show an enlargement of the corresponding gyri (Fig. 36.1). Fast fluid

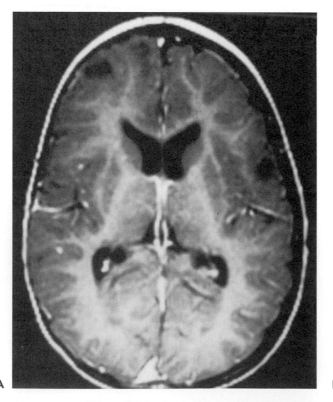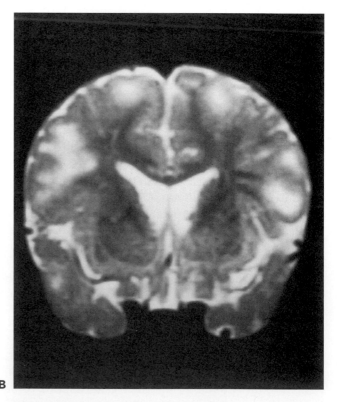

A   **B**

Figure 36.1   Magnetic resonance scan of a 6-year-old boy with tuberous sclerosis shows multiple cortical and subcortical tubers. These appear as hypointense areas on T1-weighted images (**A**) and as areas of increased signal on T2-weighted images (**B**). Also evident in **B** are subependymal nodules protruding into the lateral ventricles.

attenuated inversion recovery (FLAIR) sequences are more sensitive in picking up smaller lesions that appear as hyperintense areas (19). During early infancy, the appearance of tubers may vary, demonstrating a paradoxically increased T1 signal and a decreased T2 signal. The reason for this paradox is unclear and may be related to the immature white matter (20). The role of FLAIR sequences in the developing brain is yet to be determined. Subependymal nodules are better seen on T1-weighted sequences, whereas cortical tubers are better seen with T2-weighted sequences (21). On T1-weighted images, subependymal nodules are isointense to white matter and slightly hyperintense compared with gray matter; they are isointense or hypointense on T2-weighted images, which may show a central area of decreased signal. Tubers are further classified as sulcal islands (i.e., ring of hyperintensity surrounding an island of isointense cortex, seen on T2-weighted images) and gyral cores in which the white matter of a gyrus is hypointense, surrounded by isointense normal-appearing cortex on T1-weighted images (17). Sometimes multiple cortical tubers may give the appearance of pachygyria (22). Adjunctive imaging techniques such as magnetic resonance (MR) spectroscopy, diffusion-weighted imaging, position emission tomography (PET) scanning (with ligands such as fluoro-2-deoxyglucose, [^{11}C]-α-methyl-L-tryptophan, flumazenil, and [^{18}F]trans-4-fluoro-N-2 [4 (2-methoxyphenyl) piperazin-1-yl]ethyl]-N-(2-pyridyl) cyclohexanecarboxamide [FCWAY]), and single-photon-emission computed tomography (SPECT) scanning are newer tools used in evaluation of these patients (23,24). Their role is constantly evolving and will be clearer with additional data and improvement in techniques (25–27).

Epilepsy

The prevalence of epilepsy in patients with tuberous sclerosis has been reported in several series to be higher than 80% (14,15,28–32). These studies also found mental retardation in more than 60% of children, especially when seizures started before the age of 2 years. In a prospective study of families with tuberous sclerosis, however, Webb and coworkers (33) found a frequency of 62% for epilepsy and 38% for mental retardation. Seizures began before the age of 2 years in 71% of Westmoreland's cases (34). Infantile spasms are the most common type of seizure at presentation (36% to 69% of patients) (31,34–36), followed by focal motor (24%), grand mal (27%), and, less often, complex partial or atypical absence seizures (34). Tuberous sclerosis accounts for 25% of patients presenting with infantile spasms (37). In rare instances, patients with tuberous sclerosis may present with seizures during the neonatal period (38). Yamamoto and associates (36) found that 70% of children with tuberous sclerosis and seizures developed complex partial seizures after a follow-up period of 5 to 20 years. When seizures start after the age of 2 years, children usually have complex partial or secondarily generalized seizures (39). Roger and associates (40)

found that in patients with seizure onset after 12 months, partial seizures remained as the sole type, with one third of these children showing a favorable evolution.

The results of electroencephalography EEGare abnormal in most tuberous sclerosis patients. Westmoreland found that 88% of patients had abnormal recordings, most frequently epileptiform discharges (75%); slowing occurred in 13%. The epileptiform discharges were multifocal in 25% and focal in 23%; hypsarrhythmia occurred in 19% and generalized spike-wave discharges in 8%. Approximately 70% of focal spikes were in the temporal lobe (34). Background asymmetries have been reported in 40% of children with tuberous sclerosis, especially those with poorly controlled epilepsy (36). Cusmai and coworkers (41) reported that during follow-up, although some epileptic foci disappeared (usually occipital foci), others became evident, especially in the frontal regions (consistent with posteroanterior migration of epileptic foci in childhood [42]). Secondary bilateral synchrony appeared in 35% of children with tuberous sclerosis after the age of 2 years, especially during drowsiness and sleep (42,43). This agrees with our observations of children with multifocal spike discharges (44). Secondary bilateral synchrony was related to the presence of frontal lobe tubers. Cusmai and coworkers (41) also found that, although there was no correlation between the number of EEG foci and the number of cortical tubers, in 25 of 26 patients, there was an electroencephalographic (EEG) and MRI topographic correlation between at least one large tuber (larger than 10 mm in the axial plane and larger than 30 mm in the coronal plane) and one EEG focus. Similar results were reported by Tamaki and associates (45), who also found a higher incidence of hypsarrhythmia in patients with bilateral tubers.

Mental retardation occurs in 38% to 65% of children with tuberous sclerosis (14,15,33,40,46); approximately one third each being normal or borderline, mildly retarded, or profoundly retarded (46). They may also have dyspraxia, speech delay, visuospatial disturbance, dyscalculia, or memory problems. Marked hyperkinesia and aggressive behavior are also seen (46,47). Hunt found that the incidence of aggressive behavior was 13% and that these patients did not have a history of infantile spasms. Between 26% and 58% of children with tuberous sclerosis and infantile spasms have infantile autism (46,47), compared with 13% of patients with infantile spasms who do not have tuberous sclerosis (48). Both the number of tubers and their topography seem to play an important role in mental outcome. The persistence of epileptic foci in anterior and posterior areas is thought to be important in the development of autistic traits, such as severe disability in verbal and nonverbal communication, stereotypes, and complete indifference to social interaction (46). Patients with multiple cortical lesions are likely to have developmental delay and intractable seizures (16). The association between infantile autism and tuberous sclerosis therefore appears to be more than coincidental.

Medical management of the seizures depends on the seizure types encountered. The response of children with tuberous sclerosis and infantile spasms to corticotropin is similar to the response of children with cryptogenic infantile spasms; however, those with tuberous sclerosis have a higher relapse rate (48). Riikonen and Simell (48) suggested that these children may benefit from an extended course of corticotropin. Other generalized seizures (i.e., myoclonic, absence, and tonic-clonic) are treated with benzodiazepines (i.e., clonazepam, nitrazepam, or clorazepate) alone or in combination with valproic acid; intractable seizures may be managed with corticotropin or a ketogenic diet (1). Complex partial and focal motor seizures respond best to carbamazepine, phenytoin, or primidone. Vigabatrin is thought to be particularly effective for partial-onset and generalized seizures (i.e., infantile spasms and tonic seizures of the Lennox-Gastaut syndrome) in patients who have tuberous sclerosis (49–52). However, its ocular toxicity makes it unsuitable for long-term use.

Medical intractability is seen in approximately 50% of patients with tuberous sclerosis and partial epilepsy (36). Previously, such patients were thought to be poor candidates for epilepsy surgery owing to the presence of multifocal MRI and/or EEG abnormalities. However, this view is changing as a result of accumulating data in the past decade. In our experience, 8 of 9 patients with concordant surface EEG and MRI abnormalities were seizure free, whereas patients with less-well-localized MRI and/or EEG findings did not fare as well (3 of 8 patients were seizure free) (53). These results are similar to published reports of experience with epilepsy surgery in patients with tuberous sclerosis (54–58). Concordance in EEG and imaging abnormalities can identify potentially good surgical candidates, and seizure-free outcome in this group compares favorably with other lesional epilepsy surgery outcomes. The role of adjunctive tests (newer MRI techniques, PET, SPECT) needs to be studied further in patients with less-well-localized MRI and EEG findings. A multistaged approach involving successive removals of epileptogenic tubers has been proposed as a novel surgical strategy, further expanding the repertoire of surgical options (58).

STURGE-WEBER SYNDROME

Also known as the Sturge-Weber-Dimitri syndrome, this condition was first described in 1879 by Sturge, who thought that the neurologic features of the syndrome resulted from a nevoid condition of the brain similar to that affecting the face. Volland in 1912 and Weber in 1922 described the intracranial calcifications, and Dimitri was the first to report a case with calcifications seen on skull roentgenogram (59). The main findings are a congenital, often unilateral, nevus of the face; gyriform intracranial calcifications; and a high occurrence of epilepsy, mental retardation, hemiparesis, and glaucoma. Alexander (59)

classified Sturge-Weber variants on the basis of neurologic, ocular, and cutaneous features. Cairns and Davidson (60) reported the first Sturge-Weber patient treated by hemispherectomy. Sturge-Weber syndrome occurs sporadically, without a clear-cut inheritance pattern, although familial cases have been reported (61). It is relatively uncommon, but no precise figures regarding its incidence are known.

Clinical Features and Neuroimaging

The hallmark of Sturge-Weber syndrome is a congenital, unilateral cutaneous hemangioma (i.e., port-wine stain or nevus flammeus) affecting the upper face. In one series of 74 patients, 72% had unilateral nevi, and 28% had bilateral nevi. Nevi were found on the extremities and trunk in an unexpectedly high proportion of patients (44.6%) (62). The facial nevus is absent in approximately 5% of patients (63–65). The nevus is usually restricted to the distribution of one of the trigeminal nerve divisions; involvement of the supraorbital area is invariably accompanied by CNS meningeal involvement (59,62,66). Glaucoma, congenital (buphthalmos) or developing by the age of 2 years, was seen in 47.3% of patients.

Neurologic involvement in Sturge-Weber syndrome results from the effects of chronic ischemia of the cortex, which is produced by "vascular steal" caused by the overlying leptomeningeal venous angioma (67). Cortical atrophy and intracortical calcifications result, these may be seen histologically (68) or on skull roentgenograms—the classic tram-track appearance—as well as on CT scans. Calcifications appear on the skull roentgenogram usually between 2 and 7 years of age; they are detected earlier and found to be more extensive on CT scans. The leptomeningeal angiomatoses are more easily identified after injection of contrast during CT or MR scanning (Fig. 36.2). Angiography is abnormal in 82% of patients, showing enlargement of deep cerebral or collateral veins, decreased or absent cortical veins, or early filling of large veins (62). Although the meningeal angiomatosis is usually unilateral, bilateral involvement may occur in 15% to 26% of individuals (69–71). The meningeal angiomatosis usually is ipsilateral to the facial nevus but rarely may be contralateral to it (72). In the Klippel-Trénaunay variant of this syndrome, the nevus flammeus involves the extremities, with resulting hypertrophy of the underlying soft tissues and bone (73). Focal perfusion defects are identified on SPECT studies, and the PET scan reveals areas of hypometabolism corresponding to the location of the lesions (71). Concentrations of N-acetylaspartate are also reduced in the affected region on MR spectroscopy (74).

Progressive damage to the affected hemisphere results in hemiparesis in 30% (75) and mental retardation in 50% to 60% of patients with Sturge-Weber syndrome (69,76). As a general rule, children with Sturge-Weber syndrome do not exhibit mental retardation in the absence of

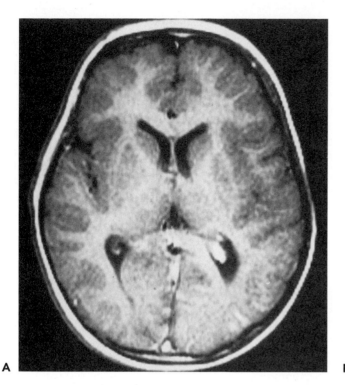
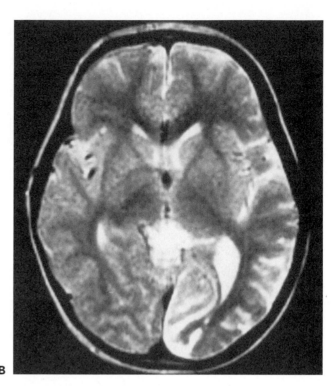

A   B

Figure 36.2 Magnetic resonance scans of a 4-year-old boy with Sturge-Weber syndrome. The unenhanced T1-weighted image (**A**) is significant only for an enlarged subarachnoid space in the left posterior quadrant. The enhanced images (**B**), however, reveal the leptomeningeal angiomatoses overlying the occipital, parietal, and posterior temporal regions, as well as a mild degree of cortical atrophy.

seizures. Hemiparesis and hemisensory loss increase in frequency with age. Hemianopsia is often present by the time hemiparesis is manifested. CT, MRI, and PET scans have documented progression of the disease. Patients who received prophylactic aspirin were found to have 65% fewer strokes than those who did not (77).

Epilepsy

Besides the facial nevus, seizures are the most common presenting feature and are seen in 71% to 89% of children (62,69,75). The seizures usually begin before the age of 2 years, most often in the first year of life, especially if angiomatosis is hemispheric, and usually before the onset of hemiparesis (62). A child with bihemispheric involvement is more likely to manifest seizures (69). The seizures are usually partial motor, affecting the contralateral limbs, or secondarily generalized; a small proportion of patients have primarily generalized tonic-clonic seizures. Temporary remission of seizures is seen in some patients, after which the seizures may return with increasing frequency. Surprisingly, few patients have a visual aura (59). The seizure type usually dictates the medical management of seizures in this syndrome. It is also important to assess and monitor vision in children with Sturge-Weber syndrome to identify and prevent the complications related to increased intraocular pressure.

Rochkind and colleagues (62) found that 96% of their patients with Sturge-Weber syndrome had abnormal elec-troencephalograms, showing attenuation of background activity on one or both sides (74%); 4% had epileptiform spikes only without background abnormalities; and 22% had epileptiform spikes in addition to background abnormalities. Epileptiform spikes were contralateral to the side of background attenuation in 8%. A small number of patients also manifest bilateral or generalized spike discharges.

Peterman and associates (75) followed 25 patients with Sturge-Weber syndrome for more than 5 years and reported spontaneous remission or controlled epilepsy in nearly half. In the Toronto series (62), 17 (32%) of 53 patients with epilepsy experienced intractable seizures and underwent surgery: 14 had a hemispherectomy and 3 had a lobectomy. Almost 65% were seizure free postoperatively, 23% had occasional seizures, and 12% had reduction of seizures. After hemispherectomy, motor function improved or was unchanged, with only 4 (23.5%) of 17 patients showing worsening of motor function (this was not a significantly worse outcome than that of the medically treated patients). Fifty-nine percent of operated patients showed intelligent quotients above 75, compared with 33% of conservatively managed patients ($p < 0.05$). The prognosis for intellectual outcome is better in patients who underwent surgery earlier (preferably before the age of 3 years) compared with those who were operated on later (78–81). In patients with bihemispheric disease and intractable generalized seizures, corpus callosotomy should be considered. However, very few patients with Sturge-Weber syndrome have undergone this procedure (82,83).

EPIDERMAL NEVUS SYNDROME

Epidermal nevi are congenital skin lesions that consist of slightly raised, ovoid, or linear plaques. In infancy, they are usually skin-colored and velvety; with age, they become more verrucous and orange or darker brown (84). Several different types have been described under the generic term *epidermal nevi*, including linear nevus sebaceous of Jadassohn, nevus verrucosus, and ichthyosis hystrix. Some investigators prefer to group them together (85,86), whereas others maintain that these are separate entities on the basis of histologic differences (87). Epidermal nevi do not involve the dermis, although such involvement is seen in the linear sebaceous nevus syndrome. The potential for malignant transformation exists after puberty. This chapter uses the generic term *epidermal nevus syndrome*, but recognizes that it can include different entities.

Insults to the developing brain during the period of neuronal migration are believed to be responsible for the associated CNS abnormalities, as are the skin lesions on the scalp and head, reflecting the close relationship between the skin structures and the developing brain (88). The skin lesions may be linear (often over the midline of the face), band-like, round, or oval (Fig. 36.3). Microscopic examination shows thickening and hyperkeratosis of the epidermis with hyperplasia of the sebaceous glands (89). Ocular and skeletal abnormalities, as well as malignancies, have been reported (86).

Solomon and Esterly (86) reported moderate to severe CNS involvement in 50% of their 60 patients. This included mental retardation; seizures; cortical atrophy; hyperkinesis; hydrocephalus; porencephaly; nonfunctioning cerebral venous sinuses (86,90); hemimacrocephaly; hemimegalencephaly (84); infantile spasms (89,91) with hypsarrhythmia or hemihypsarrhythmia (on the same side as the skin lesion); and other seizure types such as myoclonic, complex partial, partial motor, and generalized seizures. Seizure onset, especially in the linear sebaceous syndrome, is usually in the first year of life (87). Gurecki and colleagues (92) reported four new cases and reviewed the available literature through 1996. The nevi usually involved the head, although the head is spared in some patients. Ocular involvement occurs in approximately 25% of cases and includes microphthalmia, proptosis, choristomas (including dermoids and epidermoids), cataracts, and colobomas (93). A variant of the epidermal nevus syndrome with hemimegalencephaly, gyral malformation, mental retardation, facial hemihypertrophy, and seizures has been described (84). Seizures occurred in 16 of 17 patients, and infantile spasms with hypsarrhythmia or hemihypsarrhythmia were seen in 9 patients. Hemiparesis developed in 7 patients (84). Mutation of a somatic gene has been postulated. Histopathologic examination of the brain resected in epilepsy surgery cases has shown a spectrum of abnormalities, including diffuse cortical dysplasia, gyral fusion, pial glioneuronal hamartomas, cortical astrocytosis, and foci of microcalcification (94).

OTHER NEUROCUTANEOUS SYNDROMES

In neurofibromatosis type I, seizures occur in 3% to 5% of individuals, a rate that is slightly higher than in the general population (95). Korf and associates (96) found that 21 (5.4%) of 359 children with neurofibromatosis had seizures. Friedman and colleagues (97) found a higher incidence (9.4%) in a series of hospitalized patients. A variety of seizure types, including infantile spasms, absence, generalized convulsions, and complex partial seizures, have been reported. Complex partial seizures appear to be the most common type, especially in the absence of obvious structural lesions (96,97).

Incontinentia pigmenti, which occurs almost exclusively in females, presents in the neonatal period with erythematous bullous lesions that become crusted and pigmented. Children with this disorder may develop seizures (13.3%), mental retardation (12.3%), or spasticity (11.4%)

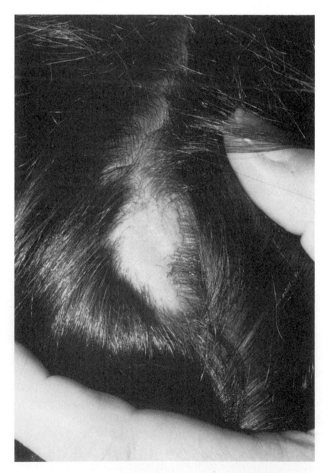

Figure 36.3 Scalp lesion in a 3-year-old girl with linear sebaceous nevus syndrome. The plaque was smooth, erythematous, and hairless; it was detected only on parting the hair and carefully searching for it.

(98). In neurocutaneous melanosis, multiple nevi are present from birth and may be hairy and pigmented (i.e., swimming-trunk nevus); meningeal melanosis and hydrocephalus are also seen. These children may have generalized or partial seizures (99). Seizures and mental retardation are also seen in approximately two-thirds of children with hypomelanosis of Ito, in which irregular, hypopigmented skin lesions with white or gray hair are seen. Seizures are more severe in early onset cases and consist of infantile spasms or myoclonic seizures. Choroidal atrophy, corneal opacities, deafness, dental anomalies, hemihypertrophy, hypotonia, and macrocephaly may also be seen (100,101). CT scans have shown cerebral atrophy, porencephaly, and low-density areas in the white matter. Autopsy showed gray matter heterotopias and abnormal cortical lamination in a patient in one series (102), indicative of abnormalities in neuronal migration. Urbach-Wiethe disease, which is recessively transmitted, manifests as yellow papules in polymorphic forms, retinal pigmentation, macular exudates, tortuous renal vessels, and malformation of the optic nerve head. Calcification of the hippocampal gyrus is associated with epilepsy in 15% to 40% of cases (103).

RELATIONSHIP OF NEUROCUTANEOUS SYNDROMES TO THE CORTICAL DYSPLASIAS

In the developing human brain between 8 and 24 weeks of gestation (104–106), neurons migrate from the ependymal surface of the ventricles to the surface of the cortex. The layers of the neocortex are formed from the inside out, so that waves of later migration pass through already formed layers (107). Neurons that do not migrate normally are at risk of stunting or early death. The neurocutaneous syndromes highlight the close association of the skin and CNS in the fetus. In Sturge-Weber syndrome, for example, the ectoderm that will form the upper face is closely apposed to the portion of the neural tube that will form the occipital lobe and adjoining cerebrum (59). Angiomatous malformation occurs between 4 and 8 weeks of gestation. Subsequent growth of the cerebral hemispheres and morphogenetic movements separate the abnormally developed vascular system of the pia mater and facial skin (68). Another theory proposes a morphogenetic link between the three cutaneous sensitive areas of the trigeminal nerve and the location of the facial staining (66). Vascular dysplasias also have been suggested as a cause of the epidermal nevus syndrome (108).

In forme fruste of tuberous sclerosis, isolated cortical tubers have been found on CT or MR scans, appearing as areas of thickened cortex or having altered signal characteristics (109,110). These patients appear to have no other stigmata of tuberous sclerosis (109,111,112). Taylor and associates (112) reported that, compared with patients with typical tuberous sclerosis, patients with the forme fruste variety had later onset of seizures (between 7 and 31 years of age), lacked a family history of the disorder, and had higher intelligence. Histologically, architectonic abnormalities of the cerebral cortex, sometimes protruding into the white matter, are seen, with disruption of normal cortical myelination and subpial clusters of giant astrocytes. Guerreiro and colleagues (55) recommended that the concept of forme fruste of tuberous sclerosis be abandoned, because these patients appear to have focal cortical dysplasia and not tuberous sclerosis. Patients with such lesions should be carefully screened to make sure they do not have any other evidence pointing to tuberous sclerosis.

REFERENCES

1. Gomez MR. *Tuberous sclerosis*, 2nd ed. New York: Raven Press, 1988.
2. Fryer A, Chalmers A, Connor JM, et al. Evidence that the gene for tuberous sclerosis is on chromosome 9. *Lancet* 1987;1:659–661.
3. Kandt RS, Haines JL, Smith M, et al. Linkage of an important gene locus for tuberous sclerosis to a chromosome 16 marker for polycystic kidney disease. *Nat Genet* 1992;2:37–41.
4. Cassidy SB. Tuberous sclerosis in children: diagnosis and course. *Comp Ther* 1984;10:43–51.
5. Fleury P, deGroot WP, Delleman JW, et al. Tuberous sclerosis: the incidence of sporadic cases versus familial cases. *Brain Dev* 1980; 2:107–117.
6. Sampson JR, Scahill SJ, Stephenson JB, et al. Genetic aspects of tuberous sclerosis in the west of Scotland. *J Med Genet* 1989;26: 28–31.
7. Ali JBM, Sepp T, Ward S, et al. Mutations in the *TSC1* gene account for a minority of patients with tuberous sclerosis. *J Med Genet* 1998;35:969–972.
8. van Slegtenhorst M, Nellist M, Nagelkerken B, et al. Interaction between hamartin and tuberin, the *TSC1* and *TSC2* gene products. *Hum Mol Genet* 1998;7:1053–1057.
9. Plank TL, Yeung RS, Henske EP. Hamartin, the product of the tuberous sclerosis 1 (*TSC1*) gene, interacts with tuberin and appears to be localized to cytoplasmic vesicles. *Cancer Res* 1998; 58:4766–4770.
10. Rennebeck G, Kleymenova EV, Anderson R, et al. Loss of function of the tuberous sclerosis 2 tumor suppressor gene results in embryonic lethality characterized by disrupted neuroepithelial growth and development. *Proc Natl Acad Sci U S A* 1998;95: 15629–15634.
11. Yeung RS. Multiple roles of the tuberous sclerosis complex genes. *Genes Chromosomes Cancer* 2003;38:368–375.
12. Johnson MW, Emelin JK, Park S-H, et al. Co-localization of TSC1 and TSC2 gene products in tubers of patients with tuberous sclerosis. *Brain Pathol* 1999;9:45–54.
13. Vinters HV, Kerfoot C, Catania M, et al. Tuberous sclerosis-related gene expression in normal and dysplastic brain. *Epilepsy Res* 1998;32:12–23.
14. Gomez MR. Criteria for diagnosis. In: Gomez MR, ed. *Tuberous sclerosis*. New York: Raven Press, 1979:9–20.
15. Gomez MR. Neurologic and psychiatric features. In: Gomez MR, ed. *Tuberous sclerosis*. New York: Raven Press, 1979:21–36.
16. Roach ES, Williams DP, Laster DW. Magnetic resonance imaging in tuberous sclerosis. *Arch Neurol* 1987;44:301–303.
17. Houser OW, Nixon JR. Central nervous system imaging. In: Gomez MR, ed. *Tuberous sclerosis*, 2nd ed. New York: Raven Press, 1988:51–62.
18. Houser OW, McLeod RA. Roentgenographic experience at the Mayo Clinic. In: Gomez MR, ed. *Tuberous sclerosis*. New York: Raven Press, 1979:27–53.
19. Takanashi J, Sugita K, Fujii K, et al. MR evaluation of tuberous sclerosis: increased sensitivity with fluid-attenuated inversion recovery and relation to severity of seizures and mental retardation. *AJNR Am J Neuroradiol* 1995;16:1923–1928.

20. Baron Y, Barkovich AJ. MR imaging of tuberous sclerosis in neonates and young infants. *AJNR Am J Neuroradiol* 1999;20: 907–916.

21. McMurdo SK Jr, Moore SH, Brant-Zawadzki M, et al. MR imaging of intracranial tuberous sclerosis. *AJR Am J Roentgenol* 1987;148: 791–796.

22. Martin N, de Broucker T, Cambier J, et al. MRI evaluation of tuberous sclerosis. *Neuroradiology* 1987;29:437–443.

23. Asano E, Chugani DC, Muzik O, et al. Multimodality imaging for improved detection of epileptogenic foci in tuberous sclerosis complex. *Neurology* 2000;54:1976–1984.

24. Jansen FE, Braun KP, van Nieuwenhuizen O, et al. Diffusion-weighted magnetic resonance imaging and identification of the epileptogenic tuber in patients with tuberous sclerosis. *Arch Neurol* 2003;60:1580–1584.

25. Fujita M, Hashikawa K, Nagai T, et al. Decrease of the central type benzodiazepine receptor in cortical tubers in a patient with tuberous sclerosis. *Clin Nucl Med* 1997;22:130–131.

26. Juhász C, Chugani DC, Muzik O, et al. Alpha-methyl-L-tryptophan PET detects epileptogenic cortex in children with intractable epilepsy. *Neurology* 2003;60:960–968.

27. Koh S, Jayakar P, Resnick T, et al. The localizing value of ictal SPECT in children with tuberous sclerosis complex and refractory partial epilepsy. *Epileptic Disord* 1999;1:41–46.

28. Bundey S, Evans K. Tuberous sclerosis: a genetic study. *J Neurol Neurosurg Psychiatry* 1969;32:591–603.

29. Donegani G, Grattarola FR, Wildi E. Tuberous sclerosis. In: Vinken PJ, Bruyn GW, eds. *The phakomatoses.* New York: Elsevier Science, 1972:340–389.

30. Nevin NC, Pearce WG. Diagnostic and genetical aspects of tuberous sclerosis. *J Med Genet* 1968;5:273–280.

31. Pampiglione G, Moynahan EJ. The tuberous sclerosis syndrome: clinical and EEG studies in 100 children. *J Neurol Neurosurg Psychiatry* 1976;39:666–673.

32. Umapathy D, Johnston AW. Tuberous sclerosis: prevalence in the Grampian region of Scotland. *J Ment Defic Res* 1989;33:349–355.

33. Webb DW, Fryer AE, Osborne JP. On the incidence of fits and mental retardation in tuberous sclerosis. *J Med Genet* 1991;28:395–397.

34. Westmoreland BF. Electroencephalographic experience at the Mayo Clinic. In: Gomez MR, ed. *Tuberous sclerosis.* New York: Raven Press, 1988:37–50.

35. Hunt A. Tuberous sclerosis: a survey of 97 cases. *Dev Med Child Neurol* 1983;25:346–357.

36. Yamamoto N, Watanabe K, Negoro T, et al. Long-term prognosis of tuberous sclerosis with epilepsy in children. *Brain Dev* 1987;9: 292–295.

37. Pampiglione G, Pugh E. Infantile spasms and subsequent appearance of tuberous sclerosis. *Lancet* 1975;2:1046.

38. Miller SP, Tasch T, Sylvain M, et al. Tuberous sclerosis complex and neonatal seizures. *J Child Neurol* 1998;13:619–623.

39. Curatolo P. Epilepsy in tuberous sclerosis. In: Ohtahara S, Roger J, eds. *New trends in pediatric epileptology.* Osaka, Japan: Dainippon Pharmaceutical, 1991:86–93.

40. Roger J, Dravet C, Boniver A, et al. L'epilepsie dans la sclerose tubereuse de Bourneville. *Boll Lega Ital Epil* 1984;45:33–38.

41. Cusmai R, Chiron C, Curatolo P, et al. Topographic comparative study of magnetic resonance imaging and electroencephalography in 34 children with tuberous sclerosis. *Epilepsia* 1990;31:747–755.

42. Gibbs EL, Gillen HW, Gibbs FA. Disappearance and migration of epileptic foci in childhood. *AMA Am J Dis Child* 1954;88:596–603.

43. Ganji S, Hellmann CD. Tuberous sclerosis: long-term follow-up and longitudinal electroencephalographic study. *Clin Electroencephalogr* 1985;16:219–224.

44. Kotagal P. Multifocal independent spike syndrome: relationship to hypsarrhythmia and the slow spike-wave (Lennox-Gastaut) syndrome. *Clin Electroencephalogr* 1995;26:23–29.

45. Tamaki K, Okuno T, Ito M, et al. Magnetic resonance imaging in relation to EEG epileptic foci in tuberous sclerosis. *Brain Dev* 1990;12:316–320.

46. Jambaqué I, Cusmai R, Curatolo P, et al. Neuropsychological aspects of tuberous sclerosis in relation to epilepsy and MRI findings. *Dev Med Child Neurol* 1991;33:698–705.

47. Hunt A, Dennis J. Psychiatric disorder among children with tuberous sclerosis. *Dev Med Child Neurol* 1987;29:190–198.

48. Riikonen R, Simell O. Tuberous sclerosis and infantile spasms. *Dev Med Child Neurol* 1990;32:203–209.

49. Chiron C, Dulac O, Beaumont D, et al. Therapeutic trial of vigabatrin in refractory infantile spasms. *J Child Neurol* 1991;6 (Suppl 2):S52–S59.

50. Curatolo P. Vigabatrin for refractory partial seizures in children with tuberous sclerosis. *Neuropediatrics* 1994;25:55.

51. Curatolo P, Chiron C, Jambaqué I, et al. Electroclinical, neuroradiological and prognostic features in childhood tuberous sclerosis. *Ann Neurol* 1994;36:519–520.

52. Dulac O, Chiron C, Luna D, et al. Vigabatrin in childhood epilepsy. *J Child Neurol* 1991;6(Suppl 2):S30–S37.

53. Lachhwani D, Pestana E, Kotagal P, et al. Epilepsy surgery in patients with tuberous sclerosis. *Epilepsia* 2003;44(Suppl 9):155.

54. Bebin EM, Kelly PJ, Gomez MR. Surgical treatment for epilepsy in cerebral tuberous sclerosis. *Epilepsia* 1993;34:651–657.

55. Guerreiro MM, Andermann F, Andermann E, et al. Surgical treatment of epilepsy in tuberous sclerosis: strategies and results in 18 patients. *Neurology* 1998;51:1263–1269.

56. Karenfort M, Kruse B, Freitag H, et al. Epilepsy surgery outcome in children with focal epilepsy due to tuberous sclerosis complex. *Neuropediatrics* 2002;33:255–261.

57. Koh S, Jayakar P, Dunoyer C, et al. Epilepsy surgery in children with tuberous sclerosis complex: presurgical evaluation and outcome. *Epilepsia* 2000;41:1206–1213.

58. Romanelli P, Najjar S, Weiner HL, et al. Epilepsy surgery in tuberous sclerosis: multistage procedures with bilateral or multilobar foci. *J Child Neurol* 2002;17:689–692.

59. Alexander GL. Sturge-Weber syndrome. In: Vinken PJ, Bruyn GW, eds. *The phakomatoses.* New York: Elsevier Science, 1972:223–240.

60. Cairns H, Davidson MA. Hemispherectomy in the treatment of infantile hemiplegia. *Lancet* 1951;2:411.

61. Koch G. Genetic aspects of the phakomatoses. In: Vinken PJ, Bruyn GW, eds. *The phakomatoses.* New York: Elsevier Science, 1972:507–512.

62. Rochkind S, Hoffman HJ, Hendrick EB. Sturge-Weber syndrome: natural history and prognosis. *J Epilepsy* 1990;3(Suppl):293–304.

63. Ambrosetto P, Ambrosetto G, Michelucci R, et al. Sturge-Weber syndrome without port-wine nevus: report of 2 cases studies by CT. *Child Brain* 1983;10:387–392.

64. Bye AM, Matheson JM, Mackenzie RA. Epilepsy surgery in Sturge-Weber syndrome. *Aust Paediatr J* 1989;25:103–105.

65. Lund M. On epilepsy in Sturge-Weber's disease. *Acta Psychiatr Neurol Scand* 1949;24:569–586.

66. Enjolras O, Riche MC, Merland JJ. Facial port-wine stains and Sturge-Weber syndrome. *Pediatrics* 1985;76:48–51.

67. Riela AR, Stump DA, Roach ES, et al. Regional cerebral blood flow characteristics of the Sturge-Weber syndrome. *Pediatr Neurol* 1985;1:85–90.

68. Wohlwill FJ, Yakovlev PL. Histopathology of meningo-facial angiomatosis (Sturge-Weber's disease): report of four cases. *J Neuropathol Exp Neurol* 1957;16:341–364.

69. Bebin EM, Gomez MR. Prognosis in Sturge-Weber disease: comparison of unihemispheric and bihemispheric involvement. *J Child Neurol* 1988;3:181–184.

70. Boltshauser E, Wilson J, Hoare RD. Sturge-Weber syndrome with bilateral intracranial calcification. *J Neurol Neurosurg Psychiatry* 1976;39:429–435.

71. Griffiths PD. Sturge-Weber syndrome revisited: the role of neuroradiology. *Neuropediatrics* 1996;27:284–294.

72. Chaudary RR, Brudricki A. Sturge-Weber syndrome with extensive intracranial calcifications contralateral to the bulk of the facial nevus, normal intelligence, and absent seizure disorder. *AJNR Am J Neuroradiol.* 1987;8:736–737.

73. Kramer W. Klippel-Trenaunay syndrome. In: Vinken PJ, Bruyn GW, eds. *The phakomatoses.* New York: Elsevier Science, 1972:390–404.

74. Moore GJ, Slovis TL, Chugani HT. Proton magnetic resonance spectroscopy in children with Sturge-Weber syndrome. *J Child Neurol* 1998;13:332–335.

75. Peterman AF, Hayles AB, Dockerty MB, et al. Encephalotrigeminal angiomatosis (Sturge-Weber disease): clinical study of thirty-five cases. *JAMA* 1958;167:2169–2176.

76. Feng YK, Yang YC. Sturge-Weber syndrome: a report of 22 cases. *Chin Med J (Engl)* 1980;93:697–708.

77. Maria BL, Neufeld JA, Rosainz LC, et al. Central nervous system structure and function in Sturge-Weber syndrome: evidence of neurologic and radiologic progression. *J Child Neurol* 1998;13: 606–618.

78. Falconer MA, Rushworth RG. Treatment of encephalotrigeminal angiomatosis (Sturge-Weber disease) by hemispherectomy. *Arch Dis Child* 1960;35:433–447.

79. Hoffman HJ, Hendrick EB, Dennis M, et al. Hemispherectomy for Sturge-Weber syndrome. *Childs Brain* 1979;5:233–248.

80. Ito M, Sato K, Ohnuki A, et al. Sturge-Weber disease: operative indications and surgical results. *Brain Dev* 1990;12:473–477.

81. Ogunmekan AO, Hwang PA, Hoffman HJ. Sturge-Weber-Dimitri disease: role of hemispherectomy in prognosis. *Can J Neurol Sci* 1989;16:78–80.

82. Nordgren RE, Reeves AG, Viguera AC, et al. Corpus callosotomy for intractable seizures in the pediatric age group. *Arch Neurol* 1991;48:364–372.

83. Rappaport ZH. Corpus callosum section in the treatment of intractable seizures in the Sturge-Weber syndrome. *Child Nerv Syst* 1988;4:231–232.

84. Pavone L, Curatolo P, Rizzo R, Micali G, et al. Epidermal nevus syndrome: a neurologic variant with hemimegalencephaly, gyral malformation, mental retardation, seizures, and facial hemihypertrophy. *Neurology* 1991;41:266–271.

85. Baker RS, Ross PA, Baumann RJ. Neurologic complications of the epidermal nevus syndrome. *Arch Neurol* 1987;44:227–232.

86. Solomon LM, Esterly NB. Epidermal and other congenital organoid nevi. *Curr Probl Pediatr* 1975;6:1–56.

87. Campbell WW, Buda FB, Sorensen G. Linear nevus sebaceous syndrome: neurological aspects documented by brain scans correlated with developmental history and radiographic studies. *Mil Med* 1978;143:175–178.

88. Choi BH, Kudo M. Abnormal neuronal migration and gliomatosis cerebri in epidermal nevus syndrome. *Acta Neuropathol (Berl)* 1981;53:319–325.

89. Herbst BA, Cohen ME. Linea nevus sebaceous: a neurocutaneous syndrome associated with infantile spasms. *Arch Neurol* 1971;24: 317–322.

90. Chalhub EG, Volpe JJ, Gado MH. Linear nevus sebaceous syndrome associated with porencephaly and nonfunctioning major cerebral venous sinuses. *Neurology* 1975;25:857–860.

91. Barth PG, Valk J, Kalsbeek GL, et al. Organoid nevus syndrome (linear nevus sebaceous of Jadassohn): clinical and radiological study of a case. *Neuropediatrics* 1977;8:418–428.

92. Gurecki PJ, Holden KR, Sahn EE, et al. Developmental neural abnormalities and seizures in epidermal nevus syndrome. *Dev Med Child Neurol* 1996;38:716–723.

93. Traboulsi EI, Zin A, Massicotte SJ, et al. Posterior scleral choristoma in the organoid nevus syndrome (linear nevus sebaceous of Jadassohn). *Ophthalmology* 1999;106:2126–2130.

94. Prayson RA, Kotagal P, Wyllie E, et al. Linear epidermal nevus syndrome and nevus sebaceous syndromes: a clinicopathologic study of 3 patients. *Arch Pathol Lab Med* 1999;123:301–305.

95. Riccardi VM, Eichner JE. *Neurofibromatosis: phenotype, natural history and pathogenesis.* Baltimore, MD: Johns Hopkins Press, 1986.

96. Korf BR, Carrazana E, Holmes GL. Patterns of seizures observed in association with neurofibromatosis 1. *Epilepsia* 1993;34: 616–620.

97. Friedman D, Rothner AD, Estes M, et al. Characterization of seizures in a hospitalized population of persons with neurofibromatosis. *Epilepsia* 1989;30:670–671.

98. Cohen BA. Incontinentia pigmenti. *Neurol Clin* 1987;5:361–377.

99. Pascual-Castroviejo I. Neurocutaneous melanosis. In: Gomez MR, ed. *Neurocutaneous diseases: a practical approach.* Boston: Butterworths, 1987:329–334.

100. Gordon N. Hypomelanosis of Ito (incontinentia pigmenti achromians). *Dev Med Child Neurol* 1994;36:271–274.

101. Hamada T, Saito T, Sugai T, et al. Incontinentia pigmenti achromians (Ito). *Arch Dermatol* 1967;96:673–676.

102. Glover MT, Brett EM, Atherton DJ. Hypomelanosis of Ito: spectrum of the disease. *J Pediatr* 1989;115:75–80.

103. Aita JA. Miscellaneous neurocutaneous diseases. In: Vinken PJ, Bruyn GW, eds. *The phakomatoses.* New York: Elsevier Science, 1972:172–206.

104. Barth PG. Disorders of neuronal migration. *Can J Neurol Sci* 1987;14:1–16.

105. Rakic P. Defects of neuronal migration and the pathogenesis of cortical malformations. In: Boer GJ, Feenstra MGP, Mirmiran M, et al., eds. *Biochemical basis of functional neuroteratology: permanent effects of chemicals on the developing brain. Progress in brain research,* vol 73. New York: Elsevier, 1988:15–37.

106. Rakic P. Specification of cerebral cortical areas. *Science* 1988;241: 170–176.

107. Epilepsy and disorders of neuronal migration [editorial]. *Lancet* 1990;336:1035.

108. Dobyns WB, Garg BP. Vascular abnormalities in epidermal nevus syndrome. *Neurology* 1991;41:276–278.

109. Andermann F, Olivier A, Melanson D, et al. Epilepsy due to focal cortical dysplasia and the forme fruste of tuberous sclerosis: a study of 15 patients. In: Wolf P, Dam M, Janz D, et al., eds. *Advances in epileptology: XVIth Epilepsy International Symposium.* New York: Raven Press, 1987:35–38.

110. Palmini A, Andermann F, Olivier A, et al. Focal neuronal migration disorders and intractable partial epilepsy: a study of 30 patients. *Ann Neurol* 1991;30:741–749.

111. Perot P, Weir B, Rasmussen T. Tuberous sclerosis: surgical therapy for seizures. *Arch Neurol* 1966;15:498–506.

112. Taylor DC, Falconer MA, Bruton CJ, et al. Focal dysplasia of the cerebral cortex in epilepsy. *J Neurol Neurosurg Psychiatry* 1971;34: 369–387.

Epilepsy in the Setting of Inherited Metabolic and Mitochondrial Disorders

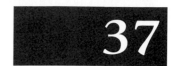

Linda D. Leary   *Douglas R. Nordli, Jr.*   *Darryl C. De Vivo*

There are more than 11,000 well-recognized and well-characterized inherited disorders in humans, with nearly 200 of these associated with seizures and epilepsy. The daunting task for the clinician is to recognize these important diagnoses in the patient with epilepsy so that optimal medical treatment, family counseling, and prognosis can be provided. Often, the presentation is not distinct enough to allow precise identification of the disorder on the basis of clinical criteria alone. Instead, the physician must observe a patient over a period of time and begin screening tests to detect abnormalities suggestive of the underlying disorder. These abnormalities point the way toward further diagnostic evaluations, which may culminate in the definitive diagnosis of the inherited disorder and actual detection of the defective gene. In other circumstances, important clues are present when a child is first seen, but these features can be easily overlooked if the clinical data are not synthesized and analyzed in an orderly way. In general, the scalp electroencephalogram has low specificity but high sensitivity for diagnosing, determining severity, and monitoring brain dysfunction over a period of time in children of all ages. Although various electroencephalographic (EEG) patterns are reported in the literature as being typical of an inborn error of metabolism, rarity of metabolic disorders, ascertainment bias, and limited repertoire of possible EEG findings in the face of enormous variability in spectrum and severity of metabolic disorders reduce the usefulness of EEG in suggesting a specific diagnosis. EEG may, however, supplement clinical assessment and other test results in shortening the list of possible diagnoses.

How can clinicians mentally organize this wealth of material? One method is to group diseases according to categories on the basis of the subcellular organelle involved: mitochondrial, lysosomal, peroxisomal, and so on. Another is to group diseases according to metabolic or catabolic pathways, such as organic aciduria, aminoaciduria, and fatty acid oxidation. However, the clinical presentation within these groups may be diverse and dissimilar. Another method of grouping is to organize diseases according to their clinical presentation. This can be performed by age, but many different disorders are responsible for seizures and epilepsy within any defined age-group. Diseases may also be organized on the basis of specific characteristics of the seizures and the epilepsy syndromes. As each metabolic and mitochondrial disorder may present along a biologic spectrum, with more severe involvement presenting earlier and in a more devastating fashion, various epilepsy syndrome presentations are consistent with the same metabolic disorder. Metabolic and mitochondrial diseases can masquerade as forms of cryptogenic epilepsy. Once the etiology is established, the epilepsy classification will change to symptomatic, generalized epilepsy caused by a specific disorder (e.g., secondary to phenylketonuria [PKU]).

In the organization of this chapter, we group the various disorders by their age at onset and list, in tabular form, the various cryptogenic or symptomatic epilepsy syndromes that might be mistaken for these disorders. In addition, we discuss clinical and EEG features of certain disorders that may provide clues to the underlying etiology. We also discuss the appropriate screening tests that may be performed, where applicable, followed by more definitive diagnostic procedures. For each condition in which a gene location is known, this is listed in parentheses with the appropriate chromosome and gene location.

METABOLIC DISORDERS IN THE NEWBORN

Seizures are a clinical feature of a number of metabolic disorders presenting in the first month of life. Although the following section does not contain a comprehensive listing of all the disorders that should be considered in this age-group, it does include those in which seizures are a prominent feature.

Nonketotic Hyperglycinemia

In the inborn error of amino acid metabolism of nonketotic hyperglycinemia (NKH), large amounts of glycine accumulate in body fluids because of a defect in the multienzyme complex for glycine cleavage. The enzyme system is confined to the mitochondria and is composed of four protein components. Defects in three of these proteins have been identified. The most common defect, affecting the P protein (a glycine decarboxylase), is encoded by a gene localized to 9p22. The majority of cases present within the first 48 hours of life with lethargy, respiratory difficulties, and seizures that are often myoclonic or characterized as infantile spasms. Cortical malformations or corpus callosum defects may be present. A burst-suppression electroencephalogram pattern is characteristic, and hypsarrhythmia has also been seen (1).

Laboratory testing reveals elevations of glycine in the plasma, urine, and cerebrospinal fluid (CSF). The absence of ketones in the blood and urine, and of organic acids in the urine, helps to differentiate NKH from other conditions associated with hyperglycinemia, such as propionic acidemia and methylmalonic acidemia. The ratio of CSF to serum glycine can also be helpful, as it is significantly elevated in patients with NKH.

The pathophysiology of NKH has not been fully elucidated, but the elevated glycine is believed to impact the central nervous system (CNS) via its role as an inhibitory transmitter in the brainstem and spinal cord, and as an excitatory transmitter in the cortex (2).

There is no long-term effective treatment for this disorder. Valproic acid should be avoided because it induces hyperglycinemia. Strychnine, an antagonist to glycine, and diazepam have been reported to blunt seizures, but have not influenced the long-term outcome (3). Using high doses of benzoate to treat patients with NKH may reduce CSF glycine and improve seizure control, but it does not appear to stop the development of mental retardation (4,5). Because benzoate treatment may deplete carnitine levels, carnitine supplementation is recommended if benzoate is used (6). Prognosis is poor, with progressive microcephaly and intractable seizures. Death often occurs within the first days to months of life.

A transient form of NKH exists with similar early clinical and biochemical findings. In this condition, however, glycine concentrations normalize between 2 and 8 weeks of life, and prognosis is favorable.

Pyridoxine Dependency

In pyridoxine dependency, refractory seizures typically develop within the first several days of life. These may be characterized by infantile spasms or a variety of partial, myoclonic, and atonic features. The disorder results from a defect on the binding site of glutamic acid decarboxylase for which pyridoxine is a cofactor. This leads to insufficient γ-aminobutyric acid (GABA) formation, which can be corrected with administration of high doses of pyridoxine. Two different genes code for glutamic acid decarboxylase in mammalian brain, *GAD1* (2q31) and *GAD2* (10p11.23) (7,8). Genetic linkage analysis of five affected families excluded these genes as mutation sites for this disorder (9). In this study, a linkage to 5q31.2-q31.3 was identified.

The EEG is characterized by generalized bursts of high-voltage delta activity interspersed with spike and sharp waves and periods of asynchronous attenuation. Treatment with high doses (100 to 200 mg intravenously) of pyridoxine can result in cessation of seizures, conversion of the EEG to a burst-suppression pattern, and later normalization of the EEG with subsequent doses (10). In some patients, doses as high as 500 mg may be necessary to elicit a response. Early treatment is critical, as it improves developmental outcome, and maintenance therapy with pyridoxine is necessary. Onset of disease may extend beyond the newborn period, making this disorder a consideration in older infants with refractory seizures as well (11,12). Therefore, a trial of pyridoxine is recommended in all infants up to 18 months of age who have refractory seizures of unclear etiology.

Molybdenum Cofactor Deficiency and Sulfite Oxidase Deficiency

The rare conditions of molybdenum cofactor deficiency and sulfite oxidase deficiency present shortly after birth with a progressive encephalopathy, feeding difficulties, hypotonia, and refractory partial, myoclonic, or apparently generalized seizures. Dysmorphic features, lens dislocation, and hepatomegaly are all characteristic findings (13).

Multifocal paroxysms and a burst-suppression pattern have been described on the electroencephalogram. Neuroimaging may show poor differentiation between the gray and white matter, severe cerebral and cerebellar atrophy, and multiple cystic cavities in the white matter.

The relatively more common molybdenum cofactor deficiency results from an absence of the hepatic cofactor leading to a combined enzyme deficiency in the three molybdenum-dependent enzymes: sulfite oxidase, xanthine dehydrogenase, and aldehyde oxidase (14). This may be caused by mutations in the gene (*MOCS1*, 6p21.3) that encodes the two enzymes for synthesis of a precursor. Mutations in molybdopterin synthase (*MOCS2*, 5q11), which converts the precursor into the organic moiety, are responsible for a second form of the disorder (15). A third type of molybdenum cofactor deficiency is caused by a mutation in the gephyrin gene (*GEPH*, 14q24) whose gene product plays a role in biosynthesis of the cofactor (16). Molybdenum cofactor deficiency and isolated sulfite oxidase deficiency both result in high levels of urinary sulfites that can be screened for by sulfite dipstick on a fresh urine sample (17,18). The two disorders can be distinguished on laboratory testing as elevations of urine xanthine and hypoxanthine, and depressions of serum uric acid seen with molybdenum cofactor deficiency that are not present with isolated sulfite oxidase deficiency (19). The enzyme deficiencies can be demonstrated in cultured fibroblasts and liver tissue. No effective treatment has been identified and prognosis is poor, with death occurring within the first days to weeks of life.

Peroxisomal Disorders

Disorders of the peroxisome have been divided into three categories: (a) disorders of peroxisomal biogenesis (Zellweger syndrome [ZS], neonatal adrenoleukodystrophy, infantile Refsum disease); (b) disorders of a single peroxisomal enzyme (X-linked adrenoleukodystrophy, acylcoenzyme A [acyl-CoA] oxidase deficiency); and (c) disorders with deficiencies of multiple peroxisomal enzymes (rhizomelic chondrodysplasia punctata). The discussion that follows is limited to ZS, acyl-CoA oxidase deficiency, and neonatal adrenoleukodystrophy.

Zellweger Syndrome

ZS is the most common peroxisomal disorder in early infancy, with an estimated incidence of 1:50,000 to 1:100,000. The ZS phenotype is caused by mutations in any of several different genes involved in peroxisome biogenesis, including peroxin-1 (7q21-q22), peroxin-2 (8q21.1), peroxin-3 (6q23-q24), peroxin-5 (12p13.3), peroxin-6 (6p21.1), and peroxin-12 (chromosome 17). In addition to these, a ZS locus on 7q11 is suspected on the basis of chromosomal aberrations.

Dysmorphic features may be noted shortly after birth. Within the first week of life, the affected child develops a severe encephalopathy, hypotonia, and hyporeflexia. Seizures occur in 80% of patients, including partial, generalized tonic-clonic (rare), and myoclonic seizures, and atypical flexor spasms. Multisystem abnormalities of the brain, kidneys, liver, skeletal system, and eyes may occur. Eye abnormalities include cataracts, glaucoma, corneal clouding, optic nerve hypoplasia, pigmentary retinal degeneration, and Brushfield spots. The presence of the latter, along with hypotonia and a mongoloid appearance, may cause confusion in the diagnosis of Down syndrome versus ZS. Findings on neuroimaging and pathologic examination are distinctive, with pachygyria or polymicrogyria localized to the opercular region and cerebellar heterotopias.

Patients with ZS have partial motor seizures originating in the arms, legs, or face. The seizures do not culminate in generalized seizures and are easily controlled with antiepileptic drugs (AEDs). The interictal electroencephalogram of patients with ZS shows infrequent bilateral independent multifocal spikes, predominantly in the frontal motor cortex and surrounding regions (20). Less frequently, hypsarrhythmia is observed.

ZS is the most severe of the peroxisomal disorders, with an apparently reduced number or absence of peroxisomes. Santos and associates (21) discovered the presence of peroxisomal ghosts that contained peroxisomal membrane proteins in patients with ZS. These ghosts lack catalase function and many or all proteins of the matrix. An accumulation of very-long-chain fatty acids occurs from a reduction in peroxisomal β-oxidation enzymes. The elevation of very-long-chain fatty acids in the serum helps determine the diagnosis. Treatment is primarily supportive, with dietary therapy being tested in milder forms of the disease.

Neonatal Adrenoleukodystrophy

Neonatal adrenoleukodystrophy, an autosomal recessive disorder with pathologic and biochemical findings resembling X-linked adrenoleukodystrophy, bears some similarity to ZS. Distinguishing features include absent or minimal facial dysmorphisms, later onset of seizures, absent or minimal cerebral malformations, and longer life span. Frequent, often intractable seizures occur that may be tonic, clonic, myoclonic, or epileptic spasms (22). No characteristic EEG pattern has been defined, but descriptions have included high-voltage slowing, polymorphic delta activity, multifocal paroxysmal discharges, burst suppression, and hypsarrhythmia. There is evidence that this disorder may be caused by a number of different gene defects, including a mutation in the peroxisomal targeting signal-1 receptor gene *PXR1*, and mutations in the peroxin-1 gene, peroxin-10 gene (chromosome 1), and peroxin-13 gene (2p15) (23).

Acyl-Coenzyme A Oxidase Deficiency

Acyl-CoA oxidase deficiency was initially described in two siblings by Poll-The and colleagues (24). Clinical features included hypotonia, pigmentary retinopathy, hearing loss, developmental delay, adrenocortical insufficiency, absence of dysmorphic features, and onset of seizures shortly after birth. A deficiency in acyl-CoA oxidase was identified, resulting from a deletion in its coding gene (17q25). In children with acyl-CoA oxidase deficiency, serum very-long-chain fatty acid levels are elevated, whereas pipecolic acid levels are normal. Cortical malformations are generally absent, and the interictal EEG may show continuous diffuse high-voltage theta activity.

Urea Cycle Disorders

Of the six enzymes in the urea cycle that are involved in the conversion of ammonia to urea, five may be defective and cause neonatal seizures. These deficiencies, with their estimated frequency in the general population are as follows: carbamoyl phosphate synthetase, 1:800,000; ornithine transcarbamoylase, 1:80,000; argininosuccinate synthetase, 1:250,000; argininosuccinate lyase, 1:70,000; and N-acetylglutamate synthetase, only a few cases reported (2). The clinical disorder resulting from a deficiency in the sixth enzyme, arginase, presents later in infancy. All these disorders are autosomal-recessive except for ornithine transcarbamoylase deficiency, which is X-linked dominant.

The clinical manifestations of the disorders are similar and result, at least in part, from ammonia elevations. Typically, affected newborns present with poor feeding, emesis, hyperventilation, lethargy, or convulsions 1 to 5 days after birth. These signs lead to deepening coma, with decorticate and decerebrate posturing and progressive loss of brainstem function. Brain imaging and pathology reveal cerebral edema with pronounced astrocytic swelling. Ammonium is taken up by the astrocytes and rapidly converted to glutamine in an energy-dependent process. The edema is associated with glutamine accumulation and energy depletion. In experimental models, blocking glutamine synthesis has prevented the occurrence of hyperammonemia-associated cerebral edema (25).

The clinical diagnosis is confirmed by elevations in serum ammonia, absence of urine ketones, and respiratory alkalosis. (In contrast, metabolic acidosis and ketosis frequently occur with disorders of organic acid or pyruvate metabolism.) Measurement of plasma citrulline and argininosuccinic acid, as well as urine orotic acid, can help differentiate the enzymatic defects. Definitive diagnosis is established via enzyme assays or deoxyribonucleic acid (DNA) analysis.

The EEG shows a low-voltage pattern, with diffuse slowing and multifocal epileptiform discharges (26). Two patients studied by Verma and coworkers (27) in 1984 demonstrated episodes of sustained monorhythmic theta activity. In patients with acute neonatal citrullinemia, a burst-suppression pattern has been described (28).

In the acute setting, hemodialysis has been used to reduce serum ammonia and can be lifesaving. Protein restriction and medical therapy aimed at lowering serum ammonia are recommended in the long-term management of these children. Liver transplantation has been successful in reducing ammonia levels in patients and in reversing neurologic deficits in adults with milder disease (29,30).

Maple Syrup Urine Disease

Maple syrup urine disease, resulting from a defect in the branched-chain α-keto acid dehydrogenase complex, was first reported by Menkes and colleagues (31) in 1954. The enzyme defect leads to accumulation of the branched-chain amino acids—valine, leucine, isoleucine—and their keto acids in body tissues and fluids. The gene locus is 19q13.1-q13.2 (32). Pathologic studies reveal diffuse myelin loss and increased total brain lipid content. Cystic degeneration of the white matter associated with gliosis is observed. Disordered neuronal migration may occur with heterotopias and disrupted cortical lamination.

Feeding difficulties and lethargy are observed during the first to second weeks of life. If left untreated, these signs may progress to stupor, apnea, opisthotonos, myoclonic jerks, and partial and generalized seizures.

A characteristic odor can be detected in the urine and cerumen, but this may not be detectable until several weeks after birth. Laboratory testing reveals a metabolic acidosis and elevated blood and urine ketones. Hypoglycemia may be present, exacerbating seizures. Ferric chloride testing of the urine causes a gray-green reaction, and the 2,4-dinitrophenylhydrazine test is positive. A marked elevation in branched-chain amino acids/branched-chain keto acids in the plasma, urine, and CSF is observed, and the presence of the abnormal metabolite L-alloisoleucine is pathognomonic for this condition. Definitive testing can be performed by enzyme assay.

The electroencephalogram shows diffuse slowing and a loss of reactivity to auditory stimuli. The "comb-like rhythm" characteristic of maple syrup urine disease was initially reported by Trottier and associates (33) in 1975, when bursts of a central mu-like rhythm were observed in four affected patients. Tharp (34) described resolution of this pattern in an affected infant when dietary therapy was initiated. Korein and coworkers (35) observed a paroxysmal spike and spike-wave response to photic stimulation in 7 of 15 affected patients. Acute treatment is aimed at counteracting the effects of hypoglycemia, acidosis, and hypotension. Dialysis or exchange transfusion rarely is necessary. Dietary therapy with protein restriction, thiamine supplementation, and elimination of branched-chain amino acids from the diet is the mainstay of treatment.

Organic Acidurias

The disorders of organic acid metabolism comprise a large number of inborn errors, including isovaleric aciduria and several ketotic hyperglycinemic syndromes (propionic acidemia, methylmalonic acidemia, and β-ketothiolase deficiency).

Symptoms develop during the neonatal period in half of the children with isovaleric aciduria (gene locus, 15q14-q15) (36), with poor feeding, vomiting, dehydration, and a progressive encephalopathy manifested by lethargy, tremors, seizures, and coma. Depressed platelets and leukocytes may be seen, and the urine odor has been described as similar to that of "sweaty feet" (37). Cerebral edema is present, and seizures are most often partial motor or generalized tonic. The electroencephalogram shows dysmature features during sleep. Distinctive biochemical findings include metabolic acidosis, ketosis, lactic acidosis, hyperammonemia, and transient bone marrow suppression. High urine concentrations of isovalerylglycine, a by-product of an alternative pathway of detoxification by glycine-N-acylase, is diagnostic.

The symptoms of propionic acidemia also appear during the neonatal period, with 20% of affected newborns having seizures as the first symptom. Characteristic features include vomiting, lethargy, ketosis, neutropenia, periodic thrombocytopenia, hypogammaglobulinemia, developmental retardation, and intolerance to protein. Patients may have very puffy cheeks and an exaggerated cupid's-bow upper lip. Mutations have been identified in both the α subunit (13q32) and β subunit (3q21-q22) of propionyl coenzyme A (CoA) carboxylase (38). Convulsions are typical, although partial seizures have also been reported. The electroencephalogram shows background disorganization, with marked frontotemporal and occipital slow-wave activity (39). In 40% of children, myoclonic seizures develop in later infancy, and older children may have atypical absence seizures. Biochemical findings include metabolic acidosis, ketosis, and elevation of branched-chain amino acids and propionic acid.

Methylmalonic acidemia may be caused by deficiencies of the enzyme methylmalonyl-CoA mutase or of adenosylcobalamin synthetic enzymes. Methylmalonic acidemia occurs in association with homocystinuria in a combined deficiency of methylmalonic-CoA mutase and methyltetrahydrofolate:homocysteine methyltransferase (40,41). Forms responsive to vitamin B_{12} have been reported (42). Stomatitis, glossitis, developmental delay, failure to thrive, and seizures are the major features. Diffuse tonic seizures and partial seizures with secondary generalization are the most frequent seizure types. Seizures may be characterized by eyelid clonus with simultaneous upward deviation of the eyes. In a review of 22 patients, Stigsby and collaborators (39) described abnormalities on the electroencephalogram in seven patients, consisting of multifocal spike discharges and depressed background activity in two, excessive generalized slowing in two, and mild background slowing with lack of sleep spindles in three. Two children were reported to have myoclonus and a hypsarrhythmic EEG pattern (43). Lesions of the globus pallidus on computed tomography or magnetic resonance imaging (MRI) are characteristic.

Fatty Acid Oxidation Defects

Deficiencies of carnitine palmitoyltransferase types I and II are common disorders of mitochondrial fatty acid oxidation and may present in the newborn period (44). The infantile type of carnitine palmitoyltransferase II deficiency presents as severe attacks of hypoketotic hypoglycemia, sometimes associated with cardiac damage, culminating in sudden death. In addition, cystic dysplasia of the brain has been noted. A deficiency in carnitine acylcarnitine translocase also may produce seizures, apnea, and bradycardia in the neonatal period. Seizures may occur in other defects of fatty acid oxidation, most notably in short-chain acyl-CoA dehydrogenase deficiency (45).

Pyruvate Dehydrogenase Deficiency, Pyruvate Carboxylase Deficiency, and Leigh Syndrome

The pyruvate dehydrogenase complex is composed of multiple copies of three enzymes: pyruvate decarboxylase (E1), dihydrolipoyl transacetylase (E2), and dihydrolipoyl dehydrogenase (E3). The core of the complex is formed by 60 E2 subunits, and the other enzymes are attached to the surface. The E1 enzyme is itself a complex structure, a heterotetramer of two α and two β subunits. The E1 α subunit is particularly important, as it contains the E1 active site; its gene locus is Xp22.2-p22.1. Pyruvate dehydrogenase deficiency has a wide variety of clinical presentations, ranging from acute lactic acidosis in infancy with severe neurologic impairment to a slowly progressive neurodegenerative disorder (46). It is one of the most common of the defined genetic defects of mitochondrial energy metabolism. Seizures frequently occur and may be manifested by infantile spasms and myoclonic seizures (47). EEG findings include multifocal slow spike-and-wave discharges. Structural abnormalities, such as agenesis of the corpus callosum, are often present on neuroimaging. The most common mutations associated with this disorder are in the E1 subunit gene located on the short arm of the X chromosome.

Two predominant clinical presentations occur with pyruvate carboxylase deficiency. The neonatal type manifests with severe lactic acidemia and death in the first few months of life. The juvenile presentation begins in the first 6 months of life with episodes of lactic acidemia precipitated by an infection. Developmental delay, failure to thrive, hypotonia, and seizures, including infantile spasms with hypsarrhythmia, may be seen. In milder forms, diffuse 1.5- to 3-Hz slowing has been noted (39). Seizures are related to the hypoglycemia that occurs secondary to Krebs cycle dysfunction. Treatment with the ketogenic diet or corticotropins may markedly exacerbate the disorder and should be avoided (48,49).

Leigh syndrome (subacute necrotizing encephalomyelopathy) may be related to various metabolic defects, including cytochrome *c* oxidase deficiency and defects in other enzymes involved in energy metabolism. Mutations in the mitochondrial DNA-encoded adenosine triphosphate (ATP)-6 subunit of ATP synthase (complex V) and any of the three catalytic subunits (E1, E2, or E3) of the pyruvate dehydrogenase complex may result in the same phenotype described by Leigh in 1951 (50,51). The syndrome may also be caused by isolated deficiency in mitochondrial complex I (nicotinamide adenine dinucleotide: ubiquinone oxidoreductase) and complex II. In addition, rare causes of Leigh syndrome include myoclonic epilepsy with ragged-red fibers (MERRF), mitochondrial encephalomyopathy with lactic acidosis and stroke-like episodes (MELAS), and mitochondrial DNA depletion (52,53). Within the first year of life, classic features include failure to thrive, lactic acidosis, and developmental delay. The disease progresses with spasticity, abnormal eye movements, and central respiratory failure. A variety of different seizures, including focal and generalized seizures, have been described (54). Cases of infantile spasms and hypsarrhythmia have been reported with Leigh syndrome (55,56). In addition, there have been several cases of epilepsia partialis continua (57). EEG features do not appear to be distinctive enough to contribute to the clinical diagnosis of Leigh syndrome (58).

Disorders of Carbohydrate Metabolism

Fructose-1,6-bisphosphatase deficiency, a rare, potentially life-threatening disorder of gluconeogenesis, presents within the first few days of life with respiratory abnormalities, hypotonia, lethargy, hepatomegaly, irritability, and convulsions. Laboratory findings reveal lactic acidosis, ketosis, hypoglycemia, elevated plasma concentrations of alanine, and the presence of abnormal urinary organic acids with glycerol and glycerol-3-phosphate. The gene location is 9q22.2-q22.3 (59). Neurologic sequelae can be prevented by avoidance of hypoglycemia.

Hereditary fructose intolerance (fructose-1,6-biphosphate aldolase deficiency) may be seen in the neonatal period in infants who are formula fed and given fructose or sucrose early in life. Symptoms include profound hypoglycemia, emesis, and convulsions. If the disease is readily diagnosed, fructose and sucrose can be eliminated from the diet before significant systemic injury occurs.

Glut-1 deficiency syndrome, a disorder of glucose transport, may present with seizures in the neonatal period. Because the disorder typically presents later in infancy, it is discussed in the section on metabolic disorders of infancy.

Early Onset Multiple Carboxylase Deficiency (Holocarboxylase Synthetase Deficiency)

The rare disorder of early onset multiple carboxylase deficiency presents in the first week of life with lethargy, respiratory abnormalities, irritability, poor feeding, and emesis. A skin rash is present in more than 50% of patients. Generalized tonic convulsions, partial motor seizures, and multifocal myoclonic jerks develop in 25% to 50% of cases.

A deficiency in the enzyme holocarboxylase synthetase leads to a decrease in holocarboxylase (60). As this enzyme links biotin to four carboxylases in the mitochondria and one in the cytosol, an inactivity of all carboxylases results. The gene location is 21q22.1. Although rare, this condition is very important to recognize because prompt treatment with biotin may result in dramatic improvement.

Laboratory findings demonstrate ketoacidosis and organic aciduria. Hyperammonemia may be seen with acute episodes. Electrographically, a burst-suppression pattern or multifocal spikes are observed. Definitive diagnosis can be made by enzyme assays, and prenatal testing is available. The gene defect has been localized to chromosome 21q22.1. Recently, Aoki and associates (61) reported seven mutations (three missense, two single-base-pair deletions, a three-base in-frame deletion, and a 68-base-pair deletion) identified in the complementary DNA (cDNA) of seven patients from Europe and the Middle East with holocarboxylase synthetase deficiency.

Treatment with biotin (10 mg/day) produces clinical improvement, and there is evidence that prenatal maternal treatment may be helpful.

METABOLIC DISORDERS OF EARLY INFANCY

Lysosomal Disorders

Tay-Sachs Disease and Sandhoff Disease

G_{M2} gangliosidosis is a lysosomal disorder that invariably includes seizures as a prominent feature. The infantile forms of G_{M2} gangliosidosis include Tay-Sachs disease, caused by a deficiency in hexosaminidase A, and Sandhoff disease, caused by a deficiency in hexosaminidase A and B. The clinical presentation is that of a progressive encephalopathy.

Tay-Sachs disease, an autosomal recessive disorder localized to chromosome 15 (15q23-q24) (62), is found in the Ashkenazi Jewish population of Eastern or Central European descent. The overall incidence in the general population (1 in 112,000 livebirths) increases to 1 in 3900 in this defined group. The enzymatic defect leads to intraneuronal accumulation of G_{M2} ganglioside. Normal development is seen until 4 to 6 months of age, when hypotonia and loss of motor skills occur. Within the next 1 to 2 years, spasticity, blindness, and macrocephaly develop. At this stage, seizures become prominent, with frequent partial motor, complex partial, and atypical absence seizures that respond poorly to medication. Myoclonic jerks are frequent and are often triggered by an exaggerated startle response to noise. The electroencephalogram is normal early in the course of disease. Gradually, background activity slows, with bursts of high-voltage delta activity and very fast central spikes (63). Diffuse spike and sharp-wave activity may be noted with acoustically induced myoclonic seizures. As the disease progresses, EEG amplitude declines. The classic cherry-red spot is present in the ocular fundi of more than 90% of patients. Enzymatic studies reveal an isolated absence or deficiency in hexosaminidase

A activity. Prenatal diagnosis and carrier detection for high-risk populations are available.

Sandhoff disease is associated with a mutation of the β-subunit of hexosaminidase, located on chromosome 5 (5q13) (64). Unlike Tay-Sachs disease, there is no association with a particular ethnic group. Clinical presentation is similar to that of Tay-Sachs; however, distinguishing features in some patients include hepatosplenomegaly and skeletal involvement. Enzymatic testing demonstrates the diminished activity of hexosaminidase A and B. Detection of N-acetylglucosamine-containing oligosaccharides in the urine and foam cells in the bone marrow is also diagnostic. As with Tay-Sachs disease, no treatment is immediately available, although one possible strategy is to deplete substrate using an inhibitor of glycosphingolipid biosynthesis, such as N-butyldeoxynojirimycin.

Krabbe Disease (Globoid Cell Leukodystrophy)

Another lysosomal disorder occurring in this age-group is globoid cell leukodystrophy (Krabbe disease). This disorder, linked to chromosome 14q31, is caused by deficient activity of galactosylceramidase. There are four forms of the disorder: (a) infantile, with onset before age 6 months; (b) late infantile, with onset between ages 6 months and 3 years; (c) juvenile, with onset between ages 3 and 7 years; and (d) adult, with onset after 7 years of age (65). The majority of cases begin within 3 to 6 months of life with irritability, poor feeding, emesis, and rigidity. Muscular spasms induced by stimulation are prominent. Blindness and optic atrophy ensue. Initially, increased tendon reflexes are present and then gradually diminish as breakdown of peripheral myelin occurs. Partial or generalized clonic or tonic seizures, as well as infantile spasms, are seen, which may be difficult to distinguish from muscular spasms (66,67). In contrast to what is observed in many classic white matter diseases, seizures occur early in the course of Krabbe disease in 50% to 75% of infants with the disorder. EEG characteristics include a hypsarrhythmia-like pattern with irregular slow activity and multifocal discharges of lower amplitude than that typically seen with West syndrome (68). In a 1969 study of seven infants by Kliemann and coworkers (68), six children had prominent β activity occurring independently in the posterior temporal regions and vertex that was superimposed over slower, high-amplitude waves. This activity was observed to be state-dependent and to occur in long runs without any apparent clinical manifestations. In the terminal stages of the disease, little electrical activity is detected. Extensive demyelination of the central and peripheral nervous systems occurs, leading to the classic laboratory features of delayed nerve conduction velocities and elevated CSF protein. The presence of multinucleated macrophages containing galactocerebroside ("globoid cells") is the pathologic hallmark of the disease. The disease is relentlessly progressive, with death by 1 to 2 years of age. Recently, bone marrow transplantation has been a promising treatment option for these patients (69).

G$_{M1}$ Gangliosidosis Types I and II

The infantile form of G$_{M1}$ gangliosidosis, type I, has been localized to chromosome 3 (3p21.33). A deficiency in β-galactosidase leads to the accumulation of G$_{M1}$ ganglioside and degradation products in nerve cells and other tissues. The affected child is initially normal and then has regression of development at 3 to 6 months of age, with rapid neurologic deterioration. Seizures develop by 2 years of age. Clinical features may include coarse facial features, hepatomegaly, bone deformities (dysostosis multiplex), visual abnormalities, hypotonia, progressive microcephaly, and hematologic abnormalities. A macular cherry-red spot can be seen. Diagnosis is determined by urine findings of galactose-containing oligosaccharides in association with elevated keratan sulfate, by characteristic vacuolization in blood lymphocytes or bone marrow, and by distinctive findings on long bone and spine radiographs. Definitive testing by enzymatic assay is available.

Neurologic deterioration in the juvenile form of G$_{M1}$ gangliosidosis type II is generally slower than in type I. Cerebral manifestations with regression of developmental milestones and visual symptoms are typically present by 2 to 4 years of age. EEG features of both forms include background slowing, with increasing, irregular slow activity as the disease progresses (70). In type II, a fluctuating 4- to 5-cycle temporal rhythmic discharge has been observed.

Disorders of Vitamin Metabolism

Disorders of vitamin metabolism with symptoms that appear in early infancy include biotinidase deficiency and folic acid disorders.

Late-Onset Multiple Carboxylase Deficiency (Biotinidase Deficiency)

Seizures are a prominent feature of late-onset multiple carboxylase deficiency, occurring in 50% to 75% of affected children. Onset of symptoms begins at 3 to 6 months of age, with hypotonia and developmental delay. Seborrheic or atopic dermatitis and alopecia are common. As the disease progresses, ataxia, optic atrophy, and sensorineural hearing loss develop. Seizures, which may be generalized tonic-clonic, partial, myoclonic, or infantile spasms, are the presenting feature in 38% of patients. EEG findings may include a suppression-burst pattern, absence of physiologic sleep patterns, poorly organized and slow waking background activity, and frequent spike and spike-and-slow-wave discharges (71). A deficiency in biotinidase, the enzyme that cleaves biotin from its precursor, can be demonstrated in the serum, leukocytes, or culture fibroblasts. Incidence is estimated at 1 in 40,000 livebirths, and the gene locus is 3p25 (72). As this is a treatable condition, therapeutic trials with high-dose oral biotin should be considered in infants with developmental delay and persistent seizures of unknown etiology.

Methylenetetrahydrofolate Reductase Deficiency

Methylenetetrahydrofolate reductase deficiency (1p36.3) (73) is the most common inborn error of folate metabolism. The metabolic defect results from insufficient production of 5-methyltetrahydrofolate, which is needed for the remethylation of homocysteine to methionine, because of a deficiency in methylenetetrahydrofolate reductase. In affected individuals, a progressive neurologic syndrome develops in infancy. Children with this disorder have acquired microcephaly and seizures characterized by intractable infantile spasms, generalized atonic and myoclonic seizures, and partial motor seizures. EEG findings vary from diffuse slowing of background activity to continuous spike-wave complexes or multifocal spikes. The early onset form differs from the late-onset form. The latter presents with progressive motor deterioration, schizophrenia-like psychiatric symptoms, and recurrent strokes; seizures are uncommon (74). Homocystinuria and elevated serum concentrations of homocystine with reduced or normal serum methionine are the main biochemical features. Dietary supplementation with folic acid, betaine, and methionine has proven beneficial (75). In the acute setting, high-dose methionine has been effective in stopping seizures.

Defects in methionine biosynthesis are also associated with seizures. Convulsions are frequent and are predominantly generalized, although myoclonic seizures with hypsarrhythmia have been reported. Diagnostic laboratory findings are megaloblastic anemia, homocystinuria, decreased methionine, and normal folate and cobalamin concentrations in the absence of methylmalonic aciduria.

Congenital Folate Malabsorption

Seizures are common in patients with congenital folate malabsorption, a rare condition believed to be caused by a defect in the folate transporter system. Folate is concentrated in the nervous system, and the CSF concentrations of folate are higher than the serum concentrations. If left untreated, a slowly progressive encephalopathy results, with intractable seizures. Other clinical and laboratory features include a female predominance, megaloblastic anemia, mouth ulceration, diarrhea, and failure to thrive. Neuroimaging studies reveal calcifications in the occipital lobes and basal ganglia (76). Treatment with high-dose oral or intravenous folate, in conjunction with methionine and vitamin B_{12}, has been successful for seizure control (77).

Inherited defects of vitamin B_{12} metabolism also may produce severe megaloblastic anemia in early infancy. Generalized tonic convulsions almost invariably occur and are refractory to conventional treatment. Methylmalonic aciduria without homocystinuria suggests this diagnosis.

Inborn Errors of Creatine Metabolism

Disorders of creatine metabolism have been identified at two points in the metabolic pathway. The first defect involves the biosynthesis of creatine and is associated with either a deficiency in guanidinoacetate N-methyltransferase deficiency (19p13.3) or in arginine:glycine amidinotransferase. The second defect occurs at the level of the creatine transporter 1. These disorders result in a depletion of brain creatine. Guanidinoacetate N-methyltransferase deficiency has a more severe phenotype and has been associated with medically refractory epilepsy (78). Normal development is followed by a developmental regression between 3 months and 2 years of age. Seizures present in the first months of life with generalized tonic-clonic, astatic, absence, myoclonic, or partial seizures. Multifocal epileptiform discharges have been reported on the electroencephalograms of affected individuals (79). Other clinical features may include dystonia, dyskinesias, microcephaly, and autistic behaviors. Supplementation with creatine monohydrate (350 mg/kg per day to 2 g/kg per day) has led to improvement in affected individuals (79). Restriction of arginine and supplementation of ornithine has been used to reduce guanidinoacetic acid accumulation (80). Diagnosis can be made by magnetic resonance spectroscopy (MRS), which demonstrates reduced brain creatine.

Glut-1 Deficiency Syndrome

The Glut-1 deficiency syndrome (Glut-1 DS), previously referred to as glucose transporter protein deficiency syndrome, was first described in 1991 (81,82). The condition results from a loss of functional glucose transporters, encoded by the GLUT-1 gene, that mediate glucose transport across the blood–brain barrier. Clinical features include developmental delay, ataxia, hypotonia, infantile seizures, and acquired microcephaly. A reduction in the CSF-to-blood glucose ratio to half of normal (typically, CSF glucose <40 mg/dL) and a low lactate concentration are diagnostic. Additional confirmation of impaired glucose transport can be performed through assays in erythrocytes (83). The GLUT-1 gene was initially mapped to the short arm of chromosome 1 (1p31.3-p35) and more recently to 1p34.2 (84). A variety of mutations in the GLUT-1 gene have been described (85,86). Families with an autosomal dominant inheritance pattern have been identified (87,88). Seizures are often the first identified feature of this syndrome. Typical seizure types include absence, myoclonic, astatic, generalized tonic-clonic, and partial seizures. A normal electroencephalogram is commonly seen between seizures, although generalized 2.5- to 4-Hz spike-wave discharges are observed in more than one-third of children older than 2 years of age (89). Affected individuals without the classic clinical features have been identified and a screening lumbar puncture should be considered in those with refractory epilepsy (87). Seizures tend to be refractory to AEDs. Initiation of the ketogenic diet is effective in the treatment of seizures as well as of the overall disease process, as it provides an alternative cerebral energy source.

Organic Acidurias

Seizures in early infancy may be the presenting symptom of branched-chain organic acidurias. These include isovaleric aciduria, 3-methylcrotonyl-CoA carboxylase deficiency, 3-methylglutaconic aciduria with normal 3-methylglutaconyl-CoA hydratase, and 3-hydroxy-3-methylglutaric aciduria. Seizures including convulsions and infantile spasms tend to be prominent in 3-methylcrotonyl-CoA carboxylase deficiency. The gene locus is at 3q25-q27. The typical abnormal organic acids include 3-hydroxyisovaleric acid and 3-methylcrotonylglycine. Serum concentrations of free carnitine are low. A biotin-responsive form has been identified (90).

Severe developmental delay, progressive encephalopathy, and seizures are features of 3-methylglutaconic aciduria with normal 3-methylglutaconyl-CoA hydratase (91). This disorder results from a mutation on chromosome 9 in the gene encoding the enzyme 3-methylglutaconyl-CoA hydratase. Seizures occur in one-third of cases, and infantile spasms have been reported early in the course of the disorder. The typical organic acid abnormality includes marked elevations in 3-methylglutaconic acid and 3-methylglutaric acid in the urine.

Seizures are the presenting symptom in 10% of patients with 3-hydroxy-3-methylglutaric aciduria, a disorder caused by a deficiency in the lyase enzyme that mediates the final step of leucine degradation and plays a pivotal role in hepatic ketone body production. This disorder is one of an increasing list of inborn errors of metabolism that clinically present as Reye syndrome or nonketotic hypoglycemia. The odor of the urine may resemble that of a cat. The chromosome location for this disorder is 1pter-p33 (92).

Infantile spasms have been reported in patients with 3-hydroxybutyric aciduria. Facial dysmorphism and brain dysgenesis are prominent manifestations. The enzyme deficiency causing this condition is unknown. Urinary excretion of 3-hydroxyisobutyric acid in the absence of ketosis is diagnostic.

Glutaric acidemia type I is a more common autosomal recessive disorder of lysine metabolism that is caused by a deficiency in glutaryl-CoA dehydrogenase (19p13.2). Seizures are often the first clinical sign of metabolic decompensation after a febrile illness. Vigabatrin, L-carnitine, baclofen, and riboflavin supplementation have been suggested (93).

Amino Acid Disorders

Phenylketonuria and Hyperphenylalaninemias

One of the most frequent inborn errors of metabolism, occurring in 1 in 10,000 to 15,000 livebirths, PKU is caused by a deficiency in hepatic phenylalanine hydroxylase (12q24.1) (94). As a consequence of the metabolic defect, toxic levels of the essential amino acid phenylalanine accumulate. If untreated, severe mental retardation, behavioral disturbances, psychosis, and acquired microcephaly can result. Seizures are present in 25% of affected children. The majority of children with PKU (80% to 95%) are found to have abnormalities on the electroencephalogram. An age-related distribution of EEG findings and seizure types has been observed since a 1957 report by Low and associates (95). Infantile spasms and hypsarrhythmia predominate in the young infant. As the children mature, tonic-clonic and myoclonic seizures become more frequent, and the electroencephalogram evolves to mild diffuse background slowing, focal sharp waves, and irregular generalized spike and slow waves (96,97). During a study by Donker and colleagues (98) in 1979, an increase in delta activity was seen as levels increased during phenylalanine loading. PKU is currently part of universal neonatal screening in most developed countries. With early detection and institution of a phenylalanine-free diet, the neurologic sequelae of hyperphenylalaninemia can be prevented.

A hyperphenylalaninemic state also occurs with disorders of phenylalanine metabolism or tetrahydrobiopterin homeostasis. In tetrahydrobiopterin deficiency, metabolism of phenylalanine, tyrosine, and tryptophan is impaired, as tetrahydrobiopterin is a cofactor for the enzyme phenylalanine hydroxylase. Three enzyme deficiencies can cause this syndrome: dihydropteridine reductase (4p15.3) (99), 6-pyruvoyltetrahydropterin synthase (11q22.3-q23.3) (100), and guanine triphosphate cyclohydrolase (14q22.1-q22.2) (181,102). This defect is present in 1 to 2 livebirths per million. Between 2 and 12 months of age, a progressive neurologic decline is observed, with acquired microcephaly and intractable seizures, including infantile spasms and myoclonic seizures. Calcification of the basal ganglia may be seen. Treatment includes restriction of phenylalanine intake, tetrahydrobiopterin supplementation, and pharmacotherapy with levodopa, carbidopa, or 5-hydroxytryptophan. If instituted in the early stages of the disorder, treatment is beneficial in some patients.

Tyrosinemia Type III

An inborn error of tyrosine metabolism, tyrosinemia type III (4-hydroxyphenylpyruvate dioxygenase deficiency) has been reported in a newborn with intractable seizures and in children who later developed infantile spasms (103). The gene locus is 12q24-qter (104). The electroencephalogram has been described as low voltage, with spike and polyspike discharges in the parietooccipital regions.

Other Amino Acid Disorders

Hyperornithinemia-hyperammonemia-homocitrullinuria syndrome, a defect of intramitochondrial ornithine transport with a gene locus at 13q14, presents with mental retardation, ataxia, spasticity, myoclonus, and chorea. Seizures, including infantile spasms, have been described with this disorder. Treatment recommendations include protein restriction and supplementation with ornithine, arginine, and citrulline.

Histidinemia or histidase deficiency is also associated with infantile spasms and myoclonic seizures. Other features include developmental delay and an exaggerated startle response. A diet low in histidine may be partially beneficial.

3-Phosphoglycerate dehydrogenase deficiency results in a defect in serine biosynthesis. The clinical presentation is intractable seizures, microcephaly, spastic tetraparesis, and profound cognitive delays (105). Reduced serine levels are found in plasma and CSF.

Urea Cycle Defects

Symptoms of urea cycle, branched-chain amino acid, and keto acid metabolism disorders may appear either in the neonatal period, as discussed previously, or during infancy.

Arginase Deficiency

A rare disorder, arginase deficiency differs from the other urea cycle defects because of its later onset. The chromosomal location is 6q23 (106). Features in affected children include a progressive spastic paraplegia, developmental delay, hyperactivity, emesis, failure to thrive, irritability, and seizures starting in the first year of life. Laboratory findings are notable for elevations of ammonia, marked hyperargininemia, and high urinary levels of arginine and orotic acid. As with the other urea cycle defects, dietary treatment is beneficial. In one refractory case, transplantation of normal erythrocytes successfully replaced the missing enzyme function (107).

Disorders of Gamma-Amino Butyric Acid (GABA) Metabolism

4-Hydroxybutyric aciduria, also known as succinic semialdehyde dehydrogenase deficiency, is an example of an inborn error of GABA metabolism (108). The gene locus is 6p22 (109). Psychomotor retardation, language delay, hypotonia, and ataxia develop between the ages of 6 months and 11 years. Fifty percent of patients present with seizures. Accumulation of 4-hydroxybutyric acid in urine, plasma, and CSF, and variable elevations of glycine, are characteristic. Although vigabatrin, an irreversible inhibitor of GABA transaminase, has been used in some individuals with positive responses (including increased socialization, behavioral improvement, increased alertness, and reduced ataxia), treatment with this agent has worsened symptoms in others (110,111).

Menkes Disease (Kinky Hair Disease)

An X-linked (Xq12-q13) disorder of copper absorption, Menkes disease was first described by Menkes and colleagues (112) in 1962. A characteristic twisting of the hair shaft, resulting in "kinky hair" of the head and eyebrows, is noted on microscopic examination of the poorly pigmented hairs. Affected boys may be premature and may have neonatal hyperbilirubinemia or hypothermia. Progressive neurologic deterioration with spasticity is present by 3 months of age, and children may have associated bone and urinary tract abnormalities as well. The disease has a rapidly fatal course.

Seizures are a prominent feature in Menkes disease, with intractable generalized or focal convulsions. Infantile spasms have also been reported (113). Stimulation-induced myoclonic jerks may be present. Multifocal spike and slow-wave activity can be seen on the electroencephalogram, sometimes resembling hypsarrhythmia (114).

Laboratory testing reveals extremely low serum copper and ceruloplasmin levels. Elevations in CSF lactate may be seen, and there is low total copper content in the brain. Neuroimaging may show brain atrophy, focal areas of necrosis, and subdural collections. Brain magnetic resonance angiography (MRA) shows dilated and tortuous intracranial blood vessels.

There is no fully effective treatment. Daily copper injections may be beneficial if administered early in the course of the disease.

Phenotypic and genotypic overlap between Menkes disease, Wilson disease, and occipital horn syndrome has been observed (115). Godwin-Austen and colleagues (116) described a disorder clinically similar to that of Wilson disease but without Kayser-Fleisher rings. Symptoms began at 12 years of age, and defective copper absorption from the distal intestine, with high copper levels in rectal mucosa, was observed. The phenotypic associations between Menkes disease and occipital horn syndrome have been thoroughly reviewed elsewhere (117).

Progressive Encephalopathy with Edema, Hypsarrhythmia, and Optic Atrophy

Progressive encephalopathy with edema, hypsarrhythmia, and optic atrophy (also known as PEHO syndrome), described by Salonen and associates (118) in 1991, is characterized by infantile spasms, arrest of psychomotor development, hypotonia, hypsarrhythmia, edema, and visual failure with optic atrophy (119). Characteristic features include epicanthal folds, midfacial hypoplasia, protruding ears, gingival hypertrophy, micrognathia, and tapering fingers. Edema develops over the limbs and face. The progressive decline seen with this disease suggests a metabolic defect, although no biochemical marker has been identified. Based on the pattern of inheritance associated with the disease, it is presumed to be an autosomal recessive disorder. Neuroimaging shows progressive brain atrophy and abnormal myelination. Hypoplasia of the corpus callosum has been reported. Seizures generally begin as infantile spasms with associated hypsarrhythmia on the electroencephalogram. Later, other seizure types may be seen, including tonic, tonic-clonic, and absence seizures. The electroencephalogram may evolve to a slow spike-and-wave pattern. Prognosis is poor in children with this disorder, with survival only into adolescence.

METABOLIC DISORDERS OF LATE INFANCY

Metachromatic Leukodystrophy

Metachromatic leukodystrophy is the result of a deficiency of arylsulfatase A (22q13.31-qter) (120). Hypotonia, weakness, and unsteady gait suggestive of a neuropathy or myopathy are the most common presenting symptoms. These are followed by a progressive decline in mental and motor skills. Partial seizures develop late in the clinical course in 25% of patients with the late-infantile form of metachromatic leukodystrophy and in 50% to 60% of patients with the juvenile-onset form (121,122). A progression from normal EEG features to diffuse slowing with epileptiform discharges correlates well with clinical decline (123). Bone marrow transplantation may be beneficial in some patients and may be accompanied by improvements in clinical neurophysiologic studies (124). It has become apparent that there may be remarkable phenotypic heterogeneity (125).

Schindler Disease

Schindler disease results from a deficiency in α-*N*-acetylgalactosaminidase (22q11) (126–128). Affected patients appear normal at birth, but progressive neurologic decline becomes evident in the second year. Manifestations include spasticity, cerebellar signs, and extrapyramidal dysfunction. Generalized tonic-clonic seizures and myoclonic jerks are common. EEG abnormalities include diffuse and multifocal spikes and spike-wave complexes.

Mucopolysaccharidoses

The mucopolysaccharidoses are a family of lysosomal storage disorders caused by a deficiency in several enzymes involved in the degradation of glycosaminoglycans. The various mucopolysaccharidoses share many clinical features, including a progressive course, multisystem involvement, organ enlargement, dysostosis multiplex, and abnormal facial features. The most common is Sanfilippo syndrome (mucopolysaccharidosis type III), in which only heparan sulfate is excreted in the urine; four different subtypes have been described, each associated with a different enzymatic defect (129). The gene locus is 17q25.3 (130). Generalized seizures develop in about 40% of patients with Sanfilippo syndrome, but these are often easily controlled with AEDs. Progressive dementia and severe behavioral disorders are other features. In a careful study of one patient, the electroencephalogram showed lack of normal sleep staging, absence of vertex waves and sleep spindles, and an unusual alteration of low-amplitude fast activity

(12 to 15 Hz) with generalized slowing (131). Bone marrow transplantation was successful in several cases but not useful in others (132).

Neuronal Ceroid Lipofuscinoses

The neuronal ceroid lipofuscinoses are a group of diseases that result in storage of lipopigments in the brain and other tissues. At least five clinical subtypes have been reported, as well as rare, atypical forms, and most are transmitted as autosomal recessive traits.

The infantile form of neuronal ceroid lipofuscinosis is found predominantly in Finland, where the incidence is 1in 20,000 of the general population. This disorder typically presents at 12 to 18 months of age with developmental regression, myoclonus, ataxia, and visual failure. Other features include incoordination of limb movements, acquired microcephaly, and optic atrophy.

Seizures are prominent, including myoclonic jerks and astatic, atonic, or generalized seizures. EEG features aid in the diagnosis, with an early attenuation and progressive loss of the background (133). Other criteria for diagnosis include characteristic neuroimaging findings of progressive cerebral and cerebellar atrophy, skin or conjunctival biopsy demonstrating typical curvilinear granular lysosomal bodies in mesenchymal cells, and DNA studies. The majority of affected patients are homozygous for a missense mutation on chromosome 1p32 (134).

Neuronal ceroid lipofuscinosis type II shares many clinical features with the infantile form. Unlike type I, no ethnic predilection exists. The gene responsible for most cases has been mapped to chromosome 11p15.5 (135). Early development is normal or may be mildly delayed. By age 2 to 4 years, insomnia, an early clinical sign, and intractable seizures develop. Multiple seizure types develop as well, with staring spells and generalized tonic-clonic, myoclonic, and atonic components. As the disease progresses, irregular myoclonic jerks evoked by proprioceptive stimuli, voluntary movement, or emotional fluctuations become prominent. Cognitive decline, ataxia, and visual failure with optic atrophy and an abnormal electroretinogram are typical (136). A characteristic EEG pattern of occipital spikes on low-frequency photic stimulation is observed (137). Giant visual evoked responses and somatosensory evoked potentials are seen as well.

Alpers Disease (Progressive Infantile Poliodystrophy)

Alpers disease, a syndrome of unknown etiology, represents a number of familial disorders characterized by a rapidly progressive encephalopathy with intractable seizures and diffuse neuronal degeneration. In the Alpers-Huttenlocher subgroup, liver involvement is present and an autosomal recessive pattern of transmission is suggested. A diagnosis of Alpers disease should be made only in the absence of known metabolic disease or an antecedent event. Along with clinical features suggestive of Alpers disease, neuroimaging should exclude other diagnostic possibilities and should show progressive brain atrophy on successive studies, with relative sparing of the white matter. Seizure types include myoclonic, focal, and generalized tonic-clonic convulsions. Brick and colleagues (138) described a continuous, anterior, high-voltage, 1-to-3-per-second spike-wave–like activity that persists despite intermittent focal seizures. The same authors noted a progressive slowing of background activity as the disease progresses. Epilepsia partialis continua and convulsive status epilepticus were observed in these patients (139). Characteristic slowing together with smaller polyspikes has also been described in individuals with this disease (140). Treatment is supportive and prognosis is poor.

Congenital Disorders of Glycosylation

Congenital disorders of glycosylation (CDG) are multisystemic diseases characterized by a defect in glycoproteins and glycolipids. CDGs can be divided into two types, depending on whether the defects impair lipid-linked oligosaccharide assembly and transfer (CDG-I) or alter trimming of the protein-bound oligosaccharide or the addition of sugars to it (CDG-II) (141). Participants at the First International Workshop on CDG in Leuven, Belgium, in November 1999, proposed a new nomenclature for CDG (142). A marker of the syndrome is a decreased number or absence of terminal trisaccharides on transferrin. CDG type Ia, phosphomannomutase-2 deficiency, is the best characterized and most common of these syndromes (16p13.3-p13.2) (143,144). During infancy, internal organ symptoms are the predominant feature and may be life-threatening. In later childhood, mental deficiency, ataxia, progressive neuropathy involving the legs, retinal degeneration, and skeletal deformities are most common. Subcutaneous tissue changes with an odd distribution of fat, retracted nipples, and odd facies, including almond-shaped eyes, have been described. Imaging studies reveal cerebellar hypoplasia (145). A unique pattern of coagulation changes is associated with the syndrome, including depression of factor XI, antithrombin III, protein C, and, to a lesser extent, protein S and heparin cofactor II. These changes may account for the stroke-like episodes observed in affected children (146). Clinical neurophysiologic studies demonstrate interictal epileptiform discharges and giant somatosensory evoked potentials (147).

The other CDG subtypes have been described in several patients each (148). Type III CDG was first described by Stibler and associates (149) in 1993 in two patients who had severe visual, motor, and mental problems, and who developed infantile spasms with hypsarrhythmia. Interestingly, these patients had patchy skin changes, similar to those of incontinentia pigmenti. The absence of polyneuropathy, pigmentary retinopathy, and cerebellar hypoplasia was felt to differentiate this disorder from the previously described CDGs. Neuroimaging showed dysmyelination and brain atrophy. A defect in glycosylation of transferrin was identified in the two children, who were both girls. Stibler and coworkers described a third child with similar clinical and biochemical features in 1999 (150). EEG findings in this child also showed hypsarrhythmia.

METABOLIC DISORDERS OF CHILDHOOD AND ADOLESCENCE

Homocystinuria

Disorders of transsulfuration include cystathionine β-synthase deficiency, the most frequent cause of homocystinuria; the gene locus is 21q22.3 (151). Mental retardation, behavioral disturbances, and seizures are manifestations of CNS involvement; ectopia lentis, osteoporosis, marfanoid habitus, and scoliosis are other common clinical findings (152,153). Some patients respond to pyridoxine therapy. Generalized seizures occur in about 20% of patients with pyridoxine-nonresponsive homocystinuria and in 16% of patients with the pyridoxine-responsive form. Electroencephalogram features are relatively nonspecific, with slowing and focal interictal epileptiform discharges that may ameliorate with treatment (154). Thromboembolism, malar flush, and livedo reticularis reflect vascular system involvement. Biochemical abnormalities include homocystinemia, methioninemia, decreased cystine concentration, and homocystinuria.

Diabetes Mellitus

In diabetes mellitus, the most common metabolic disorder, seizures are generally not a feature, except during metabolic crises with ketoacidosis and cerebral edema. Nonketotic hyperosmolar diabetic coma is associated with a high mortality rate, and generalized or partial seizures are common in this setting. Epilepsia partialis continua has been reported with NKH.

Adrenoleukodystrophy

Symptoms of the X-linked form of adrenoleukodystrophy (Xq28) classically appear in early childhood. Partial motor seizures, often with secondary generalization, and generalized tonic-clonic seizures are common features of this peroxisomal disorder. Status epilepticus has been the initial presenting symptom, and epilepsia partialis continua has also been reported. The EEG is characteristic, with high-voltage polymorphic delta activity and loss of faster frequencies over the posterior regions (155).

Lysosomal Disorders

Sialidosis Type I (Cherry-Red Spot/Myoclonus Syndrome)

Sialidosis type I, an autosomal recessive disorder of late childhood to adolescence, is characterized by progressive visual loss, polymyoclonus, and seizures. The myoclonus can be debilitating and is stimulated by voluntary movement, sensory stimulation, or excitement. Increased myoclonus with cigarette smoking and menstruation has been reported. As the disease progresses, cognitive decline, cerebellar ataxia, and blindness with optic atrophy occur. Dysmorphic features, bony abnormalities, and hepatosplenomegaly are absent. The electroencephalogram contains rhythmic spiking over the vertex, with a positive polarity overlying a low-voltage background (156). Neuroimaging shows diffuse cerebral and cerebellar atrophy. Diagnosis can be made by detection of an increase in sialic acid—containing oligosaccharides in the urine, vacuolated lymphocytes in the peripheral blood, and foamy histiocytes in bone marrow smears. Enzyme assays for deficiency of α-neuroaminidase, the structural components of which are encoded on chromosome 10, offer definitive diagnosis. The gene defect has been localized to 6p21.3 (157).

Sialidosis Type II (Galactosialidosis)

Sialidosis type II, the juvenile form of this group of disorders, has features similar to those of sialidosis type I. Distinguishing characteristics are the less prominent myoclonic activity and the additional clinical features of coarse facies, corneal clouding, dysostosis multiplex, and hearing loss. Inheritance is autosomal recessive, and a higher incidence of this form of the disease is found in Japan. In the majority of cases, a partial deficiency of β-galactosidase can be seen in addition to neuraminidase deficiency (galactosialidosis), which may be the result of a defect in protective protein; the gene locus coding for this protein is 20q13.1 (158). The electroencephalogram contains moderate-voltage generalized 4 to 6 per second paroxysms.

Gaucher Disease Type III

Three types of Gaucher disease are known: type I, a chronic form with adult onset; type II, a rare form associated with infantile demise; and type III, a chronic form with neurologic involvement. These disorders result from a mutation in the gene encoding acid β-glucosidase (1q21), which leads to accumulation of glucosylceramide in the lysosomes of cells in the reticuloendothelial system (159). In the rare type III form, hepatosplenomegaly may be present from birth or early infancy, which may cause type III to be confused with the more common type I form of Gaucher disease. When neurologic symptoms develop in childhood to early adulthood, type III can be clearly distinguished from type I, in which cerebral features are absent. Frequent myoclonic jerks and tonic-clonic seizures ultimately develop. A supranuclear palsy of horizontal gaze is present in the majority of cases and is an important diagnostic sign. Generalized rigidity, progressive cognitive decline, and facial grimacing may be present. Paroxysmal EEG abnormalities may be seen prior to the onset of convulsions, with worsening as the disease progresses; diffuse polyspikes and spike-wave discharges are also seen. The most characteristic EEG findings are rhythmic trains of spike or sharp waves at 6 to 10 per second (160). The diagnosis can be made by the clinical findings in combination with Gaucher cells detected in the bone marrow. Another laboratory abnormality is an elevated serum acid phosphatase. Unlike type I disease, which is prevalent in the Ashkenazi Jewish population, type III is reported predominantly in Sweden. A multimodal approach is suggested with enzyme replacement therapy and deoxynojirimycin analogues aimed at blocking the synthesis of glucocerebroside to lessen the systemic manifestations (161). Therapeutic trials with bone marrow transplantation have shown some success in improving CNS manifestations of Gaucher disease type III.

Neuroaxonal Dystrophies

Axonal dystrophies include infantile neuroaxonal dystrophy, pantothenate kinase-associated neurodegeneration (formerly Hallervorden-Spatz disease), and Schindler disease. Pantothenate kinase-associated neurodegeneration is not discussed here, as seizures are not a prominent feature. Information on Schindler disease is presented in the section on metabolic disorders of late infancy.

Infantile neuroaxonal dystrophy (Seitelberger disease) is an autosomal recessive disorder affecting both the central and the peripheral nervous systems. Characteristic pathologic features of axonal spheroids within the peripheral and central nervous systems are seen. Clinical features begin between 1 and 2 years of age with psychomotor regression, hypotonia, and development of a progressive motor sensory neuropathy. Seizures occur in one-third of patients, with onset of convulsions after 3 years of age. The EEG finding of high-amplitude fast activity (16 to 24 Hz), unaltered by eye opening or closure, is characteristic of all children with this disorder, regardless of the occurrence of seizures. During sleep, the fast activity may persist, and K complexes are typically absent (162). Seizure types described with infantile neuroaxonal dystrophy include myoclonic and tonic (163,164). A video-EEG case report by Wakai and associates (165) described tonic spasms and an electrographic correlate of a diffuse, 1-second, high-voltage slow complex, followed by desynchronization suggestive of infantile spasms.

Neuronal Ceroid Lipofuscinosis Type III (Spielmeyer-Vogt Disease or Late-Onset Batten Disease)

Neuronal ceroid lipofuscinosis type III, a syndrome of early childhood onset, begins between 5 and 10 years of age with visual failure, slow intellectual deterioration, and seizures; a diffuse rigidity occurs later in the course of the disease. An autosomal recessive inheritance pattern with localization to chromosome 16q12.1 is seen, and distribution is worldwide. EEG changes are nonspecific. In contrast to the Bielschowsky form of neuronal ceroid lipofuscinosis, low-frequency photic stimuli do not evoke occipital spikes.

Progressive Myoclonus Epilepsies

The progressive myoclonus epilepsies are a collection of rare disorders presenting with the triad of myoclonic seizures, tonic-clonic seizures, and progressive neurologic dysfunction that often manifests as dementia and ataxia. Onset generally begins in late childhood to adolescence. If myoclonic features are not prominent, children with this syndrome may be erroneously diagnosed with Lennox-Gastaut syndrome (166). For this reason, a careful history to detect myoclonic features is important in children with intellectual deterioration and frequent seizures.

Lafora Disease

Although the biochemical error in Lafora disease remains unknown, this autosomal recessively inherited defect has been localized to chromosome 6p24. The mean age at onset is 14 years, although symptoms may begin in adulthood. Seizures may precede other clinical signs by months to years, with multiple seizure types occurring in a previously normal individual. Cognitive decline and personality changes are prominent features. Seizure types include tonic-clonic, myoclonic, and polymyoclonus. Occipital seizures with visual phenomena have been reported in 30% to 50% of patients. Cerebellar ataxia, hypertonia, dyskinesias, and exaggerated tendon reflexes may develop later. Generalized bursts of spikes and polyspikes superimposed on a normal background may be seen initially on the electroencephalogram. The presence of spikes in the posterior quadrant is a distinguishing feature that suggests the diagnosis with the appropriate clinical scenario (167).

Spike-and-wave discharges are uncommon. As the disease progresses, the electroencephalogram becomes increasingly disorganized. A photoconvulsive response can be seen with photic stimulation (28). On neuroimaging, cerebellar atrophy is occasionally observed. The diagnosis can be made by detection of the intracytoplasmic inclusion body (Lafora body) on skin, liver, or muscle biopsy. A negative biopsy does not exclude the diagnosis, and if a high clinical suspicion is present, then a cortical biopsy may be indicated. There is no effective treatment for this disorder, and the average life span after onset is 2 to 10 years.

Unverricht-Lundborg Progressive Familial Myoclonic Epilepsy (Baltic Myoclonus)

This familial form of progressive encephalopathy is characterized by relentless myoclonus and generalized seizures. Onset is in childhood or adolescence with seizures that are predominantly myoclonic and frequently occur after awakening. Absence and atonic seizures are also observed. Although the familial pattern may initially indicate an idiopathic form of epilepsy, the severity of the myoclonus soon suggests a form of progressive myoclonus epilepsy.

Myoclonus can become quite disabling, interfering with speech and swallowing, and is often provoked by voluntary movement and excitement. Cognition is generally retained, although a mild decline may be observed later in the disease course. Cerebellar ataxia, hyporeflexia, wasting of the distal musculature, and signs of chronic denervation on electromyography may be seen. The electroencephalogram reveals progressive slowing, with generalized 3-to-5-per-second spike-wave-like bursts that are frontally predominant. Paroxysmal flicker responses and generalized spikes and polyspikes are seen with photic stimulation (168,169). Although this disorder occurs worldwide, it has an especially high incidence in Finland, Estonia, and areas of the Mediterranean. There are no specific diagnostic tests; however, DNA markers linked to the defective gene for cystatin B on the distal part of chromosome 21 were initially identified in affected individuals in Finland and the Mediterranean. The gene locus is 21q22.3 (170). Phenytoin should be avoided as it may exacerbate polymyoclonus (171). Death occurs in the third to fourth decade of life.

Myoclonic Epilepsy with Ragged-red Fibers and Mitochondrial Encephalopathy with Lactic Acidosis and Stroke-like Episodes

Onset of MERRF occurs before 20 years of age, with ataxia and seizures that are predominantly myoclonic. Affected individuals may have short stature, neurosensory hearing loss, optic atrophy, myopathy, or encephalopathy. Electroencephalogram findings may include background slowing, focal epileptiform discharges, and atypical spike or sharp and slow-wave discharges that have a variable association with the myoclonic jerks (53). Suppression of these discharges during sleep is characteristic. As with many of the progressive myoclonus epilepsies, giant somatosensory evoked potentials are observed. Lactic acidosis and the presence of ragged-red fibers on muscle biopsy are essential features of the diagnosis. The inheritance pattern is compatible with maternal transmission. In the majority of cases, a point mutation at position 8344 of the mitochondrial gene for transfer ribonucleic acid (tRNA)-lysine has been identified.

Classically, MELAS presents in childhood with the sudden onset of stroke-like episodes. Migraine-like headaches, progressive deafness, seizures, cognitive decline, and myopathic features may accompany these symptoms. In an evaluation by Berkovic and associates (172) of 12 patients with MELAS, epilepsia partialis continua was frequently seen, and seizures often evolved into partial or generalized status epilepticus. Whereas myoclonic seizures are prominent in individuals with MERRF, in an evaluation of 31 patients by Canafoglia and colleagues (173), partial seizures were seen more often in individuals with MELAS (although there was an overlap of seizure types between the two syndromes). Fujimoto and coworkers (174) reviewed 79 electroencephalograms in six patients with MELAS and two of their relatives with MELA (mitochondrial myopathy, encephalopathy, and lactic acidosis, without stroke-like episodes). In the acute stage following a stroke-like episode, 10 of 11 electroencephalograms showed focal high-voltage delta waves with polyspikes. These discharges were interpreted as ictal phenomena. Later, focal spikes or sharp waves and 14- and 6-Hz positive bursts were frequently recorded. The observed seizures were characterized by focal clonic and myoclonic movements with migrainous headache. Lactic acid is elevated in the blood, and ragged-red fibers are present on muscle biopsy. Four point mutations are predominantly seen with MELAS. Three of these (3243, 3250, and 3271) affect the mitochondrial DNA gene of tRNA-leucine. The other mutation involves a coding region of complex I of the respiratory chain.

Dentatorubral-Pallidoluysian Atrophy

Dentatorubral-pallidoluysian atrophy (DRPLA) is a rare autosomal dominant disease that is seen predominantly in the Japanese population. The disorder is related to a trinucleotide (CAG) expansion on chromosome 12p (12p13.31) (175). Clinical manifestations are dependent on the length of the unstable trinucleotide repeats and vary, from a juvenile-onset progressive myoclonus epilepsy to an adult-onset syndrome with ataxia, dementia, and choreoathetosis (176). The juvenile form can also be variable in its presentation. In general, symptoms begin in infancy to early childhood with myoclonus, ataxia, dementia, opsoclonus, or seizures that can be generalized tonic-clonic, atypical absence, or atonic (177). The electroencephalogram characteristically shows bursts of slowing, irregular spike-and-wave discharges, and multifocal paroxysmal discharges. A photoparoxysmal response is seen, and myoclonic seizures can often be triggered by photic stimulation. Pathologic features are striking, with neuronal loss and gliosis in the dentatorubral and pallidoluysian structures.

DIAGNOSTIC INVESTIGATION IN METABOLIC AND MITOCHONDRIAL DISORDERS

The diagnosis of genetically determined metabolic diseases can be complicated for many reasons. The classic aminoacidopathies and organic acidurias, once suspected, can be easily diagnosed via appropriate blood or urine measurements. However, the diagnosis of a rare condition such as CDG may require specific isoelectric focusing of the serum sialotransferrin isoform pattern in a specialized research laboratory. Before obtaining appropriate metabolic, biochemical, or tissue specimens, the physician should try to formulate a differential diagnosis. Age at onset, clinical findings, family history, ethnicity, and neurologic examination continue to be the most important considerations in initial diagnostic possibilities. Neurologists experienced in metabolic disorders can often narrow the list of possible disorders at the first clinical encounter. Therefore, a consultation

with a metabolic specialist is useful before or after initial screening tests are performed in such patients.

The presence of macular cherry-red spots, abnormal appearance of the hair, or a peculiar distribution of fat over the posterior flanks or thighs immediately suggests a diagnosis of Tay-Sachs disease, Menkes disease, or CDG, respectively. Deceleration of head growth during infancy, with consequent acquired microcephaly, implies Glut-1 deficiency syndrome or another defect of energy metabolism, the infantile form of neuronal ceroid lipofuscinosis, or Rett syndrome, among other possibilities. Dislocated lenses and a seizure followed by a stroke are characteristic of homocystinuria. Seizures with stroke-like episodes also suggest CDG, mitochondrial disorders, ornithine transcarbamoylase deficiency, and glycolytic disorders. Genetically determined metabolic diseases often have a saltatory historical pattern in contrast to neurodegenerative diseases, which are inexorably progressive.

In other circumstances, the underlying problem will not be intuitively obvious and the patient's disorder may masquerade as a form of cryptogenic epilepsy. To some extent, the differential diagnosis can be pared down by calling to mind a discrete list of diseases for each of the different epilepsy syndromes (Table 37.1). Nevertheless, it is likely that screening evaluations will need to be performed. Table 37.2 presents metabolic diseases associated with seizures and common biochemical abnormalities. A complete blood cell count with differential and platelet count should be obtained in every case. Bone marrow depression occurs in the ketotic hyperglycinemic syndromes, and the peripheral smear may reveal such important clues as a macrocytic anemia or vacuolated lymphocytes. A complete serum chemistry profile will uncover carbohydrate and electrolyte disturbances or specific organ dysfunction. Calcium and magnesium concentrations should be determined in every case. A low uric acid concentration raises the possibility of molybdenum cofactor deficiency, and low blood urea nitrogen suggests a defect involving the urea cycle. Quantitative measurement of plasma and urinary amino acids is necessary in order to identify the various aminoacidopathies. A urinary organic acid profile should be performed using the first morning urine specimen.

A lumbar puncture is required to measure various CSF metabolites. An elevated CSF protein concentration is characteristic of metachromatic leukodystrophy and globoid cell leukodystrophy. A low CSF glucose concentration is consistent with hypoglycemia caused by a defect of gluconeogenesis or a defect in the transport of glucose across the blood–brain barrier (Glut-1 deficiency syndrome). A low CSF folate concentration suggests a defect involving folate metabolism. The presence of altered levels of CSF amino acids—specifically, glycine, glutamate, serine, and GABA—may be associated with NKH, pyridoxine-dependent epilepsy, 3-phosphoglycerate dehydrogenase deficiency, or another defect in the GABA shunt. Lactate and pyruvate values are elevated in CSF disorders of cerebral

TABLE 37.1

METABOLIC DISEASES MASQUERADING AS EPILEPSY SYNDROMES

Neonatal seizures
- Urea cycle defects: argininosuccinate synthetase, ornithine transcarbamoylase, carbamoyl phosphate synthetase
- Organic acidurias: maple syrup urine disease
- Disorders of biotin metabolism: early onset multiple carboxylase deficiency (holocarboxylase synthetase deficiency)
- Peroxisomal disorders: Zellweger syndrome, acylcoenzyme A oxidase deficiency
- Other: molybdenum cofactor deficiency/sulfite oxidase deficiency, disorders of fructose metabolism, pyridoxine dependency

Early myoclonic encephalopathy/early infantile epileptogenic encephalopathy
- Nonketotic hyperglycinemia
- Propionic acidemia
- D-Glycine acidemia
- Leigh syndrome
- Creatine deficiency

Cryptogenic epilepsies other than infantile spasms and Lennox-Gastaut syndrome
- G_{M2} gangliosidoses
- G_{M1} gangliosidosis
- Infantile neuroaxonal dystrophy
- Neuronal ceroid lipofuscinosis
- Glut-1 deficiency
- Late-onset multiple carboxylase deficiency
- Disorders of folate metabolism, methylenetetrahydrofolate reductase deficiency
- Arginase deficiency (urea cycle defect)
- Tetrahydrobiopterin deficiency (aminoaciduria)
- Tyrosinemia type I (case report)

West syndrome, generalized
- Phenylketonuria/hyperphenylalaninemias
- Pyruvate dehydrogenase
- Pyruvate carboxylase
- Congenital disorder of glycosylation type III
- Organic acidurias
- Aminoacidurias

Lennox-Gastaut syndrome
- Neuronal ceroid lipofuscinosis
- Sialidoses

Progressive myoclonus epilepsies
- Lafora disease
- Unverricht-Lundborg disease
- MERRF/MELAS
- Dentatorubral-pallidoluysian atrophy
- Neuronal ceroid lipofuscinosis
- Sialidoses
- Gaucher disease

MERRF, myoclonic epilepsy with ragged-red fibers; MELAS, mitochondrial encephalomyopathy with lactic acidosis and stroke-like episodes.

energy metabolism, including pyruvate dehydrogenase deficiency, pyruvate carboxylase deficiency, numerous disturbances of the respiratory chain, and Menkes disease. A low CSF lactate value may be seen in the Glut-1 deficiency syndrome.

TABLE 37.2

METABOLIC DISEASES AND BIOCHEMICAL ABNORMALITIES

Seizures and metabolic acidosis
- Pyruvate dehydrogenase complex deficiency
- Mitochondrial encephalomyopathies
- Multiple carboxylase deficiency disorders
- Intermittent maple syrup urine disease
- Isovaleric aciduria
- Glutaric aciduria
- Propionic acidemia
- Methylmalonic acidemia

Seizures and hypoglycemia
- Glycogen storage diseases
- Fructose 1,6-bisphosphatase deficiency
- Hereditary fructose intolerance
- Organic acidemias (propionic, methylmalonic, and isovaleric)

Seizures and hyperammonemia
- Biotinidase deficiency
- Carnitine palmitoyltransferase type I deficiency
- Hyperammonemia-hyperornithinemia-homocitrullinuria disorder
- Methylmalonic aciduria
- Oxidative metabolism disorders
- Propionic acidemia
- Urea cycle defects

Abnormal CSF biogenic amines and measurement of biopterin metabolism are suggestive of several disorders associated with disturbed neurotransmission. Of these, disorders affecting dopamine and serotonin biosynthesis (tetrahydrobiopterin defects, tyrosine hydroxylase deficiency, and aromatic L-amino acid decarboxylase deficiency) may present with a well-characterized syndrome between 2 and 8 months of age. The symptoms include hypersalivation, temperature dysregulation, pinpoint pupils, ptosis, oculogyric crises, hypokinesis, rigidity, chorea, swallowing difficulties, drowsiness, myoclonic seizures, microcephaly, progressive mental retardation, and irritability. In addition, an unknown diagnostic marker compound appears on high-performance liquid chromatograms of some children with discontinuous EEG patterns and myoclonic seizures. Seizures in these children are resistant to AEDs but respond well to folinic acid (178).

Tissue biopsy specimens also provide important information in establishing a diagnosis. Specimens of skin, peripheral nerve, and skeletal muscle may provide useful clues as well. Only rarely would a liver or brain biopsy be necessary. Rectal and conjunctival biopsies are seldom performed.

At times, the EEG features may be sufficiently distinctive to suggest the diagnosis of a limited number of conditions (Table 37.3). A suppression-burst pattern is seen in patients with NKH, PKU, maple syrup urine disease, and molybdenum cofactor/sulfite oxidase deficiency, in addition to other disorders. Some distinctive EEG features include a comb-like rhythm with 7- to 9-Hz central activity, which is seen in

TABLE 37.3

ELECTROENCEPHALOGRAPHIC PATTERNS AND THEIR ASSOCIATED DISORDERS

Electroencephalogram pattern	Disorder
Comb-like rhythm	Maple syrup urine disease, propionic acidemia
Fast central spikes	Tay-Sachs disease
Rhythmic vertex-positive spikes	Sialidosis type I
Vanishing electroencephalogram	Infantile neuronal ceroid lipofuscinosis type I
High-amplitude 16- to 24-Hz activity	Infantile neuroaxonal dystrophy
Diminished spikes during sleep	Progressive myoclonus epilepsy
Giant somatosensory evoked potentials	Progressive myoclonus epilepsy
Marked photosensitivity	Progressive myoclonus epilepsy and neuronal ceroid lipofuscinosis, particularly type II
Burst-suppression pattern	Neonatal citrullinemia, nonketotic hyperglycinemia, propionic acidemia, Leigh syndrome, D-glycine acidemia, molybdenum cofactor deficiency, Menkes disease, holocarboxylase synthetase deficiency, neonatal adrenoleukodystrophy
Hypsarrhythmia	Zellweger syndrome, neonatal adrenoleukodystrophy, neuroaxonal dystrophy, nonketotic hyperglycinemia, phenylketonuria, congenital defect of glycosylation type III

patients with maple syrup urine disease and propionic acidemia; vertex-positive polyspikes, seen in sialidosis type I; biooccipital polymorphic delta activity, seen in X-linked adrenoleukodystrophy; and 16- to 24-Hz invariant activity, seen in those with infantile neuroaxonal dystrophy.

Brain imaging provides important information, although findings are rarely specific. Progressive atrophy is associated with neuronal ceroid lipofuscinosis and Alpers syndrome. White matter signal abnormalities are characteristic of metachromatic leukodystrophy, globoid cell encephalopathy, PKU, some mitochondrial diseases, Canavan disease, GABA transaminase deficiency, and some organic acidurias. Calcification of the cerebral cortex and basal ganglia is seen with many inherited metabolic diseases. Brain MRA may show abnormal dilatation and tortuosity of intracranial blood vessels in patients with Menkes disease. Brain MRS may demonstrate elevated lactate levels in those with various mitochondrial diseases, elevated *N*-acetylaspartic acid in patients with Canavan disease, or depressed creatine in those with inborn errors of creatine metabolism.

Evaluation in the Absence of Overt Clinical Clues

When the clinician is asked to evaluate a child with a progressive encephalopathy manifesting with seizures and no overt clinical clues, a screening paradigm must be used. There is seemingly no limit to the number of tests that can be performed, and the financial burden of these investigations can quickly become considerable. Accordingly, we propose the following screening tests, which should be tailored to the age and symptoms at presentation.

General

- Complete blood cell count with differential
- Electrolyte testing (SMAC-20)
- Serum amino acids
- Urine organic acids

- Serum lactate/pyruvate
- Very-long-chain fatty acids
- Serum ammonia
- Serum carnitine
- Electroencephalography
- MRI

Additional tests to consider

- Vitamin B$_6$ administration
- Lysosomal hydrolases
- Urine oligosaccharides/mucopolysaccharides
- Biotin treatment
- CSF studies
  - Glucose
  - Amino acids, including glycine and serine
  - Biogenic amines
- Serum copper/ceruloplasmin
- Serum transferrin isoelectric focusing for CDG
- Selective
  - Skin biopsy (neuronal ceroid lipofuscinoses, Lafora)
  - Muscle biopsy (MELAS, MERRF)
  - Nerve biopsy (neuroaxonal dystrophy)
  - MRS (creatine deficiency)
  - Bone marrow for Gaucher cells
  - DNA testing for MELAS, MERRF, DRPLA, Baltic myoclonus

TREATMENT OF METABOLIC AND MITOCHONDRIAL DISORDERS

The treatment of seizures associated with inherited metabolic and mitochondrial diseases should focus on the metabolic disturbance. Seizures associated with hypoglycemia, hyponatremia, hypocalcemia, and hypomagnesemia respond best to correction of these disturbances and should be treated with appropriate replacement therapy. Dietary treatment is beneficial for many inherited metabolic

TABLE 37.4

SCREENING TESTS FOR METABOLIC DISORDERS ASSOCIATED WITH EPILEPSY

Age	EEG Features	Screening Tests	Disorders
Neonatal	Burst-suppression or multifocal spikes	Vitamin B_6 administration	Vitamin B_6-responsive disorders
	Burst-suppression or multifocal spikes	CSF amino acids	Nonketotic hyperglycinemia
	Burst-suppression or multifocal spikes	Urinary sulfite dipstick/ serum uric acid	Molybdenum cofactor deficiency/sulfite oxidase deficiency
	Burst-suppression or multifocal spikes	VLCFAs	Peroxisomal disorders
	Burst-suppression or multifocal spikes	Lactate/pyruvate	Pyruvate dehydrogenase deficiency, pyruvate carboxylase deficiency, Leigh syndrome
	Burst-suppression or multifocal spikes	Serum ammonia	Early-onset multiple carboxylase deficiency
	Burst-suppression or multifocal spikes	Serum ammonia	Urea cycle defects—neonatal citrullinemia
	Low-amplitude slowing	Serum ammonia	Urea cycle defects—carbamoyl phosphate synthetase, ornithine transcarbamoylase, argininosuccinate synthetase
	Comblike rhythm	Serum amino acids	Maple syrup urine disease
	Dysmature features during sleep	Urine organic acids	Isovaleric aciduria
	Background slowing	Urine organic acids	Propionic acidemia
	Multifocal spikes, background slowing and depression	Urine organic acids	Methylmalonic acidemia
Early Infancy	Declining amplitude, very fast central spikes	Lysosomal hydrolases	Tay-Sachs disease (hexosaminidase A)
	Hypsarrhythmia	Lysosomal hydrolases	Krabbe disease (galactosylceramidase)
	Background slowing, rhythmic temporal theta in type II (juvenile form)	Urinary oligosaccharides	G_{M1} gangliosidosis (β-galactosidase)
	Burst-suppression/ multifocal spikes/slowed background	Biotin treatment/ biotinidase screen	Biotinidase deficiency
	Multifocal spikes/hypsarrhythmia	Serum amino acids	Methylenetetrahydrofolate reductase deficiency
	Hypsarrhythmia	Serum amino acids	Phenylketonuria and hyperphenylalaninemia, tyrosinemia type III, hyperammonemia-hyperornithinemia-homocitrullinuria syndrome, disorders of serine biosynthesis
	Hypsarrhythmia	Urine organic acids	Variety of organic acidurias, including 3-methylglutaconic aciduria, 3-hydroxy-3-methylglutaric aciduria, 3-hydroxybutyric aciduria, 4-hydroxybutyric aciduria
	Hypsarrhythmia	Serum copper/ ceruloplasmin	Menkes' disease
	Hypsarrhythmia	None	PEHO syndrome
	Slowing/2- to 3-Hz spike-wave discharges	CSF glucose	Glut-1 deficiency syndrome
Late Infancy	Multifocal spikes	Lysosomal hydrolases	α-N-acetylgalactosaminidase (Schindler disease)
	High-voltage, multifocal spikes	Lysosomal hydrolases	Metachromatic leukodystrophy
	Low-amplitude fast activity (12 to 15 Hz) alternating with generalized slowing	Urine mucopolysaccharides	Sanfilippo syndrome
	Vanishing EEG	Skin biopsy with EM	Infantile NCL
	Continuous anterior high-voltage 1 to 3 per second spike-wave–like activity	None	Alpers' disease
Childhood and Adolescence	Hypsarrhythmia	Serum transferrin isoelectric focusing	Congenital defects in glycosylation, CDG type III
	Background slowing with focal spikes	Urine organic acids/ serum amino acids	Homocystinuria
	EPC	Blood glucose	Diabetes mellitus with nonketotic hyperosmolar coma
	EPC and posterior attenuation/slowing	VLCFAs	Adrenoleukodystrophy
	Positive vertex spikes	Urine oligosaccharides	Sialidosis type I

TABLE 37.4
(continued)

Age	EEG Features	Screening Tests	Disorders
	4- to 6-Hz spike-wave discharges	Urine oligosaccharides	Sialidosis type II
	Rhythmic trains of spike or sharp waves at 6 to 10 per second	Gaucher cells in bone marrow	Gaucher type III
	High-amplitude fast activity (16 to 24 Hz), unaltered by eye opening	Nerve biopsy	Neuroaxonal dystrophy
	Multifocal spikes	Skin biopsy	NCL type III
	Generalized spike- and polyspike-wave discharges and occipital spikes, with photoparoxysmal response	Skin biopsy	Lafora disease
	Generalized 3- to 5-Hz spike-wave discharges with a frontal predominance	DNA testing (no screening tests)	Baltic myoclonus
	Generalized atypical spike-wave discharges	Lactate/pyruvate	MERRF
	Focal slowing and spikes, 14- and 6-Hz positive bursts	Lactate/pyruvate	MELAS
	Generalized spike-wave and photoparoxysmal response	Triplet repeats (no screening test available)	Dentatorubral-pallidoluysian atrophy

Abbreviations: CDG, congenital disorders of glycosylation; CSF, cerebrospinal fluid; EEG, electroencephalogram; EM, electron microscopy; EPC, epilepsia partialis continua; MELAS, mitochondrial encephalomyopathy with lactic acidosis and stroke-like episodes; MERRF, myoclonic epilepsy with ragged-red fibers; NCL, neuronal ceroid lipofuscinosis; PEHO, progressive encephalopathy with edema, hypsarrhythmia, and optic atrophy; VLCFAs, very-long-chain fatty acids.

diseases, including defects of the urea cycle, defects of fatty acid oxidation, gluconeogenic defects, aminoacidopathies, organic acidurias, and the Glut-1 deficiency syndrome. In particular, the ketogenic diet is effective in controlling seizures in patients with the Glut-1 deficiency syndrome, and it improves cognitive outcome in patients with pyruvate dehydrogenase deficiency (E1). PKU can be well treated with a diet low in phenylalanine. Protein restriction is recommended for defects of the urea cycle, and fat restriction is advised for defects involving fatty acid oxidation. Pyridoxine-dependent epilepsy and other vitamin-responsive syndromes can be cured by early diagnosis and prompt administration of the specific vitamin or cofactor. Enzyme protein replacement has proved effective in patients with Gaucher disease. Bone marrow transplantation has been used effectively to treat patients with mucopolysaccharidoses and adrenoleukodystrophy. Some patients with urea cycle defects, gangliosidoses, or leukodystrophies have improved with liver transplantation.

Conventional AEDs may be useful adjuncts to the specific treatment of a metabolic disorder but are often ineffective when used alone. In some circumstances, patients with metabolic derangements or neurodegenerative disorders may worsen with AED treatment that may be contraindicated—for example, phenytoin in patients with Unverricht-Lundborg disease; corticotropin and ketogenic diet in those with pyruvate carboxylase deficiency; ketogenic diet in patients with organic acidurias; and valproate in individuals with urea cycle and fatty acid oxidation defects. Metabolites of valproate interfere with β oxidation, and valproate use

depletes carnitine stores. Valproate, topiramate, zonisamide, and acetazolamide are relatively contraindicated with the ketogenic diet. Kidney stones are a complication associated with the ketogenic diet, as well as with acetazolamide, zonisamide, and topiramate use. Carnitine should be considered as a supplement in patients with any metabolic disorder that presents with seizures, particularly when valproate is used (179). An experimental report of altered glucose transport with phenobarbital raises concern for its use in patients with Glut-1 deficiency syndrome (180).

CONCLUSIONS

Seizures are often part of the clinical picture of inherited metabolic disorders, particularly when these conditions first appear during the neonatal period or infancy. Unfortunately, the clinical presentation of seizures is seldom distinctive enough to allow immediate diagnosis. Nevertheless, the timing of onset, certain characteristic clinical features, family history, and sometimes EEG findings may facilitate recognition of the more common diagnoses (Table 37.1). Why seizures commonly accompany some metabolic diseases and infrequently occur in others is only partially understood, but certain correlations are intuitively obvious. Defects in energy metabolism are commonly associated with seizures—for example, the Glut-1 deficiency syndrome, other hypoglycemic syndromes, and defects of pyruvate metabolism; the Krebs cycle; and the respiratory chain. Also, seizures frequently accompany inherited metabolic disorders that affect neurotransmission, such as NKH, pyridoxine-dependent epilepsy, and GABA transaminase deficiency. A more fundamental common mechanism may be operative in many of these conditions. For example, an alteration in the ratio of glutamic acid to GABA may exist in disorders associated with cerebral energy failure and in conditions affecting the GABA shunt. Any inherited metabolic condition in which the extracellular glutamate concentration is elevated and the extracellular GABA concentration is lowered would lower the seizure threshold. Recent studies have confirmed this speculation in patients with symptomatic hypoglycemia, NKH, and pyridoxine-dependent epilepsy.

In contrast, defects of fatty acid oxidation are less likely to be associated with epilepsy. Fatty acids do not serve as oxidizable fuels for brain metabolism. Brain function is compromised mainly when the patient is subjected to fasting and hypoketotic hypoglycemia develops. Under these conditions, the brain is deprived of its two primary fuels, glucose and ketone bodies, and disturbed consciousness and seizures may occur. An exception is short-chain acyl-CoA dehydrogenase deficiency, which is frequently associated with seizures in the absence of hypoglycemia.

Metabolic diseases provide some important insights into the neurochemical determinants of the epileptic state. Alterations of neurotransmission and ion channels are common themes in the pathophysiology of these diverse metabolic conditions. All infants and young children seen with unexplained seizure disorders (cryptogenic epilepsy) should be evaluated for an inherited metabolic disorder. A positive family history may provide an important clue, and careful studies of blood, urine, and CSF may reveal characteristic abnormalities. Table 37.4 presents an overview of possible screening tests organized according to age. Primary correction of the metabolic disturbance is the optimal treatment for the associated epilepsy, even though conventional AEDs may blunt the expression of the seizures. In certain situations, AEDs are ineffective or may actually worsen the underlying disease. Careful study of patients will continue to identify novel inherited metabolic disorders and lead to more direct and effective treatments of these conditions.

REFERENCES

1. Dalla Bernardina B, Aicardi J, Goutieres F, et al. Glycine encephalopathy. *Neuropadiatrie* 1979;10:209–225.
2. Lyon G, Adams RD, Kolodny EH. *Neurology of hereditary metabolic diseases of children*, 2nd ed. New York: McGraw-Hill, 1996.
3. Matalon R, Naidu S, Hughes JR, et al. Nonketotic hyperglycinemia: treatment with diazepam—a competitor for glycine receptors. *Pediatrics* 1983;71:581–584.
4. Hamosh A, McDonald JW, Valle D, et al. Dextromethorphan and high-dose benzoate therapy for nonketotic hyperglycinemia in an infant. *J Pediatr* 1992;121:131–135.
5. Zammarchi E, Donati MA, Ciani F, et al. Failure of early dextromethorphan and sodium benzoate therapy in an infant with nonketotic hyperglycemia. *Neuropediatrics* 1994;25:274–276.
6. Van Hove JL, Kishnani P, Muenzer J, et al. Benzoate therapy and cartinine deficiency in non-ketotic hyperglycinemia. *Am J Med Genet* 1995;59:444–453.
7. Bu DF, Erlander MG, Hitz BC, et al. Two human glutamate decarboxylases, 65-kDa GAD and 67-kDa GAD, are each encoded by a single gene. *Proc Natl Acad Sci U S A* 1992;89:2115–2119.
8. Bu DF, Tobin AJ. The exon-intron organization of the genes (GAD1 and GAD2) encoding two human glutamate decarboxylases (GAD67 and GAD65) suggests that they derive from a common ancestral GAD. *Genomics* 1994;21:222–228.
9. Cormier-Daire V, Dagoneau N, Nabbout R, et al. A gene for pyridoxine-dependent epilepsy maps to chromosome 5q31. *Am J Hum Genet* 2000;67:991–993.
10. Wang PJ, Lee WT, Hwu WL, et al. The controversy regarding diagnostic criteria for early myoclonic encephalopathy. *Brain Dev* 1998;20:530–535.
11. Chou ML, Wang HS, Hung PC, et al. Late-onset pyridoxine-dependent seizures: report of two cases. *Zhonghua Min Guo Xiao Er Ke Yi Xue Hui Za Zhi* 1995;36:434–437.
12. Goutieres F, Aicardi J. Atypical presentations of pyridoxine-dependent seizures: a treatable cause of intractable epilepsy in infants. *Ann Neurol* 1985;17:117–120.
13. Johnson JL, Waud WR, Rajagopalan KV, et al. Inborn errors of molybdenum metabolism: combined deficiencies of sulfite oxidase and xanthine dehydrogenase in a patient lacking the molybdenum cofactor. *Proc Natl Acad Sci U S A* 1980;77:3715–3719.
14. Shalata A, Mandel H, Reiss J, et al. Localization of a gene for molybdenum cofactor deficiency, on the short arm of chromosome 6, by homozygosity mapping. *Am J Hum Genet* 1998;63:148–154.
15. Reiss J, Dorche B, Stallmeyer B, et al. Human molybdopterin synthase gene: genomic structure and mutations in molybdenum cofactor deficiency type B. *Am J Hum Genet* 1999;64:706–711.
16. Reiss J, Gross-Hardt S, Christensen E, et al. A mutation in the gene for the neurotransmitter receptor-clustering protein gephyrin causes a novel form of molybdenum cofactor deficiency. *Am J Hum Genet* 2001;68:208–213.
17. Slot HM, Overweg-Plandsoen WCG, Bakker HD, et al. Molybdenum-cofactor deficiency: an easily missed cause of neonatal convulsions. *Neuropediatrics* 1993;24:139–142.
18. Wadman SK, Cats BP, de Bree PK. Sulfite oxidase deficiency and the detection of urinary sulfite [letter]. *Eur J Pediatr* 1983;141:62–63.
19. Rupar CA, Gillett J, Gordon BA, et al. Isolated sulfite oxidase deficiency. *Neuropediatrics* 1996;27:299–304.
20. Takahashi Y, Suzuki Y, Kumazaki K, et al. Epilepsy in peroxisomal diseases. *Epilepsia* 1997;38:182–188.
21. Santos MJ, Imanaka T, Shio H, et al. Peroxisomal membrane ghosts in Zellweger syndrome—aberrant organelle assembly. *Science* 1988;239:1536–1538.
22. Verma NP, Hart ZH, Nigro M. Electrophysiologic studies in neonatal adrenoleukodystrophy. *Electroencephalogr Clin Neurophysiol* 1985;60:7–15.
23. Dodt G, Braverman N, Wong C, et al. Mutations in the PTS1 receptor gene, PXR1, define complementation group 2 of the peroxisome biogenesis disorders. *Nat Genet* 1995;9:115–125.
24. Poll-The BT, Roels F, Ogier H, et al. A new peroxisomal disorder with enlarged peroxisomes and a specific deficiency of acyl-CoA oxidase (pseudo-neonatal adrenoleukodystrophy). *Am J Hum Genet* 1988;42:422–434.
25. Willard-Mack CL, Koehler RC, Hirata T, et al. Inhibition of glutamine synthetase reduces ammonia-induced astrocyte swelling in rat. *Neuroscience* 1996;71:589–599.
26. Garcia-Alvarez M, Nordli DR, De Vivo DC. Inherited metabolic disorders. In: Engel J Jr, Pedley TA, eds. *Epilepsy: a comprehensive textbook*. Philadelphia: Lippincott-Raven, 1997:2547–2562.
27. Verma NP, Hart ZH, Kooi KA. Electroencephalographic findings in urea-cycle disorders. *Electroencephalogr Clin Neurophysiol* 1984;57:105–112.
28. Naidu S, Niedermeyer E. Degenerative disorders of the central nervous system. In: Niedermeyer E, Lopes da Silva F, eds. *Electroencephalography: basic principles, clinical applications, and related fields*, 4th ed. Baltimore, MD: Williams & Wilkins, 1999:360–382.

29. Todo S, Starzl TE, Tzakis A, et al. Orthotopic liver transplantation for urea cycle enzyme deficiency. *Hepatology* 1992;15:419–422.
30. Yazaki M, Ikeda S, Takei Y, et al. Complete neurological recovery of an adult patient with type II citrullinemia after living related partial liver transplantation. *Transplantation* 1996;62:1679–1684.
31. Menkes JH, Hurst PL, Craig JM. A new syndrome: progressive familial infantile cerebral dysfunction associated with unusual urinary substance. *Pediatrics* 1954;14:462–467.
32. Fekete G, Plattner R, Crabb DW, et al. Localization of the human gene for the El alpha subunit of branched chain keto acid dehydrogenase (BCKDHA) to chromosome 19q13.1–q13.2. *Cytogenet Cell Genet* 1989;50:236–237.
33. Trottier A, Metrakos K, Geoffroy G, et al. A characteristic EEG finding in newborns with maple syrup urine disease (branched-chain keto aciduria). *Electroencephalogr Clin Neurophysiol* 1975;38:108.
34. Tharp BR. Unique EEG pattern (comb-like rhythm) in neonatal maple syrup urine disease. *Pediatr Neurol* 1992;8:65–68.
35. Korein J, Sansaricq C, Kalmijn M, et al. Maple syrup urine disease: clinical, EEG, and plasma amino acid correlations with a theoretical mechanism of acute neurotoxicity. *Int J Neurosci* 1994;79:21–45.
36. Kraus JP, Matsubara Y, Barton D, et al. Isolation of cDNA clones coding for rat isovaleryl-CoA dehydrogenase and assignment of the gene to human chromosome 15. *Genomics* 1987;1:264–269.
37. Sidbury JB Jr, Smith EK, Harlan W. An inborn error of short-chain fatty acid metabolism: the odor-of-sweaty-feet syndrome. *J Pediatr* 1967;70:8–15.
38. Kennerknecht I, Klett C, Hameister H. Assignment of the human gene propionyl coenzyme A carboxylase, alpha-chain, (PCCA) to chromosome 13q32 by in situ hybridization. *Genomics* 1992;14:550–551.
39. Stigsby B, Yarworth SM, Rahbeeni Z, et al. Neurophysiologic correlates of organic acidemias: a survey of 107 patients. *Brain Dev* 1994;16(Suppl):125–144.
40. Bartholomew DW, Batshaw ML, Allen RH, et al. Therapeutic approaches to cobalamin-C methylmalonic acidemia and homocystinuria. *J Pediatr* 1988;112:32–39.
41. Enns GM, Barkovich AJ, Rosenblatt DS, et al. Progressive neurological deterioration and MRI changes in cblC methylmalonic acidaemia treated with hydroxocobalamin. *J Inherit Metab Dis* 1999;22:599–607.
42. Mahoney MJ, Bick D. Recent advances in the inherited methylmalonic acidemias. *Acta Paediatr Scand* 1987;76:689–696.
43. Guevara-Campos J, Gonzalez-de-Guevara L, Medina-Atopo M. Methylmalonic aciduria associated with myoclonic convulsions, psychomotor retardation and hypsarrhythmia [Spanish]. *Rev Neurol* 2003;36:735–737.
44. Bonnefont JP, Demaugre F, Prip-Buus C, et al. Carnitine palmitoyltransferase deficiencies. *Mol Genet Metab* 1999;68:424–440.
45. Tein I. Role of carnitine and fatty acid oxidation and its defects in infantile epilepsy. *J Child Neurol* 2002;17(Suppl 3):3S57–3S82.
46. Brown GK, Otero LJ, LeGris M, et al. Pyruvate dehydrogenase deficiency. *J Med Genet* 1994;31:875–879.
47. Otero LJ, Brown GK, Silver K, et al. Association of cerebral dysgenesis and lactic acidemia with X-linked PDH E1 alpha subunit mutations in females. *Pediatr Neurol* 1995;13:327–332.
48. De Vivo DC, Haymond MW, Leckie MP, et al. The clinical and biochemical implications of pyruvate carboxylase deficiency. *J Clin Endocrinol Metab* 1977;45:1281–1296.
49. Rutledge SL, Snead OC III, Kelly DR, et al. Pyruvate carboxylase deficiency: acute exacerbation after ACTH treatment of infantile spasms. *Pediatr Neurol* 1989;5:249–252.
50. DiMauro S, De Vivo DC. Genetic heterogeneity in Leigh syndrome [letter]. *Ann Neurol* 1996;40:5–7.
51. Leigh D. Subacute necrotizing encephalomyelopathy in an infant. *J Neurol Neurosurg Psychiatry* 1951;14:216–221.
52. DiMauro S, Bonilla E, De Vivo DC. Does the patient have a mitochondrial encephalomyopathy? *J Child Neurol* 1999;14(Suppl 1):S23–S35.
53. So N, Kuzniecky R, Berkovic S, et al. Electrophysiological studies in myoclonus epilepsy with ragged-red fibers (MERRF) [abstract]. *Electroencephalogr Clin Neurophysiol* 1988;69:50P.
54. DiMauro S, Ricci E, Hirano M, et al. Epilepsy in mitochondrial encephalomyopathies. *Epilepsy Res Suppl* 1991;4:173–180.
55. Kamoshita S, Mizutani I, Fukuyama Y. Leigh's subacute necrotizing encephalomyelopathy in a child with infantile spasms and hypsarrhythmia. *Dev Med Child Neurol* 1970;12:430–435.
56. Tsao CY, Luquette M, Rusin JA, et al. Leigh syndrome, cytochrome C oxidase deficiency and hypsarrhythmia with infantile spasms. *Clin Electroencephalogr* 1997;28:214–217.
57. Elia M, Musumeci SA, Ferri R, et al. Leigh syndrome and partial deficit of cytochrome *c* oxidase associated with epilepsia partialis continua. *Brain Dev* 1996;18:207–211.
58. Van Erven PM, Colon EJ, Gabreels FJ, et al. Neurophysiological studies in the Leigh syndrome. *Brain Dev* 1986;8:590–595.
59. El-Maghrabi MR, Lange AJ, Jiang W, et al. Human fructose-1,6-bisphosphatase gene (FBP1): exon-intron organization, localization to chromosome bands 9q22.2-q22.3, and mutation screening in subjects with fructose-1,6-bisphosphatase deficiency. *Genomics* 1995;27:520–525.
60. Suzuki Y, Aoki Y, Ishida Y, et al. Isolation and characterization of mutations in the human holocarboxylase synthetase cDNA. *Nat Genet* 1994;8:122–128.
61. Aoki Y, Li X, Sakamoto O, et al. Identification and characterization of mutations in patients with holocarboxylase synthetase deficiency. *Hum Genet* 1999;104:143–148.
62. Nakai H, Byers MG, Nowak NJ, et al. Assignment of beta-hexosaminidase A alpha-subunit to human chromosomal region 15q23-q24. *Cytogenet Cell Genet* 1991;56:164.
63. Cobb W, Martin F, Pampiglione G. Cerebral lipidosis: an electroencephalographic study. *Brain* 1952;75:343–357.
64. Dana S, Wasmuth JJ. Selective linkage disruption in human-Chinese hamster cell hybrids: deletion mapping of the leuS, hexB, emtB, and chr genes on human chromosome 5. *Mol Cell Biol* 1982;2:1220–1228.
65. Zafeiriou DI, Anastasiou AL, Michelakaki EM, et al. Early infantile Krabbe disease: deceptively normal magnetic resonance imaging and serial neurophysiological studies. *Brain Dev* 1997;19:488–491.
66. Blom S, Hagberg B. EEG findings in late infantile metachromatic and globoid cell leucodystrophy. *Electroencephalogr Clin Neurophysiol* 1967;22:253–259.
67. Hagberg B. Krabbe's disease: clinical presentation of neurological variants. *Neuropediatrics* 1984;15(Suppl):11–15.
68. Kliemann FAD, Harden A, Pampiglione G. Some EEG observations in patients with Krabbe's disease. *Dev Med Child Neurol* 1969;11:475–484.
69. Krivit W, Shapiro EG, Peters C, et al. Hematopoietic stem-cell transplantation in globoid-cell leukodystrophy. *N Engl J Med* 1998;338:1119–1126.
70. Harden A, Martinovic Z, Pampiglione G. Neurophysiological studies in G_{M1} gangliosidosis. *Ital J Neurol Sci* 1982;3:201–206.
71. Salbert BA, Pellock JM, Wolf B. Characterization of seizures associated with biotinidase deficiency. *Neurology* 1993;43:1351–1355.
72. Cole H, Weremowicz S, Morton CC, et al. Localization of serum biotinidase (BTD) to human chromosome 3 in band p25. *Genomics* 1994;22:662–663.
73. Goyette P, Pai A, Milos R, et al. Gene structure of human and mouse methylenetetrahydrofolate reductase (MTHFR). *Mamm Genome* 1998;9:652–656.
74. Singer HS, Butler I, Rothenberg S, et al. Interrelationships among serum folate, CSF folate, neurotransmitters, and neuropsychiatric symptoms [abstract]. *Neurology* 1980;30:419.
75. Abeling NG, van Gennip AH, Blom H, et al. Rapid diagnosis and methionine administration: basis for a favourable outcome in a patient with methylene tetrahydrofolate reductase deficiency. *J Inherit Metab Dis* 1999;22:240–242.
76. Lanzkowsky P. Congenital malabsorption of folate. *Am J Med* 1970;48:580–583.
77. Corbeel L, Van den Berghe G, Jaeken J, et al. Congenital folate malabsorption. *Eur J Pediatr* 1985;143:284–290.
78. Stromberger C, Bodamer OA, Stockler-Ipsiroglu S. Clinical characteristics and diagnostic clues in inborn errors of creatine metabolism. *J Inherit Metab Dis* 2003;26:299–308.

79. Leuzzi V. Inborn errors of creatine metabolism and epilepsy: clinical features, diagnosis, and treatment. *J Child Neurol* 2002;17 (Suppl 3):3S89–3S97.

80. Schulze A. Creatine deficiency syndromes. *Mol Cell Biochem* 2003;244:143–150.

81. De Vivo DC, Trifiletti RR, Jacobson RI, et al. Defective glucose transport across the blood-brain barrier as a cause of persistent hypoglycorrhachia, seizures, and developmental delay. *N Engl J Med* 1991;325:703–709.

82. De Vivo DC, Garcia-Alvarez M, Ronen G, et al. Glucose transporter protein deficiency: an emerging syndrome with therapeutic implications. *Int Pediatr* 1995;10:51–56.

83. Klepper J, Garcia-Alvarez M, O'Driscoll KR, et al. Erythrocyte 3-O-methyl-D-glucose uptake assay for diagnosis of glucose-transporter-protein syndrome. *J Clin Lab Anal* 1999;13:116–121.

84. Shows TB, Eddy RL, Byers MG, et al. Polymorphic human glucose gene (GLUT) is on chromosome 1p31.3–p35. *Diabetes* 1987;36:546–549.

85. Seidner G, Alvarez MG, Yeh JI, et al. GLUT-1 deficiency syndrome caused by haploinsufficiency of the blood-brain barrier hexose carrier. *Nat Genet* 1998;18:188–191.

86. Wang D, Kranz-Eble P, De Vivo DC. Mutational analysis of GLUT1 (SLC2A1) in Glut-1 deficiency syndrome. *Hum Mutat* 2000;16:224–231.

87. Brockmann K, Wang D, Korenke CG, et al. Autosomal dominant glut-1 deficiency syndrome and familial epilepsy. *Ann Neurol* 2001;50:476–485.

88. Klepper J, Willemsen M, Verrips A, et al. Autosomal dominant transmission of GLUT1 deficiency. *Hum Mol Genet* 2001;10:63–68.

89. Leary LD, Wang D, Nordli DR Jr, et al. Seizure characterization and electroencephalographic features in Glut-1 deficiency syndrome. *Epilepsia* 2003;44:701–707.

90. Lehnert W, Niederhoff H, Junker A, et al. A case of biotin-responsive 3-methylcrotonylglycin- and 3-hydroxyisovaleric aciduria. *Eur J Pediatr* 1979;132:107–114.

91. Gibson KM, Wappner RS, Jooste S, et al. Variable clinical presentation in three patients with 3-methylglutaconyl-coenzyme A hydratase deficiency. *J Inherit Metab Dis* 1998;21:631–638.

92. Wang S, Nadeau JH, Duncan A, et al. 3-Hydroxy-3-methylglutaryl coenzyme A lyase (HL): cloning and characterization of a mouse liver HL cDNA and subchromosomal mapping of the human and mouse HL genes. *Mamm Genome* 1993;4:382–387.

93. Land JM, Goulder P, Johnson A, et al. Glutaric aciduria type 1 an atypical presentation together with some observations upon treatment and the possible cause of cerebral damage. *Neuropediatrics* 1992;23:322–326.

94. O'Connell P, Leppert M, Hoff M, et al. A linkage map for human chromosome 12 [abstract]. *Am J Hum Genet* 1985;37:A169.

95. Low NL, Bosma JF, Armstrong MD. Studies on phenylketonuria. VI. EEG studies on phenylketonuria. *AMA Arch Neurol Psychiatry* 1957;77:359–365.

96. Pietz J, Schmidt E, Matthis P, et al. EEGs in phenylketonuria. I: Follow-up to adulthood; II: Short-term diet-related changes in EEGs and cognitive function. *Dev Med Child Neurol* 1993;35:54–64.

97. Swaiman KF. Aminoacidopathies and organic acidemias resulting from deficiency of enzyme activity and transport abnormalities. In: Swaiman KF, Ashwal S, eds. *Pediatric neurology, principles & practice*, 3rd ed. St. Louis, MO: Mosby-Year Book, Inc. 1999:377–410.

98. Donker DN, Reits D, Van Sprang FJ, et al. Computer analysis of the EEG as an aid in the evaluation of dietetic treatment in phenylketonuria. *Electroencephalogr Clin Neurophysiol* 1979;46:205–213.

99. Romstad A, Kalkanoglu HS, Coskun T, et al. Molecular analysis of 16 Turkish families with DHPR deficiency using denaturing gradient gel electrophoresis (DGGE). *Hum Genet* 2000;107:546–553.

100. Thony B, Heizmann CW, Mattei MG. Chromosomal location of two human genes encoding tetrahydrobiopterin-metabolizing enzymes: 6-pyrovoyltetrahydrobiopterin synthase maps to 11q22.3–q23.3, and pterin-4-alpha-carbinolamine dehydratase maps to 10q22. *Genomics* 1994;19:365–368.

101. Ichinose H, Ohye T, Takahashi E, et al. Hereditary progressive dystonia with marked diurnal fluctuation caused by mutations in the GTP cyclohydrolase I gene. *Nat Genet* 1994;8:236–242.

102. Ichinose H, Ohye T, Matsuda Y, et al. Characterization of mouse and human GTP cyclohydrolase I genes: mutations in patients with GTP cyclohydrolase I deficiency. *J Biol Chem* 1995;270:10062–10071.

103. Seshia SS, Perry TL, Dakshinamurti K, et al. Tyrosinemia and intractable seizures. *Epilepsia* 1984;25:457–463.

104. Ruetschi U, Dellsen A, Sahlin P, et al. Human 4-hydroxyphenylpyruvate dioxygenase. Primary structure and chromosomal localization of the gene. *Eur J Biochem* 1993;213:1081–1089.

105. Jaeken J. Genetic disorders of gamma-aminobutyric acid, glycine, and serine as causes of epilepsy. *J Child Neurol* 2002;17(Suppl 3):3S84–3S88.

106. Takiguchi M, Haraguchi Y, Mori M. Human liver-type arginase gene: structure of the gene and analysis of the promoter region. *Nucleic Acids Res* 1988;16:8789–8802.

107. Sakiyama T, Nakabayashi H, Shimizu H, et al. A successful trial of enzyme replacement therapy in a case of argininemia. *Tohoku J Exp Med* 1984;142:239–248.

108. Jakobs C, Bojasch M, Monch E, et al. Urinary excretion of gamma-hydroxybutyric acid in a patient with neurological abnormalities. The probability of a new inborn error of metabolism. *Clin Chim Acta* 1981;111:169–178.

109. Trettel F, Malaspina P, Jodice C, et al. Human succinic semialdehyde dehydrogenase. Molecular cloning and chromosomal localization. *Adv Exp Med Biol* 1997;414:253–260.

110. Gibson KM, Doskey AE, Rabier D, et al. Differing clinical presentation of succinic semialdehyde dehydrogenase deficiency in adolescent siblings from Lifu Island, New Caledonia. *J Inherit Metab Dis* 1997;20:370–374.

111. Gropman A. Vigabatrin and newer interventions in succinic semialdehyde dehydrogenase deficiency. *Ann Neurol* 2003;54 (Suppl 6):S66–S72.

112. Menkes JH, Alter M, Steigleder GK, et al. A sex-linked recessive disorder with retardation of growth, peculiar hair, and focal cerebral and cerebellar degeneration. *Pediatrics* 1962;29:764–779.

113. Sfaello I, Castelnau P, Blanc N, et al. Infantile spasms and Menkes disease. *Epileptic Disord* 2000;2:227–230.

114. Sztriha L, Janaky M, Kiss J, et al. Electrophysiological and 99mTc-HMPAO-SPECT studies in Menkes disease. *Brain Dev* 1994;16:224–228.

115. Tumer Z, Horn N. Menkes disease: underlying genetic defect and new diagnostic possibilities. *J Inherit Metab Dis* 1998;21:604–612.

116. Godwin-Austen RB, Robinson A, Evans K, et al. An unusual neurological disorder of copper metabolism clinically resembling Wilson's disease but biochemically a distinct entity. *J Neurol Sci* 1978;39:85–98.

117. Tumer Z, Horn N. Menkes disease: recent advances and new aspects. *J Med Genet* 1997;34:265–274.

118. Salonen R, Somer M, Haltia M, et al. Progressive encephalopathy with edema, hypsarrhythmia, and optic atrophy (PEHO syndrome). *Clin Genet* 1991;39:287–293.

119. Somer M, Sainio K. Epilepsy and the electroencephalogram in progressive encephalopathy with edema, hypsarrhythmia, and optic atrophy (the PEHO syndrome). *Epilepsia* 1993;34:727–731.

120. Schindler D, Bishop DF, Wallace S, et al. Characterization of alpha-N-acetylgalactosaminidase deficiency: a new neurodegenerative lysosomal disease [abstract]. *Pediatr Res* 1988;23:333A.

121. Balslev T, Cortez MA, Blaser SI, et al. Recurrent seizures in metachromatic leukodystrophy. *Pediatr Neurol* 1997;17:150–154.

122. Fukumizu M, Matsui K, Hanaoka S, et al. Partial seizures in two cases of metachromatic leukodystrophy: electrophysiologic and neuroradiologic findings. *J Child Neurol* 1992;7:381–386.

123. Wang PJ, Hwu WL, Shen YZ. Epileptic seizures and electroencephalographic evolution in genetic leukodystrophies. *J Clin Neurophysiol* 2001;18:25–32.

124. Solders G, Celsing G, Hagenfeldt L, et al. Improved peripheral nerve conduction, EEG and verbal IQ after bone marrow transplantation for adult metachromatic leukodystrophy. *Bone Marrow Transplant* 1998;22:1119–1122.

125. Berger J, Gmach M, Mayr U, et al. Coincidence of two novel arylsulfatase A alleles and mutation 459+1G>A within a family with metachromatic leukodystrophy: molecular basis of phenotypic heterogeneity. *Hum Mutat* 1999;13:61–68.

126. Keulemans JL, Reuser AJ, Kroos MA, et al. Human alpha-*N*-acetylgalactosaminidase (alpha-NAGA) deficiency: new mutations and the paradox between genotype and phenotype. *J Med Genet* 1996;33:458–464.

127. Wang AM, Bishop DF, Desnick RJ. Human alpha-*N*-acetylgalactosaminidase—molecular cloning, nucleotide sequence, and expression of a full-length cDNA. Homology with human alpha-galactosidase A suggests evolution from a common ancestral gene. *J Biol Chem* 1990;265:21859–21866.

128. Geurts van Kessel AH, Westerveld A, de Groot PG, et al. Regional localization of the genes coding for human ACO2, ARSA, and NAGA on chromosome 22. *Cytogenet Cell Genet* 1980;28: 169–172.

129. Maroteaux P, Frezal J, Tahbaz-Zadeh NI, et al. A familial case of polydystrophic oligophrenia [French]. *J Genet Hum* 1966;15: 93–102.

130. Scott HS, Blanch L, Guo XH, et al. Cloning of the sulphamidase gene and identification of mutations in Sanfilippo A syndrome. *Nat Genet* 1995;11:465–467.

131. Kriel RL, Hauser WA, Sung JH, et al. Neuroanatomical and electroencephalographic correlations in Sanfilippo syndrome, type A. *Arch Neurol* 1978;35:838–843.

132. Sivakumur P, Wraith JE. Bone marrow transplantation in mucopolysaccharidosis type IIIA: a comparison of an early treated patient with his untreated sibling. *J Inherit Metab Dis* 1999;22:849–850.

133. Santavouri P. Neuronal ceroid lipofuscinosis in childhood. *Brain Dev* 1988;4:80–83.

134. Mole SE. Batten disease: four genes and still counting. *Neurobiol Dis* 1998;5:287–303.

135. Sleat DE, Donnelly RJ, Lackland H, et al. Association of mutations in a lysosomal protein with classical late-infantile neuronal ceroid lipofuscinosis. *Science* 1997;277:1802–1805.

136. Harden A, Pampiglione G, Picton-Robinson N. Electroretinogram and visual evoked response in a form of "neuronal lipidosis" with diagnostic EEG features. *J Neurol Neurosurg Psychiatry* 1973;36: 61–67.

137. Pampiglione G, Harden A. Neurophysiological identification of a late infantile form of "neuronal lipidosis." *J Neurol Neurosurg Psychiatry* 1973;36:68–74.

138. Brick JF, Westmoreland BF, Gomez MR. The electroencephalogram in Alper's disease [abstract]. *Electroencephalogr Clin Neurophysiol* 1984;58:31P.

139. Walton A. A case study of Alper's disease in siblings. *Am J EEG Technol* 1996;36:18–27.

140. Boyd SG, Harden A, Egger J, et al. Progressive neuronal degeneration of childhood with liver disease ("Alpers' disease"): characteristic neurophysiological features. *Neuropediatrics* 1986;17:75–80.

141. Freeze HH. Update and perspectives on congenital disorders of glycosylation. *Glycobiology* 2001;11:129R–143R.

142. Orlean P. Congenital disorders of glycosylation caused by defects in mannose addition during N-linked oligosaccharide assembly. *J Clin Invest* 2000;105:131–132.

143. Jaeken J, Stibler H, Hagberg B. The carbohydrate-deficient glycoprotein syndrome: a new inherited multisystemic disease with severe nervous system involvement. *Acta Paediatr Scand* 1991;375 (Suppl):1–71.

144. Matthijs G, Schollen E, Pardon E, et al. Mutations in PMM2, a phosphomannomutase gene on chromosome 16p13, in carbohydrate-deficient glycoprotein type I syndrome (Jaeken syndrome). *Nat Genet* 1997;16:88–92.

145. Petersen MB, Brostrom K, Stibler H, et al. Early manifestations of the carbohydrate-deficient glycoprotein syndrome. *J Pediatr* 1993;122:66–70.

146. Van Geet C, Jaeken J. A unique pattern of coagulation abnormalities in carbohydrate-deficient glycoprotein syndrome. *Pediatr Res* 1993;33:540–541.

147. Tayama M, Hashimoto T, Miyazaki M, et al. Pathophysiology of carbohydrate-deficient glycoprotein syndrome—neuroradiological and neurophysiological study [Japanese]. *No To Hattatsu* 1993;25:537–542.

148. Hagberg BA, Blennow G, Kristiansson B, et al. Carbohydrate-deficient glycoprotein syndromes: peculiar group of new disorders. *Pediatr Neurol* 1993;9:255–262.

149. Stibler H, Westerberg B, Hanefeld F, et al. Carbohydrate-deficient glycoprotein (CDG) syndrome—a new variant, type III. *Neuropediatrics* 1993;24:51–52.

150. Stibler H, Gylje H, Uller A. A neurodystrophic syndrome resembling carbohydrate-deficient glycoprotein syndrome type III. *Neuropediatrics* 1999;30:90–92.

151. Munke M, Kraus J, Watkins P, et al. Homocystinuria gene on human chromosome 21 mapped with cloned cystathionine beta-synthase probe and in situ hybridization of other chromosome 21 probes [abstract]. *Cytogenet Cell Genet* 1985;40: 706–707.

152. Gerritsen T, Vaughn JG, Waisman HA. The identification of homocystine in the urine. *Biochem Biophys Res Commun* 1962;9: 493–496.

153. Mudd SH, Skovby F, Levy HL, et al. The natural history of homocystinuria due to cystathionine beta-synthase deficiency. *Am J Hum Genet* 1985;37:1–31.

154. Del Giudice E, Striano S, Andria G. Electroencephalographic abnormalities in homocystinuria due to cystathionine synthase deficiency. *Clin Neurol Neurosurg* 1983;85:165–168.

155. Mamoli B, Graf M, Toifl K. EEG, pattern-evoked potentials and nerve conduction velocity in a family with adrenoleucodystrophy. *Electroencephalogr Clin Neurophysiol* 1979;47:411–419.

156. Engel J Jr, Rapin I, Giblin DR. Electrophysiological studies in two patients with cherry red spot—myoclonus syndrome. *Epilepsia* 1977;18:73–87.

157. Pshezhetsky AV, Richard C, Michaud L, et al. Cloning, expression and chromosomal mapping of human lysosomal sialidase and characterization of mutations in sialidosis. *Nat Genet* 1997;15: 316–320.

158. Wiegant J, Galjart NJ, Rapp AK, et al. The gene encoding human protective protein (PPGB) is on chromosome 20. *Genomics* 1991; 10:345–349.

159. Ginns EI, Choudary PV, Tsuji S, et al. Gene mapping and leader polypeptide sequence of human glucocerebrosidase: implications for Gaucher disease. *Proc Natl Acad Sci U S A* 1985;82:7101–7105.

160. Nishimura R, Omos-Lau N, Ajmone-Marsan C, et al. Electroencephalographic findings in Gaucher disease. *Neurology* 1980;30: 152–159.

161. Krivit W, Peters C, Shapiro EG. Bone marrow transplantation as effective treatment of central nervous system disease in globoid cell leukodystrophy, metachromatic leukodystrophy, adrenoleukodystrophy, mannosidosis, fucosidosis, aspartylglucosaminuria, Hurler, Maroteaux-Lamy, and Sly syndromes, and Gaucher disease type III. *Curr Opin Neurol* 1999;12:167–176.

162. Ferriss GS, Happel LT, Duncan MC. Cerebral cortical isolation in infantile neuroaxonal dystrophy. *Electroencephalogr Clin Neurophysiol* 1977;43:168–182.

163. Butzer JF, Schochet SS Jr, Bell WE. Infantile neuroaxonal dystrophy. An electron microscopic study of a case clinically resembling neuronal ceroid-lipofuscinosis. *Acta Neuropathol (Berl)* 1975;31:35–43.

164. Wakai S, Asanuma H, Tachi N, et al. Infantile neuroaxonal dystrophy: axonal changes in biopsied muscle tissue. *Pediatr Neurol* 1993;9:309–311.

165. Wakai S, Asanuma H, Hayasaka H, et al. Ictal video-EEG analysis of infantile neuroaxonal dystrophy. *Epilepsia* 1994;35:823–826.

166. Berkovic SF, Cochius J, Andermann E, et al. Progressive myoclonus epilepsies: clinical and genetic aspects. *Epilepsia* 1993;34(Suppl 3):S19–S30.

167. Ponsford S, Pye IF, Elliot EJ. Posterior paroxysmal discharge: an aid to early diagnosis in Lafora disease. *J R Soc Med* 1993;86:597–599.

168. Berkovic SF, So NK, Andermann F. Progressive myoclonus epilepsies: clinical and neurophysiological diagnosis. *J Clin Neurophysiol* 1991;8:261–274.

169. Koskiniemi M, Toivakka E, Donner M. Progressive myoclonus epilepsy. Electroencephalographical findings. *Acta Neurol Scand* 1974;50:333–359.

170. Lehesjoki AE, Eldridge R, Eldridge J, et al. Progressive myoclonus epilepsy of Unverricht-Lundborg type: a clinical and molecular genetic study of a family from the United States with four affected sibs. *Neurology* 1993;43:2384–2386.

171. Eldridge R, Iivanainen M, Stern R, et al. "Baltic" myoclonus epilepsy: hereditary disorder of childhood made worse by phenytoin. *Lancet* 1983;2:838–842.

172. Berkovic SF, Andermann F, Karpati G, et al. The epileptic syndromes associated with mitochondrial disease [abstract]. *Electroencephalogr Clin Neurophysiol* 1988;69:50P.

173. Canafoglia L, Franceschetti S, Antozzi C, et al. Epileptic phenotypes associated with mitochondrial disorders. *Neurology* 2001; 56:1340–1346.

174. Fujimoto S, Mizuno K, Shibata H, et al. Serial electroencephalographic findings in patients with MELAS. *Pediatr Neurol* 1999;20: 43–48.

175. Kuwano A, Morimoto Y, Nagai T, et al. Precise chromosomal locations of the genes for dentatorubral-pallidoluysian atrophy (DRPLA), von Willebrand factor (F8vWF) and parathyroid hormone-like hormone (PTHLH) in human chromosome 12p by deletion mapping. *Hum Genet* 1996;97:95–98.

176. Hattori H, Higuchi Y, Okuno T, et al. Early-childhood progressive myoclonus epilepsy presenting as partial seizures in dentatorubral-pallidoluysian atrophy. *Epilepsia* 1997;38:271–274.

177. Saitoh S, Momoi MY, Yamagata T, et al. Clinical and electroencephalographic findings in juvenile type DRPLA. *Pediatr Neurol* 1998;18:265–268.

178. Hyland K, Arnold LA. Value of lumbar puncture in the diagnosis of genetic metabolic encephalopathies. *J Child Neurol* 1999;14 (Suppl 1):S9–S15.

179. De Vivo DC, Bohan TP, Coulter DL, et al. L-Carnitine supplementation in childhood epilepsy: current perspectives. *Epilepsia* 1998;39:1216–1225.

180. Klepper J, Fischbarg J, Vera JC, et al. GLUT1-deficiency: barbiturates potentiate haploinsufficiency in vitro. *Pediatr Res* 1999;46:677–683.

Seizures Associated with Nonneurologic Medical Conditions

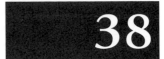

Stephan Eisenschenk   *Robin L. Gilmore*

Seizures frequently arise during the course of medical illnesses that do not primarily affect the central nervous system (CNS). The truism that appropriate treatment depends on correct diagnosis emphasizes the importance of the differential diagnosis. A patient's history, including a review of medications and physical examination should be informed by a consideration of the seizures as a symptom of CNS dysfunction. The urgency to pursue a diagnosis is related to the time of presentation following the seizure. The evaluation of a patient presenting 24 hours after a single seizure is paced by other manifestations of CNS dysfunction. In a neurologically intact patient without progressive symptoms, quick (within days), but not emergent (within hours), evaluation may be appropriate. Within the first 24 hours, vital signs, level of consciousness, and focality on examination determine urgency. The need for emergent neuroimaging studies and lumbar puncture depends on the likelihood of intracranial lesion, CNS or systemic infection, a patient's metabolic state, and the possibility of intoxication. In a patient who presents more than 1 week after an initial seizure, recurrent attacks establish the diagnosis of epilepsy.

Several factors predispose a patient to seizures, including (a) changes in blood–brain barrier permeability as a result of infection, hypoxia, dysautoregulation of cerebral blood flow, or microdeposition of hemorrhage or edema secondary to vascular endothelial damage; (b) alteration of neuronal excitability by exogenous or endogenous substances, such as excitatory and inhibitory neurotransmitters; (c) inability of glial cells to regulate the neuronal extracellular environment; (d) electrolyte imbalances; (e) hypoxia-ischemia; and (f) direct and remote effects of neoplasm (1).

Some patients without epilepsy may be genetically prone to seizures secondary to systemic factors.

Understanding the interaction of other organ systems is necessary for the appropriate management of seizures. In patients with hepatic or renal dysfunction, changes in pharmacokinetics induced by metabolic dysfunction alter treatment with antiepileptic drugs (AEDs). In cases of hepatic dysfunction, plasma concentrations must be correlated with serum albumin and protein levels and, if possible, free (unbound) levels. Patients with hepatic and renal failure may have normal serum and albumin levels, but altered protein binding, resulting in elevated concentrations of free drug (2).

METABOLIC DISORDERS

Metabolic disorders, although often suspected during outpatient evaluation of new-onset seizures, are found in <10% of patients and usually involve glucose metabolism (3). In the hospital setting, disorders of electrolytes and fluid balance predominate. Encephalopathies may be associated with electrolyte disturbances, hypocalcemia, hypercalcemia, hypoglycemia, hypothyroidism, thyrotoxic storm, adverse effects of drugs, organ failure, and many other conditions.

Hyponatremia

Because electrolyte disturbances are usually secondary processes, effective management of associated seizures begins with identification and treatment of the primary disorder in conjunction with cautious correction of the electrolyte disturbance. Hyponatremia, defined as a serum sodium level lower than 115 mEq/L, is one of the most frequently reported metabolic abnormalities, affecting 2.5% of hospitalized patients (4). Neurologic symptoms occur often in patients with acute hyponatremia (5,6), and convulsions in this setting have a mortality rate estimated to exceed 50% (7). Correction to levels higher than 120 mEq/L is essential; however, the rate of correction is controversial. Rapid correction of hyponatremia is associated with central pontine myelinolysis, manifested as pseudobulbar palsy and spastic quadriparesis (8). Originally described in patients with alcoholism and malnutrition, the condition was later observed in dehydrated patients undergoing rehydration (9) and in one small study (10) was accompanied in each patient by a recent rapid increase in serum sodium levels. Pathologic features include symmetrical, noninflammatory demyelination in the basis pontis, with relative neuronal and axonal sparing. In animal models of central pontine myelinolysis, rapid correction of sustained vasopressin-induced hyponatremia with hypertonic saline was followed by demyelination (11). Some authorities consider a correction of more than 12 mEq/L per day to be unnecessarily aggressive (10).

Levels of serum sodium are most commonly reduced as a result of either sodium depletion, water "intoxication," or both (7); these are examples of hypoosmolar hyponatremia. Hyponatremia with normal osmolality is rare, but may accompany hyperlipidemia or hyperproteinemia. Hyperosmolar hyponatremia occurs in such hyperosmolar states as hyperglycemia and is discussed later in this chapter. Hypoosmolar hyponatremia may occur with normal extracellular fluid volume, hypovolemia, or hypervolemia (12). Hypoosmolar hyponatremia with hypovolemia may follow renal (diuretic use, Addison disease) or extrarenal (vomiting, diarrhea, or "third spacing") loss. The syndrome of inappropriate antidiuretic hormone secretion, hypothyroidism, and some psychotropic agents may lead to hypoosmolar hyponatremia with normal volume. Hypoosmolar hyponatremia with hypervolemia, frequently seen with clinical edema, occurs in patients with cardiac failure, nephrotic syndrome, and acute or chronic renal failure. The therapeutic implications of these conditions are significant, because appropriate treatment for normovolemic or hypervolemic hyperosmolar hyponatremia is water restriction. Hypovolemic hyponatremia is managed by replacement of water and sodium (12).

Finally, hyponatremia is sometimes considered to be an iatrogenic effect of prescribed medications, including diuretics and serotonin reuptake inhibitors (13). Hyponatremia can also be a complication of abuse of illicit substances, such as 3,4-methylenedioxymethamphetamine (MDMA, or "Ecstasy") (14,15).

Hypocalcemia

Although seizures resulting from severe hypocalcemia (<6 mg/dL) are relatively uncommon, they occur in approximately 25% of patients who present as medical emergencies (16). Severe, acute hypocalcemia most often follows thyroid or parathyroid surgery. Late-onset hypocalcemia with seizures may appear years after extensive thyroid surgery (17); the condition is believed to be rare and is not well understood. Hypocalcemia frequently complicates renal failure and acute pancreatitis (7), and may also occur along with vitamin D deficiency and renal tubular acidosis. Nutritional rickets is still reported, although rarely in the United States, occasionally with hypocalcemic seizures (18). Tetany is the most common neuromuscular accompaniment of hypocalcemia (19). Manifesting as spontaneous, irregular, repetitive action potentials that originate in peripheral nerves, tetany is sometimes confused with seizure activity. Latent tetany may be unmasked by hyperventilation or regional ischemia (Trousseau test). In the average adult, an intravenous (IV) bolus of 15 mL of 10% calcium gluconate solution (a calcium concentration of 9 mg/mL) administered slowly, along with cardiac monitoring, followed by infusion of the equivalent of 10 mL per hour of the same solution, should relieve seizures (20).

Hypomagnesemia

Hypomagnesemia is associated with seizures, but usually only at levels lower than 0.8 mEq/L (21). Because a related hypocalcemia may be produced by a decrease in, or end-organ resistance to, circulating levels of parathyroid hormone, magnesium levels should be measured in the patient with hypocalcemia who does not respond to calcium supplementation. Convulsions are treated with intramuscular injections of 50% magnesium sulfate every 6 hours. Because transient hypermagnesemia may induce respiratory muscle paralysis (21), IV injections of calcium gluconate should be administered concurrently.

Hypophosphatemia

Profound hypophosphatemia may accompany alcohol withdrawal, diabetic ketoacidosis, long-term intake of phosphate-binding antacids, recovery from extensive burns, hyperalimentation, and severe respiratory alkalosis. A sequence of symptoms consistent with metabolic encephalopathy involves irritability, apprehension, muscle weakness, numbness, paresthesias, dysarthria, confusion, obtundation, convulsive seizures, and coma (22). Generalized tonic-clonic seizures have been noted at phosphate levels lower than 1 mg/dL, and affected patients may not respond to AED therapy (23).

Disturbances of Glucose Metabolism

Hypoglycemia and nonketotic hyperglycemia may be associated with focal seizures; such seizures do not occur with ketotic hyperglycemia, however, probably because of the anticonvulsant action of the ketosis (24). Ketosis also involves intracellular acidosis with enhanced activity of glutamic acid decarboxylase, which leads to an increase in τ-aminobutyric acid and a corresponding increase in seizure threshold.

Nonketotic hyperglycemia, with or without hyperosmolarity, may produce seizures and in animal models increases seizure frequency through brain dehydration, provided a cortical lesion is present (25). Focal motor seizures and epilepsia partialis continua, well-known complications of nonketotic hyperglycemia, occur in approximately 20% of patients (26).

Rarely, patients with focal seizures associated with nonketotic hyperglycemia may have reflex- or posture-induced epilepsy provoked by active or passive movement of an extremity (27,28) and usually have nonreflex seizures as well, related perhaps to an underlying focal cerebral ischemia. Such seizures are refractory to conventional anticonvulsant treatment. In fact, phenytoin may further increase the serum glucose level by inhibiting insulin release (29). Thus, correction of the underlying metabolic disturbance is of utmost importance.

Hypoglycemia is particularly seizure provoking and is most frequently related to insulin or oral hypoglycemic agents, although occasionally the etiology may not be obvious. Another common cause is the use of drugs that interact with oral hypoglycemic agents (30). Islet cell dysmaturation syndrome, characterized by islet cell hyperplasia, pancreatic adenomatosis, and nesidioblastosis, is associated with infantile hyperinsulinemic hypoglycemia. Bjerke and coworkers (31) reported on 11 infants with this condition, 8 of whom presented with hypoglycemic seizures. Five infants had preoperative neurologic impairment. All showed improvement postoperatively, but only one infant had normal findings on neurologic examination. Early diagnosis is a decisive factor in averting long-term complications; treatment entails resection of the pancreas.

Hypoparathyroidism

Seizures occur in 30% to 70% of patients with hypoparathyroidism, usually along with tetany and hypocalcemia. They may be generalized tonic-clonic, focal motor, or, less frequently, atypical absence and akinetic seizures. Restoration of normal calcium levels is necessary. Because AEDs may partially suppress seizures, as well as tetany and the Trousseau sign, hypocalcemia must be considered.

Thyroid Disorders

Hyperthyroidism is associated only rarely with seizures, although generalized and focal seizures have occurred in 10% of patients with thyrotoxicosis (32). Typically, thyrotoxicosis may be associated with nervousness, diaphoresis, heat intolerance, palpitations, tremor, and fatigue. Hashimoto thyroiditis often coexists with other autoimmune disorders (33), such as Hashimoto encephalopathy, a steroid-responsive relapsing condition (34) that produces seizures even in euthyroid patients (35).

Seizures have been reported in patients with myxedema. As many as 20% to 25% of patients with myxedemic coma have generalized convulsions. Patients with hypothyroidism may have obstructive sleep apnea (36) with hypoxic seizures (37).

Adrenal Disorders

Seizures are uncommon with adrenal insufficiency but may occur in patients with pheochromocytoma (38). More commonly, a pheochromocytoma-induced hypertensive crisis may trigger a hypertensive encephalopathy, characterized by altered mental status, focal neurologic signs and symptoms, and/or seizures. Other neurologic complications include stroke caused by cerebral infarction or an embolic event secondary to a mural thrombus from a dilated cardiomyopathy. Intracerebral hemorrhage may also occur because of uncontrolled hypertension. Additional symptoms are tremor, nausea, anxiety, sense of impending doom, epigastric pain, flank pain, constipation or diarrhea, and weight loss. These spells may last minutes to an hour. Blood pressure is almost always markedly elevated during the episode.

Uremia

A change in mental status is the hallmark of uremic encephalopathy, which also involves simultaneous neural depression (obtundation) and neural excitation (twitching, myoclonus, generalized seizures). Epileptic seizures occur in up to one-fourth of patients with uremia, and the reasons are quite varied.

Phenytoin is the AED usually administered to nontransplanted patients with uremia (see "Transplantation and Seizures"). Critical changes in the pharmacokinetics of AEDs include (a) increased volume of distribution, producing lowered plasma drug levels; (b) decreased protein binding, creating higher free-drug levels; and (c) increased hepatic enzyme oxygenation, yielding increased plasma elimination (2). Because patients with uremia have plasma protein-binding abnormalities and because phenytoin is highly plasma bound, drug administration is different from that in nonuremic patients. In one study, a 2-mg/kg IV dose produced a level of 1.4 μg/mL in patients with uremia, compared with 2.9 μg/mL in control patients (39). In nonuremic patients, up to 10% of phenytoin is not protein bound, whereas in uremic patients, as much as 75% may not be protein bound. Thus, free phenytoin levels (between 1 and 2 μg/mL) should be used instead of total phenytoin levels to assess therapeutic efficacy (40). With gabapentin, which is eliminated solely via renal excretion, the usual total dose should be reduced equivalently to the reduction in creatinine clearance (41).

The treatment of renal failure may also lead to dialysis dysequilibrium, characterized by headache, nausea, and irritability, which may progress to seizures, coma, and death attributable to the entry of free water into the brain, with resultant edema. Dialysis dementia, caused by the toxic effects of aluminum, is now rare. Renal transplant recipients may experience cerebrovascular disease, opportunistic infections, or malignant neoplasms, particularly primary lymphoma of the brain.

In uremic patients with renal insufficiency, adverse reactions to antibiotics are a common cause of seizures (42). Patients may have focal motor or generalized seizures, or myoclonus. In uremia, reduced protein binding increases the free fraction of highly protein-bound drugs in serum (and therefore in the CNS). Raised concentrations of neurotoxic agents, such as cephalosporins, may increase seizure susceptibility, which may be enhanced further by the altered blood–brain barrier.

The hemodialysis patient represents a special challenge because of decreased concentrations of dialyzable AEDs. Plasma protein binding determines how effectively a drug can be dialyzed. The more protein bound a drug, the less dialyzable it is (43). Hence, levels of a drug such as phenobarbital (40% to 60% protein bound) will decrease during dialysis more than will levels of valproic acid (80% to 95% bound). One way, albeit cumbersome, to avoid "losing" an agent is to dialyze against a dialysate containing the drug. Another option, if seizures occur near the time of dialysis, is to use a highly protein-bound drug, such as valproic acid. For special considerations in the kidney transplant patient, see "Transplantation and Seizures."

Inborn Errors of Metabolism

Metabolic errors, either inborn or acquired, occur most often in early childhood. Phenylketonuria is the most common of several aminoacidopathies that may be associated with infantile spasms, and myoclonic or tonic-clonic seizures occur in one-fourth of these patients (44). Evidence of hypsarrhythmia may be seen on the electroencephalogram (EEG), but a high proportion of patients have abnormal EEGs without seizures.

Although hereditary fructose intolerance does not usually involve neurologic impairment, as does untreated phenylketonuria, a small number of children experience seizures that are sometimes related to prolonged hypoglycemia (45).

Because excess ammonia is excreted as urea, disorders of the urea cycle, such as hyperammonemia, may be associated with symptoms ranging from coma and seizures to mild, nonspecific aberrations in neurologic function (44).

Various storage diseases result from abnormal accumulation of normal substrates and their catabolic products within lysosomes. The absence or inefficiency of lysosomal enzymes in such conditions as sphingolipidoses, mucopolysaccharidoses, mucolipidoses, glycogen storage diseases, and glycoproteinoses may give rise to seizures (44).

Purine syndromes and hyperuricemia are not usually associated with seizure disorders unless mental retardation or dementia coexists. Allopurinol is an important adjunctive treatment in some patients.

Porphyria

The disorders of heme biosynthesis are classified into two groups: erythropoietic and hepatic. Seizures and other neurologic manifestations occur only in the hepatic group, which comprises acute intermittent porphyria, hereditary coproporphyria, and variegate porphyria (46). Seizures affect approximately 15% of patients, usually during an acute attack (47) often precipitated by an iatrogenically introduced offending agent. The generalized (occasionally focal) seizures may begin up to 28 days after exposure to the agent. The epileptogenesis mechanism is not well understood. Some authors have suggested that δ-aminolevulinic acid and porphobilinogen, both structurally similar to the neurotransmitters glutamate and γ-aminobutyric acid (GABA), are toxic to the nervous system, although clinical evidence refutes this contention (46).

A cornerstone of treatment is the provision of a major portion of daily caloric requirements by carbohydrates to lower porphyrin excretion. Glucose prevents induction of hepatic δ-aminolevulinic acid synthetase in symptomatic patients, as does IV hematin. Porphyrogenic drugs, such as phenytoin, barbiturates, carbamazepine, succinimides, and oxazolidinediones, should be avoided. Drugs are considered unsafe if they induce experimental porphyria in animals. Using chick-embryo hepatocyte culture, Reynolds and Miska (47) found that carbamazepine, clonazepam, and valproate increased porphyrin to levels comparable with those achieved with phenobarbital and phenytoin. Bromides are recommended for the long-term management (48) and diazepam, paraldehyde, and IV magnesium sulfate therapy for the acute treatment of seizures (49). Serum bromide levels should be maintained between 60 and 90 µg/dL. Many side effects and a long half-life make bromides difficult to use. Bromides are excreted by the kidney, and paraldehyde is excreted unchanged by the lungs (the remainder by the liver). Larson and colleagues (50) reported on one patient with intractable epilepsy who was safely managed with low-dose clonazepam and a high-carbohydrate diet after phenytoin and carbamazepine use had independently precipitated attacks. In two separate studies, gabapentin controlled complex partial and secondarily generalized seizures in patients with porphyria (51,52). Because gabapentin is excreted unmetabolized by the kidneys, it does not induce hepatic microsomal enzymes (53) and should not worsen hepatic cellular dysfunction. Vigabatrin, which also does not induce hepatic metabolism, may be a useful antiseizure medication in patients with porphyria. Table 38.1 lists agents that are safe and unsafe to use in patients with porphyria (54).

<table>
<tr><td colspan="2">

TABLE 38.1

SAFE AND UNSAFE AGENTS IN PATIENTS WITH PORPHYRIA

</td></tr>
</table>

Safe Agents	Unsafe Agents
Acetaminophen	Barbiturates
Acetazolamide	Carbamazepine
Allopurinol	Chloramphenicol
Aminoglycosides	Chlordiazepoxide
Amitriptyline	Diphenhydramine
Aspirin	Enalapril
Atropine	Ergot compounds
Bromides	Erythromycin
Bupivacaine	Ethanol
Chloral hydrate	Flucloxacillin
Chlorpromazine	Flufenamic acid
Codeine	Griseofulvin
Corticosteroids	Hydrochlorothiazide
Diazepam	Imipramine
Gabapentin	Lisinopril
Heparin	Methyldopa
Insulin	Metoclopramide
Meclizine	Nifedipine
Meperidine	Oral contraceptives
Morphine	Pentazocine
Penicillins (see unsafe agents	Phenytoin
for exceptions)	Piroxicam
Procaine	Pivampicillin
Prochlorperazine	Progesterone
Promethazine	Pyrazinamide
Propoxyphene	Rifampin
Propranolol	Sulfonamides
Propylthiouracil	Theophylline
Quinidine	Valproic acid
Streptomycin	Verapamil
Temazepam	
Tetracycline	
Thyroxine	
Trifluoperazine	
Warfarin	

Adapted from Gorchein A. Drug treatment in acute porphyria. *Br J Clin Pharmacol* 1997;44:427–434, with permission.

OXYGEN DEPRIVATION

Perinatal Anoxia and Hypoxia

In utero, during delivery, or in the neonatal period, significant anoxia can extensively damage the CNS, leading to chronic, usually secondarily generalized, epilepsy most commonly associated with mental retardation or other neurologic impairment. Neonatal seizures carry a risk for increased mortality, probably from the underlying brain disease rather than from the seizures themselves (55).

In the neonatal period, subtle, frequently refractory seizures may occur, as well as tonic, focal clonic, myoclonic seizures and multifocal clonic jerks. Not all paroxysmal events are seizures, however; some are brainstem release phenomena. Continuous video-electroencephalographic monitoring has made the diagnosis of these disorders more accurate and has led to improved treatment, including the avoidance of inappropriate AED use.

Because the initial insult usually occurs *in utero*, ventilation, cerebral perfusion, and adequate glucose levels must be maintained as preventive measures. Vigorous AED treatment is recommended because of the potential for additional brain injury, but opinions vary as to the degree of vigor to be applied. Arguments for aggressive therapy have been based on the realization that seizures may compromise ventilation and increase systemic blood pressure and cerebral perfusion, leading to hemorrhagic infarction, intraventricular hemorrhage, or both (56,57). Seizures may also result in cellular starvation through exhaustion of cerebral glucose and high-energy phosphate compounds. Experimental studies demonstrate that seizures decrease brain protein levels, DNA, RNA, and cell content. Treatment of anoxic seizures in the newborn is reviewed in Chapter 32.

As the infant matures, the seizure type changes. Infantile spasms and hypsarrhythmia may occur in patients 2 to 12 months of age.

Adult Anoxia and Hypoxia

In adults, anoxic or posthypoxic seizures are residuals of cardiac arrest, respiratory failure, anesthetic misadventure, carbon monoxide poisoning, or near-drowning. Precipitating cardiac sources typically are related to embolic stroke, 13% of which involve seizures (58) or hypoperfusion or hyperperfusion of the cerebral cortex (2). Approximately 0.5% of patients who have undergone coronary bypass surgery experience seizures without evidence of focal CNS injury (59). In patients with respiratory disorder, acute hypercapnia may lower seizure threshold, whereas chronic stable hypoxia and hypercapnia rarely cause seizures. Subacute bacterial endocarditis can lead to septic emboli and intracranial mycotic aneurysms, which can produce seizures either from focal ischemia or from rupture and subarachnoid hemorrhage. Syncopal myoclonus and convulsive syncope may result from transient hypoxia.

Seizures may involve only minimal facial or axial movement (60), although nonconvulsive status epilepticus typically signifies a poor prognosis (61,62). Myoclonic status epilepticus or generalized myoclonic seizures that occur repetitively for 30 minutes are usually refractory to medical treatment (63). Concern has been raised that myoclonic status epilepticus may produce progressive neurologic injury in comatose patients resuscitated from cardiac arrest (63). When postanoxic myoclonic status epilepticus is associated with cranial areflexia, eye opening at the onset of myoclonic jerks, and EEG patterns indicating poor prognosis, the outlook for neurologic recovery is grim (64).

Treatment is directed mainly toward preventing a critical degree of hypoxic injury. Barbiturate medication and reduction of cerebral metabolic requirements by continuous hypothermia may prevent the delayed worsening (65). Frequently, the seizures cease after 3 to 5 days. Postanoxic seizures are frequently myoclonic. Phenobarbital 300 mg/day, clonazepam 8 to 12 mg/day in three divided doses, and 4-hydroxytryptophan 100 to 400 mg/day have been recommended (66), as has valproic acid (67).

ALCOHOL

Generalized tonic-clonic seizures occur during the first 48 hours of withdrawal from alcohol in intoxicated patients and are most common 12 to 24 hours after binge drinking (68). Seizures that occur more than 6 days following abstinence should not be ascribed to withdrawal. Interictal EEG findings are usually normal. Partial seizures often result from CNS infection or cerebral cicatrix caused by remote head trauma. (Recent occult head trauma, including subdural hematoma, should be considered in any alcoholic patient.) Although the incidence of alcoholism in patients with seizures is not higher than in the general population, alcoholic individuals do have a higher incidence of seizures (69).

The treatment depends on associated conditions, but replacement of alcohol is generally not recommended. To prevent the development of Wernicke-Korsakoff syndrome, thiamine should be administered prior to IV glucose. Magnesium deficiency should be corrected, as reduced levels may interfere with the action of thiamine. Preferred treatment is with benzodiazepines or paraldehyde. Paraldehyde may be administered in doses of 0.1 to 0.2 mL/kg orally or rectally every 2 to 4 hours. Diazepam, lorazepam, clorazepate, and chlordiazepoxide in conventional dosages are equally useful (70).

INFECTIONS

Infection is associated with seizures, both directly via parenchymal invasion by the pathogen and indirectly via neurotoxins. Direct parenchymal infections may be bacterial, fungal, mycobacterial, viral, spirochetal, or parasitic. Neurodegenerative disorders, such as Creutzfeldt-Jakob disease and subacute sclerosing panencephalitis, can also result from CNS infection.

Meningitis

Patients with seizures, headache, or fever (even low grade) should undergo lumbar puncture once a mass lesion has been excluded. In the infant with diffuse, very high intracranial pressure, lumbar puncture should be delayed until antibiotics and pressure-reducing measures are initiated. The pathogenic cause of bacterial meningitis varies with age: In newborns, *Escherichia coli* and group B streptococcus are most common; in children 2 months to 12 years

of age, *Haemophilus influenzae*, *Streptococcus pneumoniae*, and *Neisseria meningitidis* are usual; in children older than 12 years of age and in adults, *S. pneumoniae* and *N. meningitidis* are found most often; in adults older than 50 years of age, *H. influenzae* is increasingly being reported. In infants, geriatric patients, and the immunocompromised, *Listeria monocytogenes* must also be considered.

Encephalitis

The herpes simplex variety is the most common form of encephalitis associated with seizures (71). Fever, headache, and confusion are punctuated by both complex partial and generalized seizures. The propensity of the virus for the temporal lobe is well known. Equine encephalitides, St. Louis encephalitis, and rabies also produce seizures. Rabies is distinguished from other viruses by dysphagia, dysarthria, facial numbness, and facial muscle spasm.

Diazepam or lorazepam may be used for the acute control of seizures caused by meningitis or encephalitis. Seizures persisting for more than 1 day or the development of status epilepticus indicates the need for maintenance AED therapy—phenytoin in adults, in children, and phenobarbital in infants.

Nonbacterial Chronic Meningitis

Lyme disease, a tick-borne spirochetosis, is associated with meningitis, encephalitis, and cranial or radicular neuropathies in up to 20% of patients. Seizures are not a prominent feature. Treatment consists of high-dose IV penicillin G in addition to AEDs (72).

Neurosyphilis is another spirochetal cause of seizures, which occasionally are the initial manifestation of syphilitic meningitis. In the early 20th century, 15% of patients with adult-onset seizures had underlying neurosyphilis. The incidence decreased dramatically over the years; however, the recent upsurge in primary syphilis among younger individuals is reflected in the report that seizures occur in approximately 25% of patients with symptomatic neurosyphilis. The diagnosis rests on the demonstration of positive serologic findings and clinical symptoms, but the signs are not pathognomonic and often overlap with those of other diseases. IV penicillin remains the treatment of choice. Sarcoidosis should also be considered in patients with nonbacterial meningitis and seizures.

Opportunistic Central Nervous System Infections

Acquired immunodeficiency syndrome (AIDS) is associated with several unique neurologic disorders, and seizures may play a major role when opportunistic infections or metabolic abnormalities, especially cerebral toxoplasmosis or cryptococcal meningitis, occur. *L. monocytogenes* should also be considered in immunocompromised patients. Metabolic abnormalities, particularly uremia and hypomagnesemia, predispose patients infected with the human immunodeficiency virus (HIV) to seizures. New-onset epilepsy partialis continua as an early manifestation of progressive multifocal leukoencephalopathy in patients with HIV-1 infection has been reported (73). CNS lymphoma in HIV-infected patients may also give rise to seizures.

Parasitic Central Nervous System Infections

In some areas, neurocysticercosis is the most commonly diagnosed cause of partial seizures. The adult pork tapeworm resides in the human small bowel after ingestion of infected meat. The oncospheres (hatched ova) penetrate the gut wall and develop into encysted larval forms, usually in brain or skeletal muscle. Computed tomography (CT) scans reveal calcified lesions, cysts with little or no enhancement, and usually no sign of increased intracranial pressure. In the past, treatment involved praziquantel 50 mg/kg per day for 15 days or albendazole 15 mg/kg per day. While undergoing therapy, most patients have clinical exacerbations, including worsening seizures, attributed to inflammation with cyst expansion caused by the death of cysticerci. For this reason, steroids have been advocated during treatment.

Antihelminthic agents by themselves do not change the course of neurocysticercosis or its associated epilepsy. A trial of antihelminthic agents combined with steroids or steroids alone showed comparable efficacy in terms of patients who were cyst free at 1 year or seizure free during follow-up (74).

Hydatid disease of the CNS (echinococcal infection) may result from exposure to dogs and sheep. Echinococcal cysts destroy bone, and a large proportion of such cysts are found in vertebrae. On CT scans, echinococcal brain cysts are fewer and larger than the cysts associated with cysticercosis. Treatment is usually surgical, largely because mebendazole and flubendazole have been associated with disease progression in up to 25% of patients. Nonetheless, adjuvant chemotherapy may be warranted in some cases (75).

Trichinosis may be encountered wherever undercooked trichina-infected pork is consumed. Complications of CNS migration include seizures, meningoencephalitis, and focal neurologic signs; eosinophilia is common during acute infection. Muscle biopsy may be necessary for diagnosis (71).

Cerebral malaria is similar to neurosyphilis, in that almost every neurologic sign and symptom has been attributed to the disorder. Diagnosis requires characteristic forms in the peripheral blood smear. Treatment depends on whether chloroquine resistance is present in the geographic region of infection.

Toxoplasmosis is a parasitic infection that affects adults, children, and infants. Use of immunosuppressive agents in patients with malignancies or transplants (see related sections later in this chapter), as well as recognition of AIDS, has emphasized the need to reconsider the neurologic sequelae of toxoplasmosis. Diagnosis may be elusive. Cerebrospinal fluid may reveal normal findings or mild pleocytosis (76). Serologic data may be difficult to interpret because encephalitis caused by *Toxoplasma gondii* may occur in patients who reactivate latent organisms and do not develop the serologic response of acute infection. CT scanning may reveal typical lesions. Therapy includes pyrimethamine and sulfadiazine or trisulfapyrimidines.

Cytomegalovirus retinitis, the most common ocular opportunistic infection in patients with AIDS (77), is increasingly being treated with a combination of foscarnet and ganciclovir. Foscarnet is also used to treat cytomegalovirus esophagitis associated with AIDS, but seizures have occurred with this agent, possibly as a result of changes in ionized calcium concentrations (78).

Systemic Infections

Systemic infection involving hypoxia (e.g., pneumonia) or metabolic changes may give rise to seizures. Through an indirect, poorly understood mechanism, seizures are prominent in two serious gastrointestinal (GI) infections: shigellosis and cholera. Ashkenazi and associates (79) demonstrated that the Shiga toxin is not essential for the development of the neurologic manifestations of shigellosis and that other toxic products may play a role.

Zvulunov and colleagues (80) examined 111 children who had convulsions with shigellosis and were followed for 3 to 18 years. No deaths or persistent motor deficits occurred. Only one child developed epilepsy by the age of 8 years; 15.7% of the children had recurrent febrile seizures. Poor coordination of fine hand movements was noted in 3.3% of the 92 children who had no preexisting neurologic abnormality. The convulsions associated with shigellosis have a favorable prognosis and do not necessitate long-term follow-up or treatment.

Most clinical manifestations of cholera are caused by fluid loss. Seizures, which are the most common CNS complication, occasionally occur both before and after treatment, and may result from hypoglycemia or overcorrection of electrolyte abnormalities. The cornerstone of treatment, however, is fluid replacement. Up to 3% of body weight, or 30 mL/kg, should be administered during the first hour, followed by 7% for the next 5 to 6 hours. Lactated Ringer solution given intravenously with potassium chloride or isotonic saline and sodium lactate (in a 2:1 ratio) is used. Adjunctive treatment with a broad-spectrum antibiotic shortens the duration of diarrhea and hastens the excretion of *Vibrio cholerae*.

The seizures associated with shigellosis and cholera infection may share a common pathogenesis. Depletion of hepatic glycogen and resultant hypoglycemia are typically reported in children with these illnesses (81).

GASTROINTESTINAL DISEASE AND SEIZURES

In nontropical sprue, or celiac disease, damage to the small bowel by gluten-containing foods leads to chronic malabsorption. Approximately 10% of patients have significant neurologic manifestations, with the most frequent neurologic complication being seizures (reported in 1% to 10% of patients), which are often associated with bilateral occipital calcifications (82,83). Possible mechanisms include deficiencies of calcium, magnesium, and vitamins; genetic factors (84); and isolated CNS vasculitis (85). Malabsorption may be occult, and seizures may be the dominant feature. Strict gluten exclusion usually produces a rapid response.

Inflammatory bowel disease (ulcerative colitis and Crohn disease) is associated with a low incidence of focal or generalized seizures. Unsurprisingly, generalized seizures frequently accompany infection or dehydration. In approximately 50% of all patients with focal seizures, a vascular basis is suspected (86).

Whipple disease is a multisystem granulomatous disorder caused by *Tropheryma whippelii* (87). Approximately 10% of patients have dementia, ataxia, or oculomotor abnormalities; as many as 25% have seizures (88). Early treatment is important, as untreated patients with CNS involvement usually die within 12 months (89). Some patients develop cerebral manifestations after successful antibiotic treatment of GI symptoms (90). Although several agents that cross the blood–brain barrier, such as chloramphenicol and penicillin, have been suggested for treatment (91), a high incidence of CNS relapse led Keinath and coworkers (92) to recommend penicillin 1.2 million units and streptomycin 1.0 g per day for 10 to 14 days, followed by trimethoprim-sulfamethoxazole 1 double-strength tablet twice a day for 1 year. Treatment of the underlying disease may not prevent seizures, however, in which case AEDs in a suspension or elixir are usually required because malabsorption is a significant problem (93).

Hepatic Encephalopathy

Wilson disease, acquired hepatocerebral degeneration, Reye syndrome, and fulminant hepatic failure, among other disorders, may lead to hepatic encephalopathy. Manifestations progress through four stages. Stage 1 is incipient encephalopathy. In stage 2, mental status deteriorates and asterixis develops. In stage 3, focal or generalized seizures may occur. Stage 4 is marked by coma and decerebrate posturing.

The incidence of seizures varies from 2% to 33% (94). Hypoglycemia complicating liver failure may be responsible for some seizures. Hyperammonemia is associated with seizures and may contribute to the encephalopathy of primary hyperammonemic disorders; treatments that reduce ammonia levels also ameliorate the encephalopathy (94).

Therapy should be directed toward the etiology of the hepatic failure; levels of GI protein and lactulose must be reduced. Long-term use of AEDs is not usually required unless there is a known predisposition to seizures (e.g., previous cerebral injury). Little experience with the use of AEDs has actually been reported. Those AEDs with sedative effects may precipitate coma and are generally contraindicated. Phenytoin and gabapentin are reasonable choices, but valproic acid and its salt should be avoided.

INTOXICATION AND DRUG-RELATED SEIZURES

This section is *not* to be used as a guide to the management of drug intoxication. Rather, it reviews specific instances of intoxication during which intractable seizures sometimes develop.

Prescription Medication-Induced Seizures

Many medications provoke seizures in both epileptic and nonepileptic patients (Table 38.2). Predisposing factors include family history of seizures, concurrent illness, and

TABLE 38.2

AGENTS REPORTED TO INDUCE SEIZURES

Analgesics	Fentanyl, mefenamic acid, meperidine, pentazocine, propoxyphene, tramadol
Antibiotics	Ampicillin, carbenicillin, cephalosporins, imipenem, isoniazid, lindane, metronidazole, nalidixic acid, oxacillin, penicillin, pyrimethamine, ticarcillin
Antidepressants	Amitriptyline, bupropion, doxepin, maprotiline, mianserin, nomifensine, nortriptyline
Antineoplastic agents	Busulfan, carmustine (BCNU), chlorambucil, cytosine arabinoside, methotrexate, vincristine
Antipsychotics	Chlorpromazine, haloperidol, perphenazine, prochlorperazine, thioridazine, trifluoperazine
Bronchial agents	Aminophylline, theophylline
General anesthetics	Enflurane, ketamine, methohexital
Local anesthetics	Bupivacaine, lidocaine, procaine
Sympathomimetics	Ephedrine, phenylpropanolamine, terbutaline
Others	Alcohol, amphetamines, anticholinergics, antihistamines, aqueous iodinated contrast agents, atenolol, baclofen, cyclosporine, domperidone, ergonovine, FK506flumazenil, folic acid, foscarnet, hyperbaric oxygen, insulin, lithium, methylphenidate, methylxanthines, oxytocin, phencyclidine, tacrolimus (FK506)

high-dose intrathecal and IV administration. The convulsions are usually generalized with or without focal features; status epilepticus may occur in up to 15% of patients (95). Because many medical conditions result from polypharmacy, drug-induced seizures may be more common in geriatric patients.

Intoxication from treatment with tricyclic antidepressants (TCAs) has led to generalized tonic-clonic seizures; in fact, seizures may occur at therapeutic levels in approximately 1% of patients (93). Because desipramine is believed to have a lower risk for precipitating seizures than other drugs in this class, the agent is preferred in patients with known seizure disorders (97). Barbiturates are relatively contraindicated, and amitriptyline and imipramine depress the level of consciousness. Diazepam or paraldehyde is preferred. Physostigmine may reverse the neurologic manifestations of TCA reactions; however, because it may also cause asystole, hypotension, hypersalivation, and convulsions, this agent should not be used to treat tricyclic-induced seizures.

Fluoxetine, sertraline, and other selective serotonin reuptake inhibitors (SSRIs) have an associated seizure risk of approximately 0.2%. The SSRIs may have an antiepileptic effect at therapeutic doses (98). When combined with other serotonergic agents or monoamine oxidase inhibitors, however, they may induce the "serotonin syndrome" of delirium, tremors, and, occasionally, seizures (99). Other symptoms include agitation, myoclonus, hyperreflexia, diaphoresis, shivering, tremor, diarrhea, incoordination, and fever. Linezolid, a new synthetic antimicrobial agent, is an important weapon against methicillin-resistant *Staphylococcus aureus* (MRSA). There are reports of serotonin syndrome developing after concomitant use of linezolid and the SSRI paroxetine, as well as citalopram (100) and mirtazapine (101). Other substances used in combination with SSRIs that have precipitated the serotonin syndrome include St. John's wort (102).

Antipsychotic agents have long been known to precipitate seizures (95). Both the phenothiazines and haloperidol have been implicated, but the potential is greater with phenothiazines, and seizures occur more frequently with increasing dosage (103). Clozapine, an atypical antipsychotic agent (dibenzodiazepine class) used for the treatment of intractable schizophrenia, may also be useful for tremor and psychosis in patients with Parkinson disease (104,105). As with other antipsychotic agents, the incidence of seizures increases with increasing dosage (106). If reduction of dosage is not practical, phenytoin or valproate may be added; however, carbamazepine should be avoided because antipsychotic agents may induce agranulocytosis. Lithium may also precipitate seizures (107).

The use of theophylline and other methylxanthines may lead to generalized tonic-clonic seizures; rarely, patients may experience seizures with nontoxic levels of theophylline. Seizures resulting from overdosage are best treated with IV diazepam. Massive overdosage may induce hypocalcemia and other electrolyte abnormalities (108).

Lidocaine precipitates seizures, usually in the setting of congestive heart failure, shock, or hepatic insufficiency. General anesthetics, such as ketamine and enflurane, are also implicated (see "Central Anticholinergic Syndrome").

Verapamil intoxication may be associated with seizures through the mechanism of hypocalcemia, although hypoxia also may play a role (109). Other calcium-channel blockers have not been reported to produce this adverse effect. Meperidine, pentazocine, and propoxyphene, among other analgesic drugs, infrequently cause seizures (110).

Many antiparasitic agents and antimicrobials, particularly penicillins and cephalosporins in high concentrations, are known seizure precipitants. Lindane, an antiparasitic shampoo active against head lice (*Pediculosis capitis*), has a rare association with generalized, self-limited seizures; it is best to use another agent should reinfestation occur. Seizures have not been reported with permethrin, another antipediculosis agent.

Severe isoniazid intoxication involves coma, severe, intractable seizures, and metabolic acidosis. Ingestion of >80 mg/kg of body weight produces severe CNS symptoms that are rapidly reversed with IV administration of pyridoxine at 1 mg per every 1 mg of isoniazid (111). Conventional doses of short-acting barbiturates, phenytoin, or diazepam are also recommended to potentiate the effect of pyridoxine (112).

Recreational Drug-Induced Seizures

Alldredge and associates (113) retrospectively identified 49 cases of recreational drug-induced seizures in 47 patients seen between 1975 and 1987. Most patients experienced a single generalized tonic-clonic attack associated with acute drug intoxication, but seven patients had multiple seizures and two had status epilepticus. The recreational drugs implicated were cocaine (32 cases), amphetamines, heroin, and phencyclidine; a combination of drugs was responsible for 11 cases. Seizures occurred independently of the route of administration and were reported in both first-time and chronic abusers. Ten patients (21%) reported prior seizures, all temporally associated with drug abuse. Except for one patient who experienced prolonged status epilepticus causing a fixed neurologic deficit, most patients had no obvious short-term neurologic sequelae (113). Marijuana is unlikely to alter the seizure threshold (114). Patients with seizures who test positive for marijuana on toxicologic screening should be investigated for other illicit drug and alcohol use.

Cocaine, a biologic compound that is one of the most abused recreational drugs in the United States, commonly gives rise to tremors and generalized seizures. Seizures can develop immediately following drug administration, without other toxic signs. Convulsions and death can occur within minutes of overdose. Pascual-Leone and coworkers (115) retrospectively studied 474 patients with medical complications related to acute cocaine intoxication. Of 403 patients who had no seizure history, approximately 10% had seizures within 90 minutes of cocaine use. The majority of seizures were single and generalized, induced by IV or "crack" cocaine, and were not associated with any lasting neurologic deficits. Most of the focal or repetitive attacks involved an acute intracerebral complication or concurrent use of other drugs. Of 71 patients with previous non–cocaine-related seizures, 17% presented with cocaine-induced seizures, most of which were multiple and of the same type as they had regularly experienced (115).

The treatment of choice for recreational drug-induced seizures is diazepam or lorazepam. Bicarbonate for acidosis, artificial ventilation, and cardiac monitoring are also useful, depending on the duration of the seizures. Urinary acidification accelerates excretion of the drug. Chlorpromazine has also been recommended because it raised, rather than lowered, the seizure threshold in cocaine-intoxicated primates (116). The use of TCAs decreases vasoconstrictor and cardiac action (117).

Acute overdose of amphetamine causes excitement, chest pain, hypertension, tachycardia, and sweating, followed by delirium, hallucinations, hyperpnea, cardiac arrhythmias, hyperpyrexia, seizures, coma, and death. Because chlorpromazine prolongs the half-life of amphetamine, phenothiazines and haloperidol have been recommended; if signs of atropinization are present, neither should be used. Barbiturates can aggravate delirium. Seizures are treated with diazepam or, if long-term antiepileptic therapy is indicated, with phenytoin. Acidification of urine may enhance drug excretion.

Methamphetamine is a synthetic agent with toxic effects, including seizures, that are similar to those with amphetamine and cocaine (118). The amphetamine derivative (MDMA) stimulates the release and inhibits the reuptake of serotonin (5-HT) and other neurotransmitters, such as dopamine, to a lesser extent. Mild versions of the serotonin syndrome often develop, when hyperthermia, mental confusion, and hyperkinesia predominate (119). MDMA may also cause seizures in conjunction with rhabdomyolysis and hepatic dysfunction (120).

γ-Hydroxybutyric acid (GHB), or sodium oxybate, is an agent that is approved for use in patients with narcolepsy who experience episodes of cataplexy, a condition characterized by weak or paralyzed muscles. It is now also a popular agent among recreational drug users. GHB is a naturally occurring substance in the human brain. Its abuse potential is secondary to its ability to induce a euphoric state without a hangover effect. Additional effects of increased sensuality and disinhibition further explain the popularity of the agent. Abusers will often ingest sufficient quantities to lead to a severely depressed level of consciousness. It is not uncommon to observe seizures in these cases. With acute overdose, patients have experienced delirium and transient respiratory depression, which can be fatal (121).

GHB is believed to bind to $GABA_B$ and GHB-specific receptors. It blocks dopamine release at the synapse and produces an increase in intracellular dopamine. This is followed by a time-dependent leakage of dopamine from the neuron. GHB reportedly lengthens slow-wave sleep. The toxicity of GHB is dose-dependent and can result in nausea, vomiting, hypotonia, bradycardia, hypothermia, random clonic movements, coma, respiratory depression, and apnea. Combining GHB with other depressants or psychoactive compounds may exacerbate its effects. Other subjective effects reportedly include euphoria, hallucinations, relaxation, and disinhibition. Deaths involving solely the use of GHB appear to be rare and have involved the "recreational abuse" of the drug for its "euphoric" effects. GHB abuse frequently involves the use of other substances, such as alcohol or MDMA (122).

CENTRAL ANTICHOLINERGIC SYNDROME

Many drugs used as anesthetic agents and in the intensive care unit may cause seizures. Although a discussion of each agent is beyond the scope of this chapter, we review the central anticholinergic syndrome (123), a common disorder associated with blockade of central cholinergic neurotransmission, whose symptoms are identical to those of atropine intoxication: seizures, agitation, hallucinations, disorientation, stupor, coma, and respiratory depression. Such disturbances may be induced by opiates, ketamine, etomidate, propofol, nitrous oxide, and halogenated inhalation anesthetics, as well as by such H_2-blocking agents as cimetidine. An individual predisposition exists for central anticholinergic syndrome that is unpredictable from laboratory findings or other signs. The postanesthetic syndrome can be prevented by administration of physostigmine during anesthesia.

OTHER SEIZURE PRECIPITANTS

Heavy metal intoxication, especially with lead and mercury, is a well-known seizure precipitant. Ingestion of lead from paint and inhalation of lead oxide are specific hazards among young children. Hyperbaric oxygenation provokes seizures, possibly as a toxic effect of oxygen itself. Some antineoplastic agents, such as chlorambucil and methotrexate, precipitate seizures. Table 38.2 lists other agents reported to induce seizures.

ECLAMPSIA

A condition unique to pregnancy and puerperium, eclampsia is characterized by convulsions following a preeclamptic state involving hypertension, proteinuria, edema, and coagulopathy, as well as headache, drowsiness, and hyperreflexia. Eclampsia is associated with a maternal mortality of 1% to 2% and a rate of complications of 35% (124). In the United States, magnesium sulfate is the chosen therapy, whereas in the United Kingdom, such conventional AEDs as phenytoin and diazepam are used (125,126). The antiepileptic action of magnesium sulfate is accompanied by hypotension, weakness, ataxia, respiratory depression, and coma. The recommended "therapeutic level" is 3.29 μmol/L; however, weakness and ataxia appear at 3.5 to 5.0 μmol/L, and respiratory depression at 5.0 μmol/L (127). Kaplan and associates (128) argue that magnesium sulfate is not a proven AED; even at therapeutic levels, 12% of patients continued to have seizures in one study (129). The use of magnesium sulfate or conventional AEDs for preeclamptic or eclamptic seizures remains controversial. Because eclamptic seizures are clinically and electrographically indistinguishable from other generalized tonic-clonic attacks, the use of established AEDs, such as diazepam, lorazepam, and phenytoin, is recommended (128). In a recent randomized study of 2138 women with hypertension during labor (130), no eclamptic convulsions occurred in women receiving magnesium sulfate, whereas seizures were frequent with phenytoin use. Methodological problems, however, involved the route of administration of the second phenytoin dose after loading and the low therapeutic phenytoin level at the time of the seizure.

Magnesium sulfate has a beneficial effect on factors leading to eclampsia and can reverse cerebral arterial vasoconstriction (131). By the time a neurologist is consulted, however, the patient will have received magnesium sulfate and will require additional treatment to control seizures.

MALIGNANCY

Mechanisms for induction of seizures in patients with cancer include direct invasion of cortex or leptomeninges, metabolic derangements, opportunistic infection, and chemotherapeutic agents (132). Limbic encephalitis is a paraneoplastic syndrome seen in patients with small-cell carcinoma or, less commonly, Hodgkin disease. Patients usually present with amnestic dementia, affective disturbance, and sometimes a personality change. During the illness, both complex partial and generalized seizures may occur. Paraneoplastic limbic encephalitis associated with anti-Hu antibodies may present with seizures and precede the diagnosis of cancer (133). If the etiology of new-onset seizures is not defined in a patient with known cancer, frequent neuroimaging studies should assess the individual for metastatic disease.

Opsoclonus-myoclonus syndrome (myoclonic infantile encephalopathy) occurs most frequently in young children (mean age, 18 months). Approximately half of the cases have been reported in patients with neuroblastoma, but only approximately 3% of all neuroblastoma cases are complicated by the syndrome. Opsoclonus-myoclonus syndrome has been reported with carcinoma but occurs idiopathically as well. Because the idiopathic and paraneoplastic syndromes are indistinguishable clinically, opsoclonus-myoclonus syndrome should always prompt a search for neuroblastoma. Symptoms respond to steroid or corticotropin therapy. In the majority of cases, successful treatment of the neuroblastoma leads to remission; however, the syndrome may reappear with or without tumor recurrence (134).

VASCULITIS

Seizures as a manifestation of vasculitis may occur as a feature of encephalopathy, as a focal neurologic deficit, or in association with renal failure (135). The incidence of seizures increases with the duration and severity of the underlying vasculitis (136), and ranges from 24% to 45% (137). The relationship of the seizure disorder to the underlying disease may not always be clear, however. A confounding feature of AED therapy is the occurrence of drug-induced systemic lupus erythematosus (138). Although this association has been challenged—the seizures were believed to be an initial manifestation of lupus—phenytoin-associated lupus and spontaneous lupus do have different loci of immunoregulation (138). Systemic necrotizing vasculitis and granulomatous vasculitis rarely present with seizures. Among patients with giant-cell arteritis with nonocular signs, seizures occur in 1.5% (139). Behçet disease is associated with neurologic involvement in 10% to 25% of patients. Onset is usually acute, and seizures occasionally occur.

TRANSPLANTATION AND SEIZURES

Organ transplantation has led to newly recognized CNS disorders and new manifestations of old disorders. Seizures in patients anticipating or having undergone transplantation may be difficult to manage for several reasons: (a) these individuals are frequently metabolically stressed; (b) preexisting diseases and preceding therapies may have affected the CNS (e.g., candidates for bone marrow transplantation may have received L-asparaginase, which is associated with acute intracerebral hemorrhage and infarction, and ischemic seizures); and (c) immunosuppressive agents, particularly cyclosporine and tacrolimus (FK506), may themselves provoke seizures.

Some transplant patients appear to have an increased risk for seizures. Wijdicks and colleagues (140) concluded that most new-onset seizures in 630 patients undergoing orthotopic liver transplantation resulted from immunosuppressant neurotoxicity (cyclosporine and FK506) and did not indicate a poor outcome. Vaughn and coworkers (141) reported that of 85 patients who had received a lung transplant, 22 had seizures (including 15 of 18 patients with cystic fibrosis); in patients younger than age 25 years, particularly those given IV methylprednisolone to prevent rejection, the seizure risk was increased. Bone marrow transplant recipients with human leukocyte antigen mismatch and unrelated donor material have an enhanced risk for seizures from cyclosporine neurotoxicity (142). Foscarnet, used to treat cytomegalovirus hepatitis following bone marrow transplantation (143), may also precipitate seizures (144). For the acute management of prolonged seizures, benzodiazepines are least likely to induce the enzyme system responsible for metabolizing immunosuppressant drugs (145).

Long-term management of transplant recipients with seizures is determined after the etiology has been ascertained. Because allograft survival is decreased with phenytoin or phenobarbital and steroids (146), the use of AEDs has been discouraged (147). The half-lives of prednisolone and, probably, cyclosporine (145) are decreased when phenobarbital, phenytoin, or carbamazepine are administered. Valproic acid is a reasonable choice, except in hepatic transplantation patients and in bone marrow transplantation patients during engraftment.

Gabapentin may be useful in patients undergoing hepatic or bone marrow transplantation. The agent eliminated renally as unchanged drug from the systemic circulation, with very little gabapentin protein bound, and probably has fewer drug interactions than other AEDs. Gabapentin use in patients with renal failure must be modified, however.

Phenytoin should be considered for patients with partial seizures, except during bone marrow engraftment, when carbamazepine is also relatively contraindicated because of toxic hematologic side effects. During the 2- to 6-week period of engraftment, phenobarbital is acceptable. When AEDs other than valproic acid or gabapentin are used, the doses of immunosuppressive agents should be increased to ensure therapeutic immunosuppression. Cyclosporine levels should be determined. Experience with other AEDs, such as lamotrigine and topiramate, in these settings is limited.

REFERENCES

1. Delanty N, Vaughan CJ, French JA. Medical causes of seizures. *Lancet* 1998;352:383–390.
2. Boggs JG. Seizures in medically complex patients. *Epilepsia* 1997;38(Suppl 4):S55–S59.
3. Turnbull TL, Vanden Hoek TL, Howes DS, et al. Utility of laboratory studies in the emergency department patient with a new-onset seizure. *Ann Emerg Med* 1990;19:373–377.
4. Anderson RJ, Chung HM, Kluge R, et al. Hyponatremia: a prospective analysis of its epidemiology and the pathogenetic role of vasopressin. *Ann Intern Med* 1985;102:164–168.
5. Arieff AI, Guisardo R. Effects on the central nervous system of hypernatremic and hyponatremic states. *Kidney Int* 1976;10: 104–116.
6. Daggett P, Deanfield J, Moss F. Neurological aspects of hyponatremia. *Postgrad Med J* 1982;58:737–740.
7. Riggs JE. Neurologic manifestations of fluid and electrolyte disturbances. *Neurol Clin* 1989;7:509–523.
8. Adams RD, Victor M, Mancall EL. Central pontine myelinolysis: a hitherto undescribed disease occurring in alcoholic and malnourished patients. *AMA Arch Neurol Psychiatry* 1959;81:154–172.
9. Paguirigan A, Lefken EB. Central pontine myelinolysis. *Neurology* 1969;19:1007–1011.
10. Norenberg MD, Leslie KO, Robertson AS. Association between rise in serum sodium and central pontine myelinolysis. *Ann Neurol* 1982;11:128–135.
11. Kleinschmidt-DeMasters BK, Norenberg MD. Neuropathologic observations in electrolyte-induced myelinolysis in the rat. *J Neuropathol Exp Neurol* 1962;41:67–80.
12. Rossi NF, Schrier RW. Hyponatremic states. In: Maxwell MH, Cleeman CR, Narins RG, eds. *Clinical disorders of fluid and electrolyte metabolism*, 5th ed. New York: McGraw-Hill, 1987: 461–470.
13. Schmidt D, Sachdeo R. Oxcarbazepine for treatment of partial epilepsy: a review and recommendations for clinical use. *Epilepsy Behav* 2000;1:396–405.
14. Sue YM, Lee YL, Huang JJ. Acute hyponatremia, seizure, and rhabdomyolysis after ecstasy use. *J Toxicol Clin Toxicol* 2002;40:931–932.
15. Hartung TK, Schofield E, Short AI, et al. Hyponatraemic states following 3,4-methylenedioxymethamphetamine (MDMA, "ecstasy") ingestion. *QJM* 2002;95:431–437.
16. Gupta MM. Medical emergencies associated with disorders of calcium homeostasis. *J Assoc Physicians India* 1989;37:629–631.
17. Halperin I, Nubiola A, Vendrell J, et al. Late-onset hypocalcemia appearing years after thyroid surgery. *J Endocrinol Invest* 1989;12: 419–422.
18. Pugliese MT, Blumberg DL, Hludzinski J, et al. Nutritional rickets in suburbia. *J Am Coll Nutr* 1998;17:637–641.
19. Layzer RB. *Neuromuscular manifestations of systemic disease.* Philadelphia: FA Davis, 1985:58–62.
20. Riggs JE. Electrolyte disturbances. In: Johnson RT, ed. *Current therapy in neurologic disease.* Philadelphia: BC Decker, 1985: 325–328.
21. Whang R. Clinical disorders of magnesium metabolism. *Compr Ther* 1997;23:168–173.
22. Silvis SE, Paragas PD. Paresthesias, weakness, seizures, and hypophosphatemia in patients receiving hyperalimentation. *Gastroenterology* 1972;62:513–520.
23. Knochel JP. The pathophysiology and clinical characteristics of severe hypophosphatemia. *Arch Intern Med* 1977;137:203–220.
24. Singh BM, Strobos RJ. Epilepsia partialis continua associated with nonketotic hyperglycemia: clinical and biochemical profile of 21 patients. *Ann Neurol* 1980;8:155–160.
25. Vastola EF, Maccario M, Homan RO. Activation of epileptogenic foci by hyperosmolality. *Neurology* 1967;17:520–526.
26. Singh BM, Gupta DR, Strobos RJ. Nonketotic hyperglycemia and epilepsia partialis continua. *Arch Neurol* 1973;29:189–190.
27. Brick J, Gutrecht J, Ringel R. Reflex epilepsy and nonketotic hyperglycemia in the elderly: a specific neuroendocrine syndrome. *Neurology* 1989;39:394–399.
28. Venna N, Sabin T. Tonic focal seizures in nonketotic hyperglycemia of diabetes mellitus. *Arch Neurol* 1981;38:512–514.
29. Guisado R, Arieff AI. Neurologic manifestations of diabetic comas: correlation with biochemical alterations of the brain. *Metabolism* 1975;24:665–679.
30. Juurlink DN, Mamdani M, Kopp A, et al. Drug–drug interactions among elderly patients hospitalized for drug toxicity. *JAMA* 2003;289:1652–1658.
31. Bjerke HS, Kelly RE Jr, Geffner ME, et al. Surgical management of islet cell dysmaturation syndrome in young children. *Surg Gynecol Obstet* 1990;171:321–325.
32. Jabbari B, Huott AD. Seizures in thyrotoxicosis. *Epilepsia* 1980; 21:91–96.
33. Henderson LM, Behan PO, Aarli J, et al. Hashimoto's encephalopathy: a new neuroimmunological syndrome. *Ann Neurol* 1987:22: 140–141.
34. Shaw PJ, Walls TJ, Newman PK, et al. Hashimoto's encephalopathy: a steroid-responsive disorder associated with high antithyroid antibody titers—report of 5 cases. *Neurology* 1991;41: 228–233.
35. Henchey R, Cibula J, Helveston W, et al. Electroencephalographic findings in Hashimoto's encephalopathy. *Neurology* 1995;45: 977–981.
36. Rajagopal KR, Abbrecht PH, Derderian SS, et al. Obstructive sleep apnea in hypothyroidism. *Ann Intern Med* 1984;101:491–494.
37. Gilmore RL, Falace P, Kanga J, et al. Sleep-disordered breathing in Mobius syndrome. *J Child Neurol* 1991;6:73–77.

38. Kaplan PW. Metabolic and endocrine disorders resembling seizures. In: Engel J Jr, Pedley T, eds. *Epilepsy: a comprehensive textbook.* Philadelphia: Lippincott-Raven, 1997:2661–2770.

39. Odar-Cederlof I, Borga O. Kinetics of diphenylhydantoin in uraemic patients: consequence of decreased plasma protein binding. *Eur J Clin Pharmacol* 1974;7:31–37.

40. Lockwood AH. Neurologic complications of renal disease. *Neurol Clin* 1989;7:617–627.

41. Beydoun VA, Uthman BM, Sackellares JC. Gabapentin: pharmacokinetics, efficacy, and safety. *Clin Neuropharmacol* 1995;18:469–481.

42. Manian FA, Stone WJ, Alford RH. Adverse antibiotic effects associated with renal insufficiency. *Rev Infect Dis* 1990;12:236–249.

43. Knoben JE, Anderson PO. *Handbook of clinical drug data,* 6th ed. Hamilton, IL: Drug Intelligence, 1989:36–54.

44. Cassidy G, Corbett J. Learning disorders. In: Engel J Jr, Pedley T, eds. *Epilepsy: a comprehensive textbook.* Philadelphia: Lippincott-Raven, 1997:2053–2063.

45. Labrune P, Chatelon S, Huguet P, et al. Unusual cerebral manifestations in hereditary fructose intolerance. *Arch Neurol* 1990;47:1243–1244.

46. Sergay SM. Management of neurologic exacerbations of hepatic porphyria. *Med Clin North Am* 1979;63:453–463.

47. Reynolds NC Jr, Miska RM. Safety of anticonvulsants in hepatic porphyrias. *Neurology* 1981;31:480–484.

48. Bonkowsky HL, Sinclair PR, Emery S, et al. Seizure management in acute hepatic porphyria: risks of valproate and clonazepam. *Neurology* 1980;30:588–592.

49. Shedlofsky SI, Bonkowshy HL. Seizure management in the hepatic porphyrias: results from a cell-culture model of porphyria [letter]. *Neurology* 1984;34:399.

50. Larson AW, Wasserstrom WR, Felsher BF, et al. Posttraumatic epilepsy and acute intermittent porphyria: effects of phenytoin, carbamazepine, and clonazepam. *Neurology* 1978;28:824–828.

51. Krauss GL, Simmons-O'Brien E, Campbell M. Successful treatment of seizures and porphyria with gabapentin. *Neurology* 1995;45:594–595.

52. Zadra M, Grandi R, Erli LC, et al. Treatment of seizures in acute intermittent porphyria: safety and efficacy of gabapentin. *Seizure* 1998;7:415–416.

53. Richens A. Clinical pharmacokinetics of gabapentin. In: Chadwick D, ed. *New trends in epilepsy management: the role of gabapentin.* London: Royal Society of Medical Services, 1993:41–46.

54. Gorchein A. Drug treatment in acute porphyria. *Br J Clin Pharmacol* 1997;44:427–434.

55. Mir NA, Faquih AM, Legnain M. Perinatal risk factors in birth asphyxia: relationship of obstetric and neonatal complications to neonatal mortality in 16,365 consecutive live births. *Asia Oceania J Obstet Gynaecol* 1989;15:351–357.

56. Kreisman NR, Sick TJ, Rosenthal M. Importance of vascular responses in determining cortical oxygenation during recurrent paroxysmal events of varying duration and frequency of repetition. *J Cereb Blood Flow Metab* 1983;3:330–338.

57. Perlman JM, Herscovitch P, Kreusser KL, et al. Positron emission tomography in the newborn: effect of seizure on regional blood flow in an asphyxiated infant. *Neurology* 1985;35:244–247.

58. Easton JD, Sherman DG. Management of cerebral embolism of cardiac origin. *Stroke* 1980;11:433–442.

59. Roach GW, Kanchuger CM, Mangano CM, et al. Adverse cerebral outcomes after coronary bypass surgery. Multicenter Study of Perioperative Ischemia Research Group and the Ischemia Research and Education Foundation Investigators. *N Engl J Med* 1996;335:1857–1863.

60. Simon RP, Aminoff MJ. Electrographic status epilepticus in fatal anoxic coma. *Ann Neurol* 1986;20:351–355.

61. Boggs JG, Towne A, Smith J, et al. Frequency of potentially ictal patterns in comatose ICU patients. *Epilepsia* 1994;35(Suppl 8):135.

62. Towne AR, Pellock JM, Ko D, et al. Determinants of mortality in status epilepticus. *Epilepsia* 1994;35:27–34.

63. Krumholz A, Stern BJ, Weiss HD. Outcome from coma after cardiopulmonary resuscitation: relation to seizures and myoclonus. *Neurology* 1988;38:401–405.

64. Young GB, Gilbert JJ, Zochodne DW. The significance of myoclonic status epilepticus in postanoxic coma. *Neurology* 1990;40:1843–1848.

65. Richter JA, Holtman JR Jr. Barbiturates: their in vivo effects and potential biochemical mechanisms. *Prog Neurobiol* 1982;18:275–319.

66. Lamsback WJ, Navrozov M. The acquired metabolic disorders of the nervous system. In: Adams RD, Victor M, eds. *Principles of neurology,* 5th ed. New York: McGraw-Hill, 1993:877–902.

67. Bruni J, Willmore LJ, Wilder BJ. Treatment of post-anoxic intention myoclonus with valproic acid. *Can J Neurol Sci* 1979;6:39–42.

68. Mattson RH. Seizures associated with alcohol use and alcohol withdrawal. In: Browne TR, Feldman RG, eds. *Epilepsy: diagnosis and management.* Boston: Little, Brown, 1983:325–332.

69. Forster FM, Booker H. The epilepsies and convulsive disorders. In: Joynt R, ed. *Clinical neurology, III.* Philadelphia: JB Lippincott, 1984:1–68.

70. Engel J. *Seizures and epilepsy.* Philadelphia: FA Davis, 1989:402.

71. Labar DR, Harden C. Infection and inflammatory diseases. In: Engel J Jr, Pedley T, eds. *Epilepsy: a comprehensive textbook.* Philadelphia: Lippincott-Raven, 1997:2587–2596.

72. Garcia-Monaco JC, Benach JL. Lyme neuroborreliosis. *Ann Neurol* 1995;37:691–702.

73. Ferrari S, Monaco S, Morbin M, et al. HIV-associated PML presenting as epilepsia partialis continua. *J Neurol Sci* 1998;161:180–184.

74. Carpio A, Santillan F, Leon P, et al. Is the course of neurocysticercosis modified by treatment with antihelminthic agents? *Arch Intern Med* 1995;155:1982–1988.

75. Kammerer WS, Schantz PM. Echinococcal disease. *Infect Dis Clin North Am* 1993;7:605–618.

76. Horowitz S, Bentson JR, Benson F, et al. CNS toxoplasmosis in acquired immunodeficiency syndrome. *Arch Neurol* 1983;40:649–652.

77. Das BN, Weinberg DV, Jampol LM. Cytomegalovirus retinitis. *Br J Hosp Med* 1994;52:163–166.

78. Lor E, Liu YQ. Neurologic sequelae associated with foscarnet therapy. *Ann Pharmacother* 1994;28:1035–1037.

79. Ashkenazi S, Cleary KR, Pickering LK, et al. The association of *Shiga* toxin and other cytotoxins with the neurologic manifestations of shigellosis. *J Infect Dis* 1990;161:961–965.

80. Zvulunov A, Lerman M, Ashkenazi S, et al. The prognosis of convulsions during childhood shigellosis. *Eur J Pediatr* 1990;149:293–294.

81. Butler T, Arnold M, Islam M. Depletion of hepatic glycogen in the hypoglycaemia of fatal childhood diarrhoeal illnesses. *Trans R Soc Trop Med Hyg* 1989;83:839–843.

82. Kieslich M, Errazuriz G, Posselt HG, et al. Brain white-matter lesions in celiac disease: a prospective study of 75 diet-treated patients. *Pediatrics* 2001;108:E21.

83. Finelli PF, McEntee WJ, Ambler M, et al. Adult celiac disease presenting as cerebellar syndrome. *Neurology* 1980;30:245–249.

84. Albers JW, Nostrant TT, Riggs JE. Neurologic manifestations of gastrointestinal disease. *Neurol Clin* 1989;7:525–548.

85. Rush PJ, Inman R, Berstein M, et al. Isolated vasculitis of the central nervous system in a patient with celiac disease. *Am J Med* 1986;81:1092–1094.

86. Gendelman S, Present D, Janowitz HD. Neurological complications of inflammatory bowel disease (IBD) [abstract]. *Gastroenterology* 1982;82:1065.

87. Relman DA, Schmidt TM, MacDermott RP, et al. Identification of the uncultured bacillus of Whipple's disease. *N Engl J Med* 1992;327:293–301.

88. Louis ED, Lynch T, Kaufmann P, et al. Diagnostic guidelines in central nervous system Whipple's disease. *Ann Neurol* 1996;40:561–568.

89. Johnson L, Diamond I. Cerebral Whipple's disease. Diagnosis by brain biopsy. *Am J Clin Pathol* 1980;74:486–490.

90. Feurle GE, Volk B, Waldherr R. Cerebral Whipple's disease with negative jejunal histology. *N Engl J Med* 1979;300:907–908.

91. Ryser RJ, Locksley RM, Eng SC, et al. Reversal of dementia associated with Whipple's disease by trimethoprim-sulfamethoxazole, drugs that penetrate the blood-brain barrier. *Gastroenterology* 1984;86:745–752.

92. Keinath RD, Merrell DE, Vlietstra R, et al. Antibiotic treatment and relapse in Whipple's disease. Long-term follow-up of 88 patients. *Gastroenterology* 1985;88:1867–1873.

93. Gerard A, Sarrot-Reynauld F, Liozon E, et al. Neurologic presentation of Whipple disease: report of 12 cases and review of the literature. *Medicine (Baltimore)* 2002;81:443–457.

94. Herlong HF. Hepatic encephalopathy. In: Johnson RT, ed. *Current therapy in neurologic disease, II.* Toronto: BC Decker, 1987: 303–306.

95. Messing RO, Closson RG, Simon RP. Drug-induced seizures: a 10-year experience. *Neurology* 1984;34:1582–1586.

96. Lowry MR, Dunner FJ. Seizures during tricyclic therapy. *Am J Psychiatry* 1980;137:1461–1462.

97. Richardson JW III, Richelson R. Antidepressants: clinical update for medical practitioners. *Mayo Clin Proc* 1984;59:330–337.

98. Favale E, Rubino V, Mainardi P, et al. Anticonvulsant effect of fluoxetine in humans. *Neurology* 1995;45:1926–1927.

99. Bodner RA, Lynch T, Lewis L, et al. Serotonin syndrome. *Neurology* 1995;45:219–223.

100. Bernard L, Stern R, Lew D, et al. Serotonin syndrome after concomitant treatment with linezolid and citalopram. *Clin Infect Dis* 2003;36:1197.

101. Ubogu EE, Katirji B. Mirtazapine-induced serotonin syndrome. *Clin Neuropharmacol* 2003;26:54–57.

102. Dannawi M. Possible serotonin syndrome after combination of buspirone and St. John's wort. *J Psychopharmacol* 2002;16:401.

103. Logothetis J. Spontaneous epileptic seizures and electroencephalographic changes in the course of phenothiazine therapy. *Neurology* 1967;17:869–877.

104. Pfeiffer RF, Kang J, Graber B, et al. Clozapine for psychosis in Parkinson's disease. *Mov Disord* 1990;5:239–242.

105. Friedman JH, Lannun MC. Clozapine-responsive tremor in Parkinson's disease. *Mov Disord* 1990;5:225–229.

106. Devinsky O, Honigfeld G, Patin J. Clozapine-related seizures. *Neurology* 1991;41:369–371.

107. Julius SC, Brenner RP. Myoclonic seizures with lithium. *Biol Psychiatry* 1987;22:1184–1190.

108. Eshleman SH, Shaw LM. Massive theophylline overdose with atypical metabolic abnormalities. *Clin Chem* 1990;36:398–399.

109. Hendren WG, Schieber RS, Garrettson LK. Extracorporeal bypass for the treatment of verapamil poisoning. *Ann Emerg Med* 1989;18:984–987.

110. Blain PG, Lane RJM. Neurologic disorders. In: Davies DM, ed. *Textbook of adverse drug reactions,* 4th ed. New York: Oxford University Press, 1991:535–566.

111. Watkins RC, Hambrick EL, Benjamin G, et al. Isoniazid toxicity presenting as seizures and metabolic acidosis. *J Natl Med Assoc* 1990;2:57–64.

112. Chin L, Sievers ML, Herrier RN, et al. Potentiation of pyridoxine by depressants and anticonvulsants in the treatment of acute isoniazid intoxication in dogs. *Toxicol Appl Pharmacol* 1981;58:504–509.

113. Alldredge BK, Lowenstein DH, Simon RP. Seizures associated with recreational drug abuse. *Neurology* 1989;39:1037–1039.

114. Brust JCM, Ng SKC, Hauser AW, et al. Marijuana use and the risk of new onset seizures. *Trans Am Clin Climatol Assoc* 1992;103: 176–181.

115. Pascual-Leone A, Dhuna A, Altafullah I, et al. Cocaine-induced seizures. *Neurology* 1990;40:404–407.

116. Johnson S, O'Meara M, Young JB. Acute cocaine poisoning. Importance of treating seizures and acidosis. *Am J Med* 1983;75:1061–1064.

117. Antelman SM, Kocan D, Rowland N, et al. Amitriptyline provides long-lasting immunization against sudden cardiac death from cocaine. *Eur J Pharmacol* 1981;69:119–120.

118. Jaffe JH. Drug addiction and drug abuse. In: Gilman AG, Goodman LS, Rall TW, et al., eds. *Goodman and Gilman's the pharmacologic basis of therapeutics,* 7th ed. New York: Macmillan; 1985:550–554.

119. Parrott AC. Recreational Ecstasy/MDMA, the serotonin syndrome, and serotonergic neurotoxicity. *Pharmacol Biochem Behav* 2002;71:837–844.

120. Henry JA, Jeffreys KJ, Dawling S. Toxicity and death from 3,4-methylenedioxymethamphetamine ("ecstasy"). *Lancet* 1992;340: 384–387.

121. Li J, Stokes SA, Wockener A. A tale of novel intoxication: seven cases of gamma hydroxybutyric acid overdose. *Ann Emerg Med* 1998;31:723–728.

122. European Monitoring Centre for Drugs and Drug Addiction scientific committee report on the risk assessment of GHB in the framework of the joint action on new synthetic drugs. Lisbon, Portugal: European Center for Drugs and Drug Addiction, 2000.

123. Schneck HJ, Ruprecht J. Central anticholinergic syndrome (CAS) in anesthesia and intensive care. *Acta Anaesthesiol Belg* 1989;40: 219–228.

124. Douglas KA, Redman CWG. Eclampsia in the United Kingdom. *Br Med J* 1994;309:1395–1400.

125. Duley L, Johansen R. Magnesium sulfate for preeclampsia and eclampsia: the evidence so far. *Br J Obstet Gynaecol* 1994;101: 565–567.

126. Hutton JD, James DK, Stirrat GM, et al. Management of severe preeclampsia and eclampsia by UK consultants. *Br J Obstet Gynaecol* 1992;99:554–556.

127. Dinsdale HB. Does magnesium sulfate treat eclamptic seizures? *Arch Neurol* 1988;45:1360–1361.

128. Kaplan PW, Lesser RP, Fisher RS, et al. No, magnesium sulfate should not be used in treating eclamptic seizures. *Arch Neurol* 1988;45:1361–1364.

129. Pritchard JA, Cunningham FG, Pritchard SA. The Parkland Memorial Hospital protocol for treatment of eclampsia. Evaluation of 245 cases. *Am J Obstet Gynecol* 1984;148:951–963.

130. Lucas MJ, Leveno KJ, Cunningham FG. A comparison of magnesium sulfate with phenytoin for the prevention of eclampsia. *N Engl J Med* 1995;333:201–205.

131. Belfort MA, Mose KJ Jr. Effect of magnesium sulfate on maternal brain blood flow in preeclampsia: a randomized, placebo-controlled study. *Am J Obstet Gynecol* 1992;167:661–666.

132. Stein DA, Chamberlain MC. Evaluation and management of seizures in the patient with cancer. *Oncology* 1991;5:33–39.

133. Dalmau J, Graus F, Rosenblum MK, et al. Anti-Hu–associated paraneoplastic encephalitis/sensory neuropathy: a clinical study of 71 patients. *Medicine (Baltimore)* 1992;71:59–72.

134. Dropcho E. The remote effects of cancer on the nervous system. *Neurol Clin* 1989;7:579–603.

135. Bennahum DA, Messner RP. Recent observations on central nervous system lupus erythematosus. *Semin Arthritis Rheum* 1975;4: 253–266.

136. Adelman DC, Saltiel E, Klinenberg JR. The neuropsychiatric manifestations of systemic lupus erythematosus: an overview. *Semin Arthritis Rheum* 1986;15:185–199.

137. Ellis SG, Verity MA. Central nervous system involvement in systemic lupus erythematosus. A review of neuropathologic findings in 57 cases, 1955–1977. *Semin Arthritis Rheum* 1979;8: 212–221.

138. Alarcon-Segovia D, Palacios R. Differences in immunoregulatory T cell circuits between diphenylhydantoin-related and spontaneously occurring systemic lupus erythematosus. *Arthritis Rheum* 1981;24:1086–1092.

139. Nadeau S, Watson RT. Neurologic manifestations of vasculitis and collagen vascular syndromes. In: Joynt R, ed. *Clinical neurology,* vol 4. Philadelphia: Lippincott-Raven, 1997:1–166.

140. Wijdicks EMF, Plevak DJ, Wiesner RH, et al. Causes and outcome of seizures in liver transplant recipients. *Neurology* 1996;47: 1523–1525.

141. Vaughn BV, Ali II, Olivier KN, et al. Seizures in lung transplant recipients. *Epilepsia* 1996;37:1175–1179.

142. Zimmer WE, Hourihane JM, Wang HZ, et al. The effect of human leukocyte antigen disparity on cyclosporine neurotoxicity after allogeneic bone marrow transplantation. *AJNR Am J Neuroradiol* 1998;19:601–608.

143. Zomas A, Mehta J, Powles R, et al. Unusual infections following allogeneic bone marrow transplantation for chronic lymphocytic leukemia. *Bone Marrow Transplant* 1994;14:799–803.

144. Lor E, Liu YQ. Neurologic sequelae associated with foscarnet therapy. *Ann Pharmacother* 1994;28:1035–1037.

145. Gilmore R. Seizures and antiepileptic drug use in transplant patients. *Neurol Clin* 1988;6:279–296.

146. McEnery PT, Stempel DA. Commentary: anticonvulsant therapy and renal allograft survival. *J Pediatr* 1976;88:138–139.

147. Wassner SJ, Malekzadeh MH, Pennisi AJ, et al. Allograft survival in patients receiving anticonvulsant medications. *Clin Nephrol* 1977;8:293–297.

Epilepsy in Patients with Multiple Handicaps

39

John M. Pellock

Disabilities associated with the varying etiologies of epilepsy or with the disease itself often lead to multiple handicaps that complicate the diagnosis of epilepsy, render it refractory to treatment, and increase its morbid consequences. Some disabilities are developmental and frequently noted in children. Others are acquired disorders with accompanying behavioral, intellectual, communication, motor, and psychosocial deficits. Mental retardation and cerebral palsy are the most commonly discussed, but autism, attention deficit hyperactivity disorder, learning disabilities, depression, and psychoses all complicate epilepsy as well.

MENTAL RETARDATION

Just as epilepsy is not a solitary disease, mental retardation is not a disease, a syndrome, or a specific medical disorder. In 2002, the American Association on Mental Retardation (1) described a disability originating before age 18 years characterized by significant limitations both in intellectual functioning and adaptive behavior as expressed in conceptual, social, and practical adaptive skills. Five criteria were believed to be essential: (a) the limitation in present functioning must be considered within the context of community environments typical to the individual's age, peers, and culture; (b) to be valid an assessment must consider cultural and linguistic diversity, as well as differences in communication, sensory, motor, and behavioral factors; (c) within an individual, limitations often coexist with strengths; (d) an important purpose of describing limitations is to develop a profile of needed supports; and (e) with appropriate personalized supports over a sustained period, the life functioning of the person with mental

retardation generally will improve. These criteria do not state an intelligence quotient (IQ) measurement as a determining factor, but the 1994 (2) and 2000 (3) editions of the *Diagnostic and Statistical Manual of Mental Disorders* recognized an IQ of approximately 70 or below and further described mild (IQ 50/55 to 70), moderate (IQ 35/40 to 50/55), severe (IQ 20/25 to 35/40), and profound (IQ less than 20/25) categories. An early classification employed IQ levels for educable (50 to 75), trainable (30 to 50), and severely or profoundly retarded (less than 30). A recent trend simplifies the categories to mild (IQs from 50 to 70) and severe (IQs less than 50) (1,4,5). The abilities of a person with mental retardation depend both on intelligence, as measured by formal testing, and social adaptability, which includes interpersonal and group behaviors (4).

The comorbidities of mental retardation include cerebral palsy, autism, epilepsy, and numerous behavioral diagnoses such as attention deficit hyperactivity disorder and oppositional defiant disorder. These comorbid conditions are determined by specific etiologic diagnoses such as chromosomal disorders, neurocutaneous syndromes, central nervous system (CNS) injury, and inherited metabolic disorders (Table 39.1). The overlay of diagnostic categories and etiologies demonstrate that both epilepsy and mental retardation are symptoms of numerous conditions responsible for CNS dysfunction. Not infrequently, the specific cause remains unknown, although advances in neuroimaging, molecular genetics, and metabolic testing may remedy this lack. The relative risk of mental retardation appears to increase with decreasing socioeconomic status (1,4–6).

Severe mental retardation is found in approximately 0.3% to 0.4% of the general population, or in 10% of the mentally retarded. The mild form has an estimated

TABLE 39.1

MENTAL RETARDATION: CATEGORIES OF CAUSES

Sociocultural or environmental
- Nutritional deprivation

Developmental or cerebral dysgenesis
- Anencephaly
- Neural tube defects
- Encephalocele
- Holoprosencephaly
- Lissencephaly
- Micrencephaly
- Megalencephaly
- Hydranencephaly
- Porencephaly
- Schizencephaly

Chromosomal or genetic
- X-linked syndromes
- Multiple minor congenital anomaly syndromes
- Contiguous gene syndromes
- Single-gene disorders

Metabolic
- Perinatal and postnatal hypoxic-ischemic encephalopathy
- Hypoglycemia
- Severe hypernatremia
- Enzyme defects

Prematurity
- Intracranial hemorrhage
- Hydrocephalus
- Periventricular leukomalacia
- Periventricular hemorrhagic infarction

Traumatic brain injury
- Physical abuse, maternal trauma, birth trauma

Endocrine
- Hypothyroidism
- Hyperthyroidism
- Hypoparathyroidism

Nutritional
- Severe prenatal and postnatal protein malnutrition
- Periconceptual folate deficiency
- Vitamin and essential element deficiency

Infection
- Toxoplasmosis
- Syphilis
- Rubella
- Cytomegalovirus
- Herpes simplex virus
- Streptococcus
- Human immunodeficiency virus

Neuromuscular disorder
- Myotonic dystrophy
- Dystrophinopathy
- Cerebro-ocular muscular dystrophy

Toxic exposures
- Heavy-metal poisoning
- Alcohol-related birth defects
- Ionizing radiation
- Drug embryopathies
- Teratogens

Cerebrovascular
- Hemorrhage
- Multiple infarctions
- Venous sinus thrombosis

Neurocutaneous syndromes
- Neurofibromatoses
- Tuberous sclerosis

From Roeleveld N, Zielhuis GA, Gabreels F. The prevalence of mental retardation: a critical review of recent literature. *Dev Med Child Neurol* 1997;39:125–132.

incidence of 20 to 30 cases per 1000 livebirths, or 2% to 3% of the population, and is more frequent in males. Approximately 50% of all persons with cerebral palsy have mental retardation (7). Compared with the general population, children with developmental delay and those with a diagnosis of mental retardation are at an increased risk for epilepsy. The incidence of childhood-onset epilepsy associated with mental retardation and cerebral palsy ranges from 15% to 38% (8). The highest rates of epilepsy are found in children with severe developmental disability and multiple handicaps; coexisting cerebral palsy and mental retardation increase the likelihood of epilepsy twofold, compared with either condition alone (8). In these children, intellectual disability results primarily from the underlying brain disease, not from epilepsy (9); however, continued frequent, repetitive, and uncontrolled seizures may produce additional neuropsychological deficits.

The management of epilepsy in the multihandicapped patient begins with careful evaluation and classification. Treatment, though usually pharmacologic, may be etiologically specific in the presence of metabolic disease, involve surgery when malformations or brain foci can be localized, or use diet or vagus nerve stimulation. Practice guidelines from the American Academy of Neurology have addressed the initial evaluation of the patient with mental retardation or global developmental delay (10). Differential diagnoses to be considered will depend on clinical findings and history (Table 39.1). Some refractory epilepsy syndromes—especially encephalopathic epilepsies such as Lennox-Gastaut syndrome, infantile spasms (West syndrome), and malignant partial epilepsy—are more common in the multihandicapped patient than in the general population. Comorbid epilepsy and mental retardation is characterized by multiple, yet poorly described, seizure types, long-standing epilepsy, frequent polytherapy, increased use of sedating antiepileptic drugs (AEDs), and sometimes frequent changes in therapy. In other patients, therapy has remained unchanged for years, despite uncontrolled seizures and new drugs and modalities, increasing the risk of status epilepticus and seizure clusters. Although many etiologies of epilepsy and mental retardation are long-standing, the new onset of seizures in a person with mental retardation or other neurologic handicap requires a complete reevaluation, including brain imaging studies, because of the equivalent or heightened risk of stroke, neoplasm, and head trauma compared with the general population. Treatment of these individuals is discussed below.

CEREBRAL PALSY

Cerebral palsy frequently shares an etiology with epilepsy, and the disorders often coexist. The term *cerebral palsy* is applied to a heterogenous group of nonprogressive or static motor disorders of CNS origin that occur early in life (11). Incidence is about 2.5 cases per 1000 livebirths, higher in twins and triplets (12). Early studies suggested an approximately 28% incidence of epilepsy in persons with cerebral palsy, but more recent epidemiologic studies place the combined incidence at 0.8 cases per 1000 livebirths. Individuals with severe cerebral palsy and those with both mental retardation and cerebral palsy run a high risk of epilepsy (8).

Cerebral palsy can be classified into four clinical types: hemiplegic, diplegic, tetraplegic, and dystonic or athetoid. The hemiplegic form manifests as a motor deficit in the second to third month of life and is usually linked to porencephaly or loss of brain volume in a territory of major cerebral vessels (12). Partial epilepsy is thus frequent in these patients. Spastic diplegia is associated with prematurity; newborns or neonates weighing less than 1500 g are at greatest risk. Underlying periventricular leukomalacia is often seen. The less common tetraplegic cerebral palsy results from global ischemia or widespread brain malformation, and usually involves secondarily generalized epilepsy with multiple seizure types. Dystonic cerebral palsy is often secondary to brain injury at the basal ganglia in the last trimester of gestation; kernicterus or hypoxic ischemic damage is a frequent accompaniment (12).

The diagnostic evaluation of children with cerebral palsy parallels that for mental retardation. Perhaps the most important determination is that the motor deficit is static, nonprogressive, and long-standing. The American Academy of Neurology recommends neuroimaging studies; other testing should depend on findings from history, physical examination, and imaging (13). Worsening cerebral palsy should prompt a complete diagnostic reevaluation. Cerebral palsy and epilepsy associated with hydrocephalus managed with ventricular shunting, worsening epilepsy, motor signs, or deterioration in intellectual ability or behavior mandate reevaluation for shunt malfunction and other complications. Initiation or discontinuation of medications for spasticity, movement disorders, or maladaptive behaviors may significantly affect the frequency of seizures.

The appearance of epilepsy in the population with cerebral palsy can vary significantly. Seizures usually have an earlier onset in individuals with severe cerebral palsy than in those with milder forms. The ability to control seizures is frequently related to the severity of the motor deficit. Fewer children with symptomatic or cryptogenic epilepsy associated with cerebral palsy can eventually discontinue AEDs. In one study (12,14), 30 (54%) of 56 children with a significant neurologic handicap had recurrent seizures on withdrawal of AEDs, compared with an overall recurrence rate of 31%.

AUTISM

Autism is a heterogeneous, pervasive developmental disorder that portends lifelong debility (Table 39.2) (2,15,16). Markedly abnormal or impaired development in social interaction and communication skills, evident in the first 3 years of life, affect language and behavior (15,16). Affected children typically do not demonstrate the normal attachment to and interest in parents, caregivers, and peers and also may show little separation anxiety. Children with autistic spectrum disorders may exhibit echolalia and verbal repetition, along with abnormalities in pitch, intonation, rate, and rhythm, as well as frequent stereotypic self-stimulating movements and a fascination for toys or objects with repetitive motion (17). The more recent identification and inclusion of autism in Rett, fragile X, and Angelman syndromes suggest a higher incidence than previously reported (18,19). Epidemiologic studies indicate rates as high as 6 cases per 1000 children (18), with a 3:1 higher incidence in boys. When cases of Asperger syndrome are included, a ratio as high as 15:1 can be seen (20).

Despite multiple etiologies of autistic spectrum disorder, a specific cause is not identified in up to 90% of patients (17). Underlying diagnoses include phenylketonuria, congenital infections (rubella, cytomegalovirus), tuberous sclerosis, and fragile X and Rett syndromes. Functional abnormalities in cerebellar, cortical, and basal ganglia have been suggested. Electroencephalographic (EEG) abnormalities are present in 27% to 65% of individuals; prolonged recordings commonly demonstrate paroxysmal epileptiform activity (21,22). Correlation of EEG abnormalities and clinical seizures is not absolute, even in patients with apparent language arrest, verbal auditory agnosia, and autistic regression associated with Landau-Kleffner syndrome (23–25). Whether ongoing seizures contribute to autistic regression remains controversial (26). Approximately 70% to 75% of persons with autism have IQ scores below 70 and thus are classified as mentally retarded; 25% to 35% develop some form of epilepsy, with seizures more likely in individuals with low IQs. Hyperactivity, impulsivity, short attention span, oversensitivity to sound and touch, various preoccupations, and self-stimulatory behaviors are common. Difficulties with

TABLE 39.2
DIAGNOSTIC CRITERIA FOR AUTISTIC DISORDER (299.00)

A. A total of six (or more) items from (1), (2), and (3), with two from (1), and at least one each from (2) and (3).
  1. Qualitative impairment in social interaction, manifest by at least two of the following:
    • Marked impairment in the use of multiple nonverbal behaviors, such as eye-to-eye gaze, facial expression, body postures, and gestures, to regulate social interaction
    • Failure to develop peer relationships appropriate to developmental level
    • Lack of spontaneous seeking to share enjoyment, interests, or achievements with other people (e.g., by lack of showing, bringing, or pointing out objects of interest)
    • Lack of social or emotional reciprocity
  2. Qualitative impairment in communication, as manifest by at least one of the following:
    • Delay in, or total lack of, the development of spoken language (not accompanied by an attempt to compensate through alternative modes of communication such as gesture or mime)
    • In individuals with adequate speech, marked impairment in the ability to initiate or sustain a conversation with others
    • Stereotyped and repetitive use of language, or idiosyncratic language
    • Lack of varied, spontaneous make-believe, or social imitative play appropriate to developmental level
  3. Restrictive repetitive and stereotypic patterns of behavior, interests, and activities, as manifested by at least one of the following:
    • Encompassing preoccupation with one or more stereotyped and restricted patterns of interest that is abnormal either in intensity or focus
    • Apparently inflexible adherence to specific nonfunctional routines or rituals
    • Stereotyped and repetitive motor mannerisms (e.g., hand or finger flapping or twisting, or complex whole-body movements)
    • Persistent preoccupation with parts of objects
B. Delays or abnormal functioning in at least one of the following areas, with onset prior to age 3 years:
  1. Social interaction
  2. Language as used in social communication
  3. Symbolic or imaginative play
C. The disturbance is not better accounted for by Rett's disorder or childhood disintegrative disorder.

The other pervasive developmental disorders include Asperger's disorder, Rett syndrome, childhood disintegrative disorder, pervasive developmental disorder-not otherwise specified (PDD-NOS), or atypical autism.

Reprinted, with permission, from the *Diagnostic and statistical manual of mental disorders*, 4th ed. Washington, DC: American Psychiatric Association, 1994:70–71.

transition, along with obsessions and compulsions, frequently need specific treatments. The diagnostic evaluation of the patient with suspected autism requires detailed history taking and developmental screening, along with observation. The American Academy of Neurology evidence-based guidelines suggest extensive use of checklists for autism in toddlers, screening questionnaires, audiologic testing, and screening for lead exposure. Specific genetic and metabolic tests, and screening for other toxins or infections may be indicated. Electroencephalography may be performed if epilepsy is suspected. Brain imaging studies, although rarely helpful, may be ordered in specific cases. Psychological, developmental, and speech and language assessments, along with educational testing are critical (16).

Treatment of the autistic individual comprises behavioral approaches, education, and cognitive and language training. Early interventions may be critical. Medications that affect serotonergic and dopaminergic systems have been used, along with specific agents for abnormal behaviors or seizures. Classic and atypical neuroleptic drugs, together with selective serotonin uptake inhibitors (SSRIs), are advantageous in individual patients (18). Newer members of these classes appear not to reduce seizure threshold with fewer deleterious effects. Medications for hyperactivity and inattention may also ameliorate stereotypic behaviors. Stimulants and atomoxetine rarely exacerbate seizures; however, high doses of bupropion may aggravate epilepsy or induce new-onset seizures. The use of anticonvulsants to control behavioral outbursts and affective dysregulation has gained in popularity. The clinician who treats autistic individuals with epilepsy must be aware of the medications that can afford symptomatic relief of maladaptive behavior and consider drug interactions and toxic reactions, as well as possible decreases or exacerbations of seizures either directly or indirectly through altered sleep-wake patterns.

LANDAU-KLEFFNER SYNDROME

Landau and Kleffner first described the syndrome of acquired aphasia in childhood associated with a convulsive disorder (27), in which a previously normal child, usually male, between the ages of 3 and 7 years, deteriorates and almost seems unable to hear because of verbal auditory agnosia that may progress to mutism. Except for the language impairment, these children are intellectually normal but exhibit behavioral disturbances such as hyperactivity, attention deficit, and, rarely, psychosis. Many clinical variants have been noted, but Landau-Kleffner syndrome should be distinguished from autistic regression and disintegrative epileptiform disorder (Table 39.3) (28). Seizures occur in approximately 75% of patients before or after onset of aphasia. The EEG recording consists of a variety of nonspecific generalized and focal abnormalities that increase during sleep, progressing to continuous spike-and-wave rhythms during slow-wave sleep. Treatment includes traditional AEDs, steroids or corticotropin, immunoglobulins, and calcium-channel blockers; multiple subpial transactions may be performed. The outcome is generally poor for language recovery and normalization of behavior but seizures generally are controlled. Continuous

TABLE 39.3

COMPARISON OF LANDAU-KLEFFNER SYNDROME, AUTISTIC EPILEPTIFORM REGRESSION, AND DISINTEGRATIVE EPILEPTIFORM DISORDER

	Aphasia	Social	Cognitive	Abnormal Electro-encephalogram	Prior Normal Development
Acquired epileptiform aphasia (Landau-Kleffner syndrome)	Yes	No	No	Yes	Yes
Autistic regression	Yes	Yes	No	No	Yes or no
Autistic epileptiform regression	Yes	Yes	No	Yes	Yes or no
Disintegrative disorder	Yes	Yes	Yes	No	Yes until age 2 years
Disintegrative epileptiform disorder	Yes	Yes	Yes	Yes	Yes until age 2 years

Adapted from Nass R, Gross A. Landau-Kleffner syndrome and its variants. In: Devinsky E, Westbrook LE, eds. *Epilepsy and developmental disabilities.* Boston: Butterworth-Heinemann, 2002:79–92.

spike-and-wave rhythms in slow-wave sleep portend a less favorable outcome (29,30).

DIAGNOSTIC EVALUATION

If the patient with multiple handicaps is not young and the epilepsy is not of recent onset, the diagnostic evaluation is challenging. These patients present with numerous disabilities, multiple but poorly described, refractory seizures and frequent bouts of status epilepticus. Lifelong AED use, including polytherapy, may produce a tolerance to side effects. Documentation to help identify the interactions of all factors often is inadequate, and the ictal events are rarely witnessed. Stereotypic behaviors are frequently misinterpreted as seizures, and periods of inattention or short-lived motor activity are not recognized as ictal events or are not even noted. Re-evaluation requires a chronologic approach to determine etiology, accurate diagnosis of the epilepsy syndrome, and insight into therapeutic success and failure. Observational records noting not only total number of seizures but their characteristics, length, and time of appearance, during both wakefulness and sleep, can be useful.

If diagnostic studies are not available for review, the EEG and magnetic resonance imaging (MRI) should be repeated. The need for sedation in many of these individuals who cannot fully cooperate entails an additional risk, and the process of obtaining informed consent should include a frank explanation of risks and benefits given to the patient and legal guardian. Aberrant behavior and heavy sedation may limit the full diagnostic scope of prolonged EEG monitoring, including assessment of waking background activity; however, the actual recording of events may be impossible without the patient's cooperation or this type of record. A meticulous medical history and collaboration with caregivers may yield the most useful information about the patient during and after the ictal event. Interictal electroencephalographs and those performed as soon as possible after the presumptive seizure also may be helpful. Video recordings of events that occur at home, school, or elsewhere, are extremely valuable, even without simultaneous electroencephalography.

THERAPY

The treatment of seizures in children and adults with developmental disability and multiple handicaps follows the same principles that govern therapy for other patients with epilepsy; however, frequent comorbidity, including both motor and intellectual deficits, is a complicating factor. Epilepsy in this population is most likely cryptogenic or symptomatic, rarely idiopathic. Refractory disease is common, and only a small percentage of these patients become seizure free with or without AEDs (12,14,31–35). In addition to both partial and generalized seizures, status epilepticus and seizure clusters occur frequently. Along with long-term administration of AEDs for seizure control, plans for intermittent or acute, emergent therapy for prolonged or clustered seizures, perhaps using rectally administered diazepam or other benzodiazepines (35,36), should be in place (36–38). Medical personnel and caregivers must devise guidelines for *intermittent* use of benzodiazepines to avoid inadvertent long-term administration and consequent decreased efficacy as rescue therapy.

The AED of choice depends on its efficacy against a specific seizure type balanced by tolerability and lack of

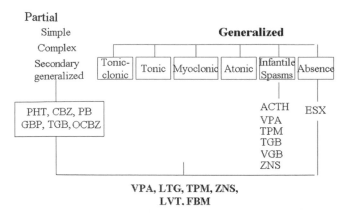

Figure 39.1 Treatment options for specific seizure types. ACTH, corticotropin; CBZ, carbamazepine; ESX, ethosuximide; FBM, felbamate; GBP, gabapentin; LTG, lamotrigine; LVT, levetiracetam; OCBZ, oxcarbazepine; PB, phenobarbital; PHT, phenytoin; TGB, tiagabine; TPM, topiramate; VGB, vigabatrin; VPA, valproic acid; ZNS, zonisamide.

adverse effects, including not exacerbating other seizure types (36). Figure 39.1 lists suggested medications for specific seizure types. Vagus nerve stimulation, ketogenic diet, and surgery should be considered when appropriate. Although most patients benefit from a reduction in drug dosage during treatment with the ketogenic diet, the interactions with drugs and metabolic effects of this nonpharmacologic method must be carefully monitored (see Chapter 70).

Behavioral disturbances are particularly difficult to manage (39). In children and adults with autistic spectrum disorder, some medications that ameliorate behavior affect serotonin and dopamine, including atypical neuroleptics, stimulants and related compounds that targeted hyperactive behavior, antidepressants, and antianxiety agents (18). Significant differences in their mechanisms of action make it difficult to explain why AEDs are efficacious in autistic spectrum disorders and other behavioral states (18). Mentally retarded individuals appear more likely than other patients to demonstrate aberrant behaviors, including significant aggressiveness, in response to a number of AEDs and psychotropic agents. Two trials in children with partial seizures demonstrate the interaction between previous behavioral states and side-effect profiles. One study of gabapentin as monotherapy for children with benign epilepsy with centrotemporal spikes reported a low incidence of behavioral side effects (36), whereas gabapentin as adjunctive therapy produced a much higher rate of negative behavior, especially in patients with mental retardation (40). Among AEDs introduced since 1990, felbamate, gabapentin, lamotrigine, topiramate, levetiracetam, oxcarbazepine, zonisamide, and vigabatrin have produced, at least in case reports, aberrant behavior in persons with behavioral comorbidity, including those with mental retardation (36). Even if comorbid conditions are not present, most AEDs can affect cognitive function and behavior, particularly with rapid titration or use of high doses (41). Careful titration and monotherapy are recommended

whenever possible. Barbiturates and benzodiazepines classically have been associated with mental obtundation, depressive symptoms, and behavioral problems, but their discontinuation will sometimes aggravate negative behaviors (42,43). Increased acting out and belligerence may appear as part of the "brightening" process that can occur with conversion to newer, less sedative AEDs. Thus, changes in therapy should be made slowly with careful clinical monitoring (36).

Polytherapy should be avoided, or, if unavoidable, reduced (34,44–46), as an excessive drug burden complicates the assessment of efficacy and tolerability. In addition to behavioral and cognitive adverse effects, drug interactions can result in cumulative toxic reactions. Complicating the reduction in polypharmacy is the belief that any change in medication will exacerbate seizure frequency. Although this occasionally may occur in an individual patient, long-term studies suggest that polypharmacy can be reduced successfully, especially when a newer AED is substituted for a traditional medication (34,36,44–46). In one study of 244 mentally retarded patients with epilepsy who were followed up for 10 years, monotherapy could be increased in 36.5% to 58.1% with no evident loss of seizure control (34). Total discontinuation of AED therapy may be more difficult (14,32,34,35), however, involving a risk of seizure recurrence that ranges from 40% to 50% (14,34). Length of seizure freedom during AED therapy and degree of mental handicap are reasonable indicators of success (14). Identification of the epilepsy syndrome may also aid in predicting successful AED withdrawal.

Therapy for the multihandicapped individual comprises several components: physical, occupational, speech, language, educational, vocational, and psychological (47–49). Unwanted effects of therapy must also be considered. In addition to specific AEDs (44), other medications may exert a negative effect on seizures. Barbiturates and benzodiazepines have a long association with rebound or withdrawal seizures; stability may return when these drugs are replaced (35). High doses of antidepressants have been linked to increased incidences of seizures in clinical trials (50): bupropion 2.2%, clomipramine 1.66%, and maprotiline 15.6% (39). The seizure risk with SSRIs is lower, ranging from 0.04% to 0.3%. For patients with epilepsy, recommended antidepressants are SSRIs, antidepressants with multiple sites of action (e.g., nefazodone and venlafaxine), monoamine oxidase inhibitors, and tricyclic antidepressants (39,50). Psychostimulants and the new agent, atomoxetine, appear unlikely to exacerbate seizures, but the subject is controversial (51); use of these agents in the management of attentional disorders and hyperactivity is not contraindicated (39,51). Sometimes, reduction in dosage of an AED prescribed primarily for a behavior disorder, such as valproate or lamotrigine used to treat bipolar symptoms, will exacerbate seizures. The physician treating a patient with multiple handicaps must appreciate this potential unwanted effect.

Adverse effects extend beyond behavioral abnormalities and neurotoxic reactions. Bone health, contracture formation, weight regulation, gastrointestinal disturbances, gynecologic concerns, and drug interactions affect not only the treatment of epilepsy but also medications prescribed for other comorbidities (42,44). Many of these patients cannot properly express or describe their complaints. Increased irritability or changes in behavior may often be the only sign of significant abnormality in this group.

CONCLUSIONS

The treatment of the multihandicapped child or adult with epilepsy must be tailored to the individual patient. A careful assessment of all comorbid conditions must be part of the intake evaluation, which should include the natural history of the epilepsy and previous treatment. New-onset seizures or seizures that have changed in type or intensity warrant a complete evaluation. Frequently, the best indicator of a good response to an AED will be past success. A medication may have been changed because of the hope for improved control of epilepsy or behavior with a newer AED. A return to tried-and-true therapy may be the best approach. The comorbid treatment and the epilepsy treatment will each affect the other. Similarly, management of comorbidities besides epilepsy will greatly improve the total outcome and quality of life. Understanding the difficulties in diagnosis and treatment of individuals with multiple handicaps and the interrelationship between epilepsy and comorbidities and their treatments is essential.

REFERENCES

1. American Association on Mental Retardation. *Mental retardation: definition, classification and systems of support*, 10th ed. Annapolis Junction, MD: AAMR Publications, 2002.
2. American Psychiatric Association. *Diagnostic and statistical manual of mental disorders*, 4th ed. Washington, DC: Author, 1994:70–71.
3. American Psychiatric Association. *Diagnostic and statistical manual of mental disorders*, 4th ed., text revision. Washington, DC: Author, 2000.
4. Roeleveld N, Zielhuis GA, Gabreels F. The prevalence of mental retardation: a critical review of recent literature. *Dev Med Child Neurol* 1997;39:125–132.
5. Weinstein B, Steedman JG, Miller G, et al. *Mental retardation*. San Diego, CA: Medlink Neurology, 2004.
6. Kiely M. The prevalence of mental retardation. *Epidemiol Rev* 1987;9:194–228.
7. Miller G. Cerebral palsies. In: Miller G, Ramer JC, eds. *Static encephalopathies of infancy and childhood*. New York: Raven Press, 1992:11–26.
8. Shinnar S, Pellock JM. Update on the epidemiology and prognosis of pediatric epilepsy. *J Child Neurol* 2002;17(Suppl 1):S4–S17.
9. Dodson WE. Epilepsy, cerebral palsy and IQ. In: Pellock JM, Dodson WE, Bourgeois BFD, eds. *Pediatric epilepsy. Diagnosis and therapy*. New York: Demos, 2002:613–627.
10. Shevell M, Aswal S, Donley D, et al. Practice parameter: evaluation of the child with global developmental delay. *Neurology* 2003; 60:367–380.
11. Badawi N, Watson L, Petterson B, et al. What constitutes cerebral palsy? *Dev Med Child Neurol* 1998;40:847–851.
12. Camfield C, Camfield P, Watson L. Cerebral palsy in children with epilepsy. In: Devinsky O, Westbrooke LE, eds. *Epilepsy and developmental disabilities*. Boston: Butterworth-Heinemann, 2002:33–40.
13. Ashwal S, Russman BS, Blaseo PA, et al. Practice parameter: diagnostic assessment of the child with cerebral palsy. *Neurology* 2004;62:851–863.
14. Camfield P, Camfield C. Initiating and discontinuing antiepileptic drugs in children with neurologic handicaps and epilepsy. In: Devinsky O, Westbrook LE, eds. *Epilepsy and developmental disabilities*. Boston: Butterworth-Heinemann, 2002:281–286.
15. Filipek PA, Accardo PJ, Baranek GT, et al. The screening and diagnosis of autistic spectrum disorders. *J Autism Dev Disord* 1999; 29:437–482.
16. Filipek PA, Accardo PJ, Ashwal S, et al. Practice parameter: screening and diagnosis of autism: report for the Quality Standards Subcommittee of the American Academy of Neurology and the Child Neurology Society. *Neurology* 2000;55:468–479.
17. Spratt EG, Macias MM, Lee DO. *Autistic spectrum disorders*. San Diego, CA: Medlink Neurology, 2004.
18. Parlermo MT, Curatolo P. Pharmacologic treatment of autism. *J Child Neurol* 2004;19:155–164.
19. Ehlers S, Gillberg C. The epidemiology of Asperger's syndrome: a total population study. *J Child Psychol Psychiatry* 1993;34: 1327–1350.
20. Baird G, Charman T, Baron-Cohen S, et al. A screening instrument for autism at 18 months of age: a 6-year follow-up study. *J Child Psychol Psychiatry* 2000;39:694–702.
21. Minshew N. Indices of neural function in autism: clinical and biologic implications. *Pediatrics* 1991;87:774–780.
22. Yaylali I, Tuchman R, Jayakar P. Comparison of the utility of routine versus prolonged EEG recordings in children with language regression [abstract]. Presented at the American Clinical Neurophysiology Society Annual Meeting, Boston, MA, September, 1996.
23. Tuchman RF. Acquired epileptiform aphasia. *Semin Pediatr Neurol* 1997;4:93–101.
24. Shinnar S, Rapin I, Arnold S, et al. Language regression in childhood. *Pediatr Neurol* 2001;24:183–189.
25. Nass R, Devinsky O. Autistic regression with rolandic spikes. *Neuropsychiatry Neuropsychol Behav Neurol* 1999;12:193–197.
26. Rapin I. Autism in search of a home in the brain. *Neurology* 1999;52:902–904.
27. Landau W. Landau-Kleffner syndrome. An eponymic badge of ignorance. *Arch Neurol* 1992;49:353.
28. Nass R, Gross A. Landau-Kleffner syndrome and its variants. In: Devinsky E, Westbrook LE, eds. *Epilepsy and developmental disabilities*. Boston: Butterworth-Heinemann, 2002:79–92.
29. Nass R, Gross A, Wisoff J, et al. Outcome of multiple subpial transections for autistic epileptiform regression. *Pediatr Neurol* 1999; 21:464–470.
30. Rossi PG, Parmeggiani A, Posar A, et al. Landau-Kleffner syndrome (LKS): long-term follow-up and links with electrical status epilepticus during sleep (ESES). *Brain Dev* 1999;21:90–98.
31. Bourgeois BFD. Controlling seizures in children with developmental disabilities: an overview. In: Devinsky E, Westbrook LE, eds. *Epilepsy and developmental disabilities*. Boston: Butterworth-Heinemann, 2002:273–280.
32. Steffenburg U, Hedstrom A, Lindroth A, et al. Intractable epilepsy in a population-based series of mentally retarded children. *Epilepsia* 1998;39:767–775.
33. Aicardi J, Shorvon SD. Intractable epilepsy. In: Engel JJ, Pedley TA, eds. *Epilepsy: a comprehensive textbook*. Philadelphia: Lippincott-Raven, 1997:1325–1331.
34. Pellock JM, Hunt PA. A decade of modern epilepsy therapy in institutionalized mentally retarded patients. *Epilepsy Res* 1996;25: 263–268.
35. Mirza EU, Credeur LH, Penry JK. Results of antiepileptic drug reduction in patients with multiple handicaps and epilepsy. *Drug Invest* 1993;5:320–326.
36. Pellock JM, Morton LD. Treatment of epilepsy in the multiply handicapped. *Ment Retard Dev Disabil Res Rev* 2000;6:309–323.
37. Dreifuss F, Rosman N, Cloyd J, et al. A comparison of rectal diazepam gel and placebo for acute repetitive seizures. *N Engl J Med* 1998;338:1869–1875.

38. Pellock JM, Leszczyszyn DJ. Status epilepticus. In: Devinsky E, Westbrook LE, eds. *Epilepsy and developmental disabilities*. Boston: Butterworth-Heinemann 2002;93–110.
39. Pellock JM. Understanding co-morbidities affecting children with epilepsy. *Neurology* 2004;62(Suppl 2):S17–S23.
40. Khurana DS, Riviello J, Helmers S, et al. Efficacy of gabapentin therapy in children with refractory seizures. *J Pediatr* 1996;128: 829–833.
41. Meador KJ. Cognitive outcomes and predictive factors in epilepsy. *Neurology* 2002;58(Suppl 5):S21–S26.
42. Brent DA, Crumrine PK, Varma RR, et al. Phenobarbital treatment and major depressive disorder in children with epilepsy. *Pediatrics* 1987;80:909–917.
43. Theodore WH, Porter RJ. Removal of sedative-hypnotic antiepileptic drugs from the regimen of patients with intractable epilepsy. *Ann Neurol* 1983;13:320–324.
44. Perucca E, Beghi E, Dulac O, et al. Assessing risk to benefit ratio in antiepileptic drug therapy. *Epilepsy Res* 2000;41:107–139.
45. Schmidt D. Reduction of two-drug therapy in intractable epilepsy. *Epilepsia* 1983;24:368–376.
46. Albright P, Bruni J. Reduction of polytherapy in epileptic patients. *Arch Neurol* 1985;42:797–799.
47. Michaud LJ, American Academy of Pediatrics Committee on Children With Disabilities. Prescribing therapy services for children with motor disabilities. *Pediatrics* 2004;113:1836–1838.
48. Tara HL, American Academy of Pediatrics Committee on School Health. School-based mental health services. *Pediatrics* 2004;113: 1839–1845.
49. Devinsky O, Westbrook LE, eds. *Epilepsy and developmental disabilities*. Boston: Butterworth-Heinemann, 2002.
50. Harden CL, Goldstein MA. Mood disorders in patients with epilepsy: epidemiology and management. *CNS Drugs* 2002;16: 291–302.
51. Feldman H, Crumrine P, Handen BL, et al. Methylphenidate in children with seizures and attention-deficit disorder. *Am J Dis Child* 1989;143:1081–1086.

Epilepsy in the Elderly

40

Ilo E. Leppik *Angela K. Birnbaum*

The elderly (persons 65 years of age and older) are the most rapidly growing segment of the population, and onset of epilepsy is higher in this group than in any other group. The incidence of a first seizure is 52 to 59 per 100,000 in persons 40 to 59 years of age but rises to 127 per 100,000 persons in those age 60 years and older (1). Approximately 1.5% of the elderly have active epilepsy, about twice the rate of younger adults. In the United States, of the approximately 181,000 persons who developed epilepsy in 1995, about 68,000 were older than age 65 years (2). In Finland, 34,453 persons had epilepsy during 1986, and 12.8% were older than age 65 years; by 2000, the number had increased to 49,003, of whom 19.7% were elderly. In persons older than age 65 years there were 396 new cases (11.2% of all new cases) in 1986, but in 2000, 597 new cases (22%) were in the elderly group (M. Sillanpaa, personal communication, 2001).

The numbers mentioned above were for the community-dwelling elderly. In nursing homes, epilepsy, seizures, and antiepileptic drug (AED) use are much more prevalent. Among 45,405 elderly residents of U.S. long-term care facilities, 4573 (10.1%) took at least one AED (3). AED use in the nursing-home population varies between 10% and 11% (4–6). Because approximately 1.5 million elderly reside in nursing homes in the United States, as many as 150,000 may be taking AEDs (7).

Approximately 7% of residents are using AEDs at admission, but approximately 3% receive their first prescription after admission. In a study of 21,551 nursing home residents in 24 states on 1 day during the spring of 1995, 10.5% had an AED order, and 9.2% of them had a seizure or epilepsy indication recorded in the physician's orders (4). (Information on how the diagnosis was made was not available.) Of the AED prescriptions, 6.2% were for phenytoin (the most commonly used AED in nursing homes), 1.8% for carbamazepine, 0.9% for valproic acid, and 1.7% for phenobarbital; 1.2% were for all other AEDs combined. Phenytoin was the most frequently initiated AED after admission if the current procedural terminology code was for seizures or epilepsy, and valproate or carbamazepine if a psychiatric or behavioral diagnosis was listed (8).

Assessment of AED efficacy and toxicity in elderly patients is challenging because seizures are sometimes difficult to observe, toxic signs and symptoms can be attributed to other causes (e.g., Alzheimer disease or stroke) or to comedications, and patients may not be able to accurately report problems. More so than younger persons, the elderly may experience more side effects, have a higher risk for drug interactions, and be less able to afford medications. Neither the benefits nor the risks of treatment have been investigated in this population, and current practices are not based on evidence.

Stroke accounts for 30% to 40% of all cases of epilepsy in the elderly (9), followed by brain tumor, head injury, and Alzheimer disease. In many cases, however, the precise cause cannot be identified, and the etiology is cryptogenic.

The most important differential diagnosis in the elderly is convulsive syncope in which a seizure is provoked by lack of circulation to the brain. Cardiac causes are common, and in the absence of a known central nervous system disorder (stroke, tumor, degeneration), syncope should be suspected. An electroencephalogram with concomitant electrocardiographic rhythm strip is essential to clarify the diagnosis.

Electrolyte imbalance, febrile illness, hypoglycemia, or hyperglycemia may also provoke seizures, but these conditions should be easily recognized by laboratory tests or physical examination and do not require long-term AED treatment.

Although the diagnosis of epilepsy is generally made only after two or more seizures, persons with a single, unprovoked seizure (no obvious cause external to the central nervous system), especially if a stroke has occurred previously, should be treated with AEDs because of the high risk of a second attack and the catastrophic consequences of a second seizure (fall, fracture, cardiac compromise).

In addition to their use in epilepsy, AEDs are prescribed for neuralgias, aggressive behavior disorders, essential tremor, and restless legs syndrome, all of which are prevalent in the elderly. When clinicians prescribe for the elderly, they must also consider the likelihood of concomitant disorders and the high individual variability in this population. As a cause of adverse reactions among the elderly, AEDs rank fifth among all drug categories (10).

CLINICAL PHARMACOLOGY OF ANTIEPILEPTIC DRUGS

Drug concentration at the site of action determines the magnitude of both desired and toxic responses. The unbound concentration in serum is in direct equilibrium with the concentration at the site of action and correlates best with drug response (11). Total serum drug concentration is useful for monitoring of therapy when the drug is not highly protein bound (<75%) or when the ratio of unbound to total drug concentration remains relatively stable. Phenytoin and valproic acid, which are the most widely used drugs in the elderly, are highly bound, and their binding is frequently altered.

The age-related physiologic changes that have the greatest effect on AED pharmacokinetics involve protein binding and the reduction in liver volume and blood flow (12–15). Reduced serum albumin and increased α_1-acid glycoprotein (AAG) concentrations in the elderly alter protein binding of some drugs (11,12,14). By age 65 years, many individuals have low-normal albumin concentrations or are frankly hypoalbuminemic (12). Albumin concentration may be further reduced by malnutrition, renal insufficiency, and rheumatoid arthritis. As serum albumin levels decline, the likelihood of reduced drug binding increases. For highly bound drugs, lower albumin levels mean a decrease in total serum drug concentration, while unbound serum drug concentration remains unchanged.

The concentration of AAG, a reactant serum protein, increases with age; further elevations occur during pathophysiologic stresses such as stroke, heart failure, trauma, infection, myocardial infarction, surgery, and chronic obstructive pulmonary disease (14). Administration of enzyme-inducing AEDs also increases AAG (16). When the concentration of AAG rises, the binding of weakly alkaline and neutral drugs such as carbamazepine (and its epoxide metabolite) to AAG can increase, causing higher total serum drug and metabolite concentrations and decreased unbound drug concentrations.

For low-clearance drugs (older AEDs), hepatic clearance is influenced primarily by the extent of protein binding and intrinsic metabolizing capacity (intrinsic clearance) of the liver. Because hepatic clearance affects steady-state drug concentrations, age-related alterations in protein binding or intrinsic clearance can affect serum drug concentrations.

The effect of age on hepatic drug metabolism remains largely unknown owing to the complexity of confounding variables and the lack of correlation between simple measures of liver function and drug metabolism (17,18). Phase I reactions (oxidation, reduction, and hydroxylation) are thought to be affected more than phase II reactions (glucuronidation, acetylation, and sulfation). In the elderly, the decrease in oxidative metabolism of some drugs is believed to be a result of changes in liver blood flow and liver mass with age (15,19). Because the enzymes for glucuronidation are also located in the hepatocytes, which decrease in number with age, a similar decrease in glucuronidation might be expected. However, limited information indicates that glucuronidation reactions appear to be spared with aging. For example, advanced age has little effect on the clearance of lorazepam, which undergoes glucuronidation; whereas, the clearance of diazepam and its active metabolite, both of which undergo oxidative metabolism, is decreased (20).

Despite the theoretical effects of age-related physiologic changes on drug disposition and the widespread use of AEDs in the elderly, few studies on AED pharmacokinetics in the elderly have been published. The available reports generally involve single-dose evaluations in small samples of the young-old (age 65 to 74 years). Data on those older than age 85 years are largely absent, even though this population may face an increased possibility of therapeutic failure and adverse reactions (21). Table 40.1 summarizes pharmacokinetic parameters in the elderly (22–39).

CHOOSING ANTIEPILEPTIC DRUGS

The paucity of information on the clinical use of AEDs in the elderly means that the "comfort level" with some drugs may play a larger role in their selection than actual experience or data. Many recommendations in this review will be modified as new knowledge is obtained.

Compared with younger adults, the elderly may represent a much more heterogeneous population. For purposes of simplification, they may be divided into three groups based on health status: the healthy elderly who have epilepsy, the elderly with multiple medical problems (EMMP), and the frail elderly in nursing homes. A drug that is optimal for the healthy elderly may be inappropriate for other groups because of differences among the groups in pharmacokinetics or pharmacodynamics. For example, total phenytoin concentrations vary widely in the frail elderly, who also use many interfering drugs in addition to AEDs (Table 40.2) (5). A study of serial blood levels in elderly nursing home residents receiving constant doses of phenytoin showed an average intrapatient variability from two- to threefold (40), complicating the interpretation of blood level data and therapeutic decisions. This large variability could not be attributed to any one factor and may be a result of absorption, which could not be addressed in the study; newer, more water-soluble drugs

TABLE 40.1

PHARMACOKINETICS OF ANTIEPILEPTIC DRUGS IN THE ELDERLY

Drug	Protein Binding (%)	Half-life (h)	Metabolism/ Route of Elimination	Comments
Carbamazepine	75–85	[a]	Hepatic	Protein binding decreased with reduced serum albumin; estimated dosage requirements 40% less than in younger adults
Felbamate	<10	[a]	Hepatic	
Gabapentin	<10	[a]	Renal	Elimination correlates with creatinine clearance; dosage may need to be reduced by 30%–50%
Lamotrigine	55	~30	Hepatic glucuronide conjugation	Dosage adjustment may not be necessary, as conjugation reactions only slightly diminished with age
Levetiracetam	<10	~12–15	Renal	Dosage may need to be reduced in elderly with diminished renal function
Oxcarbazepine	Low	[a]	Hepatic	
Phenobarbital	50	[a]	Hepatic and renal	
Phenytoin	80–93	Varies with concentration; e.g., 40–60 h at 15 mg/L	Hepatic	Protein binding decreased with reduced serum albumin; initial dosage 3–4 mg/kg; subsequent increases should be <10% of dose
Primidone		12.1 ± 4.6	Hepatic	Half-life and clearance similar to that of younger adults; dosage adjustments may not be needed
Tiagabine	95	[a]	Hepatic	
Topiramate	9–17	[a]	Hepatic and renal	Dosage may need to be reduced in elderly patients with diminished renal function
Valproic acid	87–95	[a]	Hepatic	Protein binding decreased with reduced serum albumin; dosage reduction of 30%–40% may be needed
Zonisamide	Low	[a]	Hepatic and renal	Dosage may need to be reduced in elderly with diminished renal function

[a]Half-life is longer in elderly than in younger adults, but few data are available.

may be better in this population, but this possibility needs to be investigated.

Because AEDs may affect balance, falls and fractures might be related to inappropriate use. Cost also may be a factor for many patients. Multiple medical problems

TABLE 40.2

USE OF COMEDICATIONS WITH POTENTIAL INTERACTIONS WITH ANTIEPILEPTIC DRUGS IN 4291 RESIDENTS OF NURSING HOMES

Drug Category	Percent Use with Antiepileptic Drugs
Antidepressants	18.9
Antipsychotics	12.7
Benzodiazepines	22.4
Thyroid supplements	14.0
Antacids	8.0
Calcium-channel blockers	6.9
Warfarin	5.9
Cimetidine	2.5

Data from Lackner TE, Cloyd JC, Thomas LW, et al. Antiepileptic drug use in nursing home residents: effect of age, gender, and comedication on patterns of use. *Epilepsia* 1998;39:1083–1087.

intensify these issues, and the physician must be aware of the benefits and shortcomings of all AEDs, as well as the patient's physical and fiscal health. The benefits and risks of each drug in the healthy elderly and the EMMP is discussed in the following sections (Table 40.3) (41–43).

Phenytoin

Phenytoin is effective against localization-related epilepsies and thus has an efficacy profile appropriate for the elderly; however, few studies on its ability to treat seizures in this group have been published. Evidence from the Veterans Affairs Cooperative Study suggests effectiveness equal to that of carbamazepine, phenobarbital, and primidone, although the number of subjects was small (44).

Phenytoin has a narrow therapeutic range and complex pharmacokinetics. It is absorbed slowly, is approximately 90% bound to serum albumin, and undergoes saturable metabolism, which produces nonlinear changes in steady-state serum concentrations.

Clinical studies in elderly patients show decreases in binding to albumin and increases in the free fraction (12). The protein binding of phenytoin correlates with the albumin concentration, which is typically low normal to

TABLE 40.3

ANTIEPILEPTIC DRUGS FOR THE HEALTHY ELDERLY AND FOR THE ELDERLY WITH MULTIPLE MEDICAL PROBLEMS

Drug	Safety and Side Effects[a]				Cost[b]
	Concentration Dependent	Idiosyncratic	Long-term	Drug Interactions	
Carbamazepine (Tegretol, Carbatrol)	Ataxia, diplopia, dizziness, drowsiness, headache, nausea, unsteadiness, lethargy	Blood dyscrasia, rash, hepatic failure, Stevens-Johnson syndrome	Hyponatremia	Valproate decreases carbamazepine epoxide metabolism and then increases its levels; cimetidine, erythromycin, propoxyphene, and grapefruit juice increase carbamazepine concentrations; carbamazepine also may reduce therapeutic responses to corticosteroids or thyroid hormones	$
Felbamate (Felbatol)	Anorexia, nausea, vomiting, insomnia, headache, weight loss	Aplastic anemia, acute hepatic failure	None established	Increases concentrations of phenytoin, valproic acid, and phenobarbital; carbamazepine concentration decreases, carbamazepine-epoxide metabolite increases	$$$
Gabapentin (Neurontin)	Dizziness, fatigue, somnolence, ataxia, decreased alertness	None established	Weight gain	Does not induce or inhibit liver enzymes; cimetidine reduces clearance by ≈10%; antacids reduce bioavailability by ≈20%	$$$$
Lamotrigine (Lamictal)	Diplopia, dizziness, unsteadiness, headache, ataxia	Rash, Stevens-Johnson syndrome	None established	Does not induce or inhibit liver enzymes; carbamazepine, phenobarbital, primidone, phenytoin, and oxcarbazepine increase its clearance and lower its levels; valproic acid inhibits lamotrigine clearance, increasing its levels	$$$$
Levetiracetam (Keppra)	Sedation, behavioral disturbance	None established	None established	Not an enzyme inhibitor or inducer and lacks protein binding	$$$$
Oxcarbazepine (Trileptal)	Sedation, dizziness, ataxia, nausea, somnolence, diplopia, fatigue	Rash	Hyponatremia	May increase phenytoin concentrations and decrease lamotrigine concentrations; enzyme-inducing drugs increase clearance of the active monohydrate derivative	$$$
Phenobarbital	Ataxia, drowsiness, hyperactivity, headache, unsteadiness, sedation, nausea	Blood dyscrasia, rash	Behavior changes, cognitive impairment, connective tissue disorders, intellectual blunting, metabolic bone disease, mood changes, sedation, depression	Potent enzyme inducer and decreases levels of many drugs; valproic acid, phenytoin, felbamate, cimetidine, and chloramphenicol inhibit its metabolism	$
Phenytoin (Dilantin)	Ataxia, nystagmus, behavior changes, dizziness, headache, incoordination, sedation, lethargy, cognitive impairment, fatigue, visual blurring	Rash, hepatitis, bone-marrow depression, systemic lupus erythematosus, Stevens-Johnson syndrome	Behavior changes, cerebellar syndrome, connective tissue changes, skin thickening, folate deficiency, gingival hyperplasia, hirsutism,	May reduce plasma concentration of carbamazepine, valproate, and primidone; valproate displaces phenytoin from protein binding sites and inhibits metabolism; phenylbutazone, salicylates, and tolbutamide displace phenytoin from plasma protein; chloramphenicol, cimetidine, dicumarol, isoniazid, disulfiram,	$

TABLE 40.3
(continued)

| Drug | Safety and Side Effects[a] | | | | Cost[b] |
	Concentration Dependent	Idiosyncratic	Long-term	Drug Interactions	
			coarsening of facial features, acne, cognitive impairment, metabolic bone disease, sedation	sulfonamides, and trimethoprim significantly increase phenytoin plasma concentrations; folate and rifampin may decrease phenytoin plasma concentration; phenytoin may decrease the effect of antiarrhythmic agents, digitoxin, analgesics, cyclosporine, corticosteroids, and theophylline	
Tiagabine (Gabitril)	Dizziness, somnolence, fatigue, difficulty concentrating, nervousness, tremor, blurred vision, depression, weakness	None established	None established	Carbamazepine, phenobarbital, and phenytoin increase metabolism of tiagabine and decrease its levels	$$
Topiramate (Topamax)	Somnolence, dizziness, paresthesias, difficulty concentrating, psychomotor slowing, speech or language problems, fatigue, headache	Oligohidrosis, hyperthermia, acute myopia, secondary angle-closure glaucoma	Kidney stones	Enzyme inducers, such as phenytoin and carbamazepine, decrease topiramate concentrations	$$$
Valproate (Depakote)	Gastrointestinal upset, diarrhea, abdominal cramps, constipation, sedation, drowsiness, unsteadiness, tremor, thrombocytopenia, liver enzyme elevation	Acute hepatic failure, acute pancreatitis	Hepatotoxicity, alopecia, weight gain, hyperammonemia	Enzyme inducers, such as phenytoin, phenobarbital, primidone, and carbamazepine, increase valproate clearance; topiramate may reduce its serum concentrations; highly protein-bound drugs may displace valproate; valproate inhibits metabolism of phenobarbital, carbamazepine-epoxide, and lamotrigine	$$
Zonisamide (Zonegran)	Sedation, somnolence, dizziness, cognitive impairment, nausea, fatigue, confusion	Rash, oligohidrosis	Kidney stones	Does not inhibit or induce the cytochrome P450 system; enzyme inducers can reduce zonisamide levels; lamotrigine may inhibit zonisamide clearance	$$$$$

[a]Data from Lackner TE. Strategies for optimizing AED therapy in elderly people. *Pharmacotherapy* 2002;22:329–364; Leppik IE. *Contemporary diagnosis and management of the patient with epilepsy*, 5th ed. Newtown, PA: Handbooks in Health Care, 2001; Dipiro JT, et al. *Pharmacotherapy: a pathophysiologic approach*, 5th ed. New York: McGraw-Hill, 2002.
[b]Based on cost per month (using www.Walgreens.com) and usual daily dose, which may vary from patient to patient: $ = $0–$25; $$ = $26–$100; $$$ = $101–$200; $$$$ = $201–$250; $$$$$ = $251–$300.

subnormal in the elderly. One study (22) compared the steady-state pharmacokinetics of phenytoin after oral administration in 34 elderly (age 60 to 79 years), 32 middle-aged (age 40 to 59 years), and 26 younger adults (age 20 to 39 years) with epilepsy. All patients had normal albumin concentrations and liver function and received no other medications. The maximum rate of metabolism declined with age, and values were significantly lower in the elderly than in younger adults. Other, smaller studies confirm the reduced metabolism of phenytoin in the elderly (23–25,45,46). For this reason, lower maintenance doses may be needed to attain desired unbound serum concentrations. Relatively small adjustments in dose ($\leq$10%) are recommended. Thus, rather than the 5 mg/kg per day used in younger adults, a daily dose of 3 mg/kg appears to be appropriate in the elderly (42). This translates to 160 mg/day for a 52-kg woman and 200 mg/day for a 66-kg man. Several studies revealed that although nursing home residents were taking phenytoin doses similar to those used in younger adults on a mg/kg basis (4,47), total drug concentrations were at the low end of or below the suggested therapeutic range of 10 to 20 µg/mL. In addition, women required higher doses of phenytoin to achieve serum concentrations similar to those in men (47).

Because of the drug's high protein binding, unbound concentrations may be a better indicator of efficacy and toxicity than total concentrations. Patients may achieve seizure control with "subtherapeutic" concentrations, or they may experience toxic reactions when total serum concentrations are in the "therapeutic" range. Measurement of unbound concentrations is essential for elderly patients who have (a) decreased serum albumin concentrations; (b) total phenytoin concentrations near the upper therapeutic range; (c) total concentrations that decline over time; (d) a low total concentration relative to the daily dose; or (e) total concentrations that do not correlate with clinical response. A range of 5 mg/L to 15 mg/L may be a more appropriate therapeutic range for the elderly (42).

Use of total phenytoin concentrations to manage patients may be difficult. In one study (48), total concentrations in 15 nursing home residents (46 to 90 years of age) were highly variable for reasons that could not be explained, even after chart reviews. A recent, larger study (40) of nursing home residents from 30 U.S. states showed intrapatient variability of two- to threefold (100% to 300%). Compliant younger adults exhibit only a 20% variability in phenytoin concentrations over time (49,50).

Phenytoin interacts with many drugs and should be used cautiously in the EMMP group. Valproic acid, which is also highly protein bound, competes with phenytoin for albumin binding sites and inhibits its metabolism; therefore, the elderly may need reduced phenytoin doses if valproic acid is also prescribed. Carbamazepine induces phenytoin metabolism and necessitates higher phenytoin doses. Phenobarbital is also believed to have that property, but the data are controversial (51,52). Antidepressants of the selective serotonin reuptake inhibitor class may inhibit the cytochrome P (CYP) 450 2C family of enzymes responsible for metabolizing phenytoin (53). Fluoxetine and norfluoxetine are potent CYP2C inhibitors, followed by sertraline and paroxetine; the latter two may be safer choices for the elderly. Warfarin also may alter phenytoin metabolism enough to require a dose change.

Younger adults and children generally tolerate phenytoin well, although higher levels of cognitive functioning are affected (54,55). It is not known whether the elderly are more sensitive in this regard; however, phenytoin may cause imbalance and ataxia, and EMMP patients with central nervous system disorders may be at risk (56). In a study of elderly community-dwelling women (57), phenytoin was the only drug, among the lifestyle, demographic, and health factors identified, that significantly increased the risk of nonvertebral fractures.

As a mild blocker of cardiac conduction, phenytoin should be used cautiously in persons who have heart blocks and epilepsy.

Carbamazepine

Although carbamazepine appears to control localization-related seizures in the elderly, it may produce a higher incidence of side effects than newer AEDs (58).

Young adults typically require 10 to 20 mg/kg per day taken in three or four divided doses to attain serum concentrations within the usual therapeutic range. Apparent clearance is 20% to 40% lower in the elderly than in younger adults. In one pharmacokinetic study (59), mean apparent oral clearances were 23% lower in elderly patients receiving monotherapy (57.1 $\pm$ 20.6 versus 74.6 $\pm$ 28.3 mL/h/kg; $p<0.0001$) and phenobarbital comedication (74.7 $\pm$ 25.5 versus 98.7 $\pm$ 34.9 mL/h/kg; $p<0.01$). A population analysis from three outpatient neurology clinics showed a 25% lower oral clearance of carbamazepine in patients older than 70 years of age (60). Decreases in clearance prolong elimination half-life. Lower doses and less frequent administration may be appropriate in elderly patients.

Carbamazepine interacts significantly with CYP3A4 inhibitors such as erythromycin, fluoxetine, ketoconazole, propoxyphene, and cimetidine. Grapefruit juice increases carbamazepine serum concentrations. Healthy elderly patients should inform their physician when beginning a new medication, including over-the-counter preparations. Because of additional interactions, carbamazepine needs to be used cautiously in EMMP patients. Carbamazepine can also induce the CYP3A4 system, reducing the effectiveness of other drugs.

Younger adults and children generally tolerate carbamazepine well. Whether its effects on higher levels of cognitive functioning are a problem for the elderly is not known. Imbalance and ataxia are common adverse effects.

Hyponatremia, a known phenomenon with carbamazepine use (61), may cause significant problems in young adults with polydipsia. This effect could also be a concern for patients receiving diuretics or following salt-restricted diets. Because of mild carbamazepine-induced neutropenia in the young, effects on hematopoietic parameters in the elderly require study. Carbamazepine affects cardiac rhythms and should be used cautiously, and perhaps not at all, in persons with rhythm disturbances.

The short half-life of carbamazepine entails multiple daily doses. Although half-life may be lengthened in the elderly, new slow-release formulations have overcome these limitations. Carbamazepine is moderately priced, and cost should not be a significant problem, especially if low doses are used.

Phenobarbital

Phenobarbital is effective against localization-related epilepsies. Although it is the least expensive of all AEDs, its effects on cognition and mood, demonstrated in the Veterans Affairs Cooperative Study (44), make phenobarbital an undesirable drug for the elderly. (Similar findings were noted for primidone.)

Valproic Acid

Only a few pharmacokinetic comparisons of valproic acid in young and old patients have been published (26–28). In a small study of steady-state pharmacokinetics in volunteers (ages 60 to 88 years) (26), the average unbound fraction of valproate was 10.7% in the elderly and 6.4% in the young, leading to higher absolute unbound concentrations and lower clearances in the elderly. As a result of reduced protein binding, the desired clinical response may be achieved with a lower-than-usual dose. A nationwide nursing home study (62) showed that valproic acid dose and total drug concentrations decrease within elderly age groups, being lower, for example, in an 86-year-old than in a 66-year-old. Because of the concentration-dependent binding and high protein binding of valproic acid, if the albumin concentration has decreased or if the clinical response does not correlate with total drug concentration, unbound drug should be measured.

Felbamate

Felbamate is effective against localization-related epilepsies and appears to have a broader spectrum of efficacy than some other AEDs. Felbamate undergoes primarily hepatic metabolism and has a number of drug–drug interactions, both inhibitory and inductive (29). Consequently, it may not be a good choice for EMMP patients. Elderly individuals require lower initial doses and slower titration of felbamate than do nonelderly individuals. In one study (30), healthy elderly volunteers had a lower mean clearance of felbamate (31.2 versus 25.1 mL min^{-1}; 90% confidence interval [CI] -11.4 to -0.9; $p = 0.02$) than did the younger adult group, and the elderly tolerated it less well. Aplastic anemia and hepatitis associated with felbamate are idiosyncratic, and some high-risk populations have been identified; patients without active connective tissue disorders or previous aplastic anemia may be at lower risk (63). Patients with felbamate-associated aplastic anemia may have deficiencies in erythrocyte glutathione peroxidase, superoxide dismutase, and glutathione reductase activities compared with age-matched controls (64).

Gabapentin

Gabapentin is effective against localization-related epilepsies. Renal excretion and a lack of drug–drug interactions (65) may make gabapentin especially useful for EMMP patients. As renal function decreases with age, doses may need to be adjusted in both healthy elderly and EMMP patients. Drug levels must be monitored after initiation of therapy.

Younger adults and children generally tolerate gabapentin well; however, high doses produce cognitive side effects to which the elderly may be more sensitive.

The short half-life of gabapentin necessitates multiple daily doses; in the elderly, however, the half-life may be longer. Gabapentin is expensive, and cost may be significant, especially if high doses are needed. Gabapentin is an effective treatment for neuropathic pain.

A Veterans Administration Cooperative Study comparing carbamazepine with gabapentin and lamotrigine is in progress (58) and presumably will provide further safety and efficacy information.

Lamotrigine

Lamotrigine is effective against localization related epilepsies, but few studies of its use in the elderly have been published. Metabolism occurs primarily in the liver (66). A single-dose study (67) reported a 35% decrease in clearance in healthy elderly volunteers (65 to 74 years of age) compared with younger healthy volunteers (26 to 38 years of age). In contrast, a population pharmacokinetic study (68) of 163 patients, which included 30 patients older than age 65 years, 10 between 70 and 76 years of age, and none age 85 years and older, showed no effect of age on apparent clearance of lamotrigine. In 150 elderly subjects, the dropout rate a result of adverse events was lower with lamotrigine (18%) than with carbamazepine (42%), as was the incidence of rashes (3% versus 19%) and somnolence (12% versus 29%) (69). Until further studies establish whether lamotrigine clearance decreases significantly with age, monitoring of drug levels and adjustment of doses are warranted.

Drugs, such as valproic acid, that inhibit glucuronidation reduce the elimination of lamotrigine. Clearance increases approximately two- to threefold with coadministration of phenytoin and carbamazepine but decreases twofold with coadministration of valproic acid (70); however, drug-interaction studies have included few elderly individuals. Caution may be needed when lamotrigine is used in EMMP patients.

Levetiracetam

Levetiracetam is approved as adjunctive therapy for partial-onset seizures in adults. Its extreme water solubility allows rapid and complete absorption after oral administration.

Levetiracetam is not metabolized by the liver and therefore avoids drug–drug interactions (71).

Levetiracetam's lack of protein binding (<10%) avoids the displacement of highly protein-bound drugs and the need to monitor unbound concentrations. The absence of drug interactions makes it useful for elderly epilepsy patients, particularly those taking other medications for comorbid conditions (72). The manufacturer reports a decrease of 38% in total body clearance and a half-life up to 2.5 hours longer in 61- to 88-year-old individuals with creatinine clearances ranging from 30 to 74 mL per minute. Dose adjustment depends on the patient's renal function as measured by serum creatinine and levetiracetam concentrations (73). In a recent postmarketing study (74), levetiracetam was well tolerated by the elderly.

Tiagabine

Tiagabine is effective against localization-related epilepsies. It is primarily metabolized by the liver through the CYP3A4 enzyme. Comedications that affect CYP3A4 substrates will also affect the metabolism of tiagabine, giving it a drug-interaction profile similar to that of carbamazepine. Clearance may be reduced with age. Tiagabine is highly potent; effective doses range from 20 to 60 mg per day and concentrations from 100 to 300 ng/mL or 100-fold lower than those of other AEDs (75).

Topiramate

Topiramate is effective against localization-related epilepsies. Approximately 20% bound to serum proteins, it is metabolized by the liver and excreted unchanged in the urine. The enzymes involved in its metabolism have not been identified, but the CYP450 system may be involved. Topiramate has not been studied in the elderly, but clearance may decrease with age, causing higher-than-expected serum concentrations at doses that are used in younger adults. In addition, the metabolism of topiramate can be induced by coadministered carbamazepine and phenytoin (76). Because topiramate can inhibit CYP2C19 activity (77), levels require monitoring. Effects on cognitive functioning, especially at higher levels, have been reported. It is not known whether the elderly are more sensitive to this problem.

Oxcarbazepine

Oxcarbazepine is immediately metabolized to its monohydroxy derivative. Considered the active compound, this metabolite undergoes glucuronidation and is excreted by the kidneys (78). The most extensive study in the old involved 12 young and 12 elderly, healthy, male and 12 young and 12 elderly healthy female volunteers (79). At low doses (300 to 600 mg/day), the elderly had significantly higher maximum concentrations and area-under-the-curve parameters, and a lower elimination rate constant.

Oxcarbazepine can induce the metabolism of the CYP3A4 enzyme responsible for the metabolism of dihydropyridine calcium antagonists and oral contraceptives (80,81). Plasma levels of carbamazepine (a CYP3A4 substrate) can be decreased 15% on coadministration with oxcarbazepine (82). Hyponatremia is associated with oxcarbazepine use (83) and it appears to be more pronounced with increasing age.

Benzodiazepines

Diazepam, lorazepam, clorazepate, and clonazepam are used for the treatment of epilepsy. Diazepam and lorazepam are administered intravenously as acute therapy for status epilepticus. Clorazepate and clonazepam are given orally as maintenance therapy.

Diazepam is highly protein bound (>99%) and undergoes oxidative metabolism to form the active metabolite desmethyldiazepam. Protein binding declines with age, resulting in an increased free fraction and a larger volume of distribution of the parent drug and the metabolite. Unbound clearance is reduced, prolonging the serum elimination half-life of diazepam and desmethyldiazepam. Lorazepam is less highly bound (90%) and is metabolized by conjugation to lorazepam glucuronide. The free fraction of lorazepam rises with age, and the volume of distribution increases, but less so than for diazepam. The elimination half-life of lorazepam is similar in the young and the elderly. Direct comparisons of the pharmacokinetics of clonazepam and clorazepate in the young and the elderly have not been published.

The elderly tend to be more sensitive to drugs that act on the central nervous system, but this increased sensitivity is apparently independent of drug concentration, either in the serum or at the site of action. Among such drugs, the benzodiazepines have undergone the most extensive pharmacodynamic investigation. Diazepam-induced sedation was increased in the elderly, although unbound drug concentrations did not differ from those in younger subjects (84).

Interactions with Non-Antiepileptic Drugs

Concomitant medications taken by the elderly can alter the absorption, distribution, and metabolism of AEDs, thereby increasing the risk of toxic reactions or therapeutic failure. Interfering comedications are frequently used by nursing home residents receiving AEDs (Table 40.2). No data are available for elderly outpatients. Calcium-containing antacids, sucralfate, and oral and intravenous antineoplastic drugs that damage gastrointestinal cells reduce the absorption of phenytoin (85–87). The latter agents also decrease the absorption of carbamazepine and valproate (87,88). The use of folic acid for treatment of megaloblastic anemia may decrease serum concentrations of phenytoin, and enteral feedings can also lower serum concentrations in patients receiving orally administered phenytoin (89).

Many drugs displace AEDs from plasma proteins, an effect that is especially serious when the interacting drug also inhibits the metabolism of the displaced drug; this occurs when valproate interacts with phenytoin (90). Several drugs used on a short-term basis (including propoxyphene and erythromycin) or as maintenance therapy (cimetidine, diltiazem, fluoxetine, and verapamil) significantly inhibit the metabolism of one or more AEDs that are metabolized by the CYP450 system. Phenytoin, phenobarbital, carbamazepine, and primidone can induce the CYP450 or other enzymes and increase drug metabolism. Long-term use of ethanol also induces drug metabolism (91). The interaction between antipsychotic drugs and AEDs is complex. Hepatic metabolism of haloperidol increased by carbamazepine can diminish the psychotropic response. Chlorpromazine, promazine, trifluoperazine, and perphenazine can reduce the threshold for seizures. The risk of seizures is directly proportional to the total number of psychotropic medications being taken, their doses, abrupt increases in doses, and the presence of pathologic organized brain lesions (92). The epileptic patient taking antipsychotic drugs may need a higher AED dose to control seizures. In contrast, central nervous system depressants are likely to lower the maximum dose of AEDs that can be administered before toxic symptoms occur.

CONCLUSIONS

Among major differences between newer and older AEDs are drug interactions and pharmacokinetic profiles. In general, newer AEDs have few or no drug interactions. Older AEDs, however, are much less expensive. For the healthy elderly patient, especially when cost is a consideration, older AEDs may be the first choice. The side-effect profile of older AEDs also needs to be considered. For example, valproate may not be the best AED for a patient with tremor. If sodium balance is a concern, carbamazepine may not be a first choice. For EMMP patients, lack of drug interactions and safety may be the prime concerns, and the savings realized by avoiding complications may well balance the extra cost of the AED.

Regardless of the AED chosen, doses must be appropriate to the drug's clearance, and AED levels must be monitored. Unbound (free) levels should be measured for phenytoin and valproate. The frailty and polypharmacy typical of elderly nursing home residents challenge medical management. Phenytoin, the most widely used AED, may not be the easiest or safest AED to prescribe for this group. Much more research is required, however, before better recommendations can be made.

REFERENCES

1. Hauser WA. Epidemiology of seizures in the elderly. In: Rowan AJ, Ramsay RE, eds. *Seizures and epilepsy in the elderly.* Boston: Butterworth-Heinemann, 1997:7–20.
2. Epilepsy Foundation of America. *Epilepsy, a report to the nation.* Landover, MD: Epilepsy Foundation of America, 1999.
3. Cloyd JC, Lackner TE, Leppik IE. Antiepileptics in the elderly. Pharmacoepidemiology and pharmacokinetics. *Arch Fam Med* 1994;3:589–598.
4. Garrard, J, Cloyd JC, Gross C, et al. Factors associated with antiepileptic drug use among nursing home elderly. *J Geriatr Med Sci* 2000;55:384–392.
5. Lackner TE, Cloyd JC, Thomas LW, et al. Antiepileptic drug use in nursing home residents: effect of age, gender, and comedication on patterns of use. *Epilepsia* 1998;39:1083–1087.
6. Schachter SS, Cramer GW, Thompson GD, et al. An evaluation of antiepileptic drug therapy in nursing facilities. *J Am Geriatr Soc* 1998;46:1137–1141.
7. Dey AN. Characteristics of elderly home health care users; data from the 1994 National Home and Hospice Care Survey. *Adv Data* 1996;279:1–12.
8. Garrard J, Harms S, Hardie N, et al. Antiepileptic drug use in nursing home admissions. *Ann Neurol* 2003:54:75–85.
9. Hauser WA, Hesdorffer DC, eds. *Epilepsy, frequency, causes, and consequences.* New York: Demos, 1990:1–51.
10. Moore SR, Jones JK. Adverse drug reaction surveillance in the geriatric population: a preliminary review. In: Moore SR, Teal TW, eds. *Geriatric drug use: clinical and social perspectives.* New York: Pergamon, 1985:70–77.
11. Wallace SM, Verbeeck RK. Plasma protein binding of drugs in the elderly. *Clin Pharmacokinet* 1987;12:41–72.
12. Greenblatt DJ. Reduced serum albumin concentrations in the elderly: a report from the Boston Collaborative Drug Surveillance Program. *J Am Geriatr Soc* 1979;27:20–22.
13. Rowe JW, Andres R, Tobin JD, et al. The effect of age on creatinine clearance in men: a cross-sectional and longitudinal study. *J Gerontol* 1976,31.155–163.
14. Verbeeck RK, Cardinal JA, Wallace SM. Effect of age and sex on the plasma binding of acidic and basic drugs. *Eur J Clin Pharmacol* 1984;27:91–97.
15. Wynne HA, Cope LH, Mutch E, et al. The effect of age on liver volume and apparent liver blood flow in healthy man. *Hepatology* 1989;9:297–301.
16. Tiula E, Neuvonen PJ. Antiepileptic drugs and alpha-1 acid glycoprotein. *N Engl J Med* 1982;307:1148.
17. Cusack BJ. Drug metabolism in the elderly. *J Clin Pharmacol* 1988;28:571–576.
18. Dawling S, Crome P. Clinical pharmacokinetic considerations in the elderly: an update. *Clin Pharmacokinet* 1989;17:236–263.
19. Woodhouse KW, Wynne HA. Hepatic drug metabolism and aging. *Br Med Bull* 1988;15:287–296.
20. Greenblatt DJ, Divoll M, Harmatz JS, et al. Oxazepam kinetics: effects of age and sex. *J Pharmacol Exp Ther* 1980;215:86–91.
21. Faich GA, Dreis M, Tomita D. National Adverse Drug Reaction Surveillance 1986. *Arch Intern Med* 1988;148:785–787.
22. Bauer LA, Blouin RA. Age and phenytoin kinetics in adult epileptics. *Clin Pharmacol Ther* 1982;31:301–304.
23. Bach B, Hansen JM, Kampmann JP, et al. Disposition of antipyrine and phenytoin correlated with age and liver volume in man. *Clin Pharmacokinet* 1981;6:389–396.
24. Hayes MJ, Langman MJS, Short AH. Changes in drug metabolism with increasing age, II: phenytoin clearance and protein binding. *Br J Clin Pharmacol* 1975;2:73–79.
25. Houghton GW, Richens A, Leighton M. Effects of age, height, weight and sex on serum phenytoin concentrations in epileptic patients. *Br J Clin Pharmacol* 975;2:251–256.
26. Bauer LA, Davis R, Wilensky A, et al. Valproic acid clearance: unbound fraction and diurnal variation in young and elderly adults. *Clin Pharmacol Ther* 1985;37:697–700.
27. Perucca E, Grimaldi R, Gatti G, et al. Pharmacokinetics of valproic acid in the elderly. *Br J Clin Pharmacol* 1984;17:665–669.
28. Bryson SM, Verma N, Scott PJ, et al. Pharmacokinetics of valproic acid in young and elderly subjects. *Br J Clin Pharmacol* 1983;16:104–105.
29. Graves NM. Felbamate. *Ann Pharmacother* 1993;27:1073–1081.
30. Richens A, Banfield CR, Salfi M, et al. Single and multiple dose pharmacokinetics of felbamate in the elderly. *Br J Clin Pharmacol* 1997;44:129–134.

31. Bender AD, Post A, Meier JP, et al. Plasma protein binding of drugs as a function of age in adult human subjects. *J Pharm Sci* 1975;64:1711–1713.

32. Drinka PJ, Miller J, Voeks SK, et al. Phenytoin binding in a nursing home. *J Geriatr Drug Ther* 1988;3:73–82.

33. Eadie MJ, Lander CM, Hooper WD, et al. Factors influencing plasma phenobarbitone levels in epileptic patients. *Br J Clin Pharmacol* 1977;4:41–47.

34. Edwards GB, Culberton VL, Anresen GB, et al. Free phenytoin concentrations in geriatrics. *J Geriatr Drug Ther* 1988;3:97–102.

35. Martines C, Gatti G, Sasso E, et al. The disposition of primidone in elderly patients. *Br J Clin Pharmacol* 1990;30:607–611.

36. Morselli PL. Carbamazepine: absorption, distribution and excretion. In: *Antiepileptic drugs*, 3rd ed. New York: Raven Press, 1989: 473–490.

37. Patterson M, Heazelwood R, Smithhurst B, et al. Plasma protein binding of phenytoin in the aged: *in vivo* studies. *Br J Clin Pharmacol* 1982;13:423–425.

38. Sherwin AL, Loynd JS, Bock GW, et al. Effects of age, sex, obesity, and pregnancy on plasma diphenylhydantoin levels. *Epilepsia* 1974;15:507–521.

39. Umstead GS, Morales M, McKercher PL. Comparison of total, free, and salivary phenytoin concentrations in geriatric patients. *Clin Pharm* 1986;5:59–62.

40. Birnbaum A, Hardie NA, Leppik IE, et al. Variability of total phenytoin serum concentrations within elderly nursing home residents. *Neurology* 2003;60:555–559.

41. Lackner TE. Strategies for optimizing AED therapy in elderly people. *Pharmacotherapy* 2002;22:329–364.

42. Leppik IE. *Contemporary diagnosis and management of the patient with epilepsy*, 5th ed. Newtown, PA: Handbooks in Healthcare, 2001:155–156.

43. Dipiro JT, Talbert RL, Yee GC, et al. *Pharmacotherapy: a pathophysiologic approach*, 5th ed. New York: McGraw-Hill, 2002.

44. Mattson RH, Cramer JA, Collins JF, et al. Comparison of carbamazepine, phenobarbital, phenytoin, and primidone in partial and secondarily generalized tonic-clonic seizures. *N Engl J Med* 1985;313:145–151.

45. Lambie DC, Caird FL. Phenytoin dosage in the elderly. *Age Ageing* 1977;6:133–137.

46. Troupin AS, Johannessen SI. Epilepsy in the elderly: a pharmacologic perspective. In: Smith DB, ed. *Epilepsy: current approaches to diagnosis and treatment* New York: Raven Press, 1990:141–153.

47. Birnbaum AK, Hardie NA, Leppik IE, et al. Phenytoin use in elderly nursing home residents. *Am J Geriatr Pharmacother* 2003: 1:90–95.

48. Mooradian AD, Hernandez L, Tamai IC, et al. Variability of serum phenytoin concentrations in nursing home patients. *Arch Intern Med* 1989;149:890–892.

49. Graves NM, Holmes GB, Leppik IE. Compliant populations: variability in serum concentrations. *Epilepsy Res Suppl* 1988;1: 91–99.

50. Graves NM, Leppik IE, Termond E, et al. Phenytoin clearances in a compliant population: description and application. *Ther Drug Monit* 1986;8:427–433.

51. Browne TR, Szabo GK, Evans J, et al. Phenobarbital does not alter phenytoin steady-state serum concentration or pharmacokinetics. *Neurology* 1988;38:639–642.

52. Leppik IE, Sherwin AL. Anticonvulsant activity of phenobarbital and phenytoin in combination. *J Pharmacol Exp Ther* 1977;200: 570–576.

53. Nelson MH, Birnbaum AK, Remmel RP. Inhibition of phenytoin hydroxylation in human liver microsomes by several selective serotonin re-uptake inhibitors. *Epilepsy Res* 2001;44:71–82.

54. Matthews CG, Harley JP. Cognitive and motor-sensory performances in toxic and nontoxic epileptic subjects. *Neurology* 1975;25:184–188.

55. Thompson P, Huppert FA, Trimble M. Phenytoin and cognitive function: effects on normal volunteers and implications for epilepsy. *Br J Clin Psychol* 1981;20(Pt 3):155–162.

56. Bourdet SV, Gidal BE, Alldredge BK. Pharmacologic management of epilepsy in the elderly. *J Am Pharm Assoc (Wash)* 2001;41: 421–436.

57. Bohannon AD, Hanlon JT, Landerman R, et al. Association of race and other potential risk factors with nonvertebral fractures in community-dwelling elderly women. *Am J Epidemiol* 1999;149: 1002–1009.

58. Ramsay RE, Treiman D, Walker M, et al. Treatment approaches for the elderly with epilepsy. *Epilepsy Res* 2004. In press.

59. Battino D, Croci D, Rossini A, et al. Serum carbamazepine concentrations in elderly patients: a case-matched pharmacokinetic evaluation based on therapeutic drug monitoring data. *Epilepsia* 2003;44:923–929.

60. Graves NM, Brundage RC, Wen Y, et al. Population pharmacokinetics of carbamazepine in adults with epilepsy. *Pharmacotherapy* 1998;18:273–281.

61. Henry DA, Lawson DH, Reavey P, et al. Hyponatraemia during carbamazepine treatment. *Br Med J* 1977;1:83–84.

62. Birnbaum AK, Hardie NA, Leppik IE, et al. Valproate doses and total concentrations in elderly nursing home residents. *Epilepsy Res* 2004. In press.

63. Leppik IE. Felbamate. In: Shorvon S, Perucca E, Fish D, et al., eds. *The treatment of epilepsy*, 2nd ed. Oxford, UK: Blackwell, 2004: 403–409.

64. Glauser TA. Idiosyncratic reactions: new methods of identifying high-risk patients. *Epilepsia* 2000;41(Suppl 8):S16–S29.

65. Richens A. Clinical pharmacokinetics of gabapentin. In: Chadwick D, ed. *New trends in epilepsy management: the role of gabapentin*. London: Royal Society of Medicine Services, 1993:41–46.

66. Peck AW. Clinical pharmacology of lamotrigine. *Epilepsia* 1991; 32(Suppl 2):S9–S12.

67. Posner J, Holdich T, Crome P. Comparison of lamotrigine pharmacokinetics in young and elderly healthy volunteers. *J Pharm Med* 1991;1:121–128.

68. Hussein Z, Posner J. Population pharmacokinetics of lamotrigine monotherapy in patients with epilepsy: retrospective analysis of routine monitoring data. *Br J Clin Pharmacol* 1997;43:457–465.

69. Brodie MJ, Overstall PW, Giorgi L. Multicentre, double-blind, randomised comparison between lamotrigine and carbamazepine in elderly patients with newly diagnosed epilepsy. The UK Lamotrigine Elderly Study Group. *Epilepsy Res* 1999;37:81–87.

70. Yuen AW, Land G, Weatherley BC, et al. Sodium valproate acutely inhibits lamotrigine metabolism. *Br J Clin Pharmacol* 1992;33: 511–513.

71. Leppik IE. The place of levetiracetam in the treatment of epilepsy. *Epilepsia* 2001;42:44–45.

72. Patsalos PN, Sander JW. Newer antiepileptic drugs. Towards an improved risk-benefit ratio. *Drug Saf* 1994;11:37–67.

73. French J. Use of levetiracetam in special populations. *Epilepsia* 2001;42:40–43.

74. Ferrendelli J, French J, Leppik I, et al. Levetiracetam in patients aged >65 years: a subset of the Keeper Trial. *Neurology* 2003; 60(Suppl 1):144–145.

75. Leppik IE, Gram L, Deaton R, et al. Safety of tiagabine: summary of 53 trials. *Epilepsy Res* 1999;33:235–246.

76. Sachdeo RC, Sachdeo SK, Walker SA, et al. Steady-state pharmacokinetics of topiramate and carbamazepine in patients with epilepsy during monotherapy and concomitant therapy. *Epilepsia* 1996;37:774–780.

77. Levy RH, Bishop F, Streeter AJ, et al. Explanation and prediction of drug interactions with topiramate using a CYP450 inhibition spectrum. *Epilepsia* 1995;36:47.

78. Faigle JW, Menge GP. Metabolic characteristics of oxcarbazepine (Trileptal) and their beneficial implications for enzyme induction and drug interactions. *Behav Neurol* 1990;3:21–30.

79. van Heiningen PN, Eve MD, Oosterhuis B, et al. The influence of age on the pharmacokinetics of the antiepileptic agent oxcarbazepine. *Clin Pharmacol Ther* 1991;50:410–419.

80. Klosterskov JP, Saano V, Harin P, et al. Possible interaction between oxcarbazepine and an oral contraceptive. *Epilepsia* 1992;33:1149–1152.

81. Zaccara G, Gangemi PF, Bendoni L, et al. Influence of single and repeated doses of oxcarbazepine on the pharmacokinetic profile of felodipine. *Ther Drug Monit* 1993;15:39–42.

82. Hossain M, Sallas W, Gasparini M, et al. Drug-drug interaction profile of oxcarbazepine in children and adults. *Neurology* 1999;52:A525.

83. Dong X, White JR, Leppik IE, et al. Oxcarbazepine-induced hyponatremia: a prevalence-based risk factor study. *Neurology* 2004;62:A310.

84. Cook PJ, Flanagan R, James IM. Diazepam tolerance: effect of age, regular sedation and alcohol. *Br Med J* 1984;289:351–353.

85. Hansten PD, Horn JR, eds. *Drug interactions: a clinical perspective and analysis of current developments* Vancouver, WA: Applied Therapeutics, 1993:331–371.
86. Nation RL, Evans AM, Milne RW. Pharmacokinetic drug interactions with phenytoin, I, II. *Clin Pharmacokinet* 1990;18:37–60, 131–150.
87. Neef C, de Voogd-van den Straaten I. An interaction between cytostatic and anticonvulsant drugs. *Clin Pharmacol Ther* 1988;43:372–375.
88. Bollini P, Riva R, Albani F, et al. Decreased phenytoin levels during antineoplastic therapy: a case report. *Epilepsia* 1983;24:75–78.
89. Haley CJ, Nelson J. Phenytoin-enteral feeding interaction. *Ann Pharmacother* 1989;23:796–798.
90. Cramer JA, Mattson RH. Valproic acid: in vitro plasma protein binding and interactions with phenytoin. *Ther Drug Monit* 1979;1:105–116.
91. Sandor P, Sellers EM, Dumbrell M, et al. Effect of short- and long-term alcohol use on phenytoin kinetics in chronic alcoholics. *Clin Pharmacol Ther* 1981;30:390–397.
92. Cold JA, Wells BG, Froemming JH. Seizure activity associated with antipsychotic therapy. *Ann Pharmacother* 1990;24:601–606.

Status Epilepticus

41

James J. Riviello, Jr.

Status epilepticus (SE) is a life-threatening medical emergency that requires prompt recognition and immediate treatment. SE is not a disease in itself but rather a manifestation of either a primary central nervous system (CNS) insult or a systemic disorder with secondary CNS effects. It is important to identify and specifically treat the precipitating cause to prevent ongoing neurologic injury and seizure recurrence. Basic neuroresuscitation principles—the ABCs (airway, breathing, circulation)—must be rigorously adhered to. A team approach, with an organized and systematic treatment regimen, planned in advance, is needed, including one for patients with refractory status epilepticus (RSE). Although the initial approach is standard, once a patient is stabilized, management must be individualized.

DEFINITION

Gastaut defined SE as "an epileptic seizure that is sufficiently prolonged or repeated at sufficiently brief intervals so as to produce an unvarying and enduring epileptic condition" (1). This definition, without a specific duration, at first seems vague and cumbersome, but allows a dynamic interpretation. Subsequently, a time duration was specified (2,3). The Working Group on Status Epilepticus of the Epilepsy Foundation of America (Working Group) defined SE as longer than 30 minutes of either continuous seizure activity or two or more sequential seizures without full recovery of consciousness between seizures (4).

Classification begins with seizure type, using the International Classification of Epileptic Seizures, which categorizes seizures according to onset—either partial (focal) or generalized (5–9). The revision is based on semiology (10). A modified SE system is also based on semiology (11): convulsive (generalized tonic clonic) SE, nonconvulsive SE (absence or complex partial), or simple partial (focal) SE. Nonconvulsive SE may occur with either generalized (absence) or focal (partial complex) epilepsy. SE occurs with any seizure type or epileptic syndrome. In a Netherlands study (1980–1987) of 458 patients (12), generalized convulsive SE occurred in 346 (77%), nonconvulsive SE in 65 (13%) (13), and simple partial SE in 47 (10%) (14). Of the 65 patients with nonconvulsive SE, 40 (62%) had complex partial SE and 25 (38%) had absence SE.

Generalized convulsive SE consists of continuous tonic and/or clonic motor activity, which may be symmetric or asymmetric and overt or subtle and is associated with marked impairment of consciousness with bilateral, although frequently asymmetric, electroencephalogram (EEG) ictal discharges (11,15). Subtle generalized convulsive SE has no obvious signs, despite marked impairment of consciousness and bilateral EEG discharges (15), and may evolve from prolonged convulsive SE or follow unsuccessful treatment; the division between generalized convulsive SE and nonconvulsive SE may not be obvious, because nonconvulsive SE may follow convulsive SE in the same episode. In the Netherlands study, within the nonconvulsive SE classification, focal signs occurred more often with complex partial SE, a fluctuating consciousness was more common with absence SE, and the majority of patients in both groups had prior epilepsy (13). With simple partial SE, 46 patients had somatomotor features and one had aphasia with hallucinations (14). Classification must include pseudoseizures, because pseudostatus epilepticus occurs in adults (16) and children (17,18). Pseudostatus epilepticus occurs even as an expression of Munchausen syndrome (factitious disorder by proxy) (19).

STAGES OF STATUS EPILEPTICUS

The clinical stages of SE include premonitory (prodromal) stage; incipient stage (0 to 5 minutes); early stage (5 to 30 minutes); transition to the late or established stage (30 to 60 minutes); refractory stage (longer than 60 to 90 minutes)

TABLE 41.1	
STAGES OF STATUS EPILEPTICUS	
Premonitory	
Incipient:	0 to 5 minutes
Early	5 to 30 minutes
Transition	From early to established
Established (late)	30 to 60 minutes
Refractory	After 60 minutes
Postictal	

(20); and postictal stage (Table 41.1). The premonitory stage consists of confusion, myoclonus, or increasing seizure frequency; the early stage consists of continuous seizure activity; and the refractory stage can consist of either subtle generalized convulsive SE or nonconvulsive SE. If a premonitory stage is identified, treatment should be initiated. SE should not be considered refractory if therapy has been inadequate.

A predictable sequence of EEG progression occurs during these stages in experimental models and humans: (a) discrete seizures with interictal slowing; (b) waxing and waning of ictal discharges; (c) continuous ictal discharges; (d) continuous ictal discharges punctuated by flat periods; and (e) periodic epileptiform discharges (PEDs) on a flat background (Fig. 41.1) (21). Treatment response depends on stage: In the discrete stage, all seizures were controlled with diazepam (6 of 6 patients), whereas in the PED stage, seizures stopped in only 1 of 6 patients and overt clinical seizures were converted to subtle or electrographic seizures in 5 of 6 patients (21). Every episode of SE does not pass through every one of these defined stages, however (22) (Fig. 41.2). The PED stage may also consist of either lateralized (PLED) or bilateral (PBED) patterns (23).

TRENDS IN PATIENTS WITH STATUS EPILEPTICUS

The overall trend in patients with SE has been to decrease the time duration required for diagnosis of the disorder and to treat as soon as possible when a seizure is unlikely to cease. Although the Working Group defined SE as a seizure duration of longer than 30 minutes, treatment was recommended after only 10 minutes (4). Lowenstein and colleagues proposed operational and mechanistic definitions (24). The operational definition of generalized convulsive SE in adults and older children (i.e., older than 5 years of age) is 5 minutes or longer of either a continuous seizure, or two or more discrete seizures, between which there is incomplete recovery of consciousness. In treatment studies, the Veterans Affairs Cooperative Study (25), which compared various first-line antiepileptic drugs (AEDs), used 10 minutes, and the San Francisco Prehospital Treatment study used 5 minutes (26).

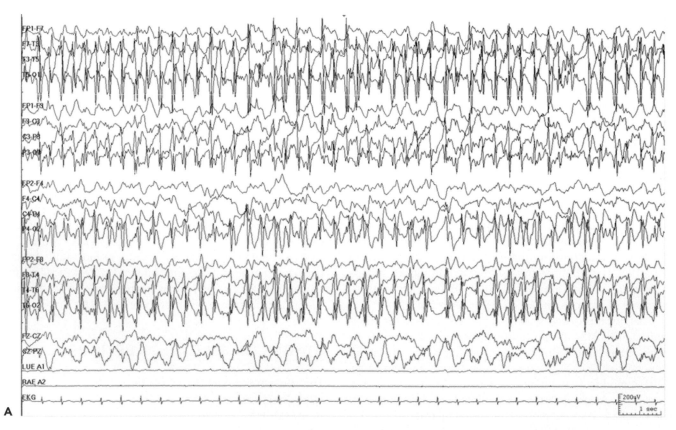

Figure 41.1 **A:** Continuous ictal discharges. **B:** Periodic epileptiform discharges on a flat background.

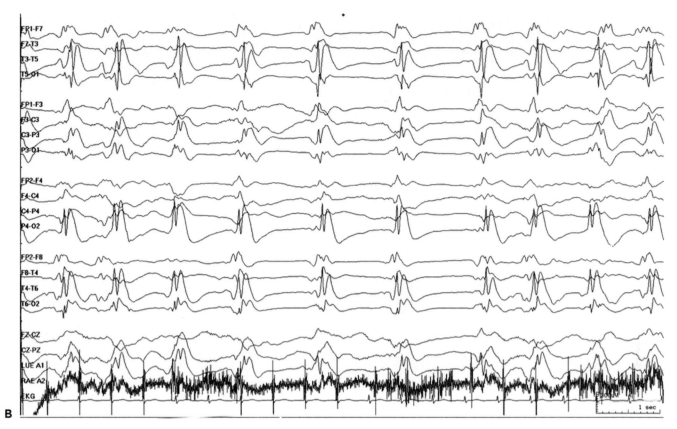

Figure 41.1   (continued)

Clinical and experimental data support these trends. A typical clinical seizure rarely lasts as long as 5 minutes. A typical generalized tonic-clonic seizure, on the other hand, lasts 31 to 51 seconds, with a postictal phase of a few seconds to 4 minutes (27). In an inpatient study, mean seizure duration was 62 seconds, with a range of 16 to 108 seconds (28). In one analysis of seizures in children, partial seizures had a duration of 97 seconds (29). In a prospective study of seizures in children, seizure duration was divided into two groups, one with a mean of 3.6 minutes (76% of cases) and the other with a mean of 31 minutes (24% of cases); if the seizure duration was 5 to 10 minutes, it was unlikely to cease spontaneously within the next few minutes (30).

In patients with SE, when first-line AEDs fail to control seizures, the Veterans Affairs Cooperative Study showed only a 5.3% response to a third AED (20), whereas in the Columbia Study, the response rate was higher (58%) when a third AED was administered earlier (31). The San Francisco Prehospital Treatment Study even showed a response to low-dose lorazepam (2 mg) administered by paramedics for out-of-hospital SE in adults (26). Experimental models also show a time-dependent treatment efficacy. In a self-sustaining model of SE induced by intermittent perforant path stimulation, both diazepam and phenytoin prevented SE when given prior to perforant path stimulation, but the efficacy of both decreased when administered

later on (32). A loss of inhibitory γ-aminobutyric acid-A (GABA$_A$) receptors occurs over time in patients with partial SE (33), and in the lithium-pilocarpine model, there is a functional change in GABA$_A$ receptors, which explains the decreased benzodiazepine response (34,35). This decreased benzodiazepine response also has been demonstrated in young animals (36).

PATHOPHYSIOLOGY

Mechanistically, SE occurs when there is a failure of factors that "normally" terminate seizures (24,37). What are the pathophysiologic mechanisms behind this? Seizures result from excessive cerebral excitation, decreased cerebral inhibition, or a combination of both. Excessive excitation itself may cause neuronal injury and cell death, referred to as excitotoxic injury. This has been demonstrated in experimental models, such as in kainic acid-induced limbic seizures (38), but its occurrence in humans had been questioned. An outbreak of poisoning from domoic acid, an excitotoxic agent, with acute symptoms, including SE, was associated with neuronal loss and astrocytosis that was greatest in the hippocampus and amygdala; this was similar to the seizures induced by kainic acid (39,40). A survivor developed epilepsy and, after death, autopsy revealed hippocampal sclerosis (41).

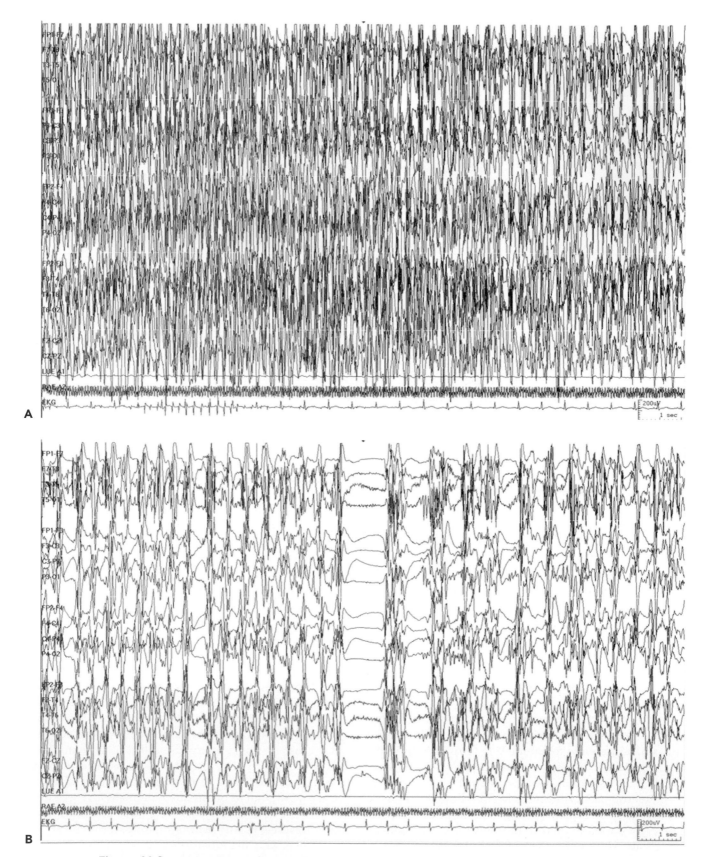

Figure 41.2 Same patient, different seizure **A:** Continuous ictal discharge. **B:** Continuous ictal discharges punctuated by flat periods.

Prolonged seizures in anesthetized baboons cause irreversible neuronal injury (42,43). Lothman outlined the alterations in systemic and brain metabolism occurring with prolonged SE (44): decreased brain oxygen tension, mismatch between the sustained increase in oxygen and glucose utilization and a fall in cerebral blood flow, and depletion of brain glucose and oxygen. Initially, brain compensatory mechanisms may protect against neuronal injury; at some point, however, there is a transition from the ability to compensate to the risk for neuronal injury. This compensation, however, requires adequate airway and good breathing, circulation, and cerebral blood flow.

EPIDEMIOLOGY OF STATUS EPILEPTICUS

There have been two large, population-based studies—from Richmond Virginia, and Rochester, Minnesota (45,46). SE accounts for 1% to 8% of hospital admissions for epilepsy. Between 4% and 16% of patients with epilepsy will have at least one episode of SE, with one-third of the cases occurring as the presenting symptom in patients with a first unprovoked seizure, one-third in patients with established epilepsy, and one-third in those with no history of epilepsy (47). These two studies estimate that 60,000 to 150,000 cases of SE occur per year (45,46). The incidence varies: in Richmond, it is 41 per 100,000 (45) and in Rochester, it is 18 per 100,000 (46), but in California, the overall rate is lower (6.2 per 100,000), with higher rates in children younger than 5 years of age (7.5 per 100,000) and the elderly (22.3 per 100,000) (48). Approximately 55,000 deaths occur per year (49). In children, SE is most common in the very young, especially those younger than 2 years of age (50); in this population, more than 80% have either a febrile or an acute symptomatic etiology. SE occurs within 2 years of the onset of epilepsy onset in most of these children (51), and recurrent SE is more likely with an underlying neurologic disorder (52).

ETIOLOGY OF STATUS EPILEPTICUS

Seizures are also classified according to etiology, and SE classification has been expanded to include symptomatic, remote symptomatic, remote symptomatic with acute precipitant, progressive encephalopathy, cryptogenic, idiopathic, and febrile SE (53).

In several studies of adult SE, trauma, tumor, and vascular disease were the most frequently identified causes, although idiopathic and unknown causes were also quite common (54–57). Etiology also differs among centers and by ages. In San Francisco, noncompliance with AEDs and alcohol withdrawal were the two most common etiologies (Table 41.2) (56,57), whereas cerebrovascular damage was the most common etiology in Richmond

TABLE 41.2
ETIOLOGY IN THE SAN FRANCISCO STUDIES: CHANGES OVER TIME

Etiology	Number of Cases	
	1980	**1993**
Anticonvulsant withdrawal	27	48
Alcohol-related	15	43
Drug intoxication	10	14
Central nervous system infection	4	12
Refractory epilepsy	—	10
Trauma	3	8
Tumor	4	7
Metabolic disorders	8	7
Stroke	15	6
Cardiac arrest	4	6
Unknown	15	8

Data from Aminoff MJ, Simon RP. Status epilepticus: causes, clinical features and consequences in 98 patients. *Am J Med* 1980;69:657–666, and Lowenstein DH, Alldredge BK. Status epilepticus at an urban public hospital in the 1980s. *Neurology* 1993;43:483–488.

(58). The Richmond study included adults and children, so etiologies were better compared (Table 41.3). In adults, cerebrovascular disease was the most common etiology, occurring in 25.2% versus only 3.3% in children, whereas in children, fever or infection was the most common cause, occurring in 35.7% versus only 4.6% in adults. Medication change was a major cause in both adults and children—20% in children versus 19% in adults (58). The incidence of tumors was higher in older studies (54,55).

TABLE 41.3
COMPARISON OF ETIOLOGY IN CHILDREN AND ADULTS IN THE RICHMOND STUDY

Etiology	% of Children (Younger than Age 16 Years)	% of Adults (Older than Age 16 Years)
Cerebrovascular	3.3	25.2
Medication change	19.8	18.9
Anoxia	5.3	10.7
Ethyl alcohol/ drug-related	2.4	12.2
Metabolic	8.2	8.8
Unknown	9.3	8.1
Fever/infection	35.7	4.6
Trauma	3.5	4.6
Tumor	0.7	4.3
Central nervous system infection	4.8	1.8
Congenital	7.0	0.8

Adapted from DeLorenzo RJ, Towne AR, Pellock JM, Ko D. Status epilepticus in children, adults, and the elderly. *Epilepsia* 1992;33 (Suppl 4):15–25.

PROGNOSIS OF PATIENT WITH STATUS EPILEPTICUS

The prognosis of SE depends on etiology, duration (3), and age (50). The mortality rate in modern, generalized convulsive SE series ranges from 4% (59) to 37% (60) and is higher with an acute precipitant (60). An acute precipitant is more likely when there is no prior history of epilepsy (60,61), but may also be responsible for death in persons with known epilepsy with SE. In one series, 63% of patients survived, 28.6% died from the underlying cause, 6.6% died from other causes, and 1.8% died from the SE itself (60). The mortality rate was 21% (14 of 85) in the Columbia study, and was higher with acute symptomatic seizures and older ages (62). A high incidence of symptomatic cases also occurs in the very young, less than age 2 years (50). The mortality was the highest—61% (25 of 41)—in *de novo* SE occurring in patients already hospitalized (63). With metabolic abnormalities, frequent precipitants—hypoxia, electrolyte imbalance, hepatic encephalopathy, and sepsis—occurred in 23 patients (56%), and 11 (27%) were being treated with theophylline at the time SE developed.

Short-term versus long-term mortality was compared using data from the Rochester study (64–66); mortality was 19% (38 of 201) within the first 30 days, but cumulative mortality was 43% over 10 years (66). The long-term mortality risk increased with an SE duration longer than 24 hours, acute symptomatic etiology, and myoclonic SE; mortality was not higher with idiopathic/cryptogenic SE (66). Specifically with respect to duration, the mortality rate in the Richmond study was 32% when the duration was longer than 60 minutes versus only 2.7% when the duration was 30 to 59 minutes (67). Other factors associated with a high mortality rate include duration longer than 1 hour, anoxia, and older age, whereas a low mortality rate was associated with alcohol and AED withdrawal (67). Elevated cerebrospinal fluid (CSF) lactate levels may indicate a poor prognosis (68).

The mortality rate in pediatric SE ranges from 4% to 11%, and is also related to etiology and age (59,69–74). In one study, the mortality was 4%, occurring only with acute symptomatic or progressive symptomatic etiologies (69). Specifically analyzing the age in children, the overall mortality rate in the Richmond study was 6%. However, within the first year, the mortality rate was 17.8%, but in the first 6 months, the mortality rate was 24%, compared with 9% in those ages 6 to 12 months, with the difference caused by a higher incidence of symptomatic SE in the youngest children (75). With respect to morbidity, a Canadian study of SE reported 34% of 40 children with an SE duration of 30 to 720 minutes had subsequent neurodevelopmental deterioration (76). Even in children with febrile SE, speech deficits have been reported (77).

In the Netherlands study (12), prognosis of patients with generalized convulsive SE was related to treatment adequacy. A favorable outcome occurred in 263 (76%) of 346 patients, with outcome related to cause, duration longer than 4 hours, more than one medical complication, and quality of care. To analyze the treatment effects, therapy was classified as insufficient when the wrong AED dose or route was used, if an unnecessary delay occurred, if mechanical ventilation was not used despite respiratory insufficiency or medical complications, or if neuromuscular paralysis was used without electroencephalograph monitoring (to detect seizure activity). The most common reason for classifying therapy as insufficient was an inadequate AED dose. In the patients with a favorable outcome (n=263), therapy was classified as good or sufficient in 85.6% and insufficient in only 10.3%; in those with sequelae (n=45), therapy was inadequate in 22.2%. When the morbidity was from SE itself, insufficient therapy occurred in 50% of patients. With the occurrence of death (n=38), therapy was sufficient in 44.7% of patients, and in cases of death caused by SE itself, therapy was considered insufficient in 62% of patients (12).

An increase in morbidity and mortality occurs with nonconvulsive SE, which is related to SE duration (36 hours to longer than 72 hours) (78). The increased morbidity with nonconvulsive SE is controversial (79–81). Following cardiopulmonary resuscitation, SE, status myoclonus, and myoclonic SE are predictive of a poor outcome (82). On the EEG, burst-suppression (83) and PEDs are predictive of a poor outcome (84), whereas a normal EEG is associated with a good prognosis (85).

MANAGEMENT OF STATUS EPILEPTICUS

The initial management of patients with SE begins with the ABCs—airway, breathing, and circulation (Table 41.4). Diagnostic studies are then selected, depending on a patient's history and physical examination (not all studies are obtained in every patient). Serum glucose should be checked immediately with Dextrostix (Bayer Corporation, West Haven, CT) to rapidly diagnose hypoglycemia. A complete blood count may be helpful for diagnosing infection, although leukocytosis may occur with SE. Electrolytes, calcium, phosphorous, and magnesium values may also be helpful. Lumbar puncture (LP) should be considered in the febrile patient. However, if concern exists about increased intracranial pressure or a structural lesion, LP can be deferred until neuroimaging is performed. If there is evidence of infection, antibiotics can be administered prior to LP, although CSF pleocytosis may occur without infection, presumably as a result of a breakdown in the blood–brain barrier (86). In one study, the highest CSF white blood cell count from SE alone (no acute insult) was 28×10^6/L (87). Low AED levels may contribute to the development of SE in both adults and children (88,89).

Neuroimaging options include cranial computed axial tomography (CAT) scan and magnetic resonance imaging (MRI). CAT scans are readily available on an emergency

TABLE 41.4
IMMEDIATE MANAGEMENT OF STATUS EPILEPTICUS

The ABCs:
Stabilize and maintain the **A**irway; position head to avoid airway obstruction
Establish **B**reathing (i.e., ventilation): administer oxygen by nasal cannula or mask
Maintain the **C**irculation: start intravenous (IV) line
Monitor the Vital Signs: pulse (electrocardiogram monitoring), respiratory rate, blood pressure, temperature, pulse oximetry, check Dextrostix
Start IV line:
Use normal saline
Consider thiamine 100 mg; followed by 50 mL of D 50W
Determine what studies are needed:
Consider complete blood cell count, electrolytes, calcium, phosphorus, magnesium; antiepileptic drug (AED) levels, toxicology
Lumbar puncture (especially if febrile)
Neuroimaging, cranial computed axial tomography scan or magnetic resonance imaging
Electroencephalography, if diagnosis initially in doubt
Points from history:
Has an AED been given (prehospital treatment or inpatient), is patient on any AEDs (especially phenobarbital or phenytoin), or does patient have any allergies?
Characteristics of past seizures: is there a history of status epilepticus?
Are treatable causes present (any acute precipitants)?
Fever or illness, head trauma, possible electrolyte imbalance, intoxications, toxin exposure?
Are chronic medical conditions present or is patient on steroid therapy? (If so, patient needs stress coverage.)

basis and should identify all disorders demanding immediate intervention, such as tumor or hydrocephalus, but may not show the early phases of infarction. CAT scan and MRI may detect focal changes, which may be transient (90), secondary to a focal seizure (suggesting the origin of the focus), with MRI the more sensitive technique. Although lesions may mimic those of ischemic stroke, they are reported to cross-vascular territories (91). Changes in diffusion-weighted images and the apparent diffusion coefficient (ADC) may occur, suggesting both cytotoxic and vasogenic edema (92). Progressive changes also occur, such as hippocampal atrophy and sclerosis, or global atrophy (93,94). In a fatal case of unexplained SE, high signal lesions in the mesial temporal lobes and hippocampal neuronal loss were reported (95). In general, neuroimaging should be performed in all patients with new-onset SE, especially if there is no prior history of epilepsy.

Intoxication with certain agents, particularly theophylline (61,63,96) and isoniazid (INH) (97), which may involve acidosis (98) and is treated with pyridoxine (vitamin B_6) (99), may predispose individuals to generalized convulsive SE or nonconvulsive SE. Cyclosporine (100) and ifosfamide (101) may predispose individuals to nonconvulsive SE, which may also occur when phenytoin or carbamazepine are used in patients with idiopathic generalized epilepsy (102); lithium (103), tiagabine (104), and amoxapine (105) might also be implicated. Fatal SE has occurred with flumazenil, therefore caution should be exercised in patients with a history of seizures, chronic benzodiazepine use, or when a mixed overdose is suspected (106).

An EEG is not initially needed for treatment. Indications for emergency EEG include unexplained altered awareness (to exclude nonconvulsive SE) (Fig. 41.3); the use of neuromuscular paralysis for SE; high-dose suppressive therapy for refractory SE; and no return to baseline or improvement in mental status following control of overt convulsive movements (to exclude ongoing SE) (107). Nonconvulsive SE may occur in 14% of patients treated for generalized convulsive SE (108). Nonconvulsive SE was detected in 8% of all comatose patients (109). Electroencephalography should be used when the diagnosis is in doubt, especially in patients with pseudoseizures (110).

ANTIEPILEPTIC DRUG THERAPY FOR STATUS EPILEPTICUS

Treatment should be aimed at controlling SE as soon as possible, particularly before brain compensatory mechanisms fail. Despite adequate oxygenation and ventilation, such failure has been reported within 30 to 60 minutes in experimental SE (44) and within 30 to 45 minutes in humans (3). Systemic and metabolic changes occur early, with increases in blood pressure, lactate, and glucose levels. Both respiratory and metabolic acidosis may develop, although the former is more common (111). Brain parenchymal oxygenation, lactate, glucose, and oxygen utilization remain stable, cerebral blood flow increases, but cerebral glucose slightly decreases. In later stages, blood pressure may be normal or decrease slightly, glucose may decrease,

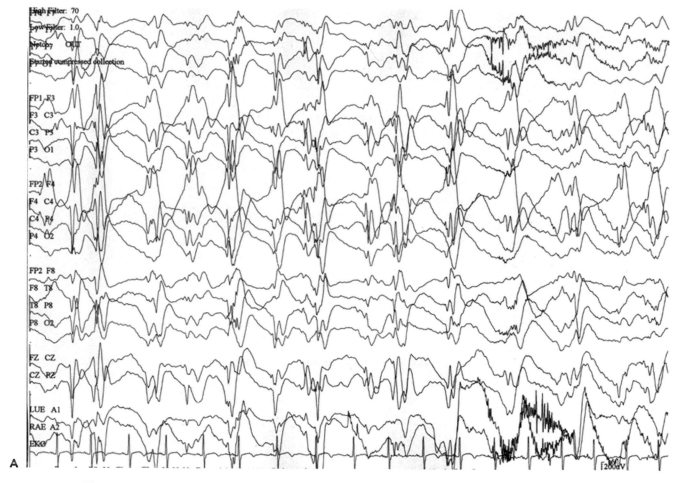

Figure 41.3 A: Nonconvulsive status epilepticus: continuous ictal discharges, slow spike and wave, with altered awareness. **B:** Nonconvulsive status epilepticus: electroencephalogram after lorazepam, now with improved awareness.

and hyperthermia and respiratory compromise may occur, leading to hypoxia and hypercarbia. Brain parenchymal oxygenation, cerebral blood flow, and brain glucose decrease all contribute to an energy mismatch (44). Neuron-specific enolase, a marker of brain injury, is elevated in the serum following both convulsive and nonconvulsive SE (112,113).

Neuronal injury may occur in the absence of metabolic derangement. In paralyzed and ventilated baboons given bicuculline, a GABA inhibitor, to induce electrographic SE (42,43), neuronal loss was observed in the neocortex and hippocampus. Flurothyl-induced brain lesions, including hypermetabolic infarction of the substantia nigra, have occurred in paralyzed and ventilated rats (114). In humans, neuronal loss was seen following SE in three patients without hypotension, hypoxemia, hypoglycemia, or hyperthermia (115).

Most of the AEDs used to treat SE have the potential for respiratory and cardiac depression, especially when administered by a loading dose (116). Therefore, protecting the airway, controlling ventilation, and monitoring cardiac and hemodynamic function are mandatory. Intravenous (IV) administration is the preferred route for the treatment of SE, especially in the inpatient setting, but if IV access is

difficult, intramuscular (IM), intrarectal, or intranasal routes have been used. The rectal route may be useful if IV access is difficult or if concern exists regarding side effects, particularly respiratory depression. Diazepam is the most widely used intrarectal AED.

Primary Antiepileptic Drugs for Status Epilepticus

Phenobarbital, phenytoin, diazepam, and lorazepam are the primary agents used as initial therapy for patients with SE (Table 41.5). Diazepam has a more rapid onset of action because of greater lipid solubility (116), but the agent must be followed by another AED because seizure recurrence is common. This is especially true with acute symptomatic SE. In one study, only 9 of 20 patients maintained seizure control for longer than 2 hours (117), and in another study, only 5 of 15 patients maintained good seizure control for 24 hours (118). Because of a smaller volume of distribution, lorazepam has longer anticonvulsant activity than diazepam (119), with less respiratory depression and sedation. In addition, the rate of seizure recurrence with lorazepam is less than that with diazepam

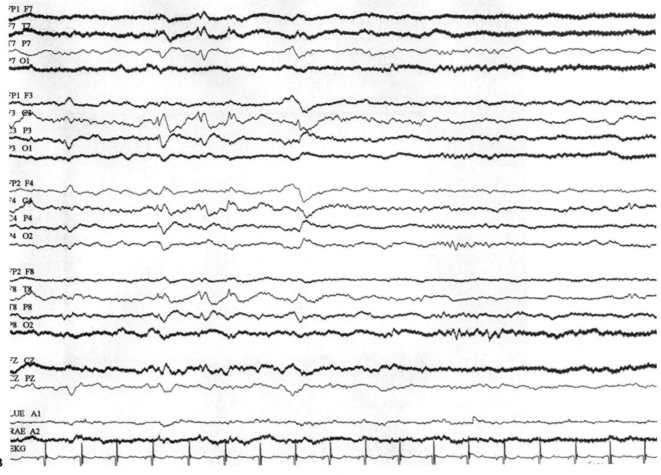

B

Figure 41.3 (continued)

(120). Lorazepam has been used in both adults and children (121,122). In a double-blind study of lorazepam 4 mg versus diazepam 10 mg, seizures were controlled in 89% of episodes with lorazepam versus 76% with diazepam, with similar times of onset and adverse events (123). Midazolam may be administered intramuscularly if there is no IV access, and has been associated with less sedation and respiratory depression (124).

Phenytoin may be administered by an IV loading dose in normal saline (it precipitates with dextrose), at 20 mg/kg (15 mg/kg in the elderly), which rapidly achieves a therapeutic level without respiratory depression or sedation and can also provide maintenance therapy (125–127). This lack of sedation is important for monitoring mental status, such as in patients with head trauma. The infusion rate should be no faster than 1 mg/kg per minute in a child

TABLE 41.5

FIRST-LINE ANTIEPILEPTIC DRUGS

Antiepileptic Drug	Dose	Rate	Maximum Dose
Lorazepam	0.1 mg/kg	2 mg/min (2–5)	8 mg
Diazepam	0.2 mg/kg	5 mg/min	16–20 mg
Fosphenytoin	20 mg PE/kg	up to 3 mg phenytoin equivalents (PE)/kg/min	150 mg/min (adult)
Phenytoin	20 mg/kg	up to 1 mg/kg/min	50 mg/min (adult) 25 mg/min (child) 20 mg/min (elderly)
Phenobarbital	20 mg/kg	1 mg/kg/min	100 mg/min (adult) 30 mg/min (child)

(not to exceed 25 mg per minute), 50 mg per minute in an adult, and 20 mg per minute in the elderly. Pulse and blood pressure should be monitored. If hypotension develops, the infusion rate should be decreased. In adults, a therapeutic level should be maintained for up to 24 hours after a loading dose has been administered (125), but not necessarily for as long in children (128). A level obtained 2 hours after loading may help guide the timing of maintenance therapy with phenytoin (128).

IV phenytoin has an alkaline pH and contains solvents that can cause vascular irritation, cardiac depression, and hypotension. The purple glove syndrome, consisting of distal limb edema, discoloration, and pain, can occur following IV phenytoin infiltration; treatment might require fasciotomies and amputation. In one series, purple glove syndrome occurred in 9 of 152 patients (129); in a prospective series, it occurred in only 3 of 179 patients (130). The syndrome has also been reported following oral dosing in a child (131). The phosphate ester prodrug of phenytoin, fosphenytoin, which is now available, is dosed as phenytoin equivalents (PE) at 20 mg PE/kg. It can be administered in a dextrose solution. Fosphenytoin is water soluble and may be given by the IM route, with paresthesias and injection-site pruritus as possible adverse effects. Bioavailability is 100% compared with that of phenytoin, and the conversion half-life is 7 to 15 minutes (132). Fosphenytoin is rapidly converted to phenytoin by serum and tissue alkaline phosphatases (133). It may be difficult to maintain therapeutic levels in infants, and additional doses may be required (134); subtherapeutic free phenytoin levels may also be seen in children older than 1 year of age (135). A 2-hour phenytoin level is suggested to ensure conversion (135). Side effects are more likely in patients with hypoalbuminemia, renal failure, or hepatic failure, and in the elderly, because of the presence of higher free phenytoin levels. In these patients; the infusion rate should be decreased by 25% to 50% (132). IV phenytoin is no longer available at Children's Hospital, Boston, Massachusetts. At other centers, IV phenytoin use is restricted to adolescents and young adults without cardiac disease who have central venous catheters. The only advantage of IV phenytoin over IV fosphenytoin is significantly lower cost.

Phenobarbital has been used to treat SE in all age groups. Although still considered the agent of choice for neonatal seizures, its efficacy is equivalent to that of phenytoin (136). Respiratory depression and sedation occur, and caution is advised, especially when phenobarbital is administered in combination with other sedative AEDs (such as benzodiazepines). However, in a randomized trial of diazepam and phenytoin versus phenobarbital (10 mg/kg IV), phenobarbital had a shorter median seizure time (5 minutes versus 9 minutes) and response latency (5.5 minutes versus 15 minutes), with a similar incidence of intubation, hypotension, and arrhythmia (137). The loading dose for phenobarbital is 20 mg/kg, administered at a rate no higher than 100 mg per minute (138) in older children and adults and 20 mg/kg in infants.

The long-awaited Veterans Affairs Cooperative Study compared the efficacy of various first-line agents—lorazepam (0.1 mg/kg), phenobarbital (15 mg/kg), diazepam (0.15 mg/kg) plus phenytoin (18 mg/kg), and phenytoin alone (18 mg/kg)—for the treatment of SE with successful treatment defined as control of seizure activity within 20 minutes (25). Treatment efficacy was similar with lorazepam (65%), phenobarbital (58%), and diazepam plus phenytoin (56%), whereas phenytoin alone was associated with lower efficacy (44%). This may be related to a 4.7-minute infusion time with lorazepam versus 33 minutes with phenytoin alone.

Second-line Agents for Status Epilepticus

Sodium valproate is available in IV form (Depacon, Abbott Laboratories, North Chicago, IL) (139); in the past, it had been administered rectally. Although the agent is not approved by the U.S. Food and Drug Administration for the treatment of SE, it is used when other agents fail. Doses of 15 to 33 mg/kg have been administered safely in adults, mostly elderly (140–149), at a rate of 20 to 50 mg per minute (141). In a review of 13 elderly patients with SE and hypotension, a mean loading dose of 25 mg/kg at 35 mg per minute was associated with no change in blood pressure (142). In one study, an infusion rate of 3 mg/kg per minute was associated with hypotension in 2 of 72 patients (145). In children, loading doses of 10 to 30 mg/kg have been used, with most using the higher-dose ranges; an infusion rate of 1 mg/kg per hour was not associated with serous side effects (146). A 20-mg/kg loading dose should produce a serum level of 75 mg/L (147). Valproate is safe in adults and children (140,145,149). Hypotension occurred in one child at an infusion rate of 30 mg/kg per hour (0.5 mg/kg per minute) (148). A loading dose of 10 to 25 mg/kg over 30 minutes has been used in neonates (150).

Standard treatment guidelines are needed in advance for all medical emergencies, to improve the quality of emergency care (151,152). Subsequent analysis of treatment can then be performed, with treatment modification, if needed. In a survey of the United Kingdom (U.K.) Intensive Care Society, only 12% of the respondents used a specific protocol (153). Few randomized clinical trials have been conducted, but treatment surveys have been performed, and the Working Group developed a timetable (4), which is currently under revision. The UK survey demonstrated that first-line therapy was frequently with a benzodiazepine plus phenytoin. In a U.S. survey of neurologists and intensivists (N=106), 76% used lorazepam first, with 95% using phenobarbital or phenytoin if lorazepam failed (154). A survey of epileptologists was conducted to establish consensus guidelines for first-line, second-line, and third-line treatment options for epilepsy syndromes (155). A treatment of choice was determined if selected by more than 50% of respondents.

Lorazepam was considered the treatment of choice for generalized convulsive, focal, and absence SE, with diazepam or phenytoin considered first-line treatment for generalized convulsive SE and focal SE; diazepam and sodium valproate were considered first-line treatment for absence epilepsy (155). Prior to the Veterans Affairs Cooperative Study, the Working Group suggested either lorazepam or diazepam as first-line therapy, but now lorazepam is initially used by many (3,154,155). We at Children's Hospital recommend lorazepam 0.1 mg/kg initially for children, at a maximum dose of 4 mg when IV access is available; if IV access is not available, diazepam or lorazepam can be administered rectally, or fosphenytoin via the IM route. However, a review of randomized clinical trials in children found no evidence that treatment with IV lorazepam was better than treatment with diazepam (156).

Treatment of Refractory Status Epilepticus

Refractory SE occurs when seizures persist despite adequate treatment. By this time, the airway should be protected, ventilation should be controlled with intubation, and transfer to the critical care unit should already be in progress. Such care requires a team approach among providers. The mortality in adults with refractory SE varies from 39% to 48% (157), and in children, from 16% to 43.5% (53,158,159). Etiology is a very important determinant, with a higher mortality among symptomatic patients (12,31,53,60,62). In children, our data demonstrate that etiology is related to prognosis (53). If convulsive activity has stopped but mental status does not improve, nonconvulsive SE must be excluded, which occurs in 14% of patients (108), and in 8% of those with unexplained coma (109). Immediate electroencephalography is performed, if available; if not available, additional empiric AED therapy must be considered.

If SE persists for longer than 1 hour despite adequate doses of conventional AEDs, then high-dose suppressive therapy with IV anesthetic agents should be used (Table 41.6). The treatment goal is to stop SE immediately and to prevent seizure recurrence. Pentobarbital has been the most widely used agent under these circumstances (160–166), administered at 2 to 10 mg/kg, followed by a continuous infusion. Midazolam has a shorter half-life and is associated with less sedation (124,167–172). High-dose phenobarbital is also used; it is associated with less cardiovascular depression than pentobarbital (173,174) but has a longer half-life.

Other agents that are used include high-dose diazepam (175,176) or lorazepam (177), thiopental (178), lidocaine (179–181), inhalational anesthetics such as isoflurane (Forane, Baxter Pharmaceuticals, Deerfield, IL) (182,183), and propofol (184). Propofol has two main advantages: a rapid onset and a short duration of action. One study with pentobarbital showed equal efficacy, but propofol con-

trolled SE in 2.6 minutes versus 123 minutes with pentobarbital (184). Propofol may cause metabolic acidosis with prolonged use in children (185,186). In adults, deaths have occurred with high propofol infusion rates (187), which is known as propofol infusion syndrome (188). Even in an adult study that showed equal efficacy for seizure control, a 57% mortality rate was reported with propofol, versus only 17% with midazolam (170). Therefore, propofol should be used with caution, especially in children and ideally for a short time only, and the infusion rate should not exceed 67 µg/kg per minute (189). Immediate control can be achieved and then another agent used if long-term suppression is needed. Ketamine may be of value, since it is a neuroprotective agent (190–192). Chlormethiazole (193), etomidate (194), and clonazepam (195) are used in Europe; paraldehyde (196) and chloral hydrate (197) may be administered rectally, although paraldehyde is no longer available in the United States. Hypothermia (198) and vagus nerve stimulation (199) have also been used.

To date, no prospective study has been conducted in patients with refractory SE. In a systematic review of refractory SE treatment with pentobarbital, propofol, or midazolam (200), pentobarbital was associated with better seizure control than the other two agents. In the UK survey (N=408), if first-line treatment failed, 142 (35%) of the respondents used a benzodiazepine infusion and 130 (32%) used a general anaesthetic. If seizures continued, 333 (82%) used thiopentone and 56 (14%) used propofol (153). Based on the consensus guidelines, the drug of choice for "therapeutic coma" in patients with generalized convulsive SE and focal SE was pentobarbital, and first-line

---

TABLE 41.6

AGENTS USED IN REFRACTORY STATUS EPILEPTICUS

Intravenous
Pentobarbital
Midazolam
Thiopental
Propofol
Phenobarbital
Diazepam
Lorazepam
Ketamine
Lidocaine
Clomethiazole
Etomidate
Magnesium (especially for eclampsia)

Rectal
Paraldehyde
Chloral hydrate

Other
Hypothermia, with pentobarbital
Inhalational agents, especially isoflurane
Vagal nerve stimulation

agents were midazolam and propofol; for absence seizures, pentobarbital was the drug of choice, with no other first-line options, and midazolam was considered second-line therapy (155). In the U.S. survey, when generalized convulsive SE was refractory to two AEDs, 43% of respondents used phenobarbital, 16% used valproate, and 19% gave one of three agents (pentobarbital, midazolam, or propofol) by continuous infusion (154).

The goal is to control refractory SE and prevent seizure recurrence. Typically, seizures are controlled within 1 hour of beginning a continuous infusion (200). The systematic review defined the following responses to treatment when seizures are not controlled: immediate (acute) treatment failure (clinical or electrographic seizures from 60 minutes to 6 hours after the initial loading dose), breakthrough seizures (any clinical or electroencephalographic seizure after the first 6 hours), withdrawal seizures (seizures occurring within 48 hours of discontinuing or tapering treatment), or changed therapy (switched AED because of poor seizure control).

Whether clinical seizures alone or both clinical and electrographic seizures need complete control is controversial (201,202). In this situation, many clinicians use high-dose suppressive therapy with a burst-suppression pattern on the EEG, aiming for complete control of both the clinical and electrographic seizures. Some aim only for control of clinical seizures (without EEG monitoring). In the U.S. survey, the titration goal with a continuous infusion was burst suppression in 56% of respondents versus elimination of seizures in 41% (154). Even if a burst-suppression pattern is the goal, the degree of suppression needed is unclear. We have used a burst-suppression pattern as the clinical end point, aiming for an interburst interval of at least 5 seconds in duration (53,203). In an analysis of the depth of electroencephalographic suppression with barbiturate anesthetics (pentobarbital or thiopental) in adults, persistent seizure control was better with electrocerebral inactivity on the EEG (17 of 20) versus a burst-suppression pattern (6 of 12 patients) (204,205). Using a midazolam infusion to eliminate all clinical and electrographic seizures and reaching burst suppression only if needed, acute treatment failure occurred in 18% of episodes, breakthrough seizures in 56%, posttreatment seizures in 68%, and treatment failure in 18% (171). In the systematic review, breakthrough seizures occurred less frequently with titration to EEG background suppression (4%) versus titration to seizure suppression only (53%). However, hypotension occurred more often with titration to background suppression (200).

TABLE 41.7

A SUGGESTED TIMETABLE FOR THE TREATMENT OF STATUS EPILEPTICUS

Time (min)	Action
0–5	Diagnose status epilepticus by observing continuing seizure activity
	Give oxygen by nasal cannula or mask; position head for optimal airway patency
	Obtain vital signs and pulse oximetry
	Establish IV line; draw venous blood samples for glucose level, serum chemistries, hematology studies, toxicology screens, and AED levels (if applicable)
	If hypoglycemia is established, or blood glucose measurement not available, administer glucose; in adults, give thiamine first (100 mg), followed by 50 mL of 50% glucose by direct push into IV line; in children, give 2 mL/kg of 25% glucose
5	If seizure continues, give lorazepam 0.1 mg/kg, at 2 mg/min
10–20	If seizure continues, give fosphenytoin 20 mg PE/kg, or if not available, phenytoin 20 mg/kg (in children, give a second dose of lorazepam 0.1 mg/kg, before giving fosphenytoin or phenytoin)
20	Give phenobarbital 20 mg/kg
30	Give additional fosphenytoin 10 mg PE/kg
40	IV valproate 40 mg/kg
40–60	Intravenous anesthesia: Pentobarbital 5 to 15 mg/kg loading dose Midazolam 0.2 mg/kg loading dose Propofol 1–2 mg/kg loading dose Thiopental 5 mg/kg All followed by IV infusions

Abbreviations: AED, antiepileptic drug; IV, intravenous; PE, phenytoin equivalents.
Modified from Delgado–Escueta AV, Wasterlain C, Treiman DM, et al. Management of status epilepticus. *N Engl J Med* 1982;306:1337–1340; Lowenstein DH, Alldredge BK. Status epilepticus. *N Engl J Med* 1998;338:970–976; and Hirsch LJ, Claassen J. The current state of treatment of status epilepticus. *Curr Neurol Neurosci Rep* 2002;2:345–356.

Prolonged high-dose suppressive therapy can be used (53,206), usually with various AED combinations. High-dose suppressive therapy is used initially for a short time (12 to 24 hours); the infusion is then tapered, and if SE recurs, the sequence restarts (3,53,203). Mirski and colleagues recommended prolonged therapy with a potentially good prognosis: a healthy patient (no premorbid illness), a self-limited disease, and with neuroimaging not indicating a poor prognosis (207). We have treated children for prolonged periods—up to 146 days (53,206)—and a 26-year-old with encephalitis was treated for 11 months (208). In our experience with children, no survivor of acute symptomatic refractory SE (n=7) returned to baseline, and all subsequently developed refractory epilepsy; seizure recurrence was reported upon drug tapering in two children, and within 1 to 16 months in the other five (206). In our entire group with refractory SE, 32% returned to baseline (53), and in the adult systematic review, only 29% (48 of 164 patients) returned to baseline (200).

Prehospital Treatment

Since the advent of intrarectal-administered AEDs, the premonitory or early stage can now be treated (209–211), although other routes of administration are also used. The prospective San Francisco Prehospital Treatment study (N=205) showed lorazepam was more effective than diazepam in terminating SE (59% response with lorazepam, versus 43% response with diazepam, and 21% response with placebo; P=0.001) (26). In a retrospective study of 38 children with generalized convulsive SE, use of prehospital diazepam (0.6 mg rectally) was associated with a shorter seizure duration (32 minutes versus 60 minutes) and a reduced likelihood of seizure recurrence in the emergency department (58% versus 85%), with no difference with respect to intubation (212). Rectal diazepam can be administered at home for the treatment of SE or serial seizures; the maximum dose is 20 mg. A new rectal gel preparation, Diastat (Xcel Pharmaceuticals, San Diego, CA), is available, which is easier to administer (213–215). Although not approved for the treatment of SE, Diastat is used as a therapeutic remedy at home; we do not advocate its use for inpatients. Lorazepam can be administered sublingually (216) and midazolam can be given by intranasal or buccal mucosa routes (217), with rapid buccal absorption documented by serum levels and EEG beta activity (218). The efficacy of intranasal midazolam (0.2 mg/kg) is equivalent to that of IV diazepam (0.3 mg/kg) for the treatment of prolonged febrile seizures (219), and buccal midazolam (10 mg) and rectal diazepam (10 mg) show equal efficacy for seizures with a duration longer than 5 minutes (217). Paraldehyde is included in a UK pediatric treatment protocol (151), but as previously noted, it is no longer available in the United States.

Emergency Department or Inpatient Treatment

Lorazepam 0.1 mg/kg should be administered initially. Table 41.7 outlines a suggested treatment sequence.

REFERENCES

1. Gastaut H. Classification of status epilepticus. *Adv Neurol* 1983; 34:15–35.
2. Delgado–Escueta AV, Wasterlain C, Treiman DM, et al. Management of status epilepticus. *N Engl J Med* 1982;306:1337–1340.
3. Lowenstein DH, Alldredge BK. Status epilepticus. *N Engl J Med* 1998;338:970–976.
4. Working Group on Status Epilepticus, Epilepsy Foundation of America. Treatment of convulsive status epilepticus. *JAMA* 1993; 270:854–859.
5. Commission on Terminology of the International League Against Epilepsy. A proposed international classification of epileptic seizures. *Epilepsia* 1964;5:297–306.
6. Gastaut H. Clinical and electroencephalographic classification of epileptic seizures. *Epilepsia* 1970;11:102–113.
7. Commission on Classification and Terminology of the International League Against Epilepsy. Proposal for a revised clinical and electroencephalographic classification of epileptic seizures. *Epilepsia* 1981;22:489–501.
8. Proposal for classification of epilepsies and epileptic syndromes. *Epilepsia* 1985;26:268–278.
9. Proposal for revised classification of epilepsies and epileptic syndromes. *Epilepsia* 1989;30:389–399.
10. Engel J Jr. A proposed diagnostic scheme for people with epileptic seizures and epilepsy: report of the ILAE task force on classification and terminology. *Epilepsia* 2001;42:796–803.
11. Treiman DM, Delgado-Escueda AV. Status epilepticus. In: Thompson RA, Green RA, Green JR, eds. *Critical care of neurological and neurosurgical emergencies.* New York: Raven Press, 1980: 53–99.
12. Scholtes FB, Renier WO, Meinardi H. Generalized convulsive status epilepticus: causes, therapy, and outcome in 346 patients. *Epilepsia* 1994;35:1104–1112.
13. Scholtes FB, Renier WO, Meinardi H. Nonconvulsive status epilepticus: causes, treatment, and outcome in 65 patients. *J Neurol Neurosurg Psychiatry* 1996;61:93–95.
14. Scholtes FB, Renier WO, Meinardi H. Simple partial status epilepticus: causes, treatment, and outcome in 65 patients. *J Neurol Neurosurg Psychiatry* 1996;61:90–92.
15. Treiman DM, DeGiorgio CM, Salisbury S, Wickboldt C. Subtle generalized convulsive status epilepticus. *Epilepsia* 1984;25: 653.
16. Pakalnis A, Drake ME Jr, Phillips B. Neuropsychiatric aspects of psychogenic status epilepticus. *Neurology* 1991;41:1104–1106.
17. Pakalnis A, Paolicchi J, Gilles E. Psychogenic status epilepticus in children: psychiatric and other risk factors. *Neurology* 2000;54: 969–970.
18. Tuxhorn IEB, Fischbach HS. Pseudostatus epilepticus in childhood. *Pediatr Neurol* 2002;27:407–409.
19. Savard G, Andermann F, Teitelbaum J, Lehmann H. Epileptic Munchausen's syndrome: a form of pseudoseizures distinct from hysteria and malingering. *Neurology* 1988;38:1628–1629.
20. Shorvon S. *Status epilepticus: its clinical features and treatment in children and adults.* Cambridge, MA: Cambridge University Press, 1994.
21. Treiman DM, Walton NY, Kendrick C. A progressive sequence of electroencephalographic changes during generalized convulsive status epilepticus. *Epilepsy Res* 1990;5:49–60.
22. Lowenstein DH, Aminoff MJ. Clinical and EEG features of status epilepticus in comatose patients. *Neurology* 1992;42:100–104.
23. Garzon E, Fernandes RM, Sakamoto AC. Serial EEG during human status epilepticus: evidence for PLED as an ictal pattern. *Neurology* 2001;57:1175–1183.
24. Lowenstein DH, Bleck T, Macdonald RL. It's time to revise the definition of status epilepticus. *Epilepsia* 1999;40:120–122.

25. Treiman DM, Meyers PD, Walton NY, et al. A comparison of four treatments for generalized convulsive status epilepticus. *N Engl J Med* 1998;339:792–798.
26. Alldredge BK, Gelb AM, Isaacs SM, et al. A comparison of lorazepam, diazepam, and placebo for the treatment of out-of-hospital status epilepticus. *N Engl J Med* 2001;345:631–637.
27. Gastaut H, Broughton R. *Epileptic seizures: clinical and electrographic features, diagnosis, and treatment.* Springfield, IL: Charles C. Thomas, 1972:25–90.
28. Theodore W, Porter R, Albert P. The secondarily generalized tonic-clonic seizure: a videotape analysis. *Neurology* 1994;44: 1403–1407.
29. Holmes GL. Partial complex seizures in children: an analysis of 69 seizures in 24 patients using EEG FM radiotelemetry and videotape recording. *Electroencephalogr Clin Neurophysiol* 1984;57:13–20.
30. Shinnar S, Berg AT, Moshe SL, et al. How long do new-onset seizures in children last? *Ann Neurol* 2001;49:659–664.
31. Mayer SA, Claassen J, Lokin J, et al. Refractory status epilepticus: frequency, risk factors, and impact on outcome. *Arch Neurol* 2002;59:205–210.
32. Mazarati AM, Baldwin RA, Sankar R, et al. Time-dependent decrease in the effectiveness of antiepileptic drugs during the course of self-sustaining status epilepticus. *Brain Res* 1998;814: 179–185.
33. Kapur J, Lothman EW, DeLorenzo RJ. Loss of GABA$_A$ receptors during partial status epilepticus. *Neurology* 1994;44:2407–2408.
34. Kapur J, Macdonald RL. Rapid seizure–induced reduction of benzodiazepine and Zn^{2+} sensitivity of hippocampal dentate granule cell GABA$_A$ receptors. *J Neurosci* 1997;17:7532–7540.
35. Jones DM, Esmaeil N, Maren S, et al. Characterization of pharmacoresistance to benzodiazepines in the rat Li-pilocarpine model of status epilepticus. *Epilepsy Res* 2002;50:301–312.
36. Goodkin HP, Liu X, Holmes GL. Diazepam terminates brief but not prolonged seizures in young, naive rats. *Epilepsia* 2003;44: 1109–1112.
37. Meldrum BS. The revised operational definition of generalized tonic-clonic (TC) status epilepticus in adults. *Epilepsia* 1999;40: 123–124.
38. Lothman EW, Collins RC, Ferrendelli JA. Kainic acid-induced limbic seizures: electrophysiologic studies. *Neurology* 1981;31: 806–812.
39. Perl TM, Bedard L, Kosatsky T, et al. An outbreak of toxic encephalopathy caused by eating mussels contaminated with domoic acid. *N Engl J Med* 1990;322:1775–1780.
40. Teitelbaum JS, Zatorre RJ, Carpenter S, et al. Neurologic sequelae of domoic acid intoxication due to the ingestion of contaminated mussels. *N Engl J Med* 1990;322:1781–1787.
41. Cendes F, Andermann F, Carpenter S, et al. Temporal lobe epilepsy caused by domoic acid intoxication: evidence for glutamate receptor-mediated excitotoxicity in humans. *Ann Neurol* 1995;37:123–126.
42. Meldrum B, Brierley JB. Prolonged epileptic seizures in primates: ischemic cell change and its relation to ictal physiological events. *Arch Neurol* 1973;28:10–17.
43. Meldrum BS. Metabolic factors during prolonged seizures and their relation to nerve cell death. *Adv Neurol* 1983;34:261–275.
44. Lothman E. The biochemical basis and pathophysiology of status epilepticus. *Neurology* 1990;40(Suppl 2):13–23.
45. DeLorenzo RJ, Hauser WA, Towne AR, et al. A prospective, population, based epidemiologic study of status epilepticus in Richmond, Virginia. *Neurology* 1996;46:1029–1035.
46. Hesdorffer DC, Logroscino G, Cascino G, et al. Incidence of status epilepticus in Rochester, Minnesota, 1965–1984. *Neurology* 1998;50:735–741.
47. Hauser WA. Status epilepticus: epidemiologic considerations. *Neurology* 1990;40(Suppl 2):9–13.
48. Wu YW, Shek DW, Garcia PA, et al. Incidence and mortality of generalized convulsive status epilepticus in California. *Neurology* 2002;58:1070–1076.
49. DeLorenzo RJ, Pellock JM, Towne AR, et al. Epidemiology of status epilepticus. *J Clin Neurophysiol* 1995;12:316–325.
50. Shinnar S, Pellock JM, Moshe SL, et al. In whom does status epilepticus occur: age–related differences in children. *Epilepsia* 1997;38:907–914.
51. Sillanpaa M, Shinnar S. Status epilepticus in a population-based cohort with childhood-onset epilepsy in Finland. *Ann Neurol* 2002;52:303–310.
52. Shinnar S, Maytal J, Krasnoff L, et al. Recurrent status epilepticus in children. *Ann Neurol* 1992;31:598–604.
53. Sahin M, Menache C, Holmes GL, et al. Outcome of severe refractory status epilepticus in children. *Epilepsia* 2001;42: 1461–1467.
54. Rowan AJ, Scott DF. Major status epilepticus: a series of 42 patients. *Acta Neurol Scand* 1970;46:573–584.
55. Oxbury JM, Whitty CWM. Causes and consequences of status epilepticus in adults: a study of 86 cases. *Brain* 1971;94: 733–744.
56. Aminoff MJ, Simon RP. Status epilepticus: causes, clinical features and consequences in 98 patients. *Am J Med* 1980;69: 657–666.
57. Lowenstein DH, Alldredge BK. Status epilepticus at an urban public hospital in the 1980s. *Neurology* 1993;43:483–488.
58. DeLorenzo RJ, Towne AR, Pellock JM, Ko D. Status epilepticus in children, adults, and the elderly. *Epilepsia* 1992;33(Suppl 4): 15–25.
59. Aicardi J, Chevrie JJ. Convulsive status epilepticus in infants and children: a study of 239 cases. *Epilepsia* 1970;11:187–197.
60. Barry E, Hauser WA. Status epilepticus: the interaction of epilepsy and acute brain disease. *Neurology* 1993;43:1473–1478.
61. Dunn DW. Status epilepticus in children: etiology, clinical features, and outcome. *J Child Neurol* 1988;3:167–173.
62. Claassen J, Lokin JK, Fitzsimmons B-FM, et al. Predictors of functional disability and mortality after status epilepticus. *Neurology* 2002;58:139–142.
63. Delanty N, French JA, Labar DR, et al. Status epilepticus arising *de novo* in hospitalized patients: an analysis of 41 patients. *Seizure* 2001;10:116–119.
64. Logroscino G, Hesdorffer DC, Cascino G, et al. Short–term mortality after a first episode of status epilepticus. *Epilepsia* 1997;38:1344–1349.
65. Logroscino G, Hesdorffer DC, Cascino G, et al. Time trends in incidence, mortality, and case-fatality after first episode of status epilepticus. *Epilepsia* 2001;42:1031–1035.
66. Logroscino G, Hesdorffer DC, Cascino GD, et al. Long-term mortality after a first episode of status epilepticus. *Neurology* 2002; 26;58:537–541.
67. Towne AR, Pellock JM, Ko D, et al. Determinants of mortality in status epilepticus. *Epilepsia* 1994;35:27–34.
68. Calabrese VP, Gruemer HD, James K, et al. Cerebrospinal fluid lactate levels and prognosis in status epilepticus. *Epilepsia* 1991;32:816–821.
69. Maytal J, Shinnar S, Moshe SL, et al. Low morbidity and mortality of status epilepticus in childhood. *Pediatrics* 1989;83:323–331.
70. Fujiwara T, Ishida S, Miyakoshi M, et al. Status epilepticus in childhood: a retrospective study of initial convulsive status and subsequent epilepsies. *Folia Psychiatr Neurol Jpn* 1979;33:337–344.
71. Phillips SA, Shanahan RJ. Etiology and mortality of status epilepticus in children: a recent update. *Arch Neurol* 1989;46: 74–76.
72. Vigevano F, DiPapua M, Fusco L, et al. Status epilepticus in infancy and childhood. *Pediatr Neurosci* 1985;1:101–112.
73. Yager JY, Cheang M, Seshia SS. Status epilepticus in childhood. *Can J Neurol Sci* 1988;15:402–405.
74. Erikkson KJ, Koivikko MJ. Status epilepticus in children: aetiology, treatment, and outcome. *Dev Med Child Neurol* 1997;39:652–658.
75. Morton LD, Garnett LK, Towne AR, et al. Mortality of status epilepticus in the first year of life. *Epilepsia* 2001;42(Suppl 7): 164–165.
76. Barnard C, Wirrell E. Does status epilepticus in children cause developmental deterioration and exacerbation of epilepsy? *J Child Neurol* 1999;14:787–794.
77. van Esch A, Ramlal IR, van Steensel-Moll HA, et al. Outcome after febrile status epilepticus. *Dev Med Child Neurol* 1996;38:19–24.
78. Krumholz A, Sung GY, Fisher RS, et al. Complex partial status epilepticus accompanied by serious morbidity and mortality. *Neurology* 1995;45:1499–1504.
79. Krumholz A. Epidemiology and evidence for morbidity of nonconvulsive status epilepticus. *J Clin Neurophysiol* 1999;16:314–322.
80. Jordan KG. Nonconvulsive status epilepticus in acute brain injury. *J Clin Neurophysiol* 1999;16:332–340.

81. Drislane FW. Evidence against permanent neurologic damage from nonconvulsive status epilepticus. *J Clin Neurophysiol* 1999; 16:323–331.

82. Krumholz A, Stern BJ, Weiss HD. Outcome from coma after cardiopulmonary resuscitation: relation to seizures and myoclonus. *Neurology* 1988;38:401–405.

83. Towne AR, Waterhouse EJ, Boggs JG, et al. Prevalence of nonconvulsive status epilepticus in comatose patients. *Neurology* 2000;54:340–345.

84. Nei M, Lee JM, Shankar VL, et al. The EEG and prognosis in status epilepticus. *Epilepsia* 1999;40:157–163.

85. Jaitly R, Sgro JA, Towne AR, et al. Prognostic value of EEG monitoring after status epilepticus: a prospective adult study. *J Clin Neurophysiol* 1997;14:326–334.

86. Schmidley JW, Simon RP. Postictal pleocytosis. *Ann Neurol* 1981; 9:81–84.

87. Barry E, Hauser WA. Pleocytosis after status epilepticus. *Arch Neurol* 1994;51:190–193.

88. Barry E, Hauser WA. Status epilepticus and antiepileptic medication levels. *Neurology* 1994;44:47–50.

89. Maytal J, Novak G, Ascher C, et al. Status epilepticus in children with epilepsy: the role of antiepileptic drug levels in prevention. *Pediatrics* 1996;98:1119–1121.

90. Kramer RE, Luders H, Lesser RP, et al. Transient focal abnormalities of neuroimaging studies during focal status epilepticus. *Epilepsia* 1987;28:528–532.

91. Lansberg MG, O'Brien MW, Norbash AM, et al. MRI abnormalities associated with partial status epilepticus. *Neurology* 1999;52: 1021–1027.

92. Senn P, Lovblad KO, Zutter D, et al. Changes on diffusion-weighted MRI with focal motor status epilepticus: case report. *Neuroradiology*. 2003;45:246–249.

93. Perez ER, Maeder P, Villemure KM, et al. Acquired hippocampal damage after temporal lobe seizures in 2 infants. *Ann Neurol* 2000;48:384–387.

94. Scott RC, Gadian DG, King MD, et al. Magnetic resonance imaging findings within 5 days of status epilepticus in childhood. *Brain* 2002;125:1951–1959.

95. Nixon J, Bateman D, Moss T. An MRI and neuropathological study of a case of fatal status epilepticus. *Seizure* 2001;10:588–591.

96. Itoh Y, Nagaki S, Kuyama N, et al. A case of acute theophylline intoxication with repeated status convulsivus [Japanese]. *No To Hattatsu* 1999;31:559–564.

97. Caksen H, Odabas D, Erol M, et al. Do not overlook acute isoniazid poisoning in children with status epilepticus. *J Child Neurol* 2003;18:142–143.

98. Hankins DG, Saxena K, Faville RJ Jr, et al. Profound acidosis caused by isoniazid ingestion. *Am J Emerg Med* 1987;5:165–166.

99. Wason S, Lacouture PG, Lovejoy FH Jr. Single high-dose pyridoxine treatment for isoniazid overdose. *JAMA* 1981;246:1102–1104.

100. Gleeson JG, duPlessis AJ, Barnes PD, et al. Cyclosporin A acute encephalopathy and seizure syndrome in childhood: clinical features and risk of seizure recurrence. *J Child Neurol* 998;13: 336–344.

101. Primavera A, Audenino D, Cocito L. Ifosfamide encephalopathy and nonconvulsive status epilepticus. *Can J Neurol Sci* 2002;29: 180–183.

102. Osorio I, Reed RC, Peltzer JN. Refractory idiopathic absence status epilepticus: a probable paradoxical effect of phenytoin and carbamazepine. *Epilepsia* 2000;41:887–894.

103. Gansaeuer M, Alsaadi TM. Lithium intoxication mimicking clinical and electrographic features of status epilepticus: a case report and review of the literature. *Clin Electroencephalogr* 2003; 34:28–31.

104. Ostrovskiy D, Spanaki MV, Morris GL III. Tiagabine overdose can induce convulsive status epilepticus. *Epilepsia* 2002;43:773–774.

105. Litovitz TL, Troutman WG. Amoxapine overdose: seizures and fatalities. *JAMA* 1983;250:1069–1071.

106. Haverkos GP, DiSalvo RP, Imhoff TE. Fatal seizures after flumazenil administration in a patient with mixed overdose. *Ann Pharmacother* 1994;28:1347–1349.

107. Privitera MD, Strawsburg RH. Electroencephalographic monitoring in the emergency department. *Emerg Med Clin North Am* 1994;12:1089–1100.

108. DeLorenzo RJ, Waterhouse EJ, Towne AR, et al. Persistent nonconvulsive status epilepticus after the control of convulsive status epilepticus. *Epilepsia* 1998;39:833–840.

109. Towne AR, Waterhouse EJ, Boggs JG, et al. Prevalence of nonconvulsive status epilepticus in comatose patients. *Neurology* 2000;54:340–345.

110. Thomas P. Status epilepticus: indications for emergency EEG [French]. *Neurophysiol Clin* 1997;27:398–405.

111. Wijdicks EF, Hubmayr RD. Acute acid-base disorders associated with status epilepticus. *Mayo Clin Proc* 1994;69:1044–1046.

112. DeGiorgio CM, Correale JD, Gott PS, et al. Serum neuron-specific enolase in human status epilepticus. *Neurology* 1995;45: 1134–1137.

113. Rabinowicz AL, Correale JD, Bracht KA, et al. Neuron-specific enolase is increased after nonconvulsive status epilepticus. *Epilepsia* 1995;36:475–479.

114. Nevander G, Ingvar M, Auer R, et al. Status epilepticus in well-oxygenated rats causes neuronal necrosis. *Ann Neurol* 1985;18: 281–290.

115. Fujikawa DG, Itabashi HH, Wu A, et al. Status epilepticus-induced neuronal loss in humans without systemic complications or epilepsy. *Epilepsia* 2000;41:981–991.

116. Browne TR. The pharmacokinetics of agents used to treat status epilepticus. *Neurology* 1990;40(Suppl 2):28–32.

117. Prensky AL, Raff MC, Moore MJ, et al. Intravenous diazepam in the treatment of prolonged seizure activity. *N Engl J Med* 1967; 276:779–784.

118. Sawyer GT, Webster DD, Schut LL. Treatment of uncontrolled seizure activity with diazepam. *JAMA* 1968;203:913–918.

119. Treiman DM. The role of benzodiazepines in the management of status epilepticus. *Neurology* 1990;40(Suppl 2):32–42.

120. Cock HR, Schapira AH. A comparison of lorazepam and diazepam as initial therapy in convulsive status epilepticus. *QJM* 2002;95: 225–231.

121. Walker JE, Homan RW, Vasko MR, et al. Lorazepam in status epilepticus. *Ann Neurol* 1979;6:207–213.

122. Lacey DJ, Singer WD, Horwitz SJ, et al. Lorazepam therapy of status epilepticus in children and adolescents. *J Pediatr* 1986; 108:771–774.

123. Leppik IE, Derivan AT, Homan RW, et al. Double-blind study of lorazepam and diazepam in status epilepticus. *JAMA* 1983; 249:1452–1454.

124. Kumar A, Bleck TP. Intravenous midazolam for the treatment of refractory status epilepticus. *Crit Care Med* 1992;20:483–488.

125. Cranford RE, Leppik IE, Patrick B, et al. Intravenous phenytoin: clinical and pharmacokinetic aspects. *Neurology* 1978;28: 874–880.

126. Cloyd JC, Gumnit RJ, McLain LW Jr. Status epilepticus. The role of intravenous phenytoin. *JAMA* 1980;244:1479–1491.

127. Salem RB, Wilder BJ, Yost RL, et al. Rapid infusion of phenytoin sodium loading doses. *Am J Hosp Pharm* 1981;38:354–357.

128. Riviello JJ Jr, Roe EJ Jr, Sapin JI, et al. Timing of maintenance phenytoin therapy after intravenous loading dose. *Pediatr Neurol* 1991;7:262–265.

129. O'Brien TJ, Cascino GD, So EL, et al. Incidence and clinical significance of the purple glove syndrome in patients receiving intravenous phenytoin. *Neurology* 1998;51:1034–1039.

130. Burneo JG, Anandan JV, Barkley GL. A prospective study of the incidence of purple glove syndrome. *Epilepsia* 2001;42: 1156–1159.

131. Yoshikawa H, Abe T, Oda Y. Purple glove syndrome caused by oral administration of phenytoin. *J Child Neurol* 2000;15:762.

132. Fischer JH, Patel TV, Fischer PA. Fosphenytoin: clinical pharmacokinetics and comparative advantages in the acute treatment of seizures. *Clin Pharmacokinet* 2003;42:33–58.

133. Browne TR. Fosphenytoin (Cerebyx). *Clin Neuropharmacol* 1997; 20:1–12.

134. Takeoka M, Krishnamoorthy KS, Soman TB, et al. Fosphenytoin in infants. *J Child Neurol* 1998;13:537–540.

135. Koul R, Deleu D. Subtherapeutic free phenytoin levels following fosphenytoin therapy in status epilepticus. *Neurology* 2002;58: 147–148.

136. Painter MJ, Scher MS, Stein AD, et al. Phenobarbital compared with phenytoin for the treatment of neonatal seizures. *N Engl J Med* 1999;341:485–489.

137. Shaner DM, McCurdy SA, Herring MO, et al. Treatment of status epilepticus: a prospective comparison of diazepam and phenytoin versus phenobarbital and optional phenytoin. *Neurology* 1988;38:202–207.

138. Holmes GL. Phenobarbital dose for status epilepticus. *Am J Hosp Pharm* 1994;51:1578.

139. Devinsky O, Leppik I, Willmore LJ, et al. Safety of intravenous valproate. *Ann Neurol* 1995;38:670–674.

140. Venkataraman V, Wheless JW. Safety of rapid intravenous infusion of valproate loading doses in epilepsy patients. *Epilepsy Res* 1999;35:147–153.

141. Naritoku DK, Mueed S. Intravenous loading of valproate for epilepsy. *Clin Neuropharmacol* 1999;22:102–106.

142. Sinha S, Naritoku DK. Intravenous valproate is well tolerated in unstable patients with status epilepticus. *Neurology* 2000;55:722–724.

143. Chez MG, Hammer MS, Loeffel M. Clinical experience of three pediatric and one adult case of spike and wave status epilepticus treated with injectable valproic acid. *J Child Neurol* 1999;14:239–242.

144. Kaplan PW. Intravenous valproate treatment of generalized nonconvulsive status epilepticus. *Clin Electroencephalogr* 1999;30:1–4.

145. Ramsay RE, Cantrell D, Collins SD, et al. Safety and tolerance of rapidly infused Depacon. A randomized trial in subjects with epilepsy. *Epilepsy Res* 2003;52:189–201.

146. Campistol J, Fernandez A, Ortega J. Status epilepticus in children. Experience with intravenous valproate. *Rev Neurol* 1999;29:359–365.

147. Hovinga CA, Chicella MF, Rose DF, et al. Use of intravenous valproate in three pediatric patients with nonconvulsive status epilepticus. *Ann Pharmacother* 1999;33:579–584.

148. White JR, Santos CS. Intravenous valproate associated with significant hypotension in the treatment of status epilepticus. *J Child Neurol* 1999;14:822–823.

149. Yu KT, Mills S, Thompson N, et al. Safety and efficacy of intravenous valproate in pediatric status epilepticus and acute repetitive seizures. *Epilepsia* 2003;44:724–726.

150. Alfonso I, Alvarez LA, Gilman J, et al. Intravenous valproate dosing in neonates. *J Child Neurol* 2000;15:827–829.

151. Shephard SM. Management of status epilepticus. *Emerg Med Clin North Am* 1994;12:941–961.

152. Appleton R, Choonara I, Martland T, et al. The treatment of convulsive status epilepticus in children. The Status Epilepticus Working Party, Members of the Status Epilepticus Working Party. *Arch Dis Child* 2000;83:415–419.

153. Walker MC, Smith SJ, Shorvon SD. The intensive care treatment of convulsive status epilepticus in the UK. Results of a national survey and recommendations. *Anaesthesia* 1995;50:130–135.

154. Claassen J, Hirsch LJ, Mayer SA. Treatment of status epilepticus: a survey of neurologists. *J Neurol Sci* 2003;211:37–41.

155. Karceski S, Morrell M, Carpenter D. The Expert Consensus Guideline Series: Treatment of Epilepsy. *Epilepsy Behav* 2001;2 (6 Suppl):A1–A50.

156. Appleton R, Martland T, Phillips B. Drug management for acute tonic-clonic convulsions including convulsive status epilepticus in children. *Cochrane Database Syst Rev* 2002:CD001905.

157. Bleck TP. Advances in the management of refractory status epilepticus. *Crit Care Med* 1993;21:955–957.

158. Gilbert DL, Gartside PS, Glauser TA. Efficacy and mortality in treatment of refractory generalized convulsive status epilepticus in children: a meta-analysis. *J Child Neurol* 1999;14:602–609.

159. Kim SJ, Lee DY, Kim JS. Neurologic outcomes of pediatric epileptic patients with pentobarbital coma. *Pediatr Neurol* 2001;25:217–220.

160. Young GB, Blume WT, Bolton CF, et al. Anesthetic barbiturates in refractory status epilepticus. *Can J Neurol Sci* 1980;7:291–292.

161. Van Ness PC. Pentobarbital and EEG burst suppression in treatment of status epilepticus refractory to benzodiazepines and phenytoin. *Epilepsia* 1990;31:61–67.

162. Young RS, Ropper AH, Hawkes D, et al. Pentobarbital in refractory status epilepticus. *Pediatr Pharmacol* 1983;3:63–67.

163. Rashkin MC, Youngs C, Penovich P. Pentobarbital treatment of refractory status epilepticus. *Neurology* 1987;37:500–503.

164. Lowenstein DH, Aminoff MJ, Simon RP. Barbiturate anesthesia in the treatment of status epilepticus: clinical experience with 14 patients. *Neurology* 1988;38:395–400.

165. Osorio I, Reed RC. Treatment of refractory generalized tonic-clonic status epilepticus with pentobarbital anesthesia after high-dose phenytoin. *Epilepsia* 1989;30:464–471.

166. Yaffe K, Lowenstein DH. Prognostic factors of pentobarbital therapy for refractory generalized status epilepticus. *Neurology* 1993;43:895–900.

167. Rivera R, Segnini M, Baltodano A, et al. Midazolam in the treatment of status epilepticus in children. *Crit Care Med* 1993;21:991–994.

168. Parent JM, Lowenstein DH. Treatment of refractory generalized status epilepticus with continuous infusion of midazolam. *Neurology* 1994;44:1837–1840.

169. Holmes GL, Riviello JJ Jr. Midazolam and pentobarbital for refractory status epilepticus. *Pediatr Neurol* 1999;20:259–264.

170. Prasad A, Worrall BB, Bertram EH, et al. Propofol and midazolam in the treatment of refractory status epilepticus. *Epilepsia* 2001;42:380–386.

171. Claassen J, Hirsch LJ, Emerson RG, et al. Continuous EEG monitoring and midazolam infusion for refractory nonconvulsive status epilepticus. *Neurology* 2001;57:1036–1042.

172. Ulvi H, Yoldas T, Mungen B, et al. Continuous infusion of midazolam in the treatment of refractory generalized convulsive status epilepticus. *Neurol Sci* 2002;23:177–182.

173. Crawford TO, Mitchell WG, Fishman LS, et al. Very-high-dose phenobarbital for refractory status epilepticus in children. *Neurology* 1988;38:1035–1040.

174. Sudoh A, Sugai K, Miyamoto T, et al. Non-intravenous high-dose phenobarbital therapy for status epilepticus refractory to continuous infusion of midazolam or pentobarbital: report of three cases [Japanese]. *No To Hattatsu* 2002;34:23–29.

175. Singhi S, Banerjee S, Singhi P. Refractory status epilepticus in children: role of continuous diazepam infusion. *J Child Neurol* 1998;13:23–26.

176. Singhi S, Murthy A, Singhi P, et al. Continuous midazolam versus diazepam infusion for refractory convulsive status epilepticus. *J Child Neurol* 2002;17:106–110.

177. Labar DR, Ali A, Root J. High-dose intravenous lorazepam for the treatment of refractory status epilepticus. *Neurology* 1994;44:1400–1403.

178. Parviainen I, Uusaro A, Kalviainen R, et al. High-dose thiopental in the treatment of refractory status epilepticus in the intensive care unit. *Neurology* 2002;59:1249–1251.

179. De Giorgio CM, Altman K, Hamilton-Byrd E, et al. Lidocaine in refractory status epilepticus: confirmation of efficacy with continuous EEG monitoring. *Epilepsia* 1992;33:913–916.

180. Pascual J, Ciudad J, Berciano J. Role of lidocaine (lignocaine) in managing status epilepticus. *J Neurol Neurosurg Psychiatry* 1992;55:49–51.

181. Sata Y, Aihara M, Hatakeyama K, et al. Efficacy and side effects of lidocaine by intravenous drip infusion in children with intractable seizures [Japanese]. *No To Hattatsu* 1997;29:39–44.

182. Kofke WA, Snider MT, Young RSK, et al. Prolonged low flow isoflurane anesthesia for status epilepticus. *Anesthesiology* 1985;62:653–656.

183. Ropper AH, Kofke WA, Bromfield EB, et al. Comparison of isoflurane, halothane, and nitrous oxide in status epilepticus. *Ann Neurol* 1986;19:98–99.

184. Stecker MM, Kramer TH, Raps EC, et al. Treatment of refractory status epilepticus with propofol: clinical and pharmacokinetic findings. *Epilepsia* 1998;39:18–26.

185. Parke TJ, Stevens JE, Rice ASC, et al. Metabolic acidosis and fatal myocardial failure after propofol infusion in children: five case reports. *BMJ* 1992;305:613–616.

186. Hanna JP, Ramundo ML. Rhabdomyolysis and hypoxia associated with prolonged propofol infusion in children. *Neurology* 1998;50:301–303.

187. Stelow EB, Johari VP, Smith SA, et al. Propofol-associated rhabdomyolysis with cardiac involvement in adults: chemical and anatomic findings. *Clin Chem* 2000;46:577–581.

188. Vasile B, Rasulo F, Candiani A, et al. The pathophysiology of propofol infusion syndrome: a simple name for a complex syndrome. *Intensive Care Med* 2003;29:1417–1425.

189. Cornfield DN, Tegtmeyer K, Nelson MD, et al. Continuous propofol infusion in 142 critically ill children. *Pediatrics* 2002;110:1177–1181.

190. Fujikawa DG. Neuroprotective effect of ketamine administered after status epilepticus onset. *Epilepsia* 1995;36:186–195.

191. Borris DJ, Bertram EH, Kapur J. Ketamine controls prolonged status epilepticus. *Epilepsy Res* 2000;42:117–122.

192. Sheth RD, Gidal BE. Refractory status epilepticus: response to ketamine. *Neurology* 1998;51:1765–1766.

193. Browne TR. Paraldehyde, chlormethiazole, and lidocaine for status epilepticus. *Adv Neurol* 1983;34:509–517.

194. Yeoman P, Hutchinson A, Byrne A, et al. Etomidate infusions for the control of refractory status epilepticus. *Intensive Care Med* 1989;15:255–259.

195. Congdon PJ, Forsythe WI. Intravenous clonazepam in the treatment of status epilepticus in children. *Epilepsia* 1980;21:97–102.

196. Curless RG, Holzman BH, Ramsay RE. Paraldehyde therapy in childhood status epilepticus. *Arch Neurol* 1983;40:477–480.

197. Lampl Y, Eshel Y, Gilad R, et al. Chloral hydrate in intractable status epilepticus. *Ann Emerg Med* 1990;19:674–676.

198. Orlowski JP, Erenberg G, Lueders H, et al. Hypothermia and barbiturate coma for refractory status epilepticus. *Crit Care Med* 1984;12:367–372.

199. Winston KR, Levisohn P, Miller BR, et al. Vagal nerve stimulation for status epilepticus. *Pediatr Neurosurg* 2001;34:190–192.

200. Claassen J, Hirsch LJ, Emerson RG, et al. Treatment of refractory status epilepticus with pentobarbital, propofol, or midazolam: a systematic review. *Epilepsia* 2002;43:146–53.

201. Bleck TP. Management approaches to prolonged seizures and status epilepticus. *Epilepsia* 1999;40(Suppl 1):S59–S63.

202. Bleck TP. Refractory status epilepticus in 2001. *Arch Neurol* 2002; 59:188–189.

203. Sahin M, Riviello JJ Jr. Prolonged treatment of refractory status epilepticus in a child. *J Child Neurol* 2001;16:147–150.

204. Krishnamurthy KB, Drislane FW. Relapse and survival after barbiturate anesthetic treatment of refractory status epilepticus. *Epilepsia* 1996;37:863–867.

205. Krishnamurthy KB, Drislane FW. Depth of EEG suppression and outcome in barbiturate anesthetic treatment for refractory status epilepticus. *Epilepsia* 1999;40:759–762.

206. Sahin M, Menache CC, Holmes GL, et al. Prolonged treatment for acute symptomatic refractory status epilepticus: outcome in children. *Neurology* 2003;61:398–401.

207. Mirski MA, Williams MA, Hanley DF. Prolonged pentobarbital and phenobarbital coma for refractory generalized status epilepticus. *Crit Care Med* 1995;23:400–404.

208. Ohori N, Fujioka Y, Ohta M. Experience in managing refractory status epilepticus caused by viral encephalitis under long-term anesthesia with barbiturate: a case report [Japanese]. *Rinsho Shinkeigaku* 1998;38:474–477.

209. Graves NM, Kriel RL. Rectal administration of antiepileptic drugs in children. *Pediatr Neurol* 1987;3:321–326.

210. Woody RC and Laney SM. Rectal anticonvulsants in pediatric practice. *Pediatr Emerg Care* 1988;4:112–116.

211. Kriel RL, Cloyd JC, Hadsall RS, et al. Home use of rectal diazepam for cluster and prolonged seizures: efficacy, adverse reactions, quality of life, and cost analysis. *Pediatr Neurol* 1991;7:13–17.

212. Alldredge BK, Wall DB, Ferriero DM. Effect of prehospital treatment on the outcome of status epilepticus in children. *Pediatr Neurol* 1995;12:213–216.

213. Cloyd JC, Lalonde RL, Beniak TE, et al. A single-blind, crossover comparison of the pharmacokinetics and cognitive effects of a new diazepam rectal gel with intravenous diazepam. *Epilepsia* 1998;39:520–526.

214. Dreifuss FE, Rosman NP, Cloyd JC, et al. A comparison of rectal diazepam gel and placebo for acute repetitive seizures. *N Engl J Med* 1998;338:1869–1875.

215. Cereghino JJ, Mitchell WG, Murphy J, et al. Treating repetitive seizures with a rectal diazepam formulation: a randomized study. *Neurology* 1998;51:1274–1282.

216. Yager JY, Seshia SS. Sublingual lorazepam in childhood serial seizures. *Am J Dis Child* 1988;142:931–932.

217. Holmes GL. Buccal route for benzodiazepines in treatment of seizures. *Lancet* 1999;353:608–609.

218. Scott RC, Besag FM, Neville BG. Buccal midazolam and rectal diazepam for treatment of prolonged seizures in childhood and adolescence: a randomised trial. *Lancet* 1999;353:623–626.

219. Lahat E, Goldman M, Barr J, et al. Comparison of intranasal midazolam with intravenous diazepam for treating febrile seizures in children: prospective randomized study. *BMJ* 2000; 321:83–86.

220. Hirsch LJ, Claassen J. The current state of treatment of status epilepticus. *Curr Neurol Neurosci Rep* 2002;2:345–356.

Psychogenic Nonepileptic Seizures

42

Selim R. Benbadis

OVERVIEW

Psychogenic nonepileptic seizures (PNES) are routinely seen at epilepsy centers, where they represent 15% to 30% of patients referred for refractory seizures (1,2). They occur fairly often in the general population, with an estimated prevalence of 2 to 33 per 100,000 persons, making this condition nearly as common as multiple sclerosis (MS) or trigeminal neuralgia. In addition to being common, PNES represent a challenge, both in diagnosis and in management.

Terminology

The terminology used to describe PNES is variable and at times confusing. A number of terms have been used, including pseudoseizures, nonepileptic seizures, nonepileptic events, psychogenic seizures, and hysterical seizures. Strictly speaking, terms such as pseudoseizures, nonepileptic seizures, and nonepileptic events include both psychogenic and nonpsychogenic (i.e., organic) episodes that mimic epileptic seizures. Examples of nonpsychogenic episodes include syncope (the most common); paroxysmal movement disorders (e.g., dystonia); cataplexy; complicated migraines; and, in children, breath-holding spells and shuddering attacks. Terms such as psychogenic or hysterical seizures, on the other hand, refer to a subset of nonepileptic seizures with the connotation of a psychological origin. Use of the term hysteria has long since fallen into disfavor. The term psychogenic seizures could possibly be interpreted as epileptic seizures triggered or exacerbated by a psychological factor. For these reasons, PNES is the preferred term (3) and is used throughout this chapter.

The Misdiagnosis of Epilepsy

The erroneous diagnosis of epilepsy is relatively common. Approximately 25% of patients previously diagnosed with epilepsy and who are not responding to antiepileptic drug (AED) therapy are found to be misdiagnosed, both in epilepsy referral clinics (4,5) and in epilepsy monitoring units (1). Most patients misdiagnosed with epilepsy are eventually shown to have PNES (1,2) or, more rarely, syncope (6,7). Occasionally, other paroxysmal conditions can be misdiagnosed as epilepsy, but PNES are by far the most common condition, followed by syncope. Often, electroencephalograms (EEGs) that are interpreted as providing evidence for epilepsy contribute to this misdiagnosis (4,6,8). As is true with other chronic conditions (e.g., MS), whenever a wrong diagnosis of epilepsy has been given, it can be very difficult to "undo." Unfortunately, once the diagnosis of "seizures" has been made, it becomes easily perpetuated without being questioned, which explains the usual diagnostic delay (9,10) and associated cost (11,12). It is disconcerting that despite the ability to render a diagnosis of PNES with near-certainty, the delay in diagnosis remains long, at about 7 to 10 years (9,10), indicating that neurologists may not have a high enough index of suspicion when AED treatment fails. This chapter begins by reviewing the steps involved in making that diagnosis and then turns to management considerations.

MAKING THE DIAGNOSIS

Suspecting the Diagnosis

PNES are initially suspected in the clinic on the basis of history and examination. A number of "red flags" are useful in clinical practice and should raise the suspicion that seizures may be psychogenic rather than epileptic. Of course, resistance to AEDs can be the first clue and is usually the reason for referral to an epilepsy center. Most (approximately 80%) of the patients with PNES have been treated with AEDs for some time before the correct diagnosis is made (13). This is because a diagnosis of epilepsy is usually based solely on history and may be difficult, especially for nonneurologists (e.g., emergency department physicians and primary care physicians). A very high frequency of episodes that are completely unaffected by AEDs (i.e., no difference whether on or off medication) should also suggest the possibility of a psychogenic etiology. The presence of specific triggers that are unusual for epilepsy can be very suggestive of PNES, and this should be asked specifically when obtaining the history. For example, emotional triggers ("stress" or "getting upset") are commonly reported in patients with PNES. Other triggers that are suggestive of PNES include pain, certain movements, sounds, and lights, especially if they are alleged to *consistently* precipitate a "seizure." The circumstances under which attacks occur can be very helpful. Like other psychogenic symptoms, PNES tend to occur in the presence of an "audience," and, for example, occurrence in a physician's office or waiting room may be predictive of a psychogenic etiology (14). Similarly, PNES tend not to occur in sleep, although they may seem to and may be reported as such (15,16).

If the historian and witnesses are astute enough, the detailed description of the spells often includes characteristics that are inconsistent with epileptic seizures. In particular, some characteristics of the motor ("convulsive") phenomena are associated with PNES (see "Electroencephalogram-Video Monitoring"). However, witnesses' accounts are rarely detailed enough to describe the episodes accurately; in fact, even seizures witnessed by physicians and thought to be epileptic often turn out to be PNES. The patient's medical history can be useful as well. Although it has not been documented, coexisting poorly defined and "fashionable" (probably psychogenic) conditions, such as fibromyalgia, chronic pain, irritable bowel, or chronic fatigue, are associated with psychogenic symptoms. In a population referred for refractory seizures, a history of fibromyalgia or chronic pain has a strong association with a diagnosis of PNES (14). Similarly, a florid review of systems suggests somatization. A psychosocial history with evidence of maladaptive behaviors or associated psychiatric diagnoses should raise the level of suspicion of PNES. The examination, paying particular attention to mental status evaluation, including general demeanor and appropriate level of concern, overdramatization, and hysterical features, can be very telling, often uncovering such histrionic behavior as "give-way" weakness or "tight-roping." Performing the examination can, in itself, act as an "induction" in suggestible patients, making a spell more likely to occur during the history taking or examination.

By contrast, the presence of certain symptoms argues in favor of epileptic seizures and should warrant caution.

These include significant postictal confusion, incontinence, and, most important, significant injury (17–21). Although some injuries have been reported in PNES, data that describe injuries in patients with PNES are based largely on patients' self-reports (22). In particular, tongue biting is highly specific to generalized tonic-clonic seizures (18) and thus is a very helpful sign when present.

Confirming the Diagnosis

EEG and Ambulatory EEG

Because of its low sensitivity, routine EEG is not very helpful in diagnosing PNES. However, the presence of repeated normal EEGs, especially in light of frequent attacks and resistance to AEDs, certainly can be viewed as a red flag (23). Ambulatory EEG is increasingly used, is cost-effective, and can contribute to the diagnosis of PNES by recording the habitual episode and documenting the absence of EEG changes. However, because of the difficulties involved in conveying this diagnosis (see "Management"), it should always be confirmed by video-EEG monitoring.

Video-Electroencephalogram Monitoring

This is the gold standard for diagnosis of PNES (2,3,9,15–19,21), and, in fact, is indicated in all patients who continue to experience frequent seizures despite the use of AEDs (24). In the hands of experienced epileptologists, the combined electroclinical analysis of both the clinical semiology of the ictus and the ictal EEG findings allows a definitive diagnosis in nearly all cases. If an attack is recorded, the diagnosis is usually easy, and it is unusual that this question (i.e., PNES versus epilepsy) cannot be answered.

The principle of video-EEG monitoring is to record an episode and demonstrate that (a) there is no change in the EEG during the clinical event, and (b) the clinical spell is not consistent with seizure types that can be unaccompanied by EEG changes. Ictal EEG has limitations because it may be negative in simple partial seizures (25,26) and in some complex partial seizures, especially frontal ones (21). Ictal EEG may also be uninterpretable or difficult if movements generate excessive artifact.

Analysis of the ictal semiology (i.e., video) is at least as important as the ictal EEG, as it often shows behaviors that are obviously nonorganic and incompatible with epileptic seizures. Certain characteristics of the motor phenomena are strongly associated with PNES, including a very gradual onset or termination; pseudosleep; discontinuous (stop-and-go) activity; and irregular or asynchronous (out-of-phase) activity side-to-side head movement, pelvic thrusting, opisthotonic posturing, stuttering, and weeping (15–17,19,21,27–30). A particularly useful sign is preserved awareness during bilateral motor activity, which is relatively specific for PNES. This is because unresponsiveness is almost always present during bilateral motor activity, with the notable exception being supplementary motor area seizures (31,32).

Inductions

Provocative techniques, also known as activation procedures, or "inductions," can be extremely useful for the diagnosis of PNES, particularly when the diagnosis remains uncertain and no spontaneous attacks occur during monitoring. Many epilepsy centers use some sort of provocative technique to aid in the diagnosis of PNES (33,34). Some variability exists among the methods used. Although intravenous (IV) saline injection has traditionally been the most common (35–38), a number of other techniques have been described (39–42), which may be preferable (see below).

The principle behind provocative techniques is suggestibility, which is a feature of somatoform disorders in general. For example, in psychogenic movement disorders, where the diagnosis rests solely on phenomenology (i.e., there is no equivalent of the EEG), response to placebo or suggestion is considered a diagnostic criterion for *definite* psychogenic mechanism (43).

There are many advantages to the use of provocative techniques. First, when carefully studied and used simultaneously with EEG, their specificity approaches 100% (44). Second, difficult situations exist in which the combination of semiology (video) and the EEG does not allow one to conclude that an episode is psychogenic in origin. As mentioned earlier, two relatively common scenarios are (a) the ictal EEG is uninterpretable because of movement-related artifacts, and (b) the ictal EEG is normal, but the symptoms are consistent with a "simple partial" seizure. In these situations, the very presence of suggestibility (i.e., suggestion triggers the episode in question) is the strongest argument to support a psychogenic etiology. Third, at least theoretically, nonepileptic is not quite synonymous with psychogenic. The combination of a recorded attack and a normal ictal EEG qualifies as a nonepileptic spell but cannot in itself be categorized as psychogenic. On the other hand, a positive induction does stamp the episode as psychogenic, and even difficult-to-convince laypersons and attorneys understand this concept. Fourth, there is a strong economic argument for the use of these techniques, especially with the constraints imposed by third-party payers. When spontaneous attacks do not occur in the allotted time for monitoring, the evaluation may be inconclusive. In such situations, provocative techniques often turn an inconclusive evaluation into a diagnostic one.

The main limitation of provocative techniques is that they introduce ethical concerns. Several valid ethical arguments against placebo induction have been raised and acknowledged, making these techniques controversial (33,34,45,46). Of primary concern is the fact that physicians cannot honestly disclose the content of the syringe (for IV saline) or cannot say that the maneuver (e.g., tuning fork or patch) induces seizures. Even if the term "seizures" is then used in a broader sense, encompassing PNES, a degree of disingenuousness persists. The problem is particularly acute when a placebo is used, which results in

deceptive "beating around the bush." Thus, techniques that do not use placebo may be preferable, which circumvents these ethical problems while retaining similar diagnostic value (42,45). The best-documented technique uses a combination of hyperventilation, photic stimulation, and strong verbal suggestion (42,47). If hyperventilation is contraindicated or ill advised, counting aloud with arms raised will work equally well. The sensitivity is comparable to that with other methods, ranging from 60% to 90% (35–39,42,44,47). One major advantage of this technique is that hyperventilation and photic stimulation truly induce seizures, so that deception is not inherent to the procedure. Indeed, these maneuvers are performed during most EEGs, so that most patients will have undergone them previously. For this reason, patients or their families are not intrigued by the induction technique and do not ask about it (42). In fact, a comparable provocative technique using "psychiatric interview" was found not to be harmful and even useful by patients (39). Provocative techniques should only be performed along with video-EEG monitoring. Without the use of a placebo, provocative techniques are similar to other clinical maneuvers performed during the neurologic examination when nonorganic symptoms are suspected.

Short-Term Outpatient Video-EEG with Activation

An extension of the use of inductions is that when patients are strongly suspected, on clinical grounds, of having PNES, they can undergo outpatient "video-EEG with activation." This can be very cost-effective, while retaining the same specificity and a reasonably high level of sensitivity. In one published series, 10 of 15 patients had their habitual nonepileptic seizures with hyperventilation plus photic stimulation plus suggestion (47). In another study, short-term outpatient video-EEG with saline induction yielded a diagnosis in 60% of patients (48). At our center this is routinely used, and in two-thirds of cases the typical episode is obtained, thus obviating the need for "long-term" video-EEG monitoring (49).

DIFFICULT AND SPECIAL ISSUES IN DIAGNOSIS

Previous Abnormal Electroencephalogram

This is a very common problem. Many patients with PNES who are seen at epilepsy centers have had previous EEGs interpreted as epileptiform activity. When carefully reviewed, the vast majority turn out to be normal variants that were overinterpreted (8). In this situation, it is essential to obtain and review the actual tracing previously read as epileptiform activity, because no amount of normal subsequent EEGs will "cancel" the previous abnormal one. Unfortunately, obtaining prior EEGs can be difficult. First, records are not always available or accessible, and second, digital electroencephalograph systems are incompatible with each other. In this regard, software that allows one to read *any* digital EEG format is very valuable and may become a necessity at referral epilepsy centers.

In children, coexisting benign focal epileptiform discharges of childhood (BFEDC) on the EEG are a common "red herring." Such discharges are frequently seen in asymptomatic children and do not necessarily confirm that the reported episodes are epileptic. When epileptic seizures do occur in patients with perirolandic BFEDC on interictal EEG, they are usually facial sensorimotor or nocturnal generalized tonic clonic in nature. When the clinical presentation is mismatched with the expected manifestations of BFEDC—for example, in children with medically refractory "convulsions" or staring spells—video-EEG is appropriate to allow examination of the EEG during clinical events. In children with nonepileptic events, the "ictal" EEG will remain normal despite the BFEDC during interictal recording.

Coexisting Epilepsy

There is a widely held belief that many or most patients with PNES also have epilepsy. A careful review of the literature shows that this belief is inaccurate. Reports that have found high percentages of patients with PNES who also have epilepsy are based on loose criteria, such as an "abnormal EEG," whereas those that required definite evidence for coexisting epilepsy found percentages between 9% and 15% (50,51).

Coexisting Organic Disease

A related phenomenon is that seizures are especially likely to be overdiagnosed as epileptic in patients with other organic neurologic diseases, such as MS, stroke, or antecedent brain surgery (52), or a history of head injury. For example, among patients in one study with traumatic brain injury diagnosed as posttraumatic epilepsy, 30% had psychogenic seizures instead (53). Thus, as is the general rule, if seizures do not respond to AEDs, a diagnosis of PNES should be considered despite the coexistence of organic disease. A diagnosis of PNES following some types of head injury may be particularly problematic if the injury involves litigation.

Psychogenic Nonepileptic Seizures After Epilepsy Surgery

PNES can occur following epilepsy surgery (54–56) and should always be considered if seizures recur and are somewhat different than they were preoperatively. In general, PNES tend to occur within 1 month after surgery (55). Risk factors include neurologic dysfunction in the right hemisphere, seizure onset after adolescence, low intelligence quotient (IQ), serious preoperative psychopathologic conditions, and major surgical complications (55,56).

Epilepsy Surgery in Patients with Psychogenic Nonepileptic Seizures

Occasionally, patients evaluated for epilepsy surgery also have PNES, triggered especially by activation procedures. Under the right circumstances, this is not a contraindication to surgery (57). If the epilepsy is refractory and the epileptic seizures are the most disabling ones, it may be appropriate to perform surgery to provide relief from the burden of seizures and high-dose AEDs, while approaching the PNES with psychiatric intervention.

PSYCHOPATHOLOGY

PNES are, by definition, a psychiatric disorder. According to the *Diagnostic and Statistical Manual of Mental Disorders* (DSM) classification (58,59), physical symptoms caused by psychological causes can fall under three categories: somatoform disorders, factitious disorders, and malingering. Somatoform disorders are, by definition, the *unconscious* production of physical symptoms caused by psychological factors, which means that the symptoms are not under voluntary control—that is, the patient is not faking and not intentionally trying to deceive. Somatoform disorders are subdivided into several disorders, depending on the characteristics of the physical symptoms and their time course. The two somatoform disorders relevant to PNES are conversion disorder and somatization disorder. In fact, the DSM-IV added a new subcategory of conversion disorder (from the DSM-III-R), specifically termed conversion disorder with seizures. In contrast to the unconscious (unintentional) production of symptoms of the somatoform disorders (including conversion), factitious disorders and malingering imply that the patient is purposely deceiving the physician—that is, faking the symptoms. The difference between the two (i.e., factitious disorder and malingering) is that in malingering, the reason for doing so is tangible and rationally understandable (albeit possibly reprehensible), whereas in factitious disorder, the motivation is a pathologic need. An important corollary, therefore, is that malingering is not considered a mental illness, whereas factitious disorder is (58,59).

It is generally accepted that most patients with PNES fall under the somatoform category (unconscious production of symptoms) rather than the intentional faking type (malingering and factitious). However, although the DSM classification is simple in theory, it is nearly impossible to know if a given patient is faking. Intentional faking can only be diagnosed in some circumstances by catching a person in the act of doing so (e.g., self-inflicting injuries, administering medications or eye drops to cause signs, putting blood in the urine to simulate hematuria). Malingering may be underdiagnosed (60), partly because the "diagnosis" of malingering is essentially an accusation.

From a practical point of view, the role of the neurologist and other medical specialists is to determine whether organic disease exists. Once the symptoms are shown to be psychogenic in nature, the exact psychiatric diagnosis and its treatment are best handled by a psychiatrist.

The role of antecedent sexual trauma or abuse is thought to be important in the psychopathology of psychogenic seizures and psychogenic symptoms in general. A history of abuse may be more common in the convulsive, rather than the limp, type of PNES (61).

PROGNOSIS

Overall, the outcome in adults is tenuous. After 10 years of symptoms, more than half of patients continue to have seizures and remain dependent on social security benefits (62,63). The outcome is better in patients with greater educational attainments, younger age at onset and diagnosis, attacks with less dramatic features, fewer additional somatoform complaints, lower dissociation scores, and lower scores on the higher-order personality dimensions "inhibitedness," "emotional dysregulation," and "compulsivity" (63). The limp or catatonic type may have a better prognosis than the convulsive or thrashing type (64). Quality of life is severely affected in patients with PNES (65).

Duration of illness is probably the single most important prognostic factor in PNES—that is, the longer patients have been treated for epilepsy, the worse the prognosis (10,64,66). Thus, obtaining a definite diagnosis of PNES early in the course is critical. Currently, the average delay in the diagnosis of PNES remains long at 7 to 10 years (9,10), indicating that the index of suspicion for psychogenic symptoms may not be high enough. In addition, an accurate diagnosis of PNES also significantly reduces subsequent health care costs (12).

Overall, the outcome in patients with PNES is better in children and adolescents (67), probably because the duration of illness is shorter and the psychopathology or stressors are different from those in adults (66,68). School refusal and family discord may be significant factors. Serious mood disorders and ongoing sexual or physical abuse are common in children with PNES and should be investigated in every case.

MANAGEMENT

Role of the Neurologist or Epileptologist

The role of the neurologist or epileptologist does not end when the diagnosis of PNES is made. In fact, perhaps the most important step in initiating treatment is in the *delivery of the diagnosis* to patients and families (10,69–71). Most patients with psychogenic symptoms have received an initial diagnosis of organic disease (e.g.,

epilepsy), so that patients' reactions typically include disbelief and denial, as well as anger and hostility ("Are you accusing me of faking?" or "Are you saying that I am crazy?"). Written information can be useful in supplementing verbal explanations, but, unfortunately, patient information on psychogenic symptoms is rather scarce. Remarkably, the American Psychiatric Association (APA) has abundant patient education materials available on diverse topics, but none on somatoform disorders (72). Patient education materials on PNES are scarce but available (73). Patient education is particularly important in psychogenic symptoms. Unless patients and families understand and accept the diagnosis, they will not comply with recommendations. Therefore, communicating the diagnosis is critical. In fact, patients' understanding and reactions to the diagnosis have an impact on outcome (10).

Communicating the diagnosis is where the failure and breakdown often occur, and this is the main obstacle to effective treatment. Typically, physicians are uncomfortable with this diagnosis and tend to be uneasy formulating a conclusion. Reports frequently remain vague and fail to give clear interpretations, leaving the clinician hanging (e.g., "there was no EEG change during the episode" or "there is no evidence for epilepsy" or "seizures were nonepileptic"), with no explanations given to patients and families. In these situations, patients often continue to be treated for epilepsy, possibly with the understanding that the test was inconclusive. The diagnosis should be explained clearly, using unambiguous terms that patients can understand, such as "psychological," "stress-induced," or "emotional." The physician communicating the diagnosis must be compassionate (remembering that most patients are not faking), but firm and confident (avoiding "wishy-washy" and confusing terms).

The neurologist should also continue to be involved and not "abandon" the patient. The neurologist can assist in weaning patients off AED therapy, and may be helpful in addressing such issues as driving and disability. With regard to driving, few data are available, and there is no evidence that patients with PNES have an increased risk for motor vehicle accidents (74), probably for the same reason that they do not usually sustain serious injuries. Nevertheless, caution is advised, and each case should be evaluated individually and jointly by the neurologist and the mental health professional. Another sensitive issue is that of disability. PNES can be truly disabling, and this should be made clear. However, logic dictates that in these cases, a disability claim should be filed and justified on the basis of a *psychiatric diagnosis*, not a neurologic one. Another reason for the neurologist to continue following these patients is that one should keep an open mind about the possibility of coexisting epilepsy.

Role of the Mental Health Professional

Psychogenic symptoms are, by definition, a psychiatric disease, and mental health professionals should treat these patients. Treatment includes psychotherapy and adjunctive medications for coexisting anxiety or depression. Unfortunately, mental health services are not always easily available, especially for the uninsured. Another obstacle is that psychiatrists tend to be skeptical about the diagnosis of psychogenic symptoms, and even in patients with PNES in whom video-EEG monitoring allows a near-certain conclusion, they tend not to believe the diagnosis (75). A useful approach to combating this skepticism is to provide the treating psychiatrist with the actual video recordings of the PNES, as these can be more convincing than written reports.

PSYCHOGENIC NONEPILEPTIC SEIZURES IN CHILDREN

Although PNES are more common in adolescence, they may occur in children as young as 5 or 6 years of age. Most of what has been emphasized here applies to children as well as to adults. However, there are certain features specific to children. First, the differential diagnosis of seizures is broader in children, with many nonepileptic, nonpsychogenic conditions to be considered (76), including tics, breath-holding spells, and shuddering attacks. In addition, children experience nonepileptic staring spells (77), which are actually episodes of behavioral inattention that are misinterpreted by adults. The gender difference of female predominance is not observed until adolescence (78), and PNES are as common in preadolescent boys as in preadolescent girls. As described above, BFEDC are a common confounding feature on the interictal EEG, and the outcome in children and adolescents with PNES is generally better than that in adults (67).

PSYCHOGENIC NONEPILEPTIC SEIZURES IN PERSPECTIVE

The literature on PNES (at least the neurology and epilepsy literature) often gives the impression that PNES represents a unique disorder. In reality, PNES are but one type of somatoform disorder. How the psychopathology is expressed (PNES, paralysis, diarrhea, or pain) is only different in the diagnostic aspects. Fundamentally, the underlying psychopathology, its prognosis, and its management are no different with PNES than with other psychogenic symptoms. Whatever the manifestations, psychogenic symptoms represent a challenge both in the diagnosis and management.

Psychogenic (nonorganic, "functional") symptoms are common in medicine. Conservative estimates are that approximately 10% of all medical services are provided for psychogenic symptoms (60). They are also common in neurology, representing approximately 9% of inpatient neurology admissions (79) and probably an even higher percentage of outpatient visits. Common neurologic symptoms that are found to be psychogenic include paralysis, mutism, visual symptoms, sensory symptoms, movement disorders, gait or balance problems, and pain (79–81). For several neurologic symptoms, signs or maneuvers have been described to help differentiate organic from nonorganic symptoms. For example, limb weakness is often evaluated by eliciting the Hoover sign, for which a quantitative version has been proposed (82). Other examples include looking for give-way weakness and alleged blindness with preserved optokinetic nystagmus. More generally, the neurologic examination often attempts to elicit signs or symptoms that do not make neuroanatomic sense (e.g., facial numbness affecting the angle of the jaw, gait with astasia-abasia, or tight-roping).

Every medical specialty has its share of symptoms that can be psychogenic. In gastroenterology, these include vomiting, dysphagia, abdominal pain, and diarrhea. In cardiology, chest pain that is noncardiac is traditionally referred to as "musculoskeletal" chest pain but is probably psychogenic. Symptoms that can be psychogenic in other medical specialties include shortness of breath and cough in pulmonary medicine, psychogenic globus or dysphonia in otolaryngology, excoriations in dermatology, erectile dysfunction in urology, and blindness or convergence spasms in ophthalmology. Pain syndromes for which a psychogenic component is likely include tension headaches, chronic back pain, limb pain, rectal pain, and pain in sexual organs. Of course, because pain is, by definition, entirely subjective, it is extremely difficult, and perhaps impossible, to ever confidently say that pain is psychogenic. It could even be argued that all pain is psychogenic, and thus psychogenic pain is one of the most "uncomfortable" diagnoses to make. In addition to isolated symptoms, some syndromes are considered to be at least partly psychogenic by some and possibly entirely psychogenic (i.e., without any organic basis) by others. These controversial but "fashionable" diagnoses include fibromyalgia, fibrositis, myofascial pain, chronic fatigue syndrome, irritable bowel syndrome, and multiple chemical sensitivity. As mentioned previously, there seems to be a relationship between fibromyalgia and PNES (14).

How are Psychogenic Nonepileptic Seizures Unique Among Psychogenic Symptoms?

Among psychogenic symptoms, PNES are unique in one main characteristic: with video-EEG monitoring, they can be diagnosed with near-certainty. This is in sharp contrast to other psychogenic symptoms, which almost always involve a diagnosis of exclusion. This feature allows a clarity and confidence of diagnosis that may assist in the critical step of convincing the patient and family of the nonorganic nature of the PNES.

REFERENCES

1. Benbadis SR, Hauser WA. An estimate of the prevalence of psychogenic non-epileptic seizures. *Seizure* 2000;9:280–281.
2. Benbadis SR, Heriaud L, O'Neill E et al. Outcome of prolonged EEG-video monitoring at a typical referral epilepsy center. *Epilepsia* 2004;45:1150–1153.
3. Gates JR. Nonepileptic seizures: time for progress. *Epilepsy Behav* 2000;1:2–6.
4. Smith D, Defalla BA, Chadwick DW. The misdiagnosis of epilepsy and the management of refractory epilepsy in a specialist clinic. *QJM* 1999;92:15–23.
5. Scheepers B, Clough P, Pickles C. The misdiagnosis of epilepsy: findings of a population study. *Seizure* 1998;7:403–406.
6. Eiris-Punal J, Rodriguez-Nunez A, Fernandez-Martinez N, et al. Usefulness of the head-upright tilt test for distinguishing syncope and epilepsy in children. *Epilepsia* 2001;42:709–713.
7. Zaidi A, Clough P, Cooper P, et al. Misdiagnosis of epilepsy: many seizure-like attacks have a cardiovascular cause. *J Am Coll Cardiol* 2000;36:181–184.
8. Benbadis SR, Tatum WO. Overintepretation of EEGs and misdiagnosis of epilepsy. *J Clin Neurophysiol* 2003;20:42–44.
9. Reuber M, Fernandez G, Bauer J, et al. Diagnostic delay in psychogenic nonepileptic seizures. *Neurology* 2002;58:493–495.
10. Carton S, Thompson PJ, Duncan JS. Non-epileptic seizures: patients' understanding and reaction to the diagnosis and impact on outcome. *Seizure* 2003;12:287–294.
11. Nowack WJ. Epilepsy: a costly misdiagnosis. *Clin Electroencephalogr* 1997;28:225–228.
12. Martin RC, Gilliam FG, Kilgore M, et al. Improved health care resource utilization following video-EEG–confirmed diagnosis of nonepileptic psychogenic seizures. *Seizure* 1998;7:385–390.
13. Benbadis SR. How many patients with pseudoseizures receive antiepileptic drugs prior to diagnosis? *Eur Neurol* 1999;41:114–115.
14. Benbadis SR. A spell in the epilepsy clinic and a history of "chronic pain" or "fibromyalgia" independently predict a diagnosis of psychogenic seizures. *Epilepsy Behav* 2005;6:264–265.
15. Benbadis SR, Lancman ME, King LM, et al. Preictal pseudosleep: a new finding in psychogenic seizures. *Neurology* 1996;47:63–67.
16. Thacker K, Devinsky O, Perrine K, et al. Nonepileptic seizures during apparent sleep. *Ann Neurol* 1993;33:414–418.
17. Desai BT, Porter RJ, Penry JK. Psychogenic seizures. A study of 42 attacks in six patients, with intensive monitoring. *Arch Neurol* 1982;39:202–209.
18. Benbadis SR, Wolgamuth BR, Goren H, et al. Value of tongue biting in the diagnosis of seizures. *Arch Intern Med* 1995;155:2346–2349.
19. Guberman A. Psychogenic pseudoseizures in non-epileptic patients. *Can J Psychiatry* 1982;27:401–404.
20. Hoefnagels WA, Padberg GW, Overweg J, et al. Transient loss of consciousness: the value of the history for distinguishing seizure from syncope. *J Neurol* 1991;238:39–43.
21. Meierkord H, Will B, Fish D, et al. The clinical features and prognosis of pseudoseizures diagnosed using video-EEG telemetry. *Neurology* 1991;41:1643–1646.
22. Peguero E, Abou-Khalil B, Fakhoury T, et al. Self-injury and incontinence in psychogenic seizures. *Epilepsia* 1995;36:586–591.
23. Davis B. Predicting nonepileptic seizures utilizing seizure frequency, EEG, and response to medication. *Eur Neurol* 2004;51:153–156.
24. Benbadis SR, Tatum WO, Vale FL. When drugs don't work: an algorithmic approach to medically intractable epilepsy. *Neurology* 2000;55:1780–1784.
25. Devinski O, Sato S, Kufta CV, et al. EEG studies of simple partial seizures with subdural electrode recordings. *Neurology* 1989;39:527–533.
26. Sperling MR, O'Connor MJ. Auras and subclinical seizures: characteristics and prognostic significance. *Ann Neurol* 1990;28:320–328.
27. Gates JR, Ramani V, Whalen S, et al. Ictal characteristics of pseudoseizures. *Arch Neurol* 1985;42:1183–1187.
28. Gulick TA, Spinks IP, King DW. Pseudoseizures: ictal phenomena. *Neurology* 1982;32:24–30.
29. Bergen D, Ristanovic R. Weeping as a common element of pseudoseizures. *Arch Neurol* 1993;50:1059–1060.
30. Vossler DG, Haltiner AM, Schepp SK, et al. Ictal stuttering: a sign suggestive of psychogenic non-epileptic seizures. *Neurology* 2004;63:516–519.
31. Kanner AM, Morris HH, Lüders H, et al. Supplementary motor seizures mimicking pseudoseizures: some clinical differences. *Neurology* 1990;40:1404–1407.
32. Morris HH 3rd, Dinner DS, Lüders H, et al. Supplementary motor seizures: clinical and EEG findings. *Neurology* 1988;38:1075–1082.
33. Schachter SC, Brown F, Rowan AJ. Provocative testing for nonepileptic seizures: attitudes and practices in the United States among American Epilepsy Society members. *J Epilepsy* 1996;9:249–252.
34. Stagno SJ, Smith ML. Use of induction procedures in diagnosing psychogenic seizures. *J Epilepsy* 1996;9:153–158.
35. Walczak TS, Williams DT, Berten W. Utility and reliability of placebo infusion in the evaluation of patients with seizures. *Neurology* 1994;44:394–399.
36. Cohen RJ, Suter C. Hysterical seizures: suggestion as a provocative EEG test. *Ann Neurol* 1982;11:391–395.
37. Bazil CW, Kothari M, Luciano D, et al. Provocation of nonepileptic seizures by suggestion in a general seizure population. *Epilepsia* 1994;35:768–770.
38. Slater JD, Brown MC, Jacobs W, et al. Induction of pseudoseizures with intravenous saline placebo. *Epilepsia* 1995;36:580–585.
39. Cohen LM, Howard GF 3rd, Bongar B. Provocation of pseudoseizures by psychiatric interview during EEG and video monitoring. *Int J Psychiatry Med* 1992;22:131–140.
40. Luther JS, McNamara JO, Carwile S, et al. Pseudoepileptic seizures: methods and video analysis to aid diagnosis. *Ann Neurol* 1982;12:458–462.
41. Riley TL, Berndt T. The role of the EEG technologist in delineating pseudoseizures. *Am J EEG Technol* 1980;20:89–96.
42. Benbadis SR, Johnson K, Anthony K, et al. Induction of psychogenic nonepileptic seizures without placebo. *Neurology* 2000;55:1904–1905.
43. Fahn S, Williams DT. Psychogenic dystonia. *Adv Neurol* 1988;50:431–455.
44. Lancman ME, Asconape JJ, Craven WJ, et al. Predictive value of induction of psychogenic seizures by suggestion. *Ann Neurol* 1994;35:359–361.
45. Benbadis SR. Provocative techniques should be used for the diagnosis of psychogenic nonepileptic seizures. *Arch Neurol* 2001;58:2063–2065.
46. Gates JR. Provocative testing should not be used for nonepileptic seizures. *Arch Neurol* 2001;58:2065–2066.
47. McGonigal A, Oto M, Russell AJ, et al. Outpatient video EEG recording in the diagnosis of non-epileptic seizures: a randomised controlled trial of simple suggestion techniques. *J Neurol Neurosurg Psychiatry* 2002;72:549–551.
48. Bhatia M, Sinha PK, Jain S, et al. Usefulness of short-term video EEG recording with saline induction in pseudoseizures. *Acta Neurol Scand* 1997;95:363–366.
49. Benbadis SR, Siegrist K, Tatum WO, Heriaud L, Anthony K. Short-term outpatient EEG video with induction in the diagnosis psychogenic seizures. *Neurology* 2004;63:1728–30.
50. Benbadis SR, Agrawal V, Tatum WO 4th. How many patients with psychogenic nonepileptic seizures also have epilepsy? *Neurology* 2001;57:915–917.
51. Lesser RP, Lueders H, Dinner DS. Evidence for epilepsy is rare in patients with psychogenic seizures. *Neurology* 1983;33:502–504.
52. Reuber M, Kral T, Kurthen M, et al. New-onset psychogenic seizures after intracranial neurosurgery. *Acta Neurochir (Wien)* 2002;144:901–907.
53. Hudak A, Agostini MA, Van Ness P, et al. Use of video-EEG monitoring in the differential diagnosis of posttraumatic seizure disorders. *Epilepsia* 2003;44(Suppl 9):5.

54. Davies KG, Blumer DP, Lobo S, et al. De novo nonepileptic seizures after cranial surgery for epilepsy: incidence and risk factors. *Epilepsy Behav* 2000;1:436–443.
55. Glosser G, Roberts D, Glosser DS. Nonepileptic seizures after resective epilepsy surgery. *Epilepsia* 1999;40:1750–1754.
56. Ney GC, Barr WB, Napolitano C, et al. New-onset psychogenic seizures after surgery for epilepsy. *Arch Neurol* 1998;55:726–730.
57. Reuber M, Kurthen M, Fernandez G, et al. Epilepsy surgery in patients with additional psychogenic seizures. *Arch Neurol* 2002;59:82–86.
58. American Psychiatric Association. *Diagnostic and statistical manual of mental disorders: DSM-III-R*, 3rd ed., rev. Washington, DC: Author,1987.
59. American Psychiatric Association. *Diagnostic and statistical manual of mental disorders: DSM-IV*, 4th ed. Washington, DC: Author, 1994.
60. Ford CV. The somatizing disorders. *Psychosomatics* 1986;27: 327–337.
61. Abubakr A, Kablinger A, Caldito G. Psychogenic seizures: clinical features and psychological analysis. *Epilepsy Behav* 2003;4:241–245.
62. Lancman ME, Brotherton TA, Asconape JJ, et al. Psychogenic seizures in adults: a longitudinal analysis. *Seizure* 1993;2:281–286.
63. Reuber M, Pukrop R, Bauer J, et al Outcome in psychogenic nonepileptic seizures: 1 to 10-year follow-up in 164 patients. *Ann Neurol* 2003;53:305–311.
64. Selwa LM, Geyer J, Nikakhtar N, et al. Nonepileptic seizure outcome varies by type of spell and duration of illness. *Epilepsia* 2000;41:1330–1334.
65. Szaflarski JP, Hughes C, Szaflarski M, et al. Quality of life in psychogenic nonepileptic seizures. *Epilepsia* 2003;44:236–242.
66. Gudmundsson O, Prendergast M, Foreman D, et al. Outcome of pseudoseizures in children and adolescents: a 6-year symptom survival analysis. *Dev Med Child Neurol* 2001;43:547–551.
67. Wyllie E, Friedman D, Lüders H, et al. Outcome of psychogenic seizures in children and adolescents compared with adults. *Neurology* 1991;41:742–744.
68. Wyllie E, Glazer JP, Benbadis S, et al. Psychiatric features of children and adolescents with pseudoseizures. *Arch Pediatr Adolesc Med* 1999;153:244–248.
69. Benbadis SR, Stagno SJ, Kosalko J, et al. Psychogenic seizures: a guide for patients and families. *J Neurosci Nurs* 1994;26:306–308.
70. McCahill ME. Somatoform and related disorders: delivery of diagnosis as first step. *Am Fam Physician* 1995;52:193–204.
71. Shen W, Bowman ES, Markand ON. Presenting the diagnosis of pseudoseizure. *Neurology* 1990;40:756–759.
72. American Psychiatric Association. 2001. Available at: http://www.psych.org/public_info/index.cfm, and http://psych.org/public_info/fact_sheets/dpa_fact.cfm. Last accessed July 11, 2005.
73. Benbadis SR, Heriaud L. Psychogenic (non-epileptic) seizures: a guide for patients & families. Available at: http://hsc.usf.edu/com/epilepsy/PNESbrochure.pdf. Last accessed July 11, 2005.
74. Benbadis SR, Blustein JN, Sunstad L. Should patients with psychogenic nonepileptic seizures be allowed to drive? *Epilepsia* 2000;41:895–897.
75. Harden CL, Burgut FT, Kanner AM. The diagnostic significance of video-EEG monitoring findings on pseudoseizure patients differs between neurologists and psychiatrists. *Epilepsia* 2003;44: 453–456.
76. Wyllie E, Benbadis S, Kotagal P. Psychogenic seizures and other nonepileptic paroxysmal events in children. *Epilepsy Behav* 2002; 3:46–50.
77. Rosenow F, Wyllie E, Kotagal P, et al. Staring spells in children: descriptive features distinguishing epileptic and nonepileptic events. *J Pediatr* 1998;133:660–663.
78. Kotagal P, Costa M, Wyllie E, et al. Paroxysmal nonepileptic events in children and adolescents. *Pediatrics* 2002;110:e46.
79. Lempert T, Dieterich M, Huppert D, et al. Psychogenic disorders in neurology: frequency and clinical spectrum. *Acta Neurol Scand* 1990;82:335–340.
80. Keane JR. Hysterical gait disorder: 60 cases. *Neurology* 1989;39: 586–589.
81. Kapfhammer HP, Dobmeier P, Mayer C, et al. Conversion syndromes in neurology. A psychopathological and psychodynamic differentiation of conversion disorder, somatization disorder and factitious disorder [German]. *Psychother Psychosom Med Psychol* 1998;48:463–474.
82. Ziv I, Djaldetti R, Zoldan Y, et al. Diagnosis of "non-organic" limb paresis by a novel objective motor assessment: the quantitative Hoover's test. *J Neurol* 1998;245:797–802.

Other Nonepileptic Paroxysmal Disorders

43

John M. Pellock

A number of conditions cause intermittent and recurring symptoms that suggest epilepsy. Although seizures must be considered in the differential diagnosis, the clinical characteristics sometimes clearly differentiate these disorders and true seizures. These so-called nonepileptic paroxysmal disorders tend to recur episodically. They must not be confused with seizures, because treatment with antiepileptic drugs is usually unnecessary and unsuccessful, drug use may risk the development of adverse effects, and alternative etiologies may be overlooked (1–6).

For the clinician dealing with a paroxysmal disorder, the patient's age and an accurate description of the event, including the time of occurrence (during wakefulness or sleep), can lead to the correct diagnosis (7). Nevertheless, some nonepileptic symptoms can be present in a patient who also has epilepsy, and unusual repetitive movements can be misdiagnosed as seizures when the actual seizures have been controlled by medication. Prensky (7) classified such symptoms as unusual movements, loss of tone or consciousness, respiratory derangements, perceptual disturbances, behavior disorders, and episodic behaviors related to disease states (Table 43.1).

The following overview of nonepileptic paroxysmal disorders is organized by age, type, and time of occurrence. Psychogenic seizures are discussed in Chapter 42.

INFANCY

Sleep

At least two paroxysmal behaviors may be confused with seizures: repetitive episodes of head banging while the infant is falling asleep and benign neonatal myoclonus usually occurring during sleep.

Head Banging (Rhythmic Movement Disorder)

Rhythmic movement disorder, such as repetitive motion of the head, trunk, or extremities, usually occurs as a parasomnia during the transition from wakefulness to sleep or from sustained sleep (8). Head banging can last from 15 to 30 minutes as the infant drifts off to sleep and, unlike similar daytime activity, is usually not related to emotional disturbance, frustration, or anger. No abnormal electroencephalographic (EEG) findings are noted. These benign movements usually disappear within 1 year of onset, typically by the second or third year of life, without treatment (7,8).

Benign Neonatal Myoclonus

Rapid and forceful myoclonic movements may involve one extremity or many parts of the body. Occurring during sleep in early infancy, these bilateral, asynchronous, and asymmetric movements usually migrate from one muscle group to another. Unlike seizures, their rhythmic jerking is not prolonged, although clusters of these movements may occur episodically in all stages of sleep. Attacks are usually only a few minutes long but may last for hours. This myoclonus is not stimulus sensitive, and EEG shows no epileptiform activity. The movements stop as the infant is awakened and should never be seen in a fully awake and alert state. No treatment is required, but clonazepam or other benzodiazepines have been suggested in children who demonstrate a large amount of benign myoclonic activity. The movements typically disappear over several months (9).

Wakefulness

Jitteriness

Neonates and young infants demonstrate this rapid generalized tremulousness, which in neonates may be severe

TABLE 43.1

COMMON SYMPTOMS OF NONEPILEPTIFORM PAROXYSMAL DISORDERS

Unusual movement	Headache
Jitteriness, tremor	Abdominal pain
Masturbation	Episodic features of specific disorders
Shuddering	Tetralogy spells
Benign sleep myoclonus	Hydrocephalic spells
Startle responses	Cardiac arrhythmias
Paroxysmal torticollis	Hypoglycemia
Self-stimulation	Hypocalcemia
Head banging (rhythmic movement	Periodic paralysis
disorder)	Hyperthyroidism
Tics (Tourette syndrome)	Gastroesophageal reflux
Paroxysmal dyskinesias	Rumination
Pseudoseizures	Drug poisoning
Eye movement	Cerebrovascular events
Head nodding	Behavior disorders
Loss of tone or consciousness	Night terrors
Syncope	Sleepwalking
Drop attacks	Nightmares
Narcolepsy/cataplexy	Rage
Attention deficit	Confusion
Acute hemiplegia	Fear
Respiratory derangements	Acute psychotic symptoms
Apnea	Fugue
Breath holding	Phobia
Hyperventilation	Panic attacks
Perceptual disturbances	Hallucinations
Dizziness	Autism
Vertigo	Munchausen by proxy

enough to be mistaken for clonic seizures. The infants are alert, and the movements may be decreased by passive flexion or repositioning of the extremities. Although jitteriness may occur spontaneously, it is typically provoked or increased by stimulation. Because neonatal jitteriness may be caused by certain pathologic states, jittery newborns are more likely than normal infants to experience seizures, and their EEG tracings may show abnormalities. Central nervous system dysfunction is the suspected etiology, but hypoxic-ischemic insults, metabolic encephalopathies such as hypoglycemia and hypocalcemia, drug intoxication or withdrawal, and intracranial hemorrhage are implicated. The more benign forms of jitteriness usually decrease without specific therapy. Prognosis depends on the etiology and in neonates with severe, prolonged jitteriness may be guarded. Nevertheless, in 38 full-term infants who were jittery after 6 weeks of age, the movements resolved at a mean age of 7.2 months; 92% had normal findings on neurodevelopmental examinations at age 3 years (10). Sedative agents may be used, but their adverse effects usually increase the irritability (10,11).

Head Banging or Rolling and Body Rocking

Head banging, head rolling, and body rocking often occur in awake infants (7). In older infants, head banging may be part of a temper tantrum. Head rolling and body rocking seemingly are pleasurable forms of self-stimulation and may be related to masturbation. If the infants are touched or their attention is diverted, the repetitive movements cease. They are more common in irritable, excessively active, mentally retarded infants (7). Nevertheless, most of this activity decreases during the second year. Particularly bothersome movements may be diminished by behavior-modification techniques, but drug treatment usually is unnecessary.

Masturbation

Infantile masturbation may mimic abdominal pain or seizures in infant girls, who may sit with their legs held tightly together or straddle the bars of the crib or playpen and rock back and forth. Distracting stimuli usually stop these movements, which disappear in several months. Masturbation in older children is less likely to be confused with seizure activity. In some mentally retarded children, however, self-stimulation can also be associated with a fugue state. Because these children are difficult to arouse during the activity, seizures are commonly suspected (12).

Benign Myoclonus of Early Infancy

Myoclonic movements occur in awake children and may resemble infantile spasms but are not associated with EEG abnormalities. Infants are usually healthy, with no evidence of neurologic deterioration. The myoclonic episodes abate without treatment after a few months (13).

Spasmodic Torticollis

Spasmodic torticollis is a disorder characterized by sudden, repetitive episodes of head tilting or turning to one side with rotation of the face to the opposite side. The episodes may last from minutes to days, during which children are irritable and uncomfortable but alert and responsive. Although behavior may be episodic while the attack continues, EEG findings remain normal. Nystagmus is not associated with this disorder. The etiology is unknown, although dystonia and labyrinthine imbalance have been proposed. A family history of torticollis or migraine may be present. Tonic or rotary movements also may be seen with gastroesophageal reflux (Sandifer syndrome), but they will be longer and less paroxysmal than torticollis without reflux (14–17).

The differential diagnosis includes congenital, inflammatory, and neoplastic conditions of the posterior fossa, cervical cord, spine, and neck in which the episodes of torticollis are sustained, lacking the usual on-and-off variability. An evaluation is necessary, but spasmodic torticollis usually subsides without treatment during the first few years of life.

Spasmus Nutans

Head nodding, head tilt, and nystagmus comprise spasmus nutans. Head nodding or intermittent nystagmus (or both) is usually noted at 4 to 12 months of age; nystagmus may be more prominent in one eye. The symptoms can vary depending on position, direction of gaze, and time of day. The children are clinically alert, and although symptoms may fluctuate throughout the day, episodic alterations in level of consciousness do not occur. Spasmus nutans usually remits spontaneously within 1 or 2 years after onset but may last as long as 8 years. Minor EEG abnormalities may be noted, but classic epileptiform paroxysms are not associated. Because mass lesions of the optic chiasm or third ventricle have been noted in a small number of these infants, computed tomography or magnetic resonance imaging studies generally should be performed (18). It is difficult to distinguish eye movements persisting into later childhood or adulthood from congenital nystagmus (18–20).

Opsoclonus

Opsoclonus is a rare abnormality characterized by rapid, conjugate, multidirectional, oscillating eye movements that are usually continuous but may vary in intensity. Because of this variation and occasionally associated myoclonic movements, generalized or partial seizures may be suspected. The children remain responsive and alert. Opsoclonus usually implies a neurologic disorder such as ataxia myoclonus or myoclonus. Children who develop these signs early in life may have a paraneoplastic syndrome caused by an underlying neuroblastoma (21–23). This triad of opsoclonus, myoclonus, and encephalopathy is termed Kinsbourne encephalopathy (dancing eyes, dancing feet) and responds to removal of the neural crest tumor or treatment with corticosteroids or corticotropin (24).

Rumination

Rumination attacks involve hyperextension of the neck, repetitive swallowing, and protrusion of the tongue and are secondary to an abnormality of esophageal peristalsis. Episodes typically follow or accompany feeding. The child is alert but sometimes seems under stress and uncomfortable. Variable feeding techniques are helpful in this disorder, which resolves as the child matures (25).

Startle Disease or Hyperexplexia

A rare familial disorder with major and minor forms, startle disease (or hyperexplexia) involves a seemingly hyperactive startle reflex, sometimes so exaggerated that it causes falling. In the major form, the infant becomes stiff when handled, and episodes of severe hypertonia cause apnea and bradycardia. Forced flexion of the neck or hips may interrupt these episodes. Also noted, along with transient hypertonia, are falling attacks without loss of consciousness, ataxia, generalized hyperreflexia, episodic shaking of the limbs resembling clonus, and excessive startle. The minor form, in which startle responses are less consistent and not associated with other findings, may represent an augmented normal startle reflex (26). The interictal electroencephalogram shows normal results, but a spike may be associated with a startle attack. Whether this discharge represents an evoked response to the stimulus or an artifact is a subject of debate. The disorder must be distinguished from so-called startle epilepsy, in which a startle is followed by a partial or generalized seizure, which suggests a defect in inhibitory regulation of brainstem centers (27,28). The prognosis in hyperexplexia is variable (26). Seizures do not develop after this benign disorder; however, clonazepam and valproic acid have been used to treat its associated startle, stiffness, jerking, and falling (29,30).

Shuddering Attacks

Shuddering attacks far exceed the normal shivering seen in most older infants and children. A very rapid tremor involves the head, arms, trunk, and even the legs; the upper extremities are adducted and flexed at the elbows or, less often, adducted and extended. The episodes may begin as early as 4 months of age, decreasing gradually in frequency and intensity before age 10 years. Treatment with antiepileptic drugs does not modify the attacks. Except for the artifact, results of electroencephalography are normal. Essential tremor may be more common in the families of children with shuddering spells than in unaffected families (31,32).

Alternating Hemiplegia

Alternating hemiplegia of childhood may be confused with epilepsy because of the paroxysmal episodes of weakness, hypertonicity, or dystonia. Presenting as tonic or dystonic events, these intermittent attacks may alternate from side to side and at times progress to quadriplegia. They usually occur at least monthly and may be part of a larger neurologic syndrome in children with delayed or retarded development who also have seizures, ataxia, and choreoathetosis. Attacks begin before 18 months of age and can be precipitated by emotional factors or fatigue. The hemiplegic episodes may last minutes or hours, and the etiology and mechanism are unknown. Although anticonvulsants and typical migraine treatments are unsuccessful, flunarizine, a calcium-channel blocker (5 mg/kg per day), has been reported to reduce recurrences (33,34).

Respiratory Derangements and Syncope

Primary breathing disorders usually occur without associated epilepsy. At times, however, respiratory symptoms may be confused with epilepsy, or, rarely, tonic stiffening, clonic jerks or seizures may follow primary apnea (35). An electroencephalogram or polysomnogram recorded during the event may easily distinguish a respiratory abnormality associated with true seizures from one completely independent of epilepsy.

Infant Apnea or Apparent Life-Threatening Events

Apnea usually occurs during sleep and may be associated with centrally mediated hypoventilation, airway obstruction, aspiration, or congenital hypoventilation. Formerly called (near) sudden infant death syndrome, these symptoms now are referred to as *apparent life-threatening events*. In central apnea, chest and abdominal movements decrease simultaneously with a drop in air flow. In obstructive apnea, movements of the chest or abdomen (or both) continue, but there is diminished air flow. Central apnea presumably results from a disturbance of the respiratory centers, whereas obstructive apnea is a peripheral event; some infants have a mixed form of the disorder. A few jerks may occur with the apneic episodes but do not represent epileptic myoclonus. The apnea that follows a seizure is a form of central apnea with postictal hypoventilation. Primary apnea, however, is only rarely followed by seizures (36,37).

The etiology and characteristics vary among infants. Apnea of prematurity responds to treatment with xanthine derivatives. In older infants with primary central apnea, elevated cerebrospinal fluid levels of β-endorphin have been reported, and treatment with the opioid antagonist naltrexone has been successful (38). The role of home cardiopulmonary monitors is controversial. Parents should be encouraged to follow the recommendations of the American Academy of Pediatrics that healthy term infants be put to sleep on their back or side to decrease the risk of apnea and possible sudden infant death syndrome (39).

Although apnea occurs less often when the child is fully awake, it may be associated with gastroesophageal reflux (40,41). Aspiration may follow. Reflux is frequently accompanied by staring or flailing or posturing of the trunk or extremities, perhaps in response to the pain of acidic contents washing back into the esophagus. Gastroesophageal reflux is more common when infants are laid supine after feeding. Diagnosis is established by radiologic demonstration of reflux or by abnormal esophageal pH levels. Reflux is treated by upright positioning of the baby during and after feeding (42), thickened feedings, the use of agents to alter sphincter tone, and fundal plication.

Cyanotic Breath-Holding Spells

Although common between the ages of 6 months and 6 years, cyanotic infant syncope (breath-holding spells) is frequently confused with tonic seizures (43). Typically precipitated by fear, frustration, or minor injury, the spells involve vigorous crying, following which the child stops breathing, often in expiration. Cyanosis occurs within several seconds, followed by loss of consciousness, limpness, and falling. Prolonged hypoxia may cause tonic stiffening or brief clonic jerking of the body. After 1 or 2 minutes of unresponsiveness, consciousness returns quickly, although the infant may be briefly tired or irritable. The crucial diagnostic point is the history of an external event, however minor, precipitating the episode. The electroencephalogram does not show interictal epileptiform discharges but may reveal slowing or suppression during the anoxic event (see Chapter 13, Figs. 13.52 and 13.53). The pathophysiologic mechanism is not well understood, but correction of any underlying anemia may reduce the attacks (44). Children with pallid breath-holding spells have autonomic dysregulation caused by parasympathetic disturbance distinct from that found in cyanotic breath-holding (45). Although the episodes appear unpleasant for the child, they do not result in neurologic damage. Antiepileptic medication may be appropriate for the rare patients with frequent postsyncopal generalized tonic-clonic seizures triggered by the anoxia.

Pallid Syncope

Precipitated by injury or fright, sometimes trivial, pallid infant syncope occurs in response to transient cardiac asystole in infants with a hypersensitive cardioinhibitory reflex. Minimal crying, perhaps only a gasp, and no obvious apnea precede loss of consciousness. The child collapses limply and subsequently may have posturing or clonic movements before regaining consciousness after a few minutes (43, 46–48). The asystolic episodes can be produced by ocular compression, but this procedure is risky and of uncertain clinical utility (see Chapter 13, Figs. 13.52 and 13.53). As with cyanotic breath-holding spells, the key to diagnosis is the association with precipitating events.

The long-term prognosis is benign. Most children require no treatment, although atropine has been recommended for frequent pallid attacks or those followed by generalized tonic-clonic seizures (49). A trial of the anticholinergic drug atropine sulfate 0.01 mg/kg every 24 hours in divided doses (maximum 0.4 mg per day) may increase heart rate by blocking vagal input. Atropine should not be prescribed during very hot weather because hyperpyrexia may occur.

CHILDREN

Sleep

Myoclonus

Nocturnal myoclonic movements, called "sleep starts" or "hypnic jerks" and associated with a sensation of falling, are less common in older children and adolescents than in infants (9). The subtle involuntary jerks of the extremities or the entire body occur while the child is falling asleep or being aroused. Repetitive rhythmic jerking is uncommon, although several series of jerks can occur during the night. The jerks are not associated with epileptiform activity, but a sensory evoked response or evidence of arousal may be present on the electroencephalogram (50–53).

Periodic repetitive movements that resemble myoclonus are seen in deeper stages of sleep and may arouse the patient so that daytime drowsiness is noted. These movements are more common in rapid eye movement (REM) than in nonrapid eye movement (NREM) sleep, and are clearly distinguished from epilepsy on sleep polysomnographic recordings.

Hypnagogic Paroxysmal Dystonia

In hypnagogic paroxysmal dystonia, an extremely rare disorder, sleep may be briefly interrupted by seemingly severe dystonic movements of the limbs lasting a few minutes and accompanied by crying out. No EEG abnormality is noted. Carbamazepine may decrease the attacks. It is not clear whether some or all patients with this clinical syndrome actually have seizures arising from the supplementary motor area (51,54).

Nightmares

Nightmares occur during REM sleep and are rarely confused with seizures. Although children may be restless during the dream, they usually do not scream out, sit up, or have the marked motor symptoms, autonomic activity, and extreme sorrow seen with night terrors. Incontinence may be present, however. Remembrance of the content of nightmares may lead to a fear of sleeping alone. An electroencephalogram recorded during these events shows no abnormalities (7).

Night Terrors (Pavor Nocturnus)

Night terrors, most common in children between the ages of 5 and 12 years, begin from 30 minutes to several hours after sleep onset, usually in stage III or IV of slow-wave sleep. Diaphoretic and with dilated pupils, the children sit up in bed, crying or screaming inconsolably for several minutes before calming down. Sleep resumes after the attack, and the event is not recalled. No treatment is recommended (55,56).

Sleepwalking

Approximately 15% of all children experience at least one episode of sleepwalking or somnambulism, which usually occurs 1 to 3 hours after sleep onset (stages III and IV). The etiology is unknown, but a familial prevalence is noted. Mumbling and sleep-talking, the child walks about in a trance and returns to bed. Semipurposeful activity such as dressing, opening doors, eating, and touching objects during an episode of somnambulism may be confused with the automatisms of complex partial seizures. The eyes are open, and the child rarely walks into objects. Amnesia follows, and no violence occurs during the event. Treatment usually is not required, except for protecting the wandering child during the night. Benzodiazepine therapy may be helpful in frequent or prolonged attacks (3,57,58).

Wakefulness

Myoclonus

In many normal, awake children, anxiety or exercise may cause an occasional isolated myoclonic jerk. Treatment is rarely necessary.

Multifocal myoclonus may occur in patients with progressive degenerative diseases or during an acute encephalopathy. It may be difficult to distinguish these movements from chorea, and these two disorders may coexist with some encephalopathic illnesses. Myoclonus persists in sleep, whereas chorea usually disappears during sleep (7).

Chorea

Usually seen as rapid jerks of the distal portions of the extremities, choreiform movements may affect muscles of the face, tongue, and proximal portions of the extremities. When associated with athetosis, chorea involves slower, more writhing movements of distal portions of the extremities. The jerks may be so fluid or continuous that they are camouflaged. Acute chorea may accompany metabolic disorders but is more likely in patients recovering from illnesses such as encephalitis. Other causes are Sydenham chorea seen with β-hemolytic streptococcal infection, drug ingestion, and mass lesions or stroke involving the basal ganglia. Treatment depends primarily on the etiology, but movements may respond to haloperidol or a benzodiazepine such as clonazepam (59,60).

Tics

Like chorea, most tics are present during wakefulness and disappear with sleep. They usually involve one or more muscle groups, are stereotypic and repetitive, and appear suddenly and intermittently. Movements may be simple or complex, rhythmic or irregular. Facial twitches, head shaking, eye blinking, sniffling, throat clearing, and shoulder shrugging are typical, although more complex facial distortions, arm swaying, and jumping have been noted. These purposeless movements cannot be completely controlled, but they may be inhibited voluntarily for brief periods and are frequently exacerbated by stress or startle (61–63).

In Tourette syndrome, complex vocal and motor tics are frequently associated with learning disabilities, hyperactivity, attention deficits, and compulsive behaviors. The incidence of simple and complex tics is high in relatives of these patients. The disorder varies in severity but tends to be lifelong, although it may stabilize or improve slightly in adolescence or early adulthood. Combinations of behavior therapy and medical treatment of tics and compulsive behavior are indicated. Haloperidol, pimozide, and clonidine have been used successfully for behavior control. Stimulants such as methylphenidate may initially exacerbate tics (61–63).

Paroxysmal Dyskinesias

Paroxysmal dyskinesias are rare disorders characterized by repetitive episodes of relatively severe dystonia or choreoathetosis (or both). Multiple brief attacks occur daily, precipitated by startle, stress, movement, or arousal from sleep (64). Consciousness is preserved, but discomfort is evident. Both sporadic and familial types have been described. Kinesigenic dyskinesia frequently is associated with the onset of movement as well as with prior hypoxic injury, hypoglycemia, and thyrotoxicosis. Alcohol, caffeine, excitement, stress, and fatigue may exacerbate attacks of paroxysmal dystonic choreoathetosis, a familial form of the disorder. Although the electroencephalogram displays normal findings during the episodes, the paroxysmal dystonic form responds to antiepileptic drugs such as carbamazepine (64–67).

Stereotypic Movements

Other repetitive movements have been mistaken for seizures, especially in neurologically impaired children. Donat and Wright (68) noted head shaking and nodding, lateral and vertical nystagmus, staring, tongue thrusting, chewing movements, periodic hyperventilation, tonic postures, tics, and excessive startle reactions in these patients, many of whom had been treated unnecessarily for epilepsy. Self-stimulatory behaviors such as rhythmic hand shaking, body rocking, and head swaying, performed during apparent unawareness of surroundings, also are common in mentally retarded children without representing or being associated with seizures. Rett syndrome should be suspected when repetitive "hand-washing" movements are noted in retarded girls (69). Deaf or blind children frequently resort to self-stimulation such as hitting their ears or poking at their eyes or ears, which has been misidentified as epilepsy. Behavior training is frequently more successful than medication in controlling these movements (68).

Head Nodding

Head nodding or head drops may be of epileptic or nonepileptic origin. A study by Brunquell and colleagues (70) showed that epileptic head drops were associated with ictal changes in facial expression and subtle myoclonic extremity movements. Rapid drops followed by slow recovery indicated seizures. When the recovery and drop phases were of similar velocity or when repetitive head bobbing occurred, nonepileptic conditions were much more common.

Staring Spells

When ordinary daydreaming or inattentive periods are repetitive and children do not respond to being called, the behaviors may be classified as absence (petit mal) attacks. During innocent daydreaming, posture is maintained and automatisms do not occur. Staring spells are usually nonepileptic in normal children with normal EEG findings, when parents report preserved responsiveness to touch, body rocking, or identification without limb twitches, upward eye movements, interrupted play, or urinary incontinence (71). Children with attention deficit hyperactivity disorder sometimes have staring spells that resemble absence or complex partial seizures. Although unresponsive to verbal stimuli, these children generally become alert immediately on being touched and frequently recall what was said during the staring spell. During these spells, the electroencephalogram pattern is normal. Attention deficit hyperactivity disorder affects 3% to 10% of children and has a male predominance. Stimulants are most widely used, but other medications may be necessary to ameliorate behavior in refractory cases. Antiepileptic drugs usually are ineffective (51,72–75).

Headaches

Recurrent headaches are rarely the sole manifestation of seizures; however, postictal headaches are not uncommon, especially following a generalized convulsion. Headaches also may precede seizures. As an isolated ictal symptom, headache occurs most frequently in children with complex partial seizures (76). Children with ictal headaches experience sudden diffuse pain, often have a history of cerebral injury, derive no relief from sleep, and lack a family history of migraine. Distinguishing headache from paroxysmal recurrent migraine may be difficult in young children when the headache's throbbing unilateral nature is absent or not readily apparent. Migraine, however, is more prevalent than epilepsy. In addition, ictal electroencephalograms during migraine usually show slowing, whereas those during epilepsy demonstrate a clear paroxysmal change. Associated gastrointestinal disturbance and a strong family history of migraine help establish the appropriate diagnosis (76–82).

Epilepsy and migraine can coexist. Children with migraine have a 3% to 7% incidence of epilepsy, and as many as 20% exhibit paroxysmal discharges on interictal electroencephalograms (79). Up to 60% of children with migraine obtain significant relief with antiepileptic medication (81,82). Other variants of migraine that may be confused with seizures include cyclic vomiting (abdominal pain), acute confusional states, and benign paroxysmal vertigo.

Recurrent Abdominal Pain

Recurrent abdominal pain may be associated with vomiting, pallor, or even fever and has been noted in migraine and epilepsy. Usually, these complaints indicate neither diagnosis, although some children with recurrent abdominal pain or vomiting may experience migraine later in life (7,83). From 7% to 76% of children with recurrent abdominal pain exhibit interictal paroxysmal EEG changes. Approximately 15% of these patients have a diagnosis of seizures, and more than 40% have recurrent headaches (7). A family history of migraine is found in approximately 20% (81). Although most of these children do not respond to antiepileptic drugs, approximately 20% obtain relief from antimigraine medications such as beta-blockers or tricyclic antidepressants (7,79,83).

Confusional Migraine

Migraine may present in an unusual and sometimes bizarre fashion as confusion, hyperactivity, partial or total amnesia, disorientation, impaired responsiveness, lethargy, and vomiting (84). These episodes must be distinguished from toxic or metabolic encephalopathy, encephalitis, acute psychosis, head trauma, and sepsis as well as from an ictal or postictal confusional state. Confusional migraine usually persists for several hours, less commonly for days, and spontaneously clears following sleep. The diagnosis is usually made following the episode when the patient or family reports severe headache or visual symptoms heralding the onset of the event or a history of similar events. During and soon after the episodes, an electroencephalogram may demonstrate regional slowing, a nondiagnostic finding.

Benign Paroxysmal Vertigo

Benign paroxysmal vertigo consists of brief recurrent episodes of disequilibrium of variable duration that may be misinterpreted as seizures. Lasting from minutes to hours, the attacks of vertigo occur as often as two to three times per week but rarely as infrequently as every 2 to 3 months. Tinnitus, hearing loss, and brainstem signs have been implicated as causes, but the onset is sudden, and the child usually is unable to walk. Extreme distress and nausea are noted, but the child remains alert and responsive during attacks. Nystagmus or torticollis is frequently observed, but between attacks, examination and electroencephalography reveal normal results. A minority of children show dysfunction on vestibular testing, but no abnormalities show on audiograms. A family history of migraine is common, and most of these children experience migraines later in life. No treatment is indicated because the attacks do not respond well to either antiepileptic or antimigraine medications. Benign paroxysmal vertigo usually subsides by ages 6 to 8 years (51,85,86).

Stool-Withholding Activity and Constipation

Children may have sudden interruption of activity and assume a motionless posture with slight truncal flexion when experiencing discomfort from withholding stool (87). The withholding behavior, which may be mistaken for absence or tonic seizures, evolves as a way to prevent the painful passage of stool that is large and hard because of chronic constipation. Small jerks of the limbs may be misperceived as myoclonus, and the child may have fecal incontinence. The behavior resolves with treatment of the chronic constipation.

Rage Attacks

The episodic dyscontrol syndrome, or recurrent attacks of rage following minimal provocation, may be seen in children with or without epilepsy. The behavior often seems completely out of character. Rage may be more common in hyperactive children or those with conduct and personality disorders. Similar dyscontrol and near rage have been seen following head injury with frontal or temporal lobe lesions. Ictal rage is rare, unprovoked, and usually not directed toward an individual. Following attacks of rage and the appearance of near psychosis, the child resumes a normal state and may recall the episode and feel remorseful. Behavior frequently can be modified during the event. Depending on the cause of the associated syndrome, beta-blockers (88), stimulant drugs, and carbamazepine along with other antiepilepsy drugs have been used to control outbursts (89).

Munchausen Syndrome by Proxy

Munchausen syndrome, or factitious disorder, describes a consistent simulation of illness leading to unnecessary investigations and treatments. When a parent or caregiver pursues such a deception using a child, the situation is called Munchausen syndrome by proxy. Infants may be brought to child neurologists with parental reports suggesting apnea, seizures, or cyanosis; older children may be described to have episodes of loss of consciousness, convulsions, ataxia, headache, hyperactivity, chorea, weakness, gait difficulties, or paralysis. Accompanying symptoms may include gastrointestinal disorders or a history of unusual accidents and injuries that are poorly explained and almost never observed by anyone but the parent(s) (Table 43.2). Sometimes the child also becomes persuaded of the reality of the "illness" and develops independent factitious symptoms such as psychogenic seizures.

The perpetrator is often the mother, who appears initially to be a model parent but has a pathologic need for

TABLE 43.2
CLINICAL FEATURES OF MUNCHAUSEN SYNDROME BY PROXY

Persistent and recurrent unexplained illness
Clinical signs at variance with the child's health status
Unusual or remarkable signs or symptoms
Signs and symptoms not recurring in parent's absence
Mother or caregiver overattentive or refuses to leave the hospital
Mother or caregiver not appropriately concerned about prognosis
Lack of anticipated response of clinical syndrome
"Rare" clinical syndrome

TABLE 43.3
CAUSES OF SYNCOPE

Vasovagal	Fear
	Pain
	Unpleasant sights
Reflex	Cough
	Micturition
	Swallowing
	Carotid sinus pressure
Decreased venous return	Orthostatic
	Soldier syncope (standing at attention)
	With Valsalva maneuver
Decreased blood volume	
No clear precipitating event	
Cardiac	Arrhythmia
	Obstructive outflow
Cerebrovascular insufficiency	
Familial	
Undetermined cause	

From Prensky AL. Migraine and migrainous variant in pediatric patients. *Pediatr Clin North Am* 1976;23:461–471, with permission.

the child to be sick (90–92). Usually young, articulate, and middle class, she has an unnatural attachment to her child, coexisting personality disorder, and somatizing behavior. The mother often has some medical training, for example, as a nurse. Families are usually dysfunctional. The parent's exaggerated and constant need for illness and medical intervention may lead to the child's death.

Treatment is similar to that of child abuse and typically involves a pediatrician, child psychiatrist, nurse, and social workers. The child is separated from the parents, and details of the history are corroborated. Medical and neurologic evaluations rule out specific disease processes. Admission of a child with paroxysmal symptoms to an epilepsy monitoring unit may help to demonstrate this behavior in both mother and child (93).

Future serious psychologic disturbances are a significant possibility. Good relationships with the nonabusive father, successful short-term foster parenting before return to the mother or long-term placement with the same foster parents, long-term treatment or successful remarriage of the mother, and early adoption are associated with more favorable outcome for the child (94).

LATE CHILDHOOD, ADOLESCENCE, AND ADULTHOOD

Wakefulness

Syncope

Syncope is common in adolescents or older children and usually can be distinguished from seizures by description. Warning signs of lightheadedness, dizziness, and visual dimming ("graying out" or "browning out") occur in most patients. Nausea is common before or after the event, and a feeling of heat or cold and profuse sweating are frequent accompaniments. A particular stimulus such as the sight of blood with vasovagal syncope, minor trauma, or being in a warm, crowded place often elicits the attack. Orthostatic syncope may follow prolonged standing or sudden change in posture. The family history may disclose similar events (95). Reflex syncope may be seen with coughing, swallowing, or micturition (96). Table 43.3 lists frequent causes of

syncope. A few clonic jerks or incontinence occurring late in syncope complicates the picture, but a full history usually elucidates the cause (80).

Physical examination frequently yields normal results, although supine and standing blood pressure measurements may implicate or rule out an orthostatic cause. A reduction in blood pressure of more than 15 points or sinus bradycardia (or both) on rapid standing is highly suggestive of orthostatic hypotension. A search for arrhythmia and murmur is warranted, as cardiac causes of syncope are primarily obstructive lesions or arrhythmias not otherwise clinically evident (96,97). Syncope associated with ophthalmoplegia, retinitis, deafness, ataxia, or seeming myopathy mandates an urgent evaluation for heart block (Kearns-Sayre syndrome) (98).

Electrocardiographic monitoring and echocardiography are frequently more valuable than electroencephalography in establishing the diagnosis. Tilt-table testing may be helpful in this regard (99,100).

Narcolepsy and Cataplexy

Narcolepsy is a state of excessive daytime drowsiness causing rapid brief sleep, sometimes during conversation or play; the patient usually awakens refreshed. Narcolepsy also includes sleep paralysis (transient episodes of inability to move on awakening) and brief hallucinations on arousal along with cataplexy, although not all patients demonstrate the complete syndrome. Measurement of sleep latency through electroencephalogram recordings reveals the appearance of REM sleep within 10 minutes in narcoleptic patients. Narcolepsy may be treated with a stimulant drug (101–103).

Cataplexy produces a sudden loss of tone with a drop to the ground in response to an unexpected touch or emotional stimulus such as laughter. Consciousness is not lost during these brief attacks. Coexistent narcolepsy is common.

Basilar Migraine

Most common in adolescent girls, basilar migraine begins with a sudden loss of consciousness followed by severe occipital or vertex headache. Dizziness, vertigo, bilateral visual loss, and, less often, diplopia, dysarthria, and bilateral paresthesias may occur. A history of headache or a family history of migraine is helpful in making the diagnosis. Of note, interictal paroxysmal EEG discharges are not uncommon in this population. Children may respond to classic migraine therapy or antiepileptic drugs (104,105). Ergot alkaloids and triptans are generally not recommended (77).

Tremor

An involuntary movement characterized by rhythmic oscillations of a particular part of the body, tremor may appear at rest or with only certain movements. Consequently, it is occasionally mistaken for seizure activity, particularly when the movement is severe and proximal such as in the "wing-beating tremor" of Wilson disease or related basal ganglia disorders. Tremors disappear during sleep. Examination at rest and during activities, possibly by manipulating the affected body part while observing the tremor, usually can define the movement by varying or obliterating the tremor. The electroencephalogram is unchanged as the tremor escalates and diminishes (106).

Panic Disorders

Panic attacks may occur as acute events associated with a chronic anxiety disorder or in patients suffering from depression or schizophrenia. These attacks last for minutes to hours and are accompanied by palpitations, sweating, dizziness or vertigo, and feelings of unreality. The following symptoms also have been noted: dyspnea or smothering sensations, unsteadiness or faintness, palpitations or tachycardia, trembling or shaking, choking, nausea or abdominal distress, depersonalization or derealization, numbness or tingling, flushes or chills, chest pain or discomfort, and fears of dying, aura, going crazy, or losing control. An electroencephalogram recorded at the time of the attacks differentiates ictal fear and nonepileptic panic attacks (107).

Panic disorders involve spontaneous panic attacks and may be associated with agoraphobia. Although they may begin in adolescence, the average age at onset is in the late twenties. Psychiatric therapy is indicated (108).

Acute fugue, phobias, hallucinations, and autistic behaviors may seem to represent seizures; however, associated features and EEG findings usually distinguish these behavioral disorders from epilepsy.

DISEASE-RELATED BEHAVIORS

Several disease states include recurrent symptoms that are misdiagnosed as epilepsy. Episodes of cyanosis, dyspnea, and unconsciousness followed by a convulsion may occur in as many as 10% to 20% of children with congenital heart disease, particularly those with significant hypoxemia. In "tet" spells, young children with tetralogy of Fallot squat nearly motionless during exercise as their cardiac reserve recovers (109).

Children and adults with shunted hydrocephalus may have seizures, although these are not usual (110). Obstruction associated with the third ventricle or aqueduct may cause the bobble-head doll syndrome (two to four head oscillations per second) in mentally retarded children (111). In hydrocephalic patients treated by ventricular shunting, acute decompensation may increase seizure frequency or give rise to symptoms misdiagnosed as seizures. So-called hydrocephalic attacks, characterized by tonic, opisthotonic postures frequently associated with a generalized tremor, are caused by increased intracranial pressure and herniation. Head tilt or dystonia also may indicate increased intracranial pressure, a posterior fossa mass, or Arnold-Chiari malformation. Urgent evaluation for malfunctioning shunt or increased intracranial pressure is warranted with any of these symptoms.

The episodic nature of periodic paralysis may lead to misidentification of the symptoms as epilepsy. Familial and sporadic cases typically are associated with disorders of sodium and potassium metabolism. Acetazolamide is useful in some forms of the disorder (112).

Cerebrovascular disorders of various types and etiologies may have transient recurrent symptoms and thus are confused with epilepsy. The exact clinical presentation of cerebrovascular disorders in both children and adults depends primarily on the size and location of the brain lesion and on the etiology of the vascular compromise (113,114). Transient ischemic attacks, episodes of ischemic neurologic deficits lasting less than 24 hours, are typically caused by small emboli or local hemodynamic factors that temporarily prevent adequate brain perfusion. Symptoms begin suddenly following an embolus, with the deficit reaching maximum severity almost immediately. Function returns several minutes or hours after the onset of symptoms. Symptomatology is characteristically separated into carotid artery syndromes with symptoms of middle cerebral artery, anterior cerebral, and lacunar deficits. The latter are most common in adults with longstanding hypertension and may be characterized by pure motor hemiparesis or monoparesis and isolated hemianesthesia. Vertebrobasilar syndromes, especially transient ischemic attacks, may be mistaken for epilepsy because of recurrence and duration and may present with ataxia, dysarthria, nausea, vomiting, vertigo, and even coma. Homonymous hemianopsia may result from posterior cerebral artery occlusion. The subclavian steal syndrome is associated with stenosis or occlusion of the subclavian artery proximal to the origin of the vertebral artery. Retrograde flow through the vertebral artery into the poststenotic subclavian artery may occur. Vertigo, ataxia, syncope, and visual disturbance occur intermittently when blood is diverted into the distal subclavian artery. Vigorous exercise of the arms tends to produce symptoms. The brachial and radial pulses in the affected extremity are absent or diminished.

The etiology of cerebral embolism includes cardiopulmonary disorders, traumatic injuries to blood vessels like dissection, and congenital or inflammatory arterial disorders. Besides blood products, air emboli, foreign-body embolism with pellets, needles, or talcum, or fat emboli may be noted. In adults, carotid and vertebrobasilar occlusion with or without embolization is typically associated with systemic cerebrovascular disease. In younger black patients, sickle cell disease always must be considered as an etiology of cerebrovascular symptoms. It is sometimes difficult to distinguish between transient ischemic attacks and brief seizures in these patients who have multiple areas of infarction. Because strokes may occur on the basis of both large- and small-vessel abnormalities associated with sickle cell disease, symptoms may vary.

Transient global amnesia deserves special mention as a symptom that may or may not be related to epilepsy. Multiple authors argue that it is either of vascular origin or related to seizures. Recurrent attacks may occur in up to 25% of cases. Attacks, however, last hours rather than minutes, and the most frequently observed EEG changes are small sharp spikes of questionable significance (115).

CONCLUSIONS

A variety of paroxysmal happenings may be confused with epilepsy. A careful medical history with description of events before, during, and after the spell, age of onset, time of occurrence, and clinical course aided by a through physical examination frequently clarify the nature of these episodes. Home video recordings of the episodes may be extremely helpful. The routine or specialized use of electroencephalography or polysomnography provides further characterization. Dual diagnoses are possible. Abnormal findings on neurologic examination are not uncommon in patients with these nonepileptic events. Previously noted interictal EEG abnormalities should be reviewed to modify the interpretation of false-positive records (116).

REFERENCES

1. Chutorian AM. Paroxysmal disorders of childhood. In: Rudolph AM, ed. *Rudolph's pediatrics*, 10th ed. Norwalk, CT: Appleton & Lange, 1991:1785–1792.
2. Gomez MR, Klass DW. Seizures and other paroxysmal disorders in infants and children. *Curr Probl Pediatr* 1972;2:2–37.
3. Pedley TA. Differential diagnosis of episodic symptoms. *Epilepsia* 1983;24(Suppl 1):S31–S44.
4. Rabe EF. Recurrent paroxysmal nonepileptic disorders. *Curr Probl Pediatr* 1974;4:3–31.
5. Rothner AD. "Not everything that shakes is epilepsy." *Cleve Clin J Med* 1989;56(Suppl 2):206–213.
6. So NK, Andermann F. Differential diagnosis. In: Engel J, Pedley TA, eds. *Differential diagnosis in epilepsy: a comprehensive textbook*. Philadelphia: Lippincott-Raven, 1998:791–797.
7. Prensky AL. An approach to the child with paroxysmal phenomenon with emphasis on nonepileptic disorders. In: Pellock JW, Dodson WE, Bourgeois B, eds. *Pediatric epilepsy: diagnosis and therapy*, 2nd ed. New York: Demos, 2001:97–116.
8. Hoban TF. Rhythmic movement disorder in children. *CNS Spectr* 2003;8:135–138.
9. Daoust-Roy J, Seshia SS. Benign neonatal sleep myoclonus. A differential diagnosis of neonatal seizures. *Am J Dis Child* 1992; 146:681.
10. Shuper A, Zalzberg J, Weitz R, et al. Jitteriness beyond the neonatal period: a benign pattern of movement in infancy. *J Child Neurol* 1991;6:243–245.
11. Parker S, Zuckerman B, Bauchner H, et al. Jitteriness in full-term neonates: prevalence and correlates. *Pediatrics* 1990;85:17–23.
12. Fleisher DR, Morrison A. Masturbation mimicking abdominal pain or seizures in young girls. *J Pediatr* 1990;116:810–814.
13. Lombroso CT, Fejerman N. Benign myoclonus of early infancy. *Ann Neurol* 1977;1:138–143.
14. Deonna T, Martin D. Benign paroxysmal torticollis in infancy. *Arch Dis Child* 1981;56:956–959.
15. Gilbert GT. Familial spasmodic torticollis. *Neurology* 1977;27: 11–13.
16. Kinsbourne M. Hiatus hernia with contortions of the neck. *Lancet* 1964;1:10–58.
17. Ramenofsky ML, Buyse M, Goldberg MJ, et al. Gastroesophageal reflux and torticollis. *J Bone Joint Surg (Am)* 1978;60:1140–1141.
18. King RA, Nelson LB, Wagner RS. Spasmus nutans. *Arch Ophthalmol* 1986;104:1501–1504.
19. Hoefnagel D, Biery B. Spasmus nutans. *Dev Med Child Neurol* 1968;10:32–35.
20. Jayalaksmi P, McNair Scott TF, Tucker SH, et al. Infantile nystagmus: a prospective study of spasmus nutans, congenital nystagmus, and unclassified nystagmus of infancy. *J Pediatr* 1970;77: 177–187.
21. Dyken P, Kolar O. Dancing eyes, dancing feet: infantile polymyoclonia. *Brain* 1968;91:305–320.
22. Moe PG, Nellhaus G. Infantile polymyoclonia-opsoclonus syndrome and neural crest tumors. *Neurology* 1970;20:756–764.
23. Soloman GE, Chutorian AM. Opsoclonus and occult neuroblastoma. *N Engl J Med* 1968;279:475–477.
24. Bienfang DC. Opsoclonus in infancy. *Arch Ophthalmol* 1974;91: 203–205.
25. Herbst JJ. Gastroesophageal reflux. *J Pediatr* 1981;98:859–870.
26. Brown P, Rothwell JC, Thompson PD, et al. The hyperexplexias and their relationship to the normal startle reflex. *Brain* 1991;114:1903–1928.
27. Aguglia U, Tinaper P, Gastaut H. Startle-induced epileptic seizures. *Epilepsia* 1984;25:720.
28. SaenzLope E, Herranz FJ, Masdue JC. Startle epilepsy: a clinical study. *Ann Neurol* 1984;16:78–81.
29. Andermann F, Andermann E. Startle disorders of man: hyperexplexia, jumping and startle epilepsy. *Brain Dev* 1988;10:213–222.
30. Andermann F, Keene DL, Andermann E, et al. Startle disease or hyperexplexia: further delineation of the syndrome. *Brain* 1980; 103:985–997.
31. Holmes GL, Russman BS. Shuddering attacks. *Am J Dis Child* 1986;140:72–74.
32. Vanasse M, Bedard P, Anderson F. Shuddering attacks in children: an early clinical manifestation of essential tremor. *Neurology* 1976;26:1027–1030.
33. Bourgeois M, Aicardi J, Goutieres F. Alternating hemiplegia of childhood. *J Pediatr* 1993;122:673–679.
34. Silver K, Andermann F. Alternating hemiplegia of childhood: a study of 10 patients and results of flunarizine treatment. *Neurology* 1993;43:36–41.
35. Watanabe K, Hara K, Hakamada S, et al. Seizures with apnea in children. *Pediatrics* 1982;79:87–90.

36. Myer EC. Infant apnea, life threatening events and sudden infant death. In: Myer EC, Pellock JM, eds. *Neurologic emergencies in infancy and childhood*, 2nd ed. New York: Demos, 1992:42–55.
37. Thach BT. Sleep apnea in infancy and childhood. *Med Clin North Am* 1985;69:1289–1315.
38. Myer EC. Naltrexone therapy of apnea in children with elevated CFS β-endorphin. *Ann Neurol* 1990;27:75–80.
39. Gibson E, Cullen JA, Spinner S, et al. Infant sleep position following new AAP guidelines. *Pediatrics* 1995;96:69–72.
40. Herbst JJ, Minton SD, Book LS. Gastroesophageal reflux causing respiratory distress and apnea in newborn infants. *J Pediatr* 1979;95:763–768.
41. Spitzer AR, Boyle JT, Tuchman DN, et al. Awake apnea associated with gastroesophageal reflux: a specific clinical syndrome. *J Pediatr* 1984;104:200–205.
42. Meyers WF, Herbst JJ. Effectiveness of positioning therapy for gastroesophageal reflux. *Pediatrics* 1982;69:768–772.
43. Lombroso CT, Lerman P. Breath-holding spells (cyanotic and pallid infantile syncope). *Pediatrics* 1967;39:563–581.
44. Colina KF, Abelson HT. Resolution of breath-holding spells with treatment of concomitant anemia. *J Pediatr* 1995;126:395–397.
45. DiMario FJ, Bauer L, Baxter D. Respiratory sinus arrhythmia in children with severe cyanotic and pallid breath-holding spells. *J Child Neurol* 1998;13:440–442.
46. Laxdal T, Gomez MR, Reiher J. Cyanotic and pallid syncopal attacks in children (breath-holding spells). *Dev Med Child Neurol* 1969;11:755–763.
47. Livingston S. Breath-holding spells in children: differentiation from epileptic attacks. *JAMA* 1970;212:2231–2235.
48. Stephenson J. Reflex anoxic seizures ("white breath-holding"): nonepileptic vagal attacks. *Arch Dis Child* 1978;53:193–200.
49. McWilliam R, Stephenson J. Atropine treatment of reflex atonic seizures. *Arch Dis Child* 1984;59:473–485.
50. Coleman RM, Pollak CP, Weitzman ED. Periodic movements in sleep (nocturnal myoclonus): relation to sleep disorders. *Ann Neurol* 1980;8:416–421.
51. Holmes GL. *Diagnosis and management of seizures in children*. Philadelphia: WB Saunders, 1987.
52. Mahowald MW, Schenck CH. NREM sleep parasomnias. *Neurol Clin* 1996;14:675–696.
53. Oswald I. Sudden bodily jerks on falling asleep. *Brain* 1959;82:92–103.
54. Godbout R, Montplaisir J, Rouleau I. Hypnogenic paroxysmal dystonia: epilepsy or sleep disorder? A case report. *Clin Electroencephalogr* 1985;16:136–142.
55. DiMario FJ, Emery ES. The natural history of night terrors. *Clin Pediatr* 1987;26:505–511.
56. Kales A, Kales JD. Sleep disorders: recent findings in the diagnosis and treatment of disturbed sleep. *N Engl J Med* 1974;290:487–499.
57. Thorpy MJ, Glovinsky PB. Parasomnias. *Psychiatr Clin North Am* 1987;10:623–639.
58. Vela-Bueno A, Soldatos CR. Episodic sleep disorders (parasomnias). *Semin Neurol* 1987;7:269–276.
59. Menkes JH. *Textbook of child neurology*. Philadelphia: Lea & Febiger, 1990.
60. Nausieda PA, Grossman BJ, Killer WC, et al. Sydenham chorea: an update. *Neurology* 1980;30:331–334.
61. Erenberg G, Rothner AD. Tourette syndrome: diagnosis and management. *Int Pediatr* 1987;2:149–153.
62. Golden GS. Tourette syndrome: recent advances. *Neurol Clin* 1990; 8:705–714.
63. Singer HS, Rosenberg LA. Development of behavioral and emotional problems in Tourette syndrome. *Pediatr Neurol* 1989;5:41–44.
64. Demirkerian M, Jankovic J. Paroxysmal dyskinesias: clinical features and classification. *Ann Neurol* 1995;38:571–579.
65. Kertesz A. Paroxysmal kinesigenic choreoathetosis. *Neurology* 1967;17:680–690.
66. Kinast M, Erenberg G, Rothner AD. Paroxysmal choreoathetosis: report of five cases and review of the literature. *Pediatrics* 1980; 65:74–77.
67. Lance JW. Familial paroxysmal dystonic choreoathetosis and its differentiation from related syndromes. *Ann Neurol* 1977;2:285–293.
68. Donat JF, Wright FS. Episodic symptoms mistaken for seizures in the neurologically impaired child. *Neurology* 1990;40:156–157.
69. Percy A, Gillberg C, Hayberg B, et al. Rett syndrome and the autistic disorder. *Neurol Clin* 1990;8:659–676.
70. Brunquell P, McKeever M, Russman BS. Differentiation of epileptic from nonepileptic head drops in children. *Epilepsia* 1990;31:401–405.
71. Rosemon F, Wyllie E, Kotagal P, et al. Staring spells in children: descriptive features distinguishing epileptic from nonepileptic events. *J Pediatr* 1998;133:660–663.
72. Barron T. The child with spells. *Pediatr Clin North Am* 1991;38:711–724.
73. Shaywitz SE, Shaywitz BA. Attention deficit disorder: current perspectives. *Pediatr Neurol* 1987;3:129–135.
74. Voeller KKS, ed. Attention deficit hyperactivity disorder (ADHD). *J Child Neurol* 1991;6(Suppl):S1–S131.
75. Weinberg WA, Brumback RA. Primary disorder of vigilance: a novel explanation of inattentiveness, daydreaming, boredom, restlessness, and sleepiness. *J Pediatr* 1990;116:720–725.
76. D'Alessandro R, Sacquengna T, Pazzaglia P, et al. Headache after partial complex seizures. In: Andermann F, Lugaresi E, eds. *Migraine and epilepsy*. London: Butterworths, 1987:273–328.
77. Annequuin D, Tourmaire B, Massiou H. Migraine and headache in childhood and adolescence. *Pediatr Clin North Am* 2000;47:617–631.
78. Barlow CF. *Headaches and migraine in children*. London: Spastics International Medical, 1984.
79. Blume WT, Young GB. Ictal pain: unilateral, cephalic and abdominal. In: Andermann F, Lugaresi E, eds. *Migraine and epilepsy*. London: Butterworths, 1987:238–248.
80. Pratt JL, Fleisher GR. Syncope in children and adolescents. *Pediatr Emerg Care* 1989;5:80–82.
81. Prensky AL. Migraine and migrainous variant in pediatric patients. *Pediatr Clin North Am* 1976;23:461–471.
82. Prensky AL, Sommer D. Diagnosis and treatment of migraine in children. *Neurology* 1979;29:506–510.
83. Hammond J. The late sequelae of recurrent vomiting of childhood. *Dev Med Child Neurol* 1974;16:15–22.
84. Gascon G, Barlow C. Juvenile migraine presenting as an acute confusional state. *J Pediatr* 1970;45:628–635.
85. Finkelhor BK, Harker LA. Benign paroxysmal vertigo of childhood. *Laryngoscope* 1987;97:1161–1163.
86. Parker W. Migraine and the vestibular system in childhood and adolescence. *Am J Otolaryngol* 1989;10:364–371.
87. Rosenberg AH. Constipation and encopresis. In: Wyllie R, Hyams JS, eds. *Pediatric gastrointestinal disease*. Philadelphia: WB Saunders, 1993:198–208.
88. Williams DT, Mehl R, Yudofsky S, et al. The effect of propranolol on uncontrolled rage outbursts in children and adolescents with organic brain dysfunction. *J Am Acad Child Psychiatry* 1982;21:129–135.
89. Elliott FA. The episodic dyscontrol syndrome and aggression. *Neurol Clin* 1984;2:113–125.
90. Folks DG. Munchausen's syndrome and other factitious disorders. *Neurol Clin* 1995;13:267–281.
91. Meadow R. Munchausen syndrome by proxy. *Arch Dis Child* 1982;57:92–98.
92. Meadow R. Neurological and developmental variants of Munchausen syndrome. *Dev Med Child Neurol* 1991;33:270–272.
93. Wyllie E, Friedman D, Rothner AD, et al. Psychogenic seizures in children and adolescents: outcome after diagnosis by ictal video and electroencephalographic recording. *Pediatrics* 1990;85:480–484.
94. Bools CN, Neale BA, Meadow SR. Follow-up of victims of fabricated illness (Munchausen syndrome by proxy). *Arch Dis Child* 1993;69:625–630.
95. Camfield PR, Camfield CS. Syncope in childhood: a case control clinical study of the familial tendency to faint. *Clin J Neurol Sci* 1990;17:306–308.
96. Katz RM. Cough syncope in children with asthma. *J Pediatr* 1970;77:48–51.
97. Ruckman RN. Cardiac causes of syncope. *Pediatr Rev* 1987;9:101–108.

98. Berenberg RA, Pellock JM, DiMauro S, et al. Lumping or splitting? Ophthalmoplegia plus or Kearns-Sayre syndrome. *Ann Neurol* 1977;1:37–54.

99. Lerman-Sagie T, Rechavia E, Strasberg B, et al. Head-up tilt for the evaluation of syncope of unknown origin in children. *J Pediatr* 1991;118:676–679.

100. Thilenius OG, Quinones JA, Husayni TS, et al. Tilt test for diagnosis of unexplained syncope in pediatric patients. *Pediatrics* 1991;87:334–338.

101. Broughton RJ. Polysomnography: principles and applications in sleep and arousal disorders. In: Niedermeyer E, Lopes da Silva F, eds. *Electroencephalography*, 2nd ed. Baltimore, MD: Urban & Schwarzenberg, 1987:687–724.

102. Kotagal S, Hartse KM, Walsh JK. Characteristics of narcolepsy in preteenaged children. *Pediatrics* 1990;85:205–209.

103. Wittig R, Zorick F, Roehrs T, et al. Narcolepsy in a 7-year-old child. *J Pediatr* 1983;102:725–727.

104. Camfield PR, Metrakos K, Andermann F. Basilar migraine, seizures, and severe epileptiform EEG abnormalities: a benign syndrome in adolescents. *Neurology* 1978;28:584.

105. Golden GS, French JH. Basilar artery migraine in young children. *Pediatrics* 1975;56:722.

106. Hallett M. Classification and treatment of tremor. *JAMA* 1991;266:1115–1117.

107. American Psychiatric Association. *Diagnostic and statistical manual of mental disorders*, 3rd ed., rev. Washington, DC: Author, 1987.

108. Kaplan HI, Sadock BJ, eds. *The comprehensive textbook of psychiatry*, 5th ed. Baltimore, MD: Williams & Wilkins, 1989.

109. Paul MH. Tetralogy of Fallot. In: Rudolph AM, ed. *Rudolph's pediatrics*, 10th ed. Norwalk, CT: Appleton & Lange, 1991:1397–1398.

110. Hack CH, Enril BG, Donat JF, et al. Seizures in relation to shunt displacement in patients with MMC. *J Pediatr* 1990;116:57–60.

111. Tomasovic JA, Nelhaus G, Moe PG. The bobblehead doll syndrome: an early sign of hydrocephalus. *Dev Med Child Neurol* 1975;17:177.

112. Meyers KR, Gilden DH, Rinaldi CF, et al. Periodic muscle weakness, normokalemia, and tubular aggregates. *Neurology* 1972;22:269.

113. Hachinski V, Norris JW. *Stroke*. Philadelphia: FA Davis, 1985.

114. Roach ES, Riela AR. *Pediatric cerebrovascular disorders*. New York: Futura, 1988.

115. Miller JW, Petersen RC, Metter EJ, et al. Transient global amnesia. *Neurology* 1987;37:733–737.

116. Metrick ME, Ritter FJ, Gates JR, et al. Nonepileptic events in children. *Epilepsia* 1991;32:322–328.

Part IV

Antiepileptic Medications

Section A **GENERAL PRINCIPLES OF ANTIEPILEPTIC DRUG THERAPY   645**

44. Antiepileptic Drug Development and Experimental Models   645
45. Pharmacokinetics and Pharmacodynamics of Antiepileptic Drugs   655
    Appendix: Selected Drug Interactions Between Antiepileptic Drugs and Other Types of Medications   665
46. Pharmacokinetics of Antiepileptic Drugs in Infants and Children   671
47. Initiation and Discontinuation of Antiepileptic Drugs   681
48. Hormones, Catamenial Epilepsy, and Reproductive and Bone Health in Epilepsy   697
49. Treatment of Epilepsy During Pregnancy   705
50. Treatment of Epilepsy in the Setting of Renal and Liver Disease   719
51. Monitoring for Adverse Effects of Antiepileptic Drugs   735
52. Pharmacogenetics of Antiepileptic Medications   747

Section B **SPECIFIC ANTIEPILEPTIC MEDICATIONS AND OTHER THERAPIES   761**

53. Carbamazepine and Oxcarbazepine   761
54. Valproate   775
55. Phenytoin and Fosphenytoin   785
56. Phenobarbital and Primidone   805
57. Ethosuximide   817
58. Benzodiazepines   829
59. Gabapentin and Pregabalin   855
60. Lamotrigine   869
61. Topiramate   877
62. Zonisamide   891
63. Levetiracetam   901
64. Tiagabine   907
65. Felbamate   913
66. Vigabatrin   921
67. Adrenocorticotropin and Steroids   931
68. Newer Antiepileptic Drugs   939
69. Less Commonly Used Antiepileptic Drugs   947
70. The Ketogenic Diet   961
71. Vagus Nerve Stimulation Therapy   969

Antiepileptic Drug Development and Experimental Models

44

Jacqueline A. French

In 1962, the Kefauver-Harris amendments to the federal Food, Drug, and Cosmetic Act ushered in the modern age of drug testing by requiring that pharmaceuticals be proved effective prior to marketing (1). At the same time, federal agencies were given the authority to determine whether the safety and efficacy of a drug had been satisfactorily demonstrated. Although this law prevented ineffective compounds from entering the market, it also significantly impeded the development of new, effective treatments. Antiepileptic drugs (AEDs) were particularly affected because of the difficulties and cost of their trials. After valproic acid was approved in 1978, no new agents were developed for a decade. Meanwhile, 50% of patients with epilepsy had either unacceptable seizure control or side effects that affected their quality of life.

From this clear need for new agents came the National Institutes of Health (NIH) Antiepileptic Drug Development (ADD) Program (2), which screens thousands of compounds against animal models of epilepsy. As of 2002, 24,000 new chemical entities have been screened (S. White, Epilepsy Research Branch NIH, personal communication 2002). A subset of these compounds is further evaluated, and in conjunction with pharmaceutical companies, the most promising agents are tested in humans via clinical trials. Mainly as a result of the efforts of the ADD Program, the 1990s saw many new AEDs approved, with even more agents entered into clinical trials. More recently, many smaller companies have entered the AED development arena. This has placed a greater emphasis on early determination of drug efficacy in order to assess potential return on investments. There is also a greater emphasis on obtaining a monotherapy indication, which is seen as advantageous in the marketplace. These corporate needs, however, must always be balanced against patient safety issues.

This chapter reviews the process by which a compound is discovered, undergoes preclinical and clinical testing, and is ultimately approved for use, with emphasis on AED development in the United States, as directed by the Food and Drug Administration (FDA).

PRECLINICAL DEVELOPMENT

Drug Discovery

Since Merritt and Putnam discovered phenytoin in 1938, identification of AEDs has depended on animal screening of anticonvulsant activity. Under the ADD Program, approximately 1000 compounds from various sources are evaluated each year for potential antiepileptic action. Sometimes pharmaceutical companies send large numbers of random compounds for screening. For example, felbamate was initially synthesized as an analogue of the tranquilizer meprobamate (3,4). Similar screening may be performed within pharmaceutical companies, often on compounds specifically designed as potential anticonvulsants. An example is vigabatrin, an irreversible inhibitor of γ-aminobutyric acid (GABA) transaminase (5). Regardless of its source, however, if a compound demonstrates no effect in animal screening, it will most likely receive no further evaluation, raising concern that agents that act via unusual mechanisms may be inappropriately rejected.

Primary Screening Models

There are two basic strategies for discovering new chemical entities that may be useful for the treatment of epilepsy. The first method is called model-based screening. In this approach, high volumes of compounds undergo chemical screens that are predictive of antiepileptic effect. Compounds that prove effective in these screens will undergo further testing to assess toxicity and to try to elucidate the mechanism of action. Topiramate and felbamate are examples of recent AEDs that were discovered in this manner. Not surprisingly, these agents are frequently determined to have multiple mechanisms of action. The second strategy used for drug discovery is known as mechanism-based screening. Here an attempt is made to synthesize a compound that will have a desired pharmacologic effect, such as GABA enhancement or N-methyl-D-aspartate (NMDA) blockade. Examples of agents recently discovered using this technique include vigabatrin and tiagabine, both of which are GABA enhancers. In most cases, compounds that are discovered based on mechanism of action will still be evaluated using standard chemical screens.

The two primary animal screens used to assess anticonvulsant activity are maximal electroshock (MES) and subcutaneous pentylenetetrazol (scMET). In the MES test, rodents receive 60-Hz alternating current for 0.2 seconds through corneal electrodes and are then observed for tonic hind-limb extension. A preadministered compound that can abolish this response is presumed to have the ability to abolish seizure propagation. In the second screen, pentylenetetrazol is administered subcutaneously. Untreated animals experience clonic spasms within 30 minutes. Compounds that increase seizure threshold can prevent this response (6). These two tests are performed at various intervals after an agent has been administered in order to assess duration of activity. If no anticonvulsant activity is evident on either test, the threshold tonic extension test—which, unlike the MES, uses submaximal rather than supramaximal electroshock stimulation—is performed before the agent is abandoned (6).

It is believed that the MES and scMET tests may, in some way, distinguish the potential utility of compounds against different seizure types. Compounds effective in the MES screen may be more useful in patients with partial and generalized tonic-clonic seizures, whereas those effective in the scMET screen may have activity against absence seizures. Unfortunately, many AEDs prove to be an exception to the rule. For example, gabapentin prevents clonic spasms after pentylenetetrazol administration but has no activity against absence seizures (7,8).

The emphasis on a small number of chemical screening models to discover new agents has been criticized by some individuals. It is possible that this method may uncover only those drugs with similar mechanisms of action and may discard novel drugs with unique properties. Although most new AEDs are effective in either MES or scMET tests, one useful compound, levetiracetam (see Chapter 63) was ineffective in either of these screens. Greater emphasis is now being placed on the use of biologic screens, including kindling models; spontaneous seizure models, such as the genetic absence epilepsy rat from Strasbourg (9) and the audiogenic seizure-prone rat, both of which model genetic spike-wave epilepsy in humans; and models of spontaneous seizures following status epilepticus, such as the perforant-path and pilocarpine-induced status models (10,11). A recent NIH workshop was held to foster identification of new models that might better predict efficacy in the human epilepsy condition (12).

Information from the three tests described is combined with results of neurotoxicity assays, including the Rotorod, positional sense, gait and stance, and muscle tone tests (6), to yield a therapeutic index (TI). The TI is the ratio of the median toxic dose (TD_{50}) to the median effective dose (ED_{50}). A high index is indicative of good tolerability at doses required to control seizures. Again, there has been a new perspective on the older model meant to elucidate toxicity. Toxicity testing is performed using acute seizure model such as MES and scMET. Recently, it was discovered that animals who have undergone kindling may be more susceptible to certain types of side effects than are normal animals. This raises the question of whether patients with epilepsy might also be prone to such side effects. In the future, it is likely that more toxicity testing will be performed in animal models of epilepsy (13,14).

Differentiation of Mechanism of Action

Tests to elucidate possible mechanisms of action include injections of the chemoconvulsants bicuculline (a GABA antagonist), picrotoxin (a chloride-channel blocker), and strychnine (a glycine antagonist). The compound can also be used to determine whether kindling can be prevented in corneally kindled rodents (indicating antiepileptogenesis) or whether seizures can be prevented in fully kindled animals (indicating antiepileptic activity). The results from these tests are becoming more critical, as investigators begin to search for agents that may prevent seizures. It has been suggested that drugs that prevent the acquisition of kindled seizures may have special properties that would prevent the development of an epileptic focus after a brain injury, such as stroke or head trauma. To date, however, such effects have not been proven. Other useful screens include the Frings audiogenic seizure-susceptible mouse, and spike-and-wave discharges provoked by γ-hydroxybutyrate (15), a possible screen for agents that have anti-absence potential (6). Genetic mouse models may also be useful for this purpose. Finally, *in vitro* tests can search for specific receptor binding and for the ability to block sodium, chloride, or calcium channels (16).

Tolerance and Pharmacokinetic Properties

Early in the evaluation of a compound some pharmacokinetic information can be obtained. Chronic dosing studies coupled with anticonvulsant screening tests can provide information on whether tolerance may develop. Liver enzyme tests can indicate toxicity and effect on hepatic metabolism, including inhibition of the cytochrome P450 enzyme. Liver tests may also help to establish the route of metabolism (e.g., oxidation or glucuronidation) (6).

Toxicity

Toxicity testing of AEDs is regulated by the FDA. Before single-dose studies in humans can be initiated, acute toxicology studies must be conducted using three dose levels in at least two animal species for a minimum of 14 days. If longer human administration is planned, subchronic studies must last 6 to 24 months (17).

Animals are observed for behavior and weight changes, eating habits, and general appearance. Full-blood analyses are performed, as well as electrocardiograms and ophthalmologic examinations. The animals are eventually killed, and all organs are closely scrutinized. Cause of death is sought in any animals that die before testing is completed. Mutagenicity by means of the Ames text and carcinogenicity in two species are determined. The full reproductive cycle is observed and analyzed—from production of eggs and sperm; through conception, delivery, and growth; to sexual maturity of the offspring (16). Preclinical testing for potential teratogenicity may be misleading, as animals may have different sensitivities than humans or may produce different metabolites. In addition, animals are exposed to much higher doses than those that will be used clinically in humans (18). Despite the uncertainty about the clinical relevance of these tests, they are used to determine the pregnancy safety labeling when a new drug is brought to market. Unique characteristics of some compounds will mandate specific studies—for example, additional toxicologic assays for NMDA-receptor blockers, which can produce neuronal death (19). On initial testing, vigabatrin was noted to produce vacuolization of central nervous system white matter in dogs and rats (2,20). Human testing was halted until, among other things, long-term studies could be performed in nonhuman primates. Fortunately, no evidence of similar toxicity was found either in primate nonhuman species or in man. Some agents are being closely scrutinized for their effects on the retina, as a result of unexpected visual changes that were associated with the GABA-antagonist vigabatrin (21). Additionally, some agents produce active metabolites, which may produce independent efficacy and toxicity. These compounds must undergo the same rigorous testing as the parent compound.

The potential of a compound to produce even frequent idiosyncratic reactions is unlikely to be revealed during preclinical testing. Moreover, metabolic pathways in humans may differ from those in other species, leading to unexpected toxic reactions. Physicians must not mistakenly believe that the TI, which assesses only dose-related neurotoxicity, indicates overall safety. For example, despite a high TI, after it was marketed, felbamate was found to be associated with a risk of inducing hematologic and hepatic disorders (22).

TESTING IN HUMANS

Once preclinical testing has been completed, human investigation of the agent, consisting of four phases, can begin.

Phase 1

During phase 1 testing, a compound is used for the first time in humans, usually healthy volunteers. Single, increasing doses are followed by long-term administration of the agent. The dose at which toxicity first appears is assessed, as well as any dose-related adverse events and the maximum tolerated dose (MTD). Half-life, time to maximum concentration, clearance, presence or absence of active metabolites, and route of elimination are all determined (23). In total, fewer than 100 normal individuals will be exposed to the agent. Phase 1 testing of AEDs usually includes patients as volunteers—a crucial point, as the MTD may be different in patients with epilepsy. In addition, most AEDs are used initially as adjunctive therapy, and drug–drug interactions should be known before efficacy testing begins.

Appropriate testing during phase 1 is critical for all phases that follow. Effective agents may appear to be ineffective if inadequate doses are administered. Conversely, selection of higher-than-optimal doses may result in an agent appearing overly toxic or being associated with excessive dropouts during clinical trials. Trial designs for efficacy testing may also be influenced by characteristics revealed during phase 1 testing.

Phases 2 and 3

During phase 2 trials, initial clinical trials determine the efficacy and toxicity of an agent. The first efficacy trial is usually termed *proof of principle*. This trial is used to obtain an initial signal of efficacy, and may be used by the sponsor of a drug to make a go/no-go business decision about continued development of the agent. Proof-of-principle trials are often open-label in design; even if they are placebo controlled, such trials may not be powered to detect a statistically significant difference. Design of the proof-of-principle trial is important, as there is great danger of discarding a potentially useful agent (24). In phase 3 trials, efficacy and safety assessments continue and may include evaluation of specialized populations, such as children, or specific seizure syndromes.

Two "adequate and well-controlled clinical trials"—so-called pivotal trials—that demonstrate efficacy must be conducted to obtain FDA approval (17). Long-term safety studies must also be completed. Of the several thousand patients who will be exposed to an AED during phases 2 and 3, several hundred will have multiple years of exposure. When these phases are complete, the sponsoring pharmaceutical company will file a New Drug Application (NDA). This document, which contains all the information obtained in preclinical and clinical testing, forms the basis on which the FDA renders its decision.

Phase 4

Once a drug is approved, phase 4, or postmarketing, testing begins, which includes surveillance studies, studies for new indications or expanded populations, and large, less tightly regulated trials.

EFFICACY AND SAFETY TRIALS

Some characteristics of patients with epilepsy and of the agents used to treat the disease make well-controlled trials very difficult to conduct. The following sections outline some major issues in the design and implementation of such trials.

Selection of Population

Epilepsy Syndrome

The term *antiepileptic drug* implies a single disease. However, epilepsy comprises a diverse group of syndromes, each with a unique clinical presentation and often with different genetics, etiology, and possibly underlying biochemical defect (25). It would be astounding if a single agent had equal efficacy in all these syndromes. In fact, most AEDs are effective either in certain seizure types or in specific seizure syndromes. As the most common seizure type in adults, partial seizures are frequently chosen for study in pivotal trials. As a result, many AEDs are approved for the treatment of partial seizures and comparatively few for other seizure types, such as absence, myoclonus, and infantile spasms. Trials in other populations have become more common. For example, lamotrigine received approval for use in seizures associated with the Lennox-Gastaut syndrome based on positive clinical trials (26). Topiramate was shown to reduce the number of seizures in a trial of patients with Lennox-Gastaut syndrome (27), as well as in a novel clinical trial of patients with primary generalized tonic-clonic convulsions (28). To date, large-scale randomized trials of the new agents have not been conducted in patients with absence or myoclonic epilepsy.

Seizure Severity

Traditionally, the most difficult-to-treat, medically refractory patients are recruited for AED trials, largely because patients may not wish to test "unproven" and "experimental" agents until conventional therapy has failed. In addition, enrollment criteria usually include frequency, such as a minimum of three to four complex partial or secondarily generalized seizures per month. These criteria ensure that there will be enough measurable seizures during a 3-month trial to obtain a statistically significant result and that only patients with the most severe epilepsy are chosen. The use of such patients may not demonstrate the true effectiveness of a new agent, and it has been hypothesized that the best conventional AEDs might fail such a difficult test (29). Even if the experimental drug can be proved effective in this challenging population, it is unclear whether the results can or should be generalized to the remainder of patients with epilepsy, who, in general, do not have intractable disease. Recently, the effort to conduct trials in patients with less intractable or even new-onset disease has attracted increasing support.

Age

Phase 2 and 3 trials are typically performed exclusively in adults; pediatric use lags far behind. For example, of the approved new agents, oxcarbazepine was the only one to receive approval at the time of launch for use in children with partial seizures; this indication has been extended to include monotherapy. Felbamate received U.S. approval in children based on its effectiveness in pediatric patients with Lennox-Gastaut syndrome (30). Gabapentin and lamotrigine have only recently been approved for pediatric use. Topiramate was approved for use in children with partial seizures in 1999, several years after its initial approval in adults levetiracetam received approval in children in 2005. Tiagabine and zonisamide are not approved for pediatric use. When drugs are approved for use in adults, they are almost immediately put to use in pediatric populations. In the past, this was carried out without any useful information on dosing schedules and pharmacokinetics. The FDA has issued new regulations requiring pediatric studies of new agents so that manufacturers can provide sufficient data in their product labeling to support pediatric use (31). Studies of new AEDs are now performed as early as infancy (32). The delay in pediatric approval is of great clinical concern. Even though most new AEDs are used in children almost immediately after approval, without adequate pediatric data, the FDA will not permit dosage or safety information to be included in a package insert. Thus, improper use may ensue.

Why are early pediatric trials of AEDs not conducted? One reason is that they cannot be performed until sufficient phase 1 pharmacokinetic data are available in appropriate-age children to permit dosage selection. Obtaining informed consent and frequent blood samples makes these phase 1 trials difficult to conduct in children.

Another complication of phase 1 pediatric trials is metabolism. An infant and young child's metabolic rate is faster than that in adults, declining gradually toward adult levels near puberty. Thus, even if pediatric efficacy trials use mg/kg dosage, resultant blood levels will be more variable than in adults. Levels that are too low may not demonstrate efficacy; levels that are too high may cause dose-related toxicity (33).

Finally, pediatric trials involve special safety issues. There is concern that AEDs with novel mechanisms of action may interfere with normal brain development or learning. Without adequate animal models, serious problems might emerge for the first time in clinical trials. In addition, lack of developmental progress or even intellectual decline may not become apparent during the short time of a controlled trial.

The NMDA antagonists are of special concern. Despite the special attention to cognitive development warranted in any trial of an NMDA antagonist, the FDA has provided no guidelines for addressing its stated concerns about this class of drugs in the context of a clinical trial. Presumably, longer trials that include comprehensive neuropsychological assessments may be necessary. Recognizing these and other issues, the NIH sponsored a consensus conference in 1994 that focused on AED development in children (34).

Women of Childbearing Potential

As recently as 1993, women of childbearing potential were excluded from clinical trials until ". . . there was preliminary evidence of efficacy from a controlled trial and appropriate animal reproduction studies have been performed" (35). In essence, this translated into restrictions during phase 1 and 2 studies. In a major shift in thinking on this important issue (36), the FDA recognized the concern that drugs may have had adequate safety and efficacy testing in only half the population (i.e., males) in which they will ultimately be used. Also, it recognized that available AEDs pose some risk in this population and may not adequately control seizures. Consequently, women of childbearing potential who use adequate birth control methods can now participate in efficacy trials. The definition of adequate birth control has changed over time. In the past, only women taking oral contraceptives were eligible for phase 2 and 3 trials. Currently, barrier methods and abstinence also are acceptable. Determining the effect of AEDs on oral contraceptive levels is now a standard part of early drug development.

There is interest in the effects of AEDs on general reproductive health. Many AEDs are known to influence the hypothalamic-pituitary axis, alter menstrual cycles, affect bone metabolism, and possibly reduce fertility (37). The newer agents may have less deleterious effects. These issues are being studied earlier and in a more rigorous fashion.

TRIAL DESIGN

Designs for clinical epilepsy studies are limited by aspects of the disease. Figure 44.1 illustrates the most common study design. Patients with complex partial seizures not controlled

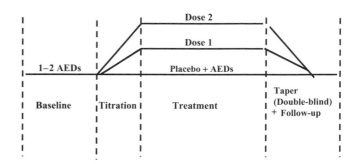

Figure 44.1 Schemata of typical randomized, placebo-controlled adjunctive trial of antiepileptic drugs.

with conventional medication serve as the experimental subjects. A minimum frequency of three to four seizures per month is required. Following a 4- to 12-week baseline period to establish the typical seizure frequency, patients are randomized in a double-blind fashion to receive placebo or study drug, which is added to their existing medication regimen. The double-blind treatment period lasts 8 to 12 weeks, after which patients have the option of continuing to take the study medication. Those randomized to the placebo arm may be converted to the study drug without interfering with the blinded nature of the trial.

The sections that follow discuss elements of protocol design as they pertain to epilepsy studies.

Blinding

Blinded comparison to a control group is a study criterion preferred by the FDA for pivotal trials (35). Traditionally, investigators have had difficulty understanding the necessity of this feature, arguing that seizures are discrete, measurable events that should not be subject to a placebo effect, particularly in patients with intractable disease who have tried multiple treatments. Yet time and again, the power of the placebo effect has been proved, even in this population. The most notable example was from an evaluation of cinromide in patients with Lennox-Gastaut syndrome. Although it was assumed that the severely retarded children in the study lacked the capacity to demonstrate a placebo effect, the greater than 50% reduction in seizures seen in an open trial of the agent was subsequently exactly matched in the placebo group of a controlled trial (38).

Choice of Control Group

In a controlled trial of an AED, investigators have three primary choices and one secondary choice for control groups, each with potential advantages and disadvantages.

Historical Control

Historical control is listed by the FDA as an acceptable form of controlled trial. With this type of study, baseline seizure counts are compared with counts during subsequent treatment; in other words, patients act as their own control. Because of the risk of a placebo effect, this design is usually unacceptable for epilepsy trials. However, there has been recent renewed interest in this type of control for monotherapy trials (39).

Placebo Control

The most traditional—and the soundest scientifically—approach compares treatment with placebo. The presence of a placebo group, however, usually mandates add-on rather than monotherapy, as ethical considerations preclude leaving patients with diagnosed epilepsy untreated. Even with adjunctive treatment, patients often express dissatisfaction with a placebo-controlled trial, which may postpone therapy for several months.

Dose Control

A dose-controlled trial has no placebo group, but rather compares low, medium, and high doses of an agent as treatment arms. In this design, all subjects receive active drug during the treatment period—a far more acceptable arrangement to patients. Problems with safety and efficacy testing are inherent to the design, however. A placebo arm is essential for determination of adverse events. In most trials, more than 90% of patients report at least one adverse event over the course of treatment. Absent a placebo group for comparison, all adverse events—not simply those that occur more often with treatment than with placebo—must be attributed to the study drug. Moreover, dose-controlled trials have a high likelihood of failure to demonstrate efficacy. For such a trial to succeed, the chosen doses must produce a statistically significant difference in efficacy. Specifically, the lowest dose must be relatively ineffective so that the higher doses will be able to demonstrate superiority. In phase 2 trials, sufficient information may not be available for appropriate dosage selection. For example, in a pivotal trial of topiramate, three doses were compared with placebo. Percent reductions in seizures with 400-, 600- and 800-mg doses were 41%, 41%, and 38%, respectively. Although results with all doses were statistically different from that with placebo, no significant differences between treatment groups were apparent (40). Dose-controlled studies are frequently conducted but usually, as in the topiramate study, include a placebo group.

Active Control

Active-control trials are common outside the United States. Because the FDA will not accept these trials as proof of efficacy, they are avoided in the United States—at least until approval has been obtained. In an active-control trial, two AEDs are directly compared. Typically, one is a conventional drug, such as carbamazepine, and the other is investigational. Clinicians like these head-to-head comparisons of efficacy and side effects because they do more than merely demonstrate the superiority of an agent over placebo. In addition, because all subjects receive active drug, these studies can use monotherapy, and the design

lends itself to evaluation of newly diagnosed patients. One of the most widely cited active-control trials was the first Veterans Administration Cooperative Study, which randomized patients with newly diagnosed partial seizures to treatment with phenobarbital, phenytoin, primidone, or carbamazepine (41). Although this study provides seminal information on the treatment of patients with epilepsy, it also offers a good example of the drawbacks of active-control trials. Efficacy was equivalent for all four drugs tested. The FDA does not accept proof of equivalence as proof of efficacy, however, even when the comparator drug is a standard agent whose effectiveness is widely accepted. The agency maintains that an agent may have been proved effective in some populations but not in the population currently under investigation (42). For example, if carbamazepine and an investigational drug were tested in a severely refractory population, neither agent might be effective yet both may cause a statistically significant seizure reduction as a result of a placebo effect. Active-control trials are acceptable, provided they are designed to demonstrate superiority of one drug over another. Several recent trials used a low therapeutic dose of valproic acid or of the comparator drug (43–45). If the comparator arm is statistically superior to the control arm, the trial is accepted as proof of efficacy.

Parallel Versus Crossover Design

A parallel-design study uses multiple patient groups that are randomly assigned to one of two or more treatments (Fig. 44.1). In a crossover-design study, the same population is exposed to each treatment in sequence and serves as its own control; therefore, fewer participants are needed to achieve statistical significance. The trial mimics clinical practice, in which patients are typically crossed over from one treatment to another. Crossover studies, however, last longer than parallel studies, and the potential exists for unblinding. This is particularly true for a placebo-controlled add-on study, in which patients may realize the order in which treatments were administered by the time they reach the second arm. Because of this risk, the FDA does not favor crossover trials.

Adjunctive Therapy Versus Monotherapy

Although monotherapy studies are difficult to design, add-on studies are intrinsically unsatisfactory. AEDs are commonly associated with drug–drug interactions that may jeopardize a clinical trial if they are not anticipated. In an early phase 2 trial, for example, felbamate was used as adjunctive therapy to the baseline drug carbamazepine (46). This study failed to demonstrate efficacy against placebo, in part because felbamate caused a reduction in carbamazepine levels, possibly leading to exacerbations of seizures. Felbamate is also known to increase phenytoin levels by 20% (47). In another felbamate trial in patients with Lennox-Gastaut syndrome (30), all patients taking phenytoin had their dose reduced by 20% from baseline and prior to randomization (30). If this had not occurred, any decrease in seizure frequency in the felbamate-treated group could have been attributed to increasing phenytoin levels rather than to direct drug efficacy, calling the validity of the trial outcome into question.

Adverse events in adjunctive trials may be magnified when drugs are combined. In such pharmacodynamic interactions, even nontoxic doses of two AEDs will produce side effects. The prevalence of this type of interaction is demonstrated by the fact that monotherapy studies almost always produce lower rates of adverse events than do polytherapy studies performed in patients of identical ages (43,48).

Even after the controlled aspect of a trial has been completed, polytherapy can confound drug evaluation. Frequency of idiosyncratic reactions is usually assessed during long-term open extensions that follow placebo-controlled trials. Because at this point there is no control group, it may be difficult to separate adverse events caused by study drugs from those associated with adjunctive standard medications. For reporting purposes, all adverse events will be attributed to the investigational agent.

A final disadvantage of conducting phase 2 and 3 trials with add-on therapy is that approval is granted only for adjunctive use, even though clinicians often wish to use a new AED as monotherapy. Of the eight recently approved AEDs, only felbamate and oxcarbazepine were indicated for use as monotherapy at the time of initial FDA approval.

The preferred method of demonstrating efficacy in monotherapy trials is to compare placebo with active drug. Concerns about patient safety preclude this approach, however. Several study designs have been devised that attempt to address safety concerns while at the same time demonstrating effectiveness of a new drug as monotherapy (49). Rather than using a true placebo, some of these designs use a "pseudoplacebo" arm. Patients in this arm receive some treatment to prevent catastrophic seizures or severe worsening, but not enough medication to prevent the occurrence of the complex partial seizures that are being evaluated in the study. Typically, either a low dose of sodium valproate or a very low dose of the study drug is used for this purpose. In one novel monotherapy protocol, known as a surgical withdrawal design, the subjects are patients whose medication is being withdrawn for the purpose of presurgical evaluation. When most or all medication use has been stopped, the experimental AED or placebo/pseudoplacebo is added in a randomized, blinded fashion. The trial ends after subjects have experienced a prespecified number of seizures (i.e., "failures") or have gone a certain time (usually 7 to 10 days) without that number of seizures having occurred (i.e., "completers"). Analysis is based on the number of completers in the placebo/pseudoplacebo group compared with the treatment group (50–53). The duration of these trials is now

considered too short for them to be useful in predicting success of a new drug as monotherapy in the outpatient setting. A second design uses an outpatient setting and randomizes patients to treatment with an experimental drug or pseudoplacebo, withdrawing baseline therapy. Outcome is assessed in terms of "failures" and "completers." Failure is determined on the basis of escape criteria, such as doubling of seizure frequency or increase in seizure severity. If more patients receiving the experimental drug at a therapeutic dose can complete the trial without fulfilling escape criteria, compared with patients receiving pseudo-placebo, the treatment is considered effective as monotherapy (48). These protocols are now in common use when a monotherapy indication is sought (43,44,48,54,55).

Monotherapy studies may also be conducted in newly diagnosed patients. In Europe, studies typically use an active-control design, in which a new drug is compared with a standard agent (56–59). Some studies compare high and low doses. For example, one study of patients with newly diagnosed epilepsy demonstrated that 900-mg and 1800-mg gabapentin doses were more effective than a 300-mg dose in preventing seizures that necessitated withdrawal from the study (60).

Monotherapy trial designs are controversial in nature. Issues have been raised about the ethics of randomizing patients to treatment arms in which dosing is known to be suboptimal (pseudoplacebo) and about the artificial nature of some of the study designs, making it difficult to translate results into real-life situations (61,62). Discussion of alternative methods of obtaining monotherapy approval is ongoing (39). It is hoped that better solutions will be found in the future.

ANALYSIS OF RESULTS

Standard Measures

Outcome Variable

In every trial, a primary outcome variable must be selected in advance and a plan for statistical analysis must be stated. Otherwise, an unsuccessful trial may be made to appear successful if an alternative analysis, which in retrospect is statistically significant, is chosen.

There are many ways in which to handle seizure data. Seizure data are nonparametric. One way to circumvent this problem is to normalize the data prior to application of a statistical treatment. Another way is to use an analysis suitable for nonparametric data. Unfortunately, not all statistical treatments are intuitively comprehensible to a clinician attempting to review data. For example, the multicenter gabapentin and pregabalin trials were analyzed with the use of response ratios (63,64), in which the difference between the treatment and baseline seizure rates is divided by the sum of the two rates. Adding to the difficulty is the fact that clinical trial results cannot be easily compared if different analyses are used. All drug treatment outcome studies should be evaluated by an "intent-to-treat" analysis. This means that all randomized patients are entered in the analysis even if they drop out early. Anything that increases the number of dropouts from a trial will reduce the likelihood of obtaining a statistically significant outcome. This includes choosing a dosage level for the trial that produces unacceptable adverse reactions in some patients, failing to foresee undesirable pharmacokinetic interactions with baseline drugs, designing a trial whose excessive procedures seem burdensome to patients, and enrolling unenthusiastic participants.

Nonstandard Outcome Measures

Seizure frequency may be a crude measure of AED effect. New methods have been used to assess improvement, although they cannot be used to obtain FDA approval. These include seizure severity measures, economic outcomes, and measurements of quality of life (65–67). Although less objective than seizure counts, some of these outcomes, such as quality of life, may better indicate whether patients find a drug beneficial. Nevertheless, they cannot distinguish among the various factors involved in "feeling better." For example, if an agent had antidepressant properties, quality of life scores might improve substantially, even though the drug had no antiepileptic effect.

CONCLUSION

What we ultimately know, or believe we know, about AEDs stems largely from information obtained through preclinical testing and clinical trials. Proper design and implementation of these investigations are crucial aspects of obtaining that information. As new and different drugs are developed, new testing procedures must also emerge to keep pace. The informed clinician must keep abreast of these innovations, so as to appropriately evaluate the results and relay the information to his or her patients.

REFERENCES

1. Drug Amendments Act of 1962. 21 USC §355 (1962).
2. Porter RJ, Cereghino JJ, Gladding GD, et al. Antiepileptic Drug Development Program. *Cleve Clin Q* 1984;51:293–305.
3. Kucharzyk N, Felbamate. Chemistry and biotransformation. In: Levy R, Mattson RJ, Meldrum BS, eds. *Antiepileptic drugs*, 4th ed. New York: Raven Press, 1995:799–806.
4. Ramsay RE, Slater JD, Antiepileptic drugs in clinical development. *Epilepsy Res Suppl* 1993;10:45–67.
5. Schechter PJ, Tranier Y, Jung MJ, et al. Audiogenic seizure protection by elevated brain GABA concentration in mice: effects of gamma-acetylenic GABA and gamma-vinyl GABA, two irreversible GABA-T inhibitors. *Eur J Pharmacol* 1977;45:319–328.
6. White H, Woodhead JS, Franklin MR, et al. Experimental selection, quantification and evaluation of antiepileptic drugs. In: Levy R, Mattson RH, Medrum BS, eds. *Antiepileptic drugs*, 4th ed. New York: Raven Press, 1995:99–110.
7. Chadwick D. Gabapentin: clinical use. In: Levy R, Mattson RH, Medrum BS, eds. *Antiepileptic drugs*, 4th ed. New York: Raven Press, 1995:851–856.
8. Taylor C. Gabapentin: mechanism of action. In: Levy R, Mattson RH, Medrum BS, eds. *Antiepileptic drugs*, 4th ed. New York: Raven Press, 1995:829–841.
9. Danober L, Deransart C, Depaulis A, et al. Pathophysiological mechanisms of genetic absence epilepsy in the rat. *Prog Neurobiol* 1998;55:27–57.
10. Coulter DA, McIntyre DC, Loscher W. Animal models of limbic epilepsies: what can they tell us? *Brain Pathol* 2002;12:240–256.
11. Loscher W. Animal models of epilepsy for the development of antiepileptogenic and disease-modifying drugs. A comparison of the pharmacology of kindling and post-status epilepticus models of temporal lobe epilepsy. *Epilepsy Res* 2002;50:105–123.
12. Stables JP, Bertram EH, White HS, et al. Models for epilepsy and epileptogenesis: report from the NIH workshop, Bethesda, Maryland. *Epilepsia* 2002;43:1410–1420.
13. Meldrum B. Do preclinical seizure models preselect certain adverse effects of antiepileptic drugs. *Epilepsy Res* 2002;50:33–40.
14. Honack D, Loscher W. Kindling increases the sensitivity of rats to adverse effects of certain antiepileptic drugs. *Epilepsia* 1995;36:763–771.
15. Snead OC III. Gamma-hydroxybutyrate model of generalized absence seizures: further characterization and comparison with other absence models. *Epilepsia* 1988;29:361–368.
16. Cereghino JJ, Kupferberg HJ. Preclinical testing. *Epilepsy Res Suppl* 1993;10:19–30.
17. Cereghino J. The Food and Drug Administration. In: Resor SR, Kutt H, eds. *The medical treatment of epilepsy*. New York: Marcel Dekker, 1993:699–712.
18. Morrell MJ. Issues for women in antiepileptic drug development. *Adv Neurol* 1998;76:149–159.
19. Olney JW, Labruyere J, Wong G, et al. NMDA antagonist neurotoxicity: mechanism and prevention. *Science* 1991;254:1515–1518.
20. Gibson JP, Yarrington JT, Loudy DE, et al. Chronic toxicity studies with vigabatrin, a GABA-transaminase inhibitor. *Toxicol Pathol* 1990;18:225–238.
21. Eke T, Talbot JF, Lawden MC. Severe persistent visual field constriction associated with vigabatrin. *BMJ* 1997;314:180–181.
22. French J, Smith M, Faught E, et al. Practice advisory: the use of felbamate in the treatment of patients with intractable epilepsy: report of the Quality Standards Subcommittee of the American Academy of Neurology and the American Epilepsy Society. *Neurology* 1999;52:1540–1545.
23. Browne TR. Clinical trials performed for the new drug approval process in the United States: standard methods and alternative methods. *Epilepsy Res Suppl* 1993;10:31–44.
24. Schmidt D. Proof of principle trials: exploratory open studies. *Epilepsy Res* 2001;45:15–18.
25. Porter RJ. New antiepileptic agents: strategies for drug development. *Lancet* 1990;336:423–424.
26. Motte J, Trevathan E, Arvidsson JF, et al. Lamotrigine for generalized seizures associated with the Lennox-Gastaut syndrome. Lamictal Lennox-Gastaut Study Group. *N Engl J Med* 1997;337:1807–1812.
27. Sachdeo RC, Glauser TA, Ritter F, et al. A double-blind, randomized trial of topiramate in Lennox-Gastaut syndrome. Topiramate YL Study Group. *Neurology* 1999;52:1882–1887.
28. Biton V, Montouris GD, Ritter F, et al. A randomized, placebo-controlled study of topiramate in primary generalized tonic-clonic seizures. Topiramate YTC Study Group. *Neurology* 1999;52:1330–1337.
29. Temkin NR, Wilensky AS. New AEDs: are the compounds or the studies ineffective? *Epilepsia* 1986;27:644–645.
30. The Felbamate Study Group in Lennox-Gastaut Syndrome. Efficacy of felbamate in childhood epileptic encephalopathy (Lennox-Gastaut syndrome). *N Engl J Med* 1993;328:29–33.
31. Brummel GL. The FDA drug approval process: focus on pediatric labeling. *Neonatal Netw* 2001;20:49–51.
32. Ouellet D, Bockbrader HN, Wesche DL, et al. Population pharmacokinetics of gabapentin in infants and children. *Epilepsy Res* 2001;47:229–241.
33. French JA, Leppik I. Testing antiepileptic drugs in children. *J Child Neurol* 1994;9(Suppl 1):S26–S32.
34. Sheridan PH, Jacobs MP. The development of antiepileptic drugs for children. Report from the NIH workshop, Bethesda, Maryland, February 17–18, 1994. *Epilepsy Res* 1996;23:87–92.

35. Katz R. The domestic drug regulatory process: why time is of the essence. *Epilepsy Res Suppl* 1993;10:91–106.
36. Merkatz RB, Temple R, Subel S, et al. Women in clinical trials of new drugs. A change in Food and Drug Administration policy. The Working Group on Women in Clinical Trials. *N Engl J Med* 1993; 329:292–296.
37. Morrell MJ. Reproductive and metabolic disorders in women with epilepsy. *Epilepsia* 2003;44(Suppl 4):11–20.
38. The Group for the Evaluation of Cinromide in the Lennox-Gastaut Syndrome. Double-blind, placebo-controlled evaluation of cinromide in patients with the Lennox-Gastaut Syndrome. *Epilepsia* 1989;30:422–429.
39. French JA, Schachter S. A workshop on antiepileptic drug monotherapy indications. *Epilepsia* 2002;4(Suppl 10):3–27.
40. Reife RA, Pledger GW. Topiramate as adjunctive therapy in refractory partial epilepsy: pooled analysis of data from five double-blind, placebo-controlled trials. *Epilepsia* 1997;38(Suppl 1):S31–S33.
41. Mattson RH, Cramer JA, Collins JF, et al. Comparison of carbamazepine, phenobarbital, phenytoin, and primidone in partial and secondarily generalized tonic-clonic seizures. *N Engl J Med* 1985;313:145–151.
42. Leber PD. Hazards of inference: the active control investigation. *Epilepsia* 1989;30(Suppl 1):S57–S63.
43. Gilliam F, Vazquez B, Sackellares JC, et al. An active-control trial of lamotrigine monotherapy for partial seizures. *Neurology* 1998;51: 1018–1025.
44. Sachdeo RC, Reife RA, Lim P, et al. Topiramate monotherapy for partial onset seizures. *Epilepsia* 1997;38:294–300.
45. Sachdeo R, Kramer LD, Rosenberg A, et al. Felbamate monotherapy: controlled trial in patients with partial onset seizures. *Ann Neurol* 1992;32:386–392.
46. Theodore WH, Raubertas RF, Porter RJ, et al. Felbamate: a clinical trial for complex partial seizures. *Epilepsia* 1991;32:392–397.
47. Sachdeo R, Wagner ML, Sachdeo S, et al. Coadministration of phenytoin and felbamate: evidence of additional phenytoin dose-reduction requirements based on pharmacokinetics and tolerability with increasing doses of felbamate. *Epilepsia* 1999;40:1122–1128.
48. Faught E, Sachdeo RC, Remler MP, et al. Felbamate monotherapy for partial-onset seizures: an active-control trial. *Neurology* 1993; 43:688–692.
49. Pledger GW, Kramer LD. Clinical trials of investigational antiepileptic drugs: monotherapy designs. *Epilepsia* 1991;32: 716–721.
50. Devinsky O, Faught RE, Wilder BJ, et al. Efficacy of felbamate monotherapy in patients undergoing presurgical evaluation of partial seizures. *Epilepsy Res* 1995;20:241–246.
51. Bergey GK, Morris HH, Rosenfeld W, et al. Gabapentin monotherapy: I. An 8-day, double-blind, dose-controlled, multicenter study in hospitalized patients with refractory complex partial or secondarily generalized seizures. The US Gabapentin Study Group 88/89. *Neurology* 1997;49:739–745.
52. Schachter SC, Vazquez B, Fisher RS, et al. Oxcarbazepine: double-blind, randomized, placebo-control, monotherapy trial for partial seizures. *Neurology* 1999;52:732–737.
53. Bourgeois B, Leppik IE, Sackellares JC, et al. Felbamate: a double-blind controlled trial in patients undergoing presurgical evaluation of partial seizures. *Neurology* 1993;43:693–696.
54. Beydoun A, Fischer J, Labar DR, et al. Gabapentin monotherapy: II. A 26-week, double-blind, dose-controlled, multicenter study of conversion from polytherapy in outpatients with refractory complex partial or secondarily generalized seizures. The US Gabapentin Study Group 82/83. *Neurology* 1997;49: 746–752.
55. Beydoun A, Sachdeo RC, Rosenfeld WE, et al. Oxcarbazepine monotherapy for partial-onset seizures: a multicenter, double-blind, clinical trial. *Neurology* 2000;54:245–251.
56. Brodie MJ, Richens A, Yuen AW. Double-blind comparison of lamotrigine and carbamazepine in newly diagnosed epilepsy. UK Lamotrigine/Carbamazepine Monotherapy Trial Group. *Lancet* 1995;345:476–479.
57. Brodie MJ, Overstall PW, Giorgi L. Multicentre, double-blind, randomised comparison between lamotrigine and carbamazepine in elderly patients with newly diagnosed epilepsy. The UK Lamotrigine Elderly Study Group. *Epilepsy Res* 1999;37;81–87.
58. Chadwick DW, Anhut H, Greiner MJ, et al. A double-blind trial of gabapentin monotherapy for newly diagnosed partial seizures. International Gabapentin Monotherapy Study Group 945–977. *Neurology* 1998;51:1282–1288.
59. Bill PA, Vigonius U, Pohlmann H, et al. A double-blind controlled clinical trial of oxcarbazepine versus phenytoin in adults with previously untreated epilepsy. *Epilepsy Res* 1997;27: 195–204.
60. Chadwick D. Safety and efficacy of vigabatrin and carbamazepine in newly diagnosed epilepsy: a multicentre randomised double-blind study. Vigabatrin European Monotherapy Study Group. *Lancet* 1999;354:13–19.
61. Chadwick D, Privitera M. Placebo-controlled studies in neurology: where do they stop? *Neurology* 1999;52:682–685.
62. Karlawish JHT, French J. The ethical and scientific shortcomings of current monotherapy epilepsy trials in newly diagnosed patients. *Epilepsy Behav* 2001;2:193–200.
63. UK Gabapentin Study Group. Gabapentin in partial epilepsy. *Lancet* 1990;335:1114–1117.
64. French JA, Kugler AR, Robbins JL, et al. Dose-response trial of pregabalin adjunctive therapy in patients with partial seizures. *Neurology* 2003;60:1631–1637.
65. Baker GA, Smith DW, Dewey M, et al. The development of a seizure severity scale as an outcome measure in epilepsy. *Epilepsy Res* 1991;8:245–251.
66. Cramer JA, French J. Quantitative assessment of seizure severity for clinical trials: a review of approaches to seizure components. *Epilepsia* 2001;42:119–129.
67. Cramer JA. Quality of life as an outcome measure for epilepsy clinical trials. *Pharm World Sci* 1997;19:227–230.

Pharmacokinetics and Pharmacodynamics of Antiepileptic Drugs

45

Blaise F. D. Bourgeois

The principles of pharmacokinetics and pharmacodynamics are heavily rooted in mathematics and may, at first, appear far removed from clinical practice. However, these disciplines of pharmacology provide powerful tools for the optimal use of antiepileptic and other drugs. Pharmacokinetics refers to drug concentrations in the body and their changes over time as a function of absorption, distribution, and elimination (what the body does to the drug). Pharmacodynamics describes the action of drugs (what the drug does to the body), especially in the target organ. Many who study these concepts do not routinely treat patients, and many involved in patient care tend to regard these concepts as less-than-useful tools for everyday clinical practice. In an effort to bridge these gaps, this chapter emphasizes the practical relevance of pharmacokinetic and pharmacodynamic principles to the treatment of patients with epilepsy.

BASIC PHARMACOKINETIC PARAMETERS

Only five or six pharmacokinetic parameters determine the blood level of a drug in a patient at any given time following a single or repeated dose by any route of administration. This concentration is a function only of extent and rate of absorption, distribution within the body, and rate of conversion or elimination (Table 45.1). Table 45.2 summarizes the main pharmacokinetic parameters, and Table 45.3 summarizes the recommended therapeutic ranges and average doses of several commonly used benzodiazepines and antiepileptic drugs (AEDs).

Absorption Parameters

Bioavailability

The amount of an administered dose that will reach the bloodstream, that is, bioavailability (F) for fraction, is a function of the route of administration and the drug preparation. Bioavailability becomes an issue in clinical practice only when one of these factors is changed, and knowing the relative bioavailability of a drug may be important. After intravenous (IV) administration, bioavailability is 1, or 100%. The absolute bioavailability can be calculated by comparing IV absorption with the absorption of a drug by any other route. If a drug cannot be administered intravenously, the relative bioavailability of two routes or two preparations can be calculated; this is often sufficient for clinical purposes. Bioavailability is usually determined by calculating the surface under the drug concentration-versus-time curve, that is, the area under the curve (AUC), following a single dose by two different routes, x and y, or for preparations x and y of the same drug, according to the following equation:

$$F_x = \frac{\text{AUC}_x}{\text{AUC}_y} = \frac{C_{SSx}}{C_{SSy}} \tag{1}$$

A correction is necessary if the doses for x and y are different. This equation also shows that F can be estimated by comparing steady-state concentrations (C_{SS}), a less precise method, because C_{SS} fluctuates throughout the day according to drug intake; and even if obtained at the same time of day, C_{SS} values are less reproducible than is the AUC. In addition, steady-state conditions must be achieved for both preparations or both routes, which can be impractical with IV or rectal administration.

TABLE 45.1
PHARMACOKINETIC PARAMETERS

Absorption parameters	Extent (bioavailability, F)
Distribution parameters	Rate (absorption constant, k_{abs})
Rate of elimination	Volume of distribution (V_d)
	Rate (distribution constant, α)
	Linear: elimination constant (β or k_{el}) or half-life ($t_{1/2}$)
	Saturable:
	Maximal elimination velocity (V_{max})
	Michaelis constant (K_m)

An example of bioavailability determination for different routes of administration is provided by a study (1) in which the relative bioavailability of sodium valproate was calculated for the oral solution, enteric-coated tablets, and suppositories by comparing AUCs over 24 hours at steady state. Bioavailability was similar for the three preparations, and only absorption rates differed. A comparison between different galenic preparations of the same drug, with C_{SS} used as a measure of bioavailability, is found in a report (2) on decreasing levels of primidone after the trademark product was replaced by the generic form. The levels returned to their initial values after reintroduction of the proprietary product. Unlike other AEDs, gabapentin has saturable dose-related bioavailability. As single doses increase, bioavailability can decrease from 60% to 30% (3). This may require fractionated four-times-daily administration at high doses.

Absorption Rate
Although the rate of absorption receives less attention from clinicians than do elimination parameters, it is just as important for optimal patient management, and the kinetic principles are the same for both. Absorption is generally a first-order (or exponential) process with a half-life, or constant (k_{abs}), that is the equivalent of the elimination constant (k_{el}). Rapid absorption is desirable when a rapid effect is necessary but is usually undesirable during long-term therapy, because it accentuates fluctuations in concentration and necessitates shorter dosage intervals with smaller doses. Ideally, every AEDs should be available as a parenteral solution for IV administration and as a slow-release preparation for long-term use. The slow-release form is not necessary if the agent has a very long elimination half-life ($t_{1/2}$), as does phenobarbital.

TABLE 45.2
PHARMACOKINETIC PARAMETERS OF ANTIEPILEPTIC DRUGS

	F (%)	T_{max} (hours)	V_d (L/kg)	Protein Binding (%)	$t_{1/2}$ (hours)	T_{ss} (days)	Therapeutic Range (mg/L)	Therapeutic Range (µmol/L)	Dose (mg/kg/day)
Bromide	>90	—	0.4	0	268	36–48	—	10–20 mEq/L	50–100
Carbamazepine	75–85	4–12	0.8–2	75	20–50[a] 5–20[a]	20–30[a]	3–12	12–50	10–30
Ethosuximide	>90	1–4	0.65	<10	30–60	7	40–100	300–700	10–40
Felbamate	>90	2–6	0.75	25	13–23	4	—	—	40–80
Gabapentin	30–60	2–3	0.85	0	5–9	2	—	—	30–40
Lamotrigine	>90	1–3	1.0	55	12–60	3–1	—	—	1–15
Levetiracetam	>95	1	0.5–0.7	0	6–8	2	—	—	30–60
Mephenytoin									5–10
Normephenytoin	—	—	—	—	70–140	15–20	15–35	70–150	
Methsuximide									10–30
Normethsuximide	—	—	—	55	30–50	7	10–50	50–250	15–30
Oxcarbazepine	>90	1–3		60			—	—	
10-OH-carbamazepine		4–6	0.7–0.8	40	10–15	2	8–20	30–80	
Phenobarbital	>90	0.5	0.55	45	65–110	15–20	10–30	40–130	2–5
Phenytoin	>90	2–12	0.75	90	10–60b	15–20	3–20	12–80	5–10
Primidone	>90	2–4	0.75	<10	8–15	—	—	—	10–20
Tiagabine	>90	1–2		96	3–8	1–2	—	—	0.1–1
Topiramate	>80	1–4	0.65	15	12–30	3–5	—	—	5–9
Valproate	>90	1–8[c]	0.16	70–93[b]	5–15	2	50–100	350–700	15–30
Vigabatrin	>80	0.5–2	0.8	0	5–8	2	—	—	40–100
Zonisamide	—	2–5	1.5	55	50–70	10–15	20–30	100–150	4–8

Abbreviations: F, indicates bioavailability; Protein binding, fraction bound to serum proteins; Therapeutic range, therapeutic range of serum concentration; $t_{1/2}$, elimination half-time; T_{max}, time interval between ingestion and maximal serum concentration; T_{ss}, steady-state time; V_d, volume or distribution.
[a]Steady-state values for half-life and serum levels are reached only after complete autoinduction.
[b]Concentration dependent.
[c]Absorption of enteric-coated tablets is delayed.

TABLE 45.3

PHARMACOKINETIC PARAMETERS OF BENZODIAZEPINES

	F (%)	T_{max} (hours)	V_d (L/kg)	Protein Binding (%)	$t_{1/2}$ (hours)	T_{ss} (days)	Therapeutic Range (μg/L)	(μmol/L)	Dose (mg/kg/day)
Clonazepam	>90	1–4	3.0	85	20–40	6	20–75	0.1–0.15	60–250
Nitrazepam	>80	1–4	1.5–3	85	20–30	5	<200	<700	0.5–1.0
Diazepam	>90	1	1–2	95	36	7	100–700	350–2,500	0.2–0.5
Nordazepam	>90	0.5–2	1–1.5	97	60–100	15	500–2,000	1,200–5,000	—
Clobazam	>90	1–4	—	—	10–30	—	—	—	0.5–2.0
Norclobazam	—	—	—	85	36–46	10	—	—	—
Lorazepam	>90	1.5–2	1.0	90	15	3	20–30	60–90	—

Abbreviations: F, indicates bioavailability; Protein binding, fraction bound to serum proteins; Therapeutic range, therapeutic range of serum concentration; $t_{1/2}$, elimination half-time; T_{max}, time interval between ingestion and maximal serum concentration; T_{ss}, steady-state time; V_d, volume or distribution.

A common misconception is that the enteric-coated form of sodium valproate, or divalproex sodium, is a slow-release preparation. Enteric-coated valproate is not absorbed before it reaches the small intestine, but once the gastric-resistant coating has been dissolved, absorption is rapid. Figure 45.1 shows serum levels of valproate after a single, first oral dose with a meal. For up to 7 hours after oral intake, valproate was not detectable in the blood, but absorption proceeded rapidly thereafter. This concentration curve indicated a delayed but fast absorption, whereas the slow-release preparations are absorbed slowly. Because of this delayed absorption of enteric-coated valproate, the lowest serum concentration of the day during long-term intake is not before the first morning dose, but usually around noon or early afternoon (1). Consequently, the morning "trough" level is a misnomer. This does not apply to the enteric-coated sprinkle capsules of divalproex sodium.

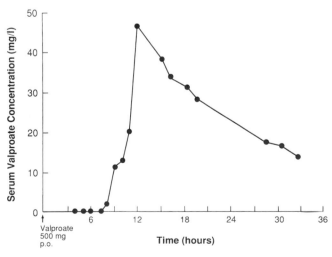

Figure 45.1 Serum concentrations of valproate after a 500-mg single, first oral dose of enteric-coated divalproex sodium in a 60.4-kg woman. The medication was taken with a meal.

Distribution Parameters

Once a drug reaches the blood, regardless of the route of administration, it will diffuse into other body fluids and various tissues until an equilibrium is reached. The extent of distribution is expressed by the volume of distribution (V_d), which often has no anatomic boundaries. The V_d is the hypothetical volume whose calculation is based on the assumption that drug concentration equals concentration in blood plasma throughout this volume (often not the case). Thus, V_d can be determined by dividing the IV dose (D_{IV}) by the increase in blood level (ΔC) associated with this dose. This is the same as the total amount of drug in the body (Q) divided by the blood concentration (C):

$$V_d = \frac{D_{IV}}{\Delta C} = \frac{Q}{C} \qquad [2]$$

The V_d is usually expressed as a relative value in liters per kilogram. In a 70-kg adult, a relative V_d of 0.5 L/kg corresponds to an absolute V_d of 35 L. Because body water represents approximately 60% of body weight, a drug with a V_d >0.6 L/kg must be assumed to be bound to certain tissue components. A decrease in serum protein binding can result in a higher value for V_d, which is based on total serum levels. Moreover, depending on the affinity of a drug for adipose tissue, V_d (L/kg) can be larger or smaller in obese individuals.

Although V_d is a theoretical concept, it has practical clinical usefulness by providing the ratio necessary to calculate the dose to load a patient rapidly to a desired blood level. Equation 2 can be solved for the dose ($D = V_d \times \Delta C$) or for the concentration ($\Delta C = D/V_d$). For example, an IV dose of 18 to 20 mg/kg phenytoin or phenobarbital is the standard treatment for status epilepticus. Because the V_d of phenytoin is about 0.75 L/kg, the concentration after the infusion will be 20/0.75 = 26.7 mg/L—adequate for a peak concentration. The V_d of phenobarbital is approximately 0.55 L/kg, yielding a peak concentration of 20/0.55 = 36.4 mg/L.

The dose for reloading to a desired level can also be calculated. Let us assume that the phenytoin level is 15 mg/L and the desired level is 25 mg/L. The necessary dose will be $(25 - 15) \times 0.75 = 7.5$ mg/kg. In nonurgent situations, loading with a drug need not be limited to the IV route and can be extended over any length of time; however, the desired level will be attained only if the maintenance dose for this level is given in addition to the loading dose during the loading period.

For example, let us assume that a 67-kg adult is estimated to require a phenytoin maintenance dose of 400 mg per day, or 6 mg/kg, to achieve a steady-state level of 18 mg/L. The patient has not yet received any phenytoin, and the goal is to reach a level of about 18 mg/L within 48 hours. This will be achieved if the patient receives a loading dose of $67 \times 0.75 \times 18 = 904.5$ mg + 800 mg, the latter being the maintenance dose for 48 hours. The total dose of approximately 1700 mg can be spread evenly over 48 hours: three 300-mg doses the first day, and 300 mg, 300 mg, and 200 mg the second day. Administering only the 900-mg loading dose over 2 days will yield a level well below 18 mg/L, because during that time, elimination of phenytoin by the liver will be ongoing.

If the final concentration equilibrium of a drug is reached rapidly following IV administration, distribution is said to occur according to a one-compartment model. If, however, a drug is rapidly distributed into one compartment but then slowly diffuses into a second and even a third compartment, distribution occurs according to a two- or three-compartment model. The total V_d will correspond to the sum of these two or three compartments. After a single IV injection, biexponential or triexponential decrease of the blood concentration will occur. Under steady-state conditions, the serum concentrations will be determined by the total, or largest, V_d; the distinction between two or three different V_d values is usually of little importance. An exception is during rapid administration and loading, because the V_d will initially be small and will increase with

time. This will require repeated administration of the agent to maintain a given blood level.

The rate at which a drug diffuses into the second or third compartment is usually expressed as the distribution half-life, or distribution constant α, as opposed to the elimination half-life, or elimination constant β. This distinction is discussed in the section "Elimination Parameters." A classic example of a two-compartment model is diazepam, which is commonly administered intravenously in patients with status epilepticus. Blood levels of diazepam decrease rapidly under these circumstances, with a half-life of 1 hour or less. This is actually a distribution half-life; the true $t_{1/2}$ of diazepam is about 36 hours.

Elimination Parameters

As soon as a drug is present in circulating blood, elimination from the bloodstream begins via enzymatic biotransformation in the liver, directly by the kidneys in an unmetabolized form, or through both processes. This elimination is clinically important because it determines both the rate at which the drug concentration will decrease once absorption is complete and the rate at which the drug will need to be replaced if a certain concentration is to be maintained.

Linear Elimination Kinetics

For most drugs, elimination is said to follow linear kinetics, which means that all processes occur in a linearly proportional fashion. For example, the number of drug molecules that will circulate through the liver or the kidneys will be twice as high for a blood concentration of 20 mg/L as for one of 10 mg/L; consequently, per unit of time, twice as many drug molecules will be metabolized by hepatic enzymes or filtrated by glomeruli at 20 mg/L as at 10 mg/L. This also means that the blood concentration will decrease twice as fast at 20mg/L as at 10 mg/L, resulting in an exponential decay curve for the drug concentration or a linear fall if the concentration is plotted on a logarithmic scale (Fig. 45.2). The slope of the second straight segment in Figure 45.2B is called β, or elimination constant k_{el}. Its units are usually

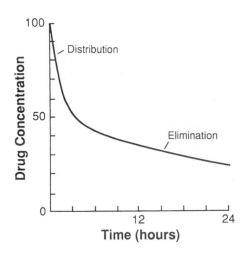

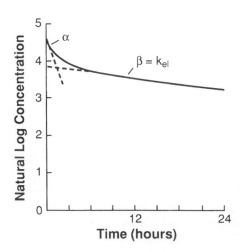

Figure 45.2 Linear elimination kinetics in a two-compartment model. **A:** Concentration and time on a linear scale; **(B)** concentration on a logarithmic scale. α, slope of the distribution phase; β, slope of the elimination phase, which is equal to k_{el}, elimination constant.

hours^{-1} or 1/hour, and it represents the fraction of drug eliminated per hour, this fraction being constant by definition. The half-life of the drug can be calculated from the value of k_{el}, the relationship being $t_{1/2} = \ln 2/k_{el} = 0.693/k_{el}$.

Following IV administration, the concentration (C_t) as a function of time is

$$C_t = C_0 \times e^{-k_{el} \times t} \qquad [3]$$

in which C_0 is the concentration at time 0 following the IV administration.

Although the basic pharmacokinetic elimination parameter is k_{el}, the concept of half-life is more useful clinically and helps to determine (a) how long it will take for a concentration to decrease from 40 to 20, from 20 to 10, or from 10 to 5; (b) how often the agent needs to be administered during long-term treatment (if possible, at least once every half-life); and (c) how long before steady-state levels are reached if the drug is introduced at a constant daily dose. The slope of the first straight segment in Figure 45.2B is the distribution constant α. With the use of this slope, the distribution half-life can be calculated as $\ln 2/\alpha$ by means of Equation 3. Drugs with rapid distribution into one compartment have a negligible distribution half-life. As discussed, drug absorption is most often a first-order process. If absorption is regarded as a linear elimination from the intestinal lumen, the same concept can be used as for elimination (Fig. 45.2), resulting in an absorption constant (k_{abs}) and an absorption half-life. The absorption half-life can be calculated only indirectly, because absorption and elimination always occur simultaneously, whereas elimination can occur alone once absorption is complete.

Nonlinear Elimination Kinetics

As noted, at a concentration of 20 mg/L, twice as many drug molecules will circulate through the liver per unit of time, and twice as many molecules will undergo enzymatic biotransformation as at a concentration of 10 mg/L. This is true as long as the corresponding enzymes are not becoming saturated and can continue to bind additional drug molecules. Phenytoin differs from other AEDs in that the enzymes responsible for most of its elimination are already partially saturated at concentrations within the recommended therapeutic range. As the concentration increases, the enzymes will no longer be able to increase the rate of biotransformation proportionally, and the linear kinetic model will no longer apply. The kinetics are now called concentration-dependent, or saturable, and there is no true half-life because the time required for the concentration to decrease by 50% of its value becomes progressively longer at higher concentrations. Steady-state levels of phenytoin increase disproportionately as the maintenance dose is increased.

The kinetics of enzymatic activity have been elucidated *in vitro* by biochemists, and no attempt will be made to elaborate on this theory. The parameters, however, can be translated into simple clinical concepts useful in the daily routine. Let us consider the patient's V_d as a huge test tube and the liver as the enzymes in the test tube that are involved in phenytoin biotransformation. Every patient has a given number of enzyme molecules in his or her liver that become progressively saturated as the phenytoin concentration increases. The patient's maximal reaction velocity (V_{max}) is reached when all enzyme molecules are continuously saturated and working at maximal capacity. Theoretically, this state of saturation is attained only at an infinitely high drug concentration. Maximum reaction velocity is not an abstract concept, but can be expressed in milligrams per day or milligrams per kilogram per day. Average adult values for V_{max} of phenytoin are about 8 mg/kg per day; this means that the liver of a normal 70-kg patient cannot metabolize more than about 560 mg phenytoin per 20 hours. If the patient ingests 600 mg per day, each day's drug intake will exceed the elimination rate, and at least 40 mg, or 0.57 mg/kg, will accumulate. With an assumed V_d of 0.75 L/kg and with the use of Equation 1, the patient's blood level will increase indefinitely by at least 0.76 mg/L every day for as long as this dose is taken. This relatively small, yet persistent increase may be overlooked for a few days, but will invariably result in toxic levels after 1 week or less than 1 month. The maintenance dose should always be lower than the V_{max}.

The second parameter for saturable kinetics is the Michaelis constant (K_m)—the blood level at which one-half of V_{max} is reached. For phenytoin, the average value in adult or pediatric patients is about 6 mg/L, or 6 µg/mL. The K_m reflects the binding affinity between the enzyme and the drug, and its value is inversely proportional to this affinity. How V_{max} and K_m can be used to calculate dose requirements or to predict a steady-state level at a given dose is discussed in the next section.

STEADY STATE AND CLEARANCE

When a drug is introduced at a constant daily dose, the levels initially will be low, the amount eliminated per day will be smaller than the daily dose, and the drug concentration will increase. As concentration increases, so does elimination, until it equals the daily maintenance dose. This final concentration is the C_{SS}. The maintenance dose is best viewed as the daily replacement dose necessary to match drug elimination and thus maintain C_{SS}. At a constant daily dose, 97% of C_{SS} is reached after five elimination half-lives of the drug. Because antiepileptic therapy is long-term in most patients, steady-state levels are particularly important in therapeutic monitoring. For any drug with linear elimination kinetics, the ratio between maintenance dose (or dose per unit of time, D/t) and the C_{SS} is constant and is equal to the clearance (Cl):

$$\frac{Cl}{Css} = D/t \qquad [4]$$

Far from being an abstract entity, clearance is probably the most clinically relevant parameter in long-term antiepileptic therapy. This ratio indicates the maintenance dose necessary to achieve a desired level, as well as the expected level at a given D/t. It can be calculated by turning Equation 4 around:

$$\frac{D}{t} = Cl \times C_{SS} \qquad [4']$$

It is best to express D/t in milligrams per kilogram per day, C_{SS} in milligrams per liter, and clearance in liters per kilogram per day. Drug clearance does not differ from creatinine clearance (24-hour urinary creatinine excretion/plasma creatinine). Plasma creatinine is a steady-state level, and 24-hour urinary excretion of creatinine is the equivalent of the maintenance (replacement) dose.

If C_{SS} is determined at a given D/t, clearance can be calculated according to Equation 4. For example, a C_{SS} of 9.6 mg/L at a daily dose of 20 mg/kg corresponds to a clearance of 2.08 L/kg per day. Because bioavailability may be incomplete, this value is more precisely called "apparent total body clearance" or "oral clearance." Clearance can also be calculated by taking population values for V_d and half-life (Table 45.2) and using the following equation (half-life should be expressed in days):

$$Cl = V_d \times k_{el} = \frac{V_d \times 0.693}{t_{1/2}} \qquad [5]$$

Using carbamazepine as an example, let us assume a V_d of 1.5 L/kg and a half-life of 12 hours, or 0.5 day. According to Equation 5, these values give a clearance of 2.08 L/kg per day. Calculated from Equation 4', the maintenance dose for a desired average concentration of 10 mg/L in a 60-kg adult is 20.8 mg/kg per day, or 1247 mg per day. Of course, the clearance of carbamazepine is not about 2 L/kg per hour for every patient, and large interindividual differences can occur, mostly because of enzymatic induction by other AEDs administered concomitantly, such as phenytoin or phenobarbital. In addition, clearance increases by a factor of 2 to 3 in any given patient during the first 2 to 3 weeks of therapy, because of the well-known enzymatic autoinduction of carbamazepine metabolism (4). For these reasons, it may often be necessary to determine carbamazepine clearance by giving a single oral dose. Clearance can also be determined after one single dose (D) by calculating the AUC from time 0 to infinity (AUC$_{0-\infty}$; Fig. 45.3):

$$Cl = \frac{D}{AUC_{0-\infty}} \qquad [6]$$

If, for example, the AUC$_{0-\infty}$ is 115 mg × hour/L after a single 10-mg/kg dose, clearance will be 0.087 L/kg per hour, or 2.09 L/kg per day. Pharmacokinetics software allows calculation of k_{abs}, V_d, k_{el}, and clearance by nonlinear regression analysis of time versus concentration points following a single drug dose.

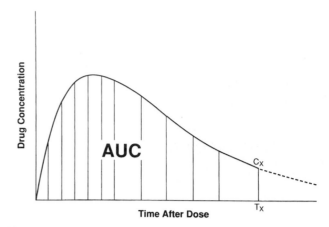

Figure 45.3 Concentration-versus-time curve after a single oral dose of a drug given at time 0. The area under the curve (AUC) can be calculated by dividing the curve into trapezoids for each interval between measured concentrations. To calculate the remaining AUC after the last sampling time x, the log/linear slope of the elimination phase (k$_{el}$) is determined, and the AUC from time x to infinity is C$_x$/k$_{el}$.

For drugs with nonlinear elimination kinetics, such as phenytoin, the concept of clearance cannot be applied as above, because clearance decreases at higher D/t values or higher concentrations (5,6). Steady-state kinetics of drugs with saturable elimination can be adequately expressed only by using the two elimination parameters V_{max} and K_m. Equations 7 and 8 summarize the relationship between D/t and steady-state blood level:

$$D/t = \frac{V_{max} \times C_{SS}}{K_m + C_{SS}} \qquad [7]$$

$$C_{SS} = \frac{K_m \times D/t}{V_{max} - D/t} \qquad [8]$$

Average values in adults are about 8 mg/kg per day for V_{max} and 6 mg/L for K_m. Let us use Equation 7 to calculate the average maintenance dose of phenytoin for an average steady-state level of 15 mg/L. The V_{max} dose of 8 mg/kg per day × 15 mg/L is divided by 6 mg/L + 15 mg/L and equals 5.7 mg/kg per day. This corresponds to a dose of 343 mg per day in a 60-kg adult and 429 mg per day in a 75-kg adult. The latter is well above the "standard" D/t of 300 mg per day, which in most adults does not provide adequate therapeutic levels.

Equation 8 can be used to calculate the steady-state phenytoin levels achieved with a dose of 300 mg per day in the same two patients. In the 60-kg patient, 300 mg per day is 5 mg/kg per day, and C_{SS} will be 6 mg/L × 5 mg/kg per day divided by 8 mg/kg per day − 5 mg/kg per day to equal 10 mg/L. In the 75-kg patient, 300 mg per day is 4 mg/kg per day and C_{SS} will be 6 mg/L. Equation 8 also expresses the nonlinearity of the dose-level relationship. A dose of 430 mg/day corresponds to a level of 15 mg/L in a 75-kg adult in this example. Changing the dose to 500 mg per day means a 16.3% increase and achieves a C_{SS} of 30 mg/L—a

100% increase over the previous steady-state level. Equation 8 also shows that when the dose is equal to V_{max}, the denominator becomes 0 and C_{SS} will be infinitely high.

Of course, not every patient has V_{max} and K_m values corresponding to the population average. For example, infants may have a V_{max} of 12 to 14 mg/kg per day, and comedication with phenobarbital can elevate the K_m value. The two unknowns, V_{max} and K_m, can be determined if C_{SS} values at two different daily doses (D/t) are available. Equation 9 can be solved for K_m as follows:

$$K_m = \frac{C_{SS1}}{D/t_1} = \left(V_{max} - \frac{D}{t_1}\right) = \frac{C_{SS2}}{D/t_2} = \left(V_{max} - \frac{D}{t_2}\right) \quad [9]$$

Equation 10 can be solved for V_{max} as follows:

$$V_{max} = \frac{C_{SS1} - C_{SS2}}{C_{SS1}/(D/t_1) - C_{SS2}/(D/t_2)} \quad [10]$$

The example of the 75-kg adult with levels of 15 mg/L at 430 mg per day (5.7 mg/kg per day) and 30 mg/L at 500 mg per day (6.67 mg/kg per day) can be used to check this equation; the calculated V_{max} value is 8 mg/kg per day. Once V_{max} is known, K_m can be determined through Equation 9. A reliable C_{SS} value for phenytoin can often be obtained only after 3 weeks of a constant dose. Changes in concentration can occur up to 2 to 3 weeks after a dosage change—the "pseudo–steady-state phenomenon" (7).

In some patients, the nonlinear relationship between phenytoin dose and steady-state levels is such that minimal changes of dose in the therapeutic range will cause major concentration jumps, making it almost impossible to stabilize the patient. Such a steep dose-level relationship within the therapeutic range is independent of V_{max} and is caused by unusually low K_m values. Figure 45.4 shows data from a patient with a V_{max} of 8 mg/kg per day and a K_m of 1.9 mg/L. A level of 10 mg/L is reached at a dose of 6.7 mg/kg per day; the level would be 20 mg/L at 7.3 mg/kg per day. The lower dose is only 8% lower. Thus, in such a patient, a change from tablets (100% phenytoin) to regular sodium phenytoin capsules (100 mg contains 92 mg phenytoin) would be sufficient to lower the phenytoin level from 20 to 10 mg/L, raising the suspicion of poor compliance.

Inversely, a high K_m will bring the dose-level relationship closer to linear kinetics. Figure 45.4 also shows data from a patient with a K_m of 12 mg/L and the same V_{max} value of 8 mg/kg per day. A dose of 5 mg/kg per day achieves a level of 20 mg/L; 10 mg/L would be reached at the 27% lower dose of 3.64 mg/kg per day. One can therefore see in Figure 45.4 that the dose-level curve becomes more linear at the higher K_m value, with the same V_{max} value.

PHARMACOKINETIC AND PHARMACODYNAMIC DRUG INTERACTIONS

Pharmacokinetic Interactions

Most kinetic interactions are caused by inhibition or induction of the enzymatic biotransformation of the AEDs (Table 45.4) (8). Inducing AEDs, which lower the level-to-dose ratio of other agents, are phenytoin, phenobarbital, primidone (either directly or through derived phenobarbital), and carbamazepine. These agents induce the metabolism of carbamazepine, oxcarbazepine monohydroxy

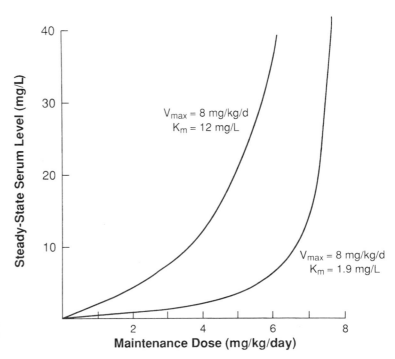

Figure 45.4 Relationship between maintenance dose and steady-state serum levels of phenytoin (see text for details).

derivative (to a lesser degree), valproate, felbamate, lamotrigine (9), topiramate (10), tiagabine, and zonisamide, thus lowering their concentrations. In addition, carbamazepine induces its own elimination (4), a process that is completed in about 3 weeks of daily intake; this autoinduction increases the elimination rate by a factor of approximately 2 to 2.5. Carbamazepine is also an inducer for valproate and an occasional inhibitor for phenytoin (11). The conversion of primidone to phenobarbital is accelerated by phenytoin (12) and carbamazepine (13). Valproate has never been shown to be an enzymatic inducer, and it is known to inhibit the biotransformation of phenobarbital (14), ethosuximide (15), and lamotrigine (9), thus raising their levels. Valproate also inhibits the metabolism of lamotrigine and of carbamazepine-epoxide, the active metabolite, increasing the epoxide concentration (16). Benzodiazepines are not included in Table 45.4, but their concentration-to-dose ratio can also be reduced by the inducing drugs (17,18). In one study, clobazam was found to reduce the clearance of valproate and primidone (19). Gabapentin, levetiracetam, and vigabatrin are neither the cause nor the object of any interactions, except for a possible elevation of felbamate levels by gabapentin (20). Levetiracetam and vigabatrin are not included in Table 45.4. Pharmacokinetic interactions with felbamate are fairly complex. Felbamate elevates levels of phenytoin (21) and valproate (22); it decreases levels of carbamazepine but increases those of its active metabolite, carbamazepine-epoxide (23). Levels of felbamate are decreased by phenytoin and carbamazepine (23); they are not significantly increased by valproate (24). Interactions involving topiramate are characterized by the induction of its elimination

by phenytoin, carbamazepine, phenobarbital, and primidone. These agents decrease the half-life of topiramate from about 24 hours to 12 to 15 hours. Topiramate may cause a modest increase in phenytoin levels. Similarly, the half-life of tiagabine is reduced by approximately 50% with the addition of enzyme-inducing agents (25).

One type of pharmacokinetic interaction not related to enzymatic activity is the displacement from serum proteins, which increases the free fraction of the drug. Although the brain concentration of a drug is assumed to be proportional to the free serum level, measuring total serum levels is appropriate as long as the ratio of free to total concentration (the free fraction) is constant. The free fraction can be altered as a result of displacement by other drugs, in infants and elderly patients, during pregnancy, and in patients with hypoalbuminemia. Displacement from serum proteins is clinically relevant only for highly bound drugs.

For example, the free fraction of serum phenytoin is normally approximately 10% (0.1), the remaining 90% being bound to serum proteins. Thus, at a total of 20 mg/L, the free level is 2.0 mg/L. If 5% of total serum phenytoin is displaced by the addition of valproate (26), the free fraction becomes 0.15, or 15%. At a total level of 20 mg/L, the free level is 3.0 mg/L—the equivalent of a total level of 30 mg/L with a normal free fraction. This 50% increase could produce toxic clinical reactions at a total level usually not associated with such effects. The displacement of phenytoin by valproate was found to be linear and predictable, each 1 mg/L of valproate increasing the free fraction of phenytoin by approximately 0.1% (i.e., at 100 mg/L of valproate, the free fraction of phenytoin is increased from approximately 10% to 20%) (27,28).

TABLE 45.4

PHARMACOKINETIC INTERACTIONS BETWEEN ANTIEPILEPTIC DRUGS

	Effects of the Addition of													
	CBZ	PHT	PB	PRM	VPA	ESM	FBM	GBP	LTG	TPM	TGB	VGB	OXC	ZNS
On Levels of														
Carbamazepine (CBZ)	↓	↓	↓	↓	↑E		↑E						↑E	↑E
Phenytoin (PHT)					↑									
Phenobarbital (PB)				↑										
Primidone (PRM)	↓	↓	↓		↑PB									
Valproate (VPA)	↓	↓	↓	↓			↑							
Ethosuximide (ESM)	↓	↓	↓	↓	↑									
Felbamate (FBM)	↓	↓	↓	↓	↑			↑						
Gabapentin (GBP)														
Lamotrigine (LTG)	↓	↓	↓	↓	↑								↓	
Topiramate (TPM)	↓	↓	↓	↓										
Tiagabine (TGB)	↓	↓	↓	↓										
Vigabatrin (VGB)														
Oxcarbazepine (OXC)	↓	↓	↓	↓										
Zonisamide (ZNS)	↓	↓								↑				

Abbreviations: E, carbamazepine-epoxide only elevated, carbamazepine may be decreased; PB, only elimination of derived phenobarbital affected.

Carbamazepine is approximately 75% bound to serum proteins; therefore, the free fraction is 0.25, or 25%. Normally, a total level of 10 mg/L corresponds to a free level of about 2.5 mg/L. If 5% of total serum carbamazepine is displaced by valproate, the free fraction increases to 0.3, or 30%, and the free level to 3.0, which is the equivalent of a total carbamazepine level of 12.0 mg/L with a normal free fraction. This 20% increase is unlikely to be clinically relevant.

Pharmacokinetic interactions between AEDs and other medications are discussed in the appendix to this chapter.

Pharmacodynamic Interactions

Discussions of drug interactions are usually limited to pharmacokinetic interactions. When two or more AEDs are administered concomitantly, however, it is just as important to consider their pharmacodynamic interaction, because this determines whether use of the combination is justifiable. When two agents are taken simultaneously, their combined effect can be additive (i.e., equal to the expected sum of the individual effects), supra-additive or potentiated (i.e., greater than the expected sum of the individual effects), or infra-additive (i.e., less than the expected additive effect). A supra-additive effect in itself is not sufficient to make a drug combination more effective than either agent used alone, because the upper dose limit of an AED is determined by its dose-related neurotoxicity. Moreover, if the neurotoxic interaction is also supra-additive, the seizure protection provided by the combination at maximal tolerated doses (MTDs) will not be greater than that from the MTD of either drug taken alone. From this quantitative point of view, a combination of two AEDs can be superior only if seizure protection is supra-additive and neurotoxicity is additive or infra-additive, or if seizure protection is additive and neurotoxicity is infra-additive.

Pharmacodynamic interactions between AEDs are more difficult to quantify than are pharmacokinetic interactions, especially in patients, and most of the limited available information was obtained from animal experiments. Table 45.5 summarizes results from some studies in which the interactions were quantified on the basis of brain concentrations in mice (29–31). Most antiepileptic interactions are purely additive, not supra-additive, as is often assumed. The neurotoxic interactions are generally either additive or infra-additive. On the basis of the concept outlined above, only a few AED combinations are potentially superior to the corresponding monotherapies: valproate plus ethosuximide, valproate plus carbamazepine, and valproate plus phenytoin. Although phenobarbital and phenytoin displayed infra-additive neurotoxicity in these experiments, the therapeutic index of phenobarbital alone was so poor that the combination still had a lower therapeutic index than that of phenytoin alone.

Two AEDs can also be more effective than one agent in patients with two seizure types responsive only to two different drugs. Many problems are associated with combination therapy including pharmacokinetic interactions, additive toxicity, a complicated drug regimen, difficulty assessing individual drug efficacy and toxicity, and higher costs. Therefore, two or more AEDs should be prescribed concomitantly only if it can be clearly demonstrated in a given patient that compared with the use of either agent alone, the combination provides better seizure protection with no additional side effects or the same seizure protection with fewer side effects. Otherwise, it is always best to return to monotherapy with the agent that has the best efficacy-to-toxicity ratio.

Only a few systematic clinical studies have suggested pharmacodynamic superiority of AED combinations. Combinations with clinically demonstrated apparent positive synergism include valproate and ethosuximide against absence seizures (32), as well as valproate and lamotrigine (33,34). These combinations appear to have the potential for superiority over use of each agent alone. Carbamazepine and vigabatrin may also have a beneficial synergistic interaction. Among 14 patients with focal epilepsy who failed to respond to monotherapy with carbamazepine and with vigabatrin, 5 (36%) became seizure free when the two agents were prescribed in combination (35). Inversely, certain drug combinations may be detrimental because of

TABLE 45.5

SUMMARY OF PHARMACODYNAMIC INTERACTIONS BETWEEN ANTIEPILEPTIC DRUGS IN ANIMAL MODELS

Drug Pair	Interaction	
	Antiepileptic	Neurotoxic
PHT + PB	Additive	Infra-additive
PHT + CBZ	Additive	Additive
CBZ + PB	Additive	Additive
VPA + BP	Additive	Additive
VPA + ESM	Additive	Infra-additive
VPA + CBZ	Additive	Infra-additive
VPA + PHT	Supra-additive	Additive
VPA + CZP	Supra-additive	Supra-additive
ESM + CZP	Supra-additive	Supra-additive
CBZ + CBZ-E	Additive	Additive
PRM + PB	Supra-additive	Infra-additive
PB + PEMA	Supra-additive	Supra-additive

Abbreviations: CBZ, carbamazepine; CBZ-E, carbamazepine-epoxide; CZP, clonazepam; ESM, ethosuximide; PB, phenobarbital; PEMA, phenylethylmalonamide; PHT, phenytoin; PRM, primidone; VPA, valproate.
Data from Bourgeois BFD, Dodson WE. Antiepileptic and neurotoxic interactions between antiepileptic drugs. In: Pitlick WH, ed. *Antiepileptic drug interactions.* New York: Demos, 1989:209–218; Bourgeois BFD, VanLente F. Effect of clonazepam on antiepileptic potency, neurotoxicity and therapeutic index of valproate and ethosuximide in mice. *Epilepsia* 1994;35(Suppl 8):142; and Chez MG, Bourgeois BFD, Pippinger CE, et al. Pharmacodynamic interactions between phenytoin and valproate: individual and combined antiepileptic and neurotoxic actions in mice. *Clin Neuropharmacol* 994;17:32–37.

exacerbation of side effects. It has been shown that the addition of lamotrigine to carbamazepine may result in symptoms suggestive of carbamazepine toxicity (i.e., diplopia, dizziness) without a change in carbamazepine levels (36).

REFERENCES

1. Issakainen J, Bourgeois BFD. Bioavailability of sodium valproate suppositories during repeated administration at steady-state in epileptic children. *Eur J Pediatr* 1987;146:404–407.
2. Wyllie E, Pippinger CE, Rothner AD. Increased seizure frequency with generic primidone. *JAMA* 1987;258:1216–1217.
3. Gidal B, DeCerce J, Bockbrader H, et al. Gabapentin bioavailability: effect of dose and frequency of administration in adult patients with epilepsy. *Epilepsy Res* 1998;31:91–99.
4. McNamara P, Colburn W, Gibaldi M. Time course of carbamazepine self-induction. *J Pharmacokinet Biopharm* 1979;7:63–68.
5. Arnold K, Gerber N. The rate of decline of diphenylhydantoin in human plasma. *Clin Pharmacol Ther* 1969;11:121–134.
6. Bourgeois BFD, Dodson WE. Phenytoin elimination in newborns. *Neurology* 1983;33:173–178.
7. Theodore W, Qu Z-P, Tsay J-Y, et al. Phenytoin: the pseudosteady-state phenomenon. *Clin Pharmacol Ther* 1984;35:822–825.
8. Bourgeois BFD. Problems of combination drug therapy in children. *Epilepsia* 1988;29(Suppl 3):S20–S24.
9. Eriksson A, Hoppu K, Nergsrdh A, et al. Pharmacokinetic interactions between lamotrigine and other antiepileptic drugs in children with intractable epilepsy. *Epilepsia* 1996;37:769–773.
10. Bourgeois BFD. Drug interaction profile of topiramate. *Epilepsia* 1996;37(Suppl 2):S14–S17.
11. Browne T, Szabo K, Evans J, et al. Carbamazepine increases phenytoin serum concentration and reduces phenytoin clearance. *Neurology* 1988;38:1146–1150.
12. Fincham RW, Schottelius DD, Sahs AL. The influence of diphenylhydantoin on primidone metabolism. *Arch Neurol* 1974;30:259–262.
13. Cloyd JC, Miller KW, Leppik IE. Primidone kinetics: effects of concurrent drugs and duration of therapy. *Clin Pharmacol Ther* 1981;29:402–407.
14. Kapetanovic I, Kupferberg H, Porter R, et al. Mechanism of valproate-phenobarbital interaction in epileptic patients. *Clin Pharmacol Ther* 1981;29:480–486.
15. Mattson RH, Cramer JA. Valproic acid and ethosuximide interaction. *Ann Neurol* 1980;7:583–584.
16. McKauge L, Tyrer H, Eadie M. Factors influencing simultaneous concentrations of carbamazepine and its epoxide in plasma. *Ther Drug Monit* 1981;3:63–70.
17. Bekersky I, Maggio A, Mattaliano VJ, et al. Influence of phenobarbital on the disposition of clonazepam and antipyrine in the dog. *J Pharmacokinet Biopharm* 1977;5:507–512.
18. Lai A, Levy R, Cutler R. Time-course of interaction between carbamazepine and clonazepam in normal man. *Clin Pharmacol Ther* 1978;24:616–323.
19. Theis JG, Koren G, Daneman R. et al. Interactions of clobazam with conventional antiepileptics in children. *J Child Neurol* 1997;12:208–213.
20. Hussein G, Troupin AS, Montouris G. Gabapentin interaction with felbamate. *Neurology* 1996;47:1106.
21. Sachdeo R, Wagner M, Sachdeo S, et al. Steady-state pharmacokinetics of phenytoin when co-administered with Felbatol (felbamate). *Epilepsia* 1992;33(Suppl 3):84.
22. Wagner ML, Graves NM, Leppik IE, et al. The effect of felbamate on valproate disposition. *Epilepsia* 1991;32(Suppl 3):15.
23. Howard J, Dix R, Shumaker R, et al. Effect of felbamate on carbamazepine pharmacokinetics. *Epilepsia* 1992;33(Suppl 3):84–85.
24. Ward D, Wagner M, Perhach J, et al. Felbamate steady-state pharmacokinetics during co-administration of valproate. *Epilepsia* 1991;32(Suppl 3):8.
25. Richens A, Gustavson L, McKelvy J, et al. Pharmacokinetics and safety of single-dose tiagabine HCl in epileptic patients chronically treated with four other antiepileptic drug regimens. *Epilepsia* 1991;32(Suppl 3):12.
26. Bruni J, Gallo J, Lee C, et al. Interactions of valproic acid with phenytoin. *Neurology* 1980;30:1233–1236.
27. Haidukewych D, Rodin EA, Zielinski JJ. Derivation and evaluation of an equation for prediction of free phenytoin concentration in patients co-medicated with valproic acid. *Ther Drug Monit* 1989;11:134–139.
28. May T, Rambeck B, Nothbaum N. Nomogram for the prediction of unbound phenytoin concentrations in patients on a combined treatment of phenytoin and valproic acid. *Eur Neurol* 1991;31:57–60.
29. Bourgeois BFD, Dodson WE. Antiepileptic and neurotoxic interactions between antiepileptic drugs. In: Pitlick WH, ed. *Antiepileptic drug interactions*. New York: Demos, 1989:209–218.
30. Bourgeois BFD, VanLente F. Effect of clonazepam on antiepileptic potency, neurotoxicity and therapeutic index of valproate and ethosuximide in mice. *Epilepsia* 1994;35(Suppl 8):142.
31. Chez MG, Bourgeois BFD, Pippinger CE, et al. Pharmacodynamic interactions between phenytoin and valproate: individual and combined antiepileptic and neurotoxic actions in mice. *Clin Neuropharmacol* 1994;17:32–37.
32. Rowan AJ, Meijer JW, de Beer-Pawlikowsky N, et al. Valproate-ethosuximide combination therapy for refractory absence seizures. *Arch Neurol* 1983;40:797–802.
33. Brodie MJ, Yuen AW. Lamotrigine substitution study: evidence for synergism with sodium valproate? 105 Study Group. *Epilepsy Res* 1997;26:423–432.
34. Pisani F, Oteri G, Russo M, et al. The efficacy of valproate-lamotrigine comedication in refractory complex partial seizures: evidence for a pharmacodynamic interaction. *Epilepsia* 1999;40:1141–1146.
35. Tanganelli P, Regesta G. Vigabatrin vs. carbamazepine monotherapy in newly diagnosed focal epilepsy: a randomized response conditional cross-over study. *Epilepsy Res* 1996;25:257–262.
36. Besag FM, Berry DJ, Pool F, et al. Carbamazepine toxicity with lamotrigine: pharmacokinetic or pharmacodynamic interaction? *Epilepsia* 1998;39:183–187.

Selected Drug Interactions Between Antiepileptic Drugs and Other Types of Medications

Kay C. Kyllonen   *Ajay Gupta*

Included in this appendix is information on drug interactions that can occur between antiepileptic drugs (AEDs) and drugs outside this class (1–13). The tables include a number of medications commonly used with AEDs but is not meant to be exhaustive. A more comprehensive list of interactions can be found in the references listed at the end of the appendix (1–4). General drug references such as *Facts and Comparisons Online, Evaluation of Drug Interactions,* and Hansten and Horn's *Drug Interactions: Analysis and Management* can also be drawn on to provide recommendations for management of potential interactions. Some programs are available for use on computers or personal data assistants (5).

ORGANIZATION OF TABLES

Drugs that affect the action or serum concentration of the AED are listed in Table 45A.1. AED effects on other types of medications are listed in Table 45A.2. A downward arrow in the impact column indicates a decreased serum concentration of the substrate or target drug likely to result in a clinically significant decreased effect. An upward arrow indicates an increased concentration likely to result in an increased effect or clinical significant toxicity.

For information on interactions between various AEDs when used together as polytherapy, the reader is referred to the tables and text in Chapter 45.

ACKNOWLEDGMENT

We thank Shelly Pedraza, Department of Neurology, the Cleveland Clinic Foundation, Cleveland, Ohio, for her help in transcribing this manuscript.

REFERENCES

1. CNS agents: anticonvulsants, and investigational drugs. *Drug facts and comparisons. EFacts* [online]. Wolters Kluwer Health, 2004. Accessed May 20, 2004.
2. Zucchero F, Hogan M, Sommer C, eds. *Evaluation of drug interactions—the standard for drug interactions.* First DataBank.
3. Hansten P, Horn J. *Drug interactions: analysis and management.* Edmonds, WA: H&H Publications.
4. Michalets EL. Update: clinically significant cytochrome P-450 drug interactions. *Pharmacotherapy* 1998;18:84–112.
5. Robinson RL, Burk MS. Identification of drug–drug interactions with personal digital assistant-based software. *Am J Med* 2004;116: 357–358.
6. Cloyd JC, Remmel RP. Antiepileptic drug pharmacokinetics and interactions: impact on treatment of epilepsy. *Pharmacotherapy* 2000;20(Part 2):139S–151S.
7. Holland KD. Efficacy, pharmacology and adverse effects of antiepileptic drugs. *Neurol Clin* 2001;19:313–345.

TABLE 45A.1
INTERACTIONS OF ANTIEPILEPTIC DRUGS WITH OTHER DRUGS

Antiepileptic Drug (AED)	Group	AED Concentration Increased by	AED Concentration Decreased by
Valproic acid	Antimicrobial	Macrolides Isoniazid	Carbapenems Rifampin
	Antineoplastic		Cisplatin Doxorubicin Methotrexate
	Gastrointestinal agents	Cimetidine	Antacids Charcoal Cholestyramine
	Pain management		Naproxen
Oxcarbazepine	Calcium-channel blocker		Verapamil
Succinimides (e.g., ethosuximide)	Antimicrobial	Isoniazid	Rifampin
Lamotrigine	Antimicrobial Pain management		Rifampin Acetaminophen multidose
Carbamazepine	Antimicrobial	Azole antifungals Isoniazid Macrolides Reverse transcriptase inhibitors Protease inhibitors	Rifampin
	Antineoplastic		Cisplatin Doxorubicin
	Cardiovascular	Calcium channel blockers	
	Gastrointestinal agents	Cimetidine	Antacids Charcoal
	Pain management	Propoxyphene	
	Psychotropic	Selective serotonin inhibitors Monoamine inhibitors Nefazodone	Bupropion
	Other	Ticlopidine	Theophylline Influenza vaccine
Barbiturates	Alkalinizing agent		Ammounium chloride
	Diuretic	Acetazolamide Furosemide	
	Gastrointestinal agent		Antacids Charcoal
	Pain management	Propoxyphene	
	Vitamin		Folic acid Pyridoxine
	Other	Methylphenidate	
Phenytoin / fosphenytoin	Antimicrobial	Azole antifungals Metionidazole Isoniazid Sulfonamides Protease inhibitors Reverse transcriptase inhibitors Trimethoprim	Oxacillin Nitrofurantoin Rifampin
	Antihistamine	Chlorpheniramine	
	Antineoplastic	5-Fluorouracil	Cisplatin Etoposide Methotrexate Vinblastine
	Cardiovascular	Amiodarone	
	Immunosuppressant		Corticosteroids
	Gastrointestinal agent	Cimetidine Omeprazole	Antacids Charcoal Sucralfate Enteral formulas
	Immunosuppressant	Allopurinol Cyclosporine	

TABLE 45A.1
(continued)

Antiepileptic Drug (AED)	Group	AED Concentration Increased by	AED Concentration Decreased by
Phenytoin / fosphenytoin (continued)	Pain management Psychotropic Vitamin	Ibuprofen Tricyclic antidepressants	Loxapine Folic acid Pryidoxine
	Other	Ticlopidine	Theophylline Influenza vaccine

TABLE 45A.2
INTERACTIONS OF ANTIEPILEPTIC DRUGS WITH OTHER DRUGS

Antiepileptic Drug (AED)	Group	Drug Decreased by AED	Drug Increased by AED
Valproic Acid	Antimicrobial Psychotropic Anticoagulant		Zidovudine Tricyclic antidepressants Warfarin
Oxcarbazepine	Calcium-channel blocker	Oral contraceptives Felodipine	
Felbamate	Anticoagulant	Oral contraceptives Warfarin	
Topiramate		Ethinyl estradiol Digoxin	
Carbamazepine	Antimicrobial	Azole antifungals Doxycycline Protease inhibitors Reverse Transcriptase inhibitors	
	Antineoplastic	Etoposide, teniposide Methotrexate Vincristine	
	Cardiovascular	Beta blockers Calcium-channel blockers	
	Endocrine	Estrogen Oral contraceptives	
	Immunosuppressant	Corticosteroids Cyclosporine Tacrolimus	
	Psychotropic	Bupropion Haloperidol Olanzepine Serotonin reuptake inhibitors Tricyclic antidepressants Ziprasidone	Lithium
	Other	Acetaminophen overdose Neuromuscular blockers Theophylline Warfarin	
	Antimicrobial	Azole antifungals	

TABLE 45A.2
(continued)

Antiepileptic Drug (AED)	Group	Drug Decreased by AED	Drug Increased by AED
Barbiturates		Doxycycline	
		Griseofulvin	
		Protease inhibitors	
		Reverse Transcriptase inhibitors	
	Antineoplastic	Etoposides, teniposide	
		Doxorubicin	
		Methotrexate	
	Cardiovascular	Digoxin	
		Lidocaine	
		Nifedipine	
		Quinidine	
	Endocrine	Estrogen/progesterone	
		Oral contraceptives	
		Corticosteroids	
	Gastrointestinal agent	Cimetidine	
	Immunosuppressant	Cyclosporine	
		Tacrolimus	
	Pain management	Acetaminophen	
		Meperidine	
		Methadone	
		Nonsteroidal anti-inflammatory drugs	
	Psychotropic	Haloperidol	
		Phenothiazines	
		Serotonin reuptake inhibitors	
		Tricyclic antidepressants	
		Tacrine	
		Risperidone	
		Ziprasidone	
	Other	Theophylline/caffeine	
		Warfarin	
Phenytoin/Fosphenytoin	Antimicrobial	Azole antifungals	Protease inhibitors
		Doxycycline	Reverse transcriptase inhibitors
	Antineoplastic	Etoposide, teniposide	
		Methotrexate	
	Cardiovascular	Digoxin	
		Calcium-channel blockers	
		Beta blockers	
		Amiodarine	
		Dopamine	
		Quinidine	
	Endocrine	Estrogen	
		Levonorqestrol	
		Oral contraceptives	
	Diuretic	Furosemide	
	Immunosuppressant	Cyclosporine	
		Tacrolimus	Meperidine
	Pain management	Acetaminophen	
		Methadone	Lithium
	Psychotropic	Haloperidol	
	Other	Levodopa	
		Theophylline	
		Warfarin	

8. Patsalos PN, Duncan JS. Antiepileptic drugs: a review of clinically significant drug interactions. *Drug Saf* 1993;9:156–184.
9. Patsalos PN, Perucca E. Clinically important drug interactions in epilepsy: general features and interactions between antiepileptic drugs. *Lancet Neurol* 2003;2:347–356.
10. Patsalos PN, Perucca E. Clinically important drug interactions in epilepsy: interactions between antiepileptic drugs and other drugs. *Lancet Neurol* 2003;2:473–481.
11. Rambeck B, Specht U, Wolf P. Pharmacokinetic interactions of the new antiepileptic drugs. *Clin Pharmacokinet* 1996;31: 309–324.
12. Vecht CJ, Wagner GL, Wilms EB. Interactions between antiepileptics and chemotherapeutic drugs. *Lancet Neurol* 2003; 2:404–409.
13. Wilbur K, Ensom MHH. Pharmacokinetic drug interactions between oral contraceptives and second-generation anticonvulsants. *Clin Pharmacokinet* 2000;38:355–365.

Pharmacokinetics of Antiepileptic Drugs in Infants and Children

46

Gail D. Anderson   *Jong M. Rho*

Over the past 20 years, the greater susceptibility to seizures of the immature brain, compared with the adult brain, as well as the effects of antiepileptic drugs (AEDs) on the developing brain, has prompted numerous scientific investigations and educational efforts. During the same period, however, far less attention has been paid to developmental pharmacokinetics, that is, factors that ultimately influence drug disposition through age-related differences in absorption, distribution, metabolism, and excretion. Clinicians have long appreciated the need for individualized pharmacotherapy because of intrinsic variations in how each patient handles drug disposition, the pharmacologic trek that begins with drug formulation, liberation, and absorption and proceeds through multiple pathways and steps to its molecular targets and clinical effects. Moreover, simplified dosing strategies are unreliable, because the growth and maturation (and, hence, presumed function) of organ systems are not linear.

Drug use in the pediatric population has been fraught with uncertainties over efficacy and tolerability. The recent increased focus on pediatric drug development has tightened regulatory requirements for conducting clinical studies in the younger patient. General principles of treatment with AEDs have been established, although detailed knowledge of developmental pharmacology remains far from complete. This chapter summarizes the features of developmental pharmacokinetics and reviews the clinical literature for traditional and newer AEDs.

DEVELOPMENTAL PHARMACOKINETICS

Many age-related differences between neonates and infants, compared with older children and adults, can affect phar-

macokinetic properties of drugs (1). For example, gastric pH is increased in neonates, infants, and young children (i.e., relative achlorhydria), decreasing to adult levels after 2 years of age, whereas gastric and intestinal motility is reduced in neonates and infants but increased in older infants and children to adult levels.

The belief that drugs are absorbed more slowly in neonates and young infants than in older children is based on the very few studies that have evaluated how the rate and extent of absorption evolve with age. In addition, little or nothing is known about the maturation of active transporters or drug-metabolizing enzymes in the gastrointestinal tract that significantly affect the bioavailability of some drugs.

Once a drug is liberated and absorbed, its distributing to various body compartments depends on its molecular size, ionization constant, and relative aqueous and lipid solubility. The increased ratio of total body water to body fat in neonates and infants helps to raise the volume of distribution (V_d) of drugs. Whether V_d increases or decreases also depends on the drug's physiochemical characteristics. Because the plasma concentration that results from a loading dose is inversely proportional to the V_d, determination of loading doses for a given drug should account for age-related changes in V_d. For example, neonates and young infants require larger loading doses of phenobarbital to attain plasma concentrations similar to those in adults.

Protein binding also affects V_d. Albumin and α_1-acid glycoprotein concentrations are decreased in the neonate and infant, and reach adult levels only by age 1 year; this alters the ratio of unbound to total plasma concentrations of AEDs. For highly protein-bound AEDs, such as phenytoin, valproate, and tiagabine, total concentrations are unreliable for therapeutic drug monitoring and underestimate the unbound, or active, concentration in neonates. Assessments of unbound plasma concentrations are required to avoid dose-dependent adverse events.

AEDs are eliminated through either renal excretion of unchanged parent drug or hepatic biotransformation to active and inactive metabolites, or to a combination of these pathways. The cytochrome P (CYP) 450 and uridine diphosphate (UDP) glucuronosyltransferase (UGT) enzymes catalyze the biotransformation of most AEDs, although some recently approved AEDs are eliminated by renal, mixed, and non-CYP or non-UGT pathways.

The CYP system represents families of multiple enzymes; each family is composed of distinct isozymes. CYP1, CYP2, and CYP3, the major CYP families, and eight primary isozymes are involved in the hepatic metabolism of most drugs: CYP1A2, CYP2A6, CYP2C8, CYP2C9, CYP2C19, CYP2D6, CYP2E1, and CYP3A4 (2). The UGT family of enzymes, UGT1 and UGT2, catalyze the transfer of a glucuronic acid moiety from a donor cosubstrate, UDP-glucuronic acid, to an aglycone. UGT1 isozymes are capable of glucuronidating a variety of drugs and endobiotics; UGT2 is more involved in the glucuronidation of steroids and bile acids in addition to some drugs.

The effect of age on hepatic metabolism depends on the types of enzymes involved (Fig. 46.1) (3). CYP-dependent metabolism is low at birth, approximately 50% to 70% of adult levels; by age 3 years, however, enzymatic activity actually exceeds that of adults. Therefore, young children have an increased ability (relative to adults) to metabolize drugs eliminated by a CYP450-dependent pathway. By puberty, CYP activity decreases to adult levels. Clinical studies suggest that the increased activity occurs with CYP1A2, CYP2C, and CYP3A4. UGT activity is deficient at birth and reaches adult levels by 4 years of age. Unfortunately, little is known about age-related pharmacokinetics of drugs metabolized predominantly by glucuronidation. Maturational difference in specific isozymes has not yet been determined.

Renal function also varies with age (Fig. 46.1). At birth, renal blood flow, glomerular filtration rates, tubular secretion, and reabsorption are approximately 25% to 30% of adult values, increase steadily by 6 months to 50% to 75%, and reach full function by approximately 1 year of age. Transporter proteins participate in renal excretion of many drugs, but data about their maturation are scant. In general, weight-normalized doses of drugs excreted unchanged by the kidneys need to be reduced only for neonates and infants.

ANTIEPILEPTIC DRUGS

Benzodiazepines

Clobazam is available as a tablet. Absorption exceeds 85%, with peak concentrations occurring in 30 minutes to 2 hours (4,5). Clobazam is eliminated predominantly by hepatic metabolism to multiple metabolites. *N*-desmethylclobazam, the primary metabolite, accumulates to approximately eightfold higher serum concentrations than clobazam after

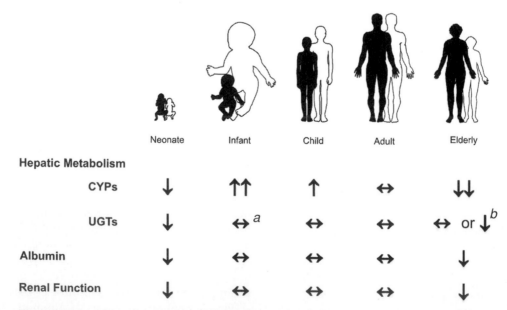

Figure 46.1 Effects of age on pharmacokinetic parameters affecting drug disposition. The shadows represent the relative rate of cytochrome P450 (CYP) activity. ªUGT (uridine diphosphate glucuronosyltransferase) activity is initially decreased in the infant and reaches adult levels by 4 years of age. ᵇUGT activity is decreased in the elderly only in some drugs but remains approximately the same with others. (From Morselli PL, Pippenger CE. Drug disposition during development: an overview. *Am Assoc Clin Chem* 1979;1–8, with permission.)

multiple doses. The polymorphically distributed CYP2C19 is primarily involved in the metabolism of N-desmethyl-clobazam. The poor-metabolizer phenotype of CYP2C19 occurs in 13% to 23% of Asians but in only 2% to 5% of whites and African Americans. Case reports have described children who had toxic reactions to normal doses of clobazam, with metabolite concentrations 10- to 27-fold higher than expected; these patients were heterozygous or homozygous for the mutant CYP2C19 alleles (6,7).

A population analysis of more than 400 epileptic patients receiving different comedications found significantly lower N-desmethylclobazam concentrations in children than in adults; the clobazam concentration-to-dose ratio did not differ with age (8). In another study of 74 children (9), clobazam and the metabolite concentrations increased with age from 1 to 18 years. Both studies showed large intersubject variability and poor correlation between plasma concentrations and efficacy. Therefore, it is unclear whether children require higher doses of clobazam than adults. Doses should be initiated with caution and titrated to effect in both populations.

Clonazepam is available as an oral or a disintegrating tablet, as drops, and in a parenteral formulation. After oral administration, bioavailability exceeds 80%, and peak concentrations occur in 1 to 4 hours (5). Clonazepam is well but variably absorbed after rectal administration; peak concentrations are reached within 10 to 30 minutes (10). After extensive metabolism to inactive metabolites, less than 1% of clonazepam is excreted unchanged in the urine. Neonates require lower weight-normalized doses than older children and adults. The elimination half-life is prolonged and clearance is significantly lower than in older children and adults (11). In small studies, the weight-normalized oral clearance was highly variable, though not significantly different from that in adults (12,13).

Diazepam is marketed as an oral solution, tablets, sustained-release capsules, and rectal suppository and gel; a parenteral formulation is also available (5). Absorption of the oral forms is complete, and peak concentrations occur within 30 to 90 minutes. Rectal administration of the solution or gel results in peak concentrations within 30 to 60 minutes (14); the suppositories exhibit slow and variable absorption and are not suitable for treatment of acute seizures (15). Diazepam is extensively metabolized to desmethyldiazepam, temazepam, and oxazepam; reactions are catalyzed by CYP2C19 and CYP3A4. The mean elimination half-life of diazepam and desmethyldiazepam is significantly prolonged in poor metabolizers of CYP2C19. Despite significant use in children, information on the age-related pharmacokinetics of diazepam is sparse. Neonates and young infants have decreased weight-normalized clearance owing to decreased formation of oxidative and conjugated metabolites (16). In a study of five children 4 to 8 years of age (16), oral clearance appeared to be twofold to threefold higher than that described in adults (17).

The recommended dosage of rectal gel for treatment of acute serial seizures in children reflects the expected increase in weight-normalized oral clearance for drugs metabolized by CYP3A4 and CYP2C19: ages 2 to 5 years, 0.5 mg/kg; 6 to 11 years, 0.3 mg/kg; children older than 11 years and adults, 0.2 mg/kg.

Lorazepam is available as oral and sublingual tablets and in a parenteral formulation. Bioavailability after oral administration is more than 90%, with peak concentrations achieved in 1 to 2 hours (5). Sublingual administration results in a bioavailability exceeding 98% and a latency before absorption of 23 minutes. Lorazepam is extensively metabolized to a glucuronide conjugate, with little renal excretion of unchanged drug. Neonates have significantly decreased oral clearance compared with children and adults (18,19). The pharmacokinetics of lorazepam are not known in children between the ages of 1 and 7 years. In children 7 to 19 years of age, the pharmacokinetics are not significantly different from values in adults. Because glucuronidation appears to reach adult levels by age 3 years, the weight-corrected dose in children after age 3 years should be the same as in adults. Infants and children younger than age 3 years should receive reduced doses.

Carbamazepine

Carbamazepine is available in oral and chewable tablets, as a suspension, and in extended-release formulations (20). The time to peak concentration is 4 to 8 hours with the tablets and extended-release formulations and 1 to 2 hours with the suspension. In six newborn and two older infants, the oral suspension was adequately absorbed from the gastrointestinal tract, with a time to peak of 7 to 15 hours (21). Rectal administration of the suspension results in equivalent blood concentration with a delayed peak concentration (22). The significantly shorter elimination half-life in children compared with adults may require three-times-daily or even four-times-daily dosing of the tablet and suspension. The controlled-release or sustained-release formulation provides significantly less fluctuation in plasma concentrations and fewer toxic reactions associated with high peak concentrations (23). Tegretol-XR loses its sustained-release properties if broken or chewed, whereas the Carbatrol capsule can be emptied onto food and maintain the sustained-release characteristics. Both can be substituted milligram for milligram for other carbamazepine products and administered twice a day.

After extensive metabolism, less than 1% of carbamazepine is excreted unchanged in the urine. Carbamazepine-epoxide accounts for approximately 25% of the dose in monotherapy and 50% in polytherapy with other inducing AEDs. Carbamazepine is a substrate for CYP3A4 (major), with minor metabolism by CYP1A2 and CYP2C8. The epoxide metabolite contributes to the drug's therapeutic effects and neurotoxicity. The effects of age on carbamazepine also must consider the active metabolite, which is rarely measured in the clinical setting. Studies have found a higher weight-adjusted total body clearance and higher carbamazepine-epoxide-to-carbamazepine ratio in children than in adults (24,25). Adult values are reached by ages 15 to 17 years with the greatest change in oral clearance occurring between 9 and 13 years of age (26). Children need weight-normalized maintenance doses approximately 50% to 100% higher than those in adults to achieve comparable serum levels.

Ethosuximide

Ethosuximide is available as capsules or syrup. Absorption is complete, with a time to peak concentration of 3 to 7 hours (27). Ethosuximide is eliminated primarily by CYP3A4-dependent metabolism, with approximately 20% excreted unchanged in the urine. The weight-adjusted oral clearance is higher in children than in adults, and the concentration-to-dose ratio is 50% higher in children 2.5 to 10 years of age than in those 15 years of age or older (28). Children need approximately 50% to 100% higher mg/kg maintenance doses than do adults to attain similar concentrations. As ethosuximide therapy is initiated primarily in young children, doses will need adjustment according to plasma concentrations to account for increased body weight and decreased clearance with age (29).

Felbamate

Felbamate is marketed as a tablet and a suspension. Absorption is nearly complete; peak concentrations occur 2 to 4 hours after administration (20). Felbamate is eliminated through renal excretion of unchanged drug (50%) and glucuronidation (20%) and is a substrate for CYP3A4 (20%) and CYP2E1. The weight-adjusted apparent clearance of felbamate is approximately 40% higher in children 2 to 12 years of age than in adults 13 to 65 years of age on monotherapy or polytherapy with other AEDs (30). A significant negative correlation in apparent clearance was noted in 17 children 2 to 12 years of age, with higher clearance in the very young decreasing to adult values by age 12 years (31). Children require weight-normalized maintenance doses approximately 40% higher than adults to attain similar concentrations.

Gabapentin

Gabapentin is available as a capsule, a tablet, and an oral solution. Absorption is less than 60% and varies significantly owing to saturation of active L-neutral amino acid transporters in the gastrointestinal tract (32). Peak concentrations occur in 2 to 3 hours. A study in two children found poor absorption of rectally administered solution (33). There is no information on the time course of maturation of the L-neutral amino acid transporter. Gabapentin is eliminated almost completely unchanged by the kidneys,

with oral clearance proportional to creatinine clearance; active tubular secretion is also involved in the renal elimination. A population analysis in subjects 2 months to 13 years of age found that children younger than 5 years had a significantly higher and more variable oral clearance than did older children (34). Infants and children younger than age 5 years required 33% higher weight-normalized doses to attain similar concentrations. The weight-normalized oral clearance in children older than age 5 years was comparable to that in adults. As creatinine clearance did not differ significantly in younger and older children, the age-related variation might be the result of decreased oral bioavailability, possibly as a result of delayed maturation of the L-neutral amino acid transporter. A small study (35) found 33% higher oral clearance in children age 10 years or younger compared with young adults. Therefore, children younger than 5 years of age will need higher weight-normalized doses than will children older than that age. After 5 years of age, weight-normalized doses higher than those in adults may be needed.

Lamotrigine

Lamotrigine is available in oral and chewable tablets. Absorption is complete, and time to peak concentration is 2 to 4 hours (20). Lamotrigine is eliminated predominantly by hepatic metabolism as glucuronide conjugates, catalyzed by UGT1A4 (36). In infants younger than 1 year of age with infantile spasms or partial seizures, concomitant medications (including enzyme inducers), increased oral clearance during the first year of life (37). During the first month, oral clearance (weight-normalized) was approximately 50% lower than in infants 2 to 12 months of age. Studies in older children have yielded conflicting results, with some reporting a trend toward a decreased concentration-to-dose ratio compared with adults; however, few of these children were receiving lamotrigine monotherapy (38–40). Whether age affects induction potential remains unclear. The lower concentration-to-dose ratios in children taking enzyme-inducing drugs may be a result of increased induction capacity. A trend toward increased oral clearance after a single dose of lamotrigine, in the absence of other AEDs, was noted in four children younger than age 6 years, compared with eight children ages 6 to 11 years, albeit with large intersubject variability (41). Overall, however, the result was not significantly different from oral clearance after a single dose of lamotrigine in normal adults (42,43). Therefore, doses in children receiving monotherapy should be similar to adult doses; whereas, higher weight-normalized doses may be needed with concomitant therapy.

Levetiracetam

Levetiracetam is available as tablets and an oral solution. Absorption is almost complete (>95%), and time to peak concentration is 1 hour. Elimination is predominantly by renal excretion of unchanged drug and by hydrolysis of the acetamide group, a reaction catalyzed by amidases, which are present in a number of tissues. Weight-normalized oral clearance is approximately 30% to 40% higher in children ages 6 to 12 years than in adults (44,45). Therefore, children older than age 6 years will require weight-normalized doses 30% to 40% higher than those in adults to achieve similar concentrations. No data are available for children younger than age 6 years.

Oxcarbazepine

The prodrug oxcarbazepine is rapidly converted to 10,11-dihydro,10-hydroxycarbazepine (MHD; monohydroxy derivative) on oral administration, a reaction catalyzed by cytosolic arylketone reductase (46). MHD is excreted unchanged in the urine or conjugated by UGT and then excreted, with only minor oxidative metabolism to dihydroxy derivative (DHD). Oxcarbazepine is available as oral tablets and a suspension. Absorption is essentially complete (>95%), with a time to peak concentration of 1 hour for the parent drug and 7 hours for MHD. In a study of 2- to 12-year-old children who received a single oral dose of oxcarbazepine, the dose and weight-normalized area under the concentration time curve (AUC) of MHD were approximately 60% less in children between 6 and 12 years than in those 2 to 6 years of age. The authors concluded that younger children should receive a higher dose than older children (20,47). Similar results were found in a population pharmacokinetic analysis (48). In addition, 6- to 12-year-old children exhibited higher weight-normalized clearance of MHD. Therefore, those younger than age 6 years and those between the ages of 6 and 11 years will require 80% higher and 30% higher weight-normalized doses, respectively, than adults to achieve similar concentrations.

Phenobarbital

Phenobarbital is available in capsule, tablet, elixir, and injectable formulations. Absorption is essentially complete, with a time to peak concentration of 1 to 4 hours. Rectal administration of the parenteral formulation results in a mean bioavailability of 90% and a time to peak concentration of 4 hours (49). Because V_d in newborns and young infants is approximately 1.5 times greater than that in older infants and children, loading doses (mg/kg) need to be at least 50% higher compared with adult doses to attain similar plasma concentrations (15 to 20 mg/kg versus 10 to 15 mg/kg).

Phenobarbital is eliminated by both renal excretion of unchanged drug and hepatic metabolism to parahydroxyphenobarbital (a reaction catalyzed primarily by CYP2C9 and CYP2C19), as well as by glucosidation to phenobarbital N-glucoside (49). Owing to the multiple pathways of elimination, CYP2C9 and CYP2C19 polymorphisms are not clinically significant (50). Newborns have a decreased clearance compared with young infants and children. During the first year of life, weight-normalized clearance is two- to threefold greater than in adults. Therefore, weight-normalized maintenance doses in children should be 50% to 100% higher than in adults.

Phenytoin

Phenytoin is available as tablets, capsules, a suspension, and a parenteral formulation. Absorption exceeds 90%; times to peak concentration are formulation dependent. Elimination is by saturable CYP2C9- and CYP2C19-dependent hepatic metabolism (51), and both children and adults who carry either mutant allele will exhibit significantly increased concentration-to-dose ratios (52–54). Phenytoin is described by a capacity-limited metabolism (i.e., Michaelis-Menten kinetics), in which V_{max} is the maximum rate of metabolic capacity. The small V_{max} in neonates results in a decreased weight-normalized unbound clearance. Also in neonates, decreased albumin reduces protein binding, so that total phenytoin concentrations do not reflect the unbound or active drug. Compared with adults, children have a significantly higher mean V_{max}, which progressively decreases until adult values are reached near puberty (55,56). Therefore, weight-normalized doses must be 50% to 100% higher in children to attain phenytoin plasma concentrations similar to those in adults.

Tiagabine

Tiagabine is available as tablets. Absorption is essentially complete, and peak concentrations occur within 1 hour. Metabolism occurs mainly by CYP3A4 and UGT pathways, with less than 2% excreted unchanged in the urine (57). The weight-corrected clearance is twofold higher in children than in adults not receiving enzyme-inducing AED polytherapy (i.e., valproate). In the presence of enzyme-inducing drugs, the weight-corrected clearance is similar in children and adults (58). Clinical evidence is insufficient to suggest that children receiving tiagabine without an enzyme inducer will need 50% higher doses than adults.

Topiramate

Topiramate is available as an oral tablet and as capsules containing sprinkles. Bioavailability is approximately 80%, with a time to peak concentration of 3 to 4 hours (59). In healthy adults, rectal administration of crushed tablet in 10 mL of water resulted in bioavailability comparable to that of the oral tablet (60). Excretion combines hepatic metabolism and renal elimination of unchanged drug. Weight-adjusted clearance is approximately 50% higher in 4- to 11-year-olds than in adults, producing concentrations approximately 33% lower (61–63). Weight-adjusted clearance is slightly higher in infants than in children and significantly higher than in adults, resulting in an increased dose requirement (64). Titration to effect, not dose, is recommended in infants and children (64). Polytherapy with inducing AEDs decreases topiramate concentrations by 50% in children and adults; therefore, the effects of age and polytherapy must be considered in topiramate dosing.

Valproate

Valproate is available in a variety of dosages, as tablets, enteric-coated capsules, an extended-release formulation, syrup, sprinkles, and parenteral preparations. Absorption is essentially complete (65). The time to peak concentration depends on the dosage form and ranges from 30 minutes to 1 hour for the syrup and from 3 to 8 hours for Depakote sprinkles and enteric-coated capsules. When the syrup is diluted 1:1 with water and given rectally, bioavailability is similar to that with oral administration (66); this strategy has been successful in the treatment of status epilepticus in children (67). Intravenous administration to children has not been sufficiently studied. A single case report of two neonates determined that the V_d was approximately 0.25 L/kg—more than 50% larger than in children and adults (68). In both neonates, each 1 mg/kg intravenous dose increased serum drug concentration by 4 μg/mL. Therefore, the loading dose must be significantly higher in neonates than in children and adults.

Hepatic metabolism is extensive, mainly by UGT-catalyzed glucuronide conjugation and β-oxidation, with minor CYP-dependent activity. Less than 5% of the dose is excreted unchanged in urine (65). Neonates receiving valproate for intractable seizures have highly variable total clearances but similar to those in adults. Because of low albumin levels in neonates, total valproate concentrations underestimate the unbound or pharmacologically active concentration. During the first 2 months of life, clearance increases significantly as hepatic enzymes mature. In infants 3 to 36 months of age, weight-normalized clearance was significantly higher than that in adults (69), and in school-age children, it was intermediate to that in infants and adults (70). Infants and young children need weight-adjusted doses 50% to 100% higher than adults to attain similar drug plasma concentrations. Polytherapy with AED inducers in children and adults significantly increases valproate clearance and lowers its concentrations; therefore, effects of age and polytherapy need to be part of dosing considerations.

Vigabatrin

Vigabatrin is administered as a racemic mixture, with the S-(+)-enantiomer responsible for pharmacologic activity. Tablets and a powder for solution or suspension are available. Peak concentrations occur in 30 minutes to 2 hours (71). Bioavailability, estimated on the basis of urinary recovery after an oral dose, is approximately 60% to 80% (72). Vigabatrin is eliminated almost completely

unchanged by the kidneys. A single-dose study in two groups of six children, ages 5 months to 2 years and 4 to 14 years, found an age-related effect only for the pharmacologically inactive R-(−)-enantiomer that was related to bioavailability, not renal elimination. In 65 adults and 114 children, the concentration-to-dose ratio of racemic vigabatrin was significantly lower in 1- to 9-year-olds, compared with 10- to 14-year-olds (73). Surprisingly, the ratio was also lower in children 10 to 14 years of age than in those older than 15 years. Children younger than age 5 years had 50% lower ratios than adults. The mechanism of this age-related difference is unknown, and its clinical significance is unclear, as no relationship between vigabatrin plasma concentrations and effect has been documented. Vigabatrin acts by irreversibly inhibiting aminobutyric acid transaminase, which results in a significantly longer biologic half-life than plasma elimination half-life. Therefore, vigabatrin is titrated slowly to clinical effect and not to therapeutic plasma concentrations.

Zonisamide

Zonisamide is available in capsules. Peak concentrations occur in 2 to 4 hours, and bioavailability is assumed to be good on the basis of urinary recovery (74). Elimination involves a combination of renal excretion of unchanged drug (approximately 35%) and metabolism through hepatic N-acetylation and reduction to 2-sulfamoylacetylphenol (SMAP). Despite considerable clinical experience in Japanese and Korean children, no formal pharmacokinetic studies in a pediatric population have been completed (75). In one report (76), doses of 8 mg/kg per day given to children ages 3 months to 15 years found peak and trough concentrations about two- to threefold higher in the older children (approximately 4 to 8 μg/mL) compared with infants and young children (approximately 2 to 4 μg/mL) (linear increase). In adults, 200 to 600 mg per day produced zonisamide concentrations of 10 μg/mL to 30 μg/mL. Children may require significantly higher doses to achieve concentrations comparable to those in adults.

CONCLUSION

Neonates, young infants, and children undergo significant (nonlinear) maturational changes in organ systems that prominently affect the absorption, distribution, metabolism, and excretion of AEDs. As a result, dosing needs to be carefully adjusted if therapeutic serum concentrations and thereby an increased likelihood of seizure freedom are to be realized (Table 46.1). In general, weight-normalized dosages of AEDs need to be increased in young infants and children, who have a greater capacity for drug disposition than do adolescents and adults. Of course, clinical judgment, combined with judicious use of serum levels and scrutiny of concomitant medications for negative drug

TABLE 46.1

AGE-SPECIFIC MAINTENANCE DOSING OF ANTIEPILEPTIC DRUGS USED IN MONOTHERAPY[a]

Drug	Average Dose			
	Neonates (mg/kg)	Infants (mg/kg)	Children (mg/kg)	Adults
Phenobarbital	3–4 qd	2.5–3.0 q12h	2–4 q12h	0.5–1.0 mg/kg q12h
Phenytoin	2.5–4.0 q12h	2–3 q8h	2.3–2.6 q8h	2 mg/kg q12h
Carbamazepine	NE	3–10 q8h	3–10 q8h	5–8 mg/kg q12h
Valproate	NE	5–10 q8h	5–10 q8h	5–10 mg/kg q12h
Ethosuximide	NE	NE	10–20 q12h	250–500 mg q12h
Felbamate	NE	NE	5–15 q8h	900–1800 mg q12h
Gabapentin	NE	NE	5–15 q8h	600–1200 mg q8h
Topiramate	NE	NE	2–5 q12h	100–200 mg q12h
Lamotrigine	NE	NE	2–5 q12h	75–150 mg q12h
Tiagabine	NE	NE	0.5–2 qd	32–56 mg qd
Oxcarbazepine	NE	NE	5–15 q8h	300–1200 mg q12h
Levetiracetam	NE	NE	5–20 q12h	500–1500 mg q12h
Zonisamide	NE	NE	2–6 q12h	100–200 mg q12h
Vigabatrin	NE	50–100 q12h	25–75 q12h	1000–1500 mg q12h

Abbreviations: NE, not established; qd, once a day.
[a]Not all antiepileptic drugs (AEDs) have FDA-approved indications for monotherapy. When AEDs are used in conjunction with other AEDs, or drugs that affect hepatic metabolism or renal function, or both, doses should be adjusted according to clinical judgment.

interactions, is required for maximum efficacy and tolerability. Expanding knowledge of pharmacokinetics, pharmacogenomics, and drug interactions will fill in gaps in data on age-dependent pharmacokinetic properties of AEDs.

REFERENCES

1. Kearns GL, Abdel-Rahman SM, Alander SW, et al. Developmental pharmacology—drug disposition, action, and therapy in infants and children. *N Engl J Med* 2003;349:1157–1167.
2. Wrighton SA, Stevens JC. The human hepatic cytochrome P450 involved in drug metabolism. *Crit Rev Toxicol* 1992;22:1–21.
3. Morselli PL, Pippenger CE. Drug disposition during development: an overview. *Am Assoc Clin Chem* 1979;1–8.
4. Rupp W, Badian M, Christ O, et al. Pharmacokinetics of single and multiple doses of clobazam in humans. *Br J Clin Pharmacol* 1979;7:51S–57S.
5. Anderson GD, Miller JW. Benzodiazepines: chemistry, biotransformation and pharmacokinetics. In: Levy RH, Mattson RH, Meldrum BS, et al., eds. *Antiepileptic drugs*, 5th ed. Philadelphia: Lippincott Williams & Wilkins, 2002:187–205.
6. Contin M, Sangiorgi S, Riva R, et al. Evidence of polymorphic CYP2C19 involvement in the human metabolism of N-desmethylclobazam. *Ther Drug Monit* 2002;24:737–741.
7. Parmeggiani A, Posar A, Sangiorgi S, et al. Unusual side-effects due to clobazam: a case report with genetic study of CYP2C19. *Brain Dev* 2004;26:63–66.
8. Bun H, Monjanel-Mouterde S, Noel F, et al. Effects of age and antiepileptic drugs on plasma levels and kinetics of clobazam and N-desmethylclobazam. *Pharmacol Toxicol* 1990;67:136–140.
9. Theis JGW, Koren G, Daneman R, et al. Interactions of clobazam with conventional antiepileptics in children. *J Child Neurol* 1997;12:208–213.
10. Rylance GW, Poulton J, Cherry RC, et al. Plasma concentrations of clonazepam after single rectal administration. *Arch Dis Child* 1986;61:186–188.
11. Andre M, Boutroy MJ, Dubruc C, et al. Clonazepam pharmacokinetics and therapeutic efficacy in neonatal seizures. *Eur J Clin Pharmacol* 1986;30:585–589.
12. Walson PD, Edge JH. Clonazepam disposition in pediatric patients. *Ther Drug Monit* 1996;18:1–5.
13. Dreifuss FE, Penry JK, Rose SW, et al. Serum clonazepam concentrations in children with absence seizures. *Neurology* 1975;25:255–258.
14. Cloyd JC, Lalonde RL, Beniak TE, et al. A single-blind, crossover comparison of the pharmacokinetics and cognitive effects of a new diazepam rectal gel with intravenous diazepam. *Epilepsia* 1998;39:520–526.
15. Knudsen FU. Plasma-diazepam in infants after rectal administration in solution and by suppository. *Acta Paediatr Scand* 1979;66:563–567.
16. Morselli PL, Principi N, Tognoni G, et al. Diazepam elimination in premature and full term infants, and children. *J Perinat Med* 1973;1:133–141.
17. Mandelli M, Tognoni G, Garattini S. Clinical pharmacokinetics of diazepam. *Clin Pharmacokinet* 1978;3:72–91.
18. McDermott CA, Kowalczyk AL, Schnitzler ER, et al. Pharmacokinetics of lorazepam in critically ill neonates with seizures. *J Pediatr* 1992;120:479–483.
19. Kearns GL, Mallory GBJ, Crom WR, et al. Enhanced hepatic drug clearance in patients with cystic fibrosis. *J Pediatr* 1990;117:972–979.
20. Battino D, Estienne M, Avanzini G. Clinical pharmacokinetics of antiepileptic drugs in paediatric patients, part II: phenytoin, carbamazepine, sulthiame, lamotrigine, vigabatrin, oxcarbazepine and felbamate. *Clin Pharmacokinet* 1995;29:341–369.
21. MacKintosh DA, Baird-Lampert J, Buchanan N. Is carbamazepine an alternative maintenance therapy for neonatal seizures? *Dev Pharmacol Ther* 1987;10:100–106.
22. Graves NM, Kriel RL, Jones-Saete C, et al. Relative bioavailability of rectally administered carbamazepine suspension in humans. *Epilepsia* 1985;26:429–433.
23. Bialer M. Pharmacokinetic evaluation of sustained release formulations of antiepileptic drugs. Clinical implications. *Clin Pharmacokinet* 1992;22:11–21.

24. Battino D, Bossi L, Croci D, et al. Carbamazepine plasma levels in children and adults: influence of age, dose, and associated therapy. *Ther Drug Monit* 1980;2:315–322.
25. Pynnonen S, Sillanpaa M, Frey H, et al. Carbamazepine and its 10,11-epoxide in children and adults with epilepsy. *Eur J Clin Pharmacol* 1977;11:129–133.
26. Albani F, Riva R, Contin M, et al. A within-subject analysis of carbamazepine disposition related to development in children with epilepsy. *Ther Drug Monit* 1992;14:457–460.
27. Battino D, Estienne M, Avanzini G. Clinical pharmacokinetics of antiepileptic drugs in paediatric patients, part I: phenobarbital, primidone, valproic acid, ethosuximide and mesuximide. *Clin Pharmacokinet* 1995;29:257–286.
28. Battino D, Cusi C, Franceschetti S, et al. Ethosuximide plasma concentrations: influence of age and associated concomitant therapy. *Clin Pharmacokinet* 1982;7:176–180.
29. Pisani F, Perucca E, Bialer M. Ethosuximide: chemistry, biotransformation, pharmacokinetics and drug interactions. In: Levy RH, Mattson RH, Meldrum BS, et al., eds. *Antiepileptic drugs*, 5th ed. Philadelphia: Lippincott Williams & Wilkins, 2002:646–651.
30. Banfield CR, Zhu GR, Jen JF, et al. The effect of age on the apparent clearance of felbamate: a retrospective analysis using nonlinear mixed-effects modeling. *Ther Drug Monit* 1996;18:19–29.
31. Carmant L, Holmes GL, Sawyer S, et al. Efficacy of felbamate in therapy for partial epilepsy in children. *J Pediatr* 1994;125:481–486.
32. Gidal BE, Radulovic LL, Kruger S, et al. Inter- and intra-subject variability in gabapentin absorption and absolute bioavailability. *Epilepsy Res* 2000;40:123–127.
33. Kriel RL, Birnbaum AK, Cloyd JC, et al. Failure of absorption of gabapentin after rectal administration. *Epilepsia* 1997;38: 1242–1244.
34. Ouellet D, Bockbrader HN, Wesche DL, et al. Population pharmacokinetics of gabapentin in infants and children. *Epilepsy Res* 2001;47:229–241.
35. Gatti G, Ferrari AR, Guerrini R, et al. Plasma gabapentin concentrations in children with epilepsy: influence of age, relationship with dosage, and preliminary observations on correlation with clinical response. *Ther Drug Monit* 2003;25:54–60.
36. Green MD, Bishop WP, Tephley TR. Expressed human UGT1.4 protein catalyzes the formation of quaternary ammonium-linked glucuronides. *Drug Metab Dispos* 1995;23:299–302.
37. Mikati MA, Fayad M, Koleilat M, et al. Efficacy, tolerability, and kinetics of lamotrigine in infants. *J Pediatr* 2002;141:31–35.
38. Battino D, Croci D, Granata T, et al. Single-dose pharmacokinetics of lamotrigine in children: influence of age and antiepileptic comedication. *Ther Drug Monit* 2001;23:217–222.
39. Bartoli A, Guerrini R, Belmonte A, et al. The influence of dosage, age and comedication on lamotrigine steady state concentrations in epileptic children: a prospective study with preliminary assessment of correlations with clinical response. *Ther Drug Monitor* 1997;19:252–260.
40. Armijo JA, Bravo J, Cuadrado A, et al. Lamotrigine serum concentration-to-dose ratio: influence of age and concomitant antiepileptic drugs and dosage implications. *Ther Drug Monit* 1999;21:182–190.
41. Chen C, Casale EJ, Duncan B, et al. Pharmacokinetics of lamotrigine in children in the absence of other antiepileptic drugs. *Pharmacotherapy* 1999;19:437–441.
42. Cohen AF, Land GS, Breimer DD, et al. Lamotrigine, a new anticonvulsant: pharmacokinetics in normal humans. *Clin Pharmacol Ther* 1987;42:535–541.
43. Posner J, Holdich T, Crome P. Comparison of lamotrigine pharmacokinetics in young and elderly healthy volunteers. *J Pharm Med* 1991;1:121–128.
44. Pellock JM, Glauser TA, Bebin EM, et al. Pharmacokinetic study of levetiracetam in children. *Epilepsia* 2001;42:1574–1579.
45. May TW, Rambeck B, Jurgens U. Serum concentrations of levetiracetam in epileptic patients: the influence of dose and co-medication. *Ther Drug Monit* 2003;25:690–699.
46. May TW, Korn-Merker E, Rambeck B. Clinical pharmacokinetics of oxcarbazepine. *Clin Pharmacokinet* 2003;42:1023–1042.
47. Pariente-Khayat A, Tran A, Vauzelle-Kervroedan F, et al. Pharmacokinetics of oxcarbazepine as add-on therapy in epileptic children. *Epilepsia* 1994;35(Suppl 8):119.
48. Sallas WM, Milosavljev S, D'Souza J, et al. Pharmacokinetic drug interactions in children taking oxcarbazepine. *Clin Pharmacol Ther* 2003;74:138–149.
49. Anderson GD. Phenobarbital: chemistry, biotransformation and pharmacokinetics. In: Levy RH, Mattson RH, Meldrum BS, Perrucca E, eds. *Antiepileptic drugs*, 5th ed. Philadelphia: Lippincott Williams & Wilkins, 2002:496–503.
50. Mamiya K, Hadama A, Yukawa E, et al. CYP2C19 polymorphism effect on phenobarbitone. Pharmacokinetics in Japanese patients with epilepsy: analysis by population pharmacokinetics. *Eur J Clin Pharmacol* 2000;55:821–825.
51. Brown TR, Leduc B. Phenytoin: chemistry and biotransformation. In: Levy RH, Mattson RH, Meldrum BS, et al., eds. *Antiepileptic drugs*, 5th ed. Philadelphia: Lippincott Williams & Wilkins, 2002:565–580.
52. Mamiya K, Ieiri I, Shimamoto J, et al. The effects of genetic polymorphisms of CYP2C9 and CYP2C19 on phenytoin metabolism in Japanese adult patients with epilepsy: studies in stereoselective hydroxylation and population pharmacokinetics. *Epilepsia* 1998;39:1317–1323.
53. Rettie AE, Haining RL, Bajpai M, et al. A common genetic basis for idiosyncratic toxicity of warfarin and phenytoin. *Epilepsy Res* 1999;35:253–255.
54. Odani A, Hashimoto Y, Otsuki Y, et al. Genetic polymorphism of the CYP2C subfamily and its effect on the pharmacokinetics of phenytoin in Japanese patients with epilepsy. *Clin Pharmacol Ther* 1997;62:287–292.
55. Dodson WE. Nonlinear kinetics of phenytoin in children. *Neurology* 1982;32:42–48.
56. Bauer LA, Blouin RA. Phenytoin Michaelis-Menten pharmacokinetics in Caucasian paediatric patients. *Clin Pharmacokinet* 1983;8:545–549.
57. Gustavson LE, Mengel HB. Pharmacokinetics of tiagabine, a gamma-aminobutyric acid-uptake inhibitor, in healthy subjects after single and multiple doses. *Epilepsia* 1995;36:605–611.
58. Gustavson LE, Boellner SW, Granneman GR, et al. A single-dose study to define tiagabine pharmacokinetics in pediatric patients with complex partial seizures. *Neurology* 1997;48:1032–1037.
59. Doose DR, Streeter AJ. Topiramate: chemistry, biotransformation and pharmacokinetics. In: Levy RH, Mattson RH, Meldrum BS, Perrucca E, eds. *Antiepileptic drugs*, 5th ed. Philadelphia: Lippincott Williams & Wilkins, 2002:727–734.
60. Conway JM, Birnbaum AK, Kriel RL, et al. Relative bioavailability of topiramate administered rectally. *Epilepsy Res* 2003;54: 91–96.
61. Rosenfeld WE, Doose DR, Walker SA, et al. A study of topiramate pharmacokinetics and tolerability in children with epilepsy. *Pediatr Neurol* 1999;20:339–344.
62. Schwabe MJ, Wheless JW. Clinical experience with topiramate dosing and serum levels in children 12 years or under with epilepsy. *J Child Neurol* 2001;16:806–808.
63. May TW, Rambeck B, Jurgens U. Serum concentrations of topiramate in patients with epilepsy: influence of dose, age, and comedication. *Ther Drug Monit* 2002;24:366–374.
64. Glauser TA, Miles MV, Tang P, et al. Topiramate pharmacokinetics in infants. *Epilepsia* 1999;40:788–791.
65. Levy RH, Shen DD, Abbott FS, et al. Valproic acid: chemistry, biotransformation and pharmacokinetics. In: Levy RH, Mattson RH, Meldrum BS, et al., eds. *Antiepileptic drugs*, 5th ed. Philadelphia: Lippincott Williams & Wilkins, 2002:780–800.
66. Cloyd JC, Kriel RL. Bioavailability of rectally administered valproic acid syrup. *Neurology* 1981;31:1348–1352.
67. Snead OC 3rd, Miles MV. Treatment of status epilepticus in children with rectal sodium valproate. *J Pediatr* 1985;106:323–325.
68. Alfonso I, Alvarez LA, Gilman J, et al. Intravenous valproate dosing in neonates. *J Child Neurol* 2000;15:827–829.
69. Hall K, Otten N, Johnston B, et al. A multivariable analysis of factors governing the steady-state pharmacokinetics of valproic acid in 52 young epileptics. *J Clin Pharmacol* 1985;25:261–268.
70. Cloyd JC, Kriel RL, Fischer JH, et al. Pharmacokinetics of valproic acid in children, I: multiple antiepileptic drug therapy. *Neurology* 1983;33:185–191.
71. Rey G, Pons G, Olive G. Vigabatrin. *Clin Pharmacokinet* 1992;23: 267–278.

72. Haegele KD, Schechter PJ. Kinetics of the enantiomers of vigabatrin after an oral dose of the racemate or the active S-enantiomer. *Clin Pharmacol Ther* 1986;40:581–586.
73. Armijo JA, Cuadrado A, Bravo J, Arteaga R. Vigabatrin serum concentration to dosage ratio: influence of age and associated antiepileptic drugs. *Ther Drug Monit* 1997;19:491–498.
74. Shah J, Shellenberger K, Canafax DM. Zonisamide: chemistry, biotransformation and pharmacokinetics. In: Levy RH, Mattson RH, Meldrum BS, Perrucca E, eds. *Antiepileptic drugs*, 5th ed. Philadelphia: Lippincott Williams & Wilkins, 2002: 873–879.
75. Glauser TA, Pellock JM. Zonisamide in pediatric epilepsy: review of the Japanese experience. *J Child Neurol* 2002;17: 87–96.
76. Miura H. Developmental and therapeutic pharmacology of antiepileptic drugs. *Epilepsia* 2000;41(Suppl 9):2–6.

Initiation and Discontinuation of Antiepileptic Drugs

47

Varda Gross Tsur   *Christine O'Dell*   *Shlomo Shinnar*

Over the past two decades there has been much information about the prognosis of seizure disorders, the effects of antiepileptic drug (AED) therapy on prognosis, and the relative risks of both seizures and of AED therapy. This chapter reviews the clinical decision making in initiating and discontinuing AEDs in children and adults, with particular emphasis on the data regarding the recurrence risk for seizures in different settings and the effect of AEDs on this risk. The risks and benefits of initiating and discontinuing AED therapy are then addressed in the context of an individualized therapeutic approach which emphasizes weighing the risks and benefits of drug therapy versus both the statistical risk of another seizure and the consequences of such an event.

RECURRENCE RISK FOLLOWING A FIRST UNPROVOKED SEIZURE

To develop a rational approach to the management of individuals who present with an initial unprovoked seizure, it is necessary to have some understanding of the natural history and prognosis of the disorder in this setting. Approximately one-third to one-half of children and adults with seizures will initially present to medical atten-

tion following a single seizure (1,2). The remainder will already have a history of prior events at the time of presentation. It is the group who present with a single seizure that are most relevant to this discussion. In accordance with the International League Against Epilepsy (ILAE) guidelines for epidemiologic research in epilepsy, a first unprovoked seizure is defined as a seizure or flurry of seizures all occurring within 24 hours in a person older than 1 month of age with no prior history of unprovoked seizures (3).

Since 1982, a number of studies have attempted to address the recurrence risk following a first unprovoked seizure using a variety of recruitment and identification techniques (4–22). The reported overall recurrence risk following a first unprovoked seizure in children and adults varies from 27% to 71%. Studies that carefully excluded those with prior seizures report recurrence risks of 27% to 52% (4–18). The higher recurrence risks are, with one exception (19), reported from studies that included subjects who already had recurrent seizures at the time of identification and who were thus more properly considered to have newly diagnosed epilepsy.

While there is considerable disparity in the absolute recurrence risk reported in the different studies, the time course of recurrence is remarkably similar among all studies (5). The majority of recurrences occur early, with approximately 50% of recurrences occurring within 6 months of the initial seizure and over 80% within 2 years of the initial seizure (5,13). Late recurrences are unusual, but they have occurred up to 10 years after the initial seizure (13,14). This time course is true both in studies that report low and high recurrence risks (4,5,7–10,12–14,19–21).

Supported in part by grant 1 R01 NS26151 (S. Shinnar) from the National Institute of Neurological Disorders and Stroke, National Institutes of Health, Bethesda, Maryland.
Portions of this chapter are reprinted from O'Dell C, Shinnar S. Initiation and discontinuation of antiepileptic drugs. *Neurol Clin* 2001;19:289–311, with permission.

A relatively small number of factors are associated with a differential recurrence risk. The most important of these are the etiology of the seizure, the electroencephalogram (EEG), and whether the first seizure occurred in wakefulness or sleep. These factors are consistent across most studies regardless of the absolute risk of recurrence reported in the individual study (4,5,7–15,18,20,21). Factors not associated with a significant change in the recurrence risk include age of onset, the number of seizures in the first 24 hours, and the duration of the initial seizure. The absolute recurrence risks appear similar in children and adults (5), although the consequences of such a recurrence are quite different. Selected risk factors are discussed below.

Etiology

In the ILAE classification, etiology of seizures is classified as remote symptomatic, cryptogenic, or idiopathic (3). Remote symptomatic seizures are those without an immediate cause but with an identifiable prior brain injury or the presence of a static encephalopathy such as mental retardation or cerebral palsy, which are known to be associated with an increased risk of seizures. Cryptogenic seizures are those occurring in otherwise normal individuals with no clear etiology. Until recently, cryptogenic seizures were also called idiopathic. In the new classification, idiopathic is reserved for seizures occurring in the context of the presumed genetic epilepsies such as benign rolandic and childhood absence (23,24). However, much of the literature on the recurrence risk following a first unprovoked seizure lumps idiopathic and cryptogenic together as idiopathic using the original classification developed by Hauser and coworkers (8).

Not surprisingly, both children and adults with a remote symptomatic first seizure have higher risk of recurrence than those with a cryptogenic first seizure. A meta-analysis of the studies published up to 1990 found that the relative risk of recurrence following a remote symptomatic first seizure was 1.8 (95% confidence interval, 1.5, 2.1) compared to those with a cryptogenic first seizure (5). Comparable findings are reported in more recent studies (13,15,21). Idiopathic first unprovoked seizures occur almost exclusively in children. Although the long-term prognosis of these children is quite favorable, the recurrence risk is actually comparable to those with a remote symptomatic first seizure (13). This is because, by definition, to meet the criteria for an idiopathic first seizure, they must have an abnormal EEG (23,24).

Electroencephalogram

The EEG is an important predictor of recurrence, particularly in cases that are not remote symptomatic and in children (5,7,8,10–13,15–18,21,25). Studies of recurrence risk following a first seizure in childhood have uniformly reported that those with an abnormal EEG have a higher recurrence risk than those with a normal EEG (5,7,12,13,15,21,25). For this reason, the American Academy of Neurology's recently published guideline on the evaluation of children with a first unprovoked seizure considers an EEG to be a standard part of the evaluation (21). Epileptiform abnormalities are more important than nonepileptiform ones, but any EEG abnormality increases the recurrence risk in cases that are not remote symptomatic (25). In our study, the risk of seizure recurrence within 24 months for children with an idiopathic/cryptogenic first seizure was 25% for those with a normal EEG, 34% for those with nonepileptiform abnormalities, and 54% for those with epileptiform abnormalities (25). Whereas in our data, any clearly abnormal electroencephalographic patterns, including generalized spike and wave, focal spikes, and focal or generalized slowing, increased the risk of recurrence, Camfield and associates (7) reported that only epileptiform abnormalities substantially increase the risk of recurrence in children. Despite minor disagreements as to which electroencephalographic patterns are most significant, the EEG appears to be the most important predictor of recurrence in children with a cryptogenic/idiopathic first seizure. In addition, it is the EEG that primarily distinguishes whether a neurologically normal child with a first seizure is classified as cryptogenic or idiopathic.

In adults, the data are more controversial. The majority of studies do find an increased recurrence risk associated with an abnormal EEG (5,9,10,18), although one study failed to find a significant effect (11). Hauser and colleagues (8) found that generalized spike-and-wave patterns are predictive of recurrence but not focal spikes. A meta-analysis of these studies concluded that the overall data do support an association between an abnormal EEG and an increased recurrence risk in adults as well (5), although which electroencephalographic patterns besides generalized spike and wave are important remains unclear (5,9,10,18).

Sleep State at Time of First Seizure

In adults, seizures that occur at night are associated with a higher recurrence risk than those that occur in the daytime (11). In children, whose sleep patterns may include daytime naps, the association is more clearly between sleep state and recurrence risk rather than time of day (13,26). Interestingly, the association is not just because nocturnal seizures tend to occur in certain epilepsy syndromes. Thus, even children whose EEG has centrotemporal spikes and who meet the criteria for benign rolandic seizures (24) have a higher recurrence risk if the first seizure occurs during sleep than if it occurs while awake (26). Furthermore, if the first seizure occurs during sleep, there is a high likelihood that the second one, should it occur, will also occur during sleep (26). In our series, the 2-year recurrence risk was 53% for children whose initial seizure occurred during sleep compared with a 30% risk for those whose initial seizure occurred while awake (13). On multivariable analysis, etiology, the EEG, and sleep state were the major significant predictors of outcome. From a therapeutic point of view, the implication of a seizure during sleep is unclear. While the recurrence risk is higher, recurrences will tend to occur in sleep. As the major risk of a brief seizure in children or adults is that it may happen at a time or place where the impairment of consciousness will have serious consequences, the morbidity of a seizure during sleep is fairly low in both cases.

Seizure Classification

In some studies, the risk of recurrence following a first unprovoked seizure is higher in subjects with a partial seizure than in those with a generalized first seizure (5). This association is mostly found on univariate analysis and disappears once the effect of etiology and the EEG are accounted for (5,8,12,13). Partial seizures are more common in those with a remote symptomatic first seizure and in children with an abnormal EEG (12). Note that some generalized seizure types, such as absence and myoclonic, very rarely present as a first seizure and so would be excluded from studies of first seizure (16,21). Generalized seizures that present to medical attention at the time of the first seizure are usually tonic-clonic (13).

Duration of Initial Seizure

In children, the duration of the first seizure is not associated with a differential recurrence risk. In our study, 48 (12%) of 407 children (38 cryptogenic/idiopathic, 10 remote symptomatic) presented with status epilepticus (duration longer than 30 minutes) as their first unprovoked seizure (13). The recurrence risk in these children was not different than in children whose first seizure was briefer. However, if a recurrence did occur it was likely to be prolonged (13,27). Of the 24 children with an initial episode of status who experienced a seizure recurrence, 5 (21%) recurred with status. Of the 147 children who presented with an initial brief seizure and experienced a seizure recurrence, only 2 (1%) recurred with status epilepticus (p <0.001). In adults there is a suggestion that a prolonged first seizure, particularly in remote symptomatic cases, is associated with a higher risk of recurrence (10).

Treatment Following a First Seizure

Four randomized clinical trials in children and adults examined the efficacy of treatment after a first unprovoked seizure (6,20,28–31). Two well-designed prospective studies which randomized subjects to treatment or placebo following a first unprovoked seizure found that treatment reduced the recurrence risk by approximately half (6,20,28). The larger Italian study included both children

and adults (20,28). However, while recurrence risk was reduced, there was no difference in long-term outcomes between the two groups. An equal proportion were in 2-year remission after 5 years of follow up (28). Although the authors of this study initially recommended treatment following a first seizure, once it became apparent that early treatment did not affect long-term prognosis, they changed their recommendation, suggesting that in the majority of cases treatment wait until the second seizure (28). In general, the accumulating evidence from a large number of studies indicates that AED therapy is effective in reducing the risk of a recurrent seizure but does not alter the underlying disorder and therefore does not change long-term prognosis (32). Based on these data and assessment of risk-to-benefit, the American Academy of Neurology has issued a practice parameter on AED therapy following a first unprovoked seizure in children and adolescents (31). This parameter recommends that (a) treatment with an AEDs is not indicated for the prevention of the development of epilepsy, and (b) treatment with an AED may be considered in circumstances where the benefits of reducing the risk of a second seizure outweigh the risks of pharmacologic and psychosocial side effects. The authors rarely prescribe AEDs after a single seizure. A practice parameter addressing this issue in adults is currently under development.

What Happens After Two Seizures?

Two studies in adults (9) and children (14) examined what happens after a second seizure. In adults, the recurrence risk after a second seizure is 70%, leading Hauser and coworkers to conclude that, in adults, once a second seizure has occurred, treatment with AEDs is appropriate (9). In children, the recurrence risk following a second seizure is also approximately 70%. Those with a remote symptomatic etiology and those whose second seizure occurs within 6 months of the first have a higher recurrence risk (14). Interestingly, factors such as an abnormal EEG and sleep state at the time of the seizure, which help to differentiate those who only have one seizure from those who experienced a recurrence, are no longer associated with a differential risk of further seizures once a second seizure occurs (14). Despite the similarities in recurrence risk, the issue of treatment following a second seizure in children is less straightforward than in adults. Many of these children have idiopathic self-limited epilepsy syndromes, such as benign rolandic, where the need for treatment has been questioned (33–35). In addition, the frequency of seizures in this group is low, with only 25% of children who had 2 seizures experiencing 10 or more seizures over a 10-year period (14). Thus, the decision regarding treatment in children with cryptogenic/idiopathic seizures who have a second seizure must be individualized and take into account whether the seizures are part of a benign self-limited syndrome, as well as the frequency of the seizures and the relative risks and benefits of treatment.

WITHDRAWAL OF ANTIEPILEPTIC DRUGS IN THOSE WHO HAVE BEEN SEIZURE FREE ON ANTIEPILEPTIC DRUG THERAPY

AED therapy effectively controls seizures in the majority of patients with epilepsy. The preponderance of evidence indicates that most patients with epilepsy will become seizure free on AEDs within a few years of diagnosis (36–43). However, the long-term use of AEDs carries with it significant morbidity. Therefore, the issue of whether one can withdraw AEDs in patients with epilepsy after a seizure-free interval becomes important in the treatment of a vast number of patients.

A large number of prospective and retrospective studies in children and adolescents, involving thousands of subjects, have been done over the past 25 years on the question of remission and relapse rates after withdrawal of AEDs. A smaller but still substantial number of studies dealing with adults have also been reported (37,44–76). A meta-analysis of the available literature reported a pooled risk of relapse of 25% at 1 year and 29% at 2 years following AED withdrawal (46).

In childhood-onset epilepsy, the majority of studies report that 60% to 75% of children and adolescents with epilepsy who have been seizure free for more than 2 to 4 years on medication will remain so after AEDs are withdrawn (44–47,53–55,57,58–61,63,68–71,74,76). Exceptionally low recurrence rates of 8% to 12% were reported in studies that limited subject entry to neurologically normal children with normal EEGs, many of whom were followed since the onset of their seizures (62,73).

In the past, it was thought that adult-onset epilepsy had a far less favorable prognosis for remission than childhood-onset epilepsy, and that withdrawal of medications was rarely feasible in this population. Although the prognosis in adults does appear to be worse than in children, newer studies suggest that the differences are smaller than was thought. Four years after onset, the majority of adults with new-onset seizures will be at least 2 years seizure free (41,42). Many adults self-discontinue their medications and are still seizure free years later (36,76). Studies of withdrawing AEDs in adults report recurrence rates of 28% to 66% (47,50,56,60,63,65,75), which is a much larger range than that reported in pediatric studies. However, it should be noted that studies that reported the lowest recurrence risks (50) limited themselves to patients followed since onset of their seizures and who had absence of other presumed risk factors. In pediatric studies, such selected populations have reported recurrence risks of less than 20%.

The preponderance of data at this time indicates that the recurrence risk following withdrawal of AEDs is somewhat higher in adult-onset epilepsy than in childhood-onset epilepsy with a relative risk of approximately 1.3 (46). However, much of the increased risk reported in some studies is a result of the higher risk of recurrence in adolescent-onset seizures (46,68). Selected populations of adults may have low recurrence risks. Two reports showed no differences in recurrence risks between children and adults (50,75). However, these studies have the highest reported recurrence risks for children (31% to 40%) and the lowest reported recurrence risks in adults (35% to 40%). In addition, their definition of children exceeds the usual limits of the term. In one study, 38% of the subjects had childhood onset but this was defined as onset before 15 years of age (50). Several studies in children have reported that an age of onset older than 10 or 12 years was associated with a higher recurrence risk, presumably because this already reflects early adult-onset epilepsy (48,67–69,73).

The data on adolescents indicate that the recurrence rate is more a function of the age at onset than the age at withdrawal of medications (46,68,69). Studies of childhood-onset epilepsy that included adolescents have reported low recurrence risk (45,46,48,54,59,62,68,69,71,73). Studies of adolescents and adults that have primarily included adolescent-onset cases have reported recurrence rates similar to those seen in adults (46,50,60,75). One retrospective study limited to adolescents with adolescent-onset seizures reported a recurrence rate of 49% (66). A recent meta-analysis found that adolescent onset epilepsy has a higher recurrence risk following AED withdrawal than either childhood- (relative risk, 1.79) or adult-onset (relative risk, 1.34) epilepsy (46).

When recurrences do occur after discontinuation of AEDs, they tend to occur early (46,68). The timing of recurrence is similar in studies of both children and adults and is independent of the absolute recurrence risk. Many occur as the medications are being tapered. At least half the recurrences occur within 6 months of medication withdrawal, 60% to 90% of recurrences occur within 1 year of withdrawal, and more than 85% of recurrences occur within 5 years (45,46,48,50,54,58–60,62,63,65,68,69,71,75). One series in adults reported that 68% of relapses were during drug withdrawal and an additional 24% occurred during the first year after discontinuation of treatment (65). Although late recurrences do occur, they are uncommon (58,68,77). There is no secondary peak in recurrence risk years after discontinuing medications.

In analyzing recurrence risks following withdrawal of AEDs, one must also consider the recurrence risk of patients who are candidates for medication withdrawal but are maintained on AEDs. Annegers and coworkers (36) found a mean relapse risk of 1.6% per year in patients who were in remission for 5 or more years. Similarly, Oller-Daurella and associates (78) reported a 12.6% recurrence rate in a group of patients who were maintained on AEDs after being in remission for 5 or more years. One large-scale, randomized trial of continued AED therapy versus slow withdrawal in 1013 patients who were seizure free for 2 or more years found a 22% recurrence rate in those maintained on medications compared with a 42% recurrence rate in those whose medications were withdrawn

(64). However, after 2 years, the subsequent recurrence risks were identical, suggesting that the increased risk of recurrence attributable to AED withdrawal occurs only in the first 2 years. Late recurrences occur but are not attributable to AED withdrawal. These relapse rates must also be considered when deciding on whether or not to continue long-term AED therapy. Interestingly, in a 30-year follow-up study of 178 patients with epilepsy, there was a slightly higher recurrence rate in those patients who remained on AEDs, although the two groups were not randomized and were, therefore, not fully comparable (43).

RISK FACTORS FOR RECURRENCE

To identify subgroups with better or less favorable prognoses for maintaining seizure remission off medications. it is important to quantify the significance of risk factors such as etiology, age of onset, type of seizure, and the EEG. Here, different studies give very different results. A discussion of potential risk factors and their significance is presented below.

Etiology and Neurologic Status

Patients with remote symptomatic epilepsy associated with a prior neurologic insult, congenital malformation, motor handicap, brain tumor, mental retardation, progressive metabolic disease, trauma, or stroke are less likely to attain complete seizure control than are those with cryptogenic or idiopathic epilepsy (36,39,43).

Even in patients with remote symptomatic epilepsy who do attain seizure remission while on medications, current data indicate that the relapse rate after discontinuation of AEDs is higher than in those with cryptogenic seizures. In one study of 264 children and adolescents, the cumulative recurrence risk 2 years following withdrawal of medications was 26% in the cryptogenic group and 42% in the neurologically abnormal group ($p < 0.005$) (68). Despite the increased risk of recurrence in the neurologically abnormal group, the majority of this population was successfully withdrawn from AEDs. The severity of mental retardation was an additional prognostic factor within this group.

Similar results have been found in other studies (46,54,58–60). A recent study of the prognosis of epilepsy in children with cerebral palsy and epilepsy (51) found that the majority of these children did not achieve remission. However, of the 69 children who achieved a 2-year seizure remission and had their medication withdrawn, 58% remained seizure free. The type of cerebral palsy was associated with a differential risk of recurrence. With one exception (61), studies that did not find such an association either had very few (69) remote symptomatic cases or were restricted to those with cryptogenic epilepsy (50,62,65,73,75). A meta-analysis estimated the relative risk

of recurrence in those with remote symptomatic epilepsy compared with cryptogenic epilepsy to be 1.55 (46).

Age

As discussed, adolescent- and adult-onset epilepsy are associated with a somewhat poorer prognosis for successful withdrawal of AED therapy (46,56,60,63,65,66,68), although selected populations may do well (50,75). The discussion that follows focuses on differences within the pediatric age group.

Many studies report that an age of onset younger than 12 years is associated with a lower recurrence risk following discontinuation of medication than an older age of onset (45,46,48,54,60,67–69,73). This corresponds to the known higher remission rates in the younger group (36,39,79).

There is some controversy as to whether a very young age of onset of younger than 2 (54,68,79) or 3 years (53,74) may be a poor prognostic factor. Studies that include large numbers of children with remote symptomatic epilepsy have found a worse prognosis in the very young (54), whereas studies of mostly cryptogenic epilepsy have produced conflicting results (53,61,69,74). In one study which examined this question (68), 73% of the children with age of onset older than 12 years and 45% of those with age of onset younger than 2 years experienced seizure recurrence compared with 26% of those with age of onset between 2 and 12 years ($p < 0.0001$). However, the poorer prognosis in those with a very young age of onset was limited to the remote symptomatic group (68). These data are consistent with the findings of Huttenlocher and coworkers (80) that neurologically abnormal children with seizure onset at younger than 2 years of age had a poor prognosis for entering remission.

There are no convincing data that withdrawing AEDs during puberty is associated with a higher risk of recurrence (34,58,59,69,81). In fact, with the exception of one isolated report (82), studies on the remission of seizures and on withdrawing AEDs (36,58,59,68,69,71) do not show a reproducible pattern that correlates with puberty. The probability of attaining remission and of maintaining remission after medication withdrawal is more a function of the age of onset and the duration of the seizure disorder, without a special role for puberty.

Electroencephalogram

An abnormal interictal EEG, particularly one with epileptiform features, is often cited as a predictor of relapse after AED withdrawal (4,46,69,82–84). Results of actual studies in children and adults, however, are conflicting.

In children, a substantial number of studies found that the EEG prior to discontinuation of AEDs was an important predictor of outcome (34,37,46,54,66–69,71). Interestingly, any electroencephalographic abnormality, not just a frankly epileptiform one, was associated with an increased risk of relapse. In a study that examined specific features of the EEG, the presence of either slowing or spikes was associated with an increased risk and the presence of both in the same patient was associated with a very high risk of recurrence (69). Two studies reported that only certain specific epileptiform patterns, such as irregular generalized spike-and-wave, were associated with an increased recurrence risk following medication withdrawal (37,83).

Further evidence for the importance of the EEG as a predictor of outcome can be inferred from three large studies (45,62,73). Because these studies excluded children with abnormal EEGs and report very low recurrence risks of 8% to 12%, they provide indirect evidence for the importance of the EEG as a predictor of recurrence. However, some studies in children did not find the EEG to be predictive (48,59). The studies which did find the EEG to be predictive were mainly of children with cryptogenic seizures. In studies that specifically analyzed the relationship between the EEG and outcome in both cryptogenic and remote symptomatic cases, the EEG was a significant predictor of outcome only in the cryptogenic group (68).

The EEG prior to treatment may also have some predictive value. Certain electroencephalographic patterns are markers for specific epileptic syndromes, such as benign rolandic epilepsy, childhood absence, or juvenile myoclonic epilepsy, which are thought to have a particularly favorable or unfavorable prognosis for remaining in remission following drug withdrawal (24,34,81,85). Changes in the EEG between the onset of seizures and time of medication withdrawal may also have a prognostic value (50,69).

The number of adult studies that have examined this issue is relatively small. Callaghan and coworkers (50) reported that an abnormal EEG was associated with an increased risk of recurrence. However, several other adult studies reported no such association (65,75). At present, the preponderance of evidence indicates that an abnormal EEG is a predictor of recurrence in children with cryptogenic epilepsy, but not in those with remote symptomatic epilepsy. In adults the data are inconclusive, but suggest that an abnormal EEG is associated with a modest increase in recurrence risk (46,47,84). Whether specific electroencephalographic patterns are associated with an increased recurrence risk is a question that requires further study.

Epilepsy Syndrome

Epilepsy syndromes are known to be associated with a differential prognosis for remission (23,24,86). Syndromes such as benign rolandic epilepsy have a particularly favorable prognosis for remission and for successfully discontinuing AEDs, even if the EEG is still abnormal (68), as EEG normalization occurs later than the clinical disappearance of seizures (24). Juvenile myoclonic epilepsy, while having a favorable prognosis for remission on medications usually requires prolonged treatment and has a high relapse rate

when medications are withdrawn (24,85). Syndromes such as Lennox-Gastaut have a poor prognosis for remission even on medications (24,43,86). Overall patients with both idiopathic and cryptogenic epilepsy syndromes have a similar prognosis (43,68,86). Interestingly, while specific idiopathic syndromes and the various other generalized epilepsy syndromes have different prognoses, the various nonidiopathic partial epilepsies do not appear to have major differences in the relapse rate following medication withdrawal (68). Unfortunately, there is a paucity of such information as few studies of AED withdrawal provide information by epilepsy syndrome. It is clear that future studies will focus on epilepsy syndrome as a major predictor of long-term prognosis and management, both at the time of diagnosis and when in remission on medications (23,38,68,86).

Other Risk Factors

Other risk factors, such as duration of epilepsy, number of seizures, seizure type, and the medication used, have not been consistently associated with a differential risk of relapse following AED withdrawal in either children or adults.

Duration of epilepsy and number of seizures are closely interrelated. A long duration of epilepsy increases the risk of recurrence, although the magnitude of the effect is small (58,59). One study also reported that having more than 30 generalized tonic-clonic seizures was associated with a high risk of recurrence after discontinuation of therapy (54). In a community-based practice, most people are easily controlled within a short time after therapy is initiated so that these factors will rarely be important (38,42,43).

The specific AED used also has not been consistently associated with the risk of recurrence, although one well-designed study reported an increased recurrence risk in adults who were on valproate compared with those on other AEDs (50). Note that all the published studies on AED withdrawal are reporting the results of AED withdrawal from the old AEDs (barbiturates, phenytoin, carbamazepine, valproate, and ethosuximide). The serum drug level does not seem to have a great impact on recurrence risk. Patients who have not had seizures for several years often have "subtherapeutic" levels, and few have high levels. Available studies show little or no correlation between drug level prior to discontinuation and seizure recurrence and outcome (69), or a very modest effect (54).

Seizure type has also not been consistently associated with recurrence risk except that children with multiple seizure types have a poorer prognosis (58,59). The data regarding partial seizures is conflicting (46,48,50,54, 58–60,63,68,69,71). Note that specific seizure types may be surrogate markers for epilepsy syndromes with a more favorable or less favorable prognosis. At this time it is not clear that any specific seizure type is associated with an increased risk of recurrence following discontinuation of medication.

HOW LONG TO TREAT AND HOW RAPIDLY TO TAPER?

Duration of Seizure-free Interval Prior to Attempting Withdrawal of Antiepileptic Drugs

The chances of remaining seizure free after medication withdrawal is similar whether a 2-year (45,48,50,60, 68,69,71) or 4-year seizure-free interval (54,58,59,63, 68,71) is used. One study that evaluated seizure-free intervals of 1 or more years did find that a longer seizure-free period was associated with a slightly lower recurrence risk (71). However, the higher relapse rates were primarily observed in those who were withdrawn after 1 year. In general, the epidemiologic data do not support the need for treatment beyond 2 years in cases where AED withdrawal is being considered.

A few investigators attempted to withdraw AEDs in children with epilepsy after a seizure-free interval of 1 year or less (52,67,83). A meta-analysis found a pooled relative risk of 1.3 for withdrawal prior to 2 years seizure free versus 2 or more years seizure free (84). While the recurrence risks in these studies are somewhat higher than in studies that used a longer seizure-free interval, they do suggest that, in selected populations, a shorter seizure-free interval may be sufficient. The higher recurrence risks reflect the fact that when a less stringent criterion for remission is used, fewer patients are actually in long-term remission. Long-term outcomes are not adversely affected by early discontinuation (67).

Duration of Medication Taper

Once the decision to withdraw AEDs has been made, the clinician needs to decide on how quickly the medications can be withdrawn. Many clinicians have used slow tapering schedules lasting many months or even years, thinking that they would reduce the risk of recurrence. Even the randomized study from the Medical Research Council (MRC) AED Drug Withdrawal Group (63) used a relatively slow taper. There is general agreement that abrupt discontinuation of AEDs is inadvisable in an outpatient setting and may increase the risk of seizure recurrence. Beyond that, there is much heated debate primarily based on mythology. A well-designed, prospective, randomized clinical trial has provided solid data on this issue (70). The study compared a rapid 6-week AED taper with a more gradual 9-month taper in children with epilepsy whose AEDs were being discontinued after a 2-year or longer seizure-free interval. There were no differences in recurrence risk at 2-years between the groups with short and long tapering regimens. This well-designed study should finally settle this long-standing controversy, although specific drugs, such as barbiturates and benzodiazepines, might require slightly longer tapering periods. Note that a long tapering period will not alter the recurrence risk at 2 years, but may delay the recurrence and,

thus, tends to prolong the period of uncertainty. Thus, a relatively short taper period is particularly important in adolescents and adults if we advise them to stop driving for 6 months to a year following AED withdrawal.

Prognosis Following Relapse

The majority of patients who relapse after medication withdrawal will become seizure free and in remission after AEDs are restarted, although not necessarily immediately (43,67,78,87,88). The prognosis for long-term remission appears to be primarily a function of the underlying epilepsy syndrome. The MRC randomized study of medication withdrawal in children and adults found that the prognosis for seizure control after recurrence in patients with previously well-controlled seizures was no different in those who were withdrawn from AED therapy and relapsed and those who relapsed while remaining on AED therapy (88).

WITHDRAWAL OF ANTIEPILEPTIC DRUGS AFTER SUCCESSFUL RESECTIVE SURGERY

Patients with intractable epilepsy who undergo resective surgery are considered a class 1 successful outcome if they are seizure free following surgery, whether or not they are on AEDs (89,90). In the past, the tendency was to maintain them on at least one AED indefinitely (90). The issue of whether and for how long patients who are seizure free following surgery need to remain on chronic AED therapy is receiving increased attention. Several retrospective studies in adults report that approximately 60% of patients with medically refractory epilepsy who become seizure free after resective surgery remain so when AEDs are withdrawn (91–93). Successful withdrawal of AEDs following resective surgery has also been reported in children (94). Generally the risks of medication withdrawal in this population appear similar to those seen in those with remote symptomatic epilepsy in remission on medications (46,68). It, therefore, appears reasonable to consider medication withdrawal in patients who are seizure free following resective surgery (90,93,94). The prognostic factors for successful medication withdrawal are not well defined but appear to be different than for those who become seizure free with medical therapy (93). The optimal timing for medication withdrawal in this population also is not clear. In principle, one can ask, following a potentially curative procedure, why wait more than a short seizure-free interval, such as 6 months or a year, before attempting withdrawal in this population (93). However, there is a real need for prospective studies to address both prognostic factors for successful medication withdrawal and whether a brief seizure-free interval is enough. Furthermore, while some patients may be eager to try coming off medication in the belief that they are cured (93), many may be unwilling to jeopardize their newly achieved seizure-free state. The decisions need to be individualized, based on the potential risks and benefits in each case and the personal preferences of the patient.

RISKS OF NOT TREATING OR OF DISCONTINUING ANTIEPILEPTIC DRUGS

The major risk associated with not treating after first seizure or of discontinuing AED therapy is having a seizure recurrence. The potential consequences of the seizure recurrence include both direct consequences and psychosocial impact. There is no convincing evidence that a brief seizure causes brain damage (31,35,95,96). Serious injury from a brief seizure is a relatively uncommon event usually related to the impairment of consciousness or loss of consciousness that occurred at an inopportune time or place (e.g., driving, riding a bicycle, swimming, on a stairway, cooking) (25,35,78). These are much less likely to occur in children who are usually in a supervised environment and are not driving, operating heavy machinery, or cooking. In a study of withdrawing AEDs in 264 children with epilepsy who were seizure free on medication, there were 100 recurrences (78). Of these, two experienced status epilepticus as their initial recurrence and have done well after reinitiation of AEDs with no long-term consequences. Five sustained an injury as a result of the initial recurrence, including four with lacerations and one with a broken arm. Thus, the rate of serious injury was quite low. Most reports of serious injuries in patients with epilepsy discuss patients with intractable epilepsy who experience injuries such as burns in the context of frequent seizures (97,98).

Status epilepticus is a concern, particularly in adults. It should be noted that the morbidity of status epilepticus in both children and adults is primarily a function of etiology and in this clinical setting will be low (96,99–101). Furthermore, the risk of status epilepticus in this population is low and essentially limited to those who have had it before (13,27). While status epilepticus is frequently reported in patients with epilepsy who are noncompliant (99,100), the occurrence of status in patients who are withdrawn from their AEDs after a seizure-free interval is very low (69,78).

Some authors, most notably Reynolds, have expressed concern that, in addition to the potential for injury, the consequences of a seizure include a worse long-term prognosis and thus argue that treatment is indicated even after a single seizure (19,102). This view is largely based on Gower's statement that "The tendency of the disease is toward self-perpetuation; each attack facilitates the occurrence of the next by increasing the instability of the nerve elements" (103), which became the basis for the popular notion that "seizures beget seizures." Current epidemiologic data and data from controlled clinical trials indicate that this is not the case (16,17,28,31,33,88,95,104). Studies

in developing countries, where treatment delays were a result of the unavailability of AEDs, show no difference in response rate in those with many prior seizures compared with new-onset patients (33,104). Prognosis is primarily a function of the underlying epilepsy syndrome, and although treatment with AEDs does reduce the risk of subsequent seizures, it does not alter the long-term prognosis for seizure control and remission (16,28,31,33,104). The decision to treat should, therefore, be made on the grounds that the patient has had a sufficient number of events to justify initiating therapy or is at sufficiently high risk for seizure recurrence to justify continued therapy, and not with the hope of somehow preventing the development of "chronic" epilepsy (31).

Although a seizure may be a dramatic and frightening event, the long-term psychosocial impact of an isolated seizure in children is minimal. In adults, the psychosocial impact can be more serious and include the loss of driving privileges and possible adverse effects on employment (105,106). Social stigma of seizures is also much more a concern in adolescents and adults.

RISKS OF INITIATING OR CONTINUING TREATMENT WITH ANTIEPILEPTIC DRUGS

Although effective in controlling seizures, antiepileptic drugs are associated with a variety of significant side effects that must be considered when deciding to initiate or to continue treatment (Table 47.1). Physicians are generally familiar with systemic side effects, including idiosyncratic, acute, and chronic. Idiosyncratic and acute adverse events sufficient to require discontinuation of the drug occur in 15% or more of patients newly treated with an AED, and need to be considered when deciding whether to initiate AED therapy. They are not generally a major concern when deciding whether to continue AEDs in patients who are seizure free as almost all those patients are on stable drug regimens without evidence of acute toxicity. Chronic toxicity is a concern in both settings. There is evidence that children may be more susceptible to chronic toxicity from AEDs (31,107). In the elderly, an additional concern is drug–drug interaction as many of these patients are on multiple other medications that also are protein bound and metabolized by the cytochrome P450 system.

It is now recognized that AED therapy is associated with a variety of both cognitive and behavioral adverse effects (107,108). These are more common in children and sometimes are difficult to recognize. In particular, children on medications since their preschool years may not be identified as having side effects from medications. Only when medications are stopped does it become apparent that the child's performance was impaired by the drug. Adults can also experience cognitive and behavioral adverse events from AED therapy. Increasingly, studies of new AEDs

TABLE 47.1

RISKS AND ADVERSE EFFECTS OF ANTIEPILEPTIC DRUG THERAPY AND OF SEIZURES[a]

RISKS OF ANTIEPILEPTIC DRUG THERAPY	RISKS OF SEIZURES
SYSTEMIC TOXICITY	**PHYSICAL INJURY**
Idiosyncratic	Loss of consciousness
Dose related	Falls
Chronic toxicity	Status epilepticus
	Children and adolescents
	Sports injuries
	Bathing/swimming: drowning
	Adolescents and adults
Teratogenicity	Driving accidents
	Bathing/shower: scalding
	Cooking injuries, burns
	HIGHER CORTICAL FUNCTIONS
Cognitive impairment	Impairment in postictal state
	Children
Adverse effects on behavior	
	PSYCHOSOCIAL
Need for daily medication	Fear of subsequent seizures
Labeling as chronic illness	Loss of privacy
	Stigma of seizures
	Children and adolescents
	Restrictions on school/social activities
	Adolescents and adults
	Restrictions on driving
	Difficulties providing childcare
	ECONOMIC/TEMPORAL
Cost of medications	Time lost because of seizure and
Cost/time of laboratory tests	recovery
Cost/time of physician visits	
	Adolescents and adults
	Discrimination in employment

[a]Some adverse effects of seizures may also occur with antiepileptic drug therapy. Adverse effects listed by age group, such as behavioral effects and bathtub drowning, are meant to indicate the predominant age group in which they occur and do not exclude their occurrence in other age groups.

include measures of neuropsychological function to help address this issue. The reason phenobarbital is no longer considered a first-line drug in adults with epilepsy is not because of its efficacy, which is excellent, but because of the impairment of cognition and behavior associated with its use. Although other agents are less of an issue, all AEDs can have adverse effects on cognition and behavior (107,108).

For women of childbearing age, including adolescents, a discussion of the risks of treatment must include consideration of the potential teratogenicity of these compounds (109–111). As the major teratogenic effects usually occur in the first few weeks of gestation, often before a woman is aware that she is pregnant, the physician must always consider this issue in advance. It impacts both on the decision to initiate or withdraw AED therapy and on the choice of AED. One must also consider that many pregnancies, par-

ticularly in adolescents, are unplanned. Furthermore, enzyme-inducing AEDs may reduce the efficacy of oral contraceptives by inducing the hepatic enzyme systems responsible for their metabolism (109–111). For this reason, we are reluctant to initiate AED therapy in adolescent females and are particularly aggressive in trying to withdraw them from medications after a 2-year seizure-free interval, even if their other risk factors are not favorable.

A hidden side effect of continued antiepileptic drug treatment is that of being labeled (Table 47.1). People with single seizures or epilepsy who have not had a seizure in many years and are off medications are considered to be healthy both by themselves and society. Those individuals can lead normal lives with very few restrictions. Unless they choose to, they rarely need to disclose that they once had seizures. In contrast, even if a patient only had a single seizure or is seizure free for many years, being on AED therapy implies chronic illness to both the patient and those around the patient (106–112). Continued use of medication requires ongoing medical care to prescribe and monitor the medication and establishes that the individual is a patient in need of treatment for a chronic condition. It also implies certain restrictions in driving, and may have an adverse impact on obtaining employment and other social issues. Labeling is a problem in both children and adults. The MRC study reported that psychosocial outcomes were improved in adults who were successfully withdrawn from AED therapy (106). In children and adolescents there is the additional problem that the perception of any chronic illness adversely affects the normal psychosocial maturation process, particularly in adolescents (34,112).

COUNSELING FAMILIES

Decisions on initiating or discontinuing AEDs ultimately depend on a relative assessment of risks and benefits. These are assessed differently by physicians and by patients and their families. Therefore, providing appropriate education and counseling to the patients and their families is critical, regardless of the final therapeutic decision. Both seizures and AED therapy are associated with some risks. Even though patients with good prognostic factors have a lower risk of recurrence, this risk is not zero even if they stay on medications. Conversely, those with poor risk factors may nevertheless maintain remission off medications. The risk of adverse events from AED therapy is essentially independent of the recurrence risk and always needs to be considered, as does the psychosocial impact of both seizures and continued AED therapy. Education assists the patient and family in making an informed decision, helps them to fully participate in the plan of care, and prepares them to deal with psychosocial consequences of the diagnosis. Informed decision making by the physician, in consultation with the family, maximizes the chances of good long-term outcomes.

Patients and families need to be reassured that the risk of a serious injury or death from an isolated seizure is low. They also need to be counseled about appropriate first aid for seizures and safety information. This is a particular problem for adults, as they are more likely to engage in activities that may predispose them to injury should a seizure occur. Places of employment may or may not be accommodating to the person at risk for a seizure.

A discussion of possible restrictions on activities is also important. Parents will need to be told that most of the child's activities can be continued, although some, such as swimming, may need closer supervision. Adolescents and adults will need specific instructions regarding activities such as swimming, cooking, and driving. Counseling often allays fears and educates the patient and family on safety precautions. This reduces the chance for injury from seizures, whether or not the patient is treated. Educational

programs are available for school personnel—teachers, nurses, and students—and information for babysitters also is readily available. Note that, in the case of the child or adult with a first seizure, this discussion is equally applicable whether or not one decides to initiate AED therapy, as therapy reduces, but does not eliminate, the risk of seizure recurrence.

The information provided must be individualized to both the situation and the sophistication level of the patient and the family. The family of a patient with epilepsy who is seizure free on medications should be familiar with the side effects of AED therapy and with seizures, and be able to discuss recurrence risks from withdrawing AEDs and the potential consequences. In the case of patients with a first seizure, the discussion needs to be more comprehensive, including first-aid measures in case of a recurrence, potential adverse effects of AEDs, risks of recurrence, impact on long-term prognosis of delaying therapy until after a second seizure, and restrictions on activity that will occur with or without therapy. It may be difficult to accomplish this in one session, especially in the emergency department where the circumstances may not be conducive to a calm discussion of the relative risks and benefits, and where key information on recurrence risks, such as the results of the electroencephalograph or an imaging study, may not be available.

Families will usually be interested in information that will help them manage the illness or specific problems. Lengthy explanations on any one issue may be confusing and are usually not helpful. Children and adults may have fear of accidents, fear of the loss of friends, fear of taking "drugs," and other less well-defined concerns. A parent's perception of the child's disorder will be an important factor in later coping and will ultimately impact on the perception of quality of life. Adults may have to make major lifestyle changes. The practitioner's prejudices regarding treatment options will undoubtedly come into play during these discussions, but the different options need to be discussed. Although more time-consuming than issuing a prescription, this counseling is necessary for both informed decision making and for favorable long-term outcomes.

A THERAPEUTIC APPROACH

Initiating Antiepileptic Drug Therapy

In children with a first seizure, there is an emerging consensus that treatment after a first unprovoked seizure is usually not indicated (6,7,12–14,31,35,46,107), particularly in neurologically normal children with a brief first seizure (31). We will rarely treat a child with a first unprovoked seizure, even in the presence of risk factors such as a remote symptomatic etiology, an abnormal EEG, or a prolonged first seizure (13,14). In children with infrequent brief seizures, particularly in the context of a self-limited benign childhood epilepsy, many clinicians do not initiate AED therapy even after a second or third seizure (14,16,33–35). This is based on an assessment of the relative risks and benefits of AED therapy in children who will most likely enter remission with or without treatment, and who will most likely continue to have only infrequent seizures (14). However, there is no consensus on this issue.

In adults, the decision to treat or not after a first seizure remains more controversial (9,17,28,102). However, prospective studies show lower recurrence risks than previously thought and a well-designed, prospective, randomized study demonstrated no impact on long-term prognosis from delaying therapy (28,31,32). Therefore, a growing number of clinicians are delaying initiating long-term AED therapy after a single seizure (9,17,28). This is particularly true in young adults who would be committing to long-term therapy and in women of childbearing potential. Following two seizures, the risk of further seizures is approximately 70%, and, in general, AED treatment is indicated (9). The major exception may be a woman who wishes to have children in the immediate future and who has had two brief seizures. In this setting there is no definite answer and the clinician and the patient must again weigh the relative risks and benefits of initiating therapy at that time or waiting (109–111).

In both children and adults, a thorough evaluation of the patient, including a detailed history and neurologic examination, as well as appropriate laboratory studies, such as an electroencephalograph and an imaging study when indicated, are important (21). Of particular importance is a careful history of prior events that may be seizures (21). A substantial proportion of patients who first come to medical attention with a seizure turn out to have had prior episodes that were also seizures (1,2,12,21). This is particularly true for patients who present with a first convulsive episode and, after a careful history is taken, are found to have had prior nonconvulsive episodes of absence or complex partial seizures. These patients fall into the category of newly diagnosed epilepsy, and not first seizure, and usually need treatment.

Withdrawing Antiepileptic Drug Therapy

The question of continuing or withdrawing AED therapy in a given patient must be considered based on an analysis of the relative risks and benefits. The goal is to achieve the best possible outcome for that patient whether it be on medication or off. In considering the risks of seizure recurrence, the statistical risk of relapse is only one piece of the puzzle. One must consider not only the mathematical probability of seizure recurrence but the consequences of such a recurrence. The risk of seizure recurrence following medication withdrawal in children is somewhat lower than in adults and, in addition, there are identifiable subgroups with a particularly favorable prognosis. Adverse effects of continued AED therapy are also clearly more an issue with children than with adults, particularly adult males. However, it

is in the area of potential consequences of a recurrence that the differences are most pronounced.

The adult who is driving and employed can suffer significant adverse social and economic consequences from having a seizure. In addition, an adult is more likely than a child to have the seizure in a setting where a physical injury may occur as a result of impaired consciousness (e.g., driving, operating machinery, cooking). Therefore, a 30% risk of recurrence, which is very acceptable in most children, may be unacceptable to adults because of the more serious consequences of a recurrence. When these are taken into account, patient preferences clearly depend on age and gender, despite similar statistical risks. In the British MRC AED withdrawal study, the psychosocial outcomes of those who successfully came off AEDs were better, and the statistical risk of recurrence was similar to those seen in children (63,64). However, when other adult patients were counseled based on the results of that study, the majority chose to remain on AED therapy (105). Nevertheless, adults who are seizure free on their AEDs for 2 or more years should have the option of AED withdrawal discussed, even if the recommendation of the clinician is to remain on medications, as some patients will find the risk-to-benefit ratio favorable (105,113). Women of childbearing age are a special category, where a more aggressive approach to AED withdrawal may be indicated for reasons already discussed (109,111,113). Another category where a more aggressive approach should be considered is young adults of either gender with childhood-onset epilepsy who are still on medications. A chance at AED withdrawal, especially if they do not need to drive, should be considered before committing them to life-long therapy (34).

The reverse argument may be made for young children. In this group, the risk of relapse is smaller and, depending on the degree of parental supervision, the consequences relatively minor, whereas the risks of side effects from medications are greater. It is much safer to withdraw AEDs in this environment than when the patient is an adult. The risk-to-benefit analysis favors attempting medication withdrawal even in those with a higher risk of relapse (34,52,83).

Adolescents are a special case with additional issues. Adolescents with any chronic illness tend to become noncompliant as part of adolescence. We would far rather withdraw AEDs in a controlled fashion and make the explicit contract that if a recurrence occurs both the patient and the clinician know that medications are needed, than have the adolescent drive and then become noncompliant. In adolescent women, issues of teratogenicity also need to be considered, especially as most pregnancies in this age group are unplanned. Even if immediate pregnancy is not a major concern, these young women will soon be entering their childbearing years and decision making needs to take this into account (109,110). On a risk-to-benefit basis, it is rational to attempt medication withdrawal at least once in adolescents, particularly young women, even if they have risk factors for recurrence. A possible exception to this discussion of adolescents is young men with juvenile myoclonic epilepsy, where there is a very high recurrence risk (24,85). This needs to be discussed with the patient. Even then, however, one attempt at withdrawal may be reasonable as the prognosis may be more variable than previously thought (24,86). In the authors' experience, the majority of adolescents who are offered the choice will choose to attempt medication withdrawal, especially if this choice is presented to them before they are driving.

The clinical data do not demonstrate any significant advantages to waiting more than 2 years before attempting AED withdrawal. The exception to this may be the child with an age-dependent epilepsy, where a longer wait may alter the recurrence risk as the underlying syndrome is more likely to be in remission. However, these are precisely the children with a favorable long-term prognosis where AED withdrawal is often successful even after a brief treatment period (33,52,68,83,84).

Once the decision to withdraw AED therapy is made, the taper should be fairly rapid, as randomized clinical studies show no advantage to a slow taper (70). A slow taper has the additional disadvantage of prolonging the period of uncertainty. In general, we taper a single AED over 4 to 6 weeks. For the patient on two AEDs, we often first taper one AED and see if the patient can be maintained on monotherapy. If the patient remains seizure free on monotherapy, then a second withdrawal is attempted with the plan of treating with monotherapy only if there is a recurrence.

CONCLUSION

Given the consequences of long-term drug therapy and its lack of effect on long-term prognosis following a first seizure, we generally do not recommend treatment following a first unprovoked seizure in either children or adults. Following a second seizure, treatment is generally indicated in adults and needs to be considered in children. In children and adolescents who are seizure free on AEDs for at least 2 years, at least one attempt should be made at medication withdrawal, even if risk factors for recurrence are present. In adults, the risk-to-benefit equation in this setting is less clear, and decisions must be individualized after discussion of the risks and benefits with the patient.

The approach presented in this chapter emphasizes that both seizures and the therapies available carry some risk and that optimal patient care requires careful balancing of these risks and benefits. Assessment of risk requires not only ascertaining the statistical risk of a seizure recurrence or of an adverse event, but also the consequences of such an event. This risk-to-benefit approach is useful not only in deciding whether to initiate or discontinue AED therapy, but also in other treatment decisions. This includes deciding whether or not to add a second drug, to try experimental drugs or therapies such as the ketogenic diet, or whether to consider epilepsy surgery. In all cases

one must balance the risks and benefits of the proposed alternatives, which may change as new information becomes available. Whatever the decision, it should be made jointly by the medical providers and the patient and family after careful discussion, including not only an assessment of the risks and benefits of treatment but also an understanding that individual patients and clinicians place different values on different outcomes and on the acceptability of certain risks.

REFERENCES

1. Groupe CAROLE (Coordination Active du Reseau Observatoire Longitudinal de l'Epilepsie). Treatment of newly diagnosed epileptic crises. A French experience. *Rev Neurol (Paris)* 2001;157: 1500–1512.
2. Sander JW, Hart YM, Johnson AL, et al. National General Practice Study of Epilepsy: newly diagnosed epileptic seizures in a general population. *Lancet* 1990;336:1267–1271.
3. Commission on Epidemiology and Prognosis, International League Against Epilepsy. Guidelines for epidemiologic studies on epilepsy. *Epilepsia* 1993;34:592–596.
4. Annegers JF, Shirts SB, Hauser WA, et al. Risk of recurrence after an initial unprovoked seizure. *Epilepsia* 1986;27:43–50.
5. Berg A, Shinnar S. The risk of seizure recurrence following a first unprovoked seizure: a quantitative review. *Neurology* 1991;41: 965–972.
6. Camfield P, Camfield C, Dooley J, et al. A randomized study of carbamazepine versus no medication following a first unprovoked seizure in childhood. *Neurology* 1989;39:851–852.
7. Camfield PR, Camfield CS, Dooley JM, et al. Epilepsy after a first unprovoked seizure in childhood. *Neurology* 1985;35: 1657–1660.
8. Hauser WA, Anderson VE, Loewenson RB, et al. Seizure recurrence after a first unprovoked seizure. *N Engl J Med* 1982;307: 522–528.
9. Hauser WA, Rich SS, Lee JR, et al. Risk of recurrent seizures after two unprovoked seizures. *N Engl J Med* 1998;338:429–434.
10. Hauser WA, Rich SS, Annegers JF, et al. Seizure recurrence after a 1st unprovoked seizure: an extended follow-up. *Neurology* 1990;40:1163–1170.
11. Hopkins A, Garman A, Clarke C. The first seizure in adult life: value of clinical features, electroencephalography and computerized tomographic scanning in prediction of seizure recurrence. *Lancet* 1988;1:721–726.
12. Shinnar S, Berg AT, Moshe SL, et al. The risk of recurrence following a first unprovoked seizure in childhood: a prospective study. *Pediatrics* 1990;85:1076–1085.
13. Shinnar S, Berg AT, Moshe SL, et al. The risk of seizure recurrence following a first unprovoked afebrile seizure in childhood: an extended follow-up. *Pediatrics* 1996;98:216–225.
14. Shinnar S, Berg AT, O'Dell C, et al. Predictors of multiple seizures in a cohort of children prospectively followed from the time of their first unprovoked seizure. *Ann Neurol* 2000;48:140–147.
15. Stroink H, Brouwer OF, Arts WF, et al. The first unprovoked seizure in childhood: a hospital based study of the accuracy of the diagnosis, rate of recurrence, and long term outcome after recurrence. Dutch Study of Epilepsy in Childhood. *J Neurol Neurosurg Psychiatry* 1998;64:595–600.
16. van Donselaar CA, Brouwer OF, Geerts AT, et al. Clinical course of untreated tonic-clonic seizures in childhood: prospective, hospital based study. *BMJ* 1997;314:401–404.
17. van Donselaar CA, Geerts AT, Schimsheimer RJ. Idiopathic first seizure in adult life: who should be treated? *BMJ* 1990;302: 620–623.
18. van Donselaar CE, Schimsheimer RJ, Geerts AT, et al. Value of the electroencephalogram in adult patients with untreated idiopathic first seizures. *Arch Neurol* 1992;49:231–237.
19. Elwes RDC, Chesterman P, Reynolds EH. Prognosis after a first untreated tonic-clonic seizure. *Lancet* 1985;2:752–753.

20. First Seizure Trial Group. Randomized clinical trial on the efficacy of antiepileptic drugs in reducing the risk of relapse after a first unprovoked tonic-clonic seizure. *Neurology* 1993;43:478–483.

21. Hirtz D, Ashwal S, Berg A, et al. Practice parameter: evaluating a first nonfebrile seizure in children: report of the Quality Standards Subcommittee of the American Academy of Neurology, the Child Neurology Society and the American Epilepsy Society. *Neurology* 2000;55:616–623.

22. Hirtz DG, Ellenberg JH, Nelson KB. The risk of recurrence of nonfebrile seizures in children. *Neurology* 1984;34:637–641.

23. Commission on Classification and Terminology of the International League Against Epilepsy. Proposal for revised classification of epilepsies and epileptic syndromes. *Epilepsia* 1989;30:389–399.

24. Roger J, Bureau M, Dravet C, et al, eds. *Epileptic syndromes in infancy, childhood and adolescence,* 3rd ed. London: John Libbey, 2002.

25. Shinnar S, Kang H, Berg AT, et al. EEG abnormalities in children with a first unprovoked seizure. *Epilepsia* 1994;35:471–476.

26. Shinnar S, Berg AT, Ptachewich Y, et al. Sleep state and the risk of seizure recurrence following a first unprovoked seizure in childhood. *Neurology* 1993;43:701–706.

27. Shinnar S, Berg AT, Moshe SL, et al. How long do new-onset seizures in children last? *Ann Neurol* 2001;49:659–664.

28. Musicco M, Beghi E, Solari A, et al. Treatment of first tonic-clonic seizure does not improve the prognosis of epilepsy. *Neurology* 1997;49:991–998.

29. Chandra B. First seizure in adults: to treat or not to treat. *Clin Neurol Neurosurg* 1992;94:S61–S63.

30. Das CP, Sawhney IMS, Lal V, et al. Risk of recurrence of seizures following single unprovoked idiopathic seizure. *Neurol India* 2000;48:357–360.

31. Hirtz D, Berg A, Bettis D, et al. Practice parameter: treatment of the child with a first unprovoked seizure. Report of the Quality Standards Subcommittee of the American Academy of Neurology and the Practice Committee of the Child Neurology Society. *Neurology* 2003;60:166–175.

32. Shinnar S, Berg AT. Does antiepileptic drug therapy prevent the development of "chronic" epilepsy? *Epilepsia* 1996;37:701–708.

33. Ambrosetto G, Tassinari CA. Antiepileptic drug treatment of benign childhood epilepsy with rolandic spikes: is it necessary? *Epilepsia* 1990;31:802–805.

34. Shinnar S, O'Dell C. Treatment decisions in childhood seizures. In: Pellock JM, Dodson WE, Bourgeois BF, eds. *Pediatric epilepsy: diagnosis and therapy,* 2nd ed. New York: Demos, 2001:291–300.

35. Freeman JM, Tibbles J, Camfield C, et al. Benign epilepsy of childhood: a speculation and its ramifications. *Pediatrics* 1987;79: 864–868.

36. Annegers JF, Hauser WA, Elveback LR. Remission of seizures and relapse in patients with epilepsy. *Epilepsia* 1979;20:729–737.

37. Andersson T, Braathen G, Persson A, et al. A comparison between one and three years of treatment in uncomplicated childhood epilepsy: a prospective study, II: the EEG as predictor of outcome after withdrawal of treatment. *Epilepsia* 1997;38:225–232.

38. Berg AT, Shinnar S, Levy SR, et al. Two-year remission and subsequent relapse in children with newly diagnosed epilepsy. *Epilepsia.* 2001;42:1553–1562.

39. Brorson LO, Wranne L. Long-term prognosis in childhood epilepsy: survival and seizure prognosis. *Epilepsia* 1987;28:324–330.

40. Callaghan N, Kenny RA, O'Neill B, et al. A prospective study between carbamazepine, phenytoin and sodium valproate as monotherapy in previously untreated and recently diagnosed patients with epilepsy. *J Neurol Neurosurg Psychiatry* 1985;48:639–644.

41. Elwes RDC, Johnson AL, Shorvon SD, et al. The prognosis for seizure control in newly diagnosed epilepsy. *N Engl J Med* 1984;311:944–947.

42. Goodridge DMG, Shorvon SD. Epileptic seizures in a population of 6000, II: treatment and prognosis. *Br Med J* 1983;287:645–647.

43. Sillanpaa M, Jalava M, Kaleva O, et al. Long-term prognosis of seizures with onset in childhood. *N Engl J Med* 1998;338:1715–1722.

44. Aldenkamp AP, Alpherts WC, Sandstedt P, et al. Antiepileptic drug-related cognitive complaints in seizure-free children with epilepsy before and after drug discontinuation. *Epilepsia* 1998;39:1070–1074.

45. Arts WFM, Visser LH, Loonen MCB, et al. Follow-up of 146 children with epilepsy after withdrawal of antiepileptic therapy. *Epilepsia* 1988;29:244–250.

46. Berg AT, Shinnar S. Relapse following discontinuation of antiepileptic drugs: a meta-analysis. *Neurology* 1994;44:601–608.

47. Berg AT, Shinnar S, Chadwick D. Discontinuing antiepileptic drugs. In: Engel J Jr, Pedley TA, eds. *Epilepsy: a comprehensive textbook.* Philadelphia: Lippincott-Raven, 1997:1275–1284.

48. Bouma PAD, Peters ACB, Arts RJHM, et al. Discontinuation of antiepileptic therapy: a prospective trial in children. *J Neurol Neurosurg Psychiatry* 1987;50:1579–1583.

49. Braathen G, Andersson T, Gylje H, et al. Comparison between one and three years of treatment in uncomplicated childhood epilepsy: a prospective study, I: outcome in different seizure types. *Epilepsia* 1996;37:822–832.

50. Callaghan N, Garrett A, Goggin T. Withdrawal of anticonvulsant drugs in patients free of seizures for two years. *N Engl J Med* 1988;318:942–946.

51. Delgado MR, Riela AR, Mills J, et al. Discontinuation of antiepileptic drug therapy after two seizure-free years in children with cerebral palsy. *Pediatrics* 1996;97:192–197.

52. Dooley J, Gordon K, Camfield P, et al. Discontinuation of anticonvulsant therapy in children free of seizures for 1 year: a prospective study. *Neurology* 1996;46:969–974.

53. Ehrhardt F, Forsythe WI. Prognosis after grand mal seizures: a study of 187 children with three year remissions. *Dev Med Child Neurol* 1989;31:633–639.

54. Emerson R, D'Souza BJ, Vining EP, et al. Stopping medication in children with epilepsy. predictors of outcome. *N Engl J Med* 1981;304:1125–1129.

55. Galimberti CA, Manni R, Parietti L, et al. Drug withdrawal in patients with epilepsy: prognostic value of the EEG. *Seizure* 1993;2:213–220.

56. Gerstle de Pasquet E, Bonnevaux de Toma S, Bainy JA, et al. Prognosis of epilepsy, remission of seizures and relapse in 808 adult patients. *Acta Neurol Latinoam* 1981;27:167–176.

57. Gherpelli JLD, Kok F, dal Forno S, et al. Discontinuing medication in epileptic children: a study of risk factors related to recurrence. *Epilepsia* 1992;33:681–686.

58. Holowach-Thurston JH, Thurston DL, Hixon BB, et al. Prognosis in childhood epilepsy: additional followup of 148 children 15 to 23 years after withdrawal of anticonvulsant therapy. *N Engl J Med* 1982;306:831–836.

59. Holowach J, Thurston DL, O'Leary J. Prognosis in childhood epilepsy: followup study of 148 cases in which therapy had been suspended after prolonged anticonvulsant control. *N Engl J Med* 1972;286:169–174.

60. Juul Jensen P. Frequency of recurrence after discontinuance of anticonvulsant therapy in patients with epileptic seizures: a new followup study after 5 years. *Epilepsia* 1968;9:11–16.

61. Mastropaolo C, Tondi M, Carboni F, et al. Prognosis after therapy discontinuation in children with epilepsy. *Neurology* 1992;32:142–145.

62. Matricardi M, Brinciott M, Benedetti P. Outcome after discontinuation of antiepileptic drug therapy in children with epilepsy. *Epilepsia* 1989;30:582–589.

63. Medical Research Council Antiepileptic Drug Withdrawal Study Group. Randomised study of antiepileptic drug withdrawal in patients with remission. *Lancet* 1991;337:1175–1180.

64. Medical Research Council Antiepileptic Drug Withdrawal Study Group. Prognostic index for recurrence of seizures after remission of epilepsy. *BMJ* 1993;306:1374–1378.

65. Overweg J, Binnie CD, Oosting J, et al. Clinical and EEG prediction of seizure recurrence following antiepileptic drug withdrawal. *Epilepsy Res* 1987;1:272–283.

66. Pestre M, Loiseau P, Dartigues JF, et al. Arret du traitement dans les crises épileptiques de l'adolescence. *Rev Neurol (Paris)* 1987;143:40–46.

67. Peters AC, Brouwer OF, Geerts AT, et al. Randomized prospective study of early discontinuation of antiepileptic drugs in children with epilepsy. *Neurology* 1998;50:724–730.

68. Shinnar S, Berg AT, Moshe SL, et al. Discontinuing antiepileptic drugs in children with epilepsy: a prospective study. *Ann Neurol* 1994;35:534–545.

69. Shinnar S, Vining EPG, Mellits ED, et al. Discontinuing antiepileptic medication in children with epilepsy after two years without seizures: a prospective study. *N Engl J Med* 1985;313:976–980.

70. Tennison M, Greenwood R, Lewis D, et al. Rate of taper of antiepileptic drugs and the risk of seizure recurrence in children. *N Engl J Med* 1994;330:1407–1410.

71. Todt H. The late prognosis of epilepsy in childhood: results of a prospective followup study. *Epilepsia* 1984;25:137–144.

72. Tonnby B, Nilsson HL, Aldenkamp AP, et al. Withdrawal of antiepileptic medication in children. Correlation of cognitive function and plasma concentration—the Multicentre "Holmfrid" Study. *Epilepsy Res* 1994;19:141–152.

73. Tsuchiya S, Maruyama H, Maruyama K, et al. A follow up study of 1007 epileptic children with anticonvulsant therapy for more than 10 years. *No To Hattatsu* 1985;17:23–28.

74. Visser LH, Arts WFM, Loonen MCB, et al. Follow-up study of 166 children with epilepsy after withdrawal of anticonvulsant therapy. *Adv Epileptol* 1987;16:401–404.

75. Wallis WE. Withdrawal of anticonvulsant drugs in seizure free epileptic patients. *Clin Neuropharmacol* 1987;10:423–433.

76. Verotti A, Morresi S, Basciani F, et al. Discontinuation of antiepileptic drugs in children with partial epilepsy. *Neurology* 2000;55:1393–1395.

77. Shinnar S, O'Dell C, Maw M, et al. Long-term prognosis of children who relapse after withdrawal of antiepileptic drug therapy. *Epilepsia* 1999;40(Suppl 7):85–86.

78. Oller-Daurella L, Pamies R, Oller FVL. Reduction or discontinuance of antiepileptic drugs in patients seizure free for more than 5 years. In: Janz D, ed. *Epileptology*. Stuttgart, Germany: Thieme, 1976:218–227.

79. Shafer SQ, Hauser WA, Annegers JF, et al. EEG and other early predictors of epilepsy remission: a community study. *Epilepsia* 1988;29:590–600.

80. Huttenlocher PR, Hapke RJ. A follow up study of intractable seizures in childhood. *Ann Neurol* 1990;28:699–705.

81. Diamantopoulos N, Crumrine PK. The effect of puberty on the course of epilepsy. *Arch Neurol* 1986;43:873–876.

82. Forster CH, Schmidberger G. Prognostische Wertigkeit von EEG verlautsuntersuchungen bei Kindern mit anfallsrezidiven nach absetzen der antikonvulsiven Therapie. In: Doose H, Gross Selbeck G, eds. *Epilepsie*. Stuttgart, Germany: Thieme, 1978:252–255.

83. Braathen G, Melander H. Early discontinuation of treatment in children with uncomplicated epilepsy: a prospective study with a model for prediction of outcome. *Epilepsia* 1997;38:561–569.

84. Sirven JI, Sperling M, Wingerchuk DM. Early versus late antiepileptic drug withdrawal for people with epilepsy in remission. *Cochrane Database Syst Rev* 2001;(3):CD001902.

85. Delgado-Escueta AV, Enrile-Bacsal F. Juvenile myoclonic epilepsy of Janz. *Neurology* 1984;34:285–294.

86. Sillanpaa M, Jalava M, Shinnar S. Epilepsy syndromes in patients with childhood-onset epilepsy. *Pediatr Neurol* 1999;21:533–537.

87. Bouma PA, Peters AC, Brouwer OF. Long term course of childhood epilepsy following relapse after antiepileptic drug withdrawal. *J Neurol Neurosurg Psychiatry* 2002;72:507–510.

88. Chadwick D, Taylor J, Johnson T. Outcomes after seizure recurrence in people with well-controlled epilepsy and the factors that influence it. The MRC Antiepileptic Drug Withdrawal Group. *Epilepsia* 1996;37:1043–1050.

89. Commission on Neurosurgery of the International League Against Epilepsy (ILAE) 1997–2001. Proposal for a new classification of outcome with respect to epileptic seizures following epilepsy surgery. *Epilepsia* 2001;42:282–286.

90. Andermann F, Bourgeois BF, Leppik IE, et al. Postoperative pharmacotherapy and discontinuation of antiepileptic drugs. In: Engel J, ed. *Surgical treatment of the epilepsies*, 2nd ed. New York: Raven Press, 1993:679–684.

91. Vickrey BG, Hay RD, Rausch R, et al. Outcome in 248 patients who had diagnostic evaluations for epilepsy surgery. *Lancet* 1995;346:1445–1449.

92. Maher J, McLachlan RS. Antiepileptic drug treatment following temporal lobectomy. *Neurology* 1997;48:1368–1374.

93. Schiller Y, Cascino GD, So EL, et al. Discontinuation of antiepileptic drugs after successful epilepsy surgery. *Neurology* 2000;54:346–349.

94. Gilliam F, Wyllie E, Kashden J, et al. Epilepsy surgery outcome: case assessment in children. *Neurology* 1997;48:1368–1374.

95. Berg AT, Shinnar S. Do seizures beget seizures? An assessment of the clinical evidence in humans. *J Clin Neurophysiol* 1997;14:102–110.

96. Shinnar S, Babb TL. Long term sequelae of status epilepticus. In: Engel J Jr, Pedley TA, eds. *Epilepsy: a comprehensive text*. Philadelphia: Lippincott-Raven, 1997:755–763.

97. Neufeld MY, Vishne T, Chistik V, et al. Life-long history of injuries related to seizures. *Epilepsy Res* 1999;34:123–127.

98. Spitz MC. Injuries and death as a consequence of seizures in people with epilepsy. *Epilepsia* 1998;39:904–907.

99. DeLorenzo RJ, Hauser WA, Towne AR, et al. A prospective population-based epidemiological study of status epilepticus in Richmond, Virginia. *Neurology* 1996;46:1029–1035.

100. Dodson WE, DeLorenzo RJ, Pedley TA, et al. The treatment of convulsive status epilepticus: recommendations of the Epilepsy Foundation of America's Working Group on Status Epilepticus. *JAMA* 1993;270:854–859.

101. Maytal J, Shinnar S, Moshe SL, et al. The low morbidity and mortality of status epilepticus in children. *Pediatrics* 1989;83:323–331.

102. Reynolds EH. Do anticonvulsants alter the natural course of epilepsy? Treatment should be started as early as possible. *BMJ* 1995;310:176–177.

103. Gowers WR. *Epilepsy and other chronic convulsive disorders*. London: J&A Churchill, 1881.

104. Sander JWAS. Some aspects of prognosis in the epilepsies: a review. *Epilepsia* 1993;34:1007–1016.

105. Jacoby A, Baker G, Chadwick D, et al. The impact of counseling with a practical statistical model on a patient's decision making about treatment for epilepsy: findings from a pilot study. *Epilepsy Res* 1993;16:207–214.

106. Jacoby A, Johnson A, Chadwick D. Psychosocial outcomes of antiepileptic drug discontinuation. *Epilepsia* 1992;33:1123–1131.

107. Committee on Drugs, American Academy of Pediatrics. Behavioral and cognitive effects of anticonvulsant therapy. *Pediatrics* 1995;96:538–540.

108. Vining EPG, Mellits ED, Dorsen MM, et al. Psychologic and behavioral effects of antiepileptic drugs in children: a double-blind comparison between phenobarbital and valproic acid. *Pediatrics* 1987;80:165–174.

109. American Academy of Neurology, Quality Standards Subcommittee. Practice parameter: management issues for women with epilepsy—summary statement. *Neurology* 1998;51:944–948.

110. Commission on Genetics, Pregnancy and the Child, International League Against Epilepsy. Guidelines for the care of women of childbearing age with epilepsy. *Epilepsia* 1993;34:588–589.

111. Yerby MS. Teratogenic effects of antiepileptic drugs: what do we advise patients. *Epilepsia* 1997;38:957–958.

112. Hoare P. Does illness foster dependency: a study of epileptic and diabetic children. *Dev Med Child Neurol* 1984;26:20–24.

113. American Academy of Neurology, Quality Standards Subcommittee. Practice parameter: a guideline for discontinuing antiepileptic drugs in seizure-free patients—summary statement. *Neurology* 1996;47:600–602.

Hormones, Catamenial Epilepsy, and Reproductive and Bone Health in Epilepsy

48

Martha J. Morrell

Steroid hormones alter the excitability of neurons of the cerebral cortex and thereby alter the seizure threshold. Seizures, in turn, change the endocrine environment, probably through actions on the hypothalamic–pituitary axis. Some antiepileptic drugs (AEDs) further complicate hormone–seizure interactions, altering the metabolism and binding of steroid hormones. This chapter discusses the clinical implications of these hormone–seizure interactions, focusing on the impact of ovarian steroid hormones on seizures and of epilepsy on reproductive and bone health.

EFFECTS OF STEROID HORMONES ON NEURONAL EXCITABILITY

Steroid and thyroid hormones influence brain excitability (1). This dynamic relationship is most clearly established for the ovarian sex steroid hormones estrogen and progesterone (2,3). Fluctuations in these hormones over a reproductive cycle change seizure susceptibility in experimental models of epilepsy (4,5).

Estrogen activates seizures in experimental models of epilepsy and in human cerebral cortex. Estrogen lowers the electroshock seizure threshold (6–8), creates new cortical seizure foci when applied topically (9), activates preexisting cortical epileptogenic foci (10), and increases the severity of chemically induced seizures (11,12). Intravenously administered estrogen activates electroencephalographic

(EEG) epileptiform activity in some women with partial epilepsy (13).

In contrast, progesterone exerts a seizure-protective effect in experimental models. High doses induce sedation and anesthesia in rats and in humans (14), primarily as a result of actions of the metabolite pregnenolone. Progesterone reduces spontaneous interictal spikes produced by cortical application of penicillin (15) and suppresses kindling (16) and focal seizures (17) in animals. It also heightens the seizure threshold to chemical convulsants (18,19), elevates the electroshock seizure threshold (8,20), and attenuates ethanol-withdrawal convulsions (18).

Steroid hormones modulate cortical excitability through several mechanisms of action. They bind to an intracellular receptor (intracytoplasmic for glucocorticoids, intranuclear for estrogen and progesterone). Binding transforms the receptor to an active form that binds to deoxyribonucleic acid (DNA), leading to gene activation and protein synthesis; this process requires 30 minutes to several hours to complete. Many neuroactive effects of steroids are evident in seconds to minutes, suggesting that some actions are also mediated at the neuronal membrane.

Gonadal and adrenocortical steroid hormones exert immediate, short effects on neuronal excitability by altering γ-aminobutyric acid (GABA)-mediated neuronal inhibition and glutamate-mediated excitation at the cell membrane (21,22). A sex steroid hormone-recognition site is present on recombinantly expressed GABA$_A$-receptor complex derived from human complementary DNA (cDNA) (23). Neurosteroids, such as those in the ovary, may act at two sites on the GABA$_A$-receptor complex: directly on the chloride channel and at a distinct site that mediates the action of GABA and benzodiazepines (24,25).

Ovarian steroids have opposing effects on neuronal excitability (26). Estrogen reduces the effectiveness of GABA-mediated neuronal inhibition by decreasing chloride conductance through the GABA$_A$-receptor complex. Longer-latency effects of estrogen on neuronal excitability are exerted through inhibition of GABA synthesis in the arcuate nucleus, the ventromedial nucleus of the hypothalamus, and the centromedial group of the amygdala (27), probably through regulation of messenger ribonucleic acid (mRNA) encoding for glutamic acid decarboxylase (GAD), the rate-limiting enzyme for GABA synthesis (28,29). Estrogen also affects mRNA encoding for GABA$_A$-receptor subunits (30). Estradiol rapidly increases responses of neurons to the excitatory neurotransmitter glutamate through agonist binding sites on the N-methyl-D-aspartate (NMDA)-receptor complex (31–34) and through a G-protein-dependent mechanism on non-NMDA glutamate receptors that activate protein kinase (35).

Woolley and colleagues demonstrated the proconvulsant effect of estrogen (2,36). Three days' exposure to elevated estradiol levels increased the density of dendritic spines and excitatory synapses on hippocampal neurons; the same also occurs with natural hormone fluctuations over the estrous cycle (37).

Progesterone and its metabolites function as allosteric-receptor antagonists or inverse agonists at the GABA$_A$-receptor complex (38), potentiating GABA-induced chloride conductance by increasing the frequency (benzodiazepine-like effects) and duration (barbiturate-like effect) of channel opening (39,40). Progesterone also modulates GAD (19), alters expression of mRNA encoding for GABA$_A$-receptor subunits (29,30), and reduces glutamate activity (32,33).

The sensitivity of neurons to the modulating effects of individual steroid hormones changes after puberty and in response to fluctuations in basal levels of steroid hormones over a reproductive cycle (19,41). The pubertal surge in estrogen appears to have a neuronal priming effect. In contrast to its effects in postpubertal rats, estrogen does not alter the rate of amygdala kindling in prepubertal male and female rats. Rats castrated prepubertally have higher seizure thresholds to minimal and maximal electroshock than do animals castrated after puberty (8,42). Several rodent models of epilepsy suggest that the sensitivity of the GABA$_A$-receptor complex to neurosteroids varies so as to maintain homeostatic regulation of brain excitability (4,25,39). In rodents, the threshold dose for seizure onset induced by chemical convulsants (bicuculline, picrotoxin, pentylenetetrazol, and strychnine)

changes over the estrus cycle. Female rats in estrus are more sensitive to chemical convulsants than are females in diestrus and males, whereas infusion of a progesterone metabolite increases the seizure threshold more for females in diestrus (25). The differential effects of estrogens on neuronal excitability also depend on cycling status. Excitability is enhanced when female rats in low-estrogen states are given estrogen (diestrus) but not when estrogen is given during a high-estrogen state (diestrus) (43).

Anatomic specificity in the cortical distribution of steroid hormone receptors may account for some of the differential effects of each steroid hormone on neuronal excitability, endocrine function, and reproductive behavior. Estrogen receptors are located primarily in the mesial temporal lobe (limbic cortex) and hypothalamus (3,44,45); progesterone and androgen receptors are also diffusely distributed over the cerebral cortex (40,45–49). Many of estrogen's effects, including the steroid-dependent suppression of GAD, are confined to the CA1 region of the hippocampus (50). Anatomic distribution also varies with development. Neocortical receptors for estrogen in the immature brain are largely absent after puberty (3,51). Anatomic specificity and varying distribution might account, in part, for changes in seizure expression with changes in reproductive function.

EFFECTS OF SEIZURES ON REPRODUCTIVE HORMONES

Seizures themselves can alter the level of some hormones, particularly hypothalamic tropic hormones and pituitary gonadotropins (52), leading ultimately to changes in secretion of gonadal steroids.

The hypothalamus regulates secretion of anterior pituitary hormones through the release of neurohormones, which in turn stimulate or inhibit release of hormones of the anterior pituitary. Gonadotropin-releasing hormone (GnRH), a hypothalamic tropic hormone, is released episodically and stimulates the pulsatile release of the pituitary gonadotropins follicle-stimulating hormone (FSH) and luteinizing hormone (LH). FSH promotes development of the primary ovarian follicle and secretion of estradiol in the female, and spermatogenesis in the male (Fig. 48.1). In females, a midcycle surge of LH stimulates ovulation and formation of the progesterone-secreting corpus luteum. In males, LH stimulates interstitial cell secretion of testosterone and other androgens.

Pituitary release of prolactin is also determined by inhibitory and stimulating factors from the hypothalamus. Prolactin initiates milk synthesis in the mammary glands and affects growth, osmoregulation, and fat and carbohydrate metabolism. Prolactin also inhibits sexual behavior (53) and promotes parental behavior (54). Elevated levels can cause impotence in human males (55).

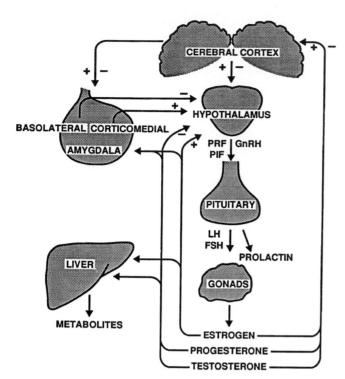

Figure 48.1 Hypothalamic–pituitary axis, illustrating amygdala interconnections to the hypothalamus. (+), excitatory feedback; (−), inhibitory feedback; FSH, follicle-stimulating hormone; GnRH, gonadotrophin-releasing hormone; LH, luteinizing hormone; PRL, prolactin.

Steroid hormones are produced by the adrenal cortex and the gonads. The principal gonadal androgens are testosterone, dihydrotestosterone, and androstenedione. Dihydroandrostenedione is produced by the adrenal cortex. Testosterone is necessary for masculinization during sexual differentiation, spermatogenesis, and development of male secondary sexual characteristics at puberty, as well as for activation of sexual and aggressive behavior and maintenance of sexual desire.

The principal female sex hormones are estrogen and progesterone. The granulosa cells of the ovarian follicle produce estrogens, including estradiol, estrone and estriol, that support the development of female secondary sexual characteristics and also affect metabolic rate, body temperature, skin texture, and fat distribution. In addition, estrogens influence sexual and parental behavior. Progesterones are produced by the corpus luteum formed from the ovarian follicle after ovulation. Progesterone is essential for uterine, vaginal, and mammary gland growth. It inhibits the menstrual cycle to maintain pregnancy and has complex effects on sexual behavior.

HORMONE DISTURBANCES IN EPILEPSY

Among the hormonal abnormalities described in persons with epilepsy are changes in the release of LH, prolactin, and gonadal testosterone that may arise as a result of seizures or treatment with AEDs.

Seizures may disturb the hypothalamic-pituitary-gonadal axis, which is modulated by the cerebral and limbic cortex. Regions of limbic cortex, particularly the amygdala, have extensive reciprocal connections with the hypothalamus (56). In the amygdala, the corticomedial nuclear group stimulates hypothalamic release of GnRH, and the basolateral nuclear group inhibits its release (57), depending on which group is affected by excitation of the amygdala. The inhibitory or stimulatory effect ultimately alters release of the corresponding pituitary hormones (58), as does seizure-precipitated release of excitatory and inhibitory neurochemicals (21), which regulate neuroendocrine function.

In men and women with epilepsy, basal concentrations of LH and LH pulse frequency are abnormal (59–63), probably from derangement of the hypothalamic GnRH pulse generator (59). Women with epilepsy not treated with AEDs had a significant increase in gonadotropin basal secretion during frequent interictal epileptiform activity. Release of LH may vary according to the epilepsy syndrome and AED exposure. LH pulsatility increased in women with a variety of untreated epilepsies (63), but diminished in those taking AEDs for temporal lobe epilepsy (62). Baseline LH levels in men receiving AEDs may be lower than normal, with an exaggerated response to GnRH (64–66).

Growth hormone and prolactin are elevated interictally in some men and women with epilepsy (45,64,67,68). Pituitary prolactin increases more than twofold after generalized convulsive seizures, most complex partial seizures, and simple partial seizures involving limbic structures but not after nonepileptic seizures (69–71). The increase occurs within 5 minutes, is maximal by 15 minutes, and persists for 1 hour (72). Other changes include elevation in corticotropin and cortisol following both convulsions and stimulation of mesial temporal lobe structures.

Levels of sex steroid hormone may be abnormal in some men and women with epilepsy, in part because of changes in steroid metabolism induced by AEDs (73). AEDs that induce the hepatic cytochrome P450 (CYP) system increase the metabolism of gonadal and adrenal steroid hormones. AEDs also induce the synthesis of sex hormone-binding globulin (SHBG), a binding protein for steroid hormones (74). Increased protein binding decreases the free, biologically active fraction of hormone. Men who receive AEDs that induce the microsomal enzyme system may have low levels of total and free testosterone and of adrenal androgens (75–78). Women taking such AEDs have low androgen and estrogen levels and elevated levels of SHBG protein (79,80). Valproate, which does not induce liver cytochrome enzymes, increases gonadal and adrenal androgen levels in women (81). Estrogen, progesterone, and androgen levels in women receiving gabapentin or lamotrigine, which do not affect on cytochrome enzymes, are not different from levels in medically normal nontreated control women. These observations suggest that changes in steroid hormones are related to AED-associated alterations in steroid metabolism and not to seizures or epilepsy (79).

EFFECTS ON SEIZURES OF CHANGES IN REPRODUCTIVE HORMONES

The frequency and severity of seizures are likely to change in concert with significant changes in reproductive status and reproductive hormones: at puberty, during the menstrual cycle, and at menopause. Juvenile myoclonic epilepsy (82) and photosensitive epilepsy (83) often arise at puberty, when a surge in pituitary gonadotropin hormones leads to production of gonadal sex steroid hormones. Conversely, absence (84) and benign rolandic epilepsy (85) may remit at this time.

Puberty exerts contradictory effects on localization-related epilepsy. Reports have described a transient worsening, attributed to a drop in AED concentrations (86), in generalized tonic-clonic seizures (87); complex partial seizures increased or deceased in frequency (88).

Interactions between hormones and seizures become clinically relevant for women experiencing catamenial exacerbations of epilepsy. In the 30% to 50% whose epileptic pattern may correspond to the menstrual cycle, vulnerability to seizures is highest about 3 days before and during flow and at ovulation (89), periods when estrogen is relatively high and progesterone is relatively low (10,89–91). This seizure exacerbation may be even more prominent in anovulatory cycles when estrogen remains high, unopposed by progesterone normally secreted by the corpus luteum (88,92).

Little is known about epilepsy at menopause, a time when ovarian failure decreases estrogen and progesterone levels and raises pituitary gonadotropic levels. Rosciszewska (87) found that seizures were likely to improve if onset had been relatively late, if a catamenial relationship existed, and if seizures were already well controlled. Women with frequent partial or tonic-clonic seizures noted worsening. Seizures beginning at menopause have been reported (93).

TREATMENT OF HORMONALLY SENSITIVE SEIZURES

The most effective treatment for any type of seizure is usually a first-line AED used alone. Women with a catamenial-associated seizures may also respond to adjunctive therapy with a carbonic anhydrase inhibitor or with hormonal therapy.

Administered orally, acetazolamide, a weak carbonic anhydrase inhibitor with mild diuretic activity, may be used as adjunctive therapy for catamenial seizures, although this is not a labeled indication. The anticonvulsant properties of acetazolamide may be related to its induction of a mild, transient metabolic acidosis; however, tolerance to its anti-convulsant properties develops quickly, necessitating use over short periods. In women with catamenial seizures and predictable menstrual cycles, acetazolamide may be given for 10 to 14 days, around the time of seizure vulnerability, in two divided doses of 250 to 1000 mg. Gastrointestinal disturbance, sedation, headache, and hypersensitivity reactions occur, particularly in those patients sensitive to sulfonamides. Bone marrow depression and renal colic arise rarely, as do electrolyte disturbances such as hypokalemia and hyperglycemia in patients with diabetes mellitus. Acetazolamide has teratogenic and embryocidal effects in rats and mice. Although this effect appears to be species specific, the drug should not be used in pregnant women.

Several small studies have evaluated the effectiveness of progesterones and antiestrogens as AEDs. Orally administered synthetic progestins are ineffective (94), although parenteral medroxyprogesterone, in doses large enough to cause amenorrhea (94,95)—120 to 150 mg intramuscularly every 6 to 12 week (96)—does reduce the seizure frequency in some women. Adverse effects include hot flashes, irregular vaginal breakthrough bleeding, breast tenderness, and a delay of 6 to 12 months before menstrual cycles resume. Natural progesterone may be given over the initial luteal phase of the cycle as 100 to 200 mg three or four times a day, with an average dose of 600 mg needed to achieve a serum level of 5 to 25 ng/mL (96,97). Reversible asthenia, emotional depression, breast tenderness, and acne have been reported. Progesterone therapy may be most advantageous in women with inadequate luteal-phase cycles, that is, serum progesterone levels of less than 5 ng/mL during the midluteal phase (96), and should be avoided during or in anticipation of a pregnancy, as well as in the absence of scrupulous contraception. Antiestrogens such as clomiphene are typically used in infertility and cancer chemotherapy. Clomiphene reduces seizures in women with intractable partial epilepsy but is associated with potentially significant hot flashes, polycystic ovaries, and unplanned pregnancy (97). New antiestrogens are under development, and some may eventually be useful in treatment of hormone-sensitive seizures. Any attempt at hormonal manipulation should be conducted in association with a gynecologist.

CONTRACEPTION IN WOMEN WITH EPILEPSY

Women taking CYP-inducing AEDs will have at least a five-fold increase in the failure rate of oral contraceptive agents (98,99), because the hormonal dosage, particularly in the mini-pill, may be insufficient to prevent ovulation or implantation.

Such women should consider using a product containing at least 50 μg of estrogen and a higher dosage of the progesterone component (100). Other forms of hormonal contraception may also carry a high risk for failure. The efficacy of subdermal levonorgestrel, a slow-release contraceptive containing progesterone only, may also be compromised in women taking CYP-inducing AEDs. In two reports (101,102), the mean progesterone concentration was significantly reduced below the level necessary to prevent ovulation and implantation.

Phenytoin, carbamazepine, and barbiturates, which induce the CYP enzyme, increase binding to SHBG, and increase steroid metabolism. Topiramate in excess of 200 mg a day and oxcarbazepine in excess of 1200 mg a day exert a modest enzyme-inducing effect. Valproate and felbamate, as inhibitors of this system, slow the metabolism of contraceptive hormones. Other marketed AEDs do not alter CYP enzymes and do not interfere with the effectiveness of hormonal contraception.

REPRODUCTIVE HEALTH IN EPILEPSY

Disturbances in reproductive health, including reduced fertility, often accompany epilepsy. Women experience an increased incidence of reproductive endocrine disturbances, polycystic ovaries, menstrual cycle disturbances, and ovulatory dysfunction (103). The American Academy of Neurology has articulated practice guidelines that address these issues in women with epilepsy (100). Men also may develop endocrine dysfunction, including abnormal spermatogenesis.

Fertility

The reduced fertility associated with epilepsy is well documented. Although a population-based incidence cohort in Iceland noted no differences in livebirth rates between patients with epilepsy and control subjects (104), other studies report fertility rates decreased by one third (105–107) to as much as two thirds (108) and a reduced likelihood to marry and have offspring in persons with epilepsy (109).

The basis for infertility is most likely physiologic. Anovulatory menstrual cycles, polycystic ovaries, and sexual dysfunction have been reported in women with epilepsy (62,63,81,97,110).

Polycystic ovary syndrome, which affects 7% of reproductive-age women (111), is characterized by frequent anovulatory cycles and phenotypic or serologic evidence for hyperandrogenism, including male-pattern hair distribution (loss of scalp hair over the crown and temporal recession), increased facial and body hair, truncal obesity, and acne. In addition, the ratio of pituitary LH to FSH is increased, as is the cholesterol concentration; the ratio of high-density to low-density lipoproteins may be reduced; and glucose intolerance and even type II diabetes may be present. Polycystic ovaries are not required for diagnosis. In fact, asymptomatic polycystic ovaries occur in 21% to 23% of healthy women (112–114). The long-term consequences of polycystic ovary syndrome and include enhanced risks for infertility, cardiovascular disease, diabetes, and endometrial cancer.

Some women with epilepsy have features of polycystic ovary syndrome (115). Approximately 25% of women with primary generalized epilepsy are likely to have anovulatory cycles compared with those with localization-related epilepsy (15%) and nonepileptic control subjects (10%) (116). Anovulatory cycles, polycystic-appearing ovaries, and hyperandrogenism appear to occur more frequently with valproate than with other AEDs (81,117); polycystic ovaries may be reversible when therapy is changed to lamotrigine (118).

Reduced fertility in men with epilepsy may stem from disturbances in pituitary gonadal hormones, similar to those in women. Men taking CYP-inducing AEDs have reduced levels of testosterone (119,120) and increased levels of sex steroid hormone-binding protein (74), and also are at risk for impaired spermatogenesis. In one study (121), 55 men with epilepsy, some treated with phenytoin monotherapy and some untreated, had reductions in seminal fluid volume, spermatozoa concentration, and total sperm count compared with control subjects.

Sexual Function

Epilepsy appears to produce a higher incidence of sexual dysfunction than other chronic neurologic illnesses, manifesting primarily as diminished sexual desire and potency (122). Studies evaluating sexual attitude and behavior noted sexual dysfunction in 30% to 66% of epileptic men (60,123–125) and 14% to 50% of women (122,123,126).

Sexual dysfunction in epilepsy is primarily physiologic not psychologic. One-third to one-half of men complain of lack of spontaneous morning penile tumescence, anorgasmia, and erectile difficulties (72,78); more than one-third of women report dyspareunia, vaginismus, and lack of vaginal lubrication in the face of normal sexual desire and experience (127).

Several studies have quantitatively evaluated physiologic sexual arousal. Fenwick and colleagues (128) found impaired nocturnal penile tumescence in men with epilepsy and low testosterone. Men with temporal lobe epilepsy achieved inadequate penile tumescence and rigidity during rapid eye movement sleep as determined by a home monitoring device (129). In an evaluation of electroencephalograph-confirmed temporal lobe partial seizures (130), both sexes had a significantly lower increase in blood flow to genital tissues in response to an erotic stimulus than did a control group, even given normal subjective sexual arousal. Sexual dysfunction in epileptic individuals thus may arise in large part from a disorder of arousal, not desire.

The cause of sexual dysfunction in this population is probably multifactorial (131). Social development is often impaired and poor self-esteem as a result of having seizures may lead individuals to feel sexually unattractive. Arousal may be negatively reinforced, particularly when sexual activity precipitates seizures or when sexual sensations or behaviors become identified with the seizure or postictal period. Realistic acceptance of the psychosomatic aspects of a chronic illness is positively correlated with sexual function, whereas poor disease acceptance is often associated with sexual dysfunction (132).

Epileptic discharges in limbic structures also may contribute to sexual dysfunction, which usually arises after the onset of seizures (72,123,133,134) and may be most common in patients with partial, rather than generalized, epilepsy (126,133–135). Some patients treated for partial epilepsy with temporal lobectomy reported postoperative improvement in sexual libido and potency, especially those with the best seizure control (123,125,136).

Sexuality in epilepsy may be adversely affected by alterations in the levels of pituitary gonadotropins, prolactin, and the sex steroid hormones (61,64,65). Reductions in LH and elevated prolactin levels are associated with sexual dysfunction, and adequate amounts of estrogen and progesterone are required for sexual behavior in females (137). Reduced testosterone levels in men and women receiving CYP-inducing AEDs are associated with deficits in sexual desire and arousal (65,78).

AEDs may contribute to sexual dysfunction through direct cortical effects. Occasional or chronic impotence is most common with barbiturate use (138); decreased libido or impotence affected 22% of men receiving primidone.

Complaints of sexual dysfunction must be judged in the context of the patient's somatic, psychologic, and social well-being, as well as the dynamics of the couple and family (132). The frequency with which sexual complaints are volunteered may depend greatly on the physician's attitude (132). A sexual history explores whether the dysfunction is chronic or situational and the etiology organic or psychogenic. The presence of precipitating factors such as acute or chronic life stresses, recent medications, illnesses, and surgery as well as depressive symptoms should be determined. A thorough physical and neurologic examination is recommended, including measurement of thyroid function; levels of testosterone, estrogen, prolactin, and LH; complete blood count and fasting glucose level; and urologic or gynecologic consultation.

Physiologic sexual dysfunction may be addressed therapeutically. If no correctable organic cause is identified, referral for the most appropriate form of intervention, such as marriage therapy, primary psychiatric therapy, sex education, behavior therapy, or psychotherapy is warranted. Vaginal dryness and dyspareunia may respond to commercially available moisturizing and lubrication products and prolongation of foreplay. Erectile difficulties may respond to therapy with selective inhibitors of cyclic guanosine-specific phosphodiesterase or with α-adrenergic blockers (5).

BONE HEALTH IN EPILEPSY

Epilepsy appears to increase the risk for bone disease. The severity of bone loss correlates with the duration of AED exposure and the number of AEDs taken, and with use of CYP-inducing AEDs. Reduced bone mineral density as measured by dual X-ray absorptiometry (DXA) is evident in the femoral neck of the hip, spine, and ribs (139). Population-based studies note that use of AEDs entails increased risks of fourfold in hip fracture and twofold in fractures overall (140).

Bone loss affects children (141) and adults, as well as both sexes. About half of men and women younger than age 50 years who had taken enzyme-inducing AEDs for at least 5 years showed DXA-documented bone loss (142), which was significant in 22- to 44-year-old men (143).

The mechanisms by which AEDs cause osteopenia (bone density between 1 and 2 standard deviations below the peak mean) and osteoporosis (more than 2 standard directions below the peak mean) are likely multifactorial. Enzyme-inducing AEDs are associated with decreased levels of serum calcium (144) and vitamin D (145) and increased levels of bone-specific alkaline phosphatase and enhanced bone turnover, as measured by serum and urine markers of osteoblast and osteoclast activity (140,146). Less information is available for other AEDs.

Treatment of AED-related bone diseases has not been clinically evaluated, but all persons should have adequate daily intake of calcium and vitamin D. The recommended daily allowances for calcium are 1200 mg per day in reproductive-age women and in men, and 1500 mg per day in children and pregnant and postmenopausal women; daily vitamin D intake should be at least 600 IU. DXA may be obtained after several years' exposure to AEDs, and bone density should be monitored at intervals of 5 years if results are normal and 2 years if osteopenia or osteoporosis is detected. Documented bone disease warrants referral to a bone specialist; gravity-resisting exercise and therapy with hormones or bisphosphonates may be appropriate.

SUMMARY

The effects of reproductive hormones on neuronal excitability may complicate seizure management in some women with epilepsy. The ovarian sex steroid hormones alter GABA-mediated inhibition and glutamate-mediated excitation, with estrogen increasing and progesterone decreasing the likelihood of a seizure. In humans, hormonal influences on seizures may become apparent at puberty and menopause. Catamenial seizures, with more frequent attacks at menstruation and ovulation, may affect 30% of women with epilepsy and be most likely in those with temporal lobe epilepsy. A greater understanding of hormonal effects on the seizure threshold should lead to the use of hormones as AEDs.

CYP-inducing AEDs increase binding and metabolism of steroid hormones and therefore the risk for failure of hormonal contraception. Women who desire hormone-based contraception should use an AED that does not induce this enzyme system or select agents with high hormone dosages.

In some men and women, seizures and AEDs alter release patterns of hypothalamic and pituitary hormones, and, ultimately, gonadal steroids. The resulting dysequilibrium of the hypothalamic–pituitary–gonadal endocrine axis may be one cause of the increased frequency of infertility, reproductive endocrine deficits, and sexual dysfunction in this population. The physician can provide appropriate referral to a urologist, gynecologist, or endocrinologist and consider the use of an alternative AED.

Adults and children with epilepsy appear at increased risk for osteopenia and osteoporosis, especially if they are taking an enzyme-inducing AED. Gravity-resisting exercise, calcium and vitamin D supplementation, and periodic DXA scans are appropriate; a bone specialist should be consulted if bone loss is detected.

REFERENCES

1. Morrell MJ. Hormones and epilepsy through the lifetime. *Epilepsia* 1992;33(Suppl 4):S49–S61.
2. Woolley CS, Schwartzkroin PA. Hormonal effects on the brain. *Epilepsia* 1998;39(Suppl 8):S2–S8.
3. Pfaff DW, McEwen BS. Actions of estrogens and progestins on nerve cells. *Science* 1983;219:808–814.
4. Finn DA, Gee KW. The influence of estrus cycle on neurosteroid potency at the gamma-aminobutyric acid receptor complex. *J Pharmacol Exp Ther* 1993;265:1374–1379.
5. Intracavernous injection of alprostadil for erectile dysfunction. *Med Lett Drugs Ther* 1995;37:83–84.
6. Stitt SL, Kinnard WJ. The effect of certain progestins and estrogens on the threshold of electrically induced seizure patterns. *Neurology* 1968;18:213–216.
7. Wooley DE, Timiras PS. Estrous and circadian periodicity and electroshock convulsions in rats. *Am J Physiol* 1962;202:379–382.
8. Wooley DE, Timiras PS. The gonad-brain relationship: effects of female sex hormones and electroshock convulsions in the rat. *Endocrinology* 1962;70:196–209.
9. Marcus EM, Watson CW, Goldman PL. Effects of steroids on cerebral electrical activity: epileptogenic effects of conjugated estrogens and related compounds in the cat and rabbit. *Arch Neurol* 1966;15:521–532.
10. Logothetis J, Harner R. Electrocortical activation by estrogens. *Arch Neurol* 1960;3:290–297.
11. Hom AC, Buterbaugh GG. Estrogen alters the acquisition of seizures kindled by repeated amygdala stimulation or pentylenetetrazol administration in ovariectomized female rats. *Epilepsia* 1986;27:103–108.
12. Woolley CS. Estradiol facilitates kainic acid-induced, but not flurothyl-induced behavioral seizure activity in adult female rats. *Epilepsia* 2000;41:510–515.
13. Logothetis J, Harner R, Morrell F, et al. The role of estrogens in catamenial exacerbation of epilepsy. *Neurology* 1959;9:352–360.
14. Harrison NL, Simmonds MA. Modulation of the GABA receptor complex by a steroid anaesthetic. *Brain Res* 1984;323:287–292.
15. Landgren S, Backstrom T, Kalistratov G. The effect of progesterone on the spontaneous interictal spike evoked by the application of penicillin to the cat's cerebral cortex. *J Neurol Sci* 1976;36: 119–133.
16. Holmes GL, Kloczko N, Weber DA, et al. Anticonvulsant effect of hormones on seizures in animals. In: Porter RJ, Mattson RH,
Ward AAM Jr, et al., eds. *Advances in epileptology. XVth Epilepsy International Symposium.* New York: Raven Press, 1984: 265–268.
17. Tauboll E, Lindstrom S. The effect of progesterone and its metabolite 5-alpha-pregnan-3-alpha-ol-20-one on focal epileptic seizures in the cat's visual cortex in vivo. *Epilepsy Res* 1993; 14:17–30.
18. Finn DA, Roberts AJ, Crabbe JC. Neuroactive steroid sensitivity in withdrawal seizure-prone and -resistant mice. *Alcohol Clin Exp Res* 1995;19:410–415.
19. Wilson MA. Influences of gender, gonadectomy, and estrous cycle on GABA/BZ receptors and benzodiazepine response in rats. *Brain Res Bull* 1992;29:165–172.
20. Spiegel E, Wycis H. Anticonvulsant effects of steroids. *J Lab Clin Med* 1945;30:947–953.
21. Brann DW, Hendry LB, Mahesh VB. Emerging diversities in the mechanism of action of steroid hormones. *J Steroid Biochem Mol Biol* 1995;52:113–133.
22. McEwen BS, Davis PG, Parsons B, et al. The brain as a target for steroid hormonal action. *Annu Rev Neurosci* 1979;2:65–112.
23. Lan NC, Chen JS, Belelli D, et al. A steroid recognition site is functionally coupled to an expressed $GABA_A$-benzodiazepine receptor. *Eur J Pharmacol* 1990;188:403–406.
24. Costa E, Auta J, Guidotti A, et al. The pharmacology of neurosteroidogenesis. *J Steroid Mol Biol* 1994;49:385–389.
25. Finn DA, Ostrom R, Gee KW. Estrus cycle and sensitivity to convulsants and the anticonvulsant effect of 3 α-hydroxy-5α-pregnan-20-one(3α,5α-P). *Neuroscience* 1993;19:1539.
26. Maggi A, Perez J. Role of female gonadal hormones in the CNS: clinical and experimental aspects. *Life Sci* 1985;37:893–906.
27. Wallis CJ, Luttge WG. Influence of estrogen and progesterone on glutamic acid decarboxylase activity in discrete regions of rat brain. *J Neurochem* 1980;34:609–613.
28. McCarthy MM, Kaufman LC, Brooks PJ, et al. Estrogen modulation of mRNA for two forms of glutamic acid decarboxylase (GAD) in rat brain. *Neuroscience* 1993;19:1191.
29. Weiland NG. Glutamic acid decarboxylase messenger ribonucleic acid is regulated by estradiol and progesterone in the hippocampus. *Endocrinology* 1992;131:2697–2702.
30. Peterson SL, Reeves A, Keller M, et al. Effects of estradiol (E_2) and progesterone (P_4) on expression of mRNA encoding $GABA_A$ receptor subunits. *Neuroscience* 1993;19:1191.
31. Weiland NG. Estradiol selectively regulates agonist binding sites on the N-methyl-D-aspartate receptor complex in the CA-1 region of the hippocampus. *Endocrinology* 1992;131:662–668.
32. Smith SS, Waterhouse BD, Chapin JK, et al. Progesterone alters GABA and glutamate responsiveness: a possible mechanism for its anxiolytic action. *Brain Res* 1987;400:353–359.
33. Smith SS, Waterhouse BD, Woodward DJ. Locally applied progesterone metabolites alter neuronal responsiveness in the cerebellum. *Brain Res Bull* 1987;18:739–747.
34. Wong M, Moss RL. Patch-clamp analysis of direct steroidal modulation of glutamate receptor-channels. *J Neuroendocrinol* 1994; 6:347–355.
35. Gu Q, Moss RL. 17 Beta-estradiol potentiates kainate-induced currents via activation of the cAMP cascade. *J Neurosci* 1996; 16:3620–3629.
36. Woolley CS, Weiland NG, McEwen BS, et al. Estradiol increases the sensitivity of hippocampal CA-1 pyramidal cells to NMDA receptor-mediated synaptic input with correlation with dendritic spine density. *J Neurosci* 1997;17:1848–1859.
37. Woolley CS, McEwen BS. Estradiol mediates fluctuation in hippocampal synapse density during the estrous cycle in the adult rat. *J Neurosci* 1992;12:2549–2554.
38. Steiger A, Trachsel L, Guldner J, et al. Neurosteroid pregnenolone induces sleep-EEG changes in man compatible with inverse agonist $GABA_A$-receptor modulation. *Brain Res* 1993;615:267–274.
39. Finn DA, Gee KW. The estrous cycle, sensitivity to convulsants and the anticonvulsant effect of a neuroactive steroid. *J Pharmacol Exp Ther* 1994;271:164–170.
40. Morrow L, Pace JR, Purdy RH, et al. Characterization of steroid interactions with gamma-aminobutyric acid receptor-gated chloride ion channels: evidence for multiple steroid recognition sites. *Mol Pharmacol* 1989;37:263–270.

41. Kawakami M, Sawyer CH. Neuroendocrine correlates of changes in brain activity thresholds by sex steroids and pituitary hormones. *Endocrinology* 1959;65:652–668.
42. Wooley DE, Timiras PS. Gonad-brain relationship: effects of castration and testosterone on convulsions in the rat. *Endocrinology* 1962;71:609–617.
43. Teyler TJ, Vardaris RM, Lewis D, et al. Gonadal steroids: effects on excitability of hippocampal pyramidal cells. *Science* 1980;209:1017–1029.
44. Pfaff DW, Keiner M. Atlas of estradiol-concentrating cells in the central nervous system of the female rat. *J Comp Neurol* 1973;151:121–158.
45. Simerly RB, Chang C, Muramatsu M, et al. Distribution of androgen and estrogen receptor mRNA-containing cells in the rat brain: an *in situ* hybridization study. *J Comp Neurol* 1990;294:76–95.
46. Sheridan PJ. The nucleus interstitialis striae terminalis and the nucleus amygdaloideus medialis: prime targets for androgen in the rat forebrain. *Endocrinology* 1979;104:130–136.
47. Michael RP, Bonsall RW, Rees HD. The uptake of [3H] testosterone and its metabolites by the brain and pituitary gland of the fetal macaque. *Endocrinology* 1989;124:1319–1326.
48. Sar M, Stumpf WE. Distribution of androgen-concentrating neurons in rat brain. In: Stumpf WE, Grant LD, eds. *Anatomical neuroendocrinology*. Basel, Switzerland: Karger, 1975:120–133.
49. Sarrieau A, Mitchell JB, Lal S, et al. Androgen binding sites in human temporal cortex. *Neuroendocrinology* 1990;51:713–716.
50. Weiland NG, Orchinik M, Brooks PJ, et al. Allopregnanolone mimics the action of progesterone on glutamate decarboxylase gene expression in the hippocampus. *Neuroscience* 1993;19:1191.
51. Stumpf WE, Sar M, Keefer DA. Atlas of estrogen target cells in rat brain. In: Stumpf WE, Grant LD, eds. *Anatomical neuroendocrinology*. Basel, Switzerland: Kanger, 1975:104–119.
52. Pritchard PB, Wannamaker BB, Sagel J, et al. Endocrine function following complex partial seizures. *Ann Neurol* 1983;14:27–32.
53. Dornan WA, Malsbury CW. Neuropeptides and male sexual behavior. *Neurosci Biobehav Rev* 1989;13:1–15.
54. Bridges RS, DiBiase R, Loundes DD, et al. Prolactin stimulation of maternal behavior in female rats. *Science* 1985;227:782–784.
55. Boyd AE, Reichlin S. Neural control of prolactin secretion in men. *Psychoneuroendocrinology* 1978;3:113–130.
56. Martin JB, Reichlin S. *Clinical neuroendocrinology*, 2nd ed. Philadelphia: FA Davis, 1987.
57. Gloor P. Physiology of the limbic system. In: Penry JK, Daly DD, eds. *Complex partial seizures and their treatment*, vol. II: *advances in neurology*. New York: Raven Press, 1975:27–55.
58. Merchenthaler I, Setalo G, Csontos C, et al. Combined retrograde tracing and immunocytochemical identification of luteinizing hormone-releasing hormone- and somatostatin-containing neurons projecting to the median eminence of the rat. *Endocrinology* 1989;125:2812–2821.
59. Herzog AG, Russell V, Vaitukaitis JL, et al. Neuroendocrine dysfunction in temporal lobe epilepsy. *Arch Neurol* 1982;39:133–135.
60. Herzog AG, Seibel MM, Schomer DL, et al. Reproductive endocrine disorders in men with partial seizures of temporal lobe origin. *Arch Neurol* 1986;43:347–350.
61. Herzog AG, Seibel MM, Schomer DL, et al. Reproductive endocrine disorders in women with partial seizures of temporal lobe origin. *Arch Neurol* 1986;43:341–346.
62. Drislane FW, Coleman AE, Schomer DL, et al. Altered pulsatile secretion of luteinizing hormone in women with epilepsy. *Neurology* 1994;44:306–310.
63. Meo R, Bilo L, Nappi C, et al. Derangement of the hypothalamic GnRH pulse generator in women with epilepsy. *Seizure* 1993;2:241–252.
64. Rodin E, Subramanian MG, Gilroy J. Investigation of sex hormones in male epileptic patients. *Epilepsia* 1984;25:690–694.
65. Spark RF, Willis CA, Royal H. Hypogonadism, hyperprolactinemia and temporal lobe epilepsy in hyposexual men. *Lancet* 1984;1:413–417.
66. Dana-Haeri J, Oxley J, Richens A. Pituitary responsiveness to gonadotrophin-releasing and thyrotrophin-releasing hormones in epileptic patients receiving carbamazepine or phenytoin. *Clin Endocrinol* 1984;20:163–168.
67. Franceschi M, Perego L, Cavagnini F, et al. Effects of long-term antiepileptic therapy in the hypothalamic-pituitary axis in man. *Epilepsia* 1984;25:46–52.
68. Pritchard PB. The effect of seizures on hormones. *Epilepsia* 1991;32(Suppl 6):S46–S50.
69. Sperling MR, Pritchard PB, Engel J, et al. Prolactin in partial epilepsy: an indicator of limbic seizures. *Ann Neurol* 1986;20:716–722.
70. Molaie M, Culebras A, Miller M. Nocturnal plasma prolactin and cortisol levels in epileptics with complex partial seizures and primary generalized seizures. *Arch Neurol* 1984;44:699–702.
71. Dana-Haeri J, Trimble MR, Oxley J. Prolactin and gonadotrophin changes following generalized and partial seizures. *J Neurol Neurosurg Psychiatry* 1983;46:331–335.
72. Pritchard PB. Hyposexuality: a complication of complex partial epilepsy. *Trans Am Neurol Assoc* 1980;105:193–195.
73. Luhdorf K. Endocrine function and antiepileptic treatment. *Acta Neurol Scand* 1983;67(Suppl 94):15–19.
74. Beastall GH, Cowan RA, Gray JMB, et al. Hormone binding globulins and anticonvulsant therapy. *Scot Med J* 1985;30:101–105.
75. Isojarvi JIT, Parakinen AJ, Rautio A, et al. Serum sex hormone levels after replacing carbamazepine with oxcarbazepine. *Eur Clin Pharmacol* 1995;47:461–464.
76. Levesque LA, Herzog AG, Seibel MM. The effect of phenytoin and carbamazepine on serum dehydroepiandrosterone sulfate in men and women who have partial seizures with temporal lobe involvement. *J Clin Endocrinol Metab* 1986;63:243–245.
77. Macphee GJ, Larkin JG, Butler E, et al. Circulating hormones and pituitary responsiveness in young epileptic men receiving long-term antiepileptic medication. *Epilepsia* 1988;29:468–475.
78. Fenwick PBC, Toone BK, Wheeler MJ, et al. Sexual behavior in a centre for epilepsy. *Acta Neurol Scand* 1985;71:428–435.
79. Morrell MJ, Flynn KL, Seale CG, et al. Reproductive dysfunction in women with epilepsy: antiepileptic drug effects on sex-steroid hormones. *CNS Spectrums* 2001; 6:771–786.
80. Stoffel-Wagner B, Bauer J, Flugel D, et al. Serum sex hormones are altered in patients with chronic temporal lobe epilepsy receiving anticonvulsant medication. *Epilepsia* 1998;39:1164–1673.
81. Isojarvi JIT, Laatikainen TJ, Pakarinen AJ, et al. Polycystic ovaries and hyperandrogenism in women taking valproate for epilepsy. *N Engl J Med* 1993;329:1383–1388.
82. Janz D, Christian W. Impulsive petit mal. *J Neurol* 1957;176:346–346.
83. Jeavons PM, Bishop A, Harding GF. The prognosis of photosensitivity. *Epilepsia* 1986;27:569–575.
84. Sato D, Dreifuss FE, Penry JK. Prognostic factors in absence seizures. *Neurology* 1976;26:788–796.
85. Lerman P, Kivity S. Benign focal epilepsy of childhood. *Arch Neurol* 1975;32:261–264.
86. Niijima S, Wallace SJ. Effects of puberty on seizure frequency. *Dev Med Child Neurol* 1989;31:174–180.
87. Rosciszewska D. Epilepsy and menstruation. In: Hopkins A, ed. *Epilepsy*. London: Chapman and Hall, 1987:373–381.
88. Diamantopoulos N, Crumrine P. The effect of puberty on the course of epilepsy. *Arch Neurol* 1986;43:873–876.
89. Herzog AG, Klein P, Ransil BJ. Three patterns of catamenial epilepsy. *Epilepsia* 1997;38:1082–1088.
90. Bäckstrom T, Jorpes P. Serum phenytoin, phenobarbital, carbamazepine, albumin, and plasma estradiol, progesterone concentration during the menstrual cycle in women with epilepsy. *Acta Neurol Scand* 1979;59:63–71.
91. Bäckstrom T, Bixo M, Hammarback S. Ovarian steroid hormones. Effects on mood, behavior and brain excitability. *Acta Obstet Gynecol Scand Suppl* 1985;130:19–24.
92. Mattson RH, Cramer JA. Epilepsy, sex hormones, and antiepileptic drugs. *Epilepsia* 1985;26(Suppl 1):S40–S49.
93. Abbasi F, Krumholz A, Kittner SJ, et al. Effects of menopause on seizures in women with epilepsy. *Epilepsia* 1999;40:205–210.
94. Mattson RH, Cramer JA, Caldwell BV, et al. Treatment of seizures with medroxyprogesterone acetate: preliminary report. *Neurology* 1984;34:1255–1258.
95. Zimmerman AW, Holden KR, Reiter EO, et al. Medroxyprogesterone acetate in the treatment of seizures associated with menstruation. *J Pediatr* 1973;83:959–963.

96. Herzog AG. Progesterone therapy in women with complex partial and secondary generalized seizures. *Neurology* 1995;45: 1660–1662.

97. Herzog AG. Reproductive endocrine considerations and hormonal therapy for women with epilepsy. *Epilepsia* 1991;32(Suppl 6):527–533.

98. Mattson RH, Cramer JA, Darney PD, et al. Use of oral contraceptives by women with epilepsy. *JAMA* 1986;256:238–240.

99. Coulam CB, Annegers JF. Do oral anticonvulsants reduce the efficacy of oral contraceptives? *Epilepsia* 1979;20:519–526.

100. Zahn CA, Morrell MJ, Collins SD, et al. Management issues for women with epilepsy: a review of the literature. American Academy of Neurology Practice guidelines. *Neurology* 1998;51:949–956.

101. Haukkamaa M. Contraception by Norplant subdermal capsules is not reliable in epileptic patients on anticonvulsant therapy. *Contraception* 1986;33:559–565.

102. Odlind V, Olsson SE. Enhanced metabolism of levonorgestrel during phenytoin treatment in a woman with Norplant implants. *Contraception* 1986;33:257–261.

103. Schachter SC. Hormonal considerations in women with seizures. *Arch Neurol* 1988;45:1267–1270.

104. Olafsson E, Hauser WA, Gudmundsson G. Fertility in patients with epilepsy: a population-based study. *Neurology* 1998;51:71–73.

105. Dansky LV, Andermann E, Andermann F. Marriage and fertility in epileptic patients. *Epilepsia* 1980;21:261–271.

106. Wallace H, Shorvon S, Tallis R. Age-specific incidence and prevalence rates of treated epilepsy in an unselected population of 2,052,922 and age-specific fertility rates of women with epilepsy. *Lancet* 1998;352:1970–1973.

107. Webber MP, Hauser WA, Ottman R, et al. Fertility in persons with epilepsy: 1935–1974. *Epilepsia* 1986;27:746–752.

108. Schupf N, Ottman R. Reproduction among individuals with idiopathic/cryptogenic epilepsy: risk factors for spontaneous abortion. *Epilepsia* 1997;38:824–829.

109. Jalava M, Sillanpaa M. Reproductive activity and offspring health of young adults with childhood-onset epilepsy: a controlled study. *Epilepsia* 1997;38:532–540.

110. Bilo L., Meo R, Valentino R, et al. Abnormal pattern of luteinizing hormone pulsatility in women with epilepsy. *Fertil Steril* 1991;55:705–711.

111. Polycystic ovary syndrome. *ACOG Pract Bull* 2002;100: 1389–1402.

112. Clayton RN, Ogden V, Hodgkinson J, et al. How common are polycystic ovaries in normal women and what is their significance for the fertility of the population? *Clin Endocrinol* 1992; 37:127–134.

113. Farquhar CM, Birdsall M, Manning P, et al. The prevalence of polycystic ovaries on ultrasound scanning in a population of randomly selected women. *Aust N Z J Obstet Gynecol* 1994;34:1–67.

114. Polson DW, Wadsworth J, Adams J, et al. Polycystic ovaries—a common finding in normal women. *Lancet* 1988;1:870–872.

115. Herzog AG, Seibel MM, Schomer D, et al. Temporal lobe epilepsy: an extrahypothalamic pathogenesis for polycystic ovarian syndrome. *Neurology* 1984;34:1389–1393.

116. Morrell MJ, Guidice L, Seale C, et al. Ovulatory dysfunction in women with epilepsy receiving antiepileptic drug monotherapy: an interaction of syndrome and treatment. *Ann Neurol* 2002;52:704–711.

117. Vainionpaa LK, Rattya J, Knip M, et al. Valproate-induced hyperandrogenism during pubertal maturation in girls with epilepsy. *Ann Neurol* 1999;45:444–450.

118. Isojarvi JIT, Rattya J, Myllyla VV, et al. Valproate, lamotrigine, and insulin-mediated risks in women with epilepsy. *Ann Neurol* 1998;43:446–451.

119. Dana-Haeri J, Oxley J. Reduction of free testosterone by antiepileptic drugs. *Br Med J* 1982;284:85–86.

120. Isojarvi JIT, Parakinen AJ, Ylipalosaari PJ, et al. Serum hormones in male epileptic patients receiving anticonvulsant medication. *Arch Neurol* 1990;47:670–676.

121. Taneja N, Kucheria K, Jain S, et al. Effect of phenytoin on semen. *Epilepsia* 1994;35:136–140.

122. Jesperson B, Nielson H. Sexual dysfunction in male and female patients with epilepsy: a study of 86 outpatients. *Arch Sex Behav* 1990;19:1–14.

123. Blumer D, Walker AE. Sexual behavior in temporal lobe epilepsy. *Arch Neurol* 1967;16:37–43.

124. Hierons R, Saunders M. Impotence in patients with temporal lobe lesions. *Lancet* 1966;2:761–764.

125. Taylor DC. Sexual behavior and temporal lobe epilepsy. *Arch Neurol* 1969;21:510–516.

126. Demerdash A, Shaalon M, Midori A, et al. Sexual behavior of a sample of females with epilepsy. *Epilepsia* 1991;32:82–85.

127. Morrell MJ, Guldner GT. Self-reported sexual function and sexual arousability in women with epilepsy. *Epilepsia* 1996;37: 1204–1210.

128. Fenwick PBC, Mercer C, Grant R, et al. Nocturnal penile tumescence and serum testosterone levels. *Arch Sex Behav* 1986;15: 13–21.

129. Guldner GT, Morrell MJ. Nocturnal penile tumescence and rigidity evaluation in men with epilepsy. *Epilepsia* 1996; 37: 1211–1214.

130. Morrell MJ, Sperling MR, Stecker M, et al. Sexual dysfunction in partial epilepsy: a deficit in physiological sexual arousal. *Neurology* 1994;44:243–247.

131. Morrell MJ. Sexuality in epilepsy. In: Engel J, Pedley TA, eds. *Epilepsy: a comprehensive textbook.* New York: Lippincott-Raven, 1997:2021–2026.

132. Jensen SB. Sexuality and chronic illness: biopsychosocial approach. *Semin Neurol* 1992;12:135–140.

133. Gastaut H, Collomb H. Etude du comportement sexuel chez les epileptiques psychomoteurs. *Ann Med Psychol (Paris)* 1956;112:657–696.

134. Saunders M, Rawson M. Sexuality in male epileptics. *J Neurol Sci* 1970;10:577–583.

135. Shukla DG, Srivastava ON, Katiyar BC. Sexual disturbances in temporal lobe epilepsy: a controlled study. *Br J Psychiatry* 1979; 134:288–292.

136. Cogen PH, Antunes JL, Correll JW. Reproductive function in temporal lobe epilepsy: the effect of temporal lobectomy. *Surg Neurol* 1979;12:243–246.

137. Sakuma Y. Brain control of female sexual behavior. In: Yokoyama A, ed. *Brain control of the reproductive system.* Tokyo: Japan Scientific Societies Press, 1992:141–155.

138. Mattson RH, Cramer JA, Collins JF, et al. Comparison of carbamazepine, phenobarbital, phenytoin and primidone in partial and secondarily generalized tonic clonic seizures. *N Engl J Med* 1985;313:145–151.

139. Valimaki M, Tiihonen M, Laitinen K, et al. Bone mineral density measured by dual-energy X-ray absorptiometry and novel markers of bone formation and resorption in patients on antiepileptic drugs. *J Bone Miner Res* 1994;9:631–637.

140. Pack AM, Morrell MJ. Epilepsy and bone health in adults. *Epilepsy Behav* 2004:5(Suppl 2):S24–S29.

141. Chung S, Ahn C. Effects of anti-epileptic drug therapy on bone mineral density in ambulatory epileptic children. *Brain Dev* 1994;16:382–385.

142. Pack AM, Olarte LS, Morrell MJ, et al. Bone mineral density in an outpatient population receiving enzyme-inducing antiepileptic drugs. *Epilepsy Behav* 2003;4:169–174.

143. Andress DL, Ozuna J, Tirschwell D, et al. Antiepileptic drug-induced bone loss in young male patients who have seizures. *Arch Neurol* 2002;59:781–786.

144. Richens A, Rowe DFJ. Disturbance of calcium metabolism by anticonvulsant drugs. *Br Med J* 1970;4:73–76.

145. Hahn TJ, Hendin BA, Scharp CR. Effect of chronic anticonvulsant therapy on serum 25-hydroxycalciferol levels in adults. *N Engl J Med* 1972;287:900–904.

146. Feldcamp J, Becker A, Witte OW, et al. Long-term anticonvulsant therapy leads to low bone mineral density—evidence for direct drug effects of phenytoin and carbamazepine on human osteoblast-like cells. *Exp Clin Endocrinol Diabetes* 2000;108: 37–43.

Treatment of Epilepsy During Pregnancy

49

Nancy Foldvary-Schaefer

Epilepsy affects nearly 1% of the population, including almost 1 million women of childbearing potential (1). The management of epilepsy during pregnancy can be challenging for neurologists as well as other health care professionals. Nearly 50% of pregnancies in the United States are unplanned, with more than half of all unplanned pregnancies ending in abortion (2). Women rarely consult health care providers for preconception planning or during the first few weeks of pregnancy (3). In a survey by the British Epilepsy Association, 51% of women with epilepsy claimed to have never received advice on contraception or the interaction between oral contraceptives (OCs) and antiepileptic drugs (AEDs) (4). Only 34% had ever discussed pregnancy with their physicians, and less than 10% had received information about the adverse effects of AEDs on fetal development (4). Of obstetricians surveyed in Scotland, 51% were unaware of the need for preconception counseling, 33% did not consider it necessary to monitor AED levels, 56% never administered vitamin K1, and nearly 15% usually or always discouraged breast-feeding (5). A U.S. survey of physician practices revealed that 4% of the neurologists and none of the obstetricians polled were aware of the effects of the six most common AEDs on OC efficacy, despite the fact that approximately 25% had reported unexpected pregnancies among patients in their practice (6). These data illustrate the magnitude of the lack of awareness on the part of health care providers of issues faced by women with epilepsy during the childbearing years. Recent guidelines and reviews on the management of women with epilepsy and numerous recent reviews of the subject are excellent resources for physicians caring for this group of patients (1,7–9).

CONTRACEPTION

In 1972, Kenyon described the first case of OC failure associated with the use of phenytoin (10). Since then, the increased risk for OC failure among women receiving drugs metabolized by the hepatic cytochrome P450 (CYP450) 3A4 (CYP3A4) enzyme, including phenytoin, primidone, carbamazepine, ethosuximide, barbiturates, and topiramate, has been documented (11–13). Drugs that induce the CYP3A4 isoenzyme accelerate the metabolism of estrogen and progesterone, reducing their concentrations by up to 50% and increasing the risk for unexpected pregnancy (11,12). Phenobarbital, primidone, phenytoin, and carbamazepine also increase the production of sex hormone-binding globulin (SHBG), to which progesterone is tightly bound (14). This further reduces the concentration of unbound (free) progesterone, increasing the likelihood of OC failure. Unexpected pregnancy has been described in women receiving phenytoin concomitantly with subdermal implants containing the synthetic progestin levonorgestrel (Norplant, Wyeth, Philadelphia, Pennsylvania) (15,16). Despite the absence of significant enzyme-inducing properties, oxcarbazepine increases the production of SHBG and significantly reduces estrogen and progesterone concentrations, suggesting that its use may be associated with an increased incidence of OC failure (17). Valproic acid, lamotrigine, gabapentin, felbamate, tiagabine, and levetiracetam do not significantly alter the metabolism of the female sex steroids (18–23). Zonisamide was found to produce small, most likely clinically insignificant, effects on ethinyl estradiol and levonorgestrel concentrations (24). The efficacy of the intramuscular progestin medroxyprogesterone (Depo-Provera, Pharmacia, Kalamazoo, Michigan) in women with epilepsy is unknown. This long-acting contraceptive is an attractive option both for noncompliant patients and for women with cognitive impairment or psychiatric disorders. Unplanned pregnancies have not been reported in women using medroxyprogesterone, although the manufacturer recommends shortening the interval between injections in women receiving enzyme-inducing drugs (25).

Less than 1% of women in the general population experience accidental pregnancy within the first year of OC use (26–28). Of 41 women receiving OCs and AEDs in one study, 3 unplanned pregnancies were reported, representing a 25-fold increase over the expected rate of 0.12 (29). The effects of AEDs on sex steroid metabolism in any given patient are unpredictable. The most reliable indicator of OC failure is midcycle bleeding, which is present in more than two-thirds of women taking AEDs prior to actual OC failure (27). Bleeding occurs more often with the use of phenytoin, phenobarbital, or carbamazepine than with valproic acid or benzodiazepines (30). Increasing the dose of estrogen restores normal bleeding patterns in the majority of cases. Previous guidelines recommend the use of OC formulations containing 50 μg ethinyl estradiol or mestranol (31). However, given the number of new formulations released in recent years, the optimal type and route of administration of hormonal contraception in women with epilepsy has not yet been elucidated. The added risk associated with the use of higher-dose estrogen should be discussed. Barrier methods are recommended if breakthrough bleeding occurs.

The effect of OCs on seizure control has not been extensively studied. Based on several small studies, a minority of women experience more frequent seizures after the initiation of OC therapy (32–34). In the only placebo-controlled study, a low-dose synthetic combination pill did not adversely affect seizure control in 20 women with epilepsy (33). More frequent laboratory monitoring is recommended at the initiation of OC therapy, because sex steroids may accelerate the metabolism of enzyme-inducing drugs. It was recently discovered that lamotrigine plasma levels were reduced by nearly 50% by OCs leading to an increase in seizures after OCs were started or signs and symptoms of toxicity after withdrawal (34a). This interaction is due to the induction of glucuronide conjugating enzymes by OCs, operative in the metabolism of lamotrigine.

OBSTETRIC COMPLICATIONS

A variety of obstetric complications occur more frequently in women with epilepsy (Table 49.1) (3,35–45). The risk for spontaneous abortion is slightly higher in women with epilepsy than in the general population, as well as in treated versus untreated women with epilepsy (35,40,46). In one study, the risk for spontaneous abortion was four times higher among women with epilepsy and more than two times higher in the wives of men with epilepsy than was the rate in the women's same-sex siblings (41). The rate of elective abortion is also higher in women with epilepsy than in the general population (35,43). Labor and delivery are uncomplicated in the majority of cases, although labor induction and cesarean section are performed at least twice as often in women with epilepsy compared with the general population (36–38,40,45,47,48). Epilepsy alone is not an indication for these procedures.

TABLE 49.1
OBSTETRIC COMPLICATIONS IN WOMEN WITH EPILEPSY

Toxemia	Abruptio placentae
Preeclampsia	Premature labor
Hemorrhage	Low Apgar scores
Anemia	Hyperemesis gravidarum
Pregnancy-induced hypertension	Perinatal mortality
Spontaneous abortion	Cesarean section
Forceps-assisted delivery	Labor induction

Cesarean section should be considered in women with neurologic or cognitive impairment that is likely to interfere with maternal cooperation during labor, women with poorly controlled seizures during the third trimester, and women with a history of stress-induced seizures. Emergency cesarean section is warranted when seizures during labor adversely affect the infant or impede maternal cooperation. The incidence of perinatal mortality is increased twofold among infants born to women with epilepsy (36,37,49–51).

SEIZURE CONTROL

The fear of more frequent seizures is a major concern among pregnant women with epilepsy. Seizure frequency appears to be unchanged in more than half of cases, whereas approximately one third of women experience more frequent seizures, and a minority are improved (Table 49.2). Seizures may increase during the first trimester (52,53) or toward the end of pregnancy and in the puerperium (47,51,54–57). Following pregnancy, seizure control reverts back to preconception levels in the majority of cases (53). Poor preconception seizure control appears to be a reliable predictor of seizure control during pregnancy. Women with monthly seizures are significantly more likely to have more frequent seizures during pregnancy than those who are seizure free or have infrequent seizures in the year before conception (43,44,47,53). Other factors leading to breakthrough seizures include declining AED concentrations as a consequence of the physiologic changes of pregnancy, noncompliance, stress, and sleep deprivation. Noncompliance and/or sleep deprivation is present in more than 50% of women with breakthrough or worsening seizures during pregnancy (58,59). Anxiety over fetal AED exposure and fears about breastfeeding are the most common reasons for noncompliance (58). The incidence of status epilepticus is comparable to that of the general epileptic population; however, morbidity and mortality for both mother and fetus are high. Eclampsia, subarachnoid hemorrhage, choriocarcinoma, pheochromocytoma, cerebral venous thrombosis, amniotic fluid embolus, and thrombotic thrombocytopenic

TABLE 49.2

SEIZURE FREQUENCY DURING PREGNANCY[a]

Series	Pregnancies	Unchanged (%)	Increased (%)	Decreased (%)	SE[b] (%)
Knight and Rhind (53)	153	51	44	5	1.3
Nakane et al. (46)	227	59	32	9	NA
Remillard et al. (56)	78	50	46	4	NA
Schmidt et al. (59)	136	50	37	13	NA
Otani (58)	125	70	23	7	NA
Bardy (55)	154	54	32	14	0
Gjerde et al. (199)	78	66	17	17	1.3
Wilhelm et al. (44)	93	63	25	6	1.0
Dravet et al. (112)	50	66	22	12	NA
Tanganelli and Regesta (43)	138	80	17	3	NA
Tomson et al. (66)	93	61	15	24	NA
Sabers et al. (51)	143	66	21	7	0
Vidovic and Della Marina (200)	50	54	22	24	0
Total	1518	61	29	10	0.6

Abbreviation: NA, data not available.
[a]Minimum of 50 pregnancies reported in the English literature.
[b]Standard error for 684 pregnancies.

purpura should be considered in women experiencing new seizure types or new onset of seizures during pregnancy.

To avoid the adverse effects of seizures on the fetus, factors leading to more frequent seizure occurrence should be minimized. Isolated, generalized motor seizures during pregnancy can produce fetal bradycardia, decelerations, and decreased variability lasting up to 30 minutes (60,61). Intracranial hemorrhage and death after isolated motor seizures have been described (62). Whether other seizure types directly harm the fetus is less clear. Nei and colleagues (63) recorded fetal decelerations lasting 3.5 minutes and pronounced fetal bradycardia during a 1-minute complex partial seizure, suggesting that nonconvulsive seizures may also be detrimental to the fetus.

PHARMACOKINETICS OF ANTIEPILEPTIC DRUGS

Changes in hepatic, renal, gastrointestinal, and cardiovascular physiology during pregnancy alter the pharmacokinetics of AEDs (64–67). As pregnancy progresses, AED concentrations tend to decrease because of reduced protein binding, greater volume of distribution, accelerated hepatic metabolism, increased renal clearance, impaired intestinal absorption, and noncompliance. Increased concentrations of estrogen and progesterone accelerate the metabolism of enzyme-inducing drugs. Serum concentrations of AEDs begin to fall in the first trimester, reaching a nadir near term and returning to their preconception levels within 4 to 12 weeks postpartum (67,68). This has been most frequently demonstrated with phenytoin (66,69–76), valproic acid (70,77), phenobarbital (68,70–72), and carbamazepine

(66,68,72). Alterations in protein binding are most marked in the third trimester, resulting in higher unbound (free) fractions of drugs that are more rapidly eliminated (78). Consequently, for the highly protein-bound drugs phenytoin, valproic acid, and, to a lesser degree, carbamazepine, free levels are more reliable during pregnancy. The percent decline in total concentrations of phenytoin, phenobarbital, carbamazepine, and valproic acid was found to be 56%, 55%, 42%, and 39%, respectively; free levels of phenytoin, phenobarbital, and carbamazepine fell by 31%, 50%, and 11%, respectively, and free valproic acid concentrations increased by 25% (67). The sharpest decline in phenytoin and phenobarbital concentrations occurs in the first trimester, whereas carbamazepine levels decline maximally in the third trimester and valproic acid concentrations appear to decline more steadily throughout pregnancy (67).

With the exception of lamotrigine, little is known of the pharmacokinetics of the newer AEDs in pregnancy. The apparent clearance of lamotrigine increases during pregnancy by as much as 330% above preconception levels, leading to breakthrough seizures and dose escalation in most cases (79,79a,80). Apparent clearance returned to baseline as early as 2 weeks postpartum, requiring dose reduction often in the first few days postpartum to prevent toxicity. Until more is known, women taking the newer AEDs should be monitored closely for breakthrough seizures during pregnancy and for signs of toxicity in the early postpartum period.

Table 49.3 shows neonatal AED pharmacokinetics. Protein binding is reduced in newborns compared with adults because of decreased albumin concentrations and increased bilirubin production. In hyperbilirubinemic states, protein binding is further reduced, resulting in increased

TABLE 49.3

PHARMACOKINETICS OF NEONATAL ANTIEPILEPTIC DRUGS

Agent	Adult Half-life (h)	Neonate Half-life (h)	Cord-to-Maternal Serum Ratio	Breast Milk-to-Plasma Ratio
Phenobarbital	75–110	42–563	0.6–1.0	0.4–0.6
Primidone	10–15	7–60	0.4–1.2	0.4–1.0
Phenytoin	9–30	9–110	0.5–1.0	0.1–0.6
Ethosuximide	30–60	41	1.0	0.8–1.0
Carbamazepine	9–15	8–36	0.5–0.8	0.2–0.7
Valproic acid	6–18	28–88	0.5–4.6	0.01–0.2
Felbamate	13–22	NA	NA	NA[a]
Gabapentin	5–7	NA	NA	0.6
Lamotrigine	12–62	NA	0.6–1.3	0.56–0.61
Topiramate	12–24	24	1.0	0.86
Tiagabine	7–9	NA	NA	NA[b]
Oxcarbazepine	8–10[c]	17[c]	0.21/0.19	0.5
Levetiracetam	6–8	NA	NA	NA
Zonisamide	50–70	61–109	0.92	0.93

Abbreviation: NA, data not available.
[a]Excreted in human breast milk; concentration unknown.
[b]Excreted in breast milk of lactating rats.
[c]For the active metabolite, 10-monohydroxy (MHD).
Data from Bossi L, Assael M, Avanzini G, et al. Plasma levels and clinical effects of antiepileptic drugs in pregnant epileptic patients and their newborns. In: Johannessen S, et al., eds. Antiepileptic therapy: advances in drug monitoring. New York: Raven Press, 1980:9–18; Nau H, Rating D, Koch S, et al. Valproic acid and its metabolites: placental transfer, neonatal pharmacokinetics, transfer via mother's milk and clinical status in neonates of epileptic mothers. J Pharmacol Exp Ther 1981;219:768–777; Bossi L. Neonatal period including drug disposition in newborn: review of the literature. In: Janz D, Dam M, Richens A, et al., eds. Epilepsy, pregnancy, and the child. New York: Raven Press, 1982:327–341; Baughman FA Jr, Randinitis EJ. Passage of diphenylhydantoin across the placenta. JAMA 1970;213:466; Briggs GG, Freeman RK, Yaffe SJ. Drugs in pregnancy and lactation: a reference guide to fetal and neonatal risk, 5th ed. Philadelphia: Lippincott Williams & Wilkins, 1998; Froescher W, Gugler R, Niesen M, et al. Protein binding of valproic acid in maternal and umbilical cord serum. Epilepsia 1984;25:244–249; Kaneko S, Sato T, Suzuki K. The levels of anticonvulsants in breast milk. Br J Clin Pharmacol 1979;7:624–627; Kuhnz W, Jager-Roman E, Rating D, et al. Carbamazepine and carbamazepine-10,11-epoxide during pregnancy and postnatal period in epileptic mother and their nursed infants: pharmacokinetics and clinical effects. Pediatr Pharmacol (New York) 1983;3:199–208; Kuhnz W, Koch S, Jakob S, et al. Ethosuximide in epileptic women during pregnancy and lactation period. Placental transfer, serum concentrations in nursed infants and clinical status. Br J Clin Pharmacol 1984;18:671–677; Kuhnz W, Koch S, Helge H, et al. Primidone and phenobarbital during lactation period in epileptic women: total and free drug serum levels in the nursed infants and their effects on neonatal behavior. Dev Pharmacol Ther 1988;11:147–154; Mirkin BL. Placental transfer and neonatal elimination of diphenylhydantoin. Am J Obstet Gynecol 1971;109:930–933; Nau H, Kuhnz W, Egger HJ, et al. Anticonvulsants during pregnancy and lactation. Transplacental, maternal and neonatal pharmacokinetics. Clin Pharmacokinet 1982;7:508–543; Pynnonen S, Kanto J, Sillanpaa M, et al. Carbamazepine: placental transport, tissue concentrations in foetus and newborn, and level in milk. Acta Pharmacol Toxicol (Copenh) 1977;41:244–253; Rane A, Bertilsson L, Palmer L. Disposition of placentally transferred carbamazepine (Tegretol) in the newborn. Eur J Clin Pharmacol 1975;8:283–284; Bulau P, Paar WD, von Unruh GE. Pharmacokinetics of oxcarbazepine and 10-hydroxy-carbazepine in the newborn child of an oxcarbazepine-treated mother. Eur J Clin Pharmacol 1988;34:311–313; Kawada K, Itoh S, Kusaka T, et al. Pharmacokinetics of zonisamide in perinatal period. Brain Dev 2002;24:95–97; Myllynen P, Pienimaki P, Jouppila P, et al. Transplacental passage of oxcarbazepine and its metabolites in vivo. Epilepsia 2001;42:1482–1485; Ohman I, Vitols S, Tomson T. Lamotrigine in pregnancy: pharmacokinetics during delivery, in the neonate, and during lactation. Epilepsia 2000;41:709–713; and Shimoyama R, Ohkubo T, Sugawara K. Monitoring of zonisamide in human breast milk and maternal plasma by solid-phase extraction HPLC method. Biomed Chromatogr 1999;13:370–372.

free fractions of such highly bound drugs as phenytoin and valproic acid. Albumin increases rapidly over the first few days of life, reaching adult levels by 5 months of age. Similarly, renal tubular function is reduced in neonates, which may have major implications on the capacity for excretion of drugs such as gabapentin, levetiracetam, and vigabatrin. Because primidone is metabolized in the newborn, levels of phenobarbital and phenylethylmalonamide may increase transiently after birth (81). Placental transfer of valproic acid is more efficient from mother to fetus, and therefore concentrations of valproic acid and its metabolites are higher in umbilical cord blood than in maternal serum (82). Serum concentrations of the other AEDs are generally lower in cord blood than in maternal serum. Drug clearance is reduced in the first few days of life; the half-life of drugs is prolonged in neonates compared with children and adults. Longer drug half-lives and slower clearance rates have been reported in premature infants compared with term infants. The activity of most enzymes involved in drug metabolism reaches that of adult levels by 2 to 3 months of age.

All of the AEDs are detectable in breast milk, usually at concentrations lower than that of maternal serum. Data on the newer AEDs are extremely limited. The primary factors influencing the excretion of drugs into breast milk include plasma protein binding, lipid binding, and ionization characteristics. For agents that are highly protein bound, excretion into breast milk tends to be low. Conversely, because breast milk has a higher triglyceride content than plasma, drugs with high lipid solubility, such as benzodiazepines, tend to accumulate in milk. Because only the un-ionized drug diffuses across biologic membranes, the degree of ionization of an agent affects its concentration in milk. Nevertheless, it is generally believed that breast-feeding need not be discouraged in women with epilepsy, because the advantages seem to outweigh the risks of adverse effects in the newborn (83). In most instances, breast-feeding is accomplished without difficulty. If irritability or sedation after feeding are observed, breast-feeding should be discontinued.

The majority of infants born to women taking AEDs have no significant AED-related adverse effects. However, neonatal sedation, hypotonia, poor sucking, feeding difficulty, and, rarely, respiratory depression have been reported. These difficulties are usually apparent at birth and disappear within 2 to 8 days. An estimated 5% to 10% of exposed infants are affected (84,85). Withdrawal symptoms have been reported in infants exposed to barbiturates, phenytoin, and benzodiazepines (85). Clinical features of neonatal AED withdrawal include hyperactivity, hyperreflexia, hyperventilation, hyperphagia, vomiting, excessive crying, disturbed sleep, seizures, tremors, myoclonus, hypertonia, sneezing, and yawning (85–88). Symptoms typically begin shortly after birth and last from days to months, although the onset may be delayed for up to 10 to 15 days (89). Transient hepatic dysfunction associated with carbamazepine exposure and paralytic ileus in a fetus exposed to clonazepam and carbamazepine have been reported (90–92).

NEONATAL OUTCOME

The incidence of a variety of adverse outcomes is increased among offspring of women with epilepsy compared with the general population. These include congenital malformations, intrauterine growth retardation, developmental delay, mental retardation, hemorrhagic disease of the newborn, isolated seizures, and epilepsy. A much better understanding of the factors affecting development of infants born to women with epilepsy is forthcoming as this is an area of intense research interest.

Developmental Outcome

Factors contributing to developmental outcome in offspring of women with epilepsy include intrauterine AED exposure,

maternal seizures, type of maternal epilepsy, underlying genetic influences, and low socioeconomic status (93). Infants born to women with epilepsy are at increased risk for cognitive impairment and developmental delay (94–98). The incidence of mental retardation is greater in offspring of treated women with epilepsy than in those of untreated women with epilepsy or in those with epileptic fathers (96). A recent study found no difference in intelligence quotient (IQ) of children born to women with epilepsy who were not treated with AEDs versus that of normal controls (99). There appears to be no correlation between IQ of offspring and presence of maternal seizures during pregnancy (94). It is unclear whether specific AEDs are more likely to produce adverse developmental outcomes. Scores on standardized measures of intelligence are slightly lower among children exposed to AEDs, particularly those exposed to polytherapy (100,101). A recent study found that infants exposed to AEDs *in utero* were significantly more likely to have special educational needs than unexposed infants (102). Additional educational needs were more common in children exposed to valproic acid, particularly if used in polytherapy (102). In a recent report of 57 children exposed to AEDs *in utero*, the majority to valproic acid monotherapy, behavioral problems were observed in 81% and hyperactivity in 39% of cases; 7% were diagnosed with attention deficit hyperactivity disorder (ADHD) (103). Prospective studies addressing the effects of specific AEDs on developmental outcome are underway.

Congenital Malformations

Major congenital malformations occur in 4% to 8% of infants born to women with epilepsy, representing a twofold increase over the incidence in the general population (Table 49.4) (1,104). Major malformations are defined as structural defects formed during organogenesis that result in significant dysfunction or death if left untreated. The malformations most commonly observed include neural tube defects (NTDs), congenital heart disease, orofacial clefts, intestinal atresia, and urogenital defects. The incidence of major malformations is highest among offspring of treated women with epilepsy (46,105–112) and, in most studies, is similar in infants born to untreated women and offspring of men with epilepsy, compared with controls. Major malformations are associated with all of the older AEDs, with the incidence highest among infants exposed to polytherapy (43,46,68,110,113–115). The risk for major malformations appears to increase with the number of AEDs, from 3.1% to 7.8% in infants exposed to one AED to 8.3% to greater than 13.5% in those exposed to three or more AEDs (111,112). Within the last 30 years, a significant increase in the use of monotherapy has resulted in an impressive decline in the incidence of major malformations in the offspring of women with epilepsy (116). In a study of nearly 1000 offspring of women with epilepsy, the risk for major malformations in women taking one AED was greater with primidone

TABLE 49.4

MAJOR MALFORMATIONS IN OFFSPRING OF WOMEN AND MEN WITH EPILEPSY VERSUS CONTROLS

Study	Treated Women with Epilepsy[a]	Untreated Women with Epilepsy[a]	Men with Epilepsy[a]	Controls[a]
Annegers et al. (104)	177 (10.7)	82 (2.4)	234 (3.8)	748 (3.5)
Bjerkedal and Bahna (36)	3,879 (4.4)	—	—	3,879 (3.5)
Holmes et al. (109)	316 (5.7)	98 (0)	—	508 (1.8)
Monson et al. (217)	205 (6)	101 (3)	—	50,591 (2.6)
Niswander and Wertelecki (218)	413 (4.1)	—	—	346,694 (0.4)
Samrén et al. (219)	1,411 (3.7)	—	—	2,000 (1.5)
Shapiro et al. (96)	305 (6.6)	186 (9.7)	396 (4.5)	49,977 (2.7)
South (220)	22 (9)	9 (0)	—	50 (0)
Speidel and Meadow (97)	305 (5.2)	62 (0)	—	448 (1.7)
Tanganelli and Regesta (43)	138 (4.9)	—	—	140 (3.1)
Watson and Spellacy (221)	51 (5.8)	—	—	50 (0)
Yerby et al. (103)	64 (4.7)	—	—	46 (4.4)

[a]Total number (% malformed).

(14.3%), valproic acid (11.1%), and phenytoin (9.1%) than with carbamazepine (5.7%) and phenobarbital (5.1%) (112). Major malformations are more common in infants exposed to high serum AED concentrations during the first trimester. This has been most consistently demonstrated with the use of valproic acid (46,56,108,112,117–119). A significant correlation between maternal serum valproic acid concentrations and congenital malformations has been observed. In one study, the authors suggested avoiding a dose greater than 1000 mg per day and a level greater than 70 μg/mL to reduce the risk for malformations. The risk for oral clefts and congenital heart disease is increased 3- to 12-fold in offspring of women with epilepsy (105,120,121). Valproic acid and carbamazepine are associated with an increased risk for spina bifida. The incidence of spina bifida in fetuses exposed to valproic acid is 1% to 2%, representing a 10- to 20-fold increase over that of the general population (122); carbamazepine is associated with a 7-fold increased risk for NTDs (123). The last decade witnessed the inception of several large, international pregnancy registries aimed at better defining the effect of AED therapy on fetal development. Over the next few years, these organizations are expected to report their findings which will likely have a major impact on treatment practices.

Minor malformations are defined as deviations from normal development that do not result in serious medical or cosmetic consequences. These include craniofacial dysmorphism, distal digit and nail hypoplasia, minor skeletal anomalies, variations in demographic patterns, and umbilical and inguinal hernias (Table 49.5). Minor anomalies are observed in 10% to 30% of offspring of parents with epilepsy, representing a two- to threefold increase over the general population (68,124–127). Offspring of treated women with epilepsy are more likely to be affected than

those of untreated women or men with epilepsy (95,125, 128–130). The number of minor anomalies appears to be highest among offspring exposed to polytherapy (68,130,131), although this has not been a consistent finding (104,125,129,132). Distal digit/nail hypoplasia is observed in 20% of offspring of treated women and in approximately 30% of infants exposed to phenytoin (125,126,130,133). Facial anthropometric measurements demonstrate predominantly midline facial abnormalities in more than 25% of offspring (132). Facial dysmorphism and distal digit/nail hypoplasia tend to improve or disappear completely in childhood (133,134).

Neonatal Vitamin K Deficiency

Infants born to women with epilepsy taking enzyme-inducing AEDs have long been thought to be at risk for hemor-

TABLE 49.5

MINOR MALFORMATIONS IN OFFSPRING OF WOMEN WITH EPILEPSY

Hypertelorism	Epicanthal folds
Up-slanted palpebral fissures	Strabismus
Broad nasal bridge	Ptosis
Short, upturned nose	Wide mouth with prominent lips
Low hairline	Long philtrum
Posteriorly rotated, low-set ears	Pinna deformities
Distal digital/nail hypoplasia	Short neck
Finger-like thumb	Head size/shape variations
Dermatoglyphic variations	Sutural ridging
Genital anomalies	Wide fontanelles
Sternal/rib anomalies	Widely spaced, hypoplastic nipples

rhagic complications because of reduced activity of vitamin K-dependent clotting factors (II, VII, IX, X) and the anticoagulation proteins C and S (135,136). Intrauterine exposure to enzyme-inducing AEDs facilitates metabolism of vitamin K through induction of the hepatic CYP450 enzymes. Neonatal manifestations range from mild prolongation of prothrombin levels to life-threatening internal bleeding in the first 24 hours of life. The disorder is believed to affect 10% of untreated infants and is associated with a 30% mortality risk.

Functionally defective coagulation factors known as PIVKAs (prothrombin induced by vitamin K absence) are detected in the plasma of patients with vitamin K deficiency. PIVKA-II (absence of factor II) is a sensitive assay for vitamin K deficiency (137). Infants of women with epilepsy taking AEDs have higher levels of PIVKA-II and lower vitamin K levels than do control infants (138–140). Treatment during the last month of pregnancy reduces bleeding and PIVKA-II levels (137). A 1992 review of the literature identified 40 cases of neonatal vitamin K deficiency in offspring exposed to AEDs *in utero* (141). Coagulation defects were present in all cases, and bleeding was reported in 30 infants. In two-thirds of the cases, bleeding was severe (intracranial, intrathoracic, intra-abdominal, or gastrointestinal). None of the nine infants who died had received vitamin K at birth. Of seven infants treated at birth, none had clinical evidence of bleeding. However, in the only prospective study of infants exposed to enzyme-inducing AEDs *in utero*, bleeding complications were not increased above controls (0.7% versus 0.4%, respectively), despite the fact that vitamin K was not administered to mothers during pregnancy or labor (142). Significant associations were found between neonatal hemorrhage and birth at less than 32 weeks' gestation or alcohol abuse, but not between neonatal hemorrhage and AED exposure.

In 1961, the American Academy of Pediatrics recommended that all infants receive vitamin K at birth because of the reduced activity of vitamin K-dependent clotting factors in newborns (143). However, the dose and method of treatment have not been standardized. Because oral vitamin K is innocuous, women taking enzyme-inducing AEDs should be treated with 10 to 20 mg per day of vitamin K_1 during the last month of pregnancy. Infants should receive 1 mg of vitamin K_1 intramuscularly and, if needed, fresh-frozen plasma at birth. Treatment of only the infant might not be effective, given the early presentation of bleeding. The absence of PIVKA in infants exposed to valproic acid suggests that treatment of women who are receiving AEDs without enzyme-inducing properties may not be necessary (138).

Seizures

The risk for seizures is greater in offspring of mothers and fathers with epilepsy than in the general population (144–146). Among 858 offspring of probands with epilepsy, the incidence of seizures was 9.3% (neonatal seizures, 1.2%; febrile seizures, 4.5%; afebrile seizures, 5%), and 4.6%

developed epilepsy (144). Of the 38 children with febrile seizures, 10 (26%) developed epilepsy, a finding that markedly exceeds the incidence in the general population. Offspring of affected mothers are 1.6 to 2.5 times more likely to have seizures than are children of affected fathers (144,145). Epilepsy is more common among offspring of probands with idiopathic epilepsy and febrile seizures than among those with symptomatic epilepsy (144,147), although this is not a universal finding (145). Seizure types in affected parents and children tend to be similar, although offspring typically have an earlier age of onset (144,147).

MECHANISMS OF TERATOGENICITY

A variety of factors contribute to the adverse outcomes seen in offspring of women with epilepsy. AEDs and folic acid deficiency are implicated most often. Other factors include genetics, socioeconomic status, maternal health, and smoking (46,52,96,119).

Antiepileptic Drugs

Meadow (148) was the first to describe distinctive craniofacial features, intrauterine growth retardation, and mental deficiency in a report of six children with intrauterine hydantoin exposure. A few years later, Hanson and Smith (134) coined "fetal hydantoin syndrome" for the constellation of physical and developmental anomalies observed in infants exposed to phenytoin. Major and minor malformations have also been reported in infants exposed to trimethadione (149,150), primidone (151,152), phenobarbital (153), valproic acid (129,154), carbamazepine (155), and benzodiazepines (156). However, the marked overlap of clinical features among offspring exposed to different AEDs challenges the existence of drug-specific fetal syndromes (125,157). In recent years, the notion of drug-specific syndromes has been replaced by the concept of "fetal antiepileptic drug syndrome." Intrauterine exposure to any of the AEDs places infants at risk for major and minor malformations, cognitive impairment, and developmental delay.

Phenytoin, phenobarbital, primidone, and valproic acid have a pregnancy risk category D rating, which is assigned to drugs in which positive evidence of human fetal risk has been demonstrated but the risk in pregnant women may be acceptable considering the benefits. A category C rating (either studies in animals revealed adverse effects on the fetus and there are no controlled studies in women, or studies in women and animals are not available) has been assigned to carbamazepine and ethosuximide. Changes in prescribing practices during the last several decades provide some support for the existence of drug-specific teratogenicity (115,158). Orofacial clefts and congenital heart defects were among the most common malformations in offspring of women with epilepsy in the 1970s because of the widespread use of phenytoin, phenobarbital, and primidone (158,159). With the increasing use of carbamazepine and valproic acid in the 1980s, a higher incidence of spina bifida aperta, hypospadias, and inguinal hernias was reported in offspring of women with epilepsy. The risk for spina bifida aperta in infants exposed to valproic acid or carbamazepine is 1% to 2% or 0.5% to 1%, respectively (158). Bilateral radial aplasia is a rare anomaly associated with valproic acid exposure (160).

The effects of the newer AEDs on fetal development are not entirely known. To date, the numbers of exposures are insufficient to make an accurate estimate of the risk to the fetus. Felbamate, gabapentin, lamotrigine, topiramate, tiagabine, oxcarbazepine, levetiracetam, and zonisamide all have a pregnancy category C rating.

Of the newer AEDs, the largest number of known outcomes is in pregnancies associated with the use of lamotrigine (161). No evidence of teratogenicity was observed in animals exposed to the maximal recommended human dose (MRHD). As of 2004, the incidence of major malformations was 2.9% among 414 monotherapy exposures, 2.7% among 182 polytherapy exposures without valproic acid, and 12.5% among 88 polytherapy exposures including valproic acid. The number of reported pregnancies is far too small to estimate the risk of malformations in infants exposed to gabapenin (161a), topiramate (162), tiagabine (163), oxcarbazepine (165–167), felbamate (168), zonisamide (169–170), and vigabatrin (172). To date, there are no reports in-utero exposure to levetiracetam.

Malformations are more common in infants exposed to multiple agents at high serum concentrations. Polytherapy increases the formation of such active metabolites as 4-en-valproic acid and epoxides that bind to embryonic and fetal nucleic acids, disrupting normal development (171). The combinations of phenobarbital, phenytoin, and primidone, as well as of carbamazepine, phenobarbital, and valproic acid with or without phenytoin, are associated with particularly high rates of abnormal development (172). These combinations produce carbamazepine-epoxide levels that are three to five times higher than those seen with the use of carbamazepine alone (173).

Genetic Predisposition

Genetic factors may predispose to the development of fetal malformations. The capacity for detoxification of oxidative metabolites appears to be genetically determined. Epoxide hydrolase is the enzyme responsible for detoxification of epoxide intermediates of phenytoin and carbamazepine. Buehler and colleagues (174) found low epoxide hydrolase levels in four infants with craniofacial dysmorphism. No anomalies were observed in infants with normal enzyme levels. Strickler and colleagues (175) discovered a defect in epoxide hydrolase activity in 14 offspring exposed to phenytoin *in utero*, 12 of whom had at least one major malformation. Similarly, low levels of glutathione peroxidase (GSH-Px), an enzyme that prevents oxidative injury

through the removal of free radicals, were found in 26 children with myelomeningocele and their parents (176). Valproic acid decreases GSH-Px activity, a finding that may underlie its association with NTDs. Recent reports of women with repeated pregnancies complicated by malformations including NTDs following valproic acid exposure suggest the presence of a genetic susceptibility to the teratogenic effects of this drug (177,178).

Folic Acid

The beneficial effects of folic acid for the prevention of NTDs were first reported in the early 1980s and have since been the subject of many reviews (179,180). Folic acid is a methyl or single-carbon donor that is necessary in many metabolic pathways, including the formation of nucleic acids and the transformation of homocysteine to methionine. Based on the presence of elevated homocysteine levels in mothers of affected fetuses, a defect in homocysteine metabolism is one proposed mechanism for the development of NTDs (181). Folic acid levels are significantly lower in women whose pregnancy results in a NTD than in those with a normal outcome (182). Folic acid deficiency is also linked to orofacial clefts, cardiovascular malformations, and urogenital and limb anomalies (179,183). However, it has not been definitively shown that folic acid supplementation reduces the risk for all major malformations in this population (184). Because of high fetal demand, folic acid levels decline in pregnancy, reaching a nadir at term (185). Serum and red blood cell folic acid levels are significantly lower in women with epilepsy than in control subjects (186–189). Subtherapeutic levels tend to be more common in women receiving polytherapy, particularly those receiving the combination of phenytoin and phenobarbital or phenytoin and primidone (187). Folic acid levels are also significantly lower in women with epilepsy who have spontaneous abortions or give birth to infants with congenital malformations than in women with normal pregnancies (187,189). The antifolate effect of some of the AEDs predisposes women with epilepsy to folic acid deficiency (187). Phenobarbital, primidone, phenytoin, and carbamazepine accelerate the metabolism of folic acid, whereas valproic acid appears to interfere with its absorption (187). The effects of the newer AEDs on folic acid metabolism are unknown.

The process of neurulation in humans begins around the 16th day of gestation (190). The anterior neuropore closes by days 23 to 26 and the posterior neuropore by days 26 to 30. Consequently, folic acid stores must be adequate during the first month of pregnancy to effectively reduce the risk for NTDs. As pregnancy is typically identified only after the first missed menstrual period, folic acid supplementation beginning prior to conception is recommended. A 1997 U.S. survey conducted revealed that only 30% of nonpregnant women take a folic acid supplement and only 23% of pregnant women had taken one within the 2 years preceding pregnancy (191).

In 1998, folate supplementation in fortified cereal grains became a requirement in the United States and Canada, to meet the recommended daily allowance (RDA) of 0.4 mg per day for women of childbearing potential. Folic acid is found in a variety of foods, including leafy green vegetables, beans, fruits, and liver. However, dietary folate has a bioavailability of only 50% (180). Consequently, 0.8 mg of dietary folic acid must be consumed to obtain the RDA of 0.4 mg (180). Only 20% to 25% of women in the United States achieve this through dietary means. Folic acid 0.4 mg per day beginning 1 month preconception and continuing through the first trimester reduces the incidence of NTDs by 50% in women with no prior history of offspring with NTDs (192). A 4-mg-per-day dose reduces the incidence of NTDs by more than 70% in women with past pregnancies complicated by NTDs (193). The recommended dose range for women with epilepsy range is 0.8 to 5 mg per day.

MANAGEMENT STRATEGIES

The management of epilepsy during pregnancy begins prior to conception. Although more than 90% of patients have uneventful pregnancies, all women with epilepsy must be counseled about the potential increased risk for obstetric complications, worsening seizure control, and adverse neonatal outcomes. AED regimens should be reassessed and optimized prior to conception to ensure appropriate treatment of seizure type(s) and epilepsy syndrome. One study found that proactive preconception counseling leads to an increase in the use of monotherapy and a significant reduction in the use of the older AEDs (194). Among 90 women with epilepsy counseled preconception, 7 were found to have serious abnormalities on screening, including two unrecognized tumors, one that proved fatal; the diagnosis of epilepsy was erroneous in 4 cases. The ideal agent during pregnancy is the one that most effectively controls seizures at serum concentrations that are well tolerated. AED discontinuation should be considered in women who have been seizure free for 2 to 5 years and have a single seizure type, normal neurologic examination, and normal electroencephalogram on treatment (1). Prior to conception, a period of observation of 6 months or longer off AEDs is recommended, because most relapses occur during this time (195). Whenever possible, polytherapy should be avoided and the lowest effective serum concentration maintained. Supplementation with a mulitvitamin and additional folic acid (0.8 to 5 mg per day) and selenium 200 μg per day, beginning preconception, is advised (196).

Pregnant women with epilepsy should be jointly managed by a team of professionals that includes a neurologist, an obstetrician/gynecologist, a pediatrician, and, in some cases, a geneticist. Major changes in AED therapy should be avoided, because the risk for seizures is usually greater than the risk for teratogenicity once pregnancy is identi-

fied. Women should be advised about the importance of proper sleep and medication compliance, particularly in the last trimester, when AED levels tend to be lowest. Seizures during labor are best treated with intravenous fosphenytoin or short-acting benzodiazepines. Serum AED concentrations should be monitored monthly, and in the postpartum period, particularly in women with seizures during pregnancy and in those taking newer AEDs, and in the postpartum period, optimally within 2 weeks of delivery and to 6 to 10 weeks later. Laboratory monitoring may need to be performed more often in women with frequent seizures, signs or symptoms of toxicity, suspected noncompliance, or a history of increased seizure frequency or status epilepticus during a prior pregnancy. Medication adjustments should be made to control seizures and maintain serum concentrations in the therapeutic range near term. Women should be monitoring clinically for signs and symptoms of toxicity beginning immediately after childbirth until serum concentrations stabilize and necessary medication adjustments should be made.

Most major malformations can be identified *in utero*. Maternal serum α-fetoprotein obtained between 16 and 18 weeks' gestation is elevated in 85% of fetuses with open NTDs and has a false-positive rate of 3% to 4% (197). Level II fetal ultrasonography should be performed between 18 and 22 weeks to identify major malformations. More than 90% of NTDs, life-threatening cardiac anomalies, and major skeletal malformations are detected by ultrasonography at this time (197). Less-severe cardiac anomalies and orofacial clefts may be identified on a second examination performed at 22 to 24 weeks' gestation. Amniocentesis should be offered to women at high risk for NTDs and to those with an elevated serum α-fetoprotein level in whom ultrasonography is nondiagnostic. Some centers advocate offering amniocentesis to all women being treated with valproic acid or carbamazepine because of the increased incidence of NTDs in exposed infants. Elevation of amniotic fluid α-fetoprotein and acetylcholinesterase can identify more than 99% of open NTDs (197). Genetic counseling should be offered to all women when fetal malformations are identified. Chromosomal analysis should be performed at the time of amniocentesis.

CONCLUSIONS

Women with epilepsy represent a challenging group for neurologists and other health care professionals. Pregnancy is uncomplicated and neonatal outcome good in the vast majority of cases. Preconception counseling, AED monotherapy, appropriate laboratory monitoring, folic acid supplementation, and appropriate prenatal testing increase the likelihood of a favorable outcome. The effects of the newer AEDs on fetal development are not entirely known. However, preliminary reports suggest that these agents may have less deleterious effects on the fetus than the older

AEDs. A variety of pregnancy registries have been established throughout the world. In North America, pregnant women with epilepsy should contact the North American Registry for Epilepsy and Pregnancy at 1-888-233-2334, so that pregnancy outcomes can be more thoroughly studied (198).

REFERENCES

1. Practice parameter: management issues for women with epilepsy (summary statement). Report of the Quality Standards Subcommittee of the American Academy of Neurology. *Neurology* 1998;51:944–948.
2. Henshaw SK. Unintended pregnancy in the United States. *Fam Plann Perspect* 1998;30:24–29, 46.
3. Seale CG, Morrell MJ, Nelson L, et al. Analysis of prenatal and gestational care given to women with epilepsy. *Neurology* 1998;51:1039–1045.
4. Crawford P, Lee P. Gender difference in management of epilepsy—what women are hearing. *Seizure* 1999;8:135–139.
5. Russell AJ, Macpherson H, Cairnie V, et al. The care of pregnant women with epilepsy—a survey of obstetricians in Scotland. *Seizure* 1996;5:271–277.
6. Krauss GL, Brandt J, Campbell M, et al. Antiepileptic medication and oral contraceptive interactions: a national survey of neurologists and obstetricians. *Neurology* 1996;46:1534–1539.
7. Zahn CA, Morrell MJ, Collins SD, et al. Management issues for women with epilepsy: a review of the literature. *Neurology* 1998;51:949–956.
8. Crawford P, Appleton R, Betts T, et al. Best practice guidelines for the management of women with epilepsy. The Women with Epilepsy Guidelines Development Group. *Seizure* 1999;8:201–217.
9. McAuley JW, Anderson GD. Treatment of epilepsy in women of reproductive age: pharmacokinetic considerations. *Clin Pharmacokinet* 2002;41:559–579.
10. Kenyon IE. Unplanned pregnancy in an epileptic. *Br Med J* 1972;1:686–687.
11. Back DJ, Bates M, Bowden A, et al. The interaction of phenobarbital and other anticonvulsants with oral contraceptive steroid therapy. *Contraception* 1980;22:495–503.
12. Crawford P, Chadwick DJ, Martin C, et al. The interaction of phenytoin and carbamazepine with combined oral contraceptive steroids. *Br J Clin Pharmacol* 1990;30:892–896.
13. Rosenfeld WE, Doose DR, Walker SA, et al. Effect of topiramate on the pharmacokinetics of an oral contraceptive containing norethindrone and ethinyl estradiol in patients with epilepsy. *Epilepsia* 1997;38:317–323.
14. Back DJ, Breckenridge AM, Crawford FE, et al. The effect of oral contraceptive steroids and enzyme inducing drugs on sex hormone binding capacity in women [proceedings]. *Br J Clin Pharmacol* 1980;9:115P.
15. Haukkamaa M. Contraception by Norplant subdermal capsules is not reliable in epileptic patients on anticonvulsant treatment. *Contraception* 1986;33:559–565.
16. Odlind V, Olsson SE. Enhanced metabolism of levonorgestrel during phenytoin treatment in a woman with Norplant implants. *Contraception* 1986;33:257–261.
17. Fattore C, Cipolla G, Gatti G, et al. Induction of ethinylestradiol and levonorgestrel metabolism by oxcarbazepine in healthy women. *Epilepsia* 1999;40:783–787.
18. Crawford P, Chadwick D, Cleland P, et al. The lack of effect of sodium valproate on the pharmacokinetics of oral contraceptive steroids. *Contraception* 1986;33:23–29.
19. Eldon MA, Underwood BA, Randinitis EJ, et al. Gabapentin does not interact with a contraceptive regimen of norethindrone acetate and ethinyl estradiol. *Neurology* 1998;50:1146–1148.
20. Molich T, Whiteman P, Orme M, et al. Effect of lamotrigine on the pharmacology of the combined oral contraceptive pill [abstract]. *Epilepsia* 1991;32:96.
21. Mengel HB, Houston A, Back DJ. An evaluation of the interaction between tiagabine and oral contraceptives in females volunteers. *J Pharm Med* 1994;4:141–150.
22. Ragueneau-Majlessi I, Levy RH, Janik F. Levetiracetam does not alter the pharmacokinetics of an oral contraceptive in healthy women. *Epilepsia* 2002;43:697–702.
23. Saano V, Glue P, Banfield CR, et al. Effects of felbamate on the pharmacokinetics of a low-dose combination oral contraceptive. *Clin Pharmacol Ther* 1995;58:523–531.
24. Data on file. Elan Pharmaceuticals, 2003.
25. Medical and drug information. Peapack, NJ: Pharmacia & Upjohn, 2003.
26. Yerby MS. Contraception, pregnancy and lactation in women with epilepsy. *Baillieres Clin Neurol* 1996;5:887–908.
27. Dam M, Gram L, Penry JK, eds. *Effect of antiepileptic drugs on estrogen and progesterone metabolism and on oral contraception.* New York: Raven Press, 1981.
28. Qureshi M, Attaran M. Review of newer contraceptive agents. *Cleve Clin J Med* 1999;66:358–366.
29. Coulam CB, Annegers JF. Do anticonvulsants reduce the efficacy of oral contraceptives? *Epilepsia* 1979;20:519–525.
30. Sonnen AEH. Sodium valproate and the contraceptive pill. *Br J Clin Pract* 1983;27(Suppl):31–36.
31. Mattson RH, Cramer JA, Darney PD, et al. Use of oral contraceptives by women with epilepsy. *JAMA* 1986;256:238–240.
32. Diamond MP, Greene JW, Thompson JM, et al. Interaction of anticonvulsants and oral contraceptives in epileptic adolescents. *Contraception* 1985;31:623–632.
33. Espir M, Walker ME, Lawson JP. Epilepsy and oral contraception. *Br Med J* 1969;1:294–295.
34. Toivakka E. Oral contraception in epileptics. *Arzneimittelforschung* 1967;17:1085.
34a. Sabers A, Buchholt JM, Uldall P, et al. Lamotrigine plasma levels reduced by oral contraceptives. *Epilepsy Research* 2001;47:151–154.
35. Andermann E, Dansky L, Linch RA. Complications of pregnancy, labour and delivery in epileptic women. In: Janz D, Dam M, Richens A, et al., eds. *Epilepsy, pregnancy, and the child.* New York: Raven Press, 1982:61–74.
36. Bjerkedal T, Bahna SL. The course and outcome of pregnancy in women with epilepsy. *Acta Obstet Gynecol Scand* 1973;52:245–248.
37. Bjerkedal T. Outcome of pregnancy in women with epilepsy, Norway 1967–1978: congenital malformations. In: Janz D, Dam M, Richens A, et al., eds. *Epilepsy, pregnancy, and the child.* New York: Raven Press, 1982:289–295.
38. Egenaes J. Outcome of pregnancy in women with epilepsy—Norway, 1967 to 1978: complications during pregnancy and delivery. In: Janz D, Dam M, Richens A, et al., eds. *Epilepsy, pregnancy, and the child.* New York: Raven Press, 1982:81–85.
39. Nelson KB, Ellenberg JH. Maternal seizure disorder, outcome of pregnancy, and neurologic abnormalities in the children. *Neurology* 1982;32:1247–1254.
40. Ogawa Y, Fukushi A, Nomura Y, et al. Complications of pregnancy, labor, and delivery in woman with epilepsy. In: Sata T, Shinagawa S, eds. *Antiepileptic drugs and pregnancy.* New York: Excerpta Medica, 1984:87–97.
41. Schupf N, Ottman R. Reproduction among individuals with idiopathic/cryptogenic epilepsy: risk factors for spontaneous abortion. *Epilepsia* 1997;38:824–829.
42. Svigos JM. Epilepsy and pregnancy. *Aust N Z J Obstet Gynaecol* 1984;24:182–185.
43. Tanganelli P, Regesta G. Epilepsy, pregnancy, and major birth anomalies: an Italian prospective, controlled study. *Neurology* 1992;42(4 Suppl 5):89–93.
44. Wilhelm J, Morris D, Hotham N. Epilepsy and pregnancy—a review of 98 pregnancies. *Aust N Z J Obstet Gynaecol* 1990;30:290–295.
45. Yerby M, Koepsell T, Daling J. Pregnancy complications and outcomes in a cohort of women with epilepsy. *Epilepsia* 1985;26:631–635.
46. Nakane Y, Okuma T, Takahashi R, et al. Multi-institutional study on the teratogenicity and fetal toxicity of antiepileptic drugs: a report of a collaborative study group in Japan. *Epilepsia* 1980;21:663–680.

47. Huhmar E, Jarvinen PA. Relation of epileptic symptoms to pregnancy, delivery and puerperium. *Ann Chir Gynaecol Fenn* 1961;50:49–64.
48. Sawhney H, Vasishta K, Suri V, et al. Pregnancy with epilepsy–a retrospective analysis. *Int J Gynaecol Obstet* 1996;54:17–22.
49. Higgins TA, Comerford JB. Epilepsy in pregnancy. *J Ir Med Assoc* 1974;67:317–320.
50. Martin PJ, Millac PA. Pregnancy, epilepsy, management and outcome: a 10-year perspective. *Seizure* 1993;2:277–280.
51. Sabers A, aRogvi-Hansen B, Dam M, et al. Pregnancy and epilepsy: a retrospective study of 151 pregnancies. *Acta Neurol Scand* 1998;97:164–170.
52. Canger R, Battino D, Canevini MP, et al. Malformations in offspring of women with epilepsy: a prospective study. *Epilepsia* 1999;40:1231–1236.
53. Knight AH, Rhind EG. Epilepsy and pregnancy: a study of 153 pregnancies in 59 patients. *Epilepsia* 1975;16:99–110.
54. Bardy AH. Seizure frequency in epileptic women during pregnancy and the puerperium: results of the prospective Helsinki study. In: Janz D, Dam M, Richens A, et al., eds. *Epilepsy, pregnancy, and the child.* New York: Raven Press, 1982:27–31.
55. Bardy AH. Incidence of seizures during pregnancy, labor and puerperium in epileptic women: a prospective study. *Acta Neurol Scand* 1987;75:356–360.
56. Remillard G, Dansky L, Andermann E, et al. Seizure frequency during pregnancy and the puerperium. In: Janz D, Dam M, Richens A, et al., eds. *Epilepsy, pregnancy, and the child.* New York: Raven Press, 1982:15–25.
57. Sabin M, Oxorn H. Epilepsy and pregnancy. *Obstet Gynecol* 1956;7:175–179.
58. Otani K. Risk factors for the increased seizure frequency during pregnancy and puerperium. *Folia Psychiatr Neurol Jpn* 1985;39:33–41.
59. Schmidt D, Canger R, Avanzini G, et al. Change of seizure frequency in pregnant epileptic women. *J Neurol Neurosurg Psychiatry* 1983;46:751–755.
60. Teramo K, Hiilesmaa V, Bardy A, et al. Fetal heart rate during a maternal grand mal epileptic seizure. *J Perinat Med* 1979;7:3–6.
61. Yerby MS. Problems and management of the pregnant woman with epilepsy. *Epilepsia* 1987;28(Suppl 3):S29–S36.
62. Minkoff H, Schaffer RM, Delke I, et al. Diagnosis of intracranial hemorrhage in utero after a maternal seizure. *Obstet Gynecol* 1985;65(Suppl 3):22S–24S.
63. Nei M, Daly S, Liporace J. A maternal complex partial seizure in labor can affect fetal heart rate. *Neurology* 1998;51:904–906.
64. Eadie MJ, Lander CM, Tyrer JH. Plasma drug level monitoring in pregnancy. *Clin Pharmacokinet* 1977;2:427–436.
65. Lander CM, Eadie MJ. Plasma antiepileptic drug concentrations during pregnancy. *Epilepsia* 1991;32:257–266.
66. Tomson T, Lindbom U, Ekqvist B, et al. Disposition of carbamazepine and phenytoin in pregnancy. *Epilepsia* 1994;35:131–135.
67. Yerby MS, Friel PN, McCormick K. Antiepileptic drug disposition during pregnancy. *Neurology* 1992;42(4 Suppl 5):12–16.
68. Lander CM, Eadie MJ. Antiepileptic drug intake during pregnancy and malformed offspring. *Epilepsy Res* 1990;7:77–82.
69. Bardy AH, Hiilesmaa VK, Teramo KA. Serum phenytoin during pregnancy, labor and puerperium. *Acta Neurol Scand* 1987;75:374–375.
70. Bardy AH, Hiilesmaa VK, Teramo K, et al. Protein binding of antiepileptic drugs during pregnancy, labor, and puerperium. *Ther Drug Monit* 1990;12:40–46.
71. Bossi L, Assael M, Avanzini G, et al. Plasma levels and clinical effects of antiepileptic drugs in pregnant epileptic patients and their newborns. In: Johannessen S, et al., eds. *Antiepileptic therapy: advances in drug monitoring.* New York: Raven Press, 1980:9–18.
72. Dam M, Christiansen J, Munck O, et al. Antiepileptic drugs: metabolism in pregnancy. *Clin Pharmacokinet* 1979;4:53–62.
73. Dansky L, Andermann E, Sherwin AL, et al. Plasma levels of phenytoin during pregnancy and the puerperium. In: Janz D, Dam M, Richens A, et al., eds. *Epilepsy, pregnancy, and the child.* New York: Raven Press, 1982:155–162.
74. Eadie MJ, McKinnon GE, Dickinson RG, et al. Phenytoin metabolism during pregnancy. *Eur J Clin Pharmacol* 1992;43:389–392.

75. Landon MJ, Kirkley M. Metabolism of diphenylhydantoin (phenytoin) during pregnancy. *Br J Obstet Gynaecol* 1979;86:125–132.
76. Mygind KI, Dam M, Christiansen J. Phenytoin and phenobarbitone plasma clearance during pregnancy. *Acta Neurol Scand* 1976;54:160–166.
77. Koerner M, Yerby M, Friel P, et al. Valproic acid disposition and protein binding in pregnancy. *Ther Drug Monit* 1989;11:228–230.
78. Ruprah M, Perucca E, Richens A. Serum protein binding of phenytoin in women: effect of pregnancy and oral contraceptives. In: Janz D, Dam M, Richens A, et al., eds. *Epilepsy, pregnancy, and the child.* New York: Raven Press, 1982:115–120.
79. Tran TA, Leppik IE, Blesi K, et al. Lamotrigine clearance during pregnancy. *Neurology* 2002;59:251–255.
79a. Pennell PB, Newport DJ, Stowe ZN, et al. The impact of pregnancy and childbirth on the metabolism of lamotrigine. *Neurology* 2004;62:292–295.
80. de Haan G-J, Edelbroek P, Segers J, et al. Gestation-induced changes in lamotrigine pharmacokinetics: A monotherapy study. *Neurology* 2004;63:571–573.
81. Nau H, Rating D, Häuser I. Placental transfer at birth and postnatal elimination of primidone and metabolites in neonates of epileptic mothers. In: Janz D, Dam M, Richens A, et al., eds. *Epilepsy, pregnancy, and the child.* New York: Raven Press, 1982:361–366.
82. Nau H, Rating D, Koch S, et al. Valproic acid and its metabolites: placental transfer, neonatal pharmacokinetics, transfer via mother's milk and clinical status in neonates of epileptic mothers. *J Pharmacol Exp Ther* 1981;219:768–777.
83. Breastfeeding and the use of human milk. American Academy of Pediatrics. Work Group on Breastfeeding. *Pediatrics* 1997;100:1035–1039.
84. Bleyer WA, Marshall RE. Barbiturate withdrawal syndrome in a passively addicted infant. *JAMA* 1972;221:185–186.
85. Bossi L. Neonatal period including drug disposition in newborn: review of the literature. In: Janz D, Dam M, Richens A, et al., eds. *Epilepsy, pregnancy, and the child.* New York: Raven Press, 1982:327–341.
86. D'Souza SW, Robertson IG, Donnai D, et al. Fetal phenytoin exposure, hypoplastic nails, and jitteriness. *Arch Dis Child* 1991;66:320–324.
87. Kaneko S, Suzuki K, Satoo T, et al. The problems of antiepileptic medication in the neonatal period: is breast-feeding advisable? In: Janz D, Dam M, Richens A, et al., eds. *Epilepsy, pregnancy, and the child.* New York: Raven Press, 1982:343–348.
88. Koch S, Jager-Roman E, Losche G, et al. Antiepileptic drug treatment in pregnancy: drug side effects in the neonate and neurological outcome. *Acta Paediatr* 1996;85:739–746.
89. Desmond MM, Schwanecke RP, Wilson GS, et al. Maternal barbiturate utilization and neonatal withdrawal symptomatology. *J Pediatr* 1972;80:190–197.
90. Frey B, Schubiger G, Musy JP. Transient cholestatic hepatitis in a neonate associated with carbamazepine exposure during pregnancy and breast-feeding. *Eur J Pediatr* 1990;150:136–138.
91. Haeusler MC, Hoellwarth ME, Holzer P. Paralytic ileus in a fetus-neonate after maternal intake of benzodiazepine. *Prenat Diagn* 1995;15:1165–1167.
92. Merlob P, Mor N, Litwin A. Transient hepatic dysfunction in an infant of an epileptic mother treated with carbamazepine during pregnancy and breastfeeding. *Ann Pharmacother* 1992;26:1563–1565.
93. Yerby MS. Pregnancy, teratogenesis, and epilepsy. *Neurol Clin* 1994;12:749–771.
94. Gaily E, Kantola-Sorsa E, Granstrom ML. Intelligence of children of epileptic mothers. *J Pediatr* 1988;113:677–684.
95. Leavitt AM, Yerby MS, Robinson N, et al. Epilepsy in pregnancy: developmental outcome of offspring at 12 months. *Neurology* 1992;42(4 Suppl 5):141–143.
96. Majewski F, Steger M, Richter B, et al. The teratogenicity of hydantoins and barbiturates in humans, with considerations on the etiology of malformations and cerebral disturbances in the children of epileptic parents. *Int J Biol Res Pregnancy* 1981;2:37–45.

97. Shapiro S, Hartz SC, Siskind V, et al. Anticonvulsants and parental epilepsy in the development of birth defects. *Lancet* 1976;1:272–275.

98. Speidel BD, Meadow SR. Maternal epilepsy and abnormalities of the fetus and newborn. *Lancet* 1972;2:839–843.

99. Holmes LB, Rosenberger PB, Harvey EA, et al. Intelligence and physical features of children of women with epilepsy. *Teratology* 2000;61:196–202.

100. Koch S, Titze K, Zimmermann RB, et al. Long-term neuropsychological consequences of maternal epilepsy and anticonvulsant treatment during pregnancy for school-age children and adolescents. *Epilepsia* 1999;40:1237–1243.

101. Vanoverloop D, Schnell RR, Harvey EA, et al. The effects of prenatal exposure to phenytoin and other anticonvulsants on intellectual function at 4 to 8 years of age. *Neurotoxicol Teratol* 1992; 14:329–335.

102. Adab N, Jacoby A, Smith D, et al. Additional educational needs in children born to mothers with epilepsy. *J Neurol Neurosurg Psychiatry* 2001;70:15–21.

103. Moore SJ, Turnpenny P, Quinn A, et al. A clinical study of 57 children with fetal anticonvulsant syndromes. *J Med Genet* 2000;37:489–497.

104. Yerby MS, Leavitt A, Erickson DM, et al. Antiepileptics and the development of congenital anomalies. *Neurology* 1992;42(4 Suppl 5):132–140.

105. Annegers JF, Hauser WA, Elveback LR, et al. Congenital malformations and seizure disorders in the offspring of parents with epilepsy. *Int J Epidemiol* 1978;7:241–247.

106. Dansky L, Andermann E, Andermann F. Major congenital malformations in the offspring of epileptic parents: genetic and environmental risk factors. In: Janz D, Dam M, Richens A, et al., eds. *Epilepsy, pregnancy, and the child*. New York: Raven Press, 1982:223–234.

107. Holmes LB, Harvey EA, Brown KS, et al. Anticonvulsant teratogenesis: I. A study design for newborn infants. *Teratology* 1994; 49:202–207.

108. Samren EB, van Duijn CM, Koch S, et al. Maternal use of antiepileptic drugs and the risk of major congenital malformations: a joint European prospective study of human teratogenesis associated with maternal epilepsy. *Epilepsia* 1997;38:981–990.

109. Waters CH, Belai Y, Gott PS, et al. Outcomes of pregnancy associated with antiepileptic drugs. *Arch Neurol* 1994;51:250–253.

110. Holmes LB, Harvey EA, Coull BA, et al. The teratogenicity of anticonvulsant drugs. *N Engl J Med* 2001;344:1132–1138.

111. Kaaja E, Kaaja R, Hiilesmaa V. Major malformations in offspring of women with epilepsy. *Neurology* 2003;60:575–579.

112. Kaneko S, Battino D, Andermann E, et al. Congenital malformations due to antiepileptic drugs. *Epilepsy Res* 1999;33:145–158.

113. Dravet C, Julian C, Legras C, et al. Epilepsy, antiepileptic drugs, and malformations in children of women with epilepsy: a French prospective cohort study. *Neurology* 1992;42(4 Suppl 5):75–82.

114. Kaneko S, Otani K, Fukushima Y, et al. Teratogenicity of antiepileptic drugs: analysis of possible risk factors. *Epilepsia* 1988;29:459–467.

115. Kaneko S, Otani K, Kondo T, et al. Malformations in infants of mothers with epilepsy receiving antiepileptic drugs. *Neurology* 1992;42(Suppl 5):68–74.

116. Lopes-Cendes I, Andermann E, Arruda F, et al. Pregnancy outcomes in epileptic women over three decades: the impact of changes in medical management of epileptic patients [abstract]. *Epilepsia* 1995;36(Suppl 4):148.

117. Lindhout D. Pharmacogenetics and drug interactions: role in antiepileptic-drug-induced teratogenesis. *Neurology* 1992;42(4 Suppl 5):43–47.

118. Omtzigt JG, Los FJ, Grobbee DE, et al. The risk of spina bifida aperta after first-trimester exposure to valproate in a prenatal cohort. *Neurology* 1992;42(4 Suppl 5):119–125.

119. Mawer G, Clayton-Smith J, Coyle H, et al. Outcome of pregnancy in women attending an outpatient epilepsy clinic: adverse features associated with higher doses of sodium valproate. *Seizure* 2002;11:512–518.

120. Abrishamchian AR, Khoury MJ, Calle EE. The contribution of maternal epilepsy and its treatment to the etiology of oral clefts:

a population based case-control study. *Genet Epidemiol* 1994; 11:343–351.

121. Hernandez-Diaz S, Werler MM, Walker AM, et al. Folic acid antagonists during pregnancy and the risk of birth defects. *N Engl J Med* 2000;343:1608–1614.

122. Lammer EJ, Sever LE, Oakley GP Jr. Teratogen update: valproic acid. *Teratology* 1987;35:465–473.

123. Hernandez-Diaz S, Werler MM, Walker AM, et al. Neural tube defects in relation to use of folic acid antagonists during pregnancy. *Am J Epidemiol* 2001;153:961–968.

124. Battino D, Granata T, Binelli S, et al. Intrauterine growth in the offspring of epileptic mothers. *Acta Neurol Scand* 1992;86: 555–557.

125. Gaily E, Granstrom ML. Minor anomalies in children of mothers with epilepsy. *Neurology* 1992;42(4 Suppl 5):128–131.

126. Kelly TE, Edwards P, Rein M, et al. Teratogenicity of anticonvulsant drugs. II: a prospective study. *Am J Med Genet* 1984;19:435–443.

127. Steegers-Theunissen RP, Renier WO, Borm GF, et al. Factors influencing the risk of abnormal pregnancy outcome in epileptic women: a multi-centre prospective study. *Epilepsy Res* 1994; 18:261–269.

128. Dieterich E, Steveling A, Lukas A, et al. Congenital anomalies in children of epileptic mothers and fathers. *Neuropediatrics* 1980; 11:274–283.

129. Jager-Roman E, Deichl A, Jakob S, et al. Fetal growth, major malformations, and minor anomalies in infants born to women receiving valproic acid. *J Pediatr* 1986;108:997–1004.

130. Wolf P, Dam M, Janz D, eds. *Major malformations and minor anomalies in infants exposed to different antiepileptic drugs during pregnancy*. New York: Raven Press, 1987.

131. Lindhout D, Omtzigt JG. Pregnancy and the risk of teratogenicity. *Epilepsia* 1992;33(Suppl 4):S41–S48.

132. Diaz-Romero RM, Garza-Morales S, Mayen-Molina DG, et al. Facial anthropometric measurements in offspring of epileptic mothers. *Arch Med Res* 1999;30:186–189.

133. Kelly TE. Teratogenicity of anticonvulsant drugs. III: Radiographic hand analysis of children exposed in utero to diphenylhydantoin. *Am J Med Genet* 1984;19:445–450.

134. Hanson JW, Smith DW. The fetal hydantoin syndrome. *J Pediatr* 1975;87:285–290.

135. Astedt B. Antenatal drugs affecting vitamin K status of the fetus and the newborn. *Semin Thromb Hemost* 1995;21:364–370.

136. Thorp JA, Gaston L, Caspers DR, et al. Current concepts and controversies in the use of vitamin K. *Drugs* 1995;49:376–387.

137. Cornelissen M, Steegers-Theunissen R, Kollee L, et al. Supplementation of vitamin K in pregnant women receiving anticonvulsant therapy prevents neonatal vitamin K deficiency. *Am J Obstet Gynecol* 1993;168(3 Pt 1):884–888.

138. Cornelissen M, Steegers-Theunissen R, Kollee L, et al. Increased incidence of neonatal vitamin K deficiency resulting from maternal anticonvulsant therapy. *Am J Obstet Gynecol* 1993;168(3 Pt 1):923–928.

139. Davies VA, Rothberg AD, Argent AC, et al. Precursor prothrombin status in patients receiving anticonvulsant drugs. *Lancet* 1985;1:126–128.

140. Howe AM, Oakes DJ, Woodman PD, et al. Prothrombin and PIVKA-II levels in cord blood from newborn exposed to anticonvulsants during pregnancy. *Epilepsia* 1999;40:980–984.

141. Moslet U, Hansen ES. A review of vitamin K, epilepsy and pregnancy. *Acta Neurol Scand* 1992;85:39–43.

142. Kaaja E, Kaaja R, Matila R, et al. Enzyme-inducing antiepileptic drugs in pregnancy and the risk of bleeding in the neonate. *Neurology* 2002;58:549–553.

143. American Academy of Pediatrics Committee on Nutrition. Vitamin K compounds and their water soluble analogues: use in therapy and prophylaxis in pediatrics. *Pediatrics* 1961;25: 501–507.

144. Beck-Mannagetta G, Janz D, Hoffmeister U, et al. Morbidity risk for seizures and epilepsy in offsprings of patients with epilepsy. In: Beck-Mannagetta G, Anderson VE, Doose H, eds. *Genetics of the epilepsies*. Berlin: Springer-Verlag, 1989:119–126.

145. Ottman R, Annegers JF, Hauser WA, et al. Higher risk of seizures in offspring of mothers than of fathers with epilepsy. *Am J Hum Genet* 1988;43:257–264.

146. U.K. Sabril Prescription Event Monitoring Study, 1999.
147. Tsuboi T. Incidence of seizures among offspring of epileptic patients. In: Janz D, Dam M, Richens A, et al., eds. *Epilepsy, pregnancy, and the child*. New York: Raven Press, 1982:503–507.
148. Meadow SR. Anticonvulsant drugs and congenital abnormalities. *Lancet* 1968;2:1296.
149. German J, Kowal A, Ehlers KH. Trimethadione and human teratogenesis. *Teratology* 1970;3:349–362.
150. Zackai EH, Mellman WJ, Neiderer B, et al. The fetal trimethadione syndrome. *J Pediatr* 1975;87:280–284.
151. Krauss CM, Holmes LB, VanLang Q, et al. Four siblings with similar malformations after exposure to phenytoin and primidone. *J Pediatr* 1984;105:750–755.
152. Rudd NL, Freedom RM. A possible primidone embryopathy. *J Pediatr* 1979;94:835–837.
153. Seip M. Growth retardation, dysmorphic facies and minor malformations following massive exposure to phenobarbitone in utero. *Acta Paediatr Scand* 1976;65:617–621.
154. DiLiberti JH, Farndon PA, Dennis NR, et al. The fetal valproate syndrome. *Am J Med Genet* 1984;19:473–481.
155. Jones KL, Lacro RV, Johnson KA, et al. Pattern of malformations in the children of women treated with carbamazepine during pregnancy. *N Engl J Med* 1989;320:1661–1666.
156. McElhatton PR. The effects of benzodiazepine use during pregnancy and lactation. *Reprod Toxicol* 1994;8:461–475.
157. Granstrom ML, Hiilesmaa VK. Malformations and minor anomalies in the children of epileptic mothers: preliminary results of prospective Helsinki study. In: Janz D, Dam M, Richens A, et al., eds. *Epilepsy, pregnancy, and the child*. New York: Raven Press, 1982:303–307.
158. Lindhout D, Meinardi H, Meijer JW, et al. Antiepileptic drugs and teratogenesis in two consecutive cohorts: changes in prescription policy paralleled by changes in pattern of malformations. *Neurology* 1992;42(4 Suppl 5):94–110.
159. Kallen B, Robert E, Mastroiacovo P, et al. Anticonvulsant drugs and malformations is there a drug specificity? *Eur J Epidemiol* 1989;5:31–36.
160. Verloes A, Frikiche A, Gremillet C, et al. Proximal phocomelia and radial ray aplasia in fetal valproic syndrome. *Eur J Pediatr* 1990;149:266–267.
161. Cunningham M, Tennis P and the International Lamotrigine Pregnancy Registry Scientific Advisory Committee. Lamotrigine and the risk of malformations in pregnancy. *Neurology* 2005;64:955–960.
161a. Montouris G. Gabapentin exposure in human pregnancy: results from the Gabapentin Pregnancy Registry. *Epilepsy Behav* 2003;4:310–317.
162. Hoyme HE, Hauck L, Quinn D. Minor anomalies accompanying prenatal exposure to topiramate [abstract]. *J Investig Med* 1998;46:119A.
163. *Integrated summary of safety*. Abbott Park, IL: Abbott Laboratories, 2003.
164. Data on file. East Hanover, NJ: Novartis Pharmaceutical, 2003.
165. Friis ML, Kristensen O, Boas J, et al. Therapeutic experiences with 947 epileptic outpatients in oxcarbazepine treatment. *Acta Neurol Scand* 1993;87:224–227.
166. Lindhout D, Omtzigt JG. Teratogenic effects of antiepileptic drugs: implications for the management of epilepsy in women of childbearing age. *Epilepsia* 1994;35(Suppl 4):S19–S28.
167. Rabinowicz A, Meischenguiser R, Ferraro SM, et al. Single-center 7-year experience of oxcarbazepine exposure during pregnancy. *Epilepsia* 2002;43(Suppl 7):208–209.
168. Felbatol package insert. Cranbury, NJ: Wallace Laboratories, 2003.
169. Kondo T, Kaneko S, Amano Y, et al. Preliminary report on teratogenic effects of zonisamide in the offspring of treated women with epilepsy. *Epilepsia* 1996;37:1242–1244.
170. Yerby M, Morrell MJ. Efficacy, safety, and tolerability of zonisamide in women [abstract]. *Epilepsia* 2000;41(Suppl 7):199.
171. Dansky LV, Rosenblatt DS, Andermann E. Mechanisms of teratogenesis: folic acid and antiepileptic therapy. *Neurology* 1992;42(4 Suppl 5):32–42.
172. Lindhout D, Meinardi H, Barth PG. Hazards of fetal exposure to drug combinations. In: Janz D, Dam M, Richens A, et al., eds. *Epilepsy, pregnancy, and the child*. New York: Raven Press, 1982:275–281.
173. Lindhout D, Hoppener RJ, Meinardi H. Teratogenicity of antiepileptic drug combinations with special emphasis on epoxidation (of carbamazepine). *Epilepsia* 1984;25:77–83.
174. Buehler BA, Delimont D, van Waes M, et al. Prenatal prediction of risk of the fetal hydantoin syndrome. *N Engl J Med* 1990;322:1567–1572.
175. Strickler SM, Dansky LV, Miller MA, et al. Genetic predisposition to phenytoin-induced birth defects. *Lancet* 1985;2:746–749.
176. Graf WD, Pippenger CE, Shurtleff DB. Erythrocyte antioxidant enzyme activities in children with myelomeningocele. *Dev Med Child Neurol* 1995;37:900–905.
177. Duncan S, Mercho S, Lopes-Cendes I, et al. Repeated neural tube defects and valproate monotherapy suggest a pharmacogenetic abnormality. *Epilepsia* 2001;42:750–753.
178. Malm H, Kajantie E, Kivirikko S, et al. Valproate embryopathy in three sets of siblings: Further proof of hereditary susceptibility. *Neurology* 2002;59:630–633.
179. Allen WP. Folic acid in the prevention of birth defects. *Curr Opin Pediatr* 1996;8:630–634.
180. Baily LB, Gregory JF III. Folate metabolism and requirements. *J Nutr* 1999;129:779–782.
181. Mills JL, McPartlin JM, Kirke PN, et al. Homocysteine metabolism in pregnancies complicated by neural-tube defects. *Lancet* 1995;345:149–151.
182. Yates JR, Ferguson-Smith MA, Shenkin A, et al. Is disordered folate metabolism the basis for the genetic predisposition to neural tube defects? *Clin Genet* 1987;31:279–287.
183. Hartridge T, Illing HM, Sandy JR. The role of folic acid in oral clefting. *Br J Orthod* 1999;26:115–120.
184. Hernandez-Diaz S, Werler MM, Walker A, et al. Folic acid antagonists during pregnancy and the risk of birth defects. *NEJM* 2000;343:1608–1614.
185. Ek J, Magnus EM. Plasma and red blood cell folate during normal pregnancies. *Acta Obstet Gynecol Scand* 1981;60:247–251.
186. Collins CS, Bailey LB, Hillier S, et al. Red blood cell uptake of supplemental folate in patients on anticonvulsant drug therapy. *Am J Clin Nutr* 1988;48:1445–1450.
187. Dansky LV, Andermann E, Rosenblatt D, et al. Anticonvulsants, folate levels, and pregnancy outcome: a prospective study. *Ann Neurol* 1987;21:176–182.
188. Goggin T, Gough H, Bissessar A, et al. A comparative study of the relative effects of anticonvulsant drugs and dietary folate on the red cell folate status of patients with epilepsy. *Q J Med* 1987;65:911–919.
189. Ogawa Y, Kaneko S, Otani K, et al. Serum folic acid levels in epileptic mothers and their relationship to congenital malformations. *Epilepsy Res* 1991;8:75–78.
190. Campbell LR, Dayton DH, Sohal GS. Neural tube defects: a review of human and animal studies on the etiology of neural tube defects. *Teratology* 1986;34:171–187.
191. From the Centers for Disease Control and Prevention. Knowledge and use of folic acid by women of childbearing age—United States, 1997. *JAMA* 1997;278:892–893.
192. Centers for Disease Control and Prevention. Recommendations for the use of folic acid to reduce the number of cases of spina bifida and other neural tube defects. *MMWR Recomm Rep* 1992;41:1–7.
193. Prevention of neural tube defects: results of the Medical Research Council Vitamin Study. MRC Vitamin Study Research Group. *Lancet* 1991;338:131–137.
194. Betts T, Fox C. Proactive pre-conception counselling for women with epilepsy—is it effective? *Seizure* 1999;8:322–327.
195. So NK. Recurrence, remission, and relapse of seizures. *Cleve Clin J Med* 1993;60:439–444.
196. Pippenger CE. Pharmacology of neural tube defects. *Epilepsia* 2003;44(Suppl 3):24–32.
197. Maternal serum screening. *Am Coll Obstet Gynecol Educ Bull* 1996;228:1–9.
198. A North American Registry for Epilepsy and Pregnancy, a unique public/private partnership of health surveillance. *Epilepsia* 1998;39:793–798.

199. Gjerde IO, Strandjord RE, Ulstein M. The course of epilepsy during pregnancy: a study of 78 cases. *Acta Neurol Scand* 1988;78:198–205.

200. Vidovic MI, Della Marina BM. Trimestral changes of seizure frequency in pregnant epileptic women. *Acta Med Croatica* 1994;48:85–87.

201. Baughman FA Jr, Randinitis EJ. Passage of diphenylhydantoin across the placenta. *JAMA* 1970;213:466.

202. Briggs GG, Freeman RK, Yaffe SJ. *Drugs in pregnancy and lactation: a reference guide to fetal and neonatal risk,* 5th ed. Philadelphia: Lippincott Williams & Wilkins, 1998.

203. Froescher W, Gugler R, Niesen M, et al. Protein binding of valproic acid in maternal and umbilical cord serum. *Epilepsia* 1984;25:244–249.

204. Kaneko S, Sato T, Suzuki K. The levels of anticonvulsants in breast milk. *Br J Clin Pharmacol* 1979;7:624–627.

205. Kuhnz W, Jager-Roman E, Rating D, et al. Carbamazepine and carbamazepine-10,11- epoxide during pregnancy and postnatal period in epileptic mother and their nursed infants: pharmacokinetics and clinical effects. *Pediatr Pharmacol (New York)* 1983; 3:199–208.

206. Kuhnz W, Koch S, Jakob S, et al. Ethosuximide in epileptic women during pregnancy and lactation period. Placental transfer, serum concentrations in nursed infants and clinical status. *Br J Clin Pharmacol* 1984;18:671–677.

207. Kuhnz W, Koch S, Helge H, et al. Primidone and phenobarbital during lactation period in epileptic women: total and free drug serum levels in the nursed infants and their effects on neonatal behavior. *Dev Pharmacol Ther* 1988;11:147–154.

208. Mirkin BL. Placental transfer and neonatal elimination of diphenylhydantoin. *Am J Obstet Gynecol* 1971;109:930–933.

209. Nau H, Kuhnz W, Egger HJ, et al. Anticonvulsants during pregnancy and lactation. Transplacental, maternal and neonatal pharmacokinetics. *Clin Pharmacokinet* 1982;7:508–543.

210. Pynnonen S, Kanto J, Sillanpaa M, et al. Carbamazepine: placental transport, tissue concentrations in foetus and newborn, and level in milk. *Acta Pharmacol Toxicol (Copenh)* 1977;41:244–253.

211. Rane A, Bertilsson L, Palmer L. Disposition of placentally transferred carbamazepine (Tegretol) in the newborn. *Eur J Clin Pharmacol* 1975;8:283–284.

212. Bulau P, Paar WD, von Unruh GE. Pharmacokinetics of oxcarbazepine and 10-hydroxy-carbazepine in the newborn child of an oxcarbazepine-treated mother. *Eur J Clin Pharmacol* 1988;34: 311–313.

213. Kawada K, Itoh S, Kusaka T, et al. Pharmacokinetics of zonisamide in perinatal period. *Brain Dev* 2002;24:95–97.

214. Myllynen P, Pienimaki P, Jouppila P, et al. Transplacental passage of oxcarbazepine and its metabolites *in vivo. Epilepsia* 2001; 42:1482–1485.

215. Ohman I, Vitols S, Tomson T. Lamotrigine in pregnancy: pharmacokinetics during delivery, in the neonate, and during lactation. *Epilepsia* 2000;41:709–713.

216. Shimoyama R, Ohkubo T, Sugawara K. Monitoring of zonisamide in human breast milk and maternal plasma by solid-phase extraction HPLC method. *Biomed Chromatogr* 1999;13:370–372.

217. Monson RR, Rosenberg L, Hartz SC, et al. Diphenylhydantoin and selected congenital malformations. *N Engl J Med* 1973;289: 1049–1052.

218. Niswander JD, Wertelecki W. Congenital malformation among offspring of epileptic women. *Lancet* 1973;1:1062.

219. Samrén EB, van Duijn CM, Christiaens GC, et al. Antiepileptic drug regimens and major congenital abnormalities in the offspring. *Ann Neurol* 1999;46:739–746.

220. South J. Teratogenic effect of anticonvulsants. *Lancet* 1972;2: 1154.

221. Watson JD, Spellacy WN. Neonatal effects of maternal treatment with the anticonvulsant drug diphenylhydantoin. *Obstet Gynecol* 1971;37:881–885.

Treatment of Epilepsy in the Setting of Renal and Liver Disease

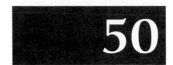

Jane G. Boggs   *Elizabeth Waterhouse*   *Robert J. DeLorenzo*

Management of seizures in the presence of renal and liver disease has become an increasingly common problem during the past several decades. Prolonged survival, achieved largely through advances in dialysis, pharmacology, and transplantation, accounts for a growing population of patients with altered metabolic capacities. The emergence of opportunistic hepatic infections in acquired immune deficiency syndrome and other immunocompromised conditions, as well as the prevalence of viral hepatitis, has increased the population with impaired liver function. Pharmacologically induced renal dysfunction and systemic diseases, such as hypertension and diabetes, continue to occur frequently in patients whom an epileptologist may encounter. Consequently, neurologists must possess a basic understanding of pharmacology and the specific pharmacokinetics of anticonvulsants in liver and renal disease.

Patients with pre-existing liver and renal disease may require transient treatment with anticonvulsants for seizures as a result of electrolyte shifts associated with worsening uremia and dialysis, as well as hepatic insufficiency caused by chronic alcohol abuse. Secondary effects of disease in either of these organs can adversely affect blood pressure and coagulation, resulting in potentially epileptogenic cerebrovascular events. In addition, patients with epilepsy are not immune to the liver and renal diseases that occur in the general population. Antiepileptic drugs (AEDs) themselves may induce such organ dysfunction, complicating or contraindicating their further use.

This chapter reviews the clinical use in liver and renal disease of the commonly prescribed AEDs and the newer anticonvulsant medications that became available between 1993 and 2004. Because the degree of debility and the response to AEDs vary significantly among patients, specific rules cannot be inferred, and practical guidelines only are offered. The general biopharmacologic principles that precede the discussion of specific agents apply not only to current anticonvulsant therapy but also to drugs potentially available in the future.

MEDICATIONS IN RENAL DISEASE: OVERVIEW

The degree to which renal disease alters the pharmacokinetics of specific drugs depends on their primary mode of elimination. Drugs excreted unchanged by the kidneys have a slower rate of elimination and longer half-life in patients with renal disease than in healthy persons, increasing drug accumulation and necessitating lower doses and longer interdose intervals to prevent toxic effects.

Drugs are divided into three classes: (a) type A, which are eliminated completely by renal excretion; (b) type B, which are eliminated by nonrenal routes; and (c) type C, which are eliminated by both renal and nonrenal routes (1,2). Because the relationship between half-life and creatinine clearance (Cl_{Cr}) is not linear, dosing predictions based on renal insufficiency are difficult. However, estimates may be determined from the following linear equation that describes the speed of drug elimination as a function of creatinine clearance:

$$K = R \times Cl_{Cr} + K_{NR} \quad (3)$$

where K is the elimination rate constant, R the slope of K against Cl_{Cr}, and K_{NR} is the rate constant for drug elimination by nonrenal routes (4).

Nomograms based on computed values of K and K_{NR} will predict new maintenance doses that are reduced proportionately to the reduction in K. However, such linear equations do not take into account the effect of renal insufficiency on drug biotransformation, elimination of metabolites with toxic properties, or decreases in plasma protein binding.

Studies show that some drug oxidations in liver endoplasmic reticulum can be accelerated in uremia (5,6). The mechanism is undefined, but several possibilities have been proposed. Poorly excreted nutritional substances that can induce microsomal drug metabolism may be present in excess quantities in renal patients. Indole-containing cruciferous plants (cabbage, cauliflower, Brussels sprouts) induce these enzymes in rats (7). Drugs with low hepatic extraction and high protein binding will have higher rates of metabolism in uremia as the free fraction increases, which, in turn, increases plasma clearance and the apparent volume of distribution (V_d):

$$V_d = VP + VT \times FP/FT \quad (8)$$

where VP is the plasma volume, VT is the extravascular volume, FP is the fraction of free drug in plasma, and FT is the fraction of free drug in tissue (9).

Protein binding of anionic acidic drugs (such as phenytoin, which is strongly bound by albumin) decreases in patients with renal dysfunction (Table 50.1). Drugs with organic bases have variable protein binding in renal disease, and those that bind primarily to one site have decreased binding, an effect described in the literature since 1938 (10). However, this reduced binding exceeds the amount that can be accounted for by a simple decrease in serum albumin. Two hypotheses relating to uremia have been proposed to resolve this discrepancy: the existence of small molecules that competitively displace drugs from normal binding sites (11) and altered binding sites of albumin molecules (12). Experimental evidence supports both mechanisms, and each probably is involved to some extent in individual patients (13). Although drug metabolism may be accelerated in uremic humans, the same drugs may exhibit slowed metabolism in uremic animals, complicating the extrapolation from experimental data (14).

Although dialysis ameliorates renal insufficiency, it alters the response to medications. The removal of drugs from serum by hemodialysis depends on numerous variables, including molecular weight, protein binding, plasma concentration, blood flow, and hematocrit, as well as on the inherent clearance characteristics of the dialyzer. Dialysis also can profoundly affect drug activity through changes in pH level, protein concentration, osmolality, electrolytes, and glucose and urea levels. Peritoneal dialysis, unlike hemodialysis, is influenced by vascular disease because the blood supply presented to the dialysate passes through arterioles. Drug additives are used more frequently in peritoneal dialysis than in hemodialysis solutions, creating a small potential for drug interactions (15). Following hemodialysis, albumin binding of such medications as phenytoin and phenobarbital is decreased, perhaps because of increased levels of nonesterified fatty

TABLE 50.1

DISPOSITION OF COMMON ANTIEPILEPTIC DRUGS IN RENAL DISEASE

Drug	Protein Binding	Total Plasma Concentration	Plasma Half-life	Risk of Intoxication	Dosage Adjustment	Removal by Dialysis
Phenytoin	↓	↓	↓	Low	Unnecessary	Negligible
Valproic acid	↓	↓	—	Low	Unnecessary	Negligible
Phenobarbital	—	—	— or ↑	High	Slight reduction	Significant
Primidone	—	—	—	High	Slight reduction	Unknown
Carbamazepine	—	—	—	Low	Unnecessary	Unknown
Ethosuximide	NA	—	—	Low	Unnecessary	Unknown
Benzodiazepines	↓	↓	—	Low	Unnecessary	Unknown
Gabapentin	—	↑	↑	Low	Reduction	Significant
Lamotrigine	Unknown	? ↑	↑	Unknown	Unknown	Moderate
Felbamate[a]	Unknown	? ↑	Unknown	Unknown	Slight reduction	Moderate
Topiramate	Unknown	↑	↑	Considerable	Reduction	Significant
Tiagabine[b]	—	—	—	Unknown	Unnecessary	Negligible
Zonisamide	Unknown	? ↑	Unknown	Unknown	Reduction	Unknown
Oxcarbazepine[c,d]	Unknown	↑	↑	Considerable	Reduction	Unknown
Levetiracetam[e]	—	↑	Unknown	Unknown	Reduction	50%

Abbreviations: ↓, reduction; —, unchanged; ↑, increased; NA, not applicable.
[a]Data on file. Wallace Laboratories.
[b]Cato et al. (110).
[c]Package insert.
[d]Rouan et al. (100)
[e]Patsalos (126).
Adapted from Asconape JJ, Penry JK. Use of antiepileptic drugs in the presence of liver and kidney disease: a review. *Epilepsia* 1982;23(Suppl 1):565–579.

acids, which bind strongly to albumin (16). This effect has been proposed for heparin, administered systemically during dialysis, with resultant activation of lipoprotein lipase (17).

MEDICATIONS IN LIVER DISEASE: OVERVIEW

Because the liver is a primary site of drug metabolism in humans, hepatic insufficiency can significantly alter biotransformation and disposition, although pathophysiologic changes will vary according to the disease or its stages. Hepatic blood inflow by the portal vein, hepatocellular mass, and functional capacity primarily determine the effects of liver disease on drug handling. Table 50.2 illustrates the major changes found in cirrhosis, acute viral hepatitis, and alcoholic hepatitis (18).

At least five categories of liver disease affect drug disposition: (a) chronic liver disease; (b) acute hepatitis; (c) drug-induced hepatotoxicity; (d) cholestasis; and (e) hepatic infiltrative/neoplastic disease. In addition, medications must be classified not only by protein binding but also by the capacity of the liver to extract drug as blood flows through the organ: flow limited, capacity limited with high protein binding, and capacity limited with low protein binding (19).

Flow-limited drugs have high extraction rates, and clearance is limited primarily by blood flow. Their rate of metabolism depends on the amount of drug presented to the liver, which is proportional to blood flow. Most anticonvulsants are capacity-limited drugs, as their extraction ratios are low (<0.2). Table 50.3 lists the extraction ratios of major antiepileptic compounds (18,20–23). The rate of metabolism of capacity-limited drugs depends on the concentration of free drug at hepatic enzyme receptor sites and thus on the extent of protein binding. Capacity-limited, binding-sensitive drugs, such as phenytoin, valproic acid, and carbamazepine, are greater than 85% bound to plasma

TABLE 50.3
EXTRACTION RATIOS OF MAJOR ANTIEPILEPTIC COMPOUNDS

Extraction Rates	Extraction Ratios	% Bound	Source
Phenytoin	0.03	90	Blaschke et al. (18)
Valproic acid	<0.05		Evans et al. (127)
Carbamazepine	<0.002		Evans et al. (127)
Benzodiazepines (diazepam)	0.03	98	Klotz et al. (21)
Hexobarbitone	0.16		Breimer et al. (20)
Amylobarbitone	0.03	61	Mawer et al. (22)

proteins at therapeutic concentrations; therefore, alterations in plasma protein concentration and binding characteristics can significantly alter their hepatic clearance (23,24). Capacity-limited, binding-insensitive drugs, such as ethosuximide, have a low affinity for plasma protein (usually less than 30% at therapeutic concentrations), and clearance is only minimally affected by changes in protein binding.

The following model, combining the principles of intrinsic metabolic capacity and blood flow, has been proposed.

$$Cl_h = Q \times F_b \times Cl_{int}/Q + F_b \times Cl_{int} \quad (25)$$

where Cl_h is the volume of blood cleared by the liver per unit time, Q is total hepatic blood flow, F_b is the fraction of drug bound to protein and cells, and Cl_{int} is the intrinsic metabolic clearance (23,24,26).

The latter term, defined as the volume of liver water cleared of drug per unit time, varies directly with the Michaelis constant. The extraction ratio (E) may be derived by dividing hepatic blood flow into total hepatic clearance:

$$Cl_h/Q = E \quad (27)$$

When combined hepatic and renal clearance occurs, clearances are additive.

TABLE 50.2
PATHOPHYSIOLOGIC CHANGES IN VARIOUS TYPES OF LIVER DISEASE

Disease	Total Hepatic Blood Flow	Hepatocellular Mass	Hepatocyte Function
Cirrhosis			
Moderate	↓	— / ↑	—
Severe	↓	↓	↓
Acute/inflammatory Liver disease			
Viral hepatitis	— / ↑	— / ↑	↓
Alcoholic hepatitis	— / ↑	— / ↑ / ↓	↓

Abbreviations: ↓, decreased; —, unchanged; ↑, increased.
From Blaschke TF, Meffin PJ, Melmon KL, et al. Influence of acute viral hepatitis on phenytoin kinetics and protein binding. *Clin Pharmacol Ther* 1975;17:685–691, with permission.

TABLE 50.4

DISPOSITION OF COMMON ANTIEPILEPTIC DRUGS IN HEPATIC DISEASE

Drug	Protein Binding	Total Plasma Concentration	Plasma Half-life	Risk of Intoxication	Dosage Adjustment
Phenytoin	↓	—	—	Considerable	Unnecessary or slight reduction
Valproic acid	↓	↓	↑	Considerable	Unnecessary or slight reduction
Phenobarbital	Unknown	—	↑	Considerable	Unnecessary or slight reduction
Primidone	Unknown	—	Unknown	Unknown	Unknown
Carbamazepine	↓	—	Unknown	Considerable?	Unknown
Benzodiazepines[a]	↓	—	↑	High	Reduction
Gabapentin	—	—	—	Low	Unnecessary
Lamotrigine	? ↓	? ↑	? ↑	Unknown	Reduction
Felbamate	? ↓	? ↑	? ↑	Contraindicated	Contraindicated
Tiagabine	↓	↑	↑	Considerable	Reduction

Abbreviations: ↓, reduced; —, unchanged; ↑, increased.
[a]Not applicable to oxazepam.
Adapted from Asconape JJ, Penry JK. Use of antiepileptic drugs in the presence of liver and kidney disease: a review. *Epilepsia* 1982;23(Suppl 1):565–579.

Although hypoalbuminemia is frequently a feature of liver disease, drug binding to plasma proteins may be decreased even without measurable changes in albumin concentration (Table 50.4). Mechanisms similar to those causing decreased protein binding in renal insufficiency have been suggested (28,29). Because intrinsic clearance varies with the type and duration of liver disease, the effects of changes in protein binding in capacity-limited, binding-sensitive drugs are complex. If hepatic disease lowers binding without changing intrinsic clearance, total drug concentration will ultimately fall because the rate of metabolism of these drugs depends on the free fraction. If liver disease reduces intrinsic clearance, total drug concentration may remain the same or increase as the free concentration increases. This can result in enhanced response or toxic effects at lower than expected drug levels and may explain the increased incidence of adverse reactions to medications such as valproic acid in liver disease (30).

Capacity-limited, binding-insensitive drugs can be considered relatively pure indicators of intrinsic clearance. However, tissue binding to substances such as ligandin may contribute to the volume of distribution of drugs and thus to their half-life. The effect of liver disease on the content and function of such binding proteins is poorly understood. Tissue binding can be affected by secondary pathologic changes of liver disease, such as alterations in tissue and plasma pH level (24,31–33) or by ascites (34,35).

Because of various types of drugs and stages of liver disease, as well as interindividual variation, predicting changes in drug kinetics in patients with hepatic insufficiency remains difficult. Studies have identified additional discrepancies between observed changes and those suggested by pharmacokinetic predictions (12,23,26). Another variable is the potential for autoinduction of microsomal enzymes after long-term drug administration. Phenobarbital and carbamazepine and their active metabolites have this potential, with resultant temporal variability in drug levels and efficacy, increased complexity of drug interactions, and the potential increased risk of liver dysfunction.

SPECIFIC DRUGS

Phenytoin

Phenytoin (5,5-diphenylhydantoin) has a dissociation constant (pK$_a$) of about 8.3 and is approximately 90% bound to plasma proteins, mainly albumin (37). A larger proportion remains free in neonates and in patients with hypoalbuminemia and uremia (38). Apparent volume of distribution is approximately 64% of body weight, as fractional binding in tissues is similar to that in plasma. Elimination occurs nearly exclusively by hepatic microsomal biotransformation, with less than 5% excreted unchanged in urine (39). The primary metabolite, 5-parahydroxyphenyl-5-phenylhydantoin, is inactive and is excreted initially in bile and subsequently in urine, mostly as glucuronide. The corresponding microsomal enzymes are saturable at usual clinical doses. For concentrations less than 10 mg/L, elimination is exponential; at high levels, it is dose dependent (40).

Effects of Renal Disease

Phenytoin is the most extensively studied anticonvulsant in renal dysfunction. Uremic plasma has lower binding capacity for phenytoin than plasma in healthy subjects, with unbound fractions as high as 30%, compared with

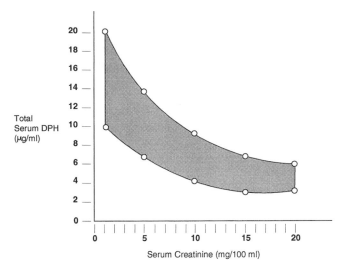

Figure 50.1 Calculated values of total serum phenytoin (diphenylhydantoin [DPH]) concentration that will produce a concentration in plasma water of 0.7 to 1.4 µg/mL. (Adapted from Rowland M, Blaschke TF, Meffin PJ, et al. Pharmacokinetics in disease states modifying hepatic and metabolic function. In: Benet LZ, ed. *Effect of disease states on drug pharmacokinetics.* Washington, DC: American Pharmaceutical Association; 1976:53–74, with permission.)

the usual 10% to 15% (28,41–43). The degree of binding impairment has been correlated with levels of albumin, blood urea nitrogen, serum creatinine, creatinine clearance, and the patient's physical disability (43,44). However, decreased binding is noted frequently in uremic patients with normal albumin levels (45), suggesting the accumulation of competitive or noncompetitive inhibiting substances (11) or altered albumin binding sites (12). Most consistently, the free fraction of phenytoin directly reflects the degree of renal failure, which can be roughly estimated by serum creatinine values. Reidenberg and Affrime (45) calculated the total phenytoin values that produce free phenytoin levels of 0.7 to 1.4 mg/L (Fig. 50.1). Decreased protein binding results in a proportionate increase in the apparent volume of distribution higher than the usual 0.6 L/kg. In chronic renal failure, this situation results in lower total plasma concentrations, reducing therapeutic ranges from 10 to 20 mg/L to as low as 5 to 10 mg/L (6,46,47).

The half-life of phenytoin is decreased in patients with uremia. Increased hepatic clearance of phenytoin observed in uremic rabbits suggests that heightened drug metabolism may account for more rapid elimination (48). However, additional studies have not demonstrated enhanced microsomal enzyme activity (49,50). Because 95% of a phenytoin dose is biotransformed, little parent drug accumulates, even in severe renal failure. Nevertheless, accumulation of the glucuronide metabolite, which is primarily excreted by the kidney, does occur in renal failure (5,51). This metabolite has no known anticonvulsant or toxic properties. Some studies suggest that it may inhibit phenytoin biotransformation (52), whereas others report no such effect (27,53).

Dialysis affects phenytoin primarily by altering protein binding. Various studies have suggested either a decrease (3) or an increase (54) in binding capacity following hemodialysis. This apparent contradiction may result from fluctuations in the free fraction of phenytoin during and after hemodialysis, leading to unexpected clinical intoxication (54). Martin and colleagues (55) reported that only 2% to 4% of intravenous phenytoin appeared in the dialysate of seven uremic patients. With a dialyzer of 4.5% efficiency, no postdialysis supplementation was necessary (55).

Finally, certain assays may give incorrect results in renally impaired patients. The enzyme-multiplied immunoassay may falsely elevate total plasma phenytoin levels in patients with severe renal insufficiency (54), tripling values obtained by gas-liquid chromatography. The cause of this discrepancy is unknown, but gas-liquid or high-performance liquid chromatography appears to be a more predictable and clinically useful method in patients with advanced renal disease (57).

Effects of Liver Disease

Plasma from patients with hepatic insufficiency also has reduced binding capacity for phenytoin (28,44,45). The degree of impairment correlates with levels of serum albumin (18,58) or total bilirubin (53), or both (29,44). It has been suggested that the total number of binding sites is reduced as a result of lower albumin concentration in competition with bilirubin (44). However, studies in alcoholic cirrhosis and acute viral hepatitis indicate that the degree of impairment is unlikely to be significant (18,25). Nevertheless, neonates with hyperbilirubinemia have substantially decreased phenytoin binding and require a reduced dose to prevent toxic effects (29).

Decreased biotransformation capacity in patients with liver disease results in accumulation of drug and increased potential for toxicity. Studies by Kutt and colleagues (14) found that in patients receiving phenytoin or phenobarbital, drug accumulated as hepatic dysfunction increased. Decreased renal excretion of metabolites was also noted.

Clinical Recommendations

Based on the shortened half-life noted in uremia, phenytoin usually should be administered no less frequently than every 8 hours. Lower loading doses may be necessary if protein binding is expected to be markedly decreased, as a high free fraction can be anticipated. Bound and free phenytoin levels should be determined for a stable level of renal function, and maintenance levels adjusted accordingly. The therapeutic range for free phenytoin remains between 1 and 2 mg/L, even in renal disease. Salivary levels closely correlate with free levels. No supplementation should be given after hemodialysis or peritoneal dialysis. Microsomal enzyme induction from long-term phenytoin administration may increase metabolism of 25-hydroxycalciferol, worsening the osteomalacia of uremia (59). Although phenytoin accumulation may accompany severe liver disease, nonlinear kinetics and difficulty in estimating hepatic metabolic capacity limit the clinician's ability to predict dose adjustments. Therefore, frequent serum determinations and gradual dose regulation are necessary.

Phenobarbital

Phenobarbital (5-ethyl-5-phenylbarbituric acid) is a weak acid with a pK_a of 7.2 that is 40% to 60% bound to plasma proteins. Its volume of distribution is approximately 0.9 L/kg (33). Up to 25% of the drug dose is eliminated by renal mechanisms, whereas the remainder is metabolized by the hepatic mixed-function oxidase system. The major metabolites, parahydroxyphenobarbital and N-hydroxyphenobarbital, are inactive and are excreted by the kidneys. Phenobarbital is a potent inducer of the microsomal enzyme system (40).

Effects of Renal Disease
Although the half-life of phenobarbital has been reported to be unchanged in uremic patients (38), some accumulation should be expected, as elimination of long-acting barbiturates depends more on renal excretion than on biotransformation. Because of this, hemodialysis and peritoneal dialysis remove a proportion of phenobarbital from the serum, thereby reducing serum levels. In impaired renal function, severe central nervous system and cardiovascular depression may result from barbiturate accumulation, further worsening the renal condition.

Effects of Liver Disease
Because a significant amount is excreted unchanged by the kidneys, phenobarbital has been promoted as a useful agent in patients with liver disease. Nevertheless, some studies have found a prolonged half-life in certain hepatic illnesses. Animal models with carbon tetrachloride-induced liver damage showed a slight reduction in plasma clearance (60). In cirrhotic patients, phenobarbital half-life was prolonged compared with that in controls (130 ± 15 hours and 86 ± 3 hours, respectively), and reduced amounts of conjugated hydroxyphenobarbital appeared in the urine (61). However, in patients with acute viral hepatitis, no statistically significant prolongation of half-life or change in metabolic excretion clearly occurred, although only one dose of phenobarbital was administered (61). In a previous study, two cirrhotic patients who chronically received phenobarbital appeared to have drug accumulation when the daily dosage exceeded 60 mg. However, this study lacked controls and was complicated by concomitant administration of other drugs (14). Biliary excretion of phenobarbital is minimal, and cholestasis does not change serum levels (61).

Clinical Recommendations
Although no short-term dosage adjustment appears necessary, lower maintenance doses of phenobarbital must be recommended. Supplementation after dialysis is probably necessary (62). The effect of liver disease on patients receiving prolonged phenobarbital therapy varies with the individual as well as with the type of liver damage. Frequent measurement of plasma concentrations will help establish dose modifications; free levels offer little additional information.

Primidone

Primidone (2-deoxyphenobarbital), structurally related to phenobarbital, is not significantly bound to plasma proteins. It is partially converted by the liver to the active forms phenobarbital and phenylethylmalonamide. Approximately 20% of a primidone dose is excreted unchanged in the urine (9).

Effects of Renal Disease
Although little information is available on the use of primidone in renal disease, accumulation with resultant toxicity has been reported, presumably from delayed renal excretion and prolongation of the phenylethylmalonamide half-life. In one report (63), phenylethylmalonamide levels were proportionately higher than those of primidone or phenobarbital and thus were hypothesized to be responsible for clinical toxicity. Another patient showed evidence of intoxication, with high phenylethylmalonamide levels and moderate elevation of phenobarbital in association with renal failure (64).

Effects of Liver Disease
As primidone is metabolized to active compounds by the liver, little difference can be anticipated in a short course of therapy in liver disease. With long-term administration, changes similar to those seen with phenobarbital may be expected. No results from experimental investigation of primidone in liver disease are available.

Clinical Recommendations
Because primidone is metabolized to three active compounds, determination of plasma concentrations may help in assessing intoxications. With very low protein binding, free levels offer little information. Although it is unclear whether primidone may be removed by dialysis, its metabolite phenobarbital certainly will be. Supplementation following dialysis may be necessary and can best be established by measuring levels of primidone, phenobarbital, and phenylethylmalonamide.

Valproic Acid

Valproic acid (2-propylpentanoic acid) is a carboxylic acid with a pK_a of 4.9. The drug is 90% bound to plasma proteins, with a resultant volume of distribution of only 0.1 to 0.4 L/kg. At higher serum concentrations, protein binding decreases (13). Elimination is mostly by hepatic biotransformation, with only 1% to 3% of the dose excreted unchanged in urine. More than 70% is present as metabolites, primarily the glucuronide of 2-propylglutaric acid. This drug has no known enzyme-inducing properties. Its metabolites show anticonvulsant activity in animal studies, particularly 3-oxovalproic acid, which has activity comparable to that of valproic acid in mice. No data on this compound's activity in humans are available (65).

Effects of Renal Disease

As with phenytoin, protein binding of valproic acid decreases in uremia (66,67). The decrease correlates with levels of blood urea nitrogen, creatinine, uric acid, and creatinine clearance but appears to have little relation to albumin and total protein levels (68). Hypoalbuminemia exerts a more significant effect in patients with a nephrotic syndrome than in healthy individuals. Hemodialysis decreased protein binding in 3 of 4 patients in one study (67). Reduced protein binding, with increased apparent volume of distribution, lowers total steady-state concentrations and unchanged free levels. As valproic acid is eliminated primarily by the liver, little accumulation in renal failure should be expected. However, its metabolites may have a prolonged effect because of delayed elimination. A single case report of valproic acid–related hepatobiliary dysfunction and reversible renal failure described decreased renal clearance of total conjugated valproic acid. *In vivo* production of rearranged valproic acid glucuronide was detected. It is unclear whether the accumulation of these altered substances is related to hepatobiliary or renal dysfunction, or both, and whether these substances are clinically active in humans (69).

Effects of Liver Disease

Valproic acid disposition studies in patients with alcoholic cirrhosis and those recovering from acute viral hepatitis (70) noted variably decreased protein binding (from 88.7% to 70.3% and 78.1%, respectively), with consequent increase in the apparent volume of distribution. Plasma half-life increased from 12.2 ± 3.7 hours in controls to 18.9 ± 5.1 hours in patients with cirrhosis and to 17 ± 3.7 hours in those with hepatitis. Total drug plasma clearance remained unimpaired in both groups, but free drug clearance decreased in cirrhotic patients. Reduced protein binding also increased the entrance of free valproic acid into blood cells and lowered metabolism by limiting substrate concentration. The investigators noted no changes in urinary excretion of valproic acid. Therefore, liver diseases studied appeared to result in reduced metabolic capacity for valproic acid that was compensated for by decreased protein binding. However, another study (68) of patients in acute stages of viral hepatitis showed increased half-life of valproic acid from 14.9 to 25.1 hours, with total drug clearance reduced from 8.6 to 3.8 mL/min.

Altered metabolic profiles of valproic acid have been described primarily in case reports of severe hepatic failure. A case resembling Reye syndrome in a 7-year-old reported significantly increased formation of three monounsaturated and four double-unsaturated metabolites in plasma (58% to 71% of valproic acid compounds compared with a maximum of 15% in controls) and in urine (34% to 61% compared with a maximum of 10% in controls) (71). Beta-oxidation, in particular, appeared suppressed, whereas omega-oxidation was increased (1). Serum-free carnitine, as well as the main beta-oxidation metabolite 3-ketovalproic acid, decreased despite serum valproic acid concentration at the upper limit of the therapeutic range in a 3-year-old with valproic acid-induced Reye syndrome (72). Autopsy of a set of twins with a progressive hepatic encephalopathy revealed hepatic necrosis only in the sibling who had received valproic acid, indicating that the drug may have aggravated preexisting hepatic pathology (73).

Rarely, valproic acid precipitates severe hepatotoxicity (74). This idiosyncratic reaction usually occurs during the first 6 months of treatment, and most cases have been reported in children. Other suggested associated risk factors for this condition include developmental delay and polytherapy. Histologic changes are variable, including cholestasis, centrilobular necrosis, and fatty changes. Clinical symptoms, such as nausea, vomiting, malaise, and breakthrough seizures, often appear before liver function tests become abnormal (75). Valproic acid causes metabolic changes because of the inhibition of enzymes involved in intermediary cell metabolism. Moderate elevations of blood ammonia are common in patients receiving valproic acid and usually do not require treatment in the absence of clinical symptoms (76).

Clinical Recommendations

Reduction of valproic acid dose generally is unnecessary in renal disease. However, decreased protein binding will lower the therapeutic range in uremic patients in proportion to the degree of renal failure. No estimated relationship has been established as it has for phenytoin, but free levels can be determined and dose adjustments should be based on clinical grounds and on the increase in free level greater than 10%. No clear evidence indicates that valproic acid must be supplemented following dialysis. Extreme caution should be exercised in the use of valproic acid in liver disease. Significant accumulation may occur as a result of increased half-life and may worsen hepatic function to a precipitous degree. The literature has little information on such cases, as valproic acid was discontinued promptly in all reported patients.

Carbamazepine

Carbamazepine (5-*H*-dibenz[*b,f*]azepine-5-carboxamide) is a neutral iminostilbene that is structurally related to imipramine. Plasma protein binding reaches 70% to 80%, and elimination depends almost entirely on hepatic biotransformation by epoxidation and hydroxylation. The most significant product is 10,11-carbamazepine epoxide, which has pharmacologic activity in animals (77). Carbamazepine can induce its own metabolism, shortening the half-life proportionately to the duration of treatment (40).

Effects of Renal Disease

Hooper and associates (78) found no evidence of reduced protein binding in patients with renal disease. Because only 1% of carbamazepine is eliminated unchanged in urine, accumulation of parent drug or the epoxide metabolite is unlikely. No studies are available on the effects of dialysis on the drug or its metabolites.

Effects of Liver Disease

Significant reduction in the percentage of carbamazepine bound to protein occurred in patients with mild liver disease (78). No clear correlation between any laboratory parameter and the degree of impairment could be determined.

Clinical Recommendations

Dose adjustment is not needed in either renal disease or dialysis. However, close monitoring of serum levels of carbamazepine and the 10,11-epoxide should be maintained, especially with long-term administration in patients with liver dysfunction.

Ethosuximide

Ethosuximide (2-ethyl-2-methylsuccinimide), a weak acid with a pK_a of 9.3, is not bound to plasma proteins. It is metabolized in the liver by hydroxylation at C-2 of the ethyl and methyl side chains with subsequent glucuronidation. Only 10% to 20% is eliminated unchanged in urine, and half-life is age dependent, increasing from approximately 30 hours in children to 60 hours in adults (40). No information is available on the pharmacokinetics of ethosuximide in renal or hepatic disease. Accumulation in renal failure is unlikely because of the small amount excreted. Significant removal during dialysis is probable, owing to the low volume of distribution and negligible protein binding. Supplementation based on serum levels following dialysis is recommended (62).

Benzodiazepines

The most commonly used benzodiazepines in epilepsy are diazepam, clonazepam, chlordiazepoxide, clorazepate, and nitrazepam. All undergo primarily hepatic biotransformation; minimal amounts appear unchanged in urine. Various metabolites such as desmethyldiazepam and oxazepam are clinically active and eliminated by the kidney in the free and glucuronidated forms. Protein binding varies among drugs (40).

Effects of Renal Disease

Although protein binding of diazepam and desmethyldiazepam declines with worsening uremia, the clinical significance of this effect remains unclear (78–80). Levels of chlordiazepoxide and diazepam have not been found to decrease following dialysis (81).

Effects of Liver Disease

Liver disease significantly alters the disposition of most benzodiazepines. Prolonged half-life of diazepam and chlordiazepoxide has been found in cirrhosis and acute viral hepatitis (82–84). Notably, oxazepam shows no evidence of altered disposition in various liver diseases (84,85). Hepatic disease reduces protein binding in all benzodiazepines studied except oxazepam (86).

Clinical Recommendations

Because renal disease has little impact on the elimination of benzodiazepines, no postdialysis supplementation or dose adjustment in uremia should be necessary. In liver disease, however, doses of diazepam, chlordiazepoxide, and probably clorazepate and clonazepam warrant reduction (87). Oxazepam appears to be an exception, as it is eliminated after glucuronidation without significant oxidative metabolism (8).

Lamotrigine

Lamotrigine [6-(2,3-dichlorophenyl)-1,2,4-triazine-3, 5-diamine] is a phenyltriazine, chemically unrelated to other AEDs. Plasma protein binding is approximately 55% at therapeutic levels. Lamotrigine is metabolized predominantly by glucuronidation, and then it is eliminated renally. It may induce its own metabolism to a modest degree when multiple doses are administered (88). When it is taken with hepatic enzyme-inducing AEDs (phenytoin, carbamazepine, phenobarbital, primidone), it is eliminated more rapidly. However, lamotrigine clearance is decreased by about 50% in the presence of valproate.

Effects of Renal Disease

Clinical experience in patients with renal dysfunction is limited, and no data are available on dosage adjustments in these patient populations. In a study of a small number of patients with renal impairment, Fillastre and colleagues (89) found that the elimination half-life of unchanged lamotrigine is prolonged in comparison with that in patients with normal renal function. Twelve volunteers with chronic renal failure and six individuals undergoing hemodialysis were given a single 100-mg dose. The mean plasma half-lives shown were 42.9 hours (chronic renal failure), 13.0 hours (during hemodialysis), and 57.4 hours (between hemodialysis treatments), compared with 26.2 hours in healthy volunteers. Approximately 20% of the amount of lamotrigine present in the body was eliminated during 4 hours of hemodialysis.

Effects of Liver Disease

The disposition of lamotrigine in patients with hepatic dysfunction has not been adequately evaluated. Posner and colleagues (90) evaluated the pharmacokinetics of a single dose of lamotrigine in seven patients with Gilbert syndrome, a benign condition associated with a deficiency in the enzyme bilirubin uridine diphosphate glucuronyl-transferase. Although the clearance of lamotrigine was lower and its half-life longer in these patients than in controls, it was felt that these differences were unlikely to be clinically significant.

Clinical Recommendations

Until more information becomes available, lamotrigine should be used with caution in patients with renal or hepatic dysfunction.

Felbamate

Felbamate (2-phenyl-1,3-propanediol dicarbamate) is a dicarbamate that is structurally similar to meprobamate. It is between 22% and 25% protein bound. Almost half of the dose is eliminated unchanged in the urine; the rest is metabolized by the liver to 2-hydroxy, *p*-hydroxy, and monocarbamate metabolites, none of which demonstrates significant antiepileptic activity (91). There is no autoinduction.

Effects of Renal Disease

Few data are available regarding the use of felbamate in patients with renal dysfunction.

Effects of Liver Disease

As of September 1999, there were 19 reported cases of hepatotoxicity associated with felbamate administration and 5 fatalities. The risk of fatal liver damage associated with felbamate is estimated to be 1 in 24,000 to 32,000 patients (92).

A detailed review of the reported cases of hepatic failure in patients treated with felbamate reveals confounding factors in up to 50% (93). Concomitant medications (valproic acid, carbamazepine, and phenytoin) or the presence of status epilepticus, acetaminophen toxicity, hepatitis, or shock liver may have played a significant role. Although no definitive diagnostic indicator has been established in unconfounded cases, research has identified a potential reactive aldehyde metabolite. Until further data are forthcoming, the clinician should consider potential risks for aplastic anemia and hepatic failure before initiating treatment with this drug.

Clinical Recommendations

Felbamate should not be prescribed for patients with a history of hepatic dysfunction. A patient who develops abnormal liver function values should be immediately withdrawn from the drug. Because felbamate is metabolized by the kidneys as well as the liver, either renal or hepatic dysfunction could decrease drug clearance. Because of the risk of aplastic anemia or hepatic failure, felbamate should not be used as a first-line AED and its use always requires careful hematologic and biochemical monitoring.

Gabapentin

Gabapentin [1-(aminomethyl)cyclohexane acetic acid] was synthesized as a γ-aminobutyric acid (GABA) analogue, although it does not act through direct GABA mechanisms. Gabapentin is not metabolized and does not inhibit or induce AED-metabolizing hepatic enzymes. It does not bind to plasma proteins and does not affect steady-state concentrations of other anticonvulsant drugs (94). It is excreted renally.

Effects of Renal Disease

Because gabapentin is excreted by the kidneys entirely, its elimination depends on renal function. Impairment of renal function decreases gabapentin clearance and increases plasma concentration in proportion to the degree of dysfunction. In 11 anuric patients given a single 400-mg oral dose of gabapentin, the half-life was 132 hours on days when hemodialysis was not performed and 3.8 hours during dialysis (95).

Effects of Liver Disease

Because of its low protein binding and renal elimination, gabapentin is theoretically a good anticonvulsant choice in patients with partial seizures and hepatic dysfunction. However, currently few data are available regarding the use of gabapentin in this population.

Clinical Recommendations

Gabapentin dosage should be decreased or the dosing interval increased in patients with renal dysfunction. The manufacturer recommends the following dosages, based on the patient's creatinine clearance: 400 mg three times a day, more than 60 mL/min; 300 mg twice a day, 30 to 60 mL/min; 300 mg once a day, 15 to 30 mL/min; and 300 mg every other day, less than 15 mL/min. A maintenance dose of 200 to 300 mg is recommended following each 4-hour session of hemodialysis, with no need for further supplementation until the next dialysis.

Oxcarbazepine

Oxcarbazepine (10,11-dihydro-10-oxocarbamazepine) is the keto analogue of carbamazepine. This compound was developed in an attempt to improve the tolerability profile of carbamazepine by elimination of metabolic production of carbamazepine 10,11-epoxide. Oxcarbazepine is rapidly and almost completely absorbed from the gastrointestinal tract after ingestion and is rapidly and nearly completely converted to the active metabolite, 10,11-dihydro-10-hydroxy-5*H*-dibenzo(*b,f*)azepine-5-carboxamide (MHD) (96). As MHD is the main compound active in the blood, pharmacokinetic data on oxcarbazepine are based on data for MHD. MHD is highly lipophilic and readily crosses the blood–brain barrier. Approximately 38% of MHD is protein bound in plasma, and its volume of distribution is approximately 0.3 to 0.8 L/kg (97–99). The half-life of MHD in plasma is approximately 8 to 10 hours. More than 95% of MHD is excreted by the kidneys. Oxcarbazepine also shows considerable placental transfer.

Effects of Renal Disease

Few studies are currently available on the effect of renal disease on oxcarbazepine levels. However, because the active, dominant metabolite is excreted by the kidneys, renal disease significantly impacts the half-life and blood levels of oxcarbazepine, and dose reductions as well as increased dosing intervals are recommended to prevent dose-dependent toxicity (100).

Effects of Liver Disease

There are no studies on the effect of liver disease on oxcarbazepine.

Clinical Recommendations

Patients with renal disease or those receiving dialysis will not eliminate oxcarbazepine as quickly as normal individuals, as noted above. Patients with liver failure may tolerate oxcarbazepine, and it may be used cautiously in this group of patients, even though no clinical studies are available at this time to guide usage. Because approximately 40% of the MHD metabolite of oxcarbazepine is protein bound, the effect of renal and liver disease on protein plasma binding may result in increased free levels of MHD.

Topiramate

Topiramate, a sulfamate-substituted monosaccharide [2,3:4, 5-bis-O-(1-methylethylidine)-β-D-fructopyranose], is structurally distinct from other anticonvulsant drugs. It is approximately 15% protein bound and not extensively metabolized. Only 20% of a single dose is metabolized by healthy adults; up to 50% of multiple doses is metabolized by patients taking other anticonvulsants. No clinically active metabolites have been identified. The drug is eliminated renally, and about 50% to 80% appears unchanged in the urine (4).

Effects of Renal and Liver Disease

As topiramate is excreted primarily via the kidneys, impaired creatinine clearance may delay elimination. In preclinical studies, topiramate was associated with a 1.5% risk of calcium renal stone formation, but this rate was not greater than that seen in placebo-treated patients (101). No increased incidence of adverse effects has been noted in patients with pre-existing renal or hepatic disease.

Clinical Recommendations

Nearly 100,000 patients have been treated with topiramate, and no significant liver abnormalities have occurred, indicating that it is unlikely that the risk of hepatotoxicity is significantly increased over that in the general population.

Renal disease is not a contraindication to the use of topiramate, although doses should be decreased and dosing intervals lengthened in patients with impaired renal function. Topiramate should be used with caution in patients with a history of probable kidney stones.

Zonisamide

Zonisamide (1,2-venzisoxazole-3-methanesulfonamide) is a new anticonvulsant that is not readily soluble in water at neutral pH but becomes more soluble as the pH increases to greater than 8. The majority of pharmacokinetic data on zonisamide has been obtained in animals, although some human data are available. In both animal and human studies, zonisamide was rapidly and essentially completely distributed throughout the body, including the brain. The metabolism of zonisamide is extensive, and it is excreted primarily in the urine. Protein binding is 50% to 60% in human sera (102–104) and is not significantly affected by usual therapeutic levels of phenytoin or phenobarbital (103). The major route of metabolism is direct acetyl or glucuronyl conjugation.

Effects of Liver and Renal Disease

There are no data on the effect of renal or liver disease on the metabolism of zonisamide. Because zonisamide is primarily excreted via the kidneys and metabolized extensively by the liver, both renal and liver disease may alter the pharmacokinetics of this drug. Further research is needed to establish the effects of zonisamide in renal and hepatic disease.

Clinical Recommendations

Because zonisamide's metabolic profile is similar to that of topiramate, it is expected that dosage adjustments similar to those required for topiramate would also be required for zonisamide when it is used in patients with liver or renal disease.

Tiagabine

Tiagabine [(−)-(R)-1-[4,4-bis(3-methyl-2-thienyl)-3-butenyl]-3-piperidinecarboxylic acid hydrochloride] increases the amount of GABA available in the extracellular space, presumably by preventing GABA uptake into presynaptic neurons. The pharmacokinetics of tiagabine had been studied in healthy individuals and patients with epilepsy, but few studies have been performed on patients with liver or renal disease. Tiagabine is rapidly absorbed and reaches maximal plasma concentrations in less than 2 hours after oral dosing (105,106). The mean elimination half-life ranges from 4 to 9 hours, and little of the drug accumulates in the plasma during multiple dosing (105,106). Hepatic metabolism is extensive, and only approximately 1% of the drug is excreted unchanged in the urine. Tiagabine does not appear to induce or inhibit hepatic microsomal enzyme systems and does not change the clearance of antipyrine, even after 14 days of administration (107,108). Initial studies suggest that tiagabine is greater than 95% protein bound.

Effects of Liver and Renal Disease

A study of 13 patients with mild or moderate impairment of hepatic function found that they had higher and more prolonged plasma concentrations of both total and unbound tiagabine after administration of tiagabine for 5 days. Hepatically impaired patients also had more neurologic side effects. Therefore, tiagabine should be used cautiously in epilepsy patients with hepatic impairment. Reduced dosages and/or longer dosing intervals may be needed, and patients should be observed closely for neurologic side effects (109). A study of 25 subjects with various degrees of renal function (ranging from normal to requiring hemodialysis) demonstrated that the pharmacokinetics of tiagabine were similar in all subjects, suggesting that dosage adjustment may be unnecessary for epilepsy patients with renal impairment (110).

Vigabatrin

Vigabatrin (γ-vinyl-GABA: ($\perp$)-4-amino-hex-5-enoic acid) is a racemate with only the S($+$) enantiomer possessing clinical efficacy. It is an irreversible inhibitor of GABA transaminase, is not protein bound, and does not induce liver enzymes. Elimination occurs principally through urinary excretion, with biotransformation accounting for less than 20% (111). Approximately 50% of the S($+$) enantiomer and 65% of the R($-$) enantiomer are excreted in the urine, and the clearance of both correlates well with creatinine clearance.

Effects of Renal Disease

Because vigabatrin is excreted renally, impaired creatinine clearance may delay elimination. Hemodialysis is expected to remove a high proportion of vigabatrin. Bachmann and coworkers reported that 60% of vigabatrin was removed from the blood pool during hemodialysis (112).

Effects of Liver Disease

Vigabatrin has not been systematically studied in patients with liver disease. Reports of use in patients with hepatic cirrhosis document reductions in plasma alanine aminotransferase (ALT) activity to normal levels after initiation of vigabatrin (113). Use of vigabatrin in patients with porphyria failed to demonstrate a desferoxamine-dependent increase in messenger RNA for 5-aminolevulinate (ALA) synthetase, the rate-limiting enzyme in porphyrin synthesis (114).

Clinical Recommendations

As plasma concentrations are likely to be elevated in patients with renal disease, a decrease in dose or increase in dosing interval may be necessary. To maintain serum concentrations and stable clinical efficacy, single doses administered only every 3 days were necessary in one case (112). As vigabatrin may reduce levels of ALT in patients with pre-existing liver disease, this liver function test may not be a useful index of liver cell damage in some cases.

Levetiracetam

Levetiracetam (S-α-ethyl-2-oxo-1-pyrolidine acetamide) is a racemically pure pyrrolidine derivative. It has rapid and nearly complete absorption, unaffected by food, with peak plasma levels reached within 1 hour of administration and steady-state plasma levels reached within 2 days of initiation. Protein binding is less than 10%, and volume of distribution is 0.7 L/kg. Levetiracetam is excreted primarily via the kidneys, with 66% of the drug appearing unchanged in the urine and the remainder metabolized to an inactive compound formed by hydrolysis of the acetamide group. Levetiracetam's half-life is 7.2 ± 1.1 hours in young, healthy subjects (115).

Effects of Renal Disease

As the major route of excretion of levetiracetam is renal, impaired creatinine clearance will delay elimination and result in accumulation of the drug. The half-life is typically 6 to 8 hours in patients under 16, but increases to 10.2 to 10.4 hours in subjects over 65, presumably because of impaired creatinine clearance (116). When the disposition of levetiracetam was studied in patients with impaired renal function, total body clearance of levetiracetam was reduced in patients with impaired renal function, as follows: 40% in the mild group (Cl_{Cr} = 50 to 80 mL/min), 50% in the moderate group (Cl_{Cr} = 30 to 50 mL/min), and 60% in the severe renal impairment group (Cl_{Cr} <30 mL/min). In anuric patients, the total body clearance decreased 70% compared with that of normal subjects. Approximately 50% of the pool of levetiracetam in the body is removed during a standard 4-hour hemodialysis procedure (see UCB Pharma package insert for Keppra levetiracetam).

Effects of Liver Disease

The lack of significant hepatic metabolism implies that primary liver disease will not impact metabolism of levetiracetam. Study of potential effects in 11 different drug-metabolizing enzymes using human liver microsomes failed to identify any pharmacokinetic interactions, even in doses exceeding expected therapeutic levels (117).

Clinical Recommendations

As with any newly approved medication, little information exists for use in patients with liver and renal disease. Such medications should be used with caution in patients with preexisting disease, and patients should be observed closely for signs of developing toxicity as clinical experience with the drug increases. Decreased doses or increased dosing intervals should be used in patients with impaired creatinine clearance. The package insert recommends the following: $Cl_{Cr} > 80$: 500 to 1500 mg every 12 hours; $Cl_{Cr} =$ 50 to 80: 500 to 1000 mg every 12 hours; $Cl_{Cr} = 30$ to 50: 250 to 750 mg every 12 hours; $Cl_{Cr} < 30$: 250 to 500 mg every 12 hours; end-stage renal disease patients using dialysis: 500 to 1000 mg every 24 hours with a 250- to 500-mg supplemental dose following dialysis.

MEDICATIONS IN LIVER AND RENAL TRANSPLANTATION

Use of AEDs in patients who are being evaluated for renal or liver transplantation is similar to that previously described for patients with renal or liver disease. Care should be taken to avoid further diminishing organ function while a patient waits for availability of a donor organ. However, this interval prior to transplantation may be the optimal time to reevaluate the diagnosis of epilepsy by video electroencephalographic monitoring or to consider revising AED therapy to reduce the likelihood of interactions with immunosuppressants and antibiotics following transplantation.

Liver transplantation is considered in patients with irreversible and progressive liver dysfunction for which no alternative therapy is available. It is rarely performed in patients older than age 70 years or in patients with coexistent active alcohol or drug abuse. Epilepsy is not a specific contraindication. Allograft donors are matched for ABO blood compatibility and liver size and should test negative for the human immunodeficiency virus (HIV) and hepatitis B and C. Immunosuppression is usually accomplished by combinations of tacrolimus or cyclosporine, steroids, azathioprine, or OKT3 (ornithine-ketoacid transaminase, monoclonal antithymocyte globulin). Other immunosuppressants are under investigation. Posttransplantation complications include liver dysfunction from primary nonfunction, acute or chronic rejection, ischemia, hepatic artery thrombosis, and biliary obstruction or leak. Bacterial, viral, fungal, and other opportunistic infections may occur, as well as renal and psychiatric disorders (118).

Renal transplantation is the treatment of choice for most patients with end-stage renal disease. Graft survival is best in living-related transplants, intermediate in living-unrelated transplants, and least in cadaveric transplants. Renal transplantation is contraindicated in patients with active glomerulonephritis, infection, malignancy, HIV, or hepatitis B, and in those with severe comorbid disease. Relative contraindications include age older than 70 years, severe psychiatric disease, moderate comorbidity, and some primary renal diseases (multiple myeloma, amyloidosis, oxalosis). Again, epilepsy is not a specific contraindication. Immunosuppression usually consists of a two- or three-drug regimen, with each drug targeted at a different stage in the immune response. Cyclosporine and prednisone

are frequently used together for the first few years after successful grafting. Azathioprine or mycophenolate mofetil is commonly used as the third drug. Tacrolimus is used less commonly than in liver transplantation, but it is used in patients with subacute or chronic rejection. Other immunosuppressive agents are under investigation. Infection is the most common complication of renal transplantation, and ganciclovir or cytomegalovirus (CMV)-immune globulin may be used prophylactically. Risk of fungal and *Pneumocystis carinii* infection increases substantially as prednisone is tapered (119).

In addition to the obvious concerns about using AEDs associated with liver or renal toxicities to treat patients with donated organs, the primary management concerns of the epileptologist are (a) AED interactions with immunosuppressants; (b) AED interactions with prophylactic antibiotics; and (c) the appropriate diagnostic and therapeutic approach to new-onset seizures following transplantation.

Antiepileptic Drug Use with Immunosuppressants

It is well documented in the literature that cyclosporine may result in neurotoxic effects, including seizures. Such effects are more frequently seen with high cyclosporine levels, but levels may be within the usual therapeutic range. Dose reduction or withdrawal of cyclosporine usually results in improvement of clinical symptoms (120). Results of animal studies suggest that cyclosporine lowers seizure threshold by inhibiting GABAergic neural activity and binding properties of the GABA receptor (121). Neoral, a newer formulation of cyclosporine, appears to reduce the potential for seizures in liver transplant recipients (122). All formulations of cyclosporine are highly protein bound, with potential for increased blood levels of unbound AEDs. Enzyme-inducing AEDs may lead to increased elimination of cyclosporine because of induction of hepatic microsomal enzymes. This interaction may precipitate or exacerbate graft-versus-host disease and lead to rejection. For this reason, AEDs with low protein binding and minimal metabolism should be considered first in patients taking cyclosporine.

Tacrolimus (FK506) has been less frequently associated with seizures than has cyclosporine (123). After reversing neurologic findings by discontinuation of cyclosporine, substitution with tacrolimus did not result in neurotoxicity (124). Like cyclosporine, however, tacrolimus is highly protein bound and is metabolized by the cytochrome P450 enzymes, with similar potential AED interactions.

Prednisone and other corticosteroids may be used before transplantation as well as chronically in combination with other immunosuppressants following transplantation. The action of corticosteroids may be blunted by enzyme-inducing AEDs, resulting in increased clearance from the circulation and prompting a need for higher steroid doses. Azathioprine is rarely associated with increased risk for seizures and has minimal potential for interaction with AEDs.

Seizures and Infections After Transplantation

Liver and renal transplant recipients are at significantly increased risk for central nervous system and systemic infections or neoplasms, both of which can significantly lower the threshold for seizures. In transplantation patients with new-onset seizures, a diligent search for localized neurologic infection or neoplasia must be conducted, especially if seizures have focal symptoms. A minimal diagnostic evaluation of such patients should include magnetic resonance imaging using fluid attenuated inversion recovery (FLAIR) sequences, usually precontrast and postcontrast, as well as carefully performed electroencephalography with appropriately selected activation procedures.

A review of interactions of AEDs with all possible antibiotic agents is beyond the scope of this chapter. However, it should be mentioned that many antibiotics, especially the beta-lactam agents, lower the threshold for seizures and that consideration of this potential is important in selecting antibiotics to treat transplant recipients, who already have a lowered threshold for seizures in comparison with that of the general population. Among the most commonly used posttransplantation prophylactic antibiotics are the antivirals, especially ganciclovir. This agent has minimal protein binding and metabolism, with clearance rate directly related to kidney function. Additive toxicity may be seen (e.g., generalized seizures in patients receiving ganciclovir with imipenem-cilastin, neutropenia in patients receiving ganciclovir with carbamazepine) and should be a consideration when selecting AEDs. Prophylactic fluconazole is sometimes used after transplantation, resulting in decreased risk for fungal colonization but higher serum cyclosporine levels and thus more potential neurotoxicity (125).

REFERENCES

1. Kuhara T, Inoue Y, Matsumoto M, et al. Altered metabolic profiles of valproic acid in a patient with Reye's syndrome. *Clin Chim Acta* 1985;145:135–142.
2. Kunin CM. A guide to use of antibiotics in patients with renal disease. *Ann Intern Med* 1967;67:151–158.
3. Adler DS, Martin E, Gambertoglio JG, et al. Hemodialysis of phenytoin in a uremic patient. *Clin Pharmacol Ther* 1975;18:65–69.
4. Dettli L, Spring P, Ryter S. Multiple dose kinetics and drug dosage in patients with kidney disease. *Acta Pharmacol Toxicol (Copenh)* 1971;29(Suppl 3):211–224.
5. Letteri JM, Mellk H, Louis S, et al. Diphenylhydantoin metabolism in uremia. *N Engl J Med* 1971;285:648–652.
6. Odar-Cederlof I, Borga O. Kinetics of diphenylhydantoin in uremia patients: consequences of decreased plasma protein binding. *Eur J Clin Pharmacol* 1974;7:31.
7. Loub WD, Wattenberg LW, Davis DW. Aryl hydrocarbon hydroxylase induction in rat tissues by naturally occurring indoles of cruciferous plants. *J Natl Cancer Inst* 1975;54:985.
8. Affrime MB, Lowenthal DT. Analgesics, sedatives, and sedative-hypnotics. In: Anderson RJ, Schrier RW, eds. *Clinical use of drugs in patients with kidney and liver disease.* Philadelphia: WB Saunders, 1981;199–210.
9. Gillette JR. Factors affecting drug metabolism. *Ann N Y Acad Sci* 1971;179:43.
10. Bennhold H. Die Vekikelfunction der Bluteiweisskorper. In: Bennhold H, Kylin E, Rusznyak S, eds. *Die Eiweisskorper des Blutplasmas.* Leipzig, Germany: Steinkopf, 1938:220–303.
11. Sjoholm I, Kober A, Odar-Cederlof I, et al. Protein binding of drugs in uremia and normal serum: the role of endogenous binding inhibitors. *Biochem Pharmacol* 1976;25:1205.
12. Shoeman DW, Azarnoff DL. The alterations of plasma proteins in uremia as reflected in their ability to bind digitoxin and diphenylhydantoin. *Pharmacology* 1972;7:169.
13. Reidenberg MM. The biotransformation of drugs in renal failure. *Am J Med* 1977;62:482.
14. Kutt H, Winters W, Scherman R, et al. Diphenylhydantoin and phenobarbital toxicity. The role of liver disease. *Arch Neurol* 1964;11:649–656.
15. Maher JF. Principles of dialysis and dialysis of drugs. *Am J Med* 1977;62:475.
16. Dromgoole SH. The effect of hemodialysis on the binding capacity of albumin. *Clin Chim Acta* 1973;46:469.
17. Dromgoole SH. The binding capacity of albumin and renal disease. *J Pharmacol Exp Ther* 1974;191:318–323.
18. Blaschke TF, Meffin PJ, Melmon KL, et al. Influence of acute viral hepatitis on phenytoin kinetics and protein binding. *Clin Pharmacol Ther* 1975;17:685–691.
19. Blaschke TF. Protein binding and kinetics of drugs in liver diseases. *Clin Pharmacokinet* 1977;2:32–44.
20. Breimer DD, Zilly W, Richter E. Pharmacokinetics of hexobarbital in acute hepatitis and after apparent recovery. *Clin Pharmacol Ther* 1975;18:433–440.
21. Klotz U, Avant GR, Hoyumpa A, et al. The effects of age and liver disease on the disposition and elimination of diazepam in adult man. *J Clin Invest* 1975;55:347–359.
22. Mawer GE, Miller NE, Turnberg LA. Metabolism of amylobarbitone in patients with chronic liver disease. *Br J Pharmacol* 1972;44:549–560.
23. Wilkinson GR, Shand DG. A physiological approach to hepatic drug clearance. *Clin Pharmacol Ther* 1975;18:377–390.
24. Rowland M, Blaschke TF, Meffin PJ, et al. Pharmacokinetics in disease states modifying hepatic and metabolic function. In: Benet LZ, ed. *Effect of disease states on drug pharmacokinetics.* Washington, DC: American Pharmaceutical Association; 1976:53–74.
25. Affrime M, Reidenberg MM. The protein binding of some drugs in plasma from patients with alcoholic liver disease. *Eur J Clin Pharmacol* 1975;8:267–269.
26. Rowland M, Benet LZ, Graham GG. Clearance concepts in pharmacokinetics. *J Pharmacokinet Biopharm* 1973;1:123–136.
27. Albert K, Hallmark M, Sakmar E, et al. Plasma concentrations of diphenylhydantoin, its parahydroxylated metabolite, and corresponding glucuronide in man. *Res Commun Chem Pathol Pharmacol* 1974;9:463–469.
28. Hooper WD, Bochner F, Endre MJ, et al. Plasma protein binding of diphenylhydantoin: effects of sex hormones, renal and hepatic disease. *Clin Pharmacol Ther* 1974;15:276–282.
29. Rane A, Lunde PKM, Jalling B, et al. Plasma protein binding of diphenylhydantoin in normal and hyperbilirubinemic infants. *J Pediatr* 1971;78:877–882.
30. Greenblatt DJ, KochWeser J. Clinical toxicity of chlordiazepoxide and diazepam in relation to serum albumin concentration: a report from the Boston Collaborative Drug Surveillance Program. *Eur J Clin Pharmacol* 1974;7:259–262.
31. Brodie BB, Mark LC, Papper EM, et al. The fate of thiopental in man and a method for its estimation in biological material. *J Pharmacol Exp Ther* 1950;98:85–96.
32. Garrett ER, Bres J, Schnelle K, et al. Pharmacokinetics of saturably metabolized amobarbital. *J Pharmacokinet Biopharmacol* 1974;2:43–103.
33. Waddell WJ, Butler TC. The distribution of phenobarbital. *J Clin Invest* 1957;36:1217–1226.
34. Branch RA, James J, Read EA. A study of factors influencing drug disposition in chronic liver disease, using the model drug (+)propranolol. *Br J Clin Pharmacol* 1976;3:243–249.
35. Lewis JP, Jusko WJ. Pharmacokinetics of ampicillin in cirrhosis. *Clin Pharmacol Ther* 1975;18:475–484.

36. Wilkinson GR, Schenker S. Drug disposition and liver disease. *Drug Metab Rev* 1975;4:139–175.
37. Booker HE, Darcey B. Serum concentrations of free diphenylhydantoin and their relationship to clinical intoxication. *Epilepsia* 1973;14:177–184.
38. Reidenberg MM, Drayer DE. Effects of renal disease upon drug disposition. *Drug Metab Rev* 1978;8:293–302.
39. Butler TC. The metabolic conversion of 5,5-diphenylhydantoin to 5-(p-hydroxyphenyl)-5-phenylhydantoin. *J Pharmacol Exp Ther* 1957;119:111.
40. Gilman AG, Goodman LS, Rall TW, et al., eds. *Goodman & Gilman's the pharmacological basis of therapeutics*, 7th ed. Elmsford, NY: Pergamon, 1985:446–472.
41. Leber HW, Schutterle G. Oxidative drug metabolism in liver microsomes from uremic rats. *Kidney Int* 1972;2:152.
42. Odar-Cederlof I, Lunde P, Sjoqvist F. Abnormal pharmacokinetics of phenytoin in a patient with uraemia. *Lancet* 1970;2:831.
43. Reidenberg MM. *Renal function and drug action.* Philadelphia: WB Saunders, 1971.
44. Olsen GD, Bennett WM, Porter GA. Morphine and phenytoin binding to plasma proteins in renal and hepatic failure. *Clin Pharmacol Ther* 1975;17:677–684.
45. Reidenberg MM, Affrime M. Influence of disease on binding of drugs to plasma proteins. *Ann N Y Acad Sci* 1973;226:115–126.
46. Ehrnebo M, Odar-Cederlof I. Binding of amobarbital, pentobarbital and diphenylhydantoin to blood cells and plasma proteins in healthy volunteers and uraemic patients. *Eur J Clin Pharmacol* 1975;8:445–453.
47. Van Peer AP, Belpaire FM, Rosseel MT, et al. Distribution of antipyrine, phenylbutazone and phenytoin in experimental renal failure. *Pharmacology* 1981;22:139–145.
48. Van Peer AP, Belpaire FM, Bogaert MG. Pharmacokinetics of drugs in rabbits with experimental acute renal failure. *Pharmacology* 1978;17:307–314.
49. Van Peer AP, Belpaire FM, Bogaert MG. In vitro hepatic oxidative metabolism of antipyrine, phenytoin and phenylbutazone in rabbits with experimental renal failure. *Arch Int Pharmacodyn Ther* 1978;234:346–347.
50. Van Peer AP, Belpaire FM, Bogaert MG. *In vitro* hepatic oxidative metabolism of antipyrine, phenytoin and phenylbutazone in uraemic rabbits. *J Pharm Pharmacol* 1980;32:135–136.
51. Borga O, Hoppel C, Odar-Cederlof I, et al. Plasma levels and renal excretion of phenytoin and its metabolites in patients with renal failure. *Clin Pharmacol Ther* 1979;26:306–314.
52. Borondy P, Chang T, Glazko AJ. Inhibition of diphenylhydantoin (DPH) hydroxylation by 5-(p-hydroxyphenyl)-5-phenylhydantoin (pHPPH) [abstract]. *Fed Proc* 1972;31:582.
53. Perucca E, Makki K, Richens A. Is phenytoin metabolism dose dependent by enzyme saturation or by feedback inhibition? *Clin Pharmacol Ther* 1978;22:46–51.
54. Steele WH, Lawrence JR, Elliott HL, et al. Alterations of phenytoin protein binding with *in vivo* haemodialysis in dialysis encephalopathy. *Eur J Clin Pharmacol* 1979;15:69–71.
55. Martin E, Gambertoglio JG, Adler DS, et al. Removal of phenytoin by hemodialysis in uremic patients. *JAMA* 1977;238:1750–1753.
56. Nandedkar A, Williamson R, Kutt H, et al. A comparison of plasma phenytoin level determinations by EMIT and gas-liquid chromatography in patients with renal insufficiency. *Ther Drug Monit* 1980;2:427–430.
57. Burgess ED, Friel PN, Blair AD, et al. Serum phenytoin concentrations in uremia. *Ann Intern Med* 1981;94:59–60.
58. Lunde PKM, Rane A, Yaffe SJ, et al. Plasma protein binding of diphenylhydantoin in man: interaction with other drugs and the effect of temperature and plasma dilution. *Clin Pharmacol Ther* 1970;11:846–855.
59. Richens A. Clinical pharmacokinetics of phenytoin. *Clin Pharmacokinet* 1979;4:153–169.
60. Breen KJ, Shaw J, Alvin J, et al. Effect of experimental hepatic injury on the clearance of phenobarbital and paraldehyde. *Gastroenterology* 1973;64:992–1004.
61. Alvin J, McHorse T, Hoyumpa A, et al. The effect of liver disease in man on the disposition of phenobarbital. *J Pharmacol Exp Ther* 1975;192:224–235.
62. Gambertoglio JG, Lauer RM. Use of neuropsychiatric drugs. In: Anderson RJ, Schrier RW, eds. *Clinical use of drugs in patients with kidney and liver disease.* Philadelphia: WB Saunders,1981:276–295.
63. Heipertz R, Guthoff A, Bernhardt W. Primidone metabolism in renal insufficiency and acute intoxication. *J Neurol* 1979;221:101–104.
64. Stern EL. Possible phenylethylmalondiamide (PEMA) intoxication. *Ann Neurol* 1977:2:356–357.
65. Gugler R, von Unruh GE. Clinical pharmacokinetics of valproic acid. *Clin Pharmacokinet* 1980;5:67–83.
66. Brewster D, Muir NC. Valproate plasma protein binding in the uremic condition. *Clin Pharmacol Ther* 1980;27:76–82.
67. Bruni J, Wang LH, Marbury TC, et al. Protein binding of valproic acid in uremic patients. *Neurology* 1980;30:557–559.
68. Gugler R, Mueller G. Plasma protein binding of valproic acid in healthy subjects and in patients with renal disease. *Br J Clin Pharmacol* 1978;5:441–446.
69. Dickinson RG, Kluck RM, Hooper WD, et al. Rearrangement of valproate glucuronide in a patient with drug associated hepatobiliary and renal dysfunction. *Epilepsia* 1985;26:589–593.
70. Klotz U, Rapp T, Mueller WA. Disposition of valproic acid in patients with liver disease. *Eur J Clin Pharmacol* 1978;13:55–60.
71. Kochen W, Schneider A, Ritz A. Abnormal metabolism of valproic acid in fatal hepatic failure. *Eur J Pediatr* 1983;141:30–35.
72. Bohles H, Richter K, Wagner-Thiessen E, et al. Decreased serum carnitine in valproate induced Reye's syndrome. *Eur J Pediatr* 1982;139:185–186.
73. Lenn NJ, Ellis WG, Washburner RB. Fatal hepatocerebral syndrome in siblings discordant for exposure to valproate. *Epilepsia* 1990;31:578–583.
74. Zafrani BS, Berthelot P. Sodium valproate in the induction of unusual hepatoxicity. *Hepatology* 1982;2:648–649.
75. Dreifuss FE, Langer WH, Moline KA, et al. Valproic acid and hepatic fatalities, II. US experience since 1984. *Neurology* 1989;39:201–207.
76. Zaret BS, Beckner RR, Marini AM, et al. Sodium valproate induced hyperammonemia without clinical hepatic dysfunction. *Neurology* 1982;32:206–208.
77. Faigle JW, Brechbuhler S, Feldman KF, et al. The biotransformation of carbamazepine. In: Birkmayer W, ed. *Epileptic seizures—behavior and pain.* Vienna: Hans Huber, 1975:127–140.
78. Hooper WD, Dubetz DK, Bochner F, et al. Plasma protein binding of carbamazepine. *Clin Pharmacol Ther* 1975;17:433–440.
79. Kangas L, Kanto J, Forsstrom J, et al. The protein binding of diazepam and N-desmethyldiazepam in patients with poor renal function. *Clin Nephrol* 1976;5:114–118.
80. Kober A, Sjoholm I, Borga O, Odar-Cederlof I. Protein binding of diazepam and digitoxin in uremic and normal serum. *Biochem Pharmacol* 1979;28:1037–1042.
81. Garella S, Lorch JA. Use of dialysis and hemoperfusion in drug overdose—an overview. In: Anderson RJ, Schrier RW, eds. *Clinical use of drugs in patients with kidney and liver disease.* Philadelphia: WB Saunders, 1981:269–309.
82. Andreasen PB, Hendel J, Greisen G, Hvidberg EF. Pharmacokinetics of diazepam in disordered liver function. *Eur J Clin Pharmacol* 1976;10:115–120.
83. Sellers EM, Greenblatt DJ, Giles HG, et al. Chlordiazepoxide and oxazepam disposition in cirrhosis. *Clin Pharmacol Ther* 1979;26:240–246.
84. Wilkinson GR. The effects of liver disease and aging on the disposition of diazepam, chlordiazepoxide, oxazepam and lorazepam in man. *Acta Psychiatr Scand* 1978;(Suppl 274):56–74.
85. Shull HJ, Wilkinson GR, Johnson R, et al. Normal disposition of oxazepam in acute viral hepatitis and cirrhosis. *Ann Intern Med* 1976;84:420–425.
86. Patwardhan RV, Schenker S. Drug use in patients with liver disease. An overview. In: Anderson RJ, Schrier RW, eds. *Clinical use of drugs in patients with kidney and liver disease.* Philadelphia: WB Saunders, 1981:166–181.
87. Asconape JJ, Penry JK. Use of antiepileptic drugs in the presence of liver and kidney disease: a review. *Epilepsia* 1982;23(Suppl 1):565–579.
88. Yau MK, Adams MA, Wargin WA, et al. A single-dose and steady-state pharmacokinetic study of lamotrigine in healthy

male volunteers. Presented at the Third International Cleveland Clinic–Bethel Epilepsy Symposium; June 16–20, 1992; Cleveland, Ohio.

89. Fillastre JP, Taburet AM, Fialaire A, et al. Pharmacokinetics of lamotrigine in patients with renal impairment: influence of hemodialysis. *Drugs Exp Clin Res* 1993;19:25–32.

90. Posner J, Cohen AF, Land G, et al. The pharmacokinetics of lamotrigine (BW 430C) in healthy subjects with unconjugated hyperbilirubinemia (Gilbert's syndrome). *Br J Clin Pharmacol* 1989;28:117–120.

91. Palmer KJ, McTavisk D. Felbamate. A review of its pharmacodynamic and pharmacokinetic properties, and therapeutic efficacy in epilepsy. *Drugs* 1993;45:1041–1065.

92. Brodie MJ, Pellock JM. Taming the brain storms: felbamate updated. *Lancet* 1995;346:918–919.

93. Pellock JM. Felbamate in epilepsy therapy: evaluating the risks. *Drug Saf* 1999;21:225–239.

94. Data on file. Ann Arbor, MI: Parke-Davis, 1995.

95. Halstenson CE, Keane WF, Tuerck D, et al. Disposition of gabapentin (GAB) in hemodialysis (HD) patients [abstract]. *J Clin Pharmacol* 1992;32:751.

96. Schutz H, Feldmann KF, Faigle JW, et al. The metabolism of 14C-oxcarbazepine in man. *Xenobiotica* 1986;16:769–778.

97. Feldmann KF, Brechbuhler S, Faigle JW, et al. Pharmacokinetics and metabolism of GP47779, the main human metabolite of oxcarbazepine (GP47680) in animals and healthy volunteers. In: Dam M, Gram L, Penry JK, eds. *Advances in epileptology. XIIth Epilepsy International Symposium.* New York: Raven Press, 1981: 89–96.

98. Kristensen O, Klitgaard NA, Jonsson B, et al. Pharmacokinetics of 10-*OH*-carbazepine, the main metabolite of the antiepileptic oxcarbazepine, from serum and saliva concentrations. *Acta Neurol Scand* 1983;68:145–150.

99. Theisohn M, Heimann G. Disposition of the antiepileptic oxcarbazepine and its metabolites in healthy volunteers. *Eur J Clin Pharmacol* 1982;22:545–551.

100. Rouan MC, Lecaillon JB, Godbillon J, et al. The effect of renal impairment on the pharmacokinetics of oxcarbazepine and its metabolites. *Eur J Clin Pharmacol* 1994;47:161–167.

101. Data on file. Philadelphia: Ortho-McNeil, 1995.

102. Kimura M, Tanaka N, Kimura Y, et al. Pharmacokinetic interaction of zonisamide in rats: effect of other antiepileptics on zonisamide. *J Pharmacobiodyn* 1992;15:631–639.

103. Matsumoto K, Miyazaki H, Fujii T, et al. Absorption, distribution and excretion of 3-(sulfamoyl[14C]methyl)-1,2-benzisoxazole (AD-810) in rats, dogs and monkeys and of AD-810 in men. *Arzneimittelforschung* 1983;33:961–968.

104. Nishiguchi K, Ohniski N, Iwakawa S, et al. Pharmacokinetics of zonisamide: saturable distribution into human and rat erythrocytes and into rat brain. *J Pharmacobiodyn* 1992;15:409–415.

105. Gustavson LE, Mengel HB. Pharmacokinetics of tiagabine, a gamma-aminobutyric acid-uptake inhibitor, in healthy subjects after single and multiple doses. *Epilepsia* 1995;36:605–611.

106. Gustavson LE, Mengel HB, Pierce MW, et al. Tiagabine, a new gamma-aminobutyric acid uptake inhibitor antiepileptic drug: pharmacokinetics after single oral doses in man. *Epilepsia* 1990;31:642.

107. Mengel HB. Tiagabine. *Epilepsia* 1994;35(Suppl 5):S81–S84.

108. Mengel HB, Pierce M, Mant T, et al. Tiagabine, a GABA-uptake inhibitor: safety and tolerance of multiple dosing in normal subjects. *Acta Neurol Scand* 1990;82(Suppl 133):35.

109. Lau AH, Gustavson LE, Sperelakis R, et al. Pharmacokinetics and safety of tiagabine in subjects with various degrees of hepatic function. *Epilepsia* 1997;38:445–451.

110. Cato A, Gustavson LE, Qian J, et al. Effect of renal impairment on the pharmacokinetics and tolerability of tiagabine. *Epilepsia* 1998;39:43–47.

111. Richens A. Pharmacology and clinical pharmacology of vigabatrin. *J Child Neurol* 1991;6:(Suppl 2):S7–S10.

112. Bachmann D, Ritz R, Wad N, et al. Vigabatrin dosing during haemodialysis. *Seizure* 1996;5:239–242.

113. Williams A, Sekaninova S, Coakly J. Suppression of elevated alanine aminotransferase activity in liver diseases by vigabatrin. *J Pediatr Child Health* 1998;34:395–397.

114. Hahn M, Gildemeister OS, Krauss GL, et al. Effects of new anticonvulsant medications on porphyrin synthesis in cultured liver cells: potential implications for patients with acute porphyria. *Neurology* 1997;49:97–106.

115. Patsalos PN. Pharmacokinetic profile of levetiracetam: toward ideal characteristics. *Pharmacol Ther* 2000;85:77–85.

116. Bialer M, Johannessen SI, Kupferberg, et al. Progress report on new antiepileptic drugs: a summary of the fourth Eilat conference (EILAT IV). *Epilepsy Res* 1999;34:1–41.

117. Nicolas JM, Collart P, Gerin B, et al. In vitro evaluation of potential drug interactions with levetiracetam, a new antiepileptic agent. *Drug Metab Dispos* 1999;27:250–254.

118. Dienstag J. Liver transplantation. In: Fauci AS, Braunwald E, Isselbacher K, et al., eds. *Harrison's principles of internal medicine*, 14th ed. New York: McGraw-Hill, 1998:1721–1725.

119. Carpenter CB, Lazarus JM. Dialysis and transplantation in the treatment of renal failure. In: Fauci AS, Braunwald E, Isselbacher K, et al., eds. *Harrison's principles of internal medicine*, 14th ed. New York: McGraw-Hill, 1988:1520–1529.

120. Gitjenbeck JM, van den Bent MJ, Vecht CJ. Cyclosporine neurotoxicity review. *J Neurol* 1999;246:339–346.

121. Shuto H, Kataoka Y, Fujisaki K, et al. Inhibition of GABA system involved in cyclosporine-induced convulsions. *Life Sci* 1999;65: 879–887.

122. Wijdicks EF, Dahlke LJ, Wiesner RH. Oral cyclosporine decreases severity of neurotoxicity in liver transplant recipients. *Neurology* 1999;12:1708–1710.

123. Neu AM, Furth SL, Case BW, et al. Evaluation of neurotoxicity in pediatric renal transplant recipients treated with tacrolimus (FK506). *Clin Transplant* 1997;11(Pt 1):412–414.

124. Wijdicks EF, Wiesner RH, Krom RA. Neurotoxicity in liver transplant recipients with cyclosporine immunosuppression. *Neurology* 1995;45:1962–1964.

125. Winston DJ, Pakrasi A, Busuttil RW. Prophylactic fluconazole in liver transplant recipients: a randomized, double blind, placebo-controlled trial. *Ann Intern Med* 1999;131:729–737.

126. Patsalos PN. Pharmacokinetic profile of levetiracetam: toward ideal characteristics. *Pharmacol Ther* 2000;85:77–85.

127. Evans WE, Schentag JJ, Jusko JW, eds. *Applied pharmacokinetics*, 3rd ed. Spokane, WA: Applied Therapeutics, 1986:542–544.

Monitoring for Adverse Effects of Antiepileptic Drugs

51

L. James Willmore   Andrew Pickens IV   John M. Pellock

Treatment of patients with epilepsy aims for complete seizure control without intolerable drug side effects (1,2). Independent of blood drug levels, toxic effects allow titration to efficacy. However, allergic reactions, metabolically or genetically determined drug-induced illnesses, and idiosyncratic effects of drugs, while rare, may be life-threatening.

Monitoring is an attempt to detect serious systemic toxic reactions of antiepileptic drugs (AEDs) in time to intervene and protect patients. The process begins with the disclosure to patients and family members of all information required for an informed decision delivered within the framework of risks and benefits. Regularly scheduled accumulation of hematologic data, routine serum chemistry values, and results of urinalysis creates an archive (3). A rational basis for this approach was thought to reside in the *Physicians' Desk Reference* (PDR) (4) and the Canadian *Compendium of Pharmaceuticals and Specialties* (5). Although these sources appear to define the standard of practice for many clinicians, they actually preserve observations about specific and well-defined groups of patients under close scrutiny during drug trials. Contrary to some clinical practices and these publications, evidence-based scientific criteria fail to support routine monitoring, and the resulting archival data rarely predict serious drug reactions. For example, two prospective studies (6,7) investigated the efficacy of routine blood and urine testing in patients receiving long-term AED treatment. One study (6) of 199 children evaluated liver, blood, and renal function at initiation of therapy and at 1, 3, and 6 months. Screening studies repeated every 6 months disclosed no serious clinical reactions from phenobarbital, phenytoin, carbamazepine, or valproate. Abnormal but clinically insignificant results prompted retesting in 12 children

(6%), and therapy was discontinued unnecessarily in 2 children. The authors concluded that routine monitoring provided no useful information and sometimes prompted unwarranted action. A second study (7) of 662 adults treated with carbamazepine, phenytoin, phenobarbital, or primidone failed to detect significant laboratory abnormalities during 6 months of monitoring and led to the conclusion that routine screening was neither cost-effective nor valuable for asymptomatic patients. Treatment of 480 patients with either carbamazepine or valproic acid in a double-blind, controlled trial also demonstrated the lack of usefulness of routine laboratory monitoring (8).

Although habits vary in the United States and elsewhere, it is good medical practice to measure biochemical function and structural circulating elements in blood at baseline before starting treatment with a new drug (9).

Efficacy and adverse effects of drugs are the foundation for treatment decisions by physicians; however, some adverse events have led to legal actions that also have affected treatment, monitoring, and the need to document patient care. Publication of such cases occurs in several circumstances. In general, a case heard in state court will be published in the official reporters for that state only if an appellate court has produced a decision marked for publication. The same is true for some trial-level decisions made by federal courts. Publication occurs when the issues determined are deemed important or significant. For example, classic cases involving AEDs have centered on medical negligence in dosage, selection of treatment, and questions about informed consent.

The approval process for drugs used in the United States is codified in the federal Food, Drug, and Cosmetic Act of

1938, as amended in 21 USC §301 et seq (2001) and the 1962 Kefauver-Harris amendment to the Food, Drug, and Cosmetic Act; both were updated with the Food, Drug, and Cosmetic Modernization Act of 1997. The Food and Drug Administration (FDA) does not regulate drug use by physicians, who may use any licensed drug to treat patients. An attempt to restrain physicians in that respect failed (*United States v Evers*, 453 F Supp 1141 [ND Ala 1978]).

U.S. standards of care are derived from expert opinion, source publications, or referred articles that underlie evidence-based medicine. Other sources are textbooks and published practice guidelines, such as those from the American Academy of Neurology and the Office of Quality Assurance and Medical Review of the American Medical Association.

In medical malpractice or negligence cases, determining the standard of care for a particular treatment is of utmost importance. The standard-of-care concept extends also to the methods used to obtain informed consent and at trial is usually established by testimony from experts citing source documents or articles from referred publications. One such reference source is the PDR (10) (Table 51.1).

As with any area of law over which a state has authority, the process for determining the standard of care can differ from state to state, particularly as regards the evidentiary force of the medication package insert and information in the PDR. States tend to use these materials in one of three ways. Although the differences among these approaches are not absolute, the categorization has educational and discussion value. In the first group are states that consider the PDR and package insert as establishing the standard of care (*Haught v Maceluch*, 681 F2d 291, *reh'ing denied*, 685 F2d 1385 [5th Cir 1985]) (10). In the second group, the package insert and PDR are considered evidence of standard of care and may establish a *prima facie* case for negligence if a physician does not follow the prescribed directions (10). Generally, however, a physician may present evidence for using a medication outside the description in the PDR and package insert (*Mulder* rule and echo of *Mulder*; see below) (Thompson v Carter, 518 So2d 609, 613 [Miss 1987]). *Mulder v Parke-Davis*, 181 NW2d 882 (Minn 1970), required a physician to explain the reason for deviating from the use of a drug as specified in the PDR. Such an explanation is best included in the patient's chart. In the third group of states, the PDR and package insert are given little credence and in some jurisdictions are inadmissible without supporting expert testimony. This is known as the echo of the *Mulder* rule (*Spensieri v Lasky*, 723 NE2d 544 [NY 1999]) (10).

These discrepancies in the handling of medical malpractice issues illustrate why it is critical to know local, regional, and national standards of practice and the idiosyncrasies of applicable law in a jurisdiction, as well as why a physician must diligently document the rationale for action in a patient's medical record.

Issues of informed consent have also required adjudication. In *Serigne v Ivker* (808 So2d 783 [La App 4th Cir 2002]), the plaintiff alleged that informed consent had not

TABLE 51.1

LEGAL ACTION REGARDING ADVERSE EFFECTS OF ANTIEPILEPTIC DRUGS

Year	Case	Drug	Issue	Outcome
2002	*Serigne v Ivker*, 808 So2d 783 (La App 4th Cir)	Dilantin (phenytoin)	Informed consent—teratogenicity	Malformation cause not connected; informed consent, established
2002	*Spano v Bertocci*	Depakote (valproic acid)	Informed consent	Patient had prior knowledge of pregnancy and effect of valproate; informed consent established
1988	*Guevara v Dorsey Laboratories*	Bellergal-S (phenobarbital)	Failure to warn physicians	Community knowledge and PDR adequate warning
1987	*Shinn v St. James Mercy Hospital*	Phenytoin	Informed consent; Stevens-Johnson syndrome	Required to disclose only common adverse effects
1984	*Menefee v Guerhing*	Phenobarbital	Informed consent; Stevens-Johnson syndrome	General warning adequate
1983	*Harbeson v Parke-Davis*	Phenytoin	Informed consent; teratogenicity	Patient not warned; malformed children—award for plaintiff
1967	*Fritz v Parke-Davis*	Phenytoin	Informed consent; hepatotoxicity	Documented serious illness and skilled care—in favor of physician
1987	*Hendricks v Charity Hospital of New Orleans*	Phenytoin	Malpractice: dose error	Found for plaintiff
1998	*Martin v Life Care Centers of America*	Phenytoin	Malpractice; failure to act on elevated plasma levels—patient death	Found for plaintiff
1992	*Pester v Graduate Hospital*	Valproate	Malpractice; failure to diagnose pancreatitis	Found for plaintiff

been obtained because teratogenicity had not been disclosed. The court found (a) that the plaintiff had failed to establish a connection between malformations and phenytoin and (b) that informed consent did exist. In *Spano v Bertocci*, a plaintiff claimed lack of informed consent based on nondisclosure of the teratogenic effects of valproic acid. At the trial and appellate court levels, informed consent was deemed to have been obtained because of the plaintiff's previous knowledge of the danger of valproate use during pregnancy.

The landmark decision of *Harbeson v Parke-Davis* (656 P.2d 483 [1983]) illustrates the diligence required in providing information for patients with childbearing potential. A woman who delivered children with fetal hydantoin syndrome claimed failure of informed consent causing wrongful birth and wrongful life. The court stated that a physician had a duty to "exercise reasonable care in disclosing 'grave risks' of (any) treatment" advocated. The physician had failed to search the literature, which would have uncovered the dangers of using phenytoin during pregnancy and would have allowed the physician to inform the patient of the risks.

Serious skin reactions, including Stevens-Johnson syndrome, have also raised issues of informed consent. *Shinn v St. James Mercy Hospital* (675 F Supp 94 [WDNY 1987]) centered on the claim that serious skin reactions to phenytoin had not been disclosed. The court decided that all adverse effects need not be disclosed to a patient, only the most common. In addition, given the patient's medical circumstance, treatment would not reasonably have been declined even if adverse effects had been delineated. Similarly, another court found that warnings in the PDR and package insert diminished the "danger-in-fact" of the medication: " . . . no reasonable trier of fact could conclude that this . . . medicine is unreasonably dangerous per se" (*Williams v Ciba-Geigy*, 686 F Supp 573 [WD La 1988]).

Documentation can be critical. A patient treated with phenytoin suffered hepatotoxic reactions, and the court originally found for the plaintiff. That decision was overturned on appeal, the appellate court stating, "Viewing the record . . . the skill and care exhibited by defendant's physicians' diagnosis and treatment were marked by devoted diligence and attention and were wholly consistent with the professional skill . . . employed by other physicians in treating and controlling . . . the complex disease of epilepsy" (*Fritz v Parke-Davis*, 152 NW2d 129 [1967]).

Errors in the use of AEDs that amount to negligence have resulted in legal action. When a patient who was to take Dilantin 500 mg per day received a prescription for 500 mg three times a day, judgment was for the plaintiff (*Hendricks v Charity Hospital of New Orleans* [La App 1987]). In *Martin v Life Care Centers of America* (No. 95-4124-B, 117th Judicial Dist Ct, Nueces County, TX, April 1998]), high plasma levels of Dilantin were associated with a patient's death, resulting in judgment for the plaintiff. One court found for the plaintiff in a case of failure to diagnose pancreatitis from the use of valproate (*Pester v Graduate Hospital*, No. 87-05-00357, Court of Common Pleas, Philadelphia, PA, Oct 1992).

Serious idiosyncratic drug reactions do not depend on dose and by their nature are unpredictable (11–13). All organs are affected, the skin most commonly (Table 51.2). Established AEDs, used in millions of patients, are known to cause agranulocytosis, aplastic anemia, blistering skin rash, hepatic necrosis, allergic dermatitis, serum sickness, and pancreatitis. Newly available drugs, used in many fewer patients, have caused allergic dermatitis and serious skin reactions (Table 51.2). With the exception of reactions to felbamate, other serious reactions have yet to be reported with any alarming frequency.

AT-RISK PROFILES

One way to minimize the risk of serious adverse effects is to identify high-risk patients by constructing clinical profiles

TABLE 51.2
IDIOSYNCRATIC REACTIONS TO ANTIEPILEPTIC DRUGS

Reaction	CBZ	ETH	FBM	GBP	LEV	LTG	PB	PHT	TPM	TGB	OXC	ZNS	VPA
Agranulocytosis	X	X	X				X	X					X
Stevens-Johnson syndrome	X	X				X	X	X					X
Aplastic anemia	X	X	X					X					X
Hepatic failure	X	X					X	X					X
Allergic dermatitis	X	X	X	X		X	X	X	X	X	X	X	X
Serum sickness	X	X					X	X					X
Pancreatitis	X												
Nephrolithiasis									X			X	

Abbreviations: CBZ, carbamazepine; ETH, ethosuximide; FBM, felbamate; GBP, gabapentin; LEV, levetiracetam; LTG, lamotrigine; PB, phenobarbital; PHT, phenytoin; TPM, topiramate.

from reports of idiopathic drug reactions (11). For example, the risk of hepatotoxic reactions from valproic acid is too nonspecific to be of much practical help; however, at-risk patients are younger than 2 years of age, being treated with several AEDs, and have known metabolic disease with developmental delay (14–16). Patients fitting this profile need detailed laboratory screening for the presence of metabolic disorders, including measurement of serum lactate, serum pyruvate, serum carnitine, and urinary organic acid levels, as well as routine hematologic and chemical tests (9). Prothrombin time, partial thromboplastin time, and determination of arterial blood gas and ammonia levels are also useful tests.

After a drug is selected, the physician must review its relative benefits and risks, documenting this discussion in the patient's record. This process forms the basis for informal informed consent. Patients should be told the criteria for success and reminded of the trial and error of drug selection and the methods for changing drugs. Because dose-related side effects aid management but interfere with treatment, negotiation defines this process. The patient must know the nature of side effects, what must be tolerated, and how side effects will influence titration. Serious, life-threatening, idiosyncratic effects must be explained clearly, but within the context of rarity. Although the patient must be ready to report symptoms, the physician must identify patients who lack advocates or who have impaired ability to communicate. Unlike most patients with epilepsy, these individuals may require a monitoring strategy. A screening program may be useful in some high-risk patients (Table 51.3).

CLINICAL MONITORING

Although routine monitoring of hepatic function revealed elevated values in 5% to 15% of patients treated with carbamazepine, fewer than 20 with significant hepatic complications were reported in the United States from 1978 to 1989 (17). Cases of pancreatitis were even rarer. Transient leukopenia occurs in up to 12% of adults and children treated with carbamazepine (18,19), and aplastic anemia or agranulocytosis, unrelated to benign leukopenia, occurs in 2 per 575,000, with an annual mortality rate of approximately 1 in 575,000 patients (17). Only 4 of 65 cases of agranulocytosis or aplastic anemia occurred in children.

Hematologic abnormalities in patients developing exfoliative dermatitis, alone or as part of systemic hypersensitivity, were not found until clinical symptoms appeared. Neither benign leukopenia nor transient elevations in hepatic enzyme predicted life-threatening reactions. A genetic abnormality in arene oxide metabolism may occur in patients at high risk for some types of adverse responses such as hepatitis (20), but a screening test for such defects is not available. Routine monitoring does not allow anticipation of life-threatening effects of carbamazepine; data for phenytoin and phenobarbital are similar (1).

Women of childbearing potential must be warned about contraceptive failure; impact on reproductive health, such as development of polycystic ovaries; and the possible effect of maternal drug treatment on a developing fetus (21). Use of AEDs that induce cytochrome P450 enzymes by women taking oral contraceptives increases the risk that contraception will fail (22–25). Gynecologists must be informed of the AED being used and of the need that the contraceptive contain at least 50 μg of estrogen (21).

Some AEDs are thought to have direct reproductive consequences for women. Whether temporal lobe epilepsy or a specific drug causes polycystic ovary syndrome has generated discussion (see ref. 26 for an up-to-date review). Either anovulatory cycles with serologic evidence or physical changes of androgen excess can define this syndrome; documentation of polycystic ovaries is not required for diagnosis. Although polycystic ovaries and hyperandrogenism are associated with valproate (27,28), high percentages of ovarian changes have been reported in women with localization-related epilepsy (29).

Pregnancy increases the number of seizures in approximately 35% of patients (30). Although changes in drug metabolism, drug absorption, or induction of metabolism may be operative, medication compliance is a major concern (31).

Women treated with AEDs have an increased risk of delivering infants with major malformations. Established drugs are associated with cleft lip and palate and serious cardiac defects (32–36). Reports from the North American Antiepileptic Drug Pregnancy Registry (35) identify phenobarbital as posing the greatest risk (a 12% rate of malformation) followed by valproate (an 8.8% rate of malformation). Carbamazepine has a 0.5% to 1.0% incidence of neural tube defects, including anencephaly and spina bifida (37). The total number of drugs used to treat a mother with epilepsy is also important. When all malformations were considered, incidence was 20.6% with one drug and 28% with two or more drugs (35). Administration of folate to women treated with AEDs is recommended in that low folate levels have been observed in women delivering malformed infants (37).

TABLE 51.3	
ASSESSMENT FOR HIGH-RISK PATIENTS TREATED WITH VALPROATE	
At risk	Younger than 2 years of age
	Treated with multiple drugs
	Known metabolic disease
	Delayed development
Specific screening studies	Serum lactate and pyruvate
	Plasma carnitine
	Urinary metabolic screen with organic acids
	Ammonia and arterial blood gases

TABLE 51.4
RECOMMENDATIONS FOR MONITORING

1. Obtain screening laboratory studies before initiation of antiepileptic drug treatment. Baseline studies provide a benchmark and could identify patients with special risk factors that could influence drug selection.
2. Blood and urine monitoring in otherwise healthy and asymptomatic patients is unnecessary.
3. Identify high-risk patients before treatment.
   a. Presumptive biochemical disorders
   b. Altered systemic health
   c. Neurodegenerative disease
   d. History of significant adverse drug reactions
   e. Patients without an advocate
      i. Those unable to communicate require a different strategy
      ii. Patients with multiple handicaps who are institutionalized
4. For newly introduced drugs, follow recommended guidelines for blood monitoring until the numbers of patients treated in this country increase and data become available.

Adapted from: Willmore LJ. Clinical risk patterns: Summary and recommendations. In: Levy RH, Penry JK, eds. Idiosyncratic reactions to valproate: Clinical risk patterns and mechanisms of toxicity. New York: Raven Press, 1991:163–165.

As new drugs become available, physicians have an obligation to review source documents for those medications and devise a strategy of treatment and for monitoring. Because data tend to be limited, a new drug should be initiated cautiously, and patients should be given as much information as possible. Although industry-produced materials may be useful, a better alternative is for physicians to provide copies of package inserts coupled with their own material describing how the drug is to be used

TABLE 51.5
SCREENING LABORATORY TESTS TO DETECT ADVERSE DRUG REACTIONS TO ANTIEPILEPTIC DRUGS

Antiepileptic Drug	Laboratory Tests
Phenytoin	CBC, liver enzymes
Phenobarbital	CBC, liver enzymes
Carbamazepine	CBC, liver enzyme
Valproate	CBC, liver enzymes, hepatic panel, serum amylase and lipase (pancreatitis), ammonia, plasma, and urine carnitine assay
Oxcarbazepine	Serum sodium
Topiramate	Urine for microscopic hematuria and renal ultrasound (renal stones), intraocular pressure (glaucoma)
Zonisamide	Urine for microscopic hematuria and renal ultrasound (renal stones)
Felbamate	CBC, reticulocyte count, liver enzymes, hepatic panel
Ethosuximide	CBC, reticulocyte count

Abbreviation: CBC, complete blood count with platelet count.

and any monitoring strategy planned. Parsimony may be the guiding principle in monitoring when established drugs are being used, but such is not necessarily the case with a newly introduced drug (Table 51.4). Baseline data should be obtained, the patient must be prepared to get in touch with the physician, and the physician must facilitate that communication. Chemical and hematologic monitoring may be recommended in the materials developed by the manufacturer in concert with the FDA. It may be wise to follow those guidelines until broader clinical experience is available. Table 51.5 summarizes screening laboratory tests that may aid in detection of adverse effects of AEDs.

SPECIFIC DRUGS

Carbamazepine

When carbamazepine is catalyzed by the hepatic monooxygenases, an epoxide is formed at the 10,11-double bond of the azepine ring (CBZ-10,11-epoxide) (38); this compound is associated with toxic symptoms (39). Hydration of the epoxide occurs through microsomal epoxide hydrolase. Inhibition of that enzyme, as with concomitant administration of valproic acid, increases the quantity of the epoxide (40). Both carbamazepine and the epoxide have anticonvulsant effects (41,42).

Severe reactions to carbamazepine can cause hematopoietic, skin, hepatic, and cardiovascular changes (18). Rash occurs in 5% to 8% of patients, and in rare cases, may progress to exfoliative dermatitis or to a bullous reaction, such as Stevens-Johnson syndrome (43). Transient leukopenia is observed in 10% to 12% of patients; however, fatal reactions, such as aplastic anemia are rare, with an annual death rate of 1.1 in 500,000 patients (44). Patients and parents must be reassured that frequent monitoring of blood counts and liver values is unnecessary (9).

Presymptomatic blood test abnormalities have not been reported in patients who develop systemic hypersensitivity reactions to carbamazepine. Genetic susceptibility as a result of a deficiency in arene oxide metabolism may be associated with hepatic injury, but pretreatment screening remains unavailable for routine patient care (20).

Ethosuximide

Ethosuximide causes nausea, gastric distress, and abdominal pain unless given with meals. Rash, severe headaches, and, on rare occasions, leukopenia, pancytopenia, and aplastic anemia have occurred (1). Neurologic effects include lethargy, agitation, aggressiveness, depression, and memory problems. Psychiatric disorders were attributed to the drug's normalization of the electroencephalographic record, but such reactions also have been described with other AEDs (45,46). Drug-induced lupus has been reported in children (47).

Felbamate

Felbamate, a dicarbamate compound related to meprobamate, involves vigorous drug interactions that may cause clinically significant toxic reactions or exacerbate seizures (48–50). Serious idiosyncratic reactions to felbamate, including aplastic anemia, occur at an incidence of approximately 1 in 4000 to 8000 persons treated (11,51–54). The death rate from aplastic anemia is more than 20 times that associated with carbamazepine (11,52,53). Some factors related to aplastic anemia during felbamate treatment are an immunologic disorder, such as lupus erythematosus, found in 33% of affected patients (11,52,53); cytopenia, found in 42% of affected patients; and an allergic or toxic reaction to another AED, found in 52% of affected patients (11,52,53).

A review of aplastic anemia cases in the United States suggested an incidence of 27 to 209 per 1 million in association with felbamate, compared with 2 to 2.5 per 1 million persons in the general population (55). Mean time to presentation was 154 days, although a few cases were reported after 6 months of treatment.

Clinical risk profiles for felbamate suggest the need for a screening strategy. Although some features such as white race, female sex, and adult status are not specific, a previous AED allergic reaction, cytopenia, an immune disorder, especially lupus erythematosus, and less than 1 year of treatment are more worrisome. Tests to measure the excretion of atopaldehyde and the ratio of monocarbamate metabolites may have screening value. Before felbamate is prescribed, manufacturer recommendations should be reviewed (56).

Hepatotoxic effects of felbamate seem less clearly associated with risk factors. The estimated incidence for all patients was 1 per 18,500 to 25,000, similar to that with valproic acid. Of the 18 patients reported in the literature, only 7 had suffered hepatic injury from felbamate; numbers are too small to construct a risk profile (11,56–58).

Guidelines now emphasize that felbamate should be used for severe epilepsy refractory to other therapy. Treatment should be preceded by a careful history to uncover indications of hematologic, hepatotoxic, and autoimmune diseases. Women with autoimmune disease account for the largest proportion of those who developed aplastic anemia. Routine hematologic and liver function tests should be performed at baseline, and patients and their families must be fully informed of the potential risks; in the United States written consent is recommended. The frequency of clinical monitoring and a specific schedule of blood tests should follow the manufacturer's recommendations, and patients should be educated about symptoms that may signify either hematologic change or hepatotoxicity.

Gabapentin

Gabapentin, 1-(aminomethyl)cyclohexane acetic acid, is structurally related to γ-aminobutyric acid (GABA). Adverse events were typically neurotoxic, but withdrawal from studies was infrequent. Use in mentally retarded children was accompanied by an increased incidence of hyperactivity and aggressive behavior (59).

Lamotrigine

Central nervous system side effects included lethargy, fatigue, and mental confusion (60–65). Serious rash appears to be correlated with the rate of dose increase (66) and may be more common in children. Current U.S. guidelines require discontinuation if a rash develops.

Morbilliform erythematous rash, urticaria, or a maculopapular pattern are most common (51,67–71); however, erythema multiforme and blistering reactions like Stevens-Johnson syndrome or toxic epidermal necrolysis can occur. Simple rashes require careful assessment to rule out a hypersensitivity syndrome. Such sensitivity reactions often include fever, lymphadenopathy, elevated liver enzyme values, and altered numbers of circulating cellular elements of blood (69).

In U.S. drug trials, rash affected approximately 10% of patients; 3.8% had to discontinue the drug, and 0.3% were hospitalized (69). Most serious rashes developed within 6 weeks of the start of treatment. In drug trials involving children, rash occurred in 12.9% and was serious in 1.1%, with half of that group having Stevens-Johnson syndrome (69). More than 80% of patients who experienced a serious rash were being treated with valproate or had been given higher-than-recommended doses (69). Rash was suspected to be a drug interaction with valproate, which inhibits the metabolism of lamotrigine, causing diminished clearance and resultant high blood levels (70). When treatment guidelines are followed, the incidence of serious rash may be reduced (69,71,72). In the United States, discontinuation is advised if rash develops. Table 51.6 lists the suggested plan for initiation of lamotrigine treatment.

Oxcarbazepine

Oxcarbazepine is a keto analogue of carbamazepine that is rapidly converted to a 10-monohydroxy active metabolite by cytosol arylketone reductase. Renal clearance of the metabolite correlates with measured creatinine clearance. Dizziness, sedation, and fatigue, possibly dose related, were reported in pivotal trials (73–77). Hyponatremia also has occurred (78,79). Oxcarbazepine was associated with malformations in a small cohort of a study that failed to identify phenytoin as causing malformations (37). Cross-reactivity in patients allergic to carbamazepine has been reported.

Phenobarbital

Idiosyncratic reactions to phenobarbital include allergic dermatitis, Stevens-Johnson syndrome, serum sickness, and hepatic failure. Agranulocytosis and aplastic anemia also have been reported (1,80). Folate deficiency in patients

TABLE 51.6

GUIDELINES FOR USE OF LAMOTRIGINE

	Weeks 1 and 2	Weeks 3 and 4	To Achieve Maintenance
Information for patients and parents about rash			
For adult patients receiving inducing drugs such as phenytoin, carbamazepine, or barbiturates (but not valproate)	50 mg each day	100 mg each day (in divided doses)	Add 50–100 mg every 1–2 weeks to 200–400 mg each day
For patients treated with valproic acid	25 mg every other day	25 mg each day	Add 25–50 mg every 1–2 weeks to 100–200 mg each day

Adapted from Willmore LJ. General principles. Safety monitoring of antiepileptic drugs. In: Levy RH, Mattson RH, Meldrum BS, et al., eds. *Antiepileptic drugs.* Philadelphia: Lippincott Williams & Wilkins, 2002:112–118.

treated with AEDs is claimed to be associated with behavioral changes (81). Phenobarbital is known to exacerbate acute intermittent porphyria (82).

Long-term treatment may cause connective tissue changes, with coarsened facial features, Dupuytren contracture, Ledderhose syndrome (plantar fibromas), and frozen shoulder (83). Sedative effects may exacerbate absence, atonic, and myoclonic seizures, although other mechanisms may be operant (84). Sudden withholding of doses of short-acting barbiturates may precipitate drug-withdrawal seizures or even status epilepticus. Phenobarbital's slow rate of clearance makes such acute seizures less of a problem, but dose tapering is recommended if discontinuation is planned. Some patients may experience mild withdrawal symptoms of tremor, sweating, restlessness, irritability, weight loss, disturbed sleep, and even psychiatric manifestations. Infants of mothers treated with phenobarbital may have irritability, hypotonia, and vomiting for several days after delivery (85).

Phenytoin

Phenytoin is a weak organic acid, poorly soluble in water, and available as free acid and a sodium salt. Because of the drug's saturation kinetics, small changes in the maintenance dose produce large changes in total serum concentration (86); thus, the half-life increases with higher plasma concentrations. Doses must be changed carefully. The steady state of phenytoin is altered by interaction with other drugs (87).

Dose-related effects of phenytoin include nystagmus, ataxia, altered coordination, cognitive changes, and dyskinesia (80). Facial features may coarsen, and body hair may change texture and darken. Acne may develop and gingival hypertrophy is common. Osteoporosis and lymphadenopathy occur with long-term use (88). Folate deficiency may be severe enough to cause megaloblastic anemia; a transient encephalopathy is said to occur by a similar mechanism (81). Prolonged exposure to high levels of plasma phenytoin has been linked to cerebellar atrophy (89,90).

Allergic dermatitis, hepatotoxicity (91), serum sickness, and aplastic anemia may be fatal (80,88). Drug-induced lupus erythematosus reactions have been observed (92).

Topiramate

Topiramate has a monosaccharide-type structure. The drug appears to influence sodium and a portion of chloride channels, blocks non–N-methyl-D-aspartate glutamate receptors, and inhibits carbonic anhydrase.

Nephrolithiasis and dose-related weight loss require discussion with patients. Many side effects in studies were caused by forced titration to high doses. Adverse cognitive effects occur at high doses in adults (93); however, slowing the pace of dose increases reduces the impact on cognitive function (94–98). Serious rashes have occurred. Reports of acute secondary angle-closure glaucoma mandate cautioning patients to report ocular pain or altered visual acuity immediately (99–101). Children should be monitored for oligohydrosis with hyperthermia, especially in hot weather (102).

Tiagabine

Tiagabine, a derivative of nipecotic acid, enhances GABA-mediated inhibition by reducing cellular uptake of GABA through an effect on transporter proteins (103,104). Although renal disease does not appear to affect tiagabine excretion (105), altered hepatic function prolongs clearance. In the pivotal trials, somnolence, asthenia, and headache occurred during dose titration. Confusion, somnolence, ataxia, and dizziness prompted withdrawal from the trials (106).

Valproate

Children younger than age 2 years who are being treated with several AEDs are at the highest risk for hepatotoxic reactions from treatment with valproate. Additional risk factors are presumed metabolic disorders or severe epilepsy complicating mental retardation and organic brain disease (14,15,107,108). Most clinicians, however, consider this pattern of incidence too restrictive or insufficiently detailed to allow identification of patients at highest risk (109). Moreover, routine laboratory monitoring does not predict fulminant and irreversible hepatic failure (110). Some patients who progressed to fatal hepatotoxic reactions never exhibited abnormalities on specific hepatic function tests. Conversely, abnormal levels of serum ammonia, carnitine, and fibrinogen, as well as hepatic function anomalies have been reported without clinically significant hepatotoxic reactions (111,112). Therefore, reporting of clinical symptoms and identification of highest-risk patients are more reliable means of monitoring. Vomiting was the most frequent initial symptom in fatal cases (14,15). Combined nausea, vomiting, and anorexia occurred in 82% of patients, whereas lethargy, drowsiness, and coma were reported in 40% (113,114). Although early drug discontinuation may reverse hepatotoxic reactions in some patients, fatalities still result (115). No biochemical markers differentiate survivors and those who die (115). Patients with hepatic failure have been rescued by administration of carnitine (116). Measurement of urinary organic acid and a metabolic evaluation are recommended in high-risk patients or in any patient without an established reason for mental retardation and seizures (109).

Dreifuss and colleagues described high-risk patients (14,15). Most fatalities occurred in the first 6 months of treatment, but some were noted up to 2 years after initiation. Children younger than age 2 years receiving polytherapy had a 1 in 500 to 800 chance of a fatal hepatotoxic event. Patients at negligible risk were those older than age 10 years who were treated with valproate alone and who were free of underlying metabolic or neurologic disorders. Intermediate-risk factors were use of monotherapy between ages 2 and 10 years and need for polytherapy at any age.

Most cases of fatal liver failure involved mental retardation, encephalopathy, and decline of neurologic function. Two of four reported patients older than age 21 years had degenerative disease of the nervous system. Nine of 16 hepatic fatalities in one report (117), and all members of the 11- to 20-year-old age group in another series were neurologically abnormal. Only 7 of 26 adults with fatal hepatic failure were considered neurologically normal (118).

Specific biochemical disorders associated with valproate-induced hepatotoxic events include urea cycle defects, organic acidurias, multiple carboxylase deficiency, mitochondrial or respiratory chain dysfunction, cytochrome aa_3 deficiency in muscle, pyruvate carboxylase deficiency, and hepatic pyruvate dehydrogenase complex deficiency (brain) (109,119,120). Clinical disorders include GM_1 gangliosidosis type 2, spinocerebellar degeneration, Friedreich ataxia, Lafora body disease, Alpers disease, and mitochondrial encephalomyelopathy with ragged red fibers (MERRF) (113).

Tremor with sustension and at rest is dose related (121). Weight gain affects from 20% to 54% of patients (122) who report appetite stimulation. Excessive weight change may require drug discontinuation. Hair loss is transient. Hair appears to be fragile, and regrowth results in a curlier shaft (123). Supplementation with zinc-containing multivitamins may be protective. Thrombocytopenia appears to be dose related. Platelet counts vary without dose changes, and are asymptomatic. Petechial hemorrhage and ecchymoses necessitate decreases in dose or even discontinuation (124,125).

Sedation and encephalopathy are less frequently encountered (126,127). Acute encephalopathy and even coma may develop on initial exposure to valproic acid (126); these patients may be severely acidotic and have elevated excretion of urinary organic acids. Because valproic acid is known to sequester coenzyme A (128), such patients are suspected of having a partially compensated defect in mitochondrial β-oxidation enzymes (127,129). Dermatologic abnormalities, although unusual, may be severe (130).

Acute hemorrhagic pancreatitis may be fatal in younger patients. Abdominal pain should lead to measurement of lipase and amylase levels (131).

Hyperammonemia may occur in the absence of hepatic dysfunction (132,133), possibly caused by inhibition of either nitrogen elimination or urea synthesis (134,135). In rare instances, an insufficiency of urea cycle enzymes such as ornithine transcarbamylase deficiency may be present (136).

Vigabatrin

Vigabatrin, also known as γ-vinyl GABA, increases tissue concentrations of GABA by irreversible inhibition of GABA-transaminase, the enzyme that degrades GABA. Vigabatrin is not approved for use in the United States, but patients may obtain it from other countries (137,138).

Severe changes in behavior with agitation, hallucinations, and altered thinking are thought to be dose related (46). Depression is a potential problem in all patients (139). Loss of peripheral retinal function is of concern (140–142). In one report (141), up to 40% of 32 adults treated with vigabatrin had concentrically constricted visual fields. These visual effects appear not to reverse after the drug is discontinued (143).

Zonisamide

Zonisamide is a sulfonamide that may cross-react in patients known to be allergic to sulfa-containing compounds (144,145). Serious skin reactions, drowsiness, and altered thinking have occurred. Patients with a history of renal stones should be informed of the risk of nephrolithiasis and advised to remain adequately hydrated. Children should be monitored for hyperthermia with oligohydrosis, especially during hot weather (146).

LEGAL AND MEDICAL DISCLAIMER

This brief review constitutes an introduction to a topic and has been prepared and provided for educational and informational purposes only; it is not intended to convey, nor should it be considered to convey, legal or medical advice. Legal and/or medical advice requires expert consultation and an in-depth knowledge of your specific situation. Although every effort has been made to provide accurate information herein, laws and precedent are always changing and will vary from state to state and jurisdiction to jurisdiction. As such, the material provided herein is not comprehensive for all legal and medical developments and may contain errors or omissions. For information regarding your particular circumstances, you should contact an attorney to confirm the current laws and how they may apply to your particular situation without delay, in that any delay may result in loss of some or all of your rights. It is hoped that this review helps you understand the need for thorough knowledge and careful documentation.

REFERENCES

1. Schmidt D. *Adverse effects of antiepileptic drugs.* New York: Raven Press, 1982.
2. Pellock JM. Efficacy and adverse effects of antiepileptic drugs. *Pediatr Clin North Am* 1989;36:435–438.
3. DeVries SI. Haematological aspects during treatment with anticonvulsant drugs. *Epilepsia* 1965;7:1–15.
4. *Physicians' desk reference,* 57th ed. Oradell, NJ: Medical Economics, 2003.
5. Krogh CME. *Compendium of pharmaceuticals and specialities.* Ottawa, Canada: Canadian Pharmaceutical Association, 1990.
6. Camfield C, Camfield P, Smith E, et al. Asymptomatic children with epilepsy: little benefit from screening for anticonvulsant-induced liver, blood or renal damage. *Neurology* 1986;36: 838–841.
7. Mattson RH, Cramer JA, Collins JF, et al. Comparison of carbamazepine, phenobarbital, phenytoin, and primidone in partial and secondarily generalized tonic-clonic seizures. *N Engl J Med* 1985;313:145–151.
8. Mattson RH, Cramer JA, Collins JF, Department of Veterans Affairs Epilepsy Cooperative Study No. 264 Group. A comparison of valproate with carbamazepine for the treatment of complex partial seizures and secondarily generalized tonic-clonic seizures in adults. *N Engl J Med* 1992;327:765–771.
9. Pellock JM, Willmore LJ. A rational guide to routine blood monitoring in patients receiving antiepileptic drugs. *Neurology* 1991; 41:961–964.
10. Bradford GE, Elben CC. The drug package insert and the PDR as establishing the standard of care in prescription drug liability cases. *J Mo Bar* 2001;57:233–242.
11. Glauser TA. Idiosyncratic reactions: new methods of identifying high-risk patients. *Epilepsia* 2000;41:S16–S29.
12. Park BK, Pirmohamed M, Kitteringham NR. Idiosyncratic drug reactions: a mechanistic evaluation of risk factors. *Br J Clin Pharmacol* 1992;34:377–395.
13. Pirmohamed M, Kitteringham NR, Park BK. The role of active metabolites in drug toxicity. *Drug Saf* 1994;11:114–144.
14. Dreifuss FE, Santilli N, Langer DH, et al. Valproic acid hepatic fatalities: a retrospective review. *Neurology* 1987;37:379–385.
15. Dreifuss FE, Langer DH, Moline KA, et al. Valproic acid hepatic fatalities, II: U.S. experience since 1984. *Neurology* 1989;39: 201–207.
16. Bryant AE, Dreifuss FE. Valproic acid hepatic fatalities, III: U.S. experience since 1986. *Neurology* 1996;46:465–469.
17. Seetharam MN, Pellock JM. Risk-benefit assessment of carbamazepine in children. *Drug Saf* 1991;6:148–158.
18. Pellock JM. Carbamazepine side effects in children and adults. *Epilepsia.* 1987;28:S64–S70.
19. Hart RG, Easton JD. Carbamazepine and hematological monitoring. *Ann Neurol* 1982;11:309–312.
20. Spielberg SP, Gordon GB, Blake DA, et al. Predisposition to phenytoin hepatotoxicity assessed in vitro. *N Engl J Med* 1981; 305:722–727.
21. Zahn CA, Morrell MJ, Collins SD, et al. Management issues for women with epilepsy: a review of the literature. American Academy of Neurology Practice Guidelines. *Neurology* 1998; 51:949–956.
22. Janz D, Schmidt D. Anti-epileptic drugs and failure of oral contraceptives. *Lancet* 1974;1:1113.
23. Schmidt D. Effect of antiepileptic drugs on estrogens and progesterone metabolism and oral contraceptives. In: Dam M, Gram L, Penry JK, eds. *Advances in epileptology: XIIth Epilepsy International Symposium.* New York: Raven Press, 1981:423–431.
24. Mattson RH, Cramer JA, Darney PD, et al. Use of oral contraceptives by women with epilepsy. *JAMA* 1986;256:238–240.
25. Coulam CB, Annegers JF. Do anticonvulsants reduce the efficacy of oral contraceptives? *Epilepsia* 1979;20:519–526.
26. Morrell MJ. Reproductive and metabolic disorders in women with epilepsy. *Epilepsia* 2003;44:11–20.
27. Isojarvi JIT, Laatikainen TJ, Pakarinen AJ. Polycystic ovaries and hyperandrogenism in women taking valproate for epilepsy. *N Engl J Med* 1993;329:1383–1388.
28. Murialdo G, Galimberti CA, Gianelli MV, et al. Effects of valproate, phenobarbital and carbamazepine on sex steroid setup in women with epilepsy. *Clin Neuropharmacol* 1998;21:52–58.
29. Morrell MJ, Giudice L, Flynn KL, et al. Predictors of ovulatory failure in women with epilepsy. *Ann Neurology* 2002;52:704–711.
30. Hauser WA, Hesdorffer DC. *Epilepsy: frequency, causes and consequences.* New York: Demos, 1990.
31. Yerby MS. Problems and management of the pregnant woman with epilepsy. *Epilepsia* 1987;28(Suppl 3):S29–S36.
32. Koch S, Loesche G, Jager-Roman E. Major birth malformations and antiepileptic drugs. *Neurology* 1992;42:83–88.
33. Annegers JF, Hauser WA, Elveback LR. Congenital malformations and seizure disorders in the offspring of parents with epilepsy. *Int J Epidemiol* 1978;7:241–247.
34. Friis ML. Facial clefts and congenital heart defects in children of parents with epilepsy: genetic and environmental etiologic factors. *Acta Neurology Scand* 1989;79:433–459.
35. Holmes LB, Harvey EA, Coull BA, et al. The teratogenicity of anticonvulsant drugs. *N Engl J Med* 2001;344:1132–1138.
36. Arpino C, Brescianini S, Robert E, et al. Teratogenic effects of antiepileptic drugs: use of an international database on malformations and drug exposure. *Epilepsia* 2000;41:1436–1443.
37. Kaaja E, Kaaja R, Hiilesmaa V. Major malformations in offspring of women with epilepsy. *Neurology* 2003;60:575–579.
38. Patsalos PN, Stephenson TJ, Krishna S, et al. Side-effects induced by carbamazepine-10,11-epoxide. *Lancet* 1985;2:496.
39. Riley RJ, Kitteringham NR, Park BK. Structural requirements for bioactivation of anticonvulsants to cytotoxic metabolites in vitro. *Br J Clin Pharmacol* 1989;28:482–487.
40. Pisani F, Caputo M, Fazio A, et al. Interaction of carbamazepine-10,11-epoxide, an active metabolite of carbamazepine, with valproate: a pharmacokinetic study. *Epilepsia* 1990;31:339–342.
41. Albright PS, Bruni J. Effects of carbamazepine and its epoxide metabolites on amygdala-kindled seizures in rats. *Neurology* 1984;34:1383–1386.
42. Bourgeois BFD, Wad N. Individual and combined antiepileptic and neurotoxic activity of carbamazepine and carbamazepine-10,11-epoxide in mice. *J Pharmacol Exp Ther* 1984; 231:411–415.
43. Coombes BW. Stevens-Johnson syndrome associated with carbamazepine. *Med J Aust* 1965;1:895–896.
44. Bertolino JG. Carbamazepine. What physicians should know about its hematologic effects. *Postgrad Med* 1990;88:183–186.
45. Wolf P, Inoue Y, Roder-Wanner U, et al. Psychiatric complications of absence therapy and their relation to alteration of sleep. *Epilepsia* 1984;25:S56–S59.
46. Brodie MJD, McKee PJW. Vigabatrin and psychosis. *Lancet* 1990; 335:1279.
47. Jacobs JC. Systemic lupus erythematosus in childhood. Report of 35 cases, with discussion of seven apparently induced by anticonvulsant medication and the prognosis and treatment. *Pediatrics* 1963;32:257.
48. Graves NM, Holmes GB, Fuerst RH, et al. Effect of felbamate on phenytoin and carbamazepine serum concentrations. *Epilepsia* 1989;30:225–229.

49. Theodore WH, Raubertas RF, Porter RJ, et al. Felbamate: a clinical trial for complex partial seizures. *Epilepsia* 1991;32:392–397.

50. Sheridan PH, Ashworth M, Milne K, et al. Open pilot study of felbamate (ADD 03055) in partial seizures. *Epilepsia* 1986;27:649–650.

51. Pellock JM. Managing pediatric epilepsy syndromes with new antiepileptic drugs. *Pediatrics* 1999;104:1106–1116.

52. Pellock JM. Felbamate. *Epilepsia* 1999;40:S57–S62.

53. Pellock JM, Brodie MJ. Felbamate: 1997 update. *Epilepsia* 1997;38:1261–1264.

54. Patton W, Duffull S. Idiosyncratic drug-induced haematological abnormalities. Incidence, pathogenesis, management and avoidance. *Drug Saf* 1994;11:445–462.

55. Kaufman DW, Kelly JP, Anderson T, et al. Evaluation of case reports of aplastic anemia among patients treated with felbamate. *Epilepsia* 1997;38:1265–1269.

56. Thompson CD, Gulden PH, Macdonald TL. Identification of modified atropaldehyde mercapturic acids in rat and human urine after felbamate administration. *Chem Res Toxicol* 1997;10:457–462.

57. Kapetanovic IM, Torchin CD, Thompson CD, et al. Potentially reactive cyclic carbamate metabolite of the antiepileptic drug felbamate produced by human liver tissue *in vitro*. *Drug Metab Dispos* 1998;26:1089–1095.

58. Thompson CD, Barthen MD, Hooper DW. Quantification in patient urine samples of felbamate and three metabolites: acid carbamate and two mercapturic acids. *Epilepsia* 1999;40:769–776.

59. Pellock JM. Utilization of new antiepileptic drugs in children. *Epilepsia* 1996;37(Suppl 1):S66–S73.

60. Binnie CD, Debets RM, Engelsman M, et al. Double-blind crossover trial of lamotrigine (Lamictal) as add-on therapy in intractable epilepsy. *Epilepsy Res* 1989;4:222–229.

61. Matsuo F, Bergen D, Faught E, et al. Placebo-controlled study of the efficacy and safety of lamotrigine in patients with partial seizures. *Neurology* 1993;43:2284–2291.

62. Warner T, Patsalos PN, Prevett M, et al. Lamotrigine-induced carbamazepine toxicity: an interaction with carbamazepine-10,11 epoxide. *Epilepsy Res* 1992;11:147–150.

63. Jawad S, Richens A, Goodwin G, et al. Controlled trial of lamotrigine (Lamictal) for refractory partial seizures. *Epilepsia* 1989;30:356–363.

64. Schapel GJ, Beran RG, Vajda FJE, et al. Double-blind, placebo-controlled, crossover study of lamotrigine in treatment resistant partial seizures. *J Neurology Neurosurg Psychiatry* 1993;56:448–453.

65. Messenheimer JA, Ramsay RA, Willmore LJ, et al. Lamotrigine therapy for partial seizures: a multicenter placebo-controlled, double-blind, crossover trial. *Epilepsia* 1994;35:113–121.

66. Wong ICK, Mawer GE, Sander JWAS. Adverse event monitoring in lamotrigine patients: a pharmacoepidemiologic study in the United Kingdom. *Epilepsia* 2001;42:237–244.

67. Schlienger RG, Shapiro LE, Shear NH. Lamotrigine-induced severe cutaneous adverse reactions. *Epilepsia* 1998;39:S22–S26.

68. Pellock JM. Overview of lamotrigine and the new antiepileptic drugs: the challenge. *J Child Neurology* 1997;12:S48–S52.

69. Guberman AH, Besag FMC, Brodie MJ, et al. Lamotrigine-associated rash: risk/benefit considerations in adults and children. *Epilepsia* 1999;40:985–991.

70. Willmore LJ, Messenheimer JA. Adult experience with lamotrigine. *J Child Neurol* 1997;12:S16–S18.

71. Messenheimer JA, Mullens EJ, Giorgi L, et al. Safety review of adult clinical trial experience with lamotrigine. *Drug Saf* 1998;18:281–296.

72. Motte J, Trevathan E, Arvidsson JFV, et al. Lamotrigine for generalized seizures associated with the Lennox-Gastaut syndrome. *N Engl J Med* 1994;337:1807–1812.

73. Friis ML, Kristensen O, Boas J, et al. Therapeutic experiences with 947 epileptic out-patients in oxcarbazepine treatment. *Acta Neurol Scand* 1993;87:224–227.

74. Schachter SC, Vasquez B, Fisher RS, et al. Oxcarbazepine: a double-blind, placebo-controlled, monotherapy trial for partial seizures. *Neurology* 1999;52:732–737.

75. Dam M, Ekberg R, Loyning Y, et al. A double-blind study comparing oxcarbazepine and carbamazepine in patients with newly diagnosed, previously untreated epilepsy. *Epilepsy Res* 1989;3:70–76.

76. Bill PA, Vigonius U, Pohlmann H, et al. A double-blind controlled clinical trial of oxcarbazepine versus phenytoin in adults with previously untreated epilepsy. *Epilepsy Res* 1997;27:195–204.

77. Christe W, Kramer G, Vigonius U, et al. A double-blind controlled clinical trial: oxcarbazepine versus sodium valproate in adults with newly diagnosed epilepsy. *Epilepsy Res* 1997;26:451–460.

78. Dam M. Practical aspects of oxcarbazepine treatment. *Epilepsia* 1994;35(Suppl 3):S23–S35.

79. Sachdeo RC, Wasserstein A, Mesenbrink PJ, et al. Effects of oxcarbazepine on sodium concentration and water handling. *Ann Neurol* 2002;51:613–620.

80. Plaa GI, Willmore LJ. General principles: toxicology. In: Levy RH, Mattson RH, Meldrum BS, eds. *Antiepileptic drugs*. New York: Raven Press, 1998:51–60.

81. Reynolds EH, Chanarin I, Milner G, et al. Anticonvulsant therapy, folic acid and vitamin B_{12} metabolism and mental symptoms. *Epilepsia* 1966;7:261–270.

82. Granick S. Hepatic porphyria and drug-induced or chemical porphyria. *Ann N Y Acad Sci* 1965;123:197.

83. Mattson RH, Cramer JA, McCutchen CB. Barbiturate-related connective tissue disorders. *Arch Intern Med* 1989;149:911–914.

84. Lerman P. Seizures induced or aggravated by anticonvulsants. *Epilepsia* 1986;27:706–710.

85. Morselli PL, Franco-Morselli R, Bossi L. Clinical pharmacokinetics in newborns and infants: age-related differences and therapeutic implications. *Clin Pharmacokinet* 1980;5:485–527.

86. Bender AD, Post A, Meier JP, et al. Plasma protein binding of drugs as a function of age in adult human subjects. *J Pharmaceut Sci* 1975;64:1711–1713.

87. Kutt H. Interactions between anticonvulsants and other commonly prescribed drugs. *Epilepsia* 1984;25(Suppl 2):S118–S131.

88. Haruda F. Phenytoin hypersensitivity: 38 cases. *Neurology* 1979;29:1480–1485.

89. Dam M. Phenytoin toxicity. In: Woodbury DM, Penry JK, Pippenger CE, eds. *Antiepileptic drugs*. New York: Raven Press, 1982;247–256.

90. Rapport RL, Shaw CM. Phenytoin-related cerebellar degeneration without seizures. *Ann Neurology* 1977;2:437.

91. Horowitz S, Patwardhan R, Marcus E. Hepatotoxic reactions associated with carbamazepine therapy. *Epilepsia* 1988;29:149–154.

92. Gleichmann H. Systemic lupus erythematosus triggered by diphenylhydantoin. *Arthritis Rheum* 1982;25:1387.

93. Stables JP, Bialer M, Johannessen SI, et al. Progress report on new antiepileptic drugs: a summary of the second Eilat conference. *Epilepsy Res* 1995;22:235–246.

94. Sharief M, Viteri C, Ben-Menachem E, et al. Double-blind, placebo controlled study of topiramate in patients with refractory partial epilepsy. *Epilepsy Res* 1996;37:217–224.

95. Tassinari CA, Michelucci R, Chauvel P, et al. Double-blind, placebo-controlled trial of topiramate (600 mg daily) for the treatment of refractory partial epilepsy. *Epilepsia* 1996;37:763–768.

96. Ben-Menachem E, Henricksen O, Dam M, et al. Double-blind, placebo-controlled trial of topiramate as add-on therapy in patients with refractory partial seizures. *Epilepsia* 1996;37:539–543.

97. Faught E, Wilder BJ, Ramsay RA, et al. Topiramate placebo-controlled dose-ranging trial in refractory partial epilepsy using 200-,400-, and 600-mg daily dosages. *Neurology* 1996;46:1648–1690.

98. Privitera M, Fincham R, Penry JK, et al. Topiramate placebo-controlled dose-ranging trial in refractory partial epilepsy using 600-, 800-, and 1,000-mg daily dosages. *Neurology* 1996;46:1678–1683.

99. Congdon NG, Friedman DS. Angle-closure glaucoma: impact, etiology, diagnosis and treatment. *Curr Opin Ophthalmol* 2003;14:70–73.

100. Sankar PS, Pasquale LR, Grosskreutz CL. Uveal effusion and secondary angle-closure glaucoma associated with topiramate use. *Arch Ophthalmol* 2001;119:2110–2111.

101. Thambi L, Kapcala LP, Chambers W, et al. Topiramate-associated secondary angle-closure glaucoma: a case series. *Arch Ophthalmol* 2002;120:1108.

102. Ben-Zeev B, Watemberg N, Augarten A, et al. Oligohydrosis and hyperthermia: pilot study of a novel topiramate adverse effect. *J Child Neurol* 2003;18:254–257.

103. Braestrup C, Nielsen EB, Sonnewald U, et al. (R)-N-[4.4-bis (3-methyl-7-thienyl)but-3-en-1-yl] nipecotic acid binds with high affinity to the brain γ-aminobutyric acid uptake carrier. *J Neurochem* 1990;54:639–647.

104. Adkins JC, Noble S. Tiagabine. A review of its pharmacodynamic and pharmacokinetic properties and therapeutic potential in the management of epilepsy. *Drugs* 1998;55:437–460.

105. Perucca E, Bialer M. The clinical pharmacokinetics of the newer antiepileptic drugs. *Clin Pharmacokinet* 1996;1:29–46.

106. Schachter SC. Tiagabine. *Epilepsia* 1999;40:S17–S22.

107. Willmore LJ. Clinical manifestations of valproate hepatotoxicity. In: Levy RH, Penry JK, eds. *Idiosyncratic reactions to valproate: clinical risk patterns and mechanisms of toxicity.* New York: Raven Press, 1991:3–7.

108. Willmore LJ. Clinical risk patterns: summary and recommendations. In: Levy RH, Penry JK, eds. *Idiosyncratic reactions to valproate: clinical risk patterns and mechanisms of toxicity.* New York: Raven Press, 1991:163–165.

109. Willmore LJ, Triggs WJ, Pellock JM. Valproate toxicity: risk-screening strategies. *J Child Neurol* 1991;6:3–6.

110. Willmore LJ, Wilder BJ, Bruni J, et al. Effect of valproic acid on hepatic function. *Neurology* 1978;28:961–964.

111. Kifune A, Kubota F, Shibata N, et al. Valproic acid-induced hyperammonemic encephalopathy with triphasic waves. *Epilepsia* 2000;41:909–912.

112. Hamer HM, Knake S, Schomburg U, et al. Valproate-induced hyperammonemic encephalopathy in the presence of topiramate. *Neurology* 2000;54:230–232.

113. van Egmond H, Degomme P, de Simpel H, et al. A suspected case of late-onset sodium valproate-induced hepatic failure. *Neuropediatrics* 1987;18:96–98.

114. Kuhara T, Inoue Y, Matsumoto M, et al. Markedly increased w-oxidation of valproate in fulminant hepatic failure. *Epilepsia* 1990;31:214–217.

115. Konig SA, Siemes H, Blaker F, et al. Severe hepatotoxicity during valproate therapy: an update and report of eight new fatalities. *Epilepsia* 1994;35:1005–1015.

116. Bohan TP, Helton E, McDonald I, et al. Effect of L-carnitine treatment for valproate-induced hepatotoxicity. *Neurology* 2001;56:1405–1409.

117. Scheffner D, Konig ST, Rauterberg-Ruland I, et al. Fatal liver failure in 16 children with valproate therapy. *Epilepsia* 1988;29:530–542.

118. Konig SA, Schenk M, Sick C, et al. Fatal liver failure associated with valproate therapy in a patient with Friedreich's disease: review of valproate hepatotoxicity in adults. *Epilepsia* 1999;40:1036–1040.

119. Lenn NJ, Ellis WG, Washburn ER, et al. Fatal hepatocerebral syndrome in siblings discordant for exposure to valproate. *Epilepsia* 1990;31:578–583.

120. Prick M, Gabreels F, Renier W, et al. Pyruvate dehydrogenase deficiency restricted to brain. *Neurology* 1981;31:398–404.

121. Hyuman NM, Dennis PD, Sinclar KG. Tremor due to sodium valproate. *Neurology* 1979;29:1177–1180.

122. Dinesen H, Gram L, Andersen T, et al. Weight gain during treatment with valproate. *Acta Neurol Scand* 1984;70:65–69.

123. Jeavons PM, Clark JE, Hirdme GA. Valproate and curly hair. *Lancet* 1977;1:359.

124. Loiseau P. Sodium valproate, platelet dysfunction and bleeding. *Epilepsia* 1981;22:141–146.

125. Sandler RM, Emberson C, Roberts GE, et al. IgM platelet autoantibody due to sodium valproate. *Br Med J* 1978;2:1683–1684.

126. Sackellares JC, Lee SI, Dreifuss FE. Stupor following administration of valproic acid to patients receiving other antiepileptic drugs. *Epilepsia* 1979;20:697–703.

127. Triggs WJ, Bohan TP, Lin S-N, et al. Valproate induced coma with ketosis and carnitine insufficiency. *Arch Neurol* 1990;47:1131–1133.

128. Millington DS, Bohan TP, Roe CR, et al. Valproylcarnitine: a novel drug metabolite identified by fast atom bombardment and thermospray liquid chromatography-mass spectrometry. *Clin Chim Acta* 1985;145:69–76.

129. Triggs WJ, Roe CR, Rhead WJ, et al. Neuropsychiatric manifestations of defect in mitochondrial beta oxidation response to riboflavin. *J Neurol Neurosurg Psychiatry* 1992;55:209–211.

130. Roujeau JC, Stern RS. Severe adverse cutaneous reactions to drugs. *N Engl J Med* 1994;331:1272–1285.

131. Wyllie E, Wyllie R, Cruse RP, et al. Pancreatitis associated with valproic acid therapy. *Am J Dis Child* 1984;138:912–914.

132. Thom H, Carter PE, Cole GF, et al. Ammonia and carnitine concentrations in children treated with sodium valproate compared with other anticonvulsant drugs. *Dev Med Child Neurol* 1991;33:795–802.

133. Zaret B, Beckner RR, Marini AM, et al. Sodium valproate-induced hyperammonemia without clinical hepatic dysfunction. *Neurology* 1982;32:206–208.

134. Hjelm M, Oberholzer V, Seakins J, et al. Valproate-induced inhibition of urea synthesis and hyperammonemia in healthy subjects. *Lancet* 1986;2:859.

135. Hjelm M, de Silva LKV, Seakins JWT, et al. Evidence of inherited urea cycle defect in a case of fatal valproate toxicity. *Br Med J* 1986;292:23–24.

136. Volzke E, Doose H. Dipropylacetate (Depakene, Ergenyl) in the treatment of epilepsy. *Epilepsia* 1973;14:185–193.

137. Haegele KD, Huebert ND, Ebel M, et al. Pharmacokinetics of vigabatrin: implications of creatinine clearance. *Clin Pharmacol Ther* 1988;44:558–565.

138. Reynolds EH. Vigabatrin. *BMJ* 1990;300:277–278.

139. Levinson DF, Devinsky O. Psychiatric adverse events during vigabatrin therapy. *Neurology* 1999;53:1503–1511.

140. Krauss GL, Johnson MA, Miller NR. Vigabatrin-associated retinal cone system dysfunction. *Neurology* 1998;50:614–618.

141. Kalviainen R, Nousiainen I, Mantyjarvi M, et al. Vigabatrin, a gabaergic antiepileptic drug, causes concentric visual field defects. *Neurology* 1999;53:922–926.

142. Eke T, Talbot J, Lawden MC. Severe persistent visual field constriction associated with vigabatrin. *BMJ* 1997;314:180–181.

143. Nousiainen I, Mantyjarvi M, Kalviainen R. No reversion in vigabatrin-associated visual field defects. *Neurology* 2001;57:1916–1917.

144. Jennett B, Teasdale G. *Management of head injuries.* Philadelphia: FA Davis, 1981:271–288.

145. Leppik IE, Willmore LJ, Homan RW, et al. Efficacy and safety of zonisamide: results of a multicenter study. *Epilepsy Res* 1993;14:165–173.

146. Knudsen JF, Thambi LR, Kapcala LP, et al. Oligohydrosis and fever in pediatric patients treated with zonisamide. *Pediatr Neurol* 2003;28:184–189.

Pharmacogenetics of Antiepileptic Medications

52

Tracy A. Glauser   *Diego A. Morita*

Marked interindividual variation in efficacy and adverse effects, a characteristic of antiepileptic drug (AED) therapy, represents the result of a delicate balance between a drug's pharmacokinetic features and its pharmacodynamic effects. As the study of "how the body affects the drug," pharmacokinetics describes the relationship of dose, concentration, and time (1). Pharmacodynamics is the study of how the drug affects the body acting on a biochemical or physiologic system (2,3).

Both genetic and nonheritable factors affect pharmacokinetic and pharmacodynamic profiles, thereby contributing to the variability in clinical response to an AED. The impact of nongenetic factors (age, weight, concomitant medications, and concurrent hepatic or renal disease) is well recognized (Fig. 52.1) (2–5).

The study of the genetic contribution to therapeutic response was first called pharmacogenetics in 1959 (6). Pharmacogenomics, a more recent term, is often used interchangeably (7) with pharmacogenetics, but it refers to the systematic study of drug effects on the entire genome. To date, pharmacogenetic research has focused on the effect of genetic polymorphisms (genotype) on a patient's clinical response to a drug (phenotype). A polymorphism is clinically relevant if two or more phenotypes occur in at least 1% of a defined population (8). These variations in DNA sequences can be single-nucleotide polymorphisms (SNPs), deletions or insertions of at least one DNA base (often hundreds or thousands), or deletions or insertions of repetitive DNA (7). Most polymorphisms are present in noncoding regions, but more than 500,000 reside in exons and can potentially change amino acids to a clinically relevant degree (8).

Genetic variation can affect a drug's pharmacokinetic and pharmacodynamic profile through alterations in any of the classic pharmacokinetic phases—absorption, distribution, metabolism, and excretion (2,5)—in drug receptor site(s), or drug transporters (Fig. 52.2). The metabolism phase exhibits the greatest potential for variability, and polymorphisms in drug-metabolizing enzyme (DME) genes are responsible for most of the more than 70 (and growing) well-described pharmacogenetic differences (7,9). Polymorphisms in the DME receptor and drug-transporter genes account for most of the rest (7,9). A molecular explanation for some of the observed pharmacogenetic differences is not yet available.

Compared with that of oncologic or psychiatric medications, anticonvulsant pharmacogenetics is in its infancy. To describe the current state of AED pharmacogenetics, this chapter is divided into three sections. The first section identifies AED-specific polymorphic candidate genes that code for AED-specific metabolizing enzymes, efflux transporters, or receptors. The second section reviews clinical data illustrating the impact of these genetic variations on each drug's pharmacokinetic or pharmacodynamic profile. The third section describes ongoing and future approaches to clarify the contribution of genetic variation to interindividual variation in AED response.

CANDIDATE GENES

Antiepileptic Drug-Metabolizing Enzymes

Metabolism of AEDs is divided into two phases (10). Phase I reactions can be oxidative (mediated by cytochrome P450

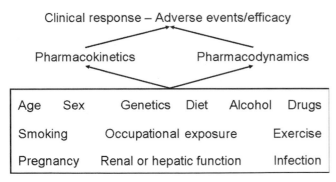

Figure 52.1 Interaction among clinical response, drug pharmacokinetics, drug pharmacodynamics, and genetic and noninheritable variables.

[CYP] enzymes) or reductive (mediated by aldoketoreductases) (10,11). Phase II reactions increase the water solubility of a drug or its phase I metabolite to improve the body's ability to excrete the compound; these reactions conjugate a drug with moieties such as glucuronic acid. Microsomal epoxide hydrolase and uridine diphosphate (UDP)-glucuronosyltransferases are examples of phase II enzymes (10,11). Phase I reactions are considered bioactivating; phase II reactions are considered a form of detoxification (10).

Genetic variability in phase I metabolizing enzymes can alter pharmacokinetic profiles and subsequently drug toxicity. The hepatic microsomal CYP enzymes, the best-studied examples, are coded by a superfamily of CYP genes and play a key role in the metabolism of phenytoin, phenobarbital, carbamazepine, diazepam, ethosuximide, zonisamide, felbamate, and tiagabine (Table 52.1) (12,13). Not all AEDs

are metabolized by this enzyme system. Some either do not undergo metabolism (gabapentin, levetiracetam) or are metabolized through alternative non-CYP pathways (lamotrigine by glucuronidation, valproic acid by β-oxidation and glucuronidation, and oxcarbazepine by aldoketoreductases).

Cytochrome P450 Genes

The CYP enzymes metabolize compounds by catalyzing the insertion of an oxygen atom from O_2 into an aromatic or aliphatic molecule to form a hydroxyl group. CYP enzymes are heme-thiolate proteins found in all living organisms (14). In mammals, for example, they are membrane bound and concentrated in the liver. The term *P450* comes from the observation that a broad-band peak occurs at a wave length of 450 nm when a difference spectrum is plotted between reduced CYP treated with nitrogen and reduced CYP treated with carbon monoxide placed in the path of a double-beam spectrometer (15).

Sequence similarities have been used to devise a standardized nomenclature for categorizing the P450 proteins into families and subfamilies (14,16). P450 proteins are in the same family if they exhibit more than 40% similarity in protein sequence; within the same family, proteins that have more than 55% sequence homology are in the same subfamily (16). Families are given a unique Arabic number; subfamilies noted by a letter after the family number and individual genes in the subfamily are denoted by a second Arabic number after the subfamily letter, for example, CYP2C9 (7,14,16,17). The website http://www.imm.ki.se/cypalleles is the most informative source for data about CYP allelic variants.

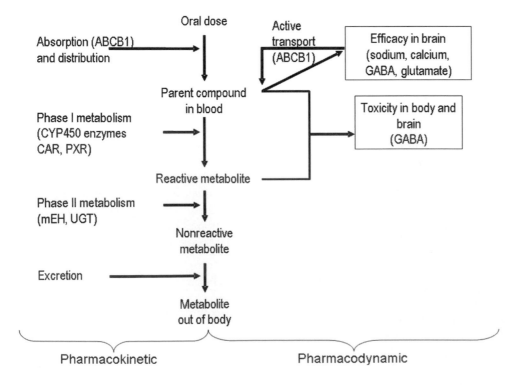

Figure 52.2 Sites of potential genetic contribution to the pharmacokinetic and pharmacodynamic profile of an antiepileptic drug.

TABLE 52.1

CYTOCHROME P450 ENZYMES INVOLVED IN THE METABOLISM OF ANTICONVULSANT MEDICATIONS

CYP	CBZ	CZP	DZP	ESM	FBM	MDZ	PB	PHT	TGB	VPA	ZNS
1A2	X										
2A6										X	
2B6			Xa			X				X	
2C8	X		X					X			
2C9			X				Xa	Xa		X	
2C18								X			
2C19			Xa				X	X		X	X
2E1					X		X				
3A4	Xa	X	Xa	X	X	Xa		X	X		Xa
3A5			Xa			X		X			X
3A7						X		X			
4B1						X					

Abbreviations: CBZ, carbamazepine; CYP, cytochrome P450; CZP, clonazepam; DZP, diazepam; ESM, ethosuximide; FBM, felbamate; MDZ, midazolam; PB, phenobarbital; PHT, phenytoin; TGB, tiagabine; VPA, valproic acid; ZNS, zonisamide.
aMajor P450 enzyme involved in metabolism.
Data from Cloyd JC, Remmel RP. Antiepileptic drug pharmacokinetics and interactions: impact on treatment of epilepsy. *Pharmacotherapy* 2000;20:139S–151S; Rendic S. Summary of information on human CYP enzymes: human P450 metabolism data. *Drug Metab Rev* 2002;34:83–448; and Glauser TA. Advancing the medical management of epilepsy: disease modification and pharmacogenetics. *J Child Neurol* 2002;17(Suppl 1):S85–S93.

In humans, 59 CYP isoenzymes have been individualized to date and distributed in 42 subfamilies and 18 CYP families. CYP2C9, CYP2C19, and CYP3A4 are particularly important to AED interactions; CYP2C9 and CYP2C19 display noteworthy pharmacogenetic polymorphisms (18). The CYP2C subfamily accounts for approximately 18% of the hepatic CYP content in humans (19).

CYP2C9

CYP2C9 is the principal CYP2C isoenzyme in the human liver (20). The CYP2C9 gene, mapped to chromosome 10q24.2, encompasses nine exons and codes for a protein of 490 amino acids (19,21). Of the 13 CYP2C9 alleles identified, CYP2C9*1, the most common, is considered the wild-type allele (19,22). Individuals homozygous for this allele are called extensive metabolizers. Four variant alleles, CYP2C9*2, CYP2C9*3, CYP2C9*4, CYP2C9*5, have been associated with significant reductions in the metabolism of CYP2C9 substrates, compared with the wild-type allele (23–26). CYP2C9*6 has been linked to inactive CYP2C9 activity (27). Individuals with at least one of these mentioned variant alleles are called poor metabolizers.

While two-thirds of whites possess the wild-type allele, one-third are heterozygous for CYP2C9*2 or CYP2C9*3 (19). CYP2C9*2 and CYP2C9*3 are much less prevalent in African Americans and Asians, more than 95% of whom express the wild-type genotype (19). To date, CYP2C9*4 has been identified exclusively in Japanese and CYP2C9*5 and CYP2C9*6 in African American populations (26–28). Six of the latest seven alleles (CYP2C9*7 through CYP2C9*12) were discovered by resequencing CYP2C9 DNA from three racial groups, whites, Asians, and Africans (African Americans and African Pygmies) (29). CYP2C9*13, the last discovered allele, was identified in the Chinese, and found to be associated with reduced plasma clearance of drugs that are substrates for CYP2C9 (30).

CYP2C19

Mapped to chromosome 10q24.1-q24.3, the CYP2C19 gene consists of 9 exons encoding a protein of 490 amino acids (18). There are 15 alleles, including the wild-type CYP2C19*1 (22). The first seven variants (CYP2C19*2 to CYP2C19*8) are inactive mutations responsible for the poor-metabolizer phenotype. The recently described CYP2C19*9 to CYP2C19*15 are potentially defective, although none has yet been studied *in vivo* (22,31).

Most individuals in all populations studied have the CYP2C19 extensive-metabolizer phenotype involving the wild-type allele. CYP2C19 poor metabolizers are much more numerous among Asians (13% to 23%) than among whites and African Americans (1% to 6%) (18). The CYP2C19*2 and CYP2C19*3 mutations are responsible for the majority of CYP2C19 poor metabolizers. The main defective allele, CYP2C19*2, occurs in 30% of Chinese, approximately 15% of whites, and approximately 17% of African Americans. CYP2C19*3 affects approximately 5% of the Chinese, and is almost nonexistent in Caucasians (32). Both alleles together can explain all Asian and approximately 80% of whites poor metabolizers (33).

CYP3A4 and CYP3A5

CYP3A4 and CYP3A5 appear to metabolize many of the same drugs, and an exclusive substrate for either has yet to be identified. The most abundant form of CYP in the human liver, CYP3A isoenzymes account for approximately 30% of the total CYP protein (34) and metabolize about half of all prescribed drugs (35). The CYP3A locus is found on 7q22.1 and consists of four members; CYP3A4 and CYP3A5 are the main isoenzymes in the liver (34,36). Each CYP3A gene contains 13 exons and encodes a 503-amino-acid protein (37).

Most of the 39 CYP3A4 variants consist of SNPs (22,38); large interethnic differences characterize the distribution of these alleles. CYP3A4*1B, which is not associated with altered catalytic activity, is present in 9% of whites and 53% of Africans and is absent in the Taiwanese population (39). CYP3A4*2 occurs in 2.7% of the Finnish population but is absent in whites from Middle and Western Europe, the Chinese, and blacks (40,41). *In vitro*, this variant showed a lower intrinsic clearance for nifedipine than the wild-type but was not significantly different for testosterone 6β-hydroxylation. CYP3A4*3 was first identified in a single Chinese individual and later found in Dutch whites with a frequency of 2.2% (40,42). The allelic variants CYP3A4*4, CYP3A4*5, and CYP3A4*6 were found in the Chinese at a frequencies of 3%, 2%, and 1% respectively (43). Measurement of the ratio of morning spot urinary 6β-hydroxycortisol to free cortisol in persons with these mutations suggests that these alleles may have a decreased activity compared with the wild type. The CYP3A4*7 through CYP3A4*13 allelic variants have been described in Middle and Western Europeans; CYP3A4*12 showed altered catalytic activity for testosterone and midazolam (41).

CYP3A4*14, CYP3A4*15, and CYP3A4*16 have been described in a study of nine different ethnic populations (38): CYP3A4*14 in a single person of unknown ancestry, CYP3A4*15 in 2% of African Americans, and CYP3A4*16 in 5% of Mexicans and Japanese. The CYP3A4*17 variant occurred in 27% of whites, whereas the CYP3A4*18 and CYP3A4*19 mutations were observed in Asians at allelic frequencies of 2% (44). *In vitro* assessments of the catalytic activity of CYP3A4 using testosterone and the insecticide chlorpyrifos demonstrated decreased activity for CYP3A4*17 and increased activity for CYP3A4*18. Overall, the heterozygous frequency of at least one nonsynonymous CYP3A4 mutant allele was 14% in whites, 10% in Japanese, and 15% in African Americans and Mexicans (38).

CYP3A5 is one of the two most important CYP3A proteins in the liver (45). Expression is variable, with reported rates in 10% to 29% of livers to at least trace presence in all liver samples, depending on the detection method used (46–49). CYP3A5 is more frequently expressed in hepatic samples of African Americans than in those from whites (60% versus 33%) (36).

Twenty-three variants of CYP3A5 have been described to date (22); however, only individuals with the wild-type

CYP3A5*1 allele produce high levels of full-length CYP3A5 messenger RNA and express the CYP3A5 protein (36). CYP3A5*1 occurs at the following frequencies: 15% in whites and Japanese, 25% in Mexicans and Southeast Asians, 33% in Pacific Islanders, 35% in Chinese, 45% in African Americans, and 60% in Southwestern American Indians (36). The CYP3A5*2 variant was described in two of five whites with no CYP3A5 protein (50) but was not found in the Chinese or African-American populations (45,51). The presence of CYP3A5*3 is the most common cause of the absence of the CYP3A5 isoenzyme, which results from alternate splicing and truncation of the protein (36). The frequency of this mutation varies from 27% in African Americans to 75% in Asians and 95% in whites (37,52). CYP3A5*4 and CYP3A5*5 were each found in 1.8% of Chinese persons (51). CYP3A5*6 was identified in 15% of African Americans and was associated with either normal or decreased enzyme activity (36). Ten percent of African Americans had the CYP3A5*7 mutation; correlation with enzymatic activity was unclear (45). The CYP3A5*8 variant occurs in African populations with a frequency of 4%; CYP3A5*9 is present in 2% of Asians; and CYP3A5*10 is found in 2% of whites (52). These three mutations exhibited decreased enzymatic activity for testosterone clearance and nifedipine oxidation, compared with the wild-type allele (52).

EPHX1

Human microsomal epoxide hydrolase (mEH), coded by the EPHX1 gene, is a major phase II enzyme involved in the detoxification of aromatic AED metabolites. This enzyme catalyzes the conversion of epoxides to less toxic *trans*-dihydrodiols that can subsequently be conjugated with glucuronic acid or glutathione and excreted. This detoxification is critical during the metabolism of phenytoin and phenobarbital (that both form arene oxide intermediates) and carbamazepine (that forms a 10,11-carbamazepine epoxide). mEH occurs abundantly in the liver, intestine, brain, kidney, lung, and adrenal gland, as well as in mononuclear leukocytes (53–55).

The EPHX1 gene is located on chromosome 1q42.1 and contains nine exons separated by eight introns (56). Two SNPs have been described in the gene's coding region. One SNP in exon 3, at amino acid position 113, changes tyrosine to histidine (His-113); the other SNP, in exon 4 at amino acid position 139, changes histidine residue to arginine (Arg-139) (56–58). Despite initial suggestions that these SNPs may alter enzyme function (57), research conducted with human liver microsomal preparations indicates "only modest impact on the enzyme's specific activity *in vivo*" (59).

UGT1 and UGT2

Glucuronidation by UDP-glucuronosyltransferase (UGT) enzymes is the major phase II reaction, which increases the polarity of target compounds by adding a glucuronic acid group to the substrate, thereby enhancing their excretion in bile or urine (60,61). UGT enzymes are membrane-bound proteins, located primarily in the liver but also found in other organs (62). The nomenclature, as recommended by Mackenzie and coworkers (63), comprises the root UGT followed by an Arabic number representing the family, followed by a letter designating the subfamily and another Arabic number denoting the individual gene.

In humans, more than 26 genes, or complementary DNAs (cDNAs), have been identified, 18 of which correspond to functional proteins. The UGT1 and UGT2 families exhibit 41% sequence homology and are further divided into three subfamilies, UGT1A, UGT2A, and UGT2B. Nine isoenzymes correspond to the UGT1 family (UGT1A1 and UGT1A3 through UGT1A10) and are encoded in a single gene locus, composed of 17 exons, on chromosome 2q37 (64). In contrast, the UGT2B subfamily members (UGT2B4, 7, 10, 11, 15, 17, and 28) are encoded by several independent genes, encompassing six exons, located on chromosome 4q13 (65). The two isoenzymes of the UGT2A subfamily (UGT2A1 and UGT2A2) also reside on chromosome 4q13 (65).

Some of the polymorphisms for UGT enzymes demonstrate altered enzymatic activity compared with the normal or wild-type allele. Of the UGT isoenzymes expressed in human liver, UGT1A1 has more than 60 identified mutations (61). UGT1A1*28, the most common mutation, is associated with Gilbert syndrome, a mild form of inherited unconjugated hyperbilirubinemia (66). It has a frequency of approximately 30% to 40% in whites, African Americans, and Hispanics, and up to 15% in Asians (61). Individuals with this polymorphism have an approximately 30% decrease in UGT1A1 protein expression and may exhibit altered lorazepam clearance compared with those with the wild-type allele (61,67). Six UGT1A3 allelic variants with different levels of enzyme activity have been identified in the Japanese population at frequencies of 5% to 12% (68). Four alleles, including the wild type, are known for UGT1A6. UGT1A6*2 has 27% to 75% lower activity toward different substrates compared with the wild type and has been recognized in 30% of American whites and 22% of Asian Americans (61,69). UGT2B15*2, an allelic variant of UGT2B15, has been identified in 50% to 55% of whites and 38% of African Americans; it exhibits increased catalytic activity for some substrates (61).

Drug Transporters

MDR1 (ABCB1, PGY1), MRP1 (ABCC1), and MRP2 (ABCC2)

Several drug-efflux transporter proteins, in particular, members of the superfamily adenosine triphosphatase (ATPase)-binding cassette (ABC) subfamilies B and C (including ABCB1, ABCC1, and ABCC2), play an important role in the absorption, tissue targeting, and elimination of drugs, thus affecting the pharmacokinetic profile and pharmacodynamic effects of AEDs.

ABCB1, also called P-glycoprotein ("P" for permeability) is an ATPase-dependent membrane transporter efflux pump, coded for by the multidrug-resistance gene 1 (MDR1 or ABCB1 or PGY1), and identified in the intestine and other human tissues as well as the blood–brain barrier (70,71). The MDR1 gene is located on chromosome 7q21.1, encompasses 28 exons, and encodes for ABCB1, a protein with an approximate length of 1280 amino acid residues (72,73). In the intestine, ABCB1 promotes the excretion of drugs in the lumen and could theoretically affect bioavailability of oral administered AEDs (74). More important, lipophilic molecules (such as the AEDs) are good substrates for the ABCB1 efflux transport system at the blood–brain barrier (Fig. 52.3).

ABCC1, also called multidrug resistance-associated protein 1 (MRP1), is coded for by the MRP1 gene located on chromosome 16p13.1. ABCC1 contains 31 exons, and the encoded protein has 1522 amino acids (75). ABCC1 is ubiquitous and as it occurs with the other MRPs its substrate specificity is partially shared with that of ABCB1 (76).

ABCC2, or MRP2, is encoded by the MRP2 gene, which contains 32 exons and is located on chromosome 10q24. ABCC2 is found primarily in the liver, kidney, and gut (76); it also has been identified in isolated capillaries from rat and pig brains (78).

The therapeutic effectiveness of AEDs could be limited by the activity of ABCB1, ABCC1, and ABCC2, which have been found to be overexpressed in the blood–brain barrier, glia, or neurons of human epileptogenic tissue (79). In one study (80) of 19 patients undergoing surgery for treatment-resistant epilepsy, 58% (11 of 19) of brain specimens had ABCB1 messenger RNA (mRNA) levels more than 10 times higher than those in normal brain. In another study (81), both ABCB1 and ABCC1 were overexpressed in reactive astrocytes in resected epileptogenic tissue from patients with dysembryoplastic neuroepithelial tumors, focal cortical dysplasia, and hippocampal sclerosis, all common causes of refractory epilepsy. ABCC1 also was overexpressed in dysplastic neurons in 5 of 14 cases of focal cortical dysplasia. Similarly, high levels of expression were found in brain tissues resected from a 4-month-old female with tuberous sclerosis and treatment-resistant epilepsy (82).

Evidence exists that carbamazepine, felbamate, gabapentin, lamotrigine, phenobarbital, phenytoin, topiramate, and valproic acid are substrates for multidrug transporters in the brain (76,79,83–88).

In a number of ethnic groups, many SNPs have been identified in the genes coding for these transporter proteins (71). Among all ABCB1 variants, the C3435T polymorphism has been found in all ethnic groups studied to date, with the following frequencies: 43% to 54% in whites, 84% in African Americans, 37% to 61% in Asians, 49% to 63% in Oceanians, 73% to 83% in Africans, and 55% in Middle Easterners (71). This polymorphism consists of a

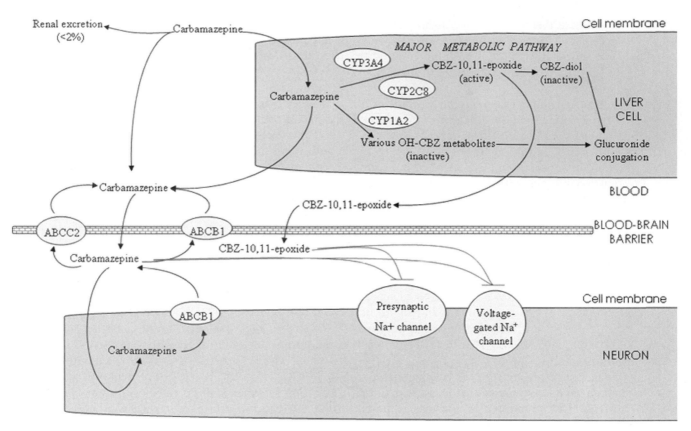

Figure 52.3 Carbamazepine pathway demonstrates all known sites for potential genetic contribution to the drug's pharmacokinetics and pharmacodynamics. (Courtesy of Brian Alldredge, PharmD.)

C → T transversion at position 3435 in exon 26; it is silent, not altering the amino-acid sequence (71). In one study (89), a single polymorphism correlated with low expression levels of ABCB1 (88). A Japanese study (90) identified 81 SNPs in the ABCC1 gene and 41 SNPs in the ABCC2 gene; no clinical associations have been recognized.

Drug Receptors

Two potential types of drug receptors could help to clarify the pharmacogenetics of AEDs: the neuronal AED ion-channel receptors (e.g., sodium, calcium channels) and the family of nuclear receptors that regulate induction of AED-specific DMEs.

SCN1A, SCN2A, SCN3A, and SCN8A
Polymorphisms in genes coding for sodium channels have been the focus of research into the genetic causes of epilepsy (91–98); however, no published human studies have examined the relationship between response to therapy and presence of polymorphisms in these genes. The sodium channel is composed of a large α subunit with auxiliary β subunits. The α subunit is the pharmacogenetic focus because the β subunits only modulate properties of the channel and are not required for its functioning.

The α subunit isoforms have slightly different electrophysiologic properties and amino acid sequences and are encoded by a family of highly conserved genes denoted by the symbols SCN1A-11A (99). SCN1A, SCN2A1, SCN3A, and SCN8A are expressed in the brain and represent potential candidate genes for pharmacogenetic studies; they map, respectively, to chromosomes 2q23-q24.3, 2q24, and 2q24, whereas SCN8A maps to chromosome 12q13.

The α subunits all have four homologous domains (I to IV), each containing six transmembrane segments (S1 to S6) (100). Site-directed mutagenesis of S6 in domains III and IV (using the *SCN2A* gene) demonstrated that these regions are important for anticonvulsant and antiarrhythmic binding (101,102). When alanine was substituted for certain amino acids in these transmembrane regions, the affinity of phenytoin and lamotrigine decreased two- to eightfold (100,101). This work clearly identified potential candidate genes for further study.

CACNA1G, CACNA1H, and CACNA1I
In an manner analogous to the neuronal sodium channels (and the genes that code for them) the α_1G, α_1H, and α_1I subunits of the T-type calcium channels are the sites of drug action against absence seizures. Voltage-dependent calcium channels in the human brain are multimeric complexes of α_1, β, and $\alpha_2\delta$ subunits (103,104); the γ subunit is expressed only in skeletal muscle. The α_1 subunit, which forms the ion-conducting pore and the channel's voltage sensor to initiate opening, is considered the most likely pharmacologic

target (103,104). Its 10 members (α_1A to α_1I and α_1S) encode six functionally distinct calcium channels (types P, Q, L, N, T, and R). Only the genes for the α_1G, α_1H and α_1I subunits encode the T-type calcium channel, supporting the belief that these three subunits are the pharmacologic targets of AEDs active against T-type calcium channels (105).

The genes that code the α_1G, α_1H, and α_1I subunits of the T-type calcium channel are designated CACNA1G, CACNA1H, and CACNA1I, respectively. CACNA1G has been mapped to 17q22, CACNA1H to 16p13.3, and CACNA1I to chromosome 22q13.1. Significant homology is seen in the membrane-spanning segments coded for by each of these genes. CACNA1H contains at least 27 exons and CACNA1I contains at least 36 exons. No polymorphisms (either naturally occurring or by site-specific mutagenesis) that alter drug binding have been described.

NR1I2 and NR1I3 (Nuclear-Receptor Subfamily 1, Group I, Members 2 and 3)

Polymorphisms in DMEs that alter enzyme activity and affect drug pharmacokinetics represent the most intensively studied area of pharmacogenetics; however, interindividual variability may exist in the extent of induction of these CYP enzymes. The constitutive androstane receptor (CAR) and the pregnane X receptor (PXR), two orphan members of the nuclear-receptor superfamily, mediate the induction of CYP2 and CYP3 enzymes, which are involved in the metabolism of many AEDs (Table 52.1) (106–108). The induction begins with exposure to an enzyme-inducing drug like phenobarbital; thereafter, CAR translocates to the nucleus, forms a dimer with the retinoid X receptor, and activates a phenobarbital responsive enhancer module. An analogous mechanism occurs with PXR (109).

The genes that code CAR and PXR are labeled NR1I3 and NR1I2, respectively. NR1I2 has been mapped to 3q13-q21 and contains nine exons. Research is under way to identify polymorphisms in humans in these and other nuclear receptors that could affect the induction of P450 enzymes that metabolize AEDs.

PHARMACOGENETICS OF INDIVIDUAL ANTIEPILEPTIC DRUGS

In this section, the effect of polymorphic variation in DMEs, drug receptors, and drug transporters is described for each AED, starting with drugs with the most extensive pharmacogenetic information available. The section ends with a discussion of pharmacogenetic associations involving drug transporters for which the epilepsy phenotype studied was not stratified by individual AEDs.

Phenytoin

Pharmacogenetic research with phenytoin has focused on the pharmacokinetic effects of polymorphisms in the CYP2C9, CYP2C19, and MDR1/ABCB1 genes. No published studies in humans have examined the association between polymorphic variation in receptor genes and clinical response to phenytoin.

Phenytoin's nonlinear metabolism accounts for its considerable interindividual pharmacokinetic variability. In humans, 4'-hydroxylation forms 5-(4'-hydroxyphenyl)-5-phenylhydantoin (4'-HPPH), which is responsible for approximately 80% of the drug's elimination. This reaction is mediated by CYP2C9 and to a lesser extent by CYP2C19 (110,111). Nonlinear pharmacokinetics, a narrow therapeutic index, and a concentration-related toxicity profile mean that small changes in CYP2C9 activity may be clinically significant for phenytoin. Studies in different populations have demonstrated that the CYP2C9*2, CYP2C9*3, CYP2C9*4, and CYP2C9*6 alleles are important *in vivo* determinants of the drug's disposition (24,25, 27,112–118). Individuals with at least one of these variant alleles are poor metabolizers, exhibiting a reduced ability to metabolize phenytoin and requiring lower-than-average doses to decrease the incidence of concentration-dependent adverse effects (116,119).

Odani and coworkers (112) observed a decrease of approximately 30% in the maximal rate of phenytoin elimination in Japanese heterozygous for CYP2C9*3, compared with those homozygous for the wild-type allele. In another study (116), the mean maintenance dose of phenytoin leading to a therapeutic serum concentration was significantly lower in patients with CYP2C9 allelic variants (199 ± 42.5 mg per day) than in those with the wild type (314 ± 61.2 mg per day; $p < 0.01$). A case report (117) concerning a heterozygous CYP2C9*3 allele carrier described a toxic concentration of phenytoin (32.6 μg/mL) despite a modest dose (187.5 mg per day); the patient showed signs of central nervous system intoxication, ataxia, and diplopia. In an African American woman with signs of neurotoxic phenytoin reactions, clearance was 17% of that in normal patients. She was homozygous for the CYP2C9*6 null polymorphism and did not carry any other known CYP2C9 or CYP2C19 allelic variants.

The activity of the CYP2C9 enzyme alone does not fully explain the large interindividual variability in phenytoin's clinical pharmacokinetics and its reported drug interactions (120). Bajpai and coworkers (121) noted that the contribution of CYP2C19 to the metabolism of phenytoin increases with an increase in drug concentration, suggesting that CYP2C19 might be important when CYP2C9 is saturated. With reported differences in K_m (Michaelis constant) values for CYP2C9-catalyzed and CYP2C19-catalyzed phenytoin hydroxylation (5.5 μmol/L versus 71.4 μmol/L), CYP2C9 is likely to become saturated at phenytoin "therapeutic concentrations" of 10 to 20 μg/mL (40–80 μmol/L) (120). This mechanism explains the increased risk of phenytoin toxic reactions with the coadministration of CYP2C19 inhibitors like ticlopidine or isoniazid. From 1% to 2% of whites are poor metabolizers for both CYP2C9 and CYP2C19, making them particularly susceptible to adverse effects of phenytoin (18).

A Japanese study (112) examining the effect of CYP2C19 polymorphisms on the pharmacokinetics of phenytoin noted an approximately 14% decrease in the maximum metabolic rate in patients with CYP2C19 variants compared with that in extensive metabolizers. In another Japanese study (113), predicted plasma concentrations with a phenytoin dose of 5 mg/kg per day were 18.7, 22.8, and 28.8 µg/mL in CYP2C19 homozygous extensive metabolizers, heterozygous extensive metabolizers, and poor metabolizers.

Following a single 300-mg dose of phenytoin, 96 healthy Turkish volunteers underwent genotyping and analyses of plasma levels of phenytoin and its metabolites (122). The ABCB1 C3435T polymorphism had no statistically significant effect on phenytoin plasma levels ($p = 0.064$); the ABCB1*TT genotype affected the metabolic ratio of p-HPPH versus phenytoin ($p = 0.026$); and the ABCB1*CC genotype was associated with low phenytoin levels ($p \leq 0.001$). On multiple regression analysis, the number of mutant CYP2C9 alleles explained 14.1% of the intrapatient variability in phenytoin plasma levels; the number of ABCB1*T alleles provided some additional explanation (1.3%); and CYP2C19*2 was not a contributory variable. Overall, the combination of CYP2C9 and ABCB1 genotyping accounted for 15.4% of the variability in phenytoin data ($r^2 = 0.154$, $p = 0.0002$). When the findings from the volunteers were applied to 35 patients with epilepsy being treated with phenytoin, the analysis of CYP2C9 and ABCB1 genotypes had "some predictive value not only in the controlled settings of a clinical trial, but also in the daily clinical practice."

Phenobarbital

Pharmacogenetic research involving phenobarbital has centered on the pharmacokinetic effect of CYP2C19 gene polymorphisms; no published human studies have examined the effect of polymorphic variation in drug-efflux transporter or receptor genes.

Approximately 20% to 30% of a dose is metabolized to p-hydroxyphenobarbital by CYP2C9 and CYP2C19 (13, 123–125). Attempts to clarify the metabolism of phenobarbital in two clinical studies from the same Japanese group reported inconsistent results (126,127). The first study (126) used a population pharmacokinetic approach to analyze the effect of CYP2C19 polymorphisms on 144 serum phenobarbital concentrations from 74 patients being treated with phenobarbital and phenytoin, but not valproic acid (126). All patients were genotyped for CYP2C19. Poor metabolizers (*2/*2 and *2/*3) had lower phenobarbital clearance values (18%; 95% confidence interval [CI], 10.6% to 27.0%) than heterozygous (*1/*2 and *1/*3) and homozygous (*1/*1) extensive metabolizers. One year later, this group administered phenobarbital 30 mg daily for 14 days to 10 healthy volunteers: five extensive metabolizers (*1/*1) and five

poor metabolizers (*2/*2 and *3/*3) (127). Cosegregation of the p-hydroxylation pathway of phenobarbital with the CYP2C19 metabolic polymorphism was confirmed, as the formation clearance (29.8 versus 21.1 mL/h) and urinary excretion (12.5% versus 7.7%) of p-hydroxyphenobarbital were significantly lower ($p < 0.05$) in the poor metabolizers than in the extensive metabolizers of CYP2C19. In contrast to the early study, however, the kinetic parameters of phenobarbital did not differ significantly in extensive and poor metabolizers, suggesting that CYP2C19 is not the main enzyme in the drug's metabolism. The authors proposed that the discrepancy may have been related to the concomitant use of phenytoin in the first study, and an interaction of these two drugs with regard to the CYP2C polymorphisms could not be ruled out.

Benzodiazepines

Pharmacogenetic research into benzodiazepines has focused on the pharmacokinetic effect of polymorphisms in the CYP2C19 gene. No human research examining the association of polymorphic variation in drug-efflux transporters or receptor genes and clinical response to benzodiazepines has been published.

At low concentrations, CYP2C19 is responsible for approximately 33% of the N-demethylation of diazepam to desmethyldiazepam (nordiazepam) and 9% of the 3-hydroxylation of diazepam to temazepam (128). CYP2C19 polymorphisms influence the rate of N-demethylation in whites and Asian populations (129–132). One study in Chinese participants (132) noted a gene-dosage effect of CYP2C19 polymorphisms on the metabolism of diazepam and desmethyldiazepam (132). In a separate study of 21 healthy Chinese males (133), serial blood samples were obtained up to 24 days after a single 5-mg oral dose of diazepam. Plasma elimination half-lives of the drug and its metabolite were significantly longer (both $p < 0.05$) and the clearance of diazepam was significantly lower ($p < 0.05$) in the four poor metabolizers than in the 17 extensive metabolizers.

Carbamazepine

The effect of EPHX1 polymorphisms on the occurrence of carbamazepine-related severe adverse reactions has been the focus of pharmacogenetic research. Published human research is lacking on the potential association of polymorphic variation in genes encoding carbamazepine-related phase I metabolizing enzymes, drug-efflux transporters or receptors, and clinical response.

Aromatic anticonvulsants like carbamazepine, phenytoin, and phenobarbital give rise to an array of severe idiosyncratic adverse events, including the anticonvulsant hypersensitivity syndrome (11,134). One of many proposed reactive metabolites of aromatic AEDs is an arene oxide intermediate (135). A series of in vitro experiments demonstrated that inherited deficiencies in mEH detoxification of arene oxides significantly increase a patient's susceptibility to severe idiosyncratic reaction from an aromatic AED (135–138).

Subsequently, a single report (139) compared EPHX1 gene polymorphisms in 10 patients with carbamazepine hypersensitivity (including toxic epidermal necrolysis, Stevens-Johnson syndrome, and hepatitis) and 10 healthy volunteers. The gene's nine exons were screened, and new mutations were sequenced. The patients showed more frequent polymorphisms, but no consistent single polymorphism or pattern was detected. In an earlier similar study (140) no EPHX1 polymorphisms were noted in patients with adverse reactions to phenytoin, phenobarbital, or carbamazepine compared with a control group. These data suggest that a single EPHX1 polymorphism "cannot be the sole determinant of the predisposition to carbamazepine hypersensitivity" (139).

Other Antiepileptic Drugs

No published human research has examined the association between response to other AEDs (ethosuximide, felbamate, gabapentin, lamotrigine, levetiracetam, tiagabine, topiramate, valproic acid, or zonisamide) and polymorphic variation in genes coding for DMEs, drug-efflux transporters, or receptor genes.

TRANSPORTERS

The incidence of the ABCB1 C3435T polymorphism was compared in 200 patients with drug-resistant epilepsy, 115 patients with drug-responsive epilepsy, and 200 control subjects without epilepsy (141). The drug-resistant epilepsy group was significantly more likely to have the CC genotype at ABCB1 3435 than the TT genotype (odds ratio, 2.66; 95% CI, 1.32 to 5.38; $p = 0.006$). Despite the statistical association, the authors cautioned that this polymorphism may not be causal. The warning is appropriate for many reasons including, but not limited to, the fact that the polymorphism itself does not alter the amino-acid sequence (142) and is within an extensive block of linkage dysequilibrium that spans most of the gene (i.e., it may be linked to the causal polymorphism) (141,142).

Two subsequent studies led to contradictory conclusions about this initial finding (143,144). One study indicated that the ABCB1 polymorphism was associated with pharmacoresistance (143), yet the second study could not confirm this finding (144).

FUTURE PHARMACOGENETIC RESEARCH

Despite their persistent use, high frequency of dose-dependent and long-term toxic reactions, and large pharmacoki-

netic and pharmacodynamic interindividual variability, AEDs, surprisingly, have not been the subject of intensive pharmacogenetic research. Understanding the genetic contribution to AED response is an opportunity to improve the drugs' efficacy and tolerability and, ultimately, the patient's quality of life.

By virtue of its continued widespread use, narrow therapeutic window, complicated pharmacokinetics, and polymorphic variation in DME genes, phenytoin was a logical starting point. Improvements in the design of pharmacogenetic association studies and assembly of large phenotype-genotype cohorts will expand the investigation to other AEDs.

Pharmacogenetic association studies traditionally have assessed the effect of one gene's polymorphic variation on the overall phenotype. In a few cases, the impact of allelic variations in one gene is large enough to alter a phenotype in an easily recognizable fashion (e.g., the relationship between polymorphisms in thiopurine S-methyltransferase and azothioprine/6-mercaptopurine–related severe hematologic toxic reactions). Generally, however, the genetic contribution to drug response is a summary of contributions from all factors that affect a drug's pharmacokinetic and pharmacodynamic profile and is best investigated through a global pathway approach that simultaneously considers polymorphic variations in all relevant genes (Fig. 52.3; personal communication, Brian Alldredge, PharmD). Once the phenotype of drug response is defined, a multivariate analysis can identify which polymorphisms contribute most to the interindividual variation in AED therapy.

To date, pharmacogenetic research has emphasized unidirectional effects (i.e., the effect of genetic polymorphisms on response to a drug); however, the interaction is actually bidirectional. Yet to be examined is the role of potential molecular factors, such as a direct AED effect on the expression of receptors, transporters, and DMEs either alone or in combination with polymorphisms in the genes encoding them. DNA microarray techniques are one way to simultaneously measure the expression levels of thousands of genes and expand research in directions previously not considered.

For example, one study (145) used oligonucleotide microarrays to assess gene expression in whole blood from 11 pediatric patients after treatment with valproic acid and compare results with those from 7 drug-free children with epilepsy. The expression of 461 genes (including downregulation of many of serine threonine kinases) was altered in the drug-treated patients compared with the drug-free patients. Eight children rendered seizure free with valproic acid demonstrated 434 upregulated genes, many in mitochondria, compared with 3 treated children with continuing seizures and 3 drug-free patients. This preliminary report concluded that valproic acid therapy was associated with two significant and unique blood gene expression patterns: one pattern for long-term monotherapy (versus the drug-free group) and a separate blood genomic profile that correlated with seizure freedom (versus the uncontrolled seizure group) (145). This type of pharmacogenomic study suggests previously undetected mechanisms of valproic acid's anticonvulsant activity that may contribute to interindividual variation and whose genetic component can be further assessed.

Our understanding of the genetic contribution to the interindividual variation in AED response will grow as more AEDs are studied and complementary methodologies are used both to generate new hypotheses and clarify systemic mechanisms underlying drug response. Additional research is needed into the cost-effectiveness of pharmacogenetic testing and the educational needs of clinicians who must incorporate these test results into actual practice.

REFERENCES

1. Dodson WE. Pharmacokinetic principles of antiepileptic therapy in children. In: Dodson WE, Pellock JM, eds. *Pediatric epilepsy: diagnosis and therapy.* New York: Demos, 1993:231–240.
2. Rowland M, Tozer TN. Clinical pharmacokinetics: concepts and applications. Philadelphia: Lippincott, Williams & Wilkins, 1995:601.
3. Shargel L, Yu A. *Applied biopharmaceutics and pharmacokinetics,* 4th ed. New York: Appleton & Lange, 1999:768.
4. Dodson WE. Pharmacokinetic principles of antiepileptic therapy in children. In: Pellock JM, Dodson WE, Bourgeois BFD, eds. *Pediatric epilepsy: diagnosis and therapy.* New York: Demos, 2001:317–327.
5. Eadie MJ. Pharmacokinetic principles of drug treatment. In: Shorvon S, Dreifuss F, Fish D, et al., eds. *The treatment of epilepsy.* London: Blackwell, 1996:138–151.
6. Kalow W. *Pharmacogenetics: heredity and the response to drugs.* Philadelphia: WB Saunders, 1962:231.
7. Nebert DW. Pharmacogenetics and pharmacogenomics: why is this relevant to the clinical geneticist? *Clin Genet* 1999;56:247–258.
8. Clancy CE, Kass RS. Pharmacogenomics in the treatment of epilepsy. *Pharmacogenomics* 2003;4:747–751.
9. Vesell ES. Advances in pharmacogenetics and pharmacogenomics. *J Clin Pharmacol* 2000;40:930–938.
10. Pirmohamed M, Kitteringham NR, Park BK. The role of active metabolites in drug toxicity. *Drug Saf* 1994;11:114–144.
11. Shapiro L, Shear N. Mechanisms of drug reactions: the metabolic track. *Semin Cutan Med Surg* 1996;15:217–227.
12. Cloyd JC, Remmel RP. Antiepileptic drug pharmacokinetics and interactions: impact on treatment of epilepsy. *Pharmacotherapy* 2000;20:139S–151S.
13. Rendic S. Summary of information on human CYP enzymes: human P450 metabolism data. *Drug Metab Rev* 2002;34:83–448.
14. Omiecinski CJ, Remmel RP, Hosagrahara VP. Concise review of the cytochrome P450s and their roles in toxicology. *Toxicol Sci* 1999;48:151–156.
15. Evans DA. Cytochrome P450—general features. In: Evans DA, ed. *Genetic factors in drug therapy: clinical and molecular pharmacogenetics.* New York: Cambridge University Press, 1993:9–18.
16. Nelson DR, Koymans L, Kamataki T, et al. P450 superfamily: update on new sequences, gene mapping, accession numbers and nomenclature. *Pharmacogenetics* 1996;6:1–42.
17. van der Weide J, Steijns LS. Cytochrome P450 enzyme system: genetic polymorphisms and impact on clinical pharmacology. *Ann Clin Biochem* 1999;36:722–729.
18. Desta Z, Zhao X, Shin JG, et al. Clinical significance of the cytochrome P450 2C19 genetic polymorphism. *Clin Pharmacokinet* 2002;41:913–958.
19. Lee CR, Goldstein JA, Pieper JA. Cytochrome P450 2C9 polymorphisms: a comprehensive review of the in-vitro and human data. *Pharmacogenetics* 2002;12:251–263.
20. Goldstein JDM, de Morais SM. Biochemistry and molecular biology of the human CYP2C subfamily. *Pharmacogenetics* 1994;4:285–299.
21. Schwarz UI. Clinical relevance of genetic polymorphisms in the human CYP2C9 gene. *Eur J Clin Invest* 2003;33(Suppl 2):23–30.
22. Human Cytochrome P450 (CYP) Allele Nomenclature Committee, 2004. Available at: http://www.imm.ki.se/cypalleles.
23. Rettie AE, Wienkers LC, Gonzalez FJ, et al. Impaired (S)-warfarin metabolism catalysed by the R144C allelic variant of CYP2C9. *Pharmacogenetics* 1994;4:39–42.
24. Kidd RS, Straughn AB, Meyer MC, et al. Pharmacokinetics of chlorpheniramine, phenytoin, glipizide and nifedipine in an individual homozygous for the CYP2C9*3 allele. *Pharmacogenetics* 1999;9:71–80.
25. Ieiri I, Tainaka H, Morita T, et al. Catalytic activity of three variants (Ile, Leu, and Thr) at amino acid residue 359 in human CYP2C9 gene and simultaneous detection using single-strand conformation polymorphism analysis. *Ther Drug Monit* 2000; 22:237–244.
26. Dickmann LJ, Rettie AE, Kneller MB, et al. Identification and functional characterization of a new CYP2C9 variant (CYP2C9*5) expressed among African Americans. *Mol Pharmacol* 2001;60:382–387.
27. Kidd RS, Curry TB, Gallagher S, et al. Identification of a null allele of CYP2C9 in an African-American exhibiting toxicity to phenytoin. *Pharmacogenetics* 2001;11:803–808.
28. Imai J, Ieiri I, Mamiya K, et al. Polymorphism of the cytochrome P450 (CYP) 2C9 gene in Japanese epileptic patients: genetic analysis of the CYP2C9 locus. *Pharmacogenetics* 2000;10:85–89.
29. Goldstein J. Polymorphisms in the human CYP2C subfamily. *Drug Metab Rev* 2002;34:5.
30. Si DG, Guo Y, Zhang Y, et al. Identification of a novel variant CYP2C9 allele in Chinese. *Pharmacogenetics* 2004;14:465–469.
31. Blaisdell J, Mohrenweiser H, Jackson J, et al. Identification and functional characterization of new potentially defective alleles of human CYP2C19. *Pharmacogenetics* 2002;12:703–711.
32. Xie HG, Kim RB, Wood AJ, et al. Molecular basis of ethnic differences in drug disposition and response. *Annu Rev Pharmacol Toxicol* 2001;41:815–850.
33. Wormhoudt LW, Commandeur JN, Vermeulen NP. Genetic polymorphisms of human N-acetyltransferase, cytochrome P450, glutathione-S-transferase, and epoxide hydrolase enzymes: relevance to xenobiotic metabolism and toxicity. *Crit Rev Toxicol* 1999;29:59–124.
34. Shimada T, Yamazaki H, Mimura M, et al. Interindividual variations in human liver cytochrome P-450 enzymes involved in the oxidation of drugs, carcinogens and toxic chemicals: studies with liver microsomes of 30 Japanese and 30 Caucasians. *J Pharmacol Exp Ther* 1994;270:414–423.
35. Wrighton SA, VandenBranden M, Ring B. The human drug metabolizing cytochromes P450. *J Pharmacokinet Biopharm* 1996;24:461–473.
36. Kuehl P, Zheng J, Lin Y, et al. Sequence diversity in CYP3A promoters and characterization of the genetic basis of polymorphic CYP3A5 expression. *Nat Genet* 2001;27:383–391.
37. Wojnowski L. Genetics of the variable expression of CYP3A in humans. *Ther Drug Monit* 2004;26:192–199.
38. Lamba JK, Lin YS, Thummel K, et al. Common allelic variants of cytochrome P4503A4 and their prevalence in different populations. *Pharmacogenetics* 2002;12:121–132.
39. Walker AH, Jaffe JM, Gunasegaram S, et al. Characterization of an allelic variant in the nifedipine-specific element of CYP3A4: ethnic distribution and implications for prostate cancer risk. *Hum Mutat* 1998;12:289.
40. Sata F, Sapone A, Elizondo G, et al. CYP3A4 allelic variants with amino acid substitutions in exons 7 and 12: evidence for an allelic variant with altered catalytic activity. *Clin Pharmacol Ther* 2000;67:48–56.
41. Eiselt R, Domanski TL, Zibat A, et al. Identification and functional characterization of eight CYP3A4 protein variants. *Pharmacogenetics* 2001;11:447–458.
42. van Schaik RH, de Wildt SN, Brosens R, et al. The CYP3A4*3 allele: is it really rare? *Clin Chem* 2001;47:1104–1106.

43. Hsieh KP, Lin YY, Cheng CL, et al. Novel mutations of CYP3A4 in Chinese. *Drug Metab Dispos* 2001;29:268–273.
44. Dai D, Tang J, Rose R, et al. Identification of variants of CYP3A4 and characterization of their abilities to metabolize testosterone and chlorpyrifos. *J Pharmacol Exp Ther* 2001;299:825–831.
45. Hustert E, Haberl M, Burk O, et al. The genetic determinants of the CYP3A5 polymorphism. *Pharmacogenetics* 2001;11:773–779.
46. Aoyama T, Yamano S, Waxman DJ, et al. Cytochrome P-450 hPCN3, a novel cytochrome P-450 IIIA gene product differentially expressed in adult human liver. *J Biol Chem* 1989;264: 10388–10395.
47. Wrighton SA, Brian WR, Sari M, et al. Studies on the expression and metabolic capabilities of human liver cytochrome P450IIIA5 (HLp3). *Mol Pharmacol* 1990;38:207–213.
48. Boobis AR, Edwards RJ, Adams DA, et al. Dissecting the function of cytochrome P450. *Br J Clin Pharmacol* 1996;42:81–89.
49. Paulussen A, Lavrijsen K, Bohets H, et al. Two linked mutations in transcriptional regulatory elements of the CYP3A5 gene constitute the major genetic determinant of polymorphic activity in humans. *Pharmacogenetics* 2000;10:415–424.
50. Jounaidi Y, Hyrailles V, Gervot L, et al. Detection of CYP3A5 allelic variant: a candidate for the polymorphic expression of the protein? *Biochem Biophys Res Commun* 1996;221:466–470.
51. Chou FC, Tzeng SJ, Huang JD. Genetic polymorphism of cytochrome P450 3A5 in Chinese. *Drug Metab Dispos* 2001;29: 1205–1209.
52. Lee SJ, Usmani KA, Chanas B, et al. Genetic findings and functional studies of human CYP3A5 single nucleotide polymorphisms in different ethnic groups. *Pharmacogenetics* 2003;13: 461–472.
53. Farin FM, Omiecinski CJ. Regiospecific expression of cytochrome P-450s and microsomal epoxide hydrolase in human brain tissue. *J Toxicol Environ Health* 1993;40:317–335.
54. de Waziers I, Cugnenc PH, Yang CS, et al. Cytochrome P 450 isoenzymes, epoxide hydrolase and glutathione transferases in rat and human hepatic and extrahepatic tissues. *J Pharmacol Exp Ther* 1990;253:387–394.
55. Seidegard J, Ekstrom G. The role of human glutathione transferases and epoxide hydrolases in the metabolism of xenobiotics. *Environ Health Perspect* 1997;105(Suppl 4):791–799.
56. Hassett C, Robinson KB, Beck NB, et al. The human microsomal epoxide hydrolase gene (EPHX1): complete nucleotide sequence and structural characterization. *Genomics* 1994;23:433–442.
57. Hassett C, Aicher L, Sidhu JS, et al. Human microsomal epoxide hydrolase: genetic polymorphism and functional expression in vitro of amino acid variants. *Hum Mol Genet* 1994;3:421–428.
58. Hassett C, Lin J, Carty CL, et al. Human hepatic microsomal epoxide hydrolase: comparative analysis of polymorphic expression. *Arch Biochem Biophys* 1997;337:275–283.
59. Omiecinski CJ, Hassett C, Hosagrahara V. Epoxide hydrolase—polymorphism and role in toxicology. *Toxicol Lett* 2000;112-113:365–370.
60. Evans WE, Relling MV. Pharmacogenomics: translating functional genomics into rational therapeutics. *Science* 1999;286:487–491.
61. Guillemette C. Pharmacogenomics of human UDP-glucuronosyltransferase enzymes. *Pharmacogenomics J* 2003;3:136–158.
62. Tukey RH, Strassburg CP. Human UDP-glucuronosyltransferases: metabolism, expression, and disease. *Annu Rev Pharmacol Toxicol* 2000;40:581–616.
63. Mackenzie PI, Miners JO, McKinnon RA. Polymorphisms in UDP glucuronosyltransferase genes: functional consequences and clinical relevance. *Clin Chem Lab Med* 2000;38:889–892.
64. Gong QH, Cho JW, Huang T, et al. Thirteen UDP glucuronosyltransferase genes are encoded at the human UGT1 gene complex locus. *Pharmacogenetics* 2001;11:357–368.
65. Wells PG, Mackenzie PI, Chowdhury JR, et al. Glucuronidation and the UDP-glucuronosyltransferases in health and disease. *Drug Metab Dispos* 2004;32:281–290.
66. Monaghan G, Ryan M, Seddon R, et al. Genetic variation in bilirubin UPD-glucuronosyltransferase gene promoter and Gilbert's syndrome. *Lancet* 1996;347:578–581.
67. Herman RJ, Chaudhary A, Szakacs CB. Disposition of lorazepam in Gilbert's syndrome: effects of fasting, feeding, and enterohepatic circulation. *J Clin Pharmacol* 1994;34:978–984.
68. Iwai M, Maruo Y, Ito M, et al. Six novel UDP-glucuronosyltransferase (UGT1A3) polymorphisms with varying activity. *J Hum Genet* 2004;49:123–128.
69. Ciotti M, Marrone A, Potter C, et al. Genetic polymorphism in the human UGT1A6 (planar phenol) UDP-glucuronosyltransferase: pharmacological implications. *Pharmacogenetics* 1997;7: 485–495.
70. Schinkel AH. P-Glycoprotein, a gatekeeper in the blood–brain barrier. *Adv Drug Deliv Rev* 1999;36:179–194.
71. Ieiri I, Takane H, Otsubo K. The MDR1 (ABCB1) gene polymorphism and its clinical implications. *Clin Pharmacokinet* 2004;43: 553–576.
72. Callen DF, Baker E, Simmers RN, et al. Localization of the human multiple drug resistance gene, MDR1, to 7q21.1. *Hum Genet* 1987;77:142–144.
73. Gottesman MM, Hrycyna CA, Schoenlein PV, et al. Genetic analysis of the multidrug transporter. *Annu Rev Genet* 1995;29: 607–649.
74. Fromm MF. Importance of P-glycoprotein for drug disposition in humans. *Eur J Clin Invest* 2003;33(Suppl 2):6–9.
75. Cole SP, Bhardwaj G, Gerlach JH, et al. Overexpression of a transporter gene in a multidrug-resistant human lung cancer cell line. *Science* 1992;258:1650–1654.
76. Borst P, Evers R, Kool M, et al. A family of drug transporters: the multidrug resistance-associated proteins. *J Natl Cancer Inst* 2000;92:1295–1302.
77. Toh S, Wada M, Uchiumi T, et al. Genomic structure of the canalicular multispecific organic anion-transporter gene (MRP2/cMOAT) and mutations in the ATP-binding-cassette region in Dubin-Johnson syndrome. *Am J Hum Genet* 1999;64:739–746.
78. Miller DS, Nobmann SN, Gutmann H, et al. Xenobiotic transport across isolated brain microvessels studied by confocal microscopy. *Mol Pharmacol* 2000;58:1357–1367.
79. Loscher W, Potschka H. Role of multidrug transporters in pharmacoresistance to antiepileptic drugs. *J Pharmacol Exp Ther* 2002;301:7–14.
80. Tishler DM, Weinberg KI, Hinton DR, et al. MDR1 gene expression in brain of patients with medically intractable epilepsy. *Epilepsia* 1995;36:1–6.
81. Sisodiya SM, Lin WR, Harding BN, et al. Drug resistance in epilepsy: expression of drug resistance proteins in common causes of refractory epilepsy. *Brain* 2002;125:22–31.
82. Lazarowski A, Sevlever G, Taratuto A, et al. Tuberous sclerosis associated with MDR1 gene expression and drug-resistant epilepsy. *Pediatr Neurol* 1999;21:731–734.
83. Huai-Yun H, Secrest DT, Mark KS, et al. Expression of multidrug resistance-associated protein (MRP) in brain microvessel endothelial cells. *Biochem Biophys Res Commun* 1998;243:816–820.
84. Adkison KD, Artru AA, Powers KM, et al. Contribution of probenecid-sensitive anion transport processes at the brain capillary endothelium and choroid plexus to the efficient efflux of valproic acid from the central nervous system. *J Pharmacol Exp Ther* 1994;268:797–805.
85. Potschka H, Fedrowitz M, Loscher W. P-glycoprotein and multidrug resistance-associated protein are involved in the regulation of extracellular levels of the major antiepileptic drug carbamazepine in the brain. *Neuroreport* 2001;12:3557–3560.
86. Potschka H, Loscher W. In vivo evidence for P-glycoprotein-mediated transport of phenytoin at the blood-brain barrier of rats. *Epilepsia* 2001;42:1231–1240.
87. Potschka H, Loscher W. Multidrug resistance-associated protein is involved in the regulation of extracellular levels of phenytoin in the brain. *Neuroreport* 2001;12:2387–2389.
88. Sills GJ, Kwan P. P-glycoprotein-mediated antiepileptic drug transport: a role in refractory epilepsy? *Epilepsia* 2001;42(Suppl 7):83.
89. Hoffmeyer S, Burk O, von Richter O, et al. Functional polymorphisms of the human multidrug-resistance gene: multiple sequence variations and correlation of one allele with P-glycoprotein expression and activity in vivo. *Proc Natl Acad Sci U S A* 2000;97:3473–3478.
90. Saito S, Iida A, Sekine A, et al. Identification of 779 genetic variations in eight genes encoding members of the ATP-binding cassette, subfamily C (ABCC/MRP/CFTR). *J Hum Genet* 2002;47: 147–171.

91. Claes L, Del-Favero J, Ceulemans B, et al. De novo mutations in the sodium-channel gene SCN1A cause severe myoclonic epilepsy of infancy. *Am J Hum Genet* 2001;68:1327–1332.

92. Escayg A, Heils A, MacDonald BT, et al. A novel SCN1A mutation associated with generalized epilepsy with febrile seizures plus—and prevalence of variants in patients with epilepsy. *Am J Hum Genet* 2001;68:866–873.

93. Kamiya K, Kaneda M, Sugawara T, et al. A nonsense mutation of the sodium channel gene SCN2A in a patient with intractable epilepsy and mental decline. *J Neurosci* 2004;24:2690–2698.

94. Sugawara T, Mazaki-Miyazaki E, Fukushima K, et al. Frequent mutations of SCN1A in severe myoclonic epilepsy in infancy. *Neurology* 2002;58:1122–1124.

95. Wallace R. Mutations in GABA-receptor genes cause human epilepsy. *Lancet Neurol* 2002;1:212.

96. Wallace RH, Scheffer IE, Parasivam G, et al. Generalized epilepsy with febrile seizures plus: mutation of the sodium channel subunit SCN1B. *Neurology* 2002;58:1426–1429.

97. Sander T, Toliat MR, Heils A, et al. Failure to replicate an allelic association between an exon 8 polymorphism of the human alpha(1A) calcium channel gene and common syndromes of idiopathic generalized epilepsy. *Epilepsy Res* 2002;49:173–177.

98. Feucht M, Fuchs K, Pichlbauer E, et al. Possible association between childhood absence epilepsy and the gene encoding GABRB3. *Biol Psychiatry* 1999;46:997–1002.

99. Goldin AL, Barchi RL, Caldwell JH, et al. Nomenclature of voltage-gated sodium channels. *Neuron* 2000;28:365–368.

100. Catterall WA. From ionic currents to molecular mechanisms: the structure and function of voltage-gated sodium channels. *Neuron* 2000;26:13–25.

101. Ragsdale DS, McPhee JC, Scheuer T, et al. Common molecular determinants of local anesthetic, antiarrhythmic, and anticonvulsant block of voltage-gated Na$^+$ channels. *Proc Natl Acad Sci U S A* 1996;93:9270–9275.

102. Yarov-Yarovoy V, Brown J, Sharp EM, et al. Molecular determinants of voltage-dependent gating and binding of pore-blocking drugs in transmembrane segment IIIS6 of the Na(+) channel alpha subunit. *J Biol Chem* 2001;276:20–27.

103. Heady TN, Gomora JC, Macdonald TL, et al. Molecular pharmacology of T-type Ca^{2+} channels. *Jpn J Pharmacol* 2001;85:339–350.

104. Felix R. Channelopathies: ion channel defects linked to heritable clinical disorders. *J Med Genet* 2000;37:729–740.

105. Sohal VS, Huguenard JR. It takes T to tango. *Neuron* 2001;31:3–4.

106. Fuhr U. Induction of drug metabolising enzymes: pharmacokinetic and toxicological consequences in humans. *Clin Pharmacokinet* 2000;38:493–504.

107. Goodwin B, Moore LB, Stoltz CM, et al. Regulation of the human CYP2B6 gene by the nuclear pregnane X receptor. *Mol Pharmacol* 2001;60:427–431.

108. Quattrochi LC, Guzelian PS. CYP3A regulation: from pharmacology to nuclear receptors. *Drug Metab Dispos* 2001;29:615–622.

109. Sueyoshi T, Negishi M. Phenobarbital response elements of cytochrome P450 genes and nuclear receptors. *Annu Rev Pharmacol Toxicol* 2001;41:123–143.

110. Dickinson R, Hooper W, Patterson M, et al. Extent of urinary excretion of p-hydroxyphenytoin in healthy subjects given phenytoin. *Ther Drug Monit* 1985;7:283–289.

111. Yasumori T, Chen LS, Li QH, et al. Human CYP2C-mediated stereoselective phenytoin hydroxylation in Japanese: difference in chiral preference of CYP2C9 and CYP2C19. *Biochem Pharmacol* 1999;57:1297–1303.

112. Odani A, Hashimoto Y, Otsuki Y, et al. Genetic polymorphism of the CYP2C subfamily and its effect on the pharmacokinetics of phenytoin in Japanese patients with epilepsy. *Clin Pharmacol Ther* 1997;62:287–292.

113. Mamiya K, Ieiri I, Shimamoto J, et al. The effects of genetic polymorphisms of CYP2C9 and CYP2C19 on phenytoin metabolism in Japanese adult patients with epilepsy: studies in stereoselective hydroxylation and population pharmacokinetics. *Epilepsia* 1998;39:1317–1323.

114. Aynacioglu AS, Brockmoller J, Bauer S, et al. Frequency of cytochrome P450 CYP2C9 variants in a Turkish population and functional relevance for phenytoin. *Br J Clin Pharmacol* 1999;48:409–415.

115. Caraco Y, Muszkat M, Wood AJ. Phenytoin metabolic ratio: a putative marker of CYP2C9 activity in vivo. *Pharmacogenetics* 2001;11:587–596.

116. van der Weide J, Steijns LS, van Weelden MJ, et al. The effect of genetic polymorphism of cytochrome P450 CYP2C9 on phenytoin dose requirement. *Pharmacogenetics* 2001;11:287–291.

117. Ninomiya H, Mamiya K, Matsuo S, et al. Genetic polymorphism of the CYP2C subfamily and excessive serum phenytoin concentration with central nervous system intoxication. *Ther Drug Monit* 2000;22:230–232.

118. Brandolese R, Scordo MG, Spina E, et al. Severe phenytoin intoxication in a subject homozygous for CYP2C9*3. *Clin Pharmacol Ther* 2001;70:391–394.

119. Goldstein JA. Clinical relevance of genetic polymorphisms in the human CYP2C subfamily. *Br J Clin Pharmacol* 2001;52:349–355.

120. Levy RH. Cytochrome P450 isozymes and antiepileptic drug interactions. *Epilepsia* 1995;36(Suppl 5):S8–S13.

121. Bajpai M, Roskos LK, Shen DD, et al. Roles of cytochrome P4502C9 and cytochrome P4502C19 in the stereoselective metabolism of phenytoin to its major metabolite. *Drug Metab Dispos* 1996;24:1401–1403.

122. Kerb R, Aynacioglu AS, Brockmoller J, et al. The predictive value of MDR1, CYP2C9, and CYP2C19 polymorphisms for phenytoin plasma levels. *Pharmacogenomics J* 2001;1:204–210.

123. Whyte MP, Dekaban AS. Metabolic fate of phenobarbital. A quantitative study of p-hydroxyphenobarbital elimination in man. *Drug Metab Dispos* 1977;5:63–70.

124. Gidal BE, Zupanc ML. Potential pharmacokinetic interaction between felbamate and phenobarbital. *Ann Pharmacother* 1994;28:455–458.

125. Reidenberg P, Glue P, Banfield CR, et al. Effects of felbamate on the pharmacokinetics of phenobarbital. *Clin Pharmacol Ther* 1995;58:279–287.

126. Mamiya K, Hadama A, Yukawa E, et al. CYP2C19 polymorphism effect on phenobarbitone. Pharmacokinetics in Japanese patients with epilepsy: analysis by population pharmacokinetics. *Eur J Clin Pharmacol* 2000;55:821–825.

127. Hadama A, Ieiri I, Morita T, et al. P-hydroxylation of phenobarbital: relationship to (S)-mephenytoin hydroxylation (CYP2C19) polymorphism. *Ther Drug Monit* 2001;23:115–118.

128. Jung F, Richardson TH, Raucy JL, et al. Diazepam metabolism by cDNA-expressed human 2C P450s: identification of P4502C18 and P4502C19 as low K(M) diazepam N-demethylases. *Drug Metab Dispos* 1997;25:133–139.

129. Andersson T, Cederberg C, Evardsson G, et al. Effect of omeprazole treatment on diazepam plasma levels in slow versus normal rapid metabolizers of omeprazole. *Clin Pharmacol Ther* 1990;47:79–85.

130. Bertilsson L, Henthorn TK, Sanz E, et al. Importance of genetic factors in the regulation of diazepam metabolism: relationship to S-mephenytoin, but not debrisoquin, hydroxylation phenotype. *Clin Pharmacol Ther* 1989;45:348–355.

131. Sohn DR, Kusaka M, Ishizaki T, et al. Incidence of S-mephenytoin hydroxylation deficiency in a Korean population and the interphenotypic differences in diazepam pharmacokinetics. *Clin Pharmacol Ther* 1992;52:160–169.

132. Qin XP, Xie HG, Wang W, et al. Effect of the gene dosage of CYP2C19 on diazepam metabolism in Chinese subjects. *Clin Pharmacol Ther* 1999;66:642–646.

133. Wan J, Xia H, He N, et al. The elimination of diazepam in Chinese subjects is dependent on the mephenytoin oxidation phenotype. *Br J Clin Pharmacol* 1996;42:471–474.

134. Dreifuss FE, Langer DH. Hepatic considerations in the use of antiepileptic drugs. *Epilepsia* 1987;28:S23–S29.

135. Spielberg SP. *In vitro* analysis of idiosyncratic drug reactions. *Clin Biochem* 1986;19:142–144.

136. Park BK, Pirmohamed M, Kitteringham NR. Idiosyncratic drug reactions: a mechanistic evaluation of risk factors. *Br J Clin Pharmacol* 1992;34:377–395.

137. Spielberg SP. In vitro assessment of pharmacogenetic susceptibility to toxic drug metabolites in humans. *Fed Proc* 1984;43:2308–2313.

138. Gibaldi M. Adverse drug effect—reactive metabolites and idiosyncratic drug reactions: part I. *Ann Pharmacother* 1992;26:416–421.
139. Green VJ, Pirmohamed M, Kitteringham NR, et al. Genetic analysis of microsomal epoxide hydrolase in patients with carbamazepine hypersensitivity. *Biochem Pharmacol* 1995;50: 1353–1359.
140. Gaedigk A, Spielberg SP, Grant DM. Characterization of the microsomal epoxide hydrolase gene in patients with anticonvulsant adverse drug reactions. *Pharmacogenetics* 1994;4:142–153.
141. Siddiqui A, Kerb R, Weale ME, et al. Association of multidrug resistance in epilepsy with a polymorphism in the drug-transporter gene ABCB1. *N Engl J Med* 2003;348:1442–1428.
142. Pedley TA, Hirano M. Is refractory epilepsy due to genetically determined resistance to antiepileptic drugs? *N Engl J Med* 2003; 348:1480–1482.
143. Zimprich F, Sunder-Plassmann R, Stogmann E, et al. Association of an ABCB1 gene haplotype with pharmacoresistance in temporal lobe epilepsy. *Neurology* 2004;63:1087–1089.
144. Tan NC, Heron SE, Scheffer IE, et al. Failure to confirm association of a polymorphism in ABCB1 with multidrug-resistant epilepsy. *Neurology* 2004;63:1090–1092.
145. Tang Y, Glauser TA, Gilbert DL, et al. Valproic acid blood genomic expression patterns in children with epilepsy—a pilot study. *Acta Neurol Scand* 2004;109:159–168.

Carbamazepine and Oxcarbazepine

53

Carlos A. M. Guerreiro   *Marilisa M. Guerreiro*

Carbamazepine (CBZ) is one of the most often prescribed drugs worldwide for the treatment of neurologic disorders. It has been used in patients with epilepsy, chronic pain syndromes, and a variety of psychiatric disorders since the early 1960s (1–3). CBZ is considered an efficacious agent for the treatment of partial and secondarily generalized seizures in children and adults, with an excellent side effect profile (4–8).

Oxcarbazepine (OXC), the 10-keto analogue of CBZ, has been used largely as an alternative for CBZ because of its more favorable pharmacologic and adverse event profiles.

CHEMISTRY AND MECHANISM OF ACTION OF CARBAMAZEPINE AND OXCARBAZEPINE

CBZ is an iminodibenzyl derivative. Both CBZ and OXC are tricyclic anticonvulsant agents that are structurally similar to antidepressants. However, unlike the tricyclic antidepressants, CBZ and OXC are neutral substances because of their carbamoyl side chains (Fig. 53.1).

OXC as a prodrug is rapidly and completely metabolized to the monohydroxy derivative (MHD). CBZ and OXC (and also their active metabolites—CBZ epoxide and MHD) share many known actions of antiepileptic drugs (AEDs). They produce blockade of voltage-dependent ionic membrane conductance (especially sodium, potassium, and calcium), resulting in stabilization of hyperexcited neural membranes and synaptic actions of such neurotransmitters as γ-aminobutyric acid (GABA), glutamate, purine, monoamine, N-methyl-D-aspartate and acetylcholine receptors; the effect is diminution of propagation of synaptic impulses (9–22). There are subtle differences in the mechanisms of action of CBZ and OXC. For instance, MHD blocks N-type calcium channels, whereas CBZ blocks L-type (19,20).

CARBAMAZEPINE

Absorption and Distribution

CBZ is absorbed from the gastrointestinal tract slowly, with an estimated bioavailability of about 80% to 90% (23). The bioavailability of the agent is similar for all formulations—that is, tablets, solution, oral suspension, chewable tablets, and extended-release tablets/capsules (24–27). However, some studies have demonstrated the advantages in reducing serum level fluctuation with controlled-release forms of CBZ (27–29). Peak plasma concentration with chronic dosing is 3 to 4 hours (30). CBZ is a lipophilic compound that crosses the blood-brain barrier readily and is rapidly distributed to various organs, including fetal tissues and amniotic fluid as well as breast milk (31–35). Pharmacokinetic parameters are shown in Table 53.1 (31,36–41). Definitions and concepts of these parameters are discussed in Chapter 45.

Metabolism

CBZ clearance is accomplished almost entirely via hepatic metabolism. The major pathways of CBZ biotransformation, consecutively or as parallel reactions, are the epoxide-diol pathway, aromatic hydroxylation, and conjugation. Metabolites from these major routes account for 80% to 90% of total urinary radioactivity. Forty percent of the main metabolites found in urine are a result of oxidation of the 10,11 double bond of the azepine rings, 25% are a

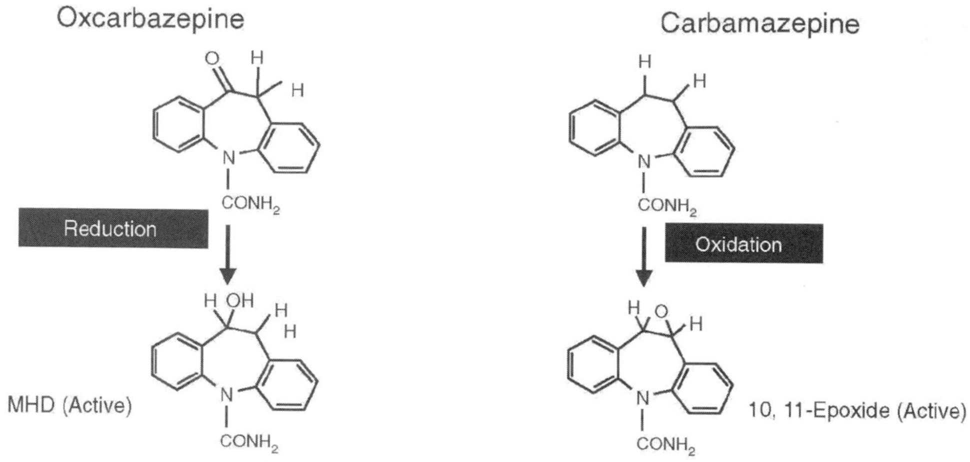

Oxcarbazepine

Carbamazepine

Figure 53.1 Chemical structure and main first-step metabolic pathways of oxcarbazepine and carbamazepine, and their active metabolites, MHD and CBZ-10,11-epoxide (CBZ-E).

result of hydroxylation of the six-membered aromatic rings, 15% are a result of direct N-glucuronidation at the carbamoyl side chain, and 5% are a result of substitution of the six-membered rings with sulfur-containing groups (42).

CBZ is oxidized by the cytochrome P450 system (CYP3A4 and CYP2C8 isoforms) (43) to CBZ-10,11-epoxide (CBZ-E), which is considered the most important product of CBZ metabolism (Figure 53.1). CBZ-E is an active metabolite that may contribute to rash and other side effects associated with CBZ use (44–46). CBZ induces the activity of CYP3A4, with the metabolic clearance of CBZ-E nearly doubled in induced patients (47).

CBZ leads to autoinduction, which increases clearance (double in monotherapy), shortens serum half-life, and decreases serum concentrations. This process takes approximately 2 to 6 weeks to occur (36,48–50).

CBZ-E is hydrolyzed primarily to trans-10,11-dihydroxy-10,11-dihydrocarbamazepine (trans-CBZ-diol). The diol is excreted in the urine and accounts for 35% of a CBZ dose (51). Another, somewhat less important metabolic pathway of CBZ is the hydroxylation at different positions of the six-membered aromatic rings (42). The third most important step in CBZ biotransformation is conjugation reactions. CBZ may be directly conjugated with glucuronic acid. Direct N-glucuronidation of CBZ and its metabolites depends on microsomal uridine diphosphate glucuronosyltransferase (UDPGT) (42). Additionally, CBZ and its phenolic metabolites can be conjugated with sulfuric acid (52).

TABLE 53.1

PHARMACOKINETIC PARAMETERS OF CBZ, OXC, AND MHD

	F (%)	T_{max} (h)	V_d (L/kg)	Protein Binding (%)	$t_{1/2}$ (h)	Tss (d)	Therapeutic Range (µg/L)	Dose (mg/kg/d)
CBZ	75–85	4–12	0.8–1.9	70–80	5–20	20–30	3–12	10–30
OXC	>95	1–2	—	—	2	—	—	10–50
MHD	—	3–5	0.75	40	8–15	2	8–20	—

Abbreviations: CBZ, carbamazepine; F, bioavailability; MHD, monohydroxy derivative; OXC, oxcarbazepine; T_{max}, time interval between ingestion and maximum serum concentration; $t_{1/2}$, elimination half-life; therapeutic range, therapeutic range of serum concentration; Tss, steady state; V_d, volume of distribution; protein binding, fraction to serum protein; .
Data from Johannessen SI, Gerna M, Bakke J, et al. CSF concentrations and serum protein binding of carbazepine and carbamazepine-10,11-epoxide in epileptic patients. *Br J Clin Pharmacol* 1976;3:575–582; Eichelbaum M, Ekbom K, Bertilsson L, et al. Plasma kinetics of carbamazepine and its epoxide in man after single and multiple doses. *Eur J Clin Pharmacol* 1975;8:337–341; Rawlins MD, Collste P, Bertilsson L, et al. Distribution and elimination kinetics of carbamazepine in man. *Eur J Clin Pharmacol* 1975;8:91–96; Hooper WD, Dubetz JK, Bochner F, et al. Plasma protein binding of carbamazepine. *Clin Pharmacol Ther* 1975;17:433–440; Bourgeois BFD. Pharmacokinetic properties of current antiepileptic drugs: what improvements are needed? *Neurology* 2000;55(Suppl 3):S11–S16; Bourgeois BFD. Pharmacokinetics and pharmacodynamics of antiepileptic drugs. In: Wyllie E, ed. *The treatment of epilepsy: principles and practice,* 3rd ed. Philadelphia: Lippincott Williams & Wilkins, 2001:729–739; and Novartis Pharmaceutical Corporation. *Trileptal (oxcarbazepine) prescription information* [online]. 2003. Available at: http://www.pharma.us.novartis.com/product/trileptal and http://www.trileptal.com/hcp/index.jsp. Last accessed July 19, 2003.

Drug Interactions

CBZ has a narrow therapeutic range, and plasma concentrations are often maximized to the upper limit of tolerance. As a low-clearance drug, CBZ is sensitive to enzyme induction or inhibition, especially by the large number of agents that induce or inhibit CYP3A4 isoenzymes (53). CBZ as well as its metabolites induce CYP3A4, CYP2C9, CYP2C19, and CYP1A2. As a result, the metabolism of other agents, including AEDs, is increased, which accounts for the decrease in blood levels (50).

The effectiveness of hormonal contraceptives, independent of preparation (oral, subcutaneous, intrauterine, implant, or injectable), can be reduced by CBZ administration. Oral contraceptives should contain ≥50 μg of estrogen. Midcycle spotting or bleeding is a sign that ovulation has not been suppressed (54–58). On the other hand, agents that interfere with the production of these isoenzymes can have a great effect on plasma levels of CBZ, leading to toxicity. Drugs that inhibit CYPA34 increase plasma concentrations of CBZ. Polytherapy that associates CBZ with inducing and inhibiting other AEDs leads to unpredictable blood levels. Pharmacokinetic interactions among CBZ, OXC, and AEDs are shown in Table 53.2 (39,59). Additional information can be found in Chapter 45.

Efficacy

The efficacy of CBZ in patients with epilepsy was first demonstrated in the early 1960s (60). The agent continues to be a first-line treatment for patients with focal-onset seizures.

Randomized, Monotherapy, Controlled Trials: CBZ versus Other Agents

Most studies (except for the 1985 investigation by Callaghan and colleagues [61]) have demonstrated no difference in efficacy between CBZ and phenytoin (PHT) as monotherapy for adults and children with epilepsy (7,62–68). No difference in efficacy was reported in trials comparing CBZ and phenobarbital (PB) in children (69), and CBZ and primidone (PRM) for the treatment of partial and generalized seizures (70). The second Veterans Administration (VA) Cooperative Study, a multicenter, randomized, double-blind, parallel-group trial, compared CBZ with valproate (VPA) for the treatment of 480 adults with complex partial (n = 206) or secondarily generalized (n = 274) seizures. The patient population comprised recently diagnosed, AED-naïve patients with epilepsy, as well as those who were being suboptimally treated. In patients with tonic-clonic seizures, there was no difference in efficacy between the two agents. However, CBZ appeared more efficacious than VPA for the treatment of patients with partial seizures, according to several outcome measures: number of seizures, seizure rate, seizure score, and time to first seizure (71,72). Other studies did not reveal any significant differences between CBZ and VPA in adults (73,74) or children (75).

Large Trials Comparing Several AEDs with CBZ

The first VA Study was a double-blind, comparative study of monotherapy with PB, PHT, PRM, and CBZ in 622 adults with partial and secondarily generalized tonic-clonic seizures (65). CBZ was found to be similarly as effective as PB, PHT, and PRM in controlling secondarily generalized tonic-clonic seizures. However, CBZ was more effective than barbiturates for the treatment of partial seizures, whether simple or complex. No difference was found between CBZ and PHT.

Other studies in the United Kingdom (68,76) did not demonstrate any differences between CBZ and PB, PHT, or VPA. However, the patients from the United Kingdom had been recently diagnosed with epilepsy, whereas half of the patients in the VA trials had been previously treated. Nevertheless, the large number of patients with complex partial seizures in the VA studies may provide the power to

---

TABLE 53.2

PHARMACOKINETIC INTERACTIONS AMONG CBZ, OXC, AND OTHER ANTIEPILEPTIC DRUGS

	Effects of the Addition of						
On Levels of	**CBZ**	**PHT**	**PB**	**PRM**	**VPA**	**OXC**	**ZNS**
CBZ	↓	↓	↓	↓	↑E	↑E	↑E
OXC	↓	↓	↓	↓			

Abbreviations: CBZ, carbamazepine; E, CBZ epoxide; OXC, oxcarbazepine; PB, phenobarbital; PHT, phenytoin; PRM, primidone; VPA, valproate; ZNS, zonisamide.
Note: Ethosuximide, felbamate, lamotrigine, gabapentin, tiagabine, and vigabatrin addition does not affect level of OXC.
Data from Bourgeois BFD. Pharmacokinetics and pharmacodynamics of antiepileptic drugs. In: Wyllie E, ed. *The treatment of epilepsy: principles and practice*, 3rd ed. Philadelphia: Lippincott Williams & Wilkins, 2001:729–739; and Bourgeois BFD. Important pharmacokinetic properties of antiepileptic drugs. *Epilepsia* 1995;36(Suppl 5):S1–S7.

detect statistically significant differences (72). Because of the above-mentioned data, CBZ has been considered a first-line AED for the treatment of partial and secondarily generalized tonic-clonic seizures, and is used as an active control in trials of all new compounds.

Carbamazepine Versus New Antiepileptic Drugs

CBZ has been tested against almost all new AEDs in monotherapy trials. The majority of these studies have shown no difference in efficacy between CBZ and lamotrigine (LTG) in adults, adolescents, and children (79–80); OXC (90); or topiramate (TPM) in children and adults (81). CBZ was significantly more efficacious than vigabatrin (VGB) (82,83), remacemide (84), and probably gabapentin (GBP) (85). The last study was not designed to compare GBP and CBZ. On the other hand, some of these studies have suggested that GBP (85), LTG (77,78), VGB (82,83), and OXC (80) are better tolerated than CBZ. There are other parameters to be considered before clinical use, however, such as the high incidence of visual field defects associated with VGB (86). These observations preclude VGB as a first-line agent for the treatment of epilepsy, except in special indications.

Based on clinical trials, it is premature to say a definitive word about AED efficacy and safety. There are several methodological limitations in many trials, with some satisfying regulatory agencies but not necessarily guaranteeing clinical use. Most studies are either undertaken with insufficient numbers of patients to demonstrate significant differences or the follow-up is relatively short, considering the seizure-free period, for a true improvement in quality of life to be realized.

According to the available data, we can conclude that CBZ is as effective as any of the other AEDs that have been investigated. More studies that assess the economic impact of epilepsy treatment are warranted to compare several therapies.

Adverse Events

Accurate determination of adverse events has been a limitation in several AED trials. Systematic active questioning of patients has revealed a completely different picture of a spontaneously self-reporting adverse event. The perception of the adverse-event profile can influence a patient's current health status (87). Although up to 50% of patients treated with CBZ experience adverse events, only 5% to 10% need to discontinue therapy (88).

Neurotoxicity

Most adverse events associated with CBZ use involve the central nervous system (CNS) and are mild, transient, and dose-related; severe idiosyncratic reactions occur rarely. The most common adverse events are nausea, gastrointestinal discomfort, headache, dizziness, incoordination, vertigo, sedation, diplopia or blurred vision (5,72,89–91),

nystagmus, tremor, and ataxia (92). Adverse events are similar in children and more common in elderly patients (88,93).

As with most AEDs, CBZ can cause several psychic disturbances, including asthenia, restlessness, insomnia, agitation, anxiety, and psychotic reactions (94). Neuropsychological adverse events associated with nontoxic, chronic CBZ use are generally minimal (7,28,95,96). Some investigators believe that the use of a sustained-release preparation can be advantageous in both children and adults (92,97).

Movement disorders, including dystonia, choreoathetosis, and tics, are associated with the use of CBZ (98–100), possibly with toxic plasma levels of the agent (72,100).

Hypersensitivity Reactions

The incidence of rash with CBZ use is approximately 10% (65,71,74,75,77). CBZ causes the anticonvulsant hypersensitivity syndrome (AHS), characterized by fever, skin rash, and internal organ involvement (101). AHS is associated with the aromatic AEDs—that is, PHT, PB, PRM, CBZ, and LTG (102,103). AHS begins within 2 to 8 weeks after AED therapy initiation; the reaction usually starts with low- or high-grade fever, and over the next 1 or 2 days a cutaneous reaction, lymphadenopathy, and pharyngitis may develop. Involvement of various internal organs may occur, resulting in hepatic, hematologic, renal, or pulmonary impairment. The most prominent manifestations are hepatitis, eosinophilia, blood dyscrasias, and nephritis. The most common cutaneous manifestation is an exanthema with or without pruritus. Rarely, severe skin reactions may occur, such as erythema multiforme, Stevens-Johnson syndrome, and toxic epidermal necrolysis (102,103). It is important to the management of the patient to be aware of acute cross-reactivity, which may be as high as 70% to 80% among CBZ, PHT, and PB (101). VPA is considered a safe, acute alternative for the treatment of patients with AHS (104).

Systemic lupus erythematosus may be induced by CBZ. Symptoms generally appear 6 to 12 months after initiation of therapy. Discontinuation of CBZ usually leads to disappearance of the symptoms (105–108).

Hair loss associated with CBZ use has been reported (109). Fatal eosinophilic myocarditis has been described as a manifestation of CBZ hypersensitivity (110).

Hematologic Effects

Transient leukopenia occurs within the first 3 months of treatment in 10% to 20% of patients taking CBZ (111,112). Persistent leukopenia, which is seen in 2% of patients, reverses with discontinuation of CBZ treatment (113). In the VA study, only one patient had a transient, clinically significant neutropenia (<1000 cells/mm^3) associated with CBZ use, and the treatment was not discontinued (72). Isolated thrombocytopenia associated with CBZ treatment has been described at a rate of 0.9 per 100,000 (114). The risk for aplastic anemia in the general population is about

2 to 2.5 per million. Aplastic anemia occurs with CBZ exposure in 5.1 per million (1 per 200,000) (88,114).

Endocrinologic Effects

Hyponatremia is an adverse event provoked by CBZ treatment (115–118). The risk for hyponatremia increases in proportion to the dose of CBZ and age of the patient; it is unusual in children (118).

Although thyroid function tests may be abnormal due to CBZ use, treated patients remain clinically euthyroid (119–124). Because of the induction effect of CBZ on the metabolism of thyroid hormones, hypothyroid patients may require higher doses of T_4 to maintain euthyroid states (125).

The effect of CBZ on metabolism of testosterone, pituitary responsiveness to gonadotrophin-releasing hormones, prolactin, follicle-stimulating hormone, and luteinizing hormone have been studied (126–133), although the clinical relevance of the findings has not been thoroughly elucidated (92).

Teratogenic Effects

As with other established AEDs, CBZ exhibits teratogenic effects (135–137). CBZ exposure has also been associated with neural tube defects (137–140). In a meta-analysis of 1,255 exposures, treatment with CBZ as monotherapy increased the risk for congenital abnormalities, but not in combination with another AED. However, polytherapy with two or more agents significantly elevates the teratogenic risk (141). Despite uncertainty about the efficacy of periconceptual folate supplementation in women with epilepsy, most authors recommend its use at the same dosage as that recommended for the general population: 0.4 to 0.6 mg per day (140,142,143). Women taking CBZ should have prenatal diagnostic ultrasonography to detect any congenital malformations (140). Breast-feeding is considered safe for women being treated with CBZ (142,144).

Miscellaneous Adverse Events

Weight gain is a common side effect associated with the use of AEDs, including CBZ, although it is not as pronounced as with VPA use (72,145–147).

Hepatic enzymes may be elevated in 5% to 22% of patients receiving CBZ treatment—mostly mild elevations with no clinical significance (148). Rarely, CBZ hepatotoxicity can be a serious adverse event that leads to death (149). Cases in pediatric patients are less common than in adults (150). Cardiac arrhythmias have also been associated with CBZ use (71,92,151,152).

CBZ may interfere with the metabolism of vitamin D, serum calcium, urine calcium, and parathyroid hormone, and may be associated with decreased bone mineral density (153–158). However, clinical manifestations of osteomalacia and osteoporosis during treatment with the agent are a complex matter due to multifactorial etiology (159–165). Dual-energy x-ray absorptiometry scanning of the hip is useful in identifying patients who are particularly susceptible to rapid bone loss while taking AEDs (166). Besides alterations in calcium and vitamin D levels, there is evidence that CBZ and PHT may have direct effects on bone cell proliferation, leading to impaired new bone formation, which may be a contributing factor in decreased bone mineral density (167). VPA, but not CBZ, was found to reduce bone mineral density in children with idiopathic epilepsy (168); other studies did not confirm these findings (169–171). The literature suggests, although not unanimously, that risk of fracture in patients with epilepsy is increased (167,172–175). Calcium and vitamin D should be supplemented when there is evidence of deficiency, abnormal investigation, or clinical findings of osteoporosis or osteomalacia.

Clinical Use

CBZ is one of the agents of choice for the treatment of cryptogenic and symptomatic localization-related epilepsies, as well as for generalized tonic-clonic seizures. Doses must be adjusted individually because of great variability in different epileptic syndromes and intra- and interindividual responses (176). When clinical condition permits, CBZ treatment should be initiated with 100 to 200 mg per day in adults and children older than 12 years of age (>40 kg). Increments up to an initial target dose of 600 to 800 mg (10 mg/kg) in adults (60 to 80 kg) (71) and changes at weekly intervals is preferred, whenever possible (177). Risk for AHS or rash is higher with rapid titration (178). Newly diagnosed patients usually require lower doses (mean dose, 7.5 mg/kg) than those with chronic epilepsy (mean dose, 10.3 mg/kg) (179). The mean effective dose in children is probably 20 mg/kg in those younger than 5 years of age and 10 mg/kg in those older than 5 years of age. If seizures cannot be controlled, doses should be gradually increased by 100- or 200-mg increments until either control is achieved or unacceptable adverse events appear (72). Control doses range from 600 to >1600 mg in adults (179,180) and 10 to >40 mg/kg per day in children. It is not possible to define any absolute therapeutic range for CBZ. Although plasma level monitoring is a useful tool for the clinician, it has no definite value. It is necessary to push the CBZ dose to the maximum clinically tolerated dose, independent of plasma level, in uncontrolled patients (60). Plasma level monitoring may be useful in patients receiving polytherapy, with usual concentrations in the range of 4 to 12 mg/L.

The dosage interval depends both on the severity of the epilepsy and on the difficulty with control. Most responsive patients, such as those newly diagnosed, need modest doses twice daily (7,177). If higher doses are necessary, however, toxicity may be avoided by taking CBZ 3 times per day. Two or 3 times per day provides similar levels, with fluctuations of 57% ± 20% and 56% ± 29%, respectively (181). In children, the interdose variation was 21% for patients receiving CBZ sustained-release and 41% for those treated with standard CBZ preparation (182). Children metabolize CBZ faster than do adults and thus may need higher doses (183). Elderly patients retain their sensitivity to dose-dependent autoinduction and heteroinduction by CBZ, but their metabolism rates remain considerably lower than those observed in matched controls. As a result, elderly individuals will require a lower dosage to achieve serum concentrations comparable to those found in nonelderly adults (184). In patients receiving doses that approximate the maximal tolerated doses, the use of sustained-release formulations of CBZ twice daily minimizes dose fluctuations and may help to adequately control seizures (185,186).

Precautions and Contraindications

CBZ should not be used in patients with a known hypersensitivity to any tricyclic antidepressant (60) or to OXC. Use of CBZ can worsen some epileptic conditions by aggravating preexisting seizures or by leading to new seizure types, particularly absence and myoclonic seizures (187,188). An increase in the number of generalized seizures has been documented in children (189–193).

OXCARBAZEPINE

Absorption, Distribution, and Metabolism

Orally administered OXC is rapidly and almost completely absorbed (194), with absorption being largely unaffected by food (195). As discussed earlier, the pharmacologic effect of OXC in humans is exerted predominantly through its main metabolite, MHD, which accounts for its unique pharmacokinetic and pharmacodynamic profile (196,197) (Fig. 53.1). OXC undergoes rapid and extensive metabolism to MHD (197). The half-life of OXC is 1 to 3.7 hours and the half-life of MHD is 8 to 10 hours (198). As a lipophilic compound, MHD is widely distributed throughout the body and easily crosses the blood-brain barrier (199,200). The plasma protein binding of MHD is approximately 40%, which is less than that of CBZ (70% to 90%). Steady state is achieved after three to four doses (176). At steady state, the pharmacokinetics of OXC are linear over the dose range of 300 to 2,400 mg per day (41,201). After oral administration of ^{14}C-labeled MHD, most of the dose is excreted in the urine within 6 days after dosing, less than 1% as unchanged drug (194). As with most AEDs, placental transfer of OXC appears to occur.

Drug Interactions

OXC exhibits no enzyme autoinduction (202) and has a limited potential for heteroinduction. Induction of the cytochrome P450 system is much less pronounced with OXC than with CBZ (203). Therefore, polytherapy is much simpler with OXC. Levels of the MHD are not significantly modified by CBZ, felbamate, LTG, PB, PHT, or VPA (204).

Whereas CBZ induces many cytochrome P450 isoenzymes (CYP1A2, CYP2C9, CYP2C19, and CYP3A4), OXC is a weak inhibitor of CYP2C19 and a weak inducer of CYP3A4. Because CYP2C19 is involved in PHT metabolism, OXC may increase plasma levels of PHT. As the CYP3A subfamily is responsible for the metabolism of estrogens, oral contraceptive levels may be lower in patients receiving OXC therapy (204). The same precautions used with CBZ therapy apply to OXC therapy, relative to coadministration with hormonal contraceptives.

Efficacy

Monotherapy

Most studies found OXC to be efficacious as monotherapy for patients with partial and generalized tonic-clonic seizures. OXC has a similar efficacy to CBZ, but with a more favorable tolerability profile (80,205).

In two large, similarly designed trials of previously untreated patients with recently diagnosed epilepsy, OXC was as effective as PHT (206) and VPA (207). A total of 287 adult patients with either partial or generalized tonic-clonic seizures, were randomized in a double-blind, parallel-group comparison of OXC and PHT (206). In the efficacy analyses, no statistically significant differences were found between the treatment groups. Seventy patients (59.3%) in the OXC group and 69 (58%) in the PHT group were seizure-free during the 48-week maintenance period (200). In the comparison of OXC and VPA (207), 249 adult patients with either partial or generalized seizures were randomized. As with OXC and PHT, no statistically significant differences were found between the treatment groups in the efficacy analyses. Sixty patients (56.6%) in the OXC group and 57 (53.8%) in the VPA group were seizure-free during the 48 weeks of maintenance treatment (207).

A multicenter, double-blind, randomized, parallel-group trial compared the efficacy of two different doses of OXC as monotherapy in a refractory epilepsy patient population (208). In the intent-to-treat analysis, 12% of patients in the higher-dose (2400 mg per day) OXC group were seizure-free, compared with 0% in the lower-dose (300 mg per day) OXC group (208).

A multicenter, double-blind, randomized, parallel-group, dose-controlled monotherapy trial compared OXC 2400 mg per day with OXC 300 mg per day in patients with uncontrolled partial-onset seizures previously receiving CBZ monotherapy (209). The trial demonstrated that OXC 2400 mg per day is efficacious when administered as monotherapy in patients with uncontrolled partial-onset seizures (209).

In another monotherapy trial (210), OXC was compared with placebo in a double-blind, randomized, two-arm, parallel-group design in hospitalized patients with refractory partial and secondarily generalized seizures. Both primary and secondary efficacy variables showed a statistically significant effect in favor of OXC (210).

A double-blind, controlled clinical trial of OXC versus PHT in children and adolescents with newly diagnosed epilepsy showed that OXC was comparable to PHT in terms of efficacy, but had significant advantages over PHT in terms of tolerability and treatment retention (211). A total of 193 patients 5 to 18 years of age with either partial or generalized tonic-clonic seizures were enrolled. In the efficacy analyses, no statistically significant differences were found between the treatment groups. Forty-nine patients (61%) in the OXC group and 46 (60%) in the PHT group were seizure-free during the 48-week maintenance period (211). A recent study has confirmed the efficacy of OXC monotherapy in children with either generalized or partial epilepsy (212).

A long-term extension phase of two multicenter, randomized, double-blind, controlled trials (206,211,213) showed that the estimated seizure-free rate after 52 weeks on open follow up was 67.2% with OXC and 62.2% with PHT. This 2-year study revealed that the majority of patients were seizure-free, suggesting an improvement in seizure control during the second year of OXC monotherapy.

Adjunctive Therapy

A multicenter, randomized, double-blind, placebo-controlled, parallel-group trial enrolled 694 patients 15 to 65 years of age, with uncontrolled partial seizures with or without secondarily generalized seizures, aiming to evaluate the efficacy of a broad OXC dosage range (600, 1200, and 2400 mg per day) as adjunctive therapy (214). Higher plasma MHD concentrations were associated with greater decreases in seizure frequency—that is, the effectiveness of OXC increased with dose increases.

Adjunctive therapy with OXC was evaluated in a multicenter, randomized, placebo-controlled trial of 267 children with inadequately controlled partial seizures taking one or two concomitant AEDs (215). Patients treated with OXC experienced a significantly greater reduction in partial seizure frequency than did those treated with placebo.

Adverse Events

Monotherapy

The main adverse events associated with OXC treatment are CNS-related effects, gastrointestinal symptoms, and idiosyncratic reactions (80,205–211,216–219). The most common adverse events are somnolence, headache, dizziness, diplopia, fatigue, nausea, vomiting, ataxia, abnormal vision, abdominal pain, tremor, dyspepsia, abnormal gait, and rash.

When OXC was compared with placebo (210), most adverse events with OXC were mild or moderate in intensity and similar to those with placebo. Adverse events reported at some time during the trial by 5% or more of all treated patients were headache, nausea, dizziness, pruritus, somnolence, diplopia, vomiting, fatigue, constipation, dyspepsia, and insomnia. Each of these adverse events

occurred with greater frequency in the OXC treatment group. Three patients in the OXC group discontinued treatment prematurely—one for a transient rash, one for postictal psychosis, and one for an administrative reason. Two patients discontinued prematurely from the placebo group, both for administrative reasons.

The trial that compared OXC with PHT (206) showed that the number of premature discontinuations due to adverse experiences with OXC was significantly lower than that with PHT. Five of 143 patients in the OXC group discontinued treatment because of tolerability reasons—rash in one case, pregnancy in one case, an astrocytoma not previously diagnosed in one case, a suicide attempt with OXC intoxication in one case, and gastrointestinal discomfort combined with depression/anxiety in one case. Sixteen of 144 patients in the PHT group discontinued treatment because of tolerability reasons—rash in 10 cases, hirsutism/gum hypertrophy in five cases, and cerebellar symptoms/sedation in the last case. Somnolence, headache, dizziness, nausea, and rash occurred in 10% or more of the patients in both groups. Gum hyperplasia, tremor, diplopia, acne, nervousness, and nystagmus occurred in less than 10% of the patients in both groups (206). When differences in the incidence of adverse events were apparent between the groups, these were nearly all in favor of OXC therapy.

The comparison of OXC and VPA (207) in 249 adults revealed no statistically significant difference between treatment groups with respect to the total number of premature discontinuations or those that are caused by adverse events. The most frequent reason for withdrawal because of adverse events in the OXC group was allergic reaction with skin symptoms (six patients); in the VPA group, it was hair loss (four patients). The most common adverse events considered to have a causal relationship to the trial treatment were somnolence, weight increase, fatigue, headache, alopecia, dizziness, nausea, tremor, abdominal pain, impaired concentration, increased appetite, and diarrhea. When differences in incidence existed between the groups, these generally favored OXC treatment. Abnormally low plasma sodium levels were reported in two OXC-treated patients. Both patients were asymptomatic with respect to their low plasma sodium levels, and neither discontinued treatment prematurely (207).

The study that compared two different doses of OXC (2,400 mg per day versus 300 mg per day) concluded that OXC was well tolerated, with fatigue, dizziness, somnolence, nausea, ataxia, and headache the most common adverse events (209). Most of the adverse events were transient and rated as mild to moderate in intensity (208).

The trial that compared the efficacy and safety of OXC with that of PHT in 193 children and adolescents (211) found that two patients in the OXC group and 14 patients in the PHT group discontinued treatment prematurely for tolerability reasons. The number of premature discontinuations due to adverse events was statistically significantly lower in the OXC group than in the PHT group. Moreover, the odds of an individual discontinuing prematurely were almost twice as high in the PHT group. Based on the findings of this trial, the authors concluded that OXC has significant advantages over PHT in terms of tolerability and treatment retention. The extension phase of this study confirmed that long-term OXC therapy (112 weeks) in children is associated with significantly fewer tolerability-related discontinuations versus PHT (220).

OXC therapy in elderly patients (65 years of age and older) seems as safe as treatment in younger adults. The four most common adverse events experienced by elderly patients were vomiting (19%), dizziness (17%), nausea (17%), and somnolence (15%). Three of 52 patients developed an asymptomatic hyponatremia, with at least one patient's serum sodium level <125 mEq/L (221).

Adjunctive Therapy

The study that evaluated the safety of a broad OXC dosage as adjunctive therapy in patients with uncontrolled partial seizures (214) found that the most common adverse events were related to the nervous and digestive systems. Rapid and fixed titration to high doses was associated with an increased risk for adverse events, which could potentially be reduced by adjusting concomitant AEDs and using a slower, flexible OXC titration schedule.

The trial that compared the safety of OXC with placebo as adjunctive therapy in children with inadequately controlled partial seizures (215) found that 91% of the OXC group and 82% of the placebo group reported at least one adverse event. Vomiting, somnolence, dizziness, and nausea occurred more frequently in the OXC-treated group. The majority of these adverse events were mild to moderate in severity. The incidence of rash was 4% in the OXC group and 5% in the placebo group. Fourteen patients (10%) in the OXC group and four patients (3%) in the placebo group discontinued treatment prematurely because of adverse events. The most common reasons for discontinuation in the OXC group were adverse events involving the digestive system (primarily nausea and vomiting), which occurred in five patients, and rash (maculopapular and erythematous), which occurred in four patients.

Hyponatremia

Hyponatremia is usually defined as a serum sodium level <135 mEq/L. Clinically significant hyponatremia (sodium level <125 mEq/L) has been observed in 2.5% of OXC-treated patients in 14 controlled trials (41,222). Acute symptoms of hyponatremia include headache, nausea, vomiting, tremors, delirium, seizures and decerebrate posturing, whereas chronic symptoms include anorexia, cramps, personality changes, gait disturbance, stupor, nausea, and vomiting (41,219). The 14 trials that evaluated 1966 patients showed that serum sodium levels increased with age, from 0% at younger than 6 years of age and 0.5% at younger than 18 years of age, to 3.4% between 18 and 64 years of age

and 7.3% at older than 65 years of age (41,219,223–226). However, in a subgroup of 27 children in whom CBZ was directly replaced with OXC, hyponatremia without symptoms was found in 1 child (3.7%) taking CBZ and in 6 children (22.2%) taking OXC (227). A recent study by Sachdeo and colleagues (228) found that OXC-induced hyponatremia is not attributable to the syndrome of inappropriate secretion of antidiuretic hormone. The authors proposed that possible mechanisms include a direct effect of OXC on the renal collecting tubules or an enhancement of their responsiveness to circulating antidiuretic hormone. Although hyponatremia has been reported, it is only rarely accompanied by clinical symptomatology and rarely leads to OXC discontinuation. The degree of hyponatremia seems to be related to the dose of OXC (226,229). Rapid titration may be another risk factor (219,226).

Other Potential Adverse Events

An analysis of 29 trials involving 2191 patients treated with OXC for up to 11.5 months showed no clinically significant weight changes in the OXC group compared with the placebo group (230). Using the same patient population, Parys and D'Souza demonstrated that OXC had no effect on blood pressure and electrocardiograms with monotherapy or combination therapy (231). In a recent study of 102 men with epilepsy, treatment with OXC or CBZ, as opposed to VPA, did not appear to have any significant effects on serum insulin or lipid levels (232).

The teratogenic potential of OXC is virtually unknown (140). Major malformations in offspring of mothers with epilepsy are associated with the use of AEDs, including OXC, during early pregnancy (233). In a preliminary report of 42 pregnant patients exposed to OXC, 25 with monotherapy and 17 in combination with other AEDs (234), there were no minor or major malformations recorded in the OXC monotherapy group. All patients received folate supplementation.

OXC does not appear to affect cognitive function in healthy volunteers or adults with newly diagnosed epilepsy. The cognitive effects of the agent in children and adolescents have not been systematically studied (235).

Clinical Use

OXC is indicated for use as monotherapy or adjunctive therapy in the treatment of partial seizures, with or without secondary generalized seizures, and primary generalized tonic-clonic seizures in adults and children with epilepsy (236). OXC is available as 150-mg, 300-mg, and 600-mg film-coated tablets for oral administration. OXC is also available as a 300-mg/5-mL (60 mg/mL) oral suspension (41). It can be taken with or without food.

In adults, treatment with OXC monotherapy should be initiated at a dose of 300 to 600 mg per day. Increases at weekly intervals are advisable and titration should be planned according to the clinical condition of the patient, because slow and gradual initiation of therapy minimizes side effects. In the case of frequent seizures, the interval may be shortened (e.g., every second day). The recommended monotherapy dosage is 600 to 1200 mg per day in two divided doses (236). OXC dosages range from 600 to 3000 mg per day. As adjunctive therapy, treatment with OXC should be initiated at a dose of 600 mg per day, administered as a twice-daily regimen. The recommended dosage for adjunctive therapy is 1200 mg per day or higher, if needed, which may be increased at weekly intervals (41).

In children, treatment should be initiated at a daily dose of 8 to 10 mg/kg, generally not to exceed 600 mg per day, administered as a twice-daily regimen. The target maintenance dose of OXC should be between 30 and 50 mg/kg per day. The pharmacokinetics of OXC are similar in children older than 8 years of age and adults. However, children younger than 8 years of age have an increased clearance compared with older children and adults; therefore, they should receive the highest maintenance doses (41).

Therapeutic drug monitoring is claimed to be of little or no value with OXC because of the linear pharmacokinetics of the agent (237), although measuring drug levels is undoubtedly useful for individualization of treatment in selected cases in a particular clinical setting. The current tentative target levels for OXC (MHD) range from 10 to 35 mg/L, or 50 to 140 μmol/L (238). Interlaboratory variability in determination of new AEDs, including MHD, was comparable to that reported with older agents (239).

Some authors feel there is no need to monitor sodium levels regularly in asymptomatic patients, unless there are special risks, such as in patients taking high doses or diuretics and in elderly individuals (240,241).

CARBAMAZEPINE VERSUS OXCARBAZEPINE

CBZ and OXC are among the most efficacious AEDs available. The literature suggests that CBZ and OXC do not differ in terms of seizure control efficacy. However, OXC has a better safety profile, including its association with fewer severe adverse events, such as idiosyncratic reactions, aplastic anemia, and agranulocytosis. Except for sodium monitoring under special circumstances with OXC treatment, laboratory monitoring of drug levels is not necessary. The OXC pharmacokinetic profile is also better than that of CBZ, with lack of autoinduction, low protein binding, linear pharmacokinetics, minimal drug interactions (except contraceptives), and no evidence of weight gain. OXC does not appear to change endogenous hormonal levels. In conclusion, OXC should be considered a first-line treatment option for patients with partial-onset seizures (236).

In some cases, a decision may be made to switch a patient from CBZ to OXC. This can either be done gradually or with a more abrupt changeover. Typically, the conversion ratio for similar efficacy is on the order of 1:1.5 (240).

REFERENCES

1. Tomson T, Ekbom K. Trigeminal neuralgia: time course of pain in relation to carbamazepine dosing. *Cephalalgia* 1981;1:91–97.
2. Dickinson RG, Eadie MJ, Vajda FJE. Carbamazepine. In: Eadie MJ, Vajda FJE, eds. *Antiepileptic drugs: pharmacology and therapeutics: handbook of experimental pharmacology*, vol 138. Berlin: Springer-Verlag, 1999:277–317.
3. Trimble MR. Carbamazepine. Clinical efficacy and use in psychiatric disorders. In: Levy RH, Mattson RH, Meldrum BS, et al., eds. *Antiepileptic drugs*, 5th ed. Philadelphia: Lippincott Williams & Wilkins, 2002:278–284.
4. Cereghino JJ, Brock JT, Van Meter JC, et al. Carbamazepine for epilepsy. A controlled prospective evaluation. *Neurology* 1974;24:401–410.
5. Rodin EA, Rim CS, Rennick PM. The effects of carbamazepine on patients with psychomotor epilepsy: results of a double-blind study. *Epilepsia* 1974;15:547–561.
6. Simonson J, Olsen IZ, Kuhl V, et al. A comparative controlled study between carbamazepine and diphenylhydantoin in psychomotor epilepsy. *Epilepsia* 1976;17:169–176.
7. Troupin A, Ojemann LM, Halpern L, et al. Carbamazepine: a double-blind comparison with phenytoin. *Neurology* 1977;27:511–519.
8. Brodie MJ, Ditcher MA. Antiepileptic drugs. *N Engl J Med* 1996;334:168–175.
9. Quattrone A, Samanin R. Decreased anticonvulsant activity of carbamazepine in 6-hydroxy-dopamine-treated rats. *Eur J Pharmacol* 1977;41:336.
10. Weiss SR, Post RM, Patel J, et al. Differential mediation of the anticonvulsant effects of carbamazepine and diazepam. *Life Sci* 1985; 36:2413–2419.
11. Macdonald RL, McLean MJ. Anticonvulsant drugs: mechanisms of action. *Adv Neurol* 1986;44:713–736.
12. McLean MJ, Macdonald RL. Carbamazepine and 10,11-epoxy-carbamazepine produce use- and voltage-dependent limitation of rapidly firing action potentials of mouse central neurons in cell culture. *J Pharmacol Exp Ther* 1986;238:727–738.
13. Macdonald RL. Seizure disorders and epilepsy. In: Johnston MV, Macdonald RL, Young AB, eds. *Principles of drug therapy in neurology*. Philadelphia: FA Davis, 1992:87–117.
14. Yan QS, Mishra PK, Burger RL, et al. Evidence that carbamazepine and antiepilepsirine may produce a component of their anticonvulsant effects by activating serotonergic neurons in genetically epilepsy-prone rats. *J Pharmacol Exp Ther* 1992;261:652–659.
15. Zona C, Tancredi V, Palma E, et al. Potassium currents in rat cortical neurons in culture are enhanced by the antiepileptic drug carbamazepine. *Can J Physiol Pharmacol* 1990;68:545–547.
16. Lampe H, Bigalke H. Carbamazepine blocks NMDA-activated currents in cultured spinal cord neurons. *Neuroreport* 1990;1:26–28.
17. Ragsdale DS, Scheuer T, Catterall WA. Frequency and voltage-dependent inhibition of type IIA Na$^+$ channels, expressed in a mammalian cell line, by local anesthetic, antiarrhythmic, and anticonvulsant drugs. *Mol Pharmacol* 1991;40:756–765.
18. Wamil A, Schmutz M, Portet C, et al. Effects of oxcarbazepine and 10-hydroxy-carbamazepine on action potential firing and generalized seizures. *Eur J Pharmacol* 1994;271:301–308.
19. Stefani A, Pisani A, De Murtas M, et al. Action of GP 47779, the active metabolite of oxcarbazepine, on the corticostriatal system. II. Modulation of high-voltage-activated calcium currents. *Epilepsia* 1995;36:997–1002.
20. Calabresi P, De Murtas M, Stefani A, et al. Action of GP 47779, the active metabolite of oxcarbazepine, on the corticostriatal system. I. Modulation of corticostriatal synaptic transmission. *Epilepsia* 1995;36:990–996.
21. Reckziegel G, Beck H, Schramm J, et al. Carbamazepine effects on Na$^+$ currents in human dentate granule cells from epileptogenic tissue. *Epilepsia* 1999;40:401–407.
22. Macdonald RL. Carbamazepine. Mechanism of action. In: Levy RH, Mattson RH, Meldrum BS, et al., eds. *Antiepileptic drugs*, 5th ed. Philadelphia: Lippincott Williams & Wilkins, 2002:227–235.

23. Pynnonen S. Pharmacokinetics of carbamazepine in man: a review. *Ther Drug Monit* 1979;1:409–431.
24. Wada JA, Troupin AS, Fried P, et al. Pharmacokinetic comparison of tablet and suspension dosage forms of carbamazepine. *Epilepsia* 1978;19:251–255.
25. Patsalos PN. A comparative pharmacokinetic study of conventional and chewable carbamazepine in epileptic patients. *Br J Clin Pharmacol* 1990;29:574–577.
26. Bialer M. Pharmacokinetic evaluation of sustained release formulations of antiepileptic drugs. *Clin Pharmacokinet* 1992;22:11–21.
27. Reunanen M, Heinonen EH, Nyman L, et al. Comparative bioavailability of carbamazepine from two slow-release preparations. *Epilepsy Res* 1992;11:61–66.
28. Aldenkamp AP, Alpherts WCJ, Moerland MC, et al. Controlled release carbamazepine: cognitive side effects in patients with epilepsy. *Epilepsia* 1987;28:507–514.
29. Persson L, Ben-Menachem E, Bengtsson E, et al. Differences in side effects between a conventional and a slow release preparation of carbamazepine. *Epilepsy Res* 1990;6:134–140.
30. Macphee GJA, Butler E, Brodie MJ. Intradose and circadian variation in circulating carbamazepine and its epoxide in epileptic patients: a consequence of autoinduction of metabolism. *Epilepsia* 1987;28:286–294.
31. Johannessen SI, Gerna M, Bakke J, et al. CSF concentrations and serum protein binding of carbazepine and carbamazepine-10,11-epoxide in epileptic patients. *Br J Clin Pharmacol* 1976;3:575–582.
32. Pynnonen S, Kanto J, Sillanpaa M, et al. Carbamazepine: placental transport, tissue concentrations in foetus and newborn, and level in milk. *Acta Pharmacol Toxicol (Copenh)* 1977;41:244–253.
33. Post RM, Uhde TW, Ballenger JC, et al. Carbamazepine and its -10,11-epoxide metabolite in plasma and CSF: Relationship to antidepressant response. *Arch Gen Psychiatry* 1983;40:673–676.
34. Froescher W, Eichelbaum M, Niesen M, et al. Carbamazepine levels in breast milk. *Ther Drug Monit* 1984;6:266–271.
35. Omtzigt JG, Los FJ, Meijer JWA, et al. The 10,11-epoxide-10,11-diol pathway of carbamazepine in early pregnancy in maternal serum, urine, and amniotic fluid: effect of dose, comedication, and relation to outcome of pregnancy. *Ther Drug Monit* 1993;15:1–10.
36. Eichelbaum M, Ekbom K, Bertilsson L, et al. Plasma kinetics of carbamazepine and its epoxide in man after single and multiple doses. *Eur J Clin Pharmacol* 1975;8:337–341.
37. Rawlins MD, Collste P, Bertilsson L, et al. Distribution and elimination kinetics of carbamazepine in man. *Eur J Clin Pharmacol* 1975;8:91–96.
38. Hooper WD, Dubetz JK, Bochner F, et al. Plasma protein binding of carbamazepine. *Clin Pharmacol Ther* 1975;17:433–440.
39. Bourgeois BFD. Pharmacokinetic properties of current antiepileptic drugs: what improvements are needed? *Neurology* 2000;55(Suppl 3):S11–S16.
40. Bourgeois BFD. Pharmacokinetics and pharmacodynamics of antiepileptic drugs. In: Wyllie E, ed. *The treatment of epilepsy: principles and practice*, 3rd ed. Philadelphia: Lippincott Williams & Wilkins, 2001:729–739.
41. Novartis Pharmaceutical Corporation. Trileptal (oxcarbazepine) prescription information [online]. 2003. Available at: http://www.trileptal.com/hcp/index.jsp. Last accessed July 19, 2003.
42. Faigle JW, Feldmann KF. Carbamazepine: chemistry and biotransformation. In: Levy RH, Mattson RH, Meldrum BS, eds. *Antiepileptic drugs*, 4th ed. New York: Raven Press, 1995:499–513.
43. Kerr BM, Thummel KE, Wurden CJ, et al. Human liver carbamazepine metabolism. Role of CYP3A4 and CYP2C8 in 10-11-epoxide formation. *Biochem Pharmacol* 1994;47:1969–1979.
44. Altafullah I, Talwar D, Loewenson R, et al. Factors influencing serum levels of carbamazepine and carbamazepine 10,11-epoxide in children. *Epilepsy Res* 1989;4:72–80.
45. Kerr BM, Levy RH. Carbamazepine. Carbamazepine epoxide. In: Levy RH, Mattson RH, Meldrum BS, eds. *Antiepileptic drugs*, 4th ed. New York: Raven Press, 1995:529–541.
46. Ramsay RE, Wilder BJ. Metabolism of tricyclic anticonvulsant drugs. *Epilepsy Behav* 2002;3:S2–S6.
47. Faigle JW, Feldmann KF. Carbamazepine: biotransformation. In: Woodbury DM, Penry JK, Pippenger CE, eds. *Antiepileptic drugs*, 2nd ed. New York: Raven Press, 1982:483–495.
48. Bertilsson L, Hojer B, Tybring G, et al. Autoinduction of carbamazepine metabolism in children examined by stable isotope technique. *Clin Pharmacol Ther* 1980;27:83–88.
49. Mikati MA, Browne TR, Collins JF. Time course of carbamazepine autoinduction. The VA Cooperative Study No. 118 Group. *Neurology* 1989;39:592–594.
50. Cloyd JC, Remmel RP. Antiepileptic drug pharmacokinetics and interactions: impact on treatment of epilepsy. *Pharmacotherapy* 2000;20(8 Pt 2):139S–151S.
51. Bourgeois BFD, Wad N. Carbamazepine-10,11-diol steady-state serum levels and renal excretion during carbamazepine therapy in adults and children. *Ther Drug Monit* 1984;6:259–265.
52. Spina E. Carbamazepine. Chemistry, biotransformation, and pharmacokinetics. In: Levy RH, Mattson RH, Meldrum BS, et al., eds. *Antiepileptic drugs*, 5th ed. Philadelphia: Lippincott Williams & Wilkins, 2002:236–246.
53. Wurden CJ, Levy RH. Carbamazepine. Interactions with other drugs. In: Levy RH, Mattson RH, Meldrum BS, et al., eds. *Antiepileptic drugs*, 5th ed. Philadelphia: Lippincott Williams & Wilkins, 2002:247–261.
54. Coulam CB, Annegers JF. Do anticonvulsants reduce the efficacy of oral contraceptives? *Epilepsia* 1979;20:519–525.
55. Mattson RH, Cramer JA, Darney PH, et al. Use of contraceptives by women with epilepsy. *JAMA* 1986;256:238–240.
56. Rapport DJ, Calabrese JR. Interactions between carbamazepine and birth control pills. *Psychosomatics* 1989;30:462–484.
57. Back DJ, Orme ML. Pharmacokinetic drug interactions with oral contraceptives. *Clin Pharmacokinet* 1990;18:472–484.
58. Liporace JD. Women's issues in epilepsy. Menses, childbearing, and more. *Postgrad Med* 1997;102:123–135.
59. Bourgeois BFD. Important pharmacokinetic properties of antiepileptic drugs. *Epilepsia* 1995;36(Suppl 5):S1–S7.
60. Loiseau P. Carbamazepine. Clinical efficacy and use in epilepsy. In: Levy RH, Mattson RH, Meldrum BS, et al., eds. *Antiepileptic drugs*, 5th ed. Philadelphia: Lippincott Williams & Wilkins, 2002:262–272.
61. Callaghan N, Kenny RA, O'Neill B, et al. A prospective study between carbamazepine, phenytoin and sodium valproate as monotherapy in previously untreated and recently diagnosed patients with epilepsy. *J Neurol Neurosurg Psychiatry* 1985;48:639–644.
62. Kosteljanetz M, Christiansen J, Dam AM, et al. Carbamazepine vs phenytoin: a controlled trial in focal motor and generalized epilepsy. *Arch Neurol* 1979;36:22–24.
63. Hakkarainen H. Carbamazepine and diphenylhydantoin as monotherapy or in combination in the treatment of adult epilepsy. *Neurology* 1980;30:354.
64. Ramsay RE, Wilder BJ, Berger JR, et al. A double-blind study comparing carbamazepine with phenytoin as initial seizure therapy in adults. *Neurology* 1983;33:904–910.
65. Mattson RH, Cramer JA, Collins JK, et al. Comparison of carbamazepine, phenobarbital, phenytoin, and primidone in partial and secondarily generalized tonic-clonic seizures. *N Engl J Med* 1985;313:145–151.
66. Stein J. Carbamazepine versus phenytoin in young epileptic children. *Drug Ther* 1989;19:76–77.
67. Forsythe I, Butler R, Berg I, et al. Cognitive impairment in new cases of epilepsy randomly assigned to carbamazepine, phenytoin, and sodium valproate. *Dev Med Child Neurol* 1991;33:524–534.
68. Heller AJ, Chesterman P, Elwes RDC, et al. Phenobarbitone, phenytoin, carbamazepine, or sodium valproate for newly diagnosed adult epilepsy: a randomized comparative monotherapy trial. *J Neurol Neurosurg Psychiatry* 1995;58:44–50.
69. Mitchell WG, Chavez JM. Carbamazepine versus phenobarbital for partial seizures in children. *Epilepsia* 1987;28:56–60.
70. Rodin EA, Rim CS, Kitano H, et al. A comparison of the effectiveness of primidone versus carbamazepine in epileptic outpatients. *J Nerv Ment Dis* 1976;163:41–46.
71. Mattson RH, Cramer JA, Collins JF. A comparison of valproate with carbamazepine for the treatment of complex partial seizures and secondarily generalized tonic-clonic seizures. *N Engl J Med* 1992;327:765–771.
72. Mattson RH. Carbamazepine. In: Engel J, Pedley T, eds. *Epilepsy: a comprehensive textbook*. Philadelphia: Lippincott-Raven, 1997:1491–1502.

73. So E, Lai CW, Pellock J, et al. Safety and efficacy of valproate and carbamazepine in the treatment of complex partial seizures. *J Epilepsy* 1992;5:149–152.

74. Richens A, Davidson DLW, Cartlidge NEF, et al. A multicentre comparative trial of sodium valproate and carbamazepine in adult onset epilepsy. Adult EPITEG Collaborative Group. *J Neurol Neurosurg Psychiatry* 1994;57:682–687.

75. Hosking G. The paediatric EPITEG trial: a comparative multicentre clinical trial of sodium valproate and carbamazepine in newly diagnosed childhood epilepsy. In: Chadwick D, ed. *Proceedings of the fourth international symposium on valproate and epilepsy.* London: Royal Society of Medicine Services, 1989;71–80.

76. De Silva M, MacArdle B, McGowan M, et al. Randomized comparative monotherapy trial of phenobarbitone, phenytoin, carbamazepine or sodium valproate for newly diagnosed childhood epilepsy. *Lancet* 1996;347:709–713.

77. Brodie MJ, Richens A, Yuen AW. Double-blind comparison of lamotrigine and carbamazepine in newly diagnosed epilepsy. UK Lamotrigine/Carbamazepine Monotherapy Group. *Lancet* 1995;345:476–479.

78. Brodie MJ, Overstall PW, Giorgi L. Multicenter, double-blind, randomized comparison between lamotrigine and carbamazepine in elderly patients with newly diagnosed epilepsy. *Epilepsy Res* 1999;37:81–87.

79. Nieto-Barrera M, Brozmanova M, Capovilla G, et al. A comparison of monotherapy with lamotrigine or carbamazepine in patients with newly diagnosed partial epilepsy. *Epilepsy Res* 2001;46:145–155.

80. Dam M, Ekberg R, Loyning Y, et al. A double-blind study comparing oxcarbazepine and carbamazepine in patients with newly diagnosed, previously untreated epilepsy. *Epilepsy Res* 1989;3:70–76.

81. Privitera MD, Brodie MJ, Mattson RH, et al. Topiramate, carbamazepine and valproate monotherapy: double-blind comparison in newly diagnosed epilepsy. *Acta Neurol Scand* 2003;107:165–175.

82. Kälviäinen R, Aikia M, Saukkonen AM, et al. Vigabatrin vs carbamazepine monotherapy in patients with newly diagnosed epilepsy. A randomized, controlled study. *Arch Neurol* 1995;52:989–996.

83. Chadwick D. Safety and efficacy of vigabatrin and carbamazepine in newly diagnosed epilepsy: a multicenter randomized double-blind study. *Lancet* 1999;354:13–19.

84. Brodie MJ, Wroe SJ, Dean AD, et al. Efficacy and safety of remacemide versus carbamazepine in newly diagnosed epilepsy: comparison by sequential analysis. *Epilepsy Behav* 2002;3:140–146.

85. Chadwick DW, Anhut H, Greiner MJ, et al. A double-blind trial of gabapentin monotherapy for newly diagnosed partial seizures. *Neurology* 1998;51:1282–1288.

86. Kälviäinen R, Nousiäinen I, Mantyjarvi M, et al. Vigabatrin, a GABAergic antiepileptic drug, causes concentric visual defect. *Neurology* 1999;53:922–926.

87. Gilliam F. Optimizing health outcomes in active epilepsy. *Neurology* 2002;58(Suppl 5):S9–S20.

88. Pellock JM. Carbamazepine side effects in children and adults. *Epilepsia* 1987;28(Suppl 3):S64–S70.

89. Livingston S, Villamater C, Sakata Y, et al. Use of carbamazepine in epilepsy. Results in 87 patients. *JAMA* 1967;200:204–208.

90. Schain RJ, Ward JW, Guthrie D. Carbamazepine as an anticonvulsant in children. *Neurology* 1977;27:476–480.

91. Schoeman JF, Elyas AA, Brett EM, et al. Correlation between plasma carbamazepine-10,11-epoxide concentration and drug side effects in children with epilepsy. *Dev Med Child Neurol* 1984;26:756–764.

92. Holmes GL. Carbamazepine. Adverse effects. In: Levy RH, Mattson RH, Meldrum BS, et al, eds. *Antiepileptic drugs,* 5th ed. Philadelphia: Lippincott Williams & Wilkins, 2002:285–297.

93. Reynolds EH. Neurotoxicity of carbamazepine. *Adv Neurol* 1975;11:345-353.

94. Sillanpää M. Carbamazepine: Pharmacology and clinical uses. *Acta Neurol Scand Suppl* 1981;88:1–220.

95. Meador KJ, Loring DW, Hug K, et al. Comparative cognitive effects of anticonvulsants. *Neurology* 1990;40:391–394.

96. Dodrill CB, Troupin AS. Neuropsychological effects of carbamazepine and phenytoin: a reanalysis. *Neurology* 1991;41:141–143.

97. van der Meyden CH, Bartel PR, Sommers DK, et al. Effect of acute doses of controlled-release carbamazepine on clinical, psychomotor, electrophysiological, and cognitive parameters of brain function. *Epilepsia* 1992;33:335–342.

98. Crosley CJ, Swender PT. Dystonia associated with carbamazepine administration: experience in brain-damaged children. *Pediatrics* 1979;63:612–615.

99. Jacome D. Carbamazepine-induced dystonia. *JAMA* 1979;241:2263.

100. Bradbury AJ, Bentick B, Todd PJ. Dystonia associated with carbamazepine toxicity. *Postgrad Med J* 1982;58:525–526.

101. Shear NH, Spielberg SP. Anticonvulsant hypersensitivity syndrome. In vitro assessment of risk. *J Clin Invest* 1988;82:1826–1832.

102. Schlienger RG, Shear NH. Antiepileptic drug hypersensitivity syndrome. *Epilepsia* 1998;39(Suppl 7):S3–S7.

103. Schlienger RG, Shapiro LE, Shear NH. Lamotrigine-induced severe cutaneous adverse reactions. *Epilepsia* 1998;39(Suppl 7):S22–S26.

104. Alldredge BK, Knutsen AP, Ferriero D. Antiepileptic drug hypersensitivity syndrome. *Pediatr Neurol* 1994;10:169–171.

105. Bateman DE. Carbamazepine induced systemic lupus erythematosus: case report. *Br Med J* 1985;291:632–633.

106. McNicholl B. Carbamazepine induced systemic lupus erythematosus. *Br Med J* 1985;291:1125–1126.

107. De Giorgio CM, Rabinowicz AL, Olivas R. Carbamazepine-induced antinuclear antibodies and systemic lupus erythematosus-like syndrome. *Epilepsia* 1991;32:128–129.

108. Toepfer M, Sitter T, Lockmüller H, et al. Drug-induced systemic lupus erythematosus after 8 years of treatment with carbamazepine. *Eur J Clin Pharmacol* 1998;54:193–194.

109. Shuper A, Stahl B, Weitz R. Carbamazepine-induced hair loss. *Drug Intell Clin Pharm* 1985;19:924.

110. Salzman MB, Valderrama E, Sood SK. Carbamazepine and fatal eosinophilic myocarditis. *N Engl J Med* 1997;336:878–879.

111. Gilhus NE, Matre R. Carbamazepine effects on mononuclear blood cells in epileptic patients. *Acta Neurol Scand* 1986;74:181–185.

112. Killian JM. Tegretol in trigeminal neuralgia with special reference to hematopoietic adverse effects. *Headache* 1969;9:58–63.

113. Hart RG, Easton JD. Carbamazepine and hematological monitoring. *Ann Neurol* 1982;11:309–312.

114. Blackburn SC, Oliart AD, Garcia Rodriguez LA, et al. Antiepileptics and blood dyscrasias: a cohort study. *Pharmacotherapy* 1998;18:1277–1283.

115. Stephens WP, Coe JY, Baylis PH. Plasma arginine vasopressin concentrations and antidiuretic action of carbamazepine. *Br Med J* 1978;1:1445–1447.

116. Perucca E, Richens A. Water intoxication produced by carbamazepine and its reversal by phenytoin. *Br J Clin Pharmacol* 1980;9:302–304.

117. Appleby L. Rapid development of hyponatremia during low-dose carbamazepine therapy. *J Neurol Neurosurg Psychiatry* 1984;47:1138.

118. Lahr MB. Hyponatremia during carbamazepine therapy. *Clin Pharmacol Ther* 1985;37:693–696.

119. Bentsen KD, Gram L, Veje A. Serum thyroid hormones and blood folic acid during monotherapy with carbamazepine or valproate. A controlled study. *Acta Neurol Scand* 1983;67:235–241.

120. Ericsson UB, Bjerre I, Forsgren M, et al. Thyroglobulin and thyroid hormones in patients on long-term treatment with phenytoin, carbamazepine, and valproic acid. *Epilepsia* 1985;26:594–596.

121. Isojärvi JI, Pakarinen AJ, Myllylä VV. Thyroid function in epileptic patients treated with carbamazepine. *Arch Neurol* 1989;46:1175–1178.

122. Isojärvi JI, Pakarinen AJ, Ylipalosaari PJ, et al. Serum hormones in male epileptic patients receiving anticonvulsant medication. *Arch Neurol* 1990;47:670–676.

123. Liewendahl K, Majuri H, Helenius T. Thyroid function tests in patients on long-term treatment with various anticonvulsant drugs. *Clin Endocrinol* 1978;8:185–191.

124. Strandjord RE, Aanerud S, Myking OL, et al. Influence of carbamazepine on serum thyroxine and triiodothyronine in patients with epilepsy. *Acta Neurol Scand* 1981;63:111–121.

125. De Luca F, Arrigo T, Pandullo E, et al. Changes in thyroid function tests induced by 2 month carbamazepine treatment in L-thyroxine-substituted hypothyroid children. *Eur J Pediatr* 1986;145:77–79.

126. Toone BK, Wheeler M, Nanjee M. Sex hormones, sexual activity and plasma anticonvulsivant levels in male epileptics. *J Neurol Neurosurg Psychiatry* 1983;46:824–826.

127. Connell JMC, Rapeport WG, Beastall GH, et al. Changes in circulating androgens during short term carbamazepine therapy. *Br J Clin Pharmacol* 1984;17:347–351.

128. Franceschi M, Perego L, Cavagnini F, et al. Effects of long-term antiepileptic therapy on the hypothalamic-pituitary axis in man. *Epilepsia* 1984;25:46–52.

129. Dana-Haeri J, Oxley J, Richens A. Pituitary responsiveness to gonadotrophin-releasing and thyrotrophin-releasing hormones in epileptic patients receiving carbamazepine or phenytoin. *Clin Endocrinol* 1984;20:163–168.

130. Bonuccelli U, Murialdo G, Martino E, et al. Effects of carbamazepine on prolactin secretion in normal subjects and in epileptic subjects. *Clin Neuropharmacol* 1985;8:165–174.

131. Isojärvi JI, Pakarinen AJ, Myllylä VV. Effects of carbamazepine therapy on serum sex hormone levels in male patients with epilepsy. *Epilepsia* 1988;29:781–786.

132. Isojärvi JI, Myllylä VV, Pakarinen AJ. Effects of carbamazepine therapy on pituitary responsiveness to luteinizing hormone-releasing hormone, thyrotropin-releasing hormone, and metoclopramide in epileptic patients. *Epilepsia* 1989;30:50–56.

133. Herzog AG, Levesque LA. Testosterone, free testosterone, non-sex hormone-binding globulin-bound testosterone, and free androgen index: which testosterone measurement is most relevant to reproductive and sexual function in men with epilepsy? *Arch Neurol* 1992;49:133–135.

134. Silveira DC, Souza EAP, Carvalho JF, et al. Interictal hyposexuality in male patients with epilepsy. *Arq Neuropsiquiatr* 2001;59:23–28.

135. Lindhoult D, Hoppener RJ, Meinardi H. Teratogenicity of antiepileptic drug combinations with special emphasis on epoxidation (of carbamazepine). *Epilepsia* 1984;25:77–83.

136. Delgado-Escueta AV, Janz D. Consensus guidelines: preconception counseling, management, and care of the pregnant woman with epilepsy. *Neurology* 1992;42(Suppl 5):149–160.

137. Rosa F. Spina bifida in infants of women treated with carbamazepine during pregnancy. *N Engl J Med* 1991;324:674–677.

138. Little BB, Santos-Ramos R, Newell JF, et al. Megadose carbamazepine during the period of neural tube closure. *Obstet Gynecol* 1993;82(4 Pt 2 Suppl):705–708.

139. Kallen B. Maternal carbamazepine and infant spina bifida. *Reprod Toxicol* 1994;8:203–205.

140. Yerby MS. Clinical care of pregnant women with epilepsy: neural tube defects and folic acid supplementation. *Epilepsia* 2003;44 (Suppl 3):S33–S40.

141. Matalon S, Schechtman S, Goldweig G, et al. The teratogenic effect of carbamazepine: a meta-analysis of 1255 exposures. *Reprod Toxicol* 2002;16:9–17.

142. Morrell MJ. Guidelines for the care of women with epilepsy. *Neurology* 1998;51(Suppl 4):S21–S27.

143. Oakley GP Jr. Folic-acid-preventable spina bifida and anencephaly. *Bull World Health Organ* 1998;76(Suppl 2):116–117.

144. Yerby MS. Problems and management of the pregnant woman with epilepsy. *Epilepsia* 1987;28(Suppl 3):S29–S36.

145. Easter D, O'Bryan-Tear CG, Verity C. Weight gain with valproate or carbamazepine–a reappraisal. *Seizure* 1997;6:121–125.

146. Hogan RE, Bertrand ME, Deaton RL, et al. Total percentage body weight changes during add-on therapy with tiagabine, carbamazepine and phenytoin. *Epilepsy Res* 2000;41:23–28.

147. Jallon P, Picard F. Bodyweight gain and anticonvulsants: a comparative review. *Drug Saf* 2001;24:969–978.

148. Cepelak I, Zanic Grubisic T, Mandusic A, et al. Valproate plus carbamazepine comedication changes hepatic enzyme activities in sera of epileptic children. *Clin Chim Acta* 1998;276:121–127.

149. Horowitz S, Patwardhan R, Marcus E. Hepatotoxic reactions associated with carbamazepine therapy. *Epilepsia* 1988;29:149–154.

150. Zucker P, Daum F, Cohen MI. Fatal carbamazepine hepatitis. *J Pediatr* 1977;91:667–668.

151. Weaver DF, Camfield R, Fraser A. Massive carbamazepine overdose: clinical and pharmacologic observations in five episodes. *Neurology* 1988;38:755–759.

152. Boesen F, Andersen EB, Jensen EK, Ladefoged SD. Cardiac conduction disturbances during carbamazepine therapy. *Acta Neurol Scand* 1983;68:49–52.

153. Pluskiewicz W, Nowakowska J. Bone status after long-term anticonvulsant therapy in epileptic patients: evaluation using quantitative ultrasound of calcaneus and phalanges. *Ultrasound Med Biol* 1997;23:553–558.

154. Valimaki MJ, Tiihonen M, Laitinen K, et al. Bone mineral density measured by dual-energy x-ray absorptiometry and novel markers of bone formation and resorption in patients on antiepileptic drugs. *J Bone Miner Res* 1994;9:631–637.

155. Stephen LJ, McLellan AR, Harrison JH, et al. Bone density and antiepileptic drugs: a case-controlled study. *Seizure* 1999;8: 339–342.

156. Pedrera JD, Canal ML, Carvajal J, et al. Influence of vitamin D administration on bone ultrasound measurements in patients on anticonvulsant therapy. *Eur J Clin Invest* 2000;30:895–899.

157. Sato Y, Kondo I, Ishida S, et al. Decreased bone mass and increased bone turnover with valproate therapy in adults with epilepsy. *Neurology* 2001;57:445–449.

158. Morrell MJ. Reproductive and metabolic disorders in women with epilepsy. *Epilepsia* 2003;44(Suppl 4):11–20.

159. Tjellesen L, Nilas L, Christiansen C. Does carbamazepine cause disturbances in calcium metabolism in epileptic patients? *Acta Neurol Scand* 1983;68:13–19.

160. Tjellesen L, Gotfredsen A, Christiansen C. Effect of vitamin D2 and D3 on bone-mineral content in carbamazepine-treated epileptic patients. *Acta Neurol Scand* 1983;68:424–428.

161. Hoikka V, Alhava EM, Karjalainen P, et al. Carbamazepine and bone mineral metabolism. *Acta Neurol Scand* 1984;70:77–80.

162. Filardi S, Guerreiro CA, Magna LA, et al. Bone mineral density, vitamin D and anticonvulsant therapy. *Arq Neuropsiquiatr* 2000; 58:616–620.

163. Valmadrid C, Voorhees C, Litt B, et al. Practice patterns of neurologists regarding bone and mineral effects of antiepileptic drug therapy. *Arch Neurol* 2001;58:1369–1374.

164. Farhat G, Yamout B, Mikati MA, et al. Effect of antiepileptic drugs on bone density in ambulatory patients. *Neurology* 2002;58: 1348–1353.

165. Tsukahara H, Kimura K, Todori Y, et al. Bone mineral status in ambulatory pediatric patients on long-term anti-epileptic drug therapy. *Pediatr Int* 2002;44:247–253.

166. Andress DL, Ozuna J, Tirschwell D, et al. Antiepileptic drug-induced bone loss in young male patients who have seizures. *Arch Neurol* 2002;59:781–786.

167. Feldkamp J, Becker A, Witte OW, et al. Long-term anticonvulsant therapy leads to low bone mineral density–evidence for direct drug effects of phenytoin and carbamazepine on human osteoblast-like cells. *Exp Clin Endocrinol Diabetes* 2000;108:37–43.

168. Sheth RD, Wesolowski CA, Jacob JC, et al. Effect of carbamazepine and valproate on bone mineral density. *J Pediatr* 1995; 127:256–262.

169. Akin R, Okutan V, Sarici U, et al. Evaluation of bone mineral density in children receiving antiepileptic drugs. *Pediatr Neurol* 1998;19:129–131.

170. Erbayat Altay E, Serdaroglu A, Tumer L, et al. Evaluation of bone mineral metabolism in children receiving carbamazepine and valproic acid. *J Pediatr Endocrinol Metab* 2000;13:933–939.

171. Rieger-Wettengl G, Tutlewski B, Stabrey A, et al. Analysis of the musculoskeletal system in children and adolescents receiving anticonvulsant monotherapy with valproic acid or carbamazepine. *Pediatrics* 2001;108:E107.

172. Lidgren L, Walloe A. Incidence of fracture in epileptics. *Acta Orthop Scand* 1977;48:356–361.

173. Annegers JF, Melton LJ III, Sun CA, et al. Risk of age-related fractures in patients with unprovoked seizures. *Epilepsia* 1989;30: 348–355.

174. Cummings SR, Nevitt MC, Browner WS, et al. Risk factors for hip fracture in white women. Study of osteoporotic fracture research group. *N Engl J Med* 1995;332:767–773.

175. Vestergaard P, Tigaran S, Rejnmark L, et al. Fracture risk is increased in epilepsy. *Acta Neurol Scand* 1999;99:269–275.

176. Sillanpää ML. Carbamazepine and oxcarbazepine. In: Wyllie E, ed. *The treatment of epilepsy: principles and practice*, 3rd ed. Philadelphia: Lippincott Williams & Wilkins, 2001:821–842.

177. Porter RJ. How to initiate and maintain carbamazepine therapy in children and adults. *Epilepsia* 1987;28(Suppl 3):S59–S63.

178. Chadwick D, Shaw MD, Foy P, et al. Serum anticonvulsant concentrations and the risk of drug induced skin eruptions. *J Neurol Neurosurg Psychiatry* 1984;47:642–644.

179. Strandjord RE, Johannessen SI. Single-drug therapy with carbamazepine in patients with epilepsy: serum levels and clinical effect. *Epilepsia* 1980;21:655–662.

180. Parsonage M. Treatment with carbamazepine: adults. *Adv Neurol* 1975;11:221–234.

181. Johannessen SI, Henriksen O. Comparison of the serum concentration profiles of Tegretol and two new slow-release preparations. *Adv Epileptol* 1987;16:421–423.

182. Ryan SW, Forsythe I, Hartley R, et al. Slow release carbamazepine in treatment of poorly controlled seizures. *Arch Dis Child* 1990; 65:930–935.

183. Dodson WE. Carbamazepine efficacy and utilization in children. *Epilepsia* 1987;28(Suppl 3):S17–S24.

184. Battino D, Croci D, Rossini A, et al. Serum carbamazepine concentrations in elderly patients: a case-matched pharmacokinetic evaluation based on therapeutic drug monitoring data. *Epilepsia* 2003;44:923–929.

185. Meyer MC, Straughn AB, Jarvi EJ, et al. The bioinequivalence of carbamazepine tablets with a history of clinical failures. *Pharm Res* 1992;9:1612–1616.

186. The Tegretol OROS Osmotic Release Delivery System Study Group. Double-blind crossover comparison of Tegretol-XR and Tegretol in patients with epilepsy. *Neurology* 1995;45: 1703–1707.

187. Perucca E, Gram L, Avanzini G, et al. Antiepileptic drugs as a cause of worsening of seizures. *Epilepsia* 1998;39:5–17.

188. Guerrini R, Belmonte A, Genton P. Antiepileptic drug-induced worsening of seizures in children. *Epilepsia* 1998;39(Suppl 3): S2–S10.

189. Shields WD, Saslow E. Myoclonic, atonic, and absence seizures following institution of carbamazepine therapy in children. *Neurology* 1983;33:1487–1489.

190. Snead OC III, Hosey LC. Exacerbation of seizures in children by carbamazepine. *N Engl J Med* 1985;313:916–921.

191. Lerman P. Seizures induced or aggravated by anticonvulsants. *Epilepsia* 1986;27:706–710.

192. Dhuna A, Pascual-Leone A, Talwar D. Exacerbation of partial seizures and onset of nonepileptic myoclonus with carbamazepine. *Epilepsia* 1991;32:275–278.

193. Liporace JD, Sperling MR, Dichter MA. Absence seizures and carbamazepine in adults. *Epilepsia* 1994;35:1026–1028.

194. Lloyd P, Flesch G, Dieterle W. Clinical pharmacology and pharmacokinetics of oxcarbazepine. *Epilepsia* 1994;35(Suppl 3): S10–S13.

195. Degen PH, Flesch G, Cardot JM, et al. The influence of food on the disposition of the antiepileptic oxcarbazepine and its major metabolites in healthy volunteers. *Biopharm Drug Dispos* 1994; 15:519–526.

196. Faigle JW, Menge GP. Metabolic characteristics of oxcarbazepine and their beneficial implications for enzyme induction and drug interactions. *Behav Neurol* 1990;3:21–30.

197. Grant SM, Faulds D. Oxcarbazepine: a review of its pharmacology and therapeutic potential in epilepsy, trigeminal neuralgia and affective disorders. *Drugs* 1992;43:873–888.

198. Theisohn M, Heimann G. Disposition of the antiepileptic oxcarbazepine and its metabolites in healthy volunteers. *Eur J Clin Pharmacol* 1982;22:545–551.

199. Kristensen O, Klitgaard NA, Jönsson B, et al. Pharmacokinetics of 10-OH-carbazepine, the main metabolite of the antiepileptic oxcarbazepine, from serum and saliva concentrations. *Acta Neurol Scand* 1983;68:145–150.

200. Gram L. Oxcarbazepine. In: Engel J Jr, Pedley TA, eds. *Epilepsy: a comprehensive textbook*. Philadelphia: Lippincott-Raven Publishers, 1997:1541–1546.

201. Hachad H, Ragueneau-Majlessi I, Levy RH. New antiepileptic drugs: review on drug interactions. *Ther Drug Monit* 2002;24: 91–103.

202. Larkin JG, McKee PJ, Forrest G, et al. Lack of enzyme induction with oxcarbazepine (600 mg daily) in healthy subjects. *Br J Clin Pharmacol* 1991;31:65–71.

203. Rabasseda X. Oxcarbazepine: anticonvulsant profile and safety. *Drugs Today* 2001;37:333–355.

204. Patsalos PN, Perucca E. Clinically important drug interactions in epilepsy: general features and interactions between antiepileptic drugs. *Lancet Neurol* 2003;2:347–356.

205. Reinikainen KJ, Keranen T, Halonen T, et al. Comparison of oxcarbazepine and carbamazepine: a double-blind study. *Epilepsy Res* 1987;1:284–289.

206. Bill PA, Vigonius U, Pohlmann H, et al. A double-blind controlled clinical trial of oxcarbazepine versus phenytoin in adults with previously untreated epilepsy. *Epilepsy Res* 1997;27: 195–204.

207. Christe W, Krämer G, Vigonius U, et al. A double-blind controlled clinical trial: oxcarbazepine versus sodium valproate in adults with newly diagnosed epilepsy. *Epilepsy Res* 1997;26: 451–460.

208. Beydoun A, Sachdeo RC, Rosenfeld WE, et al. Oxcarbazepine monotherapy for partial-onset seizures: a multicenter, double-blind, clinical trial. *Neurology* 2000;54:2245–2251.

209. Sachdeo R, Beydoun A, Schachter S, et al. Oxcarbazepine (Trileptal) as monotherapy in patients with partial seizures. *Neurology* 2001;57:864–871.

210. Schachter SC, Vazquez B, Fisher RS, et al. Oxcarbazepine: double-blind, randomized, placebo-control, monotherapy trial for partial seizures. *Neurology* 1999;52:732–737.

211. Guerreiro MM, Vigonius U, Pohlmann H, et al. A double-blind controlled clinical trial of oxcarbazepine versus phenytoin in children and adolescents with epilepsy. *Epilepsy Res* 1997;27: 205–213.

212. Serdaroglu G, Kurul S, Tutuncuoglu S, et al. Oxcarbazepine in the treatment of childhood epilepsy. *Pediatr Neurol* 2003;28:37–41.

213. Guerreiro C. Sustained seizure freedom with oxcarbazepine (Trileptal®) monotherapy over 2 years in newly diagnosed adults and children with partial and generalized tonic-clonic seizures. *Epilepsia* 2003;44(Suppl 8):116.

214. Barcs G, Walker EB, Elger CE, et al. Oxcarbazepine placebo-controlled, dose-ranging trial in refractory partial epilepsy. *Epilepsia* 2000;41:1597–1607.

215. Glauser TA, Nigro M, Sachdeo R, et al. Adjunctive therapy with oxcarbazepine in children with partial seizures. The Oxcarbazepine Pediatric Study Group. *Neurology* 2000;54:2237–2244.

216. Friis ML, Kristensen O, Boas J, et al. Therapeutic experiences with 947 epileptic out-patients in oxcarbazepine treatment. *Acta Neurol Scand* 1993;87:224–227.

217. Beran RG. Cross-reactive skin eruption with both carbamazepine and oxcarbazepine. *Epilepsia* 1993;34:163–165.

218. van Parys JAP, Meinardi H. Survey of 260 epileptic patients treated with oxcarbazepine (Trileptal) on a named-patient basis. *Epilepsy Res* 1994;19:79–85.

219. Wellington K, Goa KL. Oxcarbazepine: an update of its efficacy in the management of epilepsy. *CNS Drugs* 2001;15:137–163.

220. Guerreiro M. Better seizure control and tolerability over the long-term with oxcarbazepine (Trileptal) monotherapy compared with phenytoin in newly diagnosed children and adolescents with partial and generalized tonic-clonic seizures. *Epilepsia* 2003;44(Suppl 8):148–149.

221. Kutluay E, McCague K, D'Souza J, et al. Safety and tolerability of oxcarbazepine in elderly patients with epilepsy. *Epilepsy Behav* 2003;4:175–80.

222. Van Amelsvoort T, Bakshi R, Devaux CB, et al. Hyponatremia associated with carbamazepine and oxcarbazepine therapy: a review. *Epilepsia* 1994;35:181–188.

223. Sachdeo RC, Wasserstein AD, D'Souza J. Oxcarbazepine (Trileptal) effect on serum sodium. *Epilepsia* 1999;40(Suppl 7):103.

224. Beydoun A, Kutluay E. Oxcarbazepine. *Expert Opin Pharmacother* 2001;3:59–71.

225. Wallace SJ. Newer antiepileptic drugs: advantages and disadvantages. *Brain Dev* 2001;23:277–283.

226. Krämer G. Oxcarbazepine: adverse effects. In: Levy RH, Mattson RH, Meldrum BS, et al, eds. *Antiepileptic drugs*, 5th ed. Philadelphia: Lippincott Williams & Wilkins, 2002:479–486.

227. Holtmann M, Krause M, Opp J, et al. Oxcarbazepine-induced hyponatremia and the regulation of serum sodium after replacing carbamazepine with oxcarbazepine in children. *Neuropediatrics* 2002;33:298–300.

228. Sachdeo RC, Wasserstein A, Mesenbrink PJ, et al. Effects of oxcarbazepine on sodium concentration and water handling. *Ann Neurol* 2002;51:613–620.
229. Nielsen OA, Johannessen AC, Bardrum B. Oxcarbazepine-induced hyponatremia, a cross-sectional study. *Epilepsy Res* 1988;2:269–271.
230. Pedersen B, D'Souza J. Oxcarbazepine (Trileptal) therapy results in no clinically significant changes in weight [abstract]. *Epilepsia* 2002;43(Suppl 8):149.
231. Parys JV, D'Souza J. Oxcarbazepine (Trileptal) has no effect on vital signs and electrocardiograms [abstract]. *Epilepsia* 2002;43 (Suppl 8):149.
232. Pylvanen V, Knip M, Pakarinen AJ, et al. Fasting serum insulin and lipid levels in men with epilepsy. *Neurology* 2003;60:571–574.
233. Kaaja E, Kaaja R, Hiilesmamaa V. Major malformations in offspring of women with epilepsy. *Neurology* 2003;60: 575–579.
234. Rabinowicz A, Meischenguiser R, D'Giano CH, et al. Report of a single-centre pregnancy registry of AEDs: focus on outcomes with oxcarbazepine (Trileptal). *Epilepsia* 2002;4(Suppl 8):159.

235. Aldenkamp AP, Krom MD, Reijs R. Newer antiepileptic drugs and cognitive issues. *Epilepsia* 2003;44:21–29.
236. Schachter SC. Oxcarbazepine: clinical efficacy and use in epilepsy. In: Levy RH, Mattson RH, Meldrum BS, et al, eds. *Antiepileptic drugs*, 5th ed. Philadelphia: Lippincott Williams & Wilkins, 2002: 470–475.
237. Perucca E. Marketed new antiepileptic drugs: are they better than old-generation agents? *Ther Drug Monit* 2002;24:74–80.
238. Johannessen SI, Battino D, Berry DJ, et al. Therapeutic drug monitoring of new antiepileptic drugs. *Ther Drug Monit* 2003;25: 347–363.
239. Williams J, Bialer M, Johannessen SI, et al. Interlaboratory variability in the quantification of new generation antiepileptic drugs based on external quality assessment data. *Epilepsia* 2003; 44:40–45.
240. Shorvon S. Oxcarbazepine: a review. *Seizure* 2000;9:75–79.
241. Kalis MM, Huff NA. Oxcarbazepine, an antiepileptic agent. *Clin Ther* 2001;23:680–700.

Valproate

54

Blaise F. D. Bourgeois

HISTORICAL BACKGROUND

The anticonvulsant effect of valproic acid, or valproate (VPA), was discovered serendipitously when the agent was used as a solvent for compounds tested in an animal model of seizures (1). VPA has been used in the treatment of epilepsy for more than 30 years (2). In the United States, VPA was approved in 1978. Since then, it has been regarded as one of the major antiepileptic drugs (AEDs), distinguished from previous agents by its broad spectrum of activity against many seizure types as well as by its relatively low sedative effect. In addition to being the first agent to be highly effective against several primarily generalized seizure types, such as absences, myoclonic seizures, and tonic-clonic seizures, VPA was found to be effective in the treatment of partial seizures, Lennox-Gastaut syndrome, infantile spasms, neonatal seizures, and febrile seizures. Although VPA is also used in the treatment of affective disorders, migraine headaches, and Sydenham chorea (3), these indications will not be included in the present discussion.

CHEMISTRY AND MECHANISM OF ACTION

Valproate (MW 144.21; Fig. 54.1), a short-chain, branched fatty acid, is a colorless liquid with low solubility in water. Other forms include: (a) sodium valproate (MW 166.19), a highly water-soluble and highly hygroscopic white, crystalline material; (b) sodium hydrogen divalproate (divalproex sodium), a complex composed of equal parts of VPA and sodium valproate (Fig. 54.1); and (c) magnesium valproate, a divalproate salt. The antiepileptic activity of VPA, demonstrated in several animal models (4,5), includes protection against maximal electroshock-induced seizures; against seizures induced chemically by pentylenetetrazol, bicuculline, glutamic acid, kainic acid, strychnine, ouabain, nicotine, and intramuscular penicillin; and against seizures induced by kindling (6). This broad spectrum of efficacy of VPA in animal models suggests that the agent is effective in both preventing the spread and lowering the threshold of seizures. Although several effects of VPA have been demonstrated at the cellular level, the precise mechanism underlying the antiepileptic effect of the agent has not been identified, and more than one mechanism may be involved. Identified mechanisms include potentiation of γ-aminobutyric acid (GABA)ergic function, inhibition of γ-hydroxybutyric acid formation, reduction of excitation mediated by glutamate receptors, and inhibition of voltage-sensitive sodium channels (7). It is not known to what extent any of these actions contributes to clinical seizure protection by VPA.

ABSORPTION, DISTRIBUTION, AND METABOLISM

The main pharmacokinetic parameters of VPA are summarized in Chapter 45, Table 45.2. Different preparations of VPA are available, although not all are available in any given country. Oral preparations of VPA include VPA capsules, tablets, and syrup (immediate-release); enteric-coated tablets of sodium valproate or sodium hydrogen divalproate (divalproex sodium); divalproex sodium enteric-coated sprinkles; slow-release oral preparations; magnesium valproate; and valpromide (the amide of VPA). VPA suppositories and a parenteral formulation of sodium valproate for intravenous (IV) use are also available. The bioavailability of oral preparations of VPA is virtually complete compared with that of the IV route (8). The purpose of the enteric coating of tablets is to prevent gastric irritation associated with release of VPA in the stomach. Compared with oral syrup, the relative bioavailability of VPA suppositories was found to be 80% in volunteers (9). In a study of patients treated chronically with VPA, administration of VPA suppositories was well tolerated for several days, and the bioavailability was the same as that of the oral preparations (10).

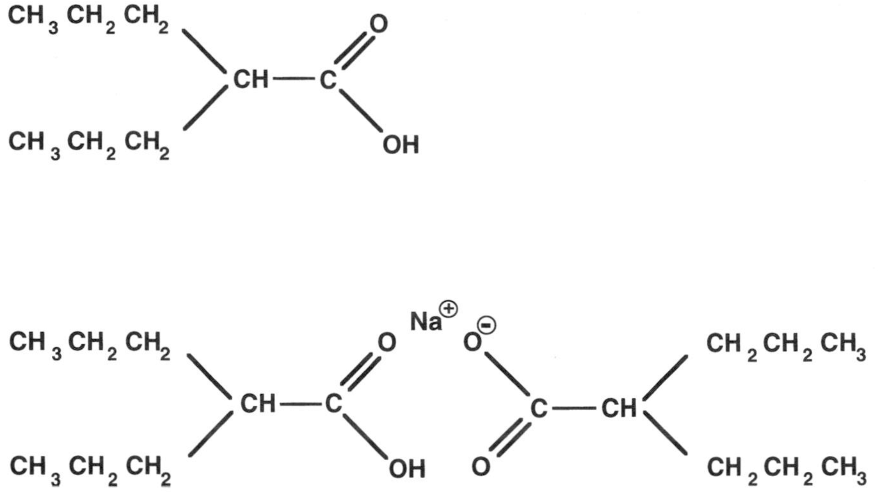

Figure 54.1 Structural formulas for valproic acid (N-dipropylacetic acid) and sodium hydrogen divalproate (divalproex sodium).

The rate of absorption of VPA after oral administration is variable, depending on the formulation. Administration of syrup or uncoated regular tablets or capsules is followed by rapid absorption and peak levels within 2 hours. Absorption from enteric-coated tablets is delayed but rapid. The onset of absorption varies as a function of the state of gastric emptying at the time of ingestion, and peak levels may be reached only 3 to 8 hours after oral ingestion of enteric-coated tablets (11-13; Chapter 45, Fig. 45.1). Therefore, in patients treated chronically with enteric-coated VPA, the true trough level may occur in the late morning or early afternoon (10). The bioavailability of enteric-coated sprinkles of divalproex sodium was compared with that of VPA syrup in 12 children, with no difference noted between the two formulations (14). However, the average time to maximal VPA concentrations was longer for sprinkles (4.2 hours) than for syrup (0.9 hours). With the IV formulation, peak VPA serum levels are reached at the end of the recommended infusion time of 60 minutes.

The volume of distribution of VPA is relatively small (0.13 to 0.19 L/kg in adults and 0.20 to 0.30 L/kg in children). VPA is highly bound to serum proteins; this binding appears to be saturable at therapeutic concentrations, with the free fraction of VPA increasing as the total concentration increases (15): 7% at 50 mg/L, 9% at 75 mg/L, 15% at 100 mg/L, 22% at 125 mg/L, and 30% at 150 mg/L. On the basis of these values, with an only three-fold increase in the total concentration of VPA, from 50 to 150 mg/L, the free level of VPA would increase more than 10 times, from 3.5 to 45 mg/L. Accordingly, a curvilinear relationship between VPA maintenance dose and total steady-state concentrations was found, with relatively smaller increases in concentrations at higher doses (16). The elimination half-life of VPA varies as a function of comedication. In the absence of inducing drugs, the half-life in adults is 13 to 16 hours (11,17), whereas in adults receiving polytherapy with inducing drugs, the average half-life is 9 hours (8). In children, the half-life is slightly shorter. Cloyd and colleagues

(18) reported an average half-life of 11.6 hours in children receiving monotherapy and 7.0 hours in those receiving polytherapy. Newborns eliminate VPA slowly; the half-life in this population is longer than 20 hours (19).

The most abundant metabolites of VPA are glucuronide and 3-oxo-VPA, which represent about 40% and 33%, respectively, of the urinary excretion of a VPA dose (20). Two desaturated metabolites of VPA, 2-ene-VPA and 4-ene-VPA, have anticonvulsant activity that is similar in potency to that of VPA itself (21). Because there is delayed but significant accumulation of 2-ene-VPA in the brain and because it is cleared more slowly than VPA (22), the formation of 2-ene-VPA provides a possible explanation for the discrepancy between the time courses of VPA concentrations and antiepileptic activity (23). It appears that 2-ene-VPA does not have the pronounced embryotoxicity (24) and hepatotoxicity (25) of 4-ene-VPA. Both are produced by the action of cytochrome P450 enzymes, which are induced by certain other AEDs (20,26). This may explain the increased risk for hepatotoxicity in patients receiving VPA concomitantly with these agents (27). However, elevation of 4-ene-VPA levels has not yet been found in patients with VPA hepatotoxicity, short-term adverse effects, or hyperammonemia (28).

DRUG INTERACTIONS

Pharmacokinetic interactions with VPA fall into three categories, based on the following features: (a) the metabolism of VPA is sensitive to enzymatic induction; (b) VPA itself can inhibit the metabolism of other agents; and (c) VPA has a high affinity for serum proteins and can displace other agents or be displaced from proteins (29–31). Concomitant administration of enzyme-inducing drugs has been repeatedly shown to lower VPA levels relative to the dose (32). Carbamazepine (33–35) and phenytoin (35) lower VPA levels by one-third to one-half, or even more, in children (36–38). When children receiving polytherapy discontinued treatment with other agents, VPA levels increased 122% after withdrawal of phenytoin, 67% after withdrawal of phenobarbital, and 50% after withdrawal of carbamazepine (39). In contrast, levels of VPA are increased by coadministration of felbamate: 28% with felbamate 1200 mg per day and 54% with felbamate 2400 mg per day (40,41). According to one study, clobazam may significantly reduce the clearance of VPA (42).

VPA affects the kinetics of other drugs either by enzymatic inhibition or by displacement from serum proteins. Phenobarbital levels have been found to increase by 57% (43) to 81% (44) after the addition of VPA. Levels of ethosuximide can also be raised by the addition of VPA, mostly in the presence of additional AEDs (45). Although VPA does not increase levels of carbamazepine itself, levels of the active metabolite carbamazepine-10,11-epoxide may double (46,47). Elimination of lamotrigine is markedly inhibited by VPA, resulting in a two-to three-fold prolongation of the lamotrigine half-life (48). Although this is a competitive interaction that is likely to be rapidly reversible upon discontinuation of VPA, the inhibition seems to persist even at low VPA concentrations (49,50). A pharmacokinetic interaction occurs between VPA and phenytoin, because both agents have a high affinity for serum proteins. VPA increases the free fraction of phenytoin (51,52). Thus, in the presence of VPA, total phenytoin concentrations in the usual therapeutic range may be associated with clinical toxicity. In contrast to inducing AEDs, VPA is not associated with oral contraceptive failure (53).

EFFICACY

Very early it became apparent that VPA is a highly effective first-line agent for the treatment of primarily generalized idiopathic seizures, such as absence seizures, generalized tonic-clonic seizures, and myoclonic seizures (54). The indication for VPA when it was first released in North America in 1978 was for treatment of absence seizures. In patients with typical and atypical absence seizures, a reduction of spike-and-wave discharges was repeatedly demonstrated (55–58). In two studies, comparison of VPA and ethosuximide for the treatment of absence seizures showed equal efficacy for the two agents (59,60). It appears that absence seizures are more likely to be fully controlled when they occur alone than when they are mixed with another seizure type (61,39). Overall, VPA appears to be somewhat less effective against atypical or "complex" absences than against simple absences (62,63). VPA can also be used effectively in patients with recurrent absence status (64).

VPA was found to be highly effective in the treatment of certain generalized convulsive seizures (65–68). Among 42 patients with intractable seizures, generalized tonic-clonic seizures were fully controlled in 14 patients by add-on VPA therapy (39). VPA was compared with phenytoin in 61 previously untreated patients with generalized tonic-clonic, clonic, or tonic seizures (69). When seizures occurring before therapeutic plasma drug levels had been reached were discounted, seizures were brought under control in 82% of VPA-treated patients, versus 76% of those treated with phenytoin. In a randomized comparison of VPA and phenytoin in patients with previously untreated tonic-clonic seizures, a 2-year remission was achieved in 27 of 37 patients receiving VPA and in 22 of 39 patients receiving phenytoin (68). Monotherapy with VPA was assessed in two studies of patients with primary (or idiopathic) generalized epilepsies (61,70). Among patients who had generalized tonic-clonic seizures only, complete seizure control was achieved in 51 of 70 patients (70) and in 39 of 44 patients (61), respectively. VPA monotherapy in children with generalized tonic-clonic seizures was also found to be highly effective (71).

Currently, VPA is the agent of first choice for most myoclonic seizures, particularly for those occurring in patients with primary or idiopathic generalized epilepsies (61,62,70). In a group of patients with primary generalized epilepsy given VPA monotherapy, 22 patients had myoclonic seizures and 20 of those experienced at least one other seizure type, either absence or tonic-clonic. The myoclonic seizures were controlled by VPA monotherapy in 18 of the 22 patients (61). Patients with juvenile myoclonic epilepsy have an excellent response to VPA (72), which remains an agent of first choice for this condition. Benign myoclonic epilepsy of infancy, which belongs to the group of primary or idiopathic generalized epilepsies, also responds well to treatment with VPA (71). Some success has been achieved with VPA in patients with postanoxic intention myoclonus (73,74). A combination of VPA and clonazepam is often used to treat the myoclonic and tonic-clonic seizures associated with severe progressive myoclonus epilepsy (75).

Like all other AEDs, VPA is less effective in the treatment of generalized encephalopathic epilepsies of infancy and childhood, such as infantile spasms and Lennox-Gastaut syndrome. In a series of patients treated with VPA, 38 had myoclonic astatic epilepsy—a term used by the authors synonymously with Lennox-Gastaut syndrome (62). Seven patients became and remained seizure free with VPA therapy. A 50% to 80% improvement was achieved in one third of patients, and other AEDs were withdrawn or reduced (62). In the same series, seizures were fully controlled in three of six patients with myoclonic absence epilepsy, all of whom were receiving combination therapy.

Reports on the use of VPA for the treatment of infantile spasms include small numbers of patients (76–78), or patients receiving corticotropin and VPA simultaneously. With VPA used as the first agent, eight of 19 infants experienced good seizure control and did not require corticotropin treatment (79). The patients who experienced an initial failure with VPA or corticotropin were switched to the other agent. Comparison of the two groups revealed a tendency toward a better response with corticotropin, but the incidence and severity of side effects was lower with VPA. A low VPA dose of 20 mg/kg per day was used in a series of 18 infants with infantile spasms not previously treated with corticotropin (80). In 12 of these patients, the short-term results were described as good to excellent. On follow-up, seven patients had residual seizure activity. The authors concluded that the efficacy of VPA was similar to that of corticotropin and that VPA was associated with fewer side effects.

The first direct comparison of VPA with carbamazepine for the treatment of partial seizures was probably an open study of 31 previously untreated adults (81). Seizure control was reported in 11 patients receiving VPA and eight patients receiving carbamazepine. In a prospective study of 79 patients with previously untreated simple partial or complex partial seizures, a comparison of carbamazepine, phenytoin, and VPA as monotherapy revealed no difference in efficacy among the three agents (82). A retrospective study of VPA monotherapy in 30 patients with simple partial and complex partial seizures in whom previous drugs had failed showed a remarkable response (83). Seizure control was achieved in 12 patients, a greater than 50% seizure reduction occurred in 10 patients, and only 9 patients showed no improvement.

Mattson and colleagues (84) reported the most comprehensive controlled comparison of VPA and carbamazepine monotherapy for the treatment of partial and secondarily generalized seizures. Several seizure indicators, as well as neurotoxicity and systemic neurotoxicity, were assessed quantitatively. Four of five efficacy indicators for partial seizures were significantly in favor of carbamazepine, and a combined composite score for efficacy and toxicity was higher for carbamazepine than for VPA at 12 months, but not at 24 months. Outcomes for secondarily generalized seizures did not differ between the two agents. Two studies—one comparing VPA and carbamazepine (85) and the other comparing VPA, carbamazepine, phenytoin, and phenobarbital (86)—were conducted in children. Equal efficacy against generalized and partial seizures was reported with all agents. Unacceptable side effects necessitating withdrawal occurred in patients receiving phenobarbital, which was prematurely eliminated from the study. More recently, VPA was evaluated in 143 adult patients with poorly controlled partial epilepsy randomized to VPA monotherapy at low plasma levels (25 to 50 mg/L) or high plasma levels (80 to 150 mg/L) (87). The reduction in frequency of both complex partial and secondarily generalized tonic-clonic seizures was significantly higher among patients in the high-level group.

Several studies have demonstrated the efficacy of VPA in the prevention of febrile seizures (88–94). Based on risk-benefit ratio considerations, VPA cannot be recommended for this indication. A small group of newborns with seizures have also been treated with VPA administered rectally (95) or orally (19). Results were favorable overall. In newborns treated with VPA, a long elimination half-life (26.4 hours) and high levels of ammonia were reported (19).

ADVERSE EFFECTS

Neurologic Effects

A dose-related tremor is relatively common in patients treated with VPA. If it does not improve sufficiently with dosage reduction, propranolol may be tried (96). Drowsiness, lethargy, and confusional states are uncommon with VPA, but may occur in some patients, usually at doses >100 mg/L. There have also been well-documented case reports of reversible dementia and pseudoatrophy of the brain (97–99). Treatment with VPA has been associated with a somewhat specific and unique adverse effect, characterized by an acute mental change that can progress to stupor or coma (100,101). It is usually associated with generalized delta slowing of the electroencephalographic tracing. The mechanism is not known with certainty, but it is probably not caused by hyperammonemia or carnitine deficiency. This encephalopathic picture is more likely to occur when VPA is added to another AED, and it is usually reversible within 2 to 3 days upon discontinuation of VPA or the other AED. Overall, VPA does not appear to have significant dose-related effects on cognition or behavior (102–106).

Gastrointestinal Effects

The most common gastrointestinal (GI) adverse effects associated with VPA use are nausea, vomiting, GI distress, and anorexia. These effects may be due, in part, to direct gastric irritation by VPA; the incidence is lower with enteric-coated tablets. Excessive weight gain is another common problem (107,108). This is not entirely attributable to increased appetite, and decreased beta oxidation of fatty acids has been postulated as a mechanism (109). Excessive weight gain seems to be less of a problem in children, and a recent report suggests that VPA is not associated with greater weight gain, compared with carbamazepine, in children (63).

Fatal hepatotoxicity remains the most feared adverse effect of VPA (22, 110–113). Two main risk factors have been clearly identified: young age and polytherapy (110). The risk for fatal hepatotoxicity in patients receiving VPA polytherapy is approximately 1:600 at younger than 3 years of age, 1:8,000 from 3 to 10 years, 1:10,000 from 11 to 20 years, 1:31,000 from 21 to 40 years, and 1:107,000 at older than 41 years of age. The risk is much lower in patients receiving monotherapy; it varies between 1:16,000 (3 to 10 years of age) and 1:230,000 (21 to 40 years of age) (110). No fatalities in patients receiving VPA monotherapy have been reported in certain age-groups (0 to 2 years, 11 to 20 years, and older than 40 years of age) (110). Because a benign elevation of liver enzymes is common during VPA therapy and because severe hepatotoxicity is not preceded by a progressive elevation of liver enzymes, laboratory monitoring is of little value despite the fact that it is often performed routinely. The diagnosis of VPA-associated hepatotoxicity depends mostly on recognition of the clinical features, which include nausea, vomiting, anorexia, lethargy, and, at times, loss of seizure control, jaundice, or edema. A recent report suggests a protective effect of L-carnitine administration in cases of established VPA-induced hepatotoxicity (114). Among 92 patients with severe, symptomatic VPA-induced hepatotoxicity, 48% of the 42 patients treated with L-carnitine survived, as opposed to 10% of the 50 patients receiving similar supportive treatment without L-carnitine. The results suggested better survival with IV, rather than enteral, L-carnitine (114).

Another serious complication of VPA treatment is the development of acute hemorrhagic pancreatitis (115–119). Suspicion should be raised by the occurrence of vomiting and abdominal pain. Serum amylase and lipase are the most helpful diagnostic tests, and abdominal ultrasonography may also be considered.

Hematologic Effects

Hematologic alterations are relatively common with VPA therapy, but they seldom lead to discontinuation of treatment (120,121). Thrombocytopenia (120,122) can fluctuate and tends to improve with dosage reduction. In conjunction with altered platelet function (123,124) and other VPA-mediated disturbances of hemostasis (125,126), it may cause excessive bleeding. Therefore, the common practice of withdrawing VPA before elective surgery is recommended despite the fact that several recent reports found no objective evidence of excessive operative bleeding in patients maintained on VPA therapy (127–129).

Hyperammonemia

Hyperammonemia is a very common finding in asymptomatic patients receiving chronic VPA therapy, particularly in those taking VPA along with an enzyme-inducing AED (130,131), and routine monitoring of ammonium levels is not warranted. Although hyperammonemia can be reduced with L-carnitine supplementation (132), there is no documentation that this is necessary or clinically beneficial (133). Chronic treatment with VPA, especially in polytherapy, tends to lower carnitine levels (134,135); however, a role for carnitine deficiency in the development of severe adverse effects of VPA has not been established. A beneficial effect of L-carnitine supplementation in acute VPA overdoses has been suggested (136,137), and a panel of pediatric neurologists has made recommendations for routine supplementation with L-carnitine in a subgroup of pediatric patients being treated with VPA (138).

Reproductive Issues

In women, VPA has been reported to cause menstrual irregularities, hormonal changes such as hyperandrogenism and hyperinsulinism, polycystic ovaries, and pubertal arrest (139–143). An additional concern has been the possible association of VPA therapy, polycystic ovaries, and elevated testosterone levels (139–141,144). The significance and reproducibility of these observations remains an open and debated issue (145,146). In a comparison of women treated with VPA, 21 with phenobarbital, 23 with carbamazepine, and 20 healthy untreated women, polycystic ovary prevalence, ovary volumes, and hirsutism scores did not differ among the groups (148). Epilepsy itself, other AEDs, and additional factors may be involved in the development of polycystic ovary syndrome (145). Treatment with VPA during the first trimester of pregnancy has been found to be associated with an estimated 1% to 2% risk of neural tube defect (148–150); a pharmacogenetic susceptibility has been suggested (151). Folate supplementation appears to reduce the risk (152), and a daily dose of at least 1 mg should be considered in all female patients of child-bearing age who are taking VPA.

Miscellaneous Effects

Excessive hair loss may be seen early during treatment with VPA, and although the hair tends to grow back, it may become different in texture (153) or color (154). Facial and limb edema can occur in the absence of VPA-induced hepatic injury (155). Children may develop secondary nocturnal enuresis after initiation of VPA therapy (81,108,156–158). Hyponatremia (159) has been reported in one patient. The occurrence of rash with VPA therapy is very rare (160).

CLINICAL USE

An initial VPA dosage of approximately 15 mg/kg/day is recommended, with subsequent increases, as necessary and tolerated, of 5 to 10 mg/kg per day at weekly intervals. The optimal VPA dose or concentration may vary according to a patient's seizure type (161). Daily doses between 10 and 20 mg/kg are often sufficient for VPA monotherapy in patients with primary generalized epilepsies (39,61, 69,70); children may require higher doses (44,62). Dosages of 30 to 60 mg/kg per day (in children, >100 mg/kg per day) may be necessary to achieve adequate VPA levels in patients being treated concomitantly with enzyme-inducing agents. If therapeutic levels of VPA are to be achieved rapidly or if patients are unable to take VPA orally, the agent can be administered intravenously (162). This route has also been suggested for the treatment of patients with status epilepticus, with an initial dose of 15 mg/kg (at 20 mg per minute) followed by 1 mg/kg per hour (163). A more rapid loading with an initial dose of 20 mg/kg has also been advocated, given at a rate of 33.3 to 555 mg per minute (164) or ≤6 mg/kg per minute (165). Rapid IV VPA loading seems to be well tolerated (166).

Because of the short half-life of VPA, it is common to divide the total daily dose into two or three doses. However, the pharmacodynamic profile of VPA may explain why equally good results have been achieved with a single daily dose (62,167,168). The value of monitoring serum levels of VPA is limited. First, there is considerable fluctuation in VPA levels because of the short half-life and variable absorption rate of the agent. Second, there seems to be a poor correlation between VPA serum levels and clinical effect, and the pharmacodynamic effect of VPA may lag behind its blood concentrations (61,169–172). Although the usual therapeutic range for VPA serum levels is 50 to 100 mg/L (350 to 700 μmol/L), levels up to 150 mg/L may be both necessary and well tolerated. In selected cases, and particularly during combination therapy with enzyme-inducing agents, VPA serum levels can be valuable, but a single measurement must be interpreted cautiously (173). Routine monitoring of liver enzymes and complete blood count with platelets is common practice; however, severe hepatotoxicity is unlikely to be detected with routine monitoring of liver enzymes.

REFERENCES

1. Meunier H, Carraz G, Neunier Y, et al. Pharmacodynamic properties of N-dipropylacetic acid [French]. *Thérapie* 1963;18:435–438.
2. Carraz G, Fau R, Chateau R, et al. Communication concerning 1st clinical tests of the anticonvulsive activity of *N*-dipropylacetic acid (sodium salt) [French]. *Ann Med Psychol (Paris)* 1964;122:577–585.
3. Daoud AS, Zaki M, Shakir R, et al. Effectiveness of sodium valproate in the treatment of Sydenham's chorea. *Neurology* 1990;40:1140–1141.
4. Frey HH, Loscher W, Reiche R, et al. Anticonvulsant potency of common antiepileptic drugs in the gerbil. *Pharmacology* 1983;27:330–335.
5. Pellegrini A, Gloor P, Sherwin AL. Effect of valproate sodium on generalized penicillin epilepsy in the cat. *Epilepsia* 1978;19:351–360.
6. Leveil V, Naquet R. A study of the action of valproic acid on the kindling effect. *Epilepsia* 1977;18:229–234.
7. Fariello RG, Varasi M, Smith MC. Valproic acid: mechanisms of action. In: Levy R, Mattson R, Meldrum B, eds. *Antiepileptic drugs*, 4th ed. New York: Raven Press, 1995:581–588.
8. Perucca E, Gatti G, Frigo GM, et al. Disposition of sodium valproate in epileptic patients. *Br J Clin Pharmacol* 1978;5:495–499.
9. Holmes GB, Rosenfeld WE, Graves NM, et al. Absorption of valproic acid suppositories in human volunteers. *Arch Neurol* 1989;46:906–909.
10. Issakainen J, Bourgeois BFD. Bioavailability of sodium valproate suppositories during repeated administration at steady state in epileptic children. *Eur J Pediatr* 1987;146:404–407.
11. Gugler R, Schell A, Eichelbaum M, et al. Disposition of valproic acid in man. *Eur J Clin Pharmacol* 1977;12:125–132.
12. Klotz U, Antonin KH. Pharmacokinetics and bioavailability of sodium valproate. *Clin Pharmacol Ther* 1977;21:736–743.
13. Levy RH, Conraud B, Loiseau P, et al. Meal-dependent absorption of enteric-coated sodium valproate. *Epilepsia* 1980;21:273–280.
14. Cloyd J, Kriel R, Jones-Saete C, et al. Comparison of sprinkle versus syrup formulations of valproate for bioavailability, tolerance, and preference. *J Pediatr* 1992;120:634–638.
15. Cramer JA, Mattson RH, Bennett DM, et al. Variable free and total valproic acid concentrations in sole- and multi-drug therapy. *Ther Drug Monit* 1986;8:411–415.
16. Gram L, Flachs H, Würtz-Jorgensen A, et al. Sodium valproate, serum level and clinical effect in epilepsy: a controlled study. *Epilepsia* 1979;20:303–312.
17. Perucca E, Grimaldi R, Gatti G, et al. Pharmacokinetics of valproic acid in the elderly. *Br J Clin Pharmacol* 1984;17:665–669.
18. Cloyd JC, Fischer JH, Kriel RL, et al. Valproic acid pharmacokinetics in children. IV. Effects of age and antiepileptic drugs on protein binding and intrinsic clearance. *Clin Pharmacol Ther* 1993;53:22–29.
19. Gal P, Oles KS, Gilman JT, et al. Valproic acid efficacy, toxicity, and pharmacokinetics in neonates with intractable seizures. *Neurology* 1988;38:467–471.
20. Levy RH, Rettenmeier AW, Anderson GD. Effects of polytherapy with phenytoin, carbamazepine, and stiripentol on formation of 4-ene-valproate, a hepatotoxic metabolite of valproic acid. *Clin Pharmacol Ther* 1990;48:225–235.
21. Löscher W, Nau H. Pharmacological evaluation of various metabolites and analogues of valproic acid. *Neuropharmacology* 1985;24:427–435.
22. Pollack GM, McHugh WB, Gengo FM, et al. Accumulation and washout kinetics of valproic acid and its active metabolites. *J Clin Pharmacol* 1986;26:668–676.
23. Nau H, Löscher W. Valproic acid: brain and plasma levels of the drug and its metabolites, anticonvulsant effects and gamma-aminobutyric acid (GABA) metabolism in the mouse. *J Pharmacol Exp Ther* 1982;220:654–659.
24. Nau H, Hauck RS, Ehlers K. Valproic acid-induced neural tube defects in mouse and human: aspects of chirality, alternative drug development, pharmacokinetics, and possible mechanisms. *Pharmacol Toxicol* 1991;69:310–321.
25. Kesterson JW, Granneman GR, Machinist JM. The hepatotoxicity of valproic acid and its metabolites in rats. I. Toxicologic, biochemical and histopathologic studies. *Hepatology* 1984;4:1143–1152.
26. Rettie AE, Rettenmeier AW, Howald WN, et al. Cytochrome P-450—catalyzed formation of delta 4-VPA, a toxic metabolite of valproic acid. *Science* 1987;235:890–893.
27. Dreifuss FE, Langer DH, Moline KA, et al. Valproic acid hepatic fatalities. II. US experience since 1984. *Neurology* 1989;39:201–207.
28. Paganini M, Zaccara G, Moroni F, et al. Lack of relationship between sodium valproate-induced adverse effects and the plasma concentration of its metabolite 2-propylpenten-4-oic acid. *Eur J Clin Pharmacol* 1987;32:219–222.
29. Bourgeois BFD. Pharmacologic interactions between valproate and other drugs. *Am J Med* 1988;84:29–33.
30. Levy RH, Koch KM. Drug interactions with valproic acid. *Drugs* 1982;24:543–556.
31. Scheyer RD, Mattson RH. Valproic acid: interactions with other drugs. In: Levy R, Mattson R, Meldrum B, eds. *Antiepileptic drugs*, 4th ed. New York: Raven Press, 1995:621–631.
32. May T, Rambeck B. Serum concentrations of valproic acid: influence of dose and comedication. *Ther Drug Monit* 1985;7:387–390.
33. Bowdle TA, Levy RH, Cutler RE. Effect of carbamazepine on valproic acid kinetics in normal subjects. *Clin Pharmacol Ther* 1979;26:629–634.
34. Hoffmann F, von Unruh GE, Jancik BC. Valproic acid disposition in epileptic patients during combined antiepileptic maintenance therapy. *Eur J Clin Pharmacol* 1981;19:383–385.
35. Reunanen MI, Luoma P, Myllyla V, et al. Low serum valproic acid concentrations in epileptic patients on combination therapy. *Curr Ther Res* 1980;28:456–462.
36. Cloyd JC, Kriel RL, Fischer JH. Valproic acid pharmacokinetics in children. II. Discontinuation of concomitant antiepileptic drug therapy. *Neurology* 1985;35:1623–1627.
37. De Wolff FA, Peters ACB, van Kempen GMJ. Serum concentrations and enzyme induction in epileptic children treated with phenytoin and valproate. *Neuropediatrics* 1982;13:10–13.
38. Sackellares JC, Sato S, Dreifuss FE, et al. Reduction of steady-state valproate levels by other antiepileptic drugs. *Epilepsia* 1981;22:437–441.
39. Henriksen O, Johannessen SI. Clinical and pharmacokinetic observations on sodium valproate: a 5-year follow-up study in 100 children with epilepsy. *Acta Neurol Scand* 1982;65:504–523.

40. Hooper WD, Franklin ME, Glue P, et al. Effect of felbamate on valproic acid disposition in healthy volunteers: inhibition of beta-oxidation. *Epilepsia* 1996;37:91–97.
41. Wagner ML, Graves NM, Leppik IE, et al. The effect of felbamate on valproate disposition. *Epilepsia* 1991;32:15.
42. Theis JG, Koren G, Daneman R, et al. Interactions of clobazam with conventional antiepileptics in children. *J Child Neurol* 1997;12:208–213.
43. Suganuma T, Ishizaki T, Chiba K, et al. The effect of concurrent administration of valproate sodium on phenobarbital plasma concentration/dosage ratio in pediatric patients. *J Pediatr* 1981; 99:314–317.
44. Redenbaugh JE, Sato S, Penry JK, et al. Sodium valproate: pharmacokinetics and effectiveness in treating intractable seizures. *Neurology* 1980;30:1–6.
45. Mattson RH, Cramer JA. Valproic acid and ethosuximide interaction. *Ann Neurol* 1980;7:583–584.
46. Levy RH, Moreland TA, Morselli PL, et al. Carbamazepine/valproic acid interaction in man and rhesus monkey. *Epilepsia* 1984;25:338–345.
47. Pisani F, Fazio A, Oteri G, et al. Sodium valproate and valpromide: differential interactions with carbamazepine in epileptic patients. *Epilepsia* 1986;27:548–552.
48. Yuen AWC, Land G, Weatherley BC, et al. Sodium valproate acutely inhibits lamotrigine metabolism. *Br J Clin Pharmacol* 1992;33:511–513.
49. Kanner AM, Frey M. Adding valproate to lamotrigine: a study of their pharmacokinetic interaction. *Neurology* 2000;55:588–591.
50. Gidal BE, Anderson GD, Rutecki PR, et al. Lack of an effect of valproate concentration on lamotrigine pharmacokinetics in developmentally disabled patients with epilepsy. *Epilepsy Res* 2000;42:23–31.
51. Pisani FD, Di Perri RG. Intravenous valproate: effects on plasma and saliva phenytoin levels. *Neurology* 1981;31:467–470.
52. Rodin EA, De Sousa G, Haidukewych D, et al. Dissociation between free and bound phenytoin levels in presence of valproate sodium. *Arch Neurol* 1981;38:240–242.
53. Mattson RH, Cramer JA, Darney PD, et al. Use of oral contraceptives by women with epilepsy. *JAMA* 1986;256:238–240.
54. Jeavons PM, Clark JE, Maheshwari MC. Treatment of generalized epilepsies of childhood and adolescence with sodium valproate ("Epilim"). *Dev Med Child Neurol* 1977;19:9–25.
55. Adams DJ, Lüders H, Pippenger CE. Sodium valproate in the treatment of intractable seizure disorders: a clinical and electroencephalographic study. *Neurology* 1978;28:152–157.
56. Maheshwari MC, Jeavons PM. Proceedings: The effect of sodium valproate (Epilim) on the EEG. *Electroencephalogr Clin Neurophysiol* 1975;39:429.
57. Braathen G, Theorell K, Persson A, et al. Valproate in the treatment of absence epilepsy in children. *Epilepsia* 1988;29:548–552.
58. Mattson RH, Cramer JA, Williamson PD, et al. Valproic acid in epilepsy: clinical and pharmacological effects. *Ann Neurol* 1978; 3:20–25.
59. Callaghan N, O'Hare J, O'Driscoll D, et al. Comparative study of ethosuximide and sodium valproate in the treatment of typical absence seizures (petit mal). *Dev Med Child Neurol* 1982;24: 830–836.
60. Sato S, White BG, Penry JK, et al. Valproic acid versus ethosuximide in the treatment of absence seizures. *Neurology* 1982;32: 157–163.
61. Bourgeois B, Beaumanoir A, Blajev B, et al. Monotherapy with valproate in primary generalized epilepsies. *Epilepsia* 1987;28: S8–S11.
62. Covanis A, Gupta AK, Jeavons PM. Sodium valproate: monotherapy and polytherapy. *Epilepsia* 1982;23:693–720.
63. Erenberg G, Rothner AD, Henry CE, et al. Valproic acid in the treatment of intractable absence seizures in children: a single-blind clinical and quantitative EEG study. *Am J Dis Child* 1982;136:526–529.
64. Berkovic SF, Andermann F, Guberman A, et al. Valproate prevents the recurrence of absence status. *Neurology* 1989;39: 1294–1297.
65. Dulac O, Steru D, Rey E, et al. Sodium valproate (Na VPa) monotherapy in childhood epilepsy [French]. *Arch Fr Pediatr* 1982;39:347–352.
66. Ramsay RE, Wilder BJ, Murphy JV, et al. Efficacy and safety of valproic acid versus phenytoin as sole therapy for newly diagnosed primary generalized tonic-clonic seizures. *J Epilepsy* 1992; 5:55–60.
67. Spitz MC, Deasy DN. Conversion to valproate monotherapy in nonretarded adults with primary generalized tonic-clonic seizures. *J Epilepsy* 1991;4:33–38.
68. Turnbull DM, Howel D, Rawlins MD, et al. Which drug for the adult epileptic patient: phenytoin or valproate? *Br Med J* 1985; 290:816–819.
69. Wilder BJ, Ramsay RE, Murphy JV, et al. Comparison of valproic acid and phenytoin in newly diagnosed tonic-clonic seizures. *Neurology* 1983;33:1474–1476.
70. Feuerstein J. A long-term study of monotherapy with sodium valproate in primary generalized epilepsy. *Br J Clin Pract* 1983; 27:17–23.
71. Dulac O, Steru D, Rey E, et al. Sodium valproate monotherapy in childhood epilepsy. *Brain Dev* 1986;8:47–52.
72. Delgado-Escueta AV, Enrile-Bacsal F. Juvenile myoclonic epilepsy of Janz. *Neurology* 1984;34:285–294.
73. Fahn S. Post-anoxic action myoclonus: improvement with valproic acid. *N Engl J Med* 1978;299:313–314.
74. Rollinson RD, Gilligan BS. Postanoxic action myoclonus (Lance-Adams syndrome) responding to valproate. *Arch Neurol* 1979; 36:44–45.
75. Iivanainen M, Himberg JJ. Valproate and clonazepam in the treatment of severe progressive myoclonus epilepsy. *Arch Neurol* 1982;39:236–238.
76. Barnes SE, Bower BD. Sodium valproate in the treatment of intractable childhood epilepsy. *Dev Med Child Neurol* 1975;17: 175–181.
77. Olive D, Tridon P, Weber M. Effect of sodium dipropylacetate on certain varieties of epileptogenic encephalopathies in infants [French]. *Schweiz Med Wochenschr* 1969;99:87–92.
78. Rohmann E, Arndt R. Effectiveness of ergenyl (dipropylacetate) in hypsarrhythmia [German]. *Kinderarztl Prax* 1976;44: 109–113.
79. Bachman DS. Use of valproic acid in treatment of infantile spasms. *Arch Neurol* 1982;39:49–52.
80. Pavone L, Incorpora G, La Rosa M, et al. Treatment of infantile spasms with sodium dipropylacetic acid. *Dev Med Child Neurol* 1981;23:454–461.
81. Loiseau P, Cohadon S, Jogeix M, et al. Efficacy of sodium valproate in partial epilepsy. Crossed study of valproate and carbamazepine [French]. *Rev Neurol (Paris)* 1984;140:434–437.
82. Callaghan N, Kenny RA, O'Neill B, et al. A prospective study between carbamazepine, phenytoin and sodium valproate as monotherapy in previously untreated and recently diagnosed patients with epilepsy. *J Neurol Neurosurg Psychiatry* 1985;48: 639–644.
83. Dean JC, Penry JK. Valproate monotherapy in 30 patients with partial seizures. *Epilepsia* 1988;29:140–144.
84. Mattson RH, Cramer JA, Collins JF, for the Department of Veterans Affairs Epilepsy Cooperative Study No. 264 Group. A comparison of valproate with carbamazepine for the treatment of complex partial seizures and secondarily generalized tonic-clonic seizures in adults. *N Engl J Med* 1992;327:765–771.
85. Verity CM, Hosking G, Easter DJ. A multicentre comparative trial of sodium valproate and carbamazepine in paediatric epilepsy. The Paediatric EPITEG Collaborative Group. *Dev Med Child Neurol* 1995;37:97–108.
86. DeSilva M, MacArdle B, McGowan M, et al. Randomised comparative monotherapy trial of phenobarbitone, phenytoin, carbamazepine, or sodium valproate for newly diagnosed childhood epilepsy. *Lancet* 1996;347:709–713.
87. Beydoun A, Sackellares JC, Shu V. Safety and efficacy of divalproex sodium monotherapy in partial epilepsy: a double-blind, concentration-response design clinical trial. Depakote Monotherapy for Partial Seizures Study Group. *Neurology* 1997;48:182–188.
88. Cavazzutti GB. Prevention of febrile convulsions with dipropylacetate (Depakine). *Epilepsia* 1975;16:647–648.
89. Herranz JL, Armijo JA, Arteaga R. Effectiveness and toxicity of phenobarbital, primidone and sodium valproate in the prevention of febrile convulsions, controlled by plasma levels. *Epilepsia* 1984;25:89–95.

90. Lee K, Melchior JC. Sodium valproate versus phenobarbital in the prophylactic treatment of febrile convulsions in childhood. *Eur J Pediatr* 1981;137:151–153.

91. Mamelle N, Mamelle JC, Plasse JC, et al. Prevention of recurrent febrile convulsions—a randomized therapeutic assay: sodium valproate, phenobarbital and placebo. *Neuropediatrics* 1984;15:37–42.

92. Minagawa K, Miura H. Phenobarbital, primidone and sodium valproate in the prophylaxis of febrile convulsions. *Brain Dev* 1981;3:385–393.

93. Ngwane E, Bower B. Continuous sodium valproate or phenobarbitone in the prevention of simple febrile convulsions. Comparison by a double-blind trial. *Arch Dis Child* 1980;55:171–174.

94. Rantala H, Tarkka R, Uhari M. A meta-analytic review of the preventive treatment of recurrences of febrile seizures. *J Pediatr* 1997;131:922–925.

95. Steinberg A, Shaley RS, Amir N. Valproic acid in neonatal status convulsion. *Brain Dev* 1986;8:278–279.

96. Karas BJ, Wilder BJ, Hammond EJ, et al. Treatment of valproate tremors. *Neurology* 1983;33:1380–1382.

97. McLachlan RS. Pseudoatrophy of the brain with valproic acid monotherapy. *Can J Neurol Sci* 1987;14:294–296.

98. Papazian O, Canizales E, Alfonso I, et al. Reversible dementia and apparent brain atrophy during valproate therapy. *Ann Neurol* 1995;38:687–691.

99. Shin C, Gray L, Armond C. Reversible cerebral atrophy: radiologic correlate of valproate-induced parkinson-dementia syndrome. *Neurology* 1992;42:277.

100. Marescaux C, Warter JM, Micheletti G, et al. Stuporous episodes during treatment with sodium valproate: report of seven cases. *Epilepsia* 1982;23:297–305.

101. Sackellares JC, Lee SI, Dreifuss FE. Stupor following administration of valproic acid to patients receiving other antiepileptic drugs. *Epilepsia* 1979;20:697–703.

102. Aman M, Werry J, Paxton JW, et al. Effect of sodium valproate on psychomotor performance in children as a function of dose, fluctuations in concentration, and diagnosis. *Epilepsia* 1987;28:115–125.

103. Gallassi R, Morreale A, Lorusso S, et al. Cognitive effects of valproate. *Epilepsy Res* 1990;5:160–164.

104. Sonnen AE, Zelvelder WH, Bruens JH. A double blind study of the influence of dipropylacetate on behaviour. *Acta Neurol Scand Suppl* 1975;60:43–47.

105. Stores G, Williams PL, Styles E, et al. Psychological effects of sodium valproate and carbamazepine in epilepsy. *Arch Dis Child* 1992;67:1330–1337.

106. Vining EPG, Mellitis ED, Dorsen MM, et al. Psychologic and behavioral effects of antiepileptic drugs in children: a double-blind comparison between phenobarbital and valproic acid. *Pediatrics* 1987;80:165–174.

107. Dean JC, Penry JK. Weight gain patterns in patients with epilepsy: comparison of antiepileptic drugs. *Epilepsia* 1995;36:72.

108. Dinesen H, Gram L, Andersen T, et al. Weight gain during treatment with valproate. *Acta Neurol Scand* 1984;70:65–69.

109. Breum L, Astrup A, Gram L, et al. Metabolic changes during treatment with valproate in humans: implications for weight gain. *Metabolism* 1992;41:666–670.

110. Bryant AE III, Dreifuss FE. Valproic acid hepatic fatalities. III. U.S. experience since 1986. *Neurology* 1996;46:465–469.

111. Dreifuss FE, Santilli N, Langer DH, et al. Valproic acid hepatic fatalities: a retrospective view. *Neurology* 1987;37:379–385.

112. König SA, Siemes H, Bläker F, et al. Severe hepatotoxicity during valproate therapy: an update and report of eight new fatalities. *Epilepsia* 1994;35:1005–1015.

113. Scheffner D, König S, Rauterberg-Ruland I, et al. Fatal liver failure in 16 children with valproate therapy. *Epilepsia* 1988;29:530–542.

114. Bohan TP, Helton E, McDonald I, et al. Effect of L-carnitine treatment for valproate-induced hepatotoxicity. *Neurology* 2001;56:1405–1409.

115. Asconapé JJ, Penry JK, Dreifuss FE, et al. Valproate-associated pancreatitis. *Epilepsia* 1993;34:177–183.

116. Camfield PR. Pancreatitis due to valproic acid. *Lancet* 1979;1:1198–1199.

117. Coulter DL, Allen RJ. Pancreatitis associated with valproic acid therapy for epilepsy. *Ann Neurol* 1980;7:693–720.

118. Williams LHP, Reynolds RP, Emery JL. Pancreatitis during sodium valproate treatment. *Arch Dis Child* 1983;58:543–544.

119. Wyllie E, Wyllie R, Cruse RP, et al. Pancreatitis associated with valproic acid therapy. *Am J Dis Child* 1984;138:912–914.

120. Hauser E, Seidl R, Freilinger M, et al. Hematologic manifestations and impaired liver synthetic function during valproate monotherapy. *Brain Dev* 1996;18:105–109.

121. May RB, Sunder TR. Hematologic manifestations of long-term valproate therapy. *Epilepsia* 1993;34:1098–1101.

122. Neophytides AN, Nutt JG, Lodish JR. Thrombocytopenia associated with sodium valproate treatment. *Ann Neurol* 1978;5:389–390.

123. Kis B, Szupera Z, Mezei Z, et al. Valproate treatment and platelet function: the role of arachidonate metabolites. *Epilepsia* 1999;40:307–310.

124. Zeller J, Schlesinger S, Runge U, et al. Influence of valproate monotherapy on platelet activation and hematologic values. *Epilepsia* 1999;40:186–189.

125. Gidal B, Spencer N, Maly M, et al. Valproate-mediated disturbances of hemostasis: relationship to dose and plasma concentration. *Neurology* 1994;44:1418–1422.

126. Kreuz W, Linde M, Funk R, et al. Valproate therapy induces von Willebrand disease type I. *Epilepsia* 1991;33:178–184.

127. Anderson GD, Lin YX, Berge C, et al. Absence of bleeding complications in patients undergoing cortical surgery while receiving valproate treatment. *J Neurosurg* 1997;87:252–256.

128. Ward MM, Barbaro NM, Laxer KD, et al. Preoperative valproate administration does not increase blood loss during temporal lobectomy. *Epilepsia* 1996;37:98–101.

129. Winter SL, Kriel RL, Novacheck TF, et al. Perioperative blood loss: the effect of valproate. *Pediatr Neurol* 1996;15:19–22.

130. Haidukewych D, John G, Zielinski JJ, et al. Chronic valproic acid therapy and incidence of increases in venous plasma ammonia. *Ther Drug Monit* 1985;7:290–294.

131. Zaccara G, Paganini M, Campostrini R, et al. Effect of associated antiepileptic treatment on valproate-induced hyperammonemia. *Ther Drug Monit* 1985;7:185–190.

132. Gidal BE, Inglese CM, Meyer JF, et al. Diet- and valproate-induced transient hyperammonemia: effect of L-carnitine. *Pediatr Neurol* 1997;16:301–305.

133. Bohles H, Sewell AC, Wenzel D. The effect of carnitine supplementation in valproate-induced hyperammonaemia. *Acta Paediatr* 1996;85:446–449.

134. Coulter DL. Carnitine deficiency in epilepsy: risk factors and treatment. *J Child Neurol* 1995;10:S32–S39.

135. Laub MC, Paetake-Brunner I, Jaeger G. Serum carnitine during valproate acid therapy. *Epilepsia* 1986;27:559–562.

136. Ishikura H, Matsuo N, Matsubara M, et al. Valproic acid overdose and L-carnitine therapy. *J Anal Toxicol* 1996;20:55–58.

137. Murakami K, Sugimoto T, Woo M, et al. Effect of L-carnitine supplementation on acute valproate intoxication. *Epilepsia* 1996;37:687–689.

138. De Vivo D, Bohan T, Coulter DL, et al. L-Carnitine supplementation in childhood epilepsy: current perspectives. *Epilepsia* 1998;39:1216–1225.

139. Isojärvi JI, Laatikainen TJ, Knip M, et al. Obesity and endocrine disorders in women taking valproate for epilepsy. *Ann Neurol* 1996;39:579–584.

140. Isojärvi JI, Laatikainen TJ, Pakarinen AJ, et al. Polycystic ovaries and hyperandrogenism in women taking valproate for epilepsy. *N Engl J Med* 1993;19:1383–1388.

141. Isojärvi JI, Rattya J, Myllyla VV, et al. Valproate, lamotrigine, and insulin-mediated risks in women with epilepsy. *Ann Neurol* 1998;43:446–451.

142. Margraf JW, Dreifuss FE. Amenorrhea following initiation of therapy with valproic acid. *Neurology* 1981;31:159.

143. Luef G, Abraham I, Trinka E, et al. Hyperandrogenism, postprandial hyperinsulinism and the risk of PCOS in a cross sectional study of women with epilepsy treated with valproate. *Epilepsy Res* 2002;48:91–102.

144. Sharma S, Jacobs HS. Polycystic ovary syndrome associated with treatment with the anticonvulsant sodium valproate. *Curr Opin Obstet Gynecol* 1997;9:391–394.

145. Genton P, Bauer J, Duncan S, et al. On the association of valproate and polycystic ovaries. *Epilepsia* 2001;42:295–304.

146. Isojärvi JI, Tauboll E, Tapanainen JS, et al. On the association between valproate and polycystic ovary syndrome: a response and an alternative view. *Epilepsia* 2001;42:305–310.

147. Murialdo G, Galimberti CA, Gianelli MV, et al. Effects of valproate, phenobarbital, and carbamazepine on sex steroid setup in women with epilepsy. *Clin Neuropharmacol* 1998;21:52–58.

148. Bjerkedal T, Czeizel A, Goujard J, et al. Valproic acid and spina bifida. *Lancet* 1982;2:1096.

149. Lindhout D, Meinardi H. Spina bifida and in-utero exposure to valproate. *Lancet* 1984;2:396.

150. Omtzigt JGC, Los FJ, Grobbee DE, et al. The risk of spina bifida aperta after first-trimester exposure to valproate in a prenatal cohort. *Neurology* 1992;42(4 Suppl 5):119–125.

151. Duncan S, Mercho S, Lopes-Cendes I, et al. Repeated neural tube defects and valproate monotherapy suggest a pharmacogenetic abnormality. *Epilepsia* 2001;42:750–753.

152. Wegner C, Nau H. Alteration of embryonic folate metabolism by valproic acid during organogenesis. *Neurology* 1992;42:17–24.

153. Jeavons PM, Clark JE, Harding GFA. Valproate and curly hair. *Lancet* 1977;1:359.

154. Herranz JL, Arteaga R, Armijo JA. Change in hair colour induced by valproic acid. *Dev Med Child Neurol* 1987;23:386–387.

155. Ettinger A, Moshe S, Shinnar S. Edema associated with long-term valproate therapy. *Epilepsia* 1990;31:211–213.

156. Choonra IA. Sodium valproate and enuresis. *Lancet* 1985;1:1276.

157. Herranz JL, Arteaga R, Armijo JA. Side effects of sodium valproate in monotherapy controlled by plasma levels: a study in 88 pediatric patients. *Epilepsia* 1982;23:203–214.

158. Panayiotopoulos CP. Nocturnal enuresis associated with sodium valproate. *Lancet* 1985;1:980–981.

159. Branten AJ, Wetzels JF, Weber AM, et al. Hyponatremia due to sodium valproate. *Ann Neurol* 1998;43:265–267.

160. Hyson C, Sadler M. Cross sensitivity of skin rashes with antiepileptic drugs. *Can J Neurol Sci* 1997;24:245–249.

161. Lundberg B, Nergardh A, Boreus LO. Plasma concentrations of valproate during maintenance therapy in epileptic children. *J Neurol* 1982;228:133–141.

162. Devinsky O, Leppik I, Willmore LJ, et al. Safety of intravenous valproate. *Ann Neurol* 1995;38:670–674.

163. Giroud M, Gras D, Escousse A, et al. Use of injectable valproic acid in status epilepticus: a pilot study. *Drug Invest* 1993;5:154–159.

164. Limdi NA, Faught E. The safety of rapid valproic acid infusion. *Epilepsia* 2000;41:1342–1345.

165. Wheless J, Venkataraman V. Safety of high intravenous valproate loading doses in epilepsy patients. *J Epilepsy* 1998;11:319–324.

166. Venkataraman V, Wheless J. Safety of rapid intravenous infusion of valproate loading doses in epilepsy patients. *Epilepsy Res* 1999;35:147–153.

167. Gjerloff I, Arentsen J, Alving J, et al. Monodose versus 3 daily doses of sodium valproate: a controlled trial. *Acta Neurol Scand* 1984;69:120–124.

168. Stefan H, Burr W, Fichsel H, et al. Intensive follow-up monitoring in patients with once daily evening administration of sodium valproate. *Epilepsia* 1974;25:152–160.

169. Brachet-Liermain A, Demarquez JL. Pharmacokinetics of dipropylacetate in infants and young children. *Pharm Weekbl* 1977;112:293–297.

170. Bruni J, Wilder BJ. Valproic acid. Review of a new antiepileptic drug. *Arch Neurol* 1979;36:393–398.

171. Burr W, Fröscher W, Hoffmann F, et al. Lack of significant correlation between circadian profiles of valproic acid serum levels and epileptiform electroencephalographic activity. *Ther Drug Monit* 1984;6:179–181.

172. Rowan AJ, Binnie CD, Warfield CA, et al. The delayed effect of sodium valproate on the photoconvulsive response in man. *Epilepsia* 1979;20:61–68.

173. Chadwick DW. Concentration-effect relationships of valproic acid. *Clin Pharmacokinet* 1985;10:155–163.

Phenytoin and Fosphenytoin

55

Diego A. Morita   *Tracy A. Glauser*

HISTORICAL BACKGROUND

Phenytoin

From the second half of the 19th century until 1938, the antiepileptic effect of commonly used medications (sodium bromide and phenobarbital) was attributed to their sedative effects (1). The landmark work of Merritt and Putnam in 1937 and 1938 (2,3) demonstrated that the antiepileptic potential of drugs could be tested in animals, the anticonvulsant effect and sedative effects could be separated, and anticonvulsant activity could be achieved without sedation. Phenytoin (compared with sodium bromide and phenobarbital) showed the greatest anticonvulsant potency with the least hypnotic activity in the cat model they devised, which compared a drug's ability to change the seizure threshold with its sedative effects.

In a subsequent series of articles, Merritt and Putnam demonstrated that phenytoin was effective in humans; the first clinical trial of phenytoin in epilepsy (4) documented freedom from seizures in 50% of 142 patients with refractory disease. This trial showed, for the first time, that a drug effective against seizures in experimental animals could be successfully used in humans. In fact, Merritt and Putnam's electroconvulsive test in animals remains the most reliable experimental indicator of antiepileptic drug (AED) efficacy in tonic-clonic and partial seizures in humans. A follow-up study described effectiveness in complex partial seizures, with or without secondarily generalized tonic-clonic seizures, but not in absence seizures (5). Today, phenytoin is one of the world's most widely prescribed AEDs (6).

Fosphenytoin

Because phenytoin is poorly soluble in water, parenteral phenytoin sodium has been formulated as an aqueous

vehicle containing propylene glycol, ethanol, and sodium hydroxide, adjusted to a pH of 12 (7,8). Unfortunately, parenteral phenytoin sodium is associated with cardiovascular complications and phlebitis (9,10). First synthesized in 1973, fosphenytoin was developed as a water-soluble phenytoin prodrug that might reduce the risks of the cardiovascular complications and phlebitis from parenteral phenytoin administration (11).

CHEMISTRY AND MECHANISM OF ACTION

Phenytoin

Phenytoin is commercially available as the free acid and the sodium salt. The molecular weight is 252.26 for the free acid and 274.25 for the sodium salt. A weak organic acid, phenytoin is poorly soluble in water. The apparent dissociation constant (pKa) ranges from 8.1 to 9.2 and requires an alkaline solution to achieve solubility in high concentrations. As a result, parenteral phenytoin sodium must be formulated as an aqueous vehicle containing 40% propylene glycol and 10% ethanol in water for injection, adjusted to a pH of 12 with sodium hydroxide (7,8,11).

Phenytoin affects ion conductance, sodium-potassium adenosine triphosphatase activity, various enzyme systems, synaptic transmission, posttetanic potentiation, neurotransmitter release, and cyclic nucleotide metabolism (12). Despite these numerous sites of action, the major anticonvulsant mechanism of action is believed to be the drug's effect on the sodium channel. Phenytoin blocks membrane channels through which sodium moves from the outside to the inside of the neuron during depolarization, suppressing the sustained repetitive firing that results from presynaptic stimulation (12–14).

**Rapid Conversion
By Phosphatase**

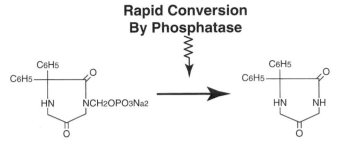

Figure 55.1 Structural formulas of fosphenytoin (*left*) and phenytoin (*right*).

Fosphenytoin

Fosphenytoin, a phenytoin prodrug, is the disodium phosphate ester of 3-hydroxymethyl-5,5-diphenylhydantoin (molecular weight 406.24) (Fig. 55.1). Following conversion, 1.5 mg of fosphenytoin yields 1 mg of phenytoin. To avoid confusion, fosphenytoin (Cerebyx) is packaged as milligram phenytoin equivalents (mg PE). Thus, 100 mg of parenteral phenytoin (Dilantin) and 100 mg PE of parenteral fosphenytoin (Cerebyx) have equal molar amounts of phenytoin.

Fosphenytoin's phosphate ester group on the basic phenytoin molecule significantly increases solubility. The water solubility of fosphenytoin at 37°C is 75,000 µg/mL, compared with 20.5 µg/mL for phenytoin (11). Thus, fosphenytoin is freely soluble in aqueous solutions and can be formulated without organic solvents (15). Fosphenytoin is formulated as a ready-mix solution of 50 mg PE/mL in water for injection, United States Pharmacopeia (USP), and tromethamine, USP (Tris) buffer adjusted to pH 8.6 to 9.0 with either hydrochloric acid, National Formulary (NF), or sodium hydroxide, NF (16). Fosphenytoin itself has no known anticonvulsant activity and derives its utility from its rapid and total conversion to phenytoin (15,16).

ABSORPTION, DISTRIBUTION, METABOLISM, AND EXCRETION

Phenytoin

Absorption

Phenytoin is available in various formulations for both oral and parenteral use (Table 55.1). Both the rate and extent of absorption may differ among the formulations, leading to clinically significant alterations in serum concentrations when switching among products.

The rate and extent of absorption of phenytoin from its site of entrance depends on pKa and lipid solubility, the pH of the medium in which it is dissolved, solubility in the medium, and concentration. These factors are frequently altered by the presence of foods or drugs in the intestinal tract and by the formulations. Little phenytoin is absorbed in the stomach because the drug is insoluble in the acidic pH of gastric juice (about 2.0), even though it is in its nonionized form in the stomach. Absorption occurs primarily in the duodenum, where the higher pH increases the solubility of phenytoin. Absorption from the jejunum and ileum is slower than from the duodenum and is poor from the colon (17,18).

In humans, the rate of absorption is variable and prolonged (19,20), and significantly influenced by the rate of elimination (21). Because dissolution is the rate-limiting process in the absorption of phenytoin, any factor that affects dissolution or solubility will affect absorption. After oral administration of a single dose, peak blood drug levels are generally reached between 4 and 8 hours later (range, 3 to 12 hours) (22,23). In patients ingesting massive amounts of phenytoin, absorption may continue for as long as 60 hours (24). Relative bioavailability increases with age, suggesting an age-dependent effect on drug absorption (25). In newborns and infants up to 3 months old, phenytoin is absorbed slowly and incompletely after both oral and

TABLE 55.1
FORMULATIONS OF PHENYTOIN AND FOSPHENYTOIN

Formulation	Preparation	Strength	Acid or Salt	Amount of Drug	Prompt or Extended
Dilantin Kapseals	Capsule	30 mg	Sodium salt	27.6 mg	Extended
Dilantin Kapseals	Capsule	100 mg	Sodium salt	92 mg	Extended
Dilantin Infatabs	Chewable tablet	50 mg	Free acid	50 mg	Prompt
Dilantin-125 suspension	Suspension	125 mg/5 mL	Free acid	125 mg/mL	Prompt
Phenytek	Capsule	200 mg	Sodium salt	184 mg	Extended
Phenytek	Capsule	300 mg	Sodium salt	276 mg	Extended
Phenytoin (generic)	Capsule	30 mg	Sodium salt	27.6 mg	Prompt and extended
Phenytoin (generic)[a]	Capsule	100 mg	Sodium salt	92 mg	Prompt and extended
Phenytoin (generic)	Suspension	125 mg/5 mL	Free acid	125 mg/mL	Prompt
Phenytoin (generic)	Injectable solution	50 mg/mL	Sodium salt	46 mg/mL	
Fosphenytoin	Injectable solution	50 mg PE/mL	Disodium salt	50 mg PE/mL	

[a]The prompt-release generic phenytoin 100-mg capsules are not bioequivalent to Dilantin 100-mg Kapseals®. The extended-release generic phenytoin 100-mg capsules are considered bioequivalent. The prescriber should be cautious when writing prescriptions.

intramuscular administration (26); absorption in older infants and children is similar to that in adults. Stable isotope tracer doses have been used to assess the bioavailability of phenytoin (27,28).

After intramuscular administration, phenytoin is absorbed slowly, as poor water solubility leads to precipitation of drug at the injection site, forming almost a depot repository (20). This prolonged absorption and pain on administration mandate use of the intravenous route if parenteral administration is required.

The reported bioavailability of rectally administered phenytoin sodium is approximately 25% (29).

Absorption of Generic Preparations

Several generic phenytoin preparations have been approved by the Food and Drug Administration (FDA) and are available in the United States; however, they are not equivalent owing to differences in their rate of absorption. Most of the generic products are not rated as bioequivalent to brand-name Dilantin because of their rapid ("prompt") absorption profile. Steady-state concentrations of the prompt formulation have been found to be either higher than those of the brand extended-release form (30), lower (31,32), or not different (33). Thus, when stable concentrations are desirable, an extended-release profile is preferred. In 1998, a 100-mg generic extended-release product (manufactured by Mylan Pharmaceuticals, Morgantown, WV) was approved as bioequivalent to Dilantin Kapseals 100 mg (34).

In contrast, the generic prompt release formulation is useful when rapid serum concentrations are desired, such as with an oral loading dose. Prompt-release phenytoin administered in three divided doses of 6 mg/kg every 3 hours reaches maximal concentrations almost 4 hours sooner than does the brand-name extended-release form given according to the same regimen (35).

Distribution

Protein Binding

Phenytoin is approximately 90% bound to plasma proteins, primarily albumin, in most healthy, ambulatory patients. Only the unbound (free) portion is pharmacologically active because protein-bound drug cannot cross the blood-brain barrier. Because unbound phenytoin distributes passively between plasma and cerebrospinal fluid, concentrations are the same in both sites (36), and the unbound plasma concentration can be used to estimate the cerebrospinal fluid concentration (18).

The generally established therapeutic range for phenytoin of 10 to 20 μg/mL includes both bound and unbound drug. As 10% is normally unbound, the equivalent unbound therapeutic range is 1 to 2 μg/mL. The extent of protein binding varies little with phenytoin plasma concentration.

The percentage of binding (70% to 95%) depends on albumin concentration and coexisting medications or illnesses. Low serum albumin, renal failure, or concomitant medications that displace phenytoin from protein-binding

sites increase the risk for changes in protein binding. Both exogenous (other highly protein-bound medications) and endogenous (increased bilirubin) substances can compete for binding sites and increase unbound phenytoin concentrations. Valproic acid significantly alters phenytoin binding to serum albumin, whereas phenobarbital, ethosuximide, diazepam, carbamazepine, and folic acid do not (37). Binding is decreased in uremia (84.2%), hepatic disease, and acquired immunodeficiency syndrome (18); in renal dysfunction, it is most apparent at creatinine clearances below 25 mL per minute (38). In patients with uremia who undergo renal transplantation, binding returns to normal when renal function recovers (39).

Total phenytoin concentrations that are below the normal range can be associated with unbound phenytoin concentrations in the therapeutic range. For example, if a patient has a subtherapeutic total phenytoin concentration of 5 μg/mL but an unbound fraction of 20%, the equivalent unbound phenytoin concentration is 1 μg/mL, which is in the "therapeutic" range. Thus patients at high risk for altered protein binding may respond to clinically subtherapeutic total concentrations and may not tolerate total serum concentrations within the therapeutic range. If such patients experience toxic reactions despite therapeutic concentrations, measurement of unbound concentrations may be warranted. Total phenytoin concentrations may be a misleading test in developing countries, where hypoalbuminemia is highly prevalent (40).

Among the methods that predict total phenytoin concentrations in the face of reduced albumin levels, the best documented is the Sheiner-Tozer method (41,42):

$$Cn = Co / (0.2 \times Alb + 0.1)$$

where Co is the measured total phenytoin concentration (mg/L), Alb is albumin concentration (g/dL), and Cn is the total phenytoin concentration that would have been observed with normal albumin concentrations.

Volume of Distribution

Phenytoin is distributed freely in the body with an average volume of distribution in humans of 0.78 L/kg (18). The volume of distribution after single intravenous doses (9.4 to 21.3 mg/kg) in children declines with age and range from 1 to 1.5 L/kg below the age of 5 years and from 0.6 to 0.8 L/kg above the age of 8 years (43). At the pH of plasma, phenytoin exists predominantly in the nonionized form, thus allowing rapid movement across cell membranes by nonionic diffusion. The volume of distribution, which correlates with body weight (44), is larger in morbidly obese patients, who may require large loading doses to achieve therapeutic concentrations (45,46).

Metabolism

In humans, the major pathway of phenytoin elimination (approximately 80%) is 4'- hydroxylation to form 5-(4'-hydroxyphenyl)-5-phenylhydantoin (4'-HPPH). This reaction is mediated mainly by the cytochrome P450

(CYP) enzyme CYP2C9, and to a lesser extent by CYP2C19 (47,48). Approximately 10% of phenytoin is eliminated to a dihydrodiol, and another 10% is metabolized to 5-(3-hydroxyphenyl)-5-phenylhydantoin (3',4'-diHPPH) (7,47,49). An arene oxide, which precedes the formation of these compounds, has been implicated in the toxicity and teratogenicity of phenytoin; however, its transient presence in patients with normally functioning arene oxide detoxification systems is unlikely to account for many of the toxic reactions (50,51).

Because phenytoin has nonlinear pharmacokinetics, a narrow therapeutic index, and a concentration-related toxicity profile, small changes in CYP2C9 activity may be clinically significant. Of the 13 CYP2C9 alleles identified to date, the most common, designated as CYP2C9*1, is considered the wild-type allele (52,53). Individuals homozygous for the wild-type allele are called extensive metabolizers. Studies in various populations demonstrated that the CYP2C9*2, CYP2C9*3, CYP2C9*4, and CYP2C9*6 alleles are important *in vivo* determinants of phenytoin disposition (54–63). Individuals with at least one of these variant alleles are called poor metabolizers and have a reduced ability to metabolize phenytoin. They may require lower-than-average phenytoin doses to decrease the incidence of concentration-dependent adverse effects (58,64).

Although two-thirds of whites possess the wild-type allele, one-third are heterozygous for the CYP2C9*2 or CYP2C9*3 allele (52). These two variant alleles are much less prevalent in African Americans and Asians, with more than 95% of these groups expressing the wild-type genotype (52). To date, the CYP2C9*4, CYP2C9*5, and CYP2C9*6 allelic variants have been identified exclusively in the Japanese (CYP2C9*4) and African-American (CYP2C9*5 and CYP2C9*6) populations (63,65,66). Six of the latest seven alleles (CYP2C9*7 through CYP2C9*12) have been discovered by resequencing CYP2C9 DNA from whites, Asians, and Africans (African Americans and African Pygmies) (67). CYP2C9*13 was identified in a Chinese population, and found to be associated with reduced plasma clearance of drugs that are substrates for CYP2C9 (68).

Odani and coworkers observed a decrease of approximately 30% in the maximal rate of phenytoin elimination in Japanese heterozygous for CYP2C9*3 compared with those homozygous for the wild-type allele (54). Moreover, the mean phenytoin maintenance dose leading to a therapeutic serum concentration was significantly lower in patients with CYP2C9 allelic variants (199 ± 42.5 mg/day) than in those with the wild-type allele (314 ± 61.2 mg/day; *p* <0.01) (58). A case report of a heterozygous CYP2C9*3 allele carrier described excessive phenytoin concentrations relative to the doses taken; a toxic level (32.6 µg/mL) was reached despite a modest dose (187.5 mg/day). The patient showed signs of central nervous system intoxication, ataxia, and diplopia (59).

The activity of CYP2C9 alone, however, does not fully explain the large interindividual variability in the clinical pharmacokinetics and reported drug interactions of phenytoin (69). Fifteen CYP2C19 alleles have been described to date (53). The first seven (CYP2C19*2 to CYP2C19*8) are inactive and are responsible for the poor-metabolizer phenotype. The recently described CYP2C19*9 to CYP2C19*15 are potentially defective, although none have yet been studied *in vivo* (70).

The majority of all populations studied have the CYP2C19 extensive-metabolizer phenotype involving the wild-type CYP2C19*1 allele. The frequency of CYP2C19 poor metabolizers is much higher in Asians (13% to 23%) than in whites and African Americans (1% to 6%) (71). The CYP2C19*2 and CYP2C19*3 mutations are responsible for most of the CYP2C19 poor metabolizers. CYP2C19*2, the main defective allele, occurs with a frequency of 30% in the Chinese population, approximately 15% in whites, and approximately 17% in African Americans. The CYP2C19*3 variant affects approximately 5% of Chinese, and is almost nonexistent in whites (72). Together, the CYP2C19*2 and CYP2C19*3 alleles can explain all Asian and approximately 80% of white poor metabolizers (73).

Because the contribution of CYP2C19 to the metabolism of phenytoin increases with an increase in drug concentration, CYP2C19 may be important when CYP2C9 is saturated. The reported differences in K_m values for CYP2C9-catalyzed and CYP2C19-catalyzed phenytoin hydroxylation (5.5 µmol/L versus 71.4 µmol/L) suggest that CYP2C9 is likely to become saturated at phenytoin therapeutic concentrations of 10 to 20 µg/mL (40 to 80 µmol/L) (74). This mechanism explains the increased risk of toxic reactions with the coadministration of CYP2C19 inhibitors such as ticlopidine or isoniazid. The 1% to 2% of white poor metabolizers for both CYP2C9 and CYP2C19 are particularly susceptible to phenytoin's adverse effects (71). Dosage adjustments based on the CYP2C9 and CYP2C19 genotypes may decrease the risk of concentration-dependent adverse effects in allelic variant carriers, particularly at the beginning of therapy.

A Japanese epilepsy study (54) noted an approximate decrease of 14% in the maximum metabolic rate in patients with CYP2C19 variants compared with those with the extensive-metabolizer phenotype. In another Japanese study (55), the predicted plasma concentrations with a phenytoin dose of 5 mg/kg per day were 18.7, 22.8, and 28.8 µg/mL in CYP2C19 homozygous extensive metabolizers, heterozygous extensive metabolizers, and poor metabolizers, respectively.

Enzyme saturation kinetics leads to phenytoin plasma concentrations increasing nonproportionally with changes in dose (Fig. 55.2) (75). The relationship between dose and concentration can be expressed by the Michaelis-Menten equation:

$$\text{Dose (mg/day)} = V_{max}C_{ss}/K_m + C_{ss}$$

where V_{max} is the maximal rate of drug metabolism, C_{ss} the steady-state serum concentration, and K_m the concentration

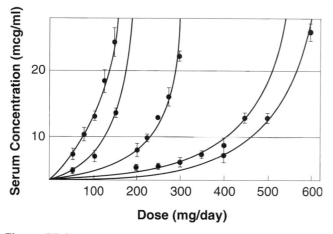

Figure 55.2 Relationship between serum phenytoin concentration and daily dose in five patients. Each point represents the mean (± standard deviation [SD]) of three to eight measurements at steady state. The curves were fitted by computer through use of the Michaelis-Menten equation. (From Richens A, Dunlop A. Serum phenytoin levels in the management of epilepsy. *Lancet* 1975;2: 247–248, with permission.)

at which V_{max} is half-maximal. The mean apparent phenytoin K_m in adults 20 to 39 years old is 5.7 µg/mL (range, 1.5 to 20.7 µg/mL); the mean V_{max} is 7.5 mg/kg/day (76). In most patients, phenytoin exhibits nonlinear pharmacokinetics because the usual therapeutic plasma concentrations exceed the usual K_m. Concomitant illnesses (77) or medications, pregnancy (78), genetic makeup (79–81), and age can significantly affect V_{max} or K_m (or both). Children have higher V_{max} values, but similar K_m values, compared with adults (82–84); elderly individuals have lower V_{max} values (mean, 6.0 mg/kg per day) (76).

Excretion

Up to 95% of phenytoin is excreted in urine and feces as metabolites, with 5% or less of unchanged phenytoin excreted in urine. Phenytoin is also excreted in breast milk (85). Some investigators have suggested that phenytoin enhances its own elimination through enzyme induction (86).

Fosphenytoin

Absorption and Bioavailability

Fosphenytoin can be administered either intravenously or intramuscularly. The values for the area under the plasma total phenytoin and free phenytoin concentration versus time curves, after either intravenous or intramuscular administration of fosphenytoin, are almost identical to that for intravenous phenytoin sodium, indicating complete bioavailability by either route (11). These findings are based on studies involving single-dose intravenous and intramuscular administration to drug-free volunteers and single-dose intravenous administration to patients with therapeutic plasma phenytoin concentrations (11,87,88).

The total and complete conversion to phenytoin presents a potential clinical problem. A mg for mg PE conversion from oral phenytoin (Dilantin) capsules to parenteral fosphenytoin (Cerebyx) solution represents a 9% increase in total dosage, because 100-mg Dilantin capsules actually contain only 92 mg of phenytoin. Dosage adjustment is not usually necessary when Cerebyx is used for up to 1 week, although a phenytoin plasma concentration should be checked after longer periods of administration.

Distribution

Protein Binding

Like phenytoin, fosphenytoin is highly bound (95% to 99%) to serum albumin in a nonlinear fashion (11). This protein binding is not affected by prior diazepam administration (89). However, in the presence of fosphenytoin, phenytoin is displaced from binding sites, rapidly increasing unbound phenytoin concentrations as a function of plasma fosphenytoin concentration. This displacement is accentuated by fosphenytoin doses of at least 15 mg PE/kg delivered at rates of 50 to 150 mg PE per minute. As plasma fosphenytoin concentrations decline, phenytoin protein binding returns to normal. There is little displacement of phenytoin after intramuscular administration of fosphenytoin (11).

Volume of Distribution

Fosphenytoin's volume of distribution is reported to be 0.13 L/kg in patients receiving 1200 mg PE fosphenytoin at 150 mg PE per minute. At lower doses and slower infusion rates, the volume of distribution is lower, 2.6 L, or approximately 0.04 L/kg for a 70-kg human (11,87,90). Fosphenytoin, a very polar molecule, achieves a rapid equilibrium between plasma and associated tissues (90).

Metabolism

After intravenous or intramuscular administration, the phosphate group of fosphenytoin is cleaved by ubiquitous nonspecific phosphatases to produce active phenytoin. The half-life of this conversion is approximately 8 to 18 minutes, is complete in a little more than an hour, and is independent of age, dose, or infusion rate (11,16,91–93). The tissue phosphatases responsible for this conversion are present at all ages; age, plasma phenytoin or fosphenytoin concentrations, and other medications do not alter their activity. The conversion of fosphenytoin to phenytoin is slightly faster in patients with hepatic or renal disease, consistent with decreased binding of fosphenytoin to plasma proteins and increased fraction of unbound fosphenytoin resulting from hypoproteinemia in these diseases (91). In addition, fosphenytoin's phosphate load of 0.0037 mmol phosphate/mg PE fosphenytoin should be considered in patients with severe renal impairment (16).

A pharmacokinetic meta-analysis of plasma total and free phenytoin concentration from seven clinical trials involving neurosurgical patients, patients with status epilepticus,

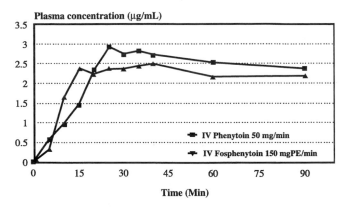

Figure 55.3 Free phenytoin concentration achieved in patients receiving an equivalent intravenous phenytoin loading dose (20 mg/kg) at 50 mg per minute and an equivalent intravenous fosphenytoin loading dose at 150 mg PE per minute. (From Eldon M, Loewen G, Voightman R, et al. Pharmacokinetics and tolerance of fosphenytoin and phenytoin administration intravenously to healthy subjects. *Can J Neurol Sci* 1993;20:5810, with permission.)

patients with stroke, and healthy volunteers demonstrated that fosphenytoin loading doses of 15 to 20 mg PE/kg administered either intravenously or intramuscularly consistently resulted in total phenytoin plasma concentrations of 10 μg/mL or more and free phenytoin concentrations of 1 μg/mL or more. These therapeutic plasma phenytoin concentrations were reached in most subjects within 10 minutes, if rapid intravenous fosphenytoin dosing (≥100 mg PE per minute) was used, or within 30 minutes, if slower intravenous (<100 mg PE per minute) or intramuscular fosphenytoin dosing was used (94).

In one study, after administration of 1200 mg of phenytoin at 50 mg per minute, peak unbound phenytoin concentrations of approximately 3 μg/mL were achieved within 0.5 hour; administration of the equivalent fosphenytoin dose, infused at a rate of 150 mg PE per minute, produced similar peak unbound phenytoin concentrations (Fig. 55.3) (95). This rapid infusion rate was well tolerated. Therefore, when rapid achievement of therapeutic phenytoin concentrations is critical, as in the treatment of status epilepticus, fosphenytoin should be administered at a rate of 150 mg PE per minute. Slower infusion rates (50 to 100 mg PE per minute) may be acceptable in nonemergencies (95).

Excretion

A clinically insignificant amount of fosphenytoin (0 % to 4% of a dose) is excreted renally (93).

PLASMA DRUG CONCENTRATIONS

Phenytoin

Most laboratories and textbooks assume a therapeutic range for phenytoin of 10 to 20 μg/mL, which clinical experience and literature have called into question.

Seizures have been controlled with concentrations lower than 10 μg/mL (96), although often, more than 20 μg/mL is needed. In one study (97), 51% of patients achieved complete control at concentrations either below or above that range. No significant association was evident between the serum phenytoin concentration and any measures of efficacy or toxicity.

Fosphenytoin

Measurement of fosphenytoin levels does not provide clinically useful information for patient care but rather has been utilized only in clinical research settings. Fosphenytoin may interfere with the ability of common laboratory immunoanalytic techniques, such as TDx/TDxFLx (fluorescence polarization) and Emit 2000 (enzyme multiplication), to measure phenytoin levels, because of cross-reactivity resulting in an artifactually elevated phenytoin concentration value. Waiting until all of the fosphenytoin to phenytoin conversion has occurred (approximately 2 hours after intravenous fosphenytoin administration, or 4 hours after intramuscular fosphenytoin administration) before attempting to measure a patient's phenytoin concentrations is recommended (11).

DRUG INTERACTIONS

Phenytoin

Phenytoin can affect, and be affected by, a number of medications (Tables 55.2 and 55.3) (98). Although these drug interactions do not preclude concomitant administration, they signal the need for more frequent determination of serum concentrations, increased monitoring for the appearance of side effects, and, if appropriate, changes in dose. Patient-specific factors, such as genetic makeup, previous exposure to other compounds, and susceptibility to the clinical outcomes of the interaction, govern the extent and clinical significance of any drug interaction. In addition, a drug may act as an inhibitor in one patient and an inducer in another (e.g., phenobarbital's effect on phenytoin).

Interactions can affect any of the four primary pharmacokinetic phases. A drug that affects absorption most likely will decrease phenytoin serum concentration. For example, administration of phenytoin with a continuous high-calorie, nitrogen liquid complete-nutrition formula through nasogastric tube feedings causes a decrease in phenytoin serum concentrations from a mean of 9.8 μg/mL to 2.72 μg/mL at the same dose (99).

Drugs that affect protein binding increase the percentage of unbound phenytoin, usually with no change in the unbound concentration and with a decrease in the total concentration. Valproic acid displaces phenytoin from protein-binding sites. When valproic acid is added to a phenytoin regimen, total phenytoin concentrations decrease, free

TABLE 55.2

BIDIRECTIONAL INTERACTIONS BETWEEN PHENYTOIN AND OTHER ANTIEPILEPTIC DRUGS

Specific Drug	Effect of AED on Phenytoin Concentration	Mechanism of AED Effect	Effect of Phenytoin on AED Concentration	Mechanism of Phenytoin Effect
Carbamazepine	↑↓	CYP2C19 induction	↓↓	CYP3A4 induction
Ethosuximide	«		↓↓	CYP3A4 induction
Felbamate	↑↑	CYP2C19 inhibition	↓↓	CYP3A4 induction
Fosphenytoin	↑ Free phenytoin	Protein-binding displacement	«	
Gabapentin	«		«	
Lamotrigine	«		↓↓	UDPGT induction
Levetiracetam	«		«	
Oxcarbazepine	↑	CYP2C19 inhibition CYP2C9 and	↓ MHD	Unknown
Phenobarbital	↑↓	CYP2C19 induction	↑	Unclear
Topiramate	↑	CYP2C19	↓↓	Unknown
Tiagabine	«		↓↓	CYP3A4 induction
Valproic acid	↓/ ? ↑ Free phenytoin	Protein-binding displacement and CYP2C9 inhibition	↓↓	CYP2C9 and CYP2C19 induction
Zonisamide	«		↓↓	CYP3A4 induction

↑↓, variable; ↑, minor increase; ↓, minor decrease; ↑↑, important increase; ↓↓, important decrease; «, no change; MHD, 10-monohydroxy derivative.

fraction increases, and free concentrations either stay the same or increase slightly. The following equation may be used to measure unbound phenytoin concentration in a patient receiving this combination (100,101):

$$\text{free PHT} = [0.095 + 0.001(\text{VPA})]\,\text{PHT}$$

where PHT = phenytoin and VPA = valproic acid.

Metabolic interactions usually cause either enzyme induction or inhibition. Addition of an inducer decreases phenytoin concentrations; addition of an inhibitor increases them. The order of addition or deletion is important. An inducer added to another compound may lead to decreases in the serum concentration of the preexisting drug; however, if that same drug is added to the inducer, the interaction would have a less noticeable clinical significance because nothing has changed—the added drug would simply require a higher dose. When an enzyme-inhibiting drug is removed from a regimen, the concentration of the remaining compound is likely to increase (102).

Fosphenytoin

As described above, in the presence of fosphenytoin, phenytoin is displaced from binding sites, rapidly increasing unbound phenytoin concentrations as a function of plasma fosphenytoin concentration (11).

EFFICACY

Phenytoin

Phenytoin is effective in the abortive treatment of acute seizures (including acute repetitive seizures and status epilepticus) or as chronic maintenance therapy to prevent seizure recurrence. As maintenance therapy, phenytoin is effective against partial-onset seizures and generalized tonic-clonic seizures but has limited efficacy in absence, clonic, myoclonic, tonic, or atonic seizures. In juvenile myoclonic epilepsy, it may be effective if tonic-clonic seizures are the sole or major seizure type. Similarly, in Lennox-Gastaut syndrome, efficacy appears limited to the tonic-clonic component (103,104).

Acute Seizures (Acute Repetitive Seizures and Status Epilepticus)

Multiple open-label series have indicated that patients with acute repetitive seizures or status epilepticus respond promptly to intravenous administration of phenytoin (103). In 60% to 80% of patients, a response was noted within 20 minutes after the initiation of an infusion (105,106). In one pediatric study (107), loading doses produced a complete or partial effect in 30 of 35 patients. The youngest children had lower concentrations and responded less favorably than did the older children.

A double-blind, randomized trial compared the efficacy of four treatments for generalized convulsive status epilepticus: diazepam (0.15 mg/kg) + phenytoin (18 mg/kg), lorazepam (0.1 mg/kg), phenobarbital (15 mg/kg), and phenytoin (18 mg/kg) (108). Success was defined as complete cessation of motor and electroencephalographic seizure activity within 20 minutes after the drug infusion began, without return of seizure activity during the next 40 minutes. Analyses were performed both on an intent-to-treat basis and including only patients with a verified diagnosis of generalized convulsive status epilepticus. Among

TABLE 55.3
BIDIRECTIONAL INTERACTIONS BETWEEN PHENYTOIN AND OTHER DRUGS

Drug	Effect on Phenytoin Concentration	Mechanism of Effect	Effect of Phenytoin on Drug Concentration	Mechanism of Effect
Antimicrobials				
Albendazole			↓	CYP3A4 induction
Isoniazid	↑	CYP2C9 inhibition		
Rifampicin	↓	CYP2C9 and CYP2C19 induction	↓	CYP3A4 induction
Sulfaphenazole	↑	CYP2C9 inhibition		
Miconazole	↑	CYP2C9 inhibition		
Fluconazole	↑	CYP2C9 inhibition		
Itraconazole	↑	CYP2C9 inhibition	↓	CYP3A4 induction
Nevirapine			↓	CYP3A4 induction
Efavirenz			↓	CYP2B6 induction
Delavirdine			↓	CYP3A4 induction
Indinavir			↓	CYP3A4 induction
Ritonavir			↓	CYP3A4 induction
Saquinavir			↓	CYP3A4 induction
Antineoplastic drugs				
Cyclophosphamide			↓	CYP2B6 and CYP2C19 induction
Ifosfamide			↓	CYP2B6 induction
Teniposide			↓	CYP3A4 and CYP2C19 induction
Etoposide			↓	CYP3A4 induction
Paclitaxel			↓	CYP3A4 induction
Methotrexate	↓	↓ Absorption		
Fluorouracil	↑	CYP2C9 inhibition		
Carmustine	↓	↓ Absorption		
Vinblastine	↓	↓ Absorption		
Vincristine	↓	↓ Absorption		
Bleomycin	↓	↓ Absorption		
Cardiovascular drugs				
Quinidine			↓	CYP3A4 induction
Amiodarone	↑	CYP2C9 inhibition	↓	CYP3A4 induction
Propranolol				CYP1A2 and CYP2C19 induction
Nifedipine			↓	CYP3A4 induction
Felodipine			↓	CYP3A4 induction
Nisoldipine			↓	CYP3A4 induction
Verapamil (oral)			↓	CYP3A4 induction
Losartan			↓ Active metabolite	CYP2C9 inhibition
Ticlopidine	↑	CYP2C19 inhibition		
Digoxin			↓	CYP3A4 induction
Atorvastatin			↓	CYP3A4 induction
Lovastatin			↓	CYP3A4 induction
Simvastatin			↓	CYP3A4 induction
Fluvastatin			↓	CYP2C9 induction
Warfarin			↑ Free warfarin (initially), then ↓	CYP2C9 induction
Gastrointestinal drugs				
Antacids	↓	↓ Absorption		
Sucralfate	↓	↓ Absorption		
Cimetidine	↑	CYP2C19 inhibition		
Omeprazole	↑	CYP2C19 inhibition		
Immunosuppressant drugs				
Cyclosporin			↓	CYP3A4 induction
Tacrolimus	↑	Protein-binding displacement	↓	CYP3A4 induction
Sirolimus			↓	CYP3A4 induction

TABLE 55.3
(continued)

Drug	Effect on Phenytoin Concentration	Mechanism of Effect	Effect of Phenytoin on Drug Concentration	Mechanism of Effect
Psychotropic drugs				
Amitriptyline	↑	CYP2C19 inhibition	↓	CYP2C19 and CYP3A4 induction
Imipramine	↑	CYP2C19 inhibition	↓	CYP1A2 and CYP2C19 induction
Clomipramine			↓	CYP1A2 and CYP2C19 induction
Mianserin			↓	CYP3A4 induction
Bupropion			↓	CYP2B6 induction
Citalopram			↓	CYP3A4 and CYP2C19 induction
Paroxetine	↑	CYP2C19 and CYP2C9 inhibition		
Fluoxetine	↑	CYP2C19 inhibition		
Fluvoxamine	↑	CYP2C19 inhibition		
Sertraline	↑	CYP2C9 inhibition		
Haloperidol			↓	CYP3A4 induction
Chlorpromazine			↓	CYP3A4 induction
Clozapine			↓	CYP1A2 induction
Quetiapine			↓	CYP3A4 induction
Diazepam			↓	CYP3A4 and CYP2C19 induction
Alprazolam			↓	CYP3A4 induction
Midazolam			↓	CYP3A4 induction
Steroids				
Hydrocortisone			↓	CYP3A4 induction
Dexamethasone			↓	CYP3A4 induction
Prednisone			↓	CYP3A4 induction
Steroidal oral contraceptives			↓	CYP3A4 induction
Miscellaneous				
Theophylline			↓	CYP3A4 induction
Fentanyl			↓	CYP3A4 induction
Methadone			↓	CYP3A4 and CYP2B6 induction

the 384 patients with verified overt generalized convulsive status epilepticus, lorazepam was the most successful treatment (64.9%, $p = 0.02$ for the overall comparison), followed by phenobarbital (58.2%), diazepam + phenytoin (55.8%), and phenytoin alone (43.6%). Lorazepam was superior to phenytoin in a direct pairwise comparison ($p = 0.002$). However, the four groups did not differ significantly either for the subgroup of verified subtle generalized convulsive status epilepticus or in the intent-to-treat analysis. The authors concluded that lorazepam is more effective than phenytoin for the treatment of overt generalized convulsive status epilepticus (108).

Controlled studies have shown that phenytoin does not prevent nonepileptic alcohol-related seizures (109,110). Ninety alcoholic patients were enrolled prospectively in a randomized, double-blind trial within 6 hours of an initial alcohol-related seizure during a withdrawal episode and

assigned to receive either 1000 mg of intravenous phenytoin or placebo. None of the patients had a history of seizures not related to alcohol withdrawal, and 71 patients had seizures during prior withdrawals. Six of 45 patients in the phenytoin group and 6 of 45 in the placebo group had at least one recurrent seizure during the postinfusion observation period. Phenytoin serum concentrations were similar in patients with and without subsequent seizures. Response rates in the two arms did not differ significantly ($p > 0.05$) (109).

Another identically designed trial (110) assigned 55 patients with alcohol withdrawal seizures and without other previous seizures to intravenous phenytoin or placebo. Of 28 patients treated with phenytoin, 6 (21%) had a seizure recurrence, compared with 5 (19%) of 27 patients given placebo. Again, response rates in the two groups did not differ significantly ($p > 0.05$) (110).

Partial-Onset and Generalized Tonic-Clonic Seizures

Multiple studies have compared the efficacy and tolerability of phenytoin with those of other AEDs (including carbamazepine, phenobarbital, primidone, valproic acid, lamotrigine, and oxcarbazepine) in the treatment of partial-onset and generalized tonic-clonic seizures. Overall, phenytoin has consistently demonstrated equal or superior efficacy compared with all other AEDs against these seizure types (111).

In the first Veterans Administration (VA) Cooperative Study (111), 622 adults were randomly assigned to treatment with phenytoin, carbamazepine, phenobarbital, or primidone and remained on therapy unless unacceptable toxic reactions or lack of efficacy was evident. Carbamazepine and phenytoin were more effective and had greater tolerability over time compared with primidone and phenobarbital in the treatment of complex partial seizures. All four AEDs were equally effective as monotherapy for generalized tonic-clonic seizures. Carbamazepine and phenytoin produced the highest rates of success, as defined by retention in the study (Fig. 55.4), and were recommended as "drugs of first-choice for single-drug therapy of adults with partial or generalized tonic-clonic seizures or with both."

In several other comparative trials, phenytoin was as effective as carbamazepine and valproic acid, with similar potential to cause major side effects (112–115). In a comparison with phenobarbital, carbamazepine, and valproic acid in 243 adults with new-onset partial or generalized tonic-clonic seizures, 27% of the patients remained seizure free and 75% had entered 1 year of remission by 3 years of follow up. No significant differences in efficacy were found among the four drugs at 1, 2, or 3 years of follow up. The incidence of unacceptable side effects necessitating withdrawal from treatment was 10% (116).

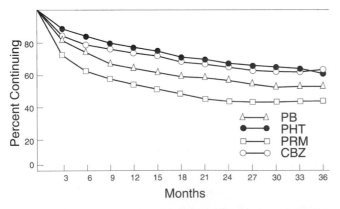

Figure 55.4 Cumulative percentage of patients remaining in the study during 36 months of follow-up. There were 275 patients at 12 months, 164 at 24 months, and 97 at 36 months. (From Mattson RH, Cramer JA, Collins JF, et al. Comparison of carbamazepine, phenobarbital, phenytoin, and primidone in partial and secondarily generalized tonic-clonic seizures. *N Engl J Med* 1985; 313:145–151, with permission.)

Two studies compared the efficacy and tolerability of oxcarbazepine and phenytoin monotherapy in patients with recent-onset partial seizures or generalized tonic-clonic seizures (117,118). Each study was a randomized (1:1 oxcarbazepine-to-phenytoin), double-blind, parallel-group trial consisting of a 14-day screening phase followed by a 56-week double-blind period (8-week flexible titration phase followed by a 48-week maintenance phase). One study (117) involving 287 adults and adolescents, ages 15 to 91 years, demonstrated no difference in the proportion of seizure-free patients during the 48 weeks of maintenance between the oxcarbazepine group (59%) and the phenytoin group (58%). The second trial (118), in 193 children and adolescents, ages 5 to 17 years, also showed no difference in the proportion of seizure-free patients during the 48-week maintenance period between the oxcarbazepine group (61%) and the phenytoin group (60%).

Lamotrigine and phenytoin monotherapy were compared in a double-blind, parallel-group study of patients with newly diagnosed untreated partial-onset seizures or generalized tonic-clonic seizures (119). After randomization to either lamotrigine ($n = 86$) or phenytoin ($n = 95$), patients entered a 6-week flexible titration phase, followed by a 48-week maintenance phase. No between-treatment difference in efficacy was detected on the basis of percentages of patients remaining on each treatment arm, those remaining seizure free during the last 24 and 40 weeks of the study, and times to first seizure after the initial 6 weeks of treatment (dose-titration period).

No monotherapy trials have compared phenytoin with felbamate, gabapentin, topiramate, tiagabine, zonisamide, or levetiracetam in the treatment of partial-onset or generalized tonic-clonic seizures.

Neonatal Seizures

Phenytoin and phenobarbital monotherapy were compared in a randomized trial of 59 neonates with seizures confirmed by electroencephalography (120). Seizures were controlled in 43% of the phenobarbital group and in 45% of the phenytoin group. Monotherapy or subsequent duotherapy controlled seizures in 59% of the neonates. The authors concluded that both drugs were "equally but incompletely effective as anticonvulsants in neonates."

Other Seizure Types

Phenytoin is considered effective for primary generalized tonic-clonic seizures (104,114); however, there is no convincing evidence that it is effective against absence, clonic, myoclonic, tonic, or atonic seizures. Phenytoin is not recommended for infantile spasms, Lennox-Gastaut syndrome, or primary generalized epilepsy syndromes such as childhood absence or juvenile myoclonic epilepsy.

Prophylaxis

For seizure prophylaxis in pregnancy-induced hypertension, phenytoin has similar (121) or inferior (122,123) efficacy to magnesium sulfate. Patients receiving phenytoin had more rapid cervical dilation, a smaller decrease in hematocrit after delivery, and a lower incidence of hot flashes (124). In addition, phenytoin did not confound the computer analysis of fetal heart rate (125).

Phenytoin is often used following neurosurgical procedures and cerebrovascular accidents. A randomized, double-blind trial compared the efficacy, tolerability, and impact on quality of life and cognitive functioning of anticonvulsant prophylaxis with phenytoin versus valproate in 100 patients following craniotomy (126). Fourteen patients (seven in each group) experienced postoperative seizures. No major between-treatment differences emerged in efficacy, tolerability, impact on quality of life, or cognitive functioning (126). A double-blind comparison of phenytoin or carbamazepine with no treatment after supratentorial craniotomy noted no significant differences but a higher incidence of side effects in the treated group (127). Thus, prophylactic anticonvulsants cannot be recommended routinely after this type of procedure.

The efficacy of phenytoin in the prevention of posttraumatic seizures was studied in a randomized, double-blind trial of 404 patients with serious head trauma (128). Patients received a phenytoin loading dose within 24 hours of injury; free phenytoin serum levels were maintained in a range from 0.75 to 1.5 μg/mL. From the time of drug loading to day 7, significantly fewer seizures occurred in the phenytoin group than in the placebo group (3.6% versus 14.2%, $p < 0.001$). No benefit was seen in the phenytoin group after day 8, however, leading to the conclusion that phenytoin had an early suppressive effect, but not a true prophylactic effect, on seizures, and that it reduced the incidence of seizures only during the first week after injury. In a secondary analysis of this study (129), no significant difference in mortality was found between patients assigned to phenytoin and those assigned to placebo (129). In a randomized, double-blind, placebo-controlled trial in children with moderate to severe blunt head injury, phenytoin did not prevent posttraumatic seizures within 48 hours of the trauma (130).

Nonepileptic Disorders

Phenytoin has been shown to be useful in neuropathic pain (131), motion sickness (132,133), cardiac arrhythmias, continuous muscle fiber activity syndrome, myotonic muscular dystrophy, and myotonia congenita (134). It may also have a role in the treatment of recessive dystrophic epidermolysis bullosa, intermittent explosive disorder, and anxiety disorder (134), and as topical therapy for burns, refractory skin ulcers (134,135), and wound healing (136).

Fosphenytoin

Fosphenytoin itself has no known anticonvulsant activity; it derives its utility from its rapid and total conversion to phenytoin (15,16).

ADVERSE EFFECTS

Phenytoin

Concentration-Dependent Effects

The most common concentration-dependent phenytoin side effects are related to the central nervous system and consist of nystagmus, ataxia, incoordination (137,138), diplopia (vestibulooccular-cerebellar syndrome), and drowsiness. Some patients may experience prominent side effects at concentrations in the lower end of the therapeutic range, while others may be free of complaints despite elevated drug concentrations. These effects are reversible with appropriate adjustments in dose. Although small decreases may completely alleviate complaints, significant dose alterations may dramatically decrease serum concentrations, leading to a recurrence of seizures. Nausea, vomiting, and epigastric pain are often improved by dividing the dose or taking it with meals (or both).

Symptoms noted at serum phenytoin concentrations higher than 30 μg/mL include dysarthria, far-lateral nystagmus, movement disorders (usually choreoathetosis and orofacial dyskinesia), exacerbation of seizures, external ophthalmoplegia, or encephalopathy (including lethargy, delirium, "psychosis," stupor, and coma) (93,138–143).

Reports of the effect of phenytoin on cognitive function vary, depending on the type of patients, presence or absence of concomitant AEDs, measurement instruments, and comparative drugs. In general, however, effects appear modest when serum concentrations are kept within standard therapeutic ranges and polypharmacy is avoided (144,145). Unfortunately, patients taking phenytoin may suffer from cognitive side effects even when these guidelines are followed (146).

Compared with carbamazepine, no difference (145, 147–151) or more changes (146,152,153) in cognition with phenytoin have been noted. In one study, phenytoin appeared to be associated with more cognitive effects than carbamazepine, although reanalysis excluding patients with elevated phenytoin concentrations showed no difference (147,154). When used as prophylaxis against seizures following head trauma, phenytoin demonstrated negative cognitive effects compared with placebo (155). No clinically significant difference in cognitive effects between phenytoin and valproate was detected in either healthy adults (156) or patients following craniotomy (126).

In one study of elderly patients, phenytoin and valproic acid had similar effects (157), whereas a second study reported no cognitive impairment resulting from modest increases in serum phenytoin concentrations (between 11 μg/mL and 16 μg/mL) (158). Motor disturbances are common in children taking phenytoin (159). In children withdrawn from AEDs, cognitive function remains unchanged, whereas psychomotor speed improves (160). Fluctuations in phenytoin serum concentrations by as much as 50% had no or an immeasurably small effect in children with well-controlled seizures receiving monotherapy with low therapeutic dosages (161). Removal of chronic phenytoin in patients receiving polypharmacy resulted in significant improvement in one test of concentration and two tests of psychomotor function (148).

Idiosyncratic Reactions

Phenytoin's idiosyncratic reactions are proposed to result from the formation of a reactive metabolite (an arene oxide) that either directly (owing to deficiencies in detoxification resulting from inadequate epoxide hydrolase activity) or indirectly (through an immune response or free radical-mediated injury) causes cell, tissue, or organ injury and, at times, death (162).

The most common idiosyncratic reaction is rash, which may occur in up to 8.5% of patients, particularly children and adolescents (163–165). The *in vivo* and *in vitro* cross-reactivity between phenytoin, phenobarbital, and carbamazepine is as high as 70% to 80% (166). A more severe dermatologic idiosyncratic reaction is the "hypersensitivity syndrome" (166). In a series of 38 affected patients, the most common manifestations were rash, fever, lymphadenopathy, eosinophilia, abnormal liver function test results, blood dyscrasias, serum sickness, renal failure, and polymyositis. Symptoms usually occur within the first 3 months of therapy (167).

Other reported idiosyncratic reactions include Stevens-Johnson syndrome, toxic epidermal necrolysis, aplastic anemia, hepatitis, pseudolymphoma, and a lupus-like reaction (138).

Adverse Effects with Long-Term Therapy

Long-term administration of phenytoin has been associated with gingival hyperplasia (168,169), hirsutism, acne, and rash. The exact incidence of gingival hyperplasia attributable to phenytoin is not known (169); reports range from 13% of patients attending general medical practices (170) to about 40% of patients taking phenytoin long term in a community-based cross-sectional study in Ferrara, Northern Italy (171). In the latter report, younger age and poorer oral hygiene seemed to predispose to the severest level of gingival involvement (171). Hyperplasia regresses after discontinuation of phenytoin (172,173).

Cerebellar atrophy has been reported after long-term (174,175) and acute use (176) of high doses, although whether the true etiologic agent was phenytoin or the seizures is unclear (177,178); single-photon-emission computed tomography scans may be a means for early detection (177).

Among other effects of long-term phenytoin therapy are alterations in laboratory values, including reduction in bone mineral density (179), low folate levels (93), macrocytosis (93), and decreases in levels of carnitine (180), low-density lipoprotein cholesterol, and apolipoprotein B (181). Levels of prolactin (182) and apolipoprotein A and A1 (181) increase, as does high-density lipoprotein cholesterol, although at doses of 100 mg/day this lipid fraction was

unchanged (183). Phenytoin may decrease levels of free testosterone and enhance its conversion to estradiol (184).

Changes in thyroid hormones have been reported (185). The thyroxine (T_4) and free T_4 index, total T_4 and triiodothyronine (T_3), free T_4, and free T_3 all decrease. Increases in serum levels of thyroid-stimulating hormone (186,187) may involve protein-binding displacement and induction of cellular metabolism (188). Phenytoin therapy may suppress immunoglobulin (Ig) production, leading to decreases in IgG (189,190) and IgA (189,191). Panhypoglobulinemia was reported in one patient infected with the human immunodeficiency virus (192). It is unclear whether these changes are a direct result of phenytoin or epilepsy (189) or if they occur with any drug with arene oxide intermediates (189,193).

Teratogenicity

"Fetal hydantoin syndrome" was described in 1975 and consisted of growth retardation, microcephaly, mental retardation, and numerous "minor" congenital anomalies (165,194). However, "fetal anticonvulsant syndrome" has replaced this term because the malformations are seen in children of mothers taking a wide variety of AEDs. Although there is agreement that anticonvulsant polypharmacy and folic acid deficiency increase the risk of malformation (195), the absolute and relative teratogenicity of phenytoin is not completely known.

Two recent studies (196,197) described the pregnancy outcomes of women with epilepsy taking AEDs. The Australian Registry of AEDs in Pregnancy monitored 292 pregnancies, 19 of which involved the use of phenytoin. The 10.5% (2 of 19) incidence of birth defects with phenytoin used in the first trimester was not significant compared with the 4.3% (1 of 23) incidence in women with epilepsy who were not taking an AED in the first trimester ($p = 0.58$). Significant increases were noted in mean birth weight (3870 versus 3395 g, $p \leq 0.01$) and length (52.7 versus 50.5 cm, $p \leq 0.0005$) of infants born to mothers taking phenytoin (196). In a study from Helsinki, Finland, of 740 fetuses exposed to maternal AEDs during the first trimester, 212 were associated with phenytoin (124 in monotherapy). The 3.3% (7 of 212) incidence of birth defects with phenytoin did not reach statistical significance in a logistic regression analysis ($p = 0.3$) (197).

Intravenous Administration

Administration of parenteral phenytoin solution is associated with local reactions, including pain and burning at the infusion site, phlebitis, and vessel cording (8,9,198). Extravasation can lead to phlebitis, chemical cellulitis, or frank necrosis (10). A unique effect of unknown etiology, purple glove syndrome (199,200), begins with discoloration and progresses to a petechial rash; severe cases may require surgical intervention. In one report (201), 9 of 152 patients (5.9%) receiving intravenous phenytoin developed purple glove syndrome.

Intravenously administered phenytoin can also lead to cardiovascular complications, such as hypotension, atrial and ventricular conduction depression, and ventricular fibrillation (9). The major risk factors for these complications include preexisting disease, advanced age, and rapid infusion (9,198). In patients without cardiovascular disease, phenytoin can be administered at 40 to 50 mg per minute (202). Rates should not exceed 25 mg per minute in patients with arteriosclerotic cardiovascular disease (203).

Fosphenytoin

Concentration-Dependent Effects

Intravenous fosphenytoin infusion has a favorable side-effect profile (8,95,204). The local reactions associated with administration of parenteral phenytoin solution (infusion-site pain, phlebitis, and vessel cording) occur significantly less often with fosphenytoin (8). Pain at the site of fosphenytoin infusion is rare, but 48.9% of patients reported pruritus or tingling (without rash) in the perianal region, elsewhere on the trunk, or on the back of the head (204). Pruritus or tingling appears soon after an infusion starts, abates rapidly when the infusion stops, and can be reduced or abolished by slowing the infusion. Decreases in systolic and diastolic blood pressure have been observed, but the changes were judged to be clinically insignificant and did not require cessation of the infusion (205). Cardiac arrhythmias have not been noted (205). Dizziness, somnolence, and ataxia were observed with a frequency similar to that after phenytoin infusion (205).

Adverse effects have been even less notable after intramuscular fosphenytoin injection (206–208). Mild local irritation occurred in only 5% of 60 patients who received intramuscular loading doses, even though the volume of injected solution was usually 15 to 20 mL (mean, 17.8 mg PE/kg or 1359.8 mg PE total) (207).

Idiosyncratic Reactions, Long-Term Adverse Reactions, Teratogenicity

No idiosyncratic reactions are associated specifically with fosphenytoin. As fosphenytoin is used only on a short-term basis, data about long-term adverse reactions are lacking. There are also no data on possible teratogenic effects with fosphenytoin.

CLINICAL USE

Phenytoin

For rapid increase in drug concentration, phenytoin doses of 15 to 20 mg/kg are used (108,209). Doses of 18 mg/kg increase phenytoin serum concentrations by approximately 23 μg/mL in adults being treated for acute seizures (210); in children with status epilepticus, similar or higher doses have been administered (107). The intravenous route is used during status epilepticus. In less acute situations,

oral administration is appropriate, but the loading dose is divided into three or four doses, given 2 to 3 hours apart to improve bioavailability and rate of absorption (211–213).

When given intravenously to adults, phenytoin should be diluted in normal saline (not in dextrose 5% in water); the infusion should not exceed 50 mg per minute and should be injected directly into a large vein through a large-gauge needle or intravenous catheter. The intramuscular route is not recommended owing to the drug's slow and erratic absorption, as well as painful local reactions likely associated with crystallization at the injection site. If, however, no other routes of administration are available, intramuscular doses 50% higher than oral doses may be needed to maintain plasma concentrations (214–216). Adjustments in dosage and monitoring of serum levels may be necessary on switching from one route to another. Therapeutic levels of phenytoin administered rectally have not been maintained in patients with seizures (217).

For maintenance therapy, the nonlinear pharmacokinetics and wide interindividual variability in metabolism and absorption necessitate individualized regimens. The typical initial dose of 300 mg/day results in concentrations between 10 and 20 μg/mL in fewer than 30% of patients, and more than 57% will achieve concentrations below 10 μg/mL (42). Doses of 6 to 8 mg/kg will produce concentrations between 10 and 20 μg/mL in approximately 45% of otherwise healthy patients, less than 10 μg/mL in 35%, and more than 20 μg/mL in 20% (42). Thereafter, adjustments should be based on clinical response, increasing dosage for lack of seizure control or lowering dosage for concentration-dependent toxic reactions.

Privitera (218) proposed the following guidelines based on initial plasma concentration: increase dosage by 100 mg/day for an initial plasma concentration of less than 7 μg/mL; increase by 50 mg/day for concentrations from 7 to 12 μg/mL; increase by 30 mg/day for concentrations greater than 12 μg/mL. This formula was tested in 129 dosage increases of 50 or 100 mg in 77 patients. All 53 increases that were within the guidelines produced plasma concentrations less than 25 μg/mL, whereas 36% of the increases that exceeded the guidelines produced plasma concentrations greater than 25 μg/mL (218).

Accurate predictions of phenytoin plasma concentrations cannot be accomplished with the Michaelis-Menten equation unless patient-specific values for V_{max} and K_m are obtainable, which is rarely possible in clinical situations. When at least some clinical data are available, numerous methods can assist in estimating an individual patient's dose (219–222) to achieve predetermined serum concentrations (223,224). The nonlinear pharmacokinetics of phenytoin not only leads to nonproportional changes in serum concentration with changes in dose but increases the apparent elimination half-life with higher concentrations. Thus, patients with "high" concentrations exhibit smaller peak-trough variability and require a longer time to achieve steady state. For most patients whose concentrations are within the therapeutic range, the peak-trough remains relatively unaffected, and steady state is reached in approximately 1 to 2 weeks. Thus, any changes in dose will require 1 to 2 weeks to achieve maximum effect. Patients receiving prompt-release phenytoin products and those with low serum concentrations and rapid phenytoin metabolism (e.g., children or patients with relatively high dose requirements) are at high risk for large peak-trough variability and often need multiple daily doses to prevent wide fluctuations in clinical response.

Children require higher milligrams per kilogram daily doses, whereas the elderly should be started on 2 to 3 mg/kg per day and doses increased carefully. Concomitant illnesses can alter phenytoin pharmacokinetics and, consequently, dosage requirements. Critically ill patients may require plasmapheresis, continuous ambulatory peritoneal dialysis, or hemofiltration. Plasmapheresis does not appear to remove a significant amount of phenytoin (225); continuous ambulatory peritoneal dialysis may not (226). In contrast, continuous hemofiltration at a high ultrafiltration rate may remove significant amounts of phenytoin in patients with renal failure with significant protein-binding changes (227). Pregnancy may necessitate an increase in phenytoin dose, especially during the third trimester (78).

Fosphenytoin

The three main situations in which fosphenytoin is used are during status epilepticus, as a temporary substitute for oral phenytoin, and in a nonemergency situation, such as in a patient undergoing a neurosurgical procedure. Fosphenytoin can be diluted in a variety of vehicles, such as dextrose 5% and 10%, lactated Ringer solution, and mannitol 20% (228).

Allen and colleagues (229) reported preliminary results of an open-label, single-dose study of intravenous fosphenytoin for treatment of status epilepticus in 54 patients. With a mean fosphenytoin dose of 967 mg PE (16.4 mg PE/kg) infused at a mean rate of 120 mg PE per minute, total and free phenytoin concentrations at or above 10 μg/mL and 1 μg/mL, respectively, were achieved within 10 to 20 minutes. No patients had cardiac arrhythmias or clinically significant hypotension. Three percent of patients reported tenderness at the infusion site 24 hours later, but no inflammation or phlebitis was observed. Seizures were controlled in 50 of the 53 patients who received an adequate dose.

Fosphenytoin (rather than phenytoin) has become part of the standard-of-care treatment protocols for convulsive status epilepticus in adults and children in many U.S. hospitals. It is preferred to phenytoin because of better tolerability at the infusion site, lack of cardiovascular complications, and overall ease of administration (230). For the treatment of convulsive status epilepticus, a fosphenytoin "loading dose" of 15 to 20 mg PE/kg can be given intravenously, with an infusion rate of at least 100 mg PE per minute and up to 150 mg PE per minute. The dose should be adjusted in patients who have hepatic impairment or hypoalbuminemia.

Fosphenytoin (given either intravenously or intramuscularly) is useful as a temporary substitute for oral phenytoin when the patient is unable to take oral medications. In this situation, the fosphenytoin dose and frequency would be the same as the patient's oral phenytoin dose and frequency.

Fosphenytoin can be useful in the prophylaxis of seizures in neurosurgical patients. A single nonemergency loading dose is given either intravenously or intramuscularly. The dose is usually 10 to 20 mg PE/kg, with an intravenous infusion rate of up to 150 mg PE per minute.

Fosphenytoin is significantly more expensive than phenytoin (231). A number of studies and editorials have reported pharmacoeconomic comparisons between fosphenytoin and intravenous phenytoin (212,231–233). The overall cost of patient care with intravenous fosphenytoin was less than with intravenous phenytoin in an emergency department setting (233). Substitution of intravenous fosphenytoin for intravenous phenytoin was associated with reduced "adverse events at a reasonable increase in total hospital costs" in a second study (232). An editorial suggested that pharmacoeconomic decisions should be based on outcome cost, not acquisition costs (231). Overall, in terms of cost effectiveness, studies in the past decade showed that despite higher acquisition cost, use of intravenous fosphenytoin appeared to be at least equivalent to, if not better than, intravenous phenytoin. However, two recent studies (212,234) have challenged this impression. The administration of intravenous fosphenytoin to adults in an emergency department did not significantly decrease the incidence of drug-related adverse effects or decrease the length of stay in the emergency department compared with the use of intravenous phenytoin. This result suggests that intravenous fosphenytoin is not more cost effective than intravenous phenytoin.

REFERENCES

1. Friedlander WJ. Putnam, Merritt, and the discovery of Dilantin. *Epilepsia* 1986;27:S1–S20.
2. Putnam T, Merritt H. Experimental determination of the anticonvulsant properties of some phenyl derivatives. *Science* 1937; 85:525–526.
3. Merritt H, Putnam T. A new series of anticonvulsant drugs tested by experiments in animals. *Arch Neurol Psychiatry* 1938;39: 1003–1015.
4. Merritt H, Putnam T. Sodium diphenyl hydantoinate in the treatment of convulsive disorders. *JAMA* 1938;111:1068–1073.
5. Merritt H, Putnam T. Further experience with the use of sodium diphenyl hydantoinate in the treatment of convulsive disorders. *Am J Psychiatry* 1940;96:1023–1027.
6. Leppik I. Antiepileptic drug selection: a view from the United States. *Epilepsia* 1995;36:S90.
7. Browne T, LeDuc B. Phenytoin: chemistry and biotransformation. In: Levy R, Mattson R, Meldrum B, eds. *Antiepileptic drugs*, 4th ed. New York: Raven Press, 1995:283–300.
8. Jamerson BD, Dukes GE, Brouwer KL, et al. Venous irritation related to intravenous administration of phenytoin versus fosphenytoin. *Pharmacotherapy* 1994;14:47–52.

9. Mattson RH. Parenteral antiepileptic/anticonvulsant drugs. *Neurology* 1996;46:S8-S13.
10. Hayes A, Chesney T. Necrosis of the hand after extravasation of intravenously administered phenytoin. *J Am Acad Dermatol* 1993;28:360–363.
11. Browne TR, Kugler AR, Eldon MA. Pharmacology and pharmacokinetics of fosphenytoin. *Neurology* 1996;46:S3–S7.
12. DeLorenzo R. Phenytoin mechanisms of action. In: Levy R, Mattson R, Meldrum B, eds. *Antiepileptic drugs,* 4th ed. New York: Raven Press, 1995:271–282.
13. Esplin D. Effects of diphenylhydantoin on synaptic transmission in cat spinal cord and stallate ganglion. *J Pharmacol Exp Ther* 1957;120:301–323.
14. Francis J, Burnham W. (3H)Phenytoin identifies a novel anticonvulsant-binding domain on voltage-dependent sodium channels. *Mol Pharmacol* 1992;42:1097–1103.
15. Knapp LE, Kugler AR. Clinical experience with fosphenytoin in adults: pharmacokinetics, safety, and efficacy. *J Child Neurol* 1998;13:S15–S18.
16. Boucher BA. Fosphenytoin: a novel phenytoin prodrug. *Pharmacotherapy* 1996;16:777–791.
17. Meinardi H, Kleijn E, Meijer Jvd, et al. Absorption and distribution of antiepileptic drugs. *Epilepsia* 1975;16:353–365.
18. Treiman DM, Woodbury DM. Phenytoin: absorption, distribution, and excretion. In: Levy RH, Mattson RH, Meldrum BS, eds. *Antiepileptic drug,* 4th ed. New York: Raven Press, 1995:301–314.
19. Davis A, Begg E, Kennedy M, et al. Application of a simplified method to determine bioavailability of an oral dose of phenytoin. *J Pharmacokinet Biopharm* 1993;21:195–208.
20. Jusko W. Bioavailability and disposition kinetics of phenytoin in man. In: Kellaway P, Petersen I, eds. *Quantitative analytic studies in epilepsy.* New York: Raven Press, 1976:115–136.
21. Irvin J, Notari R. Computer-aided dosage form design, III: feasibility assessment for an oral prolonged-release phenytoin product. *Pharm Res* 1991;8:232–237.
22. Dill W, Kazenko A, Wolff L, et al. Studies on 5,5-diphenylhydantoin (Dilantin) in animals and man. *J Pharmacol Exp Ther* 1956;118:270–279.
23. O'Malley W, Denckla M, O'Doherty D. Oral absorption of diphenylhydantoin as measured by gas liquid chromatography. *Trans Am Neurol Assoc* 1969;94:318–319.
24. Wilder B, Ramsay R. Correlation of acute diphenylhydantoin intoxication with plasma levels and metabolite excretion. *Neurology* 1976;23:1329–1332.
25. Matsukura M, Ikeda T, Higashi A, et al. Relative bioavailability of two different phenytoin preparations. Evidence for an age dependency. *Dev Pharmacol Ther* 1984;7:160–168.
26. Jalling B, Boreus L, Rane A, et al. Plasma concentrations of diphenylhydantoin in young infants. *Pharmacol Clin (Berlin)* 1970;2:200–202.
27. Browne T, Szabo G, Schumacher G, et al. Bioavailability studies of drugs with nonlinear pharmacokinetics, I: tracer dose AUC varies directly with serum concentration. *J Clin Pharmacol* 1992;32:1141–1145.
28. Kasuya Y, Mamada K, Baba S, et al. Stable-isotope methodology for the bio-availability study of phenytoin during multiple-dosing regimens. *J Pharm Sci* 1985;74:503–507.
29. Chang SW, da Silva JH, Kuhl DR. Absorption of rectally administered phenytoin: a pilot study. *Ann Pharmacother* 1999;33:781–786.
30. Mikati M, Bassett N, Schachter E. Double-blind randomized study comparing brand-name and generic phenytoin monotherapy (published erratum appears in *Epilepsia* 1992;33:1156). *Epilepsia* 1992;33:359–365.
31. Rosenbaum D, Rowan A, Tuchman L, et al. Comparative bioavailability of a generic phenytoin and Dilantin. *Epilepsia* 1994;35:656–660.
32. Tsai JJ, Lai ML, Yang YH, et al. Comparison on bioequivalence of four phenytoin preparations in patients with multiple-dose treatment. *J Clin Pharmacol* 1992;32:272–276.
33. Petker M, Morton D. Comparison of the effectiveness of two oral phenytoin products and chronopharmacokinetics of phenytoin. *J Clin Pharmacol Ther* 1993;18:213–217.
34. U.S. Food and Drug Administration. *Approval letter for phenytoin sodium, Mylan Pharmaceuticals, application number 040298.* Available at: http://www.fda.gov/cder/foi/anda/98/40-298_Phenytoin%20 Sodium_Approv.pdf.
35. Goff D, Spunt A, Jung D, et al. Absorption characteristics of three phenytoin sodium products after administration of oral loading doses. *Clin Pharm* 1984;3:634–638.
36. Woodbury D. Pharmacology of anticonvulsant drugs in CSF. In: Woods J, ed. *Neurobiology of cerebrospinal fluid,* vol 2. New York: Plenum Press, 1983:615–628.
37. Pospisil J, Perlik F. Binding parameters of phenytoin during monotherapy and polytherapy. *Int J Clin Pharmacol Ther Toxicol* 1992;30:24–28.
38. Liponi D, Winter M, Tozer T. Renal function and therapeutic concentrations of phenytoin. *Neurology* 1984;34:395–397.
39. Kang H, Leppik I. Phenytoin binding and renal transplantation. *Neurology* 1984;34:83–86.
40. Fedler C, Stewart MJ. Plasma total phenytoin: a possibly misleading test in developing countries. *Ther Drug Monit* 1999; 21:155–160.
41. Dager W, Inciardi J, Howe T. Estimating phenytoin concentrations by the Sheiner-Tozer method in adults with pronounced hypoalbuminemia. *Ann Pharmacother* 1995;29:667–670.
42. Tozer TN, Winter ME. Phenytoin. In: Evans WE, Schentag JJ, Jusko WJ, eds. *Applied pharmacokinetics. Principles of therapeutic drug monitoring.* Vancouver, WA: Applied Therapeutics, 1992:25-1–25-4.
43. Koren G, Brand N, Halkin H, et al. Kinetics of intravenous phenytoin in children. *Pediatr Pharmacol* 1984;4:31–38.
44. Vozeh S, Uematsu T, Aarons L, et al. Intravenous phenytoin loading in patients after neurosurgery and in status epilepticus. A population pharmacokinetic study. *Clin Pharmacokinet* 1988;14:122–128.
45. Abernethy D, Greenblatt D. Phenytoin disposition in obesity. Determination of loading dose. *Arch Neurol* 1985;42:468–471.
46. Oca G, Gums J, Robinson J. Phenytoin dosing in obese patients: two case reports. *Drug Intell Clin Pharm* 1988;22:708–710.
47. Dickinson R, Hooper W, Patterson M, et al. Extent of urinary excretion of *p*-hydroxyphenytoin in healthy subjects given phenytoin. *Ther Drug Monit* 1985;7:283–289.
48. Yasumori T, Chen LS, Li QH, et al. Human CYP2C-mediated stereoselective phenytoin hydroxylation in Japanese: difference in chiral preference of CYP2C9 and CYP2C19. *Biochem Pharmacol* 1999;57:1297–1303.
49. Komatsu T, Yamazaki H, Asahi S, et al. Formation of a dihydroxy metabolite of phenytoin in human liver microsomes/cytosol: roles of cytochromes P450 2C9, 2C19, and 3A4. *Drug Metab Dispos* 2000;28:1361–1368.
50. Spielberg S, Gordon G, Blake D, et al. Anticonvulsant toxicity in vitro: possible role of arene oxides. *J Pharmacol Exp Ther* 1981;217:386–389.
51. Strickler S, Dansky L, Miller M, et al. Genetic predisposition to phenytoin induced birth defects. *Lancet* 1985;1:746–749.
52. Lee CR, Goldstein JA, Pieper JA. Cytochrome P450 2C9 polymorphisms: a comprehensive review of the in-vitro and human data. *Pharmacogenetics* 2002;12:251–263.
53. Human Cytochrome P450 (CYP) Allele Nomenclature Committee, 2004. Available at: http://www.imm.ki.se/cypalleles. Last accessed October 1, 2004.
54. Odani A, Hashimoto Y, Otsuki Y, et al. Genetic polymorphism of the CYP2C subfamily and its effect on the pharmacokinetics of phenytoin in Japanese patients with epilepsy. *Clin Pharmacol Ther* 1997;62:287–292.
55. Mamiya K, Ieiri I, Shimamoto J, et al. The effects of genetic polymorphisms of CYP2C9 and CYP2C19 on phenytoin metabolism in Japanese adult patients with epilepsy: studies in stereoselective hydroxylation and population pharmacokinetics. *Epilepsia* 1998;39:1317–1323.
56. Aynacioglu AS, Brockmoller J, Bauer S, et al. Frequency of cytochrome P450 CYP2C9 variants in a Turkish population and functional relevance for phenytoin. *Br J Clin Pharmacol* 1999;48: 409–415.
57. Caraco Y, Muszkat M, Wood AJ. Phenytoin metabolic ratio: a putative marker of CYP2C9 activity *in vivo. Pharmacogenetics* 2001;11:587–596.
58. van der Weide J, Steijns LS, van Weelden MJ, et al. The effect of genetic polymorphism of cytochrome P450 CYP2C9 on phenytoin dose requirement. *Pharmacogenetics* 2001;11:287–291.

59. Ninomiya H, Mamiya K, Matsuo S, et al. Genetic polymorphism of the CYP2C subfamily and excessive serum phenytoin concentration with central nervous system intoxication. *Ther Drug Monit* 2000;22:230–232.

60. Kidd RS, Straughn AB, Meyer MC, et al. Pharmacokinetics of chlorpheniramine, phenytoin, glipizide and nifedipine in an individual homozygous for the CYP2C9*3 allele. *Pharmacogenetics* 1999;9:71–80.

61. Brandolese R, Scordo MG, Spina E, et al. Severe phenytoin intoxication in a subject homozygous for CYP2C9*3. *Clin Pharmacol Ther* 2001;70:391–394.

62. Ieiri I, Tainaka H, Morita T, et al. Catalytic activity of three variants (Ile, Leu, and Thr) at amino acid residue 359 in human CYP2C9 gene and simultaneous detection using single-strand conformation polymorphism analysis. *Ther Drug Monit* 2000;22:237–244.

63. Kidd RS, Curry TB, Gallagher S, et al. Identification of a null allele of CYP2C9 in an African-American exhibiting toxicity to phenytoin. *Pharmacogenetics* 2001;11:803–808.

64. Goldstein JA. Clinical relevance of genetic polymorphisms in the human CYP2C subfamily. *Br J Clin Pharmacol* 2001;52:349–355.

65. Imai J, Ieiri I, Mamiya K, et al. Polymorphism of the cytochrome P450 (CYP) 2C9 gene in Japanese epileptic patients: genetic analysis of the CYP2C9 locus. *Pharmacogenetics* 2000;10:85–89.

66. Dickmann LJ, Rettie AE, Kneller MB, et al. Identification and functional characterization of a new CYP2C9 variant (CYP2C9*5) expressed among African Americans. *Mol Pharmacol* 2001;60:382–387.

67. Goldstein J. Polymorphisms in the human CYP2C subfamily. *Drug Metab Rev* 2002;34:5.

68. Si D, Guo Y, Zhang Y, et al. Identification of a novel variant CYP2C9 allele in Chinese. *Pharmacogenetics* 2004;14:465–469.

69. Levy RH. Cytochrome P450 isozymes and antiepileptic drug interactions. *Epilepsia* 1995;36:S8–S13.

70. Blaisdell J, Mohrenweiser H, Jackson J, et al. Identification and functional characterization of new potentially defective alleles of human CYP2C19. *Pharmacogenetics* 2002;12:703–711.

71. Desta Z, Zhao X, Shin JG, et al. Clinical significance of the cytochrome P450 2C19 genetic polymorphism. *Clin Pharmacokinet* 2002;41:913–958.

72. Xie HG, Kim RB, Wood AJ, et al. Molecular basis of ethnic differences in drug disposition and response. *Annu Rev Pharmacol Toxicol* 2001;41:815–850.

73. Wormhoudt LW, Commandeur JN, Vermeulen NP. Genetic polymorphisms of human N-acetyltransferase, cytochrome P450, glutathione-S-transferase, and epoxide hydrolase enzymes: relevance to xenobiotic metabolism and toxicity. *Crit Rev Toxicol* 1999;29:59–124.

74. Bajpai M, Roskos LK, Shen DD, et al. Roles of cytochrome P4502C9 and cytochrome P4502C19 in the stereoselective metabolism of phenytoin to its major metabolite. *Drug Metab Dispos* 1996;24:1401–1403.

75. Richens A, Dunlop A. Serum phenytoin levels in the management of epilepsy. *Lancet* 1975;2:247–248.

76. Bauer L, Blouin R. Age and phenytoin kinetics in adult epileptics. *Clin Pharmacol Ther* 1982;31:301–304.

77. Adithan C, Srinivas B, Indhiresan J, et al. Influence of type I and type II diabetes mellitus on phenytoin steady-state levels. *Int J Clin Pharmacol Ther Toxicol* 1991;29:310–313.

78. Tomson T, Lindbom U, Ekqvist B, et al. Disposition of carbamazepine and phenytoin in pregnancy. *Epilepsia* 1994;35:131–135.

79. Grasela T, Sheiner L, Rambeck B, et al. Steady state pharmacokinetics of phenytoin from routinely collected patient data. *Clin Pharmacokinet* 1983;8:355–364.

80. Yukawa E, Higuchi S, Aoyama T. Population pharmacokinetics of phenytoin from routine clinical data in Japan. *J Clin Pharmacol Ther* 1989;14:71–77.

81. Yukawa E, Higachi S, Aoyama T. Population pharmacokinetics of phenytoin from routine clinical data in Japan: an update. *Chem Pharm Bull* 1990;38:1973–1976.

82. Bauer L, Blouin R. Phenytoin Michaelis-Menten pharmacokinetics in Caucasian paediatric patients. *Clin Pharmacokinet* 1983;8:545–549.

83. Koren G, Brand N, MacLeod S. Influence of bioavailability on the calculated Michaelis-Menten parameters of phenytoin in children. *Ther Drug Monit* 1984;6:11–14.

84. Suzuki Y, Mimaki T, Cox S, et al. Phenytoin age-dose-concentration relationship in children. *Ther Drug Monit* 1994;16:145–150.

85. Chaplin S, Smith J. Drug excretion in human breast milk. *Adverse Drug React Toxicol Rev* 1982;1:255–287.

86. Chetty M, Miller R, Seymour MA. Phenytoin auto-induction. *Ther Drug Monit* 1998;20:60–62.

87. Jamerson BD, Donn KH, Dukes GE, et al. Absolute bioavailability of phenytoin after 3-phosphoryloxymethyl phenytoin disodium (ACC-9653) administration to humans. *Epilepsia* 1990;31:592–597.

88. Browne TR, Davoudi H, Donn KH, et al. Bioavailability of ACC-9653 (phenytoin prodrug). *Epilepsia* 1989;30:S15–S21.

89. Hussey EK, Dukes GE, Messenheimer JA, et al. Evaluation of the pharmacokinetic interaction between diazepam and ACC-9653 (a phenytoin prodrug) in healthy male volunteers. *Pharm Res* 1990;7:1172–1176.

90. Leppik IE, Boucher BA, Wilder BJ, et al. Pharmacokinetics and safety of a phenytoin prodrug given i.v. or i.m. in patients. *Neurology* 1990;40:456–460.

91. Aweeka FT, Gottwald MD, Gambertoglio JG, et al. Pharmacokinetics of fosphenytoin in patients with hepatic or renal disease. *Epilepsia* 1999;40:777–782.

92. Morton LD. Clinical experience with fosphenytoin in children. *J Child Neurol* 1998;13:S19–S22.

93. Browne TR. Phenytoin and other hydantoins. In: Engel J Jr, Pedley TA, eds. *Epilepsy: a comprehensive textbook*, vol 2. Philadelphia: Lippincott-Raven, 1997:1557–1579.

94. Kugler AR, Knapp LE, Eldon MA. Rapid attainment of therapeutic phenytoin concentrations following administration of loading doses of fosphenytoin: a metaanalysis. *Neurology* 1996;46:A176.

95. Eldon M, Loewen G, Voightman R, et al. Pharmacokinetics and tolerance of fosphenytoin and phenytoin administration intravenously to healthy subjects. *Can J Neurol Sci* 1993;20:5810.

96. Hayes G, Kootsikas M. Reassessing the lower end of the phenytoin therapeutic range: a review of the literature. *Ann Pharmacother* 1993;27:1389–1392.

97. Schmidt D, Haenel F. Therapeutic plasma levels of phenytoin, phenobarbital, and carbamazepine: individual variation in relation to seizure frequency and type. *Neurology* 1984;34:1252–1255.

98. Tatro D. *Drug facts and comparisons*. St. Louis, MO: Facts & Comparisons, 1996.

99. Bauer L. Interference of oral phenytoin absorption by continuous nasogastric feedings. *Neurology* 1982;32:570–572.

100. Haidukewych D, Rodin E, Zielinski J. Derivation and evaluation of an equation for prediction of free phenytoin concentration in patients co-medicated with valproic acid. *Ther Drug Monit* 1989;11:134–139.

101. Kerrick J, Wolff D, Graves N. Predicting unbound phenytoin concentrations in patients receiving valproic acid: a comparison of two prediction methods. *Ann Pharmacother* 1995;29:470–474.

102. Duncan JS, Patsalos PN, Shorvon SD. Effects of discontinuation of phenytoin, carbamazepine, and valproate on concomitant antiepileptic medication. *Epilepsia* 1991;32:101–115.

103. Wilder B. Phenytoin: clinical use. In: Levy R, Mattson R, Meldrum B, eds. *Antiepileptic drugs*, 4th ed. New York: Raven Press, 1995:339–344.

104. Mattson RH. Efficacy and adverse effects of established and new antiepileptic drugs. *Epilepsia* 1995;36:S13–S26.

105. Leppik I, Patrick B, Crawford R. Treatment of acute seizures and status epilepticus with intravenous phenytoin. In: Delgado-Escueta A, Wasterlain C, Treiman D, et al., eds. *Status epilepticus: mechanisms of brain damage and treatment*, vol 34. New York: Raven Press, 1983:447–451.

106. Wilder B. Efficacy of phenytoin in the treatment of status epilepticus. In: Delgado-Escueta A, Wasterlain C, Treiman D, et al., eds. *Status epilepticus: mechanisms of brain damage and treatment*, vol 34. New York: Raven Press, 1983:441–446.

107. Richard M, Chiron C, d'Athis P, et al. Phenytoin monitoring in status epilepticus in infants and children. *Epilepsia* 1993;34:144–150.

108. Treiman DM, Meyers PD, Walton NY, et al. A comparison of four treatments for generalized convulsive status epilepticus. Veterans Affairs Status Epilepticus Cooperative Study Group. *N Engl J Med* 1998;339:792–798.

109. Alldredge BK, Lowenstein DH, Simon RP. Placebo-controlled trial of intravenous diphenylhydantoin for short-term treatment of alcohol withdrawal seizures. *Am J Med* 1989;87: 645–648.
110. Chance J. Emergency department treatment of alcohol withdrawal seizures with phenytoin. *Ann Emerg Med* 1991;20:520–522.
111. Mattson RH, Cramer JA, Collins JF, et al. Comparison of carbamazepine, phenobarbital, phenytoin, and primidone in partial and secondarily generalized tonic-clonic seizures. *N Engl J Med* 1985;313:145–151.
112. Callaghan N, Kenny R, O'Neill B, et al. A prospective study between carbamazepine, phenytoin, and sodium valproate as monotherapy in previously untreated and recently diagnosed patients with epilepsy. *J Neurol Neurosurg Psychiatry* 1985;48:639–644.
113. Ramsay RE, Wilder BJ, Berger JR, et al. A double-blind study comparing carbamazepine with phenytoin as initial seizure therapy in adults. *Neurology* 1983;33:904–910.
114. Wilder B, Ramsay R, Willmore L, et al. Comparison of valproic acid and phenytoin in newly diagnosed tonic-clonic seizures. *Neurology* 1983;33:1474–1476.
115. Turnbull DM, Howel D, Rawlins MD, Chadwick DW. Which drug for the adult epileptic patient: phenytoin or valproate? *Br Med J* 1985;290:815–819.
116. Heller AJ, Chesterman P, Elwes RDC, et al. Phenobarbitone, phenytoin, carbamazepine or sodium valproate for newly diagnosed adult epilepsy: a randomised comparative monotherapy trial. *J Neurol Neurosurg Psychiatry* 1995;58:44–50.
117. Bill PA, Vigonius U, Pohlmann H, et al. A double-blind controlled clinical trial of oxcarbazepine versus phenytoin in adults with previously untreated epilepsy. *Epilepsy Res* 1997;27:195–204.
118. Guerreiro MM, Vigonius U, Pohlmann H, et al. A double-blind controlled clinical trial of oxcarbazepine versus phenytoin in children and adolescents with epilepsy. *Epilepsy Res* 1997;27:205–213.
119. Steiner TJ, Dellaportas CI, Findley LJ, et al. Lamotrigine monotherapy in newly diagnosed untreated epilepsy: a double-blind comparison with phenytoin. *Epilepsia* 1999;40:601–607.
120. Painter M, Scher MS, Stein AD, et al. Phenobarbital compared with phenytoin for the treatment of neonatal seizures. *N Engl J Med* 1999;341:485–489.
121. Appleton M, Kuehl T, Raebel M, et al. Magnesium sulfate versus phenytoin for seizure prophylaxis in pregnancy-induced hypertension. *Am J Obstet Gynecol* 1991;165:907–913.
122. Anonymous. Which anticonvulsant for women with eclampsia? Evidence from the Collaborative Eclampsia Trial. *Lancet* 1995;345:1455–1463.
123. Lucas M, Leveno K, Cunningham F. A comparison of magnesium sulfate with phenytoin for the prevention of eclampsia. *N Engl J Med* 1995;333:201–205.
124. Friedman S, Lim K, Baker C, et al. Phenytoin versus magnesium sulfate in preeclampsia: a pilot study. *Am J Perinatol* 1993;10: 233–238.
125. Guzman E, Conley M, Stewart R, et al. Phenytoin and magnesium sulfate effects on fetal heart rate tracings assessed by computer analysis. *Obstet Gynecol* 1993;82:375–379.
126. Beenen LF, Lindeboom J, Trenit DG, et al. Comparative double blind clinical trial of phenytoin and sodium valproate as anticonvulsant prophylaxis after craniotomy: efficacy, tolerability, and cognitive effects. *J Neurol Neurosurg Psychiatry* 1999;67: 474–480.
127. Foy P, Chadwick D, Rajgopala N, et al. Do prophylactic anticonvulsant drugs alter the pattern of seizures after craniotomy? *J Neurol Neurosurg Psychiatry* 1992;55:753–757.
128. Temkin N, Dikmen S, Wilensky A, et al. A randomized, double-blind study of phenytoin for the prevention of post-traumatic seizures. *N Engl J Med* 1990;323:497–502.
129. Haltiner A, Newell DW, Temkin NR, et al. Side effects and mortality associated with use of phenytoin for early posttraumatic seizure prophylaxis. *J Neurosurg* 1999;91:588–592.
130. Young KD, Okada PJ, Sokolove PE, et al. A randomized, double-blinded, placebo-controlled trial of phenytoin for the prevention of early posttraumatic seizures in children with moderate to severe blunt head injury. *Ann Emerg Med* 2004;43:435–446.
131. McCleane G. Intravenous infusion of phenytoin relieves neuropathic pain: a randomized, double-blind, placebo controlled, crossover study. *Anesth Analg* 1999;89:985–988.
132. Knox G, Woodard D, Chelen W, et al. Phenytoin for motion sickness: clinical evaluation. *Laryngoscope* 1994;104:935–939.
133. Woodard D, Knox G, Myers K, et al. Phenytoin as a countermeasure for motion sickness in NASA maritime operations. *Aviat Space Environ Med* 1993;64:363–366.
134. Finkel M. Phenytoin revisited. *Clin Ther* 1984;6:577–591.
135. Pendse A, Sharma A, Sodani A, et al. Topical phenytoin in wound healing. *Int J Dermatol* 1993;32:214–217.
136. Modaghegh S, Salehian B, Tavassoli M, et al. Use of phenytoin in healing of war and non-war wounds. A pilot study of 25 cases. *Int J Dermatol* 1989;28:347–350.
137. Wilder B, Bruni J. Medical management of seizure disorders. In: *Seizure disorders: a pharmacological approach to treatment.* New York: Raven Press, 1981:35–39.
138. Bruni J. Phenytoin: toxicity. In: Levy R, Mattson R, Meldrum B, eds. *Antiepileptic drugs,* 4th ed. New York: Raven Press, 1995: 345–350.
139. Harrison MB, Lyons GR, Landow ER. Phenytoin and dyskinesias: a report of two cases and review of the literature. *Mov Disord* 1993;8:19–27.
140. Howrie D, Crumrine P. Phenytoin-induced movement disorder associated with intravenous administration for status epilepticus. *Clin Pediatr* 1985;24:467–469.
141. Micheli F, Lehkuniec E, Gatto M, et al. Hemiballism in a patient with partial motor status epilepticus treated with phenytoin. *Funct Neurol* 1993;8:103–107.
142. Moss W, Ojukwu C, Chiriboga C. Phenytoin-induced movement disorder. Unilateral presentation in a child and response to diphenhydramine. *Clin Pediatr* 1994;33:634–638.
143. Stilman N, Masdeu J. Incidence of seizures with phenytoin toxicity. *Neurology* 1985;35:1769–1772.
144. Drane DL, Meador KJ. Epilepsy, anticonvulsant drugs and cognition. *Baillieres Clin Neurol* 1996;5:877–885.
145. Devinsky O. Cognitive and behavioral effects of antiepileptic drugs. *Epilepsia* 1995;36:S46–S65.
146. Aldenkamp AP, Alpherts WC, Diepman L, et al. Cognitive side-effects of phenytoin compared with carbamazepine in patients with localization-related epilepsy. *Epilepsy Res* 1994;19:37–43.
147. Dodrill CB, Troupin AS. Neuropsychological effects of carbamazepine and phenytoin: a reanalysis. *Neurology* 1991;41: 141–143.
148. May TW, Bulmahn A, Wohlhuter M, et al. Effects of withdrawal of phenytoin on cognitive and psychomotor functions in hospitalized epileptic patients on polytherapy. *Acta Neurol Scand* 1992;86:165–170.
149. Meador KJ, Loring DW, Allen ME, et al. Comparative cognitive effects of carbamazepine and phenytoin in healthy adults. *Neurology* 1991;41:1537–1540.
150. Smith KR Jr, Goulding PM, Wilderman D, et al. Neurobehavioral effects of phenytoin and carbamazepine in patients recovering from brain trauma: a comparative study. *Arch Neurol* 1994;51: 653–660.
151. Aldenkamp AP, Vermeulen J. Phenytoin and carbamazepine: differential effects on cognitive function. *Seizure* 1995;4:95–104.
152. Pulliainen V, Jokelainen M. Effects of phenytoin and carbamazepine on cognitive functions in newly diagnosed epileptic patients. *Acta Neurol Scand* 1994;89:81–86.
153. Pulliainen V, Jokelainen M. Comparing the cognitive effects of phenytoin and carbamazepine in long-term monotherapy: a two-year follow-up. *Epilepsia* 1995;36:1195–1202.
154. Dodrill CB, Troupin AS. Psychotropic effects of carbamazepine in epilepsy: a double-blind comparison with phenytoin. *Neurology* 1977;27:1023–1028.
155. Dikmen SS, Temkin NR, Miller B, et al. Neurobehavioral effects of phenytoin prophylaxis of posttraumatic seizures. *JAMA* 1991;265:1271–1277.
156. Meador KJ, Loring DW, Moore EE, et al. Comparative cognitive effects of phenobarbital, phenytoin, and valproate in healthy adults. *Neurology* 1995;45:1494–1499.
157. Craig I, Tallis R. Impact of valproate and phenytoin on cognitive function in elderly patients: results of a single-blind randomized comparative study. *Epilepsia* 1994;35:381–390.
158. Read CL, Stephen LJ, Stolarek IH, et al. Cognitive effects of anticonvulsant monotherapy in elderly patients: a placebo-controlled study. *Seizure* 1998;7:159–162.

159. Wallace SJ. A comparative review of the adverse effects of anticonvulsants in children with epilepsy. *Drug Saf* 1996;15:378–393.
160. Aldenkamp AP, Alpherts WC, Blennow G, et al. Withdrawal of antiepileptic medication in children—effects on cognitive function: the Multicenter Holmfrid Study. *Neurology* 1993;43:41–50.
161. Aman MG, Werry JS, Paxton JW, et al. Effects of phenytoin on cognitive-motor performance in children as a function of drug concentration, seizure type, and time of medication. *Epilepsia* 1994;35:172–180.
162. Leeder JS. Mechanisms of idiosyncratic hypersensitivity reactions to antiepileptic drugs. *Epilepsia* 1998;39:S8–S16.
163. Chadwick D, Shaw M, Foy P, et al. Serum anticonvulsant concentrations and the risk of drug induced skin eruptions. *J Neurol Neurosurg Psychiatry* 1984;47:642–644.
164. Leppik I, Lapora J, Loewenson R. Seasonal incidence of phenytoin allergy unrelated to plasma levels. *Arch Neurol* 1985;42:120–122.
165. Leppik IE. Phenytoin. In: Resor SR, Kutt H, eds. *The medical treatment of epilepsy,* vol 10. New York: Marcel Dekker, 1992:279–291.
166. Schlienger RG, Shear NH. Antiepileptic drug hypersensitivity syndrome. *Epilepsia* 1998;39:S3–S7.
167. Haruda F. Phenytoin hypersensitivity: 38 cases. *Neurology* 1979;29:1480–1485.
168. Dahllof G, Preber H, Eliasson S, et al. Periodontal condition of epileptic adults treated long-term with phenytoin or carbamazepine. *Epilepsia* 1993;34:960–964.
169. Hassell T, Hefti A. Drug-induced gingival overgrowth: old problem, new problem. *Crit Rev Oral Biol Med* 1991;2:103–137.
170. Thomason J, Seymour R, Rawlins M. Incidence and severity of phenytoin-induced gingival overgrowth in epileptic patients in general medical practice. *Community Dent Oral Epidemiol* 1992;20:288–291.
171. Casetta I, Granieri E, Desidera M, et al. Phenytoin-induced gingival overgrowth: a community-based cross-sectional study in Ferrara, Italy. *Neuroepidemiology* 1997;16:296–303.
172. Brunsvold M, Tomasovic J, Ruemping D. The measured effect of phenytoin withdrawal on gingival hyperplasia. *ASDC J Dent Child* 1985;52:417–421.
173. Dahllof G, Axio E, Modeer T. Regression of phenytoin-induced gingival overgrowth after withdrawal of medication. *Swed Dent J* 1991;15:139–143.
174. Baier W, Beck U, Doose H, et al. Cerebellar atrophy following diphenylhydantoin intoxication. *Neuropediatrics* 1984;15:76–81.
175. Baier W, Beck U, Hirsch W. CT findings following diphenylhydantoin intoxication. *Pediatr Radiol* 1985;15:220–221.
176. Lindvall O, Nilsson R. Cerebellar atrophy following phenytoin intoxication. *Ann Neurol* 1984;16:258–260.
177. Jibiki I, Kido H, Matsuda H, et al. Probable cerebellar abnormality of 123I-IMP SPECT scans in epileptic patients with long-term high-dose phenytoin therapy. Based on observation of multiple cases. *Acta Neurol* 1993;15:16–24.
178. Ney G, Lantos G, Barr W, et al. Cerebellar atrophy in patients with long-term phenytoin exposure and epilepsy. *Arch Neurol* 1994;51:767–771.
179. Kubota F, Kifune A, Shibata N, et al. Bone mineral density of epileptic patients on long-term antiepileptic drug therapy: a quantitative digital radiography study. *Epilepsy Res* 1999;33:93–97.
180. Hug G, McGraw CA, Bates SR, et al. Reduction of serum carnitine concentrations during anticonvulsant therapy with phenobarbital, valproic acid, phenytoin, and carbamazepine in children. *J Pediatr* 1991;119:799–802.
181. Calandre E, Porta BS, Garcia de la Calzada D. The effect of chronic phenytoin treatment on serum lipid profile in adult epileptic patients. *Epilepsia* 1992;33:154–157.
182. Elwes R, Dellaportas C, Reynolds E, et al. Prolactin and growth hormone dynamics in epileptic patients receiving phenytoin. *Clin Endocrinol* 1985;23:263–270.
183. McKenney J, Petrizzi K, Briggs GC, et al. The effect of low-dose phenytoin on high-density lipoprotein cholesterol. *Pharmacotherapy* 1992;12:183–188.
184. Heroz A, Levesque L, Drislane F, et al. Phenytoin-induced elevation of serum estradiol and reproductive dysfunction in men with epilepsy. *Epilepsia* 1991;32:550–553.
185. Smith P, Surks M. Multiple effects of 5,5'-diphenylhydantoin on the thyroid hormone system. *Endocr Rev* 1984;5:514–524.
186. Frey B, Frey F. Phenytoin modulates the pharmacokinetics of prednisolone and the pharmacodynamics of prednisolone as assessed by the inhibition of the mixed lymphocyte reaction in humans. *Eur J Clin Invest* 1984;14:1–6.
187. Hegedus L, Hansen J, Luhdorf K, et al. Increased frequency of goitre in epileptic patients on long-term phenytoin or carbamazepine treatment. *Clin Endocrinol* 1985;23:423–429.
188. Franklyn J, Sheppard M, Ramsden D. Measurement of free thyroid hormones in patients on long-term phenytoin therapy. *Eur J Clin Pharmacol* 1984;26:633–634.
189. Basaran N, Hincal F, Kansu E, et al. Humoral and cellular immune parameters in untreated and phenytoin- or carbamazepine-treated epileptic patients. *Int J Immunopharmacol* 1994;16:1071–1077.
190. Ishizaka A, Nakaniski M, Kasahara E, et al. Phenytoin-induced IgG$_2$ and IgG$_4$ deficiencies in a patient with epilepsy. *Acta Paediatr* 1992;81:646–648.
191. Kondo N, Takao A, Tomatsu S, et al. Suppression of IgA production by lymphocytes induced by diphenylhydantoin. *J Invest Allergol Clin Immunol* 1994;4:255–257.
192. Britigan B. Diphenylhydantoin-induced hypogammaglobulinemia in a patient infected with human immunodeficiency virus. *Am J Med* 1991;90:542–527.
193. Lazoglu A, Boglioli L, Dorsett B, et al. Phenytoin-related immunodeficiency associated with Loeffler's syndrome. *Ann Allergy Asthma Immunol* 1995;74:479–482.
194. Hanson JW, Smith DW. The fetal hydantoin syndrome. *J Pediatr* 1975;87:285–290.
195. Kaneko S, Battino D, Andermann E, et al. Congenital malformations due to antiepileptic drugs. *Epilepsy Res* 1999;33:145–158.
196. Vajda FJ, O'Brien TJ, Hitchcock A, et al. The Australian Registry of Anti-Epileptic Drugs In Pregnancy: experience after 30 months. *J Clin Neurosci* 2003;10:543–549.
197. Kaaja E, Kaaja R, Hiilesmaa V. Major malformations in offspring of women with epilepsy. *Neurology* 2003;60:575–579.
198. Earnest MP, Marx JA, Drury LR. Complications of intravenous phenytoin for acute treatment of seizures. Recommendations for usage. *JAMA* 1983;249:762–765.
199. Hanna DR. Purple glove syndrome: a complication of intravenous phenytoin. *J Neurosci Nurs* 1992;24:340–345.
200. Helfaer MA, Ware C. Purple glove syndrome. *J Neurosurg Anesthesiol* 1994;6:48–49.
201. O'Brien TJ, Cascino GD, So EL, et al. Incidence and clinical consequence of the purple glove syndrome in patients receiving intravenous phenytoin. *Neurology* 1998;51:1034–1039.
202. Carducci B, Hedges J, Beal J, et al. Emergency phenytoin loading by constant intravenous infusion. *Ann Emerg Med* 1984;13:1027–1059.
203. Donovan P, Cline D. Phenytoin administration by constant intravenous infusion: selective rates of administration. *Ann Emerg Med* 1991;20:139–142.
204. Ramsay R, Philbrook B, Martinez D, et al. A double-blind, randomized safety comparison of rapidly infused intravenous loading doses of fosphenytoin vs. phenytoin. *Epilepsia* 1995;36:90.
205. Ramsay RE, DeToledo J. Intravenous administration of fosphenytoin: options for the management of seizures. *Neurology* 1996;46:S17–S19.
206. Dean J, Smith K, Boucher B, et al. Safety, tolerance and pharmacokinetics of intramuscular (IM) fosphenytoin, a phenytoin prodrug, in neurosurgery patients. *Epilepsia* 1993;34:111.
207. Ramsay R, Barkley G, Garnett W, et al. Safety and tolerance of intramuscular fosphenytoin (Cerebyx) in patients requiring a loading dose of phenytoin. *Neurology* 1995;45:A249.
208. Wilder B, Ramsay R, Marriot J, et al. Safety and tolerance on intramuscular administration of fosphenytoin, a phenytoin prodrug, for 5 days in patients with epilepsy. *Neurology* 1994;43:A308.
209. Lowenstein DH, Alldredge BK. Status epilepticus. *N Engl J Med* 1998;338:970–976.
210. Cranford R, Leppik I, Patrick B, et al. Intravenous phenytoin: clinical and pharmacokinetic aspects. *Neurology* 1978;28:874–880.
211. Jung D, Powell J, Walson P, et al. Effect of dose on phenytoin absorption. *Clin Pharmacol Ther* 1980;28:479–485.
212. Rudis MI, Touchette DR, Swadron SP, et al. Cost-effectiveness of oral phenytoin, intravenous phenytoin, and intravenous

fosphenytoin in the emergency department. *Ann Emerg Med* 2004;43:386–397.

213. Swadron SP, Rudis MI, Azimian K, et al. A comparison of phenytoin-loading techniques in the emergency department. *Acad Emerg Med* 2004;11:244–252.

214. Hvidberg EF, Dam M. Clinical pharmacokinetics of anticonvulsants. *Clin Pharmacokinet* 1976;1:161–188.

215. Serrano EE, Roye DB, Hammer RH, et al. Plasma diphenylhydantoin values after oral and intramuscular administration of diphenylhydantoin. *Neurology* 1973;23:311–317.

216. Wilensky AJ, Lowden JA. Inadequate serum levels after intramuscular administration of diphenylhydantoin. *Neurology* 1973;23:318–324.

217. Fuerst RH, Graves NM, Kriel RL, et al. Absorption and safety of rectally administered phenytoin. *Eur J Drug Metab Pharmacokinet* 1988;13:257–260.

218. Privitera M. Clinical rules for phenytoin dosing. *Ann Pharmacother* 1993;27:1169–1173.

219. Armijo J, Cavada E. Graphic estimation of phenytoin dose in adults and children. *Ther Drug Monit* 1991;13:507–510.

220. Bachmann K, Schwartz J, Forney RB Jr, et al. Single dose phenytoin clearance during erythromycin treatment. *Res Commun Chem Pathol Pharmacol* 1984;46:207–217.

221. Cai W, Chu X, Chen G. A Bayesian graphic method for predicting individual phenytoin dosage schedule. *Acta Pharmacol Sin* 1991;12:141–144.

222. Flint N, Lopez L, Robinson J, et al. Comparison of eight phenytoin dosing methods in institutionalized patients. *Ther Drug Monit* 1985;7:74–80.

223. Nakashima E, Matsushita R, Kido H, et al. Systematic approach to a dosage regimen for phenytoin based on one-point, steady-state plasma concentration. *Ther Drug Monit* 1995;17:12–18.

224. Pryka R, Rodvold K, Erdman S. An updated comparison of drug dosing methods, part I: phenytoin. *Clin Pharmacokinet* 1991;20:209–217.

225. Tobias J, Baker D, Hurwitz C. Removal of phenytoin by plasmapheresis in a patient with thrombotic thrombocytopenic purpura. *Clin Pediatr* 1992;31:105–108.

226. Hays DP, Primack WA, Abroms IF. Phenytoin clearance by continuous ambulatory peritoneal dialysis. *Drug Intell Clin Pharm* 1985;19:429–431.

227. Lau A, Kronfol N. Effect of continuous hemofiltration of phenytoin elimination. *Ther Drug Monit* 1994;16:53–57.

228. Fischer JH, Cwik MJ, Luer MS, et al. Stability of fosphenytoin sodium with intravenous solutions in glass bottles, polyvinyl chloride bags, and polypropylene syringes. *Ann Pharmacother* 1997;31:553–559.

229. Allen F, Runge J, Legarda S. Safety, tolerance, and pharmacokinetics of intravenous fosphenytoin (Cerebyx) in status epilepticus. *Epilepsia* 1995;36:90.

230. Wheless JW. Pediatric use of intravenous and intramuscular phenytoin: lessons learned. *J Child Neurol* 1998;13:S11–S14.

231. Browne TR. Intravenous phenytoin: cheap but not necessarily a bargain. *Neurology* 1998;51:942–943.

232. Armstrong EP, Sauer KA, Downey MJ. Phenytoin and fosphenytoin: a model of cost and clinical outcomes. *Pharmacotherapy* 1999;19:844–853.

233. Marchetti A, Magar R, Fischer J, et al. A pharmacoeconomic evaluation of intravenous fosphenytoin (Cerebyx) versus intravenous phenytoin (Dilantin) in hospital emergency departments. *Am J Health Syst Pharm* 1996;53:2249.

234. Coplin WM, Rhoney DH, Rebuck JA, et al. Randomized evaluation of adverse events and length-of-stay with routine emergency department use of phenytoin or fosphenytoin. *Neurol Res* 2002;24:842–848.

Phenobarbital and Primidone

56

Blaise F. D. Bourgeois

HISTORICAL BACKGROUND

Although its use has been decreasing, phenobarbital is still a major antiepileptic drug (AED). Phenobarbital (PB) has been prescribed for the treatment of epilepsy since 1912, with only bromide having been used longer. Although PB is associated with more sedative and behavioral side effects than most other AEDs, it has relatively low systemic toxicity and a long half-life, can be administered intravenously and intramuscularly, is effective in patients with status epilepticus, and is inexpensive.

Primidone (PRM) has been in clinical use since its synthesis in 1952 (1). Often referred to as a barbiturate, PRM does not strictly belong in this class; its pyrimidine ring contains only two carbonyl groups, compared with the three groups of barbituric acid (Fig. 56.1), but the remainder of the structure is identical to that of PB. Therapeutically, however, PRM is appropriately considered a barbiturate, as its effect can be attributed predominantly to the derived PB. This hepatic biotransformation has heretofore made it impossible to establish whether therapy with PRM differs clinically from that with PB or whether PRM is a PB prodrug. Complicating this issue is the experimental demonstration of independent antiepileptic activity for the other main metabolite of PRM, phenylethylmalonamide (PEMA) (Fig. 56.1).

CHEMISTRY AND MECHANISM OF ACTION

Chemically, PB is 5-ethyl-5-phenylbarbituric acid (Fig. 56.1). The molecular weight is 232.23, and the conversion factor from milligrams to micromoles is 4.31 (1 mg/L = 4.31 μmol/L). The sodium salt of PB is water soluble. PB in its free acid form is a white crystalline powder soluble in organic solvents, but with limited water and lipid solubility; it is a weak acid with a pK_a of 7.3. Many actions of PB at the cellular level have been described. Although it is not certain which are responsible for seizure protection, the available evidence seems to favor enhancement of γ-aminobutyric acid (GABA) inhibition (2). In animal models, PB protects against electroshock-induced seizures and, unlike phenytoin, carbamazepine, and PRM, against seizures induced by such chemical convulsants as pentylenetetrazol. In normal animals, PB raises the threshold and shortens the duration of afterdischarges elicited by electrical stimulation (3). Like other barbiturates, PB enhances postsynaptic $GABA_A$ receptor-mediated chloride (Cl^-) currents by prolonging the opening of the Cl^- ionophore (4). Increased flow of Cl^- into the cell decreases excitability. Presynaptically, PB can cause a concentration-dependent reduction of calcium (Ca^{2+})-dependent action potentials (5). Usually occurring at relatively high concentrations, this may contribute to seizure protection at higher therapeutic levels and, especially, to sedative and anesthetic effects.

Chemically, PRM is 5-ethyldihydro-5-phenyl-4,6(1-*H*, 5*H*) pyrimidinedione. The molecular weight is 218.264, and the conversion factor from milligrams to micromoles is 4.59 (1 mg/L = 4.59 μmol/L). PRM is very poorly soluble in water, somewhat soluble in ethanol, and virtually insoluble in organic solvents.

The basic pharmacologic mechanism of action of PRM has received relatively little attention, not least because it was uncertain for some time whether the agent itself has independent antiepileptic activity. The basic anticonvulsant action of PRM has been studied in mouse neurons in cell culture (6). PRM was compared with PB for its effect on amino acid responses and on sustained, high-frequency

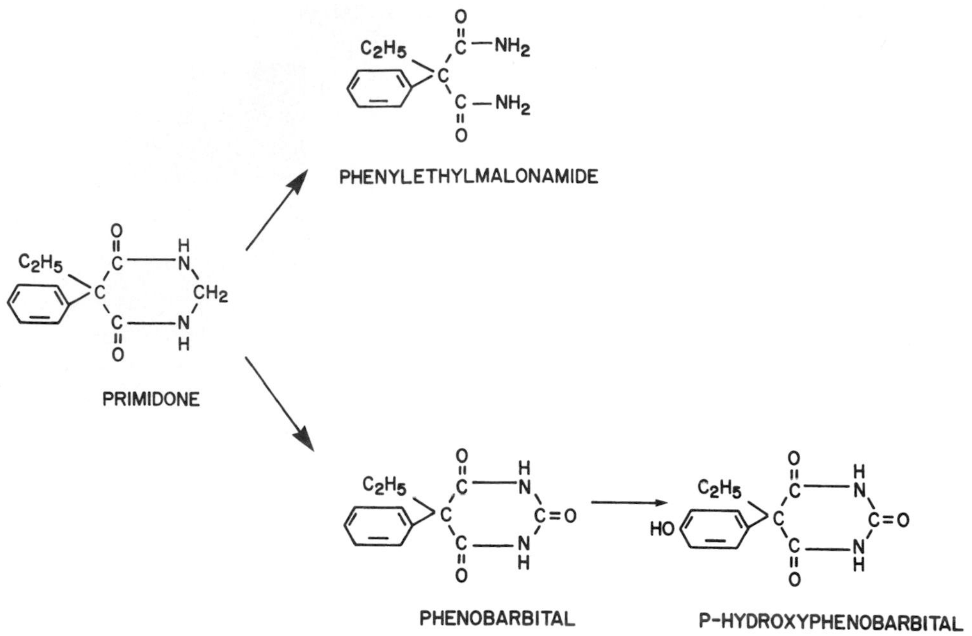

Figure 56.1 Structural formulas of primidone and its main metabolites.

firing. In contrast to PB, PRM had no effect on postsynaptic GABA and glutamate responses at concentrations up to 50 μg/mL. However, both agents limited sustained, high-frequency, repetitive firing at relatively high concentrations (>50 μg/mL). Together, PRM and PB limited sustained high-frequency, repetitive firing at clinically relevant concentrations (12 μg/mL and 20 μg/mL, respectively). The authors concluded that PRM and PB may act synergistically to reduce sustained, high-frequency, repetitive firing. These *in vitro* findings are in accordance with observations made in whole animals.

All the evidence regarding the individual antiepileptic properties of PRM, PB, and phenylethylmalonamide (PEMA) is derived from experiments in animals whose seizures were provoked, because PRM is never present alone during long-term therapy and because at least one active metabolite, PB, is present after repeated administration in humans, as well as in experimental animals. Because the metabolites accumulate a few hours after administration of the first dose, a possible long-term protection by PRM alone against spontaneously occurring seizures cannot be assessed in humans. In addition, PEMA may be involved in the overall pharmacodynamic effect of PRM. The first evidence of the independent anticonvulsant activity of PRM came from dogs who were protected against experimental seizures at a lower concentration of PB when PRM was also present than when PB alone was present (7). Rats were similarly protected against induced seizures after a single dose of PRM administered before the active metabolites could be detected (8), as were mice pretreated with a metabolic blocker that delayed the biotransformation of PRM (9,10). The anticonvulsant potency of PRM against maximal electroshock-induced seizures is similar to that of PB, but unlike PB, PRM was ineffective against

chemically induced seizures caused by pentylenetetrazol or bicuculline (9). Thus, the experimental anticonvulsant spectrum of PRM differs from that of PB and is similar to that of carbamazepine and phenytoin; therefore, PRM and PB may be two different AEDs with different mechanisms of action.

On the basis of brain concentrations in mice, PRM appears to be 2.5 times less neurotoxic than PB, with a superior therapeutic index (9). When PB and PRM were administered together in single-dose experiments in mice (11), their anticonvulsant activity was supra-additive (potentiated) and their neurotoxic effect was infra-additive. A PB-PRM brain concentration ratio of 1:1 provided the best therapeutic index. This ratio is not usually seen in patients, especially those taking PRM combined with phenytoin or carbamazepine. If PRM is different from or even better than PB for the treatment of epilepsy, its effect would be likely only when the PRM concentration equals or exceeds the PB concentration. Such a ratio is achieved only rarely with PRM monotherapy and almost never when PRM is added to phenytoin or carbamazepine, or combined with PB. The results of pharmacodynamic interactions between PRM and PB in mice were confirmed by experiments in amygdala-kindled rats. After single doses, the anticonvulsant effect of PB was potentiated by PRM, whereas side effects of PB, such as ataxia and muscle relaxation, were not increased by combined treatment with PRM (12).

In rats (13) and mice (9,10), PEMA had relatively weak anticonvulsant activity of its own. On the basis of brain concentrations in mice (9), PEMA was 16 times less potent than PB in seizure protection and 8 times less potent in neurotoxic effects, but it potentiated the anticonvulsant (11,13) and neurotoxic effects (11) of PB. Nevertheless, a quantitative analysis of these experimental results, together with the blood levels encountered in clinical practice, suggests that PEMA does not significantly add to the antiepileptic effect or neurotoxicity of PRM therapy.

ABSORPTION, DISTRIBUTION, AND METABOLISM

Phenobarbital

The main pharmacokinetic parameters of PB and PRM are summarized in Chapter 45, Table 45.2. Most formulations of PB contain sodium salt because of good aqueous solubility. The absolute bioavailability of oral preparations of PB is usually greater than 90% (14). Absorption of PB following intramuscular (IM) administration was found to be as complete as that following administration of oral tablets, compared with intravenous (IV) administration (15). Accumulation half-life for the IM route (0.73 hours) was not shorter than for the oral route (0.64 hours). Time to peak concentration is usually 2 to 4 hours. In newborns, however, peak PB plasma levels after oral administration may be reached later than after IM administration (16). A parenteral solution of PB administered rectally has a bioavailability of 89%, compared with that of IM administration (17); average time to peak concentration was 4.4 hours.

PB is not highly bound to serum proteins (45%). Protein binding of PB is lower during pregnancy and in newborns, with a bound fraction between 30% and 40% in pregnant women and their offspring (18). Reported values for the volume of distribution vary. Following IV administration, average values were 0.54 L/kg in adult volunteers and 0.61 L/kg in adult patients with epilepsy (15), both well within the reported range. The volume of distribution of PB approached 1.0 L/kg in newborns (19).

PB is eliminated mostly via renal excretion of the unchanged drug, and via hepatic metabolism and renal excretion of the metabolites. An average of 20% to 25% of PB is eliminated unchanged by the kidneys in adults, with large interindividual variability (20,21). The main metabolite of PB is *p*-hydroxyphenobarbital (Fig. 56.1). At steady state, approximately 20% to 30% of the PB dose is transformed into this metabolite, approximately 50% of which is conjugated to glucuronic acid (20,21). Nitrogen glucosidation, another relevant pathway of PB metabolism, accounts for 25% to 30% of total PB disposition (22). Other identified metabolites of PB represent a very low percentage of the total elimination.

The elimination of PB from serum follows first-order, or linear, kinetics. PB has the longest elimination half-life of the commonly used AEDs. The half-life of PB is age-dependent. The half-life is usually well above 100 hours in newborns (23) and averages 148 hours in asphyxiated newborns (24). During the neonatal period, PB elimination

accelerates markedly; thereafter, half-lives are very short, with average values of 63 hours during the first year of life and 69 hours between the ages of 1 and 5 years (25). Half-lives in adults range between 80 and 100 hours, and no evidence of autoinduction of PB metabolism has been demonstrated (15).

Primidone

PRM is supplied as 250-mg and 50-mg tablets and as syrup (1 mL = 50 mg); extremely low solubility precludes parenteral administration. After oral ingestion of tablets, the time to peak serum concentrations in adult patients with epilepsy was 2.7 (26) and 3.2 hours (27), respectively, and 4 to 6 hours after single-dose administration in children (28). In the same study, an average of 92% of the dose (range, 72% to 123%) was excreted in the urine as unchanged PRM and metabolites, probably indicating complete oral bioavailability. Concomitant administration of acetazolamide reduced the oral absorption of PRM (29). One generic preparation was found to have a lower bioavailability than the trademark product (30).

The volume of distribution of PRM ranged from 0.54 L/kg following acute intoxication (31) to 0.86 L/kg (32). The volume of distribution of PEMA after its oral administration was 0.69 L/kg (33). In human plasma, protein binding of both PRM and PEMA was less than 10% (13,27,33). Brain concentrations of PRM were found to be lower than simultaneous plasma concentrations in mice (9,10) and in rats (8). In patients undergoing surgery for intractable epilepsy, one group of investigators found an average brain-to-plasma ratio of 87% (34). In another report (10) of six patients whose mean plasma PRM concentration was 6.3 μg/mL, brain concentrations ranged between nondetectable and 2.2 μg/g. Brain concentrations of PEMA in mice were 93% (10) and 77% (9) of the plasma levels. In humans, the cerebrospinal fluid-plasma ratio for PRM ranged from 0.8 to 1.13 (27,34,35), which is similar to human saliva-to-plasma ratios (36) and which is consistent with the high free fraction of plasma PRM.

The elimination half-life of PRM varies, mainly because of enzymatic induction by comedication. In adults receiving long-term PRM monotherapy, the elimination half-life ranged from 10 to 15 hours (37–39). Therapy with additional AEDs was associated with values of 6.5 and 8.3 hours (26,27,38,39). In 12 children (four treated with PRM monotherapy, eight treated with PRM and phenytoin), half-lives ranged from 4.5 to 11 hours (mean, 8.7 hours) (28). In newborns, however, the average PRM half-life was 23 hours (range, 8 to 80 hours) (40), which were associated with a limited biotransformation to the metabolites (41).

After oral ingestion of PEMA itself, the half-life of PRM was 15.7 hours (33). The elimination rate of PEMA cannot be determined accurately in patients taking PRM, because the liver produces PEMA as long as PRM is measurable in the blood.

Because two metabolites of PRM accumulate after repeated administration of the agent and because both have independent anticonvulsant activity, an understanding of the qualitative and quantitative aspects of PRM metabolism is needed before any rational clinical use of this drug can be undertaken. Ideally, before prescribing the agent, the physician should know the relative antiepileptic potency, relative toxicity, and expected relative blood levels of PRM and its two active metabolites. Unfortunately, this information is only partially available. Although relative efficacy and relative toxicity of PRM and its metabolites have been studied acutely in animals (9,11), similar investigations are virtually impossible in humans because the three compounds are always present simultaneously during long-term therapy.

Figure 56.1 shows the relevant metabolic pathways for PRM. The first metabolite of PRM to be identified, PEMA was found initially in rats (42) and thereafter in every species studied. PB and p-hydroxyphenobarbital were discovered only 4 years later, in 1956 (43), and toxic reactions attributed to the derived PB were first reported in 1958 (44). Other metabolites of PRM, with either negligible or nondetectable blood levels during long-term therapy, have shown no practical significance. Numerous clinical studies have discussed the quantitative aspects of the biotransformation of PRM to PB and PEMA. A comparison of the ratios of PB serum levels to dose during long-term PB therapy and during long-term PRM therapy in the same patients demonstrated that 24.5% of the PRM dose is converted to PB (45). This is in accordance with the report that average PRM doses (in milligrams per kilogram per day) required to maintain a given PB level are about 5 times higher than the equivalent PB doses (46). The extent of PRM biotransformation and the ratios of the blood levels of PRM and its metabolites are very sensitive to interactions with other AEDs and are discussed separately.

INTERACTIONS WITH OTHER AGENTS

Most of the interactions of PB reflect its status as an enzymatic inducer that accelerates the biotransformation of some AEDs, as well as other agents. No clinically significant interaction with PB has been reported that involves absorption. Moreover, because PB is only 55% protein bound in serum, significant interactions involving displacement from serum proteins do not occur. Clinically, the most significant interaction affecting PB levels is the inhibition of PB elimination by valproate (47). Seen in the majority of patients, the extent of this interaction is variable, although the increase in PB concentration can reach 100%, often necessitating dosage adjustments. The concentrations of PB derived from PRM are equally affected by valproate.

In the great majority of interactions, PB affects levels of other agents. Levels of valproate (48) and carbamazepine (49) are often reduced by the addition of PB. Levels of the active metabolite of carbamazepine, the 10,11-epoxide, are less affected or may even increase, and the epoxide-carbamazepine ratio is usually higher in the presence of PB. Relative to the metabolism of phenytoin, PB appears to cause both enzymatic induction and competitive inhibition. The two effects tend to balance out in patients, and dosage adjustments of phenytoin are seldom necessary (50). PB significantly increases the clearance of lamotrigine (51), as well as that of ethosuximide, felbamate, topiramate, zonisamide, and tiagabine (52).

PB induces the metabolism of many agents besides AEDs. Among the relevant interactions, clearance and dosage requirements of theophylline (53) increase following the addition of PB. Induction of the metabolism of coumarin anticoagulants, such as warfarin (54), can cause problems when PB is introduced or discontinued. In both cases, the anticoagulant dose may require adjustment to avoid excessively long prothrombin times or loss of the desired prothrombin time prolongation. Finally, PB can accelerate the metabolism of steroids, including those contained in oral contraceptives, leading to breakthrough bleeding and contraceptive failure (55). Medium- or high-dose oral contraceptive preparations are recommended in women taking PB (56).

PRM is the cause, as well as the object, of numerous pharmacokinetic interactions (57). Because PB is invariably present during long-term PRM treatment, all of the effects of PB on other agents, described above, can be expected with PRM. The degree of enzymatic induction by other AEDs causes the extent of PRM biotransformation to vary among patients. Metabolism was analyzed in adult patients with epilepsy who received one IV dose of PRM tagged with carbon-14 (39). For 5 days, urine was assayed for PRM and its metabolites. The patients were separated into two groups: those taking no other AED (group 1) and those receiving combination therapies (group 2). Total urinary recovery was 75.5% of the PRM dose in group 1 and 77.4% in group 2. The amount of PRM excreted unchanged was 64% of the dose in group 1 but only 39.6% in group 2. Recovery of PEMA was 6.6% of the PRM dose in group 1 and 27.9% in group 2; PB recovery was 2.1% and 3.3%, respectively. The recovery of unidentified products (probably p-hydroxyphenobarbital) was 3% and 6.5%, respectively, for groups 1 and 2. After an initial dose of PRM, PEMA was detected in the blood within a few hours, whereas PB was often not measurable during the first 24 hours (26,27,37).

Pediatric data are based on 24-hour urine collections under steady-state conditions in 12 children receiving long-term PRM therapy (28): four taking PRM alone, eight taking PRM and phenytoin. On average, 92% of the daily PRM dose was recovered: 42.3% as unchanged drug, 45.2% as PEMA, and 4.9% as PB plus p-hydroxyphenobarbital.

Most reports describe enzymatic induction of the conversion of PRM to PB; some note inhibition. These interactions change not only the blood levels of PRM, PB, and PEMA

TABLE 56.1

SERUM CONCENTRATION: PRM DOSE RATIOS AND SERUM CONCENTRATION RATIOS OF PRIMIDONE, PHENOBARBITAL, AND PHENYLETHYLMALONAMIDE AT STEADY STATE[a]

	No. of Patients	Serum Concentration: PRM Dose[b]			Serum Concentration Ratio[b]	
		PRM	PB	PEMA	PB/PRM	PEMA/PRM
Monotherapy	10	0.78 ±0.25	1.47 ±0.53	0.64 ±0.39	1.65 ±0.74	0.70 ±0.36
Comedications[c]	53	0.40 ±0.15	2.40 ±0.98	0.75A ±0.42	5.83 ±2.62	1.71 ±0.75

Abbreviations: PB, phenobarbital; PEMA, phenylethylmalonamide; PRM, primidone.
[a]All blood samples were drawn before the first morning dose in hospitalized patients.
[b]Mean ± standard deviation (SD), PRM dose in mg/kg per day, serum levels in mg/L.
[c]Combination therapy included phenytoin or carbamazepine, or both.
From Bourgeois BFD. Primidone. In: Resor SR, Kutt H, eds. *Medical treatment of epilepsy*. New York: Marcel Dekker, 1992:371–378, with permission.

relative to the PRM dose, but also the ratios among the three substances. Phenytoin, a known potent inducer (38,58–60), causes the most extensive acceleration of PRM conversion, leading to a decrease in the PRM-PB serum concentration ratio. The rate of PRM biotransformation is slower with carbamazepine (38,58), which may also inhibit the conversion of PRM to PB, causing an increase in the PRM-PB serum concentration ratio (61). Table 56.1 summarizes the effect of comedication with phenytoin, carbamazepine, or both on the concentration-to-dose ratios and on the relative concentration ratios of PRM, PB, and PEMA (62). Compared with PRM monotherapy, the morning trough levels of PRM were reduced by about 50% at the same daily dose. Inversely, PB levels were increased by a factor of approximately 1.6. Thus, when patients receive concomitant phenytoin or carbamazepine, the average PRM dose required to maintain a given PB level is about 1.6 times lower than that with PRM monotherapy. Because derived PB is the product of enzymatic conversion and not the substrate, this difference is the opposite of what is usually seen with inducing interaction, namely, that the drug dose must be increased to maintain the same drug level. With PRM, such an increase often yields PB levels associated with toxic reactions.

Table 56.1 also shows that the PB-PRM concentration ratio in a morning predose blood sample was more than 3 times higher in patients taking phenytoin or carbamazepine in addition to PRM (5.83 versus 1.65, respectively). This means that at a PRM level of 10 mg/L, the corresponding average PB level would be 16.5 mg/L in a patient receiving PRM monotherapy, but 58.3 mg/L in a patient also taking phenytoin or carbamazepine.

Different effects of valproate on PRM kinetics have been described. In one study (63), transient elevations of PRM levels were observed after the addition of valproate; PB levels were not included in this analysis. Other investigators (57) found no consistent changes in PRM or PB levels after the addition of valproate to PRM therapy.

In all patients receiving long-term PRM therapy, the PB level is almost always higher than the PRM level. Attempts have been made to elevate the PRM level in relation to the PB level to obtain a greater therapeutic effect from PRM itself. Adding nicotinamide to the drug regimen (61) could achieve such a change in ratio, but the necessary doses may cause gastrointestinal side effects and hepatotoxic reactions. The antituberculosis drug isoniazid also markedly inhibits PRM biotransformation, producing relatively high PRM levels relative to PB levels (64).

EFFICACY

PB is associated with at least some degree of efficacy against every seizure type, except absence seizures, but is used mainly for the treatment of generalized convulsive seizures and partial seizures at any age. It is an agent of first choice only in neonates with seizures. In a large-scale, controlled comparison of 622 adults with partial and secondarily generalized tonic-clonic seizures (65), phenytoin, carbamazepine, PB, and PRM were equally effective in achieving complete control. PB and PRM controlled partial seizures in a lower percentage of patients than did carbamazepine; the difference in overall success rate between the agents was based mainly on their side-effect profiles. Evidence-based comparison of PB with phenytoin (66) and with carbamazepine (67) revealed no overall difference in seizure control, but PB was more likely to be withdrawn than the other two agents, presumably because of side effects. In children, PB was as effective as carbamazepine for up to 1 year in the treatment of partial seizures (36). In a randomized study of previously untreated children, PB, phenytoin, carbamazepine, and valproate were compared (68). After six of the first 10 children randomized to PB discontinued treatment mainly because of behavioral side effects, PB was eliminated from the study for ethical reasons. Generalized myoclonic seizures and, in particular, juvenile myoclonic epilepsy (69) also respond to PB, although it is not an agent of first choice. A major agent in the treatment of patients with convulsive status epilepticus, PB is usually given if seizures persist following administration of a benzodiazepine and phenytoin. The main disadvantages associated with its use are respiratory depression and pronounced sedation. In patients with status epilepticus, PB was as effective as a combination of diazepam and phenytoin (70). Very high doses of PB have been recommended for the treatment of refractory status epilepticus in children (71). This approach controlled seizures when no limits were imposed relative to maximum dose, and serum levels of 70 to 344 mg/L were achieved (71). In this series, most patients were initially intubated but recovered good spontaneous respiration despite persistently high PB levels; hypotension was uncommon. PB is the agent of first choice in newborns with any type of seizure, with control achieved in about one third of the infants (19,72,73). An efficacy rate of 85% against various neonatal seizures was noted with loading doses of up to 40 mg/kg (74); however, this high response rate cannot be explained solely on the basis of increased doses. In a recent study, newborns with seizures were randomized to initial treatment with PB or phenytoin (75). There was no difference in the percentage of neonates in whom seizure control was achieved with PB (43%) and with phenytoin (45%).

PB has been the most widely used agent for chronic prophylaxis of febrile seizures, with efficacy demonstrated at levels higher than 15 mg/L (76,77). However, such treatment is now more the exception than the rule for several reasons: improved understanding of the benign nature of simple febrile seizures; the efficacy of intermittent short-term use of rectal or oral diazepam therapy (78–80); and reservations about the possible detrimental effect on cognitive function (81,82). Failure of prophylaxis was often due to noncompliance with the regimen and subtherapeutic levels at the time of seizure recurrence.

Neurologic side effects have prevented PRM from becoming an agent of first choice for the treatment of any seizure type. Indications are similar to those for PB, except for the treatment of status epilepticus (PRM is not available in a parenteral formulation) and the prophylaxis of febrile seizures. PRM is effective against generalized tonic-clonic seizures and, when used as a primary agent, juvenile myoclonic epilepsy (83,84). However, because of its greater efficacy and lower toxicity, valproate is now preferred for the latter condition. The clinical efficacy of PRM and PB has been compared in various studies. Several demonstrated no superiority of PRM, but neither was the drug less effective (45,85,86). In one crossover study (87), the efficacy of PRM and PB was compared sequentially in the same patients. Similar PB levels were maintained during both therapies, and PRM was found to be slightly more effective than PB against generalized tonic-clonic seizures.

In partial and secondarily generalized seizures, PRM use was associated with the same degree of seizure control as phenytoin or carbamazepine (86,88). The aforementioned study by Mattson and colleagues (65), which is the most comprehensive and systematic controlled comparison of carbamazepine, phenytoin, PB, and PRM in these seizure types, showed little difference in efficacy among the agents; however, the percentage of treatment failures was highest with PRM because of an increased incidence of side effects early on. Carbamazepine and phenytoin were associated with the lowest percentage of failures. The choice between PB and PRM may depend on individual factors. After PB has failed, PRM may still be tried. However, selecting PRM before PB may save one therapeutic step, based on the assumption that PB is unlikely to be effective if maximal tolerated doses of PRM have not controlled seizures. This approach may shorten the process of documenting medical intractability for epilepsy surgery. PRM is rarely indicated against any type of seizure other than partial and secondarily generalized seizures. In particular, the agent has little or no place in the treatment of generalized epilepsies encountered in childhood, such as absence epilepsy and Lennox-Gastaut syndrome. Although some potential use has been demonstrated in the treatment of neonatal seizures (41), PRM is rarely used for this indication. PRM is contraindicated in any patient with a previous allergic or severe idiosyncratic reaction to PRM or to PB. Like PB, PRM is also contraindicated in patients with hepatic porphyria.

ADVERSE EFFECTS

Among AEDs, PB and PRM cause somewhat pronounced dose-related neurotoxic reactions, although serious systemic side effects are rare. These agents invariably produce sedation and drowsiness at high doses in adults, whereas children often become hyperactive and irritable even at levels in the normal therapeutic range. Sedation, usually present at relatively low levels during the first few days of treatment, subsides thereafter as tolerance to this effect develops. Sedation or somnolence reappears only at high therapeutic or supratherapeutic levels, usually (30 mg/L. As dose levels increase further, neurologic toxicity appears, characterized by dysarthria, ataxia, incoordination, and nystagmus. In children, sedation from PB is much less common than behavioral side effects, mainly hyperactivity, aggressiveness, and insomnia, which may be seen in almost half of all children receiving PB and can appear at levels <15 mg/L (77). Depression, particularly in the pediatric age-group, has been attributed to PB use (89). Although its effect may have been overemphasized, double-blind, controlled studies have confirmed that PB affects cognitive abilities even at levels in the therapeutic range. Children treated with PB had lower memory and concentration scores than those receiving placebo, and these differences correlated significantly with plasma levels

(90). Double-blind comparisons of PB-treated children versus untreated children (91,92) or valproate-treated children (93) demonstrated subtle but significantly lower intelligence quotient (IQ) scores in the PB groups. In an intention-to-treat analysis comparing children treated with PB or placebo for febrile seizures, the average IQ score was 8.4 points lower with PB (81) and remained 5.2 points lower 6 months after discontinuation of PB. Some differences persisted 3 to 5 years later (82). Movement disorders, such as dyskinesia, may be induced by PB, but they are rare (94). Like other AEDs, PB can exacerbate seizures or induce *de novo* seizures (95).

Allergic rashes and hypersensitivity reactions are relatively rare with PB or PRM treatment. Hematologic toxicity, mainly megaloblastic anemia, occurs even less often (less than 1%) (96). Like phenytoin and carbamazepine, PB can exacerbate acute intermittent porphyria (97) and cause osteoporosis and decreased bone mineral density, presumably through accelerated vitamin D metabolism (98,99). Vitamin K-deficient hemorrhagic disease in newborns of mothers treated with PB (100) can be prevented by administration of vitamin K to the mother before delivery. Connective tissue disorders associated with long-term PB therapy are well known (101) and have recently received renewed attention. These include Dupuytren contractures, plantar fibromatosis, heel and knuckle pads, frozen shoulder, and diffuse joint pain. Connective tissue disorders are an unusual side effect in children.

Like every AED, PB has been known to increase the risk for minor and major malformations in the offspring of mothers who were chronically exposed during pregnancy. Assessment of the specific risk for a given agent in clinical studies has been complicated by polytherapy and the underlying risk for malformation due to maternal epilepsy. No evidence suggests that PB is more teratogenic than other AEDs or that it causes a specific spectrum of malformations (102). Evidence that PB increases the risk for any type of tumor development in humans is similarly lacking (103).

Acute and chronic toxic PRM reactions can be distinguished clearly from one another, but long-term PRM side effects are difficult to separate from those associated with derived PB. Because the ratio of PRM to PB varies, toxic side effects may occur at different PRM concentrations. Moreover, reliable evidence that long-term PRM side effects differ from those with comparable PB therapy is lacking. This is also true for potential teratogenic effects. Ventriculoseptal defects, microcephaly, and poor somatic development (104) have been described in the offspring of women taking PRM, although no specific teratogenic pattern has been attributed to the agent.

The acute initial toxicity clearly differentiates PRM from PB. Even after a low initial dose of PRM, some patients experience transient side effects—usually drowsiness, dizziness, ataxia, nausea, and vomiting (65)—that are so debilitating they may be reluctant to take another dose.

Because this acute toxic reaction occurs before PB or PEMA is detected in the blood, it must be associated with PRM itself. That much larger doses of PRM are later tolerated by the same patients during long-term therapy argues for the development of tolerance to PRM probably within hours to days. The ratio of clinical toxicity score to serum PRM levels, determined in a group of patients receiving their first PRM dose (105), decreased significantly as early as 6 hours after the ingestion of drug. PB probably produces a cross-tolerance to this acute PRM toxicity, because patients on long-term PB therapy are less likely to experience the same degree of toxicity on first exposure to PRM (105,106). Cross-tolerance to PRM following PB exposure can be demonstrated in experimental animals. To achieve the same degree of seizure protection and the same level of neurotoxicity, higher brain concentrations of PRM were necessary in mice that had received PB daily for 2 weeks than in mice without any drug exposure (107).

CLINICAL USE

On the basis of its relative efficacy and toxicity profile, PB is no longer an agent of first choice for the treatment of any seizure type, except for neonates with seizures and for long-term prophylaxis of febrile seizures, if indicated. PB remains an agent of second or third choice for the treatment of generalized convulsive seizures and partial seizures at any age, and is prescribed widely for infants because it is easier to use and is associated with less systemic toxicity than phenytoin, carbamazepine, or valproate.

In adults, the daily maintenance dose of PB, between 1.5 and 4 mg/kg, achieves steady-state levels within the recommended therapeutic range of 15 to 40 mg/L. Because of its long elimination half-life and slow accumulation, the full maintenance dose can be administered on the first treatment day, although steady-state plasma levels will be reached only after 2 to 3 weeks. The daily maintenance dose of PB in children varies between 2 and 8 mg/kg; doses >8 mg/kg may be necessary in some infants to achieve high therapeutic levels. The dose is roughly inversely proportional to the child's age: 2 months to 1 year, 4 to 11 mg/kg per day; 1 to 3 years, 3 to 7 mg/kg per day; 3 to 6 years, 2 to 5 mg/kg per day (108). Given the long half-life of PB, dividing the daily dose of the agent into two or more doses appears unnecessary, even in children (109). Close monitoring of plasma levels and dosage reductions may be necessary in patients with advanced renal disease (110) and cirrhosis (111).

The IV loading dose of PB for the treatment of status epilepticus varies between 10 and 30 mg/kg; 15 to 20 mg/kg is most common. The rate of administration should not exceed 100 mg per minute (2 mg/kg per minute in children weighing less than 40 kg). PB penetrates the brain relatively slowly; however, although full equilibrium is not reached for as long as 1 hour, therapeutic brain concentrations are reached within 3 minutes (112). The initial loading dose of 15 to 20 mg/kg in newborns is similar to the dose in children and adults, and will achieve a plasma level of about 20 mg/L. This level can usually be maintained in newborns with a dose of 3 to 4 mg/kg per day (113). Loading doses up to 40 mg/kg have been used (74).

PRM should be used alone or in combination with a noninducing drug, such as gabapentin, lamotrigine, topiramate, tiagabine, vigabatrin, or a benzodiazepine. An inducing drug will shift the PRM-PB ratio to such an extent that one might just as well prescribe PB instead of PRM. For the same reason, prescribing PRM and PB simultaneously for the same patient makes no sense. Valproate may also increase PB levels, on the basis of its demonstrated inhibition of PB elimination. A low starting dose is more important with PRM than with most other AEDs because of the occurrence of transient, but severe, toxic reactions. A first dose of one-half tablet (125 mg) at bedtime is often well tolerated, but some patients initially need as little as one-quarter tablet (62.5 mg) or less. The dose can then be increased every 3 days as tolerated, to a final daily maintenance dose of 10 to 20 mg/kg. Maintenance doses are 15 to 25 mg/kg per day in newborns, 10 to 25 mg/kg per day in infants, and 10 to 20 mg/kg per day in children.

A schedule that allows rapid advancement to the full maintenance dose of PRM was devised (114) on the basis of observations in humans (105) and experimental animals (107) that PB produces cross-tolerance to the effects of PRM. After initial administration of PB, the dose is titrated as rapidly as tolerated to achieve a serum level up to 20 mg/L; abrupt switch to the full maintenance dose of PRM follows. Experimentation with various PB titration schedules revealed that most patients tolerate the following increases with minimal or no sedation: 5 mg/L after 24 hours; 10 mg/L after 48 hours; 15 mg/L after 72 hours; and 20 mg/L after 96 hours (end of day 4). These levels can be achieved in adults by administering 3 mg/kg of PB orally on day 1 (two doses of 1.5 mg/kg each, 12 hours apart); 3.5 mg/kg on day 2; 4 mg/kg on day 3, and 5 mg/kg on day 4 (Fig. 56.2). On day 5, the patient receives a full PRM maintenance dose of 12.5 to 20 mg/kg, with no significant new toxicity. This beneficial effect of PB pretreatment on initial PRM toxicity has been confirmed in a more recent study (115).

PRM monotherapy at a daily dose of 20 mg/kg will achieve, on average, PB levels of 30 mg/L (Table 56.1); however, steady-state PB levels will be reached only after 2 to 3 weeks at the same PRM dose. In patients comedicated with carbamazepine or phenytoin, the same PB level will be achieved with an average PRM dose of 10 to 15 mg/kg per day. As with most AEDs, average dosage requirements may be higher in children and lower in the elderly. Because of the relatively short half-life of PRM, usual recommendations call for dividing the daily dose into three doses, although the need to do so has never been documented. If blood levels are used to adjust the PRM dose, then PB

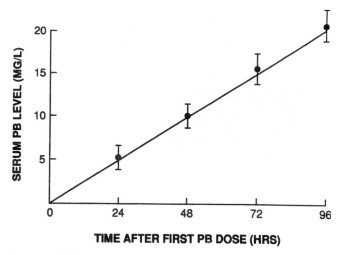

Figure 56.2 Phenobarbital (PB) loading dose over 4 days for rapid introduction of primidone. The PB values represent the average of 11 patients with standard deviation (*vertical bars*). The *solid straight line* connects the corresponding predicted values (5, 10, 15, and 20 mg/L). (Courtesy of Bourgeois BFD, unpublished data, 1991.)

rather than PRM levels are preferred, because at the usual concentration ratios the side effects from a high PB level are more likely to limit further dosage increases. Although a therapeutic range of 3 to 12 mg/L has been suggested for PRM (116), monitoring PRM levels is of little help in clinical practice. This is true for PEMA as well, which probably has no significant pharmacologic effect at levels measured in patients.

After long-term administration, PB and PRM should always be discontinued gradually over several weeks. Barbiturates and benzodiazepines are the AEDs most commonly associated with withdrawal seizures on rapid discontinuation. Unless there is a specific reason to proceed faster, it is appropriate to taper the PB or PRM dose linearly over 3 to 6 months, with reductions each month.

REFERENCES

1. Bogue JY, Carrington HC. The evaluation of "mysoline," a new anticonvulsant drug. *Br J Pharmacol* 1953;8:230–236.
2. Olson RW. Phenobarbital and other barbiturates: mechanism of action. In: Levy RH, Mattson RH, Meldrum BS, et al, eds. *Antiepileptic drugs*, 5th ed. Philadelphia: Lippincott Williams & Wilkins, 2002:489–495.
3. Straw R, Mitchell C. Effect of phenobarbital on cortical afterdischarge and overt seizure patterns in the rat. *Int J Neuropharmacol* 1966;5:323–330.
4. MacDonald R, Twyman R. Kinetic properties and regulation of GABA receptor channels. In: Narahashi R, ed. *Ion channels*. New York: Plenum, 1992:315–343.
5. Heyer E, Macdonald R. Barbiturate reduction of calcium-dependent action potentials: correlation with anesthetic action. *Brain Res* 1982;236:157–171.
6. MacDonald R, McLean M. Anticonvulsant drugs: mechanisms of action. *Adv Neurol* 1986;44:713–736.
7. Frey HH, Hahn I. Research on the significance of phenobarbital, produced by biotransformation, for the anticonvulsant action of pyrimidone [German]. *Arch Int Pharmacodyn Ther* 1960;128: 281–290.

8. Baumel IP, Gallagher BB, DiMicco D, et al. Metabolism and anti-convulsant properties of primidone in the rat. *J Pharmacol Exp Ther* 1973;186:305–314.

9. Bourgeois BFD, Dodson WE, Ferrendelli JA. Primidone, pheno-barbital, and PEMA: I. Seizure protection, neurotoxicity, and therapeutic index of individual compounds in mice. *Neurology* 1983;33:283–290.

10. Leal KW, Rapport RL, Wilensky AJ, et al. Single-dose pharmaco-kinetics and anticonvulsant efficacy of primidone in mice. *Ann Neurol* 1979;5:470–474.

11. Bourgeois BFD, Dodson WE, Ferrendelli JA. Primidone, pheno-barbital, and PEMA: II. Seizure protection, neurotoxicity, and therapeutic index of varying combinations in mice. *Neurology* 1983;33:291–295.

12. Loscher W, Honack D. Comparison of the anticonvulsant effi-cacy of primidone and phenobarbital during chronic treatment of amygdala-kindled rats. *Eur J Pharmacol* 1989;162:309–322.

13. Baumel IP, Gallagher BB, Mattson RH. Phenylethylmalonamide (PEMA). An important metabolite of primidone. *Arch Neurol* 1972;27:34–41.

14. Nelson E, Powell J, Conrad K, et al. Phenobarbital pharmacoki-netics and bioavailability in adults. *J Clin Pharmacol* 1982;18:31–42.

15. Wilensky A, Friel P, Levy R, et al. Kinetics of phenobarbital in normal subjects and epileptic patients. *Eur J Clin Pharmacol* 1982;23:87–92.

16. Jalling B. Plasma concentrations of phenobarbital in the treat-ment of seizures in the newborn. *Acta Paediatr Scand* 1975;64:514–524.

17. Graves NM, Holmes GB, Kriel RL, et al. Relative bioavailability of rectally administered phenobarbital sodium parenteral solu-tion. *DICP* 1989;23:565–568.

18. Kuhnz W, Koch S, Helge H, et al. Primidone and phenobarbital during lactation period in epileptic women: total and free drug serum levels in the nursed infants and their effects on neonatal behavior. *Dev Pharmacol Ther* 1988;1:147–154.

19. Painter MJ, Pippenger C, Wasterlain C, et al. Phenobarbital and phenytoin in neonatal seizures: metabolism and tissue distribu-tion. *Neurology* 1981;31:1107–1112.

20. Kapetanovic I, Kupferberg H, Porter R, et al. Mechanism of val-proate-phenobarbital interaction in epileptic patients. *Clin Pharmacol Ther* 1981;29:480–486.

21. Whyte M, Dekaban A. Metabolic fate of phenobarbital. A quan-titative study of p-hydroxyphenobarbital elimination in man. *Drug Metab Dispos* 1977;5:63–70.

22. Tang B, Kalow W, Grey AA. Metabolic fate of phenobarbital in man. N-glucoside formation. *Drug Metab Dispos* 1979;7:315–318.

23. Pitlick W, Painter M, Pippenger C. Phenobarbital pharmacoki-netics in neonates. *Clin Pharmacol Ther* 1978;23:346–350.

24. Gal P, Toback J, Erkan N, et al. The influence of asphyxia on phe-nobarbital dosing requirements in neonates. *Dev Pharmacol Ther* 1984;7:145–152.

25. Heimann G, Gladtke E. Pharmacokinetics of phenobarbital in childhood. *Eur J Clin Pharmacol* 1977;12:305–310.

26. Gallagher BB, Baumel IP, Mattson RH. Metabolic disposition of primidone and its metabolites in epileptic subjects after single and repeated administration. *Neurology* 1972;22:1186–1192.

27. Gallagher BB, Baumel IP. Primidone. Absorption, distribution and excretion. In: Woodbury DM, Penry JK, Schmidt RP, eds. *Antiepileptic drugs*. New York: Raven Press, 1972:357–359.

28. Kauffman RE, Habersang R, Lansky J. Kinetics of primidone metabolism and excretion in children. *Clin Pharmacol Ther* 1977;22:200–205.

29. Syverson GB, Morgan JP, Weintraub M, et al. Acetazolamide-induced interference with primidone absorption. *Arch Neurol* 1977;34:80–84.

30. Wyllie E, Pippenger CE, Rothner AD. Increased seizure fre-quency with generic primidone. *JAMA* 1987;258:1216–1217.

31. Matzke GR, Cloyd JC, Sawchuk RJ. Acute phenytoin and primi-done intoxication. A pharmacokinetic analysis. *J Clin Pharmacol* 1981;21:92–99.

32. Pisani F, Perucca E, Primerano G, et al. Single-dose kinetics of primidone in acute viral hepatitis. *Eur J Clin Pharmacol* 1984;27:465–469.

33. Pisani F, Richens A. Pharmacokinetics of phenylethylmalon-amide (PEMA) after oral and intravenous administration. *Clin Pharmacol* 1983;8:272–276.

34. Houghton GW, Richens A, Toseland PA, et al. Brain concentra-tions of phenytoin, phenobarbital and primidone in epileptic patients. *Eur J Clin Pharmacol* 1975;9:73–78.

35. Monaco F, Piredda S, Mastropaolo C, et al. Diphenylhydantoin and primidone in tears. *Epilepsia* 1981;22:185–188.

36. Mitchell W, Chavez J. Carbamazepine versus phenobarbital for partial onset seizures in children. *Epilepsia* 1987;28:56–60.

37. Booker HE, Hosokowa K, Burdette RD, et al. A clinical study of serum primidone levels. *Epilepsia* 1970;11:395–402.

38. Cloyd JC, Miller KW, Leppik IE. Primidone kinetics: effects of concurrent drugs and duration of therapy. *Clin Pharmacol Ther* 1981;29:402–407.

39. Zavadil P, Gallagher BB. Metabolism and excretion of ^{14}C-primi-done in epileptic patients. In: Janz D, ed. *Epileptology*. Stuttgart, Germany: Thieme, 1976:129–139.

40. Nau H, Rating D, Hauser I, et al. Placental transfer and pharma-cokinetics of primidone and its metabolites phenobarbital, PEMA and hydroxyphenobarbital in neonates and infants of epileptic mothers. *Eur J Clin Pharmacol* 1980;18:31–42.

41. Powell C, Painter MJ, Pippenger CC. Primidone therapy in refractory neonatal seizures. *J Pediatr* 1984;105:651–654.

42. Bogue JY, Carrington HC. Personal communication, 1952, cited by Goodman LS, Swinyard EA, Brown WC, et al. Anticonvulsant properties of 5-phenyl-5-ethyl hexahydropyrimidine-4,6-dione (Mysoline), a new antiepileptic. *J Pharmacol Exp Ther* 1953;108:428–436.

43. Butler TC, Waddell WJ. Metabolic conversion of primidone (mysoline) to phenobarbital. *Proc Soc Exp Biol Med* 1956;93:544–546.

44. Plaa GL, Fujimoto JM, Hine CH. Intoxication from primidone due to its biotransformation to phenobarbital. *JAMA* 1958;168:1769–1770.

45. Oleson OV, Dam M. The metabolic conversion of primidone to phenobarbitone in patients under long-term treatment. *Acta Neurol Scand* 1967;43:348–356.

46. Bogan J, Smith H. The relation between primidone and pheno-barbitone blood levels. *J Pharm Pharmacol* 1968;20:64–67.

47. De Gatta M, Gonzales A, Sanches M, et al. Effect of sodium val-proate on phenobarbital serum levels in children and adults. *Ther Drug Monit* 1986;8:416–420.

48. May T, Rambeck B. Serum concentrations of valproic acid: influ-ence of dose and comedication. *Ther Drug Monit* 1985;7:387–390.

49. Riva R, Contin M, Albani F, et al. Free concentration of carba-mazepine and carbamazepine-10,11-epoxide in children and adults. Influence of age and phenobarbitone co-medication. *Clin Pharmacokinet* 1985;10:524–531.

50. Browne T, Szabo G, Evan J, et al. Phenobarbital does not alter phenytoin steady-state concentration or pharmacokinetics. *Neurology* 1988;38:639–642.

51. Eriksson A, Hoppu K, Nergardh A, et al. Pharmacokinetic inter-actions between lamotrigine and other antiepileptic drugs in children with intractable epilepsy. *Epilepsia* 1996;37:769–773.

52. Riva R, Albani F, Contin M, et al. Pharmacokinetic interactions between antiepileptic drugs: clinical considerations. *Clin Pharmacokinet* 1996;31:470–493.

53. Jonkman J, Upton R. Pharmacokinetic drug interactions with theophylline. *Clin Pharmacokinet* 1984;9:309–334.

54. MacDonald M, Robinson D. Clinical observations of possible barbiturate interference with anticoagulation. *JAMA* 1968;204:97–100.

55. Hempel E, Klinger W. Drug stimulated biotransformation of hormonal steroid contraceptives: clinical implications. *Drugs* 1976;12:442–448.

56. Mattson R, Cramer J. Epilepsy, sex hormones and antiepileptic drugs. *Epilepsia* 1985;26(Suppl):S40–S55.

57. Fincham RW, Schottelius DD. Primidone: interactions with other drugs. In: Levy RH, Dreifuss F, Mattson RH, et al., eds. *Antiepileptic drugs*. New York: Raven Press, 1989:413–422.

58. Battino D, Avanzini G, Bossi L, et al. Plasma levels of primidone and its metabolite phenobarbital: effect of age and associated therapy. *Ther Drug Monit* 1983;5:73–79.

59. Fincham RW, Schottelius DD, Sahs AL. The influence of diphenylhydantoin on primidone metabolism. *Arch Neurol* 1974;30:259–262.

60. Reynolds EH, Fenton G, Fenwick P, et al. Interaction of phenytoin and primidone. *Br Med J* 1975;2:594–595.

61. Bourgeois BFD, Dodson WE, Ferrendelli JA. Interactions between primidone, carbamazepine, and nicotinamide. *Neurology* 1982;32:1122–1126.

62. Bourgeois BFD. Primidone. In: Resor SR, Kutt H, eds. *Medical treatment of epilepsy*. New York: Marcel Dekker, 1992:371–378.

63. Windorfer A, Sauer W, Gadeke R. Elevation of diphenylhydantoin and PRIMIDONE serum concentrations by addition of dipropylacetate, a new anticonvulsant drug. *Acta Paediatr* 1975;64:771–772.

64. Sutton G, Kupferberg HJ. Isoniazid as an inhibitor of primidone metabolism. *Neurology* 1975;25:1179–1181.

65. Mattson RH, Cramer JA, Collins JF, et al. Comparison of carbamazepine, phenobarbital, phenytoin and primidone in partial and secondarily generalized tonic-clonic seizures. *N Engl J Med* 1985;313:145–151.

66. Taylor S, Tudur Smith C, Williamson PR, et al. Phenobarbitone versus phenytoin monotherapy for partial onset seizures and generalized onset tonic-clonic seizures. *Cochrane Database Syst Rev* 2001;4:CD002217.

67. Tudur Smith C, Marson AG, Williamson PR. Carbamazepine versus phenobarbitone monotherapy for epilepsy. *Cochrane Database Syst Rev* 2003;1:CD001904.

68. de Silva M, MacArdle B, McGowan M, et al. Randomised comparative monotherapy trial of phenobarbitone, phenytoin, carbamazepine, or sodium valproate for newly diagnosed childhood epilepsy. *Lancet* 1996;347:709–713.

69. Resor SR, Resor LD. The neuropharmacology of juvenile myoclonic epilepsy. *Clin Neuropharmacol* 1990;6:465–491.

70. Shaner MD, McCurdy S, Herring M, et al. Treatment of status epilepticus: a prospective comparison of diazepam and phenytoin versus phenobarbital and optional phenytoin. *Neurology* 1988;38:202–207.

71. Crawford TO, Mitchell WG, Fishman LS, et al. Very-high-dose phenobarbital for refractory status epilepticus in children. *Neurology* 1988;38:1035–1040.

72. Lockman L, Kriel R, Zaske D. Phenobarbital dosage for control of neonatal seizures. *Neurology* 1979;29:1445–1449.

73. Van Orman C, Darwish HZ. Efficacy of phenobarbital in neonatal seizures. *Can J Neurol Sci* 1985;12:95–99.

74. Gal P, Toback J, Boer H, et al. Efficacy of phenobarbital monotherapy in treatment of neonatal seizures—relationship to blood vessels. *Neurology* 1982;32:1401–1404.

75. Painter MJ, Scher MS, Stein AD, et al. Phenobarbital compared with phenytoin for the treatment of neonatal seizures. *N Engl J Med* 1999;341:485–489.

76. Faero O, Kastrup K, Nielsen E, et al. Successful prophylaxis of febrile convulsions with phenobarbital. *Epilepsia* 1972;13:279–285.

77. Wolf SM, Forsythe A. Behavior disturbance, phenobarbital, and febrile seizures. *Pediatrics* 1978;61:728–731.

78. Knudsen FU. Effective short-term diazepam prophylaxis in febrile convulsions. *J Pediatr* 1985;106:487–490.

79. Rosman NP, Colton T, Labazzo J, et al. A controlled trial of diazepam administered during febrile illnesses to prevent recurrence of febrile seizures. *N Engl J Med* 1993;329:79–84.

80. Baumann RJ, Duffner PK. Treatment of children with simple febrile seizures: the AAP practice parameter. *Pediatr Neurol* 2000;23:11–17.

81. Farwell JR, Lee YJ, Hirtz DG, et al. Phenobarbital for febrile seizures—effects on intelligence and on seizure recurrence. *N Engl J Med* 1990;322:364–369.

82. Sulzbacher S, Farwell JR, Temkin N, et al. Late cognitive effects of early treatment with phenobarbital. *Clin Pediatrics* 1999;38:387–394.

83. Delgado-Escueta AV, Enrile-Bascal F. Juvenile myoclonic epilepsy of Janz. *Neurology* 1984;34:285–294.

84. Janz D. Epilepsy with impulsive petit mal (juvenile myoclonic epilepsy). *Acta Neurol Scand* 1985;72:449–459.

85. Gruber CM Jr, Brock JT, Dyken M. Comparison of the effectiveness of phenobarbital, mephobarbital, primidone, diphenylhydantoin, ethotoin, metharbital, and methylphenylethylhy-

dantoin in motor seizures. *Clin Pharmacol Ther* 1962;3:23–28.

86. White PT, Pott D, Norton J. Relative anticonvulsant potency of primidone. A double-blind comparison. *Arch Neurol* 1966;14:31–35.

87. Oxley J, Hebdige S, Laidlaw J, et al. A comparative study of phenobarbitone and primidone in the treatment of epilepsy. In: Johannessen SI, Morselli PL, Pippenger CE, et al., eds. *Antiepileptic therapy. Advances in drug monitoring*. New York: Raven Press, 1980:237–245.

88. Rodin EA, Rim CS, Kitano H, et al. A comparison of the effectiveness of primidone versus carbamazepine in epileptic outpatients. *J Nerv Ment Dis* 1976;163:41–46.

89. Brent D, Crumrine P, Varma R, et al. Phenobarbital treatment and major depressive disorder in children with epilepsy: a naturalistic follow-up. *Pediatrics* 1987;80:909–917.

90. Camfield PR. Pancreatitis due to valproic acid. *Lancet* 1979;1:1198–1199.

91. Calandre EP, Dominguez-Granados R, Gomez-Rubio M, et al. Cognitive effects of long-term treatment with phenobarbital and valproic acid in school children. *Acta Neurol Scand* 1990;81:504–506.

92. Farwell JR, Lee YJ, Hirtz DG, et al. Phenobarbital for febrile seizures—effects on intelligence and on seizure recurrence. *N Engl J Med* 1990;322:364–369.

93. Vining EP, Mellitis ED, Dorsen MM, et al. Psychologic and behavioral effects of antiepileptic drugs in children: a double-blind comparison between phenobarbital and valproic acid. *Pediatrics* 1987;80:165–174.

94. Wiznitzer M, Younkin D. Phenobarbital-induced dyskinesia in a neurologically-impaired child. *Neurology* 1984;34:1600–1601.

95. Hamano S, Mochizuki M, Morikawa T. Phenobarbital-induced absence seizure in benign childhood epilepsy with centrotemporal spikes. *Seizure* 2002;11:201–204.

96. Hawkins C, Meynell M. Macrocytosis and macrocytic anemia caused by anticonvulsant drugs. *Am J Med* 1958;27:45–63.

97. Magnussen C, Doherthy J, Hess R, et al. Grand mal seizures and acute intermittent porphyria: the problem of differential diagnosis and treatment. *Neurology* 1975;25:1121–1125.

98. Christiansen C, Rodbro P, Lund M. Incidence of anticonvulsant osteomalacia and effect of vitamin D: controlled therapeutic trial. *Br Med J* 1973;4:695–701.

99. Farhat G, Yamout B, Mikati MA, et al. Effect of antiepileptic drugs on bone density in ambulatory patients. *Neurology* 2002;58:1348–1353.

100. Deblay MF, Vert P, Andre M, et al. Transplacental vitamin K prevents hemorrhagic disease of infants of epileptic mothers. *Lancet* 1982;1:1247.

101. Cramer J, Mattson R. Phenobarbital: toxicity. In: Levy R, Mattson R, Meldrum B, eds. *Antiepileptic drugs*. New York: Raven Press, 1995:409–420.

102. Yerby M, Leavitt A, Erickson DM, et al. Antiepileptics and the development of congenital anomalies. *Neurology* 1992;42(Suppl 5):132–140.

103. Olsen H, Boice J, Jensen J, et al. Cancer among epileptic patients exposed to anticonvulsant drugs. *J Natl Cancer Inst* 1989;81:803–808.

104. Rating D, Nau H, Jager-Roman E, et al. Teratogenic and pharmacokinetic studies of primidone during pregnancy and in the offspring of epileptic women. *Acta Paediatr Scand* 1982;71:301–311.

105. Leppik IE, Cloyd JC, Miller K. Development of tolerance to the side effects of primidone. *Ther Drug Monit* 1984;6:189–191.

106. Gallagher BB, Baumel IP, Mattson RH, et al. Primidone, diphenylhydantoin and phenobarbital. Aspects of acute and chronic toxicity. *Neurology* 1973;23:145–149.

107. Bourgeois B. Individual and crossed tolerance to the anticonvulsant effect and neurotoxicity of phenobarbital and primidone in mice. In: Frey H, Froscher W, Koella WP, et al., eds. *Tolerance to beneficial and adverse effects of antiepileptic drugs*. New York: Raven Press, 1986:17–24.

108. Rossi L. Correlation between age and plasma level/dosage for phenobarbital in infants and children. *Acta Paediatr Scand* 1979;68:431–434.

109. Davis A, Mutchie K, Thompson J, et al. Once-daily dosing with phenobarbital in children with seizure disorders. *Pediatrics* 1981;68:824–827.
110. Asconape J, Penry J. Use of antiepileptic drugs in the presence of liver and kidney disease: a review. *Epilepsia* 1982;23(Suppl 1): S65–S79.
111. Alvin J, McHorse T, Hoyumpa A, et al. The effect of liver disease in man on the disposition of phenobarbital. *J Pharmacol Exp Ther* 1975;192:224–235.
112. Ramsay RE, Hammond EJ, Perchalski RJ, et al. Brain uptake of phenytoin, phenobarbital, and diazepam. *Arch Neurol* 1979;36: 535–539.
113. Painter MJ, Pippenger C, MacDonald H, et al. Phenobarbital and phenytoin blood levels in neonates. *Pediatrics* 1977;92:315–319.
114. Bourgeois BFD, Luders H, Morris H, et al. Rapid introduction of primidone using phenobarbital loading: acute primidone toxicity avoided. *Epilepsia* 1989;30:667.
115. Kanner AM, Parra J, Frey M. The "forgotten" cross-tolerance between phenobarbital and primidone: it can prevent acute primidone-related toxicity. *Epilepsia* 2000;41:1310–1314.
116. Schottelius DD, Fincham RW. Clinical application of serum primidone levels. In: Pippenger CE, Penry JK, Kutt H, eds. *Antiepileptic drugs: quantitative analysis and interpretation.* New York: Raven Press, 1978:273–282.

Ethosuximide

57

Tracy A. Glauser   *Diego A. Morita*

HISTORICAL BACKGROUND

The development of ethosuximide was a response to the need in the 1950s to develop a more effective, safer, and better tolerated anticonvulsant for the treatment of absence seizures (1). Introduced in the 1940s, trimethadione and its analogue paramethadione were the first anticonvulsants to demonstrate efficacy against absence seizures, but they were associated with significant toxicity (2–5). These toxicity issues spurred the discovery and testing in the 1950s of the succinimide family of anticonvulsants (ethosuximide, methsuximide, and phensuximide) (5). Of the succinimides, ethosuximide had the greatest efficacy and least toxicity when used against absence seizures (5). Because of this combination of efficacy and safety, ethosuximide has been considered as first-line therapy for absence seizures since its introduction in 1958 (6,7).

CHEMISTRY AND MECHANISM OF ACTION

Ethosuximide (2-ethyl-2-methylsuccinimide), with a molecular mass of 141.2, is a chiral compound containing a five-member ring, with two negatively charged carbonyl oxygen atoms with a ring nitrogen between them and one asymmetric carbon atom (8,9) (Fig. 57.1). Its chemical characteristics include a melting point of 64°C to 65°C, a weakly acidic pKa of 9.3, and a partition coefficient of 9 (chloroform-to-water; pH 7) (9). Ethosuximide is freely soluble in ethanol and water (solubility, 190 mg/5 mL) (9). A white crystalline material, ethosuximide is used clinically as a racemate and is commercially available in 250-mg capsules or 250 mg/5 mL of syrup (6,8).

The presumed mechanism of action against absence seizures is reduction of low-threshold T-type calcium currents in thalamic neurons (10,11). The spontaneous pacemaker oscillatory activity of thalamocortical neurons involves low-threshold T-type calcium currents (12). These oscillatory currents are considered to be the generators of the 3-Hz spike-and-wave rhythms in patients with absence epilepsy (12). Voltage-dependent blockade of the low-threshold T-type calcium current was demonstrated at clinically relevant ethosuximide concentrations in thalamic neurons isolated from rats and guinea pigs (10,11,13). Ethosuximide does not alter gating of these T-type Ca^{2+} channels (5,11). Combining these findings, it is proposed that ethosuximide's effect on low-threshold T-type calcium currents in thalamocortical neurons prevents the "synchronized firing associated with spike-wave discharges" (10).

There is no evidence that ethosuximide exerts an anticonvulsant effect through other common mechanisms of action (e.g., action at voltage-dependent sodium channels or postsynaptic enhancement of γ-aminobutyric acid [GABA] responses) (5,14). Single-dose administration does not alter brain GABA concentrations in mice (15). The anticonvulsant effect of ethosuximide's other actions in the brain (i.e., effects on brain enzyme physiology, membrane transport processes, and neurotransmitter processes [14]) are unclear. In cortical tissue, at concentrations significantly greater than those used for anticonvulsant effect, ethosuximide inhibits Na^+,K^+-adenosine triphosphatase (Na^+,K^+-ATPase) activity (14,16–18).

PHARMACOKINETICS

Implications of Racemic Mixture

Ethosuximide has always been used clinically as a racemate. It is theoretically possible that the two enantiomers could demonstrate different pharmacokinetic parameters or anticonvulsant effects. In rats, ethosuximide's disposition is nonstereoselective (9). Chiral gas chromatographic analysis of enantiomer concentrations in plasma samples obtained for routine monitoring, 33 patients

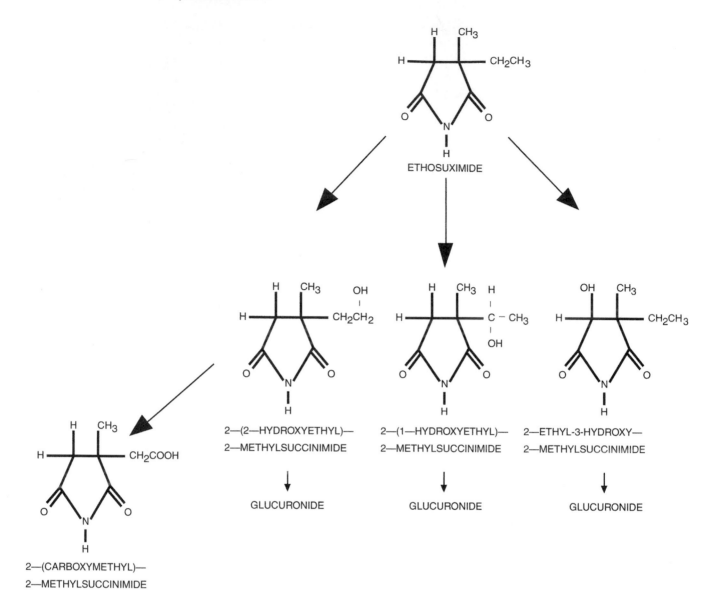

Figure 57.1 Structure and biotransformation pathways of ethosuximide (From Pisani F, Meir B. Ethosuximide: chemistry biotransformation. In: Levy R, Mattson R, Meldrum B, eds. *Antiepileptic drugs*, 4th ed. New York: Raven Press, 1995:655–658, with permission).

demonstrated that the enantiomer ratio was close to unity, and there was little interindividual variability (19). This implies that the disposition of ethosuximide in humans is nonstereoselective and that measurement of total ethosuximide for therapeutic monitoring is reasonable and appropriate (9,20). A small study (three pregnancies in two women taking ethosuximide) demonstrated that the nonstereoselective disposition was unaffected by pregnancy, placental transfer, or passage into breast milk (20).

ABSORPTION

In rats, dogs, and monkeys, absorption is rapid, with nearly complete oral bioavailability in dogs (88% to 95%) and

monkeys (93% to 97.5%) (21–26). In children and adults, absorption is considered to be rapid and nearly complete (90% to 95%), even though no intravenous formulation can be used as a reference standard to determine absolute bioavailability in humans (1,25,27,28). Absorption is reported to remain efficient over multiple administrations (25). In two single-dose capsule administration studies three volunteers given a single 1-g oral dose and four healthy adults given a 0.5-g oral dose, peak ethosuximide plasma concentrations were reached between 1 and 4 hours after administration (26,28,29). A separate study with five institutionalized children that compared capsules and syrup demonstrated peak plasma concentrations within 3 to 7 hours with either formulation (7,25–27,30). The syrup had a faster absorption rate than the capsules, but the two formulations were bioequivalent (6,7,25–27,30).

DISTRIBUTION

Tissue Distribution

In rats, ethosuximide distributes evenly to brain, plasma, and other tissues, except for adipose tissue (in which steady-state concentrations are approximately one third of those reached in plasma) (25). Ethosuximide crosses the placenta in rats (26,31), and in dog and rat studies readily passed through the blood-brain barrier (21,26). In dogs, the plasma to cerebrospinal fluid (CSF) ratio was 1.01 ± 0.15, with an estimated half-life of entry into the CSF at about 4 to 5 minutes (21,25,26,32). In one study in rats, the whole-brain to plasma ethosuximide concentrations ratio was near unity, whereas a second study in rats found uniform distribution in four discrete brain areas (cerebral cortex, cerebellum, midbrain, and pons medulla) (24,26). However, a third study in rats receiving a single intraperitoneal dose of 50 mg/kg found a decrease in brain to plasma concentrations over time, suggesting that ethosuximide may be actively transported out of the rat brain (25,33).

In humans, ethosuximide homogeneously distributes throughout the body (6). Saliva, tears, and CSF concentrations are similar to plasma concentrations (25,26,34–39). In three studies (involving 6, 15, and 19 patients), the respective correlations between saliva and serum concentrations were R = 0.99, R = 0.99, and R = 0.74 (37–39). A fourth study, which examined concentrations in paired parotid saliva and plasma samples from 10 patients, showed the average saliva to plasma ratio to be 1.04, which appeared constant over the measured time intervals (36). In light of these results, multiple studies have concluded that saliva can be used in lieu of plasma for therapeutic monitoring of ethosuximide (26,34,36–38,40).

Ethosuximide crosses the placenta in humans and has been detected in cord serum and amniotic fluid at concentrations of 104% and 111% of maternal serum concentrations, respectively (6,41). In two separate reports, ethosuximide was detected in either the urine or plasma of a newborn of a woman receiving long-term therapy (26,42, 43). The serum concentration in the newborn was similar to that in the mother (25,43). Ethosuximide is excreted in the breast milk of mothers receiving long-term therapy (25). In multiple studies, the average breast milk to maternal serum concentration ratio ranged from 0.8 to 0.94 (25,43–46). The ethosuximide serum concentration of breastfeeding infants of mothers given long-term therapy was 30% to 50% of their mother's serum concentration (25,45,46). The American Academy of Pediatrics, however, considers ethosuximide to be usually compatible with breast-feeding (47).

Volume of Distribution and Protein Building

The apparent volume of distribution in rats, dogs, and rhesus monkeys ranges from 0.7 to 0.8 L/kg (21,22,25,48). In humans, ethosuximide's apparent volume of distribution is 0.62 to 0.65 L/kg in adults and 0.69 L/kg in children, implying distribution through total body water (6,25,27,28,35).

Ethosuximide protein binding is 0% to 10% in humans, dogs, and rats (1,6,25,26,30,34,49).

METABOLISM AND EXCRETION

Animals

Metabolism is the main method of ethosuximide elimination in animals. In rhesus monkeys and rats, the drug and its metabolites are excreted predominantly by the kidney, with only a small proportion recovered in the feces (25,31). Unchanged ethosuximide accounts for only 12% of urinary recovery in rats (50).

In rats, biotransformation is catalyzed predominantly by hepatic cytochrome P450 (CYP)3A isoenzymes, with possible minor contributions by CYP2E, CYP2B, and CYP2C isoenzymes (9,25,48,51–53). These CYP enzymes are inducible, and autoinduction has been reported in rats (25,48). The major metabolite in rats and monkeys is 2-(1-hydroxyethyl)-2-methylsuccinimide, and the two minor metabolites are 2-ethyl-3-hydroxy-2-methyl-succinimide and 2-(2-hydroxyethyl)-2-methylsuccinimide (25,54). Ethosuximide provided complete protection against pentylenetetrazol-induced clonic seizures in mice at a dose of 125 mg/kg; in contrast, the major metabolite demonstrated "no significant anticonvulsant activity" (54).

Elimination appears to follow first-order kinetics in animals, except in dogs, in which Michaelis-Menten kinetics may apply (21,25,54). Studies of single- and multiple-dose ethosuximide administration in monkeys have demonstrated comparable elimination half-life and total body clearance (6,22,23). In animals, elimination half-lives range from 1 hour in mice to 9 to 26 hours in rats and 11 to 25 hours in dogs (21,25,54). Steady-state plasma concentrations are significantly higher in the morning than in the evening in rhesus monkeys receiving intravenous ethosuximide at a constant rate. These fluctuations may result from circadian changes in ethosuximide metabolizing enzymes (25,54,55).

Humans

As in animals, metabolism is the main method of ethosuximide elimination in humans. Ethosuximide undergoes extensive hepatic oxidative biotransformation (80% to 90%) to pharmacologically inactive metabolites. Although most of the remaining drug is excreted unchanged in the urine, small amounts of unchanged ethosuximide can be recovered from bile and feces (56). Ethosuximide oxidation is catalyzed mainly by enzymes of the CYP3A subfamily (6). *In vitro* studies with humanized heterologous CYP microsomal systems showed that ethosuximide is primarily oxidized by CYP3A4, with CYP2E1 playing a minor role in its metabolism (57).

The major metabolite recovered from human urine in patients receiving ethosuximide is 2-(1-hydroxyethyl)-2-methylsuccinimide, of which at least 40% is excreted as a glucuronide conjugate (9,57). Two other metabolites recovered (often as a glucuronide conjugate) from human urine, are 2-ethyl-3-hydroxy-2-methylsuccinimide and 2-(2-hydroxyethyl)-2-methylsuccinimide. The latter metabolite can undergo subsequent metabolism by the hepatic mixed-function oxidase system to form the fourth major metabolite, 2-carboxymethyl-2-methylsuccinimide (9,54, 57) (Fig. 57.1).

In humans, ethosuximide's elimination follows first-order kinetics. Total-body clearance in adults averages 0.01 L/kg per hour (28) and in two children was 0.016 and 0.013 L/kg per hour (27). This is significantly lower than hepatic plasma flow (0.9 L/kg per hour) implying that ethosuximide does not undergo a significant first-pass effect, and that drug clearance is not blood flow limited (25,26). Total-body clearance has been reported to decrease slightly after repeated dosing (25). Ethosuximide does not induce hepatic microsomal CYP enzymes or the uridine diphosphate glucuronosyltransferase (UDPGT) system (49,58,59). In humans, in contrast to rats, autoinduction does not occur (59,60).

In general, ethosuximide has a long elimination half-life that varies with age. Its mean half-life in adults reportedly ranges from 40 to 60 hours, compared with 30 to 40 hours in children (27–29,35,54,60–63). Large variations have been observed in pediatric studies, with half-lives ranging from 15 to 68 hours (27,54,61). In neonates, half-lives ranging from 32 to 41 hours have been reported (43,45). The time to reach steady-state concentration after a dosage change is 6 to 7 days for children and 12 days for adults (6,64). Ethosuximide clearance is reported to be lower in women than men (65). Dose size and repeated dosing do not affect the elimination half-life (35,61).

The effects of liver and renal disease on ethosuximide elimination have not been formally studied (25). It would seem that liver disease would impair ethosuximide elimination because of the drug's substantial hepatic oxidative metabolism, whereas renal disease would have much less impact on ethosuximide elimination (25). Hemodialysis can readily remove ethosuximide. One report estimated that approximately 50% of the body's ethosuximide was removed over a 6-hour dialysis interval and that the drug's half-life dropped to 3 to 4 hours during dialysis (25,66). In a separate case report, peritoneal dialysis decreased ethosuximide concentrations in a child taking ethosuximide and phenobarbital (67).

DRUG INTERACTIONS

Interactions with Other Antiepileptic Drugs

Ethosuximide's lack of effect on either the hepatic microsomal CYP enzymes or the UDPGT system, along with negligible protein binding, indicates a low potential for drug inter-

actions (49,64). Most investigators conclude that ethosuximide therapy does not have a clinically significant effect on the pharmacokinetics of phenytoin, phenobarbital, or carbamazepine, despite scattered reports of some changes in phenytoin or phenobarbital concentrations when ethosuximide is used in combination with phenytoin or primidone (6,68–75). There is no alteration in the plasma protein binding of carbamazepine or phenytoin when ethosuximide is used concomitantly, nor is there a change in the formation of phenobarbital from primidone (76). One study reported a significant decrease in valproic acid serum concentration after the addition of ethosuximide (120.0 ± 20.1 μg/mL before ethosuximide versus 87.0 ± 13.1 μg/mL during cotherapy with ethosuximide; $p < 0.01$). After cessation of ethosuximide, valproic acid levels rose 36.7%. The mechanism underlying this observed effect is unknown (77).

In contrast, because of ethosuximide's extensive hepatic oxidative metabolism by CYP isoenzymes, concomitant therapy with enzyme-inducing antiepileptic drugs (AEDs) would be predicted to increase ethosuximide's total clearance (75). Ethosuximide's clearance is significantly accelerated (leading to a drop in the serum concentration) when the drug is used concurrently with phenobarbital, phenytoin, or carbamazepine (49,75,78–81). In one study, discontinuation of concomitant carbamazepine therapy increased ethosuximide plasma concentrations by 48% (82). The magnitude of this effect may vary considerably among patients (78).

The effect of concomitant therapy with valproic acid on the pharmacokinetics of ethosuximide is variable, with studies showing increases, decreases, or no change in ethosuximide clearance (49,60,63,72,79,83–85). Some investigators postulate that valproic acid may inhibit the metabolism of ethosuximide leading to an increase in the plasma ethosuximide concentration (86).

Whenever an AED-ethosuximide interaction could occur, serum concentration and clinical response of both AEDs should be monitored. No formal pharmacokinetic interaction studies have examined potential ethosuximide interactions with felbamate, gabapentin, lamotrigine, tiagabine, topiramate, oxcarbazepine, levetiracetam, or zonisamide.

Interactions with Nonantiepileptic Drugs

The clearance of ethosuximide is substantially increased when it is used in combination with rifampin, an inducer of CYP3A isoenzymes (80). In contrast, concomitant use with isoniazid, a potent inhibitor of CYP isoenzymes, resulted in increased ethosuximide serum concentrations and psychotic behaviors (87).

EFFICACY

Animal Models

Ethosuximide exhibits very different efficacy profiles in the two major traditional animal models of epilepsy, the maximal electroshock test (MES) and the pentylenetetrazole seizure test. The MES is used to identify agents able to prevent the spread of seizures, and has been hypothesized to identify agents effective against partial-onset and generalized tonic-clonic seizures (5,88). Ethosuximide was ineffective against MES-induced tonic seizures, except at anesthetic doses (5,88–90), but ethosuximide blocked clonic seizures produced by subcutaneously administered pentylenetetrazol or bicuculline (5,88,90,91). These chemically induced seizure models are hypothesized to identify agents that raise the seizure threshold and may be effective against absence seizures. Ethosuximide's activity profile suggests that the drug exerts its anticonvulsant effects by raising the seizure threshold rather than by blocking the spread of seizures, and it predicts efficacy against absence rather than partial-onset or generalized tonic-clonic seizures.

Ethosuximide demonstrated activity against spontaneously occurring absence seizures in three other animal models (mutant tottering mice, Wistar rats, and spontaneously epileptic rats) (92–94), as well as activity against spike-wave seizures induced by systemic administration of γ-hydroxybutyrate (88,95–97).

Humans

Ethosuximide is an effective first-line monotherapy against typical absence seizures. Although no double-blind controlled monotherapy trials have rigorously proved this efficacy, two studies conducted in the 1970s strongly suggest it (98,99). Efficacy against typical partial seizures was examined in a study with a well-constructed method for patient selection and assessment. Each patient's absence seizures were required to meet a predetermined clinical definition and be witnessed by the principal investigator. Seizure frequency was then assessed by five separate measures: the ward's staff observation; trained observer's observation; mother's observation; physician's observation (including during patient hyperventilation); and standardized video-electroencephalographic (video-EEG) recording. These measures were combined into a "seizure index" (98). Thirty-seven patients were enrolled. By the eighth week of treatment, 19% (7 of 37 patients) were seizure free, with a 100% reduction in seizure index. Overall, during ethosuximide therapy, 49% (18 of 37) of patients demonstrated at least a 90% reduction in seizures, and 95% (35 of 37) had a 50% or more reduction. The full antiabsence effect occurred within a week for any given ethosuximide dose. Plasma ethosuximide concentrations ranged from 16.6 to 104.0 µg/mL (doses of 6.5 to 36.7 mg/kg) and, on the basis of the seizure index, the investigators suggest that the optimal ethosuximide plasma concentrations in this study were 40 to 100 µg/mL (98).

The second major study was a prospective, longitudinal, open-label investigation that used therapeutic drug monitoring to maximize clinical response (99). Seventy patients were enrolled; 54% (38 of 70) were female, with ages ranging from 4 to 28 years (median, 12 years). Thirty-eight patients (54%) had only absence seizures. The remaining patients had either absence seizures with tonic-clonic seizures (30%) or absence seizures, and one or more other generalized seizure type (16%). Approximately 50% of the patients were taking other AEDs in addition to ethosuximide. Patients received between 9.4 and 73.5 mg/kg per day of ethosuximide and were evaluated at 6-month intervals. Introduction of ethosuximide therapy completely controlled seizures in 47% (33 of 70) of the patients. None of these patients had plasma ethosuximide concentrations below 30 µg/mL; only 9% were below 40 µg/mL (99).

During the next 2.5 years, attempts were made to achieve plasma ethosuximide concentrations above 40 µg/mL in the remaining 53% (37 of 70) of patients with uncontrolled absence seizures. Improved compliance and higher dosages led to significantly higher ethosuximide plasma concentrations in 19 patients, 10 of whom became seizure free. At the 2.5-year follow-up, 61% (43 of 70) of the group was seizure free. In these patients, ethosuximide's effectiveness persisted over the next 2.5 years of follow up (total, 5 years). In contrast, ethosuximide was not able to control absence seizures in patients with both absence seizures and tonic-clonic seizures who were receiving combination AED therapy (99).

Three randomized, controlled, prospective trials have compared ethosuximide and valproic acid as monotherapy for absence seizures (100–102), and a recent Cochrane review reexamined the results (103). A parallel, open study enrolled 28 drug-naïve patients, between 4 and 15 years of age, who had typical absence seizures, and followed them up for a mean of 3 years (range, 18 months to 4 years) (100). The relative risk (RR) estimate with 95% confidence interval (CI) for seizure freedom (RR <1 favors ethosuximide) was 0.70 (95% CI, 0.32 to 1.51); the RR estimate for 50% or more reduction in seizure frequency was 1.02 (95% CI, 0.70 to 1.48). The outcomes were confirmed by 6-hour telemetry and clinical observation. Although no difference was apparent for either outcome, the confidence intervals were wide; the possibility of important differences could not be excluded, and equivalence of ethosuximide and valproic acid could not be inferred (100,103).

Another trial of similar design enrolled 20 patients between 5 and 8 years of age whose simple absence seizures had begun less than 6 months before (101). Follow up lasted for 1 to 2 years and outcomes were confirmed by clinical observation and electroencephalography. Again, wide confidence intervals and the possibility of important differences precluded confirmation of equivalence of ethosuximide and valproic acid. All patients achieved at least a 50% reduction in seizure frequency (101,103).

A double-blind, crossover study used a complex response-conditional design and recruited 45 patients between 4 and 18 years of age (102). The enrollment included both treatment-naïve patients and those with drug-resistant disease. Some had only absence seizures; others had other seizure types as well. In the first phase of this trial, patients were assigned to receive either ethosuximide with placebo valproic acid or valproic acid with placebo ethosuximide for 6 weeks. Responders continued with the randomized drug for a further 6 weeks. This group included treatment-naïve patients who became seizure free, and previously treated patients who had an 80% or more reduction in seizure frequency. Nonresponders and those with adverse effects were crossed over to the alternative treatment and followed up for another 6 weeks. No differences emerged between therapies, but the confidence intervals were wide and equivalence could not be inferred. The reduction in seizure frequency, determined by a 12-hour video-EEG telemetry, was 100% for the drug-naïve group and 80% for the drug-resistant group (102,103).

No studies have compared initial monotherapy with ethosuximide against either placebo or lamotrigine monotherapy. Controlled trials of ethosuximide's long-term efficacy or effectiveness are also lacking.

Combination therapy with ethosuximide and valproic acid for absence seizures resistant to either drug alone was reported in one open-label study of five patients (104), and many investigators subsequently recommended this combination for patients with absence seizures resistant to monotherapy (7,30,64,105). Similarly, ethosuximide in patients with both absence and tonic-clonic seizures should be combined with another AED effective against tonic-clonic seizures, such as valproic acid, carbamazepine, or phenytoin (7,64,105). Despite being reported as "highly effective" against atypical absence seizures (64,105), ethosuximide is almost always used as part of combination therapy for patients with atypical absence seizures because of the high incidence of coexisting seizure types (7).

Ethosuximide is useful in the prevention and treatment of absence status epilepticus at serum concentrations greater than 120 µg/mL (106,107), and there are reports of effectiveness in severe myoclonic epilepsy in infancy (108), childhood epileptic encephalopathy (Lennox-Gastaut syndrome) (4,109), juvenile myoclonic epilepsy (110,111), epilepsy with myoclonic absences (111), eyelid myoclonia with absences (111), epilepsy with continuous spike-and-wave during slow-wave sleep (112), photosensitive seizures (113), and gelastic seizures (30,114). No controlled studies have investigated ethosuximide's effectiveness against simple partial, complex partial, or partial secondarily generalized tonic-clonic seizures. Later reports, however, suggest that ethosuximide is effective in the treatment of epileptic negative myoclonus associated with childhood partial epilepsy (115).

ADVERSE EFFECTS

Effects That Depend on Concentration

The incidence of adverse effects due to ethosuximide in initial published reports in 1952, 1958, and 1961 was very low, ranging from 1% to 9%; subsequent studies have indicated an incidence ranging from 31% to 44% (98,116–122). Most adverse effects depend on concentration and are related to the primary and secondary pharmacologic effects of the drug. These reactions are usually predictable, dose dependent, and host independent; they resolve with dose reduction (123,124).

The most common ethosuximide concentration-dependent adverse effects involve the gastrointestinal system and include nausea (the most common), abdominal discomfort, anorexia, vomiting, and diarrhea (1,7,30,116,117,125). Between 20% and 33% of children experience these symptoms, usually at the onset of therapy (30,125). Symptoms are considered mild and respond promptly to dose reduction (30,116,117,125). Techniques to reduce the symptoms include dividing the total daily dose and administering the smaller doses at mealtime (6).

Central nervous system (CNS)-related adverse events, (e.g., drowsiness) are the second most common form of ethosuximide concentration-dependent adverse events. Drowsiness usually occurs at the onset of therapy and responds promptly to dose reduction (6,116,117,125). Other CNS-related adverse events include insomnia, nervousness (12% of children), dizziness, hiccups, lethargy, fatigue, ataxia, and behavior changes (e.g., aggression, euphoria, irritability, hyperactivity) (7,125). A direct relationship between ethosuximide therapy and these reported behavioral changes is not certain, because poor methodology (e.g., lack of reliable methods for objectively measuring behavior changes, confounding variable of polypharmacy, and lack of serum AED measurements) makes analysis of existing reports difficult at best (116,117).

Few trials have examined the potential cognitive effects of ethosuximide in a controlled fashion, accounting for confounding variables such as plasma concentrations, underlying mental retardation, concomitant AEDs, or seizure type. In one early report, psychometric testing of 25 children receiving ethosuximide for various seizure types revealed memory, speech, and emotional disturbances (126). However, no plasma concentrations were measured; all the patients were also taking barbiturates; 60% of the cohort had intelligence quotient (IQ) scores below 83; and no matched control group was used (126). In a cohort of children without epilepsy but with learning disorders, and 14- and 6-Hz positive spikes on EEG recording, administration of ethosuximide significantly improved verbal and full-scale IQ scores, without changing motor performance or personality test scores (127).

In a well-designed study, psychometric performance improved significantly over 8 weeks of ethosuximide therapy in 17 (46%) of 37 children with absence seizures (98). This improvement was significantly greater than that of a control group tested in the same fashion over the same interval (98). Only 25% of the study group had IQ scores below 83, and only 32% were receiving other AEDs (98).

Dreifuss (116,117) reported a probable dose-dependent ethosuximide-related granulocytopenia that often resolves with dose reduction without the need to terminate therapy.

Distinction between this probable adverse event and ethosuximide-associated idiosyncratic bone marrow depression (see below, Idiosyncratic Reactions) is critical. Careful clinical and laboratory monitoring is essential in making this decision.

Effects That Do Not Depend on Concentration

Some ethosuximide adverse effects do not appear to be concentration-dependent, but are also not idiosyncratic reactions in the usual sense. Headaches, reported in 14% of children, may not respond to dose reduction and may persist (6,116,117,125,128).

Episodes of psychotic behavior (i.e., anxiety, depression, visual hallucinations, auditory hallucinations, and intermittent impairment of consciousness) have been noted with ethosuximide (116,129–132) and are most likely in young adults with a history of mental disorders (6,116). The acute psychotic episodes appeared after ethosuximide-induced seizure control with associated EEG improvement, and they resolved when ethosuximide was stopped and seizures returned, illustrating the phenomenon of *forced normalization* (6,116). Psychotic symptoms have recurred when ethosuximide was restarted in patients with previous ethosuximide-related psychotic episodes (116). This forced normalization reaction is not dose dependent and, among all antiabsence AEDs, occurs with highest frequency with ethosuximide (6,133).

Most studies find no evidence of ethosuximide-associated seizure exacerbation (98,116,120,134,135); however, scattered reports describe exacerbation of myoclonic and absence seizures and transformation of absence into "grand mal" seizures in patients receiving ethosuximide (116,118, 136). Dreifuss considered this exacerbation effect to be a consequence of the high incidence of generalized tonic-clonic seizures in patients with absences seizures, coupled with ethosuximide's lack of efficacy against generalized tonic-clonic seizures (116).

Idiosyncratic Reactions

Idiosyncratic drug reactions are unpredictable, dose-independent, host-dependent reactions that are not associated with the known pharmacologic effects of the drug; they can be serious and life-threatening. Preclinical animal toxicologic testing may not detect these reactions, and often they cannot be reproduced in animal models (123,124). In general, the skin is the most commonly affected site, followed by the formed elements of the blood and liver and, to a lesser extent, the nervous system and kidneys (123, 137). These reactions may be organ specific or may manifest with generalized nonspecific symptoms, such as lymphadenopathy, arthralgias, eosinophilia, and fever (123, 138). Idiosyncratic reactions are believed to result from toxic metabolites that cause injury directly or indirectly (i.e., through an immunologic response or free radical-mediated process) (139).

Ethosuximide has been associated to various degrees with a wide array of idiosyncratic reactions (116,117,125, 140), including allergic dermatitis, rash, erythema multiforme, Stevens-Johnson syndrome (141), systemic lupus erythematosus (142–144), lupus-scleroderma syndrome (145), a lupus-like syndrome (146), blood dyscrasias (aplastic anemia, agranulocytosis) (98,122,134,147–154), dyskinesia (155,156), akathisia (155), autoimmune thyroiditis (157), and diminished renal allograft survival (158).

Mild cutaneous reactions, including allergic dermatitis and rash, are the most common ethosuximide-associated idiosyncratic reactions. They frequently resolve with withdrawal of the drug, but some patients may require steroid therapy. Patients who develop Stevens-Johnson syndrome, a potentially life-threatening condition, require more aggressive in-hospital therapy.

The symptoms of the lupus-like syndrome are described as fever, malar rash, arthritis, lymphadenopathy, and, on occasion, pleural effusions, myocarditis, and pericarditis (116). After discontinuation of ethosuximide, these patients usually fully recover, but the recovery may be prolonged (116).

The manifestations of ethosuximide-associated blood dyscrasias range from thrombocytopenia to pancytopenia and aplastic anemia (98,122,134,147–152). Between 1958 and 1994, only eight cases of ethosuximide-associated aplastic anemia were reported, with onsets of 6 weeks to 8 months after initiation of therapy (151). Six patients were receiving polypharmacy; five were taking phenytoin or ethotoin in combination with ethosuximide (151). Despite therapy, five of the eight patients died (98,122, 134,147–152).

Long-Term Effects

Adverse effects resulting from long-term therapy are related to the cumulative dose (123,124). Severe bradykinesia and parkinsonian syndrome have been reported after several years of ethosuximide treatment (121,159).

Delayed Effects

In mice, ethosuximide exhibits considerably less teratogenic effect than carbamazepine, phenytoin, phenobarbital, or primidone (160). In humans, because ethosuximide is predominantly indicated for absence seizures, which frequently remit before childbearing years, little is known about the risks that maternal use poses to the fetus (116). Not enough data are available to accurately assess the teratogenic effect of ethosuximide in humans.

CLINICAL USE

Indications

Ethosuximide, like valproic acid, is regarded as effective first-line monotherapy against typical absence seizures.

Ethosuximide may be the first choice in children younger than 10 years old with absence epilepsy, but as adolescence approaches and the risk of generalized tonic-clonic seizures increases, valproic acid clearly becomes the drug of choice (161). Ethosuximide as adjunctive therapy may be beneficial for patients whose absence seizures are not controlled by valproic acid monotherapy, patients with both absence and tonic-clonic seizures, and patients with atypical absence seizures (7,30,64,105,161). No evidence supports a role for ethosuximide as monotherapy or adjunctive therapy in patients with only simple partial, complex partial, or partial secondarily generalized tonic-clonic seizures.

Starting and Stopping

A common starting dosage for children is 10 to 15 mg/kg per day with subsequent titration to clinical response (6,7). Maintenance dosages frequently range from 15 to 40 mg/kg per day (64). In older children and adults, therapy can begin at 250 mg per day and increase by 250-mg increments until the desired clinical response is reached. The interval between dosage changes for older children and adults varies from 3 days (7) to every 12 to 15 days (6). Common maintenance doses for older children and adults are 750 to 1500 mg per day (6,7). In elderly patients, titration should involve smaller increments with longer intervals between changes (7). After a dosage change, steady-state concentration is reached in 6 to 7 days in children and 12 days in adults (6,64). Ethosuximide can be administered once, twice, or even thrice daily (with meals) for maximum seizure control with minimum adverse effects (6,7).

If intolerable side effects without seizure control or 2 or more years' freedom from absence seizures occur, discontinuation may be warranted, with gradual reduction over 4 to 8 weeks (6,7). If necessary, abrupt discontinuation is probably safe because of ethosuximide's long half-life (7).

Monitoring

Ethosuximide should always be titrated to maximal seizure control with minimal side effects. The generally accepted therapeutic range is 40 to 100 μg/mL (6,7); some patients with refractory seizures or absence status may need serum concentrations up to 150 μg/mL (7). Monitoring ethosuximide's serum concentration may help identify noncompliance and aid in maximizing seizure control (99).

There is no evidence that monitoring of blood count values during therapy anticipates the drug's idiosyncratic hematologic reactions. Patients must alert their physicians immediately if fever, sore throat, and cutaneous or other hemorrhages occur (116). However, one recommendation for monitoring is that "periodic blood counts be performed at no greater than monthly intervals for the duration of treatment with ethosuximide, and that the dosage be reduced or the drug discontinued should the total white-blood-cell count fall below 3500 or the proportion of granulocytes below 25% of the total white-blood-cell count" (116).

REFERENCES

1. Brodie M, Dichter M. Established antiepileptic drugs. *Seizure* 1997;6:159–174.
2. Lennox W. The petit mal epilepsies: their treatment with tridione. *JAMA* 1945;129:1069–1074.
3. Lennox W. Tridione in the treatment of epilepsy. *JAMA* 1947; 134:138–143.
4. Mattson RH. Efficacy and adverse effects of established and new antiepileptic drugs. *Epilepsia* 1995;36:S13–S26.
5. Rogawski M, Porter R. Antiepileptic drugs: pharmacological mechanisms and clinical efficacy with consideration of promising developmental state compounds. *Pharmacol Rev* 1990;42: 223–286.
6. Sabers A, Dam M. Ethosuximide and methsuximide. In: Shorvon S, Dreifuss F, Fish D, et al., eds. *The treatment of epilepsy*. London: Blackwell Science, 1996:414–420.
7. Bromfield E. Ethosuximide and other succinimides. In: Engel J, Pedley T, eds. *Epilepsy: a comprehensive textbook*. Philadelphia: Lippincott-Raven, 1997:1503–1508.
8. Millership JS, Mifsud J, Collier PS. The metabolism of ethosuximide. *Eur J Drug Metab Pharmacokinet* 1993;18:349–353.
9. Pisani F, Meir B. Ethosuximide: chemistry and biotransformation. In: Levy R, Mattson R, Meldrum B, eds. *Antiepileptic drugs*, 4th ed. New York: Raven Press, 1995:655–658.
10. White HS. Comparative anticonvulsant and mechanistic profile of the established and newer antiepileptic drugs. *Epilepsia* 1999; 40:S2–S10.
11. Macdonald RL, Kelly KM. Antiepileptic drug mechanisms of action. *Epilepsia* 1993;34:S1–S8.
12. Davies JA. Mechanisms of action of antiepileptic drugs. *Seizure* 1995;4:267–271.
13. Coulter C, Huguenard J, Price D. Characterization of ethosuximide reduction of low-threshold calcium current in thalamic neurons. *Ann Neurol* 1989;25:582–593.
14. Ferrendelli J, Holland K. Ethosuximide, mechanisms of action. In: Levy R, Mattson R, Meldrum B, et al., eds. *Antiepileptic drugs*, 3rd ed. New York: Raven Press, 1989:653–661.
15. Lin-Mitchell E, Chweh A. Effects of ethosuximide alone and in combination with gamma-aminobutyric acid receptor antagonists on brain gamma-aminobutyric acid concentration, anticonvulsant activity, and neurotoxicity in mice. *J Pharmacol Exp Ther* 1986;237:486–489.
16. Gilbert J, Buchan P, Scott A. Effects of anticonvulsant drug on monosaccharide transport and membrane ATPase activities of cerebral cortex. In: Harris P, Mawdsley C, eds. *Epilepsy*. Edinburgh: Churchill Livingstone, 1974:98–104.
17. Gilbert J, Scott A, Wyllie M. Effects of ethosuximide on adenosine triphosphate activities of some subcellular fractions prepared from rat cerebral cortex. *Br J Pharmacol* 1974;50:452P–453P.
18. Gilbert J, Wyllie M. The effects of the anticonvulsant ethosuximide on adenosine triphosphatase activities of synaptosomes prepared from rat cerebral cortex. *Br J Pharmacol* 1974;52:139P–140P.
19. Villen T, Bertilsson L, Sjoqvist F. Nonstereoselective disposition of ethosuximide in humans. *Ther Drug Monit* 1990;12:514–516.
20. Tomson T, Villen T. Ethosuximide enantiomers in pregnancy and lactation. *Ther Drug Monit* 1994;16:621–623.
21. El-Sayed M, Loscher W, Frey H. Pharmacokinetics of ethosuximide in the dog. *Arch Int Pharmacodyn Ther* 1978;234:180–192.
22. Patel I, Levy R, Bauer T. Pharmacokinetic properties of ethosuximide in monkeys. Single dose intravenous and oral administration. *Epilepsia* 1975;16:705–716.
23. Patel I, Levy R. Pharmacokinetic properties of ethosuximide in monkeys, II: chronic intravenous and oral administration. *Epilepsia* 1975;16:717–730.
24. Patel I, Levy R, Rapport R. Distribution characteristics of ethosuximide in discrete areas of rat brain. *Epilepsia* 1977;18:533–541.
25. Bialer M, Ziadong S, Perucca E. Ethosuximide: absorption, distribution, excretion. In: Levy R, Mattson R, Meldrum B, eds. *Antiepileptic drugs*, 4th ed. New York: Raven Press, 1995:659–665.

26. Chang T. Ethosuximide. Absorption, distribution, and excretion. In: Levy R, Mattson R, Meldrum B, et al., eds. *Antiepileptic drugs*, 3rd ed. New York: Raven Press, 1989:671–678.

27. Buchanan R, Fernandez L, Kinkel A. Absorption and elimination of ethosuximide in children. *J Clin Pharmacol* 1969;7:213–218.

28. Eadie M, Tyrer J, Smith J, McKauge L. Pharmacokinetics of drugs used for petit mal absence epilepsy. *Clin Exp Neurol* 1977;14:172–183.

29. Alvarez N, Besag F, Iivanainen M. Use of antiepileptic drugs in the treatment of epilepsy in people with intellectual disability. *J Intellect Disabil Res* 1998;42:1–15.

30. Wallace SJ. Use of ethosuximide and valproate in the treatment of epilepsy. *Neurol Clin* 1986;4:601–616.

31. Chang T, Dill W, Glazko A. Ethosuximide. Absorption, distribution and excretion. In: Woodbury D, Penry J, Schmidt R, eds. *Antiepileptic drugs*. New York: Raven Press, 1972:417–423.

32. Loscher W, Frey H. Kinetics of penetration of common anticonvulsant drugs in serum of dog and man. *Epilepsia* 1984;25: 346–352.

33. Aguilar-Veiga E, Sierra-Paredes G, Galan-Valiente J, et al. Correlations between ethosuximide brain levels measured by high performance liquid chromatography and its antiepileptic potential. *Res Comm Chem Pathol Pharmacol* 1991;7:351–364.

34. Liu H, Delgado MR. Therapeutic drug concentration monitoring using saliva samples. Focus on anticonvulsants. *Clin Pharmacokinet* 1999;36:453–470.

35. Buchanan R, Kinkel A, Smith T. The absorption and excretion of ethosuximide. *Int J Clin Pharmacol* 1973;7:213–218.

36. Horning M, Brown L, Nowlin J, et al. Use of saliva in therapeutic drug monitoring. *Clin Chem* 1977;23:157–164.

37. Piredda S, Monaco F. Ethosuximide in tears, saliva and cerebral fluid. *Ther Drug Monit* 1981;3:321–323.

38. McAuliffe J, Sherwin A, Leppik I, et al. Salivary levels of anticonvulsants: a practical approach to drug monitoring. *Neurology* 1977;27:409–413.

39. Van H. Comparative study of the levels of anticonvulsants and their free fraction in venous blood, saliva and capillary blood in man. *J Pharmacol* 1984;15:27–35.

40. Bachmann K, Schwartz J, Sullivan T, et al. Single sample estimate of ethosuximide clearance. *Int J Clin Pharmacol Ther Toxicol* 1986;24:546–550.

41. Meyer F, Quednow B, Potrafki A, et al. Pharmacokinetics of anticonvulsants in the perinatal period. *Zentralbe Gynakol* 1988;110: 1195–1205.

42. Horning M, Stratton C, Nowlin J, et al. Metabolism of 2-ethyl-2-methylsuccinimide in the rat and human. *Drug Metab Dispos* 1973;1:569–576.

43. Koup J, Rose J, Cohen M. Ethosuximide pharmacokinetics in a pregnant patient and her newborn. *Epilepsia* 1978;19:535–539.

44. Kaneko S, Sato T, Suzuki K. The levels of anticonvulsants in breast milk. *Br J Clin Pharmacol* 1979;7:624–627.

45. Kuhnz W, Koch S, Hartmann A, et al. Ethosuximide in epileptic women during pregnancy and lactation period. Placental transfer, serum concentrations in nursed infants and clinical status. *Br J Clin Pharmacol* 1984;18:671–677.

46. Hancock E, Osborne J, Milner P. Treatment of infantile spasms. *Cochrane Database Syst Rev* 2003:CD001770.

47. American Academy of Pediatrics Committee on Drugs. Transfer of drugs and other chemicals into human milk. *Pediatrics* 2001; 108:776–789.

48. Bachmann K, Jahn D, Yang C, et al. Ethosuximide disposition kinetics in rats. *Xenobiotica* 1988;18:373–380.

49. Tanaka E. Clinically significant pharmacokinetic drug interactions between antiepileptic drugs. *J Clin Pharmacol Ther* 1999;24: 87–92.

50. Burkett A, Chang T, Glazko A. A hydroxylated metabolite of ethosuximide (Zarontin) in rat urine. *Fed Proc* 1971;30:391.

51. Bachmann K. The use of single sample clearance estimates to probe hepatic drug metabolism in rats, IV: a model for possible application to phenotyping xenobiotic influences on human drug metabolism. *Xenobiotica* 1989;19:1449–1459.

52. Bachmann K, Madhira M, Rankin G. The effects of cobalt chloride, SKF-525A and N-(3,5-dichlorophenyl) succinimide on in vivo hepatic mixed function oxidase activity as determined by single-sample plasma clearances. *Xenobiotica* 1992;22:27–31.

53. Bachmann K, Chu C, Greear V. In vivo evidence that ethosuximide is a substrate for cytochrome P450IIIA. *Pharmacology* 1992;45: 121–128.

54. Chang T. Ethosuximide. Biotransformation. In: Levy R, Mattson R, Meldrum B, et al., eds. *Antiepileptic drugs*, 3rd ed. New York: Raven Press, 1989:679–683.

55. Patel I, Levy R, Bauer T. Time dependent kinetics, II: diurnal oscillations in steady state plasma ethosuximide levels in rhesus monkeys. *J Pharm Sci* 1977;66:650–653.

56. Eadie MJ. Formation of active metabolites of anticonvulsant drugs. A review of their pharmacokinetic and therapeutic significance. *Biomed Chromatogr* 1991;5:212–215.

57. Bachmann K, He Y, Sarver JG, et al. Characterization of the cytochrome P450 enzymes involved in the in vitro metabolism of ethosuximide by human hepatic microsomal enzymes. *Xenobiotica* 2003;33:265–276.

58. Gilbert J, Scott A, Galloway D, et al. Ethosuximide: liver enzyme induction and D-glucaric acid excretion. *Br J Clin Pharmacol* 1974;1:249–252.

59. Glazko A. Antiepileptic drugs: biotransformation, metabolism, and serum half-life. *Epilepsia* 1975;16:376–391.

60. Bauer L, Harris C, Wilensky A, et al. Ethosuximide kinetics: possible interaction with valproic acid. *Clin Pharmacol Ther* 1982;31: 741–745.

61. Buchanan R, Kinkel A, Turner J, et al. Ethosuximide dosage regimens. *Clin Pharmacol Ther* 1976;19:143–147.

62. Dill W, Peterson L, Chang T, et al. Physiologic disposition of alpha-methyl-alpha-ethyl succinimide (ethosuximide; Zarontin) in animals and in man. Presented at the 149th National Meeting of the American Chemical Society; Detroit, Michigan; 1965.

63. Pisani P, Narbone M, Trunfio C. Valproic acid-ethosuximide interaction: a pharmacokinetic study. *Epilepsia* 1984;25:229–233.

64. Sherwin A. Ethosuximide: clinical use. In: Levy R, Mattson R, Meldrum B, eds. *Antiepileptic drugs*, 4th ed. New York: Raven Press, 1995:667–673.

65. Bachmann KA, Schwartz J, Jauregui L, et al. Use of three probes to assess the influence of sex on hepatic drug metabolism. *Pharmacology* 1987;35:88–93.

66. Marbury T, Lee C, Perchalski R. Hemodialysis clearance of ethosuximide in patients with chronic renal failure. *Am J Hosp Pharm* 1981;38:1757–1760.

67. Marquardt E, Ishisaka D, Batra K, et al. Removal of ethosuximide and phenobarbital by peritoneal dialysis in a child. *Clin Pharm* 1992;11:1030–1031.

68. Browne T, Feldman R, Buchanan R. Methsuximide for complex seizures: efficacy, toxicity, clinical pharmacology, and drug interactions. *Neurology* 1983;33:414–418.

69. Dawson G, Brown H, Clark B. Serum phenytoin after ethosuximide. *Ann Neurol* 1978;4:583–584.

70. Frantzen E, Hansen J, Hansen O, et al. Phenytoin (Dilantin) intoxication. *Acta Neurol Scand* 1967;43:440–446.

71. Rambeck B. Pharmacological interactions of methsuximide with phenobarbital and phenytoin in hospitalized epileptic patients. *Epilepsia* 1979;20:147–156.

72. Smith G, McKauge L, Dubetz D, et al. Factors influencing plasma concentrations of ethosuximide. *Clin Pharmacokinet* 1979;4:38–52.

73. Schmidt D. The effect of phenytoin and ethosuximide on primidone metabolism in patients with epilepsy. *J Neurol* 1975;209: 115–123.

74. Battino D, Avanzini G, Bossi L. Plasma levels of primidone and its metabolite phenobarbital: effect of age and associated therapy. *Ther Drug Monit* 1983;5:73–79.

75. Riva R, Albani F, Contin M, et al. Pharmacokinetic interactions between antiepileptic drugs. Clinical considerations. *Clin Pharmacokinet* 1996;31:470–493.

76. Eadie M, Tyrer J. In: Eadie M, Tyrer J, eds. *Anticonvulsant therapy. Pharmacological basis and practice*, 2nd ed. Edinburgh: Churchill Livingstone, 1980:211–223.

77. Salke-Kellermann R, May T, Boenigk H. Influence of ethosuximide on valproic acid serum concentrations. *Epilepsy Res* 1997; 26:345–349.

78. Warren JJ, Benmaman J, Wannamaker B, et al. Kinetics of a carbamazepine-ethosuximide interaction. *Clin Pharmacol* 1980;28: 646–651.

79. Battino D, Cusi C, Franceschetti S, et al. Ethosuximide plasma concentrations: influence of age and associated concomitant therapy. *Clin Pharmacokinet* 1982;7:176–180.
80. Bachmann K, Jauregui L. Use of single sample clearance estimates of cytochrome P450 substrates to characterize human hepatic CYP status in vivo. *Xenobiotica* 1993;23:307–315.
81. Giaconne M, Bartoli A, Gatti G, et al. Effect of enyzme inducing anticonvulsants on ethosuximide pharmacokinetics in epileptic patients. *Br J Clin Pharmacol* 1996;41:575–579.
82. Duncan JS, Patsalos PN, Shorvon SD. Effects of discontinuation of phenytoin, carbamazepine, and valproate on concomitant antiepileptic medication. *Epilepsia* 1991;32:101–115.
83. Bourgeois B. Pharmacologic interactions between valproate and other drugs. *Am J Med* 1988;84:28–33.
84. Gram L, Wulff K, Rasmussen K, et al. Valproate sodium: a controlled clinical trial including monitoring of drug levels. *Epilepsia* 1977;18:141–148.
85. Mattson R, Cramer J. Valproic acid and ethosuximide interaction. *Ann Neurol* 1980;7:583–584.
86. Levy R, Koch K. Drug interactions with valproic acid. *Drugs* 1982;24:543–556.
87. van Wieringen A, Vrijlandt C. Ethosuximide intoxication caused by interaction with isoniazid. *Neurology* 1983;33:1227–1228.
88. White HS. Clinical significance of animal seizure models and mechanism of action studies of potential antiepileptic drugs. *Epilepsia* 1997;38:S9–S17.
89. Reinhard J, Reinhard J. Experimental evaluation of anticonvulsants. In: Vida J, ed. *Anticonvulsants*. New York: Academic Press, 1977:57–111.
90. Woodbury D. Applications to drug evaluations. In: Purpura P, Penry J, Tower D, et al., eds. *Experimental models of epilepsy: a manual for the laboratory worker*. New York: Raven Press, 1972: 557–583.
91. Swinyard E, Woodhead J, White H, et al. General principles. Experimental selection, quantification and evaluation of anticonvulsants. In: Levy R, Mattson R, Meldrum B, et al., eds. *Antiepileptic drugs*, 3rd ed. New York: Raven Press, 1989:85–102.
92. Heller A, Dichter M, Sidman R. Anticonvulsant sensitivity of absence seizures in the tottering mutant mouse. *Epilepsia* 1983; 25:25–34.
93. Marescaux C, Micheletti G, Vergnes M, et al. A model of chronic spontaneous petit mal-like seizures in the rat: comparison with pentylenetetrazol-induced seizures. *Epilepsia* 1984;25:326–331.
94. Sasa M, Ohno Y, Ujihara H. Effects of antiepileptic drugs on absence-like and tonic seizures in the spontaneously epileptic rat, a double mutant rat. *Epilepsia* 1988;29:505–513.
95. Godschalk M, Dzoljic M, Bonta I. Antagonism of gamma-hydroxybutyrate-induced hypersynchronization in the ECoG of the rat by anti-petit mal drugs. *Neurosci Lett* 1976;3:145–150.
96. Snead OI. Gamma-hydroxybutyrate in the monkey, II: effect of chronic oral anticonvulsant drugs. *Neurology* 1978;28:643–648.
97. Snead OI. Gamma-hydroxybutyrate model of generalized absence seizures: further characterization and comparison with other absence models. *Epilepsia* 1988;29:361–368.
98. Browne TR, Dreifuss FE, Dyken PR, et al. Ethosuximide in the treatment of absence (petit mal) seizures. *Neurology* 1975;25: 515–524.
99. Sherwin A, Robb P, Lechter M. Improved control of epilepsy by monitoring plasma ethosuximide. *Arch Neurol* 1973;28:178–181.
100. Callaghan N, O'Hara J, O'Driscoll D, et al. Comparative study of ethosuximide and sodium valproate in the treatment of typical absence seizures (petit mal). *Dev Med Child Neurol* 1982;24: 830–836.
101. Martinovic Z. Comparison of ethosuximide with sodium valproate. In: Parsonage M, Grant R, Craig AW Jr, eds. *Advances in epileptology. XIVth Epilepsy International Symposium*. New York: Raven Press, 1983:301–305.
102. Sato S, White BG, Penry JK, et al. Valproic acid versus ethosuximide in the treatment of absence seizures. *Neurology* 1982;32:157–63.
103. Posner EB, Mohamed K, Marson AG. Ethosuximide, sodium valproate or lamotrigine for absence seizures in children and adolescents. *Cochrane Database Syst Rev* 2003:CD003032.
104. Rowan A, Meijer J, deBeer-Pawlikowski N, et al. Valproate-ethosuximide combination therapy for refractory absence seizures. *Arch Neurol* 1983;40:797–802.
105. Sherwin A. Ethosuximide: clinical use. In: Levy R, Dreifuss F, Mattson R, et al., eds. *Antiepileptic drugs*, 3rd ed. New York: Raven Press, 1989:685–698.
106. Guberman A, Cantu-Reyna G, Stuss D, et al. Nonconvulsive generalized status epilepticus: clinical features, neuropsychological testing, and long-term follow-up. *Neurology* 1986;36: 1284–1291.
107. Browne TR, Dreifuss FE, Penry JK, et al. Clinical and EEG estimates of absence seizure frequency. *Arch Neurol* 1983;40:469–472.
108. Roger J, Genton P, Bureau M, et al. Less common epileptic syndromes. In: Wyllie E, ed. *The treatment of epilepsy: principles and practice*. Philadelphia: Lea & Febiger, 1993:624–635.
109. Farrell K. Secondary generalized epilepsy and Lennox-Gastaut syndrome. In: Wyllie E, ed. *The treatment of epilepsy: principles and practice*. Philadelphia: Lea & Febiger, 1993:604–613.
110. Serratosa J, Delgado-Escueta A. Juvenile myoclonic epilepsy. In: Wyllie E, ed. *The treatment of epilepsy: principles and practice*. Philadelphia: Lea & Febiger, 1993:552–570.
111. Wallace S. Myoclonus and epilepsy in childhood: a review of treatment with valproate, ethosuximide, lamotrigine and zonisamide. *Epilepsy Res* 1998;29:147–154.
112. Yasuhara A, Yoshida H, Hatanaka T, et al. Epilepsy with continuous spike-waves during slow sleep and its treatment. *Epilepsia* 1991;32:59–62.
113. Zifkin B, Andermann F. Epilepsy with reflex seizures. In: Wyllie E, ed. *The treatment of epilepsy: principles and practice*. Philadelphia: Lea & Febiger, 1993:614–623.
114. Ames F, Enderstein O. Ictal laughter: a case report with clinical, cinefilm, and EEG observations. *J Neurol Neurosurg Psychiatry* 1975;38:11–17.
115. Capovilla G, Beccaria F, Veggoiotti P, et al. Ethosuximide is effective in the treatment of epileptic negative myoclonus in childhood partial epilepsy. *J Child Neurol* 1999;14:395–400.
116. Dreifuss F. Ethosuximide: toxicity. In: Levy R, Mattson R, Meldrum B, eds. *Antiepileptic drugs*, 4th ed. New York: Raven Press, 1995: 675–679.
117. Dreifuss F. Ethosuximide: toxicity. In: Levy R, Mattson R, Meldrum B, et al., eds. *Antiepileptic drugs*, 3rd ed. New York: Raven Press, 1989:699–705.
118. Gordon N. Treatment of epilepsy with O-ethyl-o-methylsuccinimide (P.M. 671). *Neurology* 1961;11:266–268.
119. Livingston S, Pauli L, Najimabadi A. Ethosuximide in the treatment of epilepsy. *JAMA* 1952;180:104–107.
120. Zimmerman F, Bergemeister B. A new drug for petit mal epilepsy. *Neurology* 1958;8:769–776.
121. Goldensohn E, Hardie J, Borea E. Ethosuximide in the treatment of epilepsy. *JAMA* 1962;180:840–842.
122. Weinstein A, Allen R. Ethosuximide treatment of petit mal seizures. A study of 87 pediatric patients. *Am J Dis Child* 1966; 111: 63–67.
123. Park BK, Pirmohamed M, Kitteringham NR. Idiosyncratic drug reactions: a mechanistic evaluation of risk factors. *Br J Clin Pharmacol* 1992;34:377–395.
124. Pirmohamed M, Kitteringham NR, Park BK. The role of active metabolites in drug toxicity. *Drug Saf* 1994;11:114–144.
125. Wallace SJ. A comparative review of the adverse effects of anticonvulsants in children with epilepsy. *Drug Saf* 1996;15:378–393.
126. Guey J, Charles C, Coquery C, et al. Study of psychological effects of ethosuximide (Zarontin) on 25 children suffering from petit mal epilepsy. *Epilepsia* 1967;8:129–141.
127. Smith L, Phillips M, Guard H. Psychometric study of children with learning problems and 14-6 positive spike EEG patterns, treated with ethosuximide (Zarontin) and placebo. *Arch Dis Child* 1968;43:616–619.
128. Abu-Arafeh I, Wallace S. Unwanted effects of antiepileptic drugs. *Dev Med Child Neurol* 1988;30:117–121.
129. Fischer M, Korskjaer G, Pedersen E. Psychotic episodes in Zarontin treatment. Effects and side-effects in 105 patients. *Epilepsia* 1965;6:325–334.
130. Cohadon F, Loiseau P, Cohadon S. Results of treatment of certain forms of epilepsy of the petit mal type by ethosuximide. *Rev Neurol* 1964;110:201–207.
131. Lairy C. Psychotic signs in epileptics during treatment with ethosuximide. *Rev Neurol* 1964;110:225–226.

132. Sato T, Kondo Y, Matsuo T, et al. Clinical experiences of ethosuximide (Zarontin) in therapy-resistant epileptics. *Brain Nerve (Toyko)* 1965;17:958–964.
133. Wolf P, Inoue Y. Therapeutic response of absence seizures in patients of an epilepsy clinic for adolescents and adults. *J Neurol* 1984;231:225–229.
134. Buchanan R. Ethosuximide: toxicity. In: Woodbury D, Penry J, Schmidt R, eds. *Antiepileptic drugs.* New York: Raven Press, 1972: 449–454.
135. Heathfield K, Jewesbury E. Treatment of petit mal with ethosuximide. *Br Med J* 1961;2:565.
136. Todorov A, Lenn N, Gabor A. Exacerbation of generalized non-convulsive seizures with ethosuximide therapy. *Arch Neurol* 1978;35:389–391.
137. Uetrecht JP. The role of leukocyte-generated reactive metabolites in the pathogenesis of idiosyncratic drug reactions. *Drug Metab Rev* 1992;24:299–366.
138. Gibaldi M. Adverse drug effect—reactive metabolites and idiosyncratic drug reactions: part I. *Ann Pharmacother* 1992;26:416–421.
139. Glauser TA. Idiosyncratic reactions: new methods of identifying high-risk patients. *Epilepsia* 2000;41:S16–S29.
140. Pellock JM. Standard approach to antiepileptic drug treatment in the United States. *Epilepsia* 1994;35:S11–S18.
141. Taafe A, O'Brien C. A case of Stevens-Johnson syndrome associated with the anticonvulsants sulthiame and ethosuximide. *Br Dent J* 1975;138:172–174.
142. Dabbous IA, Idriss HM. Occurrence of systemic lupus erythematosus in association with ethosuccimide therapy. Case report. *J Pediatr* 1970;76:617–620.
143. Alter BP. Systemic lupus erythematosus and ethosuccimide. *J Pediatr* 1970;77:1093–1095.
144. Livingston S, Rodriguez H, Greene CA, Pauli LL. Systemic lupus erythematosus. Occurrence in association with ethosuximide therapy. *JAMA* 1968;203:731–732.
145. Teoh PC, Chan HL. Lupus-scleroderma syndrome induced by ethosuximide. *Arch Dis Child* 1975;50:658–661.
146. Singsen B, Fishman L, Hanson V. Antinuclear antibodies and lupus-like syndromes in children receiving anticonvulsants. *Pediatrics* 1976;57:529–534.
147. Cohn R. A neuropathological study of a case of petit mal epilepsy. *Electroencephalogr Clin Neurophysiol* 1968;24:282.
148. Kiorboe E, Paludan J, Trolle E, et al. Zarontin (ethosuximide) in the treatment of petit mal and related disorders. *Epilepsia* 1964; 5:83–89.
149. Kousoulieris E. Granulopenia and thrombocytopenia after ethosuximide. *Lancet* 1967;2:310–311.
150. Spittler J. Agranulocytosis due to ethosuximide with a fatal outcome. *Klin Paediatr* 1974;186:364–366.
151. Massey GV, Dunn NL, Heckel JL, et al. Aplastic anemia following therapy for absence seizures with ethosuximide [review]. *Pediatr Neurol* 1994;11:59–61.
152. Mann L, Habenicht H. Fatal bone marrow aplasia associated with administration of ethosuximide (Zarontin) for petit mal epilepsy. *Bull Los Angeles Neurol Soc* 1962;27:173–176.
153. Seip M. Aplastic anemia during ethosuximide medication. Treatment with bolus-methylprednisolone. *Acta Paediatr Scand* 1983;72:927–929.
154. Imai T, Okada H, Nanba M, et al. Ethosuximide induced agranulocytosis. *Brain Dev* 2003;25:522–524.
155. Ehyai A, Kilroy A, Fenicheal G. Dyskinesia and akathisia induced by ethosuximide. *Am J Dis Child* 1978;132:527–528.
156. Kirschberg G. Dyskinesia—an unusual reaction to ethosuximide. *Arch Neurol* 1975;32:137–138.
157. Nishiyama J, Matsukura M, Fugimoto S, et al. Reports of 2 cases of autoimmune thyroiditis while receiving anticonvulsant therapy. *Eur J Pediatr* 1983;140:116–117.
158. Wassner S, Pennisi A, Malekzadeh M, et al. The adverse effect of anticonvulsant therapy on renal allograft survival. A preliminary report. *J Pediatr* 1976;88:134–137.
159. Porter R, Penry J, Dreifuss F. Responsiveness at the onset of spike-wave bursts. *Electroencephalogr Clin Neurophysiol* 1973;34: 239–245.
160. Sullivan F, McElhatton P. A comparison of the teratogenic activity of the antiepileptic drugs carbamazepine, clonazepam, ethosuximide, phenobarbital, phenytoin, and primidone in mice. *Toxicol Appl Pharmacol* 1977;40:365–378.
161. Bourgeois BF. Important pharmacokinetic properties of antiepileptic drugs. *Epilepsia* 1995;36:S1–S7.

Benzodiazepines

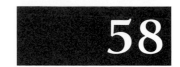

L. John Greenfield, Jr.   Howard C. Rosenberg   Richard W. Homan

Benzodiazepines were developed in 1933 from a class of heterocyclic compounds known since 1891 (1). Clinical interest initially focused on their antianxiety and sedative/hypnotic properties. Soon after the introduction of chlordiazepoxide as an anxiolytic agent in 1960, followed by diazepam (2) and nitrazepam (3), the benzodiazepines became the most widely prescribed drugs in the United States. Most have anticonvulsant properties in animal models, and in 1965 diazepam was first used to treat status epilepticus in humans (4,5). Clonazepam was introduced in the 1970s primarily as an antiepileptic drug (AED) (6), and clobazam was later developed to have a reduced sedative effect (7,8). At the turn of the 21st century, however, only a few benzodiazepines have been approved for acute or long-term use as AEDs in the United States.

The mechanism of action remained obscure until the discovery of high-affinity, saturable benzodiazepine binding to a central nervous system (CNS) receptor (9,10). The benzodiazepines also enhanced inhibitory neurotransmission mediated by γ-aminobutyric acid (GABA), the major inhibitory neurotransmitter of the mammalian brain (11). Subsequent studies confirmed that the brain benzodiazepine receptor was, in fact, a binding site on the $GABA_A$ receptor, a ligand-gated chloride channel, where these drugs act as positive allosteric modulators (12).

CHEMISTRY AND MECHANISM OF ACTION

The benzodiazepine structure consists of a benzene ring fused with a 7-member diazepine ring, with nitrogens commonly in the 1 and 4 positions (Fig. 58.1). The clinically active benzodiazepines also have a second benzene ring attached to the 5 position. For this reason, the term *benzodiazepine* now refers most often to the 5-aryl-1,4 agents. Midazolam and flumazenil have fused R1 and R2 substituents, creating further ring complexity. Most antiepileptic benzodiazepines have the 1,4 structure; however, clobazam is a 1,5-benzodiazepine (7,8,13).

Potency

Benzodiazepine potency correlates with binding affinity at the benzodiazepine sites on neuronal $GABA_A$ receptors (Table 58.1) (14,15). An electron-withdrawing group at the 7 position (chloride for diazepam, lorazepam, and clorazepate; a nitro group for clonazepam and nitrazepam) increases receptor binding affinity (16) and especially potency; all useful anticonvulsant benzodiazepines have such a group. Reducing the 7-nitro substituent of clonazepam to produce its less active metabolite (7-amino-clonazepam) greatly decreases receptor-binding affinity and anticonvulsant potency. A methyl group on the nitrogen at position 1 (as in diazepam and clobazam) increases binding affinity and potency; a hydroxyl group at position 3 (as in lorazepam) decreases potency and binding affinity. Several benzodiazepines have a halogen at the 2′ position (chloride for lorazepam and clonazepam) that increases receptor-binding affinity and potency. By itself, however, relative potency is not indicative of a drug's anticonvulsant selectivity or therapeutic usefulness.

Efficacy

Activity at the $GABA_A$ receptor is a function of the drug's affinity for the benzodiazepine binding site and its intrinsic allosteric effect on that receptor. Individual compounds have widely variable efficacy. Benzodiazepines used as AEDs are thought to be full agonists that maximally enhance $GABA_A$ receptor activity. Competitive antagonists bind to the benzodiazepine site but do not affect $GABA_A$ receptor function. The antagonist, flumazenil, is used to reverse benzodiazepine-induced sedation in anesthesia (17,18) and to treat benzodiazepine overdose (19). Several "partial agonists" at the benzodiazepine binding site—including abecarnil (20), imidazenil (21), and bretazenil

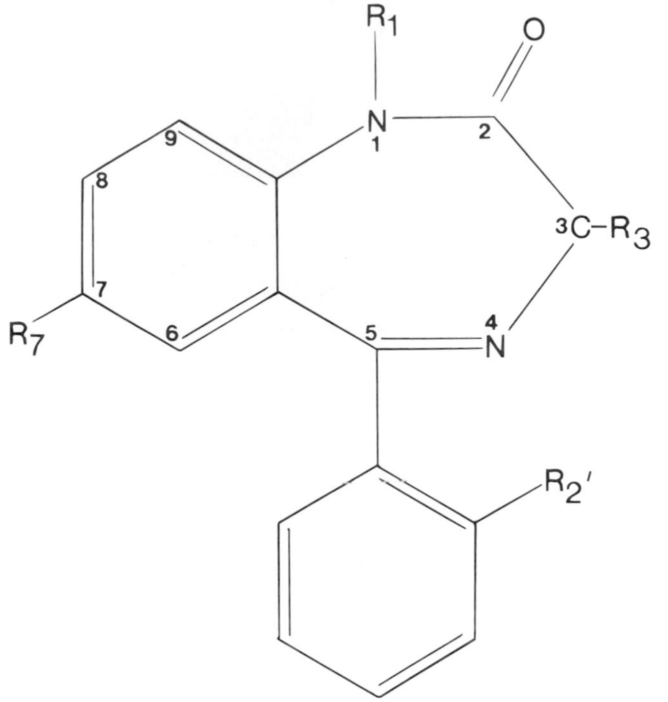

Figure 58.1 1,4-Benzodiazepine structure. For anticonvulsants, R_1 = H or CH_3; R_3 = H, OH, or COO^-; R_7 = Cl or NO_2; and R_2' = H or Cl.

(22)—although less effective than full agonists like diazepam, are anticonvulsant in animal models and appear less likely to promote tolerance (23,24). Other "inverse agonists" at the benzodiazepine site, including some β-carbolines, inhibit GABA binding or GABA-evoked currents (25). They can induce convulsive seizures or anxiety (25,26) but as yet have no clinical utility.

Anticonvulsant Activity

Benzodiazepines are effective against virtually every type of experimental seizure, but individual drugs show large quantitative differences for specific seizure models and other clinical effects (27). Benzodiazepines are particularly effective against seizures induced by the convulsant pentylenetetrazol, often considered a model of generalized absence seizures (28), but are less useful against tonic seizures induced by "maximal electroshock" (29), a model of generalized tonic-clonic convulsions. Relative doses necessary to achieve a particular effect also differ. The diazepam dose to block pentylenetetrazol seizures is 1% of that to abolish the righting response; for clonazepam, it is less than 0.02%, suggesting a larger therapeutic window. However, the dose of diazepam necessary to block maximal electroshock seizures is 11-fold higher than the dose required to suppress pentylenetetrazol seizures but is 2000-fold higher for clonazepam (27); this suggests that diazepam is more useful against generalized tonic-clonic seizures. Diazepam (30) and clorazepate (31) also slow the development of kindling, an animal model in which repeated subconvulsive electrical stimulation produces increasingly severe seizure activity (32).

GABA$_A$ Receptor Complex

The association, or "coupling," between benzodiazepine binding and GABA binding (33), demonstrated in early binding studies, suggested activity at a specific receptor associated with the bicuculline-sensitive GABA$_A$ receptor to modulate its actions on a chloride channel (33–35). Thus, a "GABA$_A$ receptor complex" appeared to incorporate binding sites for GABA, benzodiazepines, and barbiturates with a ligand-gated chloride channel. Electrophysiologic studies demonstrated that benzodiazepines increased the amplitude of GABA-mediated inhibitory postsynaptic potentials (IPSPs) (12) by raising the opening frequency of the GABA-gated chloride channel (36). This mechanism was later confirmed with single-channel studies (37).

In whole-cell patch-clamp recordings of CNS neurons, benzodiazepines shift the concentration-response curve

TABLE 58.1

ANTICONVULSANT ACTIVITY, MOTOR IMPAIRMENT, AND RECEPTOR BINDING OF SOME BENZODIAZEPINES

Benzodiazepine	ED$_{50}$ for Clonus Suppression in Kindled Rats (mg/kg)[a]	ED$_{50}$ for Ataxia (mg/kg)[a]	IC$_{50}$ for Inhibiting [³H]Flunitrazepam-Specific Binding, nM[b]
Clobazam	2.8	13.2	870
Diazepam	0.4	1.5	78
Clonazepam	0.09	0.9	16
7-Amino-clonazepam	>40	—	195

[a]Dose required to inhibit forelimb clonus or to cause ataxia in 50% of amygdala-kindled rats. (Data from Tietz EI, Rosenberg HC, Chiu TH. A comparison of the anticonvulsant effects of 1,4- and 1,5-benzodiazepines in the amygdala-kindled rat and their effects on motor function. *Epilepsy Res* 1989;3:31–40, except 7-amino-clonazepam data, which is from HC Rosenberg, EI Tietz, and TH Chiu, unpublished data, 1987.)
[b]Concentration required to displace 50% of 2 nM [³H]flunitrazepam specifically bound to rat cerebral cortical membranes. (Data from EI Tietz, TH Chiu, and HC Rosenberg, unpublished data, 1990.)

for GABA leftward (Fig. 58.2), increasing current amplitudes at lower GABA concentrations but not increasing maximal current (38). This shift is caused by an enhanced affinity for GABA at its binding site, with no change in channel-gating kinetics (37). The benzodiazepines thus increase the current produced by low GABA concentrations but have no effect at high GABA concentrations, at which receptor binding is saturated. Studies of GABAergic inhibitory postsynaptic currents (IPSCs) have suggested that GABA is present in the synaptic cleft for 1 to 3 ms at high concentrations (about 1 mM) (39,40). Thus, at individual synapses, benzodiazepines prolong the mIPSC decay phase (41,42) by slowing the dissociation of GABA from the receptor (43,44) without changing maximal mIPSP amplitude. Prolongation of the mIPSC increases the likelihood of temporal and spatial summation of multiple synaptic inputs, which, in turn, raises the amplitude of stimulus-evoked IPSCs. The benzodiazepines thus increase the inhibitory "tone" of GABAergic synapses, which prevents or limits the hypersynchronous firing of neuron populations that underlies seizure activity (45).

GABA$_A$ Receptors and Epilepsy

The anticonvulsant properties of benzodiazepines are likely related to the prominent role of GABA$_A$ receptors in epilepsy. Substantial evidence links epilepsy with dysfunction of GABAergic inhibition (45). GABA$_A$ receptors are the target not only of the benzodiazepines but also of the barbiturates and, indirectly, of tiagabine and vigabatrin, which increase GABA concentration at the synapse (45). Several animal models of epilepsy demonstrate altered numbers or functions of GABA$_A$ receptors (46). Moreover, changes in the composition or structure of the transmembrane protein subunits that make up GABA$_A$ receptors can result in epilepsy. Expression of GABA$_A$ receptor subunits is altered in the hippocampi of experimental animals with recurrent seizures (47) and in patients with temporal lobe epilepsy (48,49). Mice lacking the GABA$_A$ receptor β_3 subunit have seizures and behavioral features of Angelman syndrome (50), a neurodevelopmental disorder associated with severe mental retardation and epilepsy caused by a mutation affecting the β_3 subunit on chromosome 15q11-13 (51). In addition, two mutations in the γ_2 subunit that impair GABA$_A$ receptor function (52), K289M (53) and R43Q (54), have been linked to a syndrome of childhood absence epilepsy and febrile seizures; a loss-of-function mutation in the α_1 subunit was found in a family with autosomal dominant juvenile myoclonic epilepsy (55).

Other Benzodiazepine Actions

With a few exceptions (26), the benzodiazepines derive anticonvulsant properties from specific interaction with GABA$_A$ receptors. In one study, their high-affinity interactions with GABA$_A$ receptors did not fully explain the anticonvulsant effect, part of which occurred at concentrations much higher than necessary to saturate the GABA$_A$ receptor benzodiazepine binding site, was exponential rather than saturable, and was not antagonized by flumazenil (56). Benzodiazepines, but not GABA or muscimol, were anticonvulsant when injected into the substantia nigra pars reticulata (57,58). Pharmacodynamic issues in benzodiazepine metabolism may explain these findings (see p. 834); alternatively, other sites of action may be involved. At doses used to treat status epilepticus, benzodiazepines also inhibit voltage-gated sodium (59) and calcium channels (60) and increase GABA levels in cerebrospinal fluid (61). Benzodiazepines, however, have no interaction with the G-protein–linked GABA$_B$ receptor, which can either suppress voltage-gated Ca^{2+} channels or activate inward-rectifying K^+ channels (62).

Benzodiazepines also bind to the "peripheral benzodiazepine receptor" (PBR) (63,64), an 18-kDa protein that functions as part of the mitochondrial permeability transition pore involved in cholesterol transport (64), apoptosis, and regulation of mitochondrial function (65). Although the PBR is widely expressed throughout the body, in the central nervous system (CNS) it is restricted to ependymal cells and glia (63) and is therefore unlikely to have a role in the clinical properties of benzodiazepines.

Excitatory GABA$_A$ Currents

Benzodiazepine enhancement of GABA$_A$ receptor function may not always be anticonvulsant or even inhibitory. Early in CNS development, neurons do not express the major chloride transporters (e.g., the potassium-chloride cotransporter, KCC2) that lower intracellular chloride concentration and create the negative driving force for chloride ions found in adult neurons. As a result, activation of GABA$_A$-receptor channels can be depolarizing and excitatory and may play a trophic role in neuronal morphogenesis or synaptogenesis, or both (66,67). In fact, endogenous GABA appears to be proconvulsant in early postnatal rat hippocampal slices, as GABA$_A$ antagonists blocked epileptiform activity induced by depolarization with high external $[K^+]$ (68). However, benzodiazepine efficacy appears to be intact, likely because persistent opening of GABA channels (in the presence of benzodiazepines) may reduce the depolarizing chloride reversal potential, resulting in "shunt" inhibition or subthreshold depolarization that inactivates sodium channels and prevents firing of action potentials (69,70).

The current through GABA$_A$ receptor channels can be altered by changes in concentration of intracellular bicarbonate (71,72), which also flows though the channel (73). These changes may underlie a reduction in synaptic GABA current amplitudes during development of benzodiazepine tolerance (74,75). Depolarizing GABA$_A$ currents may also be a source of interictal spike activity, as observed in epileptic subiculum neurons in hippocampal brain slices removed from patients with temporal lobe epilepsy (76). Changes in the GABA current reversal potential might also explain why diazepam can be less effective in children with epileptic encephalopathies (77), and why, rarely, it can cause status epilepticus in patients with Lennox-Gastaut syndrome (78,79).

Molecular Biology of GABA$_A$ Receptors

The GABA$_A$ receptors have binding sites for agents that modulate receptor function, including the benzodiazepines, barbiturates, neurosteroids, general anesthetics, the novel anticonvulsant loreclezole, and the convulsant toxins picrotoxin and bicuculline. Recent research into the molecular biology of GABA$_A$ receptors has clarified the mechanisms of benzodiazepine action.

GABA$_A$ receptors belong to the ligand-gated channel superfamily that includes the nicotinic acetylcholine, glycine, and the serotonin 5HT$_3$ receptors (80). GABA$_A$ receptors are pentameric (81) transmembrane chloride channels assembled from combinations of protein subunits from several families (Fig. 58.2). Seven subunit families

have been identified (12), with 30% to 40% homology between families and about 70% homology within families. In mammals, 16 subunit subtypes have been cloned, including 6 α, 3 β, and 3 γ subtypes, single members of the δ, π (82), and ε (83) families [θ (84) may be the fourth member of the β family (85)], as well as alternatively spliced variants of the β_2 and γ_2 subtypes. Random pentomeric combinations of all of the subunits would produce tens of thousands of subunit compositions. Because GABA$_A$ receptor subtypes are differentially expressed by CNS region and cell type (86) and are developmentally regulated (87,88), the total number of possible isoforms in specific brain regions and individual neurons is reduced. The most common GABA receptor conformation contains the α_1, β_2, and γ_2 subtypes, with presumed stoichiometry of 2α, 2β and a single γ subunit; the δ subunit may in some cases substitute for γ. The subunits are arranged around a central water-filled pore that can open to conduct Cl$^-$ ions when GABA is bound (Fig. 58.2). Studies of recombinant receptors have shown that individual subunit subtypes confer different sensitivities to GABA$_A$-receptor modulators including benzodiazepines (89,90), loreclezole (91), and zinc ions (92).

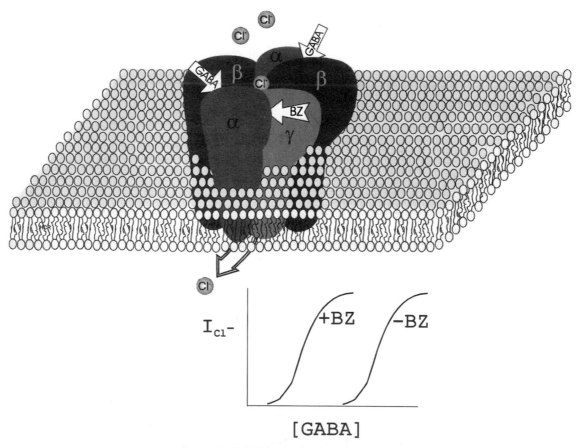

Figure 58.2 Model of a GABA$_A$ receptor in the plasma membrane. The receptor consists of five closely related subunits, each with four membrane-spanning domains. The receptor is a ligand-gated anion channel, with two binding sites for GABA (between α and β subunits) and one for benzodiazepines (between α and β subunits). In the presence of GABA, the channel becomes permeable to chloride ions, producing the fast inhibitory postsynaptic potential (IPSP). In the presence of a benzodiazepine agonist, GABA binds more efficiently, enhancing the IPSP. Benzodiazepines have no effect in the absence of GABA.

GABA$_A$ Receptor Subunits and Benzodiazepine Pharmacology

Benzodiazepine augmentation of GABA$_A$ receptor currents requires a γ subunit, and the specificity of benzodiazepine responsiveness is determined by which α subunit is present (12,93). The effect of GABA$_A$ receptor subunit composition on benzodiazepine binding has been well characterized by radioligand binding studies (94) and electrophysiology of the recombinant receptors expressed in fibroblasts (85,95). The α1 subunit results in a receptor with high affinity for the imidazopyridine hypnotic zolpidem, defining the "BZ-1" (or Ω-1) receptor type (94,96). The α$_2$ and α$_3$ subunits, combined with β and γ, result in BZ-2 receptors with moderate zolpidem affinity. GABA$_A$ receptors with the α$_5$ subunit or the γ$_3$ subunit are sensitive to diazepam but have essentially no affinity for zolpidem and are called BZ-3 receptors. GABA$_A$ receptors with the α$_4$ or α$_6$ subunits are insensitive to most benzodiazepines. Given the dependence of benzodiazepine binding and action on α and γ subunits, the benzodiazepine binding site is, not surprisingly, in a cleft between them (97).

GABA$_A$ Receptor Subunits Mediate Specific Benzodiazepine Effects

Exploration of the roles of the α subunits has been based on the discovery of a single histidine (H) residue found in all benzodiazepine-sensitive α subunits (H101 in the rat α$_1$ subunit), but not in the benzodiazepine-insensitive α$_4$ or α$_6$ subunits. Mutation of the arginine (R100) to H in α$_6$ dramatically increases benzodiazepine binding in this normally insensitive subunit, while mutation of H101 to R in α$_1$ reduces benzodiazepine sensitivity (98); this H residue was discovered in a strain of "alcohol-nontolerant" rats that had a point mutation in the α$_6$ subunit (R100Q). This spontaneous mutation made their α$_6$-containing GABA$_A$ receptors (found mostly in the cerebellum) sensitive to diazepam and likely accounted for their ethanol and benzodiazepine intolerance (99). Subsequent studies have used mice carrying "knock-in mutations" with individual α subunits mutated to be benzodiazepine insensitive. In homozygous α$_1$ (H101R) knock-in mice, the benzodiazepine anxiolytic effect was intact, but the drug did not protect against pentylenetetrazol-induced convulsions and did not produce sedation or amnesia; therefore, binding to the (wild type) α$_1$ subunit may be responsible for sedative, amnestic, and anticonvulsant actions (100,101). Moreover, the sedative-hypnotic zolpidem showed no sedative effect in α$_1$ (H101R) mice (102). Unfortunately, these findings underscore the association between sedative and anticonvulsant efficacy for the benzodiazepines at α$_1$-containing GABA$_A$ receptors. Corresponding knock-in mutations of the α$_2$ and α$_3$ subtypes (α$_2$[H101R] and α$_3$[H126R])] suggested that anxiolytic (103) and myorelaxant (104) properties of benzodiazepines derive from α$_2$- and α$_3$-containing GABA$_A$

receptors; the α$_5$ subunit is critical for amnestic effects (105).

Further underscoring the role of individual subunits in GABA$_A$ receptor function were studies that used antisense oligodeoxynucleotides (ASO) to selectively reduce the expression of specific subunits. Progesterone withdrawal results in anxiety and increased seizure susceptibility associated with an increased expression of the benzodiazepine-insensitive α$_4$ subunit (106). Pretreating rats with an ASO against the α$_4$ subunit prevented the increase in seizure susceptibility (107); this finding may have significance for catamenial epilepsy. Treatment with an ASO for the γ$_2$ subunit increased the convulsive threshold dose for methyl-β-carboline-3-carboxylate, a benzodiazepine inverse agonist, but not for picrotoxin or strychnine (108). ASO γ$_2$ treatment also reduced benzodiazepine binding but not binding to the GABA recognition site (109), indicating a reduction in benzodiazepine binding sites without a change in the number of GABA$_A$-receptor complexes. Similarly, mice lacking the γ$_2$ subunit expressed GABA$_A$ receptors with almost no benzodiazepine recognition sites and only a minor reduction in GABA binding sites (110).

Benzodiazepine Tolerance and GABA$_A$ Receptor Plasticity

Long-term benzodiazepine treatment gives rise to tolerance, decreases in sedative or anticonvulsant properties, and dependence, the continued need for drug to prevent a withdrawal syndrome (111). Tolerance requires escalation of drug doses and increases the risk of withdrawal seizures. Long-term use of benzodiazepines can also reduce their subsequent effectiveness in acute conditions (112), such as status epilepticus. Withdrawal symptoms typically involve exacerbation of the initial anxiety, insomnia, or seizures and are more common with short-acting than long-acting agents. Rebound symptoms typically return to baseline within 1 to 3 weeks after discontinuation of the drug (113). In animal studies, tolerance develops proportionally to agonist efficacy. Partial agonists produce much less tolerance than full agonists, and the antagonist flumazenil causes no tolerance-related changes in receptor number or function (24). As tolerance to one benzodiazepine may not induce tolerance to a different one, drug-specific interactions at their receptors may be operative (114). The duration of tolerance also varies among benzodiazepines (115). Several studies have noted changes in expression of GABA$_A$ receptor subunits (116–118) as well as altered synaptic physiology (119,120) that depend not only on the drug and dosage but also on the duration and method of administration; all contribute to benzodiazepine receptor occupancy. Measurements of tolerance also vary by seizure model (pentylenetetrazole, bicuculline, pilocarpine, kindling, etc.) and by the behavioral tests used to assess the other benzodiazepine clinical properties (121).

Flumazenil: Uses in Epilepsy

Flumazenil (RO15-1788) binds to the benzodiazepine site without changing GABA site binding or GABA-evoked currents; it thus meets the pharmacologic definition of an antagonist. Used primarily to reverse benzodiazepine-induced sedation (17,18), flumazenil may also reverse hepatic coma (122,123) in patients naive to benzodiazepines; this bolsters arguments for an endogenous benzodiazepine ligand or "endozapine" displaced by flumazenil (124). The role of an endogenous "diazepam binding inhibitor" peptide (125) in inhibitory neurotransmission remains unclear.

Brief exposure to flumazenil can reverse tolerance-related changes in GABA$_A$ receptor function (126,127) and subunit expression (128). The use of intermittent low doses was explored in three patients with daily seizures who had become tolerant to clonazepam (1 mg twice daily) (129). A single intravenous dose of flumazenil (1.5 mg) resulted in mild shivering lasting 30 minutes, followed by seizure freedom for an average of 13 days. Refinement of this approach may extend the use of benzodiazepines as long-term therapy for epilepsy.

Curiously, flumazenil has shown anticonvulsant efficacy in some animal models, possibly as a result of partial agonism at high doses (130,131) or antagonism of an endogenous proconvulsant (129). Epileptiform discharges in hippocampal slices were also reduced (132), and kindling was slowed (133). Doses from 0.75 to 15 mg suppressed focal epileptiform activity in six patients with temporal lobe seizures but did not affect generalized spike-and-wave activity in six patients with generalized seizures (134). Several small studies have suggested possible benefit as an AED in humans (134,135). Orally administered flumazenil reduced seizure frequency by 50% to 75% in 9 of 11 previously untreated individuals with epilepsy and in 9 of 16 patients when used adjunctively (136). Prevention of interictal epileptiform discharges on the electroencephalogram (EEG) was similar to that of diazepam (129,137).

Flumazenil can precipitate seizures in patients with hepatic encephalopathy or benzodiazepine dependence or in patients who have attempted overdose (e.g., with tricyclic antidepressants) (138). Flumazenil has been administered to patients previously treated with benzodiazepines to precipitate partial seizures during inpatient localization of seizure onset (139). [^{11}C]Flumazenil has been used in positron emission tomography studies to demonstrate regions of neuronal loss associated with epilepsy (140,141) and may aid in localizing the seizure focus in patients with dual pathologic conditions (142).

ABSORPTION, DISTRIBUTION, AND METABOLISM

The major anticonvulsant role of the benzodiazepines is as first-line therapy for status epilepticus and seizure clusters.

Intravenous administration is preferred (143) but may be difficult or impossible in very young children, necessitating use of a rectal (144–149), intraosseous (150), buccal (151,152), or nasal (153–155) route. With intravenous administration, the drug's effectiveness is determined by how fast it crosses the blood-brain barrier. The benzodiazepines are highly lipophilic and rapidly penetrate the blood-brain barrier (156), although the rate of penetration varies more than 50-fold among agents and depends on their substituent groups (157). Protein binding correlates with lipophilicity and is high for most benzodiazepines (nearly 99% for diazepam). After oral ingestion, the benzodiazepines are fully absorbed except for clorazepate, which is rapidly decarboxylated in the stomach to N-desmethyldiazepam (nordazepam) before absorption.

Despite generally long plasma half-lives, most benzodiazepines are relatively short-acting after administration of a single dose owing to rapid distribution from the brain and vascular compartment to peripheral tissues (158,159). A two-compartment model best describes their pharmacokinetics: high levels occur rapidly in the brain and other well-perfused organs, then decline rapidly with an initial brief half-life as a result of distribution into peripheral tissues and lipid stores; a much slower elimination half-life ($t_{1/2\beta}$) related to enzymatic metabolism and excretion follows. For example, the $t_{1/2\beta}$ of diazepam ranges from 20 to 54 hours (160), but the duration of action after a single intravenous injection is only 1 hour, with peak brain concentrations present for only 20 to 30 minutes (161). Distribution is fastest for the most lipophilic agents. Elimination may be prolonged by enterohepatic circulation, particularly in the elderly. These agents cross the placenta and are secreted into breast milk.

Metabolism occurs in the liver by the cytochrome P (CYP) 450 enzymes CYP3A4 and CYP2C19. Inhibitors of CYP3A4, such as erythromycin, clarithromycin, ritonavir, itraconazole, ketoconazole, nefazodone, and grapefruit juice, can slow benzodiazepine metabolism (162). Relatively little induction of hepatic enzymes occurs. Biologically active metabolites (e.g., nordazepam as a metabolite of diazepam) can significantly prolong the biologic half-lives of these agents. Figure 58.3 illustrates benzodiazepine metabolic pathways. The biotransformation and pharmacokinetics of these drugs have been extensively reviewed (56,163–165) and are presented in detail below for the individual agents.

DRUG INTERACTIONS

Benzodiazepines interact with other drugs more through pharmacodynamic than pharmacokinetic mechanisms. They are not potent enzyme inducers, nor do they strongly affect plasma protein binding of other drugs. CNS depression is increased when benzodiazepines are given with other CNS-depressant drugs (157,166).

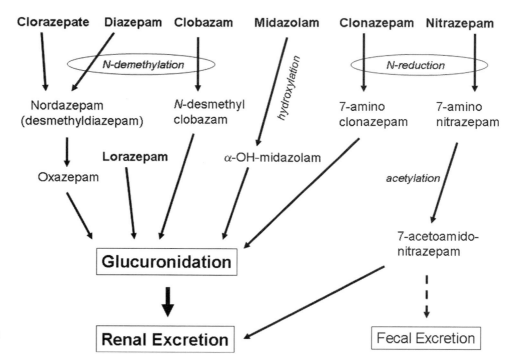

Figure 58.3 Metabolism of the anticonvulsant benzodiazepines.

Pharmacokinetic interactions with other anticonvulsants except phenobarbital are infrequent and inconsistent. Diazepam enhances phenobarbital elimination (167), and phenobarbital increases the clearance (168) and lowers plasma levels of clonazepam (169). Valproate reduces diazepam protein binding, increasing free drug levels (170), and enhances diazepam's CNS effects (167). Other AEDs may augment metabolism and clearance of N-desmethyldiazepam derived from clorazepate (171). Clobazam increases the 10-11 epoxide metabolite of carbamazepine (172).

Benzodiazepines interact little with other drugs but are affected by cytochrome P450 inhibitors. Cimetidine decreases the clearance of diazepam (173,174) and nitrazepam (175). Rifampin increases the clearance and shortens the half-life of nitrazepam (176). Probenecid markedly increases the half-life of lorazepam (177).

ANTIEPILEPTIC EFFICACY

Status Epilepticus

A cause of significant morbidity and mortality (178,179), status epilepticus requires urgent treatment to avoid neuronal damage and its neurologic consequences (180,181). The benzodiazepines have become initial therapy for status epilepticus owing to their rapid onset and proven efficacy (182), with relatively minor cardiotoxic reactions or respiratory depression compared with barbiturates (183). In the multicenter, double-blind Veterans Affairs Cooperative Status Epilepticus Trial (184), patients were randomized to receive lorazepam (0.1 mg/kg), phenytoin (18 mg/kg), phenobarbital (15 mg/kg), or diazepam (0.15 mg/kg) fol-

lowed by phenytoin (18 mg/kg). Lorazepam was effective in 64.9% of patients, phenobarbital in 58.2%, diazepam/phenytoin in 55.8%, and phenytoin in 43.6% ($p < 0.001$ lorazepam vs. phenytoin alone). Efficacy appeared to correlate with the rate at which therapeutic drug concentrations were achieved; lorazepam required the shortest time, phenytoin the longest ($p < 0.001$).

Lorazepam and diazepam were compared for treatment of simple partial, complex partial, and secondarily generalized tonic-clonic status epilepticus in a double-blind study of 78 adults with symptomatic localization-related epilepsy (182); idiopathic generalized epilepsy with absence status epilepticus was also represented. After the first injection, lorazepam (4 mg) stopped status epilepticus in 78% of patients and diazepam (10 mg) in 58%; effectiveness was 89% and 76% after the second injection ($p = NS$ between drugs). An open-label, prospective, randomized trial compared lorazepam (0.05 to 0.1 mg/kg) and diazepam (0.3 to 0.4 mg/kg) in children with acute convulsions including convulsive status epilepticus (185). Lorazepam was statistically more effective ($p < 0.01$) after the first dose and apparently safer. Its superior efficacy may be the result of a longer duration of action, based on a longer distribution half-life.

Lorazepam may replace diazepam for prehospital treatment of status epilepticus. A large clinical comparison found that status epilepticus had terminated by the time of arrival at the emergency department in 59.1% of patients treated with lorazepam (2 mg), in 42.6% treated with diazepam (5 mg), and in 21.1% given placebo (186). Rates of circulatory or ventilatory complications were similar (10.6 for lorazepam, 10.3% for diazepam) and lower than those of placebo (22.5%).

Early treatment increases the probability of seizure termination (186), most likely because prolonged seizures alter GABA$_A$ receptor susceptibility to benzodiazepines (187). Reduction in benzodiazepine sensitivity of the GABA$_A$ receptor can occur within minutes in status epilepticus (188,189) and may be responsible in part for both the persistent epileptic state and its refractoriness. Refractoriness to diazepam may be mediated by N-methyl-D-aspartate (NMDA) receptor mechanisms, as NMDA antagonists improve the response to diazepam in late pilocarpine-induced status epilepticus (190). Moreover, NMDA receptors are upregulated during benzodiazepine tolerance, and NMDA antagonists (e.g., MK801) can block benzodiazepine-withdrawal seizures (191). These findings suggest a possible strategy for treatment of late benzodiazepine-refractory status epilepticus with combinations of a benzodiazepine (e.g., intravenous midazolam) and an NMDA-receptor antagonist such as the dissociative general anesthetic, ketamine. A recent trial of oral ketamine for refractory nonconvulsive status epilepticus showed efficacy in all five children studied (192). Such approaches will require validation in controlled clinical trials.

Both lorazepam and diazepam have been approved by the U.S. Food and Drug Administration (FDA) for treatment of status epilepticus in adults; diazepam has also been approved in children more than 30 days old. Parenteral preparations of midazolam, flunitrazepam, and clonazepam expand the treatment possibilities. Clonazepam for parenteral administration is currently marketed only in Germany and the United Kingdom, and flunitrazepam is not available in the United States. Intramuscular injection and intranasal (153,154), buccal (151), endotracheal (193,194), or rectal (149,195,196) instillation also rapidly produce therapeutic levels and are effective against status epilepticus or seizure clusters.

Acute Repetitive Seizures

The need for immediate high drug levels to handle serial seizures is less urgent, and ease of administration by family or allied health workers becomes important. Diazepam rectal gel prevents subsequent seizures during seizure clusters (195,196) and can reduce the frequency of emergency department visits (145). Table 58.2 compares the clinical and pharmacologic properties of the benzodiazepines used for acute seizures. Individual agents can be selected for specific clinical situations. Repeated seizures in a patient rapidly weaned from anticonvulsants for inpatient monitoring could be treated with diazepam (rather than lorazepam), as its shorter peak duration of action may be less likely to suppress seizure activity needed later.

Long-Term Chronic Treatment of Epilepsy

Although their long-term use in epilepsy is limited by sedation and tolerance, benzodiazepines may figure in the adjunctive treatment of myoclonic and other generalized seizure types, or seizures with comorbid anxiety disorders. For example, lorazepam improved control of seizures associated with psychological stressors (197). The benzodiazepines can be an integral part of a rational polypharmaceutical regimen, defined as the minimum effective AED combination for seizure control.

Intermittent administration when seizure thresholds are transiently reduced may be the ideal strategy for benzodiazepines. Not only are they suited pharmacokinetically for such an application, but such short-term use also may avoid tolerance. For example, catamenial seizures improved with intermittent use of clobazam (198). Studies

TABLE 58.2

CLINICAL PHARMACOLOGY OF BENZODIAZEPINES USED FOR ACUTE SEIZURES

| Characteristic | Diazepam | | Lorazepam | | Midazolam | | Clonazepam |
	IV	Rectal	IV[a]	Buccal[a]	IV[a]	IM[a]	IV[b]
Initial dose (mg)	10–20	0.5–1/kg	4	2–4	0.125–0.15/kg	0.2/kg	0.01–0.09/kg
Infusion rate	8 mg/h	—	—	—	0.15–0.2 mg/kg/h	—	—
Minimum effective concentration	500 ng/mL	NA	30 ng/mL	NA	NA	NA	30 ng/mL
Onset of effect (min)	<1	2–6	<2	NA	<2	2–30	<1
Peak effect (min)	3–15	10–120	30	NA	10–50	25 ± 23	NA
Duration of effect	<20 min	NA	>360 min	NA	<50 min	20–120 min	24 h
Protein bound (%)	96–97	96–97	85–93	85–93	95 ± 2	95 ± 2	86 ± 5
Volume of distribution (L/kg)	133	133	12	12	NA	NA	NA
Distribution half-life	0.96–2.2 h	NA	2–3 h	NA	5.7 ± 2.4 min	NA	NA
Elimination half-life (h)	36 ± 4.9	36 ± 4.9	14.1	14.1	1.9 ± 0.6	1.9 ± 0.6	20–80

Abbreviations: IM, intramuscular; IV, intravenous; NA, not available.
[a]Not approved by the U.S. Food and Drug Administration for seizures.
[b]Not available in the United States.

of efficacy for specific indications with the individual agents are discussed below.

ADVERSE EVENTS

With acute treatment of status epilepticus, the primary toxic reaction is respiratory and cardiovascular depression (182,199), which is largely a result of the propylene glycol solvent (200,201). Sedation and amnesia are relatively unimportant in this setting and difficult to distinguish from the effects of status epilepticus itself. Sedation after termination of convulsive status epilepticus, however, often necessitates EEG evaluation to ensure that a conversion to nonconvulsive status epilepticus has not occurred. Administration of benzodiazepines in conjunction with other CNS-active drugs, such as phenobarbital, may enhance respiratory and cardiovascular toxic reactions (166). Rarely, parenteral administration can induce tonic status epilepticus in patients with Lennox-Gastaut syndrome (79,202). Thrombophlebitis may occur (203,204), and intra-arterial injection may produce tissue necrosis (205).

With long-term use, all benzodiazepines induce sedation and drowsiness, lightheadedness, ataxia, cognitive slowing and confusion, and anterograde amnesia. Other effects include weakness, headache, blurred vision, vertigo, nausea and vomiting, gastrointestinal distress, and diarrhea. Joint aches, chest pains, and incontinence are rare (157). The risk of tolerance, dependence, and abuse is significant but low when these agents are prescribed for appropriate indications (159,206). Abrupt withdrawal has been associated with convulsions, worsening insomnia, psychosis, and delirium tremens in nonepileptic individuals using diazepam, clonazepam, clorazepate, or nitrazepam (113,207,208). The incidence of allergic, hepatotoxic, or hematologic reactions is extremely low. Benzodiazepines can sometimes increase the frequency of seizures in epileptic patients. Specific adverse effects with the individual agents are discussed below.

INDIVIDUAL BENZODIAZEPINES

Discussion of predominantly short-term agents—diazepam, lorazepam, and midazolam—is followed by details of long-term benzodiazepines, clonazepam, clorazepate, clobazam, and nitrazepam.

Diazepam

The first benzodiazepine AED (4), diazepam (Fig. 58.4), has become standard initial therapy for status epilepticus in adults and children (182), although its primary role may be usurped by lorazepam (184,186). Oral and parenteral preparations are available. The 1993 classification of rectal diazepam as an orphan drug allowed the development of

Figure 58.4 Diazepam.

a rectal gel (Diastat) that has been effective against serial seizures (see p. 839).

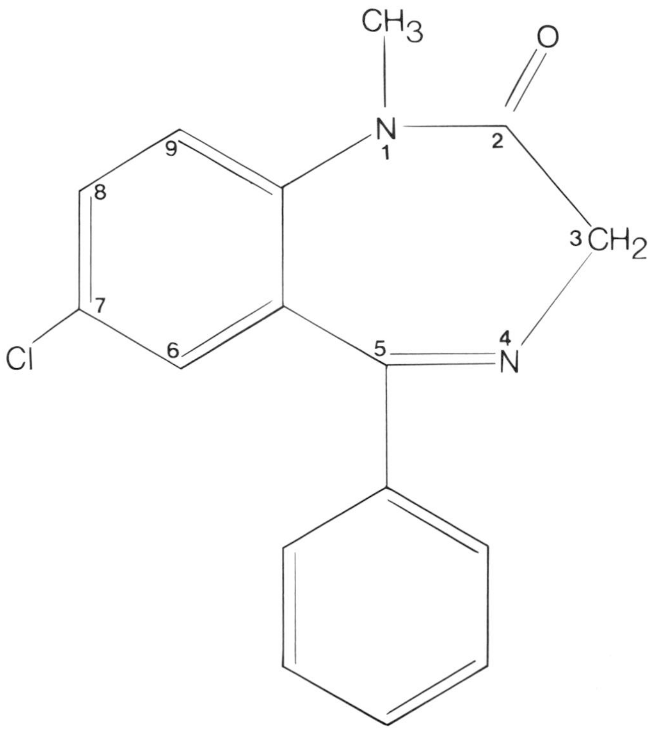

Diazepam increases β-frequency activity and background slowing on the EEG, which can be quantified by spectral analysis (209). The EEG changes may have prognostic value in seizure control; 88% (29 of 33) of patients whose EEG showed loss of abnormal activity or emergence of fast (β-frequency) activity after diazepam became seizure free or had a 50% seizure reduction (210).

Absorption, Distribution, and Metabolism

Diazepam rapidly enters the brain, but its high lipid solubility also promotes rapid redistribution into peripheral tissues. The loss of initial anticonvulsant effect is accentuated by the high degree of plasma protein binding (90% to 99%) (211). The volume of distribution is 1.1 L/kg. Plasma concentration declines rapidly during the distribution phase, with an initial half-life ($t_{1/2\alpha}$) of 1 hour (212). Diazepam undergoes demethylation to desmethyldiazepam (DMD, nordazepam), a metabolite with anticonvulsant activity and a long half-life (>20 hours), followed by slow hydroxylation (at position 3 of the diazepine ring) to oxazepam, which is also active (Fig. 58.3) (213). Small amounts of temazepam are also formed by 3-hydroxylation of diazepam. The hydroxylated metabolites are conjugated with glucuronic acid in the liver (216); renal excretion follows (213), with a $t_{1/2\beta}$ of 24 to 48 hours (167,214). Diazepam induces CYP2B (215). There is little evidence of enterohepatic circulation (216,217), but diazepam may be secreted in the gastric juices, with subsequent enterogastric circulation (218). All benzodiazepines cross the placenta and are excreted to some extent in breast milk (157,212).

Adverse Effects and Drug Interactions

Respiratory depression (219) may be exacerbated by postictal CNS depression and necessitate ventilatory support (220). Sedative side effects, including inattention and drowsiness, occur in up to 46% of patients (167) at plasma levels of about 200 ng/mL (221,222), the same level needed to suppress spikes (223) and maintain control of status epilepticus in acute studies (167). Drowsiness, fatigue, amnesia, ataxia, and falls are prominent in the elderly. The propylene glycol vehicle of intravenous diazepam can cause thrombophlebitis and lactic acidosis (203,204). In a rare paradoxical response diazepam increases seizure frequency, causes muscle spasms, or provokes status epilepticus (224). An idiosyncratic allergic interstitial nephritis has also been reported (225). Other rare adverse events include cardiac arrhythmias, hepatotoxic reactions, gynecomastia, blurred vision and diplopia, neutropenia or thrombocytopenia, rash and urticaria, and anaphylaxis (226). Despite a significant potential, abuse is rare when diazepam is prescribed for appropriate indications (159). The teratogenic effect is uncertain, but first trimester use has been linked to oral clefts (227). The teratogenic potential of valproic acid may be amplified (228).

Diazepam enhances the elimination of phenobarbital (167), probably through induction of CYP450 (215). Valproic acid displaces diazepam bound to plasma proteins, increasing free diazepam and associated sedation (170).

Clinical Applications

Status Epilepticus

Diazepam is effective initial therapy for both convulsive and nonconvulsive status epilepticus (184) and may have particular benefit in generalized absence status epilepticus, controlling 93% of patients in one study (229), as well as 89% of generalized convulsions, 88% of simple motor seizures, and 75% of complex partial status epilepticus. These numbers, higher than in the Veterans Affairs Cooperative Status Epilepticus Trial (184), may reflect differences in study populations.

Diazepam is typically administered as a single intravenous bolus of 10 to 20 mg (167). A 20-mg bolus at a rate of 2 mg/min stopped convulsions in 33% of patients within 3 minutes and in 80% within 5 minutes (230), but a single injection often does not produce lasting control and may be less effective when status results from acute CNS disease or structural brain lesions (163). This problem may be avoided by giving subsequent 5- to 10-mg intravenous doses every few hours, following diazepam with a longer-lasting anticonvulsant (e.g., phenytoin [184]), or using continuous intravenous diazepam drip. Because repeated administration decreases apparent volume of distribution and clearance, subsequent doses should be tapered to prevent toxic reactions (231). Diazepam (100 mg in 500 mL of 5% dextrose in water) infused at 40 mL/hour delivers 20 mg per hour (145) and may achieve a serum level ranging between 200 and 800 ng/mL; 500 ng/mL appears to terminate status (167,232). Complete suppression of 3-Hz spike-and-wave required 600 to 2000 ng/mL (233). Continuous infusion has been used in patients hypersensitive to anticonvulsants (234). Diazepam is adsorbed onto polyvinylchloride bags, with bioavailability reduced 50% after 8 hours (235); this should be taken into account if a long-term infusion for status epilepticus is contemplated. Because benzodiazepine efficacy decreases with duration of status epilepticus (187), higher levels or alternative treatments may be necessary in refractory status.

Pediatric Status Epilepticus

The initial recommended intravenous dose in children is 0.1 to 0.3 mg/kg by slow bolus (<5 mg per minute), repeated every 15 minutes for two doses, with a maximum of 5 mg in infants and 15 mg in older children (236,237). If intravenous administration is not possible, a solution of 0.5 to 1 mg/kg placed 3 to 6 cm into the rectum has been effective (146). In pediatric status epilepticus, a continuous infusion (0.01 to 0.03 mg/kg per minute) controlled seizures in 86% (49 of /57) of patients within an average of 40 minutes (238). Hypotension occurred in one patient (2%) and respiratory depression in six patients (12%); seven patients (14%) died. Patients in whom the infusion failed were treated with thiopental, which controlled seizures in all but necessitated ventilatory and hemodynamic support; four of these patients (44%) died. A metaanalysis of 111 patients between 1 month and 18 years of age with refractory generalized convulsive status epilepticus suggested that diazepam was less effective as continuous therapy than midazolam, thiopental, pentobarbital, or isoflurane (86% versus 100%) after stratification for etiology (239). However, all of the diazepam-treated patients were from one region in India, and none underwent continuous EEG monitoring; differences in location or details of care may have contributed to the disparate results. Mortality was 20% in symptomatic cases and 4% in idiopathic cases, and was less frequent with midazolam.

Rectal Diazepam in Pediatric Status Epilepticus

Rectal administration rapidly produces effective drug levels (240) and safely aborts status epilepticus in these patients (144,148). Paroxysmal activity ceased in 58% of children found to be in electrographic status epilepticus during EEG monitoring (241). Rectal diazepam was particularly effective for electrical status epilepticus during sleep and was less effective for hypsarrhythmia. Intraosseous injection rapidly produces plasma levels comparable to those from intravenous administration in animal studies (242), and is an alternative in children of suitable age when intravenous access is not available (150).

Febrile Convulsions

Rectal diazepam aborts febrile and nonfebrile seizures in the home (145). Although long-term prophylaxis for childhood febrile convulsions has been in disrepute, short-term benefits have remained unclear. A prospective trial randomized 289 Danish children to receive intermittent prophylaxis (diazepam at fever) or no prophylaxis (diazepam at seizure) (243). Twelve years later, there were no differences in intelligence quotient scores and motor or scholastic test results, as well as in neurologic outcome (likelihood of future seizures) between simple and complex febrile convulsions, suggesting that short-term prophylaxis did not differ from abbreviation of febrile convulsions and is probably not necessary. Moreover, the incidence of respiratory depression in children treated with intravenous or rectal diazepam, or both, is fairly high; 11 of 122 patients (9%) had a decrease in respiratory rate or oxygen saturation, with 8 requiring short-term ventilatory support (220).

Acute Repetitive Seizures

In a large multicenter, open-label trial in 149 patients older than 2 years of age, 77% of 1,578 administrations of rectal diazepam gel (Diastat) produced seizure freedom for the ensuing 12 hours (196). Response rates did not differ with infrequent (2 to 7) and frequent (8 to 78) administrations, suggesting that tolerance did not reduce effectiveness under these conditions. Sedation occurred in 17%. A 0.5-mg/kg dose (147) of diazepam rectal gel was also effective against serial seizures in adults with refractory epilepsy (149,195). Intramuscular injection may also be suitable for prophylaxis of serial seizures, but absorption is not rapid enough for status epilepticus. Intramuscular injection produced peak serum concentrations in 29 minutes in rhesus monkeys, with a volume of distribution of 1.5 L/kg and a clearance rate of 19 mL/min/kg (244). Intranasal administration is another alternative. In healthy human volunteers, peak serum concentrations of diazepam (2 mg) occurred 18 ± 11 minutes after intranasal administration, with a bioavailability of about 50% (153). A pharmacodynamic effect was seen at 5 minutes. In rabbits, bioavailability was 49% to 62% in the first 30 minutes after intranasal administration in a glycol solution; a pharmacodynamic response occurred within 1.5 and 3.5 minutes (245).

Chronic Epilepsies

Periodic courses of diazepam have been proposed for several chronic conditions for which current alternatives are often inadequate, including West syndrome, Lennox-Gastaut syndrome, Landau-Kleffner syndrome, and electrical status epilepticus during sleep (246). Oral doses (0.5 to 0.75 mg/kg per day) administered in cycles lasting 3 weeks, interrupted electrical status epilepticus and improved neuropsychological function in some cases.

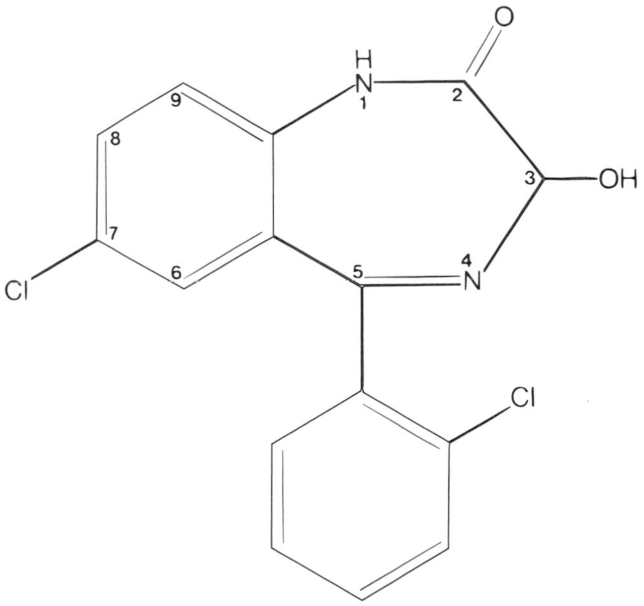

Figure 58.5 Lorazepam.

Lorazepam

With greater potency and a longer duration of action than diazepam, lorazepam (Fig. 58.5) has become the agent of choice for initial treatment of status epilepticus in adults (179). It is also less likely to produce significant respiratory depression (185) and is available in both oral and parenteral preparations.

Pharmacokinetics

Lorazepam is rapidly absorbed but is less bioavailable after oral than intravenous administration owing to enterohepatic recirculation and first-pass biotransformation in the liver (247). Peak plasma levels occur 90 to 120 minutes after oral dosing (248). Lorazepam is about 90% protein bound; cerebrospinal fluid levels are approximately equivalent to free serum levels (249). Sleep spindles on EEG recordings were observed within 30 seconds to 4 minutes after intravenous administration (250), although peak brain concentrations and maximal electroencephalographic effect did not occur until 30 minutes later (251). The volume of distribution is about 1.8 L/kg (251). After a single intravenous injection, plasma levels decrease initially owing to tissue distribution, with a $t_{1/2\alpha}$ of 2 to 3 hours. The minimal effective plasma concentration for control of status epilepticus is 30 ng/mL (252); after a 5-mg intravenous injection, plasma levels remained above that level for about 18 hours (253). Sedation, amnesia, and anxiolysis occur at plasma levels between 10 and 30 ng/mL (248).

Lorazepam is metabolized in the liver through glucuronidation at the 3-hydroxy group (254) and excreted by the kidneys (255) (Fig. 58.3). The $t_{1/2\beta}$ ranges between 8 and 25 hours (mean, 15 hours) and is the same as with oral administration (256).

Adverse Effects and Drug Interactions

Sedation, dizziness, vertigo, weakness, and unsteadiness are common; disorientation, depression, headache, sleep disturbances, agitation or restlessness, emotional disturbances, hallucinations, and delirium are less so (250,257). Impairment of psychomotor performance, dysarthria, and anterograde amnesia have also been observed. Mild respiratory depression sometimes occurs with the first intravenous dose (258). Neutropenia is rare. In a patient with Lennox-Gastaut syndrome, lorazepam precipitated tonic seizures (259). Abuse potential is relatively low. Although lorazepam is in FDA pregnancy category D, with unknown teratogenic potential, short-term use in status epilepticus may be life-saving and would likely outweigh the uncertain risks. Sudden discontinuation after long-term use has caused withdrawal seizures (260).

Valproic acid increased plasma concentrations of lorazepam (261) and decreased its clearance by 40% (262) apparently by inhibiting hepatic glucuronidation, although lorazepam does not affect valproic acid levels (261). Probenecid increased the half-life of lorazepam by inhibiting glucuronidation; toxic reactions occurred with long-term therapy (177).

Clinical Applications

Status Epilepticus

The recommended intravenous dose for status epilepticus is 0.1 mg/kg (to a maximum of 4 mg) administered at 2 mg per minute, with doses repeated after 10 to 15 minutes if necessary (184). Although less lipophilic than diazepam, lorazepam appears to cross the blood-brain barrier readily as onset of action occurred within 3 minutes in 37 cases of status epilepticus, and seizures were controlled in 89% of episodes within 10 minutes (182). In another early study, all 10 patients with generalized convulsive status epilepticus achieved control with a mean dose of 4 mg, but 9 of 11 patients with complex partial status epilepticus had problems including respiratory depression (263). Other studies have shown response rates of 80% (163) and 92% (258). Similar successes were achieved against simple partial status epilepticus (112,258). The Veterans Affairs Cooperative Status Epilepticus Trial demonstrated the superiority of lorazepam (0.1 mg/kg) to phenytoin (18 mg/kg) as initial therapy (64.9% versus 43.6%), with slightly better results for lorazepam than for diazepam (0.15 mg/kg) (184). Intravenous lorazepam (4 mg) was effective against postanoxic myoclonic status epilepticus after cardiac arrest in six patients (264). Continuous EEG monitoring during treatment is advisable, as electroclinical dissociation has been observed.

Pediatric Status Epilepticus

The usual intravenous dose is 0.05 mg/kg, repeated twice at intervals of 15 to 20 minutes (112,185). In 31 children 2 to 18 years of age, 0.05 mg/kg, repeated up to three times at 15-minute intervals terminated seizure activity in 81%

(258). Doses of 0.1 mg/kg in children and 0.07 mg/kg in adolescents terminated seizures of partial status epilepticus in 90% of patients (112). Prior treatment of status epilepticus with phenytoin, phenobarbital, or diazepam did not alter the effectiveness of lorazepam, although long-term use of clonazepam or clorazepate significantly reduced the effectiveness of lorazepam (112), indicating tolerance. When observed, respiratory depression occurred after the first injection.

Lorazepam was effective in neonatal seizures refractory to phenobarbital or phenytoin, or both. In seven neonates (gestational ages 30 to 43 weeks), 0.05 mg/kg controlled seizures within 5 minutes; 71.4% had no recurrence and the remaining patients had at least 8 hours of control (265). No respiratory depression or other adverse effects were reported. Status epilepticus in six of seven neonates was terminated with 0.05 to 0.14 mg/kg (266).

Pediatric Serial Seizures

Sublingual lorazepam (1 to 4 mg) was effective in 80% (8 of 10) and partially effective in 20% (2 of 10) of children. Clinical effect began within 15 minutes in most cases (267).

Alcohol Withdrawal Seizures

Lorazepam (2 mg) administered after a witnessed ethanol withdrawal seizure prevented a second seizure better than placebo (3% recurrence versus 24%, $p < 0.001$) and may be the agent of choice (268).

Chronic Epilepsy

Lorazepam was effective as adjunctive treatment of complex partial seizures, with an optimal dose of 5 mg/day after slow titration from 1 mg twice daily (199). Therapeutic levels ranged from 20 to 30 ng/mL. Long-term use is likely to result in tolerance and is not generally recommended.

Midazolam

Midazolam (Fig. 58.6) is a 1,4-benzodiazepine widely used for induction of anesthesia or as a preanesthetic agent. Three to four times as potent as diazepam, midazolam, either intravenously or intramuscularly, can be used in acute treatment of status epilepticus, although its short duration of action necessitates continuous intravenous maintenance or subsequent addition of another anticonvulsant. A 10-mg intramuscular injection reduced interictal spike frequency on EEG recordings similarly to 20 mg of intravenous diazepam (269), and this route is an alternative when intravenous access is unavailable.

Pharmacokinetics

Midazolam is water soluble, but at physiologic pH a conformational change in the benzodiazepine ring makes it lipid soluble (270). Serum levels after intravenous administration were best fit by a two-compartment model, with an initial tissue distribution phase (5.7 ± 2.4 minutes) and

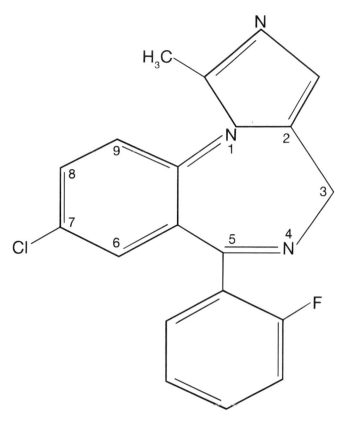

Figure 58.6 Midazolam.

an elimination phase (66 ± 37 minutes) (212). After intravenous administration of 15 to 60 mg over 5 minutes to eight healthy adult volunteers, plasma concentration for a half-maximal increase in β-frequency activity on electroencephalography was 276 ± 64 μmol/L (271). Serum concentration peaked 25 ± 23 minutes after an intramuscular injection (272). Bioavailability was 44 ± 17% after oral administration (212), ranged from 50% (273) to 83% (274) after intranasal use, was 52% after rectal administration (275), and 74.5% after buccal administration (151). Midazolam is 95 ± 2% protein bound, with a volume of distribution of 1.1 ± 0.6 L/kg and a half-life ranging from 1.9 ± 0.6 hours (212,276) to 2.8 ± 1.7 hours (272). The clearance rate is 6.6 ± 1.8 mL/min/kg, with 56 ± 26% urinary excretion.

In children 1 to 5 years of age, $t_{1/2\beta}$ of 0.2 mg/kg was 2.2 hours by the intranasal and 2.4 hours by the intravenous route (277). In critically ill neonates, the $t_{1/2\beta}$ after intravenous administration was 12.0 hours (278). The volume of distribution (3.1 L/kg) and $t_{1/2\beta}$ (5.4 hours) were significantly greater in adult intensive care patients than in healthy volunteers (0.9 L/kg and 2.3 hours) (279), although clearance did not differ significantly (6.3 versus 4.9 mL/min/kg).

Midazolam is metabolized rapidly by α-hydroxylation of the methyl group on the fused imidazole ring (Figs. 58.3 and 58.6) (270). The α-hydroxylated compound is biologically active but is eliminated with a half-life of about 1 hour after hepatic conjugation with glucuronic acid (280).

Adverse Effects and Drug Interactions

Dose-dependent sedation may be prolonged after continuous infusion despite the short half-life (281); retrograde amnesia, euphoria, confusion, and dysarthria also occur. Midazolam syrup has been associated with respiratory depression and arrest and should be given only where resuscitative drugs, equipment, and experienced personnel are immediately available. Paradoxical agitation, tremor, involuntary movements, hyperactivity, and combativeness affect about 2%; seizures and nystagmus, about 1%. Nausea (87%) and vomiting (4%) occur with midazolam syrup but are far less common with intravenous administration. Hypotension and decreased cardiac output probably result from peripheral vasodilation (270). Sudden discontinuation after long-term use can lead to withdrawal seizures (282). Midazolam is in pregnancy risk category D.

Erythromycin may prolong the half-life of midazolam to 10 to 20 hours (283). Phenytoin and carbamazepine reduce the bioavailability of oral midazolam by inducing CYP450, which enhances first-pass hepatic metabolism (284).

Clinical Applications

Status Epilepticus

Midazolam 0.2 mg/kg by slow bolus injection, followed by a maintenance infusion of 0.75 to 10 μg/kg per minute, has been recommended for treatment of refractory status epilepticus (179,285), terminating seizures within 100 seconds in seven patients in whom diazepam, lorazepam, and phenytoin with or without phenobarbital had failed (286). In general, patients should be intubated and receiving ventilatory support, as well as EEG and hemodynamic monitoring. The infusion is maintained for 12 hours and slowly tapered during continuous EEG monitoring; if seizure activity returns, the infusion is resumed for additional 12-hour periods. Tolerance may develop, and doses up to 2 mg/kg per hour have been required for control (285). Intramuscular midazolam 0.2 mg/kg has been successful in several small series (287,288). Advantages over other benzodiazepines include rapid onset of action, ease of administration and titration (with the possibility of initial intramuscular injection [287]), efficacy, and lack of serious adverse effects (285).

Pediatric Status Epilepticus

Midazolam (0.15-mg/kg bolus followed by 1- to 5-μg/kg per minute infusion) alone or with phenytoin or phenobarbital controlled status epilepticus in 19 of 20 children (mean age, 4 years) (289). In eight patients (ages 17 days to 16 years) with refractory disease treated with midazolam coma for more than 48 hours, the average dose for seizure cessation was 14 μg/kg per minute and mean duration of therapy was 192 hours; one patient could not be successfully weaned and died after 4 weeks. Midazolam was well tolerated and stopped seizures in 95% of 20 children (mean age, 4 years) (291). Intravenous midazolam

(0.1 to 0.3 mg/kg loading dose, followed by an average infusion of 2.7 μg/kg per minute for 12 hours to 6 days) was a safe and effective first-line therapy for 15 of 16 episodes in 10 children (20 months to 16 years) (292). Midazolam was also useful as a second-, third-, or fourth-line drug, controlling 34 of 38 episodes. In six neonates (1 to 9 days, 30 to 41 weeks' gestational age) 0.1 to 0.4 mg/kg per hour controlled overt seizures refractory to high-dose phenobarbital (with or without phenytoin) within 1 hour (293); electrographic seizures continued in two patients for another 12 hours. Pulse and blood pressure did not change, and no adverse reactions occurred.

Febrile Seizures

In a prospective, randomized study of 47 children, intranasal midazolam was as effective as intravenous diazepam, with shorter mean times to starting treatment and controlling seizures (3.5 versus 5.5 minutes) (155).

Pediatric Acute Repetitive Seizures

A comparison of intramuscular midazolam and intravenous diazepam for seizures lasting longer than 10 minutes found similar efficacy, although the midazolam group received medication sooner and their seizures ended sooner (294). In 26 children in the home or hospital, intranasal midazolam stopped seizures in an average of 3.6 minutes; 98% stopped within 10 minutes (295). A randomized single-site trial in 5- to 19-year-old children with Lennox-Gastaut syndrome or other symptomatic generalized epilepsies showed that midazolam (10 mg in 2 mL) administered around the buccal mucosa stopped 75% of 40 seizures, compared with 59% of 39 seizures stopped by rectal diazepam (10 mg) (152). The time to end of seizure was comparable in the two groups, and no cardiorespiratory adverse events occurred.

Clonazepam

Uniquely among the benzodiazepines, clonazepam (Fig. 58.7) is used primarily as an anticonvulsant and may be administered to treat both acute seizures and chronic epilepsy. It is effective in several types of status epilepticus (296), but is available in the United States only as an oral preparation.

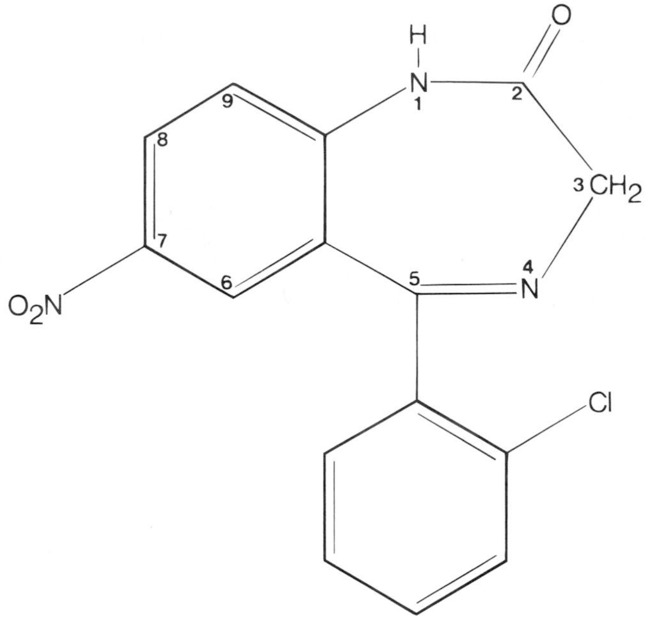

Pharmacokinetics

The $t_{1/2\alpha}$ after intravenous injection has not been studied. Absorption is 81% to 98% after oral administration; peak plasma levels occur in 1 to 4 hours (6). Clonazepam is highly lipid soluble but has relatively low plasma protein binding (86%) compared with diazepam (157). The volume of distribution is 1.5 to 4.4 L/kg (6), higher than that of diazepam or lorazepam. Primary metabolism occurs through reduction of the nitro group to form inactive 7-amino-clonazepam, which is conjugated to glucuronide and excreted by the kidneys (6). Plasma half-lives were

Figure 58.7 Clonazepam.

fairly similar in single- and multiple-dose studies, with respective ranges of 18.7 to 39 hours and 31 to 42 hours, suggesting relatively little hepatic enzyme induction (6).

Adverse Effects and Drug Interactions

Drowsiness and lethargy affect about 50% of adult patients initially, but tolerance to these symptoms occurs with continued administration (297). Up to 85% of children experienced drowsiness, which, with other side effects, necessitated drug termination in 27% (6). Respiratory and cardiovascular depression can accompany intravenous use. Nystagmus is fairly common; incoordination, ataxia, hypotonia, dysarthria, and dizziness, less so. Behavior disturbances including aggression, hyperactivity, and paranoia can be seen in up to 12% of children (298). Seizure frequency is sometimes increased, and seizures (299) or status epilepticus (300) can occur with abrupt withdrawal. Increased bronchial secretions, anorexia, or hyperphagia are possible. A "burning mouth syndrome" with painful oral dysesthesias has been described (301). Clonazepam induced obstructive sleep apnea in a narcoleptic patient (302).

Clinical Applications

Status Epilepticus

Intravenous injection of 0.01 to 0.09 mg/kg terminates most cases of status epilepticus (6), and a single 1-mg dose controlled various types of status epilepticus in 80% of 145 adults (303). Treatment succeeded as well in generalized convulsive status epilepticus (296). That study and one using oral clonazepam in children defined minimum effective plasma level as 30 ng/mL (163). In patients with absence status epilepticus, including 48 adults, 1 to 4 mg was effective in 83.3% (305).

Clonazepam was compared with lorazepam in an open-label study in 50 adults with various epilepsies (306). Clinical improvement of at least 75% occurred in 68% of lorazepam patients and in 69% of clonazepam patients. However, neither diazepam nor clonazepam was effective for status epilepticus in an open-label study of 55 patients with symptomatic generalized epilepsy, primarily Lennox-Gastaut syndrome (303).

Pediatric Status Epilepticus

Clonazepam was administered to 17 children between 2 weeks and 15 years of age, 14 of whom had generalized clonic convulsions (296). A single intravenous bolus of 0.25 mg was repeated as needed to a maximum of 0.75 mg; doses ranged from 0.01 to 0.09 mg/kg. Status epilepticus terminated in all patients. Mean clonazepam levels were 185 ng/mL 10 minutes after seizure termination and 43 ng/mL at 30 minutes, with status epilepticus still controlled. The mean drug level at seizure recurrence in eight patients was 5.1 ng/mL.

Chronic Epilepsy

The dose in children is 0.01 to 0.02 mg/kg per day and in adults may range up to 8 mg per day in two or three divided doses. A linear relationship exists between the dose and plasma concentration in children (307), with approximately 0.07 mg/kg likely to produce a serum concentration of about 40 ng/mL (304). Absence seizures were well controlled in 10 children at plasma levels of 13 to 72 ng/mL (304). Correlation between plasma levels and efficacy is relatively poor (6,307), however, owing to the development of tolerance to antiseizure effects (308). Children require higher doses than adults to maintain equivalent concentrations as a result of a higher relative clearance. Because of rapid absorption and elimination, children should receive the total daily dose in thirds (6). Clonazepam can be safely discontinued with a dosage reduction at 0.04 mg/kg per week (309).

Severe Childhood Epilepsies

Although clonazepam is effective against a variety of seizure types, side effects limit its use to the most difficult epileptic conditions. Lasting improvement occurred in 5 of 24 patients with infantile spasms and in 3 of 13 patients with Lennox-Gastaut syndrome treated with doses of 0.1 to 0.3 mg/kg per day (310). Similarly, complete control was achieved in approximately one-third of 42 cases of infantile spasms and 37 cases of Lennox-Gastaut syndrome (311).

Myoclonic Seizures

Clonazepam is effective against myoclonic atonic seizures (312), myoclonic seizures (313), Unverricht-Lundborg myoclonic epilepsy (314), and intention myoclonus (315).

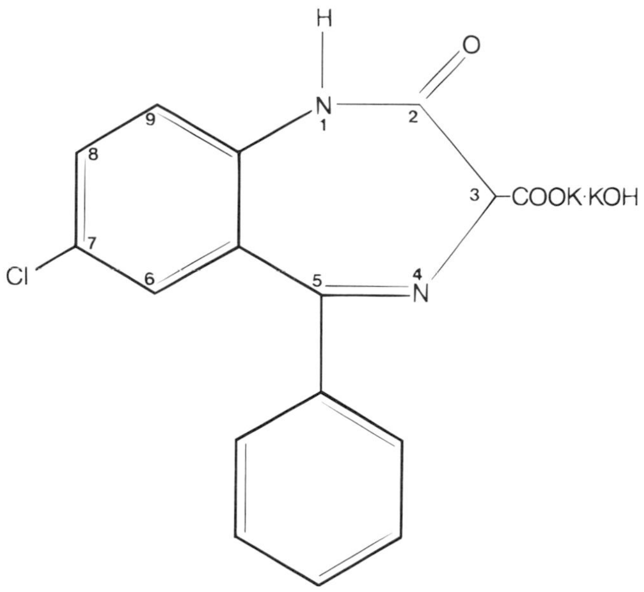

Figure 58.8 Clorazepate.

Hyperekplexia (316), acute intermittent porphyria (317), epilepsy with continuous spike-and-wave during slow-wave sleep (318), and neonatal seizures (319) have also responded.

Clorazepate

Used in adjunctive treatment of anxiety and alcohol withdrawal, clorazepate (Fig. 58.8) in epilepsy is limited to adjunctive therapy for refractory generalized or partial seizure disorders, particularly with comorbid anxiety disorders.

Pharmacokinetics

Available as a dipotassium salt, clorazepate is a prodrug that is rapidly converted to DMD, the same major active metabolite of diazepam (Fig. 58.4). Nonenzymatic decarboxylation at position 3 occurs at gastric pH, with 90% of clorazepate converted to DMD in less than 10 minutes. Conversion of absorbed drug to DMD continues more slowly in the blood. DMD is responsible for most of clorazepate's anticonvulsant effect. Bioavailability is 100% by the intramuscular route (320) and 91% (as DMD) by oral ingestion (321). Clorazepate and DMD are 97% to 98% protein bound. The time to peak DMD concentration is 0.7 to 1.5 hours, with peak response in 1 to 2.5 hours (322). Volume of distribution ranged from 0.9 to 1.5 L/kg and was greater in the elderly and the obese (323). The $t_{1/2\beta}$ for clorazepate is 2.3 hours; the 46-hour half-life of DMD (324) in elderly men and neonates (325) likely reflects impaired oxidation of DMD. DMD is further metabolized by hydroxylation to clinically active oxazepam (Fig. 58.3) (213), conjugated to glucuronic acid in the liver (214), and excreted by the kidneys, with a $t_{1/2\beta}$ of 1 to 2 days (167). As with diazepam, drugs and conditions that alter hepatic metabolism can dramatically affect the metabolism and clearance of clorazepate, DMD, and oxazepam.

Adverse Effects and Drug Interactions

Clorazepate reportedly produces less sedation than other benzodiazepine anticonvulsants, although that is still its most common side effect (326). Dizziness, ataxia, nervousness, and confusion are less often seen. Memory problems, difficulty in concentration, irritability, and depression occur in association with primidone (327). Paradoxical akathisia was reported in two patients with head trauma and seizure disorders (328). Personality changes with aggressive behavior, irritability, rage, or depression have been described (329) but may have resulted from the suppression of epileptic activity in patients with temporal lobe epilepsy (330). Hepatotoxic reactions and transient skin rashes have been noted. Withdrawal symptoms after long-term use include nervousness, insomnia, irritability, diarrhea, muscle aches, and memory impairment. Clorazepate is in pregnancy category D and has been linked to major malformations in one infant born to a mother who took the drug during the first trimester (332).

Clinical Applications

The recommended initial dose for adjunctive treatment of epilepsy is 7.5 mg three times daily (0.3 mg/kg per day), with slow increases as required, to a maximum daily dose of 90 mg (about 1 mg/kg per day) in adults and up to 3 mg/kg per day in children (326). Rapid absorption and bioconversion to DMD require twice-daily to three-times-daily dosing to avoid toxic reactions despite the long $t_{1/2\beta}$ (171). A sustained-release preparation (Tranxene-SD) delivers 22.5 mg in a single daily dose. Plasma DMD levels of 0.5 to 1.9 mg/mL may represent the therapeutic range (212). Clorazepate has not been particularly effective in prolonged treatment of any seizure type.

In 61 patients, clorazepate as adjunctive therapy slightly improved control of refractory seizures, with minimal adverse effects but no improvement on electroencephalography (333). A double-blind study that added clorazepate or phenobarbital to phenytoin reported no difference in seizure control, but patients preferred clorazepate (334). In another adjunctive trial, 12 of 31 patients with refractory epilepsy improved with clorazepate, but almost half complained of drowsiness (335). Ineffective as monotherapy, clorazepate as adjunctive therapy improved control in 59 patients with various seizure disorders (336). Refractory generalized seizures were controlled in 11 children (ages 3 to 17 years), but recurred in three, probably because of tolerance (337).

Clobazam

Clobazam (Fig. 58.9) has become the most widely used benzodiazepine for the long-term treatment of epilepsy because of effectiveness and relatively low tendency to produce sedation (338), despite a trend toward tolerance.

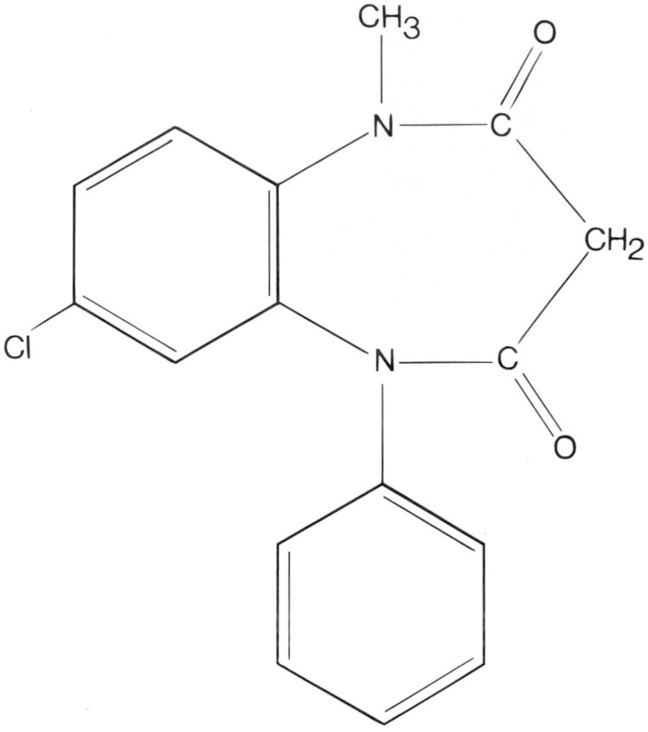

Figure 58.9 Clobazam.

After carbamazepine and phenytoin, clobazam is the third most common anticonvulsant in posttemporal lobectomy patients (339). The Canadian Study Group for Childhood Epilepsy (340) found clobazam to be effective as monotherapy in children. It is not available in the United States.

Pharmacokinetics

Clobazam is the only 1,5-benzodiazepine used clinically as an anticonvulsant. Despite a methyl group at position 1, binding affinity and potency are relatively low (Table 58.1). Peak concentrations occur in 1 to 4 hours; clobazam is highly lipid soluble and 85% protein bound.

N-desmethylclobazam, the major metabolite, is the primary anticonvulsant component in patients undergoing long-term therapy. The mean $t_{1/2\beta}$ is 18 hours for clobazam and 42 hours for the metabolite. Long-term exposure induces hepatic enzymes, leading to more rapid conversion to N-desmethylclobazam (341). Plasma levels of clobazam and N-desmethylclobazam correlated with both effect and toxicity, but therapeutic levels have not been established, probably because of the active metabolite or the development of tolerance (342).

Adverse Effects and Drug Interactions

Clobazam may have fewer or milder side effects than other benzodiazepines at equipotent doses (7,343). Psychomotor performance was not impaired after 30 mg, unlike after the 1,4-benzodiazepines nitrazepam (15 mg) and chlordiazepoxide (30 mg) (344). Levels of N-desmethylclobazam were correlated with side effects, however (345). In epileptic patients, drowsiness and fatigue predominate (341). Ataxia was described in 4 of 23 open-label studies, dizziness in 19 of 23, and vertigo in 2 of 23 studies (341). Memory disturbance, aggressiveness, dysphoria, and illusional and psychotic symptoms are relatively infrequent. An association with blurred vision has been noted; negative myoclonus occurred in addition to carbamazepine (346). Tolerance occurs with clobazam as with the 1,4-benzodiazepines (347). Seizure activity can increase on discontinuation (348).

Clinical Applications
Doses range from 10 to 50 mg per day; most studies used 10 to 30 mg per day in one or two doses. In the Canadian Clobazam Cooperative Group trial of 877 patients, the average dose was 30.8 mg in adults, and 0.86 mg/kg in children (349).

Clobazam is effective against all seizure types (350), but the benefits may be short-lived. In the Canadian study, more than 40% of patients with a single seizure type had at least a 50% or greater reduction in seizure frequency, and 60% of patients with multiple seizure types had improvement in at least one type (349). About a third had drowsiness, but this caused discontinuation in only 11%. About 9% discontinued because of seizure recurrence, thought to represent tolerance. Clobazam may be particularly useful in Lennox-Gastaut syndrome (338), but tolerance prevents its being the first choice in most epilepsies (343). Intermittent use in catamenial epilepsy apparently avoided tolerance to the anticonvulsant effect (198).

Despite reports of rapid tolerance, 40% to 50% of patients in the Canadian study (351) remained on clobazam for 4 years or longer. A seizure reduction exceeding 75% with the addition of clobazam was likely to be sustained if the epilepsy was not long-standing and had a known cause (351).

Nitrazepam

This benzodiazepine derivative (Fig. 58.10), with a nitro group at the 7 position of the benzodiazepine ring (Fig. 58.1), has been used as a hypnotic and anticonvulsant, for infantile spasms, and as adjunctive therapy for severe generalized epilepsies of childhood. Nitrazepam may be particularly effective against myoclonic seizures.

Pharmacokinetics
After oral ingestion, bioavailability is approximately 78% (352); peak concentration occurs in 1.4 hours (353). Nitrazepam is 85% to 88% protein bound (354); volume of distribution is 2.4 L/kg in healthy young adults, somewhat larger in the elderly and in women (352). In the first 24 hours after dosing, cerebrospinal fluid levels were 8% to 11% of plasma levels, with a cerebrospinal fluid $t_{1/2\beta}$ of 68 hours compared with 27 hours in plasma (352,355).

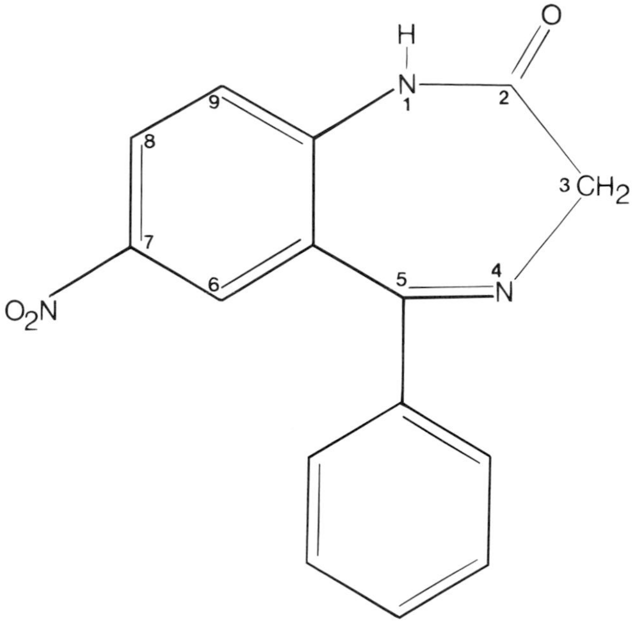

Figure 58.10 Nitrazepam.

Metabolism occurs in the liver by nitro reduction to the inactive aromatic amine 7-aminonitrazepam, followed by acetylation to 7-acetoamidonitrazepam (also inactive; Fig. 58.3) (356). Nitrazepam does not induce its own metabolism. Excretion occurs in both urine (45% to 65%) and feces (14% to 20%), with a portion apparently bound in tissues for prolonged periods (357). Metabolism is slowed in patients with hypothyroidism (358) and obesity (359).

Adverse Effects and Drug Interactions
Like most benzodiazepines, nitrazepam can produce disorientation, confusion, and drowsiness, particularly in the elderly (354). Generalized mental deterioration with dementia, inability to walk, and incontinence was observed in a 75-year-old woman; symptoms resolved on discontinuation (360). Hypotonia (357), ataxia, and driving difficulty have occurred (361), as have vivid nightmares at the onset of therapy (362). Drowsiness may be minimized by gradual upward titration from a low dose (229). Drooling and aspiration in children (363,364) were apparently caused by impaired swallowing (364); a dose less than 0.8 mg/kg per day should prevent this complication and the resulting aspiration pneumonia (364). Single 5- to 10-mg oral doses for sedation led to respiratory depression in elderly patients being treated for respiratory failure (365). Teratogenic risk, particularly oral clefts (227), is increased. More frequent seizures and new seizure types are sometimes seen (366). Tolerance can develop with long-term use. Withdrawal symptoms have included delirium (367), involuntary movements, paresthesias, confusion (207), persistent tinnitus, and opisthotonos (368).

Nitrazepam is a pregnancy category C drug. Infants born to mothers taking nitrazepam late in pregnancy have been somnolent, floppy, and poorly responsive and have required tube feeding but recovered in several days (369).

Nitrazepam appears to increase the risk of death in young patients with intractable epilepsy. In a retrospective analysis of treatment lasting from 3 days to 10 years, 21 of 302 patients died; 14 were taking nitrazepam at the time of death (370). In children younger than 3.4 years of age, the death rate was 3.98 per 100 patient-years, compared with 0.26 deaths in patients not taking nitrazepam. Nitrazepam had a slight protective effect in patients older than 3.4 years of age; death rates were 0.50 with nitrazepam and 0.86 in patients not taking the drug. Extreme caution should accompany its use in children younger than 4 years of age.

Clinical Applications

Nitrazepam is not available in the United States; in other countries, the usual daily dose is 1 mg/kg for children and 0.5 mg/kg for adults. Initial doses of 1 to 6 mg daily, with gradual increases up to 60 mg daily, have been used in pediatric seizure disorders (371–373). In 44 children enjoying satisfactory seizure control, an average dose of 0.27 mg/kg per day yielded a mean plasma concentration of 114 ng/mL (354). Levels above 220 ng/mL were likely to be toxic.

Nitrazepam was particularly effective for infantile spasms, myoclonic seizures, and Lennox-Gastaut syndrome (371,373,374). An initial daily dose of 1 to 6 mg, followed by maintenance with 0.3 to 1.1 mg/kg per day, reduced the number of daily seizures from 17.7 to 7.2 in 36 infants and children (3 months to 12 years of age) (373). Complete control of various seizure types was obtained in seven of 31 mentally retarded children (2 months to 15 years of age) and moderate control in 10; myoclonic seizures were controlled best (375).

Febrile Convulsions

Nitrazepam 0.25 to 0.5 mg/kg per day administered three times daily during fever was effective in prophylaxis (376).

Infantile Spasms and Lennox-Gastaut Syndrome

In 52 patients (1 to 24 months old) with infantile spasms and hypsarrhythmia on electroencephalography, nitrazepam (0.2 to 0.4 mg/kg per day in two divided doses) and corticotropin (40 U intramuscularly daily) were similar in efficacy and incidence of adverse effects (377). Both regimens reduced seizure frequency by 75% to 100% in 50% to 60% of patients. Of 20 children (4 to 28 months old) with infantile spasms or early Lennox-Gastaut syndrome who were treated with nitrazepam (median dose, 1.5 mg/kg per day), 5 had complete cessation of seizures, 7 had a more than 50% seizure reduction, and 8 had no response (378). Twelve children experienced pooling of oral secretions and six became sedated, but no serious side effects were reported.

FUTURE DIRECTIONS: NEW STRATEGIES FOR THE BENZODIAZEPINES

Partial benzodiazepine agonists (abecarnil, bretazenil, imidazenil) may retain anticonvulsant efficacy but be less likely to produce tolerance; their utility in human epilepsy has not been adequately explored. Therapy combining a full agonist with a partial agonist or antagonist (flumazenil), or intermittent use during periods of higher seizure risk (e.g., catamenial epilepsy), might prevent tolerance and provide new strategies for benzodiazepine use. Novel routes of administration by way of the nasal, buccal, or rectal mucosa are less invasive ways to use benzodiazepines acutely in the outpatient setting. Another novel approach is to use benzodiazepines in a device capable of detecting seizure discharges and injecting the drug at the onset of seizure activity locally onto the epileptic focus, into the cerebral ventricles, or systemically. A model for this device in rats showed decreases in seizure frequency and duration when diazepam rather than vehicle was injected onto a bicuculline-created seizure focus (379). Such innovations may expand the future role of benzodiazepines in the treatment of status epilepticus, serial seizures, and epilepsy.

REFERENCES

1. Sternbach LH. Chemistry of the 1,4-benzodiazepines and some aspects of the structure-activity relationship. In: Garattini S, Mussini R, Randall LO, eds. *The benzodiazepines.* New York: Raven Press, 1973:1–26.
2. Sternbach LH, Reeder E. Quinazolines and 1,4-benzodiazepines, IV: transformations of 7-chloro-2-methylamino-5-phenyl-^{3}H-1,4-benzodiazepine-4-oxide. *J Org Chem* 1961;26: 4936–4941.
3. Sternbach LH, Fryer RI, Keller O, et al. Quinazolines and 1,4-benzodiazepines, X: nitro-substituted 5-phenyl-1,4-benzodiazepine derivatives. *J Med Chem* 1963;6:261–265.
4. Gastaut H, Naquet R, Poire R, et al. Treatment of status epilepticus with diazepam (Valium). *Epilepsia* 1965;6:167–182.
5. Naquet R, Soulayrol R, Dolce G, et al. First attempt at treatment of experimental status epilepticus in animals and spontaneous status epilepticus in man with diazepam (Valium). *Electroencephalogr Clin Neurophysiol* 1965;18:4–27.
6. Sato S. Benzodiazepines, clonazepam. In: Levy RH, Mattson RH, Meldrum BS, eds. *Antiepileptic drugs,* 4th ed. New York: Raven Press, 1995:725–734.
7. Chapman AG, Horton RW, Meldrum BS. Anticonvulsant action of a 1,5-benzodiazepine, clobazam, in reflex epilepsy. *Epilepsia* 1978;19:293–299.
8. Robertson MM. Current status of the 1,4- and 1,5-benzodiazepines in the treatment of epilepsy: the place of clobazam. *Epilepsia* 1986;27(Suppl 1):S27–S41.
9. Braestrup C, Squires RF. Specific benzodiazepine receptors in rat brain characterized by high-affinity [^{3}H]diazepam binding. *Proc Natl Acad Sci U S A* 1977;74:3805–3809.
10. Mohler H, Okada T. Benzodiazepine receptor: demonstration in the central nervous system. *Science* 1977;198:849–851.
11. Macdonald R, Barker JL. Benzodiazepines specifically modulate GABA-mediated postsynaptic inhibition in cultured mammalian neurones. *Nature* 1978;271:563–564.
12. Macdonald RL, Olsen RW. GABA$_A$ receptor channels. *Annu Rev Neurosci* 1994;17:569–602.
13. Gastaut H, Low MD. Antiepileptic properties of clobazam, a 1,5-benzodiazepine, in man. *Epilepsia* 1979;20:437–446.

14. Braestrup C, Squires RF. Pharmacological characterization of benzodiazepine receptors in the brain. *Eur J Pharmacol* 1978;48: 263–270.
15. Mohler H, Okada T, Heitz P, et al. Biochemical identification of the site of action of benzodiazepines in human brain by ^{3}H-diazepam binding. *Life Sci* 1978;22:985–995.
16. Sieghart W, Schuster A. Affinity of various ligands for benzodiazepine receptors in rat cerebellum and hippocampus. *Biochem Pharmacol* 1984;33:4033–4038.
17. Gross JB, Blouin RT, Zandsberg S. Effect of flumazenil on ventilatory drive during sedation with midazolam and alfentanil. *Anesthesiology* 1996;85:713–720.
18. Shannon M, Albers G, Burkhardt K. Safety and efficacy of flumazenil in the reversal of benzodiazepine-induced conscious sedation. *J Pediatr* 1997;131:582–586.
19. Mullins ME. First-degree atrioventricular block in alprazolam overdose reversed by flumazenil. *J Pharm Pharmacol* 1999;51:367–370.
20. Turski L, Stephens DN, Jensen LH, et al. Anticonvulsant action of the beta-carboline abecarnil: studies in rodents and baboon, *Papio papio*. *J Pharmacol Exp Ther* 1990;253:344–352.
21. Zanotti A, Mariot R, Contarino A, et al. Lack of anticonvulsant tolerance and benzodiazepine receptor downregulation with imidazenil in rats. *Br J Pharmacol* 1996;117:647–652.
22. Rundfeldt C, Wlaz P, Honack D, et al. Anticonvulsant tolerance and withdrawal characteristics of benzodiazepine receptor ligands in different seizure models in mice. Comparison of diazepam, bretazenil and abecarnil. *J Pharmacol Exp Ther* 1995; 275:693–702.
23. Natolino F, Zanotti A, Contarino A, et al. Abecarnil, a beta-carboline derivative, does not exhibit anticonvulsant tolerance or withdrawal effects in mice. *Naunyn Schmiedebergs Arch Pharmacol* 1996;354:612–617.
24. Hernandez TD, Heninger C, Wilson MA, et al. Relationship of agonist efficacy to changes in GABA sensitivity and anticonvulsant tolerance following chronic benzodiazepine ligand exposure. *Eur J Pharmacol* 1989;170:145–155.
25. Haefely W, Kyburz E, Gerecke M, et al. Recent advances in the molecular pharmacology of benzodiazepine receptors and in the structure-activity relationships of their agonists and antagonists. *Adv Drug Res* 1985;14:165–322.
26. Polc P. Electrophysiology of benzodiazepine receptor ligands: multiple mechanisms and sites of action. *Prog Neurobiol* 1988;31:349–423.
27. Randall LO, Kappell B. Pharmacological activity of some benzodiazepines and their metabolites. In: Garattini S, Mussini E, Randall LO, eds. *The benzodiazepines*. New York: Raven Press, 1973:27–51.
28. Rogawski MA, Porter RJ. Antiepileptic drugs: pharmacological mechanisms and clinical efficacy with consideration of promising developmental stage compounds. *Pharmacol Rev* 1990;42: 223–286.
29. Swinyard EA, Castellion AW. Anticonvulsant properties of some benzodiazepines. *J Pharmacol Exp Ther* 1966;151:369–375.
30. Albertson TE, Stark LG, Derlet RW. Modification of amygdaloid kindling by diazepam in juvenile rats. *Brain Res Dev Brain Res* 1990;51:249–252.
31. Amano K, Takamatsu J, Ogata A, et al. Effect of dipotassium clorazepate on amygdaloid-kindling and comparison between amygdaloid- and hippocampal-kindled seizures. *Eur J Pharmacol* 1999;385:111–117.
32. Goddard GV, McIntyre DC, Leech CK. A permanent change in brain function resulting from daily electrical stimulation. *Exp Neurol* 1969;25:295–330.
33. Karobath M, Sperk G. Stimulation of benzodiazepine receptor binding by γ-aminobutyric acid. *Proc Natl Acad Sci U S A* 1979; 76:1004–1006.
34. Siegel E, Mamalaki C, Barnard EA. Isolation of a GABA receptor from bovine brain using a benzodiazepine affinity column. *FEBS Lett* 1982;147:45–48.
35. Martini C, Rigacci T, Lucacchini A. [^{3}H]Muscimol binding site on purified benzodiazepine receptor. *J Neurochem* 1983;41: 1183–1185.
36. Study RE, Barker JL. Diazepam and (−)-pentobarbital: fluctuation analysis reveals different mechanisms for potentiation of γ-aminobutyric acid responses in cultured central neurons. *Proc Natl Acad Sci U S A* 1981;78:7180–7184.
37. Rogers CJ, Twyman RE, Macdonald RL. Benzodiazepine and beta-carboline regulation of single GABA$_A$ receptor channels of mouse spinal neurones in culture. *J Physiol (Lond)* 1994; 475:69–82.
38. Twyman RE, Rogers CJ, Macdonald RL. Differential regulation of γ-aminobutyric acid receptor channels by diazepam and phenobarbital. *Ann Neurol* 1989;25:213–220.
39. Maconochie DJ, Zempel JM, Steinbach JH. How quickly can GABA$_A$ receptors open? *Neuron* 1994;12:61–71.
40. Jones MV, Westbrook GL. Desensitized states prolong GABA$_A$ channel responses to brief agonist pulses. *Neuron* 1995;15:181–191.
41. Edwards FA, Konnerth A, Sakmann B. Quantal analysis of inhibitory synaptic transmission in the dentate gyrus of rat hippocampal slices: a patch-clamp study. *J Physiol (Lond)* 1990; 430:213–249.
42. Puia G, Costa E, Vicini S. Functional diversity of GABA-activated Cl$^-$ currents in Purkinje versus granule neurons in rat cerebellar slices. *Neuron* 1994;12:117–126.
43. Otis TS, Mody I. Modulation of decay kinetics and frequency of GABA$_A$ receptor-mediated spontaneous inhibitory post-synaptic currents in hippocampal neurons. *Proc Natl Acad Sci U S A* 1992;78:7180–7184.
44. Mody I, De Doninck Y, Otis TS, et al. Bridging the cleft at GABA synapses in the brain. *Trends Neurosci* 1994;17:517–525.
45. Treiman DM. GABAergic mechanisms in epilepsy. *Epilepsia* 2001;42(Suppl 3):8–12.
46. Olsen RW, Wamsley JK, McCabe RT, et al. Benzodiazepine/gamma-aminobutyric acid receptor deficit in the midbrain of the seizure-susceptible gerbil. *Proc Natl Acad Sci U S A* 1985;82: 6701–6705.
47. Kokaia M, Pratt GD, Elmer E, et al. Biphasic differential changes of GABA$_A$ receptor subunit mRNA levels in dentate gyrus granule cells following recurrent kindling-induced seizures. *Mol Brain Res* 1994;23:323–332.
48. Brooks-Kayal AR, Shumate MD, Jin H, et al. Selective changes in single cell GABA$_A$ receptor subunit expression and function in temporal lobe epilepsy. *Nature Med* 1998;4:1166–1172.
49. Loup F, Weiser HG, Yonekawa Y, et al. Selective alterations in GABA$_A$ receptor subtypes in human temporal lobe epilepsy. *J Neurosci* 2000;20:5401–5419.
50. DeLorey TM, Handforth A, Anagnostaras SG, et al. Mice lacking the beta3 subunit of the GABA$_A$ receptor have the epilepsy phenotype and many of the behavioral characteristics of Angelman syndrome. *J Neurosci* 1998;18:8505–8514.
51. Matsumoto A, Kumagai T, Miura K, et al. Epilepsy in Angelman syndrome associated with chromosome 15q deletion. *Epilepsia* 1992;33:1083–1090.
52. Bianchi MT, Song L, Zhang H, et al. Two different mechanisms of disinhibition produced by GABA$_A$ receptor mutations linked to epilepsy in humans. *J Neurosci* 2002;22:5321–5327.
53. Baulac S, Huberfeld G, Gourfinkel-An I, et al. First genetic evidence of GABA$_A$ receptor dysfunction in epilepsy: a mutation in the γ$_2$-subunit gene. *Nat Genet* 2001;28:46–48.
54. Wallace RH, Marini C, Petrou S, et al. Mutant GABA(A) receptor gamma2-subunit in childhood absence epilepsy and febrile seizures. *Nat Genet* 2001;28:49–52.
55. Cossette P, Liu L, Brisebois K, et al. Mutation of GABA1 in an autosomal dominant form of juvenile myoclonic epilepsy. *Nat Genet* 2002;31:184–189.
56. Hoogerkamp A, Arends RH, Bomers AM, et al. Pharmacokinetic/pharmacodynamic relationship of benzodiazepines in the direct cortical stimulation model of anticonvulsant effect. *J Pharmacol Exp Ther* 1996;279:803–812.
57. Zhang H, Rosenberg HC, Tietz EI. Injection of benzodiazepines but not GABA or muscimol into pars reticulata of substantia nigra suppresses pentylenetetrazol seizures. *Brain Res* 1989;488:73–79.
58. Zhang H, Rosenberg HC, Tietz EI. Anticonvulsant actions and interaction of GABA agonists and a benzodiazepine in pars reticulata of substantia nigra. *Epilepsy Res* 1991;8:11–20.
59. McLean MJ, Macdonald RL. Benzodiazepines, but not beta carbolines, limit high frequency repetitive firing of action potentials of spinal cord neurons in cell culture. *J Pharmacol Exp Ther* 1988;244:789–795.

60. Skerritt JH, Werz MA, McLean MJ, et al. Diazepam and its anomalous p-chloro-derivative Ro 5-4864: comparative effects on mouse neurons in cell culture. *Brain Res* 1984;310:99–105.
61. Löscher W, Schmidt D. Diazepam increases gamma-aminobutyric acid in human cerebrospinal fluid. *J Neurochem* 1987;49:152–157.
62. Ong J, Kerr DI. Recent advances in $GABA_B$ receptors: from pharmacology to molecular biology. *Acta Pharmacol Sin* 2000;21:111–123.
63. Casellas P, Galiegue S, Basile AS. Peripheral benzodiazepine receptors and mitochondrial function. *Neurochem Int* 2002;40:475–486.
64. Papadopoulo V. Peripheral benzodiazepine receptor: structure and function in health and disease. *Ann Pharm Fr* 2003;61:30–50.
65. Galiegue S, Tinel N, Casellas P. The peripheral benzodiazepine receptor: a promising therapeutic drug target. *Curr Med Chem* 2003;10:1563–1572.
66. Ben-Ari Y. Developing networks play a similar melody. *Trends Neurosci* 2001;24:353–360.
67. Kriegstein AR, Owens DF. GABA may act as a self-limiting trophic factor at developing synapses. *Sci STKE* 2001;2001:PE1.
68. Dzhala VI, Staley KJ. Excitatory actions of endogenously released GABA contribute to initiation of ictal epileptiform activity in the developing hippocampus. *J Neurosci* 2003;23:1840–1846.
69. Thompson SM, Deisz RA, Prince DA. Relative contributions of passive equilibrium and active transport to the distribution of chloride in mammalian cortical neurons. *J Neurophysiol* 1988;60:105–124.
70. Zhang SJ, Jackson MB. $GABA_A$ receptor activation and the excitability of nerve terminals in the rat posterior pituitary. *J Physiol* 1995;483(Pt 3):583–595.
71. Staley K. Enhancement of the excitatory actions of GABA by barbiturates and benzodiazepines. *Neurosci Lett* 1992;146:105–107.
72. Staley KJ, Soldo BL, Proctor WR. Ionic mechanisms of neuronal excitation by inhibitory $GABA_A$ receptors. *Science* 1995;269:977–981.
73. Bormann J, Hamill OP, Sakmann B. Mechanism of anion permeation through channels gated by glycine and gamma-aminobutyric acid in mouse cultured spinal neurones. *J Physiol (Lond)* 1987;385:243–286.
74. Zeng X, Tietz EI. Depression of early and late monosynaptic inhibitory postsynaptic potentials in hippocampal CA1 neurons following chronic benzodiazepine administration: role of a reduction in Cl⁻ driving force. *Synapse* 1997;25:125–136.
75. Zeng XJ, Tietz EI. Role of bicarbonate ion in mediating decreased synaptic conductance in benzodiazepine tolerant hippocampal CA1 pyramidal neurons. *Brain Res* 2000;868:202–214.
76. Cohen I, Navarro V, Clemenceau S, et al. On the origin of interictal activity in human temporal lobe epilepsy in vitro. *Science* 2002;298:1418–1421.
77. Shorvon SD. *Status epilepticus. Its clinical features and treatment in children and adults.* New York: Cambridge University Press, 1994.
78. Tassinari CA, Dravet C, Roger J, et al. Tonic status epilepticus precipitated by intravenous benzodiazepine in five patients with Lennox-Gastaut syndrome. *Epilepsia* 1972;13:421–435.
79. Bittencourt PRM, Richens A. Anticonvulsant-induced status epilepticus in Lennox-Gastaut syndrome. *Epilepsia* 1981;22:129–134.
80. Schofield PR, Darlison MG, Fujita N, et al. Sequence and functional expression of the $GABA_A$ receptor shows a ligand-gated receptor super-family. *Nature* 1987;328:221–227.
81. Nayeem N, Green TP, Martin IL, et al. Quaternary structure of the native $GABA_A$ receptor determined by electron microscopic image analysis. *J Neurochem* 1994;62:815–818.
82. Hedblom E, Kirkness EF. A novel class of $GABA_A$ receptor subunit in tissues of the reproductive system. *J Biol Chem* 1997;272:15346–15350.
83. Davies PA, Hanna MC, Hales TG, et al. Insensitivity to anesthetic agents conferred by a class of $GABA_A$ receptor subunit. *Nature* 1997;385:820–823.
84. Bonnert TP, McKernan RM, Farrar S, et al. Theta, a novel gamma-aminobutyric acid type A receptor subunit. *Proc Natl Acad Sci U S A* 1999;96:9891–9896.
85. Olsen RW, Macdonald RL. $GABA_A$ receptor complex: structure and function. In: Egebjerg J, Schousboe A, Krogsgaard-Larsen P, eds. *Glutamate and GABA receptors: structure, function and pharmacology.* London: Taylor & Francis, 2002:203–235.
86. Wisden W, Laurie DJ, Monyer H, et al. The distribution of 13 $GABA_A$ receptor subunit mRNAs in the rat brain, I: telencephalon, diencephalon, mesencephalon. *J Neurosci* 1992;12:1040–1062.
87. Brooks-Kayal AR, Pritchett DB. Developmental changes in human γ-aminobutyric acid$_A$ receptor subunit composition. *Ann Neurol* 1993;34:687–693.
88. Brooks-Kayal AR, Jin H, Price M, et al. Developmental expression of $GABA_A$ receptor subunit mRNAs in individual hippocampal neurons in vitro and in vivo. *J Neurochem* 1998;70:1017–1028.
89. Pritchett DB, Sontheimer H, Shivers BD, et al. Importance of a novel $GABA_A$ subunit for benzodiazepine pharmacology. *Nature* 1989;338:582–585.
90. Wieland HA, Luddens H, Seeburg PH. A single histidine in $GABA_A$ receptors is essential for benzodiazepine agonist binding. *J Biol Chem* 1992;267:1426–1429.
91. Wingrove PB, Wafford KA, Bain C, et al. The modulatory action of loreclezole at the γ-aminobutyric acid type A receptor is determined by a single amino acid in the $β_2$ and $β_3$ subunit. *Proc Natl Acad Sci U S A* 1994;91:4569–4573.
92. Draguhn A, Verdorn TA, Ewert M, et al. Functional and molecular distinction between recombinant rat $GABA_A$ receptor subtypes by Zn^{2+}. *Neuron* 1990;5:781–788.
93. Verdoorn TA, Draguhn A, Ymer S, et al. Functional properties of recombinant rat $GABA_A$ receptors depend upon subunit composition. *Neuron* 1990;4:919–928.
94. Lüddens H, Korpi ER, Seeburg P. $GABA_A$/benzodiazepine receptor heterogeneity: neurophysiological implications. *Neuropharmacology* 1995;34:245–254.
95. Korpi ER, Gründer G, Lüddens H. Drug interactions at $GABA_A$ receptors. *Prog Neurobiol* 2002;67:113–159.
96. Doble A, Martin IL. Multiple benzodiazepine receptors—no reason for anxiety. *Trends Pharmacol Sci* 1992;13:76–81.
97. Smith GB, Olsen RW. Functional domains of $GABA_A$ receptors. *Trends Pharmacol Sci* 1995;16:162–168.
98. Dunn SMJ, Davies M, Muntoni AL, et al. Mutagenesis of the rat $α_1$ subunit of the γ-aminobutyric acid$_A$ receptor reveals the importance of residue 101 in determining the allosteric effects of benzodiazepine site ligands. *Mol Pharmacol* 1999;56:768–774.
99. Korpi ER, Kleingoor C, Kettenmann H, et al. Benzodiazepine-induced motor impairment linked to point mutation in cerebellar $GABA_A$ receptor. *Nature* 1993;361:356–359.
100. Rudolph U, Crestani F, Benke D, et al. Benzodiazepine actions mediated by specific γ-aminobutyric acid$_A$ receptor subtypes. *Nature* 2000;401:796–800.
101. McKernan RM, Rosahl TW, Reynolds DS, et al. Sedative but not anxiolytic properties of benzodiazepines are mediated by the $GABA_A$ receptor $α_1$ subunit. *Nature Neurosci* 2000;3:529–530.
102. Crestani F, Martin JR, Mohler H, et al. Mechanism of action of the hypnotic zolpidem in vivo. *Br J Pharmacol* 2000;131:1251–1254.
103. Low K, Crestani F, Keist R, et al. Molecular and neuronal substrate for the selective attenuation of anxiety. *Science* 2000;290:131–134.
104. Crestani F, Low K, Keist R, et al. Molecular targets for the myorelaxant action of diazepam. *Mol Pharmacol* 2001;59:442–445.
105. Crestani F, Keist R, Fritschy JM, et al. Trace fear conditioning involves hippocampal alpha5 GABA(A) receptors. *Proc Natl Acad Sci U S A* 2002;99:8980–8985.
106. Smith SS, Gong QH, Li X, et al. Withdrawal from 3alpha-OH-5alpha-pregnan-20-One using a pseudopregnancy model alters the kinetics of hippocampal $GABA_A$-gated current and increases the $GABA_A$ receptor alpha4 subunit in association with increased anxiety. *J Neurosci* 1998;18:5275–5284.
107. Smith SS, Gong QH, Hsu FC, et al. GABA(A) receptor alpha4 subunit suppression prevents withdrawal properties of an endogenous steroid. *Nature* 1998;392:926–930.
108. Zhao TJ, Rosenberg HC, Chiu TH. Treatment with an antisense oligodeoxynucleotide to the $GABA_A$ receptor $γ_2$ subunit increases convulsive threshold for β-CCM, a benzodiazepine "inverse agonist," in rats. *Eur J Pharmacol* 1996;306:61–66.
109. Zhao TJ, Li M, Chiu TH, et al. Decreased benzodiazepine binding with little effect on gamma-aminobutyric acid binding in rat brain after treatment with antisense oligodeoxynucleotide to the gamma-aminobutyric acid$_A$ receptor gamma-2 subunit. *J Pharmacol Exp Ther* 1998;287:752–759.

110. Gunther U, Benson J, Benke D, et al. Benzodiazepine-insensitive mice generated by targeted disruption of the gamma 2 subunit gene of gamma-aminobutyric acid type A receptors. *Proc Natl Acad Sci U S A* 1995;92:7749–7753.

111. Lader M. Withdrawal reactions after stopping hypnotics in patients with insomnia. *CNS Drugs* 1998;10:425–440.

112. Crawford TO, Mitchell WG, Snodgrass SR. Lorazepam in childhood status epilepticus and serial seizures: effectiveness and tachyphylaxis. *Neurology* 1987;37:190–195.

113. Schweitzer E, Rickels K. Benzodiazepine dependence and withdrawal: a review of the syndrome and its clinical management. *Acta Psychiatr Scand* 1998;98(Suppl 393):95–101.

114. Ramsey-Williams VA, Wu Y, Rosenberg HC. Comparison of anticonvulsant tolerance, crosstolerance, and benzodiazepine receptor binding following chronic treatment with diazepam or midazolam. *Pharmacol Biochem Behav* 1994;48:765–772.

115. Rosenberg HC. Differential expression of benzodiazepine anticonvulsant cross-tolerance according to time following flurazepam or diazepam treatment. *Pharmacol Biochem Behav* 1995;51:363–368.

116. Tietz EI, Huang X, Weng X, et al. Expression of α_1, α_5, and γ_2 GABA$_A$ receptor subunit mRNAs measured *in situ* in rat hippocampus and cortex following chronic flurazepam administration. *J Mol Neurosci* 1994;4:277–292.

117. Tietz EI, Huang X, Chen S, et al. Temporal and regional regulation of α_1, β_2 and β_3, but not α_2, α_4, α_6, β_1 or γ_2 GABA$_A$ receptor subunit messenger RNAs following one week oral flurazepam administration. *Neuroscience* 1999;91:327–341.

118. Li M, Szabo A, Rosenberg HC. Downregulation of benzodiazepine binding to α_5 subunit-containing GABA$_A$ receptors in tolerant rat brain indicates particular involvement of the hippocampal CA1 region. *J Pharmacol Exp Ther* 2000;295:689–696.

119. Xie XH, Tietz EI. Chronic benzodiazepine treatment of rats induces reduction of paired pulse inhibition in CA1 region of in vitro hippocampal slices. *Brain Res* 1991;561:69–76.

120. Zeng XJ, Tietz EI. Benzodiazepine tolerance at GABAergic synapses on hippocampal CA1 pyramidal cells. *Synapse* 1999;31:263–277.

121. Loscher W, Rundfeldt C, Honack D, et al. Long-term studies on anticonvulsant tolerance and withdrawal characteristics of benzodiazepine receptor ligands in different seizure models in mice, I: comparison of diazepam, clonazepam, clobazam and abecarnil. *J Pharmacol Exp Ther* 1996;279:561–572.

122. Grimm G, Ferenci P, Katzenschlager R, et al. Improvement of hepatic encephalopathy treated with flumazenil. *Lancet* 1988;2: 1392–1394.

123. Pomierlayrargues G, Giguere JF, Lavoie J, et al. Flumazenil in cirrhotic patients in hepatic coma—a randomized double-blind placebo-controlled crossover trial. *Hepatology* 1994;19:32–37.

124. Grimm G, Katzenschlager R, Holzner F, et al. Effect of flumazenil in hepatic encephalopathy. *Eur J Anaesthesiol Suppl* 1988;2: 147–149.

125. Alho H, Costa E, Ferrero P, et al. Diazepam-binding inhibitor: a neuropeptide located in selected neuronal populations of rat brain. *Science* 1985;229:179–182.

126. Gonsalves SF, Gallager DW. Persistent reversal of tolerance to anticonvulsant effects and GABAergic subsensitivity by a single exposure to benzodiazepine antagonist during chronic benzodiazepine administration. *J Pharmacol Exp Ther* 1987; 244:79–83.

127. Gonsalves SF, Gallager DW. Spontaneous and RO15-1788-induced reversal of subsensitivity to GABA following chronic benzodiazepines. *Eur J Pharmacol* 1985;110:163–170.

128. Tietz EI, Zeng X, Chen S, et al. Antagonist-induced reversal of functional and structural measures of hippocampal benzodiazepine tolerance. *J Pharmacol Exp Ther* 1999;291:932–942.

129. Savic I, Widen L, Stone-Elander S. Feasibility of reversing benzodiazepine tolerance with flumazenil. *Lancet* 1991;337:133–137.

130. Nutt DJ, Cowan PJ, Little HJ. Unusual interactions of benzodiazepine receptor antagonists. *Nature* 1982;295:436–438.

131. Vellucci SV, Webster RA. Is RO15-1788 a partial agonist at benzodiazepine receptors? *Eur J Pharmacol* 1983;90:263–268.

132. Polc P, Jahromi SS, Facciponte G, et al. Benzodiazepine antagonists reduce epileptiform discharges in rat hippocampal slices. *Epilepsia* 1996;37:1007–1014.

133. Robertson HA, Riives ML. A benzodiazepine antagonist is an anticonvulsant in an animal model for limbic epilepsy. *Brain Res* 1983;270:380–382.

134. Sharief MK, Sander JWAS, Shorvon S. The effects of oral flumazenil on interictal epileptic activity: results of a double-blind, placebo-controlled study. *Epilepsy Res* 1993;15:53–60.

135. Scollo-Lavizzari G. The anticonvulsant effect of the benzodiazepine antagonist, Ro15-1788: an EEG study of 4 cases. *Eur Neurol* 1984;23:1–6.

136. Scollo-Lavizzari G. The clinical anticonvulsant effects of flumazenil, a benzodiazepine antagonist. *Eur J Anaesthesiol Suppl* 1988;2:129–138.

137. Hart YM, Meinardi H, Sander JW, et al. The effect of intravenous flumazenil on interictal electroencephalographic epileptic activity: results of a placebo-controlled study. *J Neurol Neurosurg Psychiatry* 1991;54:305–309.

138. Spivey WH. Flumazenil and seizures: analysis of 43 cases. *Clin Ther* 1992;14:292–305.

139. Schulze-Bonhage A, Elger CE. Induction of partial epileptic seizures by flumazenil. *Epilepsia* 2000;41:186–192.

140. Henry TR. Functional neuroimaging with positron emission tomography. *Epilepsia* 1996;37:1141–1154.

141. Lamusuo S, Pitkanen A, Jutila L, et al. [^{11}C]Flumazenil binding in the medial temporal lobe in patients with temporal lobe epilepsy: correlation with hippocampal MR volumetry, T2 relaxometry and neuropathology. *Neurol Res* 2000;17:190–192.

142. Juhasz C, Nagy F, Muzik O, et al. [^{11}C]flumazenil PET in patients with epilepsy with dual pathology. *Epilepsia* 1999;40:566–574.

143. Delgado-Escueta AV, Wasterlain C, Treiman DM, et al. Current concepts in neurology: management of status epilepticus. *N Engl J Med* 1982;306:1337–1340.

144. Albano A, Reisdorff EJ, Wiegenstein JG. Rectal diazepam in pediatric status epilepticus. *Am J Emerg Med* 1989;7:168–172.

145. Camfield CS, Camfield PR, Smith E, et al. Home use of rectal diazepam to prevent status epilepticus in children with convulsive disorders. *J Child Neurol* 1989;4:125–126.

146. Kriel RL, Cloyd JC, Hadsall RS, et al. Home use of rectal diazepam for cluster and prolonged seizures: efficacy, adverse reactions, quality of life, and cost analysis. *Pediatr Neurol* 1991;7:13–17.

147. Remy C, Jourdil N, Villemain D, et al. Intrarectal diazepam in epileptic adults. *Epilepsia* 1992;33:353–358.

148. Dieckmann RA. Rectal diazepam for prehospital pediatric status epilepticus. *Ann Emerg Med* 1994;23:216–224.

149. Dreifuss FE, Rossman NP, Cloyd JC. A comparison of rectal diazepam gel and placebo for acute repetitive seizures. *N Engl J Med* 1998;338:1869–1875.

150. McNamara RM, Spivey WH, Unger HD, et al. Emergency applications of intraosseous infusion. *J Emerg Med* 1987;5:97–101.

151. Schwagmeier R, Alincic S, Striebel HW. Midazolam pharmacokinetics following intravenous and buccal administration. *Br J Clin Pharmacol* 1998;46:203–206.

152. Scott RC, Besag FM, Neville BG. Buccal midazolam and rectal diazepam for treatment of prolonged seizures in childhood and adolescence: a randomized trial. *Lancet* 1999;353:623–626.

153. Gizurarson S, Gudbrandsson FK, Jonsson H, et al. Intranasal administration of diazepam aiming at the treatment of acute seizures: clinical trials in healthy volunteers. *Biol Pharm Bull* 1999;22:425–427.

154. Kendall JL, Reynolds M, Goldberg R. Intranasal midazolam in patients with status epilepticus. *Ann Emerg Med* 1997;29:415–417.

155. Lahat E, Goldman M, Barr J, et al. Comparison of intranasal midazolam with intravenous diazepam for treating febrile seizures in children: prospective randomized study. *BMJ* 2000; 321:83–86.

156. Borea PA, Bonora D. Brain receptor binding and the lipophilic character of benzodiazepines. *Biochem Pharmacol* 1983;32: 603–607.

157. Charney DS, Mihic SJ, Harris RA. Hypnotics and sedatives. In: Hardman JG, Limbird LE, eds. *Goodman and Gilman's the pharmacological basis of therapeutics*, 10th ed. New York: McGraw-Hill, 2001:399–427.

158. Greenblatt DJ, Divoll M, Abernathy DR. Clinical pharmacokinetics of the newer benzodiazepines. *Clin Pharmacokinet* 1983;8: 233–252.

159. Greenblatt DJ, Shader RI, Abernethy DR. Current status of benzodiazepines (first of two parts). *N Engl J Med* 1983;309: 354–358.

160. Ochs HR, Greenblatt DJ, Divoll M. Diazepam kinetics in relation to age and sex. *Pharmacology* 1981;23:24–30.

161. Arendt RM, Greenblatt DJ, deJong RH, et al. *In vitro* correlates of benzodiazepine cerebrospinal fluid uptake, pharmacodynamic action and peripheral distribution. *J Pharmacol Exp Ther* 1993; 277:98–106.

162. Dresser GK, Spence JD, Bailey DG. Pharmacokinetic-pharmacodynamic consequences and clinical relevance of cytochrome P450 3A4 inhibition. *Clin Pharmacokinet* 2000;38:41–57.

163. Treiman DM. Pharmacokinetics and clinical use of benzodiazepines in the management of status epilepticus. *Epilepsia* 1989;30(Suppl 2):S4–10.

164. Laurijssens BE, Greenblatt DJ. Pharmacokinetic-pharmacodynamic relationships for benzodiazepines. *Clin Pharmacokinet* 1996;30:52–76.

165. Rey E, Treluyer JM, Pons G. Pharmacokinetic optimization of benzodiazepine therapy for acute seizures. Focus on delivery routes. *Clin Pharmacokinet* 1999;36:409–424.

166. Prensky AL, Raff MC, Moore MS, et al. Intravenous diazepam in the treatment of prolonged seizure activity. *N Engl J Med* 1967;276:779–786.

167. Schmidt D. Benzodiazepines, diazepam. In: Levy RH, Dreifuss FE, Mattson RH, et al., eds. *Antiepileptic drugs*, 3rd ed. New York: Raven Press, 1989:735–764.

168. Bekersky I, Maggio AC, Mattaliano V Jr, et al. Influence of phenobarbital on the disposition of clonazepam and antipyrine in the dog. *J Pharmacokinet Biopharm* 1977;5:507–512.

169. Nanda RN, Johnson RH, Keogh HJ, et al. Treatment of epilepsy with clonazepam and its effect on other anticonvulsants. *J Neurol Neurosurg Psychiatry* 1977;40:538–543.

170. Dhillon S, Richens A. Valproic acid and diazepam interaction *in vivo*. *Br J Clin Pharmacol* 1982;13:553–560.

171. Wilensky AJ, Levy RH, Troupin AS, et al. Clorazepate kinetics in treated epileptics. *Clin Pharmacol Ther* 1978;24:22–30.

172. Munoz JJ, De Salamanca RE, Diaz-Obregon C, et al. The effect of clobazam on steady state plasma concentrations of carbamazepine and its metabolites. *Br J Clin Pharmacol* 1990;29:763–765.

173. Klotz U, Reimann I. Elevation of steady-state diazepam levels by cimetidine. *Clin Pharmacol Ther* 1981;30:513–517.

174. Klotz U, Reimann I. Delayed clearance of diazepam due to cimetidine. *N Engl J Med* 1980;302:1012–1014.

175. Ochs HR, Greenblatt DJ, Gugler R, et al. Cimetidine impairs nitrazepam clearance. *Clin Pharmacol Ther* 1983;34:227–230.

176. Brockmeyer NH, Mertins L, Klimek K, et al. Comparative effects of rifampin and/or probenecid on the pharmacokinetics of temazepam and nitrazepam. *Int J Clin Pharmacol Ther Toxicol* 1990;28:387–393.

177. Abernethy DR, Greenblatt DJ, Ameer B, et al. Probenecid impairment of acetaminophen and lorazepam clearance: direct inhibition of ether glucuronide formation. *J Pharmacol Exp Ther* 1985;234:345–349.

178. Towne AR, Pellock JM, Ko D, et al. Determinants of mortality in status epilepticus. *Epilepsia* 1994;35:27–34.

179. Lowenstein DH, Alldredge BK. Status epilepticus. *N Engl J Med* 1998;338:970–976.

180. Cavazos JE, Das I, Sutula TP. Neuronal loss induced in limbic pathways by kindling: evidence for induction of hippocampal sclerosis by repeated brief seizures. *J Neurosci* 1994;14:3106–3121.

181. Lynch MW, Rutecki PA, Sutula TP. The effects of seizures on the brain. *Curr Opin Neurol Neurosurg* 1996;9:97–102.

182. Leppik IE, Derivan AT, Homan RW, et al. Double-blind study of lorazepam and diazepam in status epilepticus. *JAMA* 1983;249: 1452–1454.

183. Treiman DM. The role of benzodiazepines in the management of status epilepticus. *Neurology* 1990;40:32–42.

184. Treiman DM, Meyers PD, Walton NY, et al. A comparison of four treatments for generalized convulsive status epilepticus. Veterans Affairs Status Epilepticus Cooperative Study Group. *N Engl J Med* 1998;339:792–798.

185. Appleton R, Sweeney A, Choonara I, et al. Lorazepam versus diazepam in the acute treatment of epileptic seizures and status epilepticus. *Dev Med Child Neurol* 1995;37:682–688.

186. Alldredge BK, Gelb AM, Isaacs SM, et al. A comparison of lorazepam, diazepam, and placebo for the treatment of out-of-hospital status epilepticus. *N Engl J Med* 2001;345: 631–637.

187. Walton NY, Treiman DM. Response of status epilepticus induced by lithium and pilocarpine to treatment with diazepam. *Exp Neurol* 1988;101:267–275.

188. Kapur J, Macdonald RL. Rapid seizure-induced reduction of benzodiazepine and Zn^{2+} sensitivity of hippocampal dentate granule cell $GABA_A$ receptors. *J Neurosci* 1999;17:7532–7540.

189. Mazarati AM, Baldwin RA, Sankar R, et al. Time-dependent decrease in the effectiveness of antiepileptic drugs during the course of self-sustaining status epilepticus. *Brain Res* 1998;814: 179–185.

190. Rice AC, DeLorenzo RJ. N-methyl-D-aspartate receptor activation regulates refractoriness of status epilepticus to diazepam. *Neuroscience* 1999;93:117–123.

191. Tsuda M, Shimizu N, Yajima Y, et al. Hypersusceptibility to DMCM-induced seizures during diazepam withdrawal in mice: evidence for upregulation of NMDA receptors. *Naunyn Schmiedebergs Arch Pharmacol* 1998;357:309–315.

192. Mewasingh LD, Sekhara T, Aeby A, et al. Oral ketamine in paediatric non-convulsive status epilepticus. *Seizure* 2003;12: 483–489.

193. Pasternak SJ, Heller MB. Endotracheal diazepam in status epilepticus. *Ann Emerg Med* 1985;14:485–486.

194. Rusli M, Spivey WH, Bonner H. Endotracheal diazepam: absorption and pulmonary pathologic effects. *Ann Emerg Med* 1987; 16:314–318.

195. Kriel RL, Cloyd JC, Pellock JM, et al. Rectal diazepam gel for treatment of acute repetitive seizures. The North American Diastat Study Group. *Pediatr Neurol* 1999;20:282–288.

196. Mitchell WG, Conry JA, Crumrine PK, et al. An open-label study of repeated use of diazepam rectal gel (Diastat) for episodes of acute breakthrough seizures and clusters: safety, efficacy and tolerance. North American Diastat Group. *Epilepsia* 1999;40: 1610–1617.

197. Moffett A, Scott DF. Stress and epilepsy: the value of a benzodiazepine—lorazepam. *J Neurol Neurosurg Psychiatry* 1984;47: 165–167.

198. Feely M, Gibson J. Intermittent clobazam for catamenial epilepsy: tolerance avoided. *J Neurol Neurosurg Psychiatry* 1984; 47:1279–1282.

199. Walker JE, Homan RW, Crawford IL. Lorazepam: a controlled trial in patients with intractable partial complex seizures. *Epilepsia* 1984;25:464–466.

200. Lolin Y, Francis DA, Flanagan RJ, et al. Cerebral depression due to propylene glycol in a patient with chronic epilepsy—the value of the plasma osmolal gap in diagnosis. *Postgrad Med J* 1988;64:610–613.

201. Arbour RB. Propylene glycol toxicity related to high-dose lorazepam infusion: case report and discussion. *Am J Crit Care* 1999;8:499–506.

202. Waltregny A, Dargent J. Preliminary study of parenteral lorazepam in status epilepticus. *Acta Neurol Belg* 1975;75:219–229.

203. Graham CW, Pagano RR, Conner JT. Pain and clinical thrombophlebitis following intravenous diazepam and lorazepam. *Anaesthesia* 1978;33:188–191.

204. Parkes RB, Blanton PL, Thrash WJ. Incidence of thrombophlebitis in humans with the diazepam vehicle. *Anesth Prog* 1982;29:168–169.

205. Gould JD, Lingam S. Hazards of intra-arterial diazepam. *Br Med J* 1977;2:298–299.

206. Greenblatt DJ, Shader RI, Abernethy DR. Current status of benzodiazepines (second of two parts). *N Engl J Med* 1983;309: 410–416.

207. Busto U, Sellers EM, Naranjo CA, et al. Withdrawal reaction after long-term therapeutic use of benzodiazepines. *N Engl J Med* 1986;315:854–859.

208. Salzman C. The benzodiazepine controversy: therapeutic effects versus dependence, withdrawal, and toxicity. *Harv Rev Psychiatry* 1997;4:279–282.

209. Huang ZC, Shen DL. Studies of quantitative beta activity in EEG background changes produced by intravenous diazepam. *Clin Electroencephalogr* 1997;28:172–178.

210. Huang ZC, Shen DL. The prognostic significance of diazepam-induced EEG changes in epilepsy: a follow-up study. *Clin Electroencephalogr* 1993;24:179–187.
211. Greenblatt DJ, Divoll M. Diazepam versus lorazepam: relationship of drug distribution to duration of clinical action. In: Delgado-Escueta AV, Wasterlain C, Treiman DM, et al., eds. *Status epilepticus: mechanism of brain damage and treatment.* New York: Raven Press, 1983:487–490.
212. Hardman JG, Limbird LE, Gilman AG. Appendix II. In: Hardman JG, Limbird LE, Gilman AG, eds. *Goodman and Gilman's the pharmacological basis of therapeutics,* 10th ed. New York: McGraw-Hill, 2001:1917–2023.
213. Schwartz MA, Koechlin BA, Postma E, et al. Metabolism of diazepam in rat, dog and man. *J Pharmacol Exp Ther* 1965;149:423–435.
214. Klotz U, Antonin KH, Brügel H, et al. Disposition of diazepam and its major metabolite desmethyldiazepam in patients with liver disease. *Clin Pharmacol Ther* 1977;21:430–436.
215. Nims RW, Prough RA, Jones CR, et al. In vivo induction and in vitro inhibition of hepatic cytochrome P450 activity by the benzodiazepine anticonvulsants clonazepam and diazepam. *Drug Metab Dispos* 1997;25:750–756.
216. Eustace PW, Hailey DM, Cox AG, et al. Biliary excretion of diazepam in man. *Br J Anaesth* 1975;47:983–985.
217. Mahon WA, Inaba T, Umeda T, et al. Biliary elimination of diazepam in man. *Clin Pharmacol Ther* 1976;19:443–450.
218. Ma YM, Sun RY. Second peak of plasma diazepam concentration and enterogastric circulation. *Zhongguo Yao Li Xue Bao* 1993;14:218–221.
219. Nichol CF, Tutton IC, Smith BH. Parenteral diazepam in status epilepticus. *Neurology* 1969;19:332–343.
220. Norris E, Marzouk O, Nunn A, et al. Respiratory depression in children receiving diazepam for acute seizures: a prospective study. *Dev Med Child Neurol* 1999;41:340–343.
221. Korttila K, Linnoila M. Absorption and sedative effects of diazepam after oral administration and intramuscular administration into the vastus lateralis muscle and the deltoid muscle. *Br J Anaesth* 1975;47:857–862.
222. Korttila K, Linnoila M. Psychomotor skills related to driving after intramuscular administration of diazepam and meperidine. *Anesthesiology* 1975;42:685–691.
223. Milligan N, Dhillon S, Oxley J, et al. Absorption of diazepam from the rectum and its effect on interictal spikes in the EEG. *Epilepsia* 1982;23:323–331.
224. Al Tahan A. Paradoxic response to diazepam in complex partial status epilepticus. *Arch Med Res* 2000;31:101–104.
225. Sadjadi SA, McLaughlin K, Shah RM. Allergic interstitial nephritis due to diazepam. *Arch Intern Med* 1987;147:579.
226. Haley CJ, Haun WM, Lin S, et al. *Diazepam.* Greenwood Village, CO: Thomson Micromedex, 1974–2004.
227. Saxén I, Saxén L. Association between maternal intake of diazepam and oral clefts. *Lancet* 1975;2:498.
228. Laegreid L, Kyllerman M, Headner R, et al. Benzodiazepine amplification of valproate teratogenic effects in children of mothers with absence epilepsy. *Neuropediatrics* 1993;24:88–92.
229. Browne TR, Penry JK. Benzodiazepines in the treatment of epilepsy. A review. *Epilepsia* 1973;14:277–310.
230. Delgado-Escueta AV, Enrile-Bacsal F. Combination therapy for status epilepticus: intravenous diazepam and phenytoin. *Adv Neurol* 1983;34:477–485.
231. Walker MC, Tong X, Brown S, et al. Comparison of single- and repeated-dose pharmacokinetics of diazepam. *Epilepsia* 1998;39:283–289.
232. Ferngren HG. Diazepam treatment for acute convulsions in children. *Epilepsia* 1974;15:27–37.
233. Booker HE, Celesia GG. Serum concentrations of diazepam in subjects with epilepsy. *Arch Neurol* 1973;29:191–194.
234. Bertz RJ, Howrie DL. Diazepam by continuous intravenous infusion for status epilepticus in anticonvulsant hypersensitivity syndrome. *Ann Pharmacother* 1993;27:298–301.
235. Mahomed K, Nyamurera T, Tarumbwa A. PVC bags considerably reduce availability of diazepam. *Cent Afr J Med* 1998;44:172–173.
236. Phelps SJ, Cochran EB. Diazepam. In: *Guidelines for administration of intravenous medications to pediatric patients,* 4th ed. Bethesda, MD: Intelligence Publications, 1993.
237. Agurell S, Berlin A, Ferngren H, et al. Plasma levels of diazepam after parenteral and rectal administration. *Epilepsia* 1975;16:277–283.
238. Singhi S, Banerjee S, Singhi P. Refractory status epilepticus in children: role of continuous diazepam infusion. *J Child Neurol* 1998;13:23–26.
239. Gilbert DL, Gartside PS, Glauser T. Efficacy and mortality in treatment of refractory generalized convulsive status epilepticus. *J Child Neurol* 1999;14:602–609.
240. Meberg A, Langslet A, Bredesen JE, et al. Plasma concentration of diazepam and N-desmethyldiazepam in children after a single rectal or intramuscular dose. *Eur J Clin Pharmacol* 1978;14:273–276.
241. De Negri M, Baglietto MG, Battaglia FM, et al. Treatment of electrical status epilepticus by short diazepam (DZP) cycles after DZP rectal bolus test. *Brain Dev* 1995;17:330–333.
242. Lathers CM, Kam FJ, Spivey WH. A comparison of intraosseous and intravenous routes of administration for antiseizure agents. *Epilepsia* 1989;30:472–479.
243. Knudsen FU, Paerregaard A, Andersen R, et al. Long term outcome of prophylaxis for febrile convulsions. *Arch Dis Child* 1996;74:13–18.
244. Lukey BJ, Corcoran KD, Solana RP. Pharmacokinetics of diazepam intramuscularly administered to rhesus monkeys. *J Pharm Sci* 1991;80:918–921.
245. Bechgaard E, Gizurarson S, Hjortkjaer RK. Pharmacokinetic and pharmacodynamic response after intranasal administration of diazepam to rabbits. *J Pharmacol Exp Ther* 1997;49:747–750.
246. De Negri M, Baglietto MG, Biancheri R. Electrical status epilepticus in childhood: treatment with short cycles of high dosage benzodiazepine (preliminary note). *Brain Dev* 1993;15:311–312.
247. Herman RJ, Van Pham JD, Szakacs CB. Disposition of lorazepam in human beings: enterohepatic recirculation and first-pass effect. *Clin Pharmacol Ther* 1989;46:18–25.
248. Bradshaw EG, Ali AA, Mulley BA, et al. Plasma concentrations and clinical effects of lorazepam after oral administration. *Br J Anaesth* 1981;53:517–521.
249. Ochs HR, Busse J, Greenblatt DJ, et al. Entry of lorazepam into cerebrospinal fluid. *Br J Clin Pharmacol* 1980;10:405–406.
250. Greenblatt DJ, Joyce KA, Comer WH, et al. Clinical pharmacokinetics of lorazepam, III: intravenous injection. Preliminary results. *J Clin Pharmacol* 1977;17:490–494.
251. Greenblatt DJ, Ehrenberg BL, Gunderman J, et al. Kinetic and dynamic study of intravenous lorazepam: comparison with intravenous diazepam. *J Pharmacol Exp Ther* 1989;250:134–140.
252. Walker JE, Homan RW, Vasko MR, et al. Lorazepam in status epilepticus. *Ann Neurol* 1979;6:207–213.
253. Homan RW, Treiman DM. Lorazepam. In: Levy RH, Meldrum BS, eds. *Antiepileptic drugs,* 4th ed. New York: Raven Press, 1995;779–790.
254. Ochs HR, Greenblatt DJ, Eichelkraut W, et al. Contribution of the gastrointestinal tract to lorazepam conjugation and clonazepam nitroreduction. *Pharmacology* 1991;42:36–48.
255. Greenblatt DJ, Schillings RT, Kyriakopoulos AA, et al. Clinical pharmacokinetics of lorazepam: absorption and disposition of oral ^{14}C-lorazepam. *Clin Pharmacol Ther* 1976;21:222–230.
256. Greenblatt DJ, Shader RI, Franke K, et al. Pharmacokinetics and bioavailability of intravenous, intramuscular, and oral lorazepam in humans. *J Pharm Sci* 1979;68:57–63.
257. Ameer B, Greenblatt DJ. Lorazepam: a review of its clinical pharmacological properties and therapeutic uses. *Drugs* 1981;21:162–200.
258. Lacey DJ, Singer WD, Horwitz SJ, et al. Lorazepam therapy of status epilepticus in children and adolescents. *J Pediatr* 1986;108:771–774.
259. DiMario FJ Jr, Clancy RR. Paradoxical precipitation of tonic seizures by lorazepam in a child with atypical absence seizures. *Pediatr Neurol* 1988;4:249–251.
260. Kahan BB, Haskett RF. Lorazepam withdrawal and seizures. *Am J Psychiatry* 1984;141:1011–1012.
261. Samara EE, Granneman RG, Witt GF, et al. Effect of valproate on the pharmacokinetics and pharmacodynamics of lorazepam. *J Clin Pharmacol* 1997;37:442–450.
262. Anderson GD, Gidal BE, Kantor ED, et al. Lorazepam-valproate interaction: studies in normal subjects and isolated perfused rat liver. *Epilepsia* 1994;35:221–225.

263. Levy RJ, Krall RL. Treatment of status epilepticus with lorazepam. *Arch Neurol* 1984;41:605–611.
264. Vincent FM, Vincent T. Lorazepam in myoclonic seizures after cardiac arrest [letter]. *Ann Intern Med* 1986;104:586.
265. Deshmukh A, Wittert W, Schnitzler E, et al. Lorazepam in the treatment of refractory neonatal seizures. A pilot study. *Am J Dis Child* 1986;140:1042–1044.
266. Maytal J, Novak GP, King KC. Lorazepam in the treatment of refractory neonatal seizures. *J Child Neurol* 1991;6:319–323.
267. Yager JY, Seshia SS. Sublingual lorazepam in childhood serial seizures. *Am J Dis Child* 1988;142:931–932.
268. D'Onofrio G, Rathlev NK, Ulrich AS, et al. Lorazepam for the prevention of recurrent seizures related to alcohol. *N Engl J Med* 1999;340:915–919.
269. Jawad S, Oxley J, Wilson J, et al. A pharmacodynamic evaluation of midazolam as an antiepileptic compound. *J Neurol Neurosurg Psychiatry* 1986;49:1050–1054.
270. Dundee JW, Halliday NJ, Harper KW, et al. Midazolam. A review of its pharmacological properties and therapeutic use. *Drugs* 1984;28:519–543.
271. Breimer LT, Burm AG, Danhof M, et al. Pharmacokinetic-pharmacodynamic modelling of the interaction between flumazenil and midazolam in volunteers by aperiodic EEG analysis. *Clin Pharmacokinet* 1991;20:497–508.
272. Bell DM, Richards G, Dhillon S, et al. A comparative pharmacokinetic study of intravenous and intramuscular midazolam in patients with epilepsy. *Epilepsy Res* 1991;10:183–190.
273. Burstein AH, Modica R, Hatton M, et al. Pharmacokinetics and pharmacodynamics of midazolam after intranasal administration. *J Clin Pharmacol* 1997;37:711–718.
274. Bjorkman S, Rigemar G, Idvall J. Pharmacokinetics of midazolam given as an intranasal spray to adult surgical patients. *Br J Anaesth* 1997;79:575–580.
275. Clausen TG, Wolff J, Hansen PB, et al. Pharmacokinetics of midazolam and α-hydroxy-midazolam following rectal and intravenous administration. *Br J Clin Pharmacol* 1988;25:457–463.
276. Thummel KE, O'Shea D, Paine MF, et al. Oral first-pass elimination of midazolam involves both gastrointestinal and hepatic CYP3A-mediated metabolism. *Clin Pharmacol Ther* 1996;59:491–502.
277. Rey E, Delaunay L, Pons G, et al. Pharmacokinetics of midazolam in children: comparative study of intranasal and intravenous administration. *Eur J Clin Pharmacol* 1991;41:355–357.
278. Jacqz-Aigrain E, Oxley J, Wilson J, et al. Pharmacokinetics of midazolam during continuous infusion in critically ill neonates. *Eur J Clin Pharmacol* 1992;42:329–332.
279. Malacrida R, Fritz ME, Suter PM, et al. Pharmacokinetics of midazolam administered by continuous intravenous infusion to intensive care patients. *Crit Care Med* 1992;20:1123-1126.
280. Oldenhof H, de Jong M, Steenhoek A, et al. Clinical pharmacokinetics of midazolam in intensive care patients, a wide interpatient variability? *Clin Pharmacol Ther* 1988;43:263–269.
281. Caldwell CB, Gross JB. Physostigmine reversal of midazolam-induced sedation. *Anesthesiology* 1982;57:125–127.
282. Hantson P, Clemessy JL, Baud FJ. Withdrawal syndrome following midazolam infusion. *Intensive Care Med* 1995;21:190–194.
283. Olkkola KT, Aranko K, Luurila H, et al. A potentially hazardous interaction between erythromycin and midazolam. *Clin Pharmacol Ther* 1993;53:298–305.
284. Backman JT, Olkkola KT, Ojala M, et al. Concentrations and effects of oral midazolam are greatly reduced in patients treated with carbamazepine or phenytoin. *Epilepsia* 1996;37:253–257.
285. Hanley FD, Kross JF. Use of midazolam in the treatment of refractory status epilepticus. *Clin Ther* 1998;20:1093–1105.
286. Kumar A, Bleck TP. Intravenous midazolam for the treatment of refractory status epilepticus. *Crit Care Med* 1992;20:483–488.
287. Towne AR, DeLorenzo RJ. Use of intramuscular midazolam for status epilepticus. *J Emerg Med* 1999;17:323–328.
288. Wroblewski BA, Joseph AB. The use of intramuscular midazolam for acute seizure cessation of behavioral emergencies in patients with traumatic brain injury. *Clin Neuropharmacol* 1992;15:44–49.
289. Lal KR, Raj AG, Chacko A, et al. Continuous midazolam infusion as treatment of status epilepticus. *Arch Dis Child* 1997;76:445–448.
290. Igartua J, Silver P, Maytal J, et al. Midazolam for refractory status epilepticus in children. *Crit Care Med* 1999;27:1982–1985.
291. Koul RL, Raj AG, Chacko A, et al. Continuous midazolam infusion as treatment of status epilepticus. *Arch Dis Child* 1997;76:445–448.
292. Yoshikawa H, Yamazaki S, Abe T, et al. Midazolam as a first-line agent for status epilepticus in children. *Brain Dev* 2000;22:239–242.
293. Sheth RD, Buckley DJ, Gingold M, et al. Midazolam in the treatment of refractory neonatal seizures. *Clin Neuropharmacol* 1996;19:165–170.
294. Chamberlain JM, Altieri MA, Futterman C, et al. A prospective, randomized study comparing intramuscular midazolam with intravenous diazepam for the treatment of seizures in children. *Pediatr Emerg Care* 1997;13:92–94.
295. Jeannet PY, Roulet E, Maeder-Ingvar M, et al. Home and hospital treatment of acute seizures in children with nasal midazolam. *Eur J Paediatr Neurol* 1999;3:73–77.
296. Congdon PJ, Forsythe WI. Intravenous clonazepam in the treatment of status epilepticus in children. *Epilepsia* 1980;21:97–102.
297. Edwards VE. Side effects of clonazepam therapy. *Proc Aust Assoc Neurol* 1974;11:199–202.
298. Rothschild AJ, Shindul R, Viguera A, et al. Comparison of the frequency of behavioral disinhibition on alprazolam, clonazepam, or no benzodiazepine in hospitalized psychiatric patients. *J Clin Psychopharmacol* 2000;20:7–11.
299. Buchanan N, Sharpe C. Clonazepam withdrawal in 13 patients with active epilepsy and drug side effects. *Seizure* 1994;3:271–275.
300. Sechi GP, Zoroddu G, Rosati G. Failure of carbamazepine to prevent clonazepam withdrawal status epilepticus. *Ital J Neurol Sci* 1984;5:285–287.
301. Culhane NS, Hodle AD. Burning mouth syndrome after taking clonazepam. *Ann Pharmacother* 2001;35:874–876.
302. Schuld A, Kraus T, Haack M, et al. Obstructive sleep apnea syndrome induced by clonazepam in a narcoleptic patient with REM-sleep-behavior disorder. *J Sleep Res* 1999;8:321–322.
303. Tassinari CA, Daniele O, Michelucci R, et al. Benzodiazepines: efficacy in status epilepticus. *Adv Neurol* 1983;34:465–475.
304. Dreifuss FE, Penry JK, Rose SW, et al. Serum clonazepam concentrations in children with absence seizures. *Neurology* 1975;25:255–258.
305. Ketz E, Bernoulli C, Siegfried J. Clinical and electroencephalographic trial with clonazepam (Ro 5-4023) with special regard to status epilepticus [German]. *Acta Neurol Scand Suppl* 1973;53:47–53.
306. Sorel L, Mechler L, Harmant J. Comparative trial of intravenous lorazepam and clonazepam in status epilepticus. *Clin Ther* 1981;4:326–336.
307. Naito H, Wachi M, Nishida M. Clinical effects and plasma concentrations of long-term clonazepam monotherapy in previously untreated epileptics [German]. *Acta Neurol Scand* 1987;76:58–63.
308. McNamara JO. Drugs effective in the therapy of the epilepsies. In: Hardman JG, Limbird LE, Gilman AG, eds. *Goodman and Gilman's the pharmacological basis of therapeutics,* 10th ed. New York: McGraw-Hill, 2001:521–548.
309. Sugai K. Seizures with clonazepam: discontinuation and suggestions for safe discontinuation rates in children. *Epilepsia* 1993;34:1089–1097.
310. Vassella F, Pavlincova E, Schneider HJ, et al. Treatment of infantile spasms and Lennox-Gastaut syndrome with clonazepam (Rivotril). *Epilepsia* 1973;14:165–175.
311. Dumermuth G, Kovacs E. The effect of clonazepam (Ro 5-4023) in the syndrome of infantile spasms with hypsarrhythmia and in petit mal variant of Lennox syndrome. Preliminary report. *Acta Neurol Scand Suppl* 1973;53:26–28.
312. Mikkelsen B, Birket-Smith E, Bradt S, et al. Clonazepam in the treatment of epilepsy. A controlled clinical trial in simple absences, bilateral massive epileptic myoclonus, and atonic seizures. *Arch Neurol* 1976;33:322–325.
313. Hanson RA, Menkes JH. A new anticonvulsant in the management of minor motor seizures. *Dev Med Child Neurol* 1972;14:3–14.

314. Laitinen L, Toivakka E. Clonazepam (Ro 5-4023) in the treatment of myoclonus epilepsy. Four case reports. *Acta Neurol Scand Suppl* 1973;53:72–76.

315. Goldberg MA, Dorman JD. Intention myoclonus: successful treatment with clonazepam. *Neurology* 1976;26:24–26.

316. Ryan SG, Sherman SL, Terry JC, et al. Startle disease, or hyperekplexia: response to clonazepam and assignment of the gene (STHE) to chromosome 5q by linkage analysis. *Ann Neurol* 1992;31:663–668.

317. Suzuki A, Aso K, Ariyoshi C, et al. Acute intermittent porphyria and epilepsy: safety of clonazepam. *Epilepsia* 1992;33:108–111.

318. Yasuhara A, Yoshida H, Hatanaka T, et al. Epilepsy with continuous spike-waves during slow sleep and its treatment. *Epilepsia* 1991;32:59–62.

319. Andre M, Boutroy MJ, Bianchetti G, et al. Clonazepam in neonatal seizures: dose regimens and therapeutic efficacy. *Eur J Clin Pharmacol* 1991;40:193–195.

320. Bertler A, Lindgren S, Magnusson J-O, et al. Intramuscular bioavailability of clorazepate as compared to diazepam. *Eur J Clin Pharmacol* 1985;28:229–230.

321. Greenblatt DJ, Divoll MK, Soong MH, et al. Desmethyldiazepam pharmacokinetics: studies following intravenous and oral desmethyldiazepam, oral clorazepate, and intravenous diazepam. *J Clin Pharmacol* 1988;28:853–859.

322. Greenblatt DJ, Shader RI, Harmatz JS, et al. Self-rated sedation and plasma concentrations of desmethyldiazepam following single doses of clorazepate. *Psychopharmacology (Berl)* 1979;66:289–290.

323. Abernethy DR, Greenblatt DJ, Divoll M, et al. Prolongation of drug half-life due to obesity: studies of desmethyldiazepam (clorazepate). *J Pharm Sci* 1982;71:942–944.

324. Bertler A, Lindgren S, Magnusson J-O, et al. Pharmacokinetics of clorazepate after intravenous and intramuscular administration. *Psychopharmacology* 1983;80:236–239.

325. Shader RI, Greenblatt DJ, Ciraulo DA, et al. Effect of age and sex on disposition of desmethyldiazepam formed from its precursor clorazepate. *Psychopharmacology* 1981;75:193–197.

326. Wilensky AJ, Friel PW. Benzodiazepines, clorazepate. In: Levy RH, Mattson RH, Meldrum BS, eds. *Antiepileptic drugs*, 4th ed. New York: Raven Press, 1995:751–762.

327. Vining EP. Use of barbiturates and benzodiazepines in treatment of epilepsy. *Neurol Clin* 1986;4:617–632.

328. Joseph AB, Wroblewski BA. Paradoxical akathesia caused by clonazepam, clorazepate and lorazepam in patients with traumatic encephalopathy and seizure disorder: a subtype of benzodiazepine-induced disinhibition. *Behav Neurol* 1993;6:221–223.

329. Karch FE. Rage reaction associated with clorazepate dipotassium. *Ann Intern Med* 1979;91:61–62.

330. Livingston S, Pauli LL. Clorazepate in epilepsy. *JAMA* 1977;237:1561.

331. Parker JL. Potassium clorazepate (Tranxene)-induced jaundice. *Postgrad Med J* 1979;55:908–910.

332. Patel DA, Patel AR. Clorazepate and congenital malformations. *JAMA* 1980;244:135–136.

333. Berchou RC, Odin EA, Russell ME. Clorazepate therapy for refractory seizures. *Neurology* 1981;31:1483–1485.

334. Wilensky AJ, Ojemann LM, Temkin NR, et al. Clorazepate and phenobarbital as antiepileptic drugs: a double-blind study. *Neurology* 1981;31:1271–1276.

335. Fujii T, Okuno T, Go T, et al. Clorazepate therapy for intractable epilepsy. *Brain Dev* 1987;9:288–291.

336. Booker HE. Clorazepate dipotassium in the treatment of intractable epilepsy. *JAMA* 1974;299:552–555.

337. Naidu S, Gruener G, Brazis P. Excellent results with clorazepate in recalcitrant childhood epilepsies. *Pediatr Neurol* 1986;2:18–22.

338. Shorvon SD. The use of clobazam, midazolam and nitrazepam in epilepsy. *Epilepsia* 1998;39(Suppl 1):S15–S23.

339. Maher J, McLachlan RS. Antiepileptic drug treatment following temporal lobectomy. *Neurology* 1998;51:305–307.

340. Canadian Study Group for Childhood Epilepsy. Clobazam has equivalent efficacy to carbamazepine and phenytoin as monotherapy for childhood epilepsy. *Epilepsia* 1998;39:952–959.

341. Shorvon S. Benzodiazepines, clobazam. In: Levy RH, Mattson RH, Meldrum BS, eds. *Antiepileptic drugs*, 4th ed. New York: Raven Press, 1995:763–777.

342. Guberman A, Couture M, Blaschuk K, et al. Add-on trial of clobazam in intractable adult epilepsy with plasma level correlations. *Can J Neurol Sci* 1990;17:311–316.

343. Hanks GW. Clobazam: pharmacological and therapeutic profile. *Br J Clin Pharmacol* 1979;7(Suppl 1):151S–155S.

344. Hindmarch I. Some aspects of the effects of clobazam on human psychomotor performance. *Br J Clin Pharmacol* 1979;7(Suppl 1):77S–82S.

345. Bardy AH, Seppala T, Salokorpi T, et al. Monitoring of concentrations of clobazam and norclobazam in serum and saliva of children with epilepsy. *Brain Dev* 1991;13:174–179.

346. Genton P, Nguyen VH, Mesdjian E. Carbamazepine intoxication with negative myoclonus after the addition of clobazam. *Epilepsia* 1998;39:1115–1118.

347. Rosenberg HC, Tietz EI, Chiu TH. Tolerance to anticonvulsant effects of diazepam, clonazepam, and clobazam in amygdala-kindled rats. *Epilepsia* 1989;30:276–285.

348. Allen JW, Oxley J, Robertson MM, et al. Clobazam as adjunctive treatment in refractory epilepsy. *Br Med J (Clin Res Ed)* 1983;286:1246–1247.

349. Canadian Clobazam Cooperative Group. Clobazam in treatment of refractory epilepsy: the Canadian experience. A retrospective study. *Epilepsia* 1991;32:407–416.

350. Koeppen D, Baruzzi A, Capozza M, et al. Clobazam in therapy-resistant patients with partial epilepsy: a double-blind placebo-controlled crossover study. *Epilepsia* 1987;28:495–506.

351. Singh A, Guberman AH, Boisvert D. Clobazam in long-term epilepsy treatment: sustained responders versus those developing tolerance. *Epilepsia* 1995;36:798–803.

352. Rieder J. Plasma levels and derived pharmacokinetic characteristics of unchanged nitrazepam in man. *Arzneimittelforschung* 1973;23:212–218.

353. Nicholson AN. Hypnotics: their place in therapeutics. *Drugs* 1986;31:164–176.

354. Kangas L, Iisalo E, Kanto J, et al. Human pharmacokinetics of nitrazepam: effect of age and diseases. *Eur J Clin Pharmacol* 1979;15:163–170.

355. Kangas L, Kanto J, Siirtola T, et al. Cerebrospinal fluid concentrations of nitrazepam in man. *Acta Pharmacol Toxicol* 1977;41:74–79.

356. Breimer DD. Pharmacokinetics and metabolism of various benzodiazepines used as hypnotics. *Br J Clin Pharmacol* 1979;8:7S–13S.

357. Baruzzi A, Michelucci R, Tassinari CA. Benzodiazepines, nitrazepam. In: Levy RH, Dreifus FE, Mattson RH, et al., eds. *Antiepileptic drugs*. New York: Raven Press, 1989:785–804.

358. Kenny RA, Kafetz K, Cox M, et al. Impaired nitrazepam metabolism in hypothyroidism. *Postgrad Med* 1984;60:296–297.

359. Abernethy DR, Greenblatt DJ, Lockniskar A, et al. Obesity effects on nitrazepam disposition. *Br J Clin Pharmacol* 1986;22:551–557.

360. Evans JG, Jarvis EH. Nitrazepam and the elderly. *Br Med J* 1972;4:487.

361. Saario I, Linnoila M, Maki M. Interaction of drugs with alcohol and human psychomotor skills related to driving: effect on sleep deprivation of two weeks treatment with hypnotics. *J Clin Pharmacol* 1975;15:52–59.

362. Taylor F. Nitrazepam and the elderly. *Br Med J* 1973;1:113–114.

363. Hagberg B. The chlordiazepoxide HCl (Librium) analogue nitrazepam (Mogadon) in the treatment of epilepsy in children. *Dev Med Child Neurol* 1968;10:302–308.

364. Wyllie E, Wyllie R, Cruse RP, et al. The mechanism of nitrazepam-induced drooling and aspiration. *N Engl J Med* 1986;314:35–38.

365. Clark TJH, Collins JV, Tong D. Respiratory depression caused by nitrazepam in patients with respiratory failure. *Lancet* 1971;2:737–738.

366. Gibbs FA, Anderson EM. Treatment of hypsarrhythmia and infantile spasms with a Librium analogue. *Neurology* 1965;15:1173–1176.

367. Darcy L. Delirium tremens following withdrawal from nitrazepam. *Med J Aust* 1972;2:450.

368. Speirs CJ, Navey FL, Brooks DJ, et al. Opisthotonos and benzodiazepine withdrawal in the elderly. *Lancet* 1986;2:1101.

369. Speight AN. Floppy infant syndrome and maternal diazepam and/or nitrazepam. *Lancet* 1977;2:878.

370. Rintahaka PJ, Shewmon DA, Kyyronen P, et al. Incidence of death in patients with intractable epilepsy during nitrazepam treatment. *Epilepsia* 1999;40:492–496.

371. Baldwin R, Kenny TJ, Segal J. The effectiveness of nitrazepam in a refractory epileptic population. *Curr Ther Res* 1969;11:413–416.

372. Peterson WG. Clinical study of Mogadon, a new anticonvulsant. *Neurology* 1967;17:878–880.

373. Millichap JG, Ortiz WR. Nitrazepam in myoclonic epilepsies. *Am J Dis Child* 1966; 112:242–248.

374. Snyder CH. Myoclonic epilepsy in children: short-term comparative study of two benzodiazepine derivatives in treatment. *South Med J* 1968; 61:17–20.

375. Jan JE, Riegel JA, Crichton JU, et al. Nitrazepam in the treatment of epilepsy in childhood. *Can Med Assoc J* 1971;104:571–575.

376. Vanasse M, Masson P, Geoffroy G, et al. Intermittent treatment of febrile convulsions with nitrazepam. *Can J Neurol Sci* 1984; 11:377–379.

377. Dreifus FE, Farwell J, Holmes GL, et al. Infantile spasms: comparative trial of nitrazepam and corticotropin. *Arch Neurol* 1986;43:1107–1110.

378. Chamberlain MC. Nitrazepam for refractory infantile spasms and the Lennox Gastaut syndrome. *J Child Neurol* 1996;11:31–34.

379. Stein AG, Eder HG, Blum DE, et al. An automated drug delivery system for focal epilepsy. *Epilepsy Res* 2000;39:103–114.

380. Tietz EI, Rosenberg HC, Chiu TH. A comparison of the anticonvulsant effects of 1,4- and 1,5-benzodiazepines in the amygdala-kindled rat and their effects on motor function. *Epilepsy Res* 1989;3:31–40.

Gabapentin and Pregabalin

59

Michael J. McLean   *Barry E. Gidal*

Gabapentin (1-[aminomethyl]cyclohexaneacetic acid), or (3-cyclohexyl γ-aminobutyric acid [GABA]; see Fig. 59.1) resulted from bonding cyclohexane to the 3-position of the GABA backbone to produce a structural analogue of baclofen. Although designed as a spasmolytic agent, gabapentin was developed to treat epilepsy (1–3). Initially, gabapentin was approved by the U.S. Food and Drug Administration (FDA) at the end of 1993 as an adjunctive agent for the treatment of complex partial seizures with or without secondary generalization in patients over 12 years of age. It was approved for children 3 to 12 years of age in 2001. The agent has been approved as initial monotherapy in about 40 countries outside the United States. In 2002, gabapentin was also approved for the treatment of postherpetic neuralgia.

Broad utility of gabapentin in open use led to the development of other 3-substituted GABA analogues—a group of compounds that have been dubbed "gabapentinoids." One of these, pregabalin (3-[aminomethyl]-5-methyl-,[3S]-hexanoic acid), or (3-isobutyl-GABA; see Fig. 59.1), has been shown to be superior to placebo as add-on therapy for patients with refractory partial and secondarily generalized seizures in three pivotal trials. Anxiolytic and analgesic properties of pregabalin have also been demonstrated in placebo-controlled trials. The new drug application (NDA) containing data supporting several indications for pregabalin was submitted to the FDA in November 2003. As of July 2004, pregabalin had approval from the European Commission to market pregabalin as adjunctive treatment for partial seizures, as well as for the treatment of neuropathic pain.

CHEMISTRY

Gabapentin

Gabapentin is an amorphous crystalline substance with a molecular weight of 171.24. It is freely soluble in water

(1,4). The structure of gabapentin combines an inhibitory amino acid, GABA, and a cyclohexane ring that result in a zwitterion at physiologic pH (1,4). The agent is actively transported between body compartments by the L system amino acid transporter, which recognizes such naturally occurring, bulky, neutral amino acids as L-leucine, L-isoleucine, L-valine, and L-phenylalanine. The same carrier is presumed to mediate transport across the gut wall, the blood-brain barrier, and cell membranes (5,6). Gabapentin concentrations can be measured in protein-free plasma samples by high-performance liquid chromatography (7,8) and gas chromatography (9). Blood level assays are commercially available. Gabapentin degrades slowly to a lactam in solution as a function of pH, temperature, and buffer concentration (10). The lactam is formed during synthesis of gabapentin, and has both proconvulsant (11) and neuroprotective (12) properties in laboratory models. Presumably, the lactam does not accumulate in sufficient quantity to be clinically significant. The current proprietary synthetic methods result in a low-lactam product (13).

Pregabalin

Pregabalin is also a water-soluble compound, with a molecular weight of 159.23. It is several times more potent than gabapentin on a mg/kg basis in various animal seizure models (14). Bioavailability is 90% or more. This suggests that the L-system amino acid transporter concentrated in the duodenum is not saturated by useful doses of pregabalin (14). Additional uptake mechanisms for pregabalin may exist. Serum concentrations have been determined with high-performance liquid chromatography-ultraviolet (UV) methods (15). This suggests that commercial laboratories will offer pregabalin plasma level determinations once the agent has been approved for marketing.

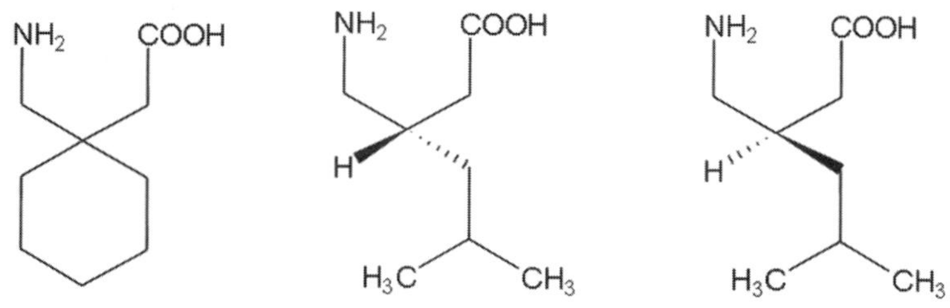

Figure 59.1 Chemical structure of gabapentin and pregabalin.

Gabapentin
(CI-945)
1-(aminomethyl)
cyclohexaneacetic acid

Pregabalin
(CI-1008)
S-(+)-3-isobutyl-GABA
active enantiomer

Pregabalin
(PD 14450)
R-(-)-isobutyl-GABA
inactive enantiomer

MECHANISMS OF ACTION

Multiple actions of gabapentin and pregabalin have been reported in animal and cell models (14,16,17), at least some of which occurred at therapeutically relevant doses or concentrations. The actions of the two agents were similar in studies of *in vitro* and animal models when compared via similar technique(s) (Table 59.1). Effects of both gabapentinoids have been noted on calcium and potassium channels, as well as on neurotransmitters, including GABA, glutamate, and serotonin.

Gabapentin is generally well tolerated, and pregabalin was well tolerated in clinical trials. This suggests that the sum of their actions is most likely modulatory, rather than highly potent. If the effects were highly potent, adverse events would limit clinical utility. Some actions may be

TABLE 59.1

EFFECTS OF GABAPENTIN AND PREGABALIN *IN VITRO* AND IN ANIMAL MODELS

	Gabapentin	Pregabalin
In vitro models		
Binding site	$\alpha_2\delta$ subunit of voltage-sensitive calcium channels	$\alpha_2\delta$ subunit of voltage-sensitive calcium channels
Voltage-sensitive Ca^{++} channels	Current through multiple types reduced	Current through multiple types reduced
Ca voltage-sensitive Na^+ channels	No direct effect	—
Voltage-sensitive K^+ channels	K_{ATP} current increased	K_{ATP} current increased
GABA	Increased concentration by MRS Increased GAD activity Increased GABA release Increased transporter expression	Inferred from animal models of decreased GABA synthesis or blockade
Glutamate	Decreased concentration	Decreased synthesis
Serotonin	Increased plasma levels associated with ↑ stage 3,4 sleep	Increase inferred from ↑ stage 3,4 sleep
Other neurotransmitters	Decreased release ($\downarrow Ca^{++}$ and $\uparrow K^+$ currents?)	Decreased release ($\downarrow Ca^{++}$ and $\downarrow K^+$ currents?)
Enzymes	Multiple effects to increase GABA, decrease glutamate; effects on PKA and PKC	—
Animal models		
Maximal electroshock model	Effective	More potent than GBP
Models of reduced GABA synthesis or blockade	Partially effective	Partially effective
Genetic absence model (GAERS)	Ineffective	Ineffective

Abbreviation: ATP, adenosine triphosphate; GABA, γ-aminobutyric acid; GAD, glutamic acid decarboxylase; GAERS, genetic absence rats from Strasbourg; MRS, magnetic resonance spectroscopy; PKA, protein kinase A; PKC, protein kinase C.

subtle under various clinical circumstances, with their relative clinical impact difficult to weigh. Thus, the mechanism(s) underlying clinical efficacy have not been determined with certainty.

PHARMACOKINETICS

The pharmacokinetic properties of gabapentin are generally favorable. However, dose-dependent bioavailability and interindividual variability in uptake require optimization on an individual basis. It is conceivable that some patients may fail to achieve desired seizure control because of inadequate absorption. This may have confounded the outcome of dose-controlled studies of gabapentin monotherapy (Vide Infra). Oral bioavailability of pregabalin, on the other hand, approaches 100% (14). This could contribute to the greater efficacy of pregabalin in clinical trials. Table 59.2 summarizes some important pharmacokinetic properties of these two agents.

Absorption

Gabapentin
Gabapentin is absorbed primarily in the small intestine, presumably because the L-amino acid transporter is concentrated there (18). Absorption of gabapentin in the colon is poor in both animals and humans (19,20).

Bioavailability of gabapentin is limited and dose-dependent. The plasma level after a single 300-mg oral dose, either as a capsule or as solution, was about 60% that

TABLE 59.2

PHARMACOKINETIC PROFILES OF GABAPENTIN AND PREGABALIN, WITH SIGNIFICANT DIFFERENCES LIMITED TO ABSORPTION

Absorption	Mediated by L-amino acid transporter
	Gabapentin: Dose-limiting bioavailability
	Increased by naproxen and morphine
	Decreased by hydrocodone
	Pregabalin: >90% bioavailability
Distribution	Water soluble
	Not extensively bound to plasma proteins
Metabolism	Not metabolized by liver
	No induction of hepatic enzymes
	No autoinduction
	No inhibition of hepatic enzymes
Elimination	Excreted intact in urine
	Excretion proportional to creatinine clearance
	Gabapentin: $t_{1/2}$ 4 to 22 hours; average, 5 to 7 hours
	Pregabalin: $t_{1/2}$ 5 to 7 hours
Interactions	No effect on other AEDs or oral contraceptives
	No effect of gabapentin on levels of other AEDs
	None with hepatic enzymes
	None with protein-binding sites

Abbreviation: AEDs, antiepileptic drugs; $t_{1/2}$, half-life;.

of an intravenous (IV) formulation (21). On a multidose regimen of 1600 mg tid, bioavailability decreased to about 35% (22).

Mean maximal plasma levels (C_{max}) were 2.7 to 2.9 µg/mL within 2 to 3 hours after oral administration of a single 300-mg capsule to healthy volunteers, and peak steady-state plasma concentrations averaged 4 µg/mL following oral administration of 300 mg every 8 hours (22–25).

A nonlinear relationship between dose and plasma levels may result from saturable absorption of gabapentin from the intestine (5). In phase 1 pharmacokinetic studies, plasma concentrations of gabapentin increased in proportion to the dose, up to 1800 mg per day. At doses from 1800 to 4800 mg per day (600 to 1600 mg q8h), plasma levels continued to rise, but less than expected (26). A nonlinear increase in plasma levels was also noted in the data from some clinical trials (27,28). Data from pharmacokinetic studies conducted in both volunteers and patients suggest that substantial interpatient variability exists for gabapentin absorption. Plasma concentrations from the open studies of patients taking 2700 to 6000 mg per day were linearly related to dose, but interindividual variability was pronounced (29,30). While apparent variability of uptake between individuals can be substantial, far less variability is noted within subjects (31).

Administration with food or typical enteral nutritional formulations does not impair absorption of gabapentin (22,31). In that gabapentin is absorbed by the L-system amino acid transporter, it may be speculated that concomitant administration with high-protein meals may interfere with absorption of the agent. Surprisingly, high-protein meals and meals rich in neutral amino acids have been reported to enhance mean plasma levels by 36% and the area under the curve (AUC) by 12% (32,33). The physiologic basis for this effect is undetermined. Enhanced amino acid transport or increased paracellular absorption could contribute. Another group of investigators also confirmed the lack of impairment in gabapentin absorption following a high-protein meal, although they did not demonstrate significantly increased oral absorption (34).

Pharmacokinetic studies suggest that patients should receive four doses per day when the total daily dose is ≥3600 mg per day (35). In one study of 36 healthy volunteers, neither C_{max} nor time to maximal serum concentration (T_{max}) were influenced by subject age, implying that absorption does not significantly change with aging (36).

Pregabalin
The absorption of pregabalin was linearly related to the dose in studies of single and multiple oral doses in patients (37). T_{max} was about 1 hour with oral bioavailability 90 percent or more (37), compared with the limited, dose-dependent uptake of gabapentin. This suggests that pregabalin absorption is not limited by a saturable process and may involve different or multiple absorption mechanisms. Pregabalin uptake was sodium-dependent and involved multiple amino

acid carriers ($b^{0,+}$, B^0, and $B^{0,+}$) in brush-border membrane vesicles prepared from duodenum, jejunum, and ileum of rats and rabbits (38). In the same model, gabapentin absorption was mediated by a sodium-independent transporter ($b^{0,+}$) and was greatest in the duodenum and ileum (38). Other mechanisms for pregabalin absorption have not been ruled out, but the short elimination half-life ($t_{1/2}$) suggests that absorption does not take place throughout the intestine.

Distribution

Gabapentinoids do not bind significantly to plasma proteins (14,39,40). Pooled data from several studies of gabapentin yield a mean volume of distribution (Vd) of 60.9 L, or 0.65 to 1.04 L/kg (22,40).

Gabapentin

Gabapentin crosses the human blood-brain barrier and is distributed to the central nervous system (CNS). Ratios of cerebrospinal fluid (CSF) to plasma concentration were 0.1 at 6 hours and 0.2 at 24 hours after a single 1,200-mg oral dose of gabapentin. After 3 months of treatment with gabapentin 900 or 1200 mg per day, concentrations in CSF varied from 6% to 34% of those in plasma (41–43). Two clearance mechanisms—passive diffusion and active transport—appear to limit accumulation (44–46).

The CNS to plasma partition ratio was 0.8:1.0 between 1 and 8 hours after a single IV dose of gabapentin (47). Assuming a partition ratio of 0.8 (47) and C_{max} ranging from 2 to 25 μg/mL at steady state, brain tissue concentrations of 1.6 to 20 μg/g are achievable.

Pregabalin

Pregabalin is not metabolized in humans, is not bound significantly to plasma proteins, and enters the brain readily (14). As in the case of gabapentin, anticonvulsant efficacy appeared with a delay after entry of pregabalin into the brain, as measured by microdialysis, and persisted to some extent as interstitial brain concentrations fell (48). Efficacy was not strictly proportional to the concentration of pregabalin in the brain, and could have been caused by delayed (e.g., biochemical) action of the agent (48).

Elimination

Gabapentin

The absorbed fraction of gabapentin is excreted unchanged in the urine (1,22). There is no evidence that gabapentin is metabolized in humans (1,22). Repeated dosing does not affect the elimination of gabapentin (39,40).

The elimination $t_{1/2}$ of gabapentin was originally estimated to be 7 to 9 hours (40,46); however, more recent data indicate a broader range of elimination $t_{1/2}$s from 4 to 22 hours (49). Whereas the oral absorption of gabapentin appears to be nonlinear, the renal clearance of the agent

has a linear relationship to creatinine clearance (ClCr) and glomerular filtration rate in both adults and children (22,49–51). Oral clearance of gabapentin appears similar between genders (36). When normalized for body weight, gabapentin oral clearance is more variable in young children (younger than 5 years of age) as compared with older children. On an mg/kg basis, younger children appear to require doses approximately 33% larger than those of older children (51).

Age- and disease-related decreases in renal function substantially reduce elimination (36,49). It is therefore reasonable to expect longer elimination $t_{1/2}$s and higher relative steady-state plasma concentrations in elderly patients compared with younger individuals. Gabapentin apparent oral clearance has been reported to range from approximately 225 mL per minute in individuals younger than 30 years of age to approximately 125 mL per minute in those older than 70 years of age. Dosage guidelines based on renal function have been generated from pharmacokinetic studies (49).

Pregabalin

Pregabalin is also excreted intact in the urine in proportion to ClCr (52). The elimination $t_{1/2}$ was approximately 9 hours for ClCr >60 mL per minute, 25 hours for ClCr 15 to 30 mL per minute, and 55 hours for hemodialysis patients (52). Renal function was the only factor that altered pregabalin pharmacokinetics; age was not an independent factor (53).

Interactions with Other Medications

Gabapentin

There is no evidence that gabapentin either induces or inhibits hepatic microsomal enzymes involved in the metabolism of other agents (40). Gabapentin does not appear to alter the metabolism of antiepileptic drugs (AEDs; carbamazepine or its epoxide, phenobarbital, phenytoin, or valproate), with the exception of felbamate (26). Hussein and associates reported that coadministration of gabapentin was associated with a 50% extension in the elimination $t_{1/2}$ of felbamate in 11 patients, presumably by a renal interaction (54). The older AEDs do not affect the pharmacokinetics of gabapentin. Similarly, no clinically significant interactions were noted with antacids (55), oral contraceptives (56), or lithium (57).

Pregabalin

Steady-state plasma levels of pregabalin were not affected significantly by carbamazepine, lamotrigine, phenobarbital, phenytoin, tiagabine, topiramate, or valproate (58). The addition of pregabalin had no effect on trough plasma levels, C_{max}, AUC, or $t_{1/2}$ of carbamazepine, lamotrigine, phenytoin, or valproate administered as monotherapy in patients with partial epilepsy (58).

Concentration-Effect Relationship

Gabapentin

The therapeutic range of gabapentin concentrations in plasma is not completely characterized. In healthy volunteers, oral dosing with 100 mg every 8 hours resulted in a mean steady-state peak plasma level of 1.91 μg/mL (22). Plasma levels $\geq 2\mu$g/mL were associated with significant clinical improvement in controlled studies (59,60). Well-tolerated, early-morning trough plasma levels exceeded 20 μg/mL in some patients receiving 4800 mg per day (50). Wilson and colleagues noted improved clinical response in a group of patients with refractory partial seizures, with gabapentin serum concentrations ranging between 6 and 20 μg/mL (30). Other studies, however, have been unable to establish a significant concentration-effect relationship (61). Nonetheless, clinical data suggest that initial plasma target concentrations between 2 and 20 μg/mL may be associated with improved clinical response. An upper limit or maximal gabapentin plasma concentration has not been identified. It is important to recognize that adequate concentration-controlled studies with gabapentin have not been conducted. Therefore, these proposed concentrations should serve as a guide, not as a conclusively established therapeutic target.

Pregabalin

Dose-related side effects predict that pregabalin will have a definable therapeutic range. Efficacy parallels oral dose in clinical trials (discussed in the next section). Although information about the relationship between dose and blood levels has not been published, the high oral bioavailability of pregabalin suggests that efficacy will parallel serum levels.

CLINICAL STUDIES OF EFFICACY AND SAFETY

Adjunctive Therapy: Placebo-Controlled Studies

The response ratio (RRatio) was the principal efficacy measure in trials of both agents. The RRatio is a measure of the percent change in seizure frequency from baseline to the end of the masked treatment period (3 months), distributed normally between ±100%. This measure is amenable to analysis with parametric statistics. A 50% reduction in seizures corresponds to an RRatio of 0.33. Also included in Tables 59.3 and 59.4 are responder rates, a secondary efficacy measure, representing the percentage of patients with a 50 percent reduction or more in the seizures.

TABLE 59.3

PIVOTAL TRIALS OF GABAPENTIN (GBP) AS ADD-ON THERAPY FOR PATIENTS WITH REFRACTORY PARTIAL AND SECONDARILY GENERALIZED TONIC-CLONIC SEIZURES

Study	Number of Subjects	Doses	Mean RRatio*	Responder Rate; % (*P* Value)
UK Gabapentin Study Group (1990)	127	GBP 1,200 mg/day vs. placebo	GBP: -0.192 Placebo: -0.060 (p = 0.0056)	GBP: 23% Placebo: 9% (p = 0.049)
US Gabapentin Study Group No. 5 (1993)	306	GBP 600, 1,200, and 1,800 mg/day vs. placebo	1,800 mg/day: -0.233 (p <0.001) 1,200 mg/day: -0.118 (p <0.023) 600 mg/day: -0.151 (p <0.007) Placebo: -0.025	1,800 mg/day: 26.4% (p <0.007) 1,200 mg/day: 17.6% (p <0.080) 600 mg/day: 18.4% (p <0.138) Placebo: 8.4%
International Gabapentin Study Group (Anhut et al., 1994)	272	GBP 900 and 1,200 mg/day vs. placebo	1,200 mg/day: -0.157 (p = 0.0055) 900 mg/day: -0.136 (p = 0.0046) Placebo: -0.025	1,200 mg/day: 28.0% (p = 0.008) 900 mg/day: 22.9% (p = 0.0046) Placebo: 10.1%

The three parallel-group studies were 12 weeks in duration, multicenter, randomized, double-blind, and placebo-controlled. Study medications were given in three divided doses. Significance is expressed as p values versus placebo.
From refs 62–64.
Abbreviation: RRatio, response ratio.

TABLE 59.4

PIVOTAL TRIALS OF PREGABALIN (PGB) AS ADD-ON THERAPY FOR PATIENTS WITH REFRACTORY PARTIAL AND SECONDARILY GENERALIZED TONIC-CLONIC SEIZURES

Study	Number of Subjects	Doses	Mean RRatio		Responder Rate, %)*: (P Value)	
1008-009	312	PGB 600 mg/day as bid or tid vs. placebo	bid: tid: Placebo:	-28 ($p \leq 0.001$) -36 ($p \leq 0.001$) -0.6	bid: tid: Placebo:	43% ($p \leq 0.001$) 48% ($p \leq 0.001$) 10%
1008-011	287	PGB 150 or 600 mg/day as tid vs. placebo	150 mg/day: 600 mg/day: Placebo:	-12 ($p \leq 0.0007$) -31 ($p \leq 0.0001$) 0.9	150 mg/day: 14% (NS) 600 mg/day: 43% ($p \leq 0.001$) Placebo: 6%	
1008-034	453	PGB 50,150,300,600 mg/day as bid vs. placebo	50 mg/day: 150 mg/day: 300 mg/day: 600 mg/day:	-6 (NS) -21 ($p \leq 0.001$) -28 ($p \leq 0.001$) -37 ($p \leq 0.001$)	50 mg/day: 14% (NS) 150 mg/day: 15% ($p \leq 0.006$) 300 mg/day: 40% ($p \leq 0.001$) 600 mg/day: 50% ($p \leq 0.001$)	

Studies were 12 weeks in duration, multicenter (United States, Canada, Europe, Australia), randomized, double-blind, and placebo-controlled. Clinically significant efficacy was present in the first week in all three studies. (Pfizer Global Research and Development, Data on file)
*Estimated from graph on poster handout by Kugler et al, 2002 (65).
Abbreviation: RRatio, response ratio; bid, twice daily; tid, three times a day; NS, not significant.

Gabapentin

Three parallel-group, placebo-controlled, double-blind, add-on trials became the basis for approval of gabapentin for the treatment of refractory partial epilepsy, with or without secondarily generalized tonic-clonic seizures (62–64; Table 59.3). These trials extended findings from two smaller dose-ranging studies that demonstrated the antiepileptic efficacy of the agent (59,60).

Pregabalin

Three pivotal, parallel-group, placebo-controlled, double-blind, add-on trials of pregabalin for the treatment of refractory partial seizures have been completed; the results have been published in abstract form (65; Table 59.4). One of these studies, which involved 453 patients with a median baseline seizure frequency of 10 seizures per month while taking one to three concomitant AEDs, revealed a trend toward a dose-response relationship when pregabalin was added at doses of 50, 150, 300, or 600 mg per day (66). Analysis of data from all three trials supported a dose-response relationship in three of four patients and indicated that treatment with pregabalin 186 mg per day should be expected to result in a 50% reduction in seizures from baseline (67). A significant reduction in seizures among patients taking pregabalin 150 to 600 mg per day was evident by study day 2 (68). Twelve percent of patients were seizure free for 6 months or more (69).

Adjunctive Therapy: Open-Label Studies

Gabapentin

Large-scale, open-label studies were conducted in the United States, Canada, Europe, and Australia to obtain additional information in the office setting on the safety, tolerability, and efficacy of gabapentin at doses up to 3600 mg per day. These studies merit review because they provide details on how gabapentin can be made to work in operational terms.

The protocol of the Study of Titration to Effect Profile of Safety (STEPS) trial in the United States allowed for dose optimization (70,71). A total of 778 physicians enrolled 2216 patients 12 years of age or older that had incompletely controlled partial seizures while taking ≤2 medications concomitantly. Seventy-four percent (n = 1639) completed the 16-week study. Of these, 17.2% (n = 281) met criteria (adequate time on doses below and above 1800 mg per day to allow comparison) for the tolerability analysis. The three most common side effects (namely, asthenia, headache, and dizziness) appeared early in the titration—that is, doses ≤1800 mg per day; the incidence was significantly lower at higher doses. The incidence of somnolence *de novo* was about the same at doses ≤1800 and >1800 mg per day (70). Approximately 11% of all study participants withdrew because of adverse events, six of which were serious (one each of sudden death, infection, overdose, ataxia, new generalized tonic-clonic seizures, and hostility).

Forty-six percent of patients who completed the STEPS trial (about 23% on an intent-to-treat basis) were seizure free in the last month of the trial on doses between 2400 and 3600 mg per day, compared with a 3-month baseline period (median frequency, 6 seizures per month) (71). About 30% of patients reached the maximal allowable dose of 3600 mg per day. A similar percentage of 198 individuals over 60 years of age became seizure free and had a similar side effect profile (72). Sixty-nine percent of patients in the STEPS study continued their medication after completion of the study; 17% withdrew because of adverse effects.

The AUS-STEPS (Australian STEPS) trial included 174 evaluable patients with partial and generalized tonic-clonic seizures inadequately controlled with one to three concomitant AEDs (73). Gabapentin was added at doses up to 4800 mg per day. Efficacy and tolerability were monitored for 6 months. Mean seizure frequency in the evaluable population decreased from about 15 to 10 seizures per month, predominantly simple and complex partial types. Fifty-three percent of patients experienced a 50% or more decrease in seizure frequency. Efficacy increased with dose. Notably, 27% (22 of 82 patients) responded at doses between 2400 and 3600 mg per day, and 30% (three of 10 patients) at doses between 3600 and 4800 mg per day. New or worsening adverse effects, similar to those reported in the US STEPS study, did not increase with higher doses, but 94% of patients reported adverse events in the course of the study. One patient committed suicide, which was thought to be unrelated to gabapentin treatment. Overall, in the AUS-STEPS trial, about 10% of patients withdrew because of adverse events.

In the 20-week Neurontin Evaluation of Outcomes in Neurological Practice (NEON) study in Canada, 114 of 190 patients who received gabapentin (Neurontin) as the first AED added to carbamazepine or phenytoin were evaluable (74). The patients had experienced 8 or more complex partial, but no tonic-clonic, seizures in the 2 months prior to the study. Gabapentin doses ranged from 300 to 3200 mg per day, with a median maintenance dose of 1,600 mg per day. The responder rate was 71%. Of those who finished the trial, 46% became seizure free; 52% were seizure free at 1 year. Eleven percent of the patients left the study before completion because of mild to moderate adverse events. Withdrawals caused by adverse events did not increase as the dose was titrated upward.

In an open, dose-optimization study in Europe, Baulac and coworkers (75) added 1200 to 2400 mg per day of gabapentin to the regimen of 610 patients already taking 2 or more AEDs for partial and tonic-clonic seizures occurring at a median baseline frequency of about 7 per month. After 6 months, 62% of patients continued taking gabapentin at a mean dose of 1739 mg per day, versus 1100 mg per day in those in the controlled trials. The overall responder rate was 33.9%. About 13% percent of patients were seizure free at the end of the study, versus 1.5% during the baseline period. Adverse effects occurred in 62% of patients, with 9.3%

discontinuing for a variety of reasons. Somnolence and asthenia were the most common reasons for study withdrawal and dose decrements. Weight gain averaging 5.4 kg occurred in 8.8% of patients and appeared to be dose-related (8% at 1200 mg per day and 15% at 2,400 mg per day). Severe adverse events (7.4%) included falls and surgery, somnolence, and personality changes.

Retrospective analyses of the efficacy of add-on gabapentin at doses of 900 to 6400 mg per day (average, 2688 mg per day) for 2 to 18 months in patients with refractory partial seizures with or without secondary generalization have been presented in preliminary form and corroborate the results of the controlled studies (75–80). Gabapentin monotherapy was achieved in 2% to 17% of individuals. A greater than 75% reduction in seizure frequency was observed in 28% of patients, and a 50% or more reduction was noted in 44%. No change was seen in 30%, and 26% of patients worsened (a greater than 50% increase in seizures). Side effects were reported in 4% to 43% of patients but were infrequent causes of discontinuation. The majority of patients tolerated the medication well. Dysphoria (aggression, irritability) and weight gain were more evident in these patients than among those in the controlled trials. In one series, 14 of 14 patients with progressive intracranial neoplasms and seizures refractory to other medications experienced a ≥50% reduction in seizures after the addition of gabapentin 900 to 2400 mg per day (81). Complete seizure control was achieved in eight of the 14. Data from open-label, extension trials have demonstrated the sustained efficacy of gabapentin (82–87).

In broad strokes, these studies of more than 3500 patients show several important points in the practice setting: Efficacy was dose-related and increased at higher doses of gabapentin than were used in the controlled trials. Sustained seizure freedom could be obtained at rates higher than expected from the controlled trials, particularly in patients who had failed less than 3 AEDs before the addition of gabapentin. Tolerability was generally good, with the majority of side effects occurring at doses ≤1800 mg per day, often being self-limited and mild to moderate in intensity. Adverse effects were not dose-related, for the most part. Withdrawal rates for adverse effects ranged from 9% to 17%. In most instances, gabapentin was administered in three or four doses per day. Some patients may benefit from twice-daily dosing, as suggested in the report by Muscas and colleagues (88). Results of large, formal studies of twice-daily gabapentin dosing have not been presented.

Pregabalin

Because pregabalin has not yet been approved for marketing, the opportunity to gather information from office practice is limited. Eighty-three percent of study patients elected to enter long-term, open-label extensions of the placebo-controlled trials (65). Interim analysis indicates sustained benefit of pregabalin 225 to 600 mg per day administered in two or three doses per day. Responder rates at different doses were in the range of 35% to 61% at 1 to 2 years. About 12% of patients withdrew because of treatment-related adverse effects.

Monotherapy Trials

Gabapentin does not have an indication for use in monotherapy, although several studies conducted in both the United States and Europe support this use. An outpatient trial of reduction to monotherapy with gabapentin involved 275 patients with refractory partial and generalized tonic-clonic seizures (27). After an 8-week baseline, gabapentin was titrated to 600, 1200, or 2400 mg per day, and other medications were discontinued over 8 weeks. The patients were then followed on gabapentin monotherapy for 16 weeks. Although 15% to 26% converted successfully to monotherapy, there was no significant difference among the three doses. In the open-label extension, gabapentin doses ≥4800 mg per day were necessary to sustain success as monotherapy in patients with refractory partial epilepsy (29). Gabapentin therapy was associated with improved cognitive function, mood, and psychosocial adjustment in this dose-controlled study without a placebo group (89).

A randomized, placebo-controlled monotherapy study lasting 8 days compared gabapentin 300 mg per day with gabapentin 3600 mg per day in 82 hospitalized patients whose other medications had been stopped during video monitoring for diagnostic purposes or presurgical evaluation (28). Gabapentin was titrated to the target dose within 24 hours. Rapid titration to 3600 mg per day was well tolerated and no patient discontinued because of side effects. Seventeen percent of the group randomized to 300 mg per day and 53% of those randomized to 3600 mg per day completed the 8-day study ($p = 0.002$). Although these types of inpatient trials do lend insight into the short-term tolerability and efficacy of a medication, they do not provide conclusive evidence of long-term effectiveness.

European monotherapy studies have been conducted with the objective of evaluating gabapentin as initial monotherapy. In the first trial, Chadwick and associates randomized 292 patients with newly diagnosed and previously untreated partial epilepsy to monotherapy with gabapentin (300, 900, or 1800 mg per day; blinded arms) or carbamazepine (600 mg per day; open-label treatment) for 6 months (90). Overall, equal percentages of patients taking gabapentin 900 or 1800 mg per day and carbamazepine 600 mg per day remained in the study at 6 months. Time to reaching an efficacy-related exit event was significantly longer in patients receiving gabapentin 900 or 1800 mg per day, compared with those receiving gabapentin 300 mg per day. This study was not designed to directly compare gabapentin and carbamazepine; however, the data suggest that although study exit rates were somewhat lower for carbamazepine, study withdrawal rates because of adverse events were higher for patients receiving carbamazepine. These results would suggest a role for gabapentin monotherapy in the newly diagnosed patient with infrequent seizures.

In another double-blind, randomized, comparative trial, Brodie and colleagues (91) evaluated gabapentin and lamotrigine in a group of newly diagnosed patients (N = 309) with partial and/or tonic-clonic seizures. In this study, patients could be titrated to gabapentin doses between 1800 and 3600 mg per day, or lamotrigine up to 300 mg per day. The primary end point was study exit because of the lack of efficacy or intolerable adverse effects. By study end (30 weeks), there was no significant difference in time to exit, proportion of patients that were seizure free, or time to first seizure, implying that gabapentin was comparable to lamotrigine in this population. The majority of patients randomized to the gabapentin arm who completed the study were receiving 1800 mg per day (74.3%), versus only 3.7% receiving 3600 mg per day. Similar proportions of patients in both study arms withdrew as result of adverse events. The most common adverse events reported in this study were dizziness, asthenia, and headache.

Results of a Veterans Affairs Cooperative Study comparing carbamazepine, gabapentin, and lamotrigine as initial monotherapy for the treatment of newly diagnosed partial epilepsy in elderly patients (≥65 years of age; N = 593) have recently been presented (92). The primary end point was retention in the study at 12 months. Secondary end points included mood, cognitive function, seizure control, tolerability, and quality of life. Patients were randomized to receive monotherapy with lamotrigine (n = 200, target dose = 150 mg per day); gabapentin (n = 195, target dose = 1500 mg per day); or carbamazepine (n = 198, target dose = 600 mg per day). Significantly more patients receiving monotherapy with lamotrigine (57.9%) or gabapentin (49.2%) remained in the study for 12 months, compared with those receiving monotherapy with carbamazepine (37%; $p = 0.010$ for gabapentin, 0.00003 for lamotrigine versus carbamazepine). The difference between lamotrigine and gabapentin for this endpoint did not reach statistical significance. Although carbamazepine was the most efficacious agent, discontinuation rates were significantly higher in carbamazepine-treated versus gabapentin-treated patients (63.5% versus 50.3%, respectively; $p = 0.0001$), with adverse effects being the main reason for study withdrawal.

Collectively, these data (open-label and European comparative studies) regarding both efficacy and tolerability tend to converge. They suggest that in the newly diagnosed patient with epilepsy, or those who are not demonstrated to be medically intractable, gabapentin appears to have comparable effectiveness to that of several other established AEDs. In addition, gabapentin may be particularly useful in the elderly patient with newly diagnosed partial seizures.

Gabapentin may have special niches. Patients with porphyria have been seizure free or nearly so with gabapentin monotherapy (93–95). In one study, refractory generalized tonic-clonic, but not absence or myoclonic, seizures tended to respond to gabapentin, but the results were not statistically significant compared with the placebo-treated group (96).

Pediatric Trials

A study of benign rolandic epilepsy (with centrotemporal spikes) demonstrated the efficacy of gabapentin over placebo (97). Several trials have now shown the safety and utility of gabapentin in children with partial seizures (98–101). Appleton and colleagues (99) evaluated 247 patients aged 3 to 12 years in a 12-week, double-blind, placebo-controlled trial of gabapentin (25 to 35 mg/kg per day) as adjunctive treatment for refractory partial seizures. The median frequency of seizures was reduced by 35% for complex partial seizures and by 28% for secondarily generalized seizures. Gabapentin was well tolerated in this population, with the most common CNS-related adverse event being somnolence (8%). Five percent of gabapentin-treated patients withdrew from the study because of adverse events. The safety and tolerability of gabapentin were also noted in a smaller study involving 52 children (2 to 17 years of age) with refractory partial seizures. In this study, gabapentin doses ranged between 24 and 70 mg/kg per day (100).

Appleton and coworkers demonstrated that gabapentin was both effective and well tolerated in children aged 3 to 12 years (101). This open-label, multicenter study examined gabapentin as add-on therapy for refractory partial seizures in 237 children over a 6-month period. All children received gabapentin 24 to 70 mg/kg per day. The overall responder rate was 34%, with 5% of the children withdrawing because of adverse events.

In a small (N = 33) placebo-controlled study evaluating the efficacy of gabapentin for the treatment of childhood absence seizures (ages 4 to 16 years), Trudeau and associates (102) reported no difference between gabapentin and placebo in either efficacy or adverse event rates. Absence seizures did not worsen. Given the small sample size, it is difficult to draw firm conclusions from this study, however.

Behavioral side effects were noted, along with increased seizures, in some children with preexisting behavioral disorders and mental retardation (103–106). Atypical absence and myoclonic seizures were reported to increase in a child with Lennox-Gastaut syndrome (107).

There are no published results of studies of pregabalin for the treatment of pediatric epilepsies.

SAFETY AND TOXICITY

Safety

Gabapentin has been prescribed for more than 12 million patients. It is widely regarded as safe and without specific organ toxicity. Status epilepticus and sudden deaths occurring in clinical trials were similar in frequency to those in the general epileptic population (108). Rare deaths have occurred because of hypersensitivity (Stevens-Johnson syndrome) in patients taking gabapentin along with other AEDs known to cause such hypersensitivity (108). In addition, abrupt discontinuation of the agent has been accomplished safely, with no reports of status epilepticus or significant increases in seizure frequency (108).

Deliberate overdoses in suicide attempts have also been reported. One individual took 49 grams of gabapentin without life-threatening complications or sequelae (109). Another patient attempting suicide took 91 grams of gabapentin, 54 grams of valproate, and had a serum ethanol level of 136 mg/dL (110). Drowsiness, dizziness, and slurred speech lasted 9 to 11 hours, without sequelae.

Overdose data are not yet available for pregabalin.

Adverse Effects

Adverse effects of gabapentin and pregabalin are similar. Table 59.5 compares the adverse effects of the two agents in pivotal trials.

Gabapentin

In controlled trials, side effects of gabapentin typically involved the CNS, began within the first few days of therapy, and lasted approximately 2 weeks, without discontinuation of therapy (109). Similar adverse effects were reported in the various studies described above. The dropout rate as a result of side effects in the different studies has been less than 15%. The most common adverse effects encountered in the add-on and monotherapy trials were somnolence and dizziness. Modest weight gain has been reported and may be somewhat dose-related (75,111–113). Abnormal movements also can occur with gabapentin therapy (114–116). Irritability and behavioral adverse effects have been noted (e.g., aggression, anger, oppositional behavior), particularly in developmentally disabled patients and those with comorbid attention-deficit hyperactivity disorder (103–106,117,118). Leg edema with or without discoloration of the skin was reported during the clinical trials and anecdotally during open use (109,119). The edema, which may be more common in the elderly, resolves with discontinuation of gabapentin. The mechanism of this side effect is not clear but may involve blockade of vascular L-type calcium channels. This speculation is based on the fact that verapamil, a prototypical L-type calcium channel blocker, also produces leg edema. Rash is relatively uncommon with gabapentin, and there are no clinical data suggesting a cross-reactivity between gabapentin and other medications. Whether patients who do experience hypersensitivity reactions to gabapentin will have similar reactions to pregabalin is unknown. It is important to recognize that the occurrence of adverse effects with gabapentin is not strictly dose related, as shown by the tolerability analysis of the STEPS study (70). Some individuals, however, do not tolerate even small doses of gabapentin.

TABLE 59.5

SOME COMMONLY OCCURRING ADVERSE EVENTS ENCOUNTERED IN CLINICAL TRIALS OF GABAPENTIN AND PREGABALIN, AND THEIR RESPECTIVE PLACEBO GROUPS

	US Gabapentin Study Group No. 5, 1993			Kugler et al, 2002 (65)		
	GBP (N=208)	PBO (N=99)	GBP/PBO	PGB (N=758)	PBO (N=294)	PGB/PBO
Somnolence	24.5	12.5	1.96	20.8	10.9	1.91
Dizziness	23.1	9.2	2.51	28.9	10.5	2.75
Ataxia	20.2	11.2	1.80	13.2	4.1	3.22
Fatigue/asthenia	11.5	7.1	1.62	11.2	8.2	1.36
Headache	14.4	12.2	1.18	9.1	11.6	0.78
Weight gain	5% to 15%*	—	—	10.4	1.4	7.43
AE-related withdrawal rate	3	1	—	15.3	6.1	

Incidence is expressed as percentage; relative incidence is expressed as the ratio of percentages in AED-treated and placebo groups.
Doses studied: GBP as 900, 1200, and 1800 mg per day in three doses per day; PGB as 50, 150, and 300 mg per day in three doses per day and 600 mg per day in two and three doses per day.
*Not given in USGBP No. 5, 1993; from Baulac et al (75).
Abbreviation: AE, adverse event; AED, antiepileptic drug; GBP, gabapentin; PBO, placebo; PGB, pregabalin.

Pregabalin

Adverse effects of pregabalin in pivotal trials were similar to those of gabapentin, with dizziness (29%), somnolence (21%), ataxia (13%), and weight gain (10%) (65). The intensity was generally mild to moderate, with withdrawal rates because of adverse effects ranging from 1.2% to 25%, depending on the dose. No deaths were reported, and the occurrence of serious adverse effects was infrequent (65). About 83% of patients in the pivotal trials elected to participate in open-label extension studies (14). The occurrence of adverse effects of pregabalin in patients (N = 257) followed for 6 months to 2 years during open-label continuation studies was somewhat different (69). The most common adverse effects were weight gain (27%), followed by dizziness (22%) and somnolence (20%); leg edema was not among the 11 most common adverse effects. About 12% of patients withdrew because of treatment-related adverse effects. Myoclonus has been reported in about 1% (120) of those treated with pregabalin. Mild, transient elevations in liver enzymes occurred in nonepileptic healthy volunteers taking pregabalin 900 mg per day during multidose pharmacokinetic studies (38). Pregabalin had minimal effects on cognitive and psychomotor function as compared to alprazolam (121).

Teratogenicity

Gabapentin

Animal studies conducted by the manufacturer revealed that gabapentin was fetotoxic in rodents (122). Gabapentin was not mutagenic *in vitro* or *in vivo* in standard assays. As a

result, gabapentin has been assigned to pregnancy category C (123).

There is little published experience with the use of gabapentin in pregnant women. A pregnancy registry has been established to gather information about the safety of gabapentin and other new AEDs in pregnancy.

Pregabalin

Data concerning the teratogenicity of pregabalin in animals and humans have not been reported.

Carcinogenicity

Gabapentin

Increased incidence of noninvasive, nonmetastasizing pancreatic acinar carcinomas in male Wistar rats taking high doses of gabapentin led to a temporary suspension of controlled trials (124). Increased incidence was not observed in female rats and mice of either gender, or in monkeys. Survival was not significantly affected. Human pancreatic cancers tend to be ductal rather than acinar. In addition, Ki-ras mutations found in human pancreatic carcinomas were not observed in gabapentin-induced pancreatic tumors in rats (125). Therefore, the relevance of the tumors in animals to human carcinogenic risk is unclear.

Male rat-specific α_{2u} globulin nephropathy is associated with many xenobiotics and increased nephrocarcinogenesis. The incidence of nephropathy increased in male rats fed high doses of gabapentin and reversed upon cessation, without significant increase in carcinomas (126). This species- and gender-specific effect has no clear relationship to human carcinogenic potential.

Pregabalin

High incidence of a specific tumor of undisclosed type in mice delayed submission of the NDA (127). The required additional toxicology studies were completed and the NDA was submitted in November 2003.

OPTIMIZING GABAPENTIN THERAPY

Given its unique pharmacokinetic profile (e.g., saturable absorption), treatment with gabapentin must be individualized (128). The initial dose and titration rate depend on urgency, comedication, and seizure frequency. Unlike the numerous AEDs that require slow initial dosage escalation schedules, many patients tolerate rapid initial dosage titration with this agent (129,130). Indeed, several clinical trials have now provided evidence of the safety and tolerability of rapid introduction of gabapentin to patients with epilepsy. Patients in one arm of the inpatient monotherapy trial received gabapentin 3600 mg in the first day, with no withdrawals for side effects (28). In another study of 574 patients with partial seizures, Fischer and colleagues compared initiation of gabapentin 900 mg per day with a more gradual regimen in which the agent was titrated upward to 900 mg per day over 3 days (131). No significant differences between the two treatment arms were detected with respect to the incidence of fatigue, ataxia, or somnolence, either on the first day of active medication or over the 5-day course of the study. Although a higher proportion of the fast-titration group experienced dizziness (10.5% versus 6.4% of slow-titration group) on day 1, dizziness was more common in the slow-titration group than in the fast-titration group during the first 3 days of treatment (15.2% versus 10.5%, respectively). The reported incidence of adverse events was similar in both titration regimens among adolescents and older patients (aged more than 60 years). Patients receiving gabapentin as the first agent for the treatment of new-onset partial seizures are likely to require the lowest doses—in the range of 900 to 1800 mg per day (90). Doses ≥3600 to 4800 mg per day may be required to benefit patients with seizures refractory to one to three AEDs prior to the addition of gabapentin (30,88).

Inadequate dosing and long intervals between doses seem to be common reasons for gabapentin treatment failure. The doses in the controlled trials are far lower than those currently used in refractory patient populations. Even though the open studies (70–74) have limited interpretability, seizure control at higher doses is probably superior to that observed in controlled trials. The STEPS study also showed that the majority of side effects were reported early in titration, at doses ≥1800 mg per day (70,71). Continued titration to doses as high as 3600 mg per day resulted in few newly emergent side effects, implying

that adverse effects tend not to be dose-dependent. Given the now well-documented safety profile of this agent, it seems reasonable to suggest that a trial of ≥3600 mg per day in three to four divided doses should be attempted before concluding that gabapentin is ineffective. An adequate trial of gabapentin can be conducted in 1 to 2 months, if necessary, so it is possible to know quickly if the agent will be useful in individual patients.

GABAPENTIN AND PREGABALIN: SUMMARY

In summary, the main advantages of gabapentin include safety, tolerability, lack of significant drug-drug interactions and protein binding, and a broad therapeutic index. The principal disadvantage seems to be marked interindividual variability in absorption because of saturation kinetics. Mixed results in monotherapy trials may have resulted from failure to incorporate strategies to compensate for variable absorption in the study designs. Twice-daily dosing has not been rigorously tested, but some patients benefit from this regimen. Pregabalin was successful in trials testing twice-daily dosing. Both agents have short $t_{1/2}$s. Effect and optimization of dosing on an individual basis are the keys to successful utilization of gabapentin.

When the results of pivotal trials based on seizure reduction were compared using the same primary outcome measure, patients treated with pregabalin (600 mg per day) achieved a greater reduction in seizures than did those treated with gabapentin at the highest dose tested (1800 mg per day). This outcome may reflect the high oral bioavailability of pregabalin, the relatively low doses of gabapentin studied compared with current open use (≥3600 mg per day), and other factors. This and the greater potency of pregabalin (4- to 6-fold greater on an mg/kg basis) mean that relatively small amounts of pregabalin must be absorbed to be efficacious and that uptake is not saturated at therapeutically relevant doses. This represents a significant advantage of pregabalin over gabapentin. Patients with a limited capacity to absorb gabapentin may benefit greatly from treatment with pregabalin.

REFERENCES

1. Schmidt B. Potential antiepileptic drugs: gabapentin. In: Levy R, Mattson R, Meldrum BS, Penry JK, Dreifuss FE, eds. *Antiepileptic drugs*, 3rd ed. New York: Raven Press. 1989:925–935.
2. Taylor CP. Mechanisms of action of new antiepileptic drugs. In: Chadwick D, ed. *New trends in epilepsy management: the role of gabapentin.* London: Royal Society of Medicine Services. 1993: 13–40.
3. Satzinger G. Antiepileptics from gamma-aminobutyric acid. *Arzneimittelforschung* 1994;44:261–266.
4. Bartoszyk GD, Meyerson N, Reimann W, et al. Gabapentin. In: Meldrum BS, Porter RJ, eds. *New anticonvulsant drugs.* London: John Libbey. 1986:147–463.
5. Stewart BH, Kugler AR, Thompson PR, Bockbrader HN. A saturable transport mechanism in the intestinal absorption of gabapentin

is the underlying cause of lack of proportionality between increasing dose and drug levels in plasma. *Pharm Res* 1993;10:276–281.

6. Su TZ, Lunney E, Campbell G, Oxender DL. Transport of gabapentin, a gamma-amino acid drug, by system L alpha-amino acid transporters: a comparative study in astrocytes, synaptosomes and CHO cells. *J Neurochem* 1995;64:2125–2131.

7. Hengy H, Kölle EU. Determination of gabapentin in plasma and urine by high-performance liquid chromatography and pre-column labelling for ultraviolet detection. *J Chromatogr* 1985; 341:473–478.

8. Lensmeyer GL, Kempf T, Gidal BE, Wiebe DA. Optimized method for determination of gabapentin in serum by high-performance liquid chromatography. *Ther Drug Monit* 1995;17:251–258.

9. Wolf CE, Saady JJ, Poklis A. Determination of gabapentin in serum using solid-phase extraction and gas-liquid chromatography. *J Analyt Toxicol* 1996;20:498–501.

10. Zour E, Lodhi SA, Nesbitt RU, et al. Stability studies of gabapentin in aqueous solutions. *Pharm Res* 1992;9:595–600.

11. Potschka H, Feuerstein TJ, Löscher W. Gabapentin-lactam, a close analogue of the anticonvulsant gabapentin, exerts convulsant activity in amygdale kindled rats. *Naunyn Schmiedebergs Archiv Pharmacol* 2000;361:200–205.

12. Jehle T, Lagreze WA, Blauth E, et al. Gabapentin-lactam (8-aza-spiro[5,4]decan-9-on; GBP-L) inhibits oxygen glucose deprivation-induced [³H]glutamate release and is a neuroprotective agent in a model of acute retinal ischemia. *Naunyn Schmiedebergs Archiv Pharmacol* 2000;362:74–81.

13. United States Patent 6,054,482, entitled Lactam-free Amino Acids. Inventors: Augart, et al, Assignee: Gödecke Aktiengesellschaft, issued April 25, 2000.

14. Ben-Menachem E, Kugler AR. Drugs in development: pregabalin. In: Levy RH, Mattson RH, Meldrum BS, Perucca E, eds. *Antiepileptic drugs*, 5th ed. New York: Raven Press. 2002:901–905.

15. Bockbrader HN, Burger PJ, Kugler AR, et al. The oral clearance (CL/F) of commonly prescribed antiepileptic drugs (AEDs) is unaffected by concomitant administration of pregabalin in adult patients with refractory partial seizures. *Neurology* 2000;54 (Suppl 3):421.

16. Taylor CP, Gee NS, Su TZ, et al. A summary of mechanistic hypotheses of gabapentin pharmacology. *Epilepsy Res* 1998; 29:233–249.

17. Taylor CP. Gabapentin: mechanisms of action. In: Levy RH, Mattson RH, Meldrum BS, Perucca E, eds. *Antiepileptic drugs*, 5th ed. New York: Raven Press. 2002:321–334.

18. Maurer HH, Rump AFE. Intestinal absorption of gabapentin in rats. *Arzneimittelforschung* 1991;41:104–106.

19. Stevenson CM, Kim JS, Fleisher D. Colonic absorption of antiepileptic agents. *Epilepsia* 1997;38:63–67.

20. Kriel RL, Birnbaum AK, Cloyd JC, et al. Failure of absorption of gabapentin after rectal administration. *Epilepsia* 1997;38: 1242–1244.

21. Vollmer KO, Anhut H, Thomann P, et al. Pharmacokinetic model and absolute bioavailability of the new anticonvulsant gabapentin. *Adv Epileptol* 1987;17:209–211.

22. Richens A. Clinical pharmacokinetics of gabapentin. In: Chadwick D, ed. *New trends in epilepsy management: the role of gabapentin.* London: Royal Society of Medicine Services. 1993:41–46.

23. Vollmer KO, Türck D, Wagner F, et al. Multiple dose pharmacokinetics of the new anticonvulsant gabapentin. *Eur J Clin Pharmacol* 1989;36(Suppl):A310.

24. Türck D, Vollmer KO, Bockbrader H, Sedman A. Dose-linearity of the new anticonvulsant gabapentin after multiple oral doses. *Eur J Clin Pharmacol* 1989;36(Suppl):A310.

25. Comstock TJ, Sica DA, Bockbrader HN, et al. Gabapentin pharmacokinetics in subjects with various degrees of renal function. *J Clin Pharmacol* 1990;30:862.

26. McLean MJ. Gabapentin. *Epilepsia* 1995;36(Suppl 2):S73–S76.

27. Beydoun A, Fischer J, Labar DR, et al. Gabapentin monotherapy: II. A 26-week, double-blind, dose-controlled, multicenter study of conversion from polytherapy in outpatients with refractory complex partial or secondarily generalized seizures. The US Gabapentin Study Group 82/83. *Neurology* 1997;49:746–752.

28. Bergey GK, Morris HH, Rosenfeld W, et al. Gabapentin monotherapy: I. An 8-day, double-blind, dose-controlled, multicenter study

29. Beydoun A, Fakhoury T, Nasreddine W, Abou-Khalil B. Conversion to high-dose gabapentin monotherapy in patients with medically refractory partial epilepsy. *Epilepsia* 1998;39:188–193.

30. Wilson EA, Sills GJ, Forrest G, et al. High-dose gabapentin in refractory epilepsy: clinical observations in 50 patients. *Epilepsy Res* 1998;29:161–166.

31. Gidal BE, Radulovic LL, Kruger S, et al. Inter- and intra-subject variability in gabapentin absorption and absolute bioavailability. *Epilepsy Res* 2000;40:123–127.

32. Gidal BE, Maly MM, Kowalski JW, et al. Gabapentin absorption: effect of mixing with foods of varying macronutrient composition. *Ann Pharmacother* 1998;32:405-408.

33. Gidal BE, Maly MM, Budde J, et al. Effect of a high-protein meal on gabapentin pharmacokinetics. *Epilepsy Res* 1996;23:71–76.

34. Benetello P, Furlanut M, Fortunato M, et al. Oral gabapentin disposition in patients with epilepsy after a high-protein meal. *Epilepsia* 1997;38:1140–1142.

35. Gidal BE, DeCerce J, Bockbrader HN, et al. Gabapentin bioavailability: effect of dose and frequency of administration in adult patients with epilepsy. *Epilepsy Res* 1998;31:91–99.

36. Boyd RA, Türck D, Sedman AJ, Bockbrader HN. Effect of age and gender on the single dose pharmacokinetics of gabapentin. *Epilepsia* 1999;40:474–479.

37. Bockbrader HN, Hunt T, Strand J, et al. Pregabalin pharmacokinetics and safety in healthy volunteers: results from two phase I studies. *Neurology* 2000;54(Suppl 3):A421.

38. Piyapolrungroj N, Li C, Bockbrader H, et al. Mucosal uptake of gabapentin vs. pregabalin in the small intestine. *Pharm Res* 2001; 18:1126–1130.

39. Vollmer KO, von Hodenberg A, Kölle EU. Pharmacokinetics and metabolism of gabapentin in rat, dog and man. *Arzneimittelforschung* 1986;36:830–839.

40. Bockbrader HN. Clinical pharmacokinetics of gabapentin. *Drugs of Today* 1995;31:19–25.

41. Ben-Menachem E, Hedner T, Persson LI. Seizure frequency and CSF gabapentin, GABA, and monoamine metabolite concentrations after 3 months' treatment with 900 mg or 1,200 mg gabapentin daily in patients with intractable complex partial seizures. *Neurology* 1990;40(Suppl 1):158.

42. Ben-Menachem E, Persson LI, Hedner T. Selected CSF biochemistry and gabapentin concentrations in the CSF and plasma in patients with partial seizures after a single oral dose of gabapentin. *Epilepsy Res* 1990;11:45–49.

43. Ben-Menachem E, Sodefelt B, Hamberger A, et al. Seizure frequency and CSF parameters in a double-blind, placebo-controlled trial of gabapentin in patients with intractable complex partial seizures. *Epilepsy Res* 1995;21:231–236.

44. Wang Y, Welty DF. The simultaneous estimation of the influx and efflux blood-brain barrier permeabilities of gabapentin using a microdialysis-pharmacokinetic approach. *Pharm Res* 1996;13: 398–403.

45. Radulovic LL, Türck D, Hodenberg AV, et al. Disposition of gabapentin (Neurontin) in mice, rats, dogs, and monkeys. *Drug Metab Disp* 1995;23:441–448.

46. Vollmer KO, Türck D, Bockbrader HN, et al. Summary of Neurontin (gabapentin) clinical pharmacokinetics. *Epilepsia* 1992;33(Suppl 3):77.

47. Ojemann LM, Friel PN, Ojemann GA. Gabapentin concentrations in human brain. *Epilepsia* 1988;29:694.

48. Feng MR, Turluck D, Burleigh J, et al. Brain microdialysis and PK/PD correlation of pregabalin in rats. *Eur J Drug Metab Pharmacokin* 2001;26:123–128.

49. Blum RA, Comstock TJ, Sica DA, et al. Pharmacokinetics of gabapentin in subjects with various degrees of renal function. *Clin Pharmacol Ther* 1994;56:154–159.

50. Callerame KJ, Toledo C, Martinez OA, et al. Gabapentin serum levels in patients on doses greater than 1,800 mg/day. *Epilepsia* 1995;36(Suppl 4):70.

51. Ouellet D, Bockbrader HN, Wesche DL, et al. Population pharmacokinetics of gabapentin in infants and children. *Epilepsy Res* 2001;47:229–241.

52. Randinitis EJ, Posvar EL, Alvey CW, et al. Pharmacokinetics of pregabalin in subjects with various degrees of renal function. *J Clin Pharmacol* 2003;43:277–283.
53. Corrigan BW, Bockbrader H, Burger PJ, et al. Pregabalin population pharmacokinetics in patients with refractory seizures. Presented at the 5th European Congress on Epileptology; October 9, 2002; Madrid, Spain.
54. Hussein G, Troupin AS, Montouris G. Gabapentin interaction with felbamate. *Neurology* 1996;47:1106.
55. Busch JA, Radulovic LL, Bockbrader HN, et al. Effect of Maalox TC on single-dose pharmacokinetics of gabapentin capsules in healthy subjects. *Pharm Res* 1992;9(Suppl):S315.
56. Eldon MA, Underwood BA, Randinitis EJ, et al. Gabapentin does not interact with a contraceptive regimen of norethindrone acetate and ethinyl estradiol. *Neurology* 1998;50:1146–1148.
57. Frye MA, Kimbrell TA, Dunn RT, et al. Gabapentin does not alter single-dose lithium pharmacokinetics. *J Clin Psychopharmacology* 1998;18:461–464.
58. Wilson E, Brodie MJ, Bockbrader HN, et al. Pregabalin drug interaction studies in patients with epilepsy maintained on either valproate (VPA), lamotrigine (LTG), phenytoin (PHY), or carbamazepine (CBZ). Presented at the 5th European Congress on Epileptology; October 9, 2002; Madrid, Spain.
59. Crawford P, Ghadualis E, Lane R, et al. Gabapentin as an antiepileptic drug in man. *J Neurol Neurosurg Psychiatry* 1987; 50:682–686.
60. Sivenius J, Kalviainen R, Ylinen A, Riekkinen P. Double-blind study of gabapentin in the treatment of partial seizures. *Epilepsia* 1991;32:539–542.
61. Lindberger M, Luhr O, Johannessen S, et al. Serum concentrations and effects of gabapentin and vigabatrin: observations from a dose titration study. *Ther Drug Monit* 2003;25:457–462.
62. UK Gabapentin Study Group. Gabapentin in partial epilepsy. *Lancet* 1990;335:1114–1117.
63. US Gabapentin Study Group, No 5. Gabapentin as add-on therapy in refractory partial epilepsy: a double-blind, placebo-controlled, parallel-group study. *Neurology* 1993;43:2292–2298.
64. Anhut H, Ashman P, Feuerstein TJ, et al. Gabapentin (Neurontin) as add-on therapy in patients with partial seizures: a double-blind, placebo-controlled study. The International Gabapentin Study Group. *Epilepsia* 1994;35:795–801.
65. Kugler AR, Robbins JL, Strand JC, et al. Pregabalin overview: a novel CNS-active compound with anticonvulsant activity. Presented at the 56th Annual Meeting of the American Epilepsy Society; December 11, 2002; Seattle, Washington.
66. French JA, Kugler AR, Robbins JL, et al. Dose-response trial of pregabalin adjunctive therapy in patients with partial seizures. *Neurology* 2003;60:1631–1637.
67. Miller R, Frame B, Corrigan B, et al. Exposure-response analysis of pregabalin add-on treatment of patients with refractory partial seizures. *Clin Pharmacol Ther* 2003;73:491–505.
68. Perucca E, Ramsay RE, Robbins JL, et al. Pregabalin demonstrates anticonvulsants activity onset by the second day. Presented at the 56th Annual Meeting of the American Epilepsy Society; December 11, 2002; Seattle, Washington.
69. Uthman BM, Beydoun A, Kugler AR, et al. Long-term efficacy and tolerability of pregabalin in patients with partial seizures. Presented at the 56th Annual Meeting of the American Epilepsy Society; December 11, 2002; Seattle, Washington.
70. McLean MJ, Morrell MJ, Willmore LJ, et al. Safety and tolerability of gabapentin as adjunctive therapy in a large multicenter study. *Epilepsia* 1999;40:965–972.
71. Morrell MJ, McLean MJ, Willmore LJ, et al. Efficacy of gabapentin as adjunctive therapy in a large multicenter study. *Seizure* 2000;9:241–248.
72. McLean MJ, Willmore LJ, Morrell MJ, et al, and the Neurontin STEPS Study Group. Efficacy of gabapentin (Neurontin) as add-on therapy for patients older than 60 with partial epilepsy [abstract]. *Epilepsia* 1997;38(Suppl 8):206.
73. Beran R, Berkovic S, Black A, et al. AUStralian study of titration to effect profile of safety (AUS-STEPS): High-dose gabapentin (Neurontin) in partial seizures. *Epilepsia* 2001;42:1335–1339.
74. Bruni J. Outcome evaluation of gabapentin as add-on therapy for partial seizures. "NEON" Study Investigators Group. Neurontin Evaluation of Outcomes in Neurological Practice. *Can J Neurol Sci* 1998;25:134–140.
75. Baulac M, Cavalcanti D, Semah F, et al. Gabapentin add-on therapy with adaptable dosages in 610 patients with partial epilepsy: an open, observational study. *Seizure* 1998;7:55–62.
76. Agomuoh TC, Barkley GL. Clinical experience with gabapentin in a tertiary referral center. *Epilepsia* 1995;36(Suppl 4):70.
77. Anderson BL, Haessly SM, Weatherford KJ, et al. An observational study of efficacy and tolerance of gabapentin. *Epilepsia* 1995;36(Suppl 4):S70.
78. Doherty KP, Gates JR, Penovich PE, Moriarty GL. Gabapentin in a medically refractory epilepsy population. Seizure response and unusual side effects. *Epilepsia* 1995;36(Suppl 4):S71.
79. Hosain S, Labar DR, Nikolov B, Harden CL. Gabapentin use in the general epileptic population. *Epilepsia* 1995;36(Suppl 4):S70.
80. Kelly KM, Kothary SP, Beydoun A. Safety and efficacy of extended gabapentin therapy for patients with complex partial or secondarily generalized seizures. *Epilepsia* 1995;36(Suppl 4):S69.
81. Piña-Garza JE, Bukhari AA, Laowattana S, et al. Treatment of patients with refractory partial epilepsies with gabapentin: a retrospective analysis. *Epilepsia* 1995;36(Suppl 4):S69.
82. Perry JR, Sawka C. Add-on gabapentin for refractory seizures in patients with brain tumours. *Can J Neurol Sci* 1996;23:128–131.
83. Ojemann LM, Wilensky AJ, Temkin NR, et al. Long-term treatment with gabapentin for partial epilepsy. *Epilepsy Res* 1992;13:159–165.
84. US Gabapentin Study Group. The long-term safety and efficacy of gabapentin (Neurontin) as add-on therapy in drug-resistant partial epilepsy. *Epilepsy Res* 1994;18:67–73.
85. Leidermann DB, Koto EM, LaMoreaux LK, McLean MJ. Long-term therapy with gabapentin (GBP; Neurontin): 5-year experience from a US open-label trial. US Gabapentin Study Group 13. *Epilepsia* 1995;36(Suppl 4):S68.
86. Handforth A, Treiman DM. Efficacy and tolerance of long-term, high-dose gabapentin: additional observations. *Epilepsia* 1994;35: 1032–1037.
87. Sivenius J, Ylinen A, Kalviainen R, Riekkinen PJ Sr. Long-term study with gabapentin in patients with drug-resistant epileptic seizures. *Arch Neurol* 1994;51:1047–1050.
88. Muscas GC, Chiroli S, Luceri F, et al. Conversion from thrice daily to twice daily administration of gabapentin (GBP) in partial epilepsy: analysis of clinical efficacy and plasma levels. *Seizure* 2000;9:47–50.
89. Leach JP, Girvan J, Paul A, Brodie MJ. Gabapentin and cognition: a double-blind, dose-ranging, placebo-controlled study in refractory epilepsy. *J Neurol Neurosurg Psychiatry* 1997;62:372–376.
90. Chadwick D, Anhut H, Murray G, et al. Gabapentin (GBP; Neurontin) monotherapy in patients with newly-diagnosed epilepsy: results of a double-blind fixed-dose study comparing three dosages of gabapentin and open-label carbamazepine. *Epilepsia* 1997;38:34.
91. Brodie MJ, Chadwick DW, Anhut H, et al. Gabapentin versus lamotrigine monotherapy: a double-blind comparison in newly diagnosed epilepsy. *Epilepsia* 2002;43:993–1000.
92. Rowan AJ, Ramsay RE. Outcome of VA Coop Study #428: Treatment of seizures in the elderly population. International Geriatric Epilepsy Symposium; September 12–14, 2003; Coral Gables, Florida.
93. Tatum WO, Zachariah SB. Gabapentin treatment of seizures in acute intermittent porphyria. *Neurology* 1995;45:1216–1217.
94. Yandel ML, Watters MR. Treatment of complex partial epilepticus unmasking acute intermittent porphyria in a patient with resected anaplastic glioma. *Clin Neurol Neurosurg* 1995;97:261–263.
95. Krauss GL, Simmons-O'Brien E, Campbell M. Successful treatment of seizures and porphyria with gabapentin. *Neurology* 1995;45:594–595.
96. Chadwick D, Leiderman DB, Sauerman W, et al. Gabapentin in generalized seizures. *Epilepsy Res* 1996;25:191–197.
97. Bourgeois B, Brown L, Pellock J, et al. Gabapentin (Neurontin) monotherapy in children with benign childhood epilepsy with centrotemporal spikes (BECTS): a 36-week, double-blind, placebo-controlled study. *Epilepsia* 1998;39(Suppl 6):163.
98. Khurana DS, Riviello J, Helmers S, et al. Efficacy of gabapentin therapy in children with refractory partial seizures. *J Pediatr* 1996;128:829–833.

99. Appleton R, Fichtner K, LaMoreaux L, et al. Gabapentin as add-on therapy in children with refractory partial seizures: a 12-week, multicentre, double-blind, placebo-controlled study. Gabapentin Paediatric Study Group. *Epilepsia* 1999;40:1147–1154.

100. Korn-Merker E, Bourusiak P, Boenigk HE. Gabapentin in childhood epilepsy: a prospective evaluation of efficacy and safety. *Epilepsy Res* 2000;38:2732.

101. Appleton R, Fichtner K, LaMoreaux L, et al. Gabapentin as add-on therapy in children with refractory partial seizures: a 24-week, multicentre, open-label study. *Dev Med Child Neurol* 2001;43:269–273.

102. Trudeau V, Myers S, LaMoreaux L, et al. Gabapentin in naive childhood absence epilepsy: results from two double-blind, placebo-controlled, multicenter studies. *J Child Neurol* 1996;11:470–475.

103. Litzinger MJ, Wiscombe N, Hanny A, et al. Increased seizures and aggression seen in persons with mental retardation and epilepsy treated with Neurontin. *Epilepsia* 1995;36(Suppl 4):S71.

104. Zupanc ML, Schroeder VM. Behavioral changes in children on gabapentin. *Epilepsia* 1995;36(Suppl 4):S73.

105. Wolf SM, Shinnar S, Kang H, et al. Gabapentin toxicity in children manifesting as behavioral changes. *Epilepsia* 1996;36:1203–1205.

106. Lee DO, Steingard RJ, Cesena M, et al. Behavioral side effects of gabapentin in children. *Epilepsia* 1996;37:87–90.

107. Vossler DG. Exacerbation of seizures in Lennox-Gastaut syndrome by gabapentin. *Neurology* 1996;46:852–853.

108. New drug application for gabapentin. Morris Plains, NJ: Parke-Davis, Division of Warner-Lambert Company.

109. Fischer JH, Barr AN, Rogers SL, et al. Lack of serious toxicity following gabapentin overdose. *Neurology* 1994;44:982–983.

110. Fernandez MC, Walter FG, Petersen LR, Walkotte SM. Gabapentin, valproic acid, and ethanol intoxication: elevated blood levels with mild clinical effects. *Clin Toxicol* 1996;34:437–439.

111. Asconape J, Collins T. Weight gain associated with the use of gabapentin. *Epilepsia* 1995;36(Suppl 4):S72.

112. Gidal BE, Maly MM, Nemire RE, Haley K. Weight gain and gabapentin therapy. *Ann Pharmacother* 1995;29:1048.

113. De Toledo JC, Toledo C, DeCerce J, Ramsay RE. Changes in body weight with chronic, high-dose gabapentin therapy. *Ther Drug Monit* 1997;19:394–396.

114. Buetefisch CM, Gutierrez A, Gutmann L. Choreoathetotic movements: a possible side effect of gabapentin. *Neurology* 1996;46:851–852.

115. Chudnow RS, Dewey RB, Lawson CR. Choreoathetosis as a side effect of gabapentin therapy in severely neurologically impaired patients. *Arch Neurol* 1997;54:910–912.

116. Reeves AL, So EL, Sharbrough FW, Krahn LE. Movement disorders associated with the use of gabapentin. *Epilepsia* 1996;37:988–990.

117. Lee DO, Steingard RJ, Cesna M, et al. Behavioral side effects of gabapentin in children. *Epilepsia* 1996;37:87–90.

118. Tallian KB, Nahata MC, Lo, W, Tsao CY. Gabapentin associated with aggressive behavior in pediatric patients with seizures. *Epilepsia* 1996;37:501–502.

119. Rowbotham M, Harden N, Stacey B, et al. Gabapentin for the treatment of postherpetic neuralgia: a randomized controlled trial. *JAMA* 1998;280:1837–1842.

120. Brigell MG, Carter CM, Smith F, Garofalo EA. Prospective evaluation of the ophthalmologic safety of pregabalin shows no evidence of toxicity. Presented at the 56th Annual Meeting of the American Epilepsy Society; December 11, 2002; Seattle, Washington.

121. Hindmarch I, Dawson J, Stanley N. Evaluation of cognitive and psychomotor profile of pregabalin compared to alprazolam in normal volunteers. Presented at the 56th Annual Meeting of the American Epilepsy Society; December 11, 2002; Seattle, Washington.

122. Data on file. Morris Plains, NJ: Parke-Davis, Division of Warner-Lambert Company, now Pfizer Inc.

123. Neurontin® prescribing information. New York: Pfizer Inc.

124. Sigler RE, Gough AW, de la Iglesia FA. Pancreatic acinar cell neoplasia in male Wistar rats following 2 years of gabapentin exposure. *Toxicology* 1995;98:73–92.

125. Fowler ML, Sigler RE, de la Iglesia FA, et al. Absence of Ki-ras mutations in exocrine pancreatic tumors from male rats chronically exposed to gabapentin. *Mutation Res* 1995;327:151–160.

126. Dominick MA, Robertson DG, Bleavins MR, et al. Alpha 2u-globulin nephropathy without nephrocarcinogenesis in male Wistar rats administered 1-(aminomethyl)cyclohexaneacetic acid. *Toxicol Appl Pharmacol* 1991;111:375–387.

127. *Datamonitor*, a publication of Pfizer Inc. August 20, 2001.

128. McLean MJ, Gidal BE. Gabapentin dosing in the treatment of epilepsy. *Clin Ther* 2003;25:1382–1406.

129. Fisher RS, Sachdeo RC, Pellock J, et al. Dose initiation of gabapentin (CI-945) add-on therapy: a multicenter, randomized, double-blind comparative study. *Epilepsia* 1996;37:158.

130. Penovich P, Fisher RS, Sachdeo RC, et al. A multicenter, randomized, double-blind, comparative, dose-initiation study of gabapentin (CI-945) in the elderly. *Epilepsia* 1996;37:158.

131. Fisher RS, Sachdeo RC, Pellock J, et al. Rapid initiation of gabapentin: a randomized, controlled trial. *Neurology* 2001;56:743–748.

Lamotrigine

60

Frank G. Gilliam   *Barry E. Gidal*

CHEMISTRY AND MECHANISM OF ACTION

Lamotrigine is a phenyltriazine, a tertiary amine derivative [3,5-diamino-6-(2,3-dichlorophenyl)-1,2,4-trizine; molecular weight, 256.09] that is poorly soluble in water or alcohol (Fig. 60.1). Lamotrigine acts through voltage and use-dependent blockade of neuronal sodium channels, with greater blockade during repetitive activation (1–4). Blockade of sodium channels activated from depolarized membrane potentials occurs at lower concentrations than those required to elicit blockade from hyperpolarized membrane but at clinically achievable concentrations (5). Lamotrigine appears to stabilize the inactivated state of the Na^+ channel. Recently, a potential binding site within the Na^+ channel pore was identified (6). In addition, lamotrigine dose-dependently inhibits high-voltage activation of Ca^{2+} currents, possibly through inhibition of presynaptic N and P/Q-type Ca^{2+} channels (3,7–9). Despite apparent activity in human absence seizures, lamotrigine does not appear to inhibit low-voltage currents mediated by T-type Ca^{2+} channels. Although these actions are mechanistically similar to those of phenytoin, important differences do exist between these agents. Phenytoin inhibits veratrine-evoked release of glutamate and γ-aminobutyric acid (GABA). At similar concentrations, lamotrigine is twice as effective in inhibiting the release of glutamate compared to the release of GABA (10). Release of excitatory amino-acid neurotransmitters such as glutamate and aspartate are blocked during sustained repetitive firing. Animal models also suggest that lamotrigine inhibits ischemia-induced release of excitatory neurotransmitters (11–14). Inhibition of nitric oxide release (15) and serotonin uptake (16) may also modestly contribute to lamotrigine's action in both epilepsy and affective disorders. Lamotrigine appears to only modestly inhibit potassium channels and is a weak inhibitor of 5-HT uptake in humans or rodents (16). Lamotrigine is not an N-methyl-D-aspartate (NMDA) receptor antagonist (17) and does not appear to alter either plasma or brain GABA concentrations in humans (18,19).

Most likely, its antiepileptic actions and clinical spectrum can be explained largely by the combination of both Na^+ and Ca^{2+} (N, P/Q) channel inhibition.

Lamotrigine prevents maximal electroshock seizures in mice, with potency and duration similar to those of phenytoin and carbamazepine, but does not prevent pentylenetetrazole-induced clonus, a model of absence seizures (20). Photically evoked afterdischarges and photoconvulsive responses are suppressed (21). Activity has been demonstrated in the genetic epilepsy-prone rat (22) and in the electrically induced electroencephalogram afterdischarge model (23). Lamotrigine does not prevent cortical kindling in rats, but it does attenuate kindled seizures in a dose-dependent manner (23–25).

ABSORPTION, DISTRIBUTION, AND METABOLISM

Lamotrigine is an orally administered drug, available in various dosage strengths and bioequivalent formulations, including dispersible tablets. Lamotrigine is completely absorbed, with a bioavailability of 98% (26). Peak serum concentrations are achieved within 1 to 3 hours after oral administration (27). Lamotrigine displays linear oral absorption, with proportionality observed after doses up to 700 mg (28,29). A secondary peak in serum concentration between 4 and 6 hours after oral or parenteral administration suggests enterohepatic recycling. Food does not significantly affect absorption (30). Systemic absorption also occurs after rectal administration, although mean areas under the curve (AUC) are approximately 50% of corresponding oral values (31).

Approximately 56% of lamotrigine is bound to plasma proteins, and moderate binding remains constant over a concentration range of 1 to 10 μg/mL (28). *In vitro*, protein

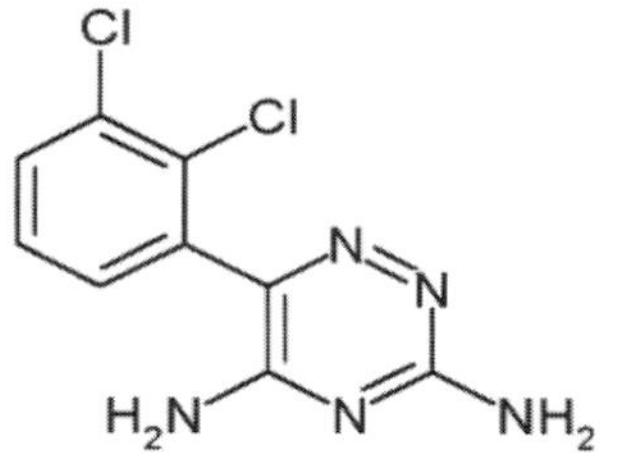

Figure 60.1 Structure of lamotrigine.

binding is unaffected by phenytoin, phenobarbital, carbamazepine, or valproate (28).

Volume of distribution is independent of dose and ranges between 0.9 and 1.2 L/kg in healthy volunteers (28,30). Data from rodents and human *ex vivo* placental perfusion studies suggest that lamotrigine easily and rapidly crosses the placenta (32) and is present in maternal milk at potentially clinically significant levels (33). In humans, lamotrigine undergoes extensive hepatic metabolism by uridine diphosphate (UDP)-glucuronosyl-transferase (UGT 1A4) (34). Glucuronide conjugation can occur at both heterocyclic nitrogen atoms to form a quaternary amine glucuronide (35). In healthy volunteers, 70% of a single dose is recovered in the urine (28), with the 5-*N* and 2-*N*-glucuronide metabolite accounting for 90% of the recovered dose. This glucuronide metabolite is pharmacologically inactive. Renal elimination of unchanged drug represents less than 10% of an administered dose.

The elimination half-life of lamotrigine monotherapy in adults is approximately 24 to 29 hours. Oral clearance averages 0.35 to 0.59 mL/kg per minute (28,36). Clearance is higher in children and lower in the elderly than in young adults. The concentration to dose ratio was approximately 30% to 50% lower in 3- to 6-year-old children than in 7- to 15-year-old children or young adults (37). In 12 children between 4 and 11 years of age receiving monotherapy, mean oral clearance was 0.64 mL/kg per minute and elimination half-life was 32 hours (38). In a group of elderly volunteers between 65 and 76 years of age, clearance was 37% lower than in a group of 26- to 38-year-old adults (27).

Evidence suggests that lamotrigine undergoes autoinduction. Population analysis of sparse data obtained retrospectively from 163 patients receiving monotherapy demonstrated a 17% increase in clearance over 48 weeks (39). This modest degree of autoinduction is not clinically meaningful, however, because initiation of lamotrigine therapy usually involves gradual dose escalation.

Severity of hepatic disease can influence lamotrigine pharmacokinetics, and patients with Child-Pugh scores of 5 to 6 (B) or 7 to 9 (C) require respective dosage reductions of 50% to 75% (40). No significant differences in plasma clearance have been noted in patients with chronic renal failure (41). Approximately 17% of a lamotrigine dose may be removed by hemodialysis, with a corresponding reduction in half-life to about 13 hours (42).

The apparent oral clearance of lamotrigine does not appear to differ significantly between men and women (39) but may increase more than 65% during pregnancy, most noticeably during the second and third trimesters. Clearance returns to prepregnancy levels postpartum (43).

A serum concentration-effect range for lamotrigine has not been defined (44,45), and patients may respond to a wide range of drug concentrations. A target range between 4 and 14 µg/mL has been suggested for patients with epilepsy (46,47). Use of serum concentration data may be used to interpret drug interactions and compliance issues.

DRUG INTERACTIONS

Effect of Other Drugs on Lamotrigine

Comedication with Inducing Antiepileptic Drugs

Substantial interpatient variability in plasma clearance of lamotrigine can be explained largely by the presence or absence of concomitant drug therapy (48,49). Lamotrigine elimination half-life is reduced approximately 50% (about 12 to 15 hours) in the presence of UGT-inducing drugs, such as carbamazepine, phenobarbital, primidone, and phenytoin (50). While the addition of an enzyme inducer to a lamotrigine-containing regimen is well established, the time course of *de-induction*, after the removal of a concomitant inducer such as phenytoin or carbamazepine, is less clear-cut. An analysis of data derived from a pivotal conversion to monotherapy trial (51) found that mean lamotrigine plasma concentrations approximately doubled after the withdrawal of concomitant phenytoin; increases of only 50% to 75% followed the withdrawal of carbamazepine cotherapy (52). These data suggested that lamotrigine concentrations did not significantly change (increase) until concentrations of phenytoin or carbamazepine approached zero (52). Similar observations came as well from a small, prospective study (53).

Lamotrigine does not interact significantly with newer antiepileptic drugs such as gabapentin, zonisamide, levetiracetam, or felbamate, although its serum concentrations have been reported to be modestly decreased when concomitantly administered with either oxcarbazepine (54–57) and may be significantly changed by felbamate (55) or topiramate (58). The clinical significance of these interactions is uncertain.

Comedication with Valproate

Because lamotrigine does not undergo cytochrome P(CYP) 450-dependent metabolism, only UGT inhibitors will decrease its clearance and increase its plasma concentrations and prolong elimination half-life to about 60 hours (59). In adult volunteers, the maximum theoretical inhibition of lamotrigine clearance by valproate is approximately 65%, with 50% occurring at valproate plasma concentrations of approximately 5 to 6 µg/mL. Valproate concentrations of approximately 50 μg/mL produce maximum theoretical inhibition, which begins at low doses of 125 to 250 mg per day and peaks at approximately 500 mg per day (60). Data from epilepsy patients who were prospectively converted from combination therapy with valproate and lamotrigine to lamotrigine monotherapy support these observations (61).

Early suggestions of modest decreases in valproate serum concentrations with concurrent lamotrigine are unlikely to be clinically significant (62,63).

Effect of Lamotrigine on Other Drugs

Lamotrigine does not induce or inhibit the mixed-function oxidase system (CYP isozymes) and is not extensively bound to plasma proteins; these properties would predict a low incidence of causing pharmacokinetic interactions. Addition of lamotrigine did not affect serum concentrations of phenytoin, phenobarbital, primidone, carbamazepine, or carbamazepine epoxide (36,64–66). Hormone concentrations were not altered in female volunteers taking oral contraceptives (67).

Effect of Nonantiepileptic Drugs on Lamotrigine

Daily doses of acetaminophen, which is 55% eliminated by glucuronide conjugation but is not a UGT inducer, unexpectedly increased lamotrigine clearance, although occasional use would not be expected to alter lamotrigine pharmacokinetics (68). One anecdotal report has suggested an increase in lamotrigine serum concentrations after the addition of the serotonin-selective reuptake inhibitor sertraline (69). Concomitant treatment with oral contraceptives may decrease lamotrigine plasma levels by approximately 40% to 50%, possibly because of UGT induction by ethinyl estradiol (70). Interestingly, this apparent induction effect appears to quickly reverse. According to the prescribing information, during the pill-free week of oral contraceptive treatment cycle, the plasma level of lamotrigine increases, reaching levels approximately twice those found during the active oral contraceptive exposure.

EFFICACY

Adjunctive Therapy for Partial Seizures

Eight premarketing, multicenter, double-blind, placebo-controlled trials defined the efficacy of lamotrigine as adjunctive treatment in adults with partial seizures (26, 71–77). Seizure frequency was reduced by more than 50% in one fourth of these patients and by 36% from baseline in the study (74) with the highest dose (500 mg). The placebo group had an 8% reduction. These studies supported the approval of lamotrigine as adjunctive therapy for partial seizures in persons 16 years of age and older.

Monotherapy for Partial Seizures

A multicenter, double-blind, randomized trial compared 500 mg of lamotrigine and 1,000 mg of valproate (51). In the protocol analysis, 56% of patients taking lamotrigine and 20% receiving low-dose valproate completed the trial by not meeting the exit criterion of a doubling of the greatest 2-day or 1-month seizure rates observed during baseline (primary end point). Lamotrigine had equivalent efficacy to carbamazepine (78) and phenytoin (79) in double-blind, randomized clinical studies of recent-onset epilepsy.

Lennox-Gastaut Syndrome in Children

A multicenter, double-blind, randomized trial (80) investigated lamotrigine as treatment for major motor seizures in patients 2 to 25 years of age with Lennox-Gastaut syndrome. The target dose of lamotrigine was 15 mg/kg for patients not taking valproate and 5 mg/kg for those taking valproate. Atonic, tonic, major myoclonic, and tonic-clinic seizures were reduced by 32% from baseline with lamotrigine; only a 9% reduction was observed with placebo. This study supported the U.S. Food and Drug Administration (FDA) indication for major motor seizures in Lennox-Gastaut syndrome in adults and children. Other studies have supported the efficacy of lamotrigine for this indication (81–84).

Idiopathic Generalized Epilepsies

The small number of patients in randomized controlled trials has precluded FDA approval of lamotrigine for use in idiopathic generalized epilepsy in the United States. Several studies (82,85–90), however, have suggested effectiveness for childhood absence epilepsy and juvenile myoclonic epilepsy. A double-blind, randomized, placebo-controlled, "responder-enriched" study (89) of recently diagnosed typical absence seizures, in which seizure frequency was confirmed by 24-hour and hyperventilation EEGs, found that 62% of patients achieved control with lamotrigine compared with 21% in the placebo group. Another add-on crossover study (85) demonstrated that lamotrigine significantly reduced seizures that were resistant to other antiepileptic drugs; 25% of the sample became seizure free. A case series suggested that severe myoclonic epilepsy may worsen with lamotrigine (91).

TOLERABILITY

Among the side effects reported with lamotrigine, rash has received the most attention (92–94), although the pathologic mechanism is unknown. The exact incidence in children and adults is difficult to determine, but a panel of

TABLE 60.1

COMMON ADVERSE EVENTS IN PIVOTAL COMPARISON OF LAMOTRIGINE MONOTHERAPY AND VALPROATE

Adverse Effects	Transition Phase (%)[a]		Monotherapy Phase (%)[a]	
	Lamotrigine	Low-Dose Valproate	Lamotrigine	Low-Dose Valproate
Dizziness	20	23	7	0
Nausea	16	19	7	2
Headache	13	13	7	14
Asthenia	12	13	2	0
Coordination abnormality	12	0	7	0
Vomiting	11	9	9	0
Rash	11	8	2	2
Somnolence	8	14	0	2
Tremor	7	10	5	7
Dyspepsia	0	14	7	2

[a]Dosages used were 500 mg per day of lamotrigine and 1,000 mg per day of valproate.
Adapted from Gilliam F, Vazquez B, Sackellares JC, et al. An active-control trial of lamotrigine monotherapy for partial seizures. *Neurology* 1998;51:1018–1025.

experts reviewing published and unpublished data concluded that "rashes leading to hospitalization, including Stevens-Johnson syndrome and hypersensitivity syndrome, occurred in approximately one of 300 adults and one of 100 children in clinical trials and appeared to be increased with overrapid titration when starting therapy and with concurrent valproate" (95). Monotherapy studies of new-onset epilepsy found no difference in occurrence of rash between lamotrigine and carbamazepine (78) or phenytoin (79), although the actual rates of serious rash when lamotrigine is initiated appropriately await additional data.

In the risk to benefit analysis cited (95), fewer than 10 deaths were attributed to lamotrigine from an estimated exposure exceeding 950000. Table 60.1 lists the most common central nervous system and systemic side effects reported with lamotrigine conversion and monotherapy in one trial (51). Some adverse events result from pharmacodynamic interactions with carbamazepine. Lamotrigine causes significantly less sedation than most other antiepileptic drugs (51,78,79). Reports of sedation ranged from 7% with lamotrigine versus 28% with phenytoin (79) to 12% versus 22% with carbamazepine (78) (both $p < 0.05$). Withdrawals as a result of adverse events were more frequent with carbamazepine (27% versus 15%) (78).

DOSING STRATEGIES

Although early clinical trials administered lamotrigine at a variety of initial dosages and titration schedules, the FDA has approved initiation schedules that support a minimum risk of rash. Recommended dosing guidelines from the FDA-approved prescribing information for specific ages and adjunctive antiepileptic drug regimens follow:

Lamotrigine Added to Enzyme-Inducing Antiepileptic Drugs in Patients Older Than 12 Years of Age

Weeks 1 and 2	50 mg per day
Weeks 3 and 4	100 mg per day in two divided doses

Usual maintenance dose: 300 to 500 mg per day (two divided doses). To achieve maintenance, doses may be increased by 100 mg per day every 1 to 2 weeks.

Lamotrigine Added to a Regimen Containing Valproate in Patients Older Than 12 Years of Age

Weeks 1 and 2	25 mg every *other* day
Weeks 3 and 4	25 mg every day

Usual maintenance dose: 100 to 400 mg per day (one or two divided doses). To achieve maintenance, doses may be increased by 25 to 50 mg per day every 1 to 2 weeks. The usual maintenance dose in patients adding lamotrigine to valproate alone ranges from 100 to 200 mg per day.

Lamotrigine Added to Enzyme-Inducing Antiepileptic Drugs in Patients 2 to 12 Years of Age

Weeks 1 and 2	0.6 mg/kg per day in two divided doses, rounded down to the nearest whole tablet
Weeks 3 and 4	1.2 mg/kg per day in two divided doses, rounded down to the nearest whole tablet

Usual maintenance dose: 5 to 15 mg/kg per day (maximum, 400 mg per day in two divided doses). To achieve maintenance, subsequent doses should be increased every 1 to 2 weeks as follows: calculate 1.2 mg/kg per day, round this amount down to the nearest whole tablet, and add this amount to the previously administered daily dose.

Maintenance doses in patients weighing less than 30 kg may need to be increased by as much as 50%, depending on clinical response.

Lamotrigine Added to a Regimen Containing Valproate in Patients 2 to 12 Years of Age

Weeks 1 and 2	0.15 mg/kg per day in one or two divided doses, rounded down to the nearest whole tablet; only whole tablets should be used for dosing
Weeks 3 and 4	0.3 mg/kg per day in one or two divided doses, rounded down to the nearest whole tablet

Weight-Based Dosing Can Be Achieved Using the Following Guide:

If patient's weight is:	Give this daily dose and use the most appropriate combination of lamotrigine 2-mg and 5-mg tablets:	
	Weeks 1 and 2	Weeks 3 and 4
6.7 to 14 kg	2 mg every *other* day	2 mg every day
14.1 to 27 kg	2 mg every day	4 mg every day
27.1 to 34 kg	4 mg every day	8 mg every day
34.1 to 40 kg	5 mg every day	10 mg every day

Usual maintenance dose: 1 to 5 mg/kg per day (maximum 200 mg per day in one or two divided doses). To achieve usual maintenance, subsequent doses must be increased every 1 to 2 weeks as follows: calculate 0.3 mg/kg per day, round this amount down to the nearest whole tablet, and add this amount to the previously administered daily dose. The usual maintenance dose in patients adding lamotrigine to valproate alone ranges from 1 to 3 mg/kg per day. Maintenance doses in patients weighing less than 30 kg may need to be increased by as much as 50%, depending on clinical response.

REFERENCES

1. Lang DG, Wang CM, Cooper BR. Lamotrigine, phenytoin and carbamazepine interactions on the sodium current present in N4TG1 mouse neuroblastoma cells. *J Pharmacol Exp Ther* 1993;266:829–835.
2. Lees G, Leach MJ. Studies on the mechanism of action of the novel anticonvulsant lamotrigine (Lamictal) using primary neurological cultures from rat cortex. *Brain Res* 1993;612:190–199.
3. Stefani A, Spadoni F, Bernardi G. Differential inhibition by riluzole, lamotrigine, and phenytoin of sodium and calcium currents in cortical neurons: implications for neuroprotective strategies. *Exp Neurol* 1997;147:115–122.
4. Xie X, Lancaster B, Peakman T, et al. Interaction of the antiepileptic drug lamotrigine with recombinant rat brain type IIA Na+ channels and with native Na+ channels in rat hippocampal neurons. *Pflugers Arch* 1995;430:437–446.
5. Coulter DA. Antiepileptic drug cellular mechanism of action: where does lamotrigine fit in? *J Child Neurol* 1997;12:S2–S9.
6. Yarov-Yarovoy V, Brown J, Sharpe EM, et al. Molecular determinants of voltage-dependent gating and binding of pore-blocking drugs in transmembrane segment IIIS6 of the Na+ channel alpha subunit. *J Biol Chem* 2001;276:20–27.
7. Stefani A, Spadoni F, Bernardi G. Voltage-activated calcium channels: targets of antiepileptic drug therapy? *Epilepsia* 1997;38:959–965.
8. Stefani A, Spadoni F, Siniscalchi A, et al. Lamotrigine inhibits Ca2+ currents in cortical neurons: functional implications. *Eur J Pharmacol* 1996;307:113–116.
9. Wang SJ, Tsai JJ, Gean PW. Lamotrigine inhibits depolarization-evoked Ca++ influx in dissociated amygdala neurons. *Synapse* 1998;29:355–362.
10. Leach MJ, Marden CM, Miller AA. Pharmacological studies on lamotrigine, a novel potential antiepileptic drug, II: neurochemical studies on the mechanism of action. *Epilepsia* 1986;27:490–497.
11. Conroy BP, Black D, Lin CY, et al. Lamotrigine attenuates cortical glutamate release during global cerebral ischemia in pigs on cardiopulmonary bypass. *Anesthesiology* 1999;90:844–854.
12. Crumrine RC, Bergstrand K, Cooper AT, et al. Lamotrigine protects hippocampal CA1 neurons from ischemic damage after cardiac arrest. *Stroke* 1997;28:2230–2236; discussion 2237.
13. Shuaib A, Mahmood RH, Wishart T, et al. Neuroprotective effects of lamotrigine in global ischemia in gerbils. A histological, in vivo microdialysis and behavioral study. *Brain Res* 1995;702:199–206.
14. Smith SE, Meldrum BS. Cerebroprotective effect of lamotrigine after focal ischemia in rats. *Stroke* 1995;26:117–121; discussion 121–122.
15. Lizasoain I, Knowles RG, Moncada S. Inhibition by lamotrigine of the generation of nitric oxide in rat forebrain slices. *J Neurochem* 1995;64:636–642.
16. Southam E, Kirkby D, Higgins GA, et al. Lamotrigine inhibits monoamine uptake in vitro and modulates 5-hydroxytryptamine uptake in rats. *Eur J Pharmacol* 1998;358:19–24.
17. McGeer EG, Zhu SG. Lamotrigine protects against kainate but not ibotenate lesions in rat striatum. *Neurosci Lett* 1990;112:348–351.
18. Shiah IS, Yatham LN, Gau YC, et al. Effect of lamotrigine on plasma GABA levels in healthy humans. *Prog Neuropsychopharmacol Biol Psychiatry* 2003;27:419–423.
19. Kuzniecky R, Ho S, Pan J, et al. Modulation of cerebral GABA by topiramate, lamotrigine and gabapentin in healthy adults. *Neurology* 2002;58:368–372.
20. Miller AA, Wheatley P, Sawyer DA, et al. Pharmacological studies on lamotrigine, a novel potential antiepileptic drug, I: anticonvulsant profile in mice and rats. *Epilepsia* 1986;27:483–489.
21. Lamb RJ, Miller AA. Effect of lamotrigine and some known anticonvulsant drugs on visually-evoked after-discharge in the conscious rat [abstract]. *Br J Pharmacol* 1985;86:765P.
22. Smith SE, al-Zubaidy ZA, Chapman AG, et al. Excitatory amino acid antagonists, lamotrigine and BW 1003C87 as anticonvulsants in the genetically epilepsy-prone rat. *Epilepsy Res* 1993;15:101–111.
23. Wheatley PL, Miller AA. Effects of lamotrigine on electrically induced afterdischarge duration in anaesthetised rat, dog, and marmoset. *Epilepsia* 1989;30:34–40.
24. O'Donnell RA, Miller AA. The effect of lamotrigine upon development of cortical kindled seizures in the rat. *Neuropharmacology* 1991;30:253–258.
25. Otsuki K, Morimoto K, Sato K, et al. Effects of lamotrigine and conventional antiepileptic drugs on amygdala- and hippocampal-kindled seizures in rats. *Epilepsy Res* 1998;31:101–112.
26. Goa KL, Ross SR, Chrisp P. Lamotrigine. A review of its pharmacological properties and clinical efficacy in epilepsy. *Drugs* 1993;46:152–176.
27. Posner J, Cohen AF, Land G, et al. The pharmacokinetics of lamotrigine (BW430C) in healthy subjects with unconjugated hyperbilirubinaemia (Gilbert's syndrome). *Br J Clin Pharmacol* 1989;28:117–120.
28. Cohen AF, Land GS, Breimer DD, et al. Lamotrigine, a new anticonvulsant: pharmacokinetics in normal humans. *Clin Pharmacol Ther* 1987;42:535–541.
29. Peck AW. Clinical pharmacology of lamotrigine. *Epilepsia* 1991;32(Suppl 2):S9–S12.
30. Ramsay RE, Pellock JM, Garnett WR, et al. Pharmacokinetics and safety of lamotrigine (Lamictal) in patients with epilepsy. *Epilepsy Res* 1991;10:191–200.
31. Birnbaum AK, Kriel RL, Burkhardt RT, et al. Rectal absorption of lamotrigine compressed tablets. *Epilepsia* 2000;41:851–853.
32. Myllynen PK, Pienimaki PK, Vahakangas KH. Transplacental passage of lamotrigine in human placental perfusion system in vitro and maternal and cord blood in vivo. *Eur J Clin Pharmacol* 2003;58:677–682.

33. Tomson T, Ohman I, Vitols S. Lamotrigine in pregnancy and lactation: a case report. *Epilepsia* 1997;38:1039–1041.
34. Magdalou J, Herber R, Bidault R, et al. In vitro N-glucuronidation of a novel antiepileptic drug, lamotrigine, by human liver microsomes. *J Pharmacol Exp Ther* 1992;260:1166–1173.
35. Hawes EM. N+-glucuronidation, a common pathway in human metabolism of drugs with a tertiary amine group. *Drug Metab Dispos* 1998;26:830–837.
36. Jawad S, Yuen WC, Peck AW, et al. Lamotrigine: single-dose pharmacokinetics and initial 1 week experience in refractory epilepsy. *Epilepsy Res* 1987;1:194–201.
37. Bartoli A, Guerrini R, Belmonte A, et al. The influence of dosage, age, and comedication on steady state plasma lamotrigine concentrations in epileptic children: a prospective study with preliminary assessment of correlations with clinical response. *Ther Drug Monit* 1997;19:252–260.
38. Chen C, Casale EJ, Duncan B, et al. Pharmacokinetics of lamotrigine in children in the absence of other antiepileptic drugs. *Pharmacotherapy* 1999;19:437–441.
39. Hussein Z, Posner J. Population pharmacokinetics of lamotrigine monotherapy in patients with epilepsy: retrospective analysis of routine monitoring data. *Br J Clin Pharmacol* 1997;43:457–645.
40. Bialer M, Johannessen SI, Kupferberg HJ, et al. Progress report on new antiepileptic drugs: a summary of the fourth Eilat conference (EILAT IV). *Epilepsy Res* 1999;34:1–41.
41. Wootton R, Soul-Lawton J, Rolan PE, et al. Comparison of the pharmacokinetics of lamotrigine in patients with chronic renal failure and healthy volunteers. *Br J Clin Pharmacol* 1997;43:23–27.
42. Fillastre JP, Taburet AM, Fialaire A, et al. Pharmacokinetics of lamotrigine in patients with renal impairment: influence of haemodialysis. *Drugs Exp Clin Res* 1993;19:25–32.
43. Tran TA, Leppik IE, Blesi K, et al. Lamotrigine clearance during pregnancy. *Neurology* 2002;59:251–255.
44. Kilpatrick C. The role of newer anticonvulsants in the management of epilepsy. *Aust N Z J Med* 1995;25:114–116.
45. Kilpatrick ES, Forrest G, Brodie MJ. Concentration-effect and concentration-toxicity relations with lamotrigine: a prospective study. *Epilepsia* 1996;37:534–538.
46. Morris RG, Black AB, Harris AL, et al. Lamotrigine and therapeutic drug monitoring: retrospective survey following the introduction of a routine service. *Br J Clin Pharmacol* 1998;46:547–551.
47. Frosher W, Keller F, Vogt H, et al. Prospective study on concentration-efficacy and concentration-toxicity: correlations with lamotrigine serum levels. *Epileptic Disord* 2002;4:49–56.
48. Battino D, Croci D, Granata T, et al. Lamotrigine plasma concentrations in children and adults: influence of age and associated therapy. *Ther Drug Monit* 1997;19:620–627.
49. Vauzelle-Kervroedan F, Rey E, Cieuta C, et al. Influence of concurrent antiepileptic medication on the pharmacokinetics of lamotrigine as add-on therapy in epileptic children. *Br J Clin Pharmacol* 1996;41:325–330.
50. Binnie CD, van Emde Boas W, Kasteleijn-Nolste-Trenite DG, et al. Acute effects of lamotrigine (BW430C) in persons with epilepsy. *Epilepsia* 1986;27:248–254.
51. Gilliam F, Vazquez B, Sackellares JC, et al. An active-control trial of lamotrigine monotherapy for partial seizures [see comments]. *Neurology* 1998;51:1018–1025.
52. Anderson GD, Gidal BE, Gilliam F, et al. Time course of lamotrigine de-induction: impact of step-wise withdrawal of carbamazepine or phenytoin. *Epilepsy Res* 2002;49:211–217.
53. Ramsay RE, Gidal BE, Pryor FM. The time course of de-induction of lamotrigine with carbamazepine and phenytoin. *Epilepsia* 2002;43:109.
54. Perucca E, Gidal BE, Baltes E. Effects of antiepileptic comedication on levetiracetam pharmacokinetics: a pooled analysis of data from randomized adjunctive therapy trials. *Epilepsy Res* 2003;53:47–56.
55. Gidal BE, Kanner A, Maly M, et al. Lamotrigine pharmacokinetics in patients receiving felbamate. *Epilepsy Res* 1997;27:1–5.
56. Berry DJ, Besag FM, Pool F, et al. Lack of effect of topiramate on lamotrigine serum concentrations. *Epilepsia* 2002;43:818–823.
57. May TW, Rambeck B, Jurgens U. Influence of oxcarbazepine and methsuximide on lamotrigine concentrations in epileptic patients with and without valproic acid comedication: results of a prospective study. *Ther Drug Monit* 1999;21:175–181.
58. Berry JD, Besage FM, Natarajan J, et al. Does topiramate change lamotrigine serum concentrations when added to treatment? An audit of a dose-escalation study [abstract]. *Epilepsia* 1998;39:56.
59. Yuen AW, Land G, Weatherley BC, et al. Sodium valproate acutely inhibits lamotrigine metabolism. *Br J Clin Pharmacol* 1992;33:511–513.
60. Gidal BE, Sheth R, Parnell J, et al. Evaluation of VPA dose and concentration effects on lamotrigine pharmacokinetics: implications for conversion to monotherapy. *Epilepsy Res* 2003;57:85–93.
61. Biton V, Natarajan S, Ramsay RE, et al. Dosing algorithm for conversion from valproate monotherapy to lamotrigine monotherapy in patients with epilepsy [abstract]. *Neurology* 2003;60:A476.
62. Anderson GD, Yau MK, Gidal BE, et al. Bidirectional interaction of valproate and lamotrigine in healthy subjects. *Clin Pharmacol Ther* 1996;60:145–156.
63. Mataringa MI, May TW, Rambeck B. Does lamotrigine influence valproate concentrations? *Ther Drug Monit* 2002;24:631–636.
64. Eriksson AS, Boreus LO. No increase in carbamazepine-10,11-epoxide during addition of lamotrigine treatment in children. *Ther Drug Monit* 1997;19:499–501.
65. Gidal BE, Rutecki P, Shaw R, et al. Effect of lamotrigine on carbamazepine epoxide/carbamazepine serum concentration ratios in adult patients with epilepsy. *Epilepsy Res* 1997;28:207–211.
66. Pisani F, Xiao B, Fazio A, et al. Single dose pharmacokinetics of carbamazepine-10,11-epoxide in patients on lamotrigine monotherapy. *Epilepsy Res* 1994;19:245–248.
67. Holdrich T, Whiteman P, Orme M, et al. Effect of lamotrigine on pharmacology of the combined oral contraceptive pill [abstract]. *Epilepsia* 1992;32(Suppl 1):96.
68. Depot M, Powell JR, Messenheimer JA Jr, et al. Kinetic effects of multiple oral doses of acetaminophen on a single oral dose of lamotrigine. *Clin Pharmacol Ther* 1990;48:346–355.
69. Kaufman KR, Gerner R. Lamotrigine toxicity secondary to sertraline. *Seizure* 1998;7:163–165.
70. Sabers A, Buchholt JM, Uldall P, et al. Lamotrigine plasma levels reduced by oral contraceptives. *Epilepsy Res* 2001;47:151–154.
71. Binnie CD, Debets RM, Engelsman M, et al. Double-blind crossover trial of lamotrigine (Lamictal) as add-on therapy in intractable epilepsy. *Epilepsy Res* 1989;4:222–229.
72. Jawad S, Richens A, Goodwin G, et al. Controlled trial of lamotrigine (Lamictal) for refractory partial seizures. *Epilepsia* 1989; 30:356–363.
73. Loiseau P, Yuen AW, Duche B, et al. A randomised double-blind placebo-controlled crossover add-on trial of lamotrigine in patients with treatment-resistant partial seizures. *Epilepsy Res* 1990;7:136–145.
74. Matsuo F, Bergen D, Faught E, et al. Placebo-controlled study of the efficacy and safety of lamotrigine in patients with partial seizures. U.S. Lamotrigine Protocol 0.5 Clinical Trial Group. *Neurology* 1993;43:2284–2291.
75. Messenheimer J, Ramsay RE, Willmore LJ, et al. Lamotrigine therapy for partial seizures: a multicenter, placebo-controlled, double-blind, cross-over trial. *Epilepsia* 1994;35:113–121.
76. Sander JW, Patsalos PN, Oxley JR, et al. A randomised double-blind placebo-controlled add-on trial of lamotrigine in patients with severe epilepsy. *Epilepsy Res* 1990;6:221–226.
77. Schapel GJ, Beran RG, Vajda FJ, et al. Double-blind, placebo controlled, crossover study of lamotrigine in treatment resistant partial seizures. *J Neurol Neurosurg Psychiatry* 1993;56:448–453.
78. Brodie MJ, Richens A, Yuen AW. Double-blind comparison of lamotrigine and carbamazepine in newly diagnosed epilepsy. UK Lamotrigine/Carbamazepine Monotherapy Trial Group [published erratum appears in *Lancet* 1995;345:662] [see comments]. *Lancet* 1995;345:476–479.
79. Steiner TJ, Dellaportas CI, Findley LJ, et al. Lamotrigine monotherapy in newly diagnosed untreated epilepsy: a double-blind comparison with phenytoin. *Epilepsia* 1999;40:601–607.
80. Motte J, Trevathan E, Arvidsson JF, et al. Lamotrigine for generalized seizures associated with the Lennox-Gastaut syndrome. Lamictal Lennox-Gastaut Study Group [published erratum appears in *N Engl J Med* 1998;339:851–852]. *N Engl J Med* 1997;337:1807–1812.
81. Donaldson JA, Glauser TA, Olberding LS. Lamotrigine adjunctive therapy in childhood epileptic encephalopathy (the Lennox Gastaut syndrome). *Epilepsia* 1997;38:68–73.

82. Mikati MA, Holmes GL. Lamotrigine in absence and primary generalized epilepsies. *J Child Neurol* 1997;12(Suppl 1):S29–S37.
83. Schlumberger E, Chavez F, Palacios L, et al. Lamotrigine in treatment of 120 children with epilepsy. *Epilepsia* 1994;35:359–367.
84. Timmings PL, Richens A. Lamotrigine as an add-on drug in the management of Lennox-Gastaut syndrome. *Eur Neurol* 1992;32:305–307.
85. Beran RG, Berkovic SF, Dunagan FM, et al. Double-blind, placebo-controlled, crossover study of lamotrigine in treatment-resistant generalised epilepsy. *Epilepsia* 1998;39:1329–1333.
86. Buchanan N. The use of lamotrigine in juvenile myoclonic epilepsy. *Seizure* 1996;5:149–151.
87. Buoni S, Grosso S, Fois A. Lamotrigine in typical absence epilepsy. *Brain Dev* 1999;21:303–306.
88. Ferrie CD, Robinson RO, Knott C, et al. Lamotrigine as an add-on drug in typical absence seizures. *Acta Neurol Scand* 1995;91:200–202.
89. Frank LM, Enlow T, Holmes GL, et al. Lamictal (lamotrigine) monotherapy for typical absence seizures in children. *Epilepsia* 1999;40:973–979.
90. Sharpe C, Buchanan N. Juvenile myoclonic epilepsy: diagnosis, management and outcome. *Med J Aust* 1995;162:133–134.
91. Guerrini R, Dravet C, Genton P, et al. Lamotrigine and seizure aggravation in severe myoclonic epilepsy. *Epilepsia* 1998;39:508–512.
92. Dooley J, Camfield P, Gordon K, et al. Lamotrigine-induced rash in children. *Neurology* 1996;46:240–242.
93. Messenheimer J, Mullens EL, Giorgi L, et al. Safety review of adult clinical trial experience with lamotrigine. *Drug Saf* 1998;18:281–296.
94. Messenheimer JA. Rash in adult and pediatric patients treated with lamotrigine. *Can J Neurol Sci* 1998;25:S14–S18.
95. Guberman AH, Besag FM, Brodie MJ, et al. Lamotrigine-associated rash: risk/benefit considerations in adults and children. *Epilepsia* 1999;40:985–991.

Topiramate

61

Michael D. Privitera

HISTORICAL BACKGROUND

Topiramate (TPM) is a highly oxygenated sulfamate-substituted monosaccharide that is structurally distinct from other anticonvulsant medications. Available in the United States as Topamax (Ortho-McNeil Pharmaceutical), it is a broad-spectrum agent that has been extensively studied in double-blind, randomized, controlled trials in adults and children. Initially approved for use as adjunctive therapy in partial-onset seizures, primary generalized tonic-clonic seizures, and multiple seizure types associated with Lennox-Gastaut syndrome, it is currently under evaluation for approval as first-line therapy in the United States.

CHEMISTRY

TPM (2,3:4,5-di-O-isopropylidene-β-D-fructopyranose sulfamate; Fig. 61.1) is a white crystalline powder, which is freely soluble in acetone, chloroform, dimethylsulfoxide, and ethanol. TPM is supplied as 25-, 50-, 100-, and 200-mg tablets and as 15- and 25-mg sprinkle capsules that can be opened and sprinkled onto soft food for children and for patients who may have difficulty swallowing tablets.

MECHANISMS OF ACTION

TPM has a unique combination of activities at various receptor sites and ion channels, which may account for its broad-spectrum profile in epilepsy and other neurologic disorders. It blocks the kainate/AMPA (α-amino-3-hydroxy-5-methylisoxazole-4-propionic acid) subtype of the glutamate receptor (1–4), with no direct effect on NMDA (N-methyl-D-aspartate) receptor activity; blocks voltage-activated sodium channels to limit sustained repetitive firing (5–9); enhances γ-aminobutyric acid (GABA)-mediated chloride flux at GABA$_A$ receptors (10,11); reduces the amplitude of high-voltage–activated calcium currents (12,13); and activates potassium conductance (14,15). It has been hypothesized that effects of TPM on voltage-activated sodium channels, high-voltage–activated calcium channels, GABA$_A$ receptors, and AMPA/kainate receptors reflect a common modulator involving protein phosphorylation (16). TPM is also a weak inhibitor of carbonic anhydrase isoenzymes (CA II and CA IV), which may modulate pH-dependent activation of voltage- and receptor-gated ion channels (17); its inhibitory effect is less than acetazolamide.

The anticonvulsant properties of TPM have been demonstrated in several animal models of epilepsy; these have been discussed elsewhere (16,18–21). Experimental studies have shown that TPM reduces seizure-induced hippocampal neuronal injury (22) and prevents spontaneous seizures following status epilepticus (23). In an experimental model of neonatal hypoxia/ischemia, TPM suppressed acute seizures and reduced subsequent susceptibility to neuronal injury and seizures induced by a second insult (kainate) (24).

PHARMACOKINETICS

Renal elimination, low protein binding, and a long half-life make TPM relatively easy to manage from a pharmacokinetic perspective.

Absorption

TPM is rapidly absorbed with peak plasma concentrations occurring in 1 to 4 hours with TPM doses of 100 to 400 mg (25). Absorption is nearly complete with less than 80% of a 100-mg dose recovered in urine (25). Coadministration with food slightly delays absorption but does not decrease bioavailability (25). TPM exhibits linear kinetics; plasma concentrations increase in proportion to dose increases (26).

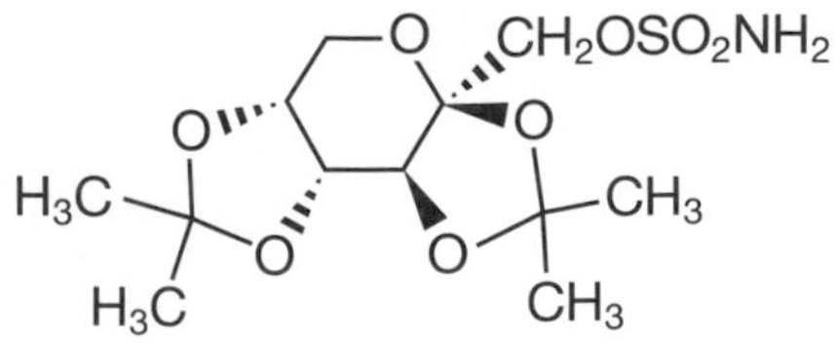

Figure 61.1 Topiramate. 2,3:4, 5-Di-*O*-isopropylidene-β-D-fructopyranose sulfamate.

Distribution and Protein Binding

The apparent volume of distribution for TPM is 38.5 to 58 L (0.6 to 0.8 L/kg, weight normalized), consistent with distribution to total body water. Binding to plasma proteins is minimal (13% to 17%) and is not considered to be a major factor in dosing and drug interactions (26).

Metabolism and Excretion

In the absence of hepatic enzyme induction, approximately 20% of a TPM dose is metabolized. When TPM is coadministered with enzyme-inducing antiepileptic drugs (AEDs), up to 50% of the TPM dose may be metabolized. Hepatic metabolism appears to involve hydroxylation, hydrolysis, and glucuronidation; none of the metabolites constitutes >5% of an administered dose, and they are quickly cleared (26).

Elimination of TPM is primarily via renal excretion, with 50% to 80% being eliminated in the urine unchanged. The half-life of TPM in adults is 20 to 30 hours in the absence of enzyme induction, allowing steady-state plasma concentrations to be reached in 4 to 8 per day. In the presence of enzyme induction, the TPM half-life in adults is 12 to 15 hours (26). In children 4 to 17 years of age, clearance is approximately 50% higher than in adults (27). Steady-state concentrations for the same mg/kg dose were correspondingly lower in children than in adults. Consistent with the higher clearance, the calculated half-life of TPM in children is approximately 15 hours without enzyme induction and 7.5 hours with enzyme induction. In young children (younger than 4 years old), clearance rates were the same or slightly higher than in older children (28). In elderly patients (65 to 85 years of age), clearance decreases only to the extent that renal function itself is reduced by age; age alone does not alter clearance in adults (29).

TPM clearance is reduced by 40% to 50% in patients with moderate (creatinine clearance, 30 to 69 mL per minute) or severe (creatinine clearance, <30 mL per minute) renal impairment compared with subjects with normal renal function (creatinine clearance, >70 mL per minute) (26). One half of the usual TPM dose is recommended in patients with moderate or severe renal impairment. Modest decreases in TPM clearance have been reported in individuals with moderate to severe hepatic impairment when compared with age- and sex-matched healthy controls; mean clearance was decreased 26% (31.8 versus 23.5 mL per minute) and half-life increased 36% (25 versus 34 hours), with parallel increases in plasma concentrations (26).

THERAPEUTIC DRUG MONITORING

Steady-state plasma concentrations of TPM are generally linear, with dose-proportional increases in plasma concentration (26). Mean plasma concentrations achieved during maintenance in randomized, controlled trials of TPM monotherapy were: 50 mg per day, 1.6 and 1.9 μg/mL; 97 mg per day, 3.8 μg/mL; 189 mg per day, 6.4 μg/mL; 313 mg per day, 11.7 μg/mL; 367 mg per day, 12.4 μg/mL (30). Studies of TPM as monotherapy have provided the opportunity to examine the relationship between TPM blood levels and clinical response. In a study comparing 50 and 500 mg per day TPM as monotherapy, plasma concentrations >9.91 μg/mL were associated with better seizure control compared with plasma concentrations of 1.77 to 9.91 μg/mL and ≤1.76 μg/mL (31). However, because of the intraindividual variations in blood levels associated with seizure control and side effects, a traditional "therapeutic range" cannot be identified. As expected, plasma concentrations are higher when TPM is administered as monotherapy (6.4 to 12.4 μg/mL with ~200 to 400 mg per day) versus its use as add-on to enzyme-inducing AEDs (1.4 to 5.3 μg/mL with ~200 to 400 mg per day). Despite the substantially higher plasma concentration with monotherapy, the incidence of central nervous system (CNS)-related adverse events, particularly cognitive effects, was substantially lower with TPM monotherapy than with adjunctive therapy. This finding underscores the contribution of pharmacodynamic interactions to the occurrence of adverse events during TPM polytherapy and the limited benefit of therapeutic drug monitoring in TPM-treated patients.

The relationship between TPM dose and plasma level was examined in children in whom TPM was titrated to clinical response or side effects (32). Among 21 children aged 6 to 12 years, TPM plasma levels were predictably related to dose (1:1 ratio). With monotherapy, a mean dose of 9.7 mg/kg per day (range, 5.5 to 16.5 mg/kg per day) resulted in a mean plasma level of 9.8 μg/mL (range, 3.4 to 16.6 μg/mL). For 20 younger children (younger than 6 years of age), however, higher monotherapy doses were needed (mean, 22.5 mg/kg per day; range, 11 to 35 mg/kg per day) to achieve seizure control; mean plasma level was 14.8 μg/mL (range, 6.1 to 23.7 μg/mL). When TPM was administered with an enzyme-inducing drug, the TPM dosage in younger children (mean, 14.2 mg/kg per day) was double that in older children (7.0 mg/kg per day) (32).

DRUG INTERACTIONS

Predominantly renal elimination and low protein binding minimize the potential for drug interactions.

Pharmacokinetic interactions between TPM and other AEDs are limited primarily to the effects of enzyme-inducing drugs on TPM. TPM plasma levels are approximately 50% lower when TPM is given with an enzyme-inducing AED (33–35) compared to TPM use alone or in combination with nonenzyme-inducing drugs (33–36). The addition of TPM does not significantly affect plasma concentrations of carbamazepine (33), valproate (36), phenobarbital/primidone (34), or lamotrigine (37). However, phenytoin plasma levels may be increased as much as 25% in some patients, particularly those in whom phenytoin metabolism may be at or near saturation (35). Studies of TPM in models designed to predict drug interactions related to the cytochrome P450 (CYP450) enzyme system have shown inhibition of only the CYP2C19 isozyme, which may account for the potential interaction with phenytoin (38). Although pharmacokinetic interactions between TPM and other AEDs are limited, the lower incidence of adverse effects with TPM monotherapy (31,39,40) suggests that pharmacodynamic interactions may affect tolerability when TPM is added to existing therapy.

Interaction studies evaluating the effect of TPM on combination oral contraceptives showed that TPM has no effect on the progestin (norethindrone, 1.0 mg) component (41,42). At doses of ≤200 mg per day, TPM has no significant effect on estrogen (ethinyl estradiol, 35 μg) concentrations (41,42). At higher doses (400 and 800 mg per day), TPM was associated with 21% and 30% reductions, respectively, in ethinyl estradiol concentrations, suggesting a modest induction of estrogen clearance (42). The level of induction is substantially less than that associated with potent enzyme-inducing agents such as carbamazepine (42% reduction in estrogen concentration) (41). The dose-related effect of TPM on estrogen clearance is consistent with the concentration-dependent induction of CYP450 CYP3A4 activity measured *in vitro* (43). TPM induced CYP3A4 enzymes only at concentrations >50 μM, a concentration that is unlikely to be achieved with dosages up to 400 mg per day; enzyme induction was still less than that associated with known inducers (phenobarbital and rifampicin) used in this study.

A slight decrease in digoxin clearance has been observed with the addition of TPM (44), but generally does not require dosage adjustments. Changes in metformin pharmacokinetics suggest that diabetic control should be monitored when TPM is added or withdrawn (45).

EFFICACY

Adjunctive Therapy

Partial-Onset Seizures

The effectiveness of TPM as adjunctive therapy across a wide range of doses (200 to 1,000 mg per day) in adults with refractory partial-onset seizures has been well documented in randomized, double-blind, placebo-controlled trials (46–54). Similarity of trial design and patient populations allowed pooled analysis of data from six of these trials (46–51). Among 743 adults (median baseline frequency, 12 seizures per month), median seizure reduction was 44% with TPM treatment versus 2% with placebo ($p \leq 0.001$); 43% of TPM-related patients (placebo, 12%; $p \leq 0.001$) achieved at least 50% seizure reduction (55). During 11 to 19 weeks of double-blind treatment, 5% of patients in the TPM group were seizure free, while no patients in the placebo group were seizure free ($p \leq 0.001$) (55). Although dosages as high as 1,000 mg per day were evaluated, the most clinically useful adjunctive therapy dosages appear to be 200 to 400 mg per day. In a 12-week, double-blind trial to further evaluate the lower end of the presumed dosing range (54), 200 mg per day TPM was added to carbamazepine. Median seizure reduction in TPM-treated patients (N = 168) was 44% (versus 20% with placebo, N = 91; $p < 0.001$); 45% of TPM-treated patients (placebo, 24%; $p = 0.001$) achieved at least 50% seizure reduction. After 2 weeks, median seizure reduction in patients receiving TPM 100 mg per day (N = 84) was 60% (placebo, 17%; $p < 0.001$), which suggests that 100 mg per day may be a target dose at which seizure control should be initially evaluated.

The initial overestimation of TPM dosage needs is evident from prospective, in-practice studies in which adults with refractory partial-onset seizures achieved good seizure control with 264 mg per day (48% of patients had 50% or more seizure reduction rate; 9% were seizure-free) (56) and 323 mg per day (68% of patients had a 50% or more seizure reduction rate) (57). When titrating to response, patients with fewer baseline seizures (less than 4 per month) required lower TPM dosages (303 mg per day) than those with higher baseline seizure frequency (341 mg per day in patients with 4 or more seizures per month) (57). In a prospective study, 17% of refractory patients had at least 50% seizure reduction and 8% were seizure-free with TPM dosages of 100 or less mg per day (58).

In treatment-resistant epilepsy patients treated at a tertiary epilepsy center, estimated long-term retention rates among 393 TPM-treated patients were 52% after 1 year, 42% at 2 years, 30% at 3 years, and 28% at 5 years (59,60). Although these rates were higher than those with another new-generation agent (lamotrigine), the low retention rate at 5 years reflects the limitations of medical therapy in patients with refractory epilepsy.

TPM was evaluated as adjunctive therapy in 86 children (2 to 16 years of age) with refractory partial-onset seizures (61). With a mean daily dose of 6 mg/kg (target dose, 5 to 9 mg/kg per day), median seizure reduction was 33% (placebo, 11%; $p = 0.03$). More TPM-treated children had at least 50% reduction in seizures (39% versus 20% with placebo; $p = 0.08$); 5% of children receiving TPM had no seizures, while no placebo-treated children were seizure free.

All 83 children completing the double-blind phase entered the long-term, open-label extension in which the dosages of TPM and concomitant AEDs could be adjusted according to clinical response (62). Mean treatment duration was 15 months, with some children being treated as long as 2.5 years; the mean TPM dosage was 9 mg/kg per day (range, 4 to 22 mg/kg per day). Among children treated for at least 6 months, 64% had at least a 50% reduction in seizures; 14% were seizure free for a minimum of 6 months. During open-label in-practice studies in children with refractory partial-onset seizures (63–66), 4% to 20% of TPM-treated children were seizure-free during treatment periods as long as 33 months.

Lennox-Gastaut Syndrome

TPM was evaluated as adjunctive therapy in 98 patients with Lennox-Gastaut syndrome confirmed by an electroencephalographic (EEG) pattern of slow spike-and-wave, multiple seizure types, including drop attacks, and a history of atypical absence episodes (67). At a maximum dose of 6 mg/kg per day, median reduction for drop attacks was 15% compared with a 5% increase with placebo; 28% of TPM-treated patients were responders (placebo, 14%). A combined measure of drop attacks and tonic-clonic seizures showed a 26% reduction with TPM and a 5% increase with placebo ($p = 0.015$); respective responder rates were 33% and 8% ($p = 0.002$). These outcomes compared favorably with those reported for lamotrigine in this population (68). The placebo-adjusted responder rate for drop attacks was 14% for TPM and 15% for lamotrigine; respective rates for major motor seizures were 25% and 17% (67,68).

During the long-term, open-label extension in which the dosages of TPM and concomitant AEDs could be adjusted according to clinical response (69), 55% of the 82 children treated with TPM for more than 6 months had at least a 50% reduction in drop attacks during the last 6 months of treatment; 15% experienced no drop attacks. Two patients were free of all seizures. The mean duration of TPM treatment was 18 months, with treatment periods as long as 3.4 years. The mean TPM dosage was 10 mg/kg per day (range, 1 to 29 mg/kg per day). Among patients treated as long as 8 years, 21% to 40% of patients had at least 50% seizure reduction, with major motor seizures being the most responsive (70,71).

Generalized Tonic-Clonic Seizures of Nonfocal Origin

Two double-blind, placebo-controlled trials (72,73) evaluated TPM in the treatment of generalized, nonfocal tonic-clonic seizures (i.e., primary generalized tonic-clonic seizures). Inclusion criteria specified tonic-clonic seizures with or without other generalized seizure types and electroencephalographic (EEG) or CCTV/EEG patterns consistent with generalized epilepsy (generalized, symmetric, synchronous spike-wave discharges and normal background activity); patients with Lennox-Gastaut syndrome or partial-onset seizures were excluded. In the two trials, more than 70% of patients had primary generalized tonic-clonic seizures plus at least one other type of generalized seizure (i.e., absence, myoclonic, or tonic).

TPM was initiated as adjunctive therapy in adults and children (at least 4 years of age) with refractory generalized tonic-clonic seizures despite treatment with one or two AEDs. The target dose was 5 to 9 mg/kg per day and the maximum daily dose was 400 mg. In one trial (72), baseline seizure frequency in the TPM-treated group (N = 39) was five generalized tonic-clonic seizures per month (placebo, 4.5 generalized tonic-clonic seizures per month; N = 41). Median seizure reduction was 57% (placebo, 9%; $p < 0.02$) for tonic-clonic seizures and 42% (placebo, 1%; $p = 0.003$) for all generalized seizures. Among TPM-treated patients, generalized tonic-clonic seizures and all generalized seizures were reduced at least 50% in 56% and 46%, respectively (respective placebo values: 20%, $p = 0.001$; 17%, $p = 0.003$). No generalized tonic-clonic seizures occurred during the 20-week study in 13% of TPM-treated patients (placebo, 5%); 5% had no generalized seizures of any type (placebo, 0% of patients).

Because the two trials were identically designed, data were pooled and analyzed. As had been observed in the single trial, TPM reduced the frequency of generalized tonic-clonic and all generalized seizures, with significantly more patients achieving 50% or greater reduction in generalized tonic-clonic (55% versus 28% with placebo; $p \leq 0.001$) and all generalized seizures (43% versus 19% with placebo; $p = 0.001$). Although small sample sizes limited analysis, TPM was also more effective than placebo in reducing the frequency of tonic and myoclonic seizures and did not exacerbate absence seizures.

All 131 patients who completed the double-blind phase entered an open-label extension phase (74). During the last 6 months of treatment, 16% had no generalized tonic-clonic seizures and 7% were seizure-free for at least 6 months. TPM was also effective against other generalized seizure types; during the last 6 months of treatment, 10% of patients with absence seizures, 33% of patients with myoclonic seizures, and 21% of patients with tonic seizures were seizure-free for at least 6 months.

In a study evaluating EEG changes and seizure control in TPM-treated patients with primary generalized epilepsies (75), more than half of patients showed reductions in epileptiform spike-wave activity, although TPM was less likely to suppress activity in patients with very high discharge frequencies at baseline. As with other broad-spectrum AEDs, seizure reduction (36% seizure-free) did not correlate with EEG response, and no correlation was observed between clinical or EEG response and TPM blood levels.

Juvenile Myoclonic Epilepsy

A small subset of patients with juvenile myoclonic epilepsy was included in the controlled trials evaluating TPM in primary generalized tonic-clonic seizures (72,73). Among 11 patients with juvenile myoclonic epilepsy receiving TPM, primary generalized tonic-clonic seizures were reduced at least 50% in 73% (versus 18% of patients receiving placebo, N = 11; p = 0.03) (76). In addition, the frequency of myoclonic seizures was reduced and the number of weeks without absence seizures was increased in TPM-treated patients. In a randomized, open-label study in patients with juvenile myoclonic epilepsy (77), TPM and valproate were similarly effective (seizure-free rates following 12 weeks' treatment: 47% and 33%, respectively). The treatment groups were similar in neurotoxicity scores; however, TPM was associated with less systemic toxicity than valproate.

West Syndrome
Eleven children with refractory West syndrome participated in a pilot study of TPM (78). At a maximum daily dose of 24 mg/kg, the frequency of infantile spasms was reduced by at least 50% in nine children, including five (45%) who were completely controlled. Ancillary seizures responded in four of six children. After 18 months of TPM (mean dosage, 29 mg/kg per per day), eight children (73%) continued on medication; four (50%) children were free of spasms, and seven (88%) children had spasms reduced by at least one half (79).

Childhood Absence Epilepsy
Five children 4 to 11 years of age with EEG-documented absence seizures and childhood absence epilepsy were treated with open-label TPM (maximum dose, 12 mg/kg per per day) (80). Three children experienced a minimum reduction of 50% at daily dosages of 5 to 6 mg/kg; two children were seizure free. Frequency was unchanged in the remaining two children, even at the maximum dosage.

Severe Myoclonic Epilepsy in Infancy
During a prospective, multicenter, open-label study in 18 patients with severe myoclonic epilepsy in infancy and refractory seizures of different types, three patients became seizure free, six patients had greater than 75% seizure reduction, and four patients had greater than 50% seizure reduction with TPM treatment (81). Seizure frequency was unchanged in five patients; no patients experienced seizure worsening. Mean treatment duration was 12 months (range, 2 to 24 months); mean TPM dose was 5.4 mg/kg per day (range, 2.8–10 mg/kg per day).

Patients with Mental Retardation, Learning Disabilities, and/or Developmental Disabilities
Among 64 patients (16 to 65 years of age) with refractory epilepsy and learning disability treated with TPM in an open-label study, 16 patients became seizure free and 29 patients had at least a 50% seizure reduction (82). Many patients, including 63% of those who were seizure free and 66% of treatment responders, were receiving TPM dosages of ≤200 mg per day. In a study evaluating the effect of TPM in 20 adults (21 to 57 years of age) with intractable mixed seizures, mental retardation, and development disabilities, two patients became seizure free and 11 patients had at least a 50% seizure reduction with TPM treatment (83). In addition, the duration and/or severity of seizures were reduced in 44% of patients. The mean duration of treatment was 42 weeks (range, 20 to 54 weeks); the mean TPM dose was 189 mg per day (range, 50 to 350 mg per day).

Refractory Status Epilepticus
In six cases of refractory status epilepticus unresponsive to sequential trials of multiple agents, including one patient who had been in a prolonged pentobarbital coma, TPM (300 to 1600 mg per day) administered via nasogastric tube successfully terminated refractory status epilepticus (84). TPM was effective against both generalized convulsive and nonconvulsive status epilepticus. All patients were subsequently discharged from the hospital.

Monotherapy

The 1990s ushered in a new era—at least in the United States—for clinical studies in newly diagnosed, previously untreated epilepsy. The use of traditional AEDs (carbamazepine, phenytoin, valproate) as first-line monotherapy is largely based on landmark Veterans' Administration Cooperative trials (85,86) and similar open-label trials in the United Kingdom (87,88). However, the U.S. Food and Drug Administration (FDA) began requiring randomized, double-blind trials demonstrating a statistically significant difference between treatments as evidence of efficacy, generating considerable debate as to how to safely and ethically accomplish this goal. One such approach is an active-control conversion-to-monotherapy design in which patients are randomized to study drug or a minimally effective active-control and preexisting AED therapy is gradually withdrawn (89). Such a design parallels the technique clinicians use to switch patients to a second trial of AED monotherapy when the first agent has failed because of ineffective seizure control or intolerable side effects. Such a design was used as a proof-of-principle trial for TPM monotherapy (90).

Monotherapy trial design becomes particularly complex when evaluating new AEDs in patients with newly or recently diagnosed epilepsy. The use of a placebo control in untreated epilepsy patients remains controversial, and only one such trial has been conducted (91). Unlike their European counterparts, regulatory authorities in the United States are unwilling to accept monotherapy equivalence trials for AEDs already approved as adjunctive therapy (89). The argument is that a trial showing equivalence of two treatments could be interpreted as meaning that both treatments were equally ineffective or that the trial simply failed to detect existing differences (89,92). Given the responsiveness of patients with newly diagnosed epilepsy, some have doubted the possibility of demonstrating a treatment effect with active-control or dose-control trials. These trial types are also controversial in relation to ethical equipoise (93).

TPM has been evaluated as first-line monotherapy in adults and children with newly or recently diagnosed epilepsy in three multicenter, randomized, double-blind trials. Two trials were dose-controlled trials (31,40), and one trial used a novel trial design to simultaneously compare TPM with two standard AEDs (i.e., carbamazepine and valproate) (39).

In the first dose-controlled trial (31), 252 adults and children who had been diagnosed with epilepsy within 3 years of study entry and who had one to six partial-onset seizures during a 3-month retrospective baseline were randomized to 50 mg per day or 500 mg per day TPM (patients weighing ≤50 kg were randomized to 25 mg per day or 200 mg per day). Patients were untreated or had been treated for more than 1 month with one AED. The primary efficacy outcome was time to exit, which was time to second seizure in 96% of patients. Time to exit was longer in patients receiving TPM 200/500 mg per day (median, 422 per day versuss 293 per day in patients receiving 25/50 mg per day), although the difference was not significant. When time to exit was analyzed using time to first seizure as a covariate, the difference between treatment groups was significant ($p = 0.01$). This finding reflected the higher seizure-free rate in patients receiving TPM 200/500 mg per day (54% versus 39% with 25/50 mg per day; $p = 0.02$) as well as the longer interval before the first seizure (median, 317 per days versus 108 per days with 25/50 mg per day; $p = 0.06$). In this study, seizure-free rates with 50 mg per day (39%) and TPM 400 mg per day (54%) were at the lower and upper ends for the range of seizure-free rates (36% to 43%) reported with therapeutic dosages of other AEDs in double-blind studies (94,95). The mean dosage among patients randomized to TPM 500 mg per day was 366 mg per day. A significant difference between treatment groups was observed for patients with one or two seizures in the 3-month baseline, but not for patients with three or more seizures in the 3-month baseline. This finding suggested that higher seizure frequency may serve as an indicator of more treatment-resistant seizures in patients with untreated epilepsy and is consistent with other reports linking higher seizure frequency before initial treatment with refractory epilepsy (96).

Results from the first dose-controlled study (31) suggested that TPM 50 mg per day was an effective dose in some patients responsive to anticonvulsant therapy and could serve as an active control to treatment with TPM 400 mg per day. Moreover, patients with one or two seizures in a 3-month baseline may represent the population of patients with newly diagnosed epilepsy who are most likely to benefit from monotherapy and not require polytherapy because of drug-resistant epilepsy. In the second dose-controlled study (40), 470 adults and children (weighing at least 25 kg) were eligible if they had untreated epilepsy diagnosed within 3 months of study entry, or if epilepsy had relapsed while they were not receiving anticonvulsant therapy. Patients could have only one or two partial-onset or generalized tonic-clonic seizures during the 3-month retrospective baseline. The primary efficacy end point was time to first seizure; seizure-free rates at 6 months and 1 year were secondary efficacy measures. Kaplan-Meier survival analyses for time to first seizure showed a significantly greater treatment effect with 400 mg per day versus 50 mg per day ($p = 0.0002$). The probability of being seizure free was 83% with 400 mg per day and 71% with 50 mg per day ($p = 0.005$) after 6 months treatment and 76% and 59% ($p = 0.001$) after 12 months. A difference between dose groups emerged within the first week after randomization when patients were receiving 25 mg per day or 50 mg per day; the between-group difference was significant after 2 weeks when patients were receiving 25 mg per day or 100 mg per day.

The effectiveness of TPM 100 mg per day as initial monotherapy in patients with newly diagnosed epilepsy was established further with a randomized, double-blind trial comparing TPM, carbamazepine, and valproate in adults and children (N = 613) with newly diagnosed epilepsy (39). No seizure types/epilepsy syndromes were excluded. During this trial, investigators selected carbamazepine (600 mg per day) or valproate (1250 mg per day) as the preferred therapy according to each patient's clinical presentation. Patients were then assigned to the carbamazepine or valproate treatment branch. Within each branch, patients were randomized to double-blind treatment with the investigator's choice of traditional AED (carbamazepine or valproate), TPM 100 mg per day, or TPM 200 mg per day. Patients continued double-blind treatment until exiting the study or until 6 months after the last patient was randomized.

The initial efficacy analysis compared time to first seizure for the two TPM dosages (100 and 200 mg per day). If TPM 200 mg per day was significantly more effective than TPM 100 mg per day, then 200 mg per day was to be compared with carbamazepine and valproate. If 200 mg per day was not significantly more effective, the protocol required TPM dosage groups to be pooled within each branch and compared with traditional therapy. For the comparison between TPM and traditional therapy, the primary efficacy measure was time to exit; secondary efficacy end points were time to first seizure and proportion of patients seizure-free during the last 6 months of double-blind treatment.

No difference was observed for the initial efficacy analysis comparing the two TPM dosages groups. Therefore, the combined TPM groups were compared with carbamazepine and valproate treatment. In both the carbamazepine and valproate branches, time to exit did not differ between the combined TPM treatment groups and traditional therapy. Because the branches were homogeneous, pooled data across branches were used to calculate 95% confidence intervals (CIs) for treatment differences. Although retention rates were higher among patients receiving TPM compared with those receiving carbamazepine or valproate,

95% CIs included zero, which indicated that between-group differences were not statistically significant. Similar results were observed for time to first seizure. The proportion of patients with no seizures during the last 6 months of double-blind treatment was 49% among patients receiving TPM 100 mg per day and 44% in each of the other three treatment groups (i.e., TPM 200 mg per day, carbamazepine, and valproate). The 95% CIs were narrow and included zero, indicating no difference among the four treatment groups.

Results from two trials showing that TPM 100 mg per day is effective in adults and children with newly diagnosed epilepsy support clinical findings suggesting that only low to moderate dosages of AEDs are required in patients with new-onset epilepsy that is responsive to treatment (97).

Other Clinical Uses

Studies suggest that TPM may prevent migraine attacks. Two randomized, double-blind, placebo-controlled trials evaluated the efficacy of TPM treatment (50, 100, and 200 mg per day) in 970 patients with migraine (98,99). The primary efficacy measure was change in mean monthly migraine frequency from baseline during double-blind treatment. Compared with placebo, significant reductions in monthly migraine frequency were reported with TPM dosages of 100 and 200 mg per day; migraine frequency was also reduced with 50 mg per day, although the difference from placebo was not statistically significant. The proportion of treatment responders with a 50% or more reduction in monthly migraine frequency was significantly greater in TPM-treated patients (36% to 54% versus 23% with placebo) (98,99). TPM may also have favorable effects in patients with cluster headache; in a case series, cluster remission occurred in nine of 10 patients (114).

TPM may have a potential role in movement disorder treatment. In a double-blind, placebo-controlled, crossover trial in 62 patients with essential tremor, TPM was associated with significant improvements in tremor severity, motor task performance, and functional disability (101), findings that were consistent with those in an earlier pilot study (102). In a retrospective chart review, TPM seemed to be effective in reducing tics in children and adolescents with Tourette syndrome (103); 59% (19/32) of patients had at least 50% reduction in tic severity scores.

Several studies suggest that TPM may be effective in various impulse control disorders. In a randomized, double-blind, placebo-controlled trial in 150 patients with alcohol dependence, TPM-treated patients had significantly fewer drinks per per day, drinks per drinking per day, and heavy drinking per days and significantly more abstinent per days compared with placebo (104). Plasma γ-glutamyl transferase, an objective index of alcohol consumption, was also significantly lower in TPM-treated patients. Among 61 obese patients with binge-eating disorder who were participating in a randomized, double-blind, placebo-controlled trial, TPM treatment was associated with significantly greater reductions in binge frequency, binge per day frequency, body mass index, body weight, and obsessive-compulsive scores (105). Open-label treatment with TPM has been reported to improve behavior, mood, weight control, compulsive eating problems, and self-mutilating behavior (notably skin picking) associated with Prader-Willi syndrome (106,107).

The observation that TPM is associated with weight loss and expected improvement in metabolic parameters (e.g., lipids, blood pressure, glucose levels) (108), led to studies of TPM (64 to 384 mg per day) in obese patients (109). After 6 months, mean percent decrease in baseline body weight was significantly greater among TPM-treated patients (range: 4.8% to 6.3%, depending on TPM dose; 2.6% with placebo). A similar pattern of weight loss was observed in patients with diabetes who participated in three double-blind, placebo-controlled trials evaluating the efficacy of TPM in painful diabetic neuropathy (110). Moreover, in these trials diabetic control, measured as HbA1c levels, improved significantly compared with placebo, with reductions in HbA1c occurring independent of weight loss. These findings are supported by data from an animal model of diabetes, in which TPM demonstrated dose-dependent decreases in blood glucose and plasma triglycerides without significant body weight changes (111).

In view of the role of glutamate and AMPA in the pathobiology of neuronal injury, attention has been focused on TPM because of its activity as an AMPA antagonist. Potential neuroprotective and disease-modifying effects of TPM have been observed in models of seizure-related neuronal injury (22), focal cerebral ischemia (112), and glutamate excitotoxicity (113). Preliminary data in patients with diabetic neuropathy suggest that TPM may improve or restore nerve function through preservation/regeneration of C-fibers, with associated improvement in functional parameters (114). Studies using a cerebral microdialysis technique in patients with traumatic brain injury showed that TPM reduced glutamate levels compared with historical controls (115). In a double-blind, placebo-controlled trial, high-dose TPM (800 mg per day) did not provide beneficial effects in patients with amyotrophic lateral sclerosis (ALS) and may have accelerated the loss of arm muscle strength. In this study, TPM treatment was associated with an increased risk of side effects (116). These findings are useful for advancing our understanding of potential therapeutic targets.

ADVERSE EFFECTS

Central Nervous System

As expected with anticonvulsants, CNS effects were the most commonly reported side effects in randomized, controlled trials with TPM. Their relatively high incidence in early double-blind, placebo-controlled trials were attributable in part to high starting doses, rapid dose escalation, and high drug load when supratherapeutic dosages of TPM were added to maximum tolerated dosages of one or more AEDs (55). Various studies showed that the incidence and severity of CNS effects, as well as premature discontinuations because of side effects, could be reduced with more gradual dose escalation, lower target doses, and reductions in the dosages of concomitant AEDs as TPM was titrated to effect (57,117,118).

Although many of the CNS effects were nonspecific complaints seen with all AEDs (e.g., somnolence, fatigue, dizziness, ataxia, confusion), the early studies were characterized by a relatively high incidence of adverse events coded to the term "abnormal thinking" per WHOART (World Health Organization Adverse Reporting Terminology) (46,47). Subsequently, neurobehavioral adverse events were coded with an expanded adverse-event term list that included psychomotor slowing, memory difficulty, concentration/attention difficulty, speech problems, language problems, and mood problems, among others. A double-blind study comparing TPM with carbamazepine and valproate as monotherapy in newly diagnosed epilepsy was the first in which the adverse events occurring with other AEDs were coded with the dictionary that is unique to TPM trials (39). The incidence of neurobehavioral side effects was low with all three medications. TPM 100 mg per day and carbamazepine 600 mg per day were indistinguishable in terms of most neurobehavioral side effects (concentration and attention difficulty, 4% in each group; psychomotor slowing, 4%; confusion, 3%; speech disorders, 2%), which occurred less frequently in patients receiving valproate 1250 mg per day (concentration and attention difficulty, 1%; psychomotor slowing, 1%; no reports of confusion or speech problems). Cognitive problems not otherwise specified, as well as memory difficulty, were slightly more common with TPM than with the other agents (cognitive problems not otherwise specified: TPM, 3%; carbamazepine and valproate, 1%; memory difficulty: TPM, 8%; valproate, 6%; carbamazepine, 5%), while language problems were somewhat more common with carbamazepine (carbamazepine, 6%; valproate, 4%; TPM, 3%).

Although TPM and carbamazepine have not been compared in terms of their effects on objective measures of cognitive function, two studies have compared TPM and valproate added to carbamazepine in patients with uncontrolled partial-onset seizures (119,120). In a double-blind study in which patients were followed for 20 weeks, one of 17 neuropsychometric variables (short-term verbal memory) showed a statistically significant difference between treatments (worsening of scores with TPM and improvement with valproate). Although the study did not include measures of language function, it used the titration schedule most commonly used in clinical practice when adding TPM to other AEDs (i.e., 25 mg per day starting dose increased

weekly in 25-mg increments to a target dose of 200–400 mg per day). In a double-blind study using a more rapid escalation schedule (50 mg per day starting dose increased weekly in 50-mg increments to a target dose of 400 mg per day) to add TPM to carbamazepine, cognitive performance was significantly worse from baseline in seven of 24 variables at the end of the 8-week titration period but in only 2 of 24 variables (controlled oral word association and symbol digit modalities) after an additional 3 months of treatment (120). Compared with valproate added to carbamazepine, TPM scores during neuropsychometric testing were slightly worse overall. In this study, it appeared that a subset of patients was more sensitive to TPM and accounted for much of the worsening in cognitive function scores. Because pharmacodynamic interactions are a major factor in the neurobehavioral adverse events that have been reported with TPM polytherapy, neuropsychometric testing during TPM monotherapy would be a better indicator of the effects of TPM on cognitive function. However, no such study in patients with epilepsy has been published. A short-term study in healthy volunteers showed that a high starting dose (100 mg per day) and escalation to 400 mg per day in 4 weeks was associated with significant decreases from baseline on measures of attention and word fluency (121). However, the results of this study have little clinical relevance since the 400 mg per day dosage was 4 times higher than the recommended target dose of 100 mg per day in newly diagnosed epilepsy.

Although the comparative study of TPM, carbamazepine, and valproate as monotherapy showed that language and speech disorders were actually no more common with TPM, at least as monotherapy, than with carbamazepine, the occurrence of word-finding difficulty during TPM therapy has generated considerable interest, as evidenced by the studies using comprehensive neuropsychometric test batteries. In addition, investigators have sought potential risk factors for adverse cognitive effects with TPM. In a prospective study from a tertiary epilepsy center, left temporal lobe epilepsy and simple partial seizures were most strongly associated with the occurrence of word-finding difficulty in the 31 of 431 patients (7%) who developed word-finding difficulty during TPM therapy (122). As in the double-blind cognitive function study (120), it appeared that the word-finding difficulty in a small subset of patients reflected a biologic vulnerability.

Carbonic Anhydrase Inhibition

Side effects that can be linked to TPM inhibition of carbonic anhydrase isozymes (CA II and CA IV) are paresthesia, renal stones, and decreased serum bicarbonate. Paresthesias are often transient, resolve with continuing treatment, and rarely lead to drug discontinuation. Paresthesias are more common with TPM monotherapy (31,39,40) than as add-on treatment (55), which is likely caused by higher TPM plasma levels in the absence of hepatic enzyme-inducing AEDs.

As in the general population, renal stone formation in TPM clinical trials was more common in men. Other risk factors for renal stone formation include personal or family history of renal stones, chronic metabolic acidosis, and coadministration of other carbonic anhydrase inhibitors or the ketogenic diet. Although chronic metabolic acidosis may increase the risk of renal stone formation, serum bicarbonate levels are not reliable predictors of renal stone formation. Patients should maintain adequate hydration to increase urinary output and lower the concentration of stone-forming substances.

In some patients, carbonic anhydrase inhibition is associated with laboratory findings of reduced serum bicarbonate levels. In clinical trials, the mean serum bicarbonate reduction was 4 mEq/L. Although reductions in serum bicarbonate levels are usually asymptomatic, nonspecific symptoms may include fatigue, anorexia, nausea, and vomiting; no correlation between these symptoms and serum bicarbonate levels was observed in TPM-treated patients. Cases of metabolic acidosis marked by hyperventilation and acute changes in mental status have been reported in patients receiving TPM, primarily children (123–125), although most cases have been asymptomatic (126–128). Reductions in serum bicarbonate levels generally occur early in treatment and tend to stabilize without progression during continued treatment. Conditions that increase bicarbonate loss (e.g., renal disease, diarrhea, other carbonic anhydrase inhibitors), interfere with carbon dioxide regulation via the lungs (e.g., severe respiratory disorders, surgery, status epilepticus), or alter acid-base balance (ketogenic diet) may have additive effects. It is prudent to monitor serum bicarbonate in patients with any of these potentially exacerbating conditions.

Weight Loss

Pooled data from double-blind, placebo-controlled trials and open-label studies showed that 85% of 1319 adults with epilepsy receiving TPM as monotherapy or as adjunctive therapy lost weight; mean body weight change was 3.8 kg loss (4.6% of baseline body weight) (129). Weight loss was a function of baseline body weight, with greater losses occurring in patients with higher pretreatment weight. Weight loss was gradual, typically began during the initial 3 months of therapy, and peaked at 12 to 18 months. Weight loss was accompanied by positive changes in lipid profile, glycemic control, and blood pressure. In a prospective study evaluating weight changes associated with TPM treatment (108), more than 80% of adults lost weight without changes in diet or exercise; obese patients (BMI $\geq$30 kg/m^2) had the greatest degree of weight loss. Reduction of body fat mass represented 60% to 70% of the absolute weight loss. In these patients, weight loss was associated with improvements in glucose, insulin, and total cholesterol levels.

Weight loss has been observed in patients receiving TPM for conditions other than epilepsy. During two double-blind, placebo-controlled trials in patients with migraine (97,98), dose-related decreases in body weight were observed; the mean percent change in body weight compared with placebo was significantly greater in patients receiving TPM. During three double-blind, placebo-controlled trials in patients with diabetic neuropathy, 18% to 40% had clinically significant weight loss (5% or more of baseline body weight) with TPM treatment (110). The observed improvement in diabetic control, measured as reduction in HbA1c levels, did not seem to correlate with TPM-induced weight loss.

Adverse Effects in Children

During controlled clinical trials with TPM adjunctive therapy, the incidence of CNS effects in children, including cognitive effects, was generally lower than that in adults, perhaps reflecting a more gradual dose-escalation schedule (55,61,67,72,73). The most common CNS effects in children were somnolence and decreased appetite. TPM did not negatively affect measures of mental status as evaluated by parents and guardians during double-blind treatment (61), although a formal study with neuropsychological testing has not been performed in children. Temporary slowing of weight gain or minor weight loss occurred with TPM treatment; however, weight gain resumed in most children with continued therapy (130). TPM does not adversely affect growth, measured as height, in children (131).

Pooled data from three randomized, double-blind trials (31,39,40) in which 245 children/adolescents as young as 3 years of age with newly or recently diagnosed epilepsy received 50 to 500 mg per day TPM as first-line monotherapy showed that the incidence of CNS effects, including neurobehavioral effects, was lower than with adjunctive therapy, even though the treatment periods were longer (median, 8 months; treatment periods as long as 2.2 years) (132). The most common CNS effects were headache, decreased appetite, and somnolence. In most children, body weight increased or did not change; among 13 patients who lost 10% or more of baseline body weight, 12 were adolescents (12 to 15 years old). No child/adolescent discontinued TPM monotherapy because of weight loss. As noted above, metabolic acidosis may be more likely to be symptomatic in children receiving TPM compared with adults.

Idiosyncratic Toxicity

No clinically significant abnormalities in hematologic or hepatic function were reported during clinical trials (55), and laboratory test values remained generally unchanged other than expected reductions in serum bicarbonate levels.

TPM has been associated with a rare ocular syndrome consisting of acute myopia with increased intraocular pressure (133). The syndrome occurs bilaterally and at any age, in contrast to primary narrow angle closure, which is rarely bilateral and rare in individuals younger than 40 years of age. Symptoms occur early in TPM therapy (within the first month) and include acute onset of blurred vision and/or ocular pain. Ophthalmologic findings were bilateral and could include severe myopia, conjunctival hyperemia, shallowing of the anterior chambers, and increased intraocular pressure. Mydriasis was an inconsistent finding. Symptoms resolve upon prompt discontinuation of TPM treatment.

Decreased sweating (oligohidrosis) and an elevation in body temperature have been reported in association with TPM use; the majority of reports were in children. Most cases occurred after exposure to hot weather (134).

Use in Pregnancy

TPM carries a category C classification (42). In animal studies, fetal abnormalities were similar to those observed with other carbonic anhydrase inhibitors such as acetazolamide, whose use has not been linked to teratogenic effects in humans. The effects of TPM in humans are unknown. Of 31 prospectively reported pregnancies with live births, TPM was the only drug exposure in 10 cases and was not associated with congenital malformations; the other 21 pregnancies involved multiple drug exposures and included two pregnancies resulting in major congenital anomalies in patients exposed to known teratogens (135). Pregnancy registries in the United States and Europe are collecting information about the use of TPM and other AEDs during pregnancy.

TPM is excreted in human breast milk and nursing infants may be exposed to small amounts of TPM (plasma concentrations in infants are 10% to 20% of maternal concentrations); the significance of this exposure is unknown (136).

CLINICAL USE

The initial randomized, controlled trials with TPM as adjunctive therapy identified TPM 200 to 400 mg per day as an appropriate target dose in adults with refractory epilepsy; subsequent studies have shown that many patients respond to TPM dosages of ≤200 mg per day. While gradual introduction improves tolerability, TPM can be added rapidly, if needed. Reducing the dose of concomitant AEDs as TPM is added also improves tolerability. In children receiving TPM as adjunctive therapy, the recommended daily dose is 5 to 9 mg/kg; the starting dose of 1 to 3 mg/kg per day can be increased in 1- to 3-mg/kg increments every 1 to 2 weeks.

As first-line monotherapy in adults with newly or recently diagnosed epilepsy, 100 mg per day is an appropriate target dose to initially assess patient response. It appears the optimal starting dose in adults is 25 mg per day, with weekly increases of 25 to 50 mg per day. As initial monotherapy in children, the recommended dose is 3 to 6 mg/kg per day, using a starting dose of 0.5 to 1 mg/kg per day and incremental increases of 0.5 to 1 mg/kg at 1- or 2-week intervals.

REFERENCES

1. Gibbs JW, Sombati S, DeLorenzo RJ, et al. Cellular actions of topiramate: blockade of kainate-evoked inward currents in cultured hippocampal neurons. *Epilepsia* 2000;41(Suppl 1):S10–S16.
2. Skradski S, White HS. Topiramate blocks kainite-evoked cobalt influx into cultured neurons. *Epilepsia* 2000;41(Suppl 1): S45–S47.
3. Coulter DA, Sombati S, DeLorenzo RJ. Topiramate effects on excitatory amino acid-mediated responses in cultured hippocampal neurons: selective blockade of kainate currents [abstract]. *Epilepsia* 1995;36(Suppl 3):S40.
4. Rogawski MA, Gryder D, Castaneda D, et al. GluR5 kainate receptors, seizures, and the amygdala. *Ann NY Acad Sci* 2003; 985:150–162.
5. DeLorenzo RJ, Sombati S, Coulter DA. Effects of topiramate on sustained repetitive firing and spontaneous recurrent seizure discharge in cultured hippocampal neurons. *Epilepsia* 2000;41 (Suppl 1):S40–S44.
6. McLean MJ, Bukhari AA, Wamil AW. Effects of topiramate on sodium-dependent action-potential firing by mouse spinal cord neurons in cell culture. *Epilepsia* 2000;41(Suppl 1):S21–S24.
7. Taverna S, Sancini G, Mantegazza M, et al. Inhibition of transient and persistent Na^+ current fractions by the new anticonvulsant topiramate. *J Pharmacol Exp Ther* 1999;288:960–968.
8. Zona C, Ciotti MT, Avoli M. Topiramate attenuates voltage-gated sodium currents in rat cerebellar granule cells. *Neurosci Lett* 1997;231:123–126.
9. Wu SP, Tsai JJ, Gean PW. Frequency-dependent inhibition of neuronal activity by topiramate in rat hippocampal slices. *Br J Pharmacol* 1998;125:826–832.
10. White HS, Brown SD, Woodhead JH, et al. Topiramate modulates GABA-evoked currents in murine cortical neurons by a non-benzodiazepine mechanism. *Epilepsia* 2000;41(Suppl 1): S17–S20.
11. White HS, Brown SD, Woodhead JH, et al. Topiramate enhances GABA-mediated chloride flux and GABA-evoked chloride currents in murine brain neurons and increases seizure threshold. *Epilepsy Res* 1997;28:167–179.
12. Zhang X-l, Velumian AA, Jones OT, et al. Modulation of high-voltage-activated calcium channels in dentate granule cells by topiramate. *Epilepsia* 2000;41(Suppl 1):S52–S60.
13. Ängehagen M, Ben-Menachem E, Rönnbäck L, Hansson E. Topiramate protects against glutamate- and kainate-induced neurotoxicity in primary neuronal-astroglial cultures. *Epilepsy Res* 2003;54:63–71.
14. Herrero AI, Del Olmo N, Gonzalez-Escalada JR, Solis JM. Two new actions of topiramate: inhibition of depolarizing GABA(A)-mediated responses and activation of a potassium conductance. *Neuropharmacology* 2002;42:210–220.
15. Russo E, Constanti A. Topiramate hyperpolarizes and modulates the slow poststimulus AHP of rat olfactory cortical neurones in vitro. *Br J Pharmacol* 2004;141:285–301.
16. Shank RP, Gardocki JF, Streeter AJ, et al. An overview of the preclinical aspects of topiramate: pharmacology, pharmacokinetics, and mechanism of action. *Epilepsia* 2000;41(Suppl 1) S3–S9.
17. Dodgson SJ, Shank RP, Maryanoff BE. Topiramate as an inhibitor of carbonic anhydrase isoenzymes. *Epilepsia* 2000;41(Suppl 1): S35–S39.
18. Nakamura J, Tamura S, Kanda T, et al. Inhibition by topiramate of seizures in spontaneously epileptic rats and DBA/2 mice. *Eur J Pharmacol* 1994;254:83–89.
19. Amano K, Hamada K, Yagi K, et al. Antiepileptic effects of topiramate on amygdaloid kindling in rats. *Epilepsy Res* 1998;31: 123–128.
20. Wauquier A, Zhou S. Topiramate: a potent anticonvulsant in the amygdala-kindled rat. *Epilepsy Res* 1996;24:73–77.

21. Edmonds HL Jr, Jiang YD, Zhang PY, et al. Anticonvulsant activity of topiramate and phenytoin in a rat model of ischemia-induced epilepsy. *Life Sci* 1996;59:PL127–PL131.

22. Niebauer M, Gruenthal M. Topiramate reduces neuronal injury after experimental status epilepticus. *Brain Res* 1999;837:263–269.

23. DeLorenzo RJ, Morris TA, Blair RE, et al. Topiramate is both neuroprotective and antiepileptogenic in the pilocarpine model of status epilepticus [abstract]. *Epilepsia* 2002;43(Suppl 7):15.

24. Koh S, Jensen FE. Topiramate blocks perinatal hypoxia-induced seizures in rat pups. *Ann Neurol* 2001;50:366–372.

25. Doose DR, Walker SA, Gisclon LG, et al. Single-dose pharmacokinetics and effect of food on the bioavailability of topiramate, a novel antiepileptic drug. *J Clin Pharmacol* 1996;36:884–891.

26. Garnett WR. Clinical pharmacology of topiramate: a review. *Epilepsia* 2002;41(Suppl 1):S61–S65.

27. Rosenfeld WE, Doose DR, Walker SA, et al. A study of topiramate pharmacokinetics and tolerability in children with epilepsy. *Pediatr Neurol* 1999;20:339–344.

28. Glauser TA, Miles MV, Tang P, et al. Topiramate pharmacokinetics in infants. *Epilepsia* 1999;40:788–791.

29. Doose DR, Larson KL, Natarajan J, et al. Comparative single-dose pharmacokinetics of topiramate in elderly versus young men and women [abstract]. *Epilepsia* 1998;39(Suppl 6):56.

30. Faught E, Squires L, Wang S, Thienel U. Tolerability and safety of topiramate as first-line monotherapy in 1,000+ epilepsy patients [abstract]. *Epilepsia* 2003;44(Suppl 9):100.

31. Gilliam FG, Veloso F, Bomhof MAM, et al. A dose-comparison trial of topiramate as monotherapy in recently diagnosed partial epilepsy. *Neurology* 2003;60:196–202.

32. Schwabe MJ, Wheless JW. Clinical experience with topiramate dosing and serum levels in children 12 years or under with epilepsy. *J Child Neurol* 2001;16:806–808.

33. Sachdeo RC, Sachdeo SK, Walker SA, et al. Steady-state pharmacokinetics of topiramate and carbamazepine in patients with epilepsy during monotherapy and concomitant therapy. *Epilepsia* 1996;37:774–780.

34. Doose DR, Walker SA, Pledger G, et al. Evaluation of phenobarbital and primidone/phenobarbital (primidone's active metabolite) plasma concentrations during administration of add-on topiramate therapy in five multicenter, double-blind, placebo-controlled trials in outpatients with partial seizures [abstract]. *Epilepsia* 1995;36(Suppl 3):S158.

35. Sachdeo RC, Sachdeo SK, Levy RH, et al. Topiramate and phenytoin pharmacokinetics during repetitive monotherapy and combination therapy to epileptic patients. *Epilepsia* 2002;43:691–696.

36. Rosenfeld WE, Liao S, Kramer LD, et al. Comparison of the steady-state pharmacokinetics of topiramate and valproate in patients with epilepsy during monotherapy and concomitant therapy. *Epilepsia* 1997;38:324–333.

37. Doose DR, Brodie ME, Wilson EA, et al. Topiramate and lamotrigine pharmacokinetics during repetitive monotherapy and combination therapy in epilepsy patients. *Epilepsia* 2003;44:917–922.

38. Levy RH, Bishop F, Streeter AJ, et al. Explanation and prediction of drug interactions with topiramate using a CYP450 inhibition spectrum [abstract]. *Epilepsia* 1995;36(Suppl 4):S47.

39. Privitera MD, Brodie MJ, Mattson RH, et al. Topiramate, carbamazepine and valproate monotherapy: double-blind comparison in newly diagnosed epilepsy. *Acta Neurol Scand* 2003;107:165–175.

40. Arroyo S, Squires L, Wang S, et al. Topiramate: effective as monotherapy in dose-response study in newly diagnosed epilepsy [abstract]. *Epilepsia* 2002;43(Suppl 7):241.

41. Doose DR, Wang S-S, Padmanabhan M, et al. Effect of topiramate or carbamazepine on the pharmacokinetics of an oral contraceptive containing norethindrone and ethinyl estradiol in healthy obese and nonobese female subjects. *Epilepsia* 2003;44:540–549.

42. Rosenfeld WE, Doose DR, Walker SA, et al. Effect of topiramate on the pharmacokinetics of an oral contraceptive containing norethindrone and ethinyl estradiol in patients with epilepsy. *Epilepsia* 1997;38:317–323.

43. Nallani SC, Glauser TA, Hariparsad N, et al. Dose-dependent induction of cytochrome P450(CYP)3A4 and activation of pregnane X receptor by topiramate. *Epilepsia* 2003;44:1521–1528.

44. Liao S, Palmer M. Digoxin and topiramate drug interaction study in male volunteers [abstract]. *Pharm Res* 1993;10(Suppl):S405.

45. Topamax® (topiramate) tablets/(topiramate capsules) Sprinkle Capsules package insert. Raritan, NJ: Ortho-McNeil Pharmaceutical, Inc, December 2003.

46. Faught E, Wilder BJ, Ramsay RE, et al. Topiramate placebo-controlled dose-ranging trial in refractory partial epilepsy using 200-, 400-, and 600-mg daily dosages. *Neurology* 1996;46:1684–1690.

47. Privitera M, Fincham R, Penry J, et al. Topiramate placebo-controlled dose-ranging trial in refractory partial epilepsy using 600-, 800-, and 1000-mg daily dosages. *Neurology* 1996;46:1678–1683.

48. Sharief M, Viteri C, Ben-Menachem E, et al. Double-blind, placebo-controlled study of topiramate in patients with refractory partial epilepsy. *Epilepsia Res* 1996;25:217–224.

49. Tassinari CA, Michelucci R, Chauvel P, et al. Double-blind, placebo-controlled trial of topiramate (600 mg daily) for the treatment of refractory partial epilepsy. *Epilepsia* 1996;37:763–768.

50. Ben-Menachem E, Henriksen O, Dam M, et al. Double-blind, placebo-controlled trial of topiramate as add-on therapy in patients with refractory partial seizures. *Epilepsia* 1996;37:539–543.

51. Rosenfeld W, Abou-Khalil B, Reife R, et al. Placebo-controlled trial of topiramate as adjunctive therapy to carbamazepine or phenytoin for partial-onset epilepsy [abstract]. *Epilepsia* 1996;37(Suppl 5):153.

52. Korean Topiramate Study Group. Topiramate in medically intractable partial epilepsies: double-blind placebo-controlled randomized parallel group trial. *Epilepsia* 1999;40:1767–1774.

53. Yen D-J, Yu H-Y, Guo Y-C, et al. A double-blind, placebo-controlled study of topiramate in adult patients with refractory partial epilepsy. *Epilepsia* 2000;41:1162–1166.

54. Guberman A, Neto W, Gassmann-Mayer C, et al. Low-dose topiramate in adults with treatment-resistant partial-onset seizures. *Acta Neurol Scand* 2002;106:183–189.

55. Reife R, Pledger G, Wu S. Topiramate as add-on therapy: pooled analysis of randomized controlled trials in adults. *Epilepsia* 2000;41(Suppl 1):S66–S71.

56. Korean Topiramate Study Group. Low dose and slow titration of topiramate as adjunctive therapy in refractory partial epilepsies: a multicentre open clinical trial. *Seizure* 2002;11:255–260.

57. Dodson WE, Kamin M, Kraut L, et al. Topiramate titration to response: analysis of individualized therapy study (TRAITS). *Ann Pharmacother* 2003;37:615–620.

58. Stephen LJ, Sills GJ, Brodie MJ. Topiramate in refractory epilepsy: a prospective observational study. *Epilepsia* 2000;41:977–980.

59. Lhatoo SD, Wong ICK, Polizzi G, et al. Long-term retention rates of lamotrigine, gabapentin, and topiramate in chronic epilepsy. *Epilepsia* 2000;41:1592–1596.

60. Lhatoo SD, Wong ICK, Sander JWAS. Prognostic factors affecting long-term retention of topiramate in patients with chronic epilepsy. *Epilepsia* 2000;41:338–341.

61. Elterman RD, Glauser TA, Wyllie E, et al. A double-blind, randomized trial of topiramate as adjunctive therapy for partial-onset seizures in children. *Neurology* 1999;52:1338–1344.

62. Ritter FJ, Glauser TA, Elterman R, et al. Effectiveness, tolerability and safety of topiramate in children with partial-onset seizures. *Epilepsia* 2000;41(Suppl 1):S82–S85.

63. Mikaeloff Y, de Saint-Martin A, Mancini J, et al. Topiramate: efficacy and tolerability in children according to epilepsy syndromes. *Epilepsy Res* 2003;53:225–232.

64. Coppola G, Caliendo G, Terracciano MM, et al. Topiramate in refractory partial-onset seizures in children, adolescents, and young adults: a multicentric open trial. *Epilepsy Res* 2001;43:255–260.

65. Mohamed K, Appleton R, Rosenbloom L. Efficacy and tolerability of topiramate in childhood and adolescent epilepsy: a clinical experience. *Seizure* 2000;9:137–141.

66. Guerreiro MM, Squires L, Mohandoss E. Topiramate as adjunctive therapy: a prospective study of 500+ children/adolescents

with refractory epilepsy [abstract]. *Epilepsia* 2002;43(Suppl 7): 58.

67. Sachdeo RC, Glauser TA, Ritter F, et al. A double-blind, randomized trial of topiramate in Lennox-Gastaut syndrome. *Neurology* 1999;52:1882–1887.

68. Motte J, Trevathan E, Arvidsson JFV, et al. Lamotrigine for generalized seizures associated with the Lennox-Gastaut syndrome. *N Engl J Med* 1997;337:1807–1812.

69. Glauser TA, Levisohn P, Ritter F, et al. Topiramate in Lennox-Gastaut syndrome: open-label treatment of patients completing a randomized controlled trial. *Epilepsia* 2000;41(Suppl 1): S86–S90.

70. Guerreiro MM, Manreza MLG, Scotoni AE, et al. A pilot study of topiramate in children with Lennox-Gastaut syndrome. *Arq Neuropsiquiatr* 1999;57:167–175.

71. Coppola G, Caliendo G, Veggiotti P, et al. Topiramate as add-on drug in children, adolescents and young adults with Lennox-Gastaut syndrome: an Italian multicentric study. *Epilepsy Res* 2002;51:147–153.

72. Biton V, Montouris GD, Ritter F, et al. A randomized, placebo-controlled study of topiramate in primary generalized tonic-clonic seizures. *Neurology* 1999;52:1330–1337.

73. Ben-Menachem E, Topiramate YTC-E Study Group. A double-blind trial of topiramate in patients with generalised tonic-clonic seizures of non-focal origin [abstract]. *Epilepsia* 1997;38(Suppl 3): 60.

74. Montouris G, Biton V, Rosenfeld WE, et al. Non-focal generalized tonic-clonic seizures: response during long-term topiramate treatment. *Epilepsia* 2000;41(Suppl 1):S77–S81.

75. Ting TY, Herman S, French JA, et al. Seizure control and EEG response in primary generalized epilepsy patients treated with topiramate [abstract]. *Epilepsia* 2002;41(Suppl 7):202.

76. Biton V, Rosenfeld WE, Twyman R, et al. Topiramate (TPM) in juvenile myoclonic epilepsy (JME): observations from randomized controlled trials in primary generalized tonic-clonic seizures (PGTCS) [abstract]. *Epilepsia* 1999;40(Suppl 7):218.

77. Levisohn PM, Holland KD, Hulihan JF, Fisher AC. Topiramate versus valproate in patients with juvenile myoclonic epilepsy [abstract]. *Epilepsia* 2003;44(Suppl 9):267–268.

78. Glauser TA, Clark PO, Strawsburg R. A pilot study of topiramate in the treatment of infantile spasms. *Epilepsia* 1998;39: 1324–1328.

79. Glauser TA, Clark PO, McGee K. Long-term response to topiramate in patients with West syndrome. *Epilepsia* 2000;41(Suppl 1): S91–S94.

80. Cross JH. Topiramate monotherapy for childhood absence seizures: an open-label pilot study. *Seizure* 2002;11:406–410.

81. Coppola G, Capovilla G, Montagnini A, et al. Topiramate as add-on drug in severe myoclonic epilepsy in infancy: an Italian multicenter open trial. *Epilepsy Res* 2002;49:45–48.

82. Kelly K, Stephen LJ, Sills GJ, et al. Topiramate in patients with learning disability and refractory epilepsy. *Epilepsia* 2002;43: 399–402.

83. Singh BK, White-Scott S. Role of topiramate in adults with intractable epilepsy, mental retardation, and developmental disabilities. *Seizure* 2002;11:47–50.

84. Towne AR, Garnett LK, Waterhouse EJ, et al. The use of topiramate in refractory status epilepticus. *Neurology* 2003;60:332–334.

85. Mattson RH, Cramer JA, Collins JF, et al. Comparison of carbamazepine, phenobarbital, phenytoin, and primidone in partial and secondarily generalized tonic-clonic seizures. *N Engl J Med* 1985;313:145–151.

86. Mattson RH, Cramaer JA, Collins JF, et al. A comparison of valproate with carbamazepine for the treatment of complex partial seizures and secondarily generalized tonic-clonic seizures in adults. *N Engl J Med* 1992;327:765–771.

87. Heller AJ, Chesterman P, Elwes RDC, et al. Phenobarbitone, phenytoin, carbamazepine, or sodium valproate for newly diagnosed adult epilepsy: a randomised comparative monotherapy trial. *J Neurol Neurosurg Psychiatry* 1995;58:44–50.

88. de Silva M, MacArdle B, McGowan M, et al. Randomised comparative monotherapy trial of phenobarbitone, phenytoin, carbamazepine, or sodium valproate for newly diagnosed childhood epilepsy. *Lancet* 1996;347:709–713.

89. Pledger GW, Kramer LD. Clinical trials of investigational antiepileptic drugs: monotherapy designs. *Epilepsia* 1991;32: 716–721.

90. Sachdeo RC, Reife RA, Lim P, et al. Topiramate monotherapy for partial onset seizures. *Epilepsia* 1997;38:294–300.

91. Sachdeo RC, Edwards K, Hasegawa H, et al. Safety and efficacy of oxcarbazepine 1200 mg per day in patients with recent-onset partial epilepsy [abstract]. *Neurology* 1999;52(Suppl 2):A391.

92. Leber P. Hazards of inference: the active control investigation. *Epilepsia* 1989;30(Suppl 1):S57–S63.

93. Chadwick D, Privitera M. Placebo-controlled trials in neurology: where do they stop? *Neurology* 1999;52:682–685.

94. Brodie MJ, Richens A, Yuen AWC, et al. Double-blind comparison of lamotrigine and carbamazepine in newly diagnosed epilepsy. *Lancet* 1995;345:476–479.

95. Steiner TJ, Dellaportas CI, Findley LJ, et al. Lamotrigine monotherapy in newly diagnosed untreated epilepsy: a double-blind comparison with phenytoin. *Epilepsia* 1999;40:601–607.

96. Kwan P, Brodie MJ. Early identification of refractory epilepsy. *N Engl J Med* 2000;342:314–319.

97. Kwan P, Brodie MJ. Effectiveness of first antiepileptic drug. *Epilepsia* 2001;42:1255–1260.

98. Brandes JL, Saper JR, Diamond M, et al. Topiramate for migraine prevention: a randomized controlled trial. *JAMA* 2004;291: 965–973.

99. Dodick DW, Neto W, Schmitt J, et al. Topiramate in migraine prevention (MIGR-001): additional efficacy measures from a randomized, double-blind, placebo-controlled trial. *Neurology* 2003;60(Suppl 1):A237–A238.

100. Wheeler SD, Carrazana EJ. Topiramate-treated cluster headache. *Neurology* 1999;53:274–276.

101. Hulihan J, Connor GS, Wu S-C, et al. Topiramate in essential tremor: pooled data from a double-blind, placebo-controlled, crossover trial [abstract]. *Neurology* 2003;60(Suppl 1):A291.

102. Connor GS. A double-blind placebo-controlled trial of topiramate treatment for essential tremor. *Neurology* 2002;59: 132–134.

103. Nelson TY, Lesser PS, Bost MT. Topiramate in children and adolescents with Tourette's syndrome [abstract]. *Ann Neurol* 2002;52(Suppl 1):S128.

104. Johnson BA, Ait-Daoud N, Bowden CL, et al. Oral topiramate for treatment of alcohol dependence: a randomized controlled trial. *Lancet* 2003;36:1677–1685.

105. McElroy SL, Arnold LM, Shapira NA, et al. Topiramate in the treatment of binge-eating disorder associated with obesity: a randomized, placebo-controlled trial. *Am J Psychiatry* 2003;160: 255–261.

106. Nigro MA, Smathers SA. An open-label trial on the efficacy of topiramate in the treatment of behavior, mood, and compulsive eating disorder of Prader Willi syndrome [abstract]. *Neurology* 2001;56(Suppl 3):A42.

107. Shapira NA, Lessig MC, Murphy TK, et al. Topiramate attenuates self-injurious behavior in Prader-Willi syndrome. *Int J Neuropsychopharmacol* 2002;5:141–145.

108. Ben-Menachem E, Axelsen M, Johanson EH, et al. Predictors of weight loss in adults with topiramate-treated epilepsy. *Obes Res* 2003;11:556–562.

109. Bray GA, Hollander P, Klein S, et al. A 6-month randomized, placebo-controlled, dose-ranging trial of topiramate for weight loss in obesity. *Obes Res* 2003;11:722–733.

110. Thienel U, Neto W, Goldstein H. Effect of topiramate on diabetic control and weight in diabetic patients [abstract]. *Epilepsia* 2002;43(Suppl 7):221–222. A

111. Demarest K, Conway B, Osborne M, et al. Topiramate improves glucose tolerance and may improve insulin sensitivity in animal models of type 2 diabetes [abstract]. *Diabetes* 2001;50(Suppl 2): A302.

112. Yang Y, Shuaib A, Li Q, et al. Neuroprotection by delayed administration of topiramate in a rat model of middle cerebral artery embolization. *Brain Res* 1998;804:169–176.

113. Angehagen M, Hansson E, Ronnback L, et al. Does topiramate (TPM) have protective effects on astroglia cells and neurons in primary cortical cultures [abstract]? *Epilepsia* 1998;39(Suppl 6): 44.

114. Vinik AI, Pittenger GL, Anderson SA, et al. Topiramate improves C-fiber neuropathy and features of the dysmetabolic syndrome in type 2 diabetes. Presented at the American Diabetes Association 63rd Scientific Sessions, June 13, 2002, New Orleans, Louisiana.

115. Alves OL, Doyle AJ, Clausen T, et al. Evaluation of topiramate neuroprotective effect in severe TBI using microdialysis. *Ann NY Acad Sci* 2003;993:25–34.

116. Cudkowicz ME, Shefner JM, Schoenfeld DA, et al, for the Northeast ALS Consortium. A randomized, placebo-controlled trial of topiramate in amyotrophic lateral sclerosis. *Neurology* 2003;61:456–464.

117. Biton V, Edwards KR, Montouris GD, et al. Topiramate titration and tolerability. *Ann Pharmacother* 2001;35:173–179.

118. Naritoku DK, Hulihan J, Karim R, et al. Reduction of antiepileptic drug (AED) co-therapy improves tolerability of add-on therapy with topiramate: a novel randomized study [abstract]. *Epilepsia* 2001;42(Suppl 7):258.

119. Aldenkamp AP, Baker G, Mulder OG, et al. A multicenter, randomized clinical study to evaluate the effect on cognitive function of topiramate compared with valproate as add-on therapy to carbamazepine in patients with partial-onset seizures. *Epilepsia* 2000;41:1167–1178.

120. Meador KJ, Loring DW, Hulihan JF, et al. Differential cognitive and behavioral effects of topiramate and valproate. *Neurology* 2003;60:1483–1488.

121. Martin R, Kuzniecky R, Ho S, et al. Cognitive effects of topiramate, gabapentin, and lamotrigine in healthy young adults. *Neurology* 1999;52:321–327.

122. Mula M, Trimble MR, Thompson P, et al. Topiramate and word-finding difficulties in patients with epilepsy. *Neurology* 2003;60:1104–1107.

123. Stowe CD, Bolliger T, James LP, et al. Acute mental status changes and hyperchloremic metabolic acidosis with long-term topiramate therapy. *Pharmacotherapy* 2000;20:105–109.

124. Ko C-h, Kong C-k. Topiramate-induced metabolic acidosis: report of two cases. *Dev Med Child Neurol* 2001;43:701–704.

125. Philippi H, Boor R, Reitter B. Topiramate and metabolic acidosis in infants and toddlers. *Epilepsia* 2002;43:744–747.

126. Wilner A, Raymond K, Pollard R. Topiramate and metabolic acidosis. *Epilepsia* 1999;40:792–795.

127. Takeoka M, Holmes GL, Thiele E, et al. Topiramate and metabolic acidosis in pediatric epilepsy. *Epilepsia* 2001;42:387–392.

128. Takeoka M, Riviello JJ, Pfeifer H, Thiele EA. Concomitant treatment with topiramate and ketogenic diet in pediatric epilepsy. *Epilepsia* 2002;43:1072–1075.

129. Rosenfeld WE, Slater J. Characterization of topiramate-associated weight changes in adults with epilepsy. *Epilepsia* 2002; 43(Suppl 7):220–221.

130. Riviello JJ, Wheless J, W SC, et al. Body weight (BW) changes during topiramate (TPM) therapy in children with epilepsy [abstract]. *Epilepsia* 1999;40(Suppl 7):127.

131. Morita DA, Glauser TA, Guo SS. Effect of topiramate on linear growth in children with refractory complex partial seizures [abstract]. *Neurology* 2000;54(Suppl 3):A193.

132. Dlugos DJ, Squires L, Wang S. Topiramate as first-line therapy: tolerability and safety in children and adolescents [abstract]. *Neurology* 2003;60(Suppl 1):A474–A475.

133. Keates E, Clark T. Acute myopia and secondary angle closure glaucoma: a rare ocular syndrome in topiramate-treated patients [abstract]. *Neurology* 2002;58:A422.

134. Ben-Zeev B, Watemberg N, Augarten A, et al. Oligohydrosis and hyperthermia: pilot study of a novel topiramate adverse effect. *J Child Neurol* 2003;18:254–257.

135. Montouris GD, Creasy G, Khan A, Neto W. Pregnancy outcomes in topiramate-treated women [abstract]. *Epilepsia* 2003;44:290.

136. Öhman I, Vitols S, Luef G, et al. Topiramate kinetics during delivery, lactation, and in the neonate: preliminary observations. *Epilepsia* 2002;43:1157–1160.

Zonisamide

62

Timothy E. Welty

Zonisamide was first synthesized in 1974 in Japan. In the early 1980s, clinical trials of zonisamide were initiated in the United States. Because of an increased risk for nephrolithiasis in patients receiving active drug, further development in the United States was halted. However, zonisamide continued to be developed in Japan, with the agent receiving marketing approval in that country in 1989. Following approval in Japan and the development of improved treatments for nephrolithiasis, additional studies in Europe and the United States were initiated, with marketing approval granted in the United States in 2000.

As a result of the gap in development of ZNS in Western nations, much information on the agent is from the Japanese experience. Language barriers have limited access to some of this information, and the available data may not always be applicable to populations and ethnic groups outside of Japan. Nevertheless, ZNS is an effective and safe antiepileptic drug (AED) that appears to have broad activity in patients with various seizure types and epilepsy syndromes.

CHEMISTRY

ZNS is classified as a sulfonamide AED that is a 1,2 benzisoxazole derivative. It is the first compound from this group of chemicals to be developed as an AED. ZNS is unrelated chemically to other AEDs (Fig. 62.1). The agent is moderately soluble in water (0.8 mg/mL) and has a pKa of 10.2. ZNS is a white powder; it has a molecular weight of 212.23.

MECHANISM OF ACTION

Several pharmacologic effects of ZNS may be responsible for its activity as an AED. Some of these activities may make ZNS useful in the treatment of other neurologic disorders as well. Results from numerous studies (1–19) demonstrate the most likely mechanism of action of ZNS to be via blockade of T-type calcium channels, inhibition of slow sodium channels, and possibly inhibition of glutamate release. In animal models of epilepsy, ZNS demonstrates activity that indicates its possible effectiveness as a broad-spectrum AED. Besides its antiepileptic activity, ZNS also has some effect as a neuroprotective agent in the treatment of ischemia (20).

PHARMACOKINETICS

Absorption

ZNS is rapidly absorbed following oral administration, with maximum concentrations achieved within 2 to 5 hours (21). The absolute bioavailability in humans is unknown because of lack of a parenteral product. Nagatomi and colleagues found the absolute bioavailability of orally administered ZNS to be 81% in rats (22). In the same study, the bioavailability of ZNS in a rectal preparation was 96%. ZNS is metabolized by the cytochrome P450 isozyme 3A4 (CYP3A4) (23). The presence of CYP3A4 in the intestine may account for the decreased bioavailability of the oral preparation.

Distribution and Protein Binding

Like many sulfonamide drugs, ZNS has a dose-dependent decrease in volume of distribution (V_d) (24). The V_d is 1.8 L/kg for a 200-mg dose and 1.2 L/kg for an 800-mg dose. Saturable binding to erythrocytes, particularly intracellular carbonic anhydrase, is the most likely explanation for this phenomenon (25–27). Additionally, 40% to 60% of ZNS is bound to plasma proteins, especially albumin (27,28).

Therefore, ZNS is concentrated in erythrocytes, not in plasma. With saturable binding to erythrocytes, the whole blood ZNS concentration is nonlinear as the dosage increases. However, the plasma ZNS concentration is linear

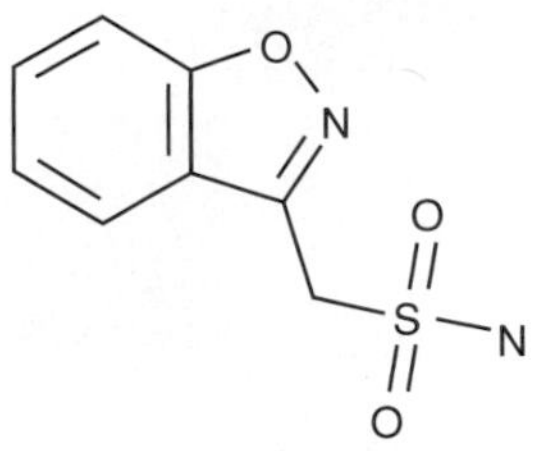

Figure 62.1   Chemistry of zonisamide.

with increased doses (21). Care must be taken in laboratory analysis and interpretation of ZNS concentrations. Results should be identified as obtained from either whole blood or plasma.

Metabolism and Clearance

Following oral administration, the half-life ($t_{1/2}$) of ZNS is estimated at 50 to 69 hours (21,29). Total clearance (Cl) following single and repeated oral doses is 0.6 to 0.71 L per hour (29). Less than 30% of ZNS is eliminated unchanged in the urine and most of the drug undergoes extensive hepatic metabolism (30). The relatively long $t_{1/2}$ and slow clearance allow for once-daily ZNS dosing.

Early studies of the pharmacokinetics of ZNS suggested that concentrations increased in a nonlinear relationship to dose (24,31). Following administration of an 800-mg dose, ZNS clearance was 22% lower than clearance estimates following 200-mg and 400-mg doses. Clearance estimates at steady state, with doses ranging from 400 to 1200 mg per day, were 40% lower than those seen following a single 400-mg dose (21,32). In a study by Wilensky and associates, although steady-state ZNS concentrations were found to be higher than predicted from single-dose data, steady-state plasma concentrations increased in a linear relationship to daily dose (33). These observations were considered to be related to the saturable, preferential binding of ZNS to erythrocytes. However, an analysis of ZNS doses and concentration in children using a nonlinear mixed effects model and population pharmacokinetic methodology demonstrated dose-dependent, Michaelis-Menten pharmacokinetics of zonisamide, with a mean maximum flow velocity (V_{max}) of 27.6 mg/day/kg and an affinity constant (K_m) of 45.9 μg/mL (34). Because the V_{max} is well above the typical range of daily ZNS doses, it is unlikely that the nonlinear nature of ZNS clearance will profoundly impact clinical practice.

The major metabolite of ZNS is 2-sulfamoylacetylphenol (SMAP), formed under anaerobic conditions by liver microsomal enzymes (23,35,36). The formation of SMAP appears to be primarily through CYP3A4 (23,35). As reported in the aforementioned studies (23,35), the metabolism of ZNS to SMAP was inhibited by cimetidine and ketoconazole, which are both known CYP3A4 inhibitors. ZNS is metabolized to a much lesser extent by CYP2C19 and CYP3A5 (37).

Plasma Concentrations and Dosing

The manufacturer's recommended dose for adults is 200 to 400 mg per day, but doses of 600 mg per day have been used in clinical trials (38). Doses >400 mg have not consistently been associated with increased efficacy. The recommended doses of ZNS are typically associated with steady-state concentrations of 10 to 30 μg/mL (29,34). However, a relationship between concentration and response has not been established. Some investigators have suggested that concentrations >30 μg/mL are associated with increased adverse effects (24,33). Therefore, it may be advisable to maintain ZNS at concentrations <30 μg/mL. The pharmacokinetics and dosing of ZNS are summarized in Table 62.1.

Special Populations

Pediatrics

No formal pharmacokinetic studies have been conducted in children. In a study of ZNS for infantile spasms by Suzuki and colleagues, daily doses of 4 to 5 mg/kg yielded plasma concentrations of 5.2 to 16.3 μg/mL (39). Additional work by the same investigators substantiated these findings, with ZNS doses of 4 to 12 mg/kg per day producing plasma concentrations of 5.2 to 30 μg/mL (40). Table 62.2 summarizes typical mean plasma concentrations related to dose and age. A comparison of pharmacokinetic parameters derived from population data in children and adults shows a similar V_d but more rapid clearance of ZNS in children (34,41). Thus, children appear to require larger doses of zonisamide, based on body weight, to achieve plasma concentrations similar to those seen in adults (42).

Three case reports have provided some documentation regarding transfer of ZNS across the placenta and into

---

TABLE 62.1

SUMMARY OF ZNS PHARMACOKINETICS AND DOSING

Parameter	Value
Oral bioavailability	81%[a]
Volume of distribution (V_d)	1.2–1.8 L/kg[b]
Protein binding	40%–60%[c]
Half-life ($t_{1/2}$)	50–69 hours
Clearance (Cl)	0.6–0.71 L per hour
Usual plasma concentrations	10–30 μg/mL[d]
Recommended dose	200–400 mg per day[e]

[a]Based on animal data.
[b]Volume of distribution is inversely related to dose because of saturable binding to erythrocytes.
[c]Additionally, ZNS is highly and preferentially bound to erythrocytes.
[d]These are typical concentrations observed with usual doses. A relationship between concentration and response has not been established.
[e]Higher doses have been used in clinical trials.

TABLE 62.2
MEAN ZNS PLASMA CONCENTRATIONS RELATED TO AGE AND DAILY DOSE

Age (y)	Mean Daily Dose (mg/kg)	Mean Plasma Concentration (μg/mL)
16	5.9	20.0
7–15	7.1	20.7
2–6	8.8	19.9
≤1	8.6	19.6

Data from reference 72.

TABLE 62.3
DRUG INTERACTIONS WITH ZONISAMIDE (ZNS)

Reduced ZNS Metabolism	Increased ZNS Metabolism	Variable Effect on ZNS Metabolism
Cyclosporine A	Phenytoin	Carbamazepine
Ketoconazole	Phenobarbital	
Dihydroergotamine	Primidone	
Triazolam		
Diazepam		
Erythromycin		

breast milk. Kawada and associates measured ZNS concentrations in umbilical cord blood, infant blood, and maternal blood in two infants born to mothers taking ZNS for the treatment of epilepsy (43). In these infants, ZNS concentrations were 92% of those in maternal blood. The investigators also measured ZNS concentrations in the breast milk of these mothers, showing these concentrations to be 41% to 57% of maternal plasma concentrations. In a separate case evaluating ZNS concentrations in breast milk up to 30 days postpartum, Shimoyama and colleagues observed breast milk concentrations that ranged from 81% to 100% of maternal plasma concentrations (44). It appears that ZNS readily crosses the placenta. ZNS also appears in breast milk at concentrations similar to maternal plasma concentrations. No clinically important adverse effects related to ZNS were documented in these case reports.

Renal Failure

A single-dose study of ZNS in individuals with moderate renal failure (creatinine clearance >0.6 L per hour) did not demonstrate any difference in pharmacokinetic parameters compared with normal individuals (45). Studies in patients with severe renal dysfunction and multiple-dose studies in patients with renal failure have not been reported.

DRUG INTERACTIONS

Because ZNS is metabolized primarily via CYP3A4 and to a lesser extent via CYP2C19, the agent is potentially prone to drug-drug interactions involving these enzyme systems. Several interactions have been studied in animals and in humans (Table 62.3). However, the exact clinical implications of these interactions have been poorly documented.

Influence of Other Agents on Zonisamide

Using *in vitro* studies of the CYP3A system, Nakasa and colleagues demonstrated that cyclosporine A, ketoconazole, dihydroergotamine, and triazolam profoundly inhibit ZNS metabolism (37). These agents reduced ZNS metabolism

by 85% to 95% compared with control. With other known inhibitors of CYP3A—diazepam, terfenadine, erythromycin, and lidocaine—the reduction in metabolism was much lower, ranging from 35% to 45%. Clinical correlates to these findings have not been documented, so recommendations for dosage adjustments in patients are not available. However, patients receiving known inhibitors of CYP3A may require lower doses of ZNS to reduce the risk for adverse events.

Inducers of CYP3A have been associated with increased ZNS metabolism (37). Phenytoin and carbamazepine have been shown to induce ZNS metabolism, with phenytoin possibly having a greater influence than carbamazepine (46,47). In a study of 12 patients receiving phenytoin or carbamazepine concomitantly with zonisamide, the mean Cl/F of ZNS was 33.9 mL per hour/kg with phenytoin and 20.6 mL per hour/kg with carbamazepine (46). However, some researchers have observed inhibition of ZNS metabolism with carbamazepine (37). Other known inducers of hepatic metabolism, particularly phenobarbital and primidone, can also increase the metabolism of ZNS (21). When ZNS is used in combination with known CYP3A inducers, ZNS doses may need to be increased to achieve seizure control. In the case of carbamazepine, care must be taken to determine if induction or inhibition is predominant in a given patient, with ZNS doses adjusted accordingly.

Influence of ZNS on Other Drugs

Studies with ZNS have shown that the agent does not induce or inhibit hepatic enzymes (48,49). It appears that ZNS does not cause any clinically significant alteration in the pharmacokinetic disposition of other drugs.

Drug-Food Interactions with Zonisamide

As a substrate for CYP3A4, ZNS is a candidate for drug-food interactions. Contained within the intestinal wall are high concentrations of CYP3A4 that can metabolize drugs before they are absorbed into systemic circulation. Several foods, particularly grapefruit juice, lime juice, and Seville orange juice, contain substances that inhibit the activity of intestinal CYP3A4. When these foods are consumed along with drugs that are metabolized by CYP3A4, there is increased absorption of the agent and a potential for adverse effects. Although this potential interaction with ZNS has not been documented, it should nonetheless be of concern. In a study of rectal ZNS administration, a route that bypasses intestinal CYP3A4, Nagatomi and colleagues consistently demonstrated increased bioavailability and absorption of the agent (22).

CLINICAL TRIALS

Clinical studies of ZNS have evaluated its use in several different types of epilepsy and epilepsy syndromes. ZNS has been used extensively in Japan and has gained increasing acceptance in much of the world elsewhere. Despite this history, there have been no direct comparisons of ZNS with other AEDs for the treatment of specific seizure types. The best published comparisons have been in two meta-analyses of clinical trials of new AEDs, including ZNS (50,51). In the first study, Marson and colleagues evaluated the odds ratio of ZNS producing a ≥50% reduction in seizure frequency compared with placebo (50). Combining data from two clinical trials, ZNS was shown to be significantly better than placebo in controlling seizures. Additionally, significantly more patients receiving ZNS stopped taking the drug compared with those treated with placebo. A comparison of ZNS with gabapentin, lamotrigine, tiagabine, topiramate, and vigabatrin failed to demonstrate any statistically significant differences among these agents. In a second meta-analysis, Marson and colleagues identified the five most common adverse effects experienced by patients treated with ZNS and showed no difference in comparison to other AED (51). This type of analysis shows that the efficacy of ZNS is equivalent to that of the other new AEDs for the treatment of seizures. However, these meta-analyses are not very helpful in determining the specific place in therapy for ZNS.

Focal-Onset Epilepsies/Partial Seizures

The earliest clinical trials in the United States and Europe of ZNS for the treatment of partial seizures were published in 1985. In an open trial of ZNS in 10 patients with refractory partial epilepsy, all but one patient had a 50% or more reduction in seizure frequency (32). ZNS doses in this study were adjusted to maintain average steady-state concentrations of 17.5 μg/mL and ranged from 3.44 to 20 mg/kg per day, administered in two divided doses. A second pilot study by Wilensky and colleagues was conducted in eight patients with refractory epilepsy (33). ZNS doses ranged from 400 to 1200 mg per day, with a mean of 475 mg per day. Patients had to be receiving phenytoin monotherapy and were then given ZNS or carbamazepine in a crossover

design. Five of the eight patients experienced improved control of their seizures compared with phenytoin monotherapy. Of these, two patients had a better response with ZNS than with phenytoin or carbamazepine; two had a better response with ZNS compared with phenytoin, but not compared with carbamazepine; and one patient had a better response with ZNS than with the other agents, but had to discontinue treatment because of a severe allergic reaction. Sufficient evidence of ZNS efficacy from these studies prompted more extensive clinical investigation.

A multicenter, placebo-controlled, double-blind, parallel-group, add-on study in Europe showed ZNS to be more effective than placebo (52). ZNS doses were increased over 4 weeks to 6 mg/kg per day in 139 patients. Further increases, depending on response, could be made, to a maximum of 20 mg/kg per day or with a plasma concentration of 40 μg/mL. At the end of the study, the mean reduction in all seizures was 16%; the mean reduction in complex partial seizures was 16.4%. Mean doses of ZNS were 7.0 mg/kg at the end of the trial and did not differ between responders and nonresponders. Nearly 30% of patients treated with ZNS had a 50% or more reduction in seizure frequency, compared with 9.4% of patients receiving placebo.

Another similar study evaluated ZNS efficacy in 167 adults over a period of 3 months (53). ZNS doses were titrated upward based on individual tolerance and ranged from 50 to 1100 mg per day, with a median dose of 500 mg per day. Compared with baseline, statistically significant reductions in seizure frequency were observed at the end of each monthly interval. The median percent reduction in seizure frequency at the end of the study was 51.8%. Among study participants, 41% had a 50% or more reduction in seizure frequency and six became seizure free while taking zonisamide. When complex partial seizures were evaluated independently, the median overall reduction was 40.6% and 43.2% of the participants had a 50% or more reduction in seizure frequency. Generalized tonic-clonic seizures were also reduced significantly during ZNS therapy. Median doses and plasma concentrations of ZNS were similar between responders and nonresponders. At the end of the study, patients were able to continue in a long-term safety trial, with 113 individuals electing to remain on ZNS therapy. Of these, only 16 patients discontinued treatment because of a perceived lack of efficacy. Two thirds of the patients choosing to continue ZNS remained on the drug for 1 year from study initiation. This study demonstrates that ZNS has good efficacy in refractory partial epilepsy and may have a prolonged benefit to patients.

A third multicenter, double-blind study used a different approach to ZNS dosing (54). In this study, patients in the placebo group were crossed over to ZNS following 12 weeks of placebo treatment. Individuals who were randomized to receive ZNS were divided into two groups: a slow initial titration and a rapid initial titration of the active drug. The dose of all patients treated with ZNS was ultimately increased to 400 mg per day. Using an intention-to-treat analysis, the median reduction in seizures for all patients initially started on ZNS was 32.3%, compared with 5.6% with placebo. Significantly more individuals taking ZNS had a 50% or more or a ≥75% or more reduction in seizure frequency. Among those who were in the placebo group and crossed over to zonisamide, the median reduction in frequency of all seizures was 40.1% and in frequency of complex partial seizures was 55%, compared with the placebo seizure frequency. The slow titration schedule in one of the ZNS groups allowed for evaluation of efficacy at 100 mg per day and 200 mg per day. At these doses the median reduction in frequency of all seizures and responder rate was statistically significantly in favor of zonisamide. Results of this study indicate that ZNS is effective in the treatment of patients with refractory partial epilepsy and that efficacy can be demonstrated at doses as low as 100 mg per day (54).

A summary of Japanese studies using ZNS in pediatric patients with partial seizures estimated that 34% of children responded to the agent (42). However, many of the studies included in this evaluation were open-label and did not have well-defined study protocols.

Generalized Epilepsies

Formal studies of ZNS in adults with primary generalized epilepsies are lacking. Henry and colleagues reported on two cases of progressive myoclonic epilepsy in which ZNS use was associated with reduced seizure frequency and improved functioning. In a case series of patients with juvenile myoclonic epilepsy, ZNS was well tolerated and associated with reduced seizures compared with valproate (55). In these patients, a comparison of ZNS with lamotrigine, topiramate, or levetiracetam demonstrated that topiramate and ZNS appeared to provide better seizure control than the other two agents.

More extensive evaluation of ZNS in primary generalized epilepsies has been conducted in children. Several studies using ZNS for the treatment of West syndrome have been published. In an open-label trial of children with newly diagnosed infantile spasms, Suzuki and coworkers used ZNS doses of 3 to 10 mg/kg per day (39). Of the 11 infants from 11 hospitals enrolled in this study, four had complete seizure control and cessation of hypsarrhythmia with ZNS doses of 4 to 5 mg/kg per day. Kishi and colleagues reported on their experience with ZNS in three children with hypsarrhythmia (56). In this small group of patients, ZNS resulted in elimination of hypsarrhythmia and seizures. A larger study in 54 patients newly diagnosed with West syndrome was conducted the following year, in 2001 (40). ZNS doses ranged from 4 to 14 mg/kg per day, with a mean dose and serum concentration of 7.2 mg/kg per day and 15.3 μg/mL, respectively. Among the participants, 11 had complete elimination of seizures and hypsarrhythmia, seven had a 50% or more reduction in seizure frequency, and 14 of those

with cryptogenic West syndrome responded. Of those whom the authors categorized as not responding, four were transiently seizure free, six had less than 50% reduction in seizure frequency, and 33 had no change in seizure frequency. The 11 individuals in this study who had elimination of seizures and hypsarrhythmia were entered into a long-term follow-up study, in which their response during a follow-up period ranging from 24 to 79 months (mean duration, 53 months) was evaluated (57). Seven of the infants who experienced an initial cessation of seizures continued to be seizure free. The presence of epileptiform activity on the electroencephalogram at the end of 3 weeks was predictive of seizure recurrence.

Although case series reports and open-label studies suggest that ZNS may be effective in patients with generalized epilepsies, the agent has not been well studied in this population. The most extensive information on ZNS use in generalized epilepsies is in children with West syndrome, with data suggesting that the agent may be a useful alternative for infants with this disorder. For other types of generalized epilepsies, ZNS may prove to be a useful alternative as well.

Monotherapy

Few clinical trials have evaluated the use of ZNS as monotherapy for the treatment of epilepsy. The most extensive studies have been conducted in children with West syndrome (39,57). Kumagai and colleagues studied ZNS monotherapy in 44 children with epilepsy (58). In this open-label trial, 30 children with various seizure types became seizure free, with six children discontinuing treatment because of adverse effects.

There is a paucity of data available on adults with epilepsy. The only published study of ZNS monotherapy was conducted by Wilensky and colleagues (33). In this study, eight adults with partial seizures who were receiving phenytoin were randomized to carbamazepine or zonisamide, then crossed over in an open-label design. Two subjects had improved seizure control with ZNS versus carbamazepine; a third individual experienced a similar response but had to discontinue treatment because of the development of Stevens-Johnson syndrome.

The limited available data on ZNS monotherapy indicate its possible effectiveness as a single agent for epilepsy. However, larger, double-blind clinical trials must be conducted before ZNS monotherapy can be recommended.

Nonepilepsy Indications

Preliminary clinical trials of ZNS in disorders other than epilepsy indicate that the agent may be effective for other indications. One study of ZNS in patients with mania and acute psychotic conditions demonstrated that 71% of subjects responded at least moderately to treatment (59). In an open-label trial of ZNS in 35 patients with neuropathic pain, mean pain scores showed little or no improvement after 8 weeks of therapy (60). In a trial of nine patients with Parkinson disease, seven of the participants showed improvement in their symptoms, especially wearing-off phenomena, when ZNS was added to their other medications (61).

ADVERSE EFFECTS

Common Adverse Effects

Several adverse effects were commonly reported (Table 62.4) in the initial and major clinical trials of ZNS (32,33,52–54). Schmidt and colleagues statistically evaluated the adverse events associated with ZNS as add-on treatment for patients with refractory partial epilepsy (52). Dizziness, somnolence, anorexia, abnormal thinking, ataxia, and confusion were more common with ZNS than with placebo. A meta-analysis that calculated the odds ratios of adverse events reported in clinical trials showed that patients taking ZNS were more likely to experience anorexia, ataxia, dizziness, and fatigue compared with those receiving placebo (51). When evaluating the reports of zonisamide-associated adverse effects, one must keep in mind that patients were receiving other AEDs, and it is not possible to entirely determine which adverse events are only caused by ZNS and which are caused by ZNS in combination with other AEDs. However, these adverse events and their frequency are similar to those reported with other, newer AEDs.

Adverse events in children appear to be similar to those in adults. The adverse events that are reported in more than 10% of children taking ZNS in combination with other AEDs include somnolence, anorexia, ataxia, fatigue, dizziness, cognitive impairment, irritability, and exanthema (42). ZNS monotherapy has been studied more extensively in children than in adults. When ZNS is used alone in children, the only adverse effect that occurs in >10% of individuals is somnolence (42). Thus, commonly reported adverse events, especially in children, may be limited by decreasing or eliminating other AEDs.

Anorexia was a commonly observed adverse event in the clinical trials. In some of these studies, this translated into a definite weight loss for many of the patients. Faught and colleagues evaluated this effect and demonstrated that significantly more patients taking ZNS (21.6%) lost more than 5 lb compared with those on placebo (54). A retrospective analysis of patients from European and American clinical trials (52–54) showed that 28.9% of individuals treated with ZNS lost more than 5 lb, compared with 8.4% of those receiving placebo—a significant difference (62). The mean weight loss for all patients taking ZNS was 4.3 lb.

These findings have prompted investigations into whether ZNS can be used to promote weight loss in individuals who are obese but not epileptic. In a double-blind, placebo-controlled study of 60 obese patients, those treated with ZNS had a mean weight loss of 9.2 kg, compared with 1.5 kg in those receiving placebo (63). This was a statistically significant difference in favor of zonisamide. A second study compared diet alone with diet plus ZNS in obese women (64). Women who took ZNS had an additional 5-lb weight loss compared with those on a diet alone.

ZNS appears to be associated with a mild to moderate weight loss. Patients who are obese or have experienced weight gain associated with the use of other AEDs may benefit from the addition of ZNS to their regimen.

Rare Adverse Effects

Early in the clinical trials of zonisamide, the formation of renal calculi was observed in some patients (53). Of the 113 patients studied by Leppik and associates, four developed kidney stones and were withdrawn. Kubota and coworkers reported three cases of nephrolithiasis in patients receiving ZNS (65), and Miyamoto and colleagues reported the case of a 10-year-old girl who developed a kidney stone after beginning ZNS therapy (66). The precise mechanism for this adverse effect has not been determined. Some have speculated that renal calculi formation is related to inhibition of carbonic anhydrase by zonisamide. However, ZNS is an extremely weak carbonic anhydrase inhibitor (65). It is important to note that all published reports on the development of renal calculi with ZNS are in patients who were taking other AEDs as well. ZNS is not contraindicated in patients with a history of kidney stones, but care should be taken when the agent is administered to these individuals. Prudent management of patients taking ZNS should include adequate hydration to maintain good urine flow.

Allergic reactions to ZNS are rare but did occur in clinical trials. Rash was the predominant allergic-type reaction

TABLE 62.4

MOST FREQUENTLY REPORTED ADVERSE EFFECTS IN CLINICAL TRIALS

Adverse Event	Percent Reporting (Range)
Fatigue	3.3%–22.5%
Ataxia	3.3%–11.3%
Nausea/vomiting	4.2%–15%
Headache	5%–15.9%
Somnolence	5.2%–18.3%
Rhinitis	5.2%–14.4%
Confusion	5.6%–10.6%
Anorexia	6.7%–15%
Dizziness	6.9%–16.9%
Nervousness	8.8%–9.9%
Abnormal thinking	9.7%–11.3%

Data from refs 32, 33, 52–54.

reported, with at least four individuals (one with Stevens-Johnson syndrome) in these studies being discontinued because of dermatologic reactions. A mild, relative neutropenia was also observed in several individuals. Because ZNS is chemically related to sulfonamide drugs, caution should be taken when using ZNS in patients with a prior allergic reaction to these agents. The exact cross-reactivity in patients known to be allergic to sulfonamides has not been determined.

Oligohidrosis is a recently recognized adverse effect of zonisamide. This side effect is marked by decreased sweating and hyperthermia. Postmarketing surveillance indicates that oligohidrosis occurs primarily in children, with all reported cases in individuals 18 years of age or younger. The estimated rate of incidence is approximately 12 cases per 10000 patient-years (67). When ZNS is used in children, parents should be instructed to carefully monitor for decreased sweating and increased body temperature. Children taking ZNS should not be exposed to extreme heat for prolonged periods.

Cognitive and behavioral effects of AEDs have received increasing attention. The cognitive effects of ZNS were examined early in its development. Berent and colleagues studied 11 patients who were on stable regimens of two to three other AEDs (68). Following a single-dose pharmacokinetic analysis, ZNS doses were calculated to maintain plasma concentrations of 15 to 40 μg/mL. A battery of neuropsychological tests was administered prior to starting and after 12 weeks of ZNS therapy. When plasma concentrations of ZNS were >30 μg/mL, the acquisition and consolidation of new information, especially verbal learning, was impaired. Miyamoto and associates reviewed 74 reported cases of psychosis associated with ZNS use between March 1984 and June 1994 (69). In their assessment, only 14 of the patients exhibited symptoms indicative of true psychosis. There were significantly more men than women, and this group was younger than the general population of patients with epilepsy. In a prospective clinical trial of ZNS monotherapy, Hirai and colleagues reported on 27 children, two of whom displayed behavioral disturbances (70). One child presented with selective mutism and the other developed obsessive-compulsive disorder. As with other AEDs, ZNS may alter cognition and behavior in some individuals. It is difficult to truly assess the incidence of these effects, however, because none of the reports accounted for the number of individuals taking zonisamide. Additionally, most of the cognitive or behavioral problems were reported in patients taking multiple AEDs.

Few data are available on the teratogenic effects of zonisamide. Kondo and colleagues surveyed 381 hospitals in Japan during June 1989 with respect to pregnancies in women using AEDs (71). Only two women exposed to ZNS during pregnancy bore children with major malformations. In both of these cases, multiple AEDs had been taken by the mothers. The authors concluded that ZNS is associated with no greater risk for teratogenicity than other AEDs.

SUMMARY

Clinical studies have proven the effectiveness of ZNS as adjunctive therapy for patients with partial seizures. These data are supported by more than a decade of use in Japan as an AED. In this experience, ZNS has been used in a variety of age-groups, seizure types, and as monotherapy. However, clinical study data outside of the primary indication are lacking. Anecdotal evidence hints that ZNS may have broad utility as an AED in both children and adults. The adverse effect and pharmacokinetic profiles of the agent are favorable, with few severe adverse effects reported and a long half-life that allows once-daily dosing.

ZNS should be considered an alternative adjunctive agent when typical AEDs have failed in the treatment of partial seizures. The agent may also be useful in patients with other seizure types and as monotherapy. Individuals who are concerned about weight gain or desire to lose weight may benefit from ZNS therapy. Care should be exercised when using ZNS in patients with a history of renal calculi and true sulfa allergies. However, these conditions do not constitute absolute contraindications to ZNS use. ZNS has been used safely and effectively in pediatric patients, but children need to be monitored carefully for oligohidrosis. Additional clinical experience and research will help to better define the role of ZNS in the management of patients with epilepsy.

REFERENCES

1. Suzuki S, Kawakami K, Nishimura S, et al. ZNS blocks T-type calcium channel in cultured neurons of rat cerebral cortex. *Epilepsy Res* 1992;12:21–27.
2. Rock DM, Macdonald RL, Taylor CP. Blockade of sustained repetitive action potentials in cultured spinal cord neurons by ZNS (AD 810, CI 912), a novel anticonvulsant. *Epilepsy Res* 1989;3:138–143.
3. Schauf CL. ZNS enhances slow sodium inactivation in Myxicola. *Brain Res* 1987;413:185–188.
4. Okada M, Kaneko S, Hirano T, et al. Effects of ZNS on dopaminergic system. *Epilepsy Res* 1995;22:193–205.
5. Okada M, Kawata Y, Mizuno K, et al. Interaction between Ca2+, K+, carbamazepine and ZNS on hippocampal extracellular glutamate monitored with a microdialysis electrode. *Br J Pharmacol* 1998;124:1277–1285.
6. Okada M, Kaneko S, Hirano T, et al. Effects of ZNS on extracellular levels of monoamine and its metabolite, and on Ca2+ dependent dopamine release. *Epilepsy Res* 1992;13:113–119.
7. Murakami T, Okada M, Kawata Y, et al. Determination of effects of antiepileptic drugs on SNAREs-mediated hippocampal monoamine release using in vivo microdialysis. *Br J Pharmacol* 2001,134:507–520.
8. Tokumaru J, Ueda Y, Yokoyama H, et al. In vivo evaluation of hippocampal antioxidant ability of ZNS in rats. *Neurochem Res* 2000;25:1107–1111.
9. Fromm GH, Shibuya T, Terrence CF. Effect of ZNS (CI-912) on a synaptic system model. *Epilepsia* 1987;28:673–679.
10. Wada Y, Hasegawa H, Yamaguchi N. Effect of a novel anticonvulsant, ZNS (AD-810, CI-912), in an experimental model of photosensitive epilepsy. *Epilepsy Res* 1990;7:117–120.
11. Masuda Y, Karasawa T, Shiraishi Y, et al. 3-Sulphamoylmethyl-1,2-benzisoxazole, a new type of anticonvulsant drug. Pharmacological profile. *Arzneimittelforschung* 1980;30:477–483.

12. Ito T, Hori M, Masuda Y, et al. 3-Sulfamoylmethyl-1,2-benzisoxazole, a new type of anticonvulsant drug: electroencephalographic profile. *Arzneimittelforschung* 1980;30:603–609.

13. Hamada K, Ishida S, Yagi K, Seino M. Anticonvulsant effects of ZNS on amygdaloid kindling in rats. *Neuroscience* 1990;16:407–412.

14. Kakegawa N. An experimental study on the modes of appearance and disappearance of suppressive effect of antiepileptic drugs on kindled seizure. *Psychiatria et Neurologia Japonica* 1986;88:81–98.

15. Takano K, Tanaka T, Fujita T, et al. Zonisamide: electrophysiological and metabolic changes in kainic acid-induced limbic seizures in rats. *Epilepsia* 1995;36:644–648.

16. Araki H, Kobayashi Y, Hashimoto Y, et al. Characteristics of flurothyl-induced seizures and the effect of antiepileptic drugs on flurothyl-induced seizures in Mongolian gerbils. *Pharmacol Biochem Behav* 2002;74:141–147.

17. Gasior M, Ungard JT, Witkin JM. Preclinical evaluation of newly approved and potential antiepileptic drugs against cocaine-induced seizures. *J Pharmacol Exp Ther* 1999;290:1148–1156.

18. Mimaki T, Tanoue H, Matsunaga Y, et al. Regional distribution of 14C-ZNS in rat brain. *Epilepsy Res* 1994;17:233–236.

19. Akaike K, Tanaka S, Tojo H, et al. Regional accumulation of 14C-ZNS in rat brain during kainic acid-induced limbic seizures. *Can J Neurol Sci* 2001;28:341–345.

20. Minato H, Kikuta C, Fujitani B, et al. Protective effect of zonisamide, an antiepileptic drug, against transient focal cerebral ischemia with middle cerebral artery occlusion-reperfusion in rats. *Epilepsia* 1997;38:975–980.

21. Perucca E, Bialer M. The clinical pharmacokinetics of the newer antiepileptic drugs. Focus on topiramate, ZNS and tiagabine. *Clin Pharmacokinet* 1996;31:29–46.

22. Nagatomi A, Mishima M, Tsuzuki O, et al. Utility of a rectal suppository containing the antiepileptic drug zonisamide. *Biol Pharm Bull* 1997;20:892–896.

23. Nakasa H, Komiya M, Ohmori S, et al. Rat liver microsomal cytochrome P-450 responsible for reductive metabolism of zonisamide. *Drug Metab Dispos* 1993;21:777–781.

24. Taylor CP, McLean JR, Bockrader HN, et al. Zonisamide. In: Meldrum BS, Porter RJ, eds. *New Anticonvulsant Drugs*. London: John Libbey; 1986:277–294.

25. Nishiguchi K, Ohnishi N, Iwakawa S, et al. Pharmacokinetics of zonisamide; saturable distribution into human and rat erythrocytes and into rat brain. *J Pharmacobiodyn* 1992;15:409–415.

26. Matsumoto K, Miyazaki H, Fujii T, et al. Binding of sulfonamides to erythrocyte proteins and possible drug-drug interaction. *Chem Pharm Bull (Tokyo)* 1989;37:2807–2810.

27. Matsumoto K, Miyazaki H, Fujii T, Hashimoto M. Binding of sulfonamides to erythrocytes and their components. *Chem Pharm Bull (Tokyo)* 1989;37:1913–1915.

28. Kimura M, Tanaka N, Kimura Y, et al. Factors influencing serum concentration of ZNS in epileptic patients. *Chem Pharm Bull (Tokyo)* 1992;40:193–195.

29. Kochak GM, Page JG, Buchanan RA, et al. Steady-state pharmacokinetics of zonisamide, an antiepileptic agent for treatment of refractory complex partial seizures. *J Clin Pharmacol* 1998;38:166–171.

30. Walker MC, Patsalos PN. Clinical pharmacokinetics of new antiepileptic drugs. *Pharmacol Ther* 1995;67:351–384.

31. Wagner JG, Sackellares JC, Donofrio PD, et al. Nonlinear pharmacokinetics of CI-912 in adult epileptic patients. *Ther Drug Monit* 1984;6:277–283.

32. Sackellares JC, Donofrio PD, Wagner JG, et al. Pilot study of ZNS (1,2-benzisoxazole-3-methanesulfonamide) in patients with refractory partial seizures. *Epilepsia* 1985;26:206–211.

33. Wilensky AJ, Friel PJ, Ojemann LM, et al. ZNS in epilepsy: a pilot study. *Epilepsia* 1985;26:212–220.

34. Hashimoto Y, Odani A, Tanigawara Y, et al. Population analysis of the dose-dependent pharmacokinetics of ZNS in epileptic patients. *Biol Pharm Bull* 1994;17:323–326.

35. Nakasa H, Komiya M, Ohmori S, et al. Characterization of human liver microsomal cytochrome P450 involved in the reductive metabolism of zonisamide. *Mol Pharmacol* 1993;44:216–221.

36. Stiff DD, Robicheau T, Zemaitis MA. Reductive metabolism of the anticonvulsant agent zonisamide, a 1,2-benzisoxazole derivative. *Xenobiotica* 1992;22:1–11.

37. Nakasa H, Nakamura H, Ono S, et al. Prediction of drug-drug interactions of ZNS metabolism in humans from in vitro data. *Eur J Clin Pharmacol* 1998;54:177–183.

38. Zonegran [package insert]. South San Francisco, Calif: Elan Pharmaceuticals, 2003.

39. Suzuki Y, Nagai T, Ono J, et al. ZNS monotherapy in newly diagnosed infantile spasms. *Epilepsia* 1997;38:1035–1038.

40. Suzuki Y. ZNS in West syndrome. *Brain Dev* 2001;23:658–661.

41. Odani A, Hashimoto Y, Takayanagi K, et al. Population pharmacokinetics of phenytoin in Japanese patients with epilepsy: analysis with a dose-dependent clearance model. *Biol Pharm Bull* 1996;19:444–448.

42. Glauser TA, Pellock JM. ZNS in pediatric epilepsy: review of the Japanese experience. *J Child Neurol* 2002;17:87–96.

43. Kawada K, Itoh S, Kusaka T, et al. Pharmacokinetics of ZNS in perinatal period. *Brain Dev* 2002;24:95–97.

44. Shimoyama R, Ohkubo T, Sugawara K. Monitoring of ZNS in human breast milk and maternal plasma by solid-phase extraction HPLC method. *Biomed Chromatogr* 1999;13:370–372.

45. Schentag JJ, Gengo FM, Wilton JH, et al. Influence of phenobarbital, cimetidine, and renal disease on ZNS kinetics. *Pharm Res* 1987;[NPE1](Suppl):S79.

46. Ojemann LM, Shastri RA, Wilensky AJ, et al. Comparative pharmacokinetics of ZNS (CI-912) in epileptic patients on carbamazepine or phenytoin monotherapy. *Ther Drug Monit* 1986;8:293–296.

47. Shinoda M, Akita M, Hasegawa M, et al. The necessity of adjusting the dosage of ZNS when coadministered with other antiepileptic drugs. *Biol Pharm Bull* 1996;19:1090–1092.

48. Mather G, Carlson S, Trager EF, et al. Prediction of ZNS interactions based on metabolic enzymes. *Epilepsia* 1997;38(Suppl 8):108.

49. Hachad H, Ragueneau-Majlessi I, Levy RH. New antiepileptic drugs: review on drug interactions. *Ther Drug Monit* 2002;24:91–103.

50. Marson AG, Kadir ZA, Chadwick DM. New antiepileptic drugs: a systematic review of their efficacy and tolerability. *BMJ* 1996;313:1169–1174.

51. Marson AG, Kadir ZA, Hutton JL, et al. The new antiepileptic drugs: a systematic review of their efficacy and tolerability. *Epilepsia* 1997;38:859–880.

52. Schmidt D, Jacob R, Loiseau P, et al. ZNS for add-on treatment of refractory partial epilepsy: a European double-blind trial. *Epilepsy Res* 1993;15:67–73.

53. Leppik IE, Wilmore LJ, Homan RW, et al. Efficacy and safety of zonisamide: results of a multicenter study. *Epilepsy Res* 1993;14:165–173.

54. Faught E, Ayala R, Montouris GG, et al. Randomized controlled trial of ZNS for the treatment of refractory partial-onset seizures. *Neurology* 2001;57:1774–1779.

55. Welty TE, Martin JN, Faught E, et al. Comparison of outcomes in patients with juvenile myoclonic epilepsy treated with lamotrigine, topiramate, zonisamide, or levetiracetam. *Epilepsia* 2002;43(Suppl 7):239.

56. Kishi T, Nejihashi Y, Kajiyama M, Ueda K. Successful ZNS treatment for infants with hypsarrhythmia. *Pediatr Neurol* 2000;23:274–277.

57. Suzuki Y, Imai K, Toribe Y, et al. Long-term response to ZNS in patients with West syndrome. *Neurology* 2002;58:1556–1559.

58. Kumagai N, Seki T, Yamawaki H, et al. Monotherapy for childhood epilepsies with zonisamide. *Jpn J Psychiatry Neurol* 1991;45:357–359.

59. Kanba S, Yagi G, Kamijima K, et al. The first open study of zonisamide, a novel anticonvulsant, shows efficacy in mania. *Prog Neuropsychopharmacol Biol Psychiatry* 1994;18:707–715.

60. Backonja MM. Use of anticonvulsants for treatment of neuropathic pain. *Neurology* 2002;59(5 Suppl 2):S14–S17.

61. Murata M, Horiuchi E, Kanazawa I. ZNS has beneficial effects on Parkinson's disease patients. *Neurosci Res* 2001;41:397–399.

62. Welty TE, Kuzniecky RI, Limdi N, Faught E. Weight loss associated with use of ZNS in European and US clinical trials. *Epilepsia* 2001;42(Suppl 7):262.

63. Gadde KM, Franciscy DM, Wagner HR 2nd, Krishnan KR. ZNS for weight loss in obese adults: a randomized controlled trial. *JAMA* 2003;289:1820–1825.

64. Kim CS. ZNS effective for weight loss in women. *J Fam Pract* 2003;52:600–601.
65. Kubota M, Nishi-Nagase M, Sakakihara Y, et al. Zonisamide-induced urinary lithiasis in patients with intractable epilepsy. *Brain Dev* 2000;22:230–233.
66. Miyamoto A, Sugai R, Okamoto T, et al. Urine stone formation during treatment with zonisamide. *Brain Dev* 2000;22:460.
67. O'Brien C. Important Drug Warning. H. Professionals, editor. 2002, Elan Pharmaceuticals.
68. Berent S, Sackellares JC, Giordani B, et al. ZNS (CI-912) and cognition: results from preliminary study. *Epilepsia* 1987;28:61–67.
69. Miyamoto T, Kohsaka M, Koyama T. Psychotic episodes during ZNS treatment. *Seizure* 2000;9:65–70.
70. Hirai K, Kimiya S, Tabata K, et al. Selective mutism and obsessive compulsive disorders associated with zonisamide. *Seizure* 2002;11:468–470.
71. Kondo T, Kaneko S, Amano Y, et al. Preliminary report on teratogenic effects of ZNS in the offspring of treated women with epilepsy. *Epilepsia* 1996;37:1242–1244.
72. Yagi K, Seino M. Methodological requirements for clinical trials in refractory epilepsies: our experience with zonisamide. In: *Symposium on Advances in Basic Research and Treatment of Refractory Epilepsy.* Kyoto, Japan: Dainippon Pharmaceutical Company Limited; 1990.

Levetiracetam

63

Joseph I. Sirven   *Joseph F. Drazkowski*

Levetiracetam (LEV) is a novel antiepileptic drug (AED) approved in 2000 by the US Food and Drug Administration as adjunctive therapy for patients with partial epilepsy. The compound was developed as a derivative of the nosotropic agent piracetam, with a wide spectrum of anticonvulsant effects in animal models of various types of epileptic seizures (1). It is chemically unrelated to existing AEDs. In addition to its unique chemical structure, LEV has a distinct mechanism of action and a favorable pharmacokinetic and safety profile, making it an attractive therapy for seizure management.

CHEMISTRY

LEV is a single enantiomer (-)-(S)-α-ethyl-2-oxo-1-pyrrolidine acetamide with a molecular weight of 170.21 (1,2). The structural formula of the agent is shown in Figure 63.1. The drug is a white to off-white crystalline powder with a faint odor and bitter taste. It is very soluble in water (104.0 g/100 mL), freely soluble in chloroform and in methanol, and soluble in ethanol. It is much less soluble to insoluble in acetonitrile and n-hexane. Keppra* (the only brand name of this compound) tablets contain LEV and the inactive ingredients silicon dioxide, cornstarch, methylcellulose, magnesium stearate, polyethylene glycol 4000, and coloring agents. LEV is supplied as 250-mg (blue), 500-mg (yellow), and 750-mg (orange) tablets (2). Currently, an oral suspension is undergoing clinical investigation for approval in the United States.

MECHANISM OF ACTION

Prior to undergoing standardized AED testing by the National Institutes of Health, LEV was found to have

---

*Keppra is a registered trademark of UCB Pharma, Inc.

antiepileptic properties. In contrast to all approved AEDs, LEV lacked conventional modulation of the acute seizure model (maximum electroshock seizure [MES] test and pentylenetetrazol [PTZ]), suggesting a novel mechanism of action (3–5). Moreover, LEV displays unique potent protection against kindled seizures in both mice and rats during kindling models (3,4). In comparative tests with established AEDs in a number of animal models of epileptic seizures, LEV displays potent protection in a broad range of animal models of chronic epilepsy, including partial and primary generalized seizures (5).

The precise mechanism by which LEV exerts its AED effect is unknown. It does not appear to derive its function from known mechanisms involved in inhibitory and excitatory neurotransmission, but it may be active at a brain-specific binding site (6). A stereoselective binding site for LEV has been shown to exist exclusively in membranes from cells in the central nervous system (CNS), but not in peripheral tissue (3,6). There is no significant displacement ($\leq$10 mM) of ligands specific for 55 different binding sites. Established AEDs, such as carbamazepine, phenytoin, valproate, phenobarbital, and clonazepam, do not possess an affinity for this binding site (6).

In studies performed to demonstrate the cellular pharmacodynamics of LEV, the agent reduces calcium current through neuron-specific, high-voltage–activated N-type calcium channels, thus reducing seizure potential (7). It does not modulate neuronal voltage-gated sodium, T-type calcium currents, or glutamate receptor-mediated neurotransmission in the spinal cord, nor does it have any conventional effects at the gamma-aminobutyric acid (GABA)a receptors (7). However, LEV does promote inhibitory neurotransmission by reducing negative allosteric effects of zinc and the beta-carbolines on GABAa and glycine receptors (8). *In vitro* and *in vivo* recordings of epileptiform activity from the hippocampus have shown that LEV inhibits burst firing without affecting normal neuronal excitability, suggesting selective suppression of hypersynchronization

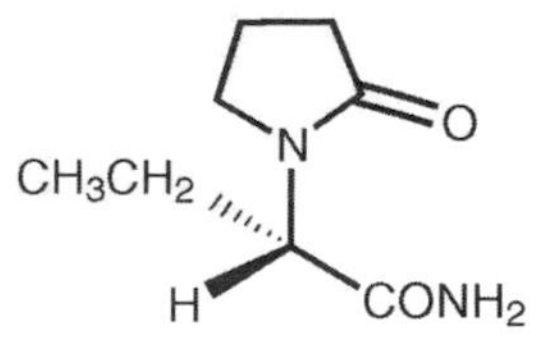

Figure 63.1 The chemical structure of levetiracetam.

of epileptiform burst firing and propagation of seizure activity (9). The only certainty regarding the mechanism of action is that further investigation is warranted to elucidate the ways in which LEV exerts its selective effects.

ABSORPTION, DISTRIBUTION, AND METABOLISM

Overview

LEV is rapidly and almost completely absorbed following oral administration. The pharmacokinetics are linear and time invariant, with low individual variability (10). LEV is not protein-bound (less than 10%), and its volume of distribution is close to the volume of intracellular and extracellular water (10,11). Sixty-six percent of the dose is unchanged as it is excreted renally (10). The major metabolic profile of LEV is an enzymatic hydrolysis of the acetamide group (10,11). LEV is not liver cytochrome P450–dependent (10). Its metabolites have no known pharmacologic activity and are renally excreted. The plasma half-life of LEV across studies is approximately 6 to 8 hours. The effects of the agent are increased in the elderly (primarily due to impaired renal clearance) and in patients with renal impairment (10,11).

Absorption and Distribution

Absorption of LEV is rapid, with peak plasma concentrations occurring about 1 hour following oral administration. Oral bioavailability is 100%, with no effect from ingestion of food. Linear pharmacokinetics characterize LEV over a dose range of 500 to 5000 mg. Steady state is achieved after 2 days of multiple twice-daily dosing. LEV is less than 10% bound to plasma proteins; clinically significant interactions with other drugs through competition for protein-binding sites are unlikely (10,11).

Metabolism and Elimination

LEV is not extensively metabolized in humans with the major metabolic pathway of enzymatic hydrolysis of the acetamide group, which produces the pharmacologically inactive carboxylic acid metabolite. There is no dependency on P450 cytochrome liver metabolism (10,11).

LEV is eliminated by renal excretion as unchanged drug, which represents 66% of the administered dose (10). The total body clearance is 0.96 mL/min/kg and the renal clearance is 0.6 mL/min/kg (10,11). The mechanism of excretion is glomerular filtration with subsequent partial tubular reabsorption. Elimination is correlated with creatinine clearance (10).

Special Populations

Pediatrics

The pharmacokinetics of LEV have been evaluated in children 6 to 12 years of age following single 20-mg/kg doses. The apparent clearance of LEV was approximately 40% higher in children than in adults. The half-life in children is 4 to 8 hours, compared with approximately 7 hours in adults. The maximum concentration of drug (C_{max}) and area under the curve (AUC) values are comparable to those in adults. There is no correlation between age and gender among pediatric patients (11).

Elderly

In older adults, total body clearance decreased by 38%, and the half-life was 2.5 hours longer compared with healthy adults (10).

Renal Impairment

Total body clearance of LEV is reduced in patients with impaired renal function by 40% in those with mild renal impairment (creatinine clearance [CrCl] 50 to 80 mL per minute), 50% in those with moderate impairment (CrCl 30 to 50 mL per minute), and 60% in those with severe renal impairment (CrCl <30 mL per minute). In patients with end-stage renal disease, total body clearance decreased by 70% compared with those with normal renal function. About 50% of LEV is removed during a standard 4-hour hemodialysis procedure. Thus, dosage should be reduced in patients with impaired renal function and supplemental doses should be given after hemodialysis (10).

Hepatic Impairment

The pharmacokinetics of LEV are unchanged in individuals with hepatic impairment. No dose adjustment is needed in patients with hepatic impairment (10).

DRUG INTERACTIONS

In vitro data on metabolic interactions indicate that LEV is unlikely to produce or be affected by pharmacokinetic interactions. Minimal plasma protein binding makes interactions due to competition for protein binding sites unlikely (12). Potential pharmacokinetic interactions were assessed, but none were reported in clinical pharmacokinetic studies with phenytoin, warfarin, digoxin, and oral contraceptives (13–16). Phase 3 studies also revealed no known interactions with other AEDs, such as phenytoin, carbamazepine, valproic acid, and phenobarbital (13).

EFFICACY

Partial-Onset Seizures

The effectiveness of LEV as adjunctive therapy in adults was established in three multicenter, randomized, double-blind, placebo-controlled clinical trials in patients with refractory partial-onset seizures with or without secondary generalization (17–19). Patients (N = 904) were randomized to one of four treatment arms: placebo, LEV 1000 mg, LEV 2000 mg, or LEV 3000 mg per day. Responder rates (50% or more reduction in seizure frequency compared with baseline) of 37.1% and 20.8%, respectively, were reported for 1000-mg per day doses for studies 1 and 2. At 2000 mg per day, a responder rate of 35.2% was reported; responder rates of 39.6% and 39.4%, respectively, were noted for 3000 mg per day (17–19). All of the response rates were statistically significant when all three LEV treatment arms were compared with placebo. Complete seizure freedom was reported to be 2% at 1000 mg and 6.7% at 3000 mg per day (17–19).

An interesting finding in study 1 was the rapid onset of efficacy of LEV (17). A significant reduction in weekly seizure frequency compared with that of the baseline period was observed during the first 2 weeks of the titration period, indicating that the agent has a rapid clinical effect at an initial dose (17). Open-label community trials confirmed the results noted in the pivotal trials, with efficacy achieved in patients at a dose of only 500 mg bid (20).

Four published studies have demonstrated the sustained efficacy of LEV as add-on epilepsy therapy for a period of at least 12 months and for as long as 54 months. The long-term tolerability of the agent is similar to that seen in the short-term, placebo-controlled trials (21–26).

Symptomatic and Idiopathic Generalized Epilepsy

An open-label trial using LEV as add-on therapy in individuals not eligible for clinical trials enrolled patients with various generalized seizure types. Twelve patients had symptomatic generalized epilepsy. One patient experienced an increase in seizures, seven had no response, and four were responders, with a 75% seizure reduction (22). Seven patients had idiopathic generalized seizures. Of these, four had refractory absence seizures with generalized tonic-clonic seizures, one had Baltic myoclonic epilepsy, one had juvenile myoclonic epilepsy, and one had Lafora body disease. The patients with progressive myoclonic epilepsy experienced a decrease in seizure frequency and myoclonic jerks. The patients with absence seizures and juvenile myoclonic epilepsy did not respond. Because of the small study size, more trials are needed to establish the efficacy of LEV in these conditions. Case reports have suggested that LEV may be beneficial for myoclonic jerks (22).

Monotherapy

Individuals with refractory partial epilepsy who completed a multicenter, double-blind, placebo-controlled, parallel-group with LEV 3000 mg per day were eligible for a monotherapy trial (19). Forty-nine patients entered the monotherapy arm. The median percent reduction in partial seizures was 73.8%, with a 50% responder rate of 59.2%. Nine patients (18.4%) remained seizure free on monotherapy (19).

Pediatrics

Two open-label trials have been conducted to assess the efficacy and safety of LEV in children with partial seizures (11,27). Twenty-three children 6 to 12 years of age with treatment-resistant partial-onset seizures who were receiving one standard AED were eligible (27). Seizure frequency in these children was evaluated and compared with a 4-week baseline seizure frequency, using a 6-week titration to a target dose of 40 mg/kg per day. Twelve children (52%) responded (50% seizure reduction), with two patients remaining seizure-free during the entire study period (27).

To date, no randomized, controlled trials have been completed in children. Open-label trials and case reports suggest that an initial lower dose and a slower dose escalation are helpful in children, with many responding to LEV doses of 1000 mg per day (11,27). Response rates at doses of 1000 mg per day are not very different from those at 2,000 mg or 3,000 mg per day. Shortly, a 10% oral grape-flavored solution (100 mg/mL) with an indication as an alternative formulation for adults with partial-onset epilepsy who have difficulty swallowing tablets will be available (Susan Peper, PharmD, UCB Pharma, personal communication). This will likely have utility both in the pediatric population and in patients who require feeding tubes.

ADVERSE EVENTS

Central Nervous System

Three main types of CNS adverse effects are associated with LEV use: fatigue, coordination difficulties, and behavioral problems (17–19,28). In the three pivotal clinical trials, 14.7% of patients reported fatigue, whereas 3.4% had coordination problems. Coordination difficulties included ataxia, abnormal gait, and incoordination. Dose reduction improved these symptoms. Fatigue and coordination problems occurred most frequently within the first 4 weeks of treatment. Of patients treated with LEV, 13% reported such behavioral symptoms as agitation, hostility, anxiety, apathy, emotional lability, depersonalization, and depression. Most of these symptoms occurred within 4 weeks of drug initiation (17–19). Dose reduction was associated with improvement in these behavioral problems, with only 0.8% of treated patients requiring hospitalization. In the

TABLE 63.1

ADVERSE EFFECTS OF LEVETIRACETAM: SYSTEMIC

Body System	Adverse Effects
Cardiac	No effect
Gastrointestinal	No significant effect
Hematologic	Minor decreases in hemoglobin, red blood cell count, and white blood cell (WBC) count
	No patients required treatment discontinuation because of these effects
Hepatic	No meaningful changes in liver function tests
Infectious	Pharyngitis, rhinitis with no relationship to WBC count
Pulmonary	No effect

open-label trial of children, there were no differences between adverse events reported in this population and those reported in adults (27).

Other Systemic Adverse Events

Table 63.1 illustrates systemic adverse effects that have been reported in clinical trials with LEV. The most frequently reported adverse events included asthenia, somnolence, and dizziness, which occurred predominantly during the first 4 weeks of treatment. In 15% of patients treated with LEV, somnolence was most often associated with discontinuation or dose reduction, followed by breakthrough seizures or dizziness (17–19).

Pregnancy

LEV is a pregnancy Category C drug, meaning that animal studies have produced evidence of developmental anomalies at doses similar to or greater than those used in humans (2). However, there are no adequate controlled studies of LEV in pregnant women. The effect of this drug on labor and delivery in humans is unknown. It is unclear whether LEV is excreted in human milk. Moreover, there is no impairment in male or female fertility (2,17–19).

CLINICAL USE

The recommended dosage of LEV is between 1000 and 3000 mg per day in two divided doses. Although in some studies there was a tendency toward greater response with higher doses, a consistent increase in response with increased dose has not been reported. Indeed, some older adults may respond to a dose as low as 500 mg per day (Susan Peper, PharmD, UCB Pharma, personal communication). Dosage should guide titration to clinical response.

LEV should be introduced gradually at 250 mg bid, in order to reduce the potential for side effects and to identify the minimum effective dose. Increases of 250 mg per day at 1- to 2-week intervals are recommended. If behavioral symptoms occur, reducing the dose may be beneficial. Although LEV has a rapid onset of effect, dose escalation that is too rapid could lead to adverse effects. A therapeutic dose range, in terms of concentration, has not been established for LEV. Dosage should be guided by clinical response. LEV may be ideally suited for individuals with seizures who are hepatically compromised or are taking multiple medications.

There are no clear guidelines established for dosing in patients younger than 16 years of age. However, open-label, postmarketing trials are attempting to fill this knowledge gap. Data from these trials suggest that children between the ages of 6 and 12 years may be initiated on a twice-daily oral regimen of 10 mg/kg per day, increased every 2 weeks by 10 mg/kg per day in divided doses up to a maximum of 40 mg/kg per day (27). In children younger than 2 years of age, initial doses of 10 mg/kg per day to 40 mg/kg per day, titrated every 2 weeks by 10 mg/kg per day to a maximal range between 15 mg/kg per day and 61 mg/kg per day, appear to be safe and well tolerated (29).

REFERENCES

1. Genton P, Van Vleyman BV. Piracetam and levetiracetam: close structural similarities but different pharmacological and clinical profiles. *Epileptic Disord* 2000;2:99–105.
2. *Physician's Desk Reference®*, 56th ed. Keppra. Montvale, New Jersey: Medical Economics, 2002.
3. Klitgaard H, Matagne A, Gobert J, et al. Evidence for a unique profile of levetiracetam in rodent models of seizures and epilepsy. *Eur J Pharmacol* 1998;353:191–206.
4. Loscher W, Honack D. Profile of ucb L059, a novel anticonvulsant drug, in models of partial and generalized epilepsy in mice and rats. *Eur J Pharmacol* 1993;232:147–158.
5. Gower AJ, Hirsch E, Boehrer A, et al. Effects of levetiracetam, a novel antiepileptic drug, on convulsant activity in two genetic rat models of epilepsy. *Epilepsy Res* 1995;22:207–213.
6. Noyer M, Gillard M, Matagne A, et al. The novel antiepileptic drug levetiracetam (ucb L059) appears to act via a specific binding site in CNS membranes. *Eur J Pharmacol* 1995;286:137–146.
7. Lukyanetz EA, Shkryl VM, Kostyuk PG. Selective blockade of N-type calcium channels by levetiracetam. *Epilepsia* 2002;43:9–18.

8. Rigo JM, Hans G, Nguyen L, et al. The anti-epileptic drug levetiracetam reverses the inhibition by negative allosteric modulators of neuronal GABA- and glycine-gated currents. *Br J Pharmacol* 2002;136:659–672.

9. Niespodziany I, Klitgaard H, Margineanu DG. Levetiracetam inhibits the high-voltage-activated Ca (2+) current in pyramidal neurones of rat hippocampal slices. *Neurosci Lett* 2001;306:5–8.

10. Patsalos PN. Pharmacokinetic profile of levetiracetam: toward ideal characteristics. *Pharmacol Ther* 2000;85:77–85.

11. Pellock JM, Glauser TA, Bebin EM, et al. Pharmacokinetic study of levetiracetam in children. *Epilepsia* 2001;42:1574–1579.

12. Nicolas JM, Collart P, Gerin B, et al. In vitro evaluation of potential drug interactions with levetiracetam, a new antiepileptic agent. *Drug Metab Dispos* 1999;27:250–254.

13. Perucca E, Gidal BE, Baltes E. Effects of antiepileptic comedication on levetiracetam pharmacokinetics: a pooled analysis of data from randomized adjunctive therapy trials. *Epilepsy Res* 2003;53:47–56.

14. Ragueneau-Majlessi I, Levy RH, Janik F. Levetiracetam does not alter the pharmacokinetics of an oral contraceptive in healthy women. *Epilepsia* 2002;43:697–702.

15. Levy RH, Ragueneau-Majlessi I, Baltes E. Repeated administration of the novel antiepileptic agent levetiracetam does not alter digoxin pharmacokinetics and pharmacodynamics in healthy volunteers. *Epilepsy Res* 2001;46:93–99.

16. Ragueneau-Majlessi I, Levy RH, Meyerhoff C. Lack of effect of repeated administration of levetiracetam on the pharmacodynamic and pharmacokinetic profiles of warfarin. *Epilepsy Res* 2001;47:55–63.

17. Cereghino JJ, Biton V, Abou-Khalil B, et al. Levetiracetam for partial seizures: results of a double-blind, randomized clinical trial. *Neurology* 2000;55:236–242.

18. Shorvon SD, Lowenthal A, Janz D, et al. Multicenter double-blind, randomized, placebo-controlled trial of levetiracetam as add-on therapy in patients with refractory partial seizures. *Epilepsia* 2000;4:1179–1186.

19. Ben-Menachem E, Falter U. Efficacy and tolerability of levetiracetam 3000 mg/d in patients with refractory partial seizures; a multicenter, double-blind, responder-selected study evaluating monotherapy. *Epilepsia* 2000;41:1276–1283.

20. Abou-Khalil B, Hemdal P, Privitera M. An open-label study of levetiracetam at individualised doses between 1000 and 3000 mg day (-1) in adult patients with refractory epilepsy. *Seizure* 2003;12:141–149.

21. Krakow K, Walker M, Otoul C, et al. Long-term continuation of levetiracetam in patients with refractory epilepsy. *Neurology* 2001;56:1772–1774.

22. Ben-Menachem E, Gilland E. Efficacy and tolerability of levetiracetam during 1-year follow-up in patients with refractory epilepsy. *Seizure* 2003;12:131–135.

23. Betts T, Waegemans T, Crawford P. A multicentre, double-blind, randomized parallel group study to evaluate the tolerability and efficacy of two oral doses of levetiracetam, 2000 mg daily and 4000 mg daily, without titration in patients with refractory epilepsy. *Seizure* 2000;9:80–87.

24. Grant R, Shorvon SD. Efficacy and tolerability of 1000-4000 mg per day of levetiracetam as add-on therapy in patients with refractory epilepsy. *Epilepsy Res* 2000;42:89–95.

25. Ben-Menachem E, Edrich P, Van Vleyman B, et al. Evidence for sustained efficacy of levetiracetam as add-on epilepsy therapy. *Epilepsy Res* 2003:53:57–64.

26. Betts T, Yarrow H, Greenhill L, et al. Clinical experience of marketed levetiracetam in an epilepsy clinic—a one year follow up study. *Seizure* 2003;12:136–140.

27. Glauser TA, Pellock JM, Bebin EM, et al. Efficacy and safety of levetiracetam in children with partial seizures: an open-label trial. *Epilepsia* 2002:43:518–524.

28. Harden C. Safety profile of levetiracetam. *Epilepsia* 2001:42 (Suppl 4):36–39.

29. Frost MD, Gustafson MC, Ritter FJ. Use of levetiracetam in children younger than 2 years [abstract]. *Epilepsia* 2002;43(Suppl 7):57.

Tiagabine

64

Steven C. Schachter

HISTORICAL BACKGROUND AND CHEMISTRY

Tiagabine (-)-(R)-1-[4,4-Bis(3-methyl-2-thienyl)-3-butenyl] nipecotic acid hydrochloride (TGB; Gabitril, Abbot Laboratories, Cephalon, Inc. West Chester, Pennsylvania) received regulatory clearance from the US Food and Drug Administration (FDA) for the adjunctive treatment of partial seizures in adults and children 12 years and older in October 1997. TGB was synthesized by using an aliphatic chain to link nipecotic acid to a lipophilic anchor (Fig. 64.1). Nipecotic acid is effective against seizures in animal models only when injected into the cerebral ventricles, because it does not cross the blood-brain barrier (BBB) (1). The lipophilic anchor allows the attached nipecotic acid to readily cross the BBB.

MECHANISM OF ACTION

TGB blocks the neuronal and glial reuptake of gamma-aminobutyric acid (GABA) after its release from postsynaptic GABA receptors, thereby enhancing GABA-mediated inhibition at central nervous system (CNS) sites (2,3). Accordingly, TGB suppresses hyperexcitability in the dentate gyrus and CA3 area in epileptic E1 mice (4).

TGB binds to the GABA uptake carrier GAT-1 in animals (5,6) and postmortem human brain tissue (7,8), but not to any other neurotransmitter uptake sites or receptors. TGB has no significant effect on sodium or calcium channels (5,9).

Animal Seizure Models

TGB reduces the severity and duration of convulsions in amygdala-kindled rats (5) and significantly retards kindling (10). In addition, TGB reduces maximal electroshock-induced seizures and bicuculline-induced seizures in rats (5), and picrotoxin-induced convulsions in mice (11). The agent partially protects against photically induced myoclonus in photosensitive baboons (5) and blocks audiogenic convulsions in genetically epilepsy-prone rats in a dose-dependent manner (12).

Efficacy in animal models of pain (13) and experimental cerebral ischemia (14–16) has also been described.

PHARMACOKINETICS

Absorption and Distribution

TGB is rapidly and almost completely absorbed (17). Oral bioavailability is approximately 90%, and the absorption of TGB is linear over the therapeutic dosage range. Maximum serum concentrations are attained within 45 to 90 minutes in the fasting state and after a mean of 2.6 hours when taken with food (9). The extent of TGB absorption is not affected by food.

Metabolism and Elimination

Extensive oxidation of TGB occurs in the liver via isoform 3A of the cytochrome P450 (CYP450) family of enzymes (18). Only 2% of the administered dose is excreted as parent drug. The E- and Z-5-oxo-tiagabine isomers are the prominent metabolites in plasma and urine. Two major metabolites in human feces remain unidentified. TGB elimination is linear over the therapeutic dosage range (19).

The half-life of TGB is 5 to 8 hours in patients with uninduced liver function (20) and 2 to 3 hours in patients taking hepatic enzyme-inducing antiepileptic drugs (AEDs) (9,19). More frequent dosing does not appear to be necessary to compensate for the shortened half-life, however. TGB 32 mg per day, as add-on therapy, is equally effective whether administered as a 16-mg dose twice daily or as an 8-mg dose four times per day (21).

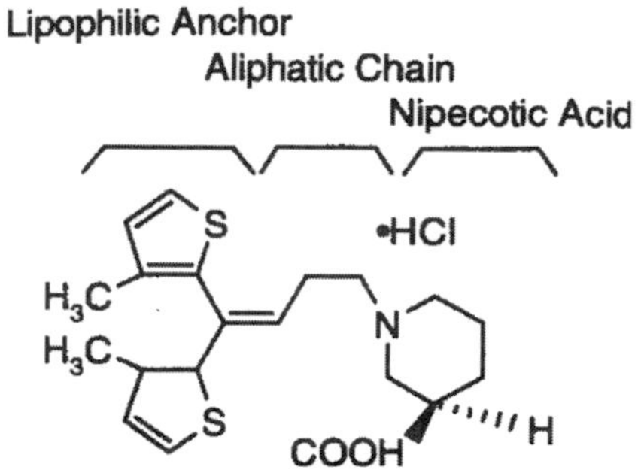

Figure 64.1 Chemical structure of tiagabine. (From Schachter SC. Tiagabine: current status and potential clinical applications. *Exp Opin Invest Drugs* 1996;5:1377–1387.)

When adjusted for body weight, TGB elimination is two times higher in children than in uninduced adults with epilepsy (22). The pharmacokinetics of TGB are similar in healthy elderly volunteers and healthy young volunteers (23).

TGB pharmacokinetics are unaffected by renal impairment (24). However, the half-life of the agent is increased to 12 to 16 hours in patients with hepatic impairment (25), necessitating dosage reductions and less frequent dosing intervals.

Drug Interactions

Concurrently administered drugs that enhance the activity of CYP3A increase the clearance of TGB and decrease the half-life of the agent. Therefore, TGB serum concentrations may increase if treatment with concomitantly administered enzyme-inducing AEDs is discontinued (26).

Because TGB neither induces nor inhibits the hepatic microsomal enzymes involved in drug metabolism, it minimally affects the serum concentrations of other agents (20). Moreover, although TGB is 96% protein bound, its serum concentration is too low to cause significant displacement of other protein-bound AEDs from albumin.

The metabolism of oral contraceptives is unaffected by TGB 8 mg per day (27), but whether higher doses of the agent have an effect on oral contraceptive metabolism is unknown.

EFFICACY

Add-on Studies of Patients with Refractory Partial Seizures

Five multicenter, double-blind, randomized, placebo-controlled studies evaluated TGB for the adjunctive treatment of partial-onset seizures in 951 patients, 675 of whom were randomly assigned to receive TGB (28–31). Three pivotal studies with parallel-group, add-on designs (21,32,33) enrolled patients taking one to three concomitant hepatic enzyme-inducing AEDs. The dose-response study com-

pared the efficacy of three different doses of TGB (16, 32, and 56 mg per day) with that of placebo (32). The thrice-daily dosing study compared the efficacy of TGB 10 mg administered three times per day with that of placebo (33).

In the dose-response study, the reduction in median seizure rates was statistically significant for both higher dosage groups (32 mg and 56 mg) compared with the placebo group (32). In the thrice-daily dosing study, TGB 10 mg administered three times per day was significantly more effective than placebo in reducing 4-week complex partial seizure (CPS) rates and simple partial seizure rates from baseline (33).

Monotherapy Trials

A dose-ranging study determined that the median tolerated dose of TGB as monotherapy for patients whose CPSs were not adequately controlled with one AED was 38.4 mg per day (range, 24 mg to 54 mg) (34).

The high- versus low-dose study randomized patients with CPS with or without secondarily generalized tonic-clonic seizures to either TGB 6 mg per day or TGB 36 mg per day (26). Median CPS rates decreased significantly in both dosage groups during TGB monotherapy in those patients who completed 12 weeks of fixed-dose treatment ($p < 0.05$). Additionally, nearly twice as many patients in the TGB 36-mg per day group as in the TGB 6-mg per day group experienced a reduction of 50% or more in CPS rates (31% versus 18%, respectively; $p = 0.038$) (34).

Long-Term Efficacy

Approximately 1200 patients received TGB for 1 year or longer in six trials. CPS rates declined by a median of 28.4% after 3 to 6 months of treatment and by 44% after treatment for 1 year or longer. Seizure reductions were maintained for up to 24 months (35).

ADVERSE EFFECTS

Add-on Studies of Patients with Refractory Partial Seizures

In the add-on trials, dizziness, asthenia (fatigue or generalized muscle weakness), nervousness, tremor, abnormal thinking (difficulty concentrating, mental lethargy, or slowness of thought), depression, aphasia (dysarthria, difficulty speaking, or speech arrest), and abdominal pain occurred significantly more often with TGB treatment than with placebo. Severe adverse effects were reported in 9% of the patients who received TGB and 5% of the patients who received placebo. Of patients treated with TGB, 13% withdrew from the study prematurely because of adverse effects, compared with 5% of those treated with placebo (38). Complex or simple partial status epilepticus occurred in four of 494 (0.8%) TGB recipients and two of 275 (0.7%) placebo recipients (36). Rash and psychosis occurred with approximately equal frequency in both groups (36). No clinically important effects attributable to TGB treatment were indicated in hematologic and biochemical test results, electrocardiograms, and vital signs. Neuropsychological testing did not reveal any evidence of worsening in mood or cognitive abilities (37).

Long-Term Studies

No new adverse events occurred in long-term studies, nor were any additional severe adverse effects reported other than those already noted with short-term therapy (38). A review of 53 clinical trials involving nearly 3100 patients treated with TGB found no clinically important effects on laboratory tests, hepatic metabolism, or concomitant AED therapy (39).

The TGB safety database was scanned for adverse effects suggestive of symptomatic visual field loss. Of the eight patients who had visual symptoms, two had visual field defects from fixed lesions (temporal lobe resection, cortical infarct) and six had transient visual complaints. Physical examination did not reveal any fixed visual defects (40).

CLINICAL USE

As of August 2003, there have been more than 39,000 patient-years of exposure to TGB. Case reports have attributed thrombocytopenia (41), convulsive status epilepticus (42), and reversible acute dystonic reactions (43) to TGB. Numerous reports have documented confusional states or nonconvulsive status epilepticus in patients with partial-onset or generalized seizures (44–54), including one patient with psychogenic nonepileptic seizures (55). Remission has been reported with decreases in the daily dose of TGB, or with the addition of clonazepam or lorazepam (47,49,50,52,55). Despite these reports, the incidence of symptoms consistent with nonconvulsive status epilepticus in blinded trials was no higher in patients treated with TGB than in those who received placebo. Since status epilepticus occurs in 5% to 10% of patients with refractory seizures, the significance of these findings is unclear (56).

Add-on TGB therapy has no effect on weight (57) and appears to have similar effects on mood as does add-on carbamazepine and phenytoin (58). The safety of TGB in pregnancy is not known.

Open case series have shown no evidence of visual field changes with long-term TGB treatment (59–61). A patient with bipolar disease treated with adjunctive TGB was reported to have asymptomatic visual field defects that reversed when the TGB was discontinued (62).

TGB continues to be used largely as an adjunctive agent in patients with partial-onset epilepsy, consistent with its FDA indication (63). An intriguing report suggests that TGB may have particular efficacy for seizures arising from glial tumors, but this awaits confirmation (64).

TGB has also been used with anecdotal success in a limited number of patients for off-label conditions, including spasticity (65,66), migraine (67), and mood and schizoaffective disorders (68–74).

TGB is available in the United States as 2-, 4-, 12-, 16-, and 20-mg tablets. Dosages should be titrated slowly to 32 to 56 mg daily in two or three divided doses in patients taking concomitant enzyme-inducing AEDs. Dosages in children have not been well established; in one pediatric trial, doses ≤ 0.4 mg/kg were used in children with uninduced hepatic function and doses ≤ 0.7 mg/kg in children taking enzyme-inducing AEDs.

The clinical utility of TGB serum concentrations is uncertain because of the short half-life of the agent in induced patients (75). Routine monitoring of liver, renal, and bone marrow function does not appear to be necessary.

CONCLUSIONS

TGB, a potent AED with linear, predictable pharmacokinetics, inhibits GABA reuptake into neurons and glia. The agent has no clinically relevant effects on hepatic metabolism or on serum concentrations of other AEDs, nor does it interact with many commonly used non-AEDs. The most common side effects associated with TGB use are CNS-related, usually mild to moderate in severity, and minimized by slow dosage titration. At doses of 32 mg to 56 mg per day, TGB has proved effective as add-on treatment in patients with partial seizures. Higher doses are well tolerated and appear to benefit some patients in open studies and in clinical experience. Additional controlled studies are needed to confirm the efficacy of TGB as monotherapy and to determine the effective dosage range.

REFERENCES

1. Krogsgaard-Larsen P, Falch E, Larsson OM, et al. GABA uptake inhibitors: relevance to antiepileptic drug research. *Epilepsy Res* 1987;1:77–93.
2. Braestrup C, Nielsen EB, Sonnewald U, et al. (R)-N-[4,4-bis (3-methyl-2-thienyl)but-3-en-1-yl]nipecotic acid binds with high affinity to the brain gamma-aminobutyric acid uptake carrier. *J Neurochem* 1990;54:639–647.
3. Giardina WJ. Anticonvulsant action of tiagabine, a new GABA-uptake inhibitor. *J Epilepsy* 1994;7:161–166.
4. Fueta Y, Schwarz W, Ohno K, et al. Selective suppression of hippocampal region hyperexcitability related to seizure susceptibility in epileptic El mice by the GABA-transporter inhibitor tiagabine. *Brain Res* 2002;947:212–217.
5. Suzdak PD, Jansen JA. A review of the preclinical pharmacology of tiagabine: a potent and selective anticonvulsant GABA uptake inhibitor. *Epilepsia* 1995;36:612–626.
6. Borden LA, Dhar TGM, Smith KE, et al. Tiagabine, SK&F 89976-A, CI-966, and NNC-711 are selective for the cloned GABA transporter GAT-1. *Eur J Pharmacol* 1994;269:219–224.
7. Eriksson IS, Allard P, Marcusson J. [3H]tiagabine binding to GABA uptake sites in human brain. *Brain Res* 1999;851:183–188.

8. Sundman-Eriksson I, Allard P. [(3)H]Tiagabine binding to GABA transporter-1 (GAT-1) in suicidal depression. *J Affect Disord* 2002;71:29–33.

9. Brodie MJ. Tiagabine pharmacology in profile. *Epilepsia* 1995;36(Suppl 6):S7–S9.

10. Morimoto K, Sato H, Yamamoto Y, et al. Antiepileptic effects of tiagabine, a selective GABA uptake inhibitor, in the rat kindling model of temporal lobe epilepsy. *Epilepsia* 1997;38:966–974.

11. Nielsen EB, Suzdak PD, Andersen KE, et al. Characterization of tiagabine (NO-328), a new potent and selective GABA uptake inhibitor. *Eur J Pharmacol* 1991;196:257–266.

12. Faingold CL, Randall ME, Anderson CA. Blockade of GABA uptake with tiagabine inhibits audiogenic seizures and reduces neuronal firing in the inferior colliculus of the genetically epilepsy-prone rat. *Exp Neurol* 1994;126:225–232.

13. Ipponi A, Lamberti C, Medica A, et al. Tiagabine antinociception in rodents depends on GABA(B) receptor activation: parallel antinociception testing and medial thalamus GABA microdialysis. *Eur J Pharmacol* 1999;368:205–211.

14. Yang Y, Li Q, Wang CX, et al. A. Dose-dependent neuroprotection with tiagabine in a focal cerebral ischemia model in rat. *Neuroreport* 2000;11:2307–2311.

15. Chen Xu W, Yi Y, Qiu L, et al. Neuroprotective activity of tiagabine in a focal embolic model of cerebral ischemia. *Brain Res* 2000;874:75–77.

16. Iqbal S, Baziany A, Gordon S, et al. Neuroprotective effect of tiagabine in transient forebrain global ischemia: an in vivo microdialysis, behavioral, and histological study. *Brain Res* 2002;946: 162–170.

17. Mengel H. Tiagabine. *Epilepsia* 1994;35(Suppl 5):S81–S84.

18. Bopp BA, Nequist GE, Rodrigues AD. Role of the cytochrome P450 3A subfamily in the metabolism of [14C] tiagabine by human hepatic microsomes. *Epilepsia* 1995;36(Suppl 3):S159.

19. Samara EE, Gustavson LE, El-Shourbagy T, et al. Population analysis of the pharmacokinetics of tiagabine in patients with epilepsy. *Epilepsia* 1998;39:868–873.

20. Gustavson LE, Mengel HB. Pharmacokinetics of tiagabine, a gamma-aminobutyric acid-uptake inhibitor, in healthy subjects after single and multiple doses. *Epilepsia* 1995;36:605–611.

21. Sachdeo RC, Leroy RF, Krauss GL, et al. Tiagabine therapy for complex partial seizures. A dose-frequency study. *Arch Neurol* 1997;54:595–601.

22. Gustavson LE, Boellner SW, Granneman GR, et al. A single-dose study to define tiagabine pharmacokinetics in pediatric patients with complex partial seizures. *Neurology* 1997;48:1032–1037.

23. Snel S, Jansen JA, Mengel HB, et al. The pharmacokinetics of tiagabine in healthy elderly volunteers and elderly patients with epilepsy. *J Clin Pharmacol* 1997;37:1015–1020.

24. Cato A, Gustavson LE, Quian J, et al. Effect of renal impairment on the pharmacokinetics and tolerability of tiagabine. *Epilepsia* 1998;39:43–47.

25. Lau AH, Gustavson LE, Sperelakis R, et al. Pharmacokinetics and safety of tiagabine in subjects with various degrees of hepatic function. *Epilepsia* 1997;38:445–451.

26. Schachter SC. Tiagabine monotherapy in the treatment of partial epilepsy. *Epilepsia* 1995;36(Suppl 6):S2–S6.

27. Mengel HB, Houston A, Back DJ. An evaluation of the interaction between tiagabine and oral contraceptives in female volunteers. *J Pharm Med* 1994;4:141–150.

28. Ostergaard LH, Gram L, Dam M. Potential antiepileptic drugs. Tiagabine. In: Levy RH, Mattson RH, Meldrum BS, eds. *Antiepileptic drugs.* New York: Raven Press. 1995;1057–1061.

29. Richens A, Chadwick DW, Duncan JS, et al. Adjunctive treatment of partial seizures with tiagabine: a placebo-controlled trial. *Epilepsy Res* 1995;21:37–42.

30. Lassen LC, Sommerville K, Mengel HB, et al. Summary of five controlled trials with tiagabine as adjunctive treatment of patients with partial seizures. *Epilepsia* 1995;36(Suppl 3):S148.

31. Crawford P, Meinardi H, Brown S, et al. Tiagabine: efficacy and safety in adjunctive treatment of partial seizures. *Epilepsia* 2001;42:531–538.

32. Uthman BM, Rowan AJ, Ahmann PA, et al. Tiagabine for complex partial seizures: a randomized, add-on, dose-response trial. *Arch Neurol* 1998;55:56–62.

33. Kalviainen R, Brodie MJ, Duncan J, et al. A double-blind, placebo-controlled trial of tiagabine given three-times daily as add-on therapy for refractory partial seizures. *Epilepsy Res* 1998;30:31–40.

34. Schachter SC, Cahill WT, Wannamaker BB, et al. Open-label dosage and tolerability study of tiagabine monotherapy in patients with refractory complex partial seizures. *J Epilepsy* 1998;11:248–255.

35. Schachter SC, Deaton R, Sommerville K. Long-term use of tiagabine for partial seizures. *Epilepsia* 1997;38(Suppl 8):S105–S106.

36. Sackellares JC, Krauss G, Sommerville KW, et al. Occurrence of psychosis in patients with epilepsy randomized to tiagabine or placebo treatment. *Epilepsia* 2002;43:394–398.

37. Dodrill CB, Arnett JL, Sommerville KW, et al. Cognitive and quality of life effects of differing dosages of tiagabine in epilepsy. *Neurology* 1997;48:1025–1031.

38. Leppik IE. Tiagabine: the safety landscape. *Epilepsia* 1995;36 (Suppl 6):S10–S13.

39. Leppik IE, Gram L, Deaton R, et al. Safety of tiagabine: summary of 53 trials. *Epilepsy Res* 1999;33:235–246.

40. Collins SD, Brun S, Kirstein YG, et al. Absence of visual field defects in patients taking tiagabine. *Epilepsia* 1998;39(Suppl 6): S146–S147.

41. Willert C, Englisch S, Schlesinger S, et al. Possible drug-induced thrombocytopenia secondary to tiagabine. *Neurology* 1999;52: 889–891.

42. Ostrovskiy D, Spanaki MV, Morris GL III. Tiagabine overdose can induce convulsive status epilepticus. *Epilepsia* 2002;43:773–774.

43. Wolanczyk T, Grabowska-Grzyb A. Transient dystonias in three patients treated with tiagabine. *Epilepsia* 2001;42:944–946.

44. Brouns R, Van Paesschen W. Recurrent complex partial status epilepticus associated with tiagabine rechallenge. *Acta Neurol Belg* 2002;102:19–20.

45. Fitzek S, Hegemann S, Sauner D, et al. Drug-induced nonconvulsive status epilepticus with low dose of tiagabine. *Epileptic Disord* 2001;3:147–150.

46. Eckardt KM, Steinhoff BJ. Nonconvulsive status epilepticus in two patients receiving tiagabine treatment. *Epilepsia* 1998;39:671–674.

47. Trinka E, Moroder T, Nagler M, et al. Clinical and EEG findings in complex partial status epilepticus with tiagabine. *Seizure* 1999;8:41–44.

48. de Borchgrave V, Lienard F, Willemart T, et al. Clinical and EEG findings in six patients with altered mental status receiving tiagabine therapy. *Epilepsy Behav* 2003;4:326–337.

49. Imperiale D, Pignatta P, Cerrato P, et al. Nonconvulsive status epilepticus due to a de novo contralateral focus during tiagabine adjunctive therapy. *Seizure* 2003;12:319–322.

50. Kellinghaus C, Dziewas R, Ludemann P. Tiagabine-related nonconvulsive status epilepticus in partial epilepsy: three case reports and a review of the literature. *Seizure* 2002;11:243–249.

51. Ettinger AB, Bernal OG, Andriola MR, et al. Two cases of nonconvulsive status epilepticus in association with tiagabine therapy. *Epilepsia* 1999;40:1159–1162.

52. Knake S, Hamer HM, Schomburg U, et al. Tiagabine-induced absence status in idiopathic generalized epilepsy. *Seizure* 1999;8:314–317.

53. Balslev T, Uldall P, Buchholt J. Provocation of non-convulsive status epilepticus by tiagabine in three adolescent patients. *Eur J Paediatr Neurol* 2000;4:169–170.

54. Skodda S, Kramer I, Spittler JF, et al. Non-convulsive status epilepticus in two patients receiving tiagabine add-on treatment. *J Neurol* 2001;248:109–112.

55. Zhu Y, Vaughn BV. Non-convulsive status epilepticus induced by tiagabine in a patient with pseudoseizure. *Seizure* 2002;11:57–59.

56. Shinnar S, Berg AT, Treiman DM, et al. Status epilepticus and tiagabine therapy: review of safety data and epidemiologic comparisons. *Epilepsia* 2001;42:372–379.

57. Hogan RE, Bertrand ME, Deaton RL, et al. Total percentage body weight changes during add-on therapy with tiagabine, carbamazepine and phenytoin. *Epilepsy Res* 2000;41:23–28.

58. Dodrill CB, Arnett JL, Deaton R, et al. Tiagabine versus phenytoin and carbamazepine as add-on therapies: effects on abilities, adjustment, and mood. *Epilepsy Res* 2000;42:123–132.

59. Krauss GL, Johnson MA, Sheth S, et al. A controlled study comparing visual function in patients treated with vigabatrin and tiagabine. *J Neurol Neurosurg Psychiatry* 2003;74:339–343.

60. Fakhoury TA, Abou-Khalil B, Lavin P. Lack of visual field defects with long-term use of tiagabine. *Neurology* 2000;54(Suppl 3): A309.

61. Nousiainen I, Mantyjarvi M, Kalviainen R. Visual function in patients treated with the GABAergic anticonvulsant drug tiagabine. *Clin Drug Invest* 2000;20:393–400.

62. Kaufman KR, Lepore FE, Keyser BJ. Visual fields and tiagabine: a quandary. *Seizure* 2001;10:525–529.

63. Schmidt D, Gram L, Brodie M, et al. Tiagabine in the treatment of epilepsy—a clinical review with a guide for the prescribing physician. *Epilepsy Res* 2000;41:245–251.

64. Striano S, Striano P, Boccella P, et al. Tiagabine in glial tumors. *Epilepsy Res* 2002;49:81–85.

65. Holden KR, Titus MO. The effect of tiagabine on spasticity in children with intractable epilepsy: a pilot study. *Pediatr Neurol* 1999;21:728–730.

66. Murinson BB, Rizzo M. Improvement of stiff-person syndrome with tiagabine. *Neurology* 2001;57:366.

67. Freitag FG, Diamond S, Diamond ML. Tiagabine in the prophylaxis of migraine. *Neurology* 1999;52(Suppl 2):A208.

68. Suppes T, Chisholm KA, Dhavale D, et al. Tiagabine in treatment refractory bipolar disorder: a clinical case series. *Bipolar Disord* 2002;4:283–289.

69. Schwartz TL. The use of tiagabine augmentation for treatment-resistant anxiety disorders: a case series. *Psychopharmacol Bull* 2002;36:53–57.

70. Kaufman KR. Adjunctive tiagabine treatment of psychiatric disorders: three cases. *Ann Clin Psychiatry* 1998;10:181–184.

71. Berigan T. Treatment of posttraumatic stress disorder with tiagabine. *Can J Psychiatry* 2002;47:788.

72. Zwanzger P, Baghai TC, Schule C, et al. Tiagabine improves panic and agoraphobia in panic disorder patients. *J Clin Psychiatry* 2001;62:656–657.

73. Schaffer LC, Schaffer CB, Howe J. An open case series on the utility of tiagabine as an augmentation in refractory bipolar outpatients. *J Affect Disord* 2002;71:259–263.

74. Carta MG, Hardoy MC, Grunze H, et al. The use of tiagabine in affective disorders. *Pharmacopsychiatry* 2002;35:33–34.

75. Perucca E. Is there a role for therapeutic drug monitoring of new anticonvulsants? *Clin Pharmacokinet* 2000;38:191–204.

Felbamate

65

Edward Faught

HISTORICAL BACKGROUND

When felbamate (FBM) was introduced to clinical practice in the United States in July 1993, there had been no major new antiepileptic drugs (AEDs) for 15 years, and enthusiasm ran high. Dangerous side effects were not anticipated based on the experience of 2100 patients enrolled in clinical trials, but in 1994, FBM was found to be associated with a high incidence of aplastic anemia (1). Compared with the 120,000 individuals who were treated with the agent in the first year, only 14,000 to 15,000 patients worldwide are now receiving FBM therapy (2). FBM remains available for patients with refractory seizures who respond poorly to other medications, with the number of treated patients remaining stable in recent years (2).

FBM is one of a series of dicarbamate compounds, including the minor tranquilizer meprobamate, synthesized in the 1950s. With no tranquilizing or sedative effects, FBM was not immediately useful. In 1986, efficacy in a wide range of experimental seizure models, with relatively low neurotoxicity, was reported (3).

Encouraging results from pharmacokinetic and pilot toxicity studies were described (4,5). Two controlled clinical trials (6,7) in patients with refractory partial seizures suggested modest efficacy of FBM as an adjunctive agent. Significant pharmacokinetic drug interactions, in part, prompted testing of FBM as a monotherapy agent. The FBM development program was characterized by the use of two innovative monotherapy clinical trial designs, which have since been applied to test several new AEDs.

CHEMISTRY AND MECHANISM OF ACTION

Chemistry

FBM (2 phenyl-1,3-propanediol dicarbamate) differs from meprobamate by having a phenyl group, rather than an aliphatic chain, at the 2-carbon position (Fig. 65.1). FBM is lipophilic and relatively insoluble in water. No parenteral preparation for humans is available, but intravenous administration in mice has been achieved by encapsulating FBM molecules with hydrophobic diketopiperazine microspheres (8). The molecular weight of the agent is 238.24 (9).

Antiepileptic Profile in Animals

FBM displayed high protective indices (toxic dose$_{50}$/effective dose$_{50}$) against both the tonic phase of maximal electroshock seizures and subcutaneous pentylenetetrazol-induced seizures in rodents (3). The agent increases seizure threshold and reduces seizure severity in fully amygdala-kindled rats (10), but it is not known whether it inhibits kindling development.

Mechanisms of Action

Evidence points to four mechanisms of antiepileptic action, all antiexcitatory. FBM interferes with voltage-gated sodium channels, resulting in blockade of sustained repetitive neuronal firing and prevention of seizure spread (11). Although earlier data suggested that FBM interfered with the function of N-methyl-D-aspartate (NMDA)-type glutamate receptors by competitive inhibition of glycine, an obligatory coagonist (12), recent studies indicate that it is noncompetitive with respect to both glycine and glutamate (13). FBM has been found to bind selectively to some NMDA-receptor subtypes, especially those containing NR2B subunits (13,14). In either case, the net effect is reduction of NMDA-receptor-modulated cationic conductance. Subtype specificity may account for the lack of side effects with FBM that are typical of such NMDA receptor blockers as MK-801 (15). The third proposed mechanism of action involves non-NMDA-excitatory amino acid receptors. Not only does FBM protect against seizures induced by quisqualate and kainate (11), but also against seizures induced by α-amino-3-hydroxy-5-methyl-4-isoxazole propionic acid (AMPA), (16). Glutamate

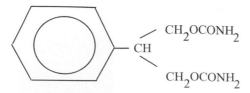

Figure 65.1   Structure of felbamate.

the natural agonist for this receptor subtype. Finally, the agent inhibits voltage-activated calcium currents at clinically relevant concentrations (17). This may inhibit release of excitatory neurotransmitters and underlie the antiabsence activity of FBM.

One or more of these antiexcitatory mechanisms may be responsible for a neuroprotective effect of FBM, which reduced neuronal damage in a rat model of hypoxia-ischemia (18), protected CA1 hippocampal neurons from apoptosis in a gerbil ischemia model (19), and exhibited neuroprotective effects in a rat model of status epilepticus (20).

FBM and related compounds have potential as treatments for status epilepticus. Fluorofelbamate, a new FBM analog, very effectively terminates seizures in the rat self-sustaining status epilepticus (SSSE) model (21). A major therapeutic problem is the relative inefficacy of phenytoin, phenobarbital, and benzodiazepines in late-stage status epilepticus. In the SSSE model, fluorofelbamate was effective but phenytoin and phenobarbital were not, even after 40 to 70 minutes of continuous seizures. Furthermore, unlike the other agents, FBM attenuated the development of recurrent, spontaneous seizures after SSSE, suggesting that it is antiepileptogenic (21).

ABSORPTION, DISTRIBUTION, AND METABOLISM

FBM is well absorbed; more than 90% of ^{14}C-labeled FBM, or its metabolites is recovered in urine and feces after oral administration (22), and the rate and extent of absorption are not affected by food or antacids (23).

FBM readily crosses the blood-brain barrier, with brain and cerebrospinal fluid concentrations in animals close to plasma concentrations (9). In human plasma, only 22% to 25% of FBM is reversibly bound to proteins (primarily albumin), independent of dosage (24), and protein-binding interactions are thus insignificant.

Of the absorbed FBM dose, 30% to 50% is excreted in the urine unchanged (22,25), with renal clearance decreasing to 9% to 22% of the total dose in patients with renal dysfunction (25). The remainder is metabolized by the liver by several pathways (26). (Fig. 65.2) Pharmacokinetic differences in patients 67 to 78 years of age were minor (27).

FBM exhibits linear first-order pharmacokinetics over a dose range of 1200 to 6000 mg per day in humans (28). Peak plasma concentration is reached 3 hours after administration of an oral dose, and concentrations increase proportionally after single and multiple doses (26). Monotherapy with FBM 3600 mg per day produced a mean trough plasma level of 78.4 μg/mL (range, 23.7 to 136.6 μg/mL) in one study (29) and a mean (± standard deviation) level of 65 (± 23) μg/mL after 112 days in another (30).

The terminal elimination half-life of 20 hours (range, 13 to 23 hours) with FBM monotherapy decreases to 13 to 14 hours in the presence of phenytoin or carbamazepine (5). The apparent volume of distribution is 0.8 L/kg (31).

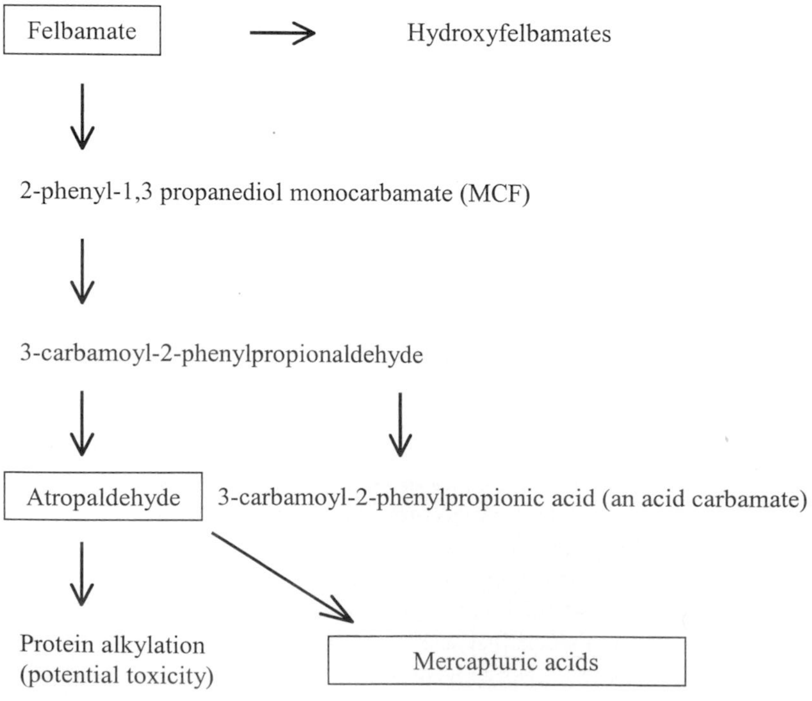

Felbamate ⟶ Hydroxyfelbamates

↓

2-phenyl-1,3 propanediol monocarbamate (MCF)

↓

3-carbamoyl-2-phenylpropionaldehyde

↓   ↓

Atropaldehyde   3-carbamoyl-2-phenylpropionic acid (an acid carbamate)

↓

Protein alkylation (potential toxicity)   Mercapturic acids

Figure 65.2   Metabolism of felbamate. Adapted from Thompson CD, Barthen MT, Hopper DW, et al. Quantification in patient urine samples of felbamate and three metabolites: acid carbamate and two mercapturic acids. *Epilepsia* 1999;40:769–776, with permission.

Steady-state plasma levels are achieved approximately 4 days following initiation of therapy (26).

EFFICACY

FBM is approved for use in the United States as either adjunctive therapy or monotherapy for patients older than 14 years of age with partial seizures, with or without generalization, and as adjunctive therapy for patients of any age with Lennox-Gastaut syndrome and its component seizure types (31).

Partial-Onset Seizures

The initial clinical trials of FBM as an adjunct to carbamazepine (6,7) or phenytoin (6) therapy used standard designs and yielded unimpressive results. Reductions in seizure frequency were either small (6) or not significantly different (7) from those with placebo. In 1998, new designs for AED trials were proposed in a workshop sponsored by the Epilepsy Branch of the National Institutes of Health (32). Clinical investigators of FBM were the first to use these designs.

In a presurgical evaluation trial (33), FBM or placebo was added to the AEDs in use at the conclusion of electroencephalogram (EEG)-video monitoring. The primary endpoint was time to occurrence of the fourth seizure or 29 days, whichever came first. Of patients randomized to placebo, 88% experienced a fourth seizure before day 29, compared with 46% taking FBM ($p = 0.03$). In outpatient monotherapy trials (29,30), standard therapy was withdrawn over 28 days, and FBM 3600 mg per day or valproate 15 mg/kg per day was substituted. The valproate dose represented a compromise between a placebo control, which might have been unsafe, and a full-dose active control, which might have called the conclusions into question (34). The end point was "escape" from treatment, defined as treatment failure according to predetermined criteria, including a doubling of seizure frequency during any 2 days or 1 month, compared with pretreatment baseline. Patients taking low-dose valproate met escape criteria more often than did FBM-treated patients (86% versus 14%, respectively, of 42 patients in the single-center study [29]; 78% versus 40%, respectively, of 95 patients in the multicenter study [30]). The "presurgical" design was also repeated as a monotherapy trial and further confirmed monotherapy efficacy (35).

Open-label experience with adjunctive FBM-therapy has been more encouraging than the original adjunctive-use controlled trials. In one open-label assessment, 20% of 111 adults had greater than 50% reductions in seizure frequency (36). Adjunctive open-label use reduced seizure frequency by 53% among a group of 30 children aged 2 to 17 years (37). No direct comparisons of FBM efficacy with that of other AEDs are available.

Lennox-Gastaut Syndrome

FBM 45 mg/kg per day was used as adjunctive therapy, usually along with valproate, in a multicenter, double-blind, controlled trial of 73 patients (38). Atonic seizures (drop attacks) were reduced by 34% and all seizures by 19%, versus a 9% decrease and a 4% increase, respectively, in these parameters with placebo. A difference in atypical absence frequency was not proved. Parents also reported increased alertness and verbal responsiveness in their children. During a 12-month, open-label follow-up, seizure frequency decreased by 50% in FBM-treated patients, compared with 15% in the placebo group (39,40). FBM may have a synergistic effect with valproate: In a study of 13 patients with Lennox-Gastaut syndrome, drop attacks were reduced by 40% and total seizures by 50% when FBM was added—effects not completely explained by the observed 12.7% increase in valproate levels (41).

Other Seizure Types

Secondarily generalized tonic-clonic seizures respond to FBM treatment (30,42). Reduction in the number of generalized tonic seizures as part of the Lennox-Gastaut syndrome has been demonstrated (38). There are reports of efficacy in small, uncontrolled series of patients with infantile spasms (43), primary generalized seizures (42,44), absence seizures (45), atypical absence seizures not part of the Lennox-Gastaut syndrome (46), and juvenile myoclonic epilepsy (47).

DRUG INTERACTIONS

Clinically significant interactions with phenytoin, carbamazepine, valproate, and phenobarbital have been established (Table 65.1). FBM is metabolized by the hepatic cytochrome P450 (CYP) system, primarily by CYP2E1 and to a minor extent by CYP3A4 (48). Thus, CYP2E1 inhibitors such as chlorzoxazone increase FBM levels, whereas CYP3A4 inhibitors such as erythromycin have little effect (49). Drugs such as carbamazepine, phenytoin, and phenobarbital, which induce CYP3A4, increase FBM clearance (48). FBM inhibits phenytoin and phenobarbital clearance by inhibiting CYP2C19 (48).

Effect on Carbamazepine

When FBM is added to carbamazepine, levels of carbamazepine decrease 20% to 30%, but carbamazepine epoxide (CBZ-E) levels increase by 50% to 60% (7,50,51). FBM induces CYP3A4-mediated carbamazepine metabolism and inhibits epoxide hydrolase, which metabolizes CBZ-E (52). These effects can cause clinical toxicity related to the elevated CBZ-E level. The carbamazepine-FBM combination

TABLE 65.1

INTERACTIONS OF FELBAMATE AND OTHER AEDS

	Effect of Felbamate on Other AEDs		Effect of Other AEDs on Felbamate Concentration (%)
	AED Change in Concentration (%)	Recommended Dose Adjustment (%)	
Phenytoin	↑ (30–50)	↓ (20–33)	↓ (15)
Carbamazepine (total)	↓ (30)	↓ (20–33)	↓ (15)
Carbamazepine (epoxide)	↑ (50–60)	—	—
Valproate	↑ (25–50)	↓ (20–33)	↔ (variable)
Phenobarbital	↑ (24)	↓ (25)	—

Abbreviation: AEDs, antiepileptic drugs.

is often associated with headache—a probable pharmaco-dynamic interaction.

Effect on Phenytoin

The addition of FBM to phenytoin reduces phenytoin clearance by 20% (4,5). Phenytoin serum levels may increase by 30% to 50%. The magnitude varies directly with the FBM dose (51) and baseline phenytoin level, and inversely with the individual phenytoin clearance rate. Typical adverse effects of phenytoin toxicity, such as dizziness and ataxia, as confirmed by measurement of total phenytoin levels, can then occur and will respond to a reduction in phenytoin dose.

Effect on Valproate

FBM increases valproate levels by inhibiting metabolism of the agent via beta-oxidation (48). In 10 patients treated with stable FBM doses, the addition of FBM 600 mg per day increased mean steady-state valproate concentrations from 69.9 mg/L to 85.5 mg/L; the addition of FBM 1200 mg per day was associated with a further increase to 103.0 mg/L (53). This 28% to 54% increase may be clinically significant and require a reduction in valproate dosage.

Effects of Other Agents on Felbamate

Both carbamazepine and phenytoin increase the metabolism of FBM, producing levels about 15% lower in the presence of either agent (50,52,54). These effects are additive. The clearance of FBM decreased by 21% as the phenytoin dose was reduced and by an additional 16.5% as the carbamazepine dose was reduced, both as consecutive maneuvers in a clinical trial (55). The addition of valproate may increase the plasma level of FBM slightly (54).

Other Drug Interactions

One patient's warfarin requirement decreased by 50% when FBM was added to the treatment regimen (56). FBM may cause elevations of phenobarbital levels by 24% (57) and increase methsuximide levels (58). There are no interactions with either lamotrigine (59) or oxcarbazepine (60).

ADVERSE EFFECTS

Common Adverse Effects

Gastrointestinal disturbances, headache, anorexia, and insomnia are frequently reported with FBM use (29,30,33). Dizziness, diplopia, and ataxia were common at low doses in the adjunctive therapy clinical trials (6), but many instances were probably related to secondary elevations in phenytoin and carbamazepine epoxide levels.

Although most adverse effects subside with monotherapy, insomnia and anorexia often persist stubbornly (29). Among 366 adults receiving monotherapy, 4.1% experienced nausea, 3.6% insomnia, 3% anorexia, 2% to 5% dizziness, and 2% weight loss (40).

During initiation of FBM therapy, adverse effects from increasing levels of other agents are managed by reduction of the concomitant drug doses. Although a rapid conversion to monotherapy was once advocated to reduce the effect of those interactions, most physicians find it easier to make a more gradual conversion. Treatment of stomachache or nausea with centrally acting antacids, and of insomnia with benzodiazepines or with a change in the timing or size of evening FBM doses, is often satisfactory. Headache is more difficult to treat without a dose reduction but may be alleviated by the reduction of a concomitant carbamazepine dose.

FBM has a stimulant effect in many patients. Although most individuals find this refreshing, it may cause insomnia, irritability, and behavioral changes. In one open-label, add-on assessment (36), behavioral problems were the leading cause of discontinuation.

At 3% to 4%, the incidence of rash did not differ between FBM and placebo in clinical trials (31). Other side effects occurring in more than 1% of patients in clinical trials were weight increase, asthenia, malaise, influenza-like symptoms, palpitation, tachycardia, agitation, psychological disturbance, aggressive reaction, and pruritus (31). Two children experienced involuntary dyskinetic movements (61).

The overall dropout rate caused by adverse effects in clinical trials was 12% (31). As expected with most drugs, this rate is higher in community practice—21% in one open-label assessment (36).

Dose-Limiting Effects

Doses in the clinical trials were limited to 3600 mg per day for adults and 45 mg/kg per day for children, with most research patients achieving these targets without dose-limiting toxicities. Higher doses may produce limiting symptoms. Among 50 patients stabilized on FBM 3600 mg or 45 mg/kg per day who received increases to 4200–7200 mg, 32% developed new or increased side effects, but only 15% required dose reductions (62). The average dose limit was 5412 mg per day or 98 mg/kg, producing an average serum concentration of 110 mg/L. The most common dose-limiting effects were dizziness, ataxia, and nausea.

Aplastic Anemia

FBM can cause severe or fatal aplastic anemia. In 1994, there were 31 cases reported to the Food and Drug Administration (63), and two additional cases were reported to the manufacturer in 1995 (64). To date, there have been 14 fatalities associated with the use of the agent. Only one additional case has been reported, but relatively few patients have been started on FBM since 1994.

Detailed review of the first 31 cases according to International Agranulocytosis and Aplastic Anemia Study criteria revealed that only 23 (74%) met criteria for a diagnosis of aplastic anemia (63). Six others had preexisting blood dyscrasias or systemic lupus erythematosus. FBM was implicated as the most likely cause in 14 patients. Nine others had at least one other plausible cause—usually the use of other medications known to cause aplastic anemia.

Based on an estimate of 110,000 patients exposed, the authors of this review (63) suggested a most probable incidence of 127 per million (one/8000 cases), compared with a population rate of two per million per year. A paucity of quantitative data on the aplastic anemia risk with other AEDs exists. Estimates for carbamazepine range from five to 39 per million per year (63). All cases were diagnosed within one year of starting felbamate, two out of three within 6 months (64). Therefore, the risk drops substantially after 1 year of therapy.

Patients developing aplastic anemia were more likely to have histories of blood dyscrasias, especially cytopenia, autoimmune disorders, and rashes or significant toxicities associated with previously used agents (64,65). It seems best to avoid FBM use in such patients. Caucasian women were the demographic group most likely to develop aplastic anemia (65).

Liver Failure

Among patients taking FBM for 25 to 959 days, 18 reported cases of liver failure resulted in nine fatalities (64). Of these, eight cases may have been a result of other factors—five associated with status epilepticus and one case each of hepatitis A, acetaminophen poisoning, and severe hypotension. Using population exposure estimates (63), this implies a risk of about one per 10,000 patient exposures. Pellock and Brodie concluded that the rate of hepatotoxicity "is within the general range of that seen with valproate and, perhaps, with other AEDs" (2).

Mechanisms of Toxicity

The mechanisms by which FBM causes aplastic anemia are unclear. Formation of a reactive, cytotoxic, intermediate metabolite, atropaldehyde (Fig. 65.2), the quantity of which may vary on a genetic basis, was proposed as the mechanism (66). Theoretically, it would be possible to identify persons at high risk by quantifying urinary metabolites in individual patients. A large prospective patient screening program failed to prove this hypothesis, however, because, fortunately, no patient enrolled in the program developed aplastic anemia attributable to FBM (67). Since atropaldehyde is detoxified by glutathione, and glutathione stores are depleted by acetaminophen, it seems prudent to advise patients on FBM therapy not to take acetaminophen.

Other mechanisms for FBM bone marrow toxicity may be important. Both felbamate and the initial metabolite 2-phenyl-1,3-propanediol monocarbamate (MCF) have been reported to cause apoptosis of bone marrow progenitor cells *in vitro* (68). Fluorofelbamate, a potent antiepileptic compound that is not metabolized to atropaldehyde, has been proposed as a safer alternative to FBM (21). However, it will be necessary to demonstrate that it does not cause bone marrow toxicity in animals by other mechanisms before it can be tested in humans.

CLINICAL USE

Patient Selection

Because of the potential for serious blood or liver reactions, FBM should not be used as initial epilepsy therapy or in patients for whom an effective alternative agent can be found. Patients with partial-onset seizures refractory to several previous drugs, especially those who have both severe epilepsy and problems with sedative effects, may be considered for treatment with FBM.

Should FBM be the agent of last choice for the refractory patient? There are now between 10 and 15 drugs available in many countries; systematic trials of all would require many years. It is becoming increasingly apparent that the likelihood of satisfactory seizure control decreases exponentially with each drug failure. The patient who fails two, and certainly three, drugs because of inefficacy may be appropriately considered to be refractory (69). Because of the unique efficacy of FBM in some refractory patients, which may relate to the unique combination of effects of the agent on cellular mechanisms, it is not unreasonable to consider FBM therapy in such patients along with other alternatives. For example, the risk for injury from atonic or tonic-clonic seizures in patients with Lennox-Gastaut syndrome refractory to other drugs indubitably exceeds the risk associated with FBM use. Valproate is usually chosen initially for the treatment of patients with this syndrome. Although lamotrigine and topiramate are also effective, comparative results suggest that FBM is more potent (38).

All patients taking FBM or their caretakers must be able to report side effects reliably, comply with blood testing, and understand the potential risks and benefits of the agent. A Quality Standards Subcommittee of the American Academy of Neurology and the American Epilepsy Society has formulated practice guidelines for the use of felbamate in specific patient populations (70) (Table 65.2).

Initial Therapy

Both children and adults may be started on FBM 15 mg/kg per day in three divided doses, taken after meals, with increases to 30 mg/kg per day and 45 mg/kg per day at 1- or 2-week intervals. Early side effects are common but usually manageable with reductions in concomitant AEDs of 20% to 33% as the FBM dose is increased. Further reductions in concomitant drug doses can be made gradually once the FBM target dose has been achieved, if FBM monotherapy is the goal. FBM is more effective and better tolerated as monotherapy than as an add-on agent, but if a seizure-free state without toxicity is achieved during the polytherapy interim, it is reasonable to defer further dose changes.

Maintenance Dosage

An average adult dose is 3600 mg per day; an average pediatric dose is 45 mg/kg per day. Some patients have tolerated doses as high as 7200 mg (adults) or 100 mg/kg per day (children) (62,71). Higher relative doses may be necessary for younger children in whom clearance is increased (37). Measurement of plasma levels is neither more nor less useful than with other agents. The average therapeutic range for FBM is approximately 50 to 110 mg/L (62,71). An inadequate response to FBM as adjunctive therapy warrants

---

TABLE 65.2

RECOMMENDATIONS FOR USE OF FELBAMATE

A. Patients for whom risk-to-benefit ratio supports use because there is class I evidence of benefit
  1. Patients with Lennox-Gastaut syndrome >4 years of age who are unresponsive to primary AEDs
  2. Intractable partial seizures in patients >18 years of age who have failed standard AEDs at therapeutic levels (monotherapy data indicate a better risk-to-benefit ratio for felbamate used as monotherapy)
  3. Patients taking felbamate >18 months
B. Patients for whom the current risk-to-benefit assessment does not support the use of felbamate
  1. New onset epilepsy in adults or children
  2. Patients who have experienced significant prior hematologic adverse events
  3. Patients in whom follow-up and compliance will not allow careful monitoring
  4. Patients unable to discuss risks to benefits (i.e., those with mental retardation, developmental disability) and for whom no parent or legal guardian is available to provide consent
C. Patients in whom risk-to-benefit ratio is unclear and based on case reports and expert opinion (class III) only, but under certain circumstances, depending on the nature and severity of the patient's seizure disorder, felbamate use may be appropriate
  1. Children with intractable partial epilepsy
  2. Patients with other generalized epilepsies unresponsive to primary agents
  3. Patients who experience unacceptable sedative or cognitive side effects with traditional AEDs
  4. Patients with Lennox-Gastaut syndrome <4 years of age who are unresponsive to other AEDs

Adapted from French J, Smith M, Faught E, et al. Practice advisory: the use of felbamate in the treatment of patients with intractable epilepsy. Report of the Quality Standards Subcommittee of the American Academy of Neurology and the American Epilepsy Society. *Neurology* 1999;52:1540–1546, with permission.

---

determination of the FBM level, as other agents may increase FBM metabolism. To sort out toxic symptoms during polytherapy, concomitant drug levels may be needed.

Monitoring for Adverse Effects

The best protection for patients is education about early symptoms of potentially serious side effects, especially unusual fatigue, pallor, dyspnea, easy bruising, and bleeding, associated with FBM therapy. Evidence suggests that these early symptoms precede laboratory confirmation of hematologic problems in most patients (72). Nausea, vomiting, or jaundice may be indicative of hepatic problems.

Periodic blood testing may not detect adverse events early enough to prevent serious illness or death, but the manufacturer recommends monitoring blood counts and liver function tests. A reasonable schedule is biweekly testing for the first 6 months and monthly for the next 6 months. The lessening of risk after 1 year of therapy requires less frequent testing, perhaps every 3 months during the second year and only if symptoms develop thereafter. At this time, there is no clinical evidence to suggest that aplastic anemia or hepatic failure is related to the FBM dose.

Withdrawal from Felbamate

Dramatic increases in seizure frequency and even status epilepticus can occur with rapid withdrawal from FBM (73). As the dose of FBM is reduced, levels of phenytoin, phenobarbital, and valproate will also decrease. Surveillance for hematologic and hepatic effects is recommended for 6 months after FBM therapy ends, because damage to bone marrow stem cells may not be manifested immediately in peripheral blood counts.

SUMMARY

FBM is especially effective as monotherapy for patients with partial-onset seizures. Animal studies and experience with Lennox-Gastaut syndrome suggest a broad spectrum of activity against generalized seizures as well. FBM is nonsedating, which is a major advantage. Nevertheless, the agent is not easy to use because of the high incidence of troublesome early side effects and many pharmacokinetic interactions.

Serious toxicities preclude FBM use except in those patients who do not achieve complete seizure control with safer agents. However, the combined risk for serious bone marrow or hepatic toxicity with FBM is only about one in 5000 patients, and for death perhaps one in 10,000. These risks are almost certainly less than the risks of continued poor seizure control. Safety may be improved by avoiding FBM use in patients with autoimmune diseases and previous histories of significant cytopenia or drug reactions, including allergic rashes.

ACKNOWLEDGMENT

I am grateful to Linda Brent for the expert preparation of this manuscript.

REFERENCES

1. Nightingale SL. Recommendation to immediately withdraw patients from treatment with felbamate. *JAMA* 1994;272:995.
2. Pellock JM, Brodie MJ. Felbamate: 1997 Update. *Epilepsia* 1997; 38:1261–1264.
3. Swinyard EA, Sofia RD, Kupferberg HJ. Comparative anticonvulsant activity and neurotoxicity of felbamate and four prototype antiepileptic drugs in mice and rats. *Epilepsia* 1986;27:27–34.
4. Sheridan PH, Ashworth M, Milne K, et al. Open pilot study of felbamate (ADD 03055) in partial seizures. *Epilepsia* 1986;27:649.
5. Wilensky AJ, Friel PN, Ojemann LM, et al. Pharmacokinetics of W-554 (ADD 03055) in epileptic patients. *Epilepsia* 1985;26:602–606.
6. Leppik IE, Dreifuss FE, Pledger GW, et al. Felbamate for partial seizures: results of a controlled clinical trial. *Neurology* 1991;141: 1785–1789.
7. Theodore WH, Raubertas RF, Porter RJ, et al. Felbamate: a clinical trial for complex partial seizures. *Epilepsia* 1991;32:392–397.
8. Lian H, Steiner SS, Sofia RD, et al. A self-complementary, self-assembling microsphere system: application for intravenous delivery of the antiepileptic and neuroprotectant compound felbamate. *J Pharm Sci* 2000;89:867–875.
9. Adusumalli VE, Yang JT, Wong KK, et al. Felbamate pharmacokinetics in the rat, rabbit, and dog. *Drug Metab Dispos* 1991;19: 1116–1125.
10. Wlaz P, Loscher W. Anticonvulsant activity of felbamate in amygdala kindling model of temporal lobe epilepsy in rats. *Epilepsia* 1997;38:1167–1172.
11. White HS, Wolf HH, Swinyard EA, et al. A neuropharmacological evaluation of felbamate as a novel anticonvulsant. *Epilepsia* 1992; 33:564–572.
12. McCabe RT, Wasterlain CG, Kucharczyk N, et al. Evidence for anticonvulsant and neuroprotectant action of felbamate mediated by strychnine-insensitive glycine receptors. *J Pharmacol Exp Ther* 1993;264:1248–1252.
13. Kleckner NW, Glazewski JC, Chen CC, et al. Subtype-selective antagonism of N-methyl-D-aspartate receptors by felbamate: insights into the mechanism of action. *J Pharmacol Exp Ther* 1999;289:886–894.
14. Harty TP, Rogawski MA. Felbamate block or recombinant N-methyl-D-aspartate receptors: selectivity for the NR2B subunit. *Epilepsy Res* 2000;39:47–55.
15. Rogawski MA, Wasterlain CG, Mazarati AM. Re: Mazarati et al. "…clinically available [antiepileptic drug] with a moderate affinity for the glycine site of the N-methyl-D-aspartate (NMDA) receptor." *Epilepsia* 2000;41:918–921.
16. DeSarro G, Ongini E, Bertorelli R, et al. Excitatory amino acid neurotransmission through both NMDA and non-NMDA receptors is involved in the anticonvulsant activity of felbamate in DBA/2 mice. *Eur J Pharmacol* 1994;262:11–19.
17. Stefani A, Spadoni F, Barnardi E. Voltage-activated calcium channels: targets of antiepileptic drug activity? *Epilepsia* 1997;38: 959–965.
18. Wasterlain CG, Adams LM, Schwartz PH, et al. Posthypoxia treatment with felbamate is neuroprotective in a rat model of hypoxia-ischemia. *Neurology* 1993;43:2303–2310.
19. Wasterlain CG, Adams LM, Wichmann JK, et al. Felbamate protects CA1 neurons from apoptosis in a gerbil model of global ischemia. *Stroke* 1996;27:1236–1240.
20. Mazarati AM, Baldwin RA, Sofia RD, et al. Felbamate in experimental model of status epilepticus. *Epilepsia* 2000;41:123–127.
21. Mazarati AM, Sofia RD, Wasterlain CG. Anticonvulsant and antiepileptogenic effects of fluorofelbamate in experimental status epilepticus. *Seizure* 2002;11:423–430.
22. Shumaker RC, Fantel C, Kelton E, et al. Evaluation of the elimination of (^{14}C) felbamate in healthy men. *Epilepsia* 1990;31:642.
23. Gudipati RM, Raymond RH, Ward DL, et al. Effect of food on the absorption of felbamate (Felbatol™) in healthy male volunteers. *Neurology* 1992;42:332.
24. Adusumalli VE, Wichmann JK, Kucharczyk N, et al. Drug concentrations in human brain tissue samples from epileptic patients treated with felbamate. *Drug Metab Dispos* 1994;22:168–170.
25. Glue P, Sulowicz W, Colucci R, et al. Single-dose pharmacokinetics of felbamate in patients with renal dysfunction. *Br J Clin Pharmacol* 1997;44:91–93.
26. Yang JT, Adusumalli VE, Wong KK, et al. Felbamate metabolism in the rat, rabbit and dog. *Drug Metab Dispos* 1991;19:1126–1134.
27. Richens A, Banfield CR, Salfi M, et al. Single and multiple dose pharmacokinetics of felbamate in the elderly. *Br J Clin Pharmacol* 1997;44:129–134.
28. Sachdeo RC, Narang-Sachdeo SK, Shumaker RC, et al. Tolerability and pharmacokinetics of monotherapy felbamate doses of 1,200-6,000 mg per day in subjects with epilepsy. *Epilepsia* 1997;38: 887–892.
29. Sachdeo R, Kramer LD, Rosenberg A, et al. Felbamate monotherapy: controlled trial in patients with partial onset seizures. *Ann Neurol* 1992;32:386–392.
30. Faught E, Sachdeo R, Remler M, et al. Felbamate monotherapy for partial onset seizures: an active-control trial. *Neurology* 1993;43: 688–692.

31. Felbatol [package insert]. Cranbury, NJ: Wallace Laboratories; 1999.
32. Pledger GW, Kramer LD. Clinical trials of investigational antiepileptic drugs: monotherapy designs. *Epilepsia* 1991;32: 716–721.
33. Bourgeois BFD, Leppik IE, Sackellares JC, et al. Felbamate double-blind efficacy trial following presurgical monitoring. *Epilepsia* 1991;32:481–486.
34. Leber P. Hazards of inference: the active control investigation. *Epilepsia* 1989;30:S57–S63.
35. Devinsky O, Faught RE, Wilder BJ, et al. Efficacy of felbamate monotherapy in patients undergoing presurgical evaluation of partial seizures. *Epilepsy Res* 1995;20:241–246.
36. Li LM, Nashef L, Moriarty J, et al. Felbamate as add-on therapy. *Eur Neurol* 1996;36:146–148.
37. Carmant L, Holmes GL, Sawyer S, et al. Efficacy of felbamate in therapy for partial epilepsy in children. *J Pediatr* 1994;125:481–486.
38. The Felbamate Study Group in Lennox-Gastaut Syndrome. Efficacy of felbamate in childhood epileptic encephalopathy (Lennox-Gastaut syndrome). *N Engl J Med* 1993;328:29–33.
39. Dodson WE. Felbamate in the treatment of Lennox-Gastaut syndrome: results of a 12-month open-label study following a randomized clinical trial. *Epilepsia* 1993;34:S18–S24.
40. Jensen PK. Felbamate in the treatment of refractory partial-onset seizures. *Epilepsia* 1993;34(Suppl 7):S25–S29.
41. Seigel H, Kelley K, Sterz B, et al. The efficacy of felbamate as add-on therapy to valproic acid in the Lennox-Gastaut syndrome. *Epilepsy Res* 1999;34:91–97.
42. Sachdeo RC, Wagner ML. Felbamate in generalized tonic-clonic seizures. *Epilepsia* 1991;32(Suppl 3):54.
43. Hurst DL, Rolan TD. The use of felbamate to treat infantile spasms. *J Child Neurol* 1995;10:134–136.
44. Leroy RF, Castain T. Pilot study of felbamate in adult medically refractory primary generalized seizure patients. *Epilepsia* 1991;32:13.
45. Devinsky O, Kothari M, Rubin R, et al. Felbamate for absence seizures. *Epilepsia* 1992;33:84.
46. Kuzniecky R, Thompson G, Faught E, et al. Felbamate add-on therapy in intractable atypical absence. *Epilepsia* 1991;32:10.
47. Sachdeo RC, Murphy JV, Kamin M. Felbamate in juvenile myoclonic epilepsy. *Epilepsia* 1992;33(Suppl 3):118.
48. Glue P, Banfield CR, Perhach JL, et al. Pharmacokinetic interactions with felbamate. In vitro-in vivo correlation. *Clin Pharmacokinet* 1997;33:214–224.
49. Sachdeo RC, Narang-Sachdeo SK, Montgomery PA, et al. Evaluation of the potential interaction between felbamate and erythromycin in patients with epilepsy. *Clin Pharmacol Ther* 1998;38:184–190.
50. Albani F, Theodore WH, Washington P, et al. Effect of felbamate on plasma levels of carbamazepine and its metabolites. *Epilepsia* 1991;32:130–132.
51. Graves NM, Holmes GB, Fuerst RH, et al. Effect of felbamate on phenytoin and carbamazepine serum concentrations. *Epilepsia* 1989;30:225–229.
52. Wagner ML, Remmel RP, Graves NM, et al. Effect of felbamate on carbamazepine and its major metabolites. *Clin Pharmacol Ther* 1993;53:536–543.
53. Wagner ML, Graves NM, Leppik IE, et al. The effect of felbamate on valproic acid disposition. *Clin Pharmacol Ther* 1994;56:494–502.
54. Wagner ML, Leppik IE, Graves NM, et al. Felbamate serum concentrations: effect of valproate, carbamazepine, phenytoin, and phenobarbital. *Epilepsia* 1990;31:642.
55. Wagner ML, Graves NM, Marienau K, et al. Discontinuation of phenytoin and carbamazepine in patients receiving felbamate. *Epilepsia* 1991;32:398–406.
56. Tisdel KA, Israel DS, Kolb KW. Warfarin-felbamate interaction: first report [letter]. *Ann Pharmacother* 1994;28:805.
57. Reidenberg P, Glue P, Banfield CR, et al. Effects of felbamate on the pharmacokinetics of phenobarbital. *Clin Pharmacol Ther* 1995;58:279–287.
58. Patrias J, Espe-Lillo J, Titter FJ. Felbamate-methosuximide interaction. *Epilepsia* 1992;33:84.
59. Gidal BE, Kanner A, Maly M, et al. Lamotrigine pharmacokinetics in patients receiving felbamate. *Epilepsy Res* 1997;27:1–5.
60. Hulsman JA, Rentmeester TW, Banfield CR, et al. Effects of felbamate on the pharmacokinetics of the monohydroxy and dihydroxy metabolites of oxcarbazepine. *Clin Pharmacol Ther* 1995;58: 383–389.
61. Kerrick JM, Kelley BJ, Maister BH, et al. Involuntary movement disorders associated with felbamate. *Neurology* 1995;45:185–187.
62. Faught E, Kuzniecky R, Thompson G. Tolerability of high-dose felbamate. *Epilepsia* 1994;35:32.
63. Kaufman DW, Kelly JP, Anderson T, et al. Evaluation of case reports of aplastic anemia among patients treated with felbamate. *Epilepsia* 1997;38:1265–1269.
64. Wallace Laboratories. Research and Development Department. *Felbatol Safety Monograph.* Cranbury, NJ, April 1999.
65. Pellock JM. Felbamate in epilepsy therapy: evaluating the risks. *Drug Saf* 1999;21:225–239.
66. Thompson CD, Barthen MT, Hopper DW, et al. Quantification in patient urine samples of felbamate and three metabolites: acid carbamate and two mercapturic acids. *Epilepsia* 1999;40:769–776.
67. Med Pointe Pharmaceuticals. Personal communication. May 2003.
68. Husain Z, Pinto C, Sofia RD, et al. Felbamate-induced apoptosis of hematopoietic cells is mediated by redox-sensitive and redox-independent pathways. *Epilepsy Res* 2002;48:57–69.
69. Kwan P, Brodie MJ. Early identification of refractory epilepsy. *N Engl J Med* 2000;342:314–319.
70. French J, Smith M, Faught E, et al. Practice advisory: the use of felbamate in the treatment of patients with intractable epilepsy. Report of the Quality Standards Subcommittee of the American Academy of Neurology and the American Epilepsy Society. *Neurology* 1999;52:1540–1546.
71. Leppik IE. Felbamate. *Epilepsia* 1995;36:S66–S72.
72. Kelly JP, Jurgelon JM, Issargrisil S, et al. An epidemiological study of aplastic anemia: relationship of drug exposures to clinical features and outcome. *Eur J Hematol* 1996;37:47–52.
73. Welty TE, Privitera M, Shukla R. Increased seizure frequency associated with felbamate withdrawal in adults. *Arch Neurol* 1998; 55:641–645.

Vigabatrin

66

Elinor Ben-Menachem

HISTORICAL BACKGROUND

Although it was known that decreases in brain gamma-aminobutyric acid (GABA) caused convulsions in animals and agents that enhanced GABA-mediated functions could have an anticonvulsant effect, the first suggestion that GABA might be an inhibitory neurotransmitter came from Elliot and van Gelder in 1958 (1).

Evidence for the anticonvulsant activity of GABA was gleaned from several observations: (a) focal agents that inhibit GABA synthesis, such as thiosemicarbazide and L-allylglycine, are proconvulsive; (b) focal agents that block the postsynaptic action of GABA, such as bicuculline and picrotoxin, are proconvulsive (2); (c) inhibition of glutamic acid decarboxylase (GAD) to block GABA synthesis causes seizures; (d) GABA receptor abnormalities are found in certain genetically determined epileptic syndromes in such animals as gerbils and audiogenic DBA/2 mice; (e) focal cortical infusion of GABA has a potent anticonvulsant effect; (f) drugs that enhance GABA-mediated inhibition are anticonvulsive in many animal models; (g) pyridoxine (i.e., the coenzyme of GAD) deficiency can cause seizures; and (h) pyridoxine or GABA itself can protect against seizures in vitamin B_6–deficient children. These observations, as well as the recognition that GABA concentrations in cerebrospinal fluid (CSF) are decreased in some epileptic syndromes, supported the idea that diminished GABAergic inhibition contributes to seizure susceptibility.

Since the 1970s, several compounds have been developed that affect GABA subtype A ($GABA_A$)-mediated inhibition at different levels and in different ways, depending on their mechanism of action. Vigabatrin (γ-vinyl-GABA) (VGB) is the only selective, irreversible GABA-transaminase (GABA-T) inhibitor that greatly increases whole-brain levels of GABA, presumably making it more available to its receptor site. It may also stimulate GABA release (3). VGB was synthesized in 1977, specifically as a substrate for GABA-T, by Jung and colleagues (4).

VGB is available worldwide, except in the United States, for use as an anticonvulsant. The agent has consistently been shown to be effective in the treatment of partial seizures and infantile spasms. The drug is not approved for use by the US Food and Drug Administration (FDA) because of the discovery of visual peripheral field defects occurring in what is likely more than 30% of patients (5).

GENERAL CHARACTERISTICS

VGB (4-amino-5-hexenoic acid, or γ-vinyl-GABA) is a structural analogue of GABA with a vinyl appendage (Fig. 66.1) rationally designed as an enzyme-activated irreversible, specific inhibitor of GABA-T (6,7). VGB is highly soluble in water, only slightly soluble in ethanol and methanol, and insoluble in hexane and toluene. This white to off-white crystalline solid has a melting point of 171°C to 177°C. The molecular mass is 129.16, and the conversion factor (CF) is 7.75 (mg/L $\times$ CF = μmol/L).

The drug exists as a racemic mixture of $R(-)$ and $S(+)$ isomers in equal proportions and exhibits no optical activity. Pharmacologic activity and toxic effects are associated only with the $S(+)$ enantiomer; the $R(\sigma)$ enantiomer is entirely inactive (8,9). No chiral inversion exists in humans. The major pharmacologic effects are determined by the half-life of the enzyme rather than by the drug or the $S(+)$ enantiomer, because GABA-T, which is the target enzyme, has a much longer half-life than VGB itself (4,10).

MECHANISMS OF ACTION

Animal Studies

VGB causes very specific effects in the brain that are probably related to its anticonvulsant activity. The brain content of GABA, GABA-T, and GAD was measured over time after intraperitoneal injection of vigabatrin 1500 mg/kg into

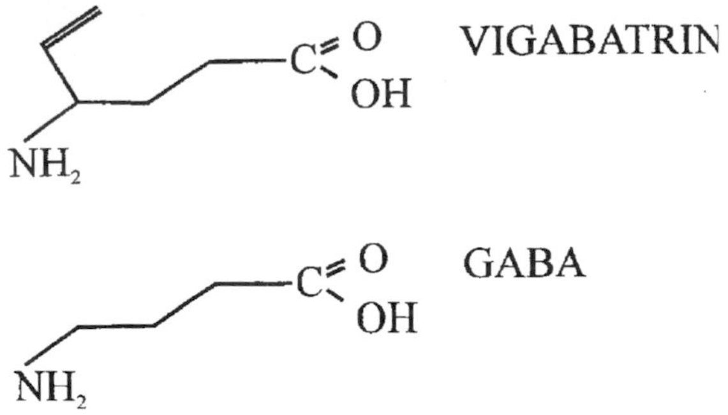

Figure 66.1 Chemical structure of vigabatrin.

mice. By 4 hours, whole-brain GABA had increased 5-fold, and GABA-T activity declined sharply. Recovery to 60% of baseline concentrations occurred after 5 days. A 30% decrease in GAD, demonstrated only at the high dose used, probably results from a feedback mechanism after the sudden increase in GABA concentration (4).

At high doses, VGB increases concentrations of β-alanine (an alternative substrate to GABA-T), homocarnosine (GABA and histidine), and hypotaurine while decreasing glutamine and threonine levels (11). Concentrations of free and total GABA and homocarnosine in the brain and CSF increase parallel to increasing doses of VGB (12).

Anticonvulsant Effects

VGB is inactive against maximal electroshock (MES)-induced seizures, bicuculline (i.e., GABA antagonist)-induced seizures, and pentylenetetrazol-induced seizures, unless injected directly into the midbrain of rats (13); however, an intravenous injection provided seizure protection after bicuculline-induced myoclonic activity (14), strychnine-induced tonic seizures (7), isoniazid-induced generalized seizures (7), audiogenic seizures in mice (15), photic-induced seizures in the baboon (16), and amygdala-kindled seizures in the rat (17).

Stereotaxic injections of small amounts of VGB into certain areas of rat brain provided seizure protection in relation to locally increased GABA levels (13). Seizure protection against MES was most prominent with local GABA increases in the midbrain tegmentum, including substantia nigra and midbrain reticular formation, but VGB injected into the thalamus, hippocampus, and cortex was not protective in this model. Seizure protection lasted up to 72 hours after a single injection to the substantia nigra. It was not until day 5 that the rats responded normally to MES. This finding supports observations that the rate of recovery of GABA-T is 5 days (4) and suggests that the anticonvulsant activity of VGB may be the result of the local increase in GABA levels rather than a direct effect of the drug.

Prevention of Epileptogenesis

Rats treated with saline or VGB were given repeated subconvulsive stimulation to the amygdala in an attempt to stimulate epileptogenesis (18). During 16 stimulations, saline-treated rats developed mild to fully developed generalized seizures, but VGB-treated animals remained seizure free. After a 10-day rest period, the rats previously treated with VGB progressed through the entire kindling procedure before developing fully kindled seizures, whereas saline-treated rats developed seizures immediately.

Neuroprotective Effects

In a Finnish study (19), rats pretreated with VGB were compared with rats pretreated with saline. Stimulation of the perforant pathway caused status epilepticus in all animals. On postmortem examination, the saline-treated rats had hippocampal cell damage and loss of somatostatin-containing interneurons in the dentate gyrus. VGB-treated rats, on the other hand, had histologically normal hippocampi. This finding suggests that VGB may have a neuroprotective effect on the hippocampus during status epilepticus (20).

Human Studies

Grove and associates (21) were the first to investigate the relationship between VGB and GABA in CSF as a means of determining the effects of this antiepileptic drug (AED) on brain neurotransmitters and amino acids. Patients with varied neurologic conditions were given VGB 0.5, 1, 2, or 6 g daily for 3 days. Free and total concentrations of GABA, β-alanine, homocarnosine, and VGB increased in a dose-responsive manner, except with 0.5 g per day, at which level no changes were noted. In another study (22), patients were treated with VGB 0.5 g twice daily, followed by VGB 1 g twice daily for 2 weeks and 2 weeks on placebo. At the end of the treatment, no changes from baseline were reported in homovanillic acid (HVA, the metabolite of dopamine) and 5-hydroxyindoleacetic acid (5-HIAA, the metabolite of serotonin), but dose-related increases were seen in free and total GABA and homocarnosine. At the end of the placebo period, GABA and homocarnosine levels had decreased to baseline values.

No consistent changes have been found in amino acids, HVA, or 5-HIAA in tissue and CSF with VGB 50 mg/kg taken for up to 3.5 years (23,24). In CSF, concentrations of acetylcholine, somatostatin, β-endorphins, prolactin, cyclic adenosine, or guanine monophosphate were also unchanged during long-term treatment (24,25). In a single-dose study, however, HVA and 5-HIAA concentrations increased initially up to 100%, but returned to baseline levels or slightly below after 1 month (10). At a 50-mg/kg dose, VGB caused a 200% to 300% increase in CSF and brain levels of GABA (26,27). A reduction in dose from 3 to 1.5 g per day proportionally decreased GABA levels in CSF (28). Dose and percentage increases in CSF GABA concentrations show a linear relationship. However, the relationship between dose increases and efficacy is more complex and may depend on the type of epilepsy. Kälviäinen and coworkers (29) suggested that responders to VGB monotherapy have higher glutamate levels (increased 14%) in the CSF before receiving the drug than do nonresponders. Nuclear magnetic resonance spectroscopy in patients treated with VGB added to conventional AEDs confirmed results of GABA analysis in CSF (30,31); however, increased levels of glutamine and corresponding decreased levels of glutamate (by 9%) were identified, compared with levels in patients receiving conventional therapy alone.

VGB also affects blood GABA and platelet GABA-T levels. At therapeutic doses of 2 to 3 g per day, platelet GABA-T is markedly reduced. A dose of 2 g per day maximally inhibits platelet GABA-T, with mean inhibition at approximately 70% (32). The concentration of plasma VGB is almost 10-fold that in CSF, and because platelets cannot regenerate GABA-T, the effect of VGB on this test system is also influenced by platelet regeneration.

ABSORPTION, DISTRIBUTION, AND METABOLISM

Absorption

Rate of Absorption

Peak VGB concentration is reached within 2 hours following administration of doses between 0.5 and 3 g (8,33,34). The absorption half-life ranges from 0.18 to 0.59 hours, and the mean terminal half-life is 5 to 7 hours. Approximately 60% to 80% of VGB can be recovered unchanged in a 24-hour urine collection, indicating a bioavailability of at least 60% to 80%. No metabolites are found in the urine, and the remaining amount of VGB probably disappears, as it is bound to GABA-T.

Effect of Food

The area under the curve (AUC) for fasted and fed volunteers was not significantly different, indicating that food does not affect the extent of absorption. The time of administration and the composition of food and time of eating should not influence clinical response (35,36).

Distribution

Body Tissues and Fluids

The apparent volume of distribution of VGB is 0.8 L/kg (total body water is 0.6 L/kg) in volunteers, with the half-life of distribution at 1 to 2 hours. A comparison of the extrapolated (or initial) volume of distribution with the steady-state volume reveals that between 50% and 75% of VGB is outside the central blood compartment at steady state (22).

In one study of patients with epilepsy, the concentration of VGB in CSF was approximately 10% of blood levels (10). In this study, patients taking concomitant AEDs were given a single dose of VGB 50 mg/kg, and CSF and blood samples were taken for up to 5 days following the treatment. The highest VGB concentrations were found in CSF after the first sample. By 24 hours, only a trace was detectable in

CSF, and no VGB was found at 72 hours or thereafter. Peak concentration in the blood was reached in 1 hour, decreasing thereafter to only small amounts detectable by 72 hours. The mean elimination half-life was 4.5 hours, and the AUC was 310 nmol/mL per hour. The VGB-CSF-to-blood ratio was 0.10. After a 3-year follow-up with doses of 50 mg/kg per day, CSF VGB levels were not significantly increased compared with the 6-month levels (23).

Protein Binding

VGB does not bind to plasma proteins and does not cause hepatic induction through cytochrome P450–dependent enzymes (33,37).

Distribution in Placenta and Breast Milk

Passage of $S(+)$ and $R(-)$ VGB across the human placenta *in vitro* showed a low level of transfer from maternal to fetal blood and was comparable to that of other α-amino acids. Clearance for both enantiomers was about 27% of phenazone (38). The maximum amount of VGB that a nursing infant would ingest per day is approximately 3.6% of the $R(-)$ and 1% of the $S(+)$ enantiomer of the maternal dose of VGB (39).

Distribution in Children

Children demonstrate a lower AUC than adults, but renal clearance is the same in both populations. Children may need higher doses of VGB to achieve the same effect seen in adults.

Metabolism

Because no metabolites have been identified, it can be assumed that VGB is not metabolized in humans. Up to 82% of the oral dose is excreted unchanged in the urine (Aventis, data on file).

Elimination

Half-Life and Rate of Excretion

The elimination half-life of VGB is 5 to 8 hours, and the total clearance is about 1.7 to 1.9 mL/kg per min, with renal clearance accounting for 70% of the total. Elimination is not influenced by dose or duration of treatment (40). The biologic half-life is measured in days, not in hours.

Elimination in the Elderly

Renal and total-body clearances are slower in the elderly. Terminal half-life showed an inverse relationship to renal function, probably because of a smaller volume of distribution in patients with lower creatinine clearance (33). In patients with low renal clearance, extrarenal clearance may be compensatory. Reduced renal clearance causes an increase in the AUC-to-body-weight ratio. Patients with renal impairment, therefore, have higher plasma concentrations of VGB and a longer terminal half-life. The half-life in the elderly with reduced creatinine clearance is approximately twice that in normal healthy volunteers. The AUC in elderly adults is 7-fold higher than in younger individuals because of reductions in renal clearance and volume of distribution. A nonlinear increase in the AUC-to-body-weight ratio occurs as creatinine clearance falls to < 60 mg per min.

EFFICACY

Adults

More than 18 years of clinical experience have confirmed the efficacy of VGB for patients with partial seizures and other specific seizure types.

Single-Blind Studies

Meta-analysis of the first 10 single-blind studies of VGB, enrolling 352 patients with highly intractable partial seizures, demonstrated that 55.8% of those treated had their seizure frequency reduced by more than 50% (22,28,41–48). Another single-blind study (49) involved less severely intractable patients who had been experiencing four partial seizures per month, but were all socially integrated and active outpatients. Of these 19 patients, 14 (73%) had a seizure reduction greater than 50%, and 10 (53%) patients had a seizure reduction greater than 70%. Two patients developed new myoclonic jerks. No deleterious effects on cognitive function were noted.

Double-Blind Studies

In Europe, six double-blind, placebo-controlled crossover studies published in the late 1980s provided the basis for registration of VGB in most countries.

In two studies, some patients experienced generalized tonic-clonic seizures (50,51); their inclusion in the efficacy analysis revealed no significant difference from the placebo groups. When these patients without partial seizures were omitted, both studies showed highly significant results in favor of VGB, as did the remaining four studies, which included only patients with partial epilepsy. In these six trials, the VGB dose ranged from 2 to 3 g per day as add-on therapy to standard AEDs. Between 0% and 7% of patients became seizure free, and between 33% and 64% had a seizure reduction greater than 50% (50–55). In another double-blind study (56) of 33 patients with refractory partial seizures, 60% had their seizures reduced by greater than 50%.

Two large, double-blind, parallel-design studies in the United States (57,58) and one in Canada (59) involved 467 patients with complex partial seizures with or without secondary generalization. VGB 1, 3, and 6 g per day was associated with a statistically significant reduction in seizures compared with placebo. In the Canadian study, 48% of the patients experienced a 50% seizure reduction, compared with 26% in the placebo group.

Monotherapy

A single-center, open-label, randomized, parallel-group study from Finland (60) compared carbamazepine and VGB as the initial agent for patients with new-onset seizures. Patients were included independent of seizure type. During the 1-year follow up, partial seizures were controlled in 21 of 50 patients taking VGB and in 25 of 50 taking carbamazepine. More carbamazepine-treated patients dropped out as a result of adverse events (12 versus 0 with VGB), and more VGB-treated patients discontinued therapy because of lack of efficacy (14 versus four with carbamazepine).

A randomized, response-conditional, crossover study (61) compared VGB and carbamazepine in 51 patients. Slightly more patients were seizure free with carbamazepine as the initial agent (51.3% versus 45.9% with VGB); only 21% of VGB-treated patients reported side effects, compared with 41% of carbamazepine-treated patients.

In an open, randomized study (62), 70 children received either carbamazepine (n = 32) or VGB (n = 38) for the treatment of new-onset partial seizures and were followed for 2 years. VGB was administered at 50 to 60 mg/kg per day and carbamazepine at 15 to 30 mg/kg per day. Efficacy variables did not differ significantly between treatments, but fewer side effects were reported with VGB.

A large, double-blind, multicenter trial of 459 adults showed that VGB was less effective than carbamazepine in controlling seizures, but as in the Finnish study, patients in the VGB group reported fewer side effects. Therefore, VGB has never received a monotherapy indication because the equivalence studies were negative (63).

Long-Term Studies

Among the numerous follow-up studies published, some reported results over more than 10 years. About 60% of initial responders showed continued benefits, suggesting that tolerance probably does not occur. Breakthrough seizures occurred, but it is not clear whether any other concomitant AED therapy had been reduced or withdrawn (43,64–70).

Children

Partial Seizures

In an open trial (71), 135 children with varied seizure types received VGB (40 to 80 mg/kg per day). Of these, 11 patients (8%) became seizure free, and 37% had a seizure reduction greater than 50%—results that are similar to those in the adult studies. Patients with partial seizures responded best. In another study (72) of 16 children with refractory epilepsy, those with partial seizures had the most favorable response. Myoclonic epilepsy tended to be aggravated.

Infantile Spasms

The first report that VGB could be effective in patients with this notoriously intractable type of seizure dates from 1991 (73). In this uncontrolled study of 70 VGB-treated children, 37 had a significant reduction in spasms. Most impressive were the patients with symptomatic infantile spasms and 71% with tuberous sclerosis became completely seizure free. In the long-term follow-up (74), 55% of the patients continued to have no seizures, including all those with tuberous sclerosis. Results from a 2-year follow-up in the United Kingdom noted that at the time of the report, 20 patients (3 to 11 months of age) had been treated with VGB as the initial AED; 14 had symptomatic disease. Starting doses of 50 to 80 mg/kg per day reached a maximum daily dose of 150 mg/kg. Of these 20 patients, 13 were free of seizures for 30 months, four children showed no response, and three had reductions of more than 75% but were not seizure free. Response to VGB occurred within 72 hours of initiation of therapy. No side effects were reported in the 20 patients.

In another long-term follow up (75) of 23 children treated with VGB for infantile spasms, 11 were seizure free at 3 months. After 5 years, 72% of 18 evaluable patients had been completely controlled for 1 year or more. Side effects were present in only 10% of patients. Of the children evaluated, 55% eventually developed other types of seizures. Mental function was normal in two children, four were moderately retarded, and 11 had severe retardation. These results are comparable to those with long-term corticotropin treatment but with fewer side effects.

Three separate VGB comparative trials have been conducted. The first study examined high-dose VGB versus low-dose VGB. In 2001, Elterman (76) found that the time to response in 67 patients randomized to high-dose VGB (100 to 148 mg/kg per day) was shorter than the time to response in 75 patients randomized to low-dose VGB (18 to 36 mg/kg per day; $p = 0.04$). A 1997 study by Chiron and colleagues (77) compared VGB with hydrocortisone in patients with West syndrome caused by tuberous sclerosis. VGB therapy stopped the occurrence of spasms in 100% of the patients with tuberous sclerosis, compared with 45% in hydrocortisone-treated patients ($p <0.01$) (77). In an open-label, response-mediated, crossover study comparing VGB and adrenocorticotrophic hormone (ACTH), there was no evidence of a difference in spasm cessation between ACTH-treated patients and VGB-treated patients in the first phase; however, ACTH was superior to VGB in stopping spasms if both phases were considered (81% versus 46%, respectively, $p <0.01$) (78).

The results of a randomized, double-blind study have now been published (79), demonstrating that VGB as the first agent to be used in infantile spasms was more effective than placebo.

Lennox-Gastaut Syndrome

Of the few published reports, some noted increases in seizure frequency following VGB therapy initiated in patients with Lennox-Gastaut syndrome and myoclonic epilepsy (80,81). Other studies described significant improvement (82,83), perhaps reflecting the dose administered. Patients with Lennox-Gastaut syndrome require lower VGB doses than those with other seizure types. Rarely, myoclonic jerks may develop during VGB treatment, necessitating withdrawal of the drug.

Interactions with Other Agents

Because VGB is not metabolized and is excreted unchanged in the urine, it does not interact significantly with other drugs. Phenytoin was the only coadministered agent with a mean decrease in serum concentration of 20% or less in two early placebo-controlled clinical trials (42,54). Phenobarbitone and primidone levels were also significantly reduced, but only in one study (32). Attempts to elucidate the nature of the phenytoin reduction (32,84) have been unsuccessful, as no changes in protein binding, or in phenytoin absorption, metabolism, or clearance, have been detected. Evidence is lacking that any loss of efficacy accompanied these lower concentrations or that the dosage of phenytoin or phenobarbitone requires alteration.

Adverse Events

Reports of adverse events are based on more than 18 years of clinical experience and marketed use. In clinical trials, sedation and fatigue were the most commonly reported side effects; about 2% of patients withdrew from treatment because of intolerability (Aventis, data on file). Seven studies on the cognitive effects of VGB treatment confirm no decline in performance and even an improvement in certain test scores (35,49,85–88).

Whether VGB can elicit psychosis has prompted intense discussion in the past 4 years. An early description of severe psychiatric reactions in 14 of 210 patients (89,90) has been followed by published case reports and warnings. Two multicenter, placebo-controlled, double-blind studies (57,58) completed in the United States analyzed psychiatric side effects to clarify the issues raised by the various nonblinded reports in the literature. In the studies, which excluded patients with severe brain damage or psychiatric disorders, 2.2% (n = 45) taking VGB 1 g per day, 6.6% (n = 135) taking VGB 3 g per day, and 7.3% (n = 41) taking VGB 6 g per day withdrew because of a psychiatric adverse event. These results support the contention that severe psychiatric adverse events occur in about 5% of VGB-treated patients with no prior psychiatric disease. A large postmarketing surveillance study (Aventis data on file) reported manifest psychosis, hallucinations, paranoia, or delusions in only 88 (0.64%) of more than 6000 patients—a rate not greater than that seen with other AEDs (91,92). Psychiatric problems are common in patients with intractable epilepsy, especially those with focal seizures. The data do not suggest that VGB elicits psychosis more often than other AEDs; however, patients with a history of severe psychiatric disturbances or severe brain damage should initially be given low doses, with upward titration proceeding with caution. Sudden withdrawal of VGB can lead to postictal psychosis.

Chronic Toxicity

Until reports of visual field defects surfaced in 1997, little information was available on the possible effects of VGB on vision or on the association of VGB with other chronic toxicities. However, it was previously noted that VGB caused an inactivation of GABA-T in the rat retina more than in other brain regions (93). Now these abnormalities are the primary reason for the FDA's lack of approval of the agent. To date, no available evidence demonstrates that visual field defects are related to the use of other AEDs.

In one of the first descriptions of this problem, in 1998 Mackenzie and Klistoner (94) reported that visual defects can be asymptomatic, which probably explains why they escaped prior observation. A reduction in the cone system may be caused by dysfunction of GABAergic cells of the inner retina (95).

The best controlled study of this problem (5), by Kälviäinen and coworkers, evaluated 19 patients taking carbamazepine and 32 patients taking VGB by analyzing the results of visual field testing. Asymptomatic concentric defects were documented in 41% of the VGB group and in none of the carbamazepine group. The defects seemed to be irreversible when VGB treatment was stopped. One report described two children (ages 10 and 15 years) with concentric visual field defects similar to those in adults (96). In another study (97), a cohort of 155 presurgical patients were retrospectively examined. All had undergone visual field analysis and 64% had been treated with VGB. Patients with visual field defects were then reexamined. It was found that the prevalence of visual field defects increased significantly with an increase in VGB dose, from 4% in those with a total life dose of <1 kg to 75% in patients with a total life dose of 3 to 4 kg. Twelve patients were reexamined 2 to 10 years after cessation of VGB therapy. All had visual field defects as before, except for 5 in whom the fields had worsened. This study has been confirmed by others (98).

Teratogenicity

No serious teratogenic effects in animals have been reported with VGB therapy, except for an increased incidence of cleft palate in rabbits receiving a high dose. As with all AEDs, VGB has a class warning against use in pregnancy because of inadequate evidence of any teratogenic effects. Information on more than 100 pregnancies in women undergoing VGB therapy notes the concomitant use of at least one additional AED in almost all patients (99). No pattern of reported abnormalities suggests that VGB has a specific teratogenic effect, but the results are inconclusive.

CLINICAL USE

Administration

Most clinical trials have used VGB dosages between 2 and 3 g daily. In the United States double-blind study, VGB 6 g per day produced a somewhat higher rate of seizure-free patients, but at the expense of more side effects (57). The consensus today is that 3 g per day is an average effective dose in adults. At 50 mg/kg per day, CSF GABA levels increase by 200% to 300%. Tapering should commence if this dose is not effective. In light of the information that cumulative doses of VGB can increase the risk for visual field defects, one should strive to treat with the lowest possible dose.

In children, dosage is determined according to body weight. Because bioavailability is lower in this patient population, the dose range is between 45 and 150 mg/kg. If 150 mg/kg is not effective, the dose should be tapered and the drug probably discontinued.

VGB can be administered once or twice per day. The tablet is tasteless, dissolves completely in fluid, and can be given to infants or children in water, juice, or milk.

Titration

In the early studies, the full VGB dose was given immediately. Today, gradual increases are recommended to prevent side effects and, especially, to reduce the frequency of such psychiatric or behavioral reactions as confusion or depression. Some patients with mild forms of epilepsy may respond to lower doses, thereby decreasing the need to titrate upward to a full dose.

For patients with severe brain damage, as in Lennox-Gastaut syndrome, it is recommended to initiate therapy at 500 mg per day, with dose titration no faster than the addition of one 500-mg tablet each week.

Discontinuation

To avoid rebound seizures, which can elicit postictal behavioral abnormalities or even status epilepticus, VGB therapy should never be stopped abruptly. A good rule is to taper the dose by 500 mg every fifth day, stabilizing the GABA level at a somewhat lower level with each reduction.

Laboratory Monitoring

Blood and CSF VGB concentrations can be measured easily through a single-step protein precipitation with subsequent precolumn derivatization with *o*-phthaldialdehyde and direct injection into a Microsorb C18 column (100). Samples spiked with other AEDs did not interfere with the assay. This type of high-pressure liquid chromatography method requires only a 50-mL sample for analysis. Other methods include a newer, and supposedly more rapid isocratic high-performance liquid chromatographic assay (101).

Clinical Monitoring

It is not necessary to monitor blood levels of VGB, which is effective only by virtue of its inhibition of GABA-T, rendering actual drug levels irrelevant. Blood levels are not even appropriate for determining compliance. A full dose of VGB taken in the morning before an appointment yields a clinically acceptable blood level.

CONCLUSION

VGB is an important treatment for complex partial seizures and infantile spasms. However, in some patients, long-term use has been associated with visual field defects and retinal changes. Except for the treatment of infantile spasms, for which it is still a first-line agent, VGB should be used cautiously, with regularly scheduled ophthalmologic examinations, including visual field tests.

REFERENCES

1. Elliot KAC, van Gelder NM. Occlusion and metabolism of gamma-aminobutyric acid by brain tissue. *J Neurochem* 1958;3: 28–40.
2. Piredda S, Lim CR, Gale K. Intracerebral site of convulsant action of bicuculline. *Life Sci* 1985;56:1295–1298.
3. Schechter PJ. Vigabatrin. In: Meldrum B, Porter RJ, eds. *New anticonvulsant drugs*. London: John Libbey, 1986;265–275.
4. Jung MF, Lippert B, Metcalf BW, et al. gamma-Vinyl GABA (4-amino-hex-5-enoic acid), a new selective irreversible inhibitor of GABA-T: effects on brain GABA metabolism in mice. *J Neurochem* 1977;29:797–802.
5. Kälviäinen R, Nousiainen I, Mantyjarvi M. Initial vigabatrin monotherapy is associated with increased risk of visual field constriction: a comparative follow-up study with patients on initial carbamazepine monotherapy and healthy controls. *Epilepsia* 1998;39(Suppl 6):72.
6. Lippert B, Metcalf B, Jung MJ, et al. 4-Amino-hex-5-enoic acid, a selective catalytic inhibitor of 4-aminobutyric acid aminotransferase in mammalian brain. *Eur J Biochem* 1977;74:441–445.
7. Schechter PJ, Tranier Y, Grove J. Attempts to correlate alterations in brain GABA metabolism by GABA-T inhibitors with their anticonvulsant effects. In: Mandel P, DeFeudes FV, eds. *GABA—Biochemistry and CNS functions*. New York: Plenum Press. 1979; 43–57.
8. Haegele KD, Schechter PJ. Kinetics of the enantiomers of vigabatrin after an oral dose of the racemate or the active S-enantiomer. *Clin Pharmacol Ther* 1986;40:581–586.
9. Rey E, Pons G, Richard MO, et al. Pharmacokinetics of the individual enantiomers of vigabatrin (gamma-vinyl GABA) in epileptic children. *Br J Clin Pharmacol* 1990;30:253–257.
10. Ben-Menachem E, Persson LI, Schechter PJ, et al. Effects of single doses of vigabatrin on CSF concentrations of GABA, homocarnosine, homovanillic acid and 5-hydroxyindoleacetic acid in patients with complex partial epilepsy. *Epilepsy Res* 1988;2: 96–101.
11. Perry TL, Kish SJ, Hansen S. Gamma-vinyl GABA: effects of chronic administration on the metabolism of GABA and other amino compounds in rat brain. *J Neurochem* 1979;32:1641–1645.
12. Palfreyman MG, Bîhlen P, Huot S, et al. The effect of gamma-vinyl GABA and gamma-acetylenic GABA on the concentration of homocarnosine in brain and CSF of the rat. *Brain Res* 1980; 190:288–292.
13. Gale K. Role of the substantia nigra in GABA-mediated anticonvulsant actions. In: Delgado-Escueta AV, Ward AA, Woodbury DM, et al, eds. *Basic mechanisms of the epilepsies. molecular and cellular approaches*. New York: Raven Press. 1986;44:343–364.
14. Kendall DA, Fox DA, Enna SJ. Effects of gamma-vinyl GABA on bicuculline-induced seizures. *Neuropharmacology* 1981;20: 351–355.
15. Schechter PJ, Tranier Y. Effect of elevated brain GABA concentrations on the actions of bicuculline and picrotoxin in mice. *Psychopharmacology* 1977;54:145–148.
16. Meldrum BS, Horton R. Blockade of epileptic responses in the photosensitive baboon, *Papio papio*, by two irreversible inhibitors of GABA-transaminase, gamma-acetylenic GABA (4-amino-hex-5-ynoic acid) and gamma-vinyl GABA (4-amino-hex-5-enoic acid). *Psychopharmacology* 1978;59:47–50.
17. Stevens JR, Phillips I, de Beaurepaire R. Gamma-vinyl GABA in endopiriform area suppresses kindled amygdala seizures. *Epilepsia* 1988;29:404–411.
18. Shin C, Rigsbee LC, McNamara JO. Anti-seizure and anti-epileptogenic effect of gamma-vinyl gamma-aminobutyric acid in amygdaloid kindling. *Brain Res* 1986;398:370–374.
19. Ylinen A, Miettinen R, Pitkänen A, et al. Enhanced GABAergic inhibition preserves hippocampal structure and function in a model of epilepsy. *Proc Natl Acad Sci U S A* 1991;88: 7650–7653.
20. Pitkänen A, Tuunanen J, Halonen T. Vigabatrin and carbamazepine have different efficacies in the prevention of status epilepticus induced neuronal damage in the hippocampus and amygdala. *Epilepsy Res* 1996;24:29–45.
21. Grove J, Fozard JR, Mamont PS. Assay of alpha-difluoromethylornithine in body fluids and tissues by automatic amino-acid analysis. *J Chromatogr* 1981;223:409–416.
22. Schechter PJ, Hanke NF, Grove J, et al. Biochemical and clinical effects of gamma-vinyl GABA in patients with epilepsy. *Neurology* 1984;34:182–186.
23. Ben-Menachem E, Persson LI, Mumford JP. Effect of long term vigabatrin therapy on selected CSF neurotransmitter concentrations. *J Child Neurol* 1991;6(Suppl 2):11–16.
24. Sivenius MRJ, Ylinen A, Murros K, et al. Double-blind dose reduction study of vigabatrin in complex partial epilepsy. *Epilepsia* 1987;28:688–692.
25. Pitkänen A, Halonen T, Ylinen A, et al. Somatostatin, beta-endorphin, and prolactin levels in human cerebrospinal fluid during the gamma-vinyl-GABA treatment of patients with complex partial seizures. *Neuropeptides* 1987;9:185–195.
26. Ben-Menachem E, Mumford J, Hamberger A. Effect of long-term vigabatrin therapy on GABA and other amino acid concentrations in the central nervous system: a case study. *Epilepsy Res* 1993;16:241–243.
27. Ben-Menachem E, Persson LI, Schechter PJ, et al. The effect of different vigabatrin treatment regimens on CSF biochemistry and seizure control in epileptic patients. *Br J Clin Pharmacol* 1989;27:79S–85S.
28. Gram L, Lyon BB, Dam M. Gamma-vinyl GABA: a single-blind trial in patients with epilepsy. *Acta Neurol Scand* 1983;68:34–39.
29. Kälviäinen R, Halonen T, Pitkänen A, et al. Amino acid levels in the cerebrospinal fluid of newly diagnosed epileptic patients: effect of vigabatrin and carbamazepine monotherapy. *J Neurochem* 1993;60:1244–1250.
30. Petroff OA, Rothman DL. Measuring human brain GABA in vivo: effects of GABA-transaminase inhibition with vigabatrin. *Mol Neurobiol* 1998;16:97–121.
31. Petroff OAC, Rothman DL, Behar KL, et al. Initial observations on effect of vigabatrin on in vivo ^{1}H spectroscopic measurements of gamma-aminobutyric acid, glutamate, and glutamine in human brain. *Epilepsia* 1995;36:457–464.
32. Richens A. Pharmacology and clinical pharmacology of vigabatrin. *J Child Neurol* 1991;6(Suppl):2S7–2S10.
33. Haegele KD, Huebert ND, Ebel M, et al. Pharmacokinetics of vigabatrin: implications of creatinine clearance. *Clin Pharmacol Ther* 1988;44:558–565.
34. Saletu B, Grunberger J, Linzmayer L, et al. Psychophysiological and psychometric studies after manipulating the GABA system by vigabatrin, a GABA-transaminase inhibitor. *Int J Psychophysiol* 1986;4:63–80.
35. Frisk-Holmberg M, Kerth P, Meyer P. Effect of food on the absorption of vigabatrin *Br J Clin Pharmacol* 1989;27:23S–25S.
36. Hoke JF, Chi EM, Antony K, et al. Effect of food on the bioavailability of vigabatrin tablets. *Epilepsia* 1991;32(Suppl 3):7.

37. Mumford JP. A profile of vigabatrin. *Br J Clin Pract* 1988; 42 (Suppl 61):7–9.

38. Challier JC, Rey E, Bintein T, et al. Passage of S(+) and R(–) gamma-vinyl-GABA across the human isolated perfused placenta. *Br J Clin Pharmacol* 1992;34:139–143.

39. Tran A, O'Mahoney T, Rey E, et al. Vigabatrin: placental transfer in vivo and excretion into breast milk of the enantiomers. *Br J Clin Pharmacol* 1998;45:409–411.

40. Grant SM, Heel RC. Vigabatrin: a review of its pharmacodynamic and pharmacokinetic properties, and therapeutic potential in epilepsy and disorders of motor control. *Drugs* 1991;41:889–926.

41. Besser R, Kramer G. Long-term efficacy and safety of vigabatrin in epileptic patients [abstract 155]. In: Program and abstracts of the 18th International Epilepsy Congress. New Delhi: India, 1989.

42. Browne TR, Mattson RH, Penry JK, et al. Vigabatrin for refractory complex partial seizures: multicenter single-blind study with long-term follow-up. *Neurology* 1987;37:184–189.

43. Cocito L, Maffini M, Perfumo P, et al. Vigabatrin in complex partial seizures: a long-term study. *Epilepsy Res* 1989;3:160–166.

44. Faedda MT, Lani C, Paris L, et al. Clinical results of vigabatrin treatment in patients with refractory epilepsy. In: Manelis J, Bental E, Loeber JN, et al, eds. *Advances in epileptology.* New York: Raven Press, 1989;170–171.

45. Michelucci R, Plasmati RM, Larmeggiani I, et al. Single-blind placebo-controlled dose modification study of vigabatrin in patients with refractory epilepsy. *Epilepsia* 1991;32(Suppl 1): S102.

46. Mumford JP, Dam M. Meta-analysis of placebo controlled studies of vigabatrin in drug resistant epilepsy. *Br J Clin Pharmacol* 1989;27:101S–107S.

47. Otto FG, Egli M. Effect of vigabatrin (gamma-vinyl GABA) on partial attacks of various localizations. In: Scheffner D, ed. *Epilepsy 90.* Reinbek, Germany: Einhoen-Presse Verlag, 1991; 230–232.

48. Ried S, Schmidt D, Stodieck SRG, et al. Vigabatrin in pharmaco-resistant epilepsies: a single-blind placebo-controlled study. In: Scheffner E, ed. *Epilepsy 90.* Reinbek: Einhorn-Presse Verlag, 1991;233–237.

49. de Bittencourt PRM, Mazer S, Marcourakis T, et al. Vigabatrin: clinical evidence supporting rational polytherapy in management of uncontrolled seizures. *Epilepsia* 1994;35:373–380.

50. Remy C, Favel P, Tell G. Double-blind, placebo-controlled, crossover study of vigabatrin in drug resistant epilepsy of the adult. *Boll Lega Ital Epil* 1986;54–55:241–243.

51. Tassinari CA, Michelucci R, Ambrosetto G, et al. Double-blind study of vigabatrin in the treatment of drug-resistant epilepsy. *Arch Neurol* 1987;44:907–910.

52. Gram L, Klosterskov P, Dam M. Gamma-vinyl GABA: a double-blind, placebo-controlled trial in partial epilepsy. *Ann Neurol* 1985;17:262–266.

53. Loiseau P, Hardenberg JP, Pestre M, et al. Double-blind, placebo-controlled study of vigabatrin (gamma-vinyl GABA) in drug-resistant epilepsy. *Epilepsia* 1986;27:115–120.

54. Rimmer EM, Richens A. Double-blind study of gamma-vinyl GABA in patients with refractory epilepsy. *Lancet* 1984;1: 189–190.

55. Tartara A, Manni R, Galimberti CA, et al. Vigabatrin in the treatment of epilepsy: a double-blind, placebo-controlled study. *Epilepsia* 1986;27:717–723.

56. Ring HA, Heller AJ, Farr IN, et al. Vigabatrin: rational treatment for chronic epilepsy. *J Neurol Neurosurg Psychiatry* 1990;53: 1051–1055.

57. Dean C, Mosier M, Penry K. Dose-response study of vigabatrin as add-on therapy in patients with uncontrolled complex partial seizures. *Epilepsia* 1999;40:74–82.

58. French JA, Mosier M, Walker S, et al. A double-blind, placebo-controlled study of vigabatrin three g/day in patients with uncontrolled complex partial seizures. Vigabatrin Protocol 024 Investigative Cohort. *Neurology* 1996;46:54–61.

59. Bruni J, Guberman A, Vachon L, et al. Vigabatrin as add-on therapy for adult complex partial seizures: a double-blind, placebo-controlled multicentre study. The Canadian Vigabatrin Study Group. *Seizure* 2000;9:224–232.

60. Kälviäinen R, Aikia M, Saukkonen AM, et al. Vigabatrin vs carbamazepine monotherapy in patients with newly diagnosed epilepsy. A randomized, controlled study. *Arch Neurol* 1995;52: 989–996.

61. Tanganelli P, Regesta G. Vigabatrin vs. carbamazepine monotherapy in newly diagnosed focal epilepsy: a randomized response conditional cross-over study. *Epilepsy Res* 1996;25:257–262.

62. Zamponi N, Cardinali C. Open comparative long-term study of vigabatrin vs carbamazepine in newly diagnosed partial seizures in children. *Arch Neurol* 1999;56:605–607.

63. Chadwick D. Safety and efficacy of vigabatrin and carbamazepine in newly diagnosed epilepsy: a multicentre randomized double-blind study. Vigabatrin European Monotherapy Study Group. *Lancet* 1999; 354:13–19.

64. Browne TR, Mattson RH, Penry JK, et al. Multicenter long-term safety and efficacy study of vigabatrin for refractory complex partial seizures: an update. *Neurology* 1991;41:363–364.

65. Michelucci R, Veri L, Passarelli D, et al. Long-term follow-up study of vigabatrin in the treatment of refractory epilepsy. *J Epilepsy* 1994;7:88–93.

66. Remy C, Beaumont D. Efficacy and safety of vigabatrin in the long-term treatment of refractory epilepsy. *Br J Clin Pharmacol* 1989;27(Suppl 1):125S–129S.

67. Reynolds EH, Ring HA, Farr IN, et al. Open, double-blind and long-term study of vigabatrin in chronic epilepsy. *Epilepsia* 1991;32:530–538.

68. Sivenius J, Ylinen A, Murros K, et al. Efficacy of vigabatrin in drug-resistant partial epilepsy during a 6-year follow-up period. *Epilepsia* 1991;32(Suppl 1):11.

69. Tartara A, Manni R, Galimberti CA, et al. Vigabatrin in the treatment of epilepsy: a long-term follow-up study. *J Neurol Neurosurg Psychiatry* 1989;52:467–471.

70. Ylinen A, Salmenoera T, Mumford JP, et al. Long-term treatment with vigabatrin—10 years of clinical experience. *Seizure* 1999;8: 181–183.

71. Livingston JH, Beaumont D, Arzimanoglou A, et al. Vigabatrin in the treatment of epilepsy in children. *Br J Clin Pharmacol* 1989;27(Suppl 1):109S–112S.

72. Luna D, Dulac O, Pajot N, et al. Vigabatrin in the treatment of childhood epilepsies: a single-blind placebo-controlled study. *Epilepsia* 1989;30:430–437.

73. Chiron C, Dulac O, Beaumont D, et al. Therapeutic trial of vigabatrin in refractory infantile spasms. *J Child Neurol* 1991;6(Suppl 2): S52–S59.

74. Appleton RE. Vigabatrin in the management of generalized seizures in children. *Seizure* 1995;4:45–48.

75. Siemes H, Brandl U, Spohr HL, et al. Long-term follow-up study of vigabatrin in pretreated children with West syndrome. *Seizure* 1998;7:293–297.

76. Elterman R. Randomized trial of vigabatrin in patients with infantile spasms. *Neurology* 2001;57:1416–1421.

77. Chiron C, Dumas C, Jambaque I, et al. Randomized trial comparing vigabatrin and hydrocortisone in infantile spasms due to tuberous sclerosis. *Epilepsy Res* 1997;26:389–395.

78. Vigevano F, Cilio MR. Vigabatrin versus ACTH as first-line treatment for infantile spasms: a randomized, prospective study. *Epilepsia* 1997;38:1270–1274.

79. Appleton RE, Peters AC, Mumford JP, et al. Randomised, placebo-controlled study of vigabatrin as first-line treatment of infantile spasms. *Epilepsia* 1999; 40:1627–1633.

80. Lortie A, Chiron C, Mumford J, et al. The potential for increasing seizure frequency, relapse, and appearance of new seizure types with vigabatrin. *Neurology* 1993;43(Suppl 5):S24–S27.

81. Michelucci R, Tassinari CA. Response to vigabatrin in relation to seizure type. *Br J Clin Pharmacol* 1989;27(Suppl 1):119S–124S.

82. Feucht M, Brantner-Inthaler S. Gamma-vinyl GABA (vigabatrin) in the therapy of Lennox-Gastaut syndrome: an open study. *Epilepsia* 1994;35:993–998.

83. Herranz JL, Arteaga R, Farr IN, et al. Dose-response study of vigabatrin in children with refractory epilepsy. *J Child Neurol* 1991;6(Suppl 2):S45–S51.

84. Rimmer EM, Richens A. Interaction between vigabatrin and phenytoin. *Br J Clin Pharmacol* 1989;27:27S–33S.

85. Dijkstra JB, McGuire AM, Trimble MR. The effect of vigabatrin on cognitive function and mood. *Hum Psychopharmacol* 1992;7:329.
86. Dodrill CB, Arnett JL, Sommerville KW, et al. Evaluation of the effects of vigabatrin on cognitive abilities and quality of life. *Neurology* 1993;43:2501–2507.
87. Grunewald RA, Thompson PJ, Corcoran R, et al. Effects of vigabatrin on partial seizures and cognitive function. *J Neurol Neurosurg Psychiatry* 1994;57:1057–1063.
88. Provinviali L, Bartolini M, Mari F, et al. Influence of vigabatrin on cognitive performance and behaviour in patients with drug-resistant epilepsy. *Acta Neurol Scand* 1996;94:12–18.
89. Sander JWAS, Hart YM. Vigabatrin and behaviour disturbances. *Lancet* 1990;335:57.
90. Sander JWAS, Hart YM, Trimble MR, et al. Behavioral disturbances associated with vigabatrin therapy. *Epilepsia* 1991; 34(Suppl 1):12.
91. Matsuo F, Bergen D, Faught E, et al. Placebo-controlled study of efficacy and safety of lamotrigine in patients with partial seizures. *Neurology* 1993;43:2284–2291.
92. Wolf P. The use of antiepileptic drugs in epileptology with respect to psychiatry. *Neuropsychobiology* 1993;27:127–131.
93. Sills GJ, Patsalos PN, Butler E, et al. Visual field constriction: accumulation of vigabatrin but not tiagabine in the retina. *Neurology* 2001;57:196–200.
94. Mackenzie R, Klistorner A. Severe persistent visual field constriction associated with vigabatrin: asymptomatic as well as symptomatic defects occur with vigabatrin. *BMJ* 1998;316:233.
95. Krauss GL, Johnson MA, Miller NR. Vigabatrin-associated retinal cone system dysfunction: electroretinogram and ophthalmologic findings. *Neurology* 1998;50:614–618.
96. Vanhatalo S, Pääkkonen L, Nousiainen I. Visual field constriction in children treated with vigabatrin. *Neurology* 1999;52: 1713–1714.
97. Malmgren K, Ben-Menachem E, Frisen L. Vigabatrin visual toxicity: evolution and dose dependence. *Epilepsia* 2001;42: 609–615.
98. Newman WD, Tocher K, Acheson JF. Vigabatrin associated visual field loss: a clinical audit to study prevalence, drug history and effects of drug withdrawal. *Eye* 2002;16:567–571.
99. Mumford JP. Epilepsy, pregnancy and vigabatrin. *Int Med Newsl* 1994;2:2–4.
100. Tsanaclis LM, Wicks J, Williams J, et al. Determination of vigabatrin in plasma by reversed-phase high-performance liquid chromatography. *Ther Drug Monit* 1991;13:251–253.
101. Chollet DF, Goumaz L, Juliano C, et al. Fast isocratic high-performance liquid chromatographic assay method for the simultaneous determination of gabapentin and vigabatrin in human serum. *J Chromatogr B Biomed Sci Appl* 2000;746:311–314.

Adrenocorticotropin and Steroids

67

Melinda A. Nolan   *O. Carter Snead III*

HISTORICAL BACKGROUND

The first report of the efficacy of adrenocorticotropin (ACTH) therapy for childhood seizures appeared in 1950, when Klein and Livingston (1) observed benefits in various types of intractable generalized seizures. Eight years later, Sorel and Dusaucy-Bauloye (2) reported control of seizures and an improvement in electroencephalographic (EEG) findings for children with infantile spasms treated with the drug. The benefit of oral steroids in this condition was established soon after that of ACTH (3–7), and since then, both drugs have been used in a number of epilepsy syndromes, including Ohtahara syndrome, Lennox-Gastaut syndrome, other myoclonic epilepsies, and Landau-Kleffner syndrome.

The epilepsy syndromes that respond uniquely to ACTH and steroid therapy have an age-related onset during a critical period of brain development, as well as a characteristic regression or plateau of acquired milestones at seizure onset and long-term cognitive impairment. In addition to beneficial effects on the convulsive state, ACTH or steroids, or both, can improve the short-term developmental trajectory and the long-term prognosis for language and cognitive development in at least some of these patients (8–12).

INFANTILE SPASMS

General Considerations

In 1841, West first described infantile spasms in his own son as "a peculiar form of infantile convulsions" (13). Later, their association with the sequelae of severe mental deficiency became clear. The EEG manifestations of infantile spasms—the high-voltage chaotic slowing with multifocal spikes and marked asynchrony—were identified in 1952 by Gibbs and Gibbs, who called the disorder *hypsarrhythmia* (14). Thus the creation of the definition of West syndrome: a triad of infantile spasms, hypsarrhythmia, and developmental regression or mental retardation.

Published studies on the efficacy of ACTH and corticosteroids in infantile spasms display considerable variability in design, complicating the establishment of research-based recommendations for optimal treatment. A few observations are generally accepted. The cumulative spontaneous remission rate over the first 12 months of seizures is about 25% (15). Seizures are almost always intractable to treatment with traditional anticonvulsant drugs. ACTH or oral steroid therapy should significantly reduce seizures in 50% to 75% of patients, but ACTH protocols, particularly those employing high-dose, long-acting synthetic formulations, are associated with a significantly high rate of side effects (16,17). The best chance for a treatment response is probably between 4 and 12 months of age in children who are neurologically normal when spasms that have no demonstrable cause begin (11,12,16,18–20). The ultimate prognosis is dismal for most patients and depends heavily on the cause of the spasms, preexisting neurologic and developmental status, the presence or absence of other seizures concomitant with the spasms, and the patient's age at seizure onset (8,12,16,21–24).

The controversies surrounding the treatment of infantile spasms outnumber the areas of agreement. Which is the most effective therapy: ACTH or steroids; other anticonvulsants such as vigabatrin, valproic acid, benzodiazepines, topiramate, or zonisamide; pyridoxine; some or all of these in combination; or yet another treatment? What is the impact of treatment with ACTH compared with steroids or anticonvulsants on long-term outcome in recurrence of spasms, evolution into other forms of intractable epilepsy, and cognitive or behavioral function? Does treatment change the outcome for a patient with preexisting mental retardation and a structurally abnormal brain? What is the optimal dosage of these drugs, and how long should treatment last? Does the ultimate outcome depend on timing of treatment? Does the efficacy of ACTH depend on the formulation (natural vs. synthetic, sustained vs. short-acting)? Most of these questions remain unanswered.

Mechanisms of Action

The pathogenesis of infantile spasms and therefore the mechanism of action of ACTH and steroids in this condition are unknown, principally because an animal model for this disorder is lacking (25). Infantile spasms begin within a narrow range of ages, and various abnormalities are causally linked; however, infantile spasms may also occur without apparent cause. The effect of ACTH and corticosteroids is frequently all or nothing, and the steroid-induced seizure-free state is often sustainable even after drug withdrawal. These observations support the theory that the developing brain experiences a significant stress response to various etiologies that results in this age-dependent epileptic encephalopathy. Within this very narrow developmental window, ACTH and steroids may be able to reset the deranged homeostatic mechanisms of the brain, thereby reducing the convulsive tendency and improving the developmental trajectory.

The Brain-Adrenal Axis

Evidence suggests that the effects of ACTH on infantile spasms may be independent of steroidogenesis. Efficacy studies have demonstrated the superiority of ACTH to corticosteroids in treating infantile spasms and its efficacy in adrenal-suppressed patients (26–29). Substantial physiologic and pharmacologic data indicate that ACTH has direct effects on brain function: increasing dendrite outsprouting in immature animals (30); stimulating myelination (31); regulating the synthesis, release, uptake, and metabolism of dopamine, norepinephrine, acetylcholine, serotonin, and γ-aminobutyric acid; regulating the binding at glutamatergic, serotonergic, muscarinic type 1, opiate, and dopaminergic receptors (32,33); and altering neuronal membrane lipid fluidity, permeability, and signal transduction (30). These neurobiologic effects can influence synaptic function and neurotransmission and may reside in fragments of the peptide devoid of corticotropic activity.

ACTH has a down-regulatory effect on corticotropin-releasing hormone (CRH), and low ACTH levels have been found in the cerebrospinal fluid of children with infantile spasms (34,35). CRH is an excitatory neuromodulator, with potent age-specific convulsant effects demonstrated in animal models (34,36). ACTH reduces CRH gene expression in specific brain regions, an effect demonstrated

in the absence of adrenal steroids and achieved with use of only the 4 to 10 fragment of ACTH, which does not release adrenal steroids (28). Melanocortin-receptor antagonists blocked this effect, suggesting that these are the targets of ACTH action (28).

An hypothesis can therefore be generated, in which a stress response enhances CRH expression, leading to neuronal hyperexcitability and seizures. By suppressing CRH expression, possibly through the action of peptide fragments of ACTH on melanocortin receptors, hyperexcitability may be reduced, ameliorating infantile spasms. Clinical trials of ACTH fragments without activity on adrenals have yielded disappointing results (37,38), but these studies used the 4 to 9 rather than the 4 to 10 peptide fragment studied in animal models (28). The events that precipitate this proposed endocrine abnormality remain unclear.

Efficacy and Dosage

Table 67.1 lists the formulations of ACTH. The biologic activity, expressed in international units (IU), permits a comparison of potency but represents the relative ability of the peptide to stimulate the adrenals and may not reflect its ability to affect brain function. The biologic activity of natural ACTH in the brain may differ from that of synthetic ACTH (12) as a result of ACTH fragments and possibly other pituitary hormones with neurobiologic activity in the brain that are present in the pituitary extracts. These compounds could enhance the therapeutic efficacy of natural ACTH (39). Any differences in the biologic effects of sustained ACTH levels provided by the depot formulations, as opposed to those of the short-acting preparations, are unknown. Given in high doses, however, long-acting depot preparations are associated with an increased incidence of severe side effects, including death from overwhelming infection (17).

Although most efficacy studies of ACTH and steroids are retrospective, an expanding body of prospective data is available (12,23,40–50). Most published literature supports the hypothesis that the natural ACTH 1 to 39 peptide (p-ACTH) is superior to oral steroids. In randomized, controlled trials, spasms ceased in 42% to 87% of children treated with ACTH, compared with 29% to 33% of children treated with prednisone (43–47). Respective relapse rates were 15% to 31% and 29% to 33%.

The most effective dose of p-ACTH for remission of spasms is, however, controversial. Notably, compared with prednisone, no major advantage was demonstrated by low doses of ACTH, whereas high doses were superior (43,44). High-dose p-ACTH (60 IU per day or 150 IU/m^2 per day) has produced excellent short-term response rates (87% to 93%) in prospective studies (43,48). In the only randomized, prospective comparison of p-ACTH, however, Hrachovy and associates (45) found no difference between high-dose and low-dose therapy. A prospective

TABLE 67.1

PREPARATIONS OF DEPOT CORTICOTROPIN

Preparation	Biologic Activity (100 IU)[a] Equivalent to	Duration of Action (h)
Short-acting forms		
Corticotropin (ACTH 1–39)—porcine pituitary extract		
Acthar gel, 80 IU/mL	0.72 mg	24–48
ACTH-carboxymethyl-cellulose	Not available	~24
Cosyntropin/tetracosactin (ACTH 1–24)—synthetic		
Cortrosyn	1.0 mg	~24
Long-acting forms		
Cosyntropin/tetracosactin (ACTH 1–24)—synthetic		
Synacthen-zinc	2.5 mg	~72
Cortrosyn-Z	2.5 mg	~72

[a]Commercial preparations are described in international units (IU), based on a potency assay in hypophysectomized rats in which depletion of adrenal ascorbic acid is measured after subcutaneous ACTH injection.

study of synthetic ACTH (47) by Yanagaki and colleagues compared very-low-dose (0.2 IU/kg per day) and low-dose (1 IU/kg per day) ACTH and found equivalent efficacy, with response and relapse rates comparable to those in other studies. Describing a stepwise increase in dosage, Heiskala and coworkers (50) demonstrated that while some patients can be controlled on lower doses of carboxymethyl-cellulose ACTH (3 IU/kg per day), others required high doses (12 IU/kg per day). Spasms were controlled initially in 65% of patients, but the rate of relapse was high.

A good response to ACTH appears to be associated with better long-term outcome (20). Some evidence supports high-dose ACTH over low-dose ACTH or oral steroids in cognitive outcome (9,11). Glaze and colleagues (40) found no difference between low-dose p-ACTH (20 to 30 IU per day) and prednisone (2 mg/kg per day). In a comparison of high-dose p-ACTH (110 IU/m² per day) and steroids, however, Lombroso (12) showed a higher rate of normal cognitive outcome in cryptogenic patients treated with ACTH than in those treated with prednisone alone (55% versus 17%). In a retrospective comparison of different ACTH dosage regimens (51), Ito and coworkers also noted a positive correlation between dose and developmental outcome.

Although data support high-dose ACTH as being more effective than low-dose ACTH, the precise dosage and duration are undetermined. The optimal dose may lie between 50 and 200 IU/m² per day. Doses of 400 IU/m² per day or higher are contraindicated because of a high incidence of life-threatening side effects (16,17,50).

In the face of controversy about the risks and benefits of high-dose ACTH therapy, an alternate approach, as outlined by Shields and Koh in [G2]Chapter 21, is to

begin with 40 IU per day for 1 to 2 weeks, increasing to 60 or 80 IU per day thereafter if the response is incomplete. If spasms and hypsarrhythmia resolve, ACTH is tapered over 1 to 4 months. If therapy at these doses is not successful, ACTH is rapidly tapered and another medication is tried.

Adverse Effects

ACTH and steroids, particularly at the high doses recommended for infantile spasms, can produce dangerous side effects. These are more frequent and more pronounced with ACTH. In prospective controlled trials, cushingoid features and extreme irritability were seen frequently; hypertension, while less common, was associated with higher doses (44–47). Vigilance is required for signs of sepsis, pneumonia, glucosuria, metabolic abnormalities involving the electrolytes calcium and phosphorus (52–54), and congestive heart failure (55,56). Of five deaths reported in prospective studies, at least two were directly attributable to ACTH (12,49).

Cerebral ventriculomegaly (47,57–61), which is not always reversible (40), can lead to subdural hematoma (62,63). The cause of the apparent cerebral atrophy is obscure, but its existence emphasizes the importance of diagnostic neuroimaging before initiation of ACTH.

Because hypothalamic-pituitary or adrenocortical dysfunction can result from ACTH therapy (64,65), morning levels of cortisol should be monitored during a taper and any medical stress treated with high-dose steroids (66). Treatment with ACTH or steroids can also be immunosuppressant and associated with infectious complications, perhaps as a result of impaired function of polymorphonuclear leukocytes (67). Both agents are therefore contraindicated in the face of serious bacterial or viral infection such as varicella or cytomegalovirus. Because of the high rate of fatal *Pneumocystis* pneumonia as an infectious complication of ACTH therapy (17,68–70), prophylaxis with trimethoprim-sulfamethoxazole, accompanied by folate supplementation and frequent blood counts, may be prudent in infants older than 2 months of age. In rare cases, ACTH can exacerbate seizures (71,72).

Vigabatrin Versus Adrenocorticotropin

Based on data from randomized controlled trials, from 23% to 65% of children treated with vigabatrin achieve short-term remission of infantile spasms, with relapse rates of 4% to 20% (46,73,74). Vigabatrin is particularly effective against infantile spasms associated with tuberous sclerosis, producing response rates up to 100% in several prospective trials (46,75,76), and is frequently advocated as a first-line therapy. Limiting its use is the characteristic concentric constriction of visual fields. This effect does occur in childhood, and the risk may be cumulative with longer duration of therapy (77–81). The incidence in very young children is not known, and perimetric testing is often impossible in this group. Electrophysiologic studies in infants, although not as sensitive as perimetry, have confirmed vigabatrin-associated abnormalities (80–82). Vigabatrin may have a place as a short-term treatment, although its safety remains uncertain.

The only published prospective comparison with ACTH (46) used depot ACTH at 10 IU per day and vigabatrin at 100 to 150 mg/kg per day. The initial response rate favored ACTH by 74% over 48% for the vigabatrin group. ACTH also normalized EEG findings more rapidly and more completely regardless of cause. Vigabatrin was better tolerated than ACTH. Prospective data on long-term outcome after vigabatrin treatment are still lacking.

Other Agents in Infantile Spasms

Valproate (83,84), nitrazepam (85), pyridoxine (86), felbamate (87), intravenous immunoglobulin (88), topiramate (89), zonisamide (90), ganaxolone (91), and the ketogenic diet (92) have been studied in small uncontrolled trials. However, there is insufficient evidence of efficacy and safety to recommend any of these therapies at this time.

Recommended Protocols for Adrenocorticotropin

The optimal dose of ACTH required to enhance short-term response and long-term cognitive outcome is unknown; however, relatively high doses given early in the disease, accompanied by a second course in the event of relapse, appear warranted. The following high-dose ACTH regimen that has been used successfully in more than 500 children (43,48,93) is recommended (Table 67.2).

The child is admitted to a daycare unit for initiation therapy. Parents are taught to administer the injection, measure urine glucose three times daily with Chemstix, and recognize spasms so as to keep an accurate seizure calendar. Any diagnostic workup indicated by clinical circumstances is also performed, including screening for occult infections. Before ACTH is started, an endocrine profile, complete blood count, urinalysis, electrolyte panel, baseline renal function tests, and calcium, phosphorus, and serum glucose levels are obtained. Blood pressure is measured and an electrocardiogram performed. The drug is not given if any of these studies show abnormal results. Diagnostic neuroimaging is indicated before initiation of ACTH or steroids because of the association with ventriculomegaly.

The initial dose of ACTH is 150 IU/m^2 per day of ACTH gel, 80 IU/mL, intramuscularly in two divided doses for 1 week. In the second week, 75 IU/m^2 per day is given, followed by 75 IU/m^2 every other day in the third week. Over the next 6 weeks, the dose is gradually tapered. The lot number of the ACTH gel is carefully recorded. Usually, a response is seen within the first 7 days; if within 2 weeks no response is noted or a steroid effect is evident, the lot is changed.

Blood pressure must be measured daily at home during the first week and three times weekly thereafter. Control of hypertension is attempted with salt restriction and amlodipine therapy rather than discontinuation of ACTH. The patient is monitored in the outpatient clinic weekly for the first month and then biweekly, with appropriate blood work at each visit. Waking and sleeping EEG patterns are obtained during and after the start of ACTH to assess treatment response. Because a response is usually noted within a week or two of initiating ACTH (42,43,45), positive results are suggested when properly trained parents report no seizures in a child whose waking and sleeping EEG patterns are normal.

If relapse occurs, the dose may be increased to the previously effective dose for 2 weeks and another tapering begun. If seizures continue, the dose may be increased to 150 IU/m^2 per day and the regimen restarted.

Recommended Protocols for Prednisone

If prednisone is chosen because of its oral formulation and lower incidence of serious side effects, the pretreatment laboratory evaluation described earlier is performed. The initial dose is 3 mg/kg per day in four divided doses for 2 weeks, followed by a 10-week taper (93). A multiple-daily-dose regimen of high-dose ACTH therapy is recommended to produce sustained elevations of plasma cortisol (42,48).

OTHER SEIZURE DISORDERS

The Ohtahara and Lennox-Gastaut syndromes are believed to represent earlier and later manifestations, respectively,

TABLE 67.2

PROTOCOL FOR ACTH THERAPY FOR INFANTILE SPASMS

Initial Assessment Before Therapy Begins

History and physical examination including Wood's light
EEG with pyridoxine injection
Blood counts, routine blood chemical analysis, urinalysis including glucose, thyroid and adrenal
   function tests
Electrocardiogram
Magnetic resonance imaging of brain
Family counseling and education for administration and monitoring of side effects

Clinical Monitoring During ACTH Therapy

Blood pressure and urine dipstick for glucose: daily first week, then thrice weekly
Blood counts, routine blood chemical analysis weekly first month, then fortnightly
EEG once during and after therapy and as indicated
Provide family with letter describing treatment and prompting urgent assessment in case of fever
   or other signs of infection

High-Dose Schedule for ACTH

Week 1	150 IU/m^2 per day IM, two divided doses
Week 2	75 IU/m^2 per day IM, single daily dose
Reassess:	If spasms stop and hypsarrhythmia resolves, continue with taper; if no clinical or EEG response, change ACTH lot or select alternative therapy and taper ACTH as appropriate
Week 3	75 IU/m^2 per day IM, alternate days
Week 4	60 IU/m^2 per day IM, alternate days
Week 5	50 IU/m^2 per day IM, alternate days
Week 6	40 IU/m^2 per day IM, alternate days
Week 7	30 IU/m^2 per day IM, alternate days
Week 8	20 IU/m^2 per day IM, alternate days
Week 9	10 IU/m^2 per day IM, alternate days
Week 10	5 IU/m^2 per day IM, alternate days, then stop ACTH

Lower-Dose Schedule for ACTH

Week 1 & 2	40 IU per day

If response is complete: taper ACTH over 1–4 months
If response is incomplete: increase to 60–80 IU per day over 1–2 weeks
If response remains incomplete: taper ACTH and try other medications

of a spectrum of infantile epileptic encephalopathies that include infantile spasms (94–97). These conditions respond poorly to traditional anticonvulsant drug therapies but are sometimes improved by the antiepileptic drugs used in infantile spasms: ACTH, steroids, benzodiazepines, and valproic acid. ACTH or steroids also may be beneficial in Landau-Kleffner syndrome.

Ohtahara Syndrome

Also known as early infantile epileptic encephalopathy, Ohtahara syndrome is characterized by spasms beginning within the first 3 months of life associated with persistent burst suppression on the EEG in all stages of the sleep-wake cycle (94). Despite reports of improvement after ACTH (94,98), vigabatrin (99), and zonisamide (94), the long-term prognosis usually is unchanged by any treatment (94,96) and involves high mortality and severely handicapped survivors. If used, ACTH should be administered as described for infantile spasms.

Lennox-Gastaut Syndrome and Other Myoclonic Disorders

ACTH and steroids have been found useful in younger children with various combinations of severe and intractable seizures, particularly atypical absence, myoclonic, tonic, and atonic seizures (1,29,93,100–105). This group includes patients with Lennox-Gastaut syndrome, a disorder characterized by mental retardation, generalized slow spike-and-wave discharges, intractable atypical absence, myoclonus, and frequent ictal falls. Several uncontrolled, retrospective studies suggest that ACTH is superior to oral steroids against these seizure types (93,100,102,103), and the regimen described in this chapter for ACTH or prednisone is recommended. Nevertheless, ACTH and steroids should be reserved for the most severe and intractable disease. Usually, the best result is temporary relief, because 70% to 90% of patients with multiple seizure types suffer a relapse during the ACTH taper (93).

In another age-dependent disorder first described by Doose (106), myoclonic astatic seizures begin between 7 months to 6 years of age in a previously normal child and are associated with generalized discharges on the EEG (107). This disorder is resistant to most conventional antiepileptic drugs; however, a retrospective study has reported response to the ketogenic diet, ACTH, and ethosuximide (107).

Landau-Kleffner Syndrome and Related Disorders

Described in 1957 (108), Landau-Kleffner syndrome, also known as acquired epileptic aphasia, is characterized by regression in receptive and expressive language associated with epileptic seizures. The usual presentation occurs between the ages of 2 and 8 years. Clinical seizures may precede, be coincident with, or develop after the onset of language deterioration, and up to 25% of patients with language loss and epileptiform EEG patterns never experience clinical seizures (109,110). Behavioral disturbances are frequent, ranging from hyperactivity and aggressiveness to autism and global cognitive deterioration. Some children display sustained agnosia and mutism; others show a waxing and waning course that parallels the EEG changes; still others demonstrate spontaneous resolution (110). The EEG typically shows 1- to 3-Hz high-amplitude spike and slow waves; these may be unilateral, bilateral, unifocal, or multifocal but often include the temporal region, with or without parietal and occipital involvement, and are activated in sleep (111).

Valproate and benzodiazepines may control the syndrome's clinical seizures but have only a partial and transient effect on the EEG abnormalities (10,112). In 1974, McKinney and McGreal described the beneficial effect of ACTH on the characteristic seizures, language regression, and behavioral change (113). Since then, although no controlled prospective trials of ACTH or steroids have been published, case reports and retrospective series have demonstrated improvements in seizure control and language in children treated with varying ACTH or corticosteroid regimens (10,110–112,114–116).

The use of ACTH or corticosteroids in patients with Landau-Kleffner syndrome appears justified; however, further study of dose and duration of therapy is warranted, as is exploration of new anticonvulsants. High-dose ACTH or prednisone, as described in this chapter for infantile spasms, may be useful, with a longer tapering schedule and concomitant use of valproic acid.

ACKNOWLEDGMENTS

This work was supported in part by the Bloorview Children's Hospital Foundation.

REFERENCES

1. Klein R, Livingston S. The effect of adrencorticotrophic hormone in epilepsy. *J Pediatr* 1950;37:733–742.
2. Sorel L, Dusaucy-Bauloye A. A propos de cas d'hypsarythmia de Gibbs: son traitement spectulaire par l'ACTH. *Acta Neurol Belg* 1958;58:130–141.
3. Dumermuth G. Über die Blitz-Nick-Salaam-Krämpfe und ihre Behandlung mit ACTH und Hydrocortison. *Mitt Helv Pediatr Acta* 1959;14:250–270.
4. Gastaut H, Salfiel J, Raybaud C, et al. A propos du traitement par l'ACTH des encéphalites myoclonique de la première enfance avec majeure (hypsarythmie). *Pediatrie* 1959;14:35–45.
5. Low N. Infantile spasms with mental retardation, I: treatment with cortisone and adrenocorticotrophin. *Pediatrics* 1958;22:1165–1169.
6. McQuarrie I, Anderson JA, Ziegler RR. Observations on the antagonistic effects of posterior pituitary and cortico-adrenal hormones in the epileptic subject. *J Clin Endocrinol* 1942;2: 406–410.
7. Stamps FW, Gibbs EL, Rosenthal IM, et al. Treatment of hypsarrhythmia with ACTH. *JAMA* 1959;171:408–411.
8. Koo B, Hwang P, Logan W. Infantile spasms: outcome and prognostic factors of cryptogenic and symptomatic groups. *Neurology* 1993;43:2322–2327.
9. Lerman P, Kivity S. The efficacy of corticotropin in primary infantile spasms. *J Pediatr* 1982;101:294–296.
10. Marescaux C, Hirsch E, Finck S, et al. Landau-Kleffner syndrome: a pharmacologic study of five cases. *Epilepsia* 1990;31:768–777.
11. Sher PK, Sheikh MR. Therapeutic efficacy of ACTH in symptomatic infantile spasms with hypsarrhythmia. *Pediatr Neurol* 1993;9:451–456.
12. Lombroso C. A prospective study of infantile spams: clinical and therapeutic correlations. *Epilepsia* 1983;24:135–158.
13. West W. On a peculiar form of infantile convulsions. *Lancet* 1841;1:724–725.
14. Gibbs FA, Gibbs EL. *Atlas of electroencephalography, II: epilepsy.* Cambridge, MA: Addison-Wesley, 1952.
15. Hrachovy RA, Glaze DG, Frost JD. A retrospective study of spontaneous remission and long-term outcome in patients with infantile spasms. *Epilepsia* 1991;32:212–214.
16. Riikonen R. A long-term follow-up study of 214 children with the syndrome of infantile spasms. *Neuropediatrics* 1982;13:14–23.
17. Riikonen R, Donner M. ACTH therapy in infantile spasms: side effects. *Arch Dis Child* 1980;55:664–672.
18. Chevrie J, Aicardi J. Le prognostic psychique des spasms infantiles traités par l'ACTH ou les corticoïdes. Analyse statistique de 78 cas suivis plus d'un an. *J Neurol Sci* 1971;12:351–368.
19. Jeavons PM, Bower BD, Dimitrakoudi M. Long-term prognosis of 150 cases of "West syndrome." *Epilepsia* 1973;14:153–164.
20. Riikonen R. Long-term outcome of West syndrome: a study of adults with a history of infantile spasms. *Epilepsia* 1996; 37:367–372.
21. Dulac O, Plouin P, Jambaque I, et al. Benign epileptic infantile spasms. *Rev Electroencephalogr Neurophysiol Clin* 1986;16:371–382.
22. Favata I, Leuzzi V, Curalto P. Mental outcome in West syndrome: prognostic value of some clinical factors. *J Ment Defic Res* 1987; 31:9–15.
23. Nolte R, Christen HJ, Doerrer J. Preliminary report of a multicenter study on the West syndrome. *Brain Dev* 1988;10:236–244.
24. Pollack MA, Zion TE, Kellaway PR. Long term prognosis of patients with infantile spasms following ACTH therapy. *Epilepsia* 1979;20:255–260.
25. Snead OC III. Neuropeptides and infantile spasms: search for an animal model. In: Porter R, ed. *Advances in epileptology: XVth Epilepsy International Symposium.* New York: Raven Press, 1984:193–196.
26. Crosley CJ, Richman RA, Thorpy MJ. Evidence for cortisol-independent anticonvulsant activity of adrenocorticotropic hormone in infantile spasms. *Ann Neurol* 1980;8:220.

27. Farwell J, Milstein J, Opheim K, et al. Adrenocorticotropic hormone controls infantile spasms independently of cortisol stimulation. *Epilepsia* 1984;25:605–608.
28. Brunson K, Khan N, Eghbal-Ahmadi M, et al. Corticotropin (ACTH) acts directly on amygdala neurons to down-regulate corticotropin-releasing hormone gene expression. *Ann Neurol* 2001;49:304–312.
29. Willig RP, Lagenstein I, Iffland E. Cortisoltagesprofile unter ACTH und Dexamethason-Therapie fruhkindlicher Anfalle (BNS- und Lennox-Syndrom). *Monatsschr Kinderheilk* 1977;126:191–197.
30. Pranzatelli MR. On the molecular mechanism of adrenocorticotrophic hormone in the CNS: neurotransmitters and receptors. *Exp Neurol* 1994;125:142–161.
31. Palo J, Savolainen H. The effect of high dose synthetic ACTH on rat brain. *Brain Res* 1974;70:313–320.
32. Pranzatelli MR. In vivo and in vitro effects of adrencorticotropic hormone on serotonin receptors in neonatal rat brain. *Dev Pharmacol Ther* 1989;12:49–56.
33. Kendall DA, McEwen BS, Enne SJ. The influence of ACTH and corticosterone on ^{3}[H]GABA receptor binding in rat brain. *Brain Res* 1982;236:365–374.
34. Baram TZ, Mitchell WG, Snead OC III, et al. Brain-adrenal axis hormones are altered in CSF of infants with massive infantile spasms. *Neurology* 1992;42:1171–1175.
35. Nagamitsu S, Matsuishi T, Yamashita Y, et al. Decreased cerebrospinal fluid levels of β-endorphin and ACTH in children with infantile spasms. *J Neural Transm* 2001;108:363–371.
36. Baram TZ, Hirsch E, Snead OC III, et al. Corticotropin-releasing hormone-induced seizures in infant rats originate in the amygdala. *Ann Neurol* 1992;31:488–494.
37. Pentella K, Bachman DS, Sandman CA. Trial of an ACTH 4 9 analog (ORG 2766) in children with intractable seizures. *Neuropediatrics* 1982;13:59–62.
38. Willig RP, Lagenstein I. Use of ACTH fragments in children with intractable seizures. *Neuropediatrics* 1982;13:55–58.
39. Snead OC III, Chiron C. Medical treatment. In: Dulac O, Chugani HT, Dalla Bernadina B, eds. *Infantile spasms and West syndrome.* London: WB Saunders. 1994:244–256.
40. Glaze DG, Hrachovy RA, Frost JD, et al. Prospective study of outcome of infants with infantile spasms treated during controlled studies of ACTH and prednisone. *J Pediatr* 1988;112:389–396.
41. Hrachovy RA, Frost JD, Kellaway PR, et al. A controlled study of prednisone therapy in infantile spasms. *Epilepsia* 1979;20:403–407.
42. Hrachovy RA, Frost JD, Kellaway P, et al. A controlled study of ACTH therapy in infantile spasms. *Epilepsia* 1980;21:631–636.
43. Baram TZ, Mitchell WG, Tournay A, et al. High-dose corticotropin (ACTH) versus prednisone for infantile spasms: a prospective, randomized, blinded study. *Pediatrics* 1996;97:375–379.
44. Hrachovy RA, Frost JD, Kellaway P, et al. Double-blind study of ACTH vs. prednisone therapy in infantile spasms. *J Pediatr* 1983;103:641–645.
45. Hrachovy RA, Frost JD, Glaze DG. High dose, long duration vs low dose, short duration corticotropin therapy in infantile spasms. *J Pediatr* 1994;124:803–806.
46. Vigevano F, Cilio MR. Vigabatrin versus ACTH as first-line treatment for infantile spasms: a randomized, prospective study. *Epilepsia* 1997;38:1270–1274.
47. Yanagaki S, Oguni H, Hayashi K, et al. A comparative study of high-dose and low-dose ACTH therapy for West syndrome. *Brain Dev* 1999;21:461–467.
48. Snead OC III, Benton JW, Hosey LC, et al. Treatment of infantile spasms with high-dose ACTH: efficacy and plasma levels of ACTH and cortisol. *Neurology* 1989;39:1027–1031.
49. Kusse MC, van Nieuwenhuizen O, van Huffelen AC, et al. The effect of non-depot ACTH(1-24) on infantile spasms. *Dev Med Child Neurol* 1993;35:1067–1073.
50. Heiskala H, Riikonen R, Santavuori P, et al. West syndrome: individualized ACTH therapy. *Brain Dev* 1996;18:456–460.
51. Ito M, Okuno T, Fujii T, et al. ACTH therapy in infantile spasms: relationship between dose of ACTH and initial effect or long-term prognosis. *Pediatr Neurol* 1990;6:240–244.
52. Hanefeld F, Sperner J, Rating D, et al. Renal and pancreatic calcification during treatment of infantile spasms with ACTH. *Lancet* 1984;1:901–904.
53. Rausch HP. Medullary nephrocalcinosis and pancreatic calcifications demonstrated by ultrasound and CT in infants after treatment with ACTH. *Radiology* 1984;153:105–107.
54. Riikonen R, Simell O, Jääskeläinen J, et al. Disturbed calcium and phosphate homeostasis during treatment with ACTH of infantile spasms. *Arch Dis Child* 1986;61:671–676.
55. Tacke E, Kupferschmid C, Lang D. Hypertrophic cardiomyopathy during ACTH treatment. *Klin Padiatr* 1983;195:124–128.
56. Alpert BS. Steroid-induced hypertrophic cardiomyopathy in an infant. *Pediatr Cardiol* 1984;5:117–118.
57. Deona T, Voumard C. Reversible cerebral atrophy and corticotropin. *Lancet* 1979;2:207–209.
58. Glaze DG, Hrachovy RA, Frost JD, et al. Computed tomography in infantile spasms: effects of hormonal therapy. *Pediatr Neurol* 1986;2:23–27.
59. Konishi Y, Yasujima M, Kuriyama M, et al. Magnetic resonance imaging in infantile spasms: effects of hormonal therapy. *Epilepsia* 1992;33:304–309.
60. Lagenstein I, Willig RP, Kuhne D. Cranial computed tomography (CCT) findings in children treated with ACTH and dexamethasone: first results. *Neuropadiatrie* 1979;10:370–384.
61. Lyen KR, Holland IM, Lyen YC. Reversible cerebral atrophy in infantile spasms caused by corticotropin. *Lancet* 1979;2:237–238.
62. Hara K, Watanabe K, Miyazaki S, et al. Apparent brain atrophy and subdural hematoma following ACTH therapy. *Brain Dev* 1981;3:45–49.
63. Okuno T, Ito M, Konishi Y, et al. Cerebral atrophy following ACTH therapy. *J Comput Assist Tomogr* 1980;4:20–23.
64. Rao JK, Willis J. Hypothalomo-pituitary-adrenal function in infantile spasms: effects of ACTH therapy. *J Child Neurol* 1987;2:220–223.
65. Ross DL. Suppressed pituitary ACTH response after ACTH treatment of infantile spasms. *J Child Neurol* 1986;1:34–37.
66. Perheentupa J, Riikonen R, Dunkel L, et al. Adrenocortical hyporesponsiveness after treatment with ACTH of infantile spasms. *Arch Dis Child* 1986;61:750–753.
67. Colleselli P, Milan M, Drigo P, et al. Impairment of polymorphonuclear leucocyte function during therapy with synthetic ACTH in children affected by epileptic encephalopathies. *Acta Paediatr Scand* 1986;75:159–169.
68. Goetting MG. Fatal *Pneumocystis* pneumonia from ACTH therapy for infantile spasms. *Ann Neurol* 1986;19:307–308.
69. Quittell LM, Fisher M, Foley CM. *Pneumocystis carinii* pneumonia in infants given adrenocorticotropic hormone for infantile spasms. *J Pediatr* 1987;110:901–903.
70. Shamir R, Garty BZ. *Pneumocystis carinii* pneumonia associated with adrenocorticotropic hormone treatment for infantile spasms. *Eur J Pediatr* 1992;151:867–895.
71. Kanayama M, Ishikawa T, Tauchi A, et al. ACTH-induced seizures in an infant with West syndrome. *Brain Dev* 1989;11:329–331.
72. Rutledge SL, Snead OC III, Kelly DR, et al. Pyruvate carboxylase deficiency: acute exacerbation after ACTH treatment of infantile spasms. *Pediatr Neurol* 1989;5:201–206.
73. Appleton RE, Peters ACB, Mumford JP, et al. Randomised, placebo-controlled study of vigabatrin as first-line treatment of infantile spasms. *Epilepsia* 1999;40:1627–1633.
74. Elterman RD, Shields WD, Mansfield KA, et al. Randomized trial of vigabatrin in patients with infantile spasms. *Neurology* 2001;57:1416–1421.
75. Wohlrab G, Boltshauser E, Schmitt B. Vigabatrin as first-line drug in West syndrome: clinical and electroencephalographic outcome. *Neuropediatrics* 1998;29:133–136.
76. Chiron C, Dumas C, Jambaque I, et al. Randomized trial comparing vigabatrin and hydrocortisone in infantile spasms due to tuberous sclerosis. *Epilepsy Res* 1997;26:389–395.
77. Wohlrab G, Boltshauser E, Schmitt B, Schriever S, Landau K. Visual field constriction is not limited to children treated with vigabatrin. *Neuropediatrics* 1999;30:130–132.
78. Vanhatalo S, Nousiainen I, Eriksson K, et al. Visual field constriction in 91 Finnish children treated with vigabatrin. *Epilepsia* 2002;43:748–756.
79. Hardus P, Verduin WM, Engelsman M, et al. Visual field loss associated with vigabatrin: quantification and relation to dosage. *Epilepsia* 2001;42:262–267.

80. Gross-Tsur V, Banin E, Shahar E, et al. Visual impairment in children with epilepsy treated with vigabatrin. *Ann Neurol* 2000;48:60–64.

81. Koul R, Chacko A, Ganesh A, et al. Vigabatrin associated retinal dysfunction in children with epilepsy. *Arch Dis Child* 2001; 85:469–473.

82. Westall C, Logan WJ, Smith K, et al. The Hospital for Sick Children, Toronto, longitudinal ERG study of children on vigabatrin. *Doc Ophthalmol* 2002;104:133–149.

83. Siemes H, Spohr HL, Michael T, et al. Therapy of infantile spasms with valproate: results of a prospective study. *Epilepsia* 1988; 29:553–560.

84. Schlumberger E, Dulac O. A simple, effective and well-tolerated treatment regime for West syndrome. *Dev Med Child Neurol* 1994;36:863–872.

85. Chamberlain MC. Nitrazepam for refractory infantile spasms and the Lennox-Gastaut syndrome. *J Child Neurol* 1996; 11:31–34.

86. Toribe Y. High-dose vitamin B6 treatment in West syndrome. *Brain Dev* 2001;23:654–657.

87. Hurst DL, Rolan TD. The use of felbamate to treat infantile spasms. *J Child Neurol* 1997;10:134–136.

88. Echenne B, Dulac O, Parayre-Chanez MJ, et al. Treatment of infantile spasms with intravenous gamma-globulins. *Brain Dev* 1991;13:313–319.

89. Glauser T, Clark PO, Strawsburg R. A pilot study of topiramate in the treatment of infantile spasms. *Epilepsia* 1998;39:1324–1328.

90. Suzuki Y, Imai K, Toribe Y, et al. Long-term response to zonisamide in patients with West syndrome. *Neurology* 2002;58: 1556–1559.

91. Kerrigan JF, Shields WD, Nelson TY, et al. Ganaxolone for treating intractable infantile spasms: a multicentre, open-label, add-on trial. *Epilepsy Res* 2000;42:133–139.

92. Kossof EH, Pyzik PL, McGrogan JR, et al. Efficacy of the ketogenic diet for infantile spasms. *Pediatrics* 2002;109:780–783.

93. Snead OC III, Benton JW, Myers GJ. ACTH and prednisone in childhood seizure disorders. *Neurology* 1983;33:966–970.

94. Yamatogi Y, Ohtahara S. Early-infantile epileptic encephalopathy with suppression-bursts, Ohtahara syndrome; its overview referring to our 16 cases. *Brain Dev* 2002;24:13–23.

95. Yamatogi Y, Ohtahara S. Age dependent epileptic encephalopathy: a longitudinal study. *Folia Psych Neurol Jpn* 1981;35:321–332.

96. Martinez BA, Roche C, Lopez-Martin V, et al. Early infantile epileptic encephalopathy. *Rev Neurol* 1995;23:297–300.

97. Donat JF. The age dependent epileptic encephalopathies. *J Child Neurol* 1992;7:7–21.

98. Campistol J, Garcia-Garcia JJ, Lobera E, et al. The Ohtahara syndrome: a special form of age dependent epilepsy. *Rev Neurol* 1997;25:212–214.

99. Baxter PS, Gardner-Medwin D, Barwick DD, et al. Vigabatrin monotherapy in resistant neonatal seizures. *Seizure* 1995;4:57–59.

100. Dobbs JM, Baird HW. The use of corticotropin and a corticosteroid in patients with minor motor seizures. *Am J Dis Child* 1960; 100:584–585.

101. Kurakawa T, Nagahide G, Fukuyama Y, et al. West syndrome and Lennox-Gastaut syndrome: a survey of natural history. *Pediatrics* 1980;65:81–88.

102. Lagenstein I, Willig RP, Iffland E. Behandlung fruhkindlicher Anfalle mit ACTH und Dexamethasone unter standardisierten Bedingungen, I: klinische Ergebnisse. *Monatsschr Kinderheilk* 1978;126:492–499.

103. Lagenstein I, Willig RP, Iffland E. Behandlung fruhkindlicher Anfalle mit ACTH und Dexamethasone unter standardisierten Bedingungen, II: elektroencephalographische Beobachtungen. *Monatsschr Kinderheilk* 1978;126:500–506.

104. Paul L, O'Neal R, Ybanez M, et al. Minor motor epilepsy. Treatment with corticotropin (ACTH) and steroid therapy. *JAMA* 1960;172:1408–1412.

105. O'Regan ME, Brown JK. Is ACTH a key to understanding anticonvulsant action? *Dev Med Child Neurol* 1998;40:82–89.

106. Doose H. Myoclonic-astatic epilepsy. *Epilepsy Res Suppl* 1992;6: 163–168.

107. Oguni H, Tanaka T, Hayashi K, et al. Treatment and long-term prognosis of myoclonic-astatic epilepsy of early childhood. *Neuropediatrics* 2002;33:122–132.

108. Landau W, Kleffner FR. Syndrome of acquired aphasia with convulsive disorder in children. *Neurology* 1957;7:523–530.

109. Appleton RE. The Landau-Kleffner Syndrome. *Arch Dis Child* 1995;72:386–387.

110. Robinson RO, Baird G, Robinson G, et al. Landau-Kleffner syndrome: course and correlates with outcome. *Dev Med Child Neurol* 2001;43:243–247.

111. Lerman P, Lerman-Sagie T, Kivity S. Effects of early corticosteroid therapy for Landau-Kleffner syndrome. *Dev Med Child Neurol* 1991;33:257–266.

112. Hirsch E, Marescaux C, Finck S, et al. Landau-Kleffner syndrome: a clinical and EEG study of five cases. *Epilepsia* 1990;31:756–767.

113. McKinney W, McGreal DA. An aphasic syndrome in children. *Can Med Assoc J* 1974;110:637–639.

114. Kellerman K. Recurrent aphasia with subclinical bioelectric status epilepticus during sleep. *Eur J Pediatr* 1978;128:207–212.

115. Van der Sandt-Koenderman WME, Smit IAC, Van Dongen HR, et al. A case of acquired aphasia and convulsive disorder. Some linguistic aspects of recovery and breakdown. *Brain Lang* 1984;21:174–183.

116. Tsuru T, Mori M, Mizuguchi M, et al. Effects of high-dose intravenous corticosteroid therapy in Landau-Kleffner syndrome. *Pediatr Neurol* 2000;22:145–147.

Newer Antiepileptic Drugs

68

Norman Delanty   *Jacqueline A. French*

Despite advances and optimal current therapy, there remains a continuing need for the development of new agents for patients with epilepsy (1–4). Among those with epilepsy, 30% to 40% continue to have seizures or experience unacceptable side effects that affect their quality of life (5,6). In a prospective study of 525 patients in a single epilepsy center between 1984 and 1997, only 63% remained seizure free for more than 1 year, with seizure-free rates being similar, regardless of whether a new or an established antiepileptic drug (AED) was used (7). Moreover, the available anticonvulsant agents suppress the symptoms of epilepsy and are not truly antiepileptic or antiepileptogenic in nature. None of these agents have been shown to influence the process of epileptogenesis in humans or to alter the underlying brain dysfunction that expresses itself as epilepsy. An ideal agent would provide complete seizure control without significant side effects or idiosyncratic life-threatening reactions; have simple, predictable pharmacokinetics; be unaffected by other drugs or medical conditions; and be nonteratogenic, affordable, and available in a parenteral formulation. An agent that prevents epilepsy (e.g., after a head injury or stroke) or that alters the underlying mechanisms of a particular epilepsy, or prevents or ameliorates its progression (8), could also be considered to be antiepileptogenic or antiepileptic.

Although nine new agents have been introduced in recent years, with attendant marketing considerations, many novel compounds with promise as useful AEDs are currently in various stages of development (Table 68.1 and Table 68.2). Some of these resulted from the Antiepileptic Drug Development (ADD) Program sponsored by the U. S. National Institutes of Health (9), which has screened more than 24,000 compounds (provided by industry and academia) for potential anticonvulsant efficacy in traditional animal models (9,10). These models have traditionally

focused mainly on the maximum electroshock (MES) test and the pentylenetetrazol (PTZ) test, which are believed to predict efficacy against tonic-clonic and absence seizures, respectively (see Chapter 44). Although this approach has identified such agents as topiramate, it does not always recognize potentially useful compounds, predict activity in humans, or test antiepileptogenic potential (11). Newer models, such as pilocarpine, kainate, or electrically induced post-status epilepsy models, are aimed at mimicking human disease and may be better suited to identify useful compounds, but are not effective for high-throughput screening of new chemical entities. Research elucidating the molecular mechanisms underlying some specific epilepsy syndromes, such as benign neonatal convulsions (12) and Unverricht-Lundborg progressive myoclonic epilepsy (13), suggests that targeted therapeutic approaches may prove more successful than mass screening techniques for some of the epilepsies. This may also be true for some of the more common forms of epilepsy, such as juvenile myoclonic epilepsy (14). Despite the limitations of screening methods, promising compounds are in development (15–18). Some are at a late stage of development (e.g., pregabalin), whereas others are at earlier stages of clinical testing (e.g., safinamide, talampanel). However, not all of these compounds will be approved for use, which is exemplified by the fact that three of the compounds discussed in the prior version of this chapter are no longer in development.

In the previous edition of this textbook, this Chapter discussed 10 anticonvulsant drugs (19). Information on harkoseride, retigabine, rufinamide, and the valproate derivatives has been updated. Zonisamide and levetiracetam, now available, are discussed in Chapters 62 and 63. Pregabalin is discussed along with gabapentin in Chapter 59. Losigamone, remacemide, and soretolide are no longer being developed and are not discussed in this chapter.

TABLE 68.1

CHEMISTRY AND POSSIBLE MECHANISM OF ACTION OF SOME NEW ANTIEPILEPTIC DRUGS

Agent	Chemistry	Possible Mechanism of Action
Carabersat	Fluorobenzoylamino benzopyran	Unknown; may have unique binding site
Fluorofelbamate	2-fluoro-2-phenyl-1,3-propanediol dicarbamate	Binds to strychnine-insensitive glycine site of NMDA receptor
Harkoseride	Trifunctional amino acid	Unknown; affinity for strychnine-insensitive glycine site of NMDA receptor; may act on novel binding site
Retigabine	Carbamic acid ethyl ester	KCNQ2/Q3 K^+ channel opener; GABA potentiation
Rufinamide	Difluorobenzyl-triazole amide	Unknown; Na^+ channel blocker; limits frequency of Na^+-dependent action potentials in neurons
Safinamide	[(S)-(+)-2-(4-(3-fluorobenzyloxy) benzylamino) propanamide, methanesulfonate]	Na^+ and Ca^{++} channel blocker
Talampanel	[(R)-7-acetyl-5-(4-aminophenyl)-8,9-dihydro-8-methyl-7H-1,3-dioxolo(4,5-h) (2,3) benzodiazepine]	AMPA-receptor blocker
Valrocemide	N-valproyl glycinamide	Valproate derivative

NMDA, N-methyl-D-aspartate; GABA, γ-aminobutyric acid; AMPA, α-amino-3-hydroxy-5-methyl-4-isoxazole-propionic acid.

CARABERSAT

Carabersat is a structurally novel fluorobenzoylamino benzopyran with anticonvulsant efficacy in *in vitro* (elevated K^+ rat hippocampal slice) and *in vivo* (MES and PTZ) models, with a greater potency than that of either carbamazepine or lamotrigine (20). The agent also has effects on the development of amygdala-kindled seizures in rats and thus may have antiepileptogenic effects. The mechanism of action of carabersat appears to be novel, depends on stereoselective activity at a unique binding site (18), and does not depend on ion channel, γ-aminobutyric acid (GABA) receptor, or glutamate modulation. In normal volunteers (136 individuals), the agent is well tolerated, reaches peak serum levels within a few hours, and has a half-life of 24 hours. Bioavailability is increased by the addition of food. In a phase 2, add-on, placebo-controlled study of 305 patients with refractory partial epilepsy, a 20% to 30% decrease in seizure frequency was reported in the high-dose carabersat (1200 mg per day) group compared with the placebo group, and the agent was well tolerated. Further studies are planned (20).

TABLE 68.2

IMPORTANT PHARMACOKINETIC PARAMETERS OF SELECTED NEW ANTIEPILEPTIC DRUGS

Agent	T_{max} (h)	Protein Binding (%)	Half-Life (h)	Metabolism
Carabersat	2–4	NA	24	Hepatic
Harkoseride	2–3	<10	12	80% renal
Retigabine	1–2	NA	8–10	Hepatic
Rufinamide	5–6	30–40	7–10	85% renal
Safinamide	1–2	NA	24	NA
Talampanel	2	65–85	7	Hepatic
Valrocemide	NA	25	6–10	5% renal to VPA

T_{max}, time to maximum serum concentration; NA, not available; VPA, valproic acid.

FLUOROFELBAMATE

The potential idiosyncratic life-threatening toxicity of felbamate has relegated this drug to use as a treatment of last resort in occasional refractory patients. Its adverse hematologic and hepatic effects are believed to be caused by formation of a reactive aldehyde intermediate metabolite (atropaldehyde or 2-phenylpropanol). To circumvent this, fluorofelbamate (2-fluoro-2-phenyl-1,3-propanediol dicarbamate), which does not have a reactive intermediate, has been developed and is currently undergoing investigation (18). A glutathione-aldehyde adduct found in the urine of rats and humans treated with felbamate has not been found in rats treated with fluorofelbamate. The mechanism of action of fluorofelbamate is likely to be similar to that of its analogue—i.e., modulation of the N-methyl-D-aspartate (NMDA) receptor by binding to its strychnine-insensitive glycine binding site. The anticonvulsant efficacy of fluorofelbamate in animal screening models appears to be at least as potent as that of felbamate. In the rat model of self-sustaining status epilepticus (SSSE) induced by 30-minute perforant path stimulation, intravenous (IV) fluorofelbamate reduced the frequency and severity of seizures, did not cause any behavioral toxicity, and protected against the evolution to chronic epilepsy (21). Fluorofelbamate is currently in phase 2 development. If the agent fulfills its promise as a safe derivative of felbamate, an IV formulation would be a welcome addition to the AED armamentarium.

HARKOSERIDE (SPM 927)

Harkoseride (SPM 927) is a novel trifunctional amino acid derivative, [R]-2-acetamido-N-benzyl-3-methoxypropionamide. The agent has potent anticonvulsant activity in several animal models of seizures, including MES and kindling paradigms (22). Harkoseride is very effective in validated models of status epilepticus, such as the cobalt homocysteine-induced generalized tonic-clonic seizure model, in which it appears to be synergistic with benzodiazepines; it also inhibits seizures in the perforant pathway model of SSSE. In addition, harkoseride is neuroprotective in several animal models of global and focal cerebral ischemia. The agent is being developed as an oral and IV treatment for patients with epilepsy and for those with neuropathic pain. Its precise mechanism of action is unclear, although harkoseride does show affinity for the strychnine-insensitive glycine site of the NMDA receptor complex, and it may also bind to an unidentified unique receptor in the brain. Radioligand binding studies of more than 100 central nervous system (CNS) proteins have revealed no significant displacement. Harkoseride is pH neutral and has good lipid solubility.

In phase 1 human studies (250 individuals), oral and IV administration caused only transient headache, fatigue, and light-headedness. Following oral administration, harkoseride exhibits near-complete absorption, which is not affected by food. The half-life of harkoseride is approximately 12 hours. The agent has linear pharmacokinetics and minimal protein binding; approximately 95% of the drug is renally excreted. No significant hemodynamic changes were observed after single IV doses of up to 300 mg in healthy volunteers. There are no significant interactions with carbamazepine, valproate, or oral contraceptives. In an initial multicenter study of 13 patients with refractory epilepsy, harkoseride was well tolerated in escalating doses of up to 600 mg per day (23). Recently, a similar study in 100 refractory patients showed a median reduction in seizures of 32% over a 12-week treatment phase, with a 50% responder rate of 33% (24). In this study, with the most common maximum tolerated dose being 600 mg per day, reported adverse effects included mild to moderate dizziness, fatigue, and somnolence. Additional studies are ongoing.

RETIGABINE

Retigabine [N-(2-amino-4-[4-fluorobenzylamino]-phenyl) carbamic acid ethyl ester] is structurally unrelated to other AEDs (25). The agent acts by opening KCNQ2/Q3 potassium channels (26,27), which mediate the potassium M-current (28), leading to neuronal hyperpolarization, without an effect on the cardiac KCNQ1 channel (29,30). Interestingly, mutations in the KCNQ2/Q3 channels have been described in benign familial neonatal convulsions (12,31,32). Retigabine also potentiates GABA-mediated currents at higher concentrations. Nontoxic doses were effective against a broad range of experimental models, including genetic models of epilepsy and the amygdala kindling model (18). The agent has demonstrated a significant antiepileptic effect in an *ex vivo* study of human neocortical slices from 17 patients who had undergone resective surgery for intractable epilepsy (33).

Retigabine has a half-life of 8 to 10 hours, has linear pharmacokinetics (in doses up to 1200 mg per day), and is metabolized primarily by glucuronidation and acetylation (34) in the liver, the kidney, and possibly the gastrointestinal (GI) tract; the N-acetylated metabolite also has anticonvulsant activity. Retigabine is not metabolized by the cytochrome P (CYP) 450 pathway. Clearance of the agent is decreased by about 30% in black individuals (35). There is also a slower elimination (by 30%) in elderly subjects, presumably on the basis of a decline in creatinine clearance (36). The parent drug and its active metabolite appear to demonstrate an interesting circadian pharmacokinetic phenomenon, with trough evening concentrations being about 30% lower than trough morning concentrations (35). Retigabine does not appear to alter the metabolism of oral contraceptives, although the agent appears to modestly increase the metabolism of lamotrigine by an unknown mechanism (37), and conversely, phenytoin and carbamazepine may increase the clearance of retigabine.

In phase 1 studies, healthy volunteers complained of fatigue, dizziness, and difficulty concentrating. In a completed 14-week, phase 2, add-on study of 396 patients that compared retigabine doses of 600, 900, and 1200 mg per day with placebo, there was a 23%, 29%, 35%, and 13% median reduction in seizure frequency, respectively. Corresponding >50% responder rates were 23%, 32%, 33%, and 16%, respectively (18). Retigabine may be administered either twice or 3 times per day, although tolerability may be better with 3-times-daily dosing. Adverse effects in patients appear to be similar to those in normal volunteers. No effect has been noted on the QT interval on the electrocardiogram.

RUFINAMIDE

Rufinamide is a structurally novel difluorobenzyl-triazole amide with broad effectiveness in the ADD animal model screening program (38). A proposed mechanism of action is blockade of the Na^+ channel, because it limits the frequency of Na^+-dependent action potentials in cultured neurons *in vitro*. Absorption is about 70% and increases with food (39); maximal plasma concentrations occur in about 6 hours. Rufinamide is only 30% to 40% protein bound, has a half-life of 7 to 10 hours, and is 85% renally excreted. Two trials have demonstrated some efficacy with the agent as add-on therapy for patients with refractory partial epilepsy. In a double-blind, 28-day study of 50 patients with partial or primary generalized seizures taking a single established AED, seizure frequency decreased by 41% in the rufinamide group and increased by 52% in the placebo group, with greater than 50% responder rates of 39% and 16%, respectively (40). No alteration in plasma levels of phenytoin, carbamazepine, or valproate was seen with the addition of rufinamide over the course of the study. Doses of 1600 to 3200 mg per day appear to be safe and well tolerated.

SAFINAMIDE

Safinamide (PNU-151774E), a structurally novel anticonvulsant, is the S-isomer of the fluorobenzyloxy-benzylamino propanamide methanesulfonate salt (41,42). It acts as a Na^+ and Ca^{++} (L- and N-type) channel blocker (43), inhibits glutamate release, and is a selective monoamine oxidase type B inhibitor. Safinamide is active in a wide range of animal models of epilepsy, including the MES model, the amygdala kindling model in the rat, and the kainate-induced model of status epilepticus. In these models, safinamide has a significantly higher protective index than such established anticonvulsants as phenytoin. The agent did not impair passive avoidance responses in rats at doses up to 40-fold the oral MES median effective dose.

Safinamide appears to be specifically concentrated in brain, with a brain to peripheral tissue ratio of 10:1. It may also be neuroprotective and has shown activity in animal models of Parkinson's disease. In phase 1 studies in humans, the agent reaches peak levels within 1 to 2 hours following absorption, has a half-life of approximately 24 hours, and appears to have linear pharmacokinetics over a range of clinically relevant doses. Safinamide appears to be well tolerated, with rare side effects of headache, somnolence, and lightheadedness at the highest dose tested (i.e., 10 mg/kg per day). Interaction studies have not yet been conducted, but *in vitro* studies indicate that the agent does not have important effects on CYP450 enzymes involved in the metabolism of other AEDs. An open-label, add-on study in patients with refractory partial epilepsy has been performed but not yet published. Safinamide is highly water soluble, which may allow for early development of an IV formulation (42).

TALAMPANEL

Talampanel [(R)-7-acetyl-5-(4-aminophenyl)-8,9-dihydro-8-methyl-7H-1,3-dioxolo(4,5-h)(2,3) benzodiazepine], or LY-300164, is a potent, selective, noncompetitive α-amino-3-hydroxy-5-methyl-4-isoxazole-propionic acid (AMPA)-receptor antagonist with potential as a mechanistically novel AED (44). It is a single R(−) stereoisomer, and its S(+) isomer is not biologically active. Talampanel does not exhibit any classic 1,4-benzodiazepine activity at the $GABA_A$ receptor. In mice, it has activity against the MES and PTZ tests, suppresses both electrically and chemically kindled seizures, and has efficacy in a model of phenytoin-resistant status epilepticus. Talampanel potentiates the anticonvulsant effects of diazepam by 10-fold in the PTZ model (45). In various species, the agent has been shown to be neuroprotective in models of cerebral ischemia and head trauma when administered subsequent to the brain insult; it has also demonstrated antiparkinsonian and antidyskinetic effects. In animal models, talampanel causes dose-dependent CNS depression and, apart from transient sedation, appears to be well tolerated at therapeutic doses.

Talampanel is well absorbed, reaches peak plasma concentrations within 2 hours, and has a half-life of approximately 7 hours; the agent is 65% to 85% protein bound. Its metabolism is partially affected by acetylator status, but a recent study suggests that this may not be a significant consideration in deciding on a dosing strategy in clinical use (46). The metabolism of talampanel is induced by the classic enzyme inducers. Interactions with valproate have not been fully elucidated. Talampanel also appears to inhibit the metabolism of valproate. The agent is metabolized via the CYP3A4 pathway, and thus has potential for further interactions with carbamazepine and tiagabine. Doses of up to 75 mg tid have been used in early clinical studies. Dose-related adverse effects include ataxia, dizziness, drowsiness, and headache. In a double-blind, crossover, controlled trial in 49 patients with refractory partial epilepsy, talampanel treatment was associated with a 21% seizure reduction from baseline, with 80% of the patients experiencing fewer seizures while on therapy (47). A phase 2, multicenter, add-on study with an open-label extension phase involving approximately 250 patients with refractory partial epilepsy is ongoing (44).

UCB 34714

UCB 34714 is an analogue of levetiracetam with high affinity for the unique levetiracetam binding site within the CNS (48). It suppresses epileptiform activity in the high K^+, low Ca^{++} model *in vitro*, and is highly potent in suppressing kindling in a number of models and in suppressing seizures in genetic models of epilepsy. UCB 34714 also has efficacy in the mouse model of SSSE. Thus far, in animal models of chronic epilepsy, the agent has been shown to be significantly more potent and at least as well tolerated as levetiracetam. Further development and investigation of this compound are warranted.

VALPROATE DERIVATIVES

Interest has centered on the search for clinically effective valproate-like compounds that lack the hepatotoxic or teratogenic potential of the parent drug (49,50) and do not inhibit the detoxifying enzyme, epoxide hydrolase (51). Structure-activity studies have yielded various series of compounds, some of which may be safer and may demonstrate more potent efficacy than valproate. Three of these agents are currently in clinical development.

Valrocemide (N-valproyl glycinamide; TV1901) (52,53) is effective in classic rodent models of seizures (i.e., MES-, PTZ-, bicuculline- and picrotoxin-induced seizures, and 6-Hz psychomotor seizures) and in kindling paradigms, and it is less toxic than its alkyl derivatives (54). At present, its precise mechanism of action is unknown. Valrocemide does not inhibit epoxide hydrolase in human liver microsomes, nor does it inhibit CYP2A6, CYP2C9, CYP2C19, CYP2D6, and CYP3A4. In studies in inbred Swiss-Vancouver mice, a strain highly susceptible to valproate-induced neural tube defects, valrocemide was nonteratogenic. The agent has a half-life of 6 to 10 hours, has linear pharmacokinetics, and is less than 25% protein bound. The clearance of valrocemide appears to be modestly increased by the concomitant use of enzyme-inducing AEDs. In phase 1 clinical trials, the agent was safe and well tolerated at doses up to 4,000 mg per day; early phase 2 assessment suggests that valrocemide is safe and effective, but additional investigation is ongoing.

NPS 1776 (3-methylbutanamide, or isovaleramide) (55) is another broad-spectrum derivative that is more potent than valproate in the MES and PTZ models. The agent has 100% bioavailability in healthy volunteers, with peak plasma levels occurring in 15 to 30 minutes. NPS 1776 is not protein bound and does not inhibit the CYP450 enzyme system.

SPD 421 (DP16; DP-VPA), a phosphatidylcholine esteric prodrug of valproic acid, is selectively activated locally by formation of intracellular phospholipase A_2, which occurs during seizures and at other times of increased oxidative stress (56). Such regulated activation of the prodrug leads to highly selective delivery of valproate to sites where it may suppress spread of seizure discharge to surrounding brain and potentially allows administration of small, but clinically effective, doses of drug, with minimal or no systemic toxic effects. A seizure or interictal discharge must occur before the agent is activated. The phospholipid moiety renders the drug inactive in the systemic circulation, enhancing its penetration through the blood-brain barrier. SPD 421 exhibits broad efficacy in animal models and is preferentially activated in genetically seizure-prone mice. It does not, however, inhibit spike-wave discharges in the Genetic Absence Epilepsy Rats from Strasbourg, perhaps because absence seizures are inhibitory in origin and do not activate phospholipase A_2. Peak plasma concentrations are attained in 6 to 8 hours after absorption from the GI tract; the half-life of SPD 421 ranges between 8 and 15 hours. In phase 1 studies (117 individuals), doses of 2400 mg have been administered for up to 2 weeks, with higher doses associated with GI side effects. Phase 2 studies are in progress.

CONCLUSIONS AND FUTURE DIRECTIONS

As in other therapeutic areas, such as the antihypertensive, antidepressant, and antipsychotic arenas, the choice of clinically effective novel compounds will likely continue to expand and help more patients with epilepsy live with fewer seizures and side effects. Continued vigilance will be needed to detect rare idiosyncratic side effects, which should include the use of postmarketing surveillance studies. Interest will also grow relative to the elucidation of optimal combination therapies using the available and upcoming agents. Perhaps surprisingly, most of the compounds discussed in this chapter do not have an *a priori*, predefined mechanistic basis of anticonvulsant activity, but have been identified mainly through screening in established animal models of seizures. Both pathways of drug discovery will likely continue. Specific mechanistic targets may include nontoxic NMDA-receptor antagonists, AMPA/kainate-receptor antagonists, glycine derivatives, and adenosine-based approaches (e.g., inhibition of adenosine kinase) (57). Advances in the recognition that many of the epilepsies are, in fact, channelopathies will also likely have significant therapeutic implications (58).

In addition, with improvement in drug-delivery systems (59) and, possibly, seizure prediction algorithms (60), the precise application of potent anticonvulsant compounds to the site of seizure focus within the brain may become a therapeutic reality (e.g., conantokin-G) (61–63). Such an approach could possibly circumvent pharmacogenomic differences in blood-brain barrier structure that may underlie intractability in some patients (64,65). An increased choice of available parenteral formulations is another reasonable expectation. The identification of compounds with antiepileptogenic neuroprotective properties remains a priority, with clinical trials enrolling high-risk patients following head injury and stroke. Finally, the ability to predict an individual's response to a particular agent, in terms of efficacy and side effects, may be enhanced by advances in pharmacogenomics.

REFERENCES

1. Delanty N, French JA. New options in epilepsy pharmacotherapy. *Formulary* 1998;33:1190–1206.
2. Marson AG, Chadwick DW. New drug treatments for epilepsy. *J Neurol Neurosurg Psychiatry* 2001;70:143–147.
3. Nguyen DK, Spencer SS. Recent advances in the treatment of epilepsy. *Arch Neurol* 2003;60:929–935.
4. Sills GJ, Brodie MJ. Update on the mechanisms of action of antiepileptic drugs. *Epileptic Disord* 2001;3:165–172.
5. Dichter MA, Brodie MJ. New antiepileptic drugs. *N Engl J Med* 1996;334:1583–1590.
6. Devinsky O. Patients with refractory seizures. *N Engl J Med* 1999;340:1565–1570.
7. Kwan P, Brodie MJ. Early identification of refractory epilepsy. *N Engl J Med* 2000;342:314–319.
8. Tasch E, Cendes F, Li LM, et al. Neuroimaging evidence of progressive neuronal loss and dysfunction in temporal lobe epilepsy. *Ann Neurol* 1999;45:568–576.
9. White HS, Wolf HH, Woodhead JH, et al. The National Institutes of Health Anticonvulsant Drug Development Program: screening for efficacy. In: French J, Leppik I, Dichter MA, eds. *Antiepileptic drug development*. Philadelphia: Lippincott–Raven, 1998:29–39.
10. White HS. Clinical significance of animal seizure models and mechanism of action studies of potential antiepileptic drugs. *Epilepsia* 1997;38(Suppl 1):S9–S17.
11. Loscher W, Leppik IE. Critical re-evaluation of previous preclinical strategies for the discovery and the development of new antiepileptic drugs. *Epilepsy Res* 2002;50:17–20.
12. Singh NA, Charlier C, Stauffer D, et al. A novel potassium channel gene, KCNQ2, is mutated in an inherited epilepsy of newborns. *Nat Genet* 1998;18:25–29.
13. Pennacchio LA, Lehesjoki AE, Stone NE, et al. Mutations in the gene encoding cystatin B in progressive myoclonic epilepsy (EPM1). *Science* 1996;271:1731–1734.
14. Cossette P, Liu L, Brisebois K, et al. Mutation of GABRA1 in an autosomal dominant form of juvenile myoclonic epilepsy. *Nat Genet* 2002;31:184–189.
15. Nicolson A, Leach JP. Future prospects for the drug treatment of epilepsy. *CNS Drugs* 2001;15:955–968.
16. Czuczwar SJ, Patsalos PN. The new generation of GABA enhancers. Potential in the treatment of epilepsy. *CNS Drugs* 2001;15:339–350.
17. Bialer M, Johannessen SI, Kupferberg HJ, et al. Progress report on new antiepileptic drugs: a summary of the Sixth Eilat Conference (EILAT VI). *Epilepsy Res* 2002;51:31–71.
18. Hovinga CA. Novel anticonvulsant medications in development. *Expert Opin Investig Drugs* 2002;11:1387–1406.
19. Delanty N, French JA. Newer antiepileptic drugs. In: Wyllie E, eds. *The treatment of epilepsy: principles and practice*, 3rd ed. Baltimore: Lippincott Williams & Wilkins, 2001:977–983.
20. Messenheimer J. Carabersat. In: Bialer M, Johannessen SI, Kupferberg HJ, et al. Progress report on new antiepileptic drugs: a summary of the Sixth Eilat Conference (EILAT VI). *Epilepsy Res* 2002;51:32–33.
21. Mazarati AM, Sofia RD, Wasterlain CG. Anticonvulsant and antiepileptogenic effects of fluorofelbamate in experimental status epilepticus. *Seizure* 2002;11:423–430.
22. Doty P, Bonn R, Horstmann R, et al. SPM 927. In: Bialer M, Johannessen SI, Kupferberg HJ, et al. Progress report on new antiepileptic drugs: a summary of the Sixth Eilat Conference (EILAT VI). *Epilepsy Res* 2002;51:42–44.
23. Fountain NB, French JA, Privetera MD. Harkoseride: safety and tolerability of a new antiepileptic drug (AED) in patients with refractory partial epilepsy. *Epilepsia* 2000;41(Suppl 7):169.
24. Sachdeo SC, Montouris GD, Beydoun A, et al. An open-label, dose titration trial to evaluate tolerability and efficacy of oral SPM 927 as adjunctive therapy in patients with partial seizures. *Neurology* 2003;60(Suppl 1):A433.
25. Hermann R, Schneider E, Menth M, et al. Retigabine. In: Bialer M, Johannessen SI, Kupferberg HJ, et al. Progress report on new antiepileptic drugs: a summary of the Sixth Eilat Conference (EILAT VI). *Epilepsy Res* 2002;51:36–38.
26. Rundfeldt C. The new anticonvulsant retigabine (D-23129) acts as an opener of K$^+$ channels in neuronal cells. *Eur J Pharmacol* 1997;336:243–249.
27. Rundfeldt C. Characterization of the K$^+$ channel opening effect of the anticonvulsant retigabine in PC12 cells. *Epilepsy Res* 1999;35:99–107.
28. Tatulian L, Delmas P, Abogadie FC, et al. Activation of expressed KCNQ potassium currents and native neuronal M-type potassium currents by the anti-convulsant drug retigabine. *J Neurosci* 2001;21:5535–5545.
29. Main MJ, Cryan JE, Dupere JRB, et al. Modulation of KCNQ2/3 potassium channels by the novel anticonvulsant retigabine. *Mol Pharmacol* 2000;58:253–262.
30. Wickenden AD, Yu W, Zou A, et al. Retigabine, a novel anti-convulsant, enhances activation of KCNQ2/Q3 potassium channels. *Mol Pharmacol* 2000;58:591–600.
31. Biervert C, Schroeder BC, Kubisch C, et al. A potassium channel mutation in neonatal human epilepsy. *Science* 1998;279:403–406.
32. Charlier C, Singh NA, Ryan SG, et al. A pore mutation in a novel KQT-like potassium channel gene in an idiopathic epilepsy family. *Nat Genet* 1998;18:53–55.
33. Straub H, Kohling R, Hohling JM, et al. Effects of retigabine on rhythmic synchronous activity of human neocortical slices. *Epilepsy Res* 2001;44:155–165.
34. Hempel R, Schupke H, McNeilly PJ, et al. Metabolism of retigabine (D-23129), a novel anticonvulsant. *Drug Metab Dispos* 1999;27:613–622.
35. Ferron GM, Paul J, Fruncillo R, et al. Multiple-dose, linear, dose-proportional pharmacokinetics of retigabine in healthy volunteers. *J Clin Pharmacol* 2002;42:175–182.
36. Hermann R, Ferron GM, Erb K, et al. Effects of age and sex on the disposition of retigabine. *Clin Pharmacol Ther* 2003;73:61–70.
37. Hermann R, Knebel NG, Niebch G, et al. Pharmacokinetic interaction between retigabine and lamotrigine in healthy subjects. *Eur J Clin Pharmacol* 2003;58:795–802.
38. Karolchyk MA, Meya U. Rufinamide: an overview [abstract 27]. Presented at: Fourth Eilat Conference on New Antiepileptic Drugs; September 6-10, 1998; Eilat, Israel.
39. Cardot JM, Lecaillon JB, Czendlik C, et al. The influence of food on the disposition of the antiepileptic rufinamide in healthy volunteers. *Biopharm Drug Dispos* 1998;19:259–262.
40. Palhagen S, Canger R, Henriksen O, et al. Rufinamide: a double-blind, placebo-controlled proof of principle trial in patients with epilepsy. *Epilepsy Res* 2001;43:115–124.
41. Fariello RG, Cattaneo C, Wischer S, et al. Safinamide. In: Bialer M, Johannessen SI, Kupferberg HJ, et al. Progress report on new antiepileptic drugs: a summary of the Sixth Eilat Conference (EILAT VI). *Epilepsy Res* 2002;51:38–40.
42. Chazot PL. Safinamide (Newron Pharmaceuticals). *Curr Opin Investig Drugs* 2001;2:809–813.
43. Salvati P, Maj R, Caccia C, et al. Biochemical and electrophysiological studies on the mechanism of action of PNU-151774E, a novel antiepileptic compound. *J Pharmacol Exp Ther* 1999;288:1151–1159.
44. Bodor N. Talampanel. In: Bialer M, Johannessen SI, Kupferberg HJ, et al. Progress report on new antiepileptic drugs: a summary of the Sixth Eilat Conference (EILAT VI). *Epilepsy Res* 2002;51:44–46.

45. Czuczwar SJ, Swiader M, Kuzniar H, et al. LY 300164, a novel antagonist of AMPA/kainate receptors, potentiates the anticonvulsive activity of antiepileptic drugs. *Eur J Pharmacol* 1998;359:103–109.
46. Langan YM, Lucas R, Jewell H, et al. Talampanel, a new antiepileptic drug: single- and multiple-dose pharmacokinetics and initial 1-week experience in patients with chronic intractable epilepsy. *Epilepsia* 2003;44:46–53.
47. Chappell AS, Sander JW, Brodie MJ, et al. A crossover, add-on trial of talampanel in patients with refractory partial seizures. *Neurology* 2002;58:1680–1682.
48. Klitgaard H. UCB Pharma. Data on file.
49. Bialer M, Haj-Yehia A, Badir K, et al. Can we develop improved derivatives of valproic acid? *Pharm World Sci* 1994;16:2–6.
50. Hadad S, Bialer M. Pharmacokinetic analysis and antiepileptic activity of N-valproyl derivatives of GABA and glycine. *Pharm Res* 1995;12:905–910.
51. Kerr BM, Levy RH. Inhibition of epoxide hydrolase by anticonvulsants and risk of teratogenicity. *Lancet* 1989;1:610–611.
52. Bialer M. Valrocemide (TV1901). In: Bialer M, Johannessen SI, Kupferberg HJ, et al. Progress report on new antiepileptic drugs: a summary of the Sixth Eilat Conference (EILAT VI). *Epilepsy Res* 2002;51:46–48.
53. Isoherranen N, Woodhead JH, White HS, et al. Anticonvulsant profile of valrocemide (TV1901): a new antiepileptic drug. *Epilepsia* 2001;42:831–836.
54. Spiegelstein O, Yagen B, Bialer M. Structure-pharmacokinetic-pharmacodynamic relationships of N-alkyl derivatives of the new antiepileptic drug valproyl glycinamide. *Epilepsia* 1999;40:545–552.
55. Isoherranen N, Yagen B, Bialer M. New CNS-active drugs which are second-generation valproic acid: can they lead to the development of a magic bullet? *Curr Opin Neurol* 2003;16:203–211.
56. Chapman D, Fletcher K, Holdich T. SPD421 (DP-VPA). In: Bialer M, Johannessen SI, Kupferberg HJ, et al. Progress report on new antiepileptic drugs: a summary of the Sixth Eilat Conference (EILAT VI). *Epilepsy Res* 2002;51:40–42.
57. Wiesner JB, Ugarkar BG, Castellino AJ, et al. Adenosine kinase inhibitors as a novel approach to anticonvulsant therapy. *J Pharmacol Exp Ther* 1999;289:1669–1677.
58. Lerche H, Jurkat-Rott K, Lehmann-Horn F. Ion channels and epilepsy. *Am J Med Genet* 2001;106:146–159.
59. Fisher RS, Ho J. Potential new methods for antiepileptic drug delivery. *CNS Drugs* 2002;16:579–593.
60. Litt B, Echauz J. Prediction of epileptic seizures. *Lancet Neurol* 2002;1:22–30.
61. McCabe T, Schachter SC. CGX-1007 (Conantokin-G). In: Bialer M, Johannessen SI, Kupferberg HJ, et al. Progress report on new antiepileptic drugs: a summary of the Sixth Eilat Conference (EILAT VI). *Epilepsy Res* 2002;51:33–34.
62. Castellino FJ, Prorok M. Conantokins: inhibitors of ion flow through the N-methyl-D-aspartate receptor channels. *Curr Drug Targets* 2000;1:219–235.
63. Heading CE. Conus peptides and neuroprotection. *Curr Opin Investig Drugs* 2002;3:915–920.
64. Sisodiya SM. Mechanisms of antiepileptic drug resistance. *Curr Opin Neurol* 2003;16:197–201.
65. Siddiqui A, Kerb R, Weale ME, et al. Association of multidrug resistance in epilepsy with a polymorphism in the drug-transporter gene ABCB1. *N Engl J Med* 2003;348:1442–1448.

Less Commonly Used Antiepileptic Drugs

69

Basim M. Uthman   *Ahmad Beydoun*

INTRODUCTION

Despite the availability of a large number of marketed antiepileptic drugs (AEDs), physicians use only a few to treat most patients with epilepsy. The six traditional AEDs used for epileptic seizures include phenytoin, carbamazepine, valproate, primidone, phenobarbital, and ethosuximide. In 1999, phenytoin (Dilantin) had a 42% market share of total AED prescriptions for epilepsy in the United States, proprietary (Tegretol) and generic carbamazepine had a 24% share, and divalproex sodium (Depakote) had captured 17% of the market (1). The remaining 17% of the market was held by all other products and generics. The availability of less-sedating AEDs led to a gradual decline in the use of primidone and phenobarbital in the United States. This prescribing pattern reflects the physician's familiarity with a particular agent, its efficacy, tolerability, pharmacokinetic profile, and cost. Results of comparative trials have led to improved objectivity in the selection of the best agent for specific seizure disorders.

Over the past decade, the introduction of new AEDs—felbamate (Felbatol[1]), gabapentin (Neurontin), lamotrigine (Lamictal), topiramate (Topamax), tiagabine (Gabitril), zonisamide (Zonegran), oxcarbazepine (Trileptal), and levetiracetam (Keppra)—has expanded the range of choices when first-line agents fail to control seizures or produce intolerable adverse events. Felbamate has been of limited use because of toxic reactions affecting the liver and bone

marrow. Because of improved tolerability, newer AEDs may replace older ones as first-line agents in the treatment of epilepsy. The availability of new AEDs has reduced the use of older AEDs over the last few years. In June 2003, the market share of Dilantin in the United States dropped to 33.3% of total AED prescriptions.

This chapter discusses less frequently used AEDs: ethotoin, methsuximide, methylphenobarbital, acetazolamide, vitamin B_6, and bromides (Table 69.1). Inferior efficacy, poor tolerability, or both have forced withdrawal of several AEDs from the market. The use of vagus nerve stimulation and the ketogenic diet is discussed elsewhere in this volume.

ETHOTOIN

Historical Background

Until phenytoin was marketed as an AED in 1938, phenobarbital was well established as the agent of choice in the treatment of seizures. Merritt and Putnam (2,3), searching for AEDs devoid of sedative effects, first reported on the anticonvulsant properties of phenyl derivatives in animal studies. They recommended clinical trials of phenytoin (Dilantin; 5,5-diphenylhydantoin; Fig. 69.1A), and soon demonstrated the superiority of the agent over phenobarbital and its lack of significant hypnotic effects (4). Phenytoin has since become the world's most commonly used agent for the treatment of patients with generalized tonic-clonic and simple and complex partial seizures. Other hydantoins were also tested, but only ethotoin is still in use today.

Chemistry and Mechanism of Action

Ethotoin (Peganone, 3-ethyl-5-phenylhydantoin; Fig. 69.1B) is similar to phenytoin, except for the deletion of one

---

[1]Tegretol and Trileptal are registered trademarks of Novartis Pharmaceuticals; Depakote is a registered trademark of Abbott Laboratories; Felbatol is a registered trademark of Wallace Laboratories; Neurontin is a registered trademark of Pfizer Inc; Lamictal is a registered trademark of GlaxoSmithKline.; Topamax is a registered trademark of Ortho-McNeil Pharmaceutical; Gabitril is a registered trademark of Cephalon, Inc.; Zonegran is a registered trademark of Elan Pharmaceuticals; Keppra is a registered trademark of UCB Pharma, Inc.

TABLE 69.1

ANTIEPILEPTIC DRUGS MARKETED IN THE UNITED STATES

Year	Nonproprietary Name[a]	Trade Name Introduced
1912	**Phenobarbital**[b]	Luminal
1935	Mephobarbital	Mebraral
1938	**Phenytoin**	Dilantin
1946	Trimethadione	Tridione
1947	Mephenytoin	Mesantoin
1949	Paramethadione	Paradione
1951	Phenacemide	Phenurone
1952	Metharbital	Gemonil
1953	Phensuximide	Milontin
1954	**Primidone**	Mysoline
1957	Methsuximide	Celontin
1957	Ethotoin	Peganone
1960	**Ethosuximide**	Zarontin
1968	Diazepam	Valium
1974	**Carbamazepine**	Tegretol
1975	Clonazepam	Clonopin
1978	**Valproate**	Depakene
1981	Clorazepate	Tranxene
1992	Felbamate	Felbatol
1994	**Gabapentin**	Neurontin
1995	**Lamotrigine**	Lamictal
1996	**Topiramate**	Topamax
1997	**Tiagabine**	Gabitril
2000	**Oxcarbazepine**	Trileptal
2000	**Zonisamide**	Zonegran
2000	**Levetiracetam**	Keppra

[a]Withdrawn AEDs are not included.
[b]Boldface indicates major AEDs.
Adapted from Levy R, Mattson R, Meldrum B, et al, eds. *Antiepileptic drugs*, 3rd ed. New York: Raven Press. 1989:xxiv.

phenyl group from position 5 and the addition of an ethyl group in position 3 of the hydantoin ring. It has a molecular mass of 204.22. Ethotoin has a broad spectrum of activity, and inhibits seizures induced by maximal electroshock and pentylenetetrazol.

Absorption, Distribution, and Metabolism

Ethotoin is slowly absorbed from the gastrointestinal (GI) tract. Absorption is dose dependent; the time to peak plasma concentration increases with increasing dose. This nonlinear metabolic profile may explain the poor correlation between daily dose and steady-state serum levels of ethotoin (5).

Ethotoin is metabolized in the liver by hydroxylation and deethylation of the hydantoin ring. It has a relatively short half-life of 6 to 9 hours.

Efficacy and Clinical Use

The clinical use of ethotoin has been limited by its hypnotic properties and low anticonvulsant potency (6). The lack of gingival hyperplasia and hirsutism, side effects of phenytoin therapy, may make ethotoin an attractive alternative AED; however, it is only one fourth as effective as phenytoin in inhibiting electrically induced convulsions in animals. Few clinical trials of ethotoin are cited in the literature. In one study (7), ethotoin reduced seizure frequency in most of the children (N = 17) with uncontrolled seizures treated with dosages of 19 to 49 mg/kg per day. Two hours after ingestion, serum levels ranged from 14 to 34 mg/mL (conversion for ethotoin: μmol/L = μg/mL $\times$ 4.90) (5). In a retrospective study of adults with medically refractory epilepsy, ethotoin as adjunctive therapy reduced overall seizure frequency, especially the frequency of tonic seizures (8). The efficacy of the agent, however, was reduced by one half within 10 months, suggesting rapid onset of tolerance. Ethotoin is ineffective in treating and may exacerbate absence seizures. Because of its short half-life, ethotoin is given in four divided doses of 20 to 40 mg/kg per day. Ethotoin is available in 250- and 500-mg tablets.

Interactions with Other Agents and Adverse Effects

No drug-drug interactions have been documented with ethotoin.

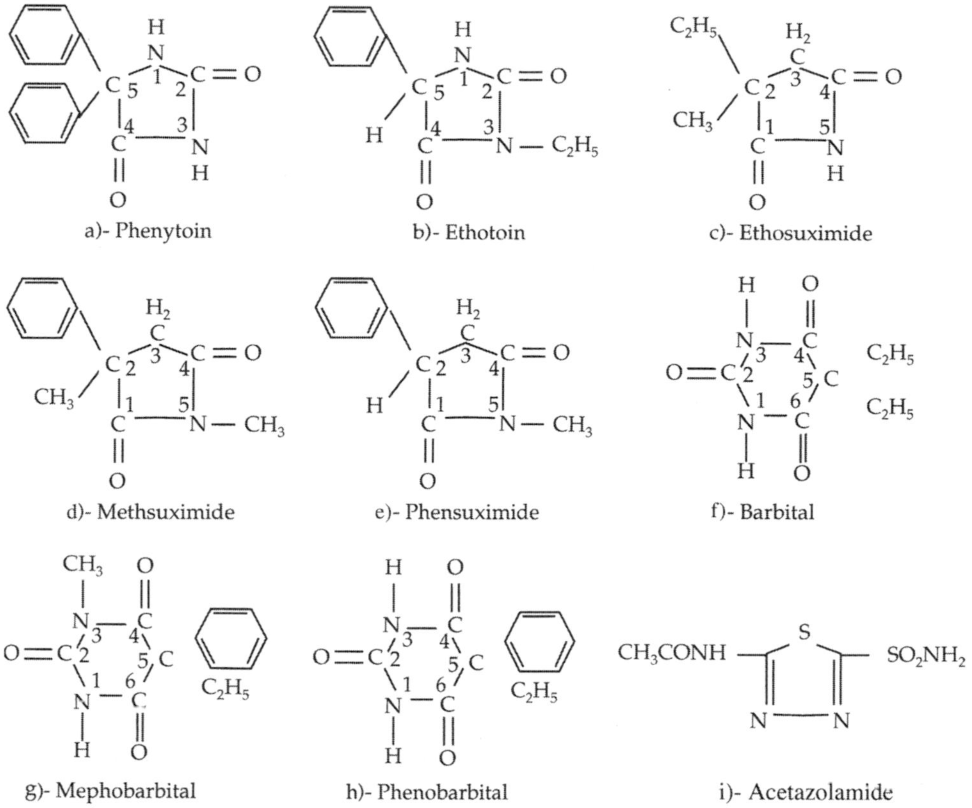

Figure 69.1 Chemical structures of selected minor and major antiepileptic drugs: **A**: Phenytoin. **B**: Ethotoin. **C–E**: Methsuximide belongs to the succinimide family (ethosuximide and phensuximide), which shares a common heterocyclic ring. **D**: Methsuximide. **F–G**: Mephobarbital is structurally similar to barbital. **H**: Phenobarbital. **I**: Acetazolamide.

Although the agent is relatively free of the common adverse effects of phenytoin, ataxia, diplopia, dizziness, insomnia, rash, and GI distress may occur during ethotoin use. Isolated cases of lymphadenopathy have been reported. Cleft lip, cleft palate, and other malformations have occurred in infants born to mothers taking ethotoin (9,10).

Ethotoin has been available for more than 3 decades, but its efficacy and safety have not been adequately established in well-controlled clinical trials, and its use in the treatment of seizures and epilepsy remains limited.

METHSUXIMIDE

Historical Background

Introduced in 1957 for the treatment of refractory absence seizures, methsuximide (Celontin²) belongs to the succinimide family (i.e., ethosuximide and phensuximide), which shares a common heterocyclic (succinimide) ring (Fig. 69.1C–E). The diverse effects of these agents in a variety of experimental and clinical seizure types are probably

related to the substitution of different chemical groups in the succinimide ring. Since phensuximide is no longer available, only methsuximide is discussed in detail in this chapter.

Chemistry and Mechanism of Action

The chemical structure of methsuximide (N-2-dimethyl-2-phenyl-succinimide) is shown in Figure 69.1D. Phenyl group substitution at the 2C position counteracts experimentally induced maximal electroshock seizures, whereas alkyl group substitution at the 2C position counteracts experimentally induced pentylenetetrazol seizures. Methyl group substitution at the 5N position adds to the antipentylenetetrazol effect and the sedative activity. Alkyl substitution at the 5N and 2C positions and phenyl substitution at the 2C position provide activity against pentylenetetrazol- and maximal electroshock-induced seizure activity (11).

Methsuximide is a nonpolar chemical compound that is water soluble and slightly lipophilic. Its exact effects on excitable membranes are unknown. Because of its effectiveness against absence and partial seizures, the agent probably has more than one mechanism of action, including effects on transmitter release, calcium uptake into

²Celontin is a registered trademark of Pfizer Inc.

presynaptic endings, and conductance of sodium, potassium, and chloride.

Absorption, Distribution, and Metabolism

Methsuximide is quickly absorbed through the GI tract, with peak plasma levels achieved in 2 to 4 hours. The agent is distributed evenly throughout the body and penetrates brain and fat tissue better than ethosuximide (12). Because of its low protein binding and poor solubility, methsuximide equilibrates with CSF (B.J. Wilder, unpublished data, 1980). It is rapidly metabolized to N-desmethyl-methsuximide or 2-methyl-2-phenyl succinimide (12–15) and has a mean half-life of 1.4 hours. Trough plasma concentrations of methsuximide are reportedly undetectable in fasting specimens (16). A major active metabolite of methsuximide, N-desmethyl-methsuximide, achieves high steady-state plasma levels and exerts a major anticonvulsant effect. The mean half-life of this metabolite is 38 hours (range, 37 to 48 hours) (13), although some investigators (16) have reported half-lives of 51.6 to 80.2 hours in patients who received maximal doses of methsuximide. Another methsuximide metabolite, N-methyl-2-hydroxymethyl-2-phenylsuccinimide, was detected by means of gas chromatography and mass spectrometry of the serum of a patient with a fatal overdose of primidone and methsuximide.

Optimal clinical effect may be achieved with a non-trough N-desmethyl-methsuximide plasma concentration of 20 to 24 µg/mL (15), near the middle of the therapeutic range of 10 to 40 µg/mL reported by Strong and colleagues (14). Browne and associates (16) reported a therapeutic range of 10 to 30 µg/mL for fasting N-desmethyl-methsuximide plasma concentrations. Steady-state plasma concentration is reached between 8.1 and 16.8 days from onset of maintenance methsuximide dose. The usual dosage increase of 150 or 300 mg per day can be made at biweekly intervals to avoid toxicity. Methsuximide is no longer available in 150-mg tablets; biweekly dosage increments of one tablet (300 mg) every other day may be used (16).

Efficacy and Clinical Use

Methsuximide has a wide spectrum of antiepileptic activity and is effective in patients with complex partial seizures (15–17), generalized tonic-clonic seizures, and absence seizures (18–21). Wilder, Buchanan, and Uthman (15,22) found methsuximide to be an effective adjunctive agent in the management of refractory complex partial seizures. Twenty-one patients taking phenytoin, phenobarbital, primidone, or carbamazepine as monotherapy or in combination were studied. Of these patients, 71% achieved good to excellent control of complex partial seizures, and a dose reduction or discontinuation of 1 or more AED was possible in 42%. Optimal plasma levels and control of complex

partial seizures were associated with daily methsuximide dosages of 9.5 to 11.0 mg/kg, with maximal seizure control observed at N-desmethyl-methsuximide plasma levels of 20 to 24 µg/mL (conversion factor for methsuximide: µmol/L = 4.92 × µg/mL). A dose-response relationship was determined after the addition of methsuximide, and seizure frequency progressively decreased as N-desmethyl-methsuximide serum levels increased.

Browne and colleagues (16) described the use of adjunctive methsuximide in 26 patients with medically refractory complex partial seizures. The maximal tolerated dose of methsuximide was maintained for 8 weeks. Of the total population, eight patients (31%) had a 50% or more reduction in seizure frequency, and four (15%) became seizure free. Eight patients withdrew from the study because of adverse events and three because of increased seizure frequency (these patients had a history of severe seizure flurries before and after initiation of methsuximide treatment). Of the eight patients who responded, five continued to have a 50% or more reduction in frequency of complex partial seizures for 3 to 34 months.

Sigler and associates (23) used methsuximide as add-on therapy in children with epilepsy refractory to first- and second-line AEDs. Forty patients (35.7%) had a 50% or more reduction in seizure frequency, and ten (8.9%) became seizure free during the short-term phase (mean, 9.1 weeks). Of the 112 patients studied, 22 (19.6%) continued to benefit from the drug (a 50% or more reduction in seizure frequency compared with baseline and absence of intolerable side effects) at long-term follow-up (mean, 3.7 years; range, 18 months to 7.1 years). In patients with good seizure control, fasting plasma levels of N-desmethyl-methsuximide were 25.3 to 44.7 mg/L (mean, 36.0 mg/L); thus, effective plasma concentrations of N-desmethyl-methsuximide in children were found to be higher than previously described. No serious or irreversible side effects were reported. Likewise, Tennison and colleagues (24) used methsuximide as add-on therapy in children with complex partial and "minor motor" seizures refractory to first- and second-line AEDs; 15 patients (60%) had a 50% or more reduction in seizure frequency, and no serious adverse events were reported.

Other reports of methsuximide as adjunctive medical therapy for complex partial seizures showed complete seizure control in 0% to 38% of patients and a 50% or more reduction in seizure frequency in 6% to 100% of patients (17,19,25–28). In one study of previously untreated patients (29), seizures were controlled in 18%, and 27% had a 50% or more reduction in seizure frequency.

Results of early studies of methsuximide showed some efficacy in patients with absence seizures (19–21). In one study (20), methsuximide was used in previously untreated patients; absences were not completely controlled in any patient, and only 20% had a greater than 50% reduction in seizure frequency. Rabe (30) reported that 10 of 16 patients became completely free of absences, and another five had seizure frequency reduced by 75%. He suggested two possible explanations for the greater effectiveness of methsuximide in his study compared with earlier work: Most of his patients had epilepsy of relatively recent onset, and he used considerably higher doses of methsuximide (1,200 to 2,100 mg per day) than did previous investigators.

Rabe also reported on the efficacy of methsuximide in four patients with juvenile myoclonic epilepsy (30). Two patients became completely free of myoclonus, and two had a reduction in frequency of at least 75%. One case report described methsuximide used with primidone to be very effective in a 17-year-old boy with drawing-induced myoclonic seizures (31). Hurst (32) described five adolescent girls with juvenile myoclonic epilepsy who became seizure free taking methsuximide; four were maintained on monotherapy.

Tolerance to the anticonvulsant effect of methsuximide develops in approximately 50% of patients treated with maximal doses, and seizure frequency returns to baseline. The low overall efficacy of methsuximide relative to that of first-line AEDs may reflect the selectively more refractory seizures in the patients studied. Failures because of toxic reactions might have occurred when the dose of methsuximide was increased too rapidly. The dose should not be increased more often than every 2 weeks in adults receiving multidrug therapy (16). Methsuximide should be considered in patients who are allergic to or whose disease is refractory to other AEDs.

Interactions with Other Agents and Adverse Effects

Methsuximide interacts with other AEDs, necessitating close monitoring of serum levels and adjustment of concurrent AED dose, especially in the face of clinical toxicity. Rambeck (33) reported that concurrent administration of methsuximide increased the mean serum concentration of phenobarbital by 37% in patients receiving this agent and by 40% in patients receiving primidone. The mean serum concentration of phenytoin increased by 78%. Patients taking phenobarbital or phenytoin had increased serum levels of N-desmethyl-methsuximide compared with patients taking methsuximide alone. These increases were attributed to competition by the drugs for a common hydroxylating enzyme system.

Conversely, the addition of methsuximide induces the metabolization of other AEDs (34,35). Methsuximide decreased the mean serum concentrations of carbamazepine (16), valproic acid (36,37), lamotrigine (35,38), and topiramate (39) when added to the treatment regimen. Methsuximide mitigated the effect of valproic acid on lamotrigine; the combination of valproic acid and lamotrigine increased the concentration of lamotrigine by 211%

compared with lamotrigine monotherapy, however, if methsuximide was added, the increased concentration of lamotrigine dropped to 8% (35).

GI disturbance, lethargy, somnolence, fatigue, and headache may be experienced, but these adverse effects are usually transient and dose-related. Other adverse experiences include hiccups, irritability, ataxia, blurred vision or diplopia, inattention, dysarthria, and psychic changes (16). In some patients, headache, photophobia, and hiccups require withdrawal of methsuximide (15). Transient leukopenia and a movement disorder have been reported (40). Delayed, profound coma following methsuximide overdose has been described (41). Charcoal hemoperfusion was successful in one case of methsuximide overdose (42).

BARBITURATES

Historical Background

Approximately 2500 barbiturate compounds have been synthesized since barbituric acid was first produced in 1864. About 25 (1%) of these compounds are licensed by the U.S. Food and Drug Administration as hypnotics, anesthetics, and anticonvulsants (11). Two barbiturates are currently marketed as AEDs: mephobarbital (Mebaral[3], methylphenobarbital, methylphenobarbitone); and phenobarbital (Luminal; Fig. 69.1H). Primidone (Mysoline) is a deoxybarbiturate metabolized to phenobarbital and phenylethyl-malonamide. All these compounds are derived from barbital, the first synthetic hypnotic barbiturate.

Phenobarbital was introduced as an AED in 1912 (43) and remains one of the major agents used worldwide for the treatment of generalized tonic-clonic and simple or complex partial seizures. It has a special use in patients with status epilepticus and is widely prescribed for prophylaxis of febrile seizures and alcohol- and drug-withdrawal seizures. Phenobarbital and primidone were reported to be less well tolerated than phenytoin and carbamazepine for the treatment of seizures of partial onset (44). A number of studies have reported on the behavioral and cognitive side effects of phenobarbital (45–49). Phenobarbital and primidone are discussed in detail in other chapters. Mephobarbital is considered here.

Chemistry and Mechanism of Action

The chemical structure of mephobarbital (5-ethyl-1-methyl-5-phenylbarbituric acid) is similar to the structure of barbital, as illustrated in Figures 69.1F and G. Mephobarbital is similar to phenobarbital except for the methyl group at the 3N position. The molecular mass of mephobarbital is 246.26. The mechanism of anticonvulsant action is probably similar to that of phenobarbital, essentially inhibiting the spread of seizure activity and elevating seizure threshold (50). All the commercially available hypnotic barbiturates exhibit anticonvulsant activity at anesthetic doses and inhibit epileptic seizures induced by electroshock, tetanus, strychnine, or pentylenetetrazol. This anticonvulsant activity is separate from the sedative or anesthetic effects and is not diminished by the concurrent administration of agents that counteract sedation (11).

Absorption, Distribution, and Metabolism

Mephobarbital is highly soluble in lipids, with lipid to water partition ratio of 100. The agent is easily absorbed and readily crosses biologic membranes. A bioavailability of 75% was found in a pharmacokinetic study of mephobarbital in two volunteers (51). It appears to be widely distributed in the body, with higher concentrations in adipose tissue and brain. In rats, brain mephobarbital levels were 8 times those simultaneously measured in blood (52). *In vitro* studies suggest that 58% to 68% of mephobarbital in highly concentrated solution is bound to human serum albumin (53).

Mephobarbital is metabolized to phenobarbital by demethylation in the liver (54–56), but a portion is excreted in human urine as a *p*-hydroxyphenyl glucuronide derivative of the parent drug (57). Phenobarbital is a known liver enzyme inducer, with this effect possibly responsible for the decrease in mephobarbital elimination half-life from approximately 50 hours initially to 12 to 24 hours during long-term therapy.

Efficacy and Clinical Use

In view of mephobarbital's metabolism, the clinical efficacy and safety of the agent could be expected to resemble those of its metabolite, phenobarbital. Use of mephobarbital began in 1932 (58). Although attempts to correlate dose and serum levels with anticonvulsant effect were made, well-controlled studies comparing the efficacy and safety of the agent with those of other AEDs for the treatment of epilepsy are not available. Nevertheless, mephobarbital is reputed to be as effective as phenobarbital in humans and less sedative (59). National Health Service prescriptions for mephobarbital in Australia have remained similar to those for phenobarbital and primidone over several years (59). There is no reason to believe that mephobarbital is more effective or has a wider anticonvulsant spectrum than the less expensive phenobarbital. It is difficult to differentiate the anticonvulsant effect of the parent drug, mephobarbital, and that of its active metabolite, phenobarbital, during long-term treatment in humans.

Because of the slower metabolism of phenobarbital, its steady-state plasma concentrations exceed those of the parent drug. Probably for that reason, the therapeutic range of mephobarbital traditionally has been expressed in terms of plasma phenobarbital concentrations. Some believe that by ignoring plasma mephobarbital levels, a measure of one active anticonvulsant substance present in the body may be overlooked (59). It is argued that because of its apparent high volume of distribution relative to that of phenobarbital and its lipid solubility, mephobarbital probably has substantially higher brain levels than plasma levels compared with phenobarbital. Usual therapeutic plasma levels of phenobarbital range from 10 to 40 μg/mL. Steady-state plasma phenobarbital levels correlate closely with mephobarbital dose.

Mephobarbital dosages of 3 to 4 mg/kg per day produce mean plasma phenobarbital levels of 15 mg/mL; a dosage of 5 mg/kg per day produces mean levels of 20 mg/mL (59). At higher mephobarbital doses and plasma levels, proportionately lower phenobarbital plasma levels are seen. This may suggest a rate-limited metabolism at high plasma mephobarbital concentrations (59). In one small study (60), plasma phenobarbital levels averaged 20 times those of mephobarbital (conversion for mephobarbital: $[\mu mol/L] = 4.06 \times [\mu g/mL]$; phenobarbital: $[\mu mol/L] = 4.31 \times [\mu g/mL]$).

Interactions with Other Agents and Adverse Effects

Any interaction that is known to occur with phenobarbital (see Chapter 56) probably will also happen with mephobarbital. Subtle adverse effects in the form of intellectual impairment and depression of cognitive abilities are of major concern in patients receiving long-term therapy with mephobarbital or metharbital (61). Other untoward reactions include hypnotic effects, irritability, hyperactivity, and alterations in sleep patterns. Up to 40% of children and probably as many elderly patients taking phenobarbital experience unpleasant side effects (11). Impairment of immediate memory and attention has been demonstrated with long-term phenobarbital use at therapeutic plasma drug levels (62,63). This effect on short-term memory and attention is a significant problem, considering the large number of school-aged children who receive phenobarbital or mephobarbital. Children who take barbiturates may experience irritability and hyperactivity. In one study (64), six of 11 children on maintenance doses of phenobarbital or mephobarbital had clear behavioral changes, including irritability, oppositional attitudes, and overactivity, compared with age-matched controls. Many of our patients reported feeling "dumb" or "mentally dull" when they received barbiturate drugs. In others already taking barbiturates when referred to us, intellectual impairment became apparent in retrospect after the drug was withdrawn. When other, safer AEDs have failed and phenobarbital or mephobarbital must be used, patients should be treated with the lowest dose that effects adequate seizure control.

Another side effect of phenobarbital that is unintentionally ignored by physicians is impotence or decreased libido. Usually, male patients are reluctant to discuss their sex lives, and physicians tend to ascribe the problem to psychosocial conflict. In a Veterans Administration Cooperative study, Mattson and colleagues (44) found that 15% of patients complained of decreased potency, decreased libido, or both. Of 56 patients who took phenobarbital for 1 year, 14% reported a transient or continuous decrease in sexual function. The problem usually disappeared when phenytoin or carbamazepine was substituted for phenobarbital, but not when phenobarbital was changed to another barbiturate.

ACETAZOLAMIDE

Historical Background

Carbonic anhydrase activity was first demonstrated in red blood cells in the early 1930s. It catalyzes reaction I:

$$\overset{\text{I}}{} \qquad \overset{\text{II}}{}$$
$$CO_2 + H_2O \leftrightarrow H_2CO_3 \leftrightarrow H^+ + HCO_3^-$$

Carbonic anhydrase has subsequently been found in many tissues, including the pancreas, gastric mucosa, renal cortex, eye, and CNS. Inhibition of carbonic anhydrase activity was observed when sulfanilamide was introduced as a chemotherapeutic agent. A large number of sulfonamides have been synthesized and tested as carbonic anhydrase inhibitors and potential diuretics. Among these, acetazolamide has been the most extensively studied. Acetazolamide was introduced as an AED by Bergstrom and coworkers (65), and later reports confirmed its effectiveness in most seizure types (66–70). Its usefulness, however, is limited by the rapid development of tolerance.

Chemistry and Mechanism of Action

Acetazolamide (Diamox[4], N-(5-sulfamoyl-1,3,4-thiadiazol-2-yl-)acetamide; Fig. 69.1I) is a weak acid with a molecular mass of 222. In the brain, acetazolamide acts through inhibition of carbonic anhydrase, causing carbon dioxide to accumulate and inducing the anticonvulsant action. Blocking carbonic anhydrase in other tissues, particularly red blood cells, causes even greater retention of carbon dioxide in the brain (71). This results in blockade of anion transport, which prevents spread of seizure activity and elevates seizure threshold. The anticonvulsant effect of acetazolamide, as measured by prevention of maximal electroshock-induced seizures (72,73), correlates with the degree of inhibition of brain carbonic anhydrase. Acetazolamide is one of the most potent carbonic anhydrase (CA) isozymes—i.e., CA I and CA II—and the agent

exhibited strong anticonvulsant properties in a maximal electroshock test in mice (74). Acetazolamide increases brain levels of GABA; however, increased carbon dioxide levels have also been shown to raise brain GABA levels. The carbonic anhydrase inhibitory effect with subsequent increase in intracellular carbon dioxide is probably responsible for the anticonvulsant properties of acetazolamide (75). Acetazolamide decreases the intracellular pH of hippocampal CA_3 neurons by 0.17 ± 0.10 within 10 minutes, and action potentials and the frequency of epileptiform bursts 10 to 15 minutes after administration (76).

High doses of acetazolamide may produce a paradoxical effect, resulting in disruption of acid-base homeostasis in the brain (77). The drug also alters choroid plexus function by its effect on carbonic anhydrase, decreasing production of CSF by limiting chloride and bicarbonate transport across the plexus (78). Woodbury (78) showed that the development of tolerance to acetazolamide is attributable to the induction of increased carbonic anhydrase synthesis in glial cells and to glial proliferation.

Absorption, Distribution, and Metabolism

Acetazolamide is rapidly absorbed from the GI tract, and peak plasma levels occur 2 to 4 hours after a single oral dose. Because acetazolamide is a weak acid, most of its absorption takes place in the duodenum and upper jejunum after some amount has been absorbed in the stomach. In humans, the agent is 90% protein bound; concentrations are lower in CSF than in plasma. The greatest concentration of acetazolamide is in red blood cells. After distribution to various tissues, it binds to carbonic anhydrase and remains in a relatively stable carbonic anhydrase–acetazolamide complex. The plasma half-life of acetazolamide is 2 to 4 days. It is eliminated in the urine unchanged through glomerular filtration, tubular filtration, and tubular secretion. Increasing urinary pH increases excretion. Acetazolamide is also excreted in bile to be resorbed from the intestinal tract.

Efficacy and Clinical Use

Acetazolamide is effective against various seizure types, particularly absence seizures, when it is used as an adjunct to other AEDs (79). After several weeks of continuous treatment, however, tolerance usually develops. Transient or intermittent use of acetazolamide is beneficial when seizures are temporarily exacerbated. This avoids the development of tolerance and may offer protection beyond that provided by AEDs administered long term. Perhaps the best application of acetazolamide is in catamenial epilepsy. The drug can be started 5 days before the expected onset of menses and continued for 11 to 14 days. With a half-life of 2 to 4 days, steady-state plasma levels occur 5 to 7 days after the initial dose, and adequate levels continue for 3 to 5 days after the agent is discontinued. This regimen

---

[4]Diamox is a registered trademark of Wyeth.

can be repeated with each menstrual cycle. In a retrospective study of 20 women with catamenial epilepsy, 40% reported a 50% or greater decrease in seizure frequency; the response rates were similar in generalized vs focal epilepsy and temporal vs extratemporal epilepsy (80). In a retrospective study of 31 patients with juvenile myoclonic epilepsy treated with long-term acetazolamide monotherapy, generalized tonic-clonic seizures were controlled in 45% (81).

Katayama and associates (82) examined the long-term effectiveness and side effects of acetazolamide when used as an adjunct to other AEDs in children with refractory epilepsy. Complete seizure control for more than 3 years was obtained in four (10.8%) of 37 patients, and six patients (16.2%) showed a greater than 50% decrease in seizure frequency for more than 6 months after the introduction of acetazolamide. None of the patients (n = 28) who were examined after long-term acetazolamide therapy, which ranged from 10 months to 14 years, showed evidence of renal calculi. A summary of the pharmacologic and pharmacokinetic properties, efficacy, and safety of acetazolamide in the treatment of epilepsy has been published (83).

The recommended daily dosage is 10 mg/kg given in a single dose or in two or three divided doses. Usual effective therapeutic plasma levels range from 8 to 14 mg/mL (conversion for acetazolamide: μmol/L = 4.5 $\times$ mg/mL). Acetazolamide is available in 125-, 250-, and 500-mg scored tablets. Delayed-release 500-mg tablets are also marketed.

Interactions with Other Agents and Adverse Effects

Elimination of acetazolamide may decrease and the half-life of the agent may increase with the concomitant use of probenecid, which blocks renal tubular secretion of acids. The absorption of salicylate may be increased and that of amphetamine may be delayed when these drugs are taken with acetazolamide. Acetazolamide is a relatively benign agent, with only a few adverse effects known. Lethargy, paresthesias, rashes, abdominal distention, and cyanosis have been reported with its use. In up to 90% of patients, acetazolamide can alter taste sensation (84) by eliminating the tingly or prickly sensation of carbonation and giving a false flat taste to carbonated beverages; we have not seen this effect in any of our patients who had been placed on intermittent treatment. Renal calculi have been reported after long-term use (81). Patients who have been taking phenytoin, barbiturates, and/or acetazolamide for 5 years or more show decreased bone mineral density (BMD) compared with healthy controls (85). A 7-year follow-up (total of $\geq$12 years of use) with these subjects revealed significantly lower BMDs when compared with their previous measurement at 5 years of treatment. In one study (86), standard height and weight scores were significantly

reduced in children receiving acetazolamide along with other AEDs. The investigators speculated that acetazolamide-induced metabolic acidosis may have been responsible for this growth suppression. Caution is advised when the agent is used in children. Teratogenic effects have been induced in animals. Although acetazolamide use may be considered if seizures are exacerbated during pregnancy, the drug should not be administered during the first trimester.

PYRIDOXINE

Historical Background

Two types of pyridoxine-related seizures occur in the newborn: those caused by pyridoxine (vitamin B_6) deficiency (87,88) and those caused by pyridoxine dependency (89,90). These rare conditions carry a poor prognosis for mental development if prompt treatment is not rendered. Pyridoxine dependency as a cause of generalized seizures in children was reported about 40 years ago (91). An autosomal recessive disorder (92), it typically manifests in neonates, but onset has been reported up to the age of 19 months (93,94). Vitamin B_6 levels are reduced in pyridoxine deficiency but are normal in pyridoxine-dependent epilepsy. In either case, vitamin B_6 is the only effective treatment; in pyridoxine deficiency, a single dose is sufficient, whereas pyridoxine dependency requires continuous vitamin B_6 administration.

Chemistry and Mechanism of Action

Pyridoxal phosphate, the active metabolite of vitamin B_6, is the coenzyme for glutamic acid decarboxylase (GAD) and GABA transaminase, the enzymes necessary for the production and metabolism of CNS GABA. In the pyridoxine dependency and deficiency states, GABA levels in CSF are significantly reduced (95). Similarly, GABA and GAD concentrations were reduced in the cortex of a patient with pyridoxine-dependent seizures (94). The underlying defect in pyridoxine-dependent epilepsy is unknown, but one theory is that it is caused by faulty GAD, which catalyzes the conversion of glutamic acid to GABA (92,96). However, glutamate and GABA studies in CSF have been contradictory, and recent genetic studies have not found any linkage between the two brain isoforms (97). Another recent hypothesis is that there may be an abnormality of pyridoxine transport, which underlies the pathophysiology of the disorder (98).

Efficacy and Clinical Use

Pyridoxine Dependency

The diagnosis is established by remission of seizures (generalized seizures or status epilepticus) with vitamin B_6 and relapse without this treatment. Given parenterally in pharmacologic amounts (50 to 100 mg), pyridoxine hydrochloride stops the seizures within minutes (89, 99–101). In pyridoxine dependency, lifelong supplementation with vitamin B_6 is needed. Withdrawal of pyridoxine even after several years of effective therapy causes seizures to reappear within days or weeks (99,101,102). Untreated patients develop intractable epilepsy, and most die within days or months (102).

Psychomotor retardation and progressive neurologic deterioration result when therapy is delayed; therefore, early diagnosis and treatment are important for stopping the seizures and preventing a chronic encephalopathy. In one study (103), serial magnetic resonance imaging (MRI) scans of the heads of children with neonatal seizures and pyridoxine dependency demonstrated progressive dilation of the ventricular system and atrophy of the cortex and subcortical white matter, which was thought to result from an imbalance of GABA and glutamic acid levels causing chronic excitotoxicity in the cerebrum. Pyridoxine-dependent seizures atypically may involve prolonged seizure-free periods with conventional AEDs before pyridoxine treatment (99,100), need for large doses before an effect is seen (104), and late onset several months after birth (100,105). Bass and coworkers (106) reported other atypical features in a child whose seizures stopped only after repeated trials of pyridoxine. The investigators warned of the possibility of decreased levels of consciousness with intravenous (IV) pyridoxine and of the need to have resuscitative equipment available.

Recommended daily oral maintenance dosages range from 2 to 300 mg, corresponding to doses from 0.2 to 30 mg/kg per day (94,95,99–102,104,105,107), with most patients becoming seizure free with doses between 20 and 100 mg per day (103). The single report of long-term follow-up suggested that the prognosis for complete seizure control is excellent (102). However, it was found that elevated cerebral glutamic acid concentrations in children with pyridoxine-dependent epilepsy may not normalize after vitamin B_6 doses sufficient to stop the seizures (108). To prevent psychomotor retardation in patients with this condition, adjustments in the vitamin B_6 dosage should be based on seizure control and on normalization of glutamate concentration in the CSF (108).

Pyridoxine-Responsive Epilepsy

The finding that CSF levels of GABA were lower in patients with infantile spasms than in controls (109,110) led to a number of trials of vitamin B_6 for the treatment of this syndrome (111–114). In the first and largest trial (113), children received daily vitamin B_6 doses of 30 to 400 mg; 13% became seizure free within 2 weeks after initiation of treatment. Vitamin B_6 as monotherapy or in combination with valproic acid was also investigated in 20 children with infantile spasms (112). Treatment began at 10 to 20 mg/kg per day, with a maintenance dose of 20 to 50 mg/kg per day in three doses. Vitamin B_6 monotherapy reduced

seizure frequency in 23% of patients, although only one patient remained seizure free during the 15-month follow-up. No statistically significant difference was identified between patients treated with vitamin B_6 monotherapy and valproate monotherapy (30 to 63 mg/kg per day); however, these agents administered in combination produced significantly better seizure reduction and electroencephalographic effects than did vitamin B_6 alone. Corticotropin was more effective than vitamin B_6 as monotherapy or in combination with valproic acid, having an excellent effect in 86% of patients who did not respond to the combination treatment; many patients, however, had later recurrences of seizures.

Blennow and Starck (111) successfully treated three children with doses ranging between 200 and 400 mg/kg per day. In another study (114), five of 17 children with infantile spasms responded to 300 mg/kg per day of vitamin B_6 within the first week of treatment, with all five becoming seizure free within 4 weeks. The investigators proposed that treatment begin with high doses for 4 to 6 weeks and be followed by a slow dosage reduction (114). In a randomized, prospective trial (115) of neonates, infants, and children younger than 12 years of age with acute recurrent seizures, adjunctive therapy with IV pyridoxine (30 to 50 mg/kg) infused over 2 to 4 hours was significantly superior to monotherapy with a conventional AED.

Adverse Effects

After IV B_6 administration, apnea, lethargy, pallor, decreased responsiveness, and hypotonia may occur immediately and persist for several hours (102,103). These reactions have also followed intramuscular administration (100,116) and the initial oral dose (117). Believed to result from a massive initial release of GABA (117), these symptoms are usually mild but on rare occasions have necessitated intubation and assisted ventilation (118). Loss of appetite, periods of restlessness and crying, vomiting, and apathy have been reported during therapy for infantile spasms with high doses of vitamin B_6 (114).

Long-term pyridoxine use can cause a peripheral neuropathy, which has been documented in animals (119) and humans (120–122), and produced experimentally in animals (123) and humans (124). The original reports suggested that doses of 2,000 to 6,000 mg per day were toxic to dorsal root ganglia, with subsequent degeneration of the peripheral sensory nerves. Later reports indicated that daily doses as low as 500 mg (125) and possibly 200 mg (121) could be neurotoxic. Early recognition of the potential toxicity of high pyridoxine doses and the complete reversal of symptoms on withdrawal of supplementation has averted permanent disability in all but two patients who received a single dose of >100 g of parenteral pyridoxine (126). Prospective studies of 70 adult patients taking daily doses of 100 to 150 mg reported no clinical or electrophysiologic evidence of neurotoxicity (127,128).

On the basis of findings in adults, high doses of pyridoxine may be potentially harmful in infants (129). Although no sensory neuropathy was observed in patients with homocystinuria who received 10 to 90 mg/kg per day during the first 10 years of life (130), nor in three children with infantile spasms treated with very high doses of vitamin B$_6$, prudence dictates (111) use of the minimum effective dosage. One case of sensory neuropathy caused by high-dose, long-term pyridoxine therapy for pyridoxine-dependent epilepsy has been reported (131).

BROMIDES

Historical Background

In 1857, at a time when seizures were linked to hysteria and masturbation, bromides, with putative antiaphrodisiac properties, were introduced for the treatment of epilepsy (132). They remained the principal AED until phenobarbital became available in 1912.

Chemistry and Mechanism of Action

The anticonvulsant mechanism of bromides is unknown, although hyperpolarization of postsynaptic membranes has been proposed. In radioligand studies, halide ions (including bromide and chloride) were found to enhance binding to benzodiazepine receptors, probably at an anion-binding site related to the GABA-gated chloride channels (133). Because bromide has a smaller hydrated diameter than chloride, it crosses cell membranes faster and tends to hyperpolarize the postsynaptic membrane, which is activated by inhibitory neurotransmitters (134).

Absorption, Distribution, and Metabolism

Bromide salts are rapidly absorbed from the GI tract and have nearly complete bioavailability (135). Not bound to plasma proteins, they can freely diffuse across membranes. The volume of distribution of bromides is similar to that of chloride ions. Tissues do not distinguish between these two anions, and their concentration in extracellular fluids depends on their relative intake and excretion. After oral administration, bromides have a half-life of approximately 12 days (135). Excretion by the kidneys occurs slowly and depends on concomitant chloride intake. A high chloride load increases the excretion of bromides and shortens the half-life. Conversely, a salt-deficient diet reduces bromide clearance and prolongs the half-life (134).

Efficacy and Clinical Use

Most reports about the efficacy of bromides include a small number of patients with a variety of seizure types treated with a number of AEDs. Bromides have generally been found to be most effective in treating patients with refractory generalized tonic-clonic seizures and to be considerably less effective in other seizure types (136–140). A retrospective, controlled clinical evaluation (139) of 60 children with medically refractory generalized tonic-clonic seizures found a 50% or more seizure reduction in 58% of patients, with 27% achieving complete control.

Bromides are usually administered as the triple bromide elixir (i.e., combination of sodium, potassium, and ammonium bromide salts) containing 240 mg/mL of bromide salt. The usual dosage in children younger than 6 years of age ranges from 300 mg twice daily to 600 mg three times daily. For children older than 6 years of age, 300 to 1,000 mg is administered 3 times daily (136). The therapeutic plasma concentration (134) ranges from 750 to 1250 mg/mL (10 to 15 mEq/L). Because toxic adverse effects may occur at a concentration of 1500 mg/mL, careful monitoring of serum is required. A steady salt intake should be maintained during treatment. Bromide treatment should be reserved for patients whose disease is refractory to other AEDs and especially for those with refractory generalized tonic-clonic seizures.

Interactions with Other Agents and Adverse Effects

No interactions of bromides with other agents have been described. Sedation is the most frequently encountered side effect of bromides. Although rare cases of acute intoxication with marked nephrotoxicity and ototoxicity have been reported, the more common adverse effects occur as a result of chronic toxicity. Referred to as bromism, these effects target the CNS, skin, and GI tract in older individuals or those with compromised renal function. Chronic intoxication is associated with weakness, tiredness, headaches, irritability, confusion, restlessness, psychosis, and sometimes coma. Dermatologic manifestations include rash, nodular or pustular lesions, and ulcerations (134,141). Anorexia, constipation, and GI distress may also occur. Bromism is treated by the administration of a large quantity of sodium chloride and a chloruretic agent. Hemodialysis or peritoneal dialysis can be used to lower bromide levels rapidly (142).

CONCLUSIONS

Major AEDs may fail because of lack of efficacy or increased toxicity and serious reactions. In these cases, less commonly used AEDs may be efficacious and may help provide better seizure control. Although these drugs are usually administered as adjunctive therapy, the physician should be encouraged to aim for monotherapy with these second-line agents if seizure frequency is reduced. Monotherapy simplifies the drug regimen, reduces cost, decreases toxic reactions, and probably further improves seizure control. Nonpharmacologic therapy, such as intermittent vagus nerve stimulation, may provide another alternative for patients with medically refractory seizures.

ACKNOWLEDGMENTS

The authors thank Dr. K.A. Abboud of the University of Florida, Department of Chemistry, who prepared Figure 69.1. The authors also thank Karen Cooper for her assistance in revising this chapter.

REFERENCES

1. Scott Levin's PPDA, MAT. February 1999.
2. Merritt HH, Putnam TJ. A new series of anticonvulsant drugs tested by experiments on animals. *Arch Neurol Psychiatry* 1938; 39:1003–1015.
3. Putnam TJ, Merritt HH. Experimental determination of anticonvulsant properties of some phenyl derivatives. *Science* 1937;85: 525–526.
4. Merritt HH, Putnam TJ. Sodium diphenylhydantoinate in treatment of convulsive disorders. *JAMA* 1938;111:1068–1073.
5. Kupferberg HJ. Other hydantoins: mephenytoin and ethotoin. In: Levy R, Mattson R, Meldrum B, et al, eds. *Antiepileptic drugs*, 3rd ed. New York: Raven Press. 1989:257–266.
6. Schwade ED, Richards RK, Everett GM. Peganone, a new anticonvulsant drug. *Dis Nerv Syst* 1956;17:155–158.
7. Carter CA, Helms RA, Boehm R. Ethotoin in seizures of childhood and adolescence. *Neurology* 1984;34:791–795.
8. Biton V, Gates JR, Ritter FJ, et al. Adjunctive therapy for intractable epilepsy with ethotoin. *Epilepsia* 1990;31:433–437.
9. Finnell RH, Dilibert JH. Hydantoin-induced teratogenesis: are arene oxide intermediates really responsible? *Helv Paediatr Acta* 1983;38:171–177.
10. Zablen M, Brand N. Cleft lip and palate with the anticonvulsant ethotoin. *N Engl J Med* 1977;297:1404.
11. Wilder BJ, Bruni J. *Seizure disorders: a pharmacological approach to treatment.* New York: Raven Press. 1981.
12. Glazko AJ, Dill WA. Other succinimides: methsuximide and phensuximide. In: Woodbury DM, Penry JK, Schmidt RP, eds. *Antiepileptic drugs.* New York: Raven Press. 1972:455–464.
13. Porter RJ, Penry JK, Lacy IR, et al. Plasma concentrations of phensuximide, methsuximide and their metabolites in relation to clinical efficacy. *Neurology* 1979;29:1509–1513.
14. Strong JM, Abe R, Gibbs EL, et al. Plasma levels of methsuximide and *N*-desmethylmethsuximide during methsuximide therapy. *Neurology* 1974;24:250–255.
15. Wilder BJ, Buchanan RB. Methsuximide for refractory complex partial seizures. *Neurology* 1981;31:741–744.
16. Browne TR, Feldman RG, Buchanan RA, et al. Methsuximide for complex partial seizures: efficacy, toxicity, clinical pharmacology, and drug interactions. *Neurology* 1983;33:414–418.
17. Coroba EF, Strobos RRJ. *N*-methyl-2-methylphenyl-succinimide, in psychomotor epilepsy. *Dis Nerv Syst* 1956;17:383–385.
18. Aird RB, Woodbury DM. *The management of epilepsy.* Springfield, IL: Charles C Thomas. 1974.
19. French EG, Rey-Bellet J, Lennox WG. Methsuximide in psychomotor and petit mal seizures. *N Engl J Med* 1958;253: 892–894.
20. Livingston S, Pauli L. Celontin in the treatment of epilepsy. *Pediatrics* 1957;19:614–618.
21. Zimmerman FT, Burgemeister BB. Use of *N*-methyl-a,-a-methylphenylsuccinimide in the treatment of petit mal epilepsy. *Arch Neurol Psychiatry* 1954;72:720–725.
22. Uthman BM, Wilder BJ. Methsuximide. In: Kutt H, Resor SR, eds. *Medical treatment of epilepsy.* New York: Marcel Dekker. 1991: 379–384.
23. Sigler M, Strassburg HM, Boenigk HE. Effective and safe but forgotten: methsuximide in intractable epilepsies in childhood. *Seizure* 2001;10:120–124.
24. Tennison MB, Greenwood RS, Miles MV. Methsuximide for intractable childhood seizures. *Pediatrics* 1991;87:186–189.
25. Carter CH, Maley MC. Use of Celontin in the treatment of mixed epilepsy. *Neurology* 1957;7:483–484.
26. Dow RW, McFarlane JP, Stevens JR. Celontin in patients with refractory epilepsy. *Neurology* 1958;8:201–204.
27. Scholl ML, Abbott JA, Schwab RS. Celontin—a new anticonvulsant. *Epilepsia* 1959;1:105–109.
28. Zimmerman FT. *N*-methyl-a,a-methylphenylsuccinimide in psychomotor epilepsy treatment. *Arch Neurol Psychiatry* 1956;76: 65–71.
29. Livingston S, Eisner V, Pauli L. Minor motor epilepsy: diagnosis, treatment and prognosis. *Pediatrics* 1958;21:916–928.
30. Rabe F. Celontin (Petinutin)—A contribution to the differential therapy of epilepsy [German]. *Nervenarzt* 1960;7:306–312.
31. Brenner RP, Seelinger DF. Drawing-induced seizures. *Arch Neurol* 1979;36:515–516.
32. Hurst DL. Methsuximide therapy of juvenile myoclonic epilepsy. *Seizure* 1996;5:47–50.
33. Rambeck B. Pharmacological interactions of methsuximide with phenobarbital and phenytoin in hospitalized epileptic patients. *Epilepsia* 1979;20:147–156.
34. Eichelbaum M, Kothe KW, Hoffmann F, et al. Kinetics and metabolism of carbamazepine during combined antiepileptic drug therapy. *Clin Pharmacol Ther* 1979;26:366–371.
35. May T, Rambeck B, Jurgens U. Influence of oxcarbazepine and methsuximide on lamotrigine concentrations in epileptic patients with and without valproic acid comedication: results of a retrospective study. *Ther Drug Monit* 1999;21: 175–181.
36. Besag FM, Berry DJ, Vasey M. Methsuximide reduces valproic acid serum levels. *Ther Drug Monit* 2001;23:694–697.
37. Mataringa MI, May TW, Rambeck B. Does lamotrigine influence valproate concentrations? *Ther Drug Monit* 2002;24: 631–636.
38. Besag FM. Methsuximide lower lamotrigine blood levels: a pharmacokinetic antiepileptic drug interaction. *Epilepsia* 2000;41: 624–627.
39. May TW, Rambeck B, Jurgens U. Serum concentrations of topiramate in patients with epilepsy: influence of dose, age, and comedication. *Ther Drug Monit* 2002;24:366–374.
40. Dooley J, Camfield P, Buckley D, et al. Methsuximide-induced movement disorder. *Pediatrics* 1991;88:1291–1292.
41. Karch SB. Methsuximide overdose: delayed onset of profound coma. *JAMA* 1973;223:1463–1465.
42. Baehler RW, Work J, Smith W, et al. Charcoal hemoperfusion in the therapy for methsuximide and phenytoin overdose. *Arch Intern Med* 1980;140:1466–1468.
43. Hauptman A. Luminal bei Epilepsie. *Munch Med Wochenschr* 1912;59:1907–1909.
44. Mattson RH, Cramer JA, Collins JF, et al. Comparison of carbamazepine, phenobarbital, phenytoin, and primidone in partial and secondary generalized tonic-clonic seizures. *N Engl J Med* 1985;313:145–151.
45. Farwell JR, Lee YJ, Hirtz DG, et al. Phenobarbital for febrile seizures: effects on intelligence and on seizure recurrence. *N Engl J Med* 1990;322:364–369.
46. Goldberg RN, Moscoso P, Bauer CR, et al. Use of barbiturate therapy in severe perinatal asphyxia: a randomized controlled trial. *J Pediatr* 1986;109:851–856.
47. Kuban KCK, Krishnamoorthy KS, Littlewood Teele R, et al. Neonatal intracranial hemorrhage and phenobarbital. *Pediatrics* 1986;77:443–450.
48. Painter MJ. How to use phenobarbital. In: Morselli PL, Pippenger CE, Penry JK, eds. *Antiepileptic drug therapy in pediatrics.* New York: Raven Press. 1983:245–250.
49. Wallin A, Boreus LO. Phenobarbital prophylaxis for hyperbilirubinemia in preterm infants: a controlled study of bilirubin disappearance and infant behavior. *Acta Pediatr Scand* 1984;73: 488–497.
50. Pritchard JW. Phenobarbital mechanisms of action. In: Woodbury D, Penry JK, Pippenger CE, eds. *Antiepileptic drugs*, 2nd ed. New York: Raven Press. 1982:1332–1335.
51. Hooper WD, Kunze HE, Eadie MJ. Qualitative and quantitative studies of methylphenobarbital metabolism in man. *Drug Metab* 1981;9:381–385.

52. Craig CR, Shideman FE. Metabolism and anticonvulsant properties of mephobarbital and phenobarbital in rats. *J Pharmacol Exp Ther* 1971;176:35–41.

53. Buch H, Knabe J, Buzello W, et al. Stereospecificity of anaesthetic activity, distribution, inactivation and protein binding of the optical antipodes of two *N*-methylated barbiturates. *J Pharmacol Exp Ther* 1970;176:709–716.

54. Pellmar TC, Wilson WA. Synaptic mechanism of pentylenetetrazol: selectivity for chloride conductance. *Science* 1977;179:912–914.

55. Smith JA, Waddell WJ, Butler TC. Demethylation of *N*-methyl derivatives of barbituric acid, hydantoin and 2,4-oxazolidinedione by rat liver microsomes. *Life Sci* 1963;7:486–492.

56. Butler TC, Mahaffee D, Mahaffee C. The role of the liver in the metabolic disposition of mephobarbital. *J Pharmacol Exp Ther* 1952;106:364–369.

57. Hooper WD, Kunze HE, Eadie MJ. Pharmacokinetics and bioavailability of methylphenobarbital in man. *Ther Drug Monit* 1981;3:39–44.

58. Blum E. Die Bekanfung epileptischer Anfalle und iher Folgeer Scheinungen mit Prominal. *Dtsch Med Wochenschr* 1932;58:230–236.

59. Eadie MJ. Other barbiturates: methyl-phenobarbital and metharbital. In: Levy R, Mattson R, Meldrum B, et al, eds. *Antiepileptic drugs*, 3rd ed. New York: Raven Press. 1989:357–378.

60. Kupferberg HJ, Longacre-Shaw J. Mephobarbital and phenobarbital plasma concentrations in epileptic patients treated with mephobarbital. *Ther Drug Monit* 1979;1:117–122.

61. Hutt SJ, Jackson PM, Belsham A, et al. Perceptual-motor behavior in relation to blood phenobarbital level: a preliminary report. *Dev Med Child Neurol* 1968;10:626–632.

62. Camfield C. Clinical trials of phenobarbital. Presented at the NIH Consensus Development Conference on Febrile Seizures. Bethesda, May 19–21, 1980.

63. McLeod CM, Dekaban AS, Hunt E. Memory impairment in epileptic patients: selective effects of phenobarbital concentrations. *Science* 1978;202:1102–1104.

64. Willis J, Nelson A, Black FW, et al. Barbiturate anticonvulsants: a neuropsychological and quantitative electroencephalographic study. *J Child Neurol* 1997;12:169–171.

65. Bergstrom WH, Carzoli RF, Lombroso C, et al. Observations on metabolic and clinical effects of carbonic anhydrase inhibitors in epileptics. *Am J Dis Child* 1952;84:771–772.

66. Ansell B, Clarke E. Acetazolamide in treatment of epilepsy. *Br Med J* 1956;1:650–661.

67. Forsythe WI, Owens JR, Toothill C. Effectiveness of acetazolamide in the treatment of carbamazepine-resistant epilepsy in children. *Dev Med Child Neurol* 1981;23:761–769.

68. Golla FL, Sessions HR. Control of petit mal by acetazolamide. *J Ment Sci* 1957;103:214–217.

69. Lombroso CT, Davidson DT Jr, Gross-Bianchi ML. Further evaluation of acetazolamide (Diamox) in treatment of epilepsy. *JAMA* 1956;160:268–272.

70. Millichap JG. Anticonvulsant action of Diamox in children. *Neurology* 1956;6:552–559.

71. Maren TH, Mayer E, Wadsworth BC. Carbonic anhydrase inhibition, I: the pharmacology of Diamox (2-acetylamino-1,3,4-thiadiazole-5-sulfonamide). *Bull Johns Hopkins Hosp* 1954;95:199–243.

72. Millichap JG, Woodbury DM, Goodman LS. Mechanism of the anticonvulsant action of acetazolamide, a carbonic anhydrase inhibitor. *J Pharmacol Exp Ther* 1955;115:251–258.

73. Velisek L, Moshé SL, Xu SG, et al. Reduced susceptibility to seizures in carbonic anhydrase II deficient mutant mice. *Epilepsy Res* 1993;14:115–121.

74. Masereel B, Rolin S, Abbate F, et al. Carbonic anhydrase inhibitors: anticonvulsant sulfonamides incorporating valproyl and other lipophilic moieties. *J Med Chem* 2002;45:312–320.

75. Woodbury DM. Pharmacology and mechanisms of action of antiepileptic drugs. In: Goldensohn ES, Appel SH, eds. *Scientific approaches to clinical neurology*. Philadelphia: Lea & Febiger. 1977:693–726.

76. Leniger T, Wiemann M, Bingmann D, et al. Carbonic anhydrase inhibitor sulthiame reduces intracellular pH and epileptiform activity of hippocampal CA3 neurons. *Epilepsia* 2002;43:469–474.

77. Woodbury DM, Kemp JW. Basic mechanisms of seizures: neurophysiological and biochemical etiology. In: Shagass C, Gerson S, Friedhoff AJ, eds. *Psychopathology and brain dysfunction*. New York: Raven Press. 1977:149–182.

78. Woodbury DM. Antiepileptic drugs: carbonic anhydrase inhibitors. In: Glaser GH, Penry JK, Woodbury DM, eds. *Antiepileptic drugs: mechanisms of action*. New York: Raven Press. 1980:617–634.

79. Panayiotopoulos CP. Treatment of typical absence seizures and related epileptic syndromes. *Paediatr Drugs* 2001;3:379–403.

80. Lim LL, Foldvary N, Mascha E, Lee J. Acetazolamide in women with catamenial epilepsy. *Epilepsia* 2001;42:746–749.

81. Resor SR Jr, Resor LD. Chronic acetazolamide monotherapy in the treatment of juvenile myoclonic epilepsy. *Neurology* 1990;40:1677–1681.

82. Katayama F, Miura H, Takanashi S. Long-term effectiveness and side effects of acetazolamide as an adjunct to other anticonvulsants in the treatment of refractory epilepsies. *Brain Dev* 2002;24:150–154.

83. Reiss WG, Oles KS. Acetazolamide in the treatment of epilepsy. *Ann Pharmacother* 1996;30:514–519.

84. Woodbury DM, Kemp JW. Other antiepileptic drugs: sulfonamides and derivatives. In: Levy R, Mattson R, Meldrum B, et al, eds. *Antiepileptic drugs*, 3rd ed. New York: Raven Press, 1989:855–876.

85. Kubota F, Kifune A, Shibata N, et al. Bone mineral density of epileptic patients on long-term antiepileptic drug therapy: a quantitative digital radiography study. *Epilepsy Res* 1999;33:93–97.

86. Futagi Y, Atani K, Abe J. Growth suppression in children receiving acetazolamide with antiepileptic drugs. *Pediatr Neurol* 1996;15:323–326.

87. Bessey OA, Adam DJD, Hansen AE. Intake of vitamin B-6 and infantile convulsions: a first approximation of requirements of pyridoxine in infants. *Pediatrics* 1957;10:33–44.

88. Livingston SJ, Hsu M, Petersen DC. Ineffectiveness of pyridoxine (vitamin B-6) in the treatment of epilepsy. *Pediatrics* 1955;16:250–251.

89. Scriver CR. Vitamin B-6–dependency infantile convulsions. *Pediatrics* 1960;26:62–74.

90. Scriver CR, Hutchison JH. The vitamin B-6 deficiency syndrome in human infancy: biochemical and clinical observations. *Pediatrics* 1963;31:240–250.

91. Hunt AD, Stokes J, McCrory WW, et al. Pyridoxine dependency: report of a case of intractable convulsions in an infant controlled by pyridoxine. *Pediatrics* 1954;13:140–145.

92. Scriver CR, Whelan DT. Glutamic acid decarboxylase (GAD) in mammalian tissue outside the central nervous system, and its possible relevance to hereditary vitamin B-6 dependency with seizures. *Ann N Y Acad Sci* 1969;166:83–96.

93. Bachmann DS. Late-onset pyridoxine-dependency convulsions. *Ann Neurol* 1983;14:692–693.

94. Coker SB. Postneonatal vitamin B-6–dependent epilepsy. *Pediatrics* 1992;90:221–223.

95. Kurleman G, Loscher W, Dominick HC, et al. Disappearance of neonatal seizures and low CSF GABA levels after treatment with vitamin B-6. *Epilepsy Res* 1987;1:152–154.

96. Yoshida T, Tada K, Arakawa T. Vitamin B 6-dependency of glutamic acid decarboxylase in the kidney from a patient with vitamin B 6 dependent convulsion. *Tohoku J Exp Med* 1971;104:195–198.

97. Baxter P. Pyridoxine-dependent seizures: a clinical and biochemical conundrum. *Biochim Biophys Acta* 2003;1647:36–41.

98. Gospe SM. Pyridoxine-dependent seizures: findings from recent studies pose new questions. *Pediatr Neurol* 2002;26:181–185.

99. Bankier A, Turner M, Hopkins IJ. Pyridoxine dependent seizures: a wider clinical spectrum. *Arch Dis Child* 1983;58:415–418.

100. Goutieres F, Aicardi J. Atypical presentations of pyridoxine-dependent seizures: a treatable cause of intractable epilepsy in infants. *Ann Neurol* 1985;17:117–120.

101. Mikati MA, Trevathan E, Krishnamoorthy KS, et al. Pyridoxine-dependent epilepsy: EEG investigations and long-term follow-up. *Electroencephalogr Clin Neurophysiol* 1991;78:215–221.

102. Haenggeli CA, Girardin E, Paunier L. Pyridoxine-dependent seizures, clinical therapeutic aspects. *Eur J Pediatr* 1991;150:452–455.

103. Gospe SM Jr, Hecht ST. Longitudinal MRI findings in pyridoxine-dependent seizures. *Neurology* 1998;51:74–78.

104. Clarke TA, Saunders BS, Feldman B. Pyridoxine-dependent seizures requiring high doses of pyridoxine for control. *Am J Dis Child* 1979;133:963–965.

105. Krishnamoorthy KS. Pyridoxine-dependency seizure: report of a rare presentation. *Ann Neurol* 1983;13:103–104.

106. Bass NE, Wyllie E, Cohen B, et al. Pyridoxine-dependent epilepsy: the need for repeated pyridoxine trials and the risk of severe electrocerebral suppression with intravenous pyridoxine infusion. *J Child Neurol* 1996;11:422–424.

107. Lott IT, Coulombe T, DiPaolo RV, et al. Vitamin B 6-dependent seizures: pathology chemical findings in brain. *Neurology* 1978;28:47–54.

108. Friedrich AM, Baumeister MD, Gsell W, et al. Glutamate in pyridoxine-dependent epilepsy: neurotoxic glutamate concentration in the cerebrospinal fluid and its normalization by pyridoxine. *Pediatrics* 1994;94:318–321.

109. Ito M, Mikawa M, Tangiguchi T. Cerebrospinal fluid GABA levels in children with infantile spasms. *Neurology* 1984;34:235–238.

110. Loscher W, Siemes H. Cerebrospinal fluid: aminobutyric acid levels in children with different types of epilepsy: effect of anticonvulsant treatment. *Epilepsia* 1985;16:314–319.

111. Blennow G, Starck L. High dose B-6 treatment in infantile spasms. *Neuropediatrics* 1986;17:7–10.

112. Ito M, Okuno T, Hattori H, et al. Vitamin B-6 and valproic acid in treatment of infantile spasms. *Pediatr Neurol* 1991;7:91–96.

113. Ohtsuka Y, Matsuda M, Kohno C, et al. Pyridoxal phosphate in the treatment of the West syndrome. In: Akimoto H, Seino M, Ward AA Jr, eds. *Advances in epileptology. XIIIth Epilepsy International Symposium.* New York: Raven Press. 1982:311–313.

114. Pietz J, Benninger C, Schafer H, et al. Treatment of infantile spasms with high-dosage vitamin B6. *Epilepsia* 1993;34:757–763.

115. Jiao FY, Takuma Y, Wu S, et al. Randomized, controlled trial of high-dose intravenous pyridoxine in the treatment of recurrent seizures in children. *Pediatr Neurol* 1997;17:54–57.

116. Garty R, Yonis Z, Braham J, et al. Pyridoxine-dependent convulsions in an infant. *Arch Dis Child* 1962;37:21–24.

117. Kroll J. Pyridoxine for neonatal seizures: an unexpected danger. *Dev Med Child Neurol* 1985;27:369–382.

118. Heeley A, Puch RJP, Clayton BE, et al. Pyridoxol metabolism in vitamin B-6 responsive convulsions of early infancy. *Arch Dis Child* 1978;53:794–802.

119. Antopol W, Tarlov IM. Experimental study of the effects produced by large doses of vitamin B-6. *J Neuropathol Exp Neurol* 1942;1:330–336.

120. Dalton K, Dalton JT. Characteristics of pyridoxine overdose neuropathy syndrome. *Acta Neurol Scand* 1987;76:8–11.

121. Parry GJ, Bredesen DE. Sensory neuropathy with low-dose pyridoxine. *Neurology* 1985;35:1466–1468.

122. Schaumburg H, Kaplan J, Windebank A, et al. Sensory neuropathy from pyridoxine abuse: a new megavitamin syndrome. *N Engl J Med* 1983;309:445–448.

123. Xu Y, Sladky JT, Brown MJ. Dose-dependent expression of neuronopathy after experimental pyridoxine intoxication. *Neurology* 1989;39:1077–1083.

124. Berger AR, Schaumburg HH, Schroeder C, et al. Dose response, coasting, and differential fibre vulnerability in human toxic neuropathy: a prospective study of pyridoxine neurotoxicity. *Neurology* 1992;42:1367–1370.

125. Berger A, Schaumburg HH. More on neuropathy from pyridoxine abuse. *N Engl J Med* 1984;311:986–987.

126. Albin R, Alpers JW, Greenberg HS, et al. Acute sensory neuropathy-neuronopathy from pyridoxine overdose. *Neurology* 1987;37:1729–1732.

127. Bernstein AL, Lobitz CS. A clinical and electrophysiologic study of the treatment of painful diabetic neuropathies with pyridoxine. In: Leklem JE, Reynolds RD, eds. *Clinical and physiological applications of vitamin B-6. Current topics in nutrition and disease.* New York: Alan R. Liss. 1988;19:415–423.

128. Del Tredici AM, Bernstein AL, Chinn K. Carpal tunnel syndrome and vitamin B-6 therapy. In: Reynolds RD, Leklem JE, eds. *Vitamin B-6: its role in health and disease. Current topics in nutrition and disease.* New York: Alan R. Liss. 1985;13:459–462.

129. Reynolds RD. Pyridoxine dependent seizures. *Arch Dis Child* 1984;59:906–907.

130. Mpofu C, Alani SM, Whitehouse C, et al. No sensory neuropathy during pyridoxine treatment in homocystinuria. *Arch Dis Child* 1991;66:1081–1082.

131. McLachlan RS, Brown WF. Pyridoxine dependent epilepsy with iatrogenic sensory neuronopathy. *Can J Neurol Sci* 1995;22:50–51.

132. Locock C. In discussion of Sieveking EH. Analysis of 52 cases of epilepsy observed by author. *Lancet.* 1857;1:527.

133. Palachios JM, Nieholt DL, Kuhar MJ. Ontogeny of GABA and benzodiazepine receptors: effects of Triton X-100, bromide and muscimol. *Brain Res* 1979;179:390–395.

134. Woodbury DM, Pippenger CE. Bromides. In: Woodbury DM, Penry JK, Pippenger CE, eds. *Antiepileptic drugs*, 2nd ed. New York: Raven Press. 1986:791–801.

135. Vaiseman N, Koren G, Pencharz P. Pharmacokinetics of oral and intravenous bromide in normal volunteers. *Clin Toxicol* 1986;24:403–413.

136. Dreifuss FE. Bromides. In: Levy R, Mattson R, Meldrum B, et al, eds. *Antiepileptic drugs*, 3rd ed. New York: Raven Press. 1989:877–879.

137. Ernst J, Doose H, Baier WK. Bromides were effective in intractable epilepsy with generalized tonic-clonic seizures and onset in early childhood. *Brain Dev* 1988;10:385–388.

138. Oguni H, Hayashi K, Oguni M, et al. Treatment of severe myoclonic epilepsy in infants with bromide and its borderline variant. *Epilepsia* 1994;35:1140–1145.

139. Steinhoff BJ, Kruse R. Bromide treatment of pharmaco-resistant epilepsies with generalized tonic-clonic seizures: a clinical study. *Brain Dev* 1992;14:144–149.

140. Stewart LS. Anticonvulsant medications. *Emerg Med Serv* 2001;30:56–66.

141. James LP, Farrar HC, Griebel ML, et al. Bromism: intoxication from a rare anticonvulsant therapy. *Pediatr Emerg Care* 1997;13:268–270.

142. Lichtenberg R, Zeller WP, Gatson R, et al. Bromate poisoning. *J Pediatr* 1989;114:891–894.

The Ketogenic Diet

70

Douglas R. Nordli, Jr.   *Darryl C. De Vivo*

INTRODUCTION

The ketogenic diet is a high-fat, low-carbohydrate, low-protein regimen that has been used for more than 70 years in thousands of patients. It is an effective and safe medical treatment for epilepsy, but it must be judiciously applied and carefully monitored.

Historical Highlights

There are biblical references to the salutary effects of starvation upon seizure control, but the earliest scientific observations were made by Geyelin at the Presbyterian Hospital in 1921 (1). Shortly thereafter, Wilder proposed a high-fat diet to mimic the effects of starvation (2). Since this high-fat diet increased the production of ketone bodies, the regimen became known as a "keto," or ketogenic diet. It was known that ketone bodies could be found in the urine of patients with diabetes and that they were produced when fatty acids were oxidized. This led to the notion that ketone bodies were potentially toxic metabolites of fatty acid degradation and that their anticonvulsant effect was caused by a sedative property, similar to the mechanisms of action of the available anticonvulsants of that era—bromides and phenobarbital.

This notion was challenged when Krebs suggested that ketone bodies were fuel for respiration in 1961 (3). In 1967, Owen and colleagues proved that ketone bodies were the major fuel for brain metabolism during starvation (4). Appleton and De Vivo (1974) developed an animal model, whereby they demonstrated that utilization of ketone bodies during starvation alters brain metabolites and increases cerebral energy reserves (5). In 1976, Huttenlocher showed that the level of ketosis correlated with efficacy (6). Livingston and associates reported extensive (41-year) experience with the ketogenic diet for the treatment of myoclonic seizures of childhood, stating that it completely controlled seizures in 54% of his patients and markedly improved control in another 26% (7). Subsequently, valproate (VPA) and other antiepileptic drugs (AEDs) effective for the control of myoclonic seizures were introduced in the United States. Yet, despite the availability of these agents, the ketogenic diet continues to be used in many centers across the country.

PRODUCTION AND UTILIZATION OF KETONE BODIES

The major precursors of ketone bodies are nonesterified fatty acids. During the fasting state, the decrease in blood glucose reduces plasma insulin production, stimulates lipolysis in fatty tissues, and increases the flux of nonesterified fatty acids to the liver. Nonesterified fatty acids can be esterified or metabolized to ketone bodies. The fate of fatty acids in the liver is determined, at least in part, by the carbohydrate status of the host (8). A critical component of this regulation is malonyl-coenzyme A (CoA), an intermediate in the pathway of lipogenesis (9,10). Malonyl-CoA inhibits carnitine acyltransferase I, which is needed to shuttle long-chain fatty acyl-CoA into the mitochondria for oxidation. The production of glucose from glycogen provides the carbon source for lipogenesis and, in particular, malonyl-CoA. If glucose is reduced, so is malonyl-CoA. The reduction in malonyl-CoA decreases the inhibition of (or increases the net activity of) carnitine acyltransferase. This allows more movement of fatty acids into the mitochondria, where fatty acyl-CoA is converted to acetyl-CoA and later to acetoacetate (AcAc). AcAc is in equilibrium with β-hydroxybutyrate, the major ketone body used by the brain.

Passage of ketone bodies into the brain may be the critical factor limiting the rate of brain utilization of these chemicals. Movement of ketone bodies into the brain relies on the monocarboxylic transporter-1 system. This is upregulated during fasting in adults and during milk feeding in neonates (11,12). Fasting studies in humans demonstrated that the brain's ability to extract ketone bodies is inversely related to the age of the subject (13). In contrast to glucose, ketone bodies can pass directly into mitochondria without being processed in the cytosol. Also in contrast to glucose, ketone bodies may be used directly by neurons for metabolism (14).

Once inside the mitochondria, β-hydroxybutyrate is converted to AcAc and then to AcAc-CoA . The enzyme that facilitates this is 3-oxoacid-CoA-transferase, or succinyl-CoA-acetoacetate-CoA-transferase. As the name implies, this conversion requires commensurate conversion of succinyl-CoA to succinate. It is possible that reduced blood glucose and increased blood ketones may be needed to induce the activity of this enzyme (15).

SCIENTIFIC BASIS OF THE DIET

Scientific studies of the ketogenic diet have revealed important biochemical and metabolic observations. The animal model designed by Appleton and De Vivo permitted study of the effect of the ketogenic diet on cerebral metabolism (5). Adult male albino rats were placed on either (a) a high-fat diet containing (by weight) 38% corn oil, 38% lard, 11% vitamin-free casein, 6.8% glucose, 4% United States Pharmacopeia salt mixture (USP), and 2.2% vitamin diet fortification mixture; or (b) a high-carbohydrate diet containing (by weight) 50% glucose, 28.8% vitamin-free casein, 7.5% corn oil, 7.5% lard, 4% USP salt mixture, and 2.2% vitamin diet fortification mixture. Parallel studies were conducted to evaluate electroconvulsive shock responses and biochemical alterations. These studies revealed that the mean voltage necessary to produce a minimal convulsion remained constant for 12 days before the high-fat diet was started and approximately 10 days after beginning the feedings (69.75 ± 1.88 volts). After 10 to 12 days on the high-fat diet, the intensity of the convulsive response to the established voltage decreased, necessitating an increase in voltage in order to reestablish a minimal convulsive response. Approximately 20 days after beginning the high-fat diet, a new convulsive threshold was achieved (81.25 ± 2.39 volts; $p < 0.01$). When the high-fat diet was replaced by the high-carbohydrate diet, a rapid change in response to the voltage was observed. Within 48 hours, the animal exhibited a maximal convulsion to the electrical stimulus that previously had produced only a minimal convulsion, and the mean voltage to produce a minimal convulsion returned to the prestudy value (70.75 ± 1.37 volts).

Blood concentrations of β-hydroxybutyrate, AcAc, chloride, esterified fatty acids, triglycerides, cholesterol, and total lipids increased in the rats fed on the high-fat diet. Brain levels of β-hydroxybutyrate and sodium were also significantly increased in the fat-fed rats.

Hori and associates studied the efficacy of the ketogenic diet in kindled animals—an appropriate model for partial seizures—and found the diet to have transient anticonvulsant properties (16). The investigators studied 32 male Sprague-Dawley rats, 20 of which were kindled and underwent behavioral testing; the 12 others underwent behavioral testing alone. Rats were kindled from P56 to 60 and then randomized (10 in each group) to treatment with either a ketogenic diet or regular rat chow. After-discharge threshold and seizure thresholds were tested at 1, 2, 4, and 5 weeks. Behavioral testing using both a water maze test and an open-field test was performed at week 3. During the period of administration of the ketogenic diet, statistically significant elevations of β-hydroxybutyrate were reported. Both the after-discharge thresholds and seizure thresholds were raised for the first 2 weeks of the diet; however, this effect disappeared by weeks 4 and 5. There was no difference in behavioral performance between the ketogenic diet rats and the controls (16).

Stafstrom and coworkers reported on electrophysiologic observations using hippocampal slices from rats treated with the ketogenic diet (17). They found that the ketogenic diet did not alter baseline electrophysiologic parameters in normal rats (excitatory postsynaptic potential [EPSP] slope, input and output relationship, responses to evoked stimulation, and Mg($++$)-free burst frequency), but that it was associated with fewer spontaneous seizures and reduced CA1 excitability in rats made chronically epileptic by administration of kainic acid. The researchers concluded that at least part of the ketogenic diet mechanism of action might involve long-term changes in network excitability. In another experiment, rats fed the ketogenic diet after kainic acid-induced status epilepticus had significantly fewer and briefer spontaneous seizures, and less supragranular mossy fiber sprouting, compared with animals on a normal diet (18). These results provide evidence that the ketogenic diet has an antiepileptogenic effect in an experimental model.

Bough and Eagles demonstrated that the ketogenic diet increases the resistance to pentylenetetrazole-induced seizures in the rat (19). In their experiment, seizures were induced by tail-vein infusion of pentylenetetrazole in rats fed either a ketogenic diet or a normal diet for 35 days. The rats fed a ketogenic diet had a significantly increased threshold for seizure induction ($p < 0.01$) compared with controls. These observations are particularly relevant because this model may mimic the condition of myoclonic seizure disorders in humans (19). In subsequent experiments, Bough and other collaborators performed recordings in the dentate gyrus of rats fed ketogenic calorie-restricted (KCR), normal calorie-restricted (NCR), or normal ad libitum (NAL) diets. *In vivo* extracellular field responses to angular bundle stimulation were recorded. Input and output curves and paired-pulse relations were used to assess network excitability, and a maximal dentate activation (MDA) protocol was used to measure electrographic seizure threshold and duration. The animals fed the KCR diet showed greater paired-pulse inhibition, elevated MDA threshold, and an absence of spreading depression-like events. Perhaps even more importantly, in the MDA model, the rate of increase in seizure duration after repeated stimuli was markedly reduced in the rats fed the KCR diet. These results agree with clinical observations made in the early 20th century that calorie restriction may be anticonvulsant, but they also show that the KCR diet has special properties and may, in fact be antiepileptogenic (20a).

De Vivo and colleagues reported on the change in cerebral metabolites in chronically ketotic rats (21), and found no changes in brain water content, electrolytes, and pH. As expected, fat-fed rats had significantly lower blood glucose concentrations and higher blood β-hydroxybutyrate and AcAc concentrations. More importantly, brain concentrations of adenosine triphosphate (ATP), glycogen, glucose-6-phosphate, pyruvate, lactate, β-hydroxybutyrate, citrate, α-ketoglutarate, and alanine were higher, and brain concentrations of fructose 1,6-diphosphate, aspartate, adenosine diphosphate (ADP), creatine, cyclic nucleotides, acid-insoluble CoA, and total CoA were lower in the fat-fed group. Cerebral energy reserves were significantly higher in the fat-fed rats (26.4 ± 0.6) compared with controls (23.6 ± 0.2; $p < 0.005$). Many of these changes in metabolites could be explained by the higher energy state of the brain cells in the fat-fed group, specifically by the ratio of ATP to ADP. In addition, the normal oxaloacetate, elevated α-ketoglutarate and decreased succinyl-CoA imply maximal tricarboxylic acid (TCA) cycle activity—quite contrary to the metabolite profile observed with anesthetic-sedative agents. Pan and associates used 31P spectroscopic imaging at 4.1T to demonstrate an elevated ratio of phosphocreatine to inorganic phosphorus in patients on the ketogenic diet and concluded that there was improvement in energy metabolism with use of the diet (22).

Another possible mechanism of action may be suggested from these biochemical alterations. Elevated α-ketoglutarate may indicate increased flux through the γ-aminobutyric acid (GABA) shunt, which may, in turn, be expected to increase cerebral GABA levels. One study of adult male rats fed a ketogenic diet, however, failed to demonstrate elevated cerebral GABA levels (23).

Finally, it is worth speculating about possible GABA mimetic effects of ketosis, given the chemical structural similarities of GABA, β-hydroxybutyrate, and AcAc. Indeed, this notion was advanced in the 1930s by Helmholz and Keith, but does not appear to have been studied further to any great extent (24,25). More recent work by Likhodii and colleagues has suggested that there may be a direct anticonvulsant action of acetone. Rats were administered acetone intraperitoneally and tested in four models: maximal electroshock, subcutaneous pentylenetetrazole, amygdala kindling, and the AY-9944 test—a model of chronic atypical absence seizures. Acetone suppressed seizures in all models (26).

These observations demonstrate that the ketogenic diet has broad anticonvulsant properties and possibly antiepileptogenic activity. In addition, the available biochemical data suggest that the diet favorably influences cerebral energetics, and that increased cerebral energy reserves and increased GABA shunt activity may be important factors bestowing an increased resistance to seizures in ketotic brain tissue (27).

ADMINISTRATION OF THE DIET

Implementation

Patients should be hospitalized for the initiation of the ketogenic diet. Close observation is important, because children with certain underlying inborn errors of metabolism, particularly ones that interfere with the utilization of ketone bodies, could quickly decompensate (28). The hospitalization also provides the opportunity for family members to be instructed on the maintenance of the diet.

The first step is to promote ketosis with a fast. This can be done by the patient fasting after dinner (6:00 PM) on the evening of admission and continuing the fast until breakfast at 8:00 AM on the third day (38 hours). This allows metabolic adaptation to the state of ketosis and an opportunity to screen the child for any severe hypoglycemic predisposition. It is typical to see a transient hypoglycemia during the first few days, which does not require any treatment unless the child demonstrates symptoms. Treatment of asymptomatic hypoglycemia delays the metabolic adaptation of the child to the state of chronic ketosis. During the fast, the patient is offered water, sugar-free beverages, and unsweetened gelatin.

The urine reveals medium to large ketones after the 38-hour fast, and the diet is started. We never have children fast any longer than this; and a shorter period of fasting (24 hours) often suffices with infants. The long-chain triglyceride (LCT) diet consists of three or four parts fat to one part nonfat (carbohydrate and protein), calculated based on weight. It is computed to provide 75 to 100 kcal/kg body weight and 1 to 2 grams of dietary protein/kg body weight per day. Caloric requirements are adjusted to minimize weight gain and to maximize ketonemia. If a 3:1 (fat-to-nonfat) ratio is insufficient to produce the required ketosis, then a ratio of 4:1 is used.

The Conventional Ketogenic Diet or Long-Chain Triglyceride Diet

Prior to initiating the conventional ketogenic or LCT diet, a dietary prescription is made. Calculation of this prescription is straightforward. For example, if a 10-kg child is to be started on a 3:1 diet, one begins by estimating the calorie requirements of the child:

$$10 \text{ kg} \times 100 \text{ kcal/day} = 1,000 \text{ kcal/day}$$

Alternatively, consulting a table of recommended daily allowances (RDAs) may derive this figure. In either case, it may require adjustment based on the child's specific metabolic needs.

The 3:1 ratio of the diet stipulates that 4 grams of food must contain 3 grams of fat and 1 gram of nonfat. The nonfat consists of both carbohydrate and protein. One gram of fat has the calorie equivalent of 9 calories, whereas 1 gram of protein or carbohydrate has the calorie equivalent of approximately 4 calories. Four grams of food (arbitrarily referred to as 1 unit here) on a 3:1 diet is then equal to 31 calories:

$$1 \text{ gram fat} = 9 \text{ calories} \times 3 = 27 \text{ calories}$$
$$1 \text{ gram protein and carbohydrate} = 4 \text{ calories} \times 1$$
$$= 4 \text{ calories}$$
$$\text{Total calories} = 27 + 4 = 31 \text{ calories/unit}$$

To calculate the daily fat intake, one first divides the daily requirements of calories by this figure of 31 calories per unit, which generates the number of units required for the day:

$$1,000 \text{ calories/day/31 calories/unit} = 32.25 \text{ units/day}$$

Next, multiplying by 27 calories of fat/unit provides the daily fat requirement:

$$32.26 \text{ units/day} \times 27 \text{ calories of fat/unit}$$
$$= 871 \text{ calories of fat/day, which is}$$
$$\text{equivalent to 96 grams.}$$

The protein requirement is 10 kg × 2 g/kg, or 20 g per day (80 calories). Alternatively, one may consult the RDA table to determine the protein requirement.

Thus far, the combination of 871 calories of fat and 80 calories of protein leaves only 49 calories (1000 − 951) not accounted for in the daily allowance. The carbohydrate intake is then calculated to supply the necessary remaining calories (49 calories), which in this case is approximately 12 grams.

The dietary prescription for this 10-kg patient on a 3:1 LCT diet is then:

Fat: 96 g/day or 32 g/meal
Protein: 20 g/day or 6.6 g/meal
Carbohydrate: 12 g/day or 4 g/meal,

Although the calculation of the calorie requirements is straightforward, the generation of the actual food prescription requires more time and effort. The approach may vary from institution to institution. In ours, the nutrition support team does the calculation and generates the prescription, and in order to provide a successful regimen, the constituents are customized to fit the individual's preferences and special needs. In so doing, the various elements of the diet may be "juggled" to conform to the nutritional requirements. A food substitution approach may be used, which is analogous to that used for diabetic diets. This approach is simple to implement and increases the flexibility of the diet (17).

Maintenance

After initiation of the diet, the patient remains in the hospital for another 2 to 3 days. This time is used to carefully instruct the parents or caretakers on the techniques of providing the diet, weighing the food, offering food substitutions, and monitoring ketosis. Patients on the ketogenic diet are often supplemented with calcium, iron, folate, and multivitamins, including vitamin D, to satisfy the RDA requirements. Protein requirements are carefully monitored and increased on an individual basis to account for weight gain and growth.

After discharge from the hospital, the child is initially seen on a monthly basis by the nutrition support team or registered dietitian. At each visit, the child's height, weight, and head circumference are charted. Electrolytes, liver function tests, serum lipids and proteins, and a complete blood count are periodically checked. On average, the calorie and nutritional needs are readjusted monthly for infants and every 6 to 12 months for children.

Termination of the Ketogenic Diet

The ketogenic diet should be stopped gradually. A sudden stop of the diet or sudden administration of glucose may aggravate seizures and precipitate status epilepticus (30). Livingston advocates maintaining the diet at a ratio 4:1 for 2 years and, if successful, weaning down to a 3:1 diet for 6 months, followed by 6 months of a 2:1 diet (31). At this point, a regular diet is given. At our institution, we have not used such a rigorous protocol.

ADVERSE EVENTS

The ketogenic diet may be lethal in certain circumstances in which cerebral energy metabolism is deranged. An example of this is pyruvate carboxylase deficiency, in which patients may present early in life with refractory myoclonic seizures (28).

Mitochondrial disorders or diseases that involve the respiratory chain, such as myoclonic epilepsy and ragged-red fiber (MERRF+) disease; mitochondrial encephalopathy, lactic acidosis, and strokelike (MELAS) syndrome, and cytochrome oxidase deficiency, would also probably be contraindications for use of the ketogenic diet, because of the increased stress on respiratory chain and TCA cycle function. Patients with fatty acid oxidation problems would also be adversely affected by use of the ketogenic diet, but such patients do not, as a rule, present with seizures.

Complications

Patients on the ketogenic diet exhibit a significantly reduced quantity of bone mass, which improves in response to vitamin D supplementation (5,000 IU per day) (32). Renal calculi may develop but the occurrence is rare. Lipemia retinalis developed in two of Dr. Livingston's patients (31). Bilateral optic neuropathy has been reported in two children who were treated with a 4:1 "classic" ketogenic diet; these patients were not originally given vitamin B supplements. After administration of vitamin B supplements, vision was restored in both patients. Thinning of hair and, rarely, alopecia may occur. Cardiovascular complications have not been observed in those adults who were examined (31). In a recent prospective study, Ballaban-Gil and associates reported serious adverse events in five of 52 children: severe hypoproteinemia (two patients), with lipemia and hemolytic anemia developing in one of these patients; renal tubular acidosis (one patient), and marked increases in liver function tests (two patients). Four of these patients were comedicated with VPA (33).

Potential Adverse Drug Interactions

Carbonic anhydrase inhibitors, such as acetazolamide and topiramate, should be avoided, particularly in the early stages of treatment with the ketogenic diet. VPA is an inhibitor of fatty acid oxidation and a mitigator of hepatic ketogenesis. At our institution, we have encountered marked elevation of liver transaminases in two patients during coadministration of VPA and the diet, as have Ballaban-Gil and colleagues (33). When possible, therefore, we avoid the use of this agent.

Carnitine supplementation is complex. The agent is often used to supplement the diet of patients with various metabolic derangements whose defects allow a build-up of undesirable intermediates. It is also not uncommon that in patients who need the ketogenic diet, a metabolic disorder of this sort is either suspected or confirmed (another reason to avoid VPA is possible). Carnitine supplementation may be desirable for these patients; however, high doses of carnitine may interfere with ketogenesis. These factors must be weighed in each patient, and the decision to use the supplement should be individualized. This topic has recently been thoroughly reviewed (34).

CLINICAL INDICATIONS FOR USE AND EFFECTIVENESS

Primary Therapy

The ketogenic diet is first-line therapy for the treatment of seizures in association with glucose transporter protein deficiency and pyruvate dehydrogenase (E1) deficiency (35,36). In both cases, the diet effectively treats seizures while providing essential fuel for brain metabolic activity. In patients with E1 deficiency, early initiation of the diet was associated with increased longevity and improved mental development.

Secondary Treatment

Multiple investigators have found the ketogenic diet to be effective in the treatment of patients with symptomatic or cryptogenic forms of generalized epilepsy. Prasad and coworkers have summarized the efficacy data (37). It is clear from the compilation that the diet may be particularly helpful when the symptomatic epilepsy manifests with myoclonic and related seizures. Dr. Livingston found that the diet completely controlled seizures in 54% of his patients with myoclonic epilepsy (7). Freeman and colleagues performed a prospective evaluation of the ketogenic diet in 150 children with refractory epilepsy. (38) At 1 year, 55% of the children remained on the diet and 27% had a greater than 90% reduction in seizure frequency. In 63 studies of 55 patients conducted by Schwartz and associates, a total of 51 studies (81%) showed a greater than 50% reduction in seizure frequency regardless of the type of diet used (39). The particular type of ketogenic diet used may not be critically important, although some investigators have found the medium chain triglyceride (MCT) diet slightly less effective. In one study, 44% of patients treated with the MCT diet achieved a greater than 50% reduction in the number of seizures (40). A corn oil ketogenic diet was found to be equally beneficial to the MCT diet (41). Regardless of the type of diet used, seizure control may be inconsistently accompanied by electroencephalographic improvement (42).

Appropriate epilepsy syndromes in which to consider early treatment with the ketogenic diet include early myoclonic epilepsy, early infantile epileptic encephalopathy, and myoclonic-absence epilepsy. Given the effectiveness of the diet in the treatment of myoclonic epilepsies, it could also be considered early for patients with severe epileptogenic myoclonic encephalopathies that are notoriously difficult to control, such as Lennox-Gastaut syndrome, myoclonic-astatic epilepsy, severe infantile myoclonic epilepsy, and early infantile epileptogenic encephalopathy. However, in our experience, most parents prefer the convenience of a medication, and it is unusual to try the ketogenic diet before at least one or two AEDs have failed. The ketogenic diet can be beneficial in infants with West syndrome who are refractory to corticosteroids and other medications (43). Based on Keith's data and our own experience, the ketogenic diet may also be useful in the treatment of children with refractory absence epilepsy without myoclonus (44). Since the brain's ability to extract ketone bodies diminishes with age, there has been concern about the use of the ketogenic diet in adolescents. However, Mady and associates have shown that the ketogenic diet can be well tolerated and effective for adolescents (45).

Preliminary evidence from Freeman's group suggests that the Atkins diet, which also induces a ketotic state, may have a therapeutic role in patients with medically resistant epilepsy. Three of the six patients (age 7 to 52 years) in their series had seizure reduction and were able to reduce their AED use (46).

Further Possible Indications

Partial Epilepsies

It is very difficult to determine precisely the efficacy of the ketogenic diet in the treatment of partial seizure disorders. Livingston stated that the diet was not effective in treating patients with partial seizures. (7,31) Keith did not classify his patients in a manner that allows one to determine its effectiveness in partial seizures (44). In current use, the diet is usually prescribed for children with other forms of refractory epilepsy.

In the study by Schwartz and coworkers, nine of the 55 children appeared to have partial seizures as their main seizure type (39). Overall, 81% of patients showed a greater than 50% reduction in seizures (39). Although the number of children in each group was small, seizure type did not seem to predict response to treatment. There has been a single report of improvement in language, behavior, and seizure control in three patients with acquired epileptic aphasia (47). Finally, the results from the kindling animal model (16) could be used to predict efficacy in localization-related epilepsies. Although these scant observations support the use of the ketogenic diet in this context, there is no compelling clinical data to favor its use over newer medications or potentially curative surgery. Therefore, children with refractory partial seizures should be evaluated to determine if they are candidates for focal resective surgery. If they are, then in our opinion, surgery need not be delayed to institute a trial of the ketogenic diet. On the other hand, if AEDs have failed and the patient is deemed to be a poor surgical candidate, then the diet should be tried. A more definitive statement would require data comparing the efficacy of the diet in patients with localization-related epilepsy versus those with generalized forms of epilepsy.

CONCLUSIONS

It is remarkable that 70 years and scores of drugs later, the ketogenic diet still retains a role in the modern treatment of children with refractory epilepsy. The diet is the treatment of choice for children with E1 deficiency and glucose transporter protein deficiency. It is an effective and safe treatment for children with refractory generalized cryptogenic or symptomatic epilepsies, but its efficacy is unclear in those with refractory localization-related epilepsy. The diet has clear anticonvulsant properties in a wide variety of animal models, including maximal electroshock, pentylenetetrazole, kindling, and kainic acid. More recent animal data suggest it also has an antiepileptogenic effect.

The ketogenic diet is generally safe but not risk-free. It may have devastating effects, particularly upon initiation,

in children with inborn errors of metabolism. For this reason, we believe it should be initiated in the hospital under the careful observation of professionals well versed in its use. Other side effects, including bone demineralization, growth failure, and kidney stones, may occur with continued administration and must be carefully followed.

Given its record of success, it is likely that the ketogenic diet will stay with us in the years to come. It deserves careful study, both by virtue of its clinical utility, as well as the potential insights to be gleaned from analyzing its effective and nonsedating mechanisms of action.

REFERENCES

1. Geyelin HR. Fasting as a method for treating epilepsy. *Medical Record* 1921;99:1037–1039.
2. Wilder RM. Effects of ketonuria on the course of epilepsy. *Mayo Clin Bull* 1921;2:307–314.
3. Krebs HA. The physiological role of the ketone bodies. *Biochem J* 1961;80:225–233.
4. Owen OE, Morgan AP, Kemp HG, et al. Brain metabolism during fasting. *J Clin Invest* 1967;46:1589–1595.
5. Appleton DB, DeVivo DC. An animal model for the ketogenic diet. *Epilepsia* 1974;15:211–227.
6. Huttenlocher PR. Ketonemia and seizures: metabolic and anticonvulsant effects of two ketogenic diets in childhood epilepsy. *Pediatr Res* 1976;10:536–540.
7. Livingston S, Pauli LL, Pruce I. Ketogenic diet in the treatment of childhood epilepsy. *Dev Med Child Neurol* 1977;19:833–834.
8. Robinson AM, Williamson DH. Physiological roles of ketone bodies as substrates and signals in mammalian tissues. *Physiol Rev* 1980;60:143–187.
9. McGarry JD, Mannaerts GP, Foster DW. A possible role for malonyl CoA in the regulation of hepatic fatty acid oxidation and ketogenesis. *J Clin Invest* 1977;60:265–270.
10. McGarry JD, Leatherman GF, Foster DW. Carnitine palmitoyltransferase I. The site of inhibition of hepatic fatty acid oxidation by malonyl-CoA. *J Biol Chem* 1978;253:4128–4136.
11. Pan JW, Telang FW, Lee JH, de Graff RA, Rothman DL, Stein DT, Hetherington HP. Measurement of beta-hydroxybutyrate in acute hyperketonemia in human brain. *J Neurochem* 2001;79:539–544.
12. Cremer JE, Braun LD, Oldendorf WH. Changes during development in transport processes of the blood-brain barrier. *Biochim Biophys Acta* 1976;448:633–637.
13. Owen OE, Morgan AP, Kemp HG, et al. Brain metabolism during fasting. *J Clin Invest* 1967;46:1589–1595.
14. Pan JW, de Graff RA, Rothman DL, Hetherington HP. 13C-[2,4]-b-hydroxybutyrate metabolism in human brain. *J Neurochem* 2002;81:45.
15. Fredericks M, Ramsey RB. 3-Oxo acid coenzyme A transferase activity in brain and tumors of the nervous system. *J Neurochem* 1978;31:1529–1531.
16. Hori A, Tandon P, Holmes GL, Stafstrom C. Ketogenic diet: effects on expression of kindled seizures and behavior in adult rats. *Epilepsia* 1997;38:750–758.
17. Stafstrom CE, Wang C, Jensen FE. Electrophysiological observations in hippocampal slices from rats treated with the ketogenic diet. *Dev Neurosci* 1999;21:393–399.
18. Muller-Schwarze AB, Tandon P, Liu Z, et al. Ketogenic diet reduces spontaneous seizures and mossy fiber sprouting in the kainic acid model. *Neuroreport* 1999;10:1517–1522.
19. Bough KJ, Eagles DA. A ketogenic diet increases the resistance to pentylenetetrazole-induced seizures in the rat. *Epilepsia* 1999;40:138–143.
20. Bough KJ, Schwartzkroin PA, Rho JM. Calorie restriction and ketogenic diet diminish neuronal excitability in rat dentate gyrus *in vivo*. *Epilepsia* 2003;44:752–760.
21. DeVivo DC, Leckie MP, Ferrendelli JS, McDougal DB. Chronic ketosis and cerebral metabolism. *Ann Neurol* 1978;3:331–337.

22. Pan JW, Bebin EM, Chu WJ, Hetherington HP. Ketosis and epilepsy: 31P spectroscopic imaging at 4.1 T. *Epilepsia* 1999;40:703–707.
23. Al-Mudallal AS, LaManna JC, Lust WD, Harik SI. Diet-induced ketosis does not cause cerebral acidosis. *Epilepsia* 1996;37:258–261.
24. Helmholz HF, Keith HM. Eight years' experience with the ketogenic diet in the treatment of epilepsy. *JAMA* 1930;95;707–709.
25. Keith HM. The effect of various factors on experimentally produced convulsions. *Am J Dis Child* 1931;41:532–543.
26. Likhodii SS, Serbanescu I, Cortez MA, et al. Anticonvulsant properties of acetone, a brain ketone elevated by the ketogenic diet. *Ann Neurol* 2003;54:219–226.
27. Nordli DR, De Vivo DC. The ketogenic diet revisited: back to the future. *Epilepsia* 1997;38:743–749.
28. DeVivo DC, Haymond MW, Leckie MP, et al. The clinical and biochemical implications of pyruvate carboxylase deficiency. *J Clin Endocrinol Metab* 1977;45:1281–1296.
29. Carroll J, Koenigsberger D. The ketogenic diet: a practical guide for caregivers. *J Am Dietetic Assoc* 1998;98:316–321.
30. Nordli DR, Koenigsberger D, Schroeder J, DeVivo DC. Ketogenic diets. In: Resor S, Kutt H, eds. *The medical treatment of epilepsy.* New York: Marcel Dekker, Inc. 1992:455–472.
31. Livingston S. *Comprehensive management of epilepsy in infancy, childhood and adolescence.* Springfield, IL: Charles C Thomas. 1972.
32. Hahn TJ, Halstead LR, DeVivo DC. Disordered mineral metabolism produced by ketogenic diet therapy. *Calcif Tissue Int* 1979;28:17–22.
33. Ballaban-Gil K, Callahan C, O'Dell C, et al. Complications of the ketogenic diet. *Epilepsia* 1998;39:744–748.
34. De Vivo DC, Bohan TP, Coulter DL, et al. L-carnitine supplementation in childhood epilepsy: current perspectives. *Epilepsia* 1998;39:1216–1225.
35. De Vivo DC, Trifiletti RR, Jacobson RI, et al. Defective glucose transport across the blood-brain barrier as a cause of persistent hypoglycorrhachia, seizures, and developmental delay. *N Engl J Med* 1991;325:713–721.
36. Wexler ID, Hemalatha SG, McConnell J, et al. Outcome of pyruvate dehydrogenase deficiency treated with ketogenic diets. Studies in patients with identical mutations. *Neurology* 1997;49:1655–1661.
37. Prasad AN, Stafstrom CE, Holmes GL. Alternative epilepsy therapies: the ketogenic diet, immunoglobulins, and steroids. *Epilepsia* 1996;37:S81–S95.
38. Freeman JM, Vining EP, Pillas DJ, et al. The efficacy of the ketogenic diet-1998: a prospective evaluation of intervention in 150 children. *Pediatrics* 1998;102:1358–1363.
39. Schwartz RH, Eaton J, Bower BD, Aynsley-Green A. Ketogenic diets in the treatment of epilepsy: short-term clinical effects. *Dev Med Child Neurol* 1989;31:145–151.
40. Sills MA, Forsythe WI, Haidukewych D, et al. The medium chain triglyceride diet and intractable epilepsy. *Arch Dis Child* 1986;61:1168–1172.
41. Woody RC, Brodie M, Hampton DK, Fiser RH Jr. Corn oil ketogenic diet for children with intractable seizures. *J Child Neurol* 1988;3:21–24.
42. Janaki S, Rashid MK, Gulati MS, et al. A clinical electroencephalographic correlation of seizures on a ketogenic diet. *Indian J Med Res* 1976;64:1057–1063.
43. Nordli DR, Koenigsberger D, Carroll J, DeVivo DC. Successful treatment of infants with the ketogenic diet [abstract]. *Ann Neurol* 1995;38:523.
44. Keith HM. Convulsive disorders in children. With reference to treatment with ketogenic diet. Boston, Mass: Little, Brown, and Company. 1963.
45. Mady MA, Kossoff EH, McGregor AL, et al. The ketogenic diet: adolescents can do it, too. *Epilepsia* 2003;44:847–851.
46. Kossoff EH, Krauss GL, McGrogan JR, Freeman JM. Efficacy of the Atkins diet as therapy for intractable epilepsy. *Neurology* 2003;61:1789–1791.
47. Bergquist AG, Chee CM, Lutchka LM, Brooks-Kayal AR. Treatment of acquired epileptic aphasia with the ketogenic diet. *J Child Neurol* 1999;14:696–701.

Vagus Nerve Stimulation Therapy

71

James W. Wheless

Epilepsy and seizures affect at least 2.3 million individuals in the United States (1). Although antiepileptic drugs (AEDs) are the primary form of treatment, recent outcome surveys reveal only mixed success even with the new AEDs that have become available over the past decade (2,3). Approximately one-third of patients have seizures that are unresponsive to pharmacologic therapy. In addition, safety and tolerability issues associated with both the acute and chronic side effects and toxicity complications further diminish the effectiveness of AEDs (4–10). Other treatment options are available for select subgroups of patients, including the ketogenic diet, which provides benefit to some children (11,12), and epilepsy surgery, which may manage or lessen poorly controlled seizures in 10% to 25% of patients (1). However, children and adults with uncontrolled seizures continue to carry a sad burden of higher mortality rates, higher rates of accidents and injuries, greater incidence of cognitive and psychiatric impairment, poor self-esteem, higher levels of anxiety and depression, and social stigmatization or isolation compared with the nonepileptic population (13). The shortcomings of AEDs, the ketogenic diet, and epilepsy surgery in improving overall outcome highlight the need for other treatments, one of which is vagus nerve stimulation (VNS) therapy.

HISTORY

The effect of VNS on central nervous system (CNS) activity has been documented, with early attempts in the 1880s linking electrical vagal nerve and cervical sympathetic stimulation and carotid artery compression to the treatment of seizures (14). In the mid-1980s, Jacob Zabara, a biophysicist at Temple University, again suggested that electrical stimulation of the vagus nerve might prevent seizures. VNS

therapy resulted from a hypothesis, formulated during his wife's Lamaze class, that the Lamaze method activated stretch receptors in the lungs, which in turn activated the vagus nerve (15). Vagus stimulation in the neck could quiet the abdominal muscle contractions that produce vomiting; Dr. Zabara likened these contractions to convulsions. Zabara believed that if VNS could alleviate vomiting and affect electroencephalographic (EEG) findings, it might ameliorate epilepsy. This theory was proved in his first canine studies (16), and a company—Cyberonics, Inc. (Houston, Texas)—was founded in 1987 to develop VNS therapy, which would be delivered by a patented method using a generator device modeled after a cardiac pacemaker.

In 1988, the first patient to have a VNS therapy device implanted became seizure free (Table 71.1) (17). Five acute-phase clinical studies analyzing the safety and effectiveness of VNS therapy followed (Table 71.2). The first two single-blind trials showed improved control in adults with intractable partial seizures who were not candidates for epilepsy surgery (17–19). The subsequent two randomized, blinded, active-control trials (E03, E05) led to approval of VNS therapy by the US Food and Drug Administration (FDA) in July 1997 for the adjunctive treatment of refractory partial-onset seizures among patients 12 years of age or older. VNS therapy is also approved for the treatment of epilepsy and depression independent of age in more than 24 countries around the world, including member nations of the European Union, Canada, and Australia. As of July 2003, more than 22,000 patients have received implants worldwide.

The VNS therapy system is made up of a pulse generator, a bipolar VNS lead, a programming wand with accompanying software for an IBM-compatible laptop or hand-held computer, a tunneling tool, and hand-held magnets (Fig. 71.1) (20,21). The pulse generator transmits electrical signals to the vagus nerve through the bipolar lead. The

TABLE 71.1
HISTORY OF VNS THERAPY

1985	First animal studies
1988	First human implant
1992	First randomized active control study (E03) completed
1994	European community approval
1996	Second randomized active control study (E05) complete
1997	US Food and Drug Administration commercial approval
July 2003	22,000+ implants worldwide

software allows placement of the programming wand over the pulse generator for reading and altering stimulation parameters (Fig. 71.2; Table 71.3). Each stimulation is preceded by 2 seconds of ramp-up time and followed by 2 seconds of ramp-down time. Two models of the VNS therapy system are currently in use: the Model 101 and the newer Model 102 (currently available only in the United States). The Model 102 titanium generator is thinner (6.9 mm), lighter (25 g), and has less volume (52.2 mm in diameter) than the previous generator models. (See the Addendum for sources of information on the VNS therapy system.)

EFFICACY

The two pivotal studies—E03 and E05—were designed to demonstrate that high (therapeutic) and low (nontherapeutic) stimulation of the vagus nerve had different effects on the frequency of partial seizures (22,23). The effects of VNS therapy during the 12-week randomized phases of the studies, which began 2 weeks after implantation, were gauged against 12- to 16-week baseline periods. E03 acute-study patients (N = 114 implanted) had epilepsy for an average of 22 years. Seizure frequency was reduced by at least half in

31% of patients in the high-stimulation group, compared with 14% in the low-stimulation group. No patients became seizure free during the acute phase, but some reported reduced seizure severity and improved postictal recovery periods. Patients in the high-stimulation group either aborted or decreased 59.8% of seizures with the magnet. No factors were identified that predicted response.

The similarly designed Study E05 was the largest prospective, controlled trial of a device for epilepsy treatment ever conducted (23). Patients (N = 199) had a median of 0.51 to 0.58 seizures per day during baseline. One patient receiving high stimulation became seizure free, and 23.4% of patients had a 50% or more reduction in seizure frequency after 3 months of treatment. The presence or absence of aura did not predict efficacy. Of the implanted patients, 99% completed the study.

Long-Term Studies

All patients exiting Study E03 were offered indefinite open-label treatment at high (effective) stimulation; 100 (88%) of the 114 patients completed an additional 12 months of VNS therapy at therapeutic stimulation levels (14 patients discontinued because of lack of efficacy but were included in the analysis as intent-to-treat). A median 20% reduction in seizure frequency occurred in the first 3 months of the extension study and improved over the ensuing months (24). In two thirds of patients, a minimum 50% reduction during the initial 3 months continued during months 10 through 12. Results among the 195 patients in the continuing long-term E05 study showed a 50% or more reduction in seizure frequency in 35% of patients and a 75% or more reduction in 20% of patients after an additional 12 months of VNS therapy at therapeutic stimulation levels (25). The median reduction in seizure frequency was 45%, with seizure frequency reductions sustained over time and only mild to moderate side effects reported.

One study of 10 adults with intractable partial seizures revealed a 10-fold increase in the mean number of 14-day

TABLE 71.2
EFFICACY OF VNS THERAPY IN CLINICAL STUDIES

Study	Design	Seizure Type	No. of Patients	Age of Patients (y)	First Implant	No. of Patients with >50% Response (%)	Mean Reduction in Seizures/Day (%)
E01	Pilot, longitudinal	Partial	11	20–58	1998	30	24[a]
E02	Pilot, longitudinal	Partial	5	18–42	1990	50	40
E04	Open, longitudinal	All types	124	3–63	1990	29	7[a]
E03	Randomized, parallel, high/low	Partial	115	13–57	1991	31/14	24[a]/6
E05	Randomized, parallel, high/low	Partial	198	13–60	1995	23/16	28[b]/15[b]

[a]$P \leq 0.05$, by student's t test.
[b]$P < 0.0001$, by analysis of variance.

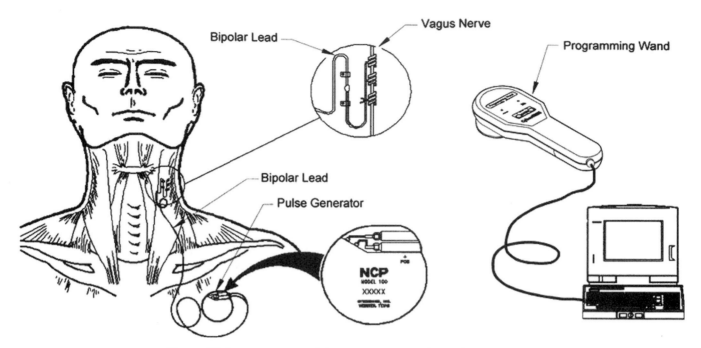

Figure 71.1   Components of the vagus nerve stimulation therapy system.

seizure-free periods after 50 months of VNS therapy with stable AED dosages (26). Seizure-free periods increased every year; one patient continued to be seizure free after 36.5 months. A prospective, open evaluation of 64 patients reported results for up to 5 years of follow up (27). No change in AED dosages occurred during the first 6 months of VNS therapy, which lasted an average of 20 months. Nineteen of 47 patients with partial seizures, five of nine with idiopathic generalized seizures, and five of eight with Lennox-Gastaut syndrome had a seizure reduction of greater than 50% or more. In this population with refractory seizures, 44% experienced a substantial reduction in severity and frequency over a long period. A recent report on long-term outcomes of 30 patients receiving VNS therapy (28) showed continued improvements over time, with 54% of patients at 1 year and 61% at 2 years exhibiting seizure frequency reductions of 50% or more compared with baseline. The mechanisms underlying the gradual improvements in response to VNS therapy seen over time in these long-term studies, however, have yet to be elucidated.

Pediatric, Elderly, and Special Populations

Studies indicate that response to VNS therapy is independent of age, seizure type, or syndrome. The largest retrospective pediatric study to date showed the same median reduction in seizure frequency of 51% at 6 months among patients aged 12 to 18 years (n = 56) and among those less than 12 years of age (n = 20) (29). Particularly favorable results, including reduced seizure frequency and severity and improved quality of life (QoL), have been reported among patients in open studies of Lennox-Gastaut syndrome and other refractory childhood epilepsies, such as hypothalamic hamartomas, epileptic encephalopathies, and tuberous sclerosis complex (29–41). Verbal performance, alertness, motor and cognitive functions, and general behavior improved, sometimes dramatically (33,36,42,43). A retrospective study (44) showed that improved QoL (particularly in the area of alertness) was associated with VNS therapy in patients with autism (n = 59) or Landau-Kleffner syndrome (LKS; n = 6), with more than half of the patients

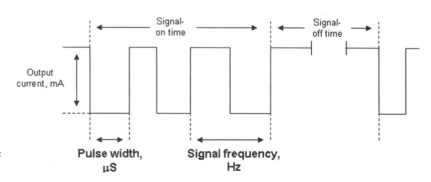

Figure 71.2   Therapy stimulation parameters of vagus nerve stimulation.

TABLE 71.3

VNS THERAPY PARAMETERS

	High	Low	Rapid Cycling[a]
VNS current (mA)	Up to **3.5**	**1.2** (0.25–2.75)	Up to **3.5**
Frequency (Hz)	**30** (20–50)	**1** (to 2)	**30**
Pulse width (ms)	**500**	**130**	**500**
On time (s)	**30** (to 90)	**30**	**7**
Off time (min)	**5** (to 10)	**180** (60–180)	**0.2**
Magnet current (mA)	**Same as VNS**	**0**	**Same as VNS**
On time (s)	**30** (to 90)	**30**	**30**
Pulse width (μs)	**500**	**130**	**500**

Values in bold type are the most common settings from the E03 and E05 studies.
[a]From refs. 27, 33, and 109 with permission.
VNS = vagus nerve stimulation.

in each group also experiencing a 50% or more reduction in seizure frequency at follow-up (12 months of follow up for autism and 6 months for LKS patients). Studies have also shown both seizure frequency reductions and improved QoL among both institutionalized and noninstitutionalized patients with mental retardation/developmental delay (MRDD) (45,46). Small open studies of VNS in patients with symptomatic generalized epilepsy demonstrated reductions in seizure frequency of 41% (median) (47) and 46% (mean) (48). VNS therapy also successfully stopped a case of refractory generalized convulsive status epilepticus in a patient 13 years of age (49).

In a study of VNS therapy among patients 50 years of age or more, 21 of 31 patients experienced a 50% or greater decrease in seizure frequency at 1 year, accompanied by significant improvements in QoL from baseline over time (50). These studies indicate that age and seizure type or syndrome are not contraindications for the use of VNS therapy. A recent review (51) also indicated that VNS therapy is well tolerated among various patient populations, with rare withdrawals from treatment. A study of stimulation parameters among patients of different ages (52) recommended age-related stimulation adjustments based on age-related changes seen in vagus nerve characteristics. Early studies indicated that children might respond more rapidly than adults, with reductions in the interval between stimulations resulting in improved control (Table 71.3) (33,42). Additional pediatric studies reported that higher output currents might be required, particularly when lower pulse durations are used (53–55). Optimal stimulus parameter settings for patients of various ages or with specific seizure types or syndromes, however, have not yet been defined.

MECHANISM OF ACTION

The mechanisms by which VNS reduces seizure activity in humans were not known at the time VNS therapy was approved by the FDA. However, considerable progress in mechanistic VNS research has been made over the last 6 years. Electrical stimulation of the peripheral vagus nerve requires polysynaptic transmission to mediate the antiseizure effect. The anatomical distribution of vagal projections underlies the therapeutic actions of VNS therapy. Vagal visceral afferents have a diffuse CNS projection, with activation of these pathways broadly affecting neuronal excitability (21,56,57). A recent review (57) examined the vagus nerve projections and CNS connections, as well as the current animal and human imaging studies, which indicate that VNS exerts both acute and long-term antiepileptic effects.

EXPERIMENTAL STUDIES

The first studies of the antiepileptic effects of VNS were conducted in 1937 (56). Subsequent experiments in cats showed that vagal stimulation produced EEG desynchronization (58) or synchronization, depending on the parameters used (59,60). Stimulation of the slow-conducting fibers most effectively resulted in EEG desynchronization. Hypersynchronized cortical and thalamocortical neuronal interactions characterize seizures; therefore, it was postulated that desynchronizing these activities would lead to antiseizure effects of VNS.

Initial work in cats and recent studies of strychnine-induced seizures in the dog, maximal electroshock and pentylenetetrazol-induced seizures in the rat, and the alumina-gel monkey model (16,58,61–64) showed that cervical vagal stimulation decreased interictal epileptiform discharges and shortened or aborted seizures; the antiepileptic effects outlasted the stimulus (16,61,62,65) and depended on its frequency and cumulative duration (62–64). These effects are now known to be mediated by activation of myelinated A and B fibers (66–68). Most central projections of the vagus nerve terminate in the nucleus of the solitary tract, with extensions to brain stem nuclei, thalamus, amygdala, and hypothalamus. Increased release of γ-aminobutyric acid (GABA) and glycine by brain stem and subcortical nuclei was proposed as the antiepileptic mechanism of VNS therapy (63,64). Brain stem nuclei are known to influence seizure susceptibility (69–73); based on animal studies, the nucleus of the tractus solitarius is likely the key brain stem structure involved in transmitting and modulating VNS antiseizure effects.

Also unknown are the processes that mediate the sustained anticonvulsant effect of VNS therapy, but this effect, which outlasts the stimulation, suggests long-term changes in neural activity. Expression of *fos* immunoreactivity was induced by VNS in regions of the rat brain important in epileptogenesis (74); *fos* immunolabeling in the locus ceruleus suggested VNS modulation of norepinephrine release. Increased norepinephrine release by the locus ceruleus is antiepileptogenic. In rats with chronic or acute locus ceruleus lesions, VNS-induced seizure suppression was attenuated, supporting a noradrenergic mechanism (72). This first evidence of a structure mediating the anticonvulsant action of VNS may have pharmacologic implications for clinical practice. Drugs that activate the locus ceruleus or potentiate norepinephrine effects may enhance the efficacy of VNS. Pending the results of further animal testing, it is likely that the antiepileptic action of VNS is mediated through neuronal networks that project from brain stem to forebrain structures. Vagal projections to noradrenergic and serotonergic neuromodulatory systems of the brain may also explain the positive effects of VNS in improving mood disorders.

In summary, animal studies have established three distinct temporal patterns for the antiseizure effects of VNS: (a) acute abortive effects, in which an ongoing seizure is attenuated by VNS; (b) acute prophylactic effects, in which seizure-inducing agents are less effective in provoking seizures when applied at the end of VNS; and (c) chronic progressive prophylactic effects, in which total seizure counts are reduced more following chronic VNS stimulation. In addition, animal studies have shown that VNS can antagonize the development of epilepsy in the kindling model of epileptogenesis (75). Based on these studies, the mechanism of action of VNS therapy appears to be largely distinct from that of AED therapies (57).

CLINICAL STUDIES

Initial scalp recording performed in a small number of adults did not demonstrate a significant effect of VNS on EEG total power, median frequency, power in any of the conventional frequency bands (76), interictal epileptiform activity, or the waking or sleep background rhythms (17,76–78). At seizure onset, however, VNS has terminated both the clinical and the EEG seizure activity (77). Studies that are more recent have suggested that some patients may

have a change in interictal epileptiform discharges (IEDs) with VNS. Fifteen adults with refractory partial-onset seizure disorders showed a significant reduction in IEDs during stimulation and the interstimulation period immediately following stimulation, compared with baseline, with the reduction in IEDs greater among patients whose seizures decreased by more than 50% on VNS. Additionally, the patients who had a significant decrease in IEDs experienced the positive effect of magnetic extra stimulation in abolishing seizures (79). A single adult patient undergoing presurgical evaluation with intrahippocampal depth electrodes showed alteration of IEDs by VNS (increased spikes at 5 Hz, decreased at 30 Hz) (80). Chronic VNS in children was recently reported to reduce IEDs (81). However, this population was quite different from that in the earlier adult series. Included were patients with generalized and partial-onset seizures, greater frequency of IEDs, and younger age. During 12 months of VNS therapy, both generalized and focal spikes were diminished; however, this did not correlate well with seizure reduction. Pattern-reversal visual-evoked potentials, brain stem auditory-evoked potentials, and cognitive (P300) potentials were all unaffected by VNS (82).

Release of anticonvulsant neurotransmitters at the projection sites of vagus nerve afferent fibers was hypothesized as a mechanism of action (83,84). Cerebrospinal fluid samples assayed for amino acid and neurotransmitter metabolites in 16 patients before and after 3 months of VNS therapy showed a treatment-induced increase in GABA (an inhibitory amino acid), a decrease in aspartate (an excitatory amino acid), and an increase in ethanolamine (a membrane lipid precursor) (83).

Positron emission tomography (PET) $H_2^{15}O$ cerebral blood flow (CBF) imaging identifies the neuroanatomical structures recruited by VNS in humans. A pilot study of three adults showed activation of the right thalamus, right posterotemporal cortex, left putamen, and left inferior cerebellum (85). Localization to the thalamus may explain the therapeutic benefit of VNS and is consistent with the role of that structure as a generator and modulator of cerebral activity. In a study of high and low stimulation (43), PET demonstrated CBF alterations at sites that receive vagal afferents and projections, including dorsal medulla, right postcentral gyrus, thalamus, cerebellum bilaterally, and limbic structures (bilateral hippocampus and amygdala). The high-stimulation group had more activation and deactivation sites, although the anatomical patterns during VNS were similar in both groups. Finally, acute CBF alterations were correlated with long-term therapeutic response, in an attempt to exclude those regions that show changes in VNS-induced synaptic activity but may not participate in VNS-related antiseizure actions (86). Decreased seizure frequency was associated with increased CBF only in the right and left thalami. Studies of chronic VNS therapy have shown the same anatomical distribution of CBF (85,87). Demonstration of these acute regional alterations does not clarify the mechanism of action of long-term, intermittent VNS, which may involve neurotransmitters or neurochemicals at those sites that outlast the stimulation.

Functional magnetic resonance imaging (fMRI) evaluating the time course of regional CBF alterations during VNS therapy can be performed safely in patients implanted with a vagal nerve stimulator (88). Preliminary fMRI studies have agreed with the PET studies, with the most robust activation observed in the thalami and insular cortices, with some activation also seen in ipsilateral basal ganglia, anterior parietal cortex, and other cortical areas (88,89).

SELECTION OF CANDIDATES

In the United States, VNS therapy is indicated as an adjunctive treatment for adults and adolescents 12 years of age or older with refractory partial-onset seizures (20). In the European Union, VNS therapy is indicated as an adjunctive treatment for patients with partial- or generalized-onset seizures without an age limitation. However, indications for VNS therapy were derived from the clinical trial experience, not from an understanding of its physiologic action. Age, sex, and frequency of seizures, secondarily generalized seizures, or interictal EEG spikes do not predict response to VNS therapy. The type or number of coadministered AEDs also do not predict response (48,90). Therefore, children may benefit considerably from VNS therapy, but randomized, controlled studies have not been completed. Patients with other seizure types or epilepsy syndromes also may benefit from VNS therapy.

Although optimal use parameters continue to be defined, candidates should meet the following criteria: (a) medically refractory seizures, (b) adequate trials of at least two AEDs, (c) exclusion of nonepileptic events, and (d) ineligibility for epilepsy surgery (Fig. 71.3). Focal resective surgery (temporal lobectomy or lesional neocortical epilepsy) is preferred for appropriate patients because of its superior seizure-free rate (91–93). Recent open studies suggest that VNS therapy may be used among patients considered for corpus callosotomy, producing lower rates of morbidity (94–96), and among those who have previously undergone epilepsy surgery (29,97). Earlier use (within 2 years of seizure onset or after failure of two or three AEDs) of VNS therapy may also produce a higher response rate, as well as reduce the negative side effects associated with long-term epilepsy and AED therapy, which hinder development (98,99).

Use of VNS therapy is contraindicated in patients with prior bilateral or left cervical vagotomy, and safety and efficacy have not been established for stimulation of the right vagus nerve. Patients with existing pulmonary or cardiac disease should be evaluated carefully before implantation; chronic obstructive pulmonary disease may increase the risk for dyspnea. Patients with cardiac conduction disorders were not studied in the controlled trials. A cardiologist's evaluation should precede implantation, with postprocedural Holter monitoring performed if clinically indicated. Patients with a history of obstructive sleep apnea should be treated with care, as an increase in apneic events during stimulation is possible. Lowering stimulation frequency (i.e., pulse width and signal frequency to 250 μs and 20 Hz, respectively) may prevent exacerbation of this condition (100).

INITIATION AND MAINTENANCE

Hospitalization for implantation of the device is preceded by evaluations by a neurologist and by a surgeon with experience in the carotid sheath. With the patient typically under general anesthesia (although local or regional anesthesia has been used successfully as well [101]), the lead wires are placed on the left cervical vagus nerve and the generator is placed in a subcutaneous pocket in the left upper chest (102,103). Intraoperative electrical impedance testing ensures integrity of the system. Rare cases of bradycardia, asystole, or both mandate initial lead testing in the

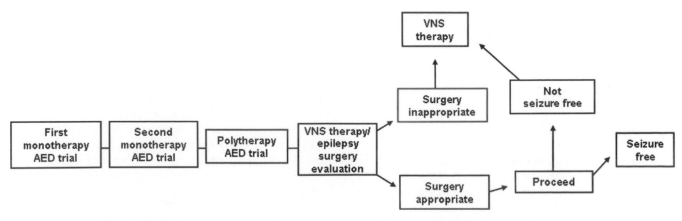

Figure 71.3   Treatment selection flow chart. AED = antiepileptic drug; VNS = vagus nerve stimulation. Used with permission from Wheless JW, Maggio V. *Neurology* 2002;59(Suppl 4):S21–S25.

operating room (20,104,105); the anesthesiologist should be notified immediately before this test. Correct placement of the lead electrodes around the vagus nerve is critical. Two methods have been developed to help confirm correct placement of the electrodes intraoperatively (106), depending on the type of anesthesia used for the procedure. For patients receiving general anesthesia, the larynx and vocal cords can be monitored by fiberoptic endoscopy for contraction of the left lateral larynx wall and vocal cord tightening. For patients being implanted under local and regional anesthesia, stimulation intensities can be increased until a voice alteration is noticed. Neither procedure is harmful to the patient nor greatly extends the length of the surgery.

Prophylactic antibiotics may be administered both in the operating room and postoperatively. The patient can be discharged after the procedure, which usually lasts for less than 1 hour, or can be observed overnight. Discharge education should include care of the incisions and use of the magnet. In clinical studies, the generator's output current was kept at 0 mA for the first 2 weeks; however, programmed stimulation is now being initiated at 0.25 mA in some operating rooms (29). Dosages of AEDs are generally kept stable for the first 3 months of stimulation unless an early response is noted.

A few weeks after implantation, the patient is examined to confirm wound healing and proper generator operation, either to begin or to continue programming. Output current is increased in 0.25-mA increments until stimulation is comfortable (Table 71.1). The subsequent stimulation schedule is determined by patient response. Standard parameter settings range from 20 to 30 Hz at a pulse width of 250 to 500 μs and an output current of 0.25 to 3.5 mA for 30 seconds "on" time and 5 minutes "off" time (55). At each visit, the generator and the battery are assessed for end of service; the battery's life expectancy of 7 to 10 years depends on the programmed stimulation parameters. If VNS therapy is to be continued, the generator can be replaced at the appropriate time in less than 20 minutes.

VNS may be continued indefinitely and without damage to the vagus nerve as long as the stimulation is less than 50 Hz and the duty cycle operates less than 50% of the time (20,107,108). Two safety features that protect patients from continuous stimulation or uncomfortable side effects are the magnet and the watchdog timer. The magnet can act as an "off" switch when held or taped over the generator. The watchdog timer is an internal monitor that limits the number of pulses to be delivered without an "off" time to prevent excess stimulation.

COMPLICATIONS AND ADVERSE EFFECTS

Surgical complications and difficulties are rare. Fracture of the electrode, related to fatigue at the junction between contact and the lead wire, was a common problem with early devices (19,109–112). Substitution of a quadrifilar wire improved electrode tolerance that had been compromised by repetitive neck motion. Incisional infections are unusual and generally respond to antibiotic therapy. Fluid accumulation at the pulse generator site with or without infection occurs in 1% to 2% of implantations and resolves with aspiration and antibiotics; the rare cases of refractory infection require removal of the generator. However, one case of deep wound infection associated with implantation of the generator was reported to be managed successfully with open wound treatment without removal of the device, an alternative option if removal of the device appears hazardous (113). Unilateral vocal cord paralysis, which accompanies approximately 1% of implants, may be caused by excess manipulation of the vagus nerve, and subsequent damage to the vagal artery and its reinforcing arterioles (114); in most cases, it remits completely over several weeks.

Common side effects, which occur primarily when the stimulator is actually delivering a pulse (Table 71.4), are dose dependent and usually mild or absent when VNS

TABLE 71.4

ADVERSE EVENTS WITH VAGUS NERVE STIMULATION[a]

Adverse Event	E03 and E05 Patients (n = 314; 591 device years) >3 Months' Follow-up No. of Patients (%)	E03 and E05 Patients with High Stimulation (n = 152) >3 Months' Follow-up No. of Patients (%)
Voice alteration	156 (50)	91 (60)
Increased coughing	129 (41)	57 (38)
Paresthesia	87 (28)	32 (21)
Dyspnea	55 (18)	32 (21)
Dyspepsia	36 (12)	22 (15)
Laryngismus	10 (3.2)	9 (5.9)

[a]Number of patients reporting the adverse event at least once in the E03 and E05 randomized studies.

parameters are appropriately programmed (22,23,115); many patients become accustomed to them with time. Most patients experience hoarseness or a change in vocal quality and tingling over the left cervical region on delivery of the electrical pulse. Subjective dyspnea or a sensation of muscle tightening in the neck may occur, without changes on pulmonary function testing (23). Cough or throat pain during stimulus delivery sometimes necessitates a reduction in current or pulse width (116).

Despite the widespread visceral efferent projections of the vagus nerve, systemic effects are rare. Pulmonary function does not change significantly in patients without concomitant lung disease (23,117), but may deteriorate in the face of intense stimulation and obstructive lung disease (117). Inhalation of ipratropium bromide or lowering of the stimulus frequency or current is recommended. No substantial effects on cardiac function were reported during clinical studies (20,22,23,115,118). An analysis of total mortality and sudden death in epileptic patients (to August 1996) revealed the expected rate in individuals with severe, intractable epilepsy (119). The clinical studies demonstrated no clinically relevant effects on the gastrointestinal system, serum chemistries, AED concentrations, vital signs, or weight.

Rare reported side effects associated with VNS therapy include diarrhea (120), sternocleidomastoid muscle spasm (121), phrenic nerve stimulation (122), tonsillar pain (123), and emergent psychiatric disorders (124,125). Of seven patients treated with VNS therapy who developed a major psychiatric disorder (124), all had a history of a dysphoric disorder and most had daily seizures before treatment with VNS. The severe dysphoric or psychotic conditions emerged once seizure frequency was reduced by 75% or more, but remitted or improved satisfactorily with psychotropic medication, with two patients also requiring a decrease or interruption of VNS therapy. Children with a history of dysphagia may experience swallowing difficulties during VNS therapy (126,127); using a magnet to turn off the stimulator during mealtime may help. The majority of side effects, including many of the rare incidents reported, are amenable to stimulus modifications, which could include changes in output current and/or pulse width.

ADVANTAGES AND DISADVANTAGES

Many patients maintained on VNS therapy can decrease their total AED burden, which typically results in a more alert patient who, while still receiving polytherapy, is without the cognitive or systemic side effects typically associated with multiple therapies. Therefore, use of AED monotherapy with VNS therapy may produce a better risk to benefit ratio than that with two AEDs. Even when AEDs cannot be substantially decreased or withdrawn, however, VNS therapy may allow amelioration of seizures with no

risk of toxic organ reactions, drug interactions or failures, allergies, rashes, and other systemic adverse effects or cognitive side effects (128,129); in some patients, memory, alertness, mood, and communication have been shown to improve (78,130–133). Improvements in QoL independent of treatment effect on seizure frequency, as well as increased daytime vigilance, have also been reported (134–136). In addition, because the beneficial results are maintained without active patient participation, VNS therapy may be an ideal treatment for the partially compliant. Data on VNS therapy in pregnancy are limited, but teratogenesis is not expected. Two patients who became pregnant while on VNS therapy both gave birth to healthy babies (27). Finally, VNS therapy can both prevent and abort seizures. The ability to trigger the device externally (with the magnet) and to interrupt the seizure or improve the postictal phase empowers the patient and provides a sense of control over epilepsy.

On the other hand, VNS is an empiric therapy, with no way to predict response except by trial. The initial cost (often between $15,000 and $20,000) can be prohibitive without coverage by a third-party payer. Over the life of the system, however, this cost approximates that of many of the new AEDs (137). In addition, although weeks to months may elapse before seizure frequency decreases, cost-effectiveness studies indicate that VNS therapy provides a substantial cost-savings benefit to hospitals over the long-term course of treatment (138,139). These cost benefits are sustained over time and are sufficient to cover or exceed the cost of the device.

According to the manufacturer of the device, a transmit-and-receive head coil MRI should be performed rather than a full-body MRI, with the generator programmed to 0 mA for the procedure and returned to the original settings thereafter (20). However, successful head coil MRIs have been performed among patients both with and without the device turned off (140). If the device does remain on during the MRI, the device should be interrogated postprocedure to ensure that the magnetic field did not deactivate the device or change the pre-MRI settings. Although not recommended by the manufacturer, successful body-coil MRIs with the use of an ice pack over the area of the device leads have been reported among three patients (141). Diathermy, which could heat the system above safe levels and thereby cause either temporary or permanent tissue or nerve damage, should be avoided in patients receiving VNS therapy.

FUTURE DEVELOPMENTS

Since the first device implantation more than 10 years ago, the number of AEDs has increased yet uncontrolled seizures continue. The question not answered in clinical studies is, when should VNS therapy be used? Currently,

VNS is not used until multiple medications have failed and surgery is not an option. However, preliminary studies indicate that VNS therapy may be more effective when used earlier in the treatment process, particularly within 2 years of diagnosis after two or three AEDs have failed to control seizures (98).

Other research questions, if answered, have the potential to dramatically improve the overall treatment of all patients with epilepsy. Are there unique stimulation parameters for certain seizure types (e.g., partial versus generalized), syndromes (e.g., Lennox-Gastaut), or age groups? Might some AEDs or other medications enhance the effectiveness of VNS therapy? What are the psychosocial effects of VNS therapy on the families of individuals with epilepsy? Answers to such questions and improvements in technology will expand the role of VNS therapy for uncontrolled epilepsy.

Finally, VNS has raised interest in the role of neurostimulation as a treatment for epilepsy. Cooper and colleagues described cerebellar stimulation for treatment of epilepsy in the 1970s (142–144). Unfortunately, their results could not be consistently reproduced (145,146), but following these studies, other investigators began to explore direct stimulation therapy in the CNS as a treatment for epilepsy. Single-patient reports and small series have described antiepileptic effects with stimulation of the caudate nucleus (147), hippocampus (148,149), subthalamic nucleus (150–152), anterior nucleus (153–156), and centromedian nucleus (157–161) of the thalamus. However, efficacy reports have not been consistent. Currently, efficacy and indications are under investigation. The future of direct brain neurostimulation (DBS) therapy for the treatment of epilepsy will depend on its efficacy compared with that of VNS. In order for DBS to emerge as a treatment option for patients with intractable epilepsy, future studies will need to document specific indications for which DBS has superior efficacy compared with VNS, as the former will always be associated with increased morbidity. Peripheral nerve stimulation of the trigeminal nerve is a promising new treatment (162) with the potential advantage of being minimally invasive.

ADDENDUM

Videotapes and information on the VNS therapy system are available free to patients, nurses, and physicians from Cyberonics, Inc.

REFERENCES

1. *Epilepsy: a report to the nation.* Landover, Md: Epilepsy Foundation of America; 1999.
2. Brodie MJ, Kwan P. Staged approach to epilepsy management. *Neurology* 2002;58:S2–S8.
3. Schmidt D. The clinical impact of new antiepileptic drugs after a decade of use in epilepsy. *Epilepsy Res* 2002;50:21–32.
4. Kwan P, Brodie MJ. Effectiveness of first antiepileptic drug. *Epilepsia* 2001;42:1255–1260.
5. Camfield P, Camfield C. Acute and chronic toxicity of antiepileptic medications: a selective review. *Can J Neurol Sci* 1994;21: S7–S11.
6. Jallon P. The problem of intractability: the continuing need for new medical therapies in epilepsy. *Epilepsia* 1997;38(Suppl 9): S37–S42.
7. Pellock JM. Antiepileptic drug therapy in the United States: a review of clinical studies and unmet needs. *Neurology* 1995;45: S17–S24.
8. Pellock JM, Pippenger CE. Adverse effects of antiepileptic drugs. In: Dodson WE, Pellock JM, eds. *Pediatric epilepsy: diagnosis and therapy.* New York: Demos, 1993;253–264.
9. Patsalos PN, Duncan JS. Antiepileptic drugs. A review of clinically significant drug interactions. *Drug Saf* 1993;9:156–184.
10. Schmidt D. *Adverse effects of antiepileptic drugs.* New York: Raven Press, 1982.
11. Vining EP, Freeman JM, Ballaban-Gil K, et al. A multicenter study of the efficacy of the ketogenic diet. *Arch Neurol* 1998;55: 1433–1437.
12. Wheless JW, Ashwal S. The ketogenic diet. In: Swaiman KF, Ashwal S, eds. *Pediatric neurology: principles and practice,* 3rd ed. Philadelphia: CV Mosby Co, 1999:719–728.
13. Fisher RS, Parks-Trusz SL, Lehman C. Social issues in epilepsy. In: Shorvon S, Dreifus F, Fish D, et al, eds. *The treatment of epilepsy.* Cambridge: Blackwell Science, 1996:357–369.
14. Lanska DJ. J.L. Corning and vagal nerve stimulation for seizures in the 1880s. *Neurology* 2002;58:452–459.
15. Lesser RP. Unexpected places: how did vagus nerve stimulation become a treatment for epilepsy? *Neurology* 1999;52:1117–1118.
16. Zabara J. Inhibition of experimental seizures in canines by repetitive vagal stimulation. *Epilepsia* 1992;33:1005–1012.
17. Penry JK, Dean JC. Prevention of intractable partial seizures by intermittent vagal stimulation in humans: preliminary results. *Epilepsia* 1990;31(Suppl 2):S40–S43.
18. Uthman BM, Wilder BJ, Hammond EJ, et al. Efficacy and safety of vagus nerve stimulation in patients with complex partial seizures. *Epilepsia* 1990;31(Suppl 2):S44–S50.
19. Uthman BM, Wilder BJ, Penry JK, et al. Treatment of epilepsy by stimulation of the vagus nerve. *Neurology* 1993;43:1338–1345.
20. Physician's manual for the VNS therapy pulse model 102 generator. Houston, Texas: Cyberonics, Inc, 2002.
21. Schachter SC, Saper CB. Vagus nerve stimulation. *Epilepsia* 1998;39:677–686.
22. A randomized controlled trial of chronic vagus nerve stimulation for treatment of medically intractable seizures. The Vagus Nerve Stimulation Study Group. *Neurology* 1995;45:224–230.
23. Handforth A, DeGiorgio CM, Schachter SC, et al. Vagus nerve stimulation therapy for partial-onset seizures: a randomized active-control trial. *Neurology* 1998;51:48–55.
24. Salinsky MC, Uthman BM, Ristanovic RK, et al. Vagus nerve stimulation for the treatment of medically intractable seizures. Results of a 1-year open-extension trial. Vagus Nerve Stimulation Study Group. *Arch Neurol* 1996;53:1176–1180.
25. DeGiorgio CM, Schachter SC, Handforth A, et al. Prospective long-term study of vagus nerve stimulation for the treatment of refractory seizures. *Epilepsia* 2000;41:1195–1200.
26. Clarke BM, Upton AR, Griffin H, et al. Seizure control after stimulation of the vagus nerve: clinical outcome measures. *Can J Neurol Sci* 1997;24:222–225.
27. Ben-Menachem E, Hellstrom K, Waldton C, et al. Evaluation of refractory epilepsy treated with vagus nerve stimulation for up to 5 years. *Neurology* 1999;52:1265–1267.
28. Chavel SM, Westereld M, Spencer S. Long-term outcome of vagus nerve stimulation for refractory partial epilepsy. *Epilepsy Behav* 2003;4:302–309.
29. Helmers SL, Wheless JW, Frost M, et al. Vagus nerve stimulation therapy in pediatric patients with refractory epilepsy: retrospective study. *J Child Neurol* 2001;16:843–848.
30. Aicardi J. Vagal nerve stimulation in epileptic encephalopathies. *Pediatrics* 1999;103:821–822.
31. Frost M, Gates J, Helmers SL, et al. Vagus nerve stimulation in children with refractory seizures associated with Lennox-Gastaut syndrome. *Epilepsia* 2001;42:1148–1152.

32. Hornig G, Murphy JV. Vagal nerve stimulation: updated experience in 60 pediatric patients. *Epilepsia* 1998;39:169.

33. Hornig GW, Murphy JV, Schallert G, et al. Left vagus nerve stimulation in children with refractory epilepsy: an update. *South Med J* 1997;90:484–488.

34. Lundgren J, Amark P, Blennow G, et al. Vagus nerve stimulation in 16 children with refractory epilepsy. *Epilepsia* 1998;39:809–813.

35. Murphy JV. Left vagal nerve stimulation in children with medically refractory epilepsy. The Pediatric VNS Study Group. *J Pediatr* 1999;134:563–566.

36. Parker AP, Polkey CE, Binnie CD, et al. Vagal nerve stimulation in epileptic encephalopathies. *Pediatrics* 1999;103:778–782.

37. Schallert G, Murphy J. Vagal nerve stimulation: experience in 60 children. *Neurology* 1998;50:A14.

38. Aldenkamp AP , Majoie HJM, Berfelo MW, et al. Long-term effects of 24-month treatment with vagus nerve stimulation on behaviour in children with Lennox-Gastaut syndrome. *Epilepsy Behav* 2002;3:475–479.

39. Murphy JV, Wheless JW, Schmoll CM. Left vagal nerve stimulation in six patients with hypothalamic hamartomas. *Pediatr Neurol* 2000;23:167–168.

40. Hosain S, Nikalov B, Harden C, et al. Vagus nerve stimulation treatment for Lennox-Gastaut syndrome. *J Child Neurol* 2000;15:509–512.

41. Parain D, Penniello MJ, Berquen P, et al. Vagal nerve stimulation in tuberous sclerosis complex patients. *Pediatr Neurol* 2001;25:213–216.

42. Murphy JV, Hornig G, Schallert G. Left vagal nerve stimulation in children with refractory epilepsy. Preliminary observations. *Arch Neurol* 1995;52:886–889.

43. Henry TR, Bakay RA, Votaw JR, et al. Brain blood flow alterations induced by therapeutic vagus nerve stimulation in partial epilepsy: I. Acute effects at high and low levels of stimulation. *Epilepsia* 1998;39:983–990.

44. Park YD. The effects of vagus nerve stimulation therapy on patients with intractable seizures and either Landau-Kleffner syndrome or autism. *Epilepsy Behav* 2003;4:286–290.

45. Andriola MR, Vitale SA. Vagus nerve stimulation in the developmentally disabled. *Epilepsy Behav* 2001;2:129–134.

46. Gates J, Huf R, Frost M. Vagus nerve stimulation for patients in residential treatment facilities. *Epilepsy Behav* 2001;2:563–567.

47. Labar D, Nikolov B, Tarver B, et al. Vagus nerve stimulation for symptomatic generalized epilepsy: a pilot study. *Epilepsia* 1998;39:201–205.

48. Labar D, Murphy J, Tecoma E. Vagus nerve stimulation for medication-resistant generalized epilepsy. E04 VNS Study Group. *Neurology* 1999;52:1510–1512.

49. Winston KR, Levisohn P, Miller BR, et al. Vagal nerve stimulation for status epilepticus. *Pediatr Neurosurg* 2001;34:190–192.

50. Sirven JI, Sperling M, Naritoku D, et al. Vagus nerve stimulation therapy for epilepsy in older adults. *Neurology* 2000;54:1179–1182.

51. Privitera MD, Welty TE, Ficker DM, et al. Vagus nerve stimulation for partial seizures. *Cochrane Database Syst Rev* 2002;CD002896.

52. Koo B, Ham SD, Sood S, et al. Human vagus nerve electrophysiology: a guide to vagus nerve stimulation parameters. *J Clin Neurophysiol* 2001;18:429–433.

53. Crumrine PK. Vagal nerve stimulation in children. *Semin Pediatr Neurol* 2000;7:216–223.

54. Majoie HJ, Berfelo MW, Aldenkamp AP, et al. Vagus nerve stimulation in children with therapy-resistant epilepsy diagnosed as Lennox-Gastaut syndrome: clinical results, neuropsychological effects, and cost-effectiveness. *J Clin Neurophysiol* 2001;18:419–428.

55. Heck C, Helmers SL, DeGiorgio CM. Vagus nerve stimulation therapy, epilepsy, and device parameters: scientific basis and recommendations for use. *Neurology* 2002;59:S31–S37.

56. Rutecki P. Anatomical, physiological, and theoretical basis for the antiepileptic effect of vagus nerve stimulation. *Epilepsia* 1990;31(Suppl 2):S1–S6.

57. Henry TR. Therapeutic mechanisms of vagus nerve stimulation. *Neurology* 2002;59:S3–S14.

58. Zanchetti A, Wang SC, Moruzzi G. The effect of vagal afferent stimulation on the EEG pattern of the cat. *Electroencephalogr Clin Neurophysiol* 1952;4:357–361.

59. Chase MH, Sterman MB, Clemente CD. Cortical and subcortical patterns of response to afferent vagal stimulation. *Exp Neurol* 1966;16:36–49.

60. Chase MH, Nakamura Y, Clemente CD, et al. Afferent vagal stimulation: neurographic correlates of induced EEG synchronization and desynchronization. *Brain Res* 1967;5:236–249.

61. Lockard JS, Congdon WC, DuCharme LL. Feasibility and safety of vagal stimulation in monkey model. *Epilepsia* 1990;31(Suppl 2):S20–S26.

62. Takaya M, Terry WJ, Naritoku DK. Vagus nerve stimulation induces a sustained anticonvulsant effect. *Epilepsia* 1996;37:1111–1116.

63. Woodbury DM, Woodbury JW. Effects of vagal stimulation on experimentally induced seizures in rats. *Epilepsia* 1990;31(Suppl 2):S7–S19.

64. Woodbury JW, Woodbury DM. Vagal stimulation reduces the severity of maximal electroshock seizures in intact rats: use of a cuff electrode for stimulating and recording. *Pacing Clin Electrophysiol* 1991;14:94–107.

65. McLachlan RS. Suppression of interictal spikes and seizures by stimulation of the vagus nerve. *Epilepsia* 1993;34:918–923.

66. Zagon A, Kemeny AA. Slow hyperpolarization in cortical neurons: a possible mechanism behind vagus nerve simulation therapy for refractory epilepsy? *Epilepsia* 2000;41:1382–1389.

67. Krahl SE, Senanayake SS, Handforth A. Destruction of peripheral C-fibers does not alter subsequent vagus nerve stimulation-induced seizure suppression in rats. *Epilepsia* 2001;42:586–589.

68. Banzett RB, Guz A, Paydarfar D, et al. Cardiorespiratory variables and sensation during stimulation of the left vagus in patients with epilepsy. *Epilepsy Res* 1999;35:1–11.

69. Depaulis A, Vergnes M, Liu Z, et al. Involvement of the nigral output pathways in the inhibitory control of the substantia nigra over generalized non-convulsive seizures in the rat. *Neuroscience* 1990;39:339–349.

70. Walker BR, Easton A, Gale K. Regulation of limbic motor seizures by GABA and glutamate transmission in nucleus tractus solitarius. *Epilepsia* 1999;40:1051–1057.

71. Magdaleno-Madrigal VM, Valdes-Cruz A, Martinez-Vargas D, et al. Effect of electrical stimulation of the nucleus of the solitary tract on the development of electrical amygdaloid kindling in the cat. *Epilepsia* 2002;43:964–969.

72. Krahl SE, Clark KB, Smith DC, et al. Locus coeruleus lesions suppress the seizure-attenuating effects of vagus nerve stimulation. *Epilepsia* 1998;39:709–714.

73. Miller JW. The role of mesencephalic and thalamic arousal systems in experimental seizures. *Prog Neurobiol* 1992;39:155–178.

74. Naritoku DK, Terry WJ, Helfert RH. Regional induction of fos immunoreactivity in the brain by anticonvulsant stimulation of the vagus nerve. *Epilepsy Res* 1995;22:53–62.

75. Fernandez-Guardiola A, Martinez A, Valdes-Cruz A, et al. Vagus nerve prolonged stimulation in cats: effects on epileptogenesis (amygdala electrical kindling): behavioral and electrographic changes. *Epilepsia* 1999;40:822–829.

76. Salinsky MC, Burchiel KJ. Vagus nerve stimulation has no effect on awake EEG rhythms in humans. *Epilepsia* 1993;34:299–304.

77. Hammond EJ, Uthman BM, Reid SA, et al. Vagus nerve stimulation in humans: neurophysiological studies and electrophysiological monitoring. *Epilepsia* 1990;31(Suppl 2):S51–S59.

78. Hammond EJ, Uthman BM, Reid SA, et al. Electrophysiological studies of cervical vagus nerve stimulation in humans: I. EEG effects. *Epilepsia* 1992;33:1013–1020.

79. Kuba R, Guzaninova M, Brazdil M, et al. Effect of vagal nerve stimulation on interictal epileptiform discharges: a scalp EEG study. *Epilepsia* 2002;43:1181–1188.

80. Olejniczak PW, Fisch BJ, Carey M, et al. The effect of vagus nerve stimulation on epileptiform activity recorded from hippocampal depth electrodes. *Epilepsia* 2001;42:423–429.

81. Koo B. EEG changes with vagus nerve stimulation. *J Clin Neurophysiol* 2001;18:434–441.

82. Hammond EJ, Uthman BM, Reid SA, et al. Electrophysiologic studies of cervical vagus nerve stimulation in humans: II. Evoked potentials. *Epilepsia* 1992;33:1021–1028.

83. Ben-Menachem E, Hamberger A, Hedner T, et al. Effects of vagus nerve stimulation on amino acids and other metabolites in the CSF of patients with partial seizures. *Epilepsy Res* 1995;20:221–227.

84. Hammond EJ, Uthman BM, Wilder BJ, et al. Neurochemical effects of vagus nerve stimulation in humans. *Brain Res* 1992; 583:300–303.

85. Ko D, Heck C, Grafton S, et al. Vagus nerve stimulation activates central nervous system structures in epileptic patients during PET H2(15)O blood flow imaging. *Neurosurgery* 1996;39:426–430; discussion 430–431.

86. Henry TR, Votaw JR, Pennell PB, et al. Acute blood flow changes and efficacy of vagus nerve stimulation in partial epilepsy. *Neurology* 1999;52:1166–1173.

87. Henry TR, Votaw JR, Bakay RAE, et al. Vagus nerve stimulation-indcued cerebral blood flow changes differ in acute and chronic therapy of complex partial seizures. *Epilepsia* 1998;39:92.

88. Sucholeiki R , Alsaadi TM, Morris GL 3rd, et al. fMRI in patients implanted with a vagal nerve stimulator. *Seizure* 2002;11:157–162.

89. Narayanan JT, Watts R, Haddad N, et al. Cerebral activation during vagus nerve stimulation: a functional MR study. *Epilepsia* 2002;43:1509–1514.

90. Labar DR. Antiepileptic drug use during the first 12 months of vagus nerve stimulation therapy: a registry study. *Neurology* 2002;59:S38–S43.

91. Sperling MR, O'Connor MF, Saykin AJ, et al. Temporal lobectomy for refractory epilepsy. *JAMA* 1996;276:470–475.

92. Van Ness PC. Surgical outcome for neocortical (extrahippocampal) focal epilepsy. In: Luders HO, ed. *Epilepsy surgery.* New York: Raven Press, 1992:613–624.

93. Fisher RS, Handforth A. Reassessment: vagus nerve stimulation for epilepsy: a report of the Therapeutics and Technology Assessment Subcommittee of the American Academy of Neurology. *Neurology* 1999;53:666–669.

94. Baumgartner JE, Clifton GL, Wheless JW, et al. Corpus callosotomy. *Techniques Neurosurg* 1995;1:45–51.

95. Sorenson JM, Wheless JW, Baumgartner JE, et al. Corpus callosotomy for medically intractable seizures. *Pediatr Neurosurg* 1997; 27:260–267.

96. Camfield PR, Camfield CS. Vagal nerve stimulation for treatment of children with epilepsy. *J Pediatr* 1999;134:532–533.

97. Schwartz TH, Spencer DD. Strategies for reoperation after comprehensive epilepsy surgery. *J Neurosurg* 2001;95:615–623.

98. Renfroe JB, Wheless JW. Earlier use of adjunctive vagus nerve stimulation therapy for refractory epilepsy. *Neurology* 2002;59: S26–S30.

99. Scherrmann J, Hoppe C, Kral T, et al. Vagus nerve stimulation: clinical experience in a large patient series. *J Clin Neurophysiol* 2001;18:408–414.

100. Malow BA, Edwards J, Marzec M, et al. Effects of vagus nerve stimulation on respiration during sleep: a pilot study. *Neurology* 2000;55:1450–1454.

101. Bernard EJ, Passannante AN, Mann B, et al. Insertion of vagal nerve stimulator using local and regional anesthesia. *Surg Neurol* 2002;57:94–98.

102. Amar AP, Heck CN, Levy ML, et al. An institutional experience with cervical vagus nerve trunk stimulation for medically refractory epilepsy: rationale, technique, and outcome. *Neurosurgery* 1998;43:1265–1276; discussion 1276–1280.

103. Reid SA. Surgical technique for implantation of the neurocybernetic prosthesis. *Epilepsia* 1990;31(Suppl 2):S38–S39.

104. Asconape JJ, Moore DD, Zipes DP, et al. Early experience with vagus nerve stimulation for the treatment of epilepsy: cardiac complications. *Epilepsia* 1998;39:193.

105. Tatum WO 4th, Moore DB, Stecker MM, et al. Ventricular asystole during vagus nerve stimulation for epilepsy in humans. *Neurology* 1999;52:1267–1269.

106. Vaughn BV, Bernard E, Lannon S, et al. Intraoperative methods for confirmation of correct placement of the vagus nerve stimulator. *Epileptic Disord* 2001;3:75–78.

107. Agnew WF, McCreery DB. Considerations for safety with chronically implanted nerve electrodes. *Epilepsia* 1990;31(Suppl 2): S27–S32.

108. Agnew WF, McCreery DB, Yuen TG, et al. Histologic and physiologic evaluation of electrically stimulated peripheral nerve: considerations for the selection of parameters. *Ann Biomed Eng* 1989;17:39–60.

109. Murphy JV, Hornig GW, Schallert GS, et al. Adverse events in children receiving intermittent left vagal nerve stimulation. *Pediatr Neurol* 1998;19:42–44.

110. Landy HJ, Ramsay RE, Slater J, et al. Vagus nerve stimulation for complex partial seizures: surgical technique, safety, and efficacy. *J Neurosurg* 1993;78:26–31.

111. Terry R, Tarver WB, Zabara J. An implantable neurocybernetic prosthesis system. *Epilepsia* 1990;31(Suppl 2):S33–S37.

112. Terry RS, Tarver WB, Zabara J. The implantable neurocybernetic prosthesis system. *Pacing Clin Electrophysiol* 1991;14:86–93.

113. Ortler M, Luef G, Kofler A, et al. Deep wound infection after vagus nerve stimulator implantation: treatment without removal of the device. *Epilepsia* 2001;42:133–135.

114. Fernando DA, Lord RS. The blood supply of vagus nerve in the human: its implication in carotid endarterectomy, thyroidectomy and carotid arch aneurectomy. *Anat Anz* 1994;176:333–337.

115. Ramsay RE, Uthman BM, Augustinson LE, et al. Vagus nerve stimulation for treatment of partial seizures: 2. Safety, side effects, and tolerability. First International Vagus Nerve Stimulation Study Group. *Epilepsia* 1994;35:627–636.

116. Liporace J, Hucko D, Morrow R, et al. Vagal nerve stimulation: adjustments to reduce painful side effects. *Neurology* 2001;57:885–886.

117. Lotvall J, Lunde H, Augustinson LE, et al. Airway effects of direct left-sided cervical vagal stimulation in patients with complex partial seizures. *Epilepsy Res* 1994;18:149–154.

118. Setty AB, Vaughn BV, Quint SR, et al. Heart period variability during vagal nerve stimulation. *Seizure* 1998;7:213–217.

119. Annegers JF , Coan SP, Hauser WA, et al. Epilepsy, vagal nerve stimulation by the NCP system, mortality, and sudden, unexpected, unexplained death. *Epilepsia* 1998;39:206–212.

120. Sanossian N, Haut S. Chronic diarrhea associated with vagal nerve stimulation. *Neurology* 2002;58:330.

121. Iriarte J, Artieda J, Alegre M, et al. Spasm of the sternocleidomastoid muscle induced by vagal nerve stimulation. *Neurology* 2001; 57:2319–2320.

122. Leijten FS, Van Rijen PC. Stimulation of the phrenic nerve as a complication of vagus nerve pacing in a patient with epilepsy. *Neurology* 1998;51:1224–1225.

123. Duhaime AC, Melamed S, Clancy RR. Tonsillar pain mimicking glossopharyngeal neuralgia as a complication of vagus nerve stimulation: case report. *Epilepsia* 2000;41:903–905.

124. Blumer D, Davies K, Alexander A, et al. Major psychiatric disorders subsequent to treating epilepsy by vagus nerve stimulation. *Epilepsy Behav* 2001;2:466–472.

125. Klein JP, Jean-Baptiste M, Thompson JL, et al. A case report of hypomania following vagus nerve stimulation for refractory epilepsy. *J Clin Psychiatry* 2003;64:485.

126. Lundgren J, Ekberg O, Olsson R. Aspiration: a potential complication to vagus nerve stimulation. *Epilepsia* 1998;39:998–1000.

127. Schallert G , Foster J, Lindquist N, et al. Chronic stimulation of the left vagal nerve in children: effect on swallowing. *Epilepsia* 1998; 39:1113–1114.

128. Ben-Menachem E. Vagus-nerve stimulation for the treatment of epilepsy. *Lancet Neurology* 2002;1:477–482.

129. Hoppe C, Helmstaedter C, Scherrmann J, et al. No evidence for cognitive side effects after 6 months of vagus nerve stimulation in epilepsy patients. *Epilepsy Behav* 2001;2:351–356.

130. Clark KB, Naritoku DK, Smith DC, et al. Enhanced recognition memory following vagus nerve stimulation in human subjects. *Nat Neurosci* 1999;2:94–98.

131. Harden CL. Mood changes in epilepsy patients treated with vagus nerve stimulation. *Epilepsy Behav* 2001;2:S17–S20.

132. Clarke BM, Upton AR, Griffin H, et al. Chronic stimulation of the left vagus nerve: cognitive motor effects. *Can J Neurol Sci* 1997;24:226–229.

133. Clarke BM, Upton AR, Griffin H, et al. Chronic stimulation of the left vagus nerve in epilepsy: balance effects. *Can J Neurol Sci* 1997;24:230–234.

134. Cramer JA. Exploration of changes in health-related quality of life after 3 months of vagus nerve stimulation. *Epilepsy Behav* 2001;2:460–465.

135. Galli R, Bonanni E, Pizzanelli C, et al. Daytime vigilance and quality of life in epileptic patients treated with vagus nerve stimulation. *Epilepsy Behav* 2003;4:185–191.

136. Malow BA, Edwards J, Marzec M, et al. Vagus nerve stimulation reduces daytime sleepiness in epilepsy patients. *Neurology* 2001;57: 879–884.

137. Graves N. Anticonvulsants: choices and costs. *Am J Manage Care* 1998;49:S463–S474.

138. Boon P, D'Have M, Van Walleghem P, et al. Direct medical costs of refractory epilepsy incurred by three different treatment modalities: a prospective assessment. *Epilepsia* 2002;43:96–102.

139. Ben-Menachem E, Hellstrom K, Verstappen D. Analysis of direct hospital costs before and 18 months after treatment with vagus nerve stimulation therapy in 43 patients. *Neurology* 2002;59: S44–S47.

140. Benbadis SR, Nyhenhuis J, Tatum WO 4th, et al. MRI of the brain is safe in patients implanted with the vagus nerve stimulator. *Seizure* 2001;10:512–515.

141. Wilfong AA. Body MRI and vagus nerve stimulation. *Epilepsia* 2002;43:347.

142. Cooper IS, Amin I, Riklan M, et al. Chronic cerebellar stimulation in epilepsy. Clinical and anatomic studies. *Arch Neurol* 1976;33:559–570.

143. Cooper IS, Amin I, Gilman S. The effect of chronic cerebellar stimulation upon epilepsy in man. *Trans Am Neurol Assoc* 1973;98:192–196.

144. Cooper IS, Amin I, Upton A, et al. Safety and efficacy of chronic cerebellar stimulation. *Appl Neurophysiol* 1977/78;40:124–134.

145. Van Buren JM, Wood JH, Oakley J, Hambrecht F. Preliminary evaluation of cerebellar stimulation by double-blind stimulation and biologic criteria in the treatment of epilepsy. *J Neurosurg* 1978;48:407–416.

146. Wright GD, McLellan DL, Brice JG. A double-blind trial of chronic cerebellar stimulation in twelve patients with severe epilepsy. *J Neurol Neurosurg Psychiatry* 1984;47:769–774.

147. Chkhenkeli SA, Chkhenkeli IS. Effects of therapeutic stimulation of nucleus caudatus on epileptic electrical activity of brain in patients with intractable epilepsy. *Stereotact Funct Neurosurg* 1997;69:221–224.

148. Velasco M, Velasco F, Velasco AL, et al. Subacute electrical stimulation of the hippocampus blocks intractable temporal lobe seizures and paroxysmal EEG activities. *Epilepsia* 2000;41:158–169.

149. Yamamoto J, Ikeda A, Satow T, et al. Low-frequency electrical cortical stimulation has an inhibitory effect on epileptic focus in mesial temporal lobe epilepsy. *Epilepsia* 2002;43:491–495.

150. Charbardes S, Kahane P, Minotti L, et al. Deep brain stimulation in epilepsy with particular reference to the subthalamic nucleus. *Epileptic Disord* 2002;44(Suppl 3):S83–S93.

151. Benabid AL, Minotti L, Koudsie A, et al. Antiepileptic effect of high-frequency stimulation of the subthalamic nucleus (corpus luysi) in a case of medically intractable epilepsy caused by focal dysplasia: a 30-month follow-up. Technical case report. *Neurosurgery* 2002;50: 1385–1392.

152. Loddenkemper T, Pan A, Neme S, et al. Deep brain stimulation in epilepsy. *J Clin Neurophysiol* 2001;18:512–532.

153. Cooper IS, Upton ARM, Amin I. Reversibility of chronic neurologic deficits. Some effects of electrical stimulation of the thalamus and internal capsule in man. *Appl Neurophysiol* 1980;43:244–258.

154. Upton ARM, Cooper IS, Springman M, Amin I. Suppression of seizures and psychosis of limbic system origin by chronic stimulation of anterior nucleus of the thalamus. *Intl J Neurol* 1985/86; 19–20:223–228.

155. Hodaie M, Wennberg RA, Dostrovsky JO, Lozano AM. Chronic anterior thalamus stimulation for intractable epilepsy. *Epilepsia* 2002;43:603–608.

156. Mirski MA, Tsai YC, Rossell LA, et al. Anterior thalamic mediation of experimental seizures: selective EEG spectral coherence. *Epilepsia* 2003;44:355–365.

157. Fisher RS, Uematsu S, Krauss GL, et al. Placebo-controlled pilot study of centromedian thalamic stimulation in treatment of intractable seizures. *Epilepsia* 1992;33:841–851.

158. Velasco F, Velasco M, Velasco AL, Jimenez F. Effect of chronic electrical stimulation of the centromedian thalamic nuclei on various intractable seizure patterns: I. Clinical seizures and paroxysmal EEG activity. *Epilepsia* 1993;34:1052–1064.

159. Velasco M, Velasco F, Velasco AL, et al. Effect of chronic electrical stimulation of the centromedian thalamic nuclei on various intractable seizure patterns: II. Psychological performance and background EEG activity. *Epilepsia* 1993;34:1065–1074.

160. Velasco F, Velasco M, Velasco AL, et al. Electrical stimulation of the centromedian thalamic nucleus in control of seizures: long-term studies. *Epilepsia* 1995;36:63–71.

161. Velasco M, Velasco F, Velasco AL. Centromedian-thalamic and hippocampal electrical stimulation for the control of intractable epileptic seizures. *J Clin Neurophysiol* 2001;18:495–513.

162. DeGiorgio CM, Shewmon A, Whitehurst T. Trigeminal nerve stimulation for epilepsy. *Neurology* 2003;61:421–422.

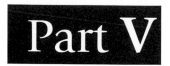

Epilepsy Surgery

Section A IDENTIFICATION OF CANDIDATES AND PRESURGICAL EVALUATION 983

72. Issues of Medical Intractability for Surgical Candidacy 983
73. Recognition of Potential Surgical Candidates and Video-Electroencephalographic Evaluation 993
74. Magnetic Resonance Imaging Techniques in the Evaluation for Epilepsy Surgery 1009
75. The Intracarotid Amobarbital Procedure 1031
76. Metabolic and Functional Neuroimaging 1041
77. Intracranial Electroencephalography and Localization Studies 1059

Section B EPILEPSY SURGERY IN SPECIFIC SETTINGS 1069

78. Hippocampal Sclerosis and Dual Pathology 1069
79. Resection for Uncontrolled Epilepsy in the Setting of Focal Lesions on MRI: Tumor, Vascular Malformation, Trauma, and Infarction 1087
80. Epilepsy Surgery in Focal Malformations of Cortical Development 1103
81. Hemispherectomy: Medications, Technical Approaches, and Results 1111
82. Epilepsy Surgery in the Absence of a Lesion on MRI 1125
83. Epilepsy Surgery in Infants and Children 1143
84. Corpus Callosotomy and Multiple Subpial Transections 1159
85. Newer Operative and Stereotactic Techniques and Their Application to Hypothalamic Hamartoma 1169
86. Outcome and Complications of Epilepsy Surgery 1175

Issues of Medical Intractability for Surgical Candidacy

72

Patrick Kwan   *Martin J. Brodie*

INTRODUCTION

Although the effectiveness of epilepsy surgery for patients with surgically remediable syndromes refractory to antiepileptic drug (AED) treatment, in particular anterior temporal lobectomy for mesial temporal lobe epilepsy, has been demonstrated in uncontrolled studies (1,2) and confirmed in a double-blind, randomized, controlled setting (3), controversies over the selection criteria for surgical candidacy continue. One of the prerequisites for epilepsy surgery is demonstrated "medical intractability" (4). The term is often used interchangeably with "medical refractoriness" or "pharmacoresistance." The *Oxford English Dictionary* defines "intractable" as "not easily treated or dealt with; resisting treatment effort." Although the concept may appear to be self-explanatory and intuitive at first glance, the precise definition of "medical intractability" has remained elusive (5,6). This chapter aims to explore the issues surrounding the definition of intractable epilepsy, with particular reference to its relevance to selection of surgical candidacy.

PSEUDORESISTANCE

The term "pseudoresistance" has been introduced to describe the condition in which seizures persist because the disorder has not been adequately or appropriately treated (5). It may arise in a number of situations, and must be excluded or corrected before AED treatment can be declared as having failed.

Incorrect Diagnosis

If a patient does not have epilepsy, AED therapy is unlikely to be helpful. A wide range of conditions can mimic epileptic seizures and must be considered in the differential diagnosis. Syncopal attacks, during which there may be clonic movements and incontinence, are commonly misdiagnosed as epileptic seizures (7). Pseudoseizures or nonepileptic psychogenic seizures are estimated to account for 10% to 45% of patients with apparently refractory epilepsy (8). Diagnosis can be challenging, as nonepileptic attacks often coexist with epilepsy or may develop as a substitute for seizures once the epilepsy is controlled (9). Mistaking other conditions for epilepsy can lead to unnecessary and potentially harmful treatments and delays in initiating appropriate therapy (7).

Incorrect Drug Choice or Inadequate Dosage

Incorrect classification of syndrome/seizure type is another common cause of drug failure. The profile of activity against different seizure types varies among the AEDs (10,11). Certain epilepsy syndromes and seizures have been found to be particularly responsive to specific AEDs, whereas others may be exacerbated by incorrectly chosen agents (12,13). A notable example is juvenile myoclonic epilepsy, which responds well to sodium valproate even at low doses (14). The syndrome is often misdiagnosed (15), however, leading to an erroneous choice of drug (e.g., carbamazepine or phenytoin), which can exacerbate myoclonic jerks and absence seizures (16). It is not uncommon at an initial clinic visit to be uncertain whether a young patient is reporting generalized absence or short-lived complex partial seizures.

In some circumstances, failure of an AED is not due to an incorrect drug choice for a particular seizure type(s), but rather because the agent is not prescribed at optimal dosage. Because of genetic and environmental factors, wide interindividual variability exists in the dosages at which beneficial and toxic effects are observed (17). Patients are often switched to an alternative treatment before the maximum tolerated dose (MTD) of their current AED is reached, resulting in persistent seizures that could have been controlled at higher dosages. One of the reasons for failure to optimize the dose in an individual patient is injudicious reliance on monitoring serum drug concentration, including a "therapeutic range" that can be interpreted as dictating dosage adjustment without adequate clinical correlation (18). Although "therapeutic" or "target" ranges are often quoted for established AEDs in standard textbooks (19), these should only be used as an aid in dosage adjustment. The treating clinician must realize that some patients will do well below the lower limit of the range, whereas others will tolerate higher levels with benefits and without toxicity.

In a study of 30 patients with serum phenytoin concentrations >20 mg/L (the widely quoted upper level of the target range), 17 patients became seizure free or had a significant reduction in seizure frequency from a baseline of one or more seizures per week when their dose was increased to achieve this high serum level (20). In another study of 74 consecutive patients referred for epilepsy surgery for presumed drug resistance, a systematic protocol to titrate their AED to the MTD, regardless of serum levels, resulted in a greater than 80% reduction in seizure frequency and cancellation of planned surgery in seven patients (9.5%) (21). An individualized approach must, therefore, be adopted when titrating an AED to the MTD before being declared a failure.

Imperfect Compliance or Inappropriate Lifestyle

As with other chronic medical conditions, imperfect adherence to the therapeutic regimen is one of the most common factors resulting in epilepsy treatment failure. AED noncompliance remains the most frequently identified etiology of status epilepticus in adults (22). The reasons for noncompliance are multifactorial, including socioeconomic, racial, and family factors (23). A survey of 232 adolescents identified support from the treating physician as the most powerful predictor of compliance with treatment regimens (24). Adherence to treatment may also be improved by simplifying the dosing regimen. Cramer and colleagues found that compliance rates in patients with epilepsy decreased as the frequency of drug administration increased, from 89% with once-daily dosing to 81% with twice-daily drug administration, 77% with 3-times-daily administration, dropping to only 39% with 4-times-daily administration (25).

Abuse of alcohol and recreational drugs can cause seizures and nonadherence to AED treatment. Similarly, sleep deprivation and stress are common precipitants. Social and lifestyle factors should, therefore, be considered when evaluating the efficacy of pharmacologic treatment.

INTENDED CONTEXT OF DEFINITION

Before the criteria for defining medical intractability are discussed, it should be emphasized that, by default, intractability is a relative concept rather than an absolute designation, which is influenced by the context in which it is intended to apply. A practical definition of medical intractability is required for three main purposes: (a) selection of patients for epilepsy surgery, (b) recruitment in experimental drug trials, and (c) identification for inclusion in epidemiologic studies. Because of these varying purposes, the definition may vary widely in different settings. For instance, since industry-sponsored regulatory add-on trials of experimental agents are typically of relatively short duration, the definition of refractory epilepsy for enrollment purposes usually requires high baseline monthly seizure frequency in order to achieve adequate statistical power with minimum sample size (26). In epidemiologic studies, the definition of medical intractability should reflect the outcome of epilepsy in response to treatment—that is, the likelihood of success or failure with successive AED regimens. This requires an understanding of the natural history of treated and untreated epilepsy, which remains poorly documented (27).

The relativity of any definition of medical intractability is particularly poignant in the context of candidacy for potentially "curative" resective epilepsy surgery. Aided by technical advances in neuroimaging and video electroencephalographic (EEG) monitoring, improvements in technique, and a better understanding of the anatomic and pathophysiologic bases of the epilepsies, resective surgery has become a highly effective and safe treatment modality for certain remediable syndromes, the prototype of which is mesial temporal lobe epilepsy (28,29). With a reported remission rate of 60% to 70% from centers across the world, mortality close to zero, and permanent neurologic morbidity less than 5%, anterior temporal lobectomy has made mesial temporal lobe epilepsy, an often medically intractable condition, highly surgically treatable in appropriately selected patients (30). A clinically relevant, pragmatic definition of drug resistance for patients with this epilepsy syndrome must, therefore, take into account the potential success of surgical treatment. Indeed, since the effectiveness of surgery may vary for different types of epilepsy, syndrome-specific predictive models may be required (31). Such definitions will have to be updated periodically with the availability of new AEDs and improvement in surgical techniques and outcomes.

ELEMENTS OF THE DEFINITION

Bearing in mind the aforementioned considerations, a discussion of the criteria used in defining medical intractability, with particular reference to epilepsy surgery, will follow. Although the definitions of medical intractability found in the medical literature seem to be highly variable (Table 72.1), sometimes even from the same authors, three key elements need to be incorporated: number of AEDs failed, frequency of seizures, and duration of treatment (3,32–42).

Number of Drugs Failed

An implicit assumption in any definition of medical intractability is that remission will not or is very unlikely to be attained with further manipulation of AED treatment. Therefore, the most important element in defining medical intractability is the number of AEDs failed at optimal dosage. Any definition must be based on an assessment of the probability of subsequent remission after each drug failure. Until recently, clinicians have had a relatively limited therapeutic armamentarium with which to treat epilepsy. With the approval of ten new AEDs in the past decade, the choice has been substantially widened and the number of possible combinations is now almost limitless. No patient will be able to try all AED regimens. A number of questions remain to be answered: How many trials of single AEDs should be used before a patient is treated with polytherapy? How many AEDs, either singly or in combination (and in how many combinations), have to fail before a seizure disorder can be recognized as medically refractory and surgery considered? At what stage does epilepsy become pharmacoresistant to AED treatment? Are there clinical features that will allow prediction of subsequent refractoriness? Answers to these questions depend on an understanding of the natural history of treated epilepsy, in particular its progress in response to treatment.

TABLE 72.1

SELECTED DEFINITIONS OF MEDICALLY INTRACTABLE EPILEPSY FROM MEDICAL LITERATURE

Reference	Type of Study	Definition
32	Epidemiology	One or more seizure per month for a period of at least 2 years, treated with at least three AEDs either singly or in combination
33	Epidemiology	Failure of two AEDs for seizure control or failure of one AED for seizure control and two others for intolerable side effects, with at least one seizure per month over an 18-month period
34	Surgery	20 complex partial seizures during the 24 months preceding surgical evaluation and a history of failure of two first-line AEDs
35	Epidemiology	One or more seizures every 2 months during the first 5 years of treatment or at least one seizure per year for longer treatment duration
36	Epidemiology	One or more seizures per month during the final 12 months of follow-up despite history of treatment with three or more AEDs
37	Phase 3 drug trial	At least 12 seizures within 12 weeks despite the use of at least two AEDs simultaneously or consecutively
38	Epidemiology (temporal lobe epilepsy)	Persistence of any seizures involving impairment of consciousness between 18 and 24 months after epilepsy onset despite at least two maximally tolerated AED trials
39	Epidemiology	One or more seizures per month for at least 2 years despite appropriate anticonvulsant agents at maximum tolerated blood levels
40	Epidemiology	Failure of two AEDs due to lack of efficacy, with one or more seizures over the past year
41	Epidemiology	At least one seizure per year during the last 10 years of observation
42	Phase 3 drug trial	An average of at least four seizures per month for 3 months prior to enrollment while taking one or two AEDs
3	Surgery	At least one seizure per month on average during the preceding year despite the use of two or more AEDs, one of which was phenytoin, carbamazepine, or valproic acid

Abbreviation: AED, antiepileptic drug.

TABLE 72.2

SUCCESS OF AED REGIMENS IN 470 PATIENTS WITH NEWLY DIAGNOSED, PREVIOUSLY UNTREATED EPILEPSY

Variable	No. of Patients	% of Patients
Seizure free on first monotherapy agent	222	47
Seizure free on second monotherapy agent	61	13
Seizure free on third monotherapy agent	6	1
Seizure free on two agents	12	3
Total seizure free	301	64

Data from ref. 40.

Outcome With Respect to Treatment Course

Although modern population-based epidemiologic studies have demonstrated that 30% to 40% of patients with epilepsy do not enter remission (43–47), it remains unclear what factors contribute to the development of pharmacoresistance. Studies have focused on the two ends of the process—that is, at diagnosis, and when remission is attained or refractory epilepsy has developed, with little documentation on how patients get from one end to the other. Yet, the great majority of patients, at least in developed countries, will be started on an AED when the diagnosis of epilepsy is made. From a practical point of view, it would be useful to gauge the chance of success with the first-ever AED, as well as with successive regimens. When the first agent fails to control the epilepsy, as is often the case, little is known about the proportion of patients responding to subsequent monotherapy or AED combinations, and whether there is any difference in effectiveness between these treatment strategies. Understanding the likely response to successive treatment regimens can also shed important light on the biologic mechanisms underpinning drug resistance.

In a Veterans Affairs study, among the 82 patients who received polytherapy after failure of the first drug, only nine (11%) became seizure free (48). In a relatively small cohort of 59 adult patients with chronic epilepsy poorly controlled on monotherapy, Schmidt and Richter (49) reported that substitution of another agent resulted in remission in only 12%.

The relationship between outcome and course of AED treatment has been specifically addressed in an ongoing, long-term study of patients with newly diagnosed epilepsy, conducted in Glasgow, Scotland, since 1982. In the first analysis reported in 2000, 525 unselected adolescent and adult patients (median age at onset, 26 years) were given a diagnosis of epilepsy, commenced on AED therapy, and followed for up to 16 years, with a median of 5 years (40). Among the 470 patients who had never before received AED treatment, 64% entered remission for at least 1 year. Forty-seven percent of patients became and remained

seizure free on their first drug, 13% on the second drug, but only 4% on the third drug or a combination of two drugs (Table 72.2). Among those who became seizure free on their first drug, greater than 90% did so at moderate daily dosing (≤800 mg carbamazepine, ≤1,500 mg sodium valproate, ≤300 mg lamotrigine) (50). Thirty-five patients (7% of the total population) who responded to the first or second monotherapy agent were able to withdraw from treatment and remained seizure free.

Response to the first AED was the most powerful predictor of prognosis. Among the 248 patients in whom treatment with the first agent was unsuccessful, only 79 (32%) subsequently became seizure free. Indeed, only 11% of the 113 patients in whom the first drug failed primarily due to lack of efficacy (as opposed to adverse events or other causes) later reported complete seizure control.

Among the patients in whom the first drug was substituted due to inadequate efficacy, only 17% entered remission on the second monotherapy agent and 26% became seizure free when another AED was added. No patient became seizure free when combination therapy was used after failure of two consecutive monotherapy agents. The probability of seizure freedom diminished progressively with successive AED regimens, whether substitution or add-on therapy, particularly after failure of two regimens (Fig. 72.1) (51). In a more recent updated analysis of 780 previously AED-naïve patients, only 7% of patients failing two well-tolerated regimens achieved remission; for those failing their first three regimens, this figure fell further to only 3.3%. If adverse events prevented titration to target doses with at least one of the first two regimens, the prognosis for remission was better, at 19%.

Existing data on pediatric epilepsy are encouraging and enable us to predict medical intractability early in the disease course. Camfield and colleagues (36) conducted an

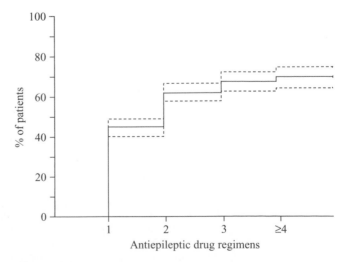

Figure 72.1 Probability of seizure freedom in patients with newly diagnosed epilepsy, according to the number of antiepileptic drug regimens. Dotted lines represent 95% confidence intervals. (From ref 12, with permission).

elegant population-based study that included 417 children (seizure onset between 1 month and 16 years), with an average follow up of 8 years. Of the participants, 83% of the children received only one AED in the first year of treatment, which rendered 61% seizure free. These patients did not require AEDs at the end of their follow up—that is, they achieved remission. Only 4% of the children receiving a single AED during the first year went on to develop intractable epilepsy. Of those patients (17%) who had inadequate seizure control with the first AED, only 42% achieved complete remission of their epilepsy, whereas 29% developed intractable epilepsy. However, the authors did not specify the number of successive AEDs tried in these children. Specifically, this study did not provide information about responsiveness, or lack thereof, to the second AED.

Based on their findings, the investigators concluded that a patient's outcome is less favorable if the first AED is not efficacious, and that failure of at least two AEDs should be an indication to consider surgical or other treatment modalities. Their study period was between 1977 and 1985, when most of the newer AEDs had not yet been approved for the treatment of epilepsy. Nevertheless, given the equivalent efficacy of most AEDs, it is unlikely that a repeat study with the newer AEDs would significantly alter the prediction of intractability after two failed AEDs.

In another retrospective analysis of 120 patients in Philadelphia aged 1 to 18 years with recent-onset temporal lobe epilepsy, the only identified predictor of intractability at 2 years was "failure of the first AED trial" (38).

Operational Definition

Observations from these outcome studies support the hypothesis that patients with newly diagnosed epilepsy comprise two distinct populations, who can often be identified early in the course of the treatment paradigm (12). Approximately 60% of patients will have a favorable prognosis. They will become seizure free on a modest or moderate dose of the first- or second-choice AED as monotherapy, without developing intolerable side effects. In some patients, treatment may be subsequently withdrawn without relapse, suggesting that the "seizure generator" had, indeed, remitted. The remaining patients (40%) will have "difficult-to-control" epilepsy, usually from the outset. Predictors of poor prognosis include syndromic classification, symptomatic etiology of epilepsy, high initial number or frequency of seizures, presence of psychiatric comorbidity, and family history of epilepsy (5,40,52–55), all of which can be recognized early in the course of the disorder.

Many authors have empirically used the failure of two or three AEDs as a cutoff for the definition of medical intractability (Table 72.1). Data from the Glasgow studies lend further support to an operational definition of refractory epilepsy as failure of two appropriately chosen AEDs in adequate doses, or one monotherapy and one combination regimen, due to lack of efficacy.

Seizure Frequency

There is no universal agreement as to how frequent and over what period of time seizures must be occurring to constitute intractability. Seizure frequency used by different authors in defining intractability ranges from one per month to one per year, in an almost arbitrary fashion (Table 72.1). Such variability stems from the semantic difficulty involved in defining a concept opposite that of remission. Remission may be defined simply as absence of seizures with (or without) the use of AED therapy for a particular period of time (56). Many researchers maintain that intractability is not the reverse of remission (57,58). However, studies including patients treated surgically (59–62) and medically (63) suggest that absolute seizure freedom is the only relevant outcome consistently associated with improvement in quality of life. In a community-based survey of 696 patients with epilepsy, subjects with one or more seizures over the past 2 years had higher levels of anxiety and depression, greater perceived stigma and impact of epilepsy, and lower employment rates than did those in remission (64). In many countries, having even one seizure per year poses restrictions on driving (65,66). It may, therefore, be argued that in terms of the effect on psychosocial functioning, a patient's epilepsy may be considered intractable when one or more seizures per year are occurring (40). The impact of these seizures on a patient's lifestyle and the likely outcome of surgical treatment must be taken into consideration.

Duration of Treatment

Some authors have incorporated the duration of AED treatment when defining intractability, arguing that patients with a few seizures per year in the first 2 years following epilepsy onset should not be viewed in the same light as those in whom seizures persist after 10 or 15 years of treatment (58). This assumption depends on how often patients "cross" from one prognostic group to the other over time, an issue that has been prospectively investigated by Berg and colleagues in 613 newly diagnosed children with a range of epilepsy syndromes (33). At the 2-year follow-up of 595 patients, 53% had been seizure free for at least 1 year ("good" outcome); 8% were defined as "intractable/bad outcome" (failure of two or more AEDs, one or more seizures per month over 18 months or longer); and the rest were "indeterminate." When 390 of these patients were reviewed at 4 years, the good and bad outcomes persisted in greater than 80% of cases. Of those patients in the indeterminate group, 8% had become intractable. In a separate analysis, the authors found that among the 442 children who had entered the 2-year remission, 107 (74%) relapsed, but only 31 (7%) did so "spontaneously" while receiving a stable AED regimen (67). In an updated analysis of the Glasgow database, only 6% of 780 patients with newly diagnosed epilepsy relapsed after at least 1 year of seizure freedom, with a median relapse duration of 25 months (55). The relapse rate was time-dependent, with 9% of the patients starting on AED therapy before 1995 subsequently developing refractory epilepsy after an initial positive response.

These observations suggest that in most patients, the prognosis of epilepsy can be determined early in the course of the disorder (i.e., after 2 years of treatment), following a favorable trial of two AEDs or one monotherapy and one combination regimen. In a small proportion of patients, the condition appears to "progress" with time to a drug-resistant state after a period of seizure freedom. Therefore, in general, defining medical intractability as a function of the number of AEDs failed represents a more consistent criterion than duration of illness, which is more arbitrary.

The natural history of individual epilepsy types and syndromes is highly variable. A notable example is mesial temporal lobe epilepsy associated with hippocampal sclerosis, for which accumulating evidence suggests a progressive course in some patients (68) but not in others (69). In a retrospective survey of 333 patients who underwent resective surgery for medically refractory epilepsy (88% of whom had anterior temporal lobectomy), the average time to failure of two first-line AEDs was 9.1 years (median, 5 years). Of 284 patients from the cohort, 26% recalled a previous period of at least 1 year of seizure freedom since the onset of their epilepsy (34). This suggests that for some patients with temporal lobe epilepsy, medical intractability may not declare itself in the early stages of the disorder. Indeed, an initial apparently benign course seems to be one of the characteristics of this condition (70), but how often such a pattern is observed can only be accurately determined in a prospective study in which all patients with temporal lobe epilepsy are followed from the point of presentation with epileptic seizures. In the Glasgow cohort, patients with underlying hippocampal sclerosis differed little in outcome from those with other localization-related epilepsies (71,72). Clearly, since epilepsy is not a single disease, syndrome and etiology-specific prospective prognostic studies are needed if individual patients are to be managed more appropriately.

Pediatric Issues

The timing of epilepsy surgery in children is further complicated by the need to consider the potential consequences of the insults from repeated seizures and from surgical intervention on the developing brain (73). This issue is particularly notable and sensitive when evaluating infants with catastrophic localization-related epilepsies, who may have many seizures per day. A large number of AEDs might have been tried and might have failed over a relatively short period. Although controlled studies are lacking, resumption of developmental progression after early surgery has been observed. For instance, Wyllie and colleagues (74) performed various forms of epilepsy surgery in 12 children with a variety of pathologies at a mean age

of 15.3 months, with all but one becoming seizure free or having at least worthwhile improvement. In addition, "catch-up" developmental progress was noted in these infants. Therefore, the decision about the timing of surgery in children is strongly affected by the severity and natural history of the specific syndrome, taking into account the potential detrimental effects of continued seizures on neural plasticity, as well as on developmental and psychosocial outcomes. In some cases of catastrophic epilepsy, surgery should be considered even earlier than 2 years of onset following thorough, individualized evaluation (75,76).

FUTURE RESEARCH DIRECTIONS

It should be apparent from the previous discussion that the development of a valid, clinically relevant definition of medical intractability requires a better understanding of the natural history of each epilepsy syndrome. To this end, there is no substitution for population-based, long-term studies following patients from the point of presentation and diagnosis. With an ever-expanding list of AEDs, more well-designed prospective studies are needed to document the course of epilepsy in response to treatment and to provide data on the chance of remission with each successive drug regimen, so that a practical cutoff point of number of drugs failed may be applied when labeling a seizure disorder pharmacoresistant. Complicating the matter is the use of AED polytherapy, which is often instituted when monotherapy fails. Whether this would be a more effective management strategy if used earlier and in what situations remain to be determined (12,77).

Outcome studies should also address the fundamental question of what constitutes drug failure. For example, should it be defined objectively by persistence of seizures despite attaining a target serum drug concentration, or dosage and duration of the AED regimen? Alternatively, should it be judged according to the individual circumstances of each drug trial? Whether drug withdrawal due to intolerability should be regarded as failure in defining drug resistance has not been thoroughly explored. In the Glasgow studies, withdrawal of the first AED due to intolerability was itself a predictive factor of poorer long-term outcome, compared with withdrawal due to idiosyncratic reactions or other factors unrelated to treatment (40). However, these studies and more recent data suggest that the eventual outcome is slightly more favorable if treatment failure is due to poor tolerability rather than to lack of efficacy. Some authors consider failure of two AEDs due to intolerable side effects equivalent to failure of one drug due to inadequate efficacy for the purposes of defining intractability (33).

Among the three key elements included in the definition of medical intractability, the greatest variation seems to exist for seizure frequency. To be clinically relevant, the frequency incorporated should reflect the impact on a patient's quality of life. More studies are needed to evaluate the relationship between seizure frequency and severity on quality-of-life measurements (78), and their clinical significance (79,80). The hypothesis that medical intractability may be identified in most patients within 1 to 2 years after initiating treatment raises the question of whether surgery should be offered early to those patients with surgically remediable syndromes, in particular those with mesial temporal lobe epilepsy. A National Institutes of Health–funded, multicenter, randomized, controlled trial of patients 12 years of age or older with refractory mesial temporal lobe epilepsy, despite treatment with two AEDs for less than 2 years, is currently underway to examine whether surgery results in better outcome compared with an additional 2 years of medication (81). Similar pediatric studies are needed to address whether early surgery might result in improved long-term developmental outcome, particularly in infants with catastrophic focal epilepsies.

As in other disciplines of medicine, the impact of pharmacogenetics is increasingly being felt in epileptology (82). The influence of genetic variation in drug metabolizing genes, in particular those encoding the cytochrome P450 enzymes, on susceptibility to drug toxicity has long been recognized (83,84). There is recent conflicting evidence that polymorphisms of the *ABCB1* (or *MDR1*) gene may be associated with resistance to AED therapy in patients with epilepsy via the effect on expression of the drug transporter P-glycoprotein at the blood-brain barrier (85). A Brazilian study showed that a variant allele *Asn171Ser* of the cellular prion protein gene was more common in patients who underwent surgery for refractory mesial temporal lobe epilepsy associated with hippocampal sclerosis than in the general population and was related to a poorer outcome after temporal lobectomy (86). As the complexity of genetic influence on treatment responsiveness becomes better understood, pharmacogenetic profiling may, in the future, be recognized as a practical determinant of medical intractability.

CONCLUSIONS

A definition of medical intractability that has broad recognition among the epilepsy community will have particular relevance to the selection of surgical candidates and is essential for establishing the acceptable standard of care, as well as for the valid comparison of treatment results among different centers. In practice, different definitions may be used in different contexts (surgical candidacy, experimental drug trials, epidemiologic studies), and pseudoresistance must be excluded before a seizure disorder is deemed intractable.

Recent long-term prospective studies of newly diagnosed patients represent an important step in improved documentation of the natural history of treated epilepsy. A consensus is being reached that, for operational purposes, medical refractoriness should be suspected when two appropriately chosen, well-tolerated, first-line AEDs or one

monotherapy and one combination regimen have failed due to lack of efficacy (13). However, the period may vary from syndrome to syndrome and from patient to patient. There is a need to conduct syndrome-specific prognostic studies.

In a patient with apparently medically intractable epilepsy, the decision to pursue epilepsy surgery and not continue pharmacologic manipulation must be made on a case-by-case basis, taking into consideration the patient's wishes, the likely prognosis with treatment modalities, the available medical and surgical expertise, and the potential risks and benefits of resective surgery. The challenge facing the clinician is to develop individualized protocols that maximize the likelihood of successful drug therapy but that also efficiently identify patients suitable for curative resective surgery.

REFERENCES

1. Engel J Jr. Update on surgical treatment of the epilepsies: summary of the Second International Palm Desert Conference on the Surgical Treatment of the Epilepsies (1992). *Neurology* 1993;43: 1612–1617.
2. McIntosh AM, Wilson SJ, Berkovic SF. Seizure outcome after temporal lobectomy: current research practice and findings. *Epilepsia* 2001;42:1288–1307.
3. Wiebe S, Blume WT, Girvin JP, et al. A randomized, controlled trial of surgery for temporal-lobe epilepsy. *N Engl J Med* 2001;345: 311–318.
4. Bourgeois BFD. General concepts of medical intractability. In: Lüders HO, Comair YG, eds. *Epilepsy surgery*. Philadelphia: Lippincott Williams & Wilkins, 2001:63–68.
5. Perucca E. Pharmacoresistance in epilepsy: how should it be defined? *CNS Drugs* 1998:10:171–179.
6. Regesta G, Tanganelli P. Clinical aspects and biological bases of drug-resistant epilepsies. *Epilepsy Res* 1999;34:109–122.
7. Smith D, Defalla BA, Chadwick DW. The misdiagnosis of epilepsy and the management of refractory epilepsy in a specialist clinic. *QJM* 1999;92:15–23.
8. Devinsky O. Patients with refractory seizures. *N Engl J Med* 1999;340:1565–1570.
9. Kuyk J, Leijten F, Meinardi H, et al. The diagnosis of psychogenic non-epileptic seizures: a review. *Seizure* 1997;6:243–253.
10. Brodie MJ, Dichter MA. Antiepileptic drugs. *N Engl J Med* 1996; 334:168–175.
11. Dichter MA, Brodie MJ. New antiepileptic drugs. *N Engl J Med* 1996;334:1583–1590.
12. Brodie MJ, Kwan P. Staged approach to epilepsy management. *Neurology* 2002;58(Suppl 5):S2–S8.
13. Kwan P, Brodie MJ. Drug treatment of epilepsy: when does it fail and how to optimize its use? *CNS Spectr* 2004;9:110–119.
14. Karlovassitou-Koniari A, Alexiou D, Angelopoulos P, et al. Low dose sodium valproate in the treatment of juvenile myoclonic epilepsy. *J Neurol* 2002;249:396–399.
15. Renganathan R, Delanty N. Juvenile myoclonic epilepsy: underappreciated and under-diagnosed. *Postgrad Med J* 2003;79: 78–80.
16. Perucca E, Gram L, Avanzini G, et al. Antiepileptic drugs as a cause of worsening seizures. *Epilepsia* 1998;39:5–17.
17. Perucca E, Dulac O, Shorvon S, et al. Harnessing the clinical potential of antiepileptic drug therapy: dosage optimisation. *CNS Drugs* 2001;15:609–621.
18. McKee PJW, Brodie MJ. Therapeutic drug monitoring. In: Engel J Jr, Pedley TA, eds. *Epilepsy: a comprehensive textbook*. Philadelphia: Lippincott-Raven, 1997:1181–1194.
19. Johannessen SI, Tomson T. Laboratory monitoring of antiepileptic drugs. In: Levy RH, Mattson RH, Meldrum BS, et al, eds. *Antiepileptic drugs*, 4th ed. Philadelphia, Lippincott Williams & Wilkins, 2002:103–111.

20. Cobos JE. High-dose phenytoin in the treatment of refractory epilepsy. *Epilepsia* 1987;28:111–114.
21. Hermanns G, Noachtar S, Tuxhorn I, et al. Systematic testing of medical intractability for carbamazepine, phenytoin, and phenobarbital or primidone in monotherapy for patients considered for epilepsy surgery. *Epilepsia* 1996;37:675–679.
22. DeLorenzo RJ, Pellock JM, Towne AR, et al. Epidemiology of status epilepticus. *J Clin Neurophysiol* 1995;12:316–325.
23. Snodgrass SR, Vedanarayanan VV, Parker CC, et al. Pediatric patients with undetectable anticonvulsant blood levels: comparison with compliant patients. *J Child Neurol* 2001;16: 164–168.
24. Kyngas H. Predictors of good compliance in adolescents with epilepsy. *Seizure* 2001;10:549–553.
25. Cramer JA, Mattson RH, Prevey ML, et al. How often is medication taken as prescribed? A novel assessment technique. *JAMA* 1989;261:3273–3277.
26. Committee for Proprietary Medicinal Products. The European Agency for the Evaluation of Medicinal Products. Note for guidance on clinical investigation of medicinal products in the treatment of epileptic disorders. London, November 16, 2000.
27. Kwan P, Sander JW. The natural history of epilepsy: an epidemiological view. *J Neurol Neuro Surg Psychiatry* 2004;75:1376–1381.
28. Engel J Jr. Surgery for seizures. *N Engl J Med* 1996;334:647–652.
29. Wieser HG. Epilepsy surgery: past, present and future. *Seizure* 1998;7:173–184.
30. Engel J Jr, Wiebe S, French J, et al. Practice parameter: temporal lobe and localized neocortical resections for epilepsy: report of the Quality Standards Subcommittee of the American Academy of Neurology, in Association with the American Epilepsy Society and the American Association of Neurological Surgeons. *Neurology* 2003;60:538–547.
31. Dlugos DJ. The early identification of candidates for epilepsy surgery. *Arch Neurol* 2001;58:1543–1546.
32. Berg AT, Levy SR, Novotny EJ, et al. Predictors of intractable epilepsy in childhood: a case-control study. *Epilepsia* 1996;37:24–30.
33. Berg AT, Shinnar S, Levy SR, et al. Defining early seizure outcomes in pediatric epilepsy: the good, the bad and the in-between. *Epilepsy Res* 2001;43:75–84.
34. Berg AT, Langfitt J, Shinnar S, et al. How long does it take for partial epilepsy to become intractable? *Neurology* 2003;60: 186–190.
35. Camfield PR, Camfield CS. Antiepileptic drug therapy: when is epilepsy truly intractable? *Epilepsia* 1996;37(Suppl 1):S60–S65.
36. Camfield PR, Camfield CS, Gordon K, et al. If a first antiepileptic drug fails to control a child's epilepsy, what are the chances of success with the next drug? *J Pediatr* 1997;131:821–824.
37. Cereghino JJ, Biton V, Abou-Khalil B, et al. Levetiracetam for partial seizures: results of a double-blind, randomized clinical trial. *Neurology* 2000;55:236–242.
38. Dlugos DJ, Sammel MD, Strom BL, et al. Response to first drug trial predicts outcome in childhood temporal lobe epilepsy. *Neurology* 2001;57:2259–2264.
39. Huttenlocher PR, Hapke RJ. A follow-up study of intractable seizures in childhood. *Ann Neurol* 1990;28:699–705.
40. Kwan P, Brodie MJ. Early identification of refractory epilepsy. *N Engl J Med* 2000;342:314–319.
41. Sillanpää M. Remission of seizures and predictors of intractability in long-term follow-up. *Epilepsia* 1993;34:930–936.
42. US Gabapentin Study Group No. 5. Gabapentin as add-on therapy in refractory partial epilepsy: a double-blind, placebo-controlled, parallel-group study. *Neurology* 1993;43:2292–2298.
43. Elwes RD, Johnson AL, Shorvon SD, et al. The prognosis for seizure control in newly diagnosed epilepsy. *N Engl J Med* 1984; 311:944–947.
44. Shafer SQ, Hauser WA, Annegers JF, et al. EEG and other early predictors of epilepsy remission: a community study. *Epilepsia* 1988; 29:590–600.
45. Cockerell OC, Johnson AL, Sander JW, et al. Remission of epilepsy: results from the National General Practice Study of Epilepsy. *Lancet* 1995;346:140–144.
46. Collaborative Group for the Study of Epilepsy. Prognosis of epilepsy in newly referred patients: a multicenter prospective study of the effects of monotherapy on the long-term course of epilepsy. *Epilepsia* 1992;33:45–51.
47. Sillanpää M, Jalava M, Kaleva O, et al. Long-term prognosis of seizures with onset in childhood. *N Engl J Med* 1998;338: 1715–1722.
48. Mattson RH, Cramer JA, Collins JF, et al. Comparison of carbamazepine, phenobarbital, phenytoin, and primidone in partial and secondarily generalized tonic-clonic seizures. *N Engl J Med* 1985;313:145–151.
49. Schmidt D, Richter K. Alternative single anticonvulsant drug therapy for refractory epilepsy. *Ann Neurol* 1986;19:85–87.
50. Kwan P, Brodie MJ. Effectiveness of first antiepileptic drug. *Epilepsia* 2001;42:1255–1260.
51. Kwan P, Brodie MJ. Epilepsy after the first drug fails: substitution or add-on? *Seizure* 2000;9:464–468.
52. Arts WF, Geerts AT, Brouwer OF, et al. The early prognosis of epilepsy in childhood: the prediction of a poor outcome. *Epilepsia* 1999;40:726–734.
53. MacDonald BK, Johnson AL, Goodridge DM, et al. Factors predicting prognosis of epilepsy after presentation with seizures. *Ann Neurol* 2000;48:833–841.
54. Berg AT, Shinnar S, Levy SR, et al. Early development of intractable epilepsy in children: a prospective study. *Neurology* 2001;56: 1445–1452.
55. Mohanraj R, Brodie MJ. Prediction of refractory epilepsy. *Epilepsia* 2003;44(Suppl 8):156.
56. Commission on Epidemiology and Prognosis, International League Against Epilepsy. Guidelines for epidemiologic studies on epilepsy. *Epilepsia* 1993;34:592–596.
57. Hauser WA, Hesdorffer D. Epidemiology of intractable epilepsy. In: Lüders HO, Comair YG, eds. *Epilepsy surgery.* Philadelphia: Lippincott Williams & Wilkins, 2001:55–61.
58. Berg AT. Understanding the delay before epilepsy surgery: who develops intractable focal epilepsy and when? *CNS Spectr* 2004;9: 136–144.
59. Vickrey BG, Hays RD, Engel J Jr, et al. Outcome assessment for epilepsy surgery: the impact of measuring health-related quality of life. *Ann Neurol* 1995;37:158–166.
60. Wheelock I, Peterson C, Buchtel HA. Presurgery expectations, postsurgery satisfaction, and psychosocial adjustment after epilepsy surgery. *Epilepsia* 1998;39:487–494.
61. Gilliam F, Kuzniecky R, Meador K, et al. Patient-oriented outcome assessment after temporal lobectomy for refractory epilepsy. *Neurology* 1999;53:687–694.
62. Markand ON, Salanova V, Whelihan E, et al. Health-related quality of life outcome in medically refractory epilepsy treated with anterior temporal lobectomy. *Epilepsia* 2000;41:749–759.
63. Birbeck GL, Hays RD, Cui X, et al. Seizure reduction and quality of life improvements in people with epilepsy. *Epilepsia* 2002;43: 535–538.
64. Jacoby A, Baker GA, Steen N, et al. The clinical course of epilepsy and its psychosocial correlates: findings from a U.K. Community study. *Epilepsia* 1996;37:148–161.
65. Fisher RS, Parsonage M, Beaussart M, et al. Epilepsy and driving: an international perspective. *Epilepsia* 1994;35:675–684.
66. Berg AT, Engel J Jr. Restricted driving for people with epilepsy. *Neurology* 1999;52:1306–1307.
67. Berg AT, Shinnar S, Levy SR, et al. Two-year remission and subsequent relapse in children with newly diagnosed epilepsy. *Epilepsia* 2001;42:1553–1562.
68. Fuerst D, Shah J, Shah A, et al. Hippocampal sclerosis is a progressive disorder: a longitudinal volumetric MRI study. *Ann Neurol* 2003;53:413–416.
69. Kobayashi E, Lopes-Cendes I, Guerreiro CA, et al. Seizure outcome and hippocampal atrophy in familial mesial temporal lobe epilepsy. *Neurology* 2001;56:166–172.
70. Engel J Jr. Introduction to temporal lobe epilepsy. *Epilepsy Res* 1996;26:141–150.
71. Stephen LJ, Kwan P, Brodie MJ. Does the cause of localisation-related epilepsy influence the response to antiepileptic drug treatment? *Epilepsia* 2001;42:357–362.
72. Brodie MJ, Mohanraj R. Pharmacological outcomes in newly diagnosed epilepsy. *Epilepsia* 2003;44(Suppl 8):84.

73. Oguni H, Mukahira K, Tanaka T, et al. Surgical indication for refractory childhood epilepsy. *Epilepsia* 2000;41(Suppl 9): 21–25.

74. Wyllie E, Comair YG, Kotagal P, et al. Epilepsy surgery in infants. *Epilepsia* 1996;37:625–637.

75. Wyllie E. Surgical treatment of epilepsy in children. *Pediatr Neurol* 1998;19:179–188.

76. Cross JH. Epilepsy surgery in childhood. *Epilepsia* 2002;43(Suppl 3): 65–70.

77. Deckers CL, Czuczwar SJ, Hekster YA, et al. Selection of antiepileptic drug polytherapy based on mechanisms of action: the evidence reviewed. *Epilepsia* 2000;41:1364–1374.

78. Vickrey BG, Berg AT, Sperling MR, et al. Relationships between seizure severity and health-related quality of life in refractory localization-related epilepsy. *Epilepsia* 2000;41:760–764.

79. Baker GA, Camfield C, Camfield P, et al. Commission on Outcome Measurement in Epilepsy, 1994–1997: final report. *Epilepsia* 1998; 39:213–231.

80. Wiebe S, Matijevic S, Eliasziw M, et al. Clinically important change in quality of life in epilepsy. *J Neurol Neurosurg Psychiatry* 2002;73:116–120.

81. Engel J Jr, Erba G, Kieburtz K. Early randomized surgical epilepsy trial. Available at: http://www.erset.org. Accessed on August 1,2005.

82. Ball S, Borman N. Pharmacogenetics and drug metabolism. *Nat Biotechnol* 1998;16:S4–S5.

83. Pirmohamed M, Park BK. Genetic susceptibility to adverse drug reactions. *Trends Pharmacol Sci* 2001;22:298–305.

84. Holmes GL. The interface of preclinical evaluation with clinical testing of antiepileptic drugs: role of pharmacogenomics and pharmacogenetics. *Epilepsy Res* 2002;50:41–54.

85. Kwan P, Brodie MJ. Potential role of drug transporters in the pathogenesis of medically intractable epilepsy. *Epilepsia* 2005; 46:224–235.

86. Walz R, Castro RM, Velasco TR, et al. Surgical outcome in mesial temporal sclerosis correlates with prion protein gene variant. *Neurology* 2003;61:1204–1210.

Recognition of Potential Surgical Candidates and Video-Electroencephalographic Evaluation

73

Gregory D. Cascino

In the United States, 1% to 4% of the population has epilepsy—i.e., two or more unprovoked seizures, and approximately 180 000 patients are newly diagnosed each year (1,2). Worldwide, epilepsy affects an estimated 50 million people (1,2). Rates of unprovoked seizure activity are highest in early childhood and increase again with age (1,2). Partial or localization-related epilepsy characterized by *focal seizure activity* is most common in adults with recurrent, unprovoked seizures (1–3), with more than 90% of the incident cases of epilepsy in adults involving focal seizures (1,2). The most frequently occurring seizure type is a complex partial seizure of medial temporal lobe origin (1–3). Approximately 45% of patients with partial epilepsy have medically refractory disorders (3). A minority who fail to respond to first-line therapy will be rendered seizure free with antiepileptic medications approved since 1993 (4–6). In one population-based study, approximately 10% of 470 newly diagnosed patients whose initial antiepileptic drug was unsuccessful achieved control with subsequent medical therapies, but nearly one third of those who were followed up for 5 years developed medically refractory seizures (6). The early response to antiepileptic drug therapy is highly predictive of long-term medical outcome, and the most "effective" drug for partial epilepsy is often the first medication used (6). A seizure disorder is likely to be considered "refractory" after the first two drug regimens (6).

INTRACTABLE EPILEPSY

Approximately 20% to 30% of all patients with epilepsy have seizures that are physically and socially disabling (1–10), and these individuals are at significantly greater risk for long-term morbidity and mortality than a control population (11). Intractable epilepsy may be associated with psychosocial deprivation, inability to operate a motor vehicle, unemployment or underemployment, limited educational opportunities, and need for a caregiver. Often, it may be a "catastrophic" disorder accompanied by progressive neurocognitive impairment and behavioral alterations (3–6). Unfavorable seizure control significantly increases the cost of epilepsy (12,13). Each year, prevalent cases of epilepsy cost the United States approximately $12 billion, and almost 90% of these mostly indirect expenses are related to the care of patients with recurrent seizures and intractable epilepsy (13). Treatment of intractable partial epilepsy includes antiepileptic drugs, vagus nerve stimulation (VNS), and epilepsy surgery (6,14,15). The rate of response, i.e., at least a 50% reduction in seizures, with medical therapy and VNS is approximately 30% to 40% (14); complete control occurs in fewer than 10% of patients (6,14). Surgical ablation of the epileptic brain tissue in patients with a localization-related epilepsy is the most effective way to significantly reduce seizure activity and improve quality of life (7–10,15–17). Epilepsy surgery may be appropriate for patients who have failed to respond to "two well-tolerated treatment regimens" (6). This chapter emphasizes the importance of preoperative electrophysiologic findings in the evaluation of potential surgical candidates.

SURGICAL TREATMENT OF EPILEPSY

Identification of Patients

Epilepsy surgery is a highly effective and safe alternative for selected patients with intractable partial epilepsy (7–10, 15–17) that aims to reduce seizure tendency and allow the individual to become a participating and productive member of society (3,7). Other goals include avoidance of neurologic morbidity and reduced exposure to toxic reactions of antiepileptic drugs. Potential candidates have physically and medically disabling seizures that significantly impair quality of life, and these patients should be identified early in medical treatment and selected for diagnostic evaluation (7–10). Focal corticectomy, the most common operative procedure in the adult patient, involves resection of the epileptic brain tissue in the anterior temporal lobe (17). In patients with intractable partial epilepsy, a focal cortical resection includes the site of seizure onset and initial seizure propagation, with excision of the pathologic lesion (15–17). Patients with medial temporal lobe epilepsy and substrate-directed or lesional epilepsy may achieve a significant reduction in seizures (10,17) but are less likely to respond to antiepileptic drugs and may have a pathologic substrate underlying the epileptogenic zone. Magnetic resonance imaging (MRI) may demonstrate structural abnormalities and plays a pivotal role in the selection and evaluation of patients for alternative forms of therapy (7,18–21). Its sensitivity and specificity in identifying posttraumatic alterations, vascular anomalies, tumors, malformation of cortical development (MCD), and mesial temporal sclerosis (MTS) have been confirmed (18–21). The preoperative evaluation is designed to identify the site of seizure onset and to localize functional cerebral cortex by means of scalp-recorded ictal EEG monitoring and neuropsychological studies; visual perimetry and cerebral arteriography (Wada test) are performed as needed.

Medial Temporal Lobe Epilepsy

Epilepsy surgery has been compared favorably to antiepileptic drug therapy as regards seizure outcome and quality of life in patients with intractable temporal lobe epilepsy (17). The most common localization of the epileptogenic zone in adults is the mesial temporal lobe.

Approximately 70% of patients who undergo a temporal lobe resection become seizure free during long-term follow-up (8,17). More than 90% of patients with concordant unilateral temporal lobe epileptiform discharges and a neuroimaging alteration experience an excellent outcome after anterior temporal lobectomy (8). Partial seizures involving the "detonator structures" of the temporal lobe, i.e., amygdalohippocampal formation, may be associated with a characteristic aura and ictal behavior (3,15–17) and involve neurocognitive impairment (3,8). The hallmark lesion of medial temporal lobe epilepsy is MTS (18–21), and the surgically excised hippocampus almost invariably shows focal cell loss and gliosis (7,8,18–21). Optimally, MRI in adults with partial epilepsy should include temporal lobe coronal or oblique coronal images using T1-weighted and T2-weighted sequences (18–21). MRI usually reveals atrophy of the hippocampal formation, reflecting neuronal loss, with a signal intensity change in patients with MTS. Fluid-attenuated inversion recovery sequences increase the sensitivity of MRI to detect a signal change (20).

Substrate-Directed or Lesional Epilepsy

Patients with lesional epilepsy may have a primary brain tumor, vascular anomaly, MCD, or a structural intra-axial abnormality, e.g., posttraumatic encephalomalacia, as the etiology of the seizure disorder (7,9,10,16). A low-grade glial neoplasm, cavernous hemangioma, and focal cortical dysplasia are commonly encountered (7,9,10,16). The MRI almost invariably shows an abnormal structure, and the seizure types are classified as substrate-directed partial epilepsy. The diagnostic yield of MRI in substrate-directed epilepsy depends on the underlying pathologic findings (7,9,10,16,18–21); however, the test's high sensitivity and specificity for identifying tumors and vascular malformations have been demonstrated (7,9,10,16). In patients with MCD, the MRI may detect an intra-axial structural abnormality suggesting the likely site of seizure onset and the pathologic lesion (7,9,10). In patients with an MRI-identified foreign-tissue lesion, the electroclinical correlation essentially confirms the epileptogenicity of the structural abnormality (9,10). Concordance between the pathologic substrate and the ictal-onset zone indicates a highly favorable operative outcome in selected individuals, with more than 80% of patients with a low-grade glial neoplasm or a cavernous hemangioma becoming seizure free after surgery (9,10). In contrast, fewer than 40% of patients with focal cortical dysplasia have an excellent operative outcome (22).

VIDEO-EEG EVALUATION

The gold standard for surgical localization in intractable epilepsy is the ictal electroencephalographic (EEG) pattern

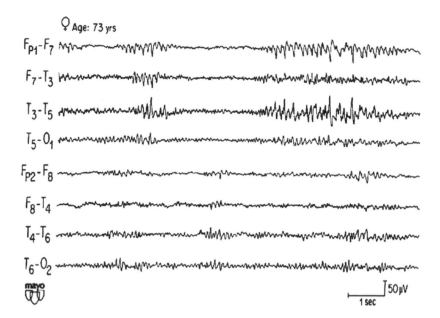

Figure 73.1   Left temporal wicket waves.

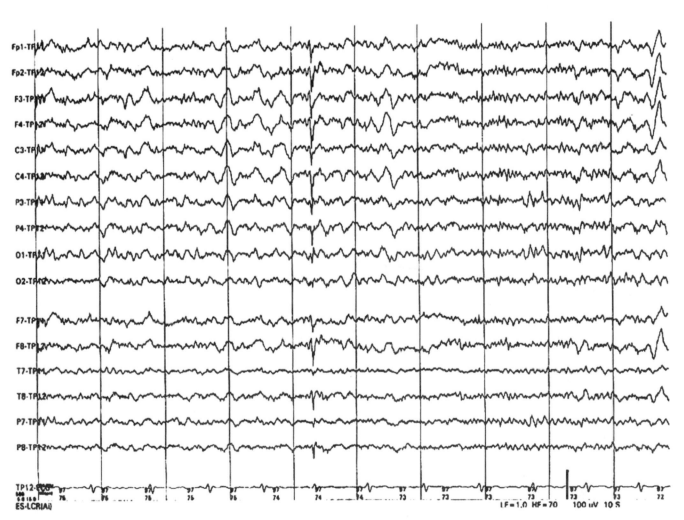

Figure 73.2   Benign sporadic sleep spike or small sharp spike.

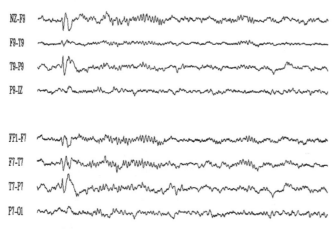

Figure 73.3   Interictal EEG shows left temporal spike discharges in a patient with left temporal lobe epilepsy.

identified on long-term scalp-recorded video-EEG monitoring (23–32). The electroclinical correlation during the typical ictal behavior is a critical part of the preoperative investigation (23–33). The presence of a peri-ictal neurologic deficit may also aid in localizing and/or lateralizing the site of seizure onset (33). With digital video-EEG, or computer-assisted EEG monitoring, less time is needed to review data (24,28,29), and paper storage is no longer a concern. The EEG is recorded on a disc and is available for immediate analysis (29). Montage reformatting is also possible (29). Seizures and epileptiform discharges are automatically detected by the on-line program or manual use of the event-recorder button. Off-line analysis may include the spatial and temporal extent of a seizure discharge, e.g., time delays between various regions (interhemispheric time difference), and use of a sharp digital filter to remove electromyographic artifacts (28,29). The EEG data are archived on a helical-scan magnetic tape. The high cost is a disadvantage.

Limitations of the Interictal EEG Recording

The outpatient awake and sleep EEG is the most common neurodiagnostic procedure for the patient with recurrent, unprovoked seizures or epilepsy and is usually sufficient for classifying seizure type and initiating medical therapy (27,30–33). A minority of patients with epilepsy will require video-EEG monitoring for diagnostic classification (27). The study usually lasts approximately 45 minutes to 1 hour, and requires minimal preparation (30). The patient may be sleep deprived to facilitate the recording of sleep activity, as epileptiform discharges may be present exclusively during non–rapid eye movement sleep (27,30). Provocative maneuvers like hyperventilation and photic stimulation during the EEG also may activate epileptiform activity. Use of supplementary scalp electrodes, sphenoidal, or zygomatic electrodes may increase the diagnostic yield (30–33). Interictal epilepti-

form discharges are used to localize the "irritative zone" in patients with partial seizure disorders. The routine EEG may not predict the response to medical therapy or indicate the likelihood of a seizure remission (30–33).

In patients with intractable seizures being considered for surgical treatment (33), the routine EEG may be repetitively "normal" and not identify epileptiform discharges owing to a sampling phenomenon or the presence of a partial seizure disorder not associated with interictal epileptiform discharges, as occurs in the "oligospikers" (30,33). The absence of epileptiform discharges may be more common in patients with extratemporal seizure disorders (30). The EEG may also be altered by antiepileptic drugs (27,30). Nonspecific findings, including benign variants, may incorrectly suggest a potential epileptiform pattern (30–33) (Figs. 73.1 and 73.2). The sensitivity and specificity of EEG recordings during clinical episodes, i.e., ictal EEG pattern, are superior to those of the routine EEG (30–33). The irritative zone may be remote or not contiguous with the epileptogenic zone (33).

In patients with a surgically remediable epileptic syndrome, interictal EEG findings may predict ictal origin and postoperative outcome (19,34–36) (Fig. 73.3). Strictly unilateral epileptiform discharges that are concordant with results of other noninvasive preoperative studies, such as neuroimaging or neuropsychological tests, may indicate a favorable long-term operative outcome (8,19,34,35). Bitemporal interictal epileptiform discharges may serve to indicate bitemporal *epileptogenicity* in selected patients who lack lateralizing predominance and to predict a less favorable seizure outcome postoperatively (36). Importantly, interictal EEG findings, both epileptiform discharges and focal slow-wave activity, that are concordant with structural lesions on MRI may help in selection of potential surgical candidates and design of an operative strategy, and preclude the need for long-term intracranial EEG monitoring (8–10,19,34,35).

Limitations of Video-EEG Monitoring

Scalp-recorded ictal EEG also has important diagnostic limitations. The absence of ictal EEG changes, i.e., no extracranial EEG correlate, may occur in patients with simple partial seizures and auras and, rarely, during complex partial seizures (23,26). Patients with partial seizures of extratemporal, mainly frontal lobe, origin may experience repetitive seizures without an associated scalp-recorded ictal EEG pattern (23–33). The diagnosis of epilepsy in these individuals is based on the ictal semiology and on results of interictal EEG recordings and neuroimaging studies (23,31–33). Myogenic and electrode artifacts during seizures may also obscure an ictal electrographic seizure pattern (23). Unfortunately, a potential hazard of video-EEG monitoring is the occurrence of a secondarily generalized tonic-clonic seizure following a reduction in antiepileptic drug on

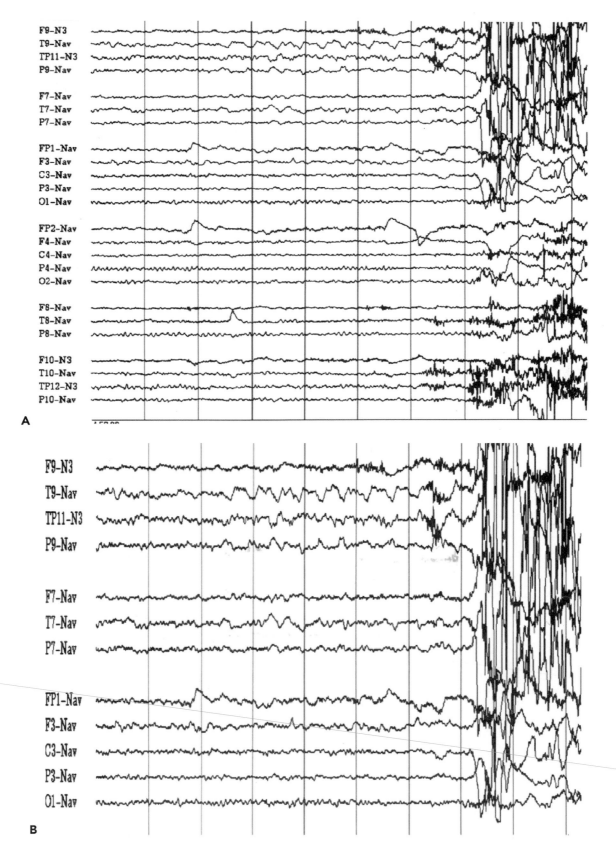

Figure 73.4   **A,B.** The EEG during a complex partial seizure reveals a rhythmic discharge over the left temporal head region most prominent at T9-Nav and T7-Nav. The ictal pattern is better identified in Figure B, which excludes the right central and temporal electrodes. Note the preservation of posterior alpha activity at seizure onset over the left posterior head region.

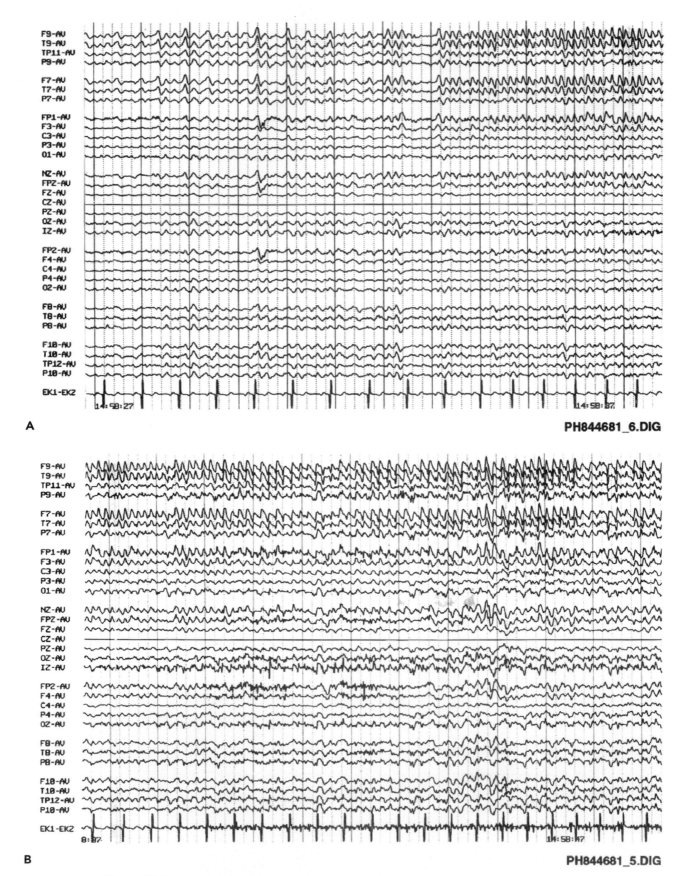

Figure 73.5   A,B. The EEG during a complex partial seizure reveals a rhythmic discharge over the left temporal head region most prominent at F7-AV, F9-AV, and T9-AV.

admission. Finally, patients may not have a typical, habitual seizure during prolonged EEG recordings despite the withdrawal of antiepileptic drugs.

Video-EEG Monitoring for Surgical Localization

The rationale for ictal EEG recordings includes confirmation of seizure type, evaluation of ictal semiology, and surgical localization (Figs. 73.4 and 73.5). The electroclinical correlation is used to lateralize or localize the epileptic brain tissue (23,31–33). Most patients are admitted to an epilepsy-monitoring unit, and their antiepileptic drug is tapered or withdrawn, as appropriate. Video-EEG monitoring follows a neurologic history and examination as well as an outpatient EEG. Obtaining the structural MRI monitoring may be helpful because identifying a neuroimaging abnormality is important in selecting patients for surgical treatment (8–10,18–21) (Figs. 73.3 and 73.5). Continuous computer-assisted, long-term video-EEG

monitoring is performed throughout the hospitalization. Trained personnel perform peri-ictal speech and memory testing and insure the patient's safety. Inability to localize the epileptogenic area with noninvasive monitoring is an indication for long-term intracranial EEG monitoring with a subdural grid or implanted depth electrodes (37) (Fig. 73.6). Ictal scalp recordings alone may suffice if results are concordant with other neurodiagnostic studies (7–10,18–21) (Fig. 73.5). The selection of surgical patients, however, must consider more than the preoperative electrophysiologic results and reveal a broad consensus on the localization of the epileptogenic zone and the underlying pathologic findings (Figs. 73.7 and 73.8). Patients with a concordant neurologic evaluation are more likely to achieve a significant reduction in seizure tendency (34–36). The EEG recordings must be interpreted in conjunction with the remainder of the presurgical evaluation (Fig. 73.9). Electrocorticography can also be performed at surgery to further define the irritative zone and amend the focal cortical resection (38).

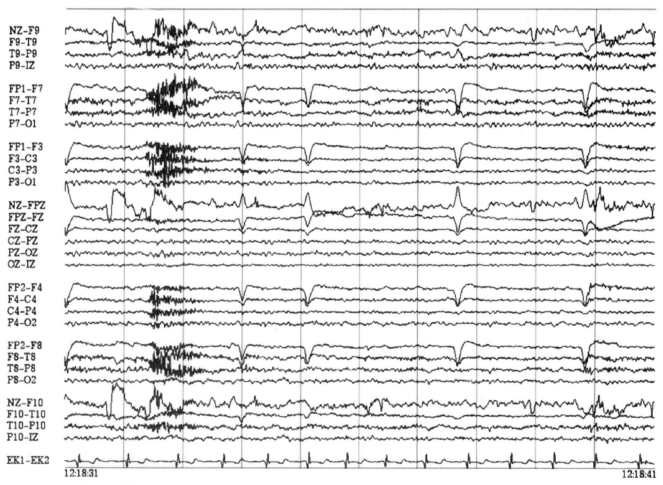

Figure 73.6 **A–E.** The ictal EEG pattern during a complex partial seizure of right temporal lobe origin. **A.** No obvious alteration is noted during the aura. **B–E.** A progressive seizure discharge is present over the right temporal lobe head region during the complex partial seizure (F10, T10). **C–E.** Involvement of the left temporal region during the electrographic seizure is also seen.

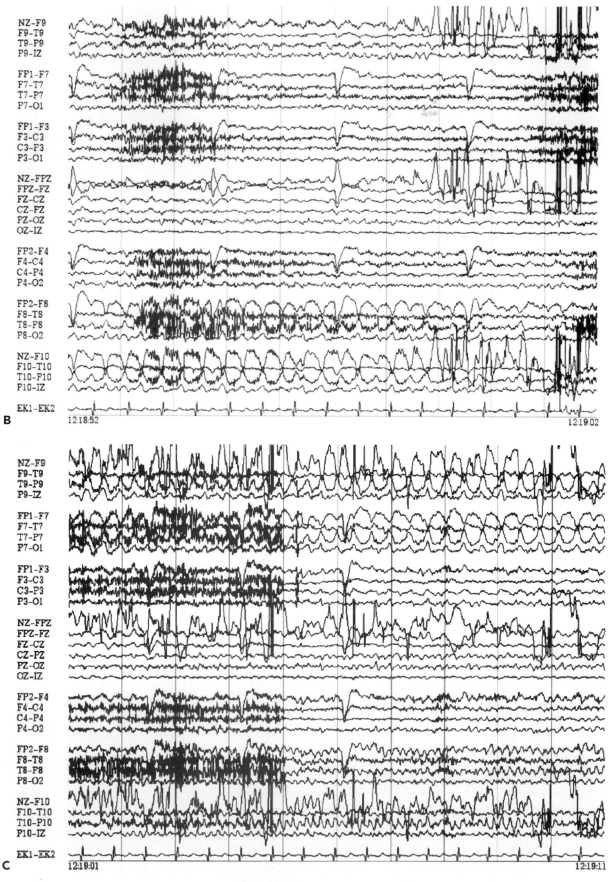

Figure 73.6   *(continued)*

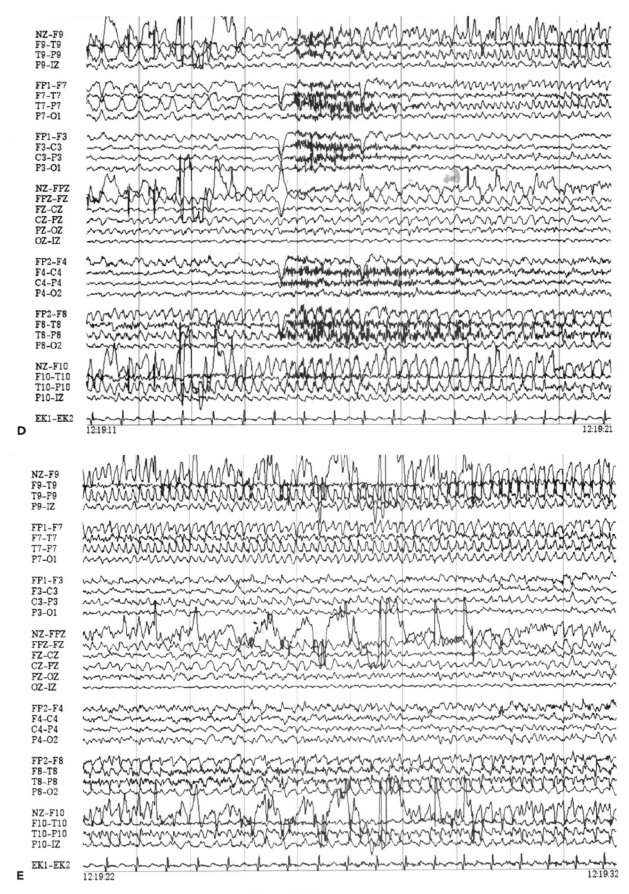

Figure 73.6 (continued)

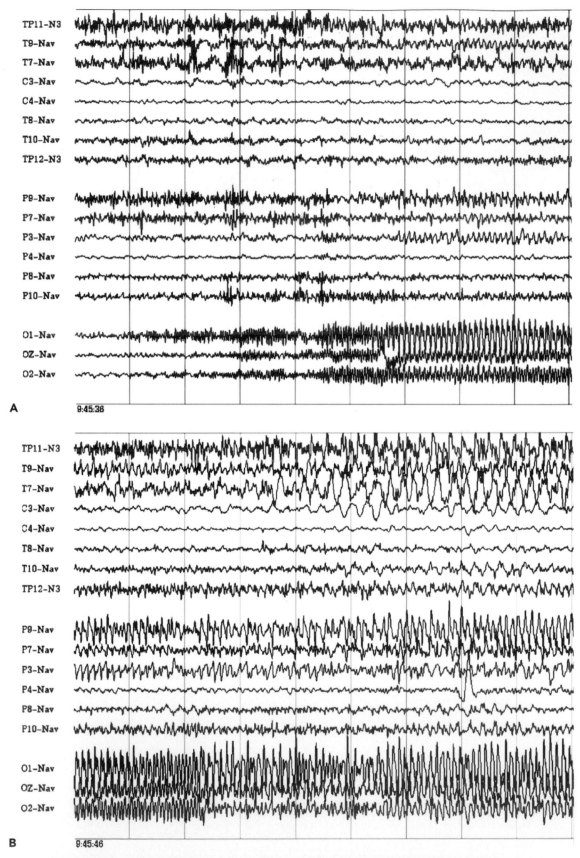

Figure 73.7 **A.** EEG pattern during a partial seizure of left occipital origin shows a high-frequency discharge most prominent at O1-Nav. **B.** The progressive seizure pattern involves both occipital regions and propagates into the left temporal and left parietal regions.

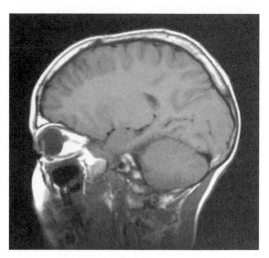

Figure 73.8 MRI of the head shows a malformation of cortical development over the left occipital region. There was pathologic evidence for focal cortical dysplasia.

SISCOM

Peri-ictal functional imaging with the use of computer-aided subtraction ictal single-photon emission tomography (SPECT) coregistered to MRI (SISCOM) may help in localizing the epileptogenic zone in patients with intractable partial epilepsy (39–41). At the Mayo Clinic, the interictal study is coregistered to the ictal SPECT study by matching the surface points on the cerebral binary images of the two procedures. The normalized interictal image is subtracted from the normalized ictal image to derive the difference (subtraction) in cerebral blood flow related to the partial seizure. Thresholding of the subtraction image displays only the pixels with intensities greater than two standard deviations above zero (39), and these images are coregistered onto the structural MRI. After subdural electrodes have been implanted for long-term intracranial EEG monitoring, their positions can be segmented from a spiral computed tomography

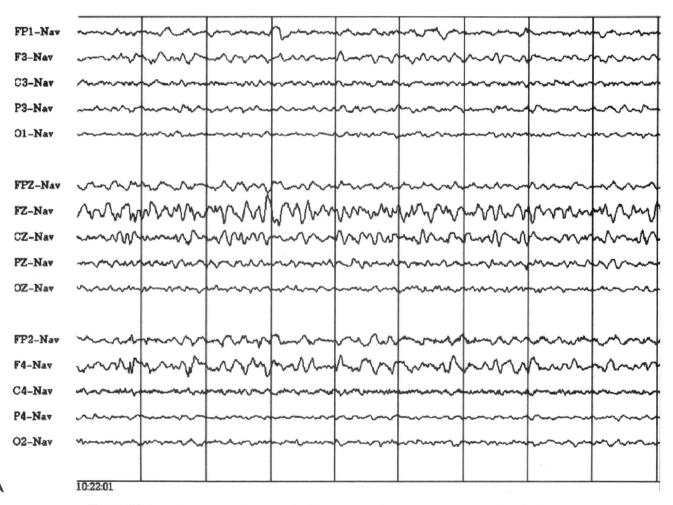

A   10:22:01

Figure 73.9 **A.** Subtle right frontal and midline seizure discharge in a patient with right frontal lobe seizures; muscle artifact has been filtered out. **B.** A midline spike discharge is prominent at FZ-Nav. **C.** Despite the movement artifact, a high-frequency midline and bilateral frontocentral seizure discharge can be identified. Long-term intracranial EEG monitoring confirmed the right mesial frontal lobe onset of seizure activity.

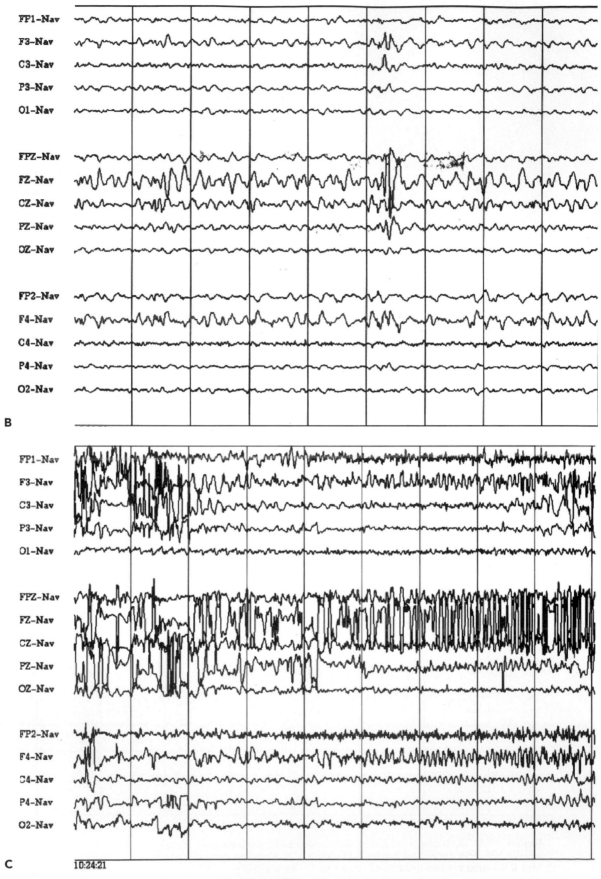

Figure 73.9 (continued)

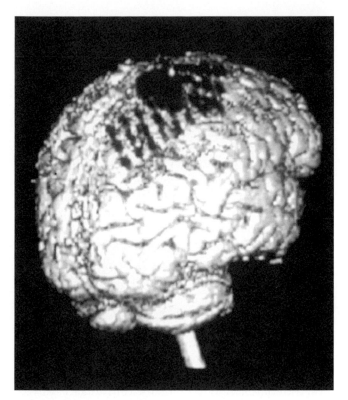

Figure 73.10 A SISCOM study in a patient with right mesial frontal lobe seizures. The region of SISCOM-identified hyperperfusion is depicted in red. The subdural grid of electrodes (blue) was placed for surgical localization. Please see the color insert.

scan and coregistered with the SISCOM image to determine the relationship between the localized alteration in peri-ictal blood flow and the ictal-onset zone (Fig. 73.10). SISCOM may be useful in the evaluation of patients with non–substrate-directed partial epilepsy (39). The localized blood flow alteration usually is intimately associated with the epileptogenic zone (39–41). SISCOM is indicated primarily when there is difficulty in localizing the epileptogenic zone. Such clinical situations include a normal structural MRI, conflicting preoperative evaluation, or a unilateral, widespread intra-axial lesion (39–41).

In a study (40) in 36 patients with extratemporal epilepsy who underwent SISCOM preoperatively, a localizing SISCOM alteration concordant with the epileptogenic zone predicted an excellent surgical outcome ($p < 0.05$). Eleven of 19 patients (57.9%) with a concordant SISCOM *focus*, and 3 of 17 patients (17.6%) with a nonlocalizing or discordant SISCOM, became seizure free or experienced only nondisabling seizures. Approximately three fourths of the patients with a localized SISCOM abnormality had a normal structural MRI. In addition, the extent of resection of the SISCOM *focus* had prognostic importance ($p < 0.05$). Failure to resect the neocortical region intimately associated with the localized blood flow change concordant with the ictal-onset zone predicted an unfavorable outcome (40).

ILLUSTRATED CASE REPORTS

Case 1

A 33-year-old patient was admitted to the epilepsy-monitoring unit for surgical localization. The patient had a prolonged febrile seizure during childhood. Unprovoked partial seizures were associated with an abdominal aura that consisted of a "rising sensation." Behavioral arrest, lip smacking, and right-hand dystonic posturing occurred during ictus; peri-ictal dysphasia was prominent. The neurologic history and examination were otherwise unremarkable. The seizures had been refractory to many trials of antiepileptic drugs. Prominent left temporal spike discharges were noted during sleep (Fig. 73.3). During video-EEG monitoring, the patient had several observed seizures. The ictal pattern indicated a progressive seizure of left temporal lobe origin (Fig. 73.5). MRI of the head showed atrophy of the left hippocampal formation (Fig. 73.11). The patient ultimately underwent a successful left anterior temporal lobectomy. Severe focal hippocampal neuronal loss with mesial temporal lobe gliosis was present.

Comment

In this patient with left medial temporal lobe epilepsy, unilateral temporal lobe epileptiform discharges, a unilateral hippocampal lesion on MRI, and MTS predicted an excellent operative outcome.

Case 2

A 23-year-old patient was admitted for video-EEG monitoring to evaluate surgical candidacy after 10 years of medically refractory partial seizures. There was no history of a remote symptomatic neurologic disorder. An aura associated with a

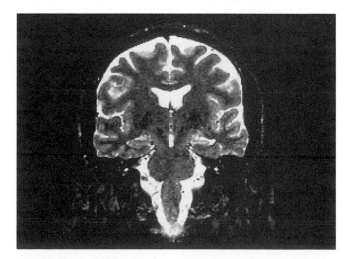

Figure 73.11 MRI of the head (oblique-coronal, T2-weighted) shows left hippocampal atrophy and a prominent, increased hippocampal signal change. There was pathologic evidence for mesial temporal sclerosis.

"panic sensation" occurred at seizure onset. Routine EEG revealed bilateral, independent, temporal lobe spike discharges, maximal on the right. MRI of the head was normal. Ictal semiology included posturing of the left upper extremity. The scalp-recorded ictal EEG revealed a rhythmic right temporal lobe seizure discharge during onset of the complex partial seizure and a subsequent prolonged and sustained left temporal lobe seizure (Fig. 73.6) with prominent postictal aphasia. Chronic intracranial EEG monitoring confirmed the right medial temporal lobe onset of the habitual seizures with rapid propagation to the left temporal lobe. There were frequent bitemporal, independent spike discharges without lateralized predominance. The patient is considering a right anterior temporal lobectomy if subsequent antiepileptic drug trials are ineffective.

Comment

This patient with partial epilepsy of temporal lobe origin may not be a highly favorable surgical candidate because of the normal MRI results and prominent bitemporal epileptogenicity (34–36).

Case 3

A 7-year-old child was admitted for video-EEG monitoring to evaluate surgical localization. Beginning at 1 year of age, recurrent seizures consisted of elevation of the right upper extremity, turning of the head and eyes to the right, and loss of consciousness. The patient often fell during a seizure. Evidence supported pervasive developmental delay and an intractable seizure disorder. Bioccipital, independent spike discharges, maximal on the left, were seen on routine EEG. The scalp-recorded ictal EEG revealed a rhythmic discharge over the left occipital region at seizure onset, with spread predominantly to the left temporal and left parietal regions and contralateral posterior head region (Fig. 73.7). MRI of the head showed a lesion in the left occipital lobe consistent with an MCD (Fig. 73.8). After long-term intracranial EEG monitoring with a subdural electrode grid to locate the ictal-onset zone, resection included the focal cortical dysplasia. After a few acute postoperative seizures, the patient has remained under control.

Comment

This patient's substrate-directed partial seizure disorder was related to an MCD. Seizure tendency decreased significantly after resection of the lesion and epileptic brain tissue. Proceeding with surgery without intracranial EEG monitoring was an alternative in this patient.

Case 4

A 22-year-old patient underwent long-term video-EEG monitoring to assess surgical candidacy. Stereotypical clinical events were associated with behavioral arrest and staring, and a vague, ill-defined aura consisted of a cephalic sensation. The seizures began after an episode of presumed malaria in childhood and were refractory to antiepileptic drugs. The routine EEG revealed mild diffuse slowing and no interictal epileptiform discharges. MRI of the head was normal. On scalp-recorded ictal EEG, a midline and right frontal rhythmic discharge was variably present (Fig. 73.9). Considerable muscle and movement artifact was noted during the seizures. There was no EEG correlate during the aura. A SISCOM study showed a right mesial frontal lobe region of hyperperfusion (Fig. 73.10). Intracranial EEG monitoring with a subdural grid of electrodes showed the ictal-onset zone to be intimately related to the SISCOM region of hyperperfusion. A focal cortical resection revealed only gliosis. The patient has remained seizure free after surgery.

Comment

This patient had nonlesional extratemporal seizures. Peri-ictal functional imaging demonstrated a focal abnormality that altered the preoperative strategy. The patient was subsequently shown to be a favorable candidate for a focal cortical resection based on the concordance between the SISCOM-identified abnormality and the ictal onset zone (40).

CONCLUSIONS

Video-EEG monitoring is an essential preoperative investigation in patients with intractable epilepsy being considered for surgical treatment. In addition to classifying seizure type(s) and localizing the epileptogenic zone, the results of interictal and ictal EEG recordings have prognostic importance. Scalp-recorded ictal EEG may be sufficient to localize the site of seizure onset in selected patients with surgically remediable epileptic syndromes. The results of video-EEG monitoring need to be correlated with other components of a comprehensive neurologic evaluation before an operative strategy is determined. Ultimately, the selection of candidates for epilepsy surgery depends on the disabling effect of the seizure disorder, the localization of the epileptic brain tissue, results of the preoperative evaluation, the "suspected" underlying lesion, and the putative benefits of a reduction in seizure tendency.

REFERENCES

1. Hauser W. The natural history of drug resistant epilepsy: epidemiologic considerations. *Epilepsy Res Suppl* 1992;5:25–28.
2. Hauser A, Hesdorffer D. Prognosis. In: Hauser WA, Hesdorffer DC, eds. *Epilepsy: frequency, causes and consequences.* New York: Demos. 1990:197–243.
3. Dreifuss FE. Goals of surgery for epilepsy. In: Engel J Jr, ed. *Surgical treatment of the epilepsies,* 1st ed. New York: Raven Press. 1987:31–49.
4. Mattson RH. Drug treatment of uncontrolled seizures. *Epilepsy Res Suppl* 1992;5:29–35.

5. Camfield P, Camfield C. Antiepileptic drug therapy: when is epilepsy truly intractable? *Epilepsia* 1996;37(Suppl 1):S60–S65.

6. Brodie MJ, Kwan P. Staged approach to epilepsy management. *Neurology* 2002;58:S2–S8.

7. Cascino GD. Selection of candidates for surgical treatment of epilepsy. In: Cascino GD, Jack CR Jr, eds. *Neuroimaging in epilepsy: principles and practice.* Boston: Butterworth-Heinemann. 1996: 209–218.

8. Radhakrishnan K, So EL, Silbert PL, et al. Predictors of outcome of anterior temporal lobectomy for intractable epilepsy: a multivariate study. *Neurology* 1998;51:465–471.

9. Cascino GD, Boon PAJM, Fish DR. Surgically remediable lesional syndromes. In: Engel J Jr, ed. *Surgical treatment of the epilepsies,* 2nd ed. New York: Raven Press. 1993:77–86.

10. Awad IA, Rosenfeld J, Ahl H, et al. Intractable epilepsy and structural lesions of the brain: mapping, resection strategies, and seizure outcome. *Epilepsia* 1991;32:179–186.

11. Lhatoo SD, Johnson AL, Goodridge DM, et al. Mortality in epilepsy in the first 11 to 14 years after diagnosis: multivariate analysis of a long-term, prospective, population-based cohort. *Ann Neurol* 2001;49:336–344.

12. Begley CE, Lairson DR, Reynolds TF, et al. Early treatment cost in epilepsy and how it varies with seizure type and frequency. *Epilepsy Res* 2001;47:205–215.

13. Begley CE, Famulari M, Annegers JF, et al. The cost of epilepsy in the United States: an estimate from population-based clinical and survey data. *Epilepsia* 2000;41:342–351.

14. The Vagus Nerve Stimulation Study Group. A randomized trial of chronic vagus nerve stimulation for treatment of medically intractable seizures. *Neurology* 1995;45:224–230.

15. Engel J, Wiebe S, French J, et al. Practice parameter: temporal lobe and localized neocortical resections for epilepsy (an evidence-based review). *Neurology* 2003;60:538–547.

16. Mosewich RK, So EL, O'Brien TJ, et al. Factors predictive of the outcome of frontal lobe epilepsy surgery. *Epilepsia* 2000;41: 843–849.

17. Wiebe S, Blume WT, Girvin JP, et al, and the Effectiveness and Efficiency of Surgery for Temporal Lobe Epilepsy Study Group. A randomized, controlled trial of surgery for temporal-lobe epilepsy. *N Engl J Med* 2001;345:311–318.

18. Cascino GD, Trenerry MR, So E, et al. Routine EEG and temporal lobe epilepsy: relation to long-term EEG monitoring, quantitative MRI, and operative outcome. *Epilepsia* 1996;37: 651–656.

19. Cambier DM, Cascino GD, So EL, et al. Video-EEG monitoring in patients with hippocampal atrophy. *Acta Neurol Scand* 2001; 103:1–7.

20. Jackson GD. Visual analysis in mesial temporal sclerosis. In: Cascino GD, Jack CR, eds. *Neuroimaging in epilepsy: principles and practice.* Boston: Butterworth-Heinemann. 1996:73–110.

21. Cascino GD, Jack CR Jr, Parisi JE, et al. MRI in the presurgical evaluation of patients with frontal lobe epilepsy and children with temporal lobe epilepsy: pathological correlation and prognostic importance. *Epilepsy Res* 1992;11:51–59.

22. Palmini A, Andermann F, Olivier A, et al. Focal neuronal migrational disorders and intractable partial epilepsy: results of surgical treatment. *Ann Neurol* 1991;30:750–757.

23. Quesney LF, Gloor P. Localization of epileptogenic foci. In: Gotman J, Ives JR, Gloor P, eds. *Long-term monitoring in epilepsy.* Amsterdam: Elsevier. 1985:165–200.

24. Gotman J. Seizure recognition and analysis. In: Gotman J, Ives JR, Gloor P, eds. *Long-term monitoring in epilepsy.* Amsterdam: Elsevier. 1985:133–145.

25. Ives JR. Video recording during long-term EEG monitoring of epileptic patients. In: Gumnit R, ed. *Intensive neurodiagnostic monitoring.* New York: Raven Press. 1987:1–11.

26. Devinsky O, Sato S, Kufta CV, et al. Electroencephalographic studies of simple partial seizures with subdural electrode recordings. *Neurology* 1989;39:527–533.

27. Daly DD. Epilepsy and syncope. In: Daly DD, Pedley TA, eds. *Current practice of clinical electroencephalography.* New York: Raven Press. 1990:269–334.

28. Gotman J, Levtova V, Farine B. Graphic representation of the EEG during epileptic seizures. *Electroencephalogr Clin Neurophysiol* 1993;87:206–214.

29. Gotman J, Ives JR. Computer-assisted data collection and analysis. In: Wyllie E, ed. *The treatment of epilepsy: principles and practice.* Baltimore: Williams and Wilkins. 1996:280–291.

30. Chabolla DR, Cascino GD. Interpretation of extracranial EEG. In: Wyllie E, ed. *The treatment of epilepsy: principles and practice.* Baltimore: Williams and Wilkins. 1996:264–279.

31. Fish DR. The role of scalp electroencephalography in presurgical evaluation. In: Shorvon S, Dreifuss F, Fish D, et al, eds. *The treatment of epilepsy.* London: Blackwell. 1996:542–561.

32. Cascino GD. Use of routine and video electroencephalography. In: Wyllie E, ed. *Neurologic clinics: epilepsy.* Philadelphia: WB Saunders. 2001:271–287.

33. Cascino GD. Clinical indications and diagnostic yield of video-electroencephalographic monitoring in patients with seizures and spells. *Mayo Clin Proc* 2002;77:1111–1120.

34. Holmes MD, Kutsy RL, Ojemann GA, et al. Interictal, unifocal spikes in refractory extratemporal epilepsy predict ictal origin and postsurgical outcome. *Clin Neurophysiol* 2000;111: 1802–1808.

35. Schulz R, Luders HO, Hoppe M, et al. Interictal EEG and ictal scalp EEG propagation are highly predictive of surgical outcome in mesial temporal lobe epilepsy. *Epilepsia* 2000;41: 564–570.

36. Holmes MD, Miles AN, Dodrill CB, et al. Identifying potential surgical candidates in patients with evidence of bitemporal epilepsy. *Epilepsia* 2003;44:1075–1079.

37. Schiller Y, Cascino GD, Sharbrough FW. Chronic intracranial EEG monitoring for localizing the epileptogenic zone: an electroclinical correlation. *Epilepsia* 1998;39:1302–1308.

38. Cascino GD, Trenerry MR, Jack CR, et al. Electrocorticography and temporal lobe epilepsy: relationship to quantitative MRI and operative outcome. *Epilepsia* 1995;36:692–696.

39. O'Brien TJ, O'Connor MK, Mullan BP, et al. Subtraction ictal SPECT co-registered to MRI in partial epilepsy: description and technical validation of the method with phantom and patients studies. *Nucl Med Commun* 1998;19:31–45.

40. O'Brien TJ, So EL, Mullan BP, et al. Subtraction peri-ictal SPECT is predictive of extratemporal epilepsy surgery outcome. *Neurology* 2000;55:1668–1677.

41. So EL. Integration of EEG, MRI and SPECT in localizing the seizure focus for epilepsy surgery. *Epilepsia* 2000;41(Suppl 3): S48–S54.

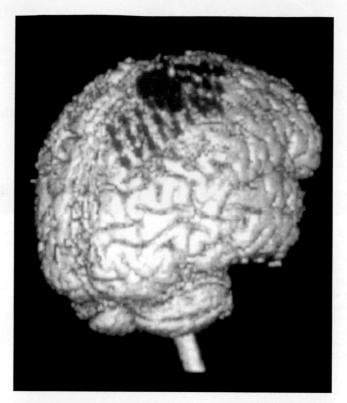

Figure 73.10 A SISCOM study in a patient with right mesial frontal lobe seizures. The region of SISCOM-identified hyperperfusion is depicted in red. The subdural grid of electrodes (blue) was placed for surgical localization.

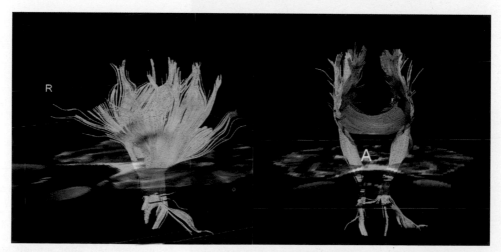

Figure 74.15 Diffusion tractology image. Bilateral corticospinal tracts (left and right, yellow) and interhemispheric connections (right, orange) calculated from high-resolution diffusion tensor sequence at 3T that used custom-built software by Drs. Ruopeng Wang and Greg Sorensen and colleagues at the Division of Health Sciences & Technology, Athinoula A. Martinos Center for Biomedical Imaging. The directional bias of the diffusion can inform about the structure of underlying white-matter tracts. Analysis techniques in development may enable statistical measures of connectivity and enhance understanding of cerebral malformations and seizure propagation.

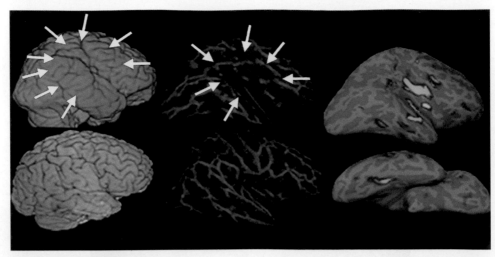

Figure 74.16 T-test comparison of abnormal and normal hemispheric structure. The top row shows a surface rendering of the abnormal left hemisphere (left, top image) with an area of abnormal gyral folding (*arrows*). Inflated surface representation with color coding of sulcal depth: red represents sulcal depth; green, gyral height in the abnormal hemisphere (middle, top). T-test statistics detected significant differences in sulcal depth and gyral height compared with the normal representation (not shown) in the colored areas on the right images (top and bottom). The bottom left and middle images are the surface and inflated representations of the normal right hemisphere in the same individual. Although the statistical map underrepresents the region involved, it shows the potential of quantitative techniques in phenotyping cerebral malformations. Images were created from a 3D SPGR sequence (a thin-section volumetric T1-weighted sequence) obtained with a standard head coil at 1.5T.

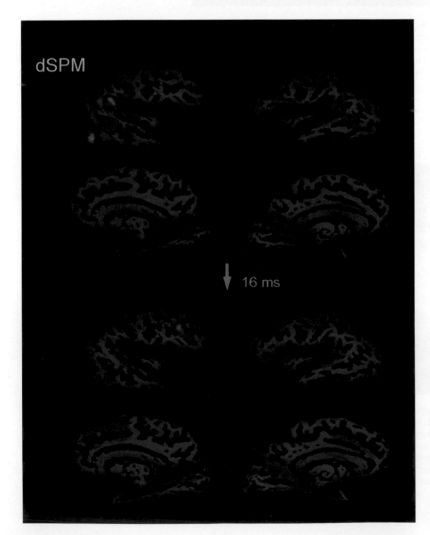

Figure 74.17 MEG activity of a spike constrained by anatomic MRI represented on the inflated brain in a 16-year-old right-handed patient with right temporal lobe epilepsy. The top four images show lateral (top row) and medial views (second row) of the right hemisphere (left side) and left hemisphere (right side). Areas in red represent increased neuronal MEG activity at the beginning of the spike, which is more marked in the right temporal lobe. The spike propagated from the right temporal to the right frontal area (bottom four images) within 16 msec. This image shows snapshots of a movie calculated for MEG activity by means of dynamic statistic parametric mapping (196). Courtesy of Dr. Hideaki Shiraishi, Division of Health Sciences & Technology, Athinoula A. Martinos Center for Biomedical Imaging.

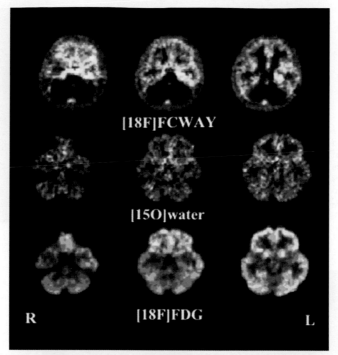

Figure 76.1 [¹⁸F]FDG-PET (*bottom row*) in a 43-year-old patient with right temporal lobe epilepsy and right mesial temporal sclerosis. Glucose uptake is decreased in right mesial and lateral temporal regions. [¹⁵O]Water PET (*middle row*) shows nearly normal perfusion; only 30% to 40% of patients with temporal hypometabolism also demonstrate decreased perfusion in the epileptogenic zone. [¹⁸F]trans-4-fluoro-N-2-[4-(2-methoxyphenyl)piperazin-1-yl]ethyl]-N-(2-pyridyl)cyclohexane carboxamide [¹⁸F](FCWAY)-PET (*top row*) shows decreased binding in right temporal lobe, most pronounced in the amygdala and hippocampus. Absent ligand binding in the cerebellum reflects absence of serotonin 5HT 1A receptors in cerebellar tissue. Raphe nucleus ligand binding is seen. Left image is right brain. (From Toczek MT, Carson RE, Lang L, et al. PET imaging of 5-HT1A receptor binding in patients with temporal lobe epilepsy. *Neurology* 2003;60:749–756. Courtesy of William H. Theodore, National Institutes of Health, Bethesda, Maryland.)

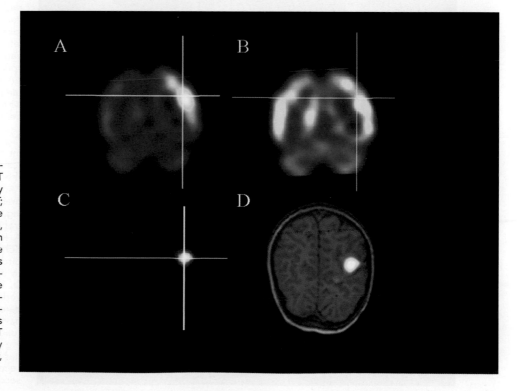

Figure 76.4 Ictal ⁹⁹ᵐTc-hexam-ethyl-propyleneamine oxime SPECT in a young adult with refractory partial seizures. **A**, interictal SPECT; **B**, ictal SPECT; **C**, subtraction image of interictal from ictal SPECT; **D**, subtraction SPECT coregistration with magnetic resonance image (SISCOM). Study demonstrates increased ictal perfusion in the parietal lobe. Here, the right side of the image is the left brain. Chronic invasive recording and surgery subsequently confirmed the ictal focus identified by subtraction SPECT techniques. (Courtesy of Gregory Cascino, Mayo Clinic, Rochester, Minnesota.)

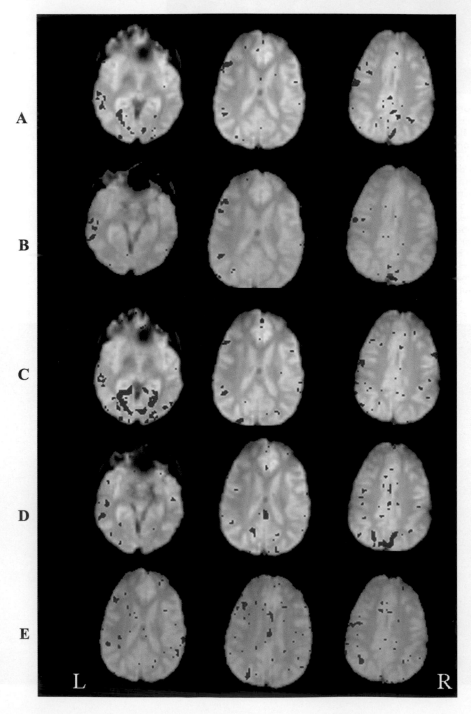

Figure 76.5 10-year-old with a right mesial mass seen as increased signal. fMRI of motor tapping of left hand, compared to rest, yields activation (red), which identifies primary motor cortex posterior to the lesion. Mirror activation ipsilateral to tapping hand is also seen. Supplementary motor cortex activation is adjacent to the lesion.

L   R

Figure 76.6 MRI (echo planar imaging, blood oxygenation level–dependent) panel of tasks. **I.** A 14-year-old girl with left temporal lobe focus; panel of tasks shows left frontal and left temporal activation demonstrating left hemisphere dominance for language. **II.** An 11-year-old with left superior temporal glioma resected at 2 years with recurrent seizures; all tasks demonstrate right-hemisphere activation in temporal and frontal regions. Microscopic metal fragments from burr hole placement results in artifact. The left side of the image is the left brain. "Activated" voxels representing brain regions involved in performing the task compared with a control condition (rest) appear in red. **A.** Reading task, naming to description. (e.g., "What is a large pink bird?"); **B.** auditory task, naming to description; **C.** reading stories; **D.** listening to stories; **E.** covert verbal fluency to categories compared to silent rest. Auditory tasks have a reverse speech control; reading paradigm control is viewing dot patterns. Each paradigm has six cycles, consisting of a 32-second control condition and a 32-second task condition.

A

B

C

D

E

L   R

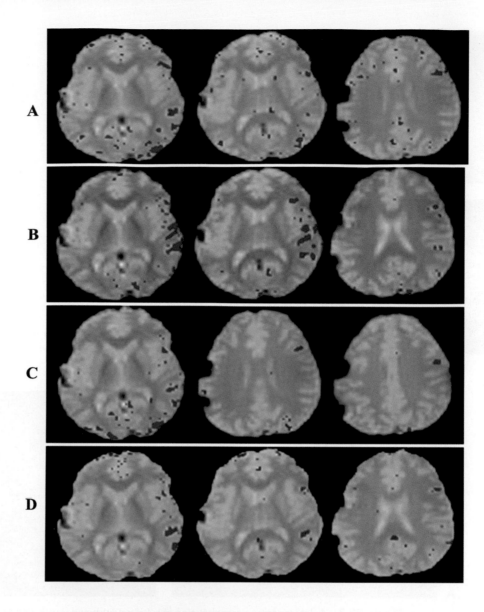

Figure 76.6 (continued)

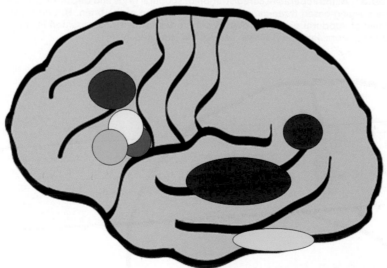

Figure 76.7 Schema showing areas activated with different paradigms advocated in individual studies. Areas adjacent to and along the superior temporal sulcus (blue) are activated by tasks that stress phrase or sentence comprehension such as listening to stories, or reading stories or sentences. Supramarginal gyrus (and sometimes angular gyrus) (purple) may also be activated in auditory sentence-processing tasks. Fusiform gyrus (light blue), is activated by tasks that require feature search or identification, such as identifying written characters or naming objects. Middle frontal gyrus (red) is implicated in verbal working memory for reading, grammatical decipherment, or verbal recall. Inferior frontal gyrus subregions are activated by a variety of tasks: phonologic fluency (orange), syntactic/semantic decision (green), semantic fluency, or recall (yellow).

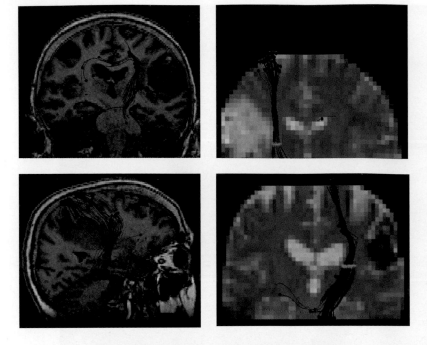

Figure 79.2 Fiber tracking with diffusion tensor MRI acquisition.

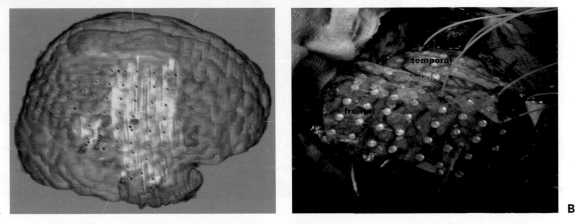

A
B

Figure 80.3 **A:** Intraoperative coregistration of subdural grids and depth electrodes on magnetic resonance imaging-based three-dimensional reconstruction of the brain. **B:** Corresponding intraoperative view of subdural grids and depths electrodes in their final position in the same patient. Frontal and temporal lobes and sylvian fissures are indicated.

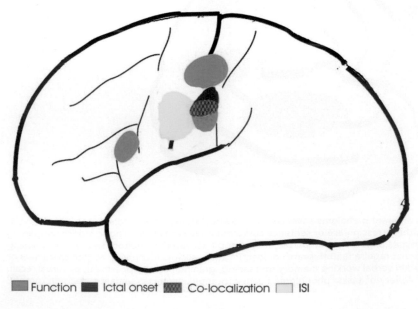

■ Function ■ Ictal onset ▨ Co-localization ▢ ISI

Figure 80.4 Illustration showing a case of malformations caused by abnormal cortical development with significant signal fluid attenuated inversion recovery increase (*yellow*). Note the lack of overlap of the epileptic area (*red*) and the lesion (*yellow*).

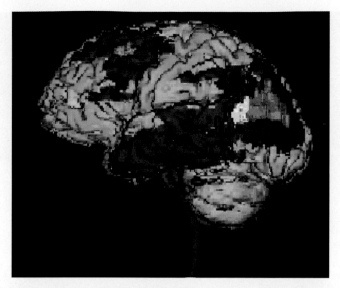

Figure 82.3 Surface distribution of marked 2-deoxy-2-[¹⁸F] fluoro-2-deoxy-D-glucose (FDG)-positron emission tomography (PET) (red) and [¹¹C]flumazenil (FMZ)-PET (white) abnormalities, as well as the region of cortical resection (black), in a patient with left posterior parietal seizure focus. The bulk of the cortex with decreased FMZ binding was removed, whereas the majority of the hypometabolic cortex was not resected. The patient has been seizure free for 40 months. (From Juhasz C, Chugani D, Muzik O, et al. Relationship of flumazenil and glucose PET abnormalities to neocortical epilepsy surgery outcome. *Neurology* 2001;56:1650–1658, with permission.)

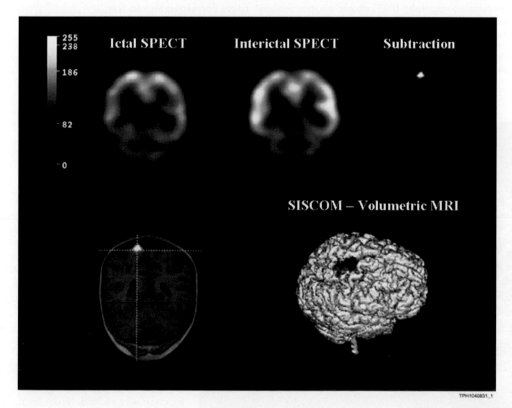

Figure 82.4 Steps to obtaining subtraction ictal SPECT (single-photon emission computed tomography) coregistered to MRI (magnetic resonance imaging) (SISCOM) image. Ictal (*upper left*) and interictal (*upper middle*) SPECT images are obtained. After normalization of their mean intensities and coregistration with each other, subtraction is performed to obtain a "difference" image (*upper right*). The difference image is then coregistered with MRI images at specific planes (*lower left*) or on the surface of a three-dimensional MRI image (*lower right*). (From So E. Role of neuroimaging in the management of seizure disorders. *Mayo Clin Proc* 2002;77:1251–1264, with permission.)

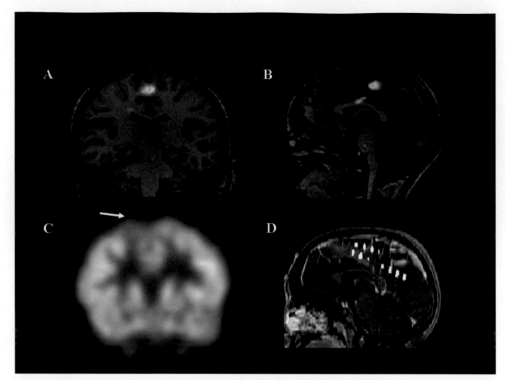

Figure 82.6 **A:** Coronal view of subtraction ictal SPECT (single-photon emission computed tomography) coregistered to magnetic resonance imaging (MRI) (SISCOM) showing an apparently midline hyperperfusion focus in a 13-year-old male who had between 1 and 10 attacks per night of bilateral extremity movements and facial grimacing. Epilepsy-protocol MRI was normal and scalp ictal electroencephalogram was nonlocalizing. **B:** Sagittal view of SISCOM shows that the hyperperfusion focus was at the right posterior mesial frontal region. **C:** 2-[18F]fluoro-2-deoxy-D-glucose (FDG)-positron emission tomography (PET) shows a hypometabolic focus corresponding to the SISCOM hyperperfusion focus. **D:** MRI with coregistered CT (computed tomography)-derived images of subdural electrode contacts (white marks) on the SISCOM and PET abnormalities. The intracranial EEG recording confirmed ictal onset at the SISCOM and PET abnormalities. Surgical resection of the region rendered the patient free of seizures, with minimal weakness in the left toes. Pathologic examination of the specimen revealed cortical dysplasia.

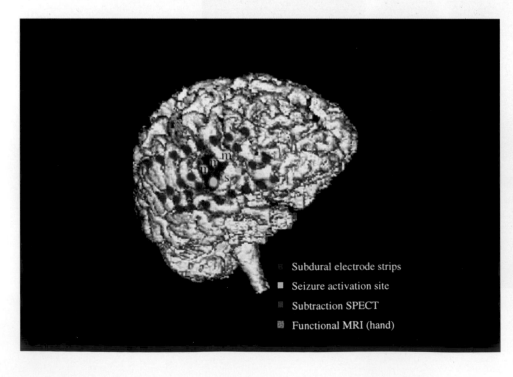

Subdural electrode strips

Seizure activation site

Subtraction SPECT

Functional MRI (hand)

Figure 82.7 Three-dimensional rendition of MRI (magnetic resonance imaging) of brain with coregistration of sensory area of the hand identified with functional MRI (green), subtraction ictal SPECT (single-photon emission computed tomography) coregistered to MRI (SISCOM) hyperperfusion focus (red), subdural electrodes (blue), and electrodes where electroencephalograph-detected seizures commenced (yellow). m = electrode sites where facial motor activity was elicited with electrocortical stimulation; s = electrode site where sensory function was elicited. (From So E. Role of neuroimaging in the management of seizure disorders. *Mayo Clin Proc* 2002;77: 1251–1264, with permission.)

Magnetic Resonance Imaging Techniques in the Evaluation for Epilepsy Surgery

74

Susanne Knake   *P. Ellen Grant*

Approximately 60% of all patients with epilepsy (0.4% of the population in industrialized countries) suffer from focal epilepsy syndromes. About 15% of these patients have medically intractable seizures and might be candidates for surgical epilepsy treatment (1,2). The goal of surgical treatment is seizure control by complete disconnection of the epileptogenic zone, which is defined as the area of tissue indispensable for the generation of clinical seizures under preservation of the eloquent cortex (2). Magnetic resonance imaging (MRI) enables the detection of anatomic lesions that are candidates for the epileptogenic zone (3). A focal anatomic abnormality involving cortex (either neocortex or hippocampus) that is identified in a region consistent with clinical semiology or electroencephalographic (EEG) findings is the probable cause of the epileptic seizures (4). In temporal lobe epilepsy, the probability of a seizure-free outcome is 82% with concordant lesions and 56% with an unremarkable MRI (5). Respective figures in frontal lobe epilepsy are 72% and 41% (6). MRI detects surgically relevant lesions in up to 80% of patients who undergo temporal lobectomy (6–9) and in about 60% of those undergoing frontal lobe surgeries (6). MRI also detects cerebral malformations associated with epilepsy syndromes, thereby helping to guide medical therapy. When coregistered, MRI can illustrate the topographic relationship between lesions and eloquent cortex defined by functional MRI, EEG, single-photon-emission computed tomography (SPECT), positron emission tomography (PET), or magnetoencephalography (MEG).

This chapter reviews the criteria for use of an MRI and the type of MRI that should be used, outlines the imaging sequences to evaluate mesial temporal and neocortical epilepsies, and describes the imaging findings in associated conditions.

WHO SHOULD HAVE AN MRI?

The International League Against Epilepsy recommends one nonemergent MRI for all patients except those with idiopathic generalized epilepsies (10,11). MRI is often normal in IGE (12,13), but most of these studies did not include high-resolution techniques. In addition, the differences between focal epilepsy and IGE may not be distinct, and some seizures that appear to be generalized by clinical and EEG criteria are actually rapidly spreading partial seizures (14). Because MRI might help to exclude an unusual but potentially treatable cause, one state-of-the-art examination may be reasonable in every epilepsy patient.

WHAT TYPE OF MRI SHOULD BE ORDERED?

MRI should be performed on a state-of-the-art 1.5- or 3-T scanner. The poor image quality of low-field or open systems could miss subtle abnormalities despite interpretation by experienced neuroradiologists. Even if performed

3T PROTOCOL[a]

Sequence	Direction	Slices (no.)	TR (ms)	TE (ms)	Matrix (mm)	Slice Thickness (mm)	Gap (%)	Min (~)	iPAT
MPRAGE	Sagittal (coronal and axial reformats)	160	2000	3.71	256 × 256	1	0	4:40	2
High-resolution T2 TSE	Coronal or axial	27	6000	96	512 × 384	3	0	6:08	0
FLAIR	Coronal or axial	28	10,000 TI = 2500	70 10 degrees	384 × 288	5	20	3:32	0
Gradient echo T2	Coronal or axial	24	359	12	256 × 252	5	0	3:21	2

[a]In addition to routine brain sequences, for patients with focal seizures. For mesial temporal sclerosis, the high-resolution T2 and FLAIR sequences should be angled perpendicular to the axis of the hippocampi. For neocortical epilepsy, the optimal imaging plane for the lobe of interest is chosen. Abbreviations: FLAIR, fluid-attenuated inversion recovery; MPRAGE, magnetization-prepared rapid gradient echo; TE, echo time; TI, inversion time; T2 TSE, T2-turbo-spin-echo; TR, repetition time; iPAT, integrated parallel acquisition technique.

on a 1.5-T system, older MRI techniques may not include all of the modern sequences. Phased-array imaging at 1.5 T or 3 T, can increase lesion detection and should be considered for patients with focal epilepsies, particularly medically refractory seizures, in whom 1.5-T studies with a standard head coil yield normal or discordant results (15,16). The imaging sequences performed will depend on the duration and type of epilepsy as well as the age of the patient because the differential diagnosis differs in each of these categories (Table 74.1). The protocol for new-onset seizures in adults typically includes postcontrast studies; in children, whose seizures are less often secondary to neoplasms, a high-resolution protocol with contrast is used only on identification of a lesion. High-resolution T1-weighted and T2-weighted images through the hippocampi are recommended for mesial temporal lobe epilepsy. The same type of weighted images are appropriate for focal neocortical epilepsies but through the lobe of interest if no lesion is obvious and including in adults a gradient-echo T2 sequence. Therefore, when MRI studies are requested, new-onset seizures should be distinguished from epilepsy syndromes and the type of epilepsy should be described. Imaging protocols are discussed below.

MESIAL TEMPORAL LOBE EPILEPSY

A tailored MRI protocol is important for diagnosing mesial temporal sclerosis (MTS) and predicting surgical outcome. Assessment by an experienced observer is also crucial (17) as MTS especially is often missed by the inexperienced reader (18). Radiographically proven unilateral hippocampal sclerosis is closely correlated with seizure-free outcome in up to 80% of patients after temporal lobe resections (5,19–22). MRI also detects dual pathology, which occurs in about 15% of patients with hippocampal sclerosis (23),

involves a less favorable outcome, and usually requires resection of both abnormalities for control (24,25). Dual pathology is common in patients with developmental disorders of the temporal lobe and may be associated with bilateral hippocampal abnormalities (26,27).

Protocol

High-resolution images through the hippocampi can detect the primary findings that establish a diagnosis of MTS as well as secondary abnormalities (Table 74.1). Images through the rest of the brain allow detection of dual pathology. Although imaging sequences may vary slightly from center to center, essential components are thin-section high-matrix T2 fast spin echo (FSE), thin-section fluid-attenuated inversion recovery (FLAIR) images angled perpendicular to the long axis of the hippocampus, and volumetric T1-weighted images with a partition size not exceeding 2 mm through the entire brain; a gradient-echo T2 sequence is a high priority in adults. Symmetric alignment of the head improves the accuracy of visual assessments of asymmetric hippocampal volume. Some centers obtain short tau inversion recovery (STIR) sequences because of the excellent gray-white contrast and ability to assess the hippocampal signal. Our volumetric T1-weighted sequence provides higher resolution of the gray-white junction, and T2 FSE and FLAIR images evaluate the hippocampal signal. Spin-echo T2-weighted sequences are probably more sensitive to subtle increases in T2 signal but the long imaging times often necessitate cardiac gating to obtain adequate images.

Qualitative Assessment

The assessment usually begins with a close inspection of the hippocampi on oblique T2 FSE images, preferably with

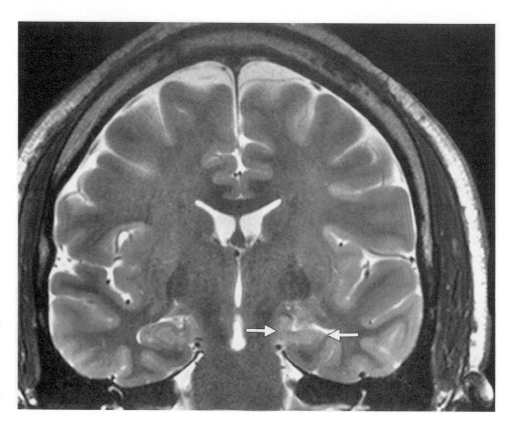

Figure 74.1 Coronal T2 FSE obtained with an 8-channel phased-array coil at 3T. The left hippocampus is smaller than the right, T2 signal is increased, and the internal architecture is blurred (*arrows*). These are primary imaging features of mesial temporal sclerosis.

magnification. Increased T2 signal, which reportedly has a sensitivity of 93% and a specificity of 74% (28), can be detected in specific sectors, along with blurring of the internal architecture (Fig. 74.1). In more severe cases, decreased undulations in the hippocampal head can often be identified (29). T2-signal increases in the collateral white matter and blurring of the gray-white junction are also visible on this sequence. Table 74.2 summarizes the radiographic findings of MTS (5,9,29,30–44).

Close inspection of the FLAIR images confirms T2 signal asymmetry. On FLAIR images, the hippocampus normally is brighter than neocortex, and the choroid plexus just superior to the hippocampi is bright. A comparison with T2 FSE images can avoid misdiagnosing bilateral disease or mistaking choroid plexus for hippocampal hyperintensity. Scrutiny of the coronal volumetric T1 images allows comparison of hippocampal and temporal lobe volumes. Secondary MTS findings such as volume loss in the circuit of Papez are best detected on this sequence, as are temporal lobe polymicrogyria and heterotopia. A gradient-echo T2 sequence may also detect dual pathology such as subtle cavernous venous, or cryptic venous, malformations or old hemorrhagic shear injury that would otherwise be missed. A normal or small T2-bright hippocampus makes the diagnosis in the appropriate clinical setting. In asymptomatic individuals, an increased T2 signal in the hippocampus (45,46) and a small hippocampus without signal abnormality (45) have uncertain significance. Increased hippocampal volume associated

with increased T2 signal may suggest acute swelling because of recent severe seizure activity (47,48), infiltrating glioma, or cortical dysplasia. Although such acute swelling can progress to MTS, the differential diagnosis of an enlarged hippocampus does not include MTS (48,49). Normal variants not associated with seizures are hippocampal sulcal remnants and choroidal fissure cysts (29,50,51); both are equal to cerebrospinal fluid in signal

TABLE 74.2

PRIMARY AND SECONDARY RADIOGRAPHIC FINDINGS OF MESIAL TEMPORAL SCLEROSIS

Finding

Primary
   Increased hippocampal signal intensity (5,9,30)
   Hippocampal atrophy (31–34)
   Loss of the internal architecture (33,35–37)
Secondary (temporal lobe)
   Thinning of collateral white matter in adjacent parahippocampal gyrus (38)
   Loss of hippocampal head digitizations (29)
   Diminished demarcation between gray and white matter in temporal lobe neocortex (38–40)
   Temporal lobe atrophy and enlarged temporal horn (41)
Secondary (extratemporal)
   Atrophy of the mamillary body (42)
   Atrophy of fornix/amygdale (43)
   Thalamic and caudate atrophy (44)

intensity on all sequences. Occurring in about 10% of the population, hippocampal sulcal remnants are 1- to 2-mm structures between the dentate gyrus and the cornu ammonis that represent a failure of normal embryogenic involution of the hippocampal sulcus. Choroidal fissure cysts, located just above the hippocampus, become more frequent with age (29,51).

Magnetic Resonance Spectroscopy

MRS noninvasively measures the integrity and function of neuronal tissue; ^{31}P-MRS evaluates cerebral energetics and pH. Studies at 1.5 T and 4.1 T have shown reductions of 50% in the ratio of phosphocreatine/inorganic phosphate (PCr/Pi) in the affected lobe of patients with temporal lobe epilepsy and of 24% in the contralateral temporal lobe (52–54), thought to indicate persistent impairment of energy metabolism. Despite these intriguing changes, a low signal-to-noise ratio, poor spatial resolution, and widespread unavailability for routine clinical studies limit the clinical application of ^{31}P-MRS. ^{1}H-MRS, in contrast, can be performed on most clinical 1.5-T scanners with spatial resolutions between approximately 1 and 8 cc, depending on whether multivoxel or single-voxel techniques are used. ^{1}H-MRS provides biochemical information about neuronal function (*N*-acetyl aspartate [NAA]), membrane turnover (choline), and total energy stores (creatine [Cr]) as well as the presence of cerebral lactate. Its sensitivity and specificity in temporal lobe epilepsy ranges from 60% (55) to 97% (56) and is greater with higher-spatial-resolution techniques (57). High-quality routine MRI of the hippocampus and ^{1}H-MRS for localization have not been directly compared but are probably complementary. Because absolute quantification of NAA, choline, and Cr is difficult, the sum of creatine and phosphocreatinine is assumed to be constant in adults and ratios of NAA and choline to Cr are usually calculated. Ipsilateral decreases in NAA/Cr occur in about 90% of MTS cases, and the side of functional abnormality corresponds highly with the side of seizure onset on EEG (58). The loss of NAA and the decreased NAA/Cr ratio are associated with dysfunctional mitochondrial metabolism and neuronal loss (38,39,59–61) but reflect neuronal as well as glial function (62). Combined with MRI findings, MRS improves predictions of surgical outcomes (63) and may help with lateralization in MRI-negative patients with temporal lobe epilepsy (64). With voxels typically including at most only part of the hippocampus, these MRS findings probably characterize the extrahippocampal, temporal lobe metabolic abnormalities in patients with mesial temporal lobe epilepsy. In fact, although NAA/Cr levels and ipsilateral hippocampal volumes can be statistically related, they share only a small percentage of variance and may be related but distinct (65,66). Temporal lobe MRS findings may also indicate a more widespread underlying pathologic condition (67). NAA/Cr decreases in the contralateral hemisphere may

predict a poor surgical outcome (68). Lactate levels are normally absent in the brain or present in very low levels. The lactate resonance consists of two distinct peaks at 1.3 ppm and indicates a disturbance of the cellular oxidative mechanism. Lactate has been identified in the region of seizure activity during status epilepticus and epilepsia partialis continua and in the hippocampus within 24 hours after temporal lobe seizures (69–72). Lactate may also alter the excitability of local neurons (73).

Because acute and transient changes have also been reported in MRS (71,74), results should be interpreted in conjunction with recent seizure activity. The ^{1}H-MRS signal also may be influenced by antiepileptic medication and even by metabolic interventions such as a ketogenic diet (57,75,76).

Quantitative Assessment

Hippocampal volumetry and T2-relaxometry show increased sensitivity over visual analysis in the detection of hippocampal sclerosis ranging from about 80%–90% to 90%–95% (29,38,39,60,77–79). However, T2-relaxometry requires an additional imaging sequence that lengthens an already protracted protocol, and both techniques require manual segmentation of the hippocampus and postprocessing to calculate T2 values and volumes. Although the added sensitivity has not yet prompted their incorporation into clinical protocols for mesial temporal lobe epilepsy, these techniques have enhanced our understanding of MTS. Hippocampal volumetry has disclosed a spectrum of volume loss in MTS (80,81), and total loss of volume has been correlated with reduced neuronal density (82–84). Longitudinal volumetric MRI studies have shown progressive hippocampal volume loss in patients with intractable mesial temporal lobe seizures, whereas patients with new-onset well-controlled temporal lobe epilepsy exhibited no change over the same period (85). No volume loss had been identified in extratemporal epilepsy, emphasizing the specificity of volumetric studies. Automated methods for calculating hippocampal volumes are being developed (86,87) and, if validated, could be used routinely.

T2-relaxometry measures the decay in signal intensity at different echo times in a series of T2-weighted images acquired at the same slice. Techniques range from the use of a 16-echo sequence (88,89) or two echoes (90–92) and time-efficient sequences (79,91); all reliably measured the T2 signal in the hippocampus and the amygdala (93). Boundaries with cerebrospinal fluid must be carefully avoided in this operator-dependent technique. During measurement of the T2-relaxation time along the long axis of the hippocampus in healthy individuals, a study described a characteristic profile that is disturbed in patients with hippocampal sclerosis (94). The hippocampal relaxation time correlates well with the glial and neuronal ratio, particularly in the CA1 subregion (80,84).

New MRI Techniques for Temporal Lobe Epilepsies

Diffusion-Weighted Imaging

Apparent diffusion coefficients (ADC) are elevated interictally in the involved hippocampus and to a lesser extent the uninvolved hippocampus (63,95). Injection of flumazenil significantly decreases the ADC in the seizure-onset zone, as defined by EEG and structural MRI (96). If imaging was performed within 15 minutes of a seizure lasting at least 60 seconds, the most pronounced ADC decreases (up to 25% to 31%) were observed in the epileptogenic zone but were only transient (97). In prolonged status, more persistent decreases may correlate with hippocampal injury and the development of MTS (47,98).

Hippocampal Shape Analysis

Hippocampal shape analysis may suggest a typical three-dimensional pattern of volume loss in patients with mesial temporal epilepsy (99).

Arterial Spin Labeling Perfusion MRI

Arterial spin labeling (ASL) uses electromagnetic fields to label the nuclear spins of hydrogen in the water of inflowing blood, making blood itself an endogenous tracer (100). In patients with temporal lobe epilepsy, ASL can show interictal asymmetries in mesial temporal lobe cerebral blood flow (100,101); its role in neocortical epilepsy is unclear. Significant improvements in signal-to-noise ratio (SNR) at higher field strengths will optimize this technique (102).

FOCAL NEOCORTICAL EPILEPSIES

Less common than mesial temporal epilepsy in adults, focal neocortical epilepsy involves more variable and subtle abnormalities that may be located anywhere in the neocortex. For this reason, routine MRI is often interpreted as normal in neocortical epilepsy.

MRI plays a central role. Although a pathologic substrate portends a poor long-term response to medical treatment (103), a lesion corresponding to the ictal-onset zone may improve surgical prognosis. For example, 72% of patients with identifiable lesions have good surgical outcomes compared with 41% of patients with no lesions (6). Surgical outcomes improve if the entire lesion is resected, making precise anatomic delineation important (2). Evaluation of the images by an experienced reader is also critical, particularly in the absence of an obvious lesion (18). Surgical success is much lower than in mesial temporal epilepsy, often because brain MRI may show no lesion or one too extensive for complete resection (104). Among neocortical lobe epilepsies, temporal and frontal lobe syndromes are most common, followed by parietal and occipital lobe epilepsy

(105,106). Frontal lobe epilepsy is less frequently treated surgically than temporal lobe epilepsy—between 5.5% and 18% in large series (107,108).

Given the large number of MRI-negative studies in neocortical epilepsy, the priority becomes thin-section imaging, with contrast reserved for new-onset epilepsy. Lengthy protocols give rise to movement artifact, degrading image quality; therefore, the study must be tailored. The structural anomalies associated with chronic partial neocortical epilepsy (107) can be grouped into mass lesions, encephalomalacia, and malformations of cortical development (MCD).

This section describes our neocortical imaging protocol and characterizes the most common lesions in the three categories. Discussions of normal imaging, the relationship between MRI-detected lesions and ictal onset, and future perspectives follow.

Protocol

Essential components are 3-mm or less high-matrix T2 FSE images obtained through the lobe of highest suspicion, coronal volumetric T1-weighted images no larger than 2 mm through the entire brain, and a gradient-echo T2 sequence (Table 74.1). Contrast should be used in all adults and in children with obvious lesions, but if time is an issue, the high-resolution sequences take precedence. A patient can always return for a contrast study if a small lesion is identified; however, if omitting the thin sections misses a small nonenhancing lesion, the disease may be labeled nonlesional. Positioning is important; symmetric alignment of the head enhances the visual assessments of gyral asymmetries. STIR sequences may be obtained, but our center uses a volumetric T1-weighted sequence to evaluate the gray-white junction. Spin-echo T2-weighted sequences can detect a subtle increased signal in the cortex or white matter associated with cortical dysplasias, but time constraints preclude their routine use.

Qualitative Assessment

When a lesion is identified, an associated positive or negative mass effect or no mass effect must be established. These categories correspond to the three types of lesion.

Positive Mass Effect/Mass Lesion

Mass lesions linked to neocortical epilepsy take the form of neoplasms, vascular malformations, and central nervous system infections. As the last are unlikely to concern the epileptologist, the discussion is limited to neoplasms and vascular malformations.

Neoplasms that present as seizure disorders and without focal neurologic signs or symptoms are typically lower grade and involve the cortex (Table 74.3) (75,109–128). Higher-grade tumors, typically centered in the white matter,

TABLE 74.3

LOW-GRADE NEOPLASMS ASSOCIATED WITH EPILEPSY

	DNT	Ganglioglioma/ Gangliocytoma	PXA	Oligodendro-glioma
T2 contrast	Hyperintense	Hyperintense	Hyperintense	Isointense to cortex
T1 contrast	Hypointense	Hypointense	Hypointense	Usually hypointense, variable
Contrast enhancement	Variable	Common, in solid portion	Common in solid portion	About 50%
Contour	Well circumscribed, peripheral	Well circumscribed, solid, and cystic, peripheral	Solid mass, +/− cyst peripheral	Peripheral
Surrounding edema	Rare	Rare	Uncommon	In 50%
Hemorrhage	Rare	Rare	Rare	Frequent
Calcification	Common	Common (best on CT)	Uncommon	Common
Age at onset	Usually before age 20	Young adults, children	Young adults	30–50 y
Most common location	Temporal lobe	Temporal lobe	Temporal lobe	Frontal lobe
Prognosis postsurgery	Excellent; rare reports of malignant transformation	Excellent	Variable; 10%–25% recurrence or malignant transformation	Poor
Other features	Cortical malformations	Cortical malformations in up to 5%	Typically involve cortex, questionable origin, associated with cortical malformations (rare)	Tendency to invade cortex; cortical thickening
References	(109–117)	(75,118–122)	(123–126)	(127,128)

have more acute presentations and require rapid neuro-oncologic assessment.

Neoplasms are found in about 12% of medically intractable patients, usually children and young adults, who have a structural lesion on MRI (105). Most often located in the temporal lobe (129,130), the neoplasms include ganglion-cell masses (ganglioglioma and gangliocytoma) (Fig. 74.2), dysembryoplastic neuroepithelial tumors (DNT) (Fig. 74.3), and pleomorphic xanthoastrocytoma. All are peripheral or superficial. Ganglion-cell neoplasms and DNTs have neuronal elements and excellent surgical outcomes if the entire lesion can be excised. Outcomes of pleomorphic xanthoastrocytoma vary owing to recurrence and malignant transformation in 10% to 25%. Occasionally, an oligodendroglioma in an adult may present as a seizure disorder because the tumor tends to secondarily invade cortex; differentiation from other benign neoplasms allows initiation of oncologic treatment.

There are four types of cerebral parenchymal vascular malformations: (1) cavernous malformations (also known as cryptic venous malformations or cavernous venous malformations) (CM); (2) developmental venous anomalies (DVA); (3) capillary telangiectasias; and (4) arterial venous malformations (AVM). CMs have the strongest association with epilepsy and occur in 4% of the population. Seizures are a common presenting symptom (131,132) and focal ictal onsets are often identified on EEG. CMs can be very small and difficult, if not impossible, to identify on routine brain MRI studies and on thin-section FSE sequences (Fig. 74.4). Associated hemosiderin causes marked "blooming" on gradient-echo sequences, increasing the sensitivity for lesion detection and making these sequences essential to the presurgical evaluation of focal epilepsies. CMs contain cysts filled with blood products of various ages and various signal intensities on T1- and T2-weighted imaging. A well-defined hemosiderin rim should also be identified. Contrast enhancement is mild, and no surrounding edema is present unless a recent parenchymal hemorrhage has occurred. Because they replace and do not displace normal tissue, CMs typically have no mass effect on the surrounding brain. A contrast examination is recommended to identify an adjacent DVA, which may alter the surgical approach.

Best identified on postcontrast studies, DVAs appear as a "Medusa head" of multiple small veins draining into a single large vein without a mass effect. They drain regions of

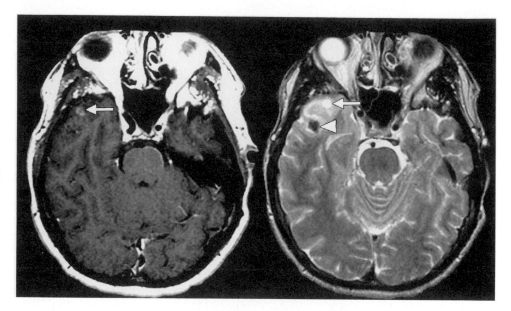

Figure 74.2 Ganglioglioma. Axial postcontrast T1 (left) and axial T2 FSE (right) obtained with a routine head coil at 1.5T. An enhancing nodule (*arrow*, left) is associated with a focus of high T2 signal representing a cyptic component (*arrow*, right). Also noted is a focus of low T2 signal representing calcification (*arrowhead*, right). Note the lack of surrounding edema.

normal brain and are the most common vascular anomaly. The epilepsy sometimes reported with DVAs is likely caused by CM or malformations, as the vast majority of patients with DVAs do not have a seizure disorder (133). Capillary telangiectasias have no known link to seizures. Seizures that accompany AVMs are most likely caused by ischemic damage/encephalomalacia and hemorrhage of the surrounding cortex (134,135). Treatment centers on the AVM.

Negative Mass Effect

Encephalomalacia

Encephalomalacia resulting in seizure disorders appears as cortical thinning and increased T2 signal in the subcortical white matter, often associated with volume loss. Encephalomalacia can result from embolic or thrombotic strokes, hypoxic/hypoperfusion events, traumatic brain injury, or prior infection. The seizure disorder typically begins months to years after the acute event; alternatively, the acute event may have been occult (136). Outcomes are

good if the area of cortical injury can be excised (137,138). Not all regions of encephalomalacia are or will become epileptogenic, and imaging cannot make that distinction. Extratemporal encephalomalacia has been reported in patients successfully treated for temporal lobe epilepsy with temporal lobe resections (139).

Rasmussen Encephalitis

Rasmussen encephalitis can produce focal swelling within the first 4 months of onset, but by the time an MRI is obtained, focal volume loss with increased T2 signal in the cortex and subcortical white matter is noted. Early changes are most prominent in the peri-insular region. Ipsilateral caudate volume loss or ipsilateral ventriculomegaly are noted occasionally (140,141). Volume loss and T2-signal changes often progress (142).

Sturge-Weber Syndrome

Focal atrophy with abnormal leptomeningeal enhancement representing an angioma (143,144) characterizes

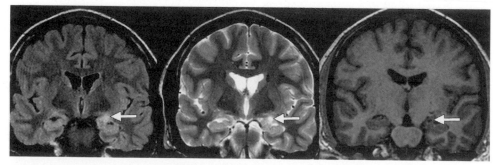

Figure 74.3 Dysembryoplastic neuroepithelial tumor. Coronal FLAIR (left), T2 FSE (middle), and coronal three-dimensional SPGR (spoiled gradient recalled echo), a thin-section volumetric T1 sequence (right) obtained with a routine head coil at 1.5T. A small mass lesion with increased FLAIR signal (*arrow*, left), well-defined increased T2 signal (*arrow*, middle), and well-defined low T1 signal (left) has the typical appearance, although much smaller than most. No enhancement was identified on post contrast images (not shown).

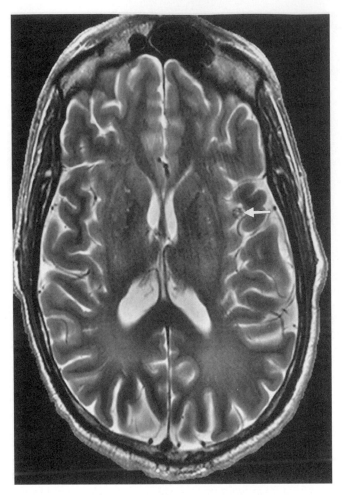

Figure 74.4 Cavernous angioma. Axial T2 FSE obtained with an 8-channel phased-array coil at 3T. A small multicystic lesion with well-defined margins and low T2 signal is present in the left insular cortex.

Sturge-Weber syndrome. A port-wine stain suggests the diagnosis, and warrants a contrast examination. Infrequently, seizures are severe enough to warrant visually guided resection of the pial angioma and underlying cortex (145). Bilateral or extensive involvement may alter surgical management.

No Mass Effect/Malformations of Cortical Development

In MRI series, MCDs have been reported in about 4% to 25% of the adults or 10% to 50% of children (29,146–148). Errors in stem cell proliferation and differentiation, neuronal migration, or cortical organization or their combination with errors in later developmental steps may result in MCD (149). Barkovich and colleagues (150) classify malformations in this manner. This section focuses on the detection and diagnosis of MCD on MRI. The classification and genetics of MCD are discussed elsewhere in this book. Some mass effect can be present, but dysmorphic gyral structure, not gyral displacement, is the dominant finding.

TABLE 74.4
IMAGING APPROACH TO DETECT AND CHARACTERIZE MALFORMATIONS OF CORTICAL DEVELOPMENT

Axial T2, coronal thin section T2, and axial FLAIR
   Symmetry of size: normal or asymmetric?
   Gyral folding pattern: normal, simplified, or increased?
   Gray-white junction: smooth, irregular, or blurred?
   Symmetry of white-matter signal?
   Uniformity of cortical signal?
Volumetric T1
   Gyral folding pattern: normal, simplified, or increased?
   Gray-white junction: smooth, irregular, or blurred?
   Uniformity of cortical signal?
   Subcortical or periventricular gray-matter lesions?

Table 74.4 lists a way to detect and document the imaging features of an MCD. Following is a summary of the imaging findings in the most common MCDs associated with epilepsy, organized by appearance.

Asymmetry in Size

Increased Volume/Hemimegalencephaly Cerebral or lobar asymmetry should prompt evaluation for other features of hemimegalencephaly (Fig. 74.5) that may range from absence of any normal gyral structure to subtle changes. If myelination is complete, the involved white matter appears normal on T1 and is increased on T2. Ipsilateral lateral ventriculomegaly is characteristic but in exceptional cases may not be present. The frontal horn of the ipsilateral lateral ventricle is always dysmorphic and points anteriorly (151,152). These patients may benefit from a surgery (153), although overall outcomes remain guarded (154,155).

Decreased Volume A dysmorphic, small hemisphere with ipsilateral ventricular enlargement caused by decreased white-matter volume should raise suspicions of subcortical heterotopia. MRI discloses curvilinear regions of gray-matter signal intensity extending from the cortex to the ventricular margin. The overlying cortex is typically thinned and has a simplified gyral folding pattern. The corpus callosum is absent or partially absent in 70% of patients (156,157).

Simplified Gyral Folding and Smooth Gray-White Junction

Classic Lissencephaly The essential features are a highly simplified gyral folding pattern to complete agyria, a thick band of heterotopic gray matter, and a cell-sparse white-matter band between the heterotopic gray matter and the cortex. Prominent findings posteriorly have been linked to defects in *LIS1* (17q13.3), with some patients exhibiting the full Miller-Dieker syndrome. Prominent findings anteriorly accompany defects in *XLIS* or *DCX* (Xq22.3-23) (158). Presurgical evaluation is not performed.

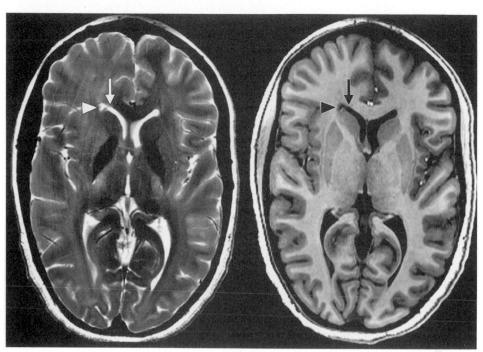

Figure 74.5 Hemimegalencephaly. Axial T2 FSE (left) and axial magnetization-prepared rapid gradient echo (MPRAGE), a thin-section volumetric T1-weighted sequence (right) obtained with an 8-channel phased-array coil at 3T. In this subtle case the right hemisphere is larger, but the typical ipsilateral ventriculomegaly is absent; however, anterior pointing of the ipsilateral frontal horn of the lateral ventricle is noted (*arrow*, left and right). The T2 signal is diffusely increased, but the T1 signal is normal in the ipsilateral hemispheric white matter. Ipsilateral abnormal gyral folding is present in the right frontal lobe in the region of most severe seizure activity. A nonspecific, probably incidental, right periventricular cyst is noted (*arrowhead*).

Lissencephaly/Pachygyria A simplified gyral folding pattern with a smooth gray-white junction but no cell-sparse zone best describes lissencephaly or pachygyria. Among the genes that cause or contribute to human lissencephaly are *14-3-3 epsilon*, *RELN*, and *ARX* (159), each of which is associated with a characteristic malformation of the cerebral cortex and sometimes other brain structures. These patients do not typically present for surgical evaluation (160).

Irregular Gray-White Junction

Cobblestone Lissencephaly Abnormalities in radial organization result in radial bands of gray matter that extend perpendicular to the cortical surface into the subcortical white matter, which, in turn, produces an irregular gray-white junction. Marked hypomyelination with a markedly increased T2 signal in the white matter is also seen. Cobblestone lissencephaly may present as Walker-Warburg syndrome (POMT1 gene) (161) and Fukuyama congenital muscular dystrophy (chromosome 9q31-32) (162). These patients rarely seek presurgical evaluation.

Polymicrogyria Polymicrogyria may appear as thickened cortex but serrations of the gray-white junctions distinguish it from lissencephaly and pachygria (Fig. 74.6). Polymicrogyria can be unilateral and focal or bilateral and multifocal. If a single focus is identified, the similar region

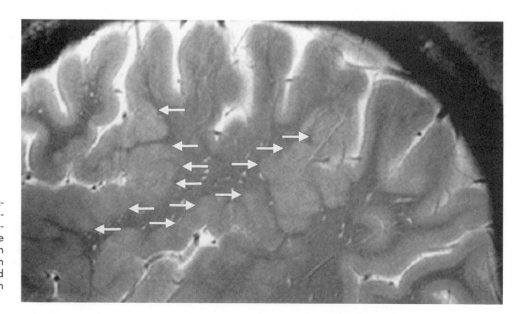

Figure 74.6 Polymicrogyria. Sagittal T2 FSE obtained with phased-array surface coils at 1.5T. In addition to the irregular gray-white junction, the multiple small gyri can be seen on this high-resolution image (*arrows*). This patient also had a much smaller contralateral region of polymicrogyria (not shown).

in the contralateral hemisphere should be scrutinized, as multiple foci will influence surgical outcome and may necessitate invasive monitoring. The pattern of lobar involvement in bilateral syndromes may also determine the likely genetic defect. Bilateral frontal, perisylvian, medial parieto-occipital, and lateral parietal perisylvian syndromes have been described (163). The gene for bilateral frontoparietal polymicrogyria has been identified on chromosome 16 (16q12.2-21) (164,165). These patients are rarely considered for surgery (160).

Schizencephaly A direct communication between the subarachnoid space and the ventricle is lined by gray matter with an irregular gray-white junction. Schizencephaly may be unilateral, and associated with contralateral polymicrogyria, or bilateral and is classified as either open- or closed-lip, depending on the size of the communicating tract (Fig. 74.7). No characteristic pattern of inheritance has yet been described (158). These patients are rarely surgical candidates (160).

Focal Asymmetry in White-Matter Signal

Focal Cortical Dysplasia with White-Matter Signal Abnormalities In the mature brain, many focal cortical dysplasias involve increased white-matter T2 signal and either an increased or a decreased T1 signal; these changes have been correlated with the presence of balloon cells (166). In some cases, a diffusely increased T2 signal in white matter is the only abnormality detectable on MRI (Fig. 74.8). In transmantle dysplasia (Fig. 74.9), only a small cone-shaped region of increased T2 extends from the ventricular margin to the cortex, with the cortical involvement identifiable superficial to the white-matter abnormality. As the tubers of tuberous sclerosis look similar, a full evaluation for that disorder is prudent in patients with transmantle dysplasias (167). Occasionally, very focal, cystic lesions in the subcortical white matter may be the only abnormality on MR. In unmyelinated brains, involved white matter appears as areas of decreased T2 and increased T1 signal, probably as a result of early myelination. Ictal SPECT and fluoro-2-deoxyglucose (FDG)-PET studies correctly localize the pathologic lobe in up to 65% of patients (168). Surgery is appropriate if the entire lesion can be resected (169); however, not all patients become seizure free (160,170).

Focal Cortical Signal Abnormality on T1 or T2

Cortical Dysplasia Small focal cortical dysplasias without white-matter changes require high-resolution techniques for detection (Fig. 74.10). These patients are good surgical candidates.

Subcortical Band or Periventricular Nodules Isointense to Cortex on T1

Volumetric T1-weighted sequences are indispensable in the search for heterotopic gray matter, as these lesions may be difficult, if not impossible, to identify on other sequences.

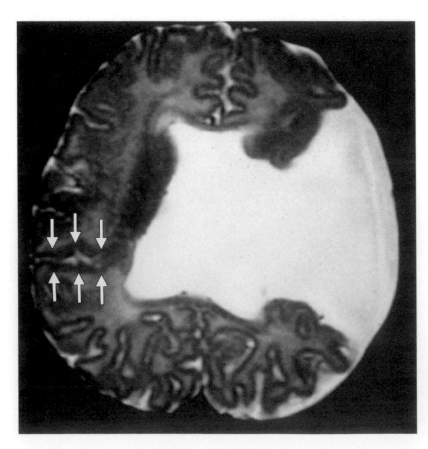

Figure 74.7 Schizencephaly. Axial T2 FSE obtained with a routine head coil at 1.5T. In this immature brain, an open-lip schizencephaly is on the left and a closed-lip form on the right (*arrows*). Communication between the subarachnoid space and the ventricle can be seen on the left. The right cleft communicated with the ventricle on the next slice (not shown).

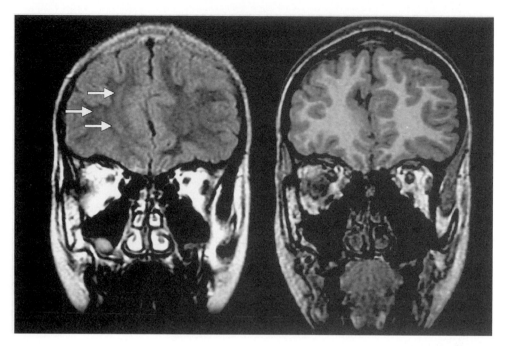

Figure 74.8 Focal cortical dysplasia with only white-matter involvement identified on MRI. Coronal FLAIR (left) and coronal 3D SPGR, a thin-section volumetric T1 sequence (right), obtained with a routine head coil at 1.5T. Ill-defined increased T2 signal occurs throughout the white matter of the visualized right frontal lobe (*arrows*, left), but no obvious abnormality is identified on the T1-weighted sequence. This case emphasizes the importance of reviewing FLAIR (and T2 FSE) images on narrow windows for areas of white-matter signal asymmetry.

Band Heterotopia Bands of cortical signal intensity in the subcortical gray matter with undulations lower in frequency than those in overlying cortex describe band heterotopias (Fig. 74.11). They can be either unilateral or bilateral and when bilateral may be asymmetric. Frontal or posterior predominance may hint at the underlying genetic abnormality. Subcortical band heterotopia, or double-cortex syndrome, occurs very rarely in males; in a recent review, at least 110 females but only 11 males were affected. The syndrome usually involves mutations in the doublecortin (DCX) (Xq22.3-q23) gene when frontally predominant, much less frequently in the LIS1 (17p13.3) gene when posteriorly predominant (171). The patients are poor surgical candidates (160).

Periventricular Nodular Heterotopia Close scrutiny of the occipital horn, a common location for isolated lesions

(Fig. 74.12), is needed to rule out small heterotopia. This condition is poorly amenable to surgery, because either the nodules are too diffuse for complete resection or the site of ictal onset is unclear (160,172).

Hypothalamic Hamartoma Large lesions are easy to identify, but subtle hamartomas are often sessile and project into the third ventricle (Fig. 74.13). The lesions are isointense to gray matter on T1 and isointense to hyperintense on T2. Patients have benefited from surgery or stereotactic radiosurgery (173–176), but one series (173) reported a high rate of complications.

Initial MR Negative

If initial MRI results are negative but a focal lesion is highly suspected, the following questions should be asked:

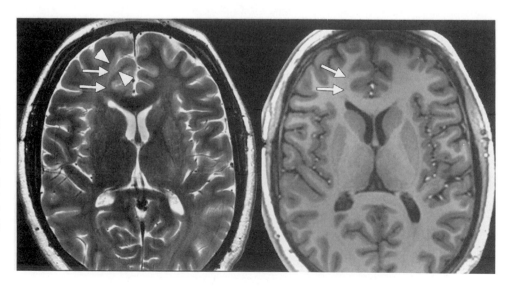

Figure 74.9 Transmantle focal cortical dysplasia. Axial T2 FSE (left) and axial MPRAGE, a thin-section volumetric T1-weighted sequence (right), obtained with an 8-channel phased-array coil at 3T. A cone-shaped region of increased T2 signal begins at the ventricular margin, extends to the depth of a sulcus (*arrows*, left), and corresponds to a more subtle region of decreased T1 signal (*arrows*, right). Increases in T2 (*arrowhead*, left) signal is seen in the overlying cortex.

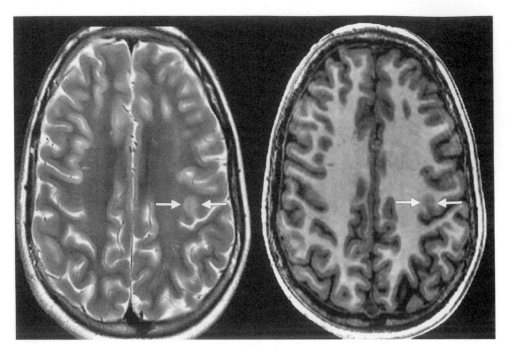

Figure 74.10 Focal cortical dysplasia with only cortical involvement on MRI. Axial T2 FSE (left) and axial MPRAGE, a thin-section volumetric T1-weighted sequence (right), obtained with an 8-channel phased-array coil at 3T. A blurred gray-white junction, cortical increased T2 signal (*arrow*, left), and increased T1 signal (*arrow*, right) are identified. Lesion location corresponded to seizure semiology.

1. Did artifacts degrade image quality?

Movement and braces and other dental hardware can significantly degrade image quality. Mild sedation or general anesthesia may sometimes be needed. Braces may have to be removed.

2. Were all recommended sequences performed?

Gradient-echo T2 sequences are important in adults, as FSE T2 sequences are insensitive to hemosiderin and CVA can be missed. A thin-section volumetric T1 can detect periventricular and band heterotopias that can be over-looked on T2 and FLAIR sequences. Thin-section T2 images through the lobe or suspicious region are essential for detecting small DNTs, especially in the mesial temporal region.

3. Was a subtle lesion overlooked?

The most commonly overlooked lesions are small focal cortical dysplasias, transmantle dysplasias, and periventricular and band heterotopias. To avoid this problem, (1) perform axial T2 and FLAIR images first, looking for sulci that are either too deep or too straight or disorganized

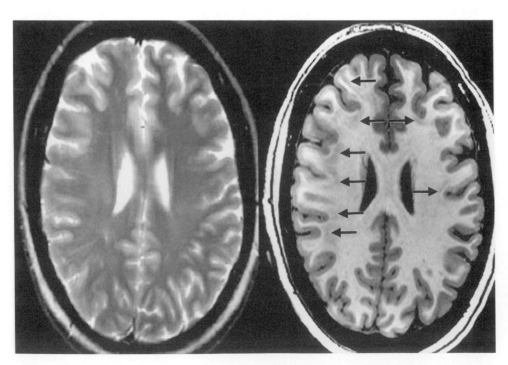

Figure 74.11 Band heterotopia. Axial T2 FSE (left) and axial MPRAGE, a thin-section volumetric T1-weighted sequence (right), obtained with an 8-channel phased array coil at 3T. Bilateral subcortical bands of heterotopic gray matter, right larger than left, are identified on the T1-weighted sequence (*arrows*, right) but are impossible to detect on the T2 FSE sequence (left). This case emphasizes the importance of a thin-section T1-weighted sequence in seizure evaluation.

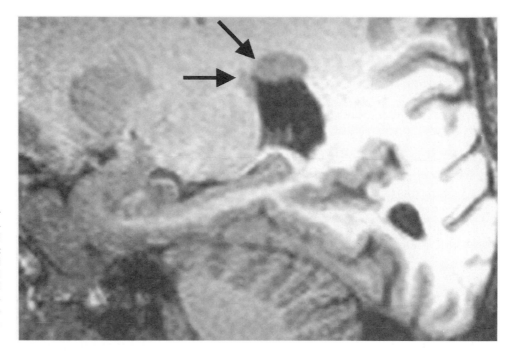

Figure 74.12 Periventricular nodular heterotopia in two gray-matter regions (*arrows*). Sagittal MPRAGE, a thin-section volumetric T1-weighted sequence obtained with an 8-channel phased-array coil at 3T. The lesions are best detected by systematic study of the periventricular regions adjacent to the atria of the lateral ventricles on thin-section T1-weighted images.

gyral folding; (2) narrow the viewing windows so that the images are high contrast and compare white-matter signal on both sides. Subtle focal increases in T2 may be the only finding of a focal cortical dysplasia (Fig. 74.8). Check for small tracts of increased T2 signal extending from the periventricular region to the cortex (hallmark of transmantle dysplasias) and for increased T2 in involved cortex. The smallest of the lesions we detected was less than 5 mm in diameter at the cortex and only a few millimeters wide in the white matter; (3) finally, scrutinize the volumetric T1 sequence for abnormally increased signal in the cortex and regions of cortical signal intensity

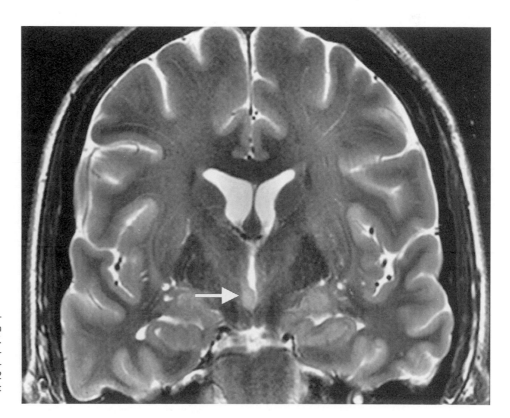

Figure 74.13 Hypothalamic hamartoma. Coronal T2 FSE obtained with an 8-channel phased-array coil at 3T. A small sessile hamartoma protruding into the floor of the third ventricle is hyperintense to cortex on T2 and isointense to cortex on T1 (not shown).

in the subcortical and periventricular white matter. If the tailored epilepsy MRI at 1.5 T is still normal and the EEG or semiology strongly suggests a focal onset, consider thin-section spin-echo T2 and proton density–weighted imaging at 1.5 T or phased-array imaging at 1.5 T or 3 T. Phased-array studies provide increased signal to noise, improving spatial resolution and image contrast (16) and enhancing the detection of small lesions (15).

Epileptogenic Zone and Epileptogenic Lesion

The epileptogenic lesion is the radiographically identified one that presumably caused the epileptic seizures. Not all lesions seen in patients with epilepsy are epileptogenic, however (2), and an epileptogenic lesion detected on MRI does not necessarily represent the epileptogenic zone, the area indispensable for generating seizures (25,29,148,177). Correlation with semiology, EEG, MEG, and grid or depth electrode recordings is necessary, as the entire epileptogenic zone cannot now be directly measured (2). In patients with epilepsy caused by developmental malformations, epileptogenicity may be intrinsic (170) because of excitability of the surrounding, more normal cortex. The two theories are not discordant with the observation that complete resection of the anatomic lesion and a rim of relatively normal marginal tissue predicts a good seizure outcome (169,177). Intraoperative stereotactic devices may facilitate complete resection of small or sulcus-deep focal lesions that are difficult to visualize intraoperatively. Apparently focal lesions also may be part of a larger malformation. There will be better documentation of which MR-visible lesions do well with complete resection and which ones are markers of more widespread abnormalities.

FUTURE IMAGING PERSPECTIVES/EVOLVING TRENDS

Postictal and Interictal Imaging

Diffusion-weighted imaging (DWI) and perfusion-weighted imaging (PWI) have raised interest in acute epilepsy imaging (Fig. 74.14) (98,178–180). With the development of MRI-compatible EEG leads, some sites have tested blood oxygen level–dependent (BOLD) fMRI to detect focal blood flow changes associated with interictal spikes (181–184). Despite initial promise, however, logistical problems and general unavailability of simultaneous EEG recording limit these techniques to research applications.

Diffusion Tensor Imaging

Diffusion tensor imaging (DTI) may aid in evaluating white-matter integrity. It has been used to estimate the integrity of large fiber bundles (Fig. 74.15) and to detect white-matter organizational disturbances characterized by alterations in fractional anisotropy and ADC compared with healthy matched controls. The affected subcortical white matter extended beyond the visible cortical abnormality in patients with cortical dysplasia (185–187) and temporal lobe epilepsy (188). The technique remains investigational, however, and awaits pathologic correlation to prove its accuracy.

Magnetization Transfer Imaging

Magnetic transfer imaging evaluates the macromolecular environment of mobile water protons. Used for many years to assess white-matter changes in multiple sclerosis, it has identified abnormal white-matter areas in patients

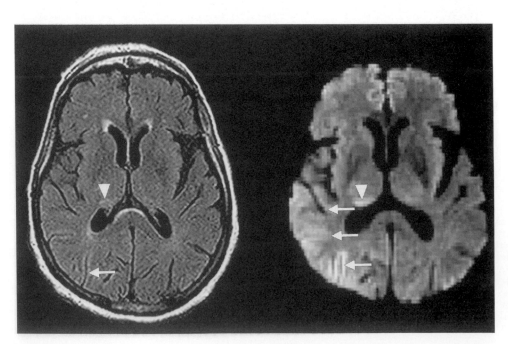

Figure 74.14 Status epilepticus. Axial FLAIR (left) and axial DWI (right) obtained with a routine head coil at 1.5T. Increased cortical T2 signal (*arrows*, left) and widespread increased DWI signal (*arrows*, right) as well as increased thalamic T2 and DWI signal (*arrowhead*, left and right) are seen. Note the normal-appearing white matter.

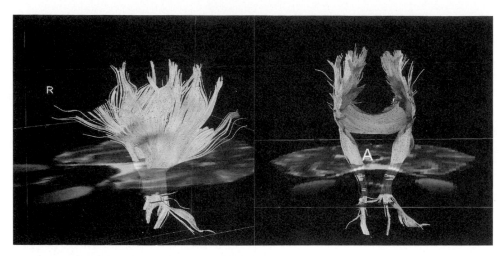

Figure 74.15 Diffusion tractology image. Bilateral corticospinal tracts (left and right, yellow) and interhemispheric connections (right, orange) calculated from high-resolution diffusion tensor sequence at 3T that used custom-built software by Drs. Ruopeng Wang and Greg Sorensen and colleagues at the Division of Health Sciences & Technology, Athinoula A. Martinos Center for Biomedical Imaging. The directional bias of the diffusion can inform about the structure of underlying white-matter tracts. Analysis techniques in development may enable statistical measures of connectivity and enhance understanding of cerebral malformations and seizure propagation. Please see color insert.

with focal epilepsies that correspond to the EEG abnormality, even when MRI showed negative results (189).

Semiautomated Voxel-Based Morphometry

Semiautomated techniques for analyzing cortical thickness and automated methods for calculating subcortical volumes are in development (86,87). Accurate manual segmentation is labor intensive, time-consuming, and tedious (190). Automation can make cerebral volumetrics part of a routine clinical assessment but currently requires validation and standardization (87). Recently, semiautomated voxel-based techniques for measuring cortical thickness have detected gray-matter changes (Fig. 74.16) (191–193). If validated, these techniques would allow greater accuracy in describing normal and abnormal

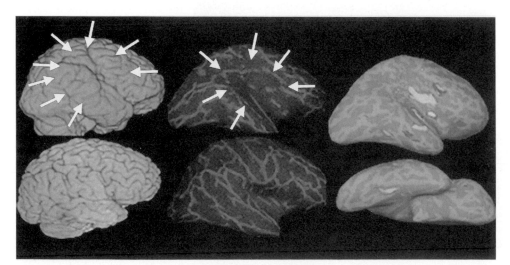

Figure 74.16 T-test comparison of abnormal and normal hemispheric structure. The top row shows a surface rendering of the abnormal left hemisphere (left, top image) with an area of abnormal gyral folding (*arrows*). Inflated surface representation with color coding of sulcal depth: red represents sulcal depth; green, gyral height in the abnormal hemisphere (middle, top). T-test statistics detected significant differences in sulcal depth and gyral height compared with the normal representation (not shown) in the colored areas on the right images (top and bottom). The bottom left and middle images are the surface and inflated representations of the normal right hemisphere in the same individual. Although the statistical map underrepresents the region involved, it shows the potential of quantitative techniques in phenotyping cerebral malformations. Images were created from a 3D SPGR sequence (a thin-section volumetric T1-weighted sequence) obtained with a standard head coil at 1.5T. Please see color insert.

cerebral structure and in analyzing the association between cerebral structure (phenotype) and genotype.

Curvilinear Reconstructions/ Three-Dimensional Rendering

Surface-based three-dimensional (3D) rendering of the brain has allowed evaluation of the gyri (194). Curvilinear reconstruction of the brain surface presents information about large parts of the gyral pattern by producing symmetric views of the cortex and detecting small abnormalities through a comparison of the two hemispheres (60,195).

High-Field MRI

MRI at field strengths of 3 T or higher increases the signal-to-noise ratio for similar imaging times, decreases scan time, increases spatial resolution, and improves contrast-to-noise ratio. A heightened ability to detect subtle small lesions of focal epilepsy at 3 T (196) provides an incentive for imaging in these patients (102). At high field strengths, magnetic resonance spectroscopy (MRS) increases the signal-to-noise

ratio up to 80% and improves separation of metabolite peaks, allowing better resolution of glutamine and glutamate and detection of γ-aminobutyric acid. Diffusion, perfusion, and fMRI studies also enhance the SNR at higher field strengths. In the scanning of ex vivo pathologic specimens at 7 T using long averaging times and small surface coils, a voxel size of 0.002 mm³ can be achieved. Whether these gains in spatial resolution allow detection of microdysgenesis, leptomeningeal glioneuronal heterotopia, and nodular cortical dysplasias awaits further research.

Multimodal Imaging

The combination of fMRI, MEG, and EEG may elucidate the onset and spread of seizure activity (28,171). MEG and EEG data combined with structural MRI through the distributed solution method of dynamic statistic parametric mapping can show activity at all recorded sensors at a given time and therefore the spread of brain activity with high temporal resolution (Fig. 74.17) (197,198). MEG and EEG-guided MRI interpretation aids in detecting subtle structural abnormalities (199,200) and may as well

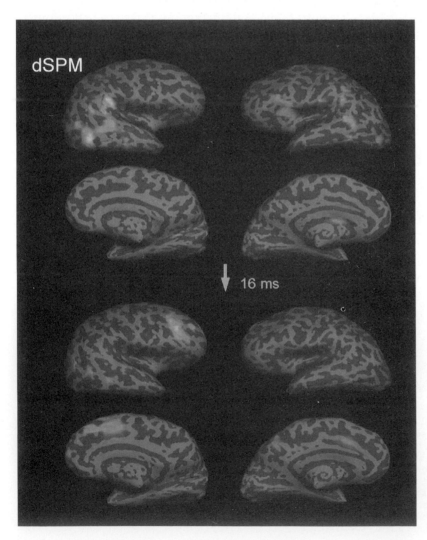

Figure 74.17 MEG activity of a spike constrained by anatomic MRI represented on the inflated brain in a 16-year-old right-handed patient with right temporal lobe epilepsy. The top four images show lateral (top row) and medial views (second row) of the right hemisphere (left side) and left hemisphere (right side). Areas in red represent increased neuronal MEG activity at the beginning of the spike, which is more marked in the right temporal lobe. The spike propagated from the right temporal to the right frontal area (bottom four images) within 16 msec. This image shows snapshots of a movie calculated for MEG activity by means of dynamic statistic parametric mapping (196). Courtesy of Dr. Hideaki Shiraishi, Division of Health Sciences & Technology, Athinoula A. Martinos Center for Biomedical Imaging. Please see color insert.

help interpreting magnetoencephalograph (MEG) and EEG findings.

Ultimately, we hope to combine functional information about neural activity obtained by EEG and MEG, about blood flow obtained by ASL, and about metabolism obtained by spike-triggered fMRI, ADC, and MRS with structural information from high-resolution 3D imaging and DTI. This would improve our understanding of epileptogenicity and pathways of epileptic spread and would be invaluable in the presurgical assessment and differentiation of the epileptogenic lesion and the irritative and seizure-onset zones and their relationships to the eloquent cortex.

ACKNOWLEDGMENTS

This work was supported in part by the National Center for Research Resources (P41RR14075) and the Mental Illness and Neuroscience Discovery (MIND) Institute. We thank Larry Wald, John Pitts, Andreas Potthast, Christina Triantafyllou, Chris Wiggins, and Graham Wiggins for technical support of our 8-channel head coil for 3T, as well as Mary Foley for helping to acquire and maintain our images. We also thank Anders Dale, Bruce Fischl, David Salat, Dave Tuch, and Ruopeng Wang for the use of their image analysis tools and Ji-Kyung Choi for her MRS expertise. Thanks also to Eric Halgren, Bruce Rosen, Hideaki Shiraishi, Greg Sorensen, and Steve Stufflebeam for their support of the epilepsy program. Finally, we are indebted to our clinical collaborators who provide us with interesting and challenging patients: Ann Bergin, Peter Black, Blaise Bourgeois, Edward Bromfield, Keith Chiappa, Andrew Cole, Rees Cosgrove, Barbara Dworetzky, Dan Hoch, Greg Holmes, Pal Larsson, Joseph Madsen, James Riviello, Donald Schomer, and Elizabeth Thiele.

REFERENCES

1. Engel J Jr. Update on surgical treatment of the epilepsies. *Clin Exp Neurol* 1992;29:32–48.
2. Rosenow F, Luders H. Presurgical evaluation of epilepsy. *Brain* 2001;124:1683–1700.
3. Foldvary N, Bingaman WE, Wyllie E. Surgical treatment of epilepsy. *Neurol Clin* 2001;19:491–515.
4. Luders H, Awad I. Conceptual considerations. In: Luders HO, ed. *Epilepsy surgery.* New York: Raven Press, 1992:51–62.
5. Kuzniecky R, Burgard S, Faught E, et al. Predictive value of magnetic resonance imaging in temporal lobe epilepsy surgery. *Arch Neurol* 1993;50:65–69.
6. Mosewich RK, So EL, O'Brien TJ, et al. Factors predictive of the outcome of frontal lobe epilepsy surgery. *Epilepsia* 2000;41:843–849.
7. Berkovic SF, McIntosh AM, Kalnins RM, et al. Preoperative MRI predicts outcome of temporal lobectomy: an actuarial analysis. *Neurology* 1995;45:1358–1363.
8. Bronen RA, Fulbright RK, Spencer DD, et al. Refractory epilepsy: comparison of MR imaging, CT, and histopathologic findings in 117 patients. *Radiology* 1996;201:97–105.
9. So EL. Role of neuroimaging in the management of seizure disorders. *Mayo Clin Proc* 2002;77:1251–1264.
10. Commission on Neuroimaging of the International League Against Epilepsy. Guidelines for neuroimaging evaluation of patients with uncontrolled epilepsy considered for surgery. *Epilepsia* 1998;39:1375–1376.
11. Commission on Neuroimaging of the International League Against Epilepsy. Recommendations for neuroimaging of patients with epilepsy. *Epilepsia* 1997;38:1255–1256.
12. Lee BI, Heo K, Kim JS, et al. Syndromic diagnosis at the epilepsy clinic: role of MRI in lobar epilepsies. *Epilepsia* 2002;43:496–504.
13. Wieshmann UC. Clinical application of neuroimaging in epilepsy. *J Neurol Neurosurg Psychiatry* 2003;74:466–470.
14. Kobayashi K, Ohtsuka Y, Oka E, et al. Primary and secondary bilateral synchrony in epilepsy: differentiation by estimation of interhemispheric small time differences during short spike-wave activity. *Electroencephalogr Clin Neurophysiol* 1992;83:93–103.
15. Grant PE, Barkovich AJ, Wald LL, et al. High-resolution surface-coil MR of cortical lesions in medically refractory epilepsy: a prospective study. *Am J Neuroradiol* 1997;18:291–301.
16. Wald LL, Carvajal L, Moyher SE, et al. Phased array detectors and an automated intensity-correction algorithm for high-resolution MR imaging of the human brain. *Magn Reson Med* 1995;34:433–439.
17. Duncan JS. Neuroimaging for epilepsy: quality and not just quantity is important. *J Neurol Neurosurg Psychiatry* 2002;73:612–613.
18. Von Oertzen J, Urbach H, Jungbluth S, et al. Standard magnetic resonance imaging is inadequate for patients with refractory focal epilepsy. *J Neurol Neurosurg Psychiatry* 2002;73:643–647.
19. Hardy SG, Miller JW, Holmes MD, et al. Factors predicting outcome of surgery for intractable epilepsy with pathologically verified mesial temporal sclerosis. *Epilepsia* 2003;44:565–568.
20. Jutila L, Immonen A, Mervaala E, et al. Long term outcome of temporal lobe epilepsy surgery: analyses of 140 consecutive patients. *J Neurol Neurosurg Psychiatry* 2002;73:486–494.
21. Kim JH, Tien RD, Felsberg GJ, et al. Fast spin-echo MR in hippocampal sclerosis: correlation with pathology and surgery. *Am J Neuroradiol* 1995;16:627–636.
22. Radhakrishnan K, So EL, Silbert PL, et al. Predictors of outcome of anterior temporal lobectomy for intractable epilepsy: a multivariate study. *Neurology* 1998;51:465–471.
23. Cendes F, Cook MJ, Watson C, et al. Frequency and characteristics of dual pathology in patients with lesional epilepsy. *Neurology* 1995;45:2058–2064.
24. Li LM, Cendes F, Andermann F, et al. Surgical outcome in patients with epilepsy and dual pathology. *Brain* 1999;122(Pt 5):799–805.
25. Sisodiya SM, Moran N, Free SL, et al. Correlation of widespread preoperative magnetic resonance imaging changes with unsuccessful surgery for hippocampal sclerosis. *Ann Neurol* 1997;41:490–496.
26. Ho SS, Kuzniecky RI, Gilliam F, et al. Temporal lobe developmental malformations and epilepsy: dual pathology and bilateral hippocampal abnormalities. *Neurology* 1998;50:748–754.
27. Mohamed A, Wyllie E, Ruggieri P, et al. Temporal lobe epilepsy due to hippocampal sclerosis in pediatric candidates for epilepsy surgery. *Neurology* 2001;56:1643–1649.
28. Lee DH, Gao FQ, Rogers JM, et al. MR in temporal lobe epilepsy: analysis with pathologic confirmation. *Am J Neuroradiol* 1998;19: 19–27.
29. Bronen RA, Gupta V. Epilepsy. In: Atlas SW, ed. *Magnetic resonance imaging of brain and spine,* 3rd ed. Philadelphia: Lippincott Williams & Wilkins, 2002:415–455.
30. Jackson GD, Kuzniecky RI, Cascino GD. Hippocampal sclerosis without detectable hippocampal atrophy. *Neurology* 1994;44: 42–46.
31. Cascino GD. Clinical correlations with hippocampal atrophy. *Magn Reson Imaging* 1995;13:1133–1136.
32. Jackson GD. The diagnosis of hippocampal sclerosis: other techniques. *Magn Reson Imaging* 1995;13:1081–1093.
33. Jackson GD, Berkovic SF, Duncan JS, et al. Optimizing the diagnosis of hippocampal sclerosis using MR imaging. *Am J Neuroradiol* 1993;14:753–762.
34. Jackson GD, Berkovic SF, Tress BM, et al. Hippocampal sclerosis can be reliably detected by magnetic resonance imaging. *Neurology* 1990;40:1869–1875.
35. Berkovic SF, Andermann F, Olivier A, et al. Hippocampal sclerosis in temporal lobe epilepsy demonstrated by magnetic resonance imaging. *Ann Neurol* 1991;29.175–182.
36. Kuzniecky R, de la Sayette V, Ethier R, et al. Magnetic resonance imaging in temporal lobe epilepsy: pathological correlations. *Ann Neurol* 1987;22:341–347.
37. Oppenheim C, Dormont D, Biondi A, et al. Loss of digitations of the hippocampal head on high-resolution fast spin-echo MR: a sign of mesial temporal sclerosis. *Am J Neuroradiol* 1998;19: 457–463.
38. Meiners LC, van Gils A, Jansen GH, et al. Temporal lobe epilepsy: the various MR appearances of histologically proven mesial temporal sclerosis. *Am J Neuroradiol* 1994;15:1547–1555.
39. Meiners LC, Witkamp TD, de Kort GA, et al. Relevance of temporal lobe white matter changes in hippocampal sclerosis.

Magnetic resonance imaging and histology. *Invest Radiol* 1999; 34:38–45.

40. Ryvlin P, Coste S, Hermier M, et al. Temporal pole MRI abnormalities in temporal lobe epilepsy. *Epileptic Disord* 2002;4(Suppl 1): S33–S39.
41. Bronen RA, Cheung G, Charles JT, et al. Imaging findings in hippocampal sclerosis: correlation with pathology. *Am J Neuroradiol* 1991;12:933–940.
42. Kim JH, Tien RD, Felsberg GJ, et al. Clinical significance of asymmetry of the fornix and mamillary body on MR in hippocampal sclerosis. *Am J Neuroradiol* 1995;16:509–515.
43. Cendes F, Andermann F, Gloor P, et al. Atrophy of mesial structures in patients with temporal lobe epilepsy: cause or consequence of repeated seizures? *Ann Neurol* 1993;34:795–801.
44. Moran NF, Lemieux L, Kitchen ND, et al. Extrahippocampal temporal lobe atrophy in temporal lobe epilepsy and mesial temporal sclerosis. *Brain* 2001;124:167–175.
45. Mamourian A. Incidental detection of hippocampal sclerosis. *Am J Neuroradiol* 1999;20:1575–1576.
46. Moore KR, Swallow CE, Tsuruda JS. Incidental detection of hippocampal sclerosis on MR images: is it significant? *Am J Neuroradiol* 1999;20:1609–1612.
47. Kim JA, Chung JI, Yoon PH, et al. Transient MR signal changes in patients with generalized tonicoclonic seizure or status epilepticus: periictal diffusion-weighted imaging. *Am J Neuroradiol* 2001; 22:1149–1160.
48. Sokol DK, Demyer WE, Edwards-Brown M, et al. From swelling to sclerosis: acute change in mesial hippocampus after prolonged febrile seizure. *Seizure* 2003;12:237–240.
49. Van Paesschen W, Duncan JS, Stevens JM, et al. Longitudinal quantitative hippocampal magnetic resonance imaging study of adults with newly diagnosed partial seizures: one-year follow-up results. *Epilepsia* 1998;39:633–639.
50. Sasaki M, Sone M, Ehara S, et al. Hippocampal sulcus remnant: potential cause of change in signal intensity in the hippocampus. *Radiology* 1993;188:743–746.
51. Yoneoka Y, Kwee IL, Fujii Y, et al. Criteria for normalcy of cavities observed within the adult hippocampus: high-resolution magnetic resonance imaging study on a 3.0-T system. *J Neuroimaging* 2002;12:231–235.
52. Chu WJ, Hetherington HP, Kuzniecky RI, et al. Lateralization of human temporal lobe epilepsy by 31P NMR spectroscopic imaging at 4.1 T. *Neurology* 1998;51:472–479.
53. Knowlton RC, Abou-Khalil B, Sawrie SM, et al. In vivo hippocampal metabolic dysfunction in human temporal lobe epilepsy. *Arch Neurol* 2002;59:1882–1886.
54. Kuzniecky R, Hetherington H, Pan J, et al. Proton spectroscopic imaging at 4.1 tesla in patients with malformations of cortical development and epilepsy. *Neurology* 1997;48:1018–1024.
55. Connelly A, Van Paesschen W, Porter DA, et al. Proton magnetic resonance spectroscopy in MRI-negative temporal lobe epilepsy. *Neurology* 1998;51:61–66.
56. Kuzniecky R, Hetherington H, Ho S, et al. Topiramate increases cerebral GABA in healthy humans. *Neurology* 1998;51:627–629.
57. Hetherington HP, Pan J, Jullie W, et al. 1H and 31P spectroscopy and bioenergetics in the lateralization of seizures in temporal lobe epilepsy. *J Magn Reson Imaging* 2002;16:477–483.
58. Cendes F, Caramanos Z, Andermann F, et al. Proton magnetic resonance spectroscopic imaging and magnetic resonance imaging volumetry in the lateralization of temporal lobe epilepsy: a series of 100 patients. *Ann Neurol* 1997;42:737–746.
59. Kuzniecky RI, Burgard S, Bilir E, et al. Qualitative MRI segmentation in mesial temporal sclerosis: clinical correlations. *Epilepsia* 1996;37:433–439.
60. Meiners LC, Scheffers JM, De Kort GA, et al. Curved reconstructions versus three-dimensional surface rendering in the demonstration of cortical lesions in patients with extratemporal epilepsy. *Invest Radiol* 2001;36:225–233.
61. Petroff OA, Errante LD, Kim JH, et al. N-acetyl-aspartate, total creatine, and myo-inositol in the epileptogenic human hippocampus. *Neurology* 2003;60:1646–1651.
62. Kuzniecky R, Palmer C, Hugg J, et al. Magnetic resonance spectroscopic imaging in temporal lobe epilepsy: neuronal dysfunction or cell loss? *Arch Neurol* 2001;58:2048–2053.

63. Kantarci K, Shin C, Britton JW, et al. Comparative diagnostic utility of 1H MRS and DWI in evaluation of temporal lobe epilepsy. *Neurology* 2002;58:1745–1753.
64. Woermann FG, Free SL, Koepp MJ, et al. Voxel-by-voxel comparison of automatically segmented cerebral gray matter—a rater-independent comparison of structural MRI in patients with epilepsy. *Neuroimage* 1999;10:373–384.
65. Kuzniecky R, Hugg JW, Hetherington H, et al. Relative utility of 1H spectroscopic imaging and hippocampal volumetry in the lateralization of mesial temporal lobe epilepsy. *Neurology* 1998; 51:66–71.
66. Sawrie SM, Martin RC, Knowlton R, et al. Relationships among hippocampal volumetry, proton magnetic resonance spectroscopy, and verbal memory in temporal lobe epilepsy. *Epilepsia* 2001;42:1403–1407.
67. Mueller SG, Suhy J, Laxer KD, et al. Reduced extrahippocampal NAA in mesial temporal lobe epilepsy. *Epilepsia* 2002;43:1210–1216.
68. Martin RC, Sawrie S, Hugg J, et al. Cognitive correlates of 1H MRSI-detected hippocampal abnormalities in temporal lobe epilepsy. *Neurology* 1999;53:2052–2058.
69. Castillo M, Smith JK, Kwock L. Proton MR spectroscopy in patients with acute temporal lobe seizures. *Am J Neuroradiol* 2001;22:152–157.
70. Lazeyras F, Blanke O, Zimine I, et al. MRI, (1)H-MRS, and functional MRI during and after prolonged nonconvulsive seizure activity. *Neurology* 2000;55:1677–1682.
71. Mueller SG, Kollias SS, Trabesinger AH, et al. Proton magnetic resonance spectroscopy characteristics of a focal cortical dysgenesis during status epilepticus and in the interictal state. *Seizure* 2001;10:518–524.
72. Park YD, Allison JD, Weiss KL, et al. Proton magnetic resonance spectroscopic observations of epilepsia partialis continua in children. *J Child Neurol* 2000;15:729–733.
73. Castillo M, Kwock L, Scatliff J, et al. Proton MR spectroscopy in neoplastic and non-neoplastic brain disorders. *Magn Reson Imaging Clin North Am* 1998;6:1–20.
74. Ende GR, Laxer KD, Knowlton RC, et al. Temporal lobe epilepsy: bilateral hippocampal metabolite changes revealed at proton MR spectroscopic imaging. *Radiology* 1997;202:809–817.
75. Otsubo H, Hoffman HJ, et al. Evaluation, surgical approach and outcome of seizure patients with gangliogliomas. *Pediatr Neurosurg* 1990;16:208–212.
76. Pan JW, Bebin EM, Chu WJ, et al. Ketosis and epilepsy: 31P spectroscopic imaging at 4.1 T. *Epilepsia* 1999;40:703–707.
77. Bronen RA, Anderson AW, Spencer DD. Quantitative MR for epilepsy: a clinical and research tool? *Am J Neuroradiol* 1994;15: 1157–1160.
78. Jack CR Jr, Sharbrough FW, Twomey CK, et al. Temporal lobe seizures: lateralization with MR volume measurements of the hippocampal formation. *Radiology* 1990;175:423–429.
79. Okujava M, Schulz R, Ebner A, et al. Measurement of temporal lobe T2 relaxation times using a routine diagnostic MR imaging protocol in epilepsy. *Epilepsy Res* 2002;48:131–142.
80. Duncan JS. Neuroimaging methods to evaluate the etiology and consequences of epilepsy. *Epilepsy Res* 2002;50:131–140.
81. Jack CR Jr, Sharbrough FW, Cascino GD, et al. Magnetic resonance image-based hippocampal volumetry: correlation with outcome after temporal lobectomy. *Ann Neurol* 1992;31:138–146.
82. Lee N, Tien RD, Lewis DV, et al. Fast spin-echo, magnetic resonance imaging-measured hippocampal volume: correlation with neuronal density in anterior temporal lobectomy patients. *Epilepsia* 1995;36:899–904.
83. Van Paesschen W, Connelly A, King MD, et al. The spectrum of hippocampal sclerosis: a quantitative magnetic resonance imaging study. *Ann Neurol* 1997;41:41–51.
84. Van Paesschen W, Revesz T, Duncan JS, et al. Quantitative neuropathology and quantitative magnetic resonance imaging of the hippocampus in temporal lobe epilepsy. *Ann Neurol* 1997;42: 756–766.
85. Fuerst D, Shah J, Shah A, et al. Hippocampal sclerosis is a progressive disorder: a longitudinal volumetric MRI study. *Ann Neurol* 2003;53:413–416.
86. Dale AM, Fischl B, Sereno MI. Cortical surface-based analysis, I: segmentation and surface reconstruction. *Neuroimage* 1999;9:179–194.

87. Fischl B, Salat DH, Busa E, et al. Whole brain segmentation: automated labeling of neuroanatomical structures in the human brain. *Neuron* 2002;33:341–355.

88. Jack CR Jr. Hippocampal T2 relaxometry in epilepsy: past, present, and future. *Am J Neuroradiol* 1996;17:1811–1814.

89. Jackson GD, Connelly A, Duncan JS, et al. Detection of hippocampal pathology in intractable partial epilepsy: increased sensitivity with quantitative magnetic resonance T2 relaxometry. *Neurology* 1993;43:1793–1799.

90. Duncan JS, Bartlett P, Barker GJ. Technique for measuring hippocampal T2 relaxation time. *Am J Neuroradiol* 1996;17:1805–1810.

91. von Oertzen J, Urbach H, Blumcke I, et al. Time-efficient T2 relaxometry of the entire hippocampus is feasible in temporal lobe epilepsy. *Neurology* 2002;58:257–264.

92. Woermann FG, Steiner H, Barker GJ, et al. A fast FLAIR dual-echo technique for hippocampal T2 relaxometry: first experiences in patients with temporal lobe epilepsy. *J Magn Reson Imaging* 2001;13:547–552.

93. Van Paesschen W, Sisodiya S, Connelly A, et al. Quantitative hippocampal MRI and intractable temporal lobe epilepsy. *Neurology* 1995;45:2233–2240.

94. Woermann FG, Barker GJ, Birnie KD, et al. Regional changes in hippocampal T2 relaxation and volume: a quantitative magnetic resonance imaging study of hippocampal sclerosis. *J Neurol Neurosurg Psychiatry* 1998;65:656–664.

95. Yoo SY, Chang KH, Song IC, et al. Apparent diffusion coefficient value of the hippocampus in patients with hippocampal sclerosis and in healthy volunteers. *Am J Neuroradiol* 2002;23:809–812.

96. Konermann S, Marks S, Ludwig T, et al. Presurgical evaluation of epilepsy by brain diffusion: MR-detected effects of flumazenil on the epileptogenic focus. *Epilepsia* 2003;44:399–407.

97. Hufnagel A, Weber J, Marks S, et al. Brain diffusion after single seizures. *Epilepsia* 2003;44:54–63.

98. Diehl B, Najm I, Ruggieri P, et al. Postictal diffusion-weighted imaging for the localization of focal epileptic areas in temporal lobe epilepsy. *Epilepsia* 2001;42:21–28.

99. Hogan RE, Bucholz RD, Choudhuri I, et al. Shape analysis of hippocampal surface structure in patients with unilateral mesial temporal sclerosis. *J Digit Imaging* 2000;13:39–42.

100. Wolf RL, Alsop DC, Levy-Reis I, et al. Detection of mesial temporal lobe hypoperfusion in patients with temporal lobe epilepsy by use of arterial spin labeled perfusion MR imaging. *Am J Neuroradiol* 2001;22:1334–1341.

101. Detre JA, Alsop DC. Perfusion magnetic resonance imaging with continuous arterial spin labeling: methods and clinical applications in the central nervous system. *Eur J Radiol* 1999;30:115–124.

102. Briellmann RS, Pell GS, Wellard RM, et al. MR imaging of epilepsy: state of the art at 1.5 T and potential of 3 T. *Epileptic Disord* 2003;5:3–20.

103. Engel J Jr. Overview: who should be considered a surgical candidate? In: *Surgical pathology of the nervous system and its coverings.* New York: Churchill Livingstone, 1991:23–26.

104. Kral T, Kuczaty S, Blumcke I, et al. Postsurgical outcome of children and adolescents with medically refractory frontal lobe epilepsies. *Childs Nerv Syst* 2001;17:595–601.

105. Li LM, Fish DR, Sisodiya SM, et al. High resolution magnetic resonance imaging in adults with partial or secondary generalised epilepsy attending a tertiary referral unit. *J Neurol Neurosurg Psychiatry* 1995;59:384–387.

106. Spencer DD, Spencer SS, Mattson RH, et al. Intracerebral masses in patients with intractable partial epilepsy. *Neurology* 1984;34:432–436.

107. Comair YG, Choi HY, Van Ness PC. Neocortical resections. In: Engel J Jr, ed. *Epilepsy. The comprehensive CD-ROM.* Philadelphia: Lippincott Williams & Wilkins, 1999:30170–30317.

108. Olivier A. Extratemporal resections. In: Engel J Jr, ed. *Surgical treatment of the epilepsies.* New York: Raven Press, 1993:489–500.

109. Daumas-Duport C, Scheithauer BW, Chodkiewicz JP, et al. Dysembryoplastic neuroepithelial tumor: a surgically curable tumor of young patients with intractable partial seizures. Report of thirty-nine cases. *Neurosurgery* 1988;23:545–556.

110. Daumas-Duport C, Varlet P, Bacha S, et al. Dysembryoplastic neuroepithelial tumors: nonspecific histological forms—a study of 40 cases. *J Neurooncol* 1999;41:267–280.

111. Fernandez C, Girard N, Paz Paredes A, et al. The usefulness of MR imaging in the diagnosis of dysembryoplastic neuroepithelial tumor in children: a study of 14 cases. *Am J Neuroradiol* 2003;24:829–834.

112. Hammond RR, Duggal N, Woulfe JM, et al. Malignant transformation of a dysembryoplastic neuroepithelial tumor. Case report. *J Neurosurg* 2000;92:722–725.

113. Koeller KK, Dillon WP. Dysembryoplastic neuroepithelial tumors: MR appearance. *Am J Neuroradiol* 1992;13:1319–1325.

114. Ostertun B, Wolf HK, Campos MG, et al. Dysembryoplastic neuroepithelial tumors: MR and CT evaluation. *Am J Neuroradiol* 1996;17:419–430.

115. Pasquier B, Peoc HM, Fabre-Bocquentin B, et al. Surgical pathology of drug-resistant partial epilepsy. A 10-year experience with a series of 327 consecutive resections. *Epileptic Disord* 2002;4:99–119.

116. Prayson RA. Bcl-2, bcl-x, and bax expression in dysembryoplastic neuroepithelial tumors. *Clin Neuropathol* 2000;19:57–62.

117. Raymond AA, Halpin SF, Alsanjari N, et al. Dysembryoplastic neuroepithelial tumor. Features in 16 patients. *Brain* 1994;117(Pt 3):461–475.

118. Morris HH, Matkovic Z, Estes ML, et al. Ganglioglioma and intractable epilepsy: clinical and neurophysiologic features and predictors of outcome after surgery. *Epilepsia* 1998;39:307–313.

119. Prayson RA, Estes ML, Morris HH. Coexistence of neoplasia and cortical dysplasia in patients presenting with seizures. *Epilepsia* 1993;34:609–615.

120. Prayson RA, Frater JL. Cortical dysplasia in extratemporal lobe intractable epilepsy: a study of 52 cases. *Ann Diagn Pathol* 2003;7:139–146.

121. Prayson RA, Khajavi K, Comair YG. Cortical architectural abnormalities and MIB1 immunoreactivity in gangliogliomas: a study of 60 patients with intracranial tumors. *J Neuropathol Exp Neurol* 1995;4:513–520.

122. Zentner J, Hufnagel A, Ostertun B, et al. Surgical treatment of extratemporal epilepsy: clinical, radiologic, and histopathologic findings in 60 patients. *Epilepsia* 1996;37:1072–1080.

123. Davies KG, Maxwell RE, Seljeskog E, et al. Pleomorphic xanthoastrocytoma—report of four cases, with MRI scan appearances and literature review. *Br J Neurosurg* 1994;8:681–689.

124. Lach B, Duggal N, DaSilva VF, et al. Association of pleomorphic xanthoastrocytoma with cortical dysplasia and neuronal tumors. A report of three cases. *Cancer* 1996;78:2551–2563.

125. Mascalchi M, Muscas GC, Galli C, et al. MRI of pleomorphic xanthoastrocytoma: case report. *Neuroradiology* 1994;36:446–447.

126. van Roost D, Kristof R, Zentner J, et al. Clinical, radiological, and therapeutic features of pleomorphic xanthoastrocytoma: report of three patients and review of the literature. *J Neurol Neurosurg Psychiatry* 1996;60:690–692.

127. Daumas-Duport C, Varlet P, Tucker ML, et al. Oligodendrogliomas. Part I: patterns of growth, histological diagnosis, clinical and imaging correlations: a study of 153 cases. *J Neurooncol* 1997;34:37–59.

128. Lee YY, Van Tassel P. Intracranial oligodendrogliomas: imaging findings in 35 untreated cases. *Am J Roentgenol* 1989;152:361–369.

129. Khajavi K, Comair YG, Wyllie E, et al. Surgical management of pediatric tumor-associated epilepsy. *J Child Neurol* 1999;14:15–25.

130. Luyken C, Blumcke I, Fimmers R, et al. The spectrum of long-term epilepsy-associated tumors: long-term seizure and tumor outcome and neurosurgical aspects. *Epilepsia* 2003;44:822–830.

131. Houtteville JP. Brain cavernoma: a dynamic lesion. *Surg Neurol* 1997;48:610–614.

132. Maggi G, Aliberti F, Ruggiero C, et al. Cerebral cavernous angiomas in critical areas. Reports of three cases in children. *J Neurosurg Sci* 1997;41:353–357.

133. Topper R, Jurgens E, Reul J, et al. Clinical significance of intracranial developmental venous anomalies. *J Neurol Neurosurg Psychiatry* 1999;67:234–238.

134. Heikkinen ER, Konnov B, Melnikov L, et al. Relief of epilepsy by radiosurgery of cerebral arteriovenous malformations. *Stereotact Funct Neurosurg* 1989;53:157–166.

135. Yeh HS, Tew JM Jr, Gartner M. Seizure control after surgery on cerebral arteriovenous malformations. *J Neurosurg* 1993;78:12–18.

136. Annegers JF, Coan SP. The risks of epilepsy after traumatic brain injury. *Seizure* 2000;9:453–457.

137. Kazemi NJ, So EL, Mosewich RK, et al. Resection of frontal encephalomalacias for intractable epilepsy: outcome and prognostic factors. *Epilepsia* 1997;38:670–677.

138. Wyllie E, Comair Y, Ruggieri P, et al. Epilepsy surgery in the setting of periventricular leukomalacia and focal cortical dysplasia. *Neurology* 1996;46:839–841.

139. Alsaadi TM, Bateman LM, Laxer KD, et al. Potentially misleading extratemporal lobe lesions in patients with temporal lobe epilepsy. *J Neurol Neurosurg Psychiatry* 2003;74:566–569.

140. Chiapparini L, Granata T, Farina L, et al. Diagnostic imaging in 13 cases of Rasmussen's encephalitis: can early MRI suggest the diagnosis? *Neuroradiology* 2003;45:171–183.

141. Granata T, Gobbi G, Spreafico R, et al. Rasmussen's encephalitis: early characteristics allow diagnosis. *Neurology* 2003;60:422–425.

142. Takeoka M, Kim F, Caviness VS Jr, et al. MRI volumetric analysis in Rasmussen encephalitis: a longitudinal study. *Epilepsia* 2003;44:247–251.

143. Marti-Bonmati L, Menor F, Poyatos C, et al. Diagnosis of Sturge-Weber syndrome: comparison of the efficacy of CT and MR imaging in 14 cases. *Am J Roentgenol* 1992;158:867–871.

144. Sugama S, Yoshimura H, Ashimine K, et al. Enhanced magnetic resonance imaging of leptomeningeal angiomatosis. *Pediatr Neurol* 1997;17:262–265.

145. Arzimanoglou AA, Andermann F, Aicardi J, et al. Sturge-Weber syndrome: indications and results of surgery in 20 patients. *Neurology* 2000;55:1472–1479.

146. Brodtkorb E, Nilsen G, Smevik O, et al. Epilepsy and anomalies of neuronal migration: MRI and clinical aspects. *Acta Neurol Scand* 1992;86:24–32.

147. Jackson GD. New techniques in magnetic resonance and epilepsy. *Epilepsia* 1994;35(Suppl 6):S2–13.

148. Raymond AA, Fish DR, Sisodiya SM, et al. Abnormalities of gyration, heterotopias, tuberous sclerosis, focal cortical dysplasia, microdysgenesis, dysembryoplastic neuroepithelial tumour and dysgenesis of the archicortex in epilepsy. Clinical, EEG and neuroimaging features in 100 adult patients. *Brain* 1995;118(Pt 3):629–660.

149. Robertson R, Caruso PA, Truwit CL, et al. Disorders of brain development. In: Atlas SW, ed. *Magnetic resonance imaging of the brain and spine*, 3rd ed. Philadelphia: Lippincott Williams & Wilkins, 2002.

150. Barkovich AJ, Kuzniecky RI, Dobyns WB, et al. A classification scheme for malformations of cortical development. *Neuropediatrics* 1996;27:59–63.

151. Flores-Sarnat L. Hemimegalencephaly. Part 1: genetic, clinical, and imaging aspects [discussion 384]. *J Child Neurol* 2002;17:373–384.

152. Pavone L, Curatolo P, Rizzo R, et al. Epidermal nevus syndrome: a neurologic variant with hemimegalencephaly, gyral malformation, mental retardation, seizures, and facial hemihypertrophy. *Neurology* 1991;41:266–271.

153. Devlin AM, Cross JH, Harkness W, et al. Clinical outcomes of hemispherectomy for epilepsy in childhood and adolescence. *Brain* 2003;126:556–566.

154. Carreno M, Wyllie E, Bingaman W, et al. Seizure outcome after functional hemispherectomy for malformations of cortical development. *Neurology* 2001;57:331–333.

155. Edwards JC, Wyllie E, Ruggeri PM, et al. Seizure outcome after surgery for epilepsy due to malformation of cortical development. *Neurology* 2000;55:1110–1114.

156. Barkovich AJ. Morphologic characteristics of subcortical heterotopia: MR imaging study. *Am J Neuroradiol* 2000;21:290–295.

157. Barkovich AJ. Subcortical heterotopia: a distinct clinicoradiologic entity. *Am J Neuroradiol* 1996;17:1315–1322.

158. Guerrini R, Carrozzo R. Epileptogenic brain malformations: clinical presentation, malformative patterns and indications for genetic testing. *Seizure* 2001;10:532–543.

159. Kato M, Dobyns WB. Lissencephaly and the molecular basis of neuronal migration. *Hum Mol Genet* 2003;12:R89–96.

160. Sisodiya SM. Surgery for malformations of cortical development causing epilepsy. *Brain* 2000;123(Pt 6):1075–1091.

161. Beltran-Valero de Bernabe D, Currier S, Steinbrecher A, et al. Mutations in the O-mannosyltransferase gene POMT1 give rise to the severe neuronal migration disorder Walker-Warburg syndrome. *Am J Hum Genet* 2002;71:1033–1043.

162. Dobyns WB, Patton MA, Stratton RF, et al. Cobblestone lissencephaly with normal eyes and muscle. *Neuropediatrics* 1996;27:70–75.

163. Barkovich AJ, Hevner R, Guerrini R. Syndromes of bilateral symmetrical polymicrogyria. *Am J Neuroradiol* 1999;20:1814–1821.

164. Chang BS, Piao X, Bodell A, et al. Bilateral frontoparietal polymicrogyria: clinical and radiological features in 10 families with linkage to chromosome 16. *Ann Neurol* 2003;53:596–606.

165. Piao X, Basel-Vanagaite L, Straussberg R, et al. An autosomal recessive form of bilateral frontoparietal polymicrogyria maps to chromosome 16q12.2-21. *Am J Hum Genet* 2002;70:1028–1033.

166. Urbach H, Scheffler B, Heinrichsmeier T, et al. Focal cortical dysplasia of Taylor's balloon cell type: a clinicopathological entity with characteristic neuroimaging and histopathological features, and favorable postsurgical outcome. *Epilepsia* 2002;43: 33–40.

167. Barkovich AJ, Kuzniecky RI, Bollen AW, et al. Focal transmantle dysplasia: a specific malformation of cortical development. *Neurology* 1997;49:1148–1152.

168. Lee SK, Choe G, Hong KS, et al. Neuroimaging findings of cortical dyslamination with cytomegaly. *Epilepsia* 2001;42: 850–856.

169. Kloss S, Pieper T, Pannek H, et al. Epilepsy surgery in children with focal cortical dysplasia (FCD): results of long-term seizure outcome. *Neuropediatrics* 2002;33:21–26.

170. Palmini A, Gambardella A, Andermann F, et al. Intrinsic epileptogenicity of human dysplastic cortex as suggested by corticography and surgical results. *Ann Neurol* 1995;37:476–487.

171. D'Agostino MD, Bernasconi A, Das S, et al. Subcortical band heterotopia (SBH) in males: clinical, imaging and genetic findings in comparison with females. *Brain* 2002;125:2507–2522.

172. Raymond AA, Fish DR, Stevens JM, et al. Subependymal heterotopia: a distinct neuronal migration disorder associated with epilepsy. *J Neurol Neurosurg Psychiatry* 1994;57:1195–1202.

173. Palmini A, Chandler C, Andermann F, et al. Resection of the lesion in patients with hypothalamic hamartomas and catastrophic epilepsy. *Neurology* 2002;58:1338–1347.

174. Rosenfeld JV. James IV lecture. Epilepsy surgery, hypothalamic hamartomas and the quest for a cure. *J R Coll Surg Edinb* 2002; 47:653–659.

175. Rosenfeld JV, Harvey AS, Wrennall J, et al. Transcallosal resection of hypothalamic hamartomas, with control of seizures, in children with gelastic epilepsy. *Neurosurgery* 2001;48: 108–118.

176. Unger F, Schrottner O, Feichtinger M, et al. Stereotactic radiosurgery for hypothalamic hamartomas. *Acta Neurochir Suppl* 2002; 84:57–63.

177. Palmini A, Gambardella A, Andermann F, et al. Operative strategies for patients with cortical dysplastic lesions and intractable epilepsy. *Epilepsia* 1994;35(Suppl 6):S57–71.

178. Flacke S, Wullner U, Keller E, et al. Reversible changes in echo planar perfusion- and diffusion-weighted MRI in status epilepticus. *Neuroradiology* 2000;42:92–95.

179. Oster J, Doherty C, Grant PE, et al. Diffusion-weighted imaging abnormalities in the splenium after seizures. *Epilepsia* 2003;44: 852–854.

180. Warach S, Levin JM, Schomer DL, et al. Hyperperfusion of ictal seizure focus demonstrated by MR perfusion imaging. *Am J Neuroradiol* 1994;15:965–968.

181. Bonmassar G, Purdon PL, Jaaskelainen IP, et al. Motion and ballistocardiogram artifact removal for interleaved recording of EEG and EPs during MRI. *Neuroimage* 2002;16:1127–1141.

182. Krakow K, Messina D, Lemieux L, et al. Functional MRI activation of individual interictal epileptiform spikes. *Neuroimage* 2001;13:502–505.

183. Schomer DL, Bonmassar G, Lazeyras F, et al. EEG-linked functional magnetic resonance imaging in epilepsy and cognitive neurophysiology. *J Clin Neurophysiol* 2000;17:43–58.

184. Seeck M, Lazeyras F, Michel CM, et al. Non-invasive epileptic focus localization using EEG-triggered functional MRI and

electromagnetic tomography. *Electroencephalogr Clin Neurophysiol* 1998;106:508–512.

185. Eriksson SH, Rugg-Gunn FJ, Symms MR, et al. Diffusion tensor imaging in patients with epilepsy and malformations of cortical development. *Brain* 2001;124:617–626.

186. Rugg-Gunn FJ, Eriksson SH, Symms MR, et al. Diffusion tensor imaging of cryptogenic and acquired partial epilepsies. *Brain* 2001;124:627–636.

187. Wieshmann UC, Clark CA, Symms MR, et al. Reduced anisotropy of water diffusion in structural cerebral abnormalities demonstrated with diffusion tensor imaging. *Magn Reson Imaging* 1999; 17:1269–1274.

188. Arfanakis K, Hermann BP, Rogers BP, et al. Diffusion tensor MRI in temporal lobe epilepsy. *Magn Reson Imaging* 2002;20:511–519.

189. Rugg-Gunn FJ, Eriksson SH, Boulby PA, et al. Magnetization transfer imaging in focal epilepsy. *Neurology* 2003;60:1638–1645.

190. Kennedy DN, Lange N, Makris N, et al. Gyri of the human neo-cortex: an MRI-based analysis of volume and variance. *Cereb Cortex* 1998;8:372–384.

191. Fischl B, Dale AM. Measuring the thickness of the human cerebral cortex from magnetic resonance images. *Proc Natl Acad Sci U S A* 2000;97:11050–11055.

192. Rosas HD, Liu AK, Hersch S, et al. Regional and progressive thinning of the cortical ribbon in Huntington's disease. *Neurology* 2002;58:695–701.

193. Sailer M, Fischl B, Salat D, et al. Focal thinning of the cerebral cortex in multiple sclerosis. *Brain* 2003;126:1734–1744.

194. Sisodiya SM, Fish DR, Shorvon SD. Increasing the yield from volumetric MRI in patients with epilepsy. *Magn Reson Imaging* 1995;13:1147–1152.

195. Bastos AC, Comeau RM, Andermann F, et al. Diagnosis of subtle focal dysplastic lesions: curvilinear reformatting from three-dimensional magnetic resonance imaging. *Ann Neurol* 1999;46: 88–94.

196. Knake SWL, Triantafyllou C, Stufflebeam S, et al. High-resolution surface-coil MRI in focal epilepsies—a prospective study at 3 T. 2003.

197. Dale AM, Halgren E. Spatiotemporal mapping of brain activity by integration of multiple imaging modalities. *Curr Opin Neurobiol* 2001;11:202–208.

198. Dale AM, Liu AK, Fischl BR, et al. Dynamic statistical parametric mapping: combining fMRI and MEG for high-resolution imaging of cortical activity. *Neuron* 2000;26:55–67.

199. Moore KR, Funke ME, Constantino T, et al. Magnetoencephalographically directed review of high-spatial-resolution surface-coil MR images improves lesion detection in patients with extratemporal epilepsy. *Radiology* 2002;225:880–887.

200. Zhang W, Simos PG, Ishibashi H, et al. Multimodality neuroimaging evaluation improves the detection of subtle cortical dysplasia in seizure patients. *Neurol Res* 2003;25:53–57.

The Intracarotid Amobarbital Procedure

75

Max R. Trenerry   David W. Loring

The preoperative evaluation of patients for epilepsy surgery typically includes electroencephalographic (EEG) monitoring, magnetic resonance imaging (MRI), neurologic examination, neuropsychological examination, and Wada (intracarotid amobarbital) testing. This chapter reviews Wada testing and its use in the evaluation of candidates for temporal lobectomy. A brief review of the history of Wada testing is followed by a discussion of Wada language and memory testing, use of the procedure in children, and attentional and emotional correlates.

HISTORY

The first attempt to functionally inactivate cerebral language regions pharmacologically was made by Gardiner (1), who injected procaine directly into the cerebral cortex before neurosurgical intervention. Harris and Snyder (2) provide a historical review of Gardiner's contributions to speech localization using this approach. Wada used intracarotid amobarbital injection to lateralize language before electroconvulsive treatment. Originally published in Japanese in 1949, Wada's seminal paper has been translated into English (3). Wada also describes initially using a carotid injection of amobarbital in a young boy with partial seizures, which is recounted in the historical context of postwar Japan (4). Wada later adapted this procedure to identify cerebral language laterality in candidates for epilepsy surgery while he was a Rockefeller Fellow at the Montreal Neurologic Institute (5). Milner and associates (6) subsequently modified the procedure to include a memory component to assess risk of postoperative amnesia and its relation to seizure onset laterality, likelihood of significant memory loss, and seizure outcome.

Concern about posttemporal lobectomy amnesia arose after experience at the Montreal Neurologic Institute with several early patients, including two who underwent bilateral temporal lobectomy (such as HM), as well as others with contralateral hippocampal lesions who underwent unilateral temporal lobectomy (7,8). The Wada test is used to functionally inactivate a single hemisphere; this allows the assessment of whether language and memory abilities are supported by the nonperfused contralateral hemisphere.

METHODOLOGY

Surveys of epilepsy surgery centers (9,10) suggest great procedural variability. In most approaches, however, a cerebral angiogram is conducted before Wada testing to evaluate cerebral vasculature, assess hemispheric cross-flow, verify a patent posterior communicating artery, and assess perfusion of the posterior cerebral artery. The importance of the angiogram becomes especially clear in the rare instance of a unilateral or bilateral persistent trigeminal artery, which often perfuses vital brainstem structures. Ordinarily, Wada testing should not be conducted when there is evidence of brainstem perfusion.

In most Wada procedures, patients hold their arms straight up in the air and begin counting. A bolus injection of an amobarbital solution, in saline or bacteriostatic water, is then administered into the internal carotid artery over a 4- to 5-second interval through a transfemoral catheter placed above the carotid bifurcation. Onset of contralateral arm paresis is readily evident, and disruption of automatic verbal activity (i.e., counting) typically provides the first indication of language dominance. Interruption of automatic activity, however, may be caused by the acute effect of the amobarbital bolus. Language is assessed and memory items are presented during the hemiparesis. Memory for information presented during the drug effect is evaluated on return to baseline, which usually occurs after approximately 10 minutes. The second hemisphere is usually perfused in a similar manner, although some centers wait 30 minutes between injections and others perform the second study on a different day.

Beyond these generalities, however, similarities between Wada procedures across various surgery centers are limited. Some centers use preinjection testing similar to that used during the procedure to obtain a detailed baseline. Other centers may use only preinjection hand strength as a means of gauging the hemiparesis. Use of the EEG is variable, and a wide range of stimuli are used for language and memory assessment. Moreover, the Wada test is not performed on all patients in some centers. For example, candidates for right temporal lobectomy who are right-handed and do not have ictal or postictal aphasia during EEG monitoring may not undergo Wada testing at some centers. The amobarbital dose also has been reported to vary from center to center, from about 70 mg to as high as 225 mg per injection (9), although there is a more recent trend toward lower dosing.

LANGUAGE ASSESSMENT

Criteria for determining language dominance vary across centers; this limits comparability of study results. Snyder and colleagues (10) found that centers reporting 10% to 60% impairment versus those reporting 0% to 6% used different criteria to detect speech or language impairment. Centers reporting low prevalence of mixed-hemisphere language representation generally did not use criteria involving production of partial phonemes, impairment of serial rote speech, or impaired ability to express familiar words. Ability to name objects, however, was used to determine speech lateralization by more than 90% of the responding centers in the Snyder survey (10). Six or more objects are usually presented for naming during amobarbital-induced hemiparesis. Estimates are in general agreement that 90% or more of right-handed individuals are left-hemisphere language dominant (11,12).

Benson (11) reviewed studies of aphasia in left- and right-handed persons after various types of left- or right-hemisphere insult (e.g., surgical, traumatic). Thirty-two percent of the non–right-handed patients developed aphasia after left-hemisphere insult, whereas 60% of right-handed patients developed aphasia after left-hemisphere insult. Twenty-four percent of the non–right-handed patients developed language disorders after right-hemisphere insult, and only 2% of right-handed patients developed aphasia after right-hemisphere insult. Mixed language dominance has been reported in 0% to 60% of temporal lobectomy patients, with about half of the epilepsy surgery centers in one survey reporting a 0% to 20% incidence (10). In one series, two of 103 patients evaluated with Wada testing had exclusive right-hemisphere language,

and another 22 patients had bilateral representation (13). Language representation was asymmetric in 17 of the 22 patients with bilateral language, and 13 of these had more left- than right-hemisphere representation. Exclusive right-hemisphere language, therefore, seems to be relatively rare, a finding supported by functional MRI studies (14). Language representation might best be conceptualized as a continuous rather than a dichotomous variable (13).

Two other studies (15,16) describe the results of Wada language lateralization testing in groups of 368 and 167 epilepsy surgery patients. Risse and coworkers (16) reported that, of 304 right-handed patients, 87% were left-hemisphere language dominant and 13% had right or bilateral representation. Of 64 left-handed patients, 62% were left-hemisphere language dominant and 38% had right or bilateral language representation. Similarly, Helmstaedter and colleagues (15) found that 82% of 137 right-handed patients had left-hemisphere language dominance and 18% had "atypical" dominance. However, only 30% of 30 left-handed patients had left-hemisphere language dominance; the other 70% had atypical language dominance (15). This apparent difference may be caused by sample composition, as Risse and associates may have included more nontemporal surgical candidates in their group; alternatively, it may be related to differences in classification systems (16). Both reports indicated that right-hemisphere language dominance is associated with early onset of seizures, injury, or lesion in the left hemisphere. Women with left-hemisphere ictal onset are more likely to have atypical language representation (17).

There is generally good agreement between language results of Wada testing and operative or extraoperative cortical language mapping (18–20). Both hemispheres, however, are rarely studied with stimulation mapping, which severely limits opportunities to compare stimulation with amobarbital data.

The rate and pattern of language and memory recovery after sodium amobarbital injection are potential confounding factors that affect interpretation. Ravdin and associates (21) reported on the serial recovery of language in candidates for right (15) and left (22) temporal lobectomy. After injection in the language-dominant hemisphere, "intelligible vocalization" occurred on average at 3 minutes 27 seconds. Paraphasias were common, and language function returned to baseline in a stereotyped order. Average time for return of naming ability was 8 minutes 29 seconds; average time to comprehension return was 9 minutes 58 seconds; and average recovery of repetition ability was 12 minutes 30 seconds. Thirty-six of the 39 patients with left-hemisphere language dominance were initially mute, and 28 of the 39 recovered language in the order presented above, with some variation of order in the other 11 patients.

Morris and colleagues (23) studied language and memory recovery during the Wada test in 49 patients with left-hemisphere language dominance who were candidates for temporal lobectomy; doses averaged 120 mg. Language began to recover rapidly within about 3 minutes after injection of the language-dominant hemisphere. Language testing included reading words, naming line drawings, and responding to faces. Capacity to encode and later recognize the same items, however, was not associated with the language impairment. The investigators concluded that induced aphasia does not significantly affect recognition memory, even though patients may not be able to name or read stimulus items. A separate study (24) reported similar findings. In general, there is a tendency to perform more poorly when the language-dominant hemisphere is perfused, and some centers employ an "aphasia correction" when calculating memory results in the language-dominant hemisphere. However, this correction does not necessarily improve diagnostic accuracy (25).

WADA MEMORY TESTING

Memory testing was added to the Wada test for language lateralization to provide information about the risk of profound postoperative amnesia. The Wada memory test was not originally intended to predict risk for degrees of memory decline after temporal lobectomy, but it has gradually assumed this purpose. Most Wada protocols involve presentation of objects, photographs, or line drawings during the induced hemiparesis; the patient is asked to recall this information after neurologic status has returned to baseline. This usually occurs in about 10 minutes. An exception is the University of Washington protocol, which requires patients to name items and, after a brief interference task, to recall the item that had just been displayed (26).

Wada memory results have been used to aid in confirming seizure onset laterality, to predict postoperative seizure control, and to predict memory outcome. The underlying assumption is that pharmacologic ablation of an abnormal hippocampus, which supports only limited memory function, will result in little change in the ability to recall material presented during hemispheric anesthesia. Chelune (27) has conceptualized this in terms of determining the functional reserve of the contralateral hippocampus and the functional adequacy of the hippocampus ipsilateral to seizure onset in candidates for temporal lobectomy.

CRITICISM OF WADA MEMORY TESTING

The capacity of Wada testing to determine risk for memory decline has been debated. In one series (28), 10 patients who performed poorly on Wada testing underwent anterior temporal lobectomy without becoming amnestic and experienced improved seizure control. This suggests that some patients could needlessly be denied surgery if the Wada test were the only measure of the contralateral hemisphere's ability to sustain memory function.

The capacity of a Wada procedure to test mesial temporal function has been criticized. Dasheiff and coworkers (29) reported that patients with frontal lobe or generalized epilepsy had poorer Wada performances than temporal lobectomy patients. They suggested that this is contrary to expectation if the Wada test, in fact, measures mesial temporal function. Yet these findings are consistent with temporal lobectomy patients having greater mesial temporal dysfunction than patients with frontal generalized epilepsy. Temporary amobarbital ablation of neurocognitive function supported by abnormal mesial temporal structures in patients with temporal lobe epilepsy should result in little compromise or change of memory function during Wada testing. Ablation of healthier mesial temporal structures in patients with frontal generalized epilepsy would result in greater Wada memory test deficits.

A large number of independently conducted studies support the validity of Wada testing, typically based on comparison of hemispheric memory asymmetry, to lateralize pathology consistent with the hemisphere of ictal onset (24–26,30–44). Although these reports support the validity of the Wada test in lateralizing cerebral pathology in candidates for epilepsy surgery, particularly temporal lobectomy, differences in Wada protocols involving stimulus presentation and amobarbital dosage confound direct comparison of these studies. Wada testing has been reported to correctly classify 45% to 75% of patients with left temporal epilepsy and 67% to 79% of patients with right temporal epilepsy. Patients with right temporal epilepsy have been more accurately identified in these studies; incorrect classification ranges from about 6% to 11% for patients with left temporal epilepsy and from 4% to 9% for patients with right temporal epilepsy (31,35,36).

Interestingly, two studies address the meaning of nonlateralizing Wada tests. Swearer and associates (44) reported on 23 patients with temporal lobe epilepsy, 19 of whom underwent surgery. The four patients who did not have surgery were considered poor candidates because bihemispheric seizures occurred during intracranial monitoring. These four patients had a significantly lower difference between their Wada memory scores than the other patients, and the authors proposed that lack of a significant Wada memory asymmetry suggests bihemispheric onset. Hamberger and colleagues (34) reported on 20 patients with lateral or neocortical onset and 22 patients with mesiobasal-onset temporal lobectomy. Histopathologic analysis, intracranial EEG, or presence of a temporal neocortical lesion was used to determine region of ictal onset. The investigators correctly classified 18 of the 22 patients with mesial temporal onset and seven of the 10 patients with lateral cortical onset. The patients with lateral onset had a significantly smaller memory asymmetry than the patients with mesial onset. Taken together, these studies further support the notion that Wada test memory asymmetries are associated with mesial temporal pathology and ictal onset in candidates for temporal lobectomy and that lack of asymmetry is associated with a nonmesial temporal region of onset.

Several investigations have demonstrated that Wada memory performance is associated with the nature and extent of pathology. Rausch and coworkers (45) found that Wada memory performance was associated with the extent of hippocampal neuronal loss, which was measured as a composite of cell counts across five hippocampal regions. Sass and colleagues (46) demonstrated that temporal lobectomy patients with poor memory performance after injection of the hemisphere contralateral to the seizure focus had lower cell counts in the CA3 hippocampal subfield. CA3 hippocampal cell counts also correlated with the amount of information recalled following contralateral amobarbital injection.

Davies and associates (32) reported on their experience with Wada testing in 30 temporal lobectomy patients with adequate Wada, MRI, and histopathologic results. They demonstrated that recognition memory was asymmetric by comparing right and left hemisphere injections; a difference of at least ±2 (of a possible 8) occurred in 73% of the patients. Lateralization was correct in 91% of the 22 patients; two cases were incorrectly lateralized, and eight patients had indeterminate asymmetry scores. Quantitative MRI hippocampal volumes and T2 values are correlated with Wada memory asymmetry scores (30,47). Baxendale and coworkers (30) studied data from 48 patients with temporal lobe epilepsy and they found that unilateral Wada memory scores were not correlated with individual hippocampal volumes or T2. However, a significant correlation was shown in the difference between hippocampal volumes or T2 and the difference between Wada memory scores.

Amobarbital injection by way of the internal carotid artery has also been criticized because that vascular distribution does not supply the posterior three fourths of the hippocampus in most patients (48,49). Hart and colleagues (50) used technetium ^{99m}Tc-hexamethyl-propyleneamine oxime (HMPAO) single-photon-emission computed tomography (SPECT) to study the distribution of amobarbital delivered through the internal carotid artery. The distribution of amobarbital was unpredictable. A review of SPECT films demonstrated perfusion of regions by amobarbital that were not shown on angiographic films. These authors also found that medial temporal regions were perfused by amobarbital in only 28% of the patients studied. They proposed that both medial and lateral temporal regions play a role in memory and proposed that a tracer such as HMPAO accompany amobarbital injection. Use of combined ^{99m}Tc-HMPAO SPECT and amobarbital demonstrated that mesial temporal structures were rarely perfused and suggested that hippocampal function may not be affected during intracarotid amobarbital injection (51). Castillo and colleagues (52) reported that SPECT results were not associated with Wada test performance and so did not alter interpretation. Soucy and associates (53) also noted a lack of correlation between SPECT-determined perfusion and recall of information learned during Wada testing.

In a well-designed study, Morton and colleagues (38) showed that temporal lobectomy patients who demonstrated filling of the posterior cerebral artery on internal carotid angiography had a larger Wada memory deficit; this effect was greater for right-hemisphere injection. Significant posterior cerebral artery filling on angiography may alter Wada test interpretation; more conservative interpretive criteria could be used if posterior cerebral artery filling were absent, more liberal criteria, if it were present.

Electrographic data have supported functional hippocampal inactivation during Wada testing. Gotman and colleagues (54) found hippocampal EEG slowing from depth electrodes on the injected side that persisted along with electrographic changes in other portions of the injected hemisphere. Intracarotid injection of amobarbital may therefore effectively denervate the hippocampus, even though that structure is not directly perfused. Ahern and associates (55) noted bilateral but asymmetric EEG changes during intracarotid testing, regardless of whether the side of seizure onset or the contralateral hemisphere was injected. EEG changes were maximal in the injected hemisphere. These investigators suggested that the EEG changes in the noninjected hemisphere result from cessation of neuronal input from the injected regions, a position similar to that of Gotman and colleagues (54). The Ahern team also suggested sequentially injecting each hemisphere by way of the internal carotid artery and comparing the memory results from each study (55).

McMackin and associates (22) studied the relationship between depth-recorded EEG and HMPAO SPECT in 10 patients undergoing Wada testing. HMPAO was injected 25 to 30 seconds after injection of amobarbital, and the SPECT scan was coregistered with MRI. An equal regional cerebral blood flow change in anterior and posterior hippocampal regions was observed on SPECT, although only three patients had posterior cerebral artery filling on angiographic studies. Delta activity increased and regional cerebral blood flow decreased during the amobarbital injection. These findings are consistent with those of Gotman and colleagues (54). Both anterior and posterior hippocampal regions undergo deafferentation with internal carotid amobarbital injection, as demonstrated by the reduced blood flow there despite lack of direct posterior cerebral perfusion.

The degree of sedation is also associated with memory performance. Greater impairment of consciousness evaluated with a modified Glasgow Coma Scale was associated with poorer recognition memory in 97 patients and was most prominent following left-hemisphere injections and injections contralateral to the seizure focus (56). It has been argued that this effect occurs when the dominant cerebral hemisphere is injected (57).

SUPPORT FOR PREDICTION OF MEMORY OUTCOME AND SEIZURE CONTROL OUTCOME

Multiple studies support the Wada test's validity for predicting of postoperative memory change. Jones-Gotman (58) reported that temporal lobectomy patients who performed poorly on Wada testing at the Montreal Neurologic Institute had poorer memory outcomes than patients whose results suggested memory support by the contralateral (unoperated) hemisphere. However, Wyllie and colleagues (59) found that failure to recall more than 67% of information presented during amobarbital perfusion of the intended operative hemisphere was not significantly associated with poorer postoperative memory. Comparison of ipsilateral with contralateral Wada memory performances yielded a trend suggesting that patients with lower ipsilateral Wada memory performances were at greater risk for memory decline. Postoperative memory may not be associated with unilateral Wada memory performance from either left- or right-hemisphere injection alone. Asymmetric Wada memory performance based on comparison of the ipsilateral and contralateral hemisphere injections, however, may predict verbal memory decline following left temporal lobectomy (60). Lee and colleagues (61) reported that Wada memory asymmetries, regardless of their magnitude, predict seizure control 12 months after surgery in children who undergo temporal or nontemporal procedures.

As discussed, Wada memory testing may also aid in lateralizing seizure onset. Alpherts and coworkers (62) reported correct lateralization of ictal onset in 85% of patients with various neuropathologies. Consequently, some patients with EEG patterns that suggest a lateralized seizure onset, but who also have some inconsistencies in their evaluations may be spared invasive monitoring with depth electrodes if strong Wada memory asymmetries are present. Timing of memory stimulus presentation after amobarbital injection influences recall performance; recall for items presented shortly after injection was better for lateralizing the side of seizure onset than was recall for items presented after partial return of language function (37,63). Wada memory test asymmetries (ipsilateral/contralateral), which are based on comparison of memory performance after each injection, are related to postoperative seizure control (40,43,64,65). The type of stimuli used in memory testing is also important. Use of real objects is better than use of line drawings for lateralizing seizure onset (24,36,66). The Wada test was not useful in predicting postoperative seizure control in patients with ganglioglioma (67).

Bilateral Wada testing may not be essential. Soucy and colleagues (53) reported that temporal lobectomy candidates had poorer recall for information learned during the injection of the hemisphere contralateral to seizure onset. The contralateral injection has also been shown to predict postoperative verbal memory change in these patients (68).

WADA TESTING WITH CHILDREN

Invasive procedures in children present special medical— and often behavioral—management problems. Hinz and associates (18) demonstrated that Wada testing and intraoperative mapping results are similar to language lateralization findings. However, mapping was accomplished only for the operated hemisphere. Wada testing methods for children have been described in detail (18,19,69). These protocols used a baseline assessment before the study. While many adult Wada protocols include baseline assessment, it is more important in young children to familiarize them with the procedure and reduce their anxiety. Szabo and Wyllie (69) and Williams and Rausch (19) also simplified the protocol items on the basis of baseline assessment. Doses were frequently reduced for many patients in these reports and ranged from 50 to 125 mg per injection (18,19,69). Williams and Rausch (19) gave less amobarbital to children 13 years of age or younger (mean, 90.28 mg) than to older children (119.74 mg).

Szabo and Wyllie (69) suggested that children with an intelligence quotient below 70 may perform poorly on Wada testing. Williams and Rausch (19) reported that children 13 years or younger were more likely to fail testing during the ipsilateral (with respect to seizure onset) testing, regardless of the amobarbital dosage. They also noted that injection of the hemisphere contralateral to the seizure focus was likely to produce memory failure (recollection or recognition of less than 67% of memory stimuli on return to baseline), regardless of age or language dominance. This latter finding enhances the validity of the procedure for lateralizing seizure onset. Poor Wada test performance should be expected after injection of the contralateral, and relatively healthier, hemisphere compared with the hemisphere ipsilateral to the seizure onset.

Discussing problems in anesthesia management during pediatric Wada testing, Binner and coworkers (70) described a 16-year-old boy who was anesthetized with alfentanil and propofol during placement of the femoral catheter. The fast-acting anesthetics allowed the patient to return to neurologic baseline in only about 5 minutes, so that testing could proceed without additional medication side effects. This strategy may be useful in younger or more apprehensive children; however, the patient, may derive more benefit from the use of a pediatric psychologist to administer behavioral interventions designed to reduce anxiety and discomfort and increase the child's sense of being able to cope with the situation (3,71). Reporting the results of a multicenter study, Lee and associates (61) noted that, in general, children under 10 years of age were given less amobarbital, but this policy varied somewhat across centers. Wada memory performance was best after amobarbital injection of the side of ictal onset in patients undergoing temporal and nontemporal surgeries.

ATTENTION AND EMOTION

Attention

Effects on cognitive functions in addition to language and memory have been studied during Wada testing (72,73). At the Medical College of Georgia, patients were trained to perform a nonverbal tactile attention task and were then evaluated by means of this task during Wada testing. Inattention and extinction occurred more often after amobarbital injection of the right internal carotid artery. The investigators concluded that suppressed function of either hemisphere can result in contralateral neglect but that the right hemisphere has greater capacity to direct attention toward the contralateral hemispace (72).

Several reports (74–76) have described anosognosia—the inability to recognize the presence of a deficit—after Wada testing. This defect tends to be seen more often in patients with trauma to the right hemisphere. Gilmore and colleagues (76) used methohexital, rather than amobarbital, for Wada testing of eight consecutive patients. All the patients recalled right hemiparesis after injection of methohexital into the left internal carotid artery; none recalled the induced left hemiparesis that followed the injection into the right internal carotid artery. Failure to recall weakness after right-hemisphere Wada testing may not represent a generalized memory failure but instead may demonstrate a hemisphere-specific memory deficit (76).

Durkin and colleagues (75) described on 115 left-hemisphere language-dominant patients who underwent Wada testing with amobarbital. Over three fourths reported no unilateral weakness after either left or right injection. Among the patients who reported only left or right hemiparesis, 74% recalled the effect after left internal carotid injection and 26%, after right internal carotid injection. Thus, these data provide some support for the Gilmore findings. The Durkin group suggests that this is because they used longer-acting amobarbital rather than methohexital. In a follow-up study to the Gilmore report, Adair and associates (74) noted anosognosia after 30 of 31 right internal carotid injections and after 15 of 31 left internal carotid injections ($p < 0.001$). Confabulation does not appear to explain anosognosia for hemiparesis (77).

Emotion

Cerebral localization of emotion has been controversial. Some investigators have reported that lesions in the language-dominant hemisphere produced symptoms of depression, but others suggest that the nondominant hemisphere modulates affective behavior (78–82). Ahern and Schwartz (83) proposed that posterior right-hemisphere regions are involved in emotional perception and that frontal regions are differentially lateralized with regard to involvement in emotional expression. Specifically, they posited that the left hemisphere has a greater role in expression of positive emotion, whereas the right hemisphere is involved in expression of negative affect.

In another study (84), 59% of 44 epilepsy surgery patients had changes in emotional expression during Wada testing. Slightly more euphoric reactions (laughter and elevated mood) followed right-hemisphere (44%) than left-hemisphere (32%) injection. Crying was more likely after left-hemisphere injection.

Difficulty in rating photographs of faces depicting positive, negative, or neutral emotions increased after non-dominant-hemisphere injection (85). Wada testing was also found to influence the internal affective state (77). Self-rated mood was lower with inactivation of the left hemisphere than during right-hemisphere injection, when no change was reported. The latter result might appear strange in view of previous reports that euphoric affect is more likely during right-hemisphere inactivation. However, the Ahern study (78) used patient self-reporting without observer assessments. Given the data on anosognosia during and after right-hemisphere injection, it may be that patients generally cannot recognize changes in their mood during amobarbital injection into the right hemisphere.

MEDICAL COLLEGE OF GEORGIA WADA PROTOCOL: CLINICAL CORE

Aided by a neurologist, the neuropsychologist conducts the Wada test immediately after cerebral angiography; both hemispheres are studied on the same day.

Patients count repeatedly from 1 to 20 with hands raised, palms turned rostrally, and fingers spread. A 100-mg injection of amobarbital sodium is administered by hand over 4 to 5 seconds through a percutaneous transfemoral catheter. After demonstration of hemiplegia and evaluation of eye-gaze deviation, the patient executes a simple midline command (e.g., "touch your nose"). Beginning approximately 30 to 45 seconds after the injection, eight common objects are presented for 4 to 8 seconds each, and the object names are repeated twice to the patient. Examples of the Wada memory items include ordinary household objects (e.g., fork, mousetrap), small toys (e.g., troll doll), and plastic food (e.g., hot dog, pizza). If confusion, inattention, or nonresponsiveness occurs, the patient's eyes may be held open. After presentation of memory items, language is assessed in detail.

Recognition memory of material presented during the procedure is tested after the effects of amobarbital have worn off, as demonstrated by a return to baseline language performance on all tasks (described below), return of 5/5 strength, and absence of pronator drift, asterixis, and bradykinesia.

Language

Language rating is based on performance of five linguistic tasks (counting disruption, comprehension, naming, repetition, and reading). Our formal approach to calculating a language laterality ratio is for research purposes and is not routinely used clinically.

Expressive Language/Counting

The expressive language score (0 to 4) is based on disruption of counting ability at the initiation of the Wada test (4 = normal, slowed, or brief pause of approximately 20 seconds or less; 3 = counting perseveration with normal sequencing; 2 = sequencing errors; 1 = single number or word perseveration; 0 = arrest of more than 20 seconds). We chose this duration of speech arrest to ensure that a counting interruption is not caused by the medication's acute generalized disruptive effects. If speech arrest occurs, patients are repeatedly urged to begin counting again starting with "1," as the more overlearned portion of the sequence will be less likely disrupted from medication effects. Speech arrest by itself is a poor measure of language laterality (86).

Comprehension

Initially, the patient executes a simple midline command (e.g., "open your mouth"). After presentation of the object memory stimulus, a modified token test is used for more systematic testing. The token test consists of four geometric shapes of different colors that are presented vertically to the subject's ipsilateral visual field. The rating is based on the level of syntactic complexity in the correctly executed command: (1) "point to the red circle after the green square"; (2) "point to the red circle and then point to the green square"; (3) "point to the red triangle." A score of 3 is awarded for completion of the complex two-stage command with inverted syntax, a score of 2 for the successful simple two-stage command, 1 for the one-stage command, and 0 if the subject could not perform any commands.

Confrontation Naming

Two line drawings of common objects (e.g., watch, jacket) are presented, and the subject is asked to name the objects and their parts (e.g., watchband, collar). Performance is qualitatively scored on a 0- to 3-point scale.

Repetition

After object naming, the patient repeats phrases (e.g., "No ifs, ands, or buts"), and the repetition is graded on a scale of 0 to 3. If unable to provide any response, the patient is asked to repeat "Mary had a little lamb."

Reading

Patients are asked to read either "The car backed over the curb" or "The rabbit hopped down the lane." Performance is rated on a scale of 0 to 3.

General Language Considerations

When language impairments are present, language stimuli are presented throughout the recovery phase to monitor drug effects, and the time of complete language recovery is noted. The same stimuli as used in the initial assessment, or alternative stimuli, are used, except for repetition. Additional repetition items such as "Methodist-Episcopal" and sentences from the Boston Diagnostic Aphasia Examination (e.g., "The spy fled to Greece") are used to monitor recovery, because repetition is a highly sensitive measure of mild language impairment. Positive paraphasic responses are considered the strongest evidence of language representation in the hemisphere being studied.

Memory

After amobarbital injection, a minimum of 10 minutes is required before memory testing. Although free recall of object memory stimuli may be obtained, interpretation of Wada memory performance is based solely on object recognition.

Ipsilateral Performance

The eight objects are presented randomly, interspersed with 16 foils, and a forced-choice recognition is obtained. A correction of one-half the number of false-positive responses is subtracted from the number of objects correctly recognized to correct for possible response bias and guessing. Thus, the expected score in the absence of true recognition would be 0.

Laterality Scores

Because Wada memory scores assist in lateralizing seizure onset by demonstrating lateralized dysfunction, the order of injection is randomized across subjects and memory results are interpreted in a blinded fashion. To assess lateralized asymmetries, interhemispheric Wada memory difference scores (i.e., left injection score minus right injection score) derived from corrected memory performances are computed; positive scores suggest left temporal lobe dysfunction and negative scores, right temporal lobe impairment.

General Memory Considerations

Fixed pass/fail criteria are not used for memory performance after injection ipsilateral to the seizure onset. In general, however, if a score is lower than two of eight correct, the Wada memory assessment is repeated; scores of at least three are preferred. Interhemispheric performance asymmetries of at least two are interpreted as evidence of lateralized impairment, although greater asymmetries are interpreted with more confidence. As with the ipsilateral performance, the asymmetry scores are not absolute, and memory performance is always considered in the context of other clinical factors, including consistency of seizure onset, presence of a structural lesion such as tumor, and hippocampal atrophy shown on MRI. Asymmetries in the "wrong" direction are cause for particular concern. In these cases, the procedure may be repeated bilaterally with a 75-mg dose, beginning on the side ipsilateral to the presumed seizure onset.

SUMMARY

Wada testing has been a standard part of temporal lobectomy evaluation since the early 1960s. The procedure was initially used to lateralize language function but was soon modified to assess risk for postoperative amnesia. Its use has now evolved to predict degrees of memory decline. Numerous studies support the validity of Wada testing for lateralization of pathologic findings in temporal lobectomy patients. The validity of Wada test results has also been supported by correlations between Wada memory performance and hippocampal pyramidal cell loss or MRI-determined hippocampal volumes. The Wada test predicts seizure control and memory outcome after temporal lobectomy and has also been used to study emotion and attention. Interpretation of Wada memory data could be influenced by the nature and extent of the pathology and the degree of sedation during testing. Although there is evidence that a large posterior cerebral artery may alter memory performance, perfusion of the hippocampus by way of the posterior cerebral artery is not necessary for valid Wada memory testing. The Wada test lateralizes seizure onset and predicts postoperative seizure control and the degree of verbal memory decline after left temporal lobectomy. It remains to be seen, however, whether Wada memory performance and data from other sources such as MRI, ictal SPECT, positron emission tomography, or functional MRI are redundant or independently contribute to diagnosis and treatment.

ACKNOWLEDGMENTS

Portions of this chapter are reprinted from Trenerry MR, Loring DW. Intracarotid amobarbital procedure: the Wada test. In: Latchaw R, Jack CR Jr, eds. *Neuroimaging clinics of North America.* Philadelphia: WB Saunders. 1995. This work was supported by NIH grant NS28374 awarded to C. R. Jack, Jr.

REFERENCES

1. Gardiner WJ. Injection of procaine into the brain to locate speech area in left-handed persons. *Arch Neurol Psychiatry* 1941;46: 1035–1038.
2. Harris LJ, Snyder PJ. Cerebral anesthesia for localization of speech: the contribution of W. James Gardner. *Brain Lang* 1997;56:377–396.
3. Wada J. Clinical experimental observations of carotid artery injections of sodium amytal. *Brain Cogn* 1997;33:211–213.
4. Wada J. Youthful season revisited. *Brain Cogn* 1997;33:7–10.
5. Wada J, Rasmussen T. Intracarotid injection of sodium amytal for the lateralization of cerebral speech dominance: experimental and clinical observations. *J Neurosurg* 1960;17:266–282.
6. Milner B, Branch C, Rasmussen T. Study of short-term memory after intracarotid injection of sodium amytal. *Trans Am Neurol Assoc* 1962;87:224–226.
7. Penfield W, Mathieson G. Memory: autopsy findings and comments on the role of the hippocampus in experimental recall. *Arch Neurol* 1974;31:145–154.
8. Penfield W, Milner B. Memory deficit produced by bilateral lesions in the hippocampal zone. *Arch Neurol Psychiatry* 1958;79: 475–497.
9. Rausch R. Psychological evaluation. In: Engel J Jr, ed. *Surgical treatment of the epilepsies.* New York, NY: Raven Press, 1987: 181–195.
10. Snyder PJ, Novelly RA, Harris LJ. Mixed speech dominance in the intracarotid sodium amytal procedure: validity and criteria issues. *J Clin Exp Neuropsychol* 1990;12:629–643.
11. Benson DF. Language in the left hemisphere. In: Benson DF, Zaidel E, eds. *The dual brain: hemispheric specialization in humans.* New York, NY: Guilford Press, 1985:193–203.
12. Branch C, Milner B, Rasmussen T. Intracarotid sodium amytal for the lateralization of cerebral speech dominance: observations in 123 patients. *J Neurosurg* 1964;21:399–405.
13. Loring DW, Meador KJ, Lee GP, et al. Cerebral language lateralization: evidence from intracarotid amobarbital testing. *Neuropsychologia* 1990;28:831–838.
14. Binder JR, Swanson SJ, Hammeke TA, et al. Determination of language dominance using functional MRI: a comparison with the Wada test. *Neurology* 1996;46:978–984.
15. Helmstaedter C, Kurthen M, Linke DB, et al. Patterns of language dominance in focal left and right hemisphere epilepsies: relation to MRI findings, EEG, sex, and age at onset of epilepsy. *Brain Cogn* 1997;33:135–150.
16. Risse GL, Gates JR, Fangman MC. A reconsideration of bilateral language representation based on the intracarotid amobarbital procedure. *Brain Cogn* 1997;33:118–132.
17. Kurthen M, Helmstaedter C, Elger CE, et al. Sex differences in cerebral language dominance in complex-partial epilepsy. *Naturwissenschaften* 1997;84:131–133.
18. Hinz AC, Berger MS, Ojemann GA, et al. The utility of the intracarotid amytal procedure in determining hemispheric speech lateralization in pediatric epilepsy patients undergoing surgery. *Child Nerv Syst* 1994;10:239–243.
19. Williams JM, Rausch R. Factors in children that predict performance on the intracarotid amobarbital procedure. *Epilepsia* 1992;33:1036–1041.
20. Wyllie E, Lüders H, Murphy D, et al. Intracarotid amobarbital (Wada) test for language dominance: correlation with results of cortical stimulation. *Epilepsia* 1990;31:156–161.
21. Ravdin LD, Perrine K, Haywood CS, et al. Serial recovery of language during the intracarotid amobarbital procedure. *Brain Cogn* 1997;33:151–160.
22. McMackin D, Dubeau F, Jones-Gotman M, et al. Assessment of the functional effect of the intracarotid sodium amobarbital procedure using co-registered MRI/HMPAO-SPECT and SEEG. *Brain Cogn* 1997;33:50–70.
23. Morris RG, Polkey CE, Cox T. Independent recovery of memory and language functioning during the intracarotid sodium amytal test. *J Clin Exp Neuropsychol* 1998;20:433–444.
24. Carpenter K, Oxbury JM, Oxbury S, et al. Memory for objects presented early after intracarotid sodium amytal: a sensitive clinical neuropsychological indicator of temporal lobe pathology. *Seizure* 1996;5:103–108.
25. Hamberger MJ, Hirsch LJ. Effects of incorporating memory confidence ratings and language handicap modifications on intracarotid amobarbital procedure (Wada test) memory asymmetry scores. *Epilepsia* 1999;40:1286–1291.
26. Dodrill CB, Ojemann GA. An exploratory comparison of three methods of memory assessment with the intracarotid amobarbital procedure. *Brain Cogn* 1997;33:210–223.
27. Chelune G. Hippocampal adequacy versus functional reserve: predicting memory functions following temporal lobectomy. *Arch Clin Neuropsychol* 1995;10:413–432.
28. Loring DW, Lee GP, Meador KJ, et al. The intracarotid amobarbital procedure as a predictor of memory failure following unilateral temporal lobectomy. *Neurology* 1990;40:605–610.
29. Dasheiff RM, Shelton J, Ryan C. Memory performance during the Amytal test in patients with non-temporal lobe epilepsy. *Arch Neurol* 1993;50:701–705.

30. Baxendale SA, Van Paesschen W, Thompson PJ, et al. The relation between quantitative MRI measures of hippocampal structure and the intracarotid amobarbital test. *Epilepsia* 1997;38:998–1007.
31. Breier JJ, Thomas AB, Plenger PM, et al. Asymmetries in the effect of side of seizure onset on recognition memory following intracarotid amobarbital injection. *Epilepsia* 1997;38:1209–1215.
32. Davies KG, Hermann BP, Foley KT. Relation between intracarotid amobarbital memory asymmetry scores and hippocampal sclerosis in patients undergoing anterior temporal lobe resections. *Epilepsia* 1996;37:522–525.
33. Glosser G, Deutsch GK, Cole LC, et al. Differential lateralization of memory discrimination and response bias in temporal lobe epilepsy patients. *J Int Neuropsychol Soc* 1998;4:502–511.
34. Hamberger MJ, Walczak TS, Goodman RR. Intracarotid amobarbital procedure memory performance and age at first risk for seizures distinguish between lateral neocortical and mesial temporal lobe epilepsy. *Epilepsia* 1996;37:1088–1092.
35. Kneebone AC, Chelune GJ, Lüders H. Individual patient prediction of seizure lateralization in temporal lobe epilepsy: a comparison between neuropsychological memory measures and the intracarotid amobarbital procedure. *J Int Neuropsychol Soc* 1997;3:159–168.
36. Loring DW, Hermann BP, Perrine K, et al. Effect of Wada memory stimulus type in discriminating lateralized temporal lobe impairment. *Epilepsia* 1997;38:219–224.
37. Loring DW, Meador KJ, Lee GP, et al. Wada memory and timing of stimulus presentation. *Epilepsy Res* 1997;26:461–464.
38. Morton N, Polkey CE, Cox T, et al. Episodic memory dysfunction during sodium amytal testing of epileptic patients in relation to posterior cerebral artery perfusion. *J Clin Exp Neuropsychol* 1996;18:24–37.
39. Perrine K, Donofrio N, Devinsky O, et al. Interhemispheric memory transfer in the intracarotid amobarbital procedure. *Neuropsychiatry Neuropsychol Behav Neurol* 1998;11:8–11.
40. Perrine K, Westerveld M, Sass KJ, et al. Wada memory disparities predict seizure laterality and postoperative seizure control. *Epilepsia* 1995;36:851–856.
41. Roman DD, Beniak TE, Nugent S. Memory performance on the intracarotid amobarbital procedure as a predictor of seizure focus. *Epilepsy Res* 1996;25:243–248.
42. Rouleau I, Robidoux J, Labrecque R, et al. Effect of focus lateralization on memory assessment during the intracarotid amobarbital procedure. *Brain Cogn* 1997;33:224–241.
43. Sperling MR, Saykin AJ, Glosser G, et al. Predictors of outcome after anterior temporal lobectomy: the internal carotid amobarbital test. *Neurology* 1994;44:2325–2330.
44. Swearer JM, Kane KJ, Phillips CA, et al. Predictive value of the intracarotid amobarbital test in bihemispheric seizure onset. *Neurology* 1999;52:409–411.
45. Rausch R, Babb TL, Engel J Jr, et al. Memory following intracarotid amobarbital injection contralateral to hippocampal damage. *Arch Neurol* 1989;46:783–788.
46. Sass KJ, Lencz T, Westerveld M, et al. The neural substrate of memory impairment demonstrated by the intracarotid amobarbital procedure. *Arch Neurol* 1991;48:48–52.
47. Loring DW, Murro AM, Meador KJ, et al. Wada memory testing and hippocampal volume measurements in the evaluation for temporal lobectomy. *Neurology* 1993;43:1789–1793.
48. Jack C Jr, Nichols DA, Sharbrough FW, et al. Selective posterior cerebral artery amytal test for evaluating memory function before surgery for temporal lobe seizure. *Radiology* .
49. Jack CR Jr, Nichols DA, Sharbrough FW, et al. Selective posterior cerebral artery injection of amytal: new method of preoperative memory testing. *Mayo Clin Proc* 1989;64:965–975.
50. Hart J, Lewis PJ, Lesser RP, et al. Anatomic correlates of memory from intracarotid amobarbital injections with technetium Tc-99m hexamethylpropyleneamine oxime SPECT. *Arch Neurol* 1993;50:745–750.
51. Jeffery PJ, Monsein LH, Szabo Z, et al. Mapping the distribution of amobarbital sodium in the intracarotid Wada test by use of Tc-99m HMPAO with SPECT. *Radiology* 1991;178:847–850.
52. Castillo M, Mukherji SK, McCartney WH. Cerebral amobarbital sodium distribution during Wada testing: utility of digital subtraction angiography and single-photon emission tomography. *Neuroradiology* 2000;42:814–817.
53. Soucy JP, Rouleau I, Roy D, et al. Absence of correlation between amobarbital distribution as assessed with SPECT brain perfusion imaging and behavioral manifestations during the intracarotid amobarbital procedure (Wada test). *Prog Neuropsychopharmacol Biol Psychiatry* 1999;23:259–274.
54. Gotman J, Bouwer MS, Jones-Gotman M. Intracranial EEG study of brain structures affected by internal carotid injection of amobarbital. *Neurology* 1992;42:2136–2143.
55. Ahern GL, Labiner DM, Hutzler R, et al. Quantitative analysis of the EEG in the intracarotid amobarbital procedure, I: amplitude analysis. *Electroencephalogr Clin Neurophysiol* 1994;91:21–32.
56. Meador KJ, Loring DW, Lee GP, et al. Level of consciousness and memory during the intracarotid sodium amobarbital procedure. *Brain Cogn* 1997;33:178–188.
57. Serafetinides EA. Wada testing [letter]. *Neurology* 1995;45:396.
58. Jones-Gotman M. Neuropsychological techniques in the identification of epileptic foci. *Epilepsy Res Suppl* 1992;5:87–94.
59. Wyllie E, Naugle R, Awad I, et al. Intracarotid amobarbital procedure, I: prediction of decreased modality-specific memory scores after transient lobectomy. *Epilepsia* 1991;32:857–864.
60. Loring DW, Meador KJ, Lee GP, et al. Wada memory asymmetries predict verbal memory decline after anterior temporal lobectomy. *Neurology* 1995;45:1329–1333.
61. Lee GP, Park YD, Westerveld M, et al. Wada memory performance predicts seizure outcome after epilepsy surgery in children. *Epilepsia* 2003;44:936–943.
62. Alpherts WCJ, Vermeulen J, van Veelen CWM. The Wada test: prediction of focus lateralization by asymmetric and symmetric recall. *Epilepsy Res* 2000;39:239–249.
63. Loring DW, Meador KJ, Lee GP, et al. Stimulus timing effects on Wada memory testing. *Arch Neurol* 1994;51:806–810.
64. Lancman ME, Benbadis S, Geller E, et al. Sensitivity and specificity of asymmetric recall on WADA test to predict outcome after temporal lobectomy. *Neurology* 1998;50:455–459.
65. Loring DW, Meador KL, Lee GP, et al. Wada memory performance predicts seizure outcome following anterior temporal lobectomy. *Neurology* 1994;44:2322–2324.
66. Loring DW, Hermann BP, Perrine K, et al. Memory for real objects is superior to line drawing recognition in discriminating lateralized temporal lobe impairment during the Wada test. *J Int Neuropsychol Soc* 1995;1:134.
67. Morris HH, Matkovic Z, Estes ML, et al. Ganglioglioma and intractable epilepsy: clinical and neurophysiologic features and predictors of outcome after surgery. *Epilepsia* 1998;39:307–313.
68. Stroup E, Langfitt J, Berg M, et al. Predicting verbal memory decline following anterior temporal lobectomy. *Neurology* 2003;60:1266–1273.
69. Szabo CA, Wyllie E. Intracarotid amobarbital testing for language and memory dominance in children. *Epilepsy Res* 1993;15:239–246.
70. Binner RA, Ginsberg B, Bloch EC, et al. Anesthetic management of a pediatric Wada test. *Anesth Analg* 1992;74:619–623.
71. Melamed BG, Robbins RL, Graves S. Preparation for surgery and medical procedures. In: Russo DC, Varni JW, eds. *Behavioral pediatrics: research and practice*. New York, NY: Plenum Press, 1982:225–267.
72. Meador KJ, Loring DW, Lee GP, et al. Right cerebral specialization for tactile attention as evidenced by intracarotid sodium amytal. *Neurology* 1988;38:1763–1766.
73. Spiers PA, Schomer DL, Blume HW, et al. Visual neglect during intracarotid amobarbital testing. *Neurology* 1990;40:1600–1606.
74. Adair JC, Gilmore RL, Fennell EB, et al. Anosognosia during intracarotid barbiturate anesthesia: unawareness or amnesia for weakness. *Neurology* 1995;45:241–243.
75. Durkin MW, Meador KJ, Nichols ME, et al. Anosognosia and the intracarotid amobarbital procedure (Wada test). *Neurology* 1994;44:978.
76. Gilmore RL, Heilman KM, Schmidt RP, et al. Anosognosia during Wada testing. *Neurology* 1992;42:925–927.
77. Lu LH, Barrett AM, Schwartz RL, et al. Anosognosia and confabulation during the Wada test. *Neurology* 1997;49:1316–1322.
78. Ahern GL, Herring AM, Tackenberg JN, et al. Affective self-report during the intracarotid sodium amobarbital test. *J Clin Exp Neuropsychol* 1994;16:372–376.

79. Folstein MF, Maiberger R, McHugh PR. Mood disorder as a specific complication of stroke. *J Neurol Neurosurg Psychiatry* 1977;40: 1018–1020.

80. Hecaen H. Clinical symptomatology in right and left hemispheric lesions. In: Mountcastle VB, ed. *Interhemispheric relations and cerebral dominance.* Baltimore, Md: Johns Hopkins Press, 1962:1062: 215–243.

81. Robinson RG, Kubos KL, Starr LB, et al. Mood disorders in stroke patients: importance of location of lesion. *Brain* 1984;107: 81–93.

82. Williams JM, Little MM, Klein K. Depression and hemispheric site of cerebral vascular accident. *Arch Clin Neuropsychol* 1986;1: 393–398.

83. Ahern GL, Schwartz GE. Differential lateralization for positive and negative emotion in the human brain: EEG spectral analysis. *Neuropsychologia* 1985;23:745–755.

84. Lee GP, Loring DW, Meador KJ, et al. Hemispheric specialization for emotional expression: a re-examination of results from intracarotid administration of sodium amobarbital. *Brain Cogn* 1990;12: 267–280.

85. Ahern GL, Schomer DL, Kleefield J. Right hemisphere advantage for evaluating emotional facial expressions. *Cortex* 1991;27:193–202.

86. Benbadis SR, Binder JR, Swanson SJ, et al. Is speech arrest during Wada testing a valid method for determining hemispheric representation of language? *Brain Lang* 1998;65:441–446.

Metabolic and Functional Neuroimaging

76

William D. Gaillard

Functional imaging studies using radiotracers, such as positron emission tomography (PET) and single-photon-emission computed tomography (SPECT), are performed to identify or confirm the ictal focus in preparation for surgery, to identify eloquent cortical regions to be spared during epilepsy surgery, and to investigate the pathophysiology of partial and generalized seizure disorders. In contrast to PET and SPECT, functional magnetic resonance imaging (fMRI) has been used primarily to identify eloquent cortex to be spared during epilepsy surgery: primary motor and sensory cortex as well as areas of "higher-ordered" cortical function such as those involved in language and memory.

PRINCIPLES: PET AND SPECT

Radiotracer studies using PET or SPECT allow for the *in vivo* assessment of physiologic function in humans. Such studies include glucose consumption ([^{18}F]fluoro-2-deoxyglucose; [^{18}F]FDG), cerebral blood flow ([^{15}O]water), and neurotransmitter synthesis (dopamine and serotonin) or receptor ligand binding (agonists or antagonists to benzodiazepine, opiate, serotonin, and N-methyl-D-aspartate [NMDA] receptors). A physiologic probe designed to assess a targeted function is labeled with a radioactive tag. The decay of the radioactive tag is associated with the emission of high-energy particles, or gamma rays, that are subsequently detected by the scanner; their origin is then computed. PET has a theoretical and practical resolution of 2 to 3 mm, which is superior to that of SPECT. Furthermore, unlike SPECT, PET studies can be quantitated. Use and application

of PET ligands are in part determined by compound half-lives: ^{18}F-tagged compounds have a 110-minute half-life, ^{11}C a 20-minute half-life, and ^{15}O a 2-minute half-life. As a consequence of its longer half-life, [^{18}F]FDG cannot be used to assess short-lived physiologic phenomena such as ictal states, whereas the very short half-life of [^{15}O]water renders it suitable for capturing the brief activity of cognitive processes. Given the relatively short half-life of PET ligands, data acquisition must occur shortly or immediately after injection.

In contrast, SPECT ligands have a longer half-life. ^{99m}Tc-Hexamethyl-propyleneamine oxime (^{99m}Tc-HMPAO) or ^{99m}Tc-ethyl cysteinate dimer (^{99m}Tc-ECD) for cerebral perfusion has replaced ^{123}I-based ligands such as [^{123}I]iodoamphetamine and [^{123}I]trimethyl-hydroxymethyl-iodobenzylpropane diamine, so that data can be collected hours after injection. SPECT is less expensive and more readily available than PET, but the basic premises are similar. SPECT ligands used in epilepsy are primarily markers of perfusion, though some receptor ligands are also available, such as [^{123}I]iomazenil ([^{123}I]IMZ) for benzodiazepine receptor studies. The compounds that mark blood flow, HMPAO and ECD, have a distribution in the brain that is proportional to cerebral blood flow. Both ligands are lipophilic; they generally cross the blood-brain barrier on their first pass through brain tissue, become trapped, and exhibit little subsequent redistribution. Neither ligand has linear uptake at high cerebral blood flow rates, and thus cerebral blood flow is underestimated in certain circumstances (1). Although there are some individual differences in tracer distribution (1,2), HMPAO and ECD have comparable efficacy in epilepsy studies (3).

PET IN THE EVALUATION OF EPILEPSY

[^{18}F]FDG-PET and Temporal Lobe Epilepsy

The greatest clinical experience in evaluating patients with partial epilepsy has been gained with [^{18}F]FDG-PET. Several studies have identified interictal regional decreases in glucose consumption that are invariably ipsilateral to the seizure focus—typically, but not always, most pronounced in the temporal lobe (Fig. 76.1) (4–6).

Regional hypometabolism is seen in 65% to 90% of patients with temporal lobe epilepsy; the figure is closer to 90% on recent-generation scanners and to 60% for patients who show normal findings on MRI (7–10). The area of decreased glucose utilization is often more extensive than the epileptogenic zone; it may extend into adjacent inferior frontal or parietal lobe neocortex (6,11–13) and occasionally into ipsilateral thalamus (12,14) and contralateral cerebellum (6,11,12). The regional abnormalities are invariably unilateral to the ictal focus; however,

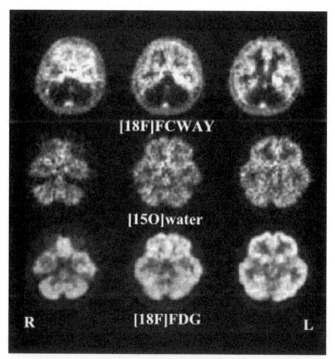

Figure 76.1 [^{18}F]FDG-PET (*bottom row*) in a 43-year-old patient with right temporal lobe epilepsy and right mesial temporal sclerosis. Glucose uptake is decreased in right mesial and lateral temporal regions. [^{15}O]Water PET (*middle row*) shows nearly normal perfusion; only 30% to 40% of patients with temporal hypometabolism also demonstrate decreased perfusion in the epileptogenic zone. [^{18}F]trans-4-fluoro-*N*-2-[4-(2-methoxyphenyl)piperazin-1-yl]ethyl]-*N*-(2-pyridyl)cyclohexane carboxamide [^{18}F](FCWAY)-PET (*top row*) shows decreased binding in right temporal lobe, most pronounced in the amygdala and hippocampus. Absent ligand binding in the cerebellum reflects absence of serotonin 5HT 1A receptors in cerebellar tissue. Raphe nucleus ligand binding is seen. Left image is right brain. (From Toczek MT, Carson RE, Lang L, et al. PET imaging of 5-HT1A receptor binding in patients with temporal lobe epilepsy. *Neurology* 2003;60:749–756. Courtesy of William H. Theodore, National Institutes of Health, Bethesda, Maryland.) Please see color insert.

lobar localization is somewhat less reliable, about 80% to 90%. The few reports of false lateralization have occurred after surgery (5), when interpretation relied on nonquantitative analysis, or during subclinical seizures (5,15,16). Focal interictal regional hypometabolism also predicts a good surgical outcome (8,17–19). Different investigators using different methods and regional analyses have found different regional hypometabolism predictive of good outcome: inferior lateral temporal, anterior lateral, and uncus (8,17,19). Bilateral temporal hypometabolism portends a less optimistic surgical outcome and in half of patients reflects bilateral foci (20). Patients with focal temporal abnormalities have a 93% chance of good surgical outcome; those without have only a 63% chance (18,19). The ability to confirm the focus and predict surgical outcome improves with quantitative means, typically when asymmetry indexes [AI; e.g., AI = 2(left − right)/(left + right)] are greater than two standard deviations from normative data, or about 10% to 15% (18). Lesser degrees of asymmetry, though visually apparent, may result in misleading information and erroneous conclusions (7,18). Voxel-based statistical methods, performed in a standard anatomic atlas that allows comparison of individual patient images to normal control group data, have been advocated as an alternative means of reliable analysis (21,22). Given that [^{18}F]FDG-PET is often performed to confirm the focus, focal abnormalities may reduce the need for, or extent of, invasive monitoring when laterality of the focus is in doubt (5,18,19). Issues of frontal versus temporal focus may not always be reliably resolved by interictal [^{18}F]FDG-PET studies, and invasive studies or other PET ligand studies may be needed. Conflicting localizing or lateralization data nearly always merit invasive monitoring.

Ictal [^{18}F]FDG-PET studies are uncommon because of technical constraints such as ligand availability and unpredictability of seizures. They may show profound focal increases in glucose consumption but may also demonstrate normal results or decreased consumption. The results depend on the delivery of ligand, time and duration of the seizure, and degree of offsetting postictal hypometabolism. Although interesting, they have limited clinical use (23).

The reasons for regional hypometabolism are incompletely understood. Glucose consumption occurs primarily at the synapse. Regional hypometabolism appears to reflect a decrease in glucose influx from reduced glucose transport across the blood-brain barrier, which correlates with subsequent reduced phosphorylation (24). Cell loss with ensuing synaptic loss and altered remote projections, as occurs with hippocampal atrophy in mesial temporal sclerosis, may account for a portion, but not all of regional hypometabolism in temporal lobe epilepsy. (25–31). Hypometabolism does not correlate with lifetime generalized tonic-clonic seizures or frequency of complex partial seizures (32). Dysplastic tissue with aberrant synaptic connectivity can have either decreased or normal glucose consumption (33,34). The abnormalities in some circumstances appear to be functional, as some patients have profound decreases in glucose uptake and no discernible pathologic lesion; regional decreased glucose uptake may vary with relation to previous ictal events (35) and clinical manifestations of the previous seizure (13). In patients with mesial temporal sclerosis, the predominant regions that may manifest decreased glucose consumption are the lateral neocortex and, to a lesser extent, the frontal cortex. This may reflect the distant projection of functional loss in mesial structures. Frontal and contralateral hypometabolism appear to be reversible with successful temporal lobectomy (26,36,37).

Studies differ in the extent to which patients with mesial temporal seizures show pronounced lateral hypometabolism: Mesial greater than lateral, lateral greater than mesial, and equal mesial and lateral temporal reductions in glucose uptake have been reported (6,7,38–40). Patients with neocortical temporal epilepsy may have greater lateral than mesial metabolic abnormalities (39). There is sufficient variability among patients that individual predictions of seizure focus within the temporal lobe cannot be based on [18F]FDG-PET.

[18F]FDG-PET will be abnormal when MRI shows significant abnormalities, for example, in mesial temporal sclerosis, tumor, vascular malformation, infarct, and most instances of cortical dysplasia. In this setting, [18F]FDG-PET provides little additional information beyond that of MRI. [18F]FDG-PET may be more sensitive than MRI in temporal lobe epilepsy in some circumstances. Current PET techniques are helpful in 85% to 90% of patients, volumetric MRI in 60% to 70%, and magnetic resonance spectroscopy (MRS) in 55%. Higher-resolution scanning techniques, including high-resolution fast spin echo, fluid-attenuated inversion recovery, T2 relaxometry, magnetization transfer, and high-resolution thin-cut spoiled gradient recall anatomic sequences, have reduced the utility of [18F]FDG-PET (9,27). Comparison studies report varying efficacy results with different imaging modalities, which generally reflect the particular research strengths of the investigators rather than the intrinsic advantages of the techniques studied.

Although glucose consumption in temporal cortex is decreased, perfusion is often maintained, especially in lateral neocortex (7,41,42). Interictal studies of cerebral blood flow using [15O]water find a decrease in perfusion in only 50% of patients, but one fifth of these provide falsely localizing information (7) (Fig. 76.1). This experience is similar to that in interictal SPECT studies and quantitative perfusion ascertained by arterial spin-labeled fMRI (8,43,44). These data suggest that vascular tone may be impaired in temporal lobe epilepsy and that the relationship between metabolism and perfusion is altered. For these reasons, interictal blood flow studies are unreliable markers of the epileptogenic zone and do not predict surgical outcome (7,45).

Metabolic abnormalities are less common in patients with recent-onset, nonrefractory, or well-controlled partial epilepsy. Within less than 3 years of seizure onset, 30% of adults with nonlesional epilepsy have focal findings on [18F]FDG-PET (46). From 40% to 50% of adults without refractory seizures of limited duration (more than 5 years) have focal abnormalities (46,47). In other studies, 20% of adults with well-controlled partial seizures had regional metabolic abnormalities (48). In these adult populations, localization of seizures is less certain than in patients with refractory epilepsy—an important consideration because patients with extratemporal lobe epilepsy are less likely to have abnormal [18F]FDG-PET studies (49).

Chronic partial epilepsy typically begins during childhood. In a study of 40 children with recent-onset partial epilepsy (mean duration, 1 year) and normal MRI (except for mesial temporal sclerosis), 20% demonstrated regional hypometabolism, all ipsilateral to the presumed focus. All the abnormalities were found among the 32 children with a suspected temporal lobe focus. Although this population is at high risk for continued seizures, not all the children will ultimately develop refractory epilepsy; it remains to be seen whether [18F]FDG-PET can predict epilepsy prognosis (50). In contrast, 70% of children with chronic partial epilepsy (duration 10 years) have focal metabolic abnormalities. There is evidence that adult patients with a longer duration of epilepsy are more likely to have focal [18F]FDG-PET abnormalities (6,41,50). Partial seizures of longer duration are also associated with a greater dissociation between metabolism and blood flow (7,41). These [18F]FDG and cerebral blood flow studies, along with cross-sectional studies using volumetric MRI, may be taken as evidence that temporal lobe epilepsy in some patients is associated with chronic and continued neuronal injury (41,51–53).

Other PET Ligands in Temporal Lobe Epilepsy

In addition to widespread reduction in glucose utilization in cortical projection areas, with relatively preserved perfusion, ligand-binding studies reveal other functional abnormalities in patients with temporal lobe epilepsy (Table 76.1). These findings reflect hippocampal atrophy, loss of neuron populations, or a neuronal response to epilepsy.

GABA-A Receptor Studies

Unlike [18F]FDG-PET, which typically demonstrates hypometabolism that is more widespread than the epileptogenic zone, PET with [11C]flumazenil ([11C]FMZ), a benzodiazepine antagonist of the γ-aminobutyric acid (GABA)-A receptor, shows focal abnormalities confined to the hippocampal formation (10,54–57). Autoradiographic study of pathologic tissue indicates that most decreased [11C]FMZ binding is proportional to cell loss (10,55,58). In contrast, some [11C]FMZ binding studies performed in patients with mesial temporal sclerosis argue for an absence or downregulation of GABA receptors beyond that expected by

TABLE 76.1

PET LIGANDS IN TEMPORAL AND NEOCORTICAL (NONLESIONAL) EPILEPSY

Ligand	Tracer	Action	Temporal Lobe Epilepsy	Neocortical
FDG	[18]F	Glucose uptake and consumption	Decreased mesial, lateral	Decreased
FMZ	[11]C	GABA A-receptor benzodiazepine-site antagonist	Decreased hippocampal formation, amygdala	Mixed
FCWAY	[18]F	5HT1A-receptor antagonist	Decreased hippocampal formation, amygdala	
AMT	[11]C	Precursor, 5HT/kynurenine synthesis	Increased normal hippocampal formation	Increased dysplasia; epileptogenic tubers
Carfentanil	[11]C	Opiate mu-receptor agonist	Increased temporal lobe neocortex, decreased amygdala	
Cyclofoxy	[18]F	Opiate mu-, kappa-receptor antagonist	Increased ipsilateral temporal lobe	
Diprenorphine	[11]C	Opiate mu-, kappa-, delta-receptor agonist	No change	
Methyl ketamine	[11]C	NMDA-receptor antagonist	Decreased	
Doxepin	[11]C	H1-receptor agonist	Decreased	
Deprenyl	[11]C	MAO B inhibitor (glial)	Increased	

atrophy alone. After accounting for partial volume effect, a 38% reduction in [11C]FMZ binding is found in sclerotic hippocampus beyond reduction in hippocampal formation volume (56,59,60). In partial epilepsy, a greater degree and extent of decreased [11C]FMZ binding are seen in patients with more frequent seizures, and decreased binding may extend to projection areas of the epileptogenic region (61,62). In one third of patients with mesial temporal sclerosis, there is decreased [11C]FMZ binding in the contralateral hippocampal formation but to a lesser extent than in the epileptogenic hippocampus. This finding is similar to those in MRS studies (9,60,63). In patients with a temporal focus and normal MRI, however, [11C]FMZ-PET is less useful (10). SPECT with [123I]IMZ, a benzodiazepine ligand (64,65), shows results similar to those of the PET ligand.

Serotonin Receptor and Synthesis Studies

Serotonin (5HT) IA-receptor binding is reduced, to a greater degree than reduced glucose uptake, in epileptogenic mesial temporal lobe, as deduced by the selective antagonist [18F]trans-4-fluoro-N-2-[4-(2-methoxyphenyl)piperazin-1-yl]ethyl]-N-(2-pyridyl)cyclohexanecarboxamide ([18F]FCWAY) (66) (Fig. 76.1). Alpha-[11C]methyl-L-tryptophan ([11C]AMT) is increased in the hippocampus ipsilateral to mesial temporal lobe epilepsy in patients with normal hippocampal formation volumes but not mesial temporal sclerosis (67). [11C]AMT, designed as a serotonin precursor, may also be a marker for quinolinic or kynurenic acid, compounds implicated in excitatory neurotransmission (67–69).

Opiate-Receptor–Binding Studies

Mu-opiate binding determined by [11C]carfentanil, a selective mu agonist, is increased in temporal lobe neocortex ipsilateral to the seizure focus and decreased in amygdala, supporting either an increase in empty receptors or altered receptor affinity (70). [18F]Cyclofoxy, a mu and kappa antagonist, has higher binding in the ipsilateral temporal lobe but shows no significant change in asymmetry index (71). Further studies using [11C]diprenorphine, which labels mu-, kappa-, and delta-opiate receptors, do not show any significant changes.

NMDA, Histamine, and MAO-B Ligand Studies

In one study, (S)-[N-methyl-11C]ketamine, an NMDA-receptor antagonist, showed a 9% to 34% decrease in the ipsilateral temporal lobe in eight patients with temporal lobe epilepsy (72). This observation may reflect either lowered NMDA receptor density or neuronal cell loss. [11C]Doxepin demonstrates an increase in H1-receptor binding in the epileptogenic zone that is hypometabolic, as shown with [18F]FDG-PET (73). The ligand deuterium-L-[11C]deprenyl measures the increased expression of monoamine oxidase B and is thought to be a hallmark of gliosis. In patients with temporal lobe epilepsy, but not neocortical epilepsy, there is a lower initial distribution in the ipsilateral temporal lobe but subsequent enhanced accumulation in the temporal lobe ipsilateral to the focus (74,75). This observation complements findings of MRS employed to detect changes in choline signal, which also reflect gliosis (9,76). Similar results have been found in nine patients with temporal lobe epilepsy using the SPECT ligand and monoamine oxidase B inhibitor [123I]Ro 43-0463 (77).

PET in Extratemporal Lobe Epilepsy

[18F]FDG-PET is less efficacious in identifying the epileptogenic zone in extratemporal lobe epilepsy than in temporal lobe epilepsy. Most extratemporal lobe epilepsy series include patients with structural lesions that, not surprisingly, show concordant hypometabolism. When patients with abnormal MRI findings are excluded, 20% to 50% of the relatively small populations remaining show regional decreases in glucose consumption (10,49,78–81). Some investigators have found a good correlation between regional hypometabolism and the epileptogenic zone; others have found a reasonable correlation with side, but not site, of ictal origin.

[^{11}C]FMZ-PET studies yield mixed and inconsistent results (10,82,83). [^{11}C]FMZ binding may be reduced and is more restricted in cortical extent than are [^{18}F]FDG-PET abnormalities, when present; appears to correlate with the site of ictal activity; and, if resected, is associated with improved outcome (83–86). Patients with acquired lesions may have regional focal reductions in [^{11}C]FMZ binding concordant with the lesion but most marked at the margins (82,85). In other studies, two thirds of patients with neocortical epilepsy and normal MRI had [^{11}C]FMZ abnormalities, either increased or decreased, that were bilateral in half the subjects (82,87). Techniques that correct for gray-matter volume averaging may help in identifying abnormal [^{11}C]FMZ binding in cortical dysplasia or ectopic neurons in white matter, as well as in avoiding false-positive interpretations (87–90). In view of these mixed findings, the role of [^{11}C]FMZ in nonlesional epilepsy remains unclear. In patients with extratemporal lobe partial epilepsy, ictal SPECT may be a better identifier of epileptogenic cortex (see below).

PET in Generalized Epilepsy

PET has been used to explore generalized, predominantly absence, epilepsies. Glucose consumption and perfusion are globally increased (91,92). [^{15}O]Water studies performed during electroencephalographic (EEG) bursts of spike and wave demonstrate not only an increase in global perfusion but also a preferential increase in the thalamic regions, supporting the notion of the thalamus as the facilitator of absence events (93). There are no reported differences in [^{11}C]FMZ binding in the interictal or ictal state in absence epilepsy (94). However, valproate reduces [^{11}C]FMZ binding in patients with childhood or juvenile absence epilepsy. [^{11}C]Diprenorphine, the nonspecific opiate ligand, does not show any differences between patients with absence epilepsy and normal control subjects, especially in the thalamus (95).

PET in Children with Epilepsy

[^{18}F]FDG-PET studies of normal development show increased glucose utilization in all brain areas, peaking around 5 to 8 years of age that parallels synaptic density (96–98). Mature patterns of glucose uptake are established in primary motor and sensory cortex before they are consolidated in association cortex. [^{18}F]FDG-PET studies of children with partial epilepsy show regional abnormalities similar to those seen in adults with temporal or extratemporal lobe epilepsy (discussed above) (Fig. 76.2). Although the primary generalized epilepsies are typically viewed as pediatric disorders, imaging studies have been performed only in adults (see above). Pediatric epilepsy syndromes including infantile spasms, Lennox-Gastaut syndrome, Landau-Klefner syndrome, Rasmussen's encephalitis, and several of the cortical dysplasias, including tuberous sclerosis, have been studied.

Although children with infantile spasms may show extensive hypometabolism, usually in posterior brain regions (33,99), these abnormalities often correspond to MRI abnormalities and may identify areas of dysgenesis not readily apparent with older MRI techniques. However, some children with a generalized EEG and normal MRI exhibit regional metabolic abnormalities (100). PET has been used in these cases to remove the epileptogenic zone in children with catastrophic epilepsy (101). In some children, however, the metabolic abnormalities seen at onset of infantile spasms may resolve with time and thus may

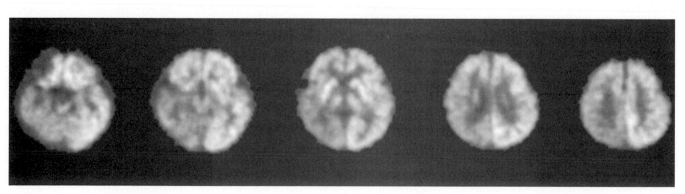

R   L

Figure 76.2 [^{18}F]FDG-PET scan in a 14-month-old with focal seizures (right posterior quadrant focus), secondary generalization, and normal MRI. Hypometabolism in the right posterior quadrant is seen.

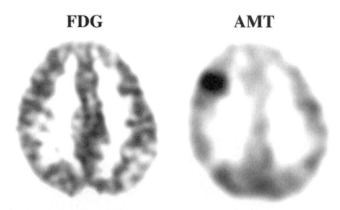

FDG   AMT

Figure 76.3 [^{18}F]FDG-PET (left) and [^{11}C] AMT-PET (right) in a 3.2-year-old child with frontal lobe epilepsy and normal MRI. [^{18}F]FDG-PET is normal. [^{11}C] AMT-PET shows markedly increased ligand uptake in the epileptogenic area; pathologic review of resected tissue demonstrated focal cortical dysplasia. (From Juhasz C, Chugani DC, Muzik O, et al. Alpha-methyl-L-tryptophan PET detects epileptogenic cortex in children with intractable epilepsy. *Neurology* 2003;60:960–968. Courtesy of Csaba Juhaz, Detroit Children's Hospital.)

represent a functional state that is potentially reversible with successful medical therapy (102–104). In children with Rasmussen encephalitis and hemimegalencephaly (105,106), widespread hemispheric hypometabolism is typical. PET has been advocated in some circumstances to assess the integrity of the good hemisphere before extensive cortical resection (33,99).

In tuberous sclerosis, tubers are often hypometabolic (107), whereas there is some evidence that the more epileptogenic tubers have increased serotonin or kynurenic acid synthesis, reflected by increased [^{11}C]AMT uptake (69,108). [^{11}C]AMT uptake is also enhanced in focal cortical dysplasia; MRI (especially in children less than 2 years) and [^{18}F]FDG-PET may be normal. (68,69,108) (Fig. 76.3).

PET studies in Lennox-Gastaut and Landau-Klefner syndromes have yielded mixed results. Children with Lennox-Gastaut syndrome may have focal or multifocal abnormalities or diffuse cortical hypometabolism, or normal results (109–111). In children with generalized EEG findings, nonfocal examinations, longer-duration seizures, and normal MRI, studies are normal or diffusely hypometabolic. A minority exhibit regional metabolic abnormalities, either hypometabolic or hypermetabolic, but many of these children have focal findings on neurologic examination or have partial seizures (109,111). In Landau-Kleffner syndrome and electrical status epilepticus of sleep, [^{18}F]FDG-PET has yielded inconsistent results, mostly involving temporal hypometabolism, although other areas may be hypometabolic or hypermetabolic (112–114).

PET and Antiepileptic Drugs

Several studies have examined the effect of antiepileptic drugs on glucose consumption and to a lesser extent on cerebral perfusion. The GABAergic-receptor agonists phenobarbital and benzodiazepine reduce glucose consumption by 20% to 30% (115,116). In contrast, vigabatrin, an inhibitor of GABA degradation that increases cerebrospinal fluid GABA, reduces glucose uptake by only 8.1% (117). The sodium-channel blockers carbamazepine and phenytoin reduce glucose uptake by 9.5% and 11.5%, respectively (118,119). Valproate, when used in conjunction with carbamazepine in patients with epilepsy, results in a 22% reduction; however, with monotherapy in normal volunteers, the reduction is only 9.5% (120,121) with a decrease in perfusion of 14.9% (120). Although the effects of antiepileptic drugs appear to be global, some evidence with valproate of greater decreases in cerebral blood flow in the thalamus may reflect an effect of valproate in controlling the generalized epilepsies (120).

CEREBRAL BLOOD FLOW STUDIES USING SPECT

SPECT and Seizure Focus Identification

Interictal SPECT studies demonstrate regional hypoperfusion in 40% to 50% of patients with partial epilepsy of temporal lobe origin that is ipsilateral to a proven epileptogenic area. However, approximately 5% to 10% of studies are falsely lateralizing (7,8,10,43,122). These findings are similar to those of interictal perfusion studies performed with [^{15}O]water PET (discussed above). SPECT is more suitable for ictal studies than either [^{15}O]water or [^{18}F]FDG-PET and has provided both useful and reliable information. This is possible because both ^{99m}Tc-HMPAO and ^{99m}Tc-ECD have a rapid first-pass uptake but a long half-life; the latter makes possible ligand availability for bedside injection at ictus as well as time to arrange for data-acquisition scanning within 4 to 6 hours after injection. Ictal SPECT, compared with an interictal study, demonstrates regional hyperperfusion in 67% to 90% of patients (Fig. 76.4) that in a large majority of patients correlates with the ictal focus and has been validated with simultaneous invasive video-EEG (123). These findings hold true for temporal as well as extratemporal lobe epilepsy in both children and adults (3,8,43,124–127). The usefulness of ictal studies approaches that of [^{18}F]FDG-PET in patients with temporal lobe epilepsy, and ictal studies are probably superior to PET for extratemporal focus localization. Results are often more reliable for partial seizures than for generalized seizures. False localization is reported in 3% to 4% of studies, presumably because of seizure propagation, and is more likely with later injection times (8,126,128). Subtraction techniques with MRI coregistration provide enhanced comparison and semiquantitation of perfusion changes between the interictal and ictal states compared with visual comparison alone (32% to 39% versus 83% to 85%) (128–130) (Fig. 76.4). Focal ictal SPECT

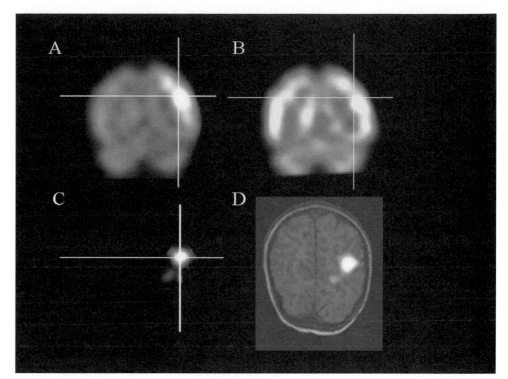

Figure 76.4 Ictal ^{99m}Tc-hexam-ethyl-propyleneamine oxime SPECT in a young adult with refractory partial seizures. **A**, ictal SPECT; **B**, ictal SPECT; **C**, subtraction image of interictal from ictal SPECT; **D**, subtraction SPECT coregistration with magnetic resonance image (SISCOM). Study demonstrates increased ictal perfusion in the parietal lobe. Here, the right side of the image is the left brain. Chronic invasive recording and surgery subsequently confirmed the ictal focus identified by subtraction SPECT techniques. (Courtesy of Gregory Cascino, Mayo Clinic, Rochester, Minnesota.) Please see color insert.

also predicts surgical outcome (126,131,132). Many SPECT studies have included patients with clear structural abnormalities such as tumor, mesial temporal sclerosis, and vascular malformations. As with [^{18}F]FDG-PET, it is unclear whether SPECT contributes to the evaluation in this setting. It is most useful in evaluating patients with nonlesional partial epilepsy, especially extratemporal partial epilepsy.

Ictal SPECT findings are related to the timing of injection and the clinical manifestations of seizure propagation (133). For an ictal SPECT study to be useful, the ligand must be injected during the ictus and no later than 30 seconds after the seizure ends. The earlier the injection, the more reliable the study results. During the ictus, there is focal increase in cerebral blood flow to involved cortex, often with a surround of decreased perfusion. After the seizure, a postictal hypoperfusion may return rapidly to an interictal state (127). Postictal hypoperfusion abnormalities are more reliable than interictal hypoperfusion (60% to 70% versus 40% to 50%) (123,126). After ligand injection, lorazepam is sometimes administered to diminish the likelihood of subsequent seizures. Data from the scan can be acquired up to 6 hours after the injection. Moreover, if a patient has multiple seizure types, each type must be captured. Automated systems may help to improve timing of ligand delivery (134); video-EEG monitoring is critical for interpretation of SPECT studies. Newer SPECT ligands (^{99m}Tc-HMPAO and ^{99m}Tc-ECD) have greater stability and offer a longer window of injectability (from 30 minutes to 4 hours after composition).

fMRI, [^{15}O]WATER PET, AND BRAIN MAPPING OF CORTICAL FUNCTION

Although interictal [^{15}O]water PET has not been useful in identifying the epileptogenic zone and the short half-life of [^{15}O]water makes ictal studies impracticable, [^{15}O]water PET and fMRI have proved useful in identifying eloquent cortex. Both tools have been used in surgical planning to identify areas to be spared during surgery, serve as a replacement for the intracarotid amobarbital procedure, and aid in understanding how chronic epilepsy affects cerebral organization or higher-ordered cognitive function. Brain mapping of language processing is focused predominantly on language lateralization and localization, as chronic partial epilepsy is associated with altered cerebral representation of language functions. The cerebral location of language function, is often difficult to predict, and may involve transfer of language capacity partially or wholly to the typically nondominant hemisphere (135,136) or involve intrahemispheric redistribution of language function (137,138).

Similar principles underlie brain evaluation with [^{15}O]water PET and fMRI. Both techniques rely on the observation that increased neuronal activity, primarily at the synapse, is associated with regional increases in cerebral blood flow (139–141). Detecting the location of changes in blood flow that occur during cognitive tasks (e.g., involving language and memory) allows the mapping of neural networks involved in these tasks. PET measures capillary rather than venous blood flow, is less sensitive to motion—thus allowing spoken and overt responses—and may be more suitable for patients who are less cooperative or cognitively impaired.

[^{15}O]Water PET and Brain Mapping

Although [^{15}O]water PET studies of language and cognition are typically analyzed and presented as group rather than as individual data sets, advances in PET technology allow for repeated injections of [^{15}O]water, resulting in less radiation exposure and making feasible reliable individual perfusion maps of cognitive processes (142,143). Such methods are reliable for lateralization and, unlike the intracarotid amobarbital procedure, localization of language function. Most of these studies rely on verbal fluency or naming tasks, similar to fMRI studies reviewed below, which readily identify anterior language areas.

Using an auditory comprehension and naming task, Bookheimer and colleagues (144) compared individual activation patterns with PET and subdural grid stimulation and found excellent correlation between the disruption elicited by cortical stimulation and the cerebral blood flow activation elicited by task performance. Their study is the first to confirm the assumed reciprocal relationship between activation as defined by local increase in blood flow and the disruption of function elicited by cortical stimulation. Like other functional studies, these studies are valid only for specific aspects of language assessed by the experimental paradigm. Not all activated areas may be critical to language function. For example, the cingulate and supplementary motor cortex are often identified because of their role in sustaining attention and motor planning rather than language processing *per se*. Furthermore, what is crucial may not exceed statistical threshold and may not be apparent. Other studies using PET to identify motor sensory cortex find good correlation (less than 5 mm) with corticography (145,146).

fMRI PRINCIPLES

fMRI relies primarily on blood oxygenation level-dependent (BOLD) contrast techniques, which take advantage of MRI signal changes that differ when hemoglobin is in a deoxygenated versus an oxygenated state. Increased neural activity is associated with tightly regulated increases in blood flow that often exceed local metabolic demand. This physiologic epiphenomenon of luxury hyperperfusion can be ascertained by BOLD fMRI. The phenomenon is most pronounced on the venous side of the capillary bed, where there is a relative increase in quantity, and hence ratio, of oxygenated to deoxygenated hemoglobin. The change in MRI signal is proportional to this effect. Because the signal change is small (0.5% to 5%), multiple observations are necessary to reliably detect it. Optical imaging studies show that the vascular response follows the stimulus onset by 2 seconds and reaches a peak effect in 5 to 7 seconds

(141). The reasons for vascular response are unknown but may include ensuring adequate oxygen and glucose to meet anticipated demand and driving oxygen diffusion in view of increased cerebral blood flow; alternatively, vascular response may be a means of removing metabolic and potentially toxic waste products (147).

The fMRI signal is nonquantitative; it measures a relative signal change between two conditions. Choice of task and control conditions is critical to an effective study. Stimuli must be sufficiently distinct to initiate a hemodynamic response, and the control tasks should not elicit blood flow changes in the brain regions studied. In addition, the temporal resolution (4 seconds) is considerably slower than neuronal firing frequency but is superior to that of [^{15}O]water PET (60 seconds). Fast MRI techniques, such as echo planar or spiral imaging, detect signal change over time by obtaining whole-brain data every 2 to 5 seconds. Spatial resolution is typically 3 to 5 mm, but recent advances in coil design may achieve whole-brain resolution of 1 mm.

Different statistical methods have been used to determine the significance of signal change in a voxel between control and task conditions, identified as "activated." The results are similar using t maps, z maps, cross-correlation, linear regression, and nonparametric maps (147). Most methods involve overly rigorous thresholds in an attempt to mitigate spurious activation that may not identify brain areas truly involved in the experimental task. Many cognitive studies are performed with group analysis; however, for evaluation of epilepsy patients, individual rather than group studies are important. The practical statistical threshold appears to vary among individuals (148,149). As with PET, activated regions may not be critical to the task, and not all critical areas may be activated.

For any patient-oriented functional brain-mapping studies, neuropsychological testing ensures that the tasks are appropriate for the individual. Multiple tasks, multiple repetitions of a task, and well-characterized control conditions are important. Tasks that cannot be performed will not activate brain regions of interest. Cognitive deficits, common among epilepsy populations, may affect fMRI or [^{15}O]water PET activation patterns. If activation maps are atypical, repeat studies are needed to ensure replicability. Studies that cannot be rationally interpreted are not diagnostic and may require confirmation from cortical mapping or the intracarotid amobarbital procedure. fMRI studies are sensitive to motion and require subject cooperation, which is problematic in cognitively impaired, claustrophobic, or very young patients (younger than 5 years). In scan monitoring of a task, response may ensure task performance but may also change cognitive aspects of the paradigm and involve additional cognitive networks.

fMRI Motor and Sensory Mapping

fMRI studies readily identify primary motor and sensory cortex (150–153), as signal changes in these brain areas are

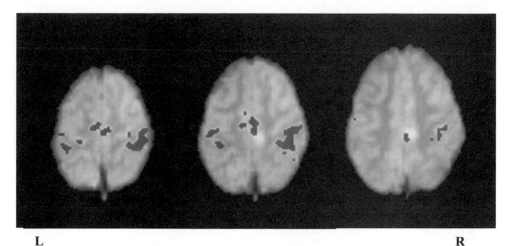

Figure 76.5 10-year-old with a right mesial mass seen as increased signal. fMRI of motor tapping of left hand, compared to rest, yields activation (red), which identifies primary motor cortex posterior to the lesion. Mirror activation ipsilateral to tapping hand is also seen. Supplementary motor cortex activation is adjacent to the lesion. Please see color insert.

L   R

5% on a 1.5-T scanner. In contrast, a 0.5% to 1.5% signal change is seen in cognitive studies in association cortex. Surgery in patients with parietal or frontal lobe epilepsy often requires identification of the sensory or motor cortex. Most reports of motor and sensory fMRI involve patients evaluated for surgical resection of tumor, vascular malformation, dysplasia, or encephalomalacia. Several large series demonstrate the capacity of fMRI to readily and reliably identify motor and sensory cortex (146,154–156) (Fig. 76.5). Motor cortex representing tongue, hand, finger, arm, and foot areas can be identified with tongue movement, finger tapping, and toe wiggling; analogous sensory areas are identified with brushing or an air puff. The supplementary motor area can be identified with complex finger movements (157). Correlation at the time of resection, confirmed with corticography or evoked-potential mapping in these patients, has been excellent. Cortical stimulation and fMRI activation typically lie within 3 to 5 mm of each other. Dysplastic tissue can also demonstrate activation (158).

fMRI LANGUAGE LATERALIZATION AND LOCALIZATION

A number of studies demonstrate that fMRI language paradigms reliably identify hemispheric dominance for language, including bilateral and right-hemisphere language representation in adults and in children 5 years of age and older (Fig. 76.6). As with [15O]water PET paradigms, these studies typically rely on tests of verbal fluency: word generation to letters or generating a rhyming word, word stem completion (phonetic tasks), and word generation to categories or verb generation from nouns (both semantic tasks) (146,149,155,159–161). Verbal fluency paradigms reliably activate inferior frontal cortex (Brodmann areas 44 and 45) and midfrontal cortex (Brodmann areas 9 and 46; dorsolateral prefrontal cortex). Semantic decision tasks (determining whether a word pair is abstract or concrete or whether a presented word falls into a previously stated

category) activate the same midfrontal brain regions as well as Brodmann area 47 (148,162,163). Verbal fluency and semantic decision tasks show marked activation in frontal cortex, 67% to 90% of which occurs in the dominant hemisphere (Fig. 76.7). A limitation, especially for evaluating patients with temporal lobe epilepsy, is the relatively limited ability to activate temporal language cortex (164) (Figs. 76.6 and 76.7).

Paradigms designed to identify receptive language fields in the temporal lobe in individual subjects use more linguistically complex auditory or visual language stimuli—sentences or phrases rather than single words (Figs. 76.6 and 76.7). Reading paradigms using sentences and stories are potent identifiers of dominant superior and middle temporal cortex (164–166). As with fluency and semantic decision tasks, there is some bilateral activation, but 70% to 90% of the activation is found in the dominant hemisphere. These tasks may also engage dominant middle frontal and, to a lesser extent, inferior frontal lobes. Listening to sentences activates the left superior temporal gyrus, with minor activation in right regions, when control tasks involving unfamiliar languages or reverse speech are used to control for primary and secondary auditory processing (167,168). Reading and auditory language processing reliably identify dominant language cortex in the temporal lobe, as well as the dorsolateral prefrontal cortex, in patients with refractory partial epilepsy confirmed by the intracarotid amobarbital procedure (164,169). Tasks may be designed to combine both language comprehension and expression: deciding whether a three-word sentence is syntactically and semantically correct (169) or naming to description (164).

There is excellent agreement between results of intracarotid amobarbital testing and fMRI when the above-mentioned tasks are used to identify left, bilateral, and right language dominance (148,156,161,164,169,170). Most studies, however, report partial disparity in 10% to 15% of patients regardless of the paradigm employed — in these instances, one method shows unilateral findings, the other

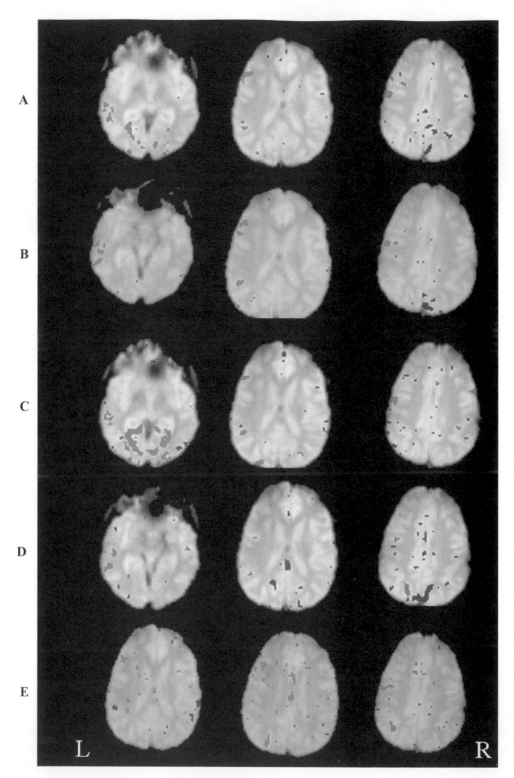

Figure 76.6 (Case I). MRI (echo planar imaging, blood oxygenation level– dependent) panel of tasks. **I.** A 14-year-old girl with left temporal lobe focus; panel of tasks shows left frontal and left temporal activation demonstrating left hemisphere dominance for language. **II.** An 11-year-old with left superior temporal glioma resected at 2 years with recurrent seizures; all tasks demonstrate right-hemisphere activation in temporal and frontal regions. Microscopic metal fragments from burr hole placement results in artifact. The left side of the image is the left brain. "Activated" voxels representing brain regions involved in performing the task compared with a control condition (rest) appear in red. **A.** Reading task, naming to description. (e.g., "What is a large pink bird?"); **B.** auditory task, naming to description; **C.** reading stories; **D.** listening to stories; **E.** covert verbal fluency to categories compared to silent rest. Auditory tasks have a reverse speech control; reading paradigm control is viewing dot patterns. Each paradigm has six cycles, consisting of a 32-second control condition and a 32-second task condition. Please see color insert.

bilateral (156,161,164,169,170). It is difficult to know whether fMRI or intracarotid amobarbital testing is correct, as both have defined limitations. Direct comparisons are imperfect: intracarotid amobarbital testing relies heavily on object naming, which has not proved useful in individual fMRI series (170,171). Partial disparity may be reduced to 5% to 8% if a panel of tasks is used (164,172) (Fig. 76.7). This strategy may employ similar paradigms targeted at one

process to increase reliability (160,171,173), or tasks to assess varied aspects of language in frontal and temporal regions (164,174). Complete discordance is uncommon, but when described, either intracarotid amobarbital testing or fMRI (or [^{15}O]water PET), depending on circumstances, has proved correct (142,143) (see below). Asymmetry indices are higher when region-of-interest analyses targeted at language cortex are used, in comparison to hemispheric asymmetry

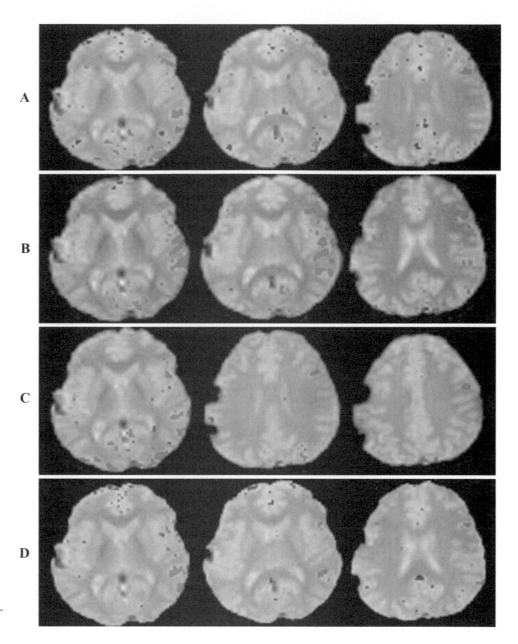

Figure 76.6 (Case II). *(continued)*. Please see color insert.

indices (164,175), although visual and region-of-interest analyses yield similar findings (164,176). fMRI results also predict language deficits following epilepsy surgery (177).

In rare circumstances, fMRI yields falsely lateralizing information, mostly derived from activation seen in homologous regions, because "true" activation is obscured by physiologic factors that alter the BOLD response: large tumors with edema and mass effect (178); vascular malformations that induce a steal effect (179); and studies performed postictally (180).

The evidence suggests good correspondence between cortical stimulation and fMRI activation, but results do not entirely overlap. fMRI–electrocortical stimulation (ECS) comparison studies for language find that 65% to 70% of activated areas lie within 10 mm of positive ECS (closer to 5 mm for frontal lobe); fMRI-negative sites in 90% of patients are never falsely negative (the other 10% were

performed when BOLD response may have been impaired) (146,171,173). Minor differences usually amount to less than 5 mm and may arise from coregistration program error, BOLD identification of draining veins rather than capillaries, or the loss of true positives with overly stringent thresholds. Several language tasks during mapping are necessary, because different aspects of language are variously expressed (171,173).

fMRI Memory Studies

From a practical perspective, the ability to assess the integrity of hippocampal function is desirable for planning mesial temporal tissue resection. Memory is difficult to study, however, because almost everything humans do requires memory, and presumably the hippocampus, in some capacity (181). Designing paradigms to achieve

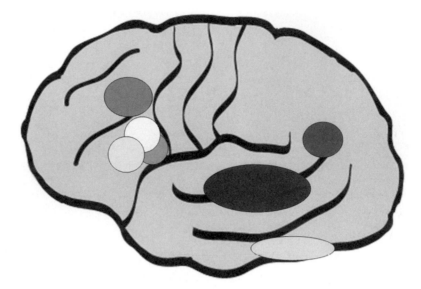

Figure 76.7   Schema showing areas activated with different paradigms advocated in individual studies. Areas adjacent to and along the superior temporal sulcus (blue) are activated by tasks that stress phrase or sentence comprehension such as listening to stories, or reading stories or sentences. Supramarginal gyrus (and sometimes angular gyrus) (purple) may also be activated in auditory sentence-processing tasks. Fusiform gyrus (light blue), is activated by tasks that require feature search or identification, such as identifying written characters or naming objects. Middle frontal gyrus (red) is implicated in verbal working memory for reading, grammatical decipherment, or verbal recall. Inferior frontal gyrus subregions are activated by a variety of tasks: phonologic fluency (orange), syntactic/semantic decision (green), semantic fluency, or recall (yellow). Please see the color insert.

signal differences between task and control conditions is therefore difficult. Paradigms using encoding and retrieval of complex images demonstrate activation of posterior and bilateral hippocampus and parahippocampal gyrus (181,182), whereas retrieval using verbal identifiers of encoded memory for pictures appears to involve the anterior subiculum bilaterally. Encoding of novel stimuli followed by recall is associated with activation of the posterior parahippocampus (183). Verbal encoding appears to preferentially activate left parahippocampal gyrus, whereas nonverbal stimuli, such as patterns, preferentially activate the right parahippocampus. Complex pictures, which may involve verbal encoding as well as visual imagery, activate bilateral parahippocampal regions; face encoding is bilateral with a right bias; and mental navigation yields similar patterns as picture encoding (183–188). Unlike language studies, in which several paradigms have been successfully studied in normal individuals and patients, too few normal volunteers have been evaluated to establish normative data for memory tasks. These techniques have not been extensively used to evaluate patients, and predictive paradigms have not yet been validated.

Activation of the middle left parahippocampal gyrus and hippocampus was found during the verbal encoding of the semantic decision task described previously (148) in patients with right temporal lobe, but not left temporal lobe, epilepsy (189). The analysis was reported as a group study, however, and individual variation may have been lost in the group with left temporal lobe epilepsy. A mental navigation task predicted side of seizure onset, but data

were insufficient to correlate with individual results of intracarotid amobarbital testing (188). Patients with temporal lobe epilepsy have substantially greater activation in the dorsolateral prefrontal cortex than MTS patients have in the hippocampus, suggesting compensatory strategies and networks for verbal encoding (186,187).

A few small series have explored application of memory techniques in individual patients with epilepsy (174,186, 190). Using a visual encoding paradigm based on those described by Stern and colleagues (182,190), one study found bilateral parahippocampal activation, albeit with slightly greater activation in the right posterior parahippocampus in normal individuals. Furthermore, an asymmetry index involving activation in posterior mesial temporal regions matched lateralization by the intracarotid amobarbital procedure in patients with temporal lobe epilepsy (190). Extensions of this study yielded good, but not excellent, agreement with intracarotid amobarbital testing. fMRI activation predicted postsurgical outcome for that specific encoding task (191). A paradigm that compared indoor and outdoor scene decision with a scrambled-image match decision control also found good, but incomplete, correlation with intracarotid amobarbital testing (191). Another study in 10 patients used a panel of encoding tasks—verbal, face, scene, and pattern—and found encouraging preliminary findings relative to intracarotid amobarbital testing (186). To be efficacious, memory fMRI paradigms must establish memory capacity of the side not targeted for resection as well as predict postoperative memory performance. As with language mapping strategies, a panel of different memory probes will likely be required.

fMRI: Ictal and Interictal Localization

In rare and serendipitous circumstances, fMRI can identify regional blood flow changes that accompany partial seizures (158,192,193). All instances of ictal fMRI have involved patients with frequent seizures (epilepsia partialis continua in two patients), accompanied by minimal head movement and confirmed either by interictal and ictal SPECT studies or by cortical ictal recordings. Moreover, the time-course analysis can demonstrate the anatomic distribution of seizure onset and propagation (193). In this instance, the superior temporal resolution of fMRI provides additional information beyond SPECT or PET cerebral blood flow–based studies. fMRI of patients with absence seizures shows increased thalamic signal and decreased cortical signal and thus provides supporting human evidence implicating the thalamus in the pathophysiology of these seizures (194). Time-locked fMRI data acquisition of spikes detected by EEG can measure regional increases in MRI signal associated with interictal activity in mesial temporal structures, neocortex, and structural lesions (195–197). Such methods may ultimately prove to be reliable ways of localizing epileptogenic cortex and do not rely on the chance occurrence of seizures during scanning.

fMRI Advantages and Limitations

Unlike PET, fMRI technology is common and relatively inexpensive and studies can be performed with little risk and no radiation. Most important, studies can be repeated to confirm findings, especially if no or unusual activation patterns are found. A number of paradigms can map different aspects of language—often more than can be performed in the operating room. Additionally, fMRI identifies language areas deep in sulcal areas that are often inaccessible to cortical stimulation (198). It can also be used to reliably study children over the age of 5 years.

fMRI is restricted to patients who will be medically safe in the scanner. To be studied successfully, patients must be awake and cooperative and must lie still. Motion artifact remains the principal cause of failed studies, a particular issue in very young, fidgety, or cognitively impaired patients. Activation is task and control specific; a given task may not be optimal for identifying targeted cortex.

As a clinical tool, fMRI can reliably lateralize language function and identify motor or sensory strip in anticipation of surgery. It can also localize language function and therefore is a useful guide for sparing eloquent cortex. Activated areas are likely to be involved in task processing, although not all activated areas may be critical for language function. The statistical threshold used may underestimate the extent of area activated. In certain clinical circumstances (tumor, vascular malformation, postictal

state), fMRI may be unreliable. Memory paradigms are not yet well established. Application for seizure mapping is limited with current technology, is almost entirely fortuitous, and cannot be used reliably, except in rare circumstances.

CLINICAL RECOMMENDATIONS FOR USE OF METABOLIC AND FUNCTIONAL IMAGING IN EVALUATION OF PATIENTS WITH PARTIAL EPILEPSY

MRI, MRS, PET, and SPECT provide complementary information. When a structural lesion is present, for example, with a tumor or mesial temporal sclerosis, further imaging, though of interest, usually does not provide information relevant to clinical care. MRS and PET may add information in patients with temporal lobe epilepsy when routine MRI is normal. [^{18}F]FDG-PET provides excellent lateralization of seizure focus but less reliable localization and a lower yield in patients with extratemporal epilepsy. Ictal SPECT is most useful in extratemporal lobe epilepsy in which other modalities are less helpful or unavailable; without EEG confirmation, invasive studies are usually indicated in these settings. The contribution of new PET ligands is not well established, but [^{11}C]FMZ, [^{18}F]FCWAY, and [^{11}C]AMT may provide additional localizing information. fMRI and [^{15}O]water PET are reliable techniques for lateralization and localization of language function, particularly when a panel of tasks is used. Memory assessment with fMRI may ultimately also prove reliable. Information obtained by functional mapping can be used to direct surgery and cortical mapping necessary for anatomic confirmation and resection.

REFERENCES

1. Asenbaum S, Brucke T, Pirker W, et al. Imaging of cerebral blood flow with technetium-99m-HMPAO and technetium-99m-ECD: a comparison. *J Nucl Med* 1998;39:613–618.
2. Oku N, Matsumoto M, Hashikawa K, et al. Intra-individual differences between technetium-99m-HMPAO and technetium-99m-ECD in the normal medial temporal lobe. *J Nucl Med* 1997;38:1109–1111.
3. O'Brien TJ, Brinkmann BH, Mullan BP, et al. Comparative study of 99mTc-ECD and 99mTc-HMPAO for peri-ictal SPECT: qualitative and quantitative analysis. *J Neurol Neurosurg Psychiatry* 1999;66:331–339.
4. Engel J Jr, Brown WJ, Kuhl DE, et al. Pathological findings underlying focal temporal lobe hypometabolism in partial epilepsy. *Ann Neurol* 1982;12:518–529.
5. Engel J Jr, Henry TR, Risinger MW, et al. Presurgical evaluation for partial epilepsy: relative contributions of chronic depth-electrode recordings versus FDG-PET and scalp-sphenoidal ictal EEG. *Neurology* 1990;40:1670–1677.
6. Theodore WH, Fishbein D, Dubinsky R. Patterns of cerebral glucose metabolism in patients with partial seizures. *Neurology* 1988; 38:1201–1206.
7. Gaillard WD, Fazilat S, White S, et al. Interictal metabolism and blood flow are uncoupled in temporal lobe cortex of patients with partial epilepsy. *Neurology* 1995;45:1841–1848.
8. Ho SS, Berkovic SF, Berlangieri SU, et al. Comparison of ictal SPECT and interictal PET in the presurgical evaluation of temporal lobe epilepsy. *Ann Neurol* 1995;37:738–745.

9. Knowlton RC, Laxer KD, Ende G, et al. Presurgical multimodality neuroimaging in electroencephalographic lateralized temporal lobe epilepsy. *Ann Neurol* 1997;42:829–837.

10. Ryvlin P, Bouvard S, Le Bars D, et al. Clinical utility of flumazenil-PET versus [18F]fluorodeoxyglucose-PET and MRI in refractory partial epilepsy. A prospective study in 100 patients. *Brain* 1998; 121:2067–2081.

11. DeCarli C, McIntosh AR, Blaxton TA. Use of positron emission tomography for the evaluation of epilepsy. *Neuroimaging Clin North Am* 1995;5:623–645.

12. Henry TR, Mazziotta JC, Engel JJ, et al. Quantifying interictal metabolic activity in human temporal lobe epilepsy. *J Cereb Blood Flow Metab* 1990;10:748–757.

13. Savic I, Altshuler L, Baxter L. Pattern of interictal hypometabolism in PET scans with fluorodeoxyglucose F18 reflects prior seizure types in patients with mesial temporal lobe seizures. *Arch Neurol* 1997;54:129–136.

14. Khan N, Leenders KL, Hajek M, et al. Thalamic glucose metabolism in temporal lobe epilepsy measured with 18F-FDG positron emission tomography (PET). *Epilepsy Res* 1997;28:233–243.

15. Nagarajan L, Schaul N, Eidelberg D, et al. Contralateral temporal hypometabolism on positron emission tomography in temporal lobe epilepsy. *Acta Neurol Scand* 1996;93:81–84.

16. Sperling MR, Alavi A, Reivich M, et al. False lateralization of temporal lobe epilepsy with FDG positron emission tomography. *Epilepsia* 1995;36:722–727.

17. Manno EM, Sperling MR, Ding X, et al. Predictors of outcome after temporal lobectomy: positron emission tomography. *Neurology* 1994;44:2331–2336.

18. Theodore WH, Gaillard WD, Sato S, et al. PET measurement of cerebral blood flow and temporal lobectomy. *Ann Neurol* 1994; 36:241–244.

19. Theodore WH, Sato S, Kufta CV, et al. FDG-positron emission tomography and invasive EEG: seizure focus detection and surgical outcome. *Epilepsia* 1997;38:81–86.

20. Koutroumanidis M, Hennessy MJ, Seed PT, et al. Significance of interictal bilateral temporal hypometabolism in temporal lobe epilepsy. *Neurology* 2000;54:1811–1821.

21. Van Bogaert P, Massager N, Tugendhaft P, et al. Statistical parametric mapping of regional glucose metabolism in mesial temporal lobe epilepsy. *Neuroimage* 2000;12:129–138.

22. Lee SK, Lee DS, Yeo JS, et al. FDG-PET images quantified by probabilistic atlas of brain and surgical prognosis of temporal lobe epilepsy. *Epilepsia* 2002;43:1032–1038.

23. Engel J, Kuhl DE, Phelps M. Local cerebral metabolism during partial seizures. *Neurology* 1983;33:400–413.

24. Cornford EM, Gee MN, Swartz BE, et al. Dynamic [18F]fluorodeoxyglucose positron emission tomography and hypometabolic zones in seizures: reduced capillary influx. *Ann Neurol* 1998;43:801–808.

25. Foldvary N, Lee N, Hanson MW, et al. Correlation of hippocampal neuronal density and FDG-PET in mesial temporal lobe epilepsy. *Epilepsia* 1999;40:26–29.

26. Dupont S, Croize AC, Semah F, et al. Is amygdalohippocampectomy really selective in medial temporal lobe epilepsy? A study using positron emission tomography with (18)fluorodeoxyglucose. *Epilepsia* 2001;42:731–740.

27. Gaillard WD, Bhatia S, Bookheimer SY, et al. FDG-PET and volumetric MRI in the evaluation of patients with partial epilepsy. *Neurology* 1995;45:123–126.

28. Semah F, Baulac M, Hasboun D, et al. Is interictal temporal hypometabolism related to mesial temporal sclerosis? A positron emission tomography/magnetic resonance imaging confrontation. *Epilepsia* 1995;36:447–456.

29. Theodore WH, Gaillard WD, De Carli C, et al. Hippocampal volume and glucose metabolism in temporal lobe epileptic foci. *Epilepsia* 2001;42:130–132.

30. Knowlton RC, Laxer KD, Klein G, et al. In vivo hippocampal glucose metabolism in mesial temporal lobe epilepsy. *Neurology* 2001;57:1184–1190.

31. O'Brien TJ, Newton MR, Cook MJ, et al. Hippocampal atrophy is not a major determinant of regional hypometabolism in temporal lobe epilepsy. *Epilepsia* 1997;38:74–80.

32. Spanaki MV, Kopylev L, Liow K, et al. Relationship of seizure frequency to hippocampus volume in temporal lobe epilepsy. *Epilepsia* 2000;41:1227–1229.

33. Chugani HT, Shields WD, Shewmon DA, et al. Infantile spasms; I: PET identifies focal cortical dysgenesis in cryptogenic cases for surgical treatment. *Ann Neurol* 1990;27:406–413.

34. Lee N, Radtke RA, Gray L, et al. Neuronal migration disorders: positron emission tomography correlations. *Ann Neurol* 1994; 35:290–297.

35. Leiderman DB, Albert P, Balish M, et al. The dynamics of metabolic change following seizures as measured by positron emission tomography with fludeoxyglucose F18. *Arch Neurol* 1994; 51:932–936.

36. Akimura T, Yeh HS, Mantil JC, et al. Cerebral metabolism of the remote area after epilepsy surgery. *Neurol Med Chir* 1999;39: 16–25.

37. Spanaki MV, Kopylev L, DeCarli C, et al. Postoperative changes in cerebral metabolism in temporal lobe epilepsy. *Arch Neurol* 2000;57:1447–1452.

38. Arnold S, Schlaug G, Niemann H, et al. Topography of interictal glucose hypometabolism in unilateral mesiotemporal epilepsy. *Neurology* 1996;46:1422–1430.

39. Hajek M, Antonini A, Leenders KL, et al. Mesiobasal versus lateral temporal lobe epilepsy: metabolic differences in the temporal lobe shown by interictal 18F-FDG positron emission tomography. *Neurology* 1993;43:79–86.

40. Sackellares JC, Siegal GJ, Abou-Khalil BW, et al. Differences between lateral and mesial temporal metabolism interictally in epilepsy of temporal lobe origin. *Neurology* 1990;40:1420–1426.

41. Breier JI, Mullani NA, Thomas AB, et al. Effects of duration of epilepsy on the uncoupling of metabolism and blood flow in complex partial seizures. *Neurology* 1997;48:1047–1053.

42. Fink GR, Pawlik G, Stefan H, et al. Temporal lobe epilepsy—evidence for interictal uncoupling of blood-flow and glucose-metabolism in temporomesial structures. *J Neurol Sci* 1996;137: 28–34.

43. Rowe CC, Berkovic SF, Sia ST. Localization of epileptic foci with postictal single photon emission computed tomography. *Ann Neurol* 1989;26:660–668.

44. Ryvlin P, Philippon B, Cinotti L, et al. Functional neuroimaging strategy in temporal lobe epilepsy: a comparative study of 18FDG-PET and 99mTc-HMPAO-SPECT. *Ann Neurol* 1992;31: 650–656.

45. Lee DS, Lee JS, Kang KW, et al. Disparity of perfusion and glucose metabolism of epileptogenic zones in temporal lobe epilepsy demonstrated by SPM/SPAM analysis on 15O water PET, [18F]FDG-PET, and [99mTc]-HMPAO SPECT. *Epilepsia* 2001; 42:1515–1522.

46. Matheja P, Kuwert T, Ludemann P, et al. Temporal hypometabolism at the onset of cryptogenic temporal lobe epilepsy. *Eur J Nucl Med* 2001;28:625–632.

47. Matheja P, Kuwert T, Stodieck SR, et al. PET and SPECT in medically non-refractory complex partial seizures. Temporal asymmetries of glucose consumption, benzodiazepine receptor density, and blood flow. *Nuklearmedizin* 1998;37:221–226.

48. Hosokawa S, Kato M, Otsuka M, et al. Positron emission tomography in epilepsy: correlative study. *Jpn J Psychiatry Neurol* 1989; 43:349–353.

49. Theodore WH, Gaillard WD. PET studies in neocortical epilepsy. In: Williamson PD, Siegel AM, Thadani VM, et al, eds. *Neocortical epilepsy*. Baltimore: Lippincott Williams & Wilkins, 2000:435–446.

50. Gaillard WD, Kopylev L, Weinstein S, et al. Low incidence of abnormal 18FDG-PET in children with new onset partial epilepsy: a prospective study. *Neurology* 2002;58:717–722.

51. Kalviainen R, Salmenpera T, Partanen K, et al. Recurrent seizures may cause hippocampal damage in temporal lobe epilepsy. *Neurology* 1998;50:1377–1382.

52. Tasch E, Cendes F, Li LM, et al. Neuroimaging evidence of progressive neuronal loss and dysfunction in temporal lobe epilepsy. *Ann Neurol* 1999;45:568–576.

53. Theodore WH, Gaillard WD. Neuroimaging and the progression of epilepsy. *Prog Brain Res* 2002;135:305–313.

54. Debets RM, Sadzot B, van Isselt JW, et al. Is 11C-flumazenil PET superior to 18FDG PET and 123I-iomazenil SPECT in presurgical evaluation of temporal lobe epilepsy? *J Neurol Neurosurg Psychiatry* 1997;62:141–150.

55. Henry TR, Frey KA, Sackellares JC, et al. In vivo cerebral metabolism and central benzodiazepine-receptor binding in temporal lobe epilepsy. *Neurology* 1993;43:1998–2006.

56. Koepp MJ, Richardson MP, Brooks DJ, et al. Cerebral benzodiazepine receptors in hippocampal sclerosis. An objective in vivo analysis. *Brain* 1996;119:1677–1687.

57. Savic I, Ingvar M, Stone-Elander S. Comparison of [11 C] flumazenil and [18F] FDG as PET markers of epileptic foci. *J Neurol Neurosurg Psychiatry* 1993;56:615–621.

58. Burdette DE, Sakurai SY, Henry TR, et al. Temporal lobe central benzodiazepine binding in unilateral mesial temporal lobe epilepsy. *Neurology* 1995;45:934–941.

59. Koepp MJ, Hand KS, Labbe C, et al. In vivo [11C]flumazenil-PET correlates with ex vivo [3H]flumazenil autoradiography in hippocampal sclerosis. *Ann Neurol* 1998;43:618–626.

60. Koepp MJ, Labbe C, Richardson MP, et al. Regional hippocampal [11C]flumazenil PET in temporal lobe epilepsy with unilateral and bilateral hippocampal sclerosis. *Brain* 1997;120:1865–1876.

61. Savic I, Svanborg E, Thorell JO. Cortical benzodiazepine receptor changes are related to frequency of partial seizures: a positron emission tomography study. *Epilepsia* 1996;37:236–244.

62. Hammers A, Koepp MJ, Labbe C, et al. Neocortical abnormalities of [11C]-flumazenil PET in mesial temporal lobe epilepsy. *Neurology* 2001;56:897–906.

63. Cendes F, Andermann F, Dubeau F. Normalization of neuronal metabolic dysfunction after surgery for temporal lobe epilepsy. Evidence from proton MR spectroscopic imaging. *Neurology* 1997;49:1525–1533.

64. Lamusuo S, Ruottinen HM, Knuuti J, et al. Comparison of [18F]FDG-PET, [99mTc]-HMPAO-SPECT, and [123I]-iomazenil-SPECT in localising the epileptogenic cortex. *J Neurol Neurosurg Psychiatry* 1997;63:743–748.

65. Tanaka S, Yonekura Y, Ikeda A. Presurgical identification of epileptic foci with iodine-123 iomazenil SPECT: comparison with brain perfusion SPECT and FDG-PET. *Eur J Nucl Med* 1997;24:27–34.

66. Toczek MT, Carson RE, Lang L, et al. PET imaging of 5-HT1A receptor binding in patients with temporal lobe epilepsy. *Neurology* 2003;60:749–756.

67. Natsume J, Kumakura Y, Bernasconi N, et al. Alpha-[11C] methyl-L-tryptophan and glucose metabolism in patients with temporal lobe epilepsy. *Neurology* 2003;60:756–761.

68. Juhasz C, Chugani DC, Muzik O, et al. Alpha-methyl-L-tryptophan PET detects epileptogenic cortex in children with intractable epilepsy. *Neurology* 2003;60:960–968.

69. Fedi M, Reutens DC, Andermann F, et al. Alpha-[11C]-methyl-L-tryptophan PET identifies the epileptogenic tuber and correlates with interictal spike frequency. *Epilepsy Res* 2003;52:203–213.

70. Frost JJ, Mayberg HS, Fisher RS. Mu-opiate receptors measured by positron emission tomography are increased in temporal lobe epilepsy. *Ann Neurol* 1988;23:231–237.

71. Theodore WH, Carson RE, Andreasen P, et al. PET imaging of opiate receptor binding in human epilepsy using [18F]cyclofoxy. *Epilepsy Res* 1992;13:129–139.

72. Kumlien E, Hartvig P, Valind S, et al. NMDA-receptor activity visualized with (S)-[N-methyl-11C]ketamine and positron emission tomography in patients with medial temporal lobe epilepsy. *Epilepsia* 1999;40:30–37.

73. Itoh M, Yanai K, Yamaguchi S, et al. In vivo visualization of neurotransmitter function in the human brain by PET. *No To Hattatsu* 1995;27:146–152. Japanese.

74. Bergstrom M, Kumlien E, Lilja A, et al. Temporal lobe epilepsy visualized with PET with 11C-L-deuterium-deprenyl-analysis of kinetic data. *Acta Neurol Scand* 1998;98:224–231.

75. Kumlien E, Nilsson A, Hagberg G, et al. PET with 11C-deuterium-deprenyl and 18F-FDG in focal epilepsy. *Acta Neurol Scand* 2001;103:360–366.

76. Hugg JW, Laxer KD, Matsun CB, et al. Neuron loss localizes human temporal lobe epilepsy by in vivo proton magnetic spectroscopy imaging. *Ann Neurol* 1993;34:788–794.

77. Buck A, Frey LD, Blauenstein P, et al. Monoamine oxidase B single-photon emission tomography with [123I]Ro 43-0463: imaging in volunteers and patients with temporal lobe epilepsy. *Eur J Nucl Med* 1998;25:464–470.

78. Henry TR, Sutherling W, Engel J. Interictal cerebral metabolism in partial epilepsies of neocortical origin. *Epilepsy Res* 1991;10: 174–182.

79. Swartz B, Delgado-Escueta AV, Walsh GO. Surgical outcomes in pure frontal lobe epilepsy and foci that mimic them. *Epilepsy Res* 1998;29:97–108.

80. Kim YK, Lee DS, Lee SK, et al. (18)F-FDG PET in localization of frontal lobe epilepsy: comparison of visual and SPM analysis. *J Nucl Med* 2002;43:1167–1174.

81. Hong KS, Lee SK, Kim JY, et al. Pre-surgical evaluation and surgical outcome of 41 patients with non-lesional neocortical epilepsy. *Seizure* 2002;11:184–192.

82. Richardson MP, Koepp MJ, Brooks DJ. 11C-Flumazenil PET in neocortical epilepsy. *Neurology* 1998;51:485–492.

83. Savic I, Thorell JO, Roland P. [11C] Flumazenil positron emission tomography visualizes frontal epileptogenic regions. *Epilepsia* 1995;36:1225–1232.

84. Muzik O, da Silva EA, Juhasz C, et al. Intracranial EEG versus flumazenil and glucose PET in children with extratemporal lobe epilepsy. *Neurology* 2000;54:171–179.

85. Juhasz C, Chugani DC, Muzik O, et al. Electroclinical correlates of flumazenil and fluorodeoxyglucose PET abnormalities in lesional epilepsy. *Neurology* 2000;55:825–835.

86. Juhasz C, Chugani DC, Muzik O, et al. Relationship of flumazenil and glucose PET abnormalities to neocortical epilepsy surgery outcome. *Neurology* 2001;56:1650–1658.

87. Hammers A, Koepp MJ, Richardson MP, et al. Central benzodiazepine receptors in malformations of cortical development: a quantitative study. *Brain* 2001;124:1555–1565.

88. Richardson MP, Friston KJ, Sisodiya S, et al. Cortical grey matter and benzodiazepine receptors in malformations of cortical development. A voxel-based comparison of structural and functional imaging data. *Brain* 1997;120:1961–1973.

89. Richardson MP, Koepp MJ, Brooks DJ, et al. Benzodiazepine receptors in focal epilepsy with cortical dysgenesis: an 11C-flumazenil PET study. *Ann Neurol* 1996;40:188–198.

90. Hammers A, Koepp MJ, Hurlemann R, et al. Abnormalities of grey and white matter [11C]flumazenil binding in temporal lobe epilepsy with normal MRI. *Brain* 2002;125:2257–2271.

91. Engel J Jr, Lubens P, Kuhl DE, et al. Local cerebral metabolic rate for glucose during petit mal absences. *Ann Neurol* 1985;17:121–128.

92. Theodore WH, Brooks R, Margolin R, et al. Positron emission tomography in generalized seizures. *Neurology* 1985;35: 684–690.

93. Prevett MC, Duncan JS, Jones T, et al. Demonstration of thalamic activation during typical absence seizures using H2(15)O and PET. *Neurology* 1995;45:1396–1402.

94. Prevett MC, Lammertsma AA, Brooks DJ, et al. Benzodiazepine-GABAA receptor binding during absence seizures. *Epilepsia* 1995;36:592–599.

95. Prevett MC, Cunningham VJ, Brooks DJ, et al. Opiate receptors in idiopathic generalized epilepsy measured with [11C] diprenorphine and positron emission tomography. *Epilepsy Res* 1994;19: 71–77.

96. Bentourkia M, Michel C, Ferriere G, et al. Evolution of brain glucose metabolism with age in epileptic infants, children and adolescents. *Brain Dev* 1998;20:524–529.

97. Chugani HT, Phelps ME, Mazziotta JC. Positron emission tomography study of human brain functional development. *Ann Neurol* 1987;22:487–497.

98. Van Bogaert P, Wikler D, Damhaut P. Regional changes in glucose metabolism during brain development from the age of 6 years. *Neuroimage* 1998;8:62–68.

99. Chugani HT, Shewmon DA, Shields WD, et al. Surgery for intractable infantile spasms: neuroimaging perspectives. *Epilepsia* 1993;34:764–771.

100. Chugani HT, Conti JR. Etiologic classification of infantile spasms in 140 cases: role of positron emission tomography. *J Child Neurol* 1996;11:44–48.

101. Chugani HT, Shewmon DA, Peacock WJ, et al. Surgical treatment of intractable neonatal-onset seizures: the role of positron emission tomography. *Neurology* 1988;38:1178–1188.

102. Maeda N, Watanabe K, Negoro T. Transient focal cortical hypometabolism in idiopathic West's syndrome. *Pediatr Neurol* 1993;9:430–434.

103. Metsahonkala L, Gaily E, Rantala H, et al. Focal and global cortical hypometabolism in patients with newly diagnosed infantile spasms. *Neurology* 2002;58:1646–1651.

104. Itomi K, Okumura A, Negoro T, et al. Prognostic value of positron emission tomography in cryptogenic West syndrome. *Dev Med Child Neurol* 2002;44:107–111.

105. DeCarli C, Gaillard WD, Ko D. Cerebral metabolism in epilepsy partialis continua. *Epilepsia* 1994;35:147.

106. Rintahaka PJ, Chugani HT, Messa C, et al. Hemimegalencephaly: evaluation with positron emission tomography. *Pediatr Neurol* 1993;9:21–28.

107. Rintahaka PJ, Chugani HT. Clinical role of positron emission tomography in children with tuberous sclerosis complex. *J Child Neurol* 1997;12:42–52.

108. Chugani DC, Chugani HT, Muzik O, et al. Imaging epileptogenic tubers in children with tuberous sclerosis complex using alpha-[11C]methyl-L-tryptophan positron emission tomography. *Ann Neurol* 1998;44:858–866.

109. Chugani HT, Mazziotta JC, Engel J Jr , et al. The Lennox-Gastaut syndrome: metabolic subtypes determined by 2-deoxy-2[18F]fluoro-D-glucose positron emission tomography. *Ann Neurol* 1987; 21:4–13.

110. Gaillard WD, Leiderman DB, White S. FDG-PET in children with seizures. *Epilepsia* 1991;32:72.

111. Theodore W, Rose D, Patronas N, et al. Cerebral glucose metabolism in the Lennox-Gastaut syndrome. *Ann Neurol* 1987;21:14–21.

112. da Silva EA, Chugani DC, Muzik O, et al. Landau-Kleffner syndrome: metabolic abnormalities in temporal lobe are a common feature. *J Child Neurol* 1997;12:489–495.

113. Maquet P, Hirsch E, Metz-Lutz MN, et al. Regional cerebral glucose metabolism in children with deterioration of one or more cognitive functions and continuous spike-and-wave discharges during sleep. *Brain* 1995;118:1497–1520.

114. Rintahaka PJ, Chugani HT, Sankar R. Landau-Kleffner syndrome with continuous spikes and waves during slow-wave sleep. *J Child Neurol* 1995;10:127–133.

115. Foster NL, VanDerSpek AF, Aldrich MS, et al. The effect of diazepam sedation on cerebral glucose metabolism in Alzheimer's disease as measured using positron emission tomography. *J Cereb Blood Flow Metab* 1987;7:415–420.

116. Theodore W, DiChiro G, Margolin R. Barbiturates reduce human cerebral glucose metabolism. *Neurology* 1986;36:60–64.

117. Spanaki MV, Siegel H, Kopylev L, et al. The effect of vigabatrin on cerebral blood flow and metabolism. *Neurology* 1999;53:1518–1522.

118. Theodore W, Bairamian D, Newmark ME, et al. Effect of phenytoin on human cerebral glucose metabolism. *J Cereb Blood Flow Metab* 1986;6:315–320.

119. Theodore WH, Bromfield E, Onorati L. The effect of carbamazepine on cerebral glucose metabolism. *Ann Neurol* 1989;25:516–520.

120. Gaillard WD, Zeffiro TA, Fazilat S, et al. Effect of valproate on cerebral glucose metabolism and cerebral blood flow as determined by 18-FDG and O-15 water PET. *Epilepsia* 1996;37:515–521.

121. Leiderman DB, Balish M, Bromfield EB, et al. Effect of valproate on human cerebral glucose metabolism. *Epilepsia* 1991;32:417–422.

122. Markand ON, Salanova V, Worth R, et al. Comparative study of interictal PET and ictal SPECT in complex partial seizures. *Acta Neurol Scand* 1997;95:129–136.

123. Spanaki MV, Zubal IG, MacMullan J, et al. Periictal SPECT localization verified by simultaneous intracranial EEG. *Epilepsia* 1999;40:267–274.

124. Harvey AS, Bowe JM, Hopkins IJ, et al. Ictal 99mTc-HMPAO single photon emission computed tomography in children with temporal lobe epilepsy. *Epilepsia* 1993;34:869–877.

125. Harvey AS, Hopkin IJ, Bowe JM, et al. Frontal lobe epilepsy: clinical seizure characteristics and localization with ictal 99mTc HMPAO SPECT. *Neurology* 1993;43:1966–1980.

126. O'Brien TJ, So EL, Mullan BP, et al. Subtraction ictal SPECT co-registered to MRI improves clinical usefulness of SPECT in localizing the surgical seizure focus. *Neurology* 1998;50:445–454.

127. Rowe CC, Berkovic SF, Austin MC, et al. Patterns of postictal cerebral blood flow in temporal lobe epilepsy: qualitative and quantitative analysis. *Neurology* 1991;41:1096–1103.

128. Lewis PJ, Siegel A, Siegel AM, et al. Does performing image registration and subtraction in ictal brain SPECT help localize neocortical seizures? *J Nucl Med* 2000;41:1619–1626.

129. Chang DJ, Zubal IG, Gottschalk C, et al. Comparison of statistical parametric mapping and SPECT difference imaging in patients with temporal lobe epilepsy. *Epilepsia* 2002;43:68–74.

130. Lee SK, Lee SH, Kim SK, et al. The clinical usefulness of ictal SPECT in temporal lobe epilepsy: the lateralization of seizure focus and correlation with EEG. *Epilepsia* 2000;41:955–962.

131. O'Brien TJ, So EL, Mullan BP, et al. Subtraction SPECT co-registered to MRI improves postictal SPECT localization of seizure foci. *Neurology* 1999;52:137–146.

132. Spanaki MV, Spencer SS, Corsi M, et al. Sensitivity and specificity of quantitative difference SPECT analysis in seizure localization. *J Nucl Med* 1999;40:730–736.

133. Shin WC, Hong SB, Tae WS, et al. Ictal hyperperfusion patterns according to the progression of temporal lobe seizures. *Neurology* 2002;58:373–380.

134. Sepkuty JP, Lesser RP, Civelek CA, et al. An automated injection system (with patient selection) for SPECT imaging in seizure localization. *Epilepsia* 1998;39:1350–1356.

135. Loring DW, Strauss E, Hermann BP, et al. Effects of anomalous language representation on neuropsychological performance in temporal lobe epilepsy. *Neurology* 1999;53:260–264.

136. Rasmussen T, Milner B. The role of early left-brain injury in determining lateralization of cerebral speech functions. *Ann N Y Acad Sci* 1977;299:355–369.

137. Devinsky O, Perrine K, Llinas R, et al. Anterior temporal language areas in patients with early onset of temporal lobe epilepsy. *Ann Neurol* 1993;34:727–732.

138. Ojemann G, Ojemann J, Lettich E, et al. Cortical language localization in left, dominant hemisphere. An electrical stimulation mapping investigation in 117 patients. *J Neurosurg* 1989;71:316–326.

139. Fox PT, Raichle ME. Focal physiological uncoupling of cerebral blood flow and oxidative metabolism during somatosensory stimulation of human subjects. *Proc Natl Acad Sci USA* 1986;323:806–809.

140. Roy CS, Sherrington CS. On the regulation of blood flow to the brain. *J Physiol* 1890;11:85–108.

141. Logothetis NK. The underpinnings of the BOLD functional magnetic resonance imaging signal. *J Neurosci* 2003;23:3963–3971.

142. Hunter K, Blaxton T, Bookheimer SY, et al. 15O Water positron emission tomography in language localization: a study comparing positron emission tomography visual and computerized region of interest analysis with the Wada test. *Ann Neurol* 1999;45:662–665.

143. Pardo JV, Fox PT. Preoperative assessment of the cerebral hemispheric dominance for language with CBF PET. *Hum Brain Mapp* 1993;1:57–68.

144. Bookheimer SY, Zeffiro T, Blaxton T, et al. A direct comparison of PET activation and electrocortical stimulation mapping for language localization. *Neurology* 1997;48:1056–1065.

145. Bittar RG, Olivier A, Sadikot AF, et al. Localization of somatosensory function by using positron emission tomography scanning: a comparison with intraoperative cortical stimulation. *J Neurosurg* 1999;90:478–483.

146. Fitzgerald DB, Cosgrove GR, Ronner S, et al. Location of language in the cortex: a comparison between functional MR imaging and electrocortical stimulation. *Am J Neuroradiol* 1997;18:1529–1539.

147. Moonen CTW, Bandettini PA. *Functional MRI.* Heidelberg: Springer, 2000.
148. Binder JR, Swanson SJ, Hammeke TA, et al. Determination of language dominance using functional MRI: a comparison with the Wada test. *Neurology* 1996;46:978–984.
149. Hertz-Pannier L, Gaillard WD, Mott S, et al. Assessment of language hemispheric dominance in children with epilepsy using functional MRI. *Neurology* 1997;48:1003–1012.
150. Hammeke TA, Yetkin FZ, Mueller WM, et al. Functional magnetic resonance imaging of somatosensory stimulation. *Neurosurgery* 1994;35:677–681.
151. Kim SG, Ashe J, Georgopoulos AP, et al. Functional imaging of human motor cortex at high magnetic field. *J Neurophysiol* 1993;69:297–302.
152. Kwong K, Belliveau J, Chesler D, et al. Dynamic magnetic resonance imaging of human brain activity during primary sensory stimulation. *Proc Natl Acad Sci USA* 1992;89:5675–5679.
153. Rao SM, Binder JR, Bandettini PA, et al. Functional magnetic resonance imaging of complex human movements. *Neurology* 1993;43:2311–2318.
154. Jack CR, Thompson RM, Butts RK, et al. Sensory motor cortex: correlation of presurgical mapping with functional MR imaging and invasive cortical mapping. *Radiology* 1994;190:85–92.
155. Stapleton SR, Kiriakipoulos E, Mikulis D, et al. Combined utility of functional MRI, cortical mapping, and frameless stereotaxy in the resection of lesions in eloquent areas of brain in children. *Pediatr Neurosurg* 1997;26:68–82.
156. Lehericy S, Duffau H, Cornu P, et al. Correspondence between functional magnetic resonance imaging somatotopy and individual brain anatomy of the central region: comparison with intraoperative stimulation in patients with brain tumors. *J Neurosurg* 2000;92:589–598.
157. Nelson L, Lapsiwala S, Haughton VM, et al. Preoperative mapping of the supplementary motor area in patients harboring tumors in the medial frontal lobe. *J Neurosurg* 2002;97:1108–1114.
158. Schwartz TH, Resor SR, De La Paz R, et al. Functional magnetic resonance imaging localization of ictal onset to a dysplastic cleft with simultaneous sensorimotor mapping: intraoperative electrophysiological confirmation and postoperative follow-up: technical note. *Neurosurgery* 1998;43:639–645.
159. Gaillard WD, Sachs BC, Whitnah JR, et al. Developmental aspects of language processing: fMRI of verbal fluency in children and adults. *Hum Brain Mapp* 2003;18:176–185.
160. Ramsey NF, Sommer I, Rutten GJ, et al. Combined analysis of language tasks in fMRI improves assessment of hemispheric dominance for language functions in individual subjects. *Neuroimage* 2001;13:719–733.
161. Yetkin FZ, Swanson S, Fischer M, et al. Functional MR of frontal lobe activation: comparison with Wada language results. *Am J Neuroradiol* 1998;19:1095–1098.
162. Binder JR, Rao SM, Hammeke TA, et al. Functional magnetic resonance imaging of human auditory cortex. *Ann Neurol* 1994;35:662–672.
163. Desmond JE, Sum JM, Wagner AD, et al. Language lateralization in WADA-tested patients using functional MRI. *Brain* 1995;118:1411–1419.
164. Gaillard WD, Balsamo L, Xu B, et al. Language dominance in partial epilepsy patients identified with an fMRI reading task. *Neurology* 2002;59:256–265.
165. Gaillard WD, Balsamo LM, Ibrahim Z, et al. fMRI identifies regional specialization of neural networks for reading in young children. *Neurology* 2003;60:94–100.
166. Gaillard WD, Pugliese M, Grandin CB, et al. Cortical localization of reading in normal children: an fMRI language study. *Neurology* 2001;57:47–54.
167. Schlosser MJ, Aoyagi N, Fulbright RK, et al. Functional MRI studies of auditory comprehension. *Hum Brain Mapp* 1998;6:1–13.
168. Ahmad Z, Balsamo LM, Sachs BC, et al. Auditory comprehension of language in young children: neural networks identified with fMRI. *Neurology* 2003;60:1598–1605.
169. Carpentier A, Pugh KR, Westerveld M, et al. Functional MRI of language processing: dependence on input modality and temporal lobe epilepsy. *Epilepsia* 2001;42:1241–1254.
170. Benson RR, FitzGerald DB, LeSeuer LL, et al. Language dominance determined by whole brain functional MRI in patients with brain lesions. *Neurology* 1999;52:798–809.
171. Rutten GJ, Ramsey NF, van Rijen PC, et al. fMRI-determined language lateralization in patients with unilateral or mixed language dominance according to the Wada test. *Neuroimage* 2002;17:447–460.
172. Gaillard WD, Balsamo L, Xu B, et al. fMRI language task panel improves determination of language dominance. *Neurology* 2004;63:1403–1408.
173. Pouratian N, Bookheimer S, Rex D, et al. Utility of preoperative functional magnetic resonance imaging for identifying language cortices in patients with vascular malformations. *J Neurosurg* 2002;97:21–32.
174. Deblaere K, Backes WH, Hofman P, et al. Developing a comprehensive presurgical functional MRI protocol for patients with intractable temporal lobe epilepsy: a pilot study. *Neuroradiology* 2002;44:667–673.
175. Spreer J, Arnold S, Quiske A, et al. Determination of hemisphere dominance for language: comparison of frontal and temporal fMRI activation with intracarotid amytal testing. *Neuroradiology* 2002;44:467–474.
176. Fernandez G, de Greiff A, von Oertzen J, et al. Language mapping in less than 15 minutes: real-time functional MRI during routine clinical investigation. *Neuroimage* 2001;14:585–594.
177. Sabsevitz DS, Swanson SJ, Hammeke TA, et al. Use of preoperative functional neuroimaging to predict language deficits from epilepsy surgery. *Neurology* 2003;60:1788–1792.
178. Gaillard WD, Bookheimer SY, Cohen M. The use of fMRI in neocortical epilepsy. In: Williamson PD, Siegal AM, Roberts DE, Thudani VM, et al. eds. *Advances in Neurology vol. 84 Neocortical Epilepsy.* Philadelphia: Lippincott Williams & Wilkins, 2000:391–404.
179. Lehericy S, Biondi A, Sourour N, et al. Arteriovenous brain malformations: is functional MR imaging reliable for studying language reorganization in patients? Initial observations. *Radiology* 2002;223:672–682.
180. Jayakar P, Bernal B, Santiago Medina L, et al. False lateralization of language cortex on functional MRI after a cluster of focal seizures. *Neurology* 2002;58:490–492.
181. Gabrieli JDE, Brewer JB, Desmond JE, et al. Separate neural bases of two fundamental memory processes in the human medial temporal lobe. *Science* 1997;276:264–266.
182. Stern CE, Corkin S, González RG, et al. The hippocampal formation participates in novel picture encoding: evidence from functional magnetic resonance imaging. *Proc Natl Acad Sci U S A* 1996;93:8660–8665.
183. Brewer JB, Zhao Z, Desmond JE, et al. Making memories: brain activity that predicts how well visual experience will be remembered. *Science* 1998;281:1185–1187.
184. Kelley WM, Miezin FM, McDermott KB, et al. Hemispheric specialization in human dorsal frontal cortex and medial temporal lobe for verbal and nonverbal memory encoding. *Neuron* 1998;20:927–936.
185. Golby AJ, Poldrack RA, Brewer JB, et al. Material-specific lateralization in the medial temporal lobe and prefrontal cortex during memory encoding. *Brain* 2001;124:1841–1854.
186. Golby AJ, Poldrack RA, Illes J, et al. Memory lateralization in medial temporal lobe epilepsy assessed by functional MRI. *Epilepsia* 2002;43:855–863.
187. Dupont S, Van de Moortele PF, Samson S, et al. Episodic memory in left temporal lobe epilepsy: a functional MRI study. *Brain* 2000;123(Pt 8):1722–1732.
188. Jokeit H, Okujava M, Woermann FG. Memory fMRI lateralizes temporal lobe epilepsy. *Neurology* 2001;57:1786–1793.
189. Bellgowan PSF, Binder JR, Swanson SJ, et al. Side of seizure focus predicts left medial temporal lobe activation during verbal encoding. *Neurology* 1998;51:479–484.
190. Detre JA, Maccotta L, King D, et al. Functional MRI lateralization of memory in temporal lobe epilepsy. *Neurology* 1998;50:926–932.

191. Binder JR, Detre JA, Jones-Gotman M, et al. Functional MRI of episodic memory in temporal lobe epilepsy. *Epilepsia* 2002; 43(Suppl 7).

192. Detre JA, Sirven JI, Alsop DC, et al. Localization of subclinical ictal activity by functional magnetic resonance imaging: correlation with invasive monitoring. *Ann Neurol* 1995;38: 618–624.

193. Jackson GD, Connelly A, Cross JH, et al. Functional magnetic resonance imaging of focal seizures. *Neurology* 1994;44: 850–856.

194. Salek-Haddadi A, Lemieux L, Merschhemke M, et al. Functional magnetic resonance imaging of human absence seizures. *Ann Neurol* 2003;53:663–667.

195. Krakow K, Woermann FG, Symms MR, et al. EEG-triggered functional MRI of interictal epileptiform activity in patients with partial seizures. *Brain* 1999;122:1679–1688.

196. Symms MR, Allen PJ, Woermann FG, et al. Reproductive localization of interictal epileptiform discharges using EEG-triggered fMRI. *Phys Med Biol* 1999;44:N161–N168.

197. Krakow K, Lemieux L, Messina D, et al. Spatio-temporal imaging of focal interictal epileptiform activity using EEG-triggered functional MRI. *Epileptic Disord* 2001;3:67–74.

198. Rutten GJM, van Rijen PC, van Veelen CWM, et al. Language area localization with three-dimensional functional magnetic resonance imaging matches intrasulcal electrosimulation in Broca's area. *Ann Neurol* 1999;46:405–415.

Intracranial Electroencephalography and Localization Studies

77

Selim R. Benbadis   *Elaine Wyllie*   *William E. Bingaman*

In recent years, as new neuroimaging techniques have revealed hippocampal sclerosis, focal cortical dysplasia, and other subtle epileptogenic lesions, the use of chronically implanted invasive electrodes has decreased at many epilepsy surgery centers. The risks of invasive electrodes are not warranted when magnetic resonance imaging (MRI) and extracranial electroencephalography (EEG) disclose concordant evidence of an epileptogenic zone in a safely resectable area. Neuroimaging is now so advanced that the majority of patients who undergo resective epilepsy surgery do not require invasive EEG studies. In some cases, however, invasive techniques remain important because of discordant or poorly defined results from noninvasive testing or close proximity of the epileptogenic zone to eloquent cortex.

EXTRACRANIAL ELECTROENCEPHALOGRAPHY: THE STARTING POINT

The questions to be answered with intracranial electrodes are shaped by the results of the noninvasive evaluation, including extracranial EEG (1–3). Ideal for the initial identification of a suspected region of epileptogenesis, extracranial EEG provides a broad survey of EEG rhythms throughout both hemispheres and should be designed to yield the maximum localizing information about the epileptogenic zone (3). Sphenoidal electrodes (Fig. 77.1) may be helpful when mesial temporal lobe epilepsy is suspected. Generally, surface EEG-video monitoring is the initial test for any patient with frequent seizures despite medications, as 20% to 30% of adults will turn out to have psychogenic seizures (see Chapter 42).

The main limitation of extracranial EEG is decreased sensitivity to cortical generators (4,5). Intracranial electrodes overcome the sensitivity limitations of extracranial electrodes because they are closer to the cortical focus and free of the dampening effect of the skull and scalp. This increased sensitivity, however, is at the expense of more restricted sampling, or "vision," and involves an enhanced risk of complications.

Intracranial EEG may fail to define further the epileptogenic zone if problem areas are insufficiently covered, but the use of large numbers of electrodes is limited by the proportional increase in the rate of complications. For this reason, intracranial electrodes should be used only after noninvasive testing (i.e., EEG, video semiology, and imaging) has "narrowed down" the epileptogenic zone to a limited brain region that can be covered safely and adequately by the chosen invasive technique.

The strength of the hypothesis based on the results of the noninvasive evaluation is a key to successful use of invasive techniques. The clearer the question formulated for testing, the greater the chance of success with the invasive evaluation.

This chapter provides an overview of the invasive techniques available for these difficult cases and reviews the major clinical situations and how they can be approached.

INTRACRANIAL ELECTRODES: AN OVERVIEW

Depth and subdural electrodes are the most commonly used intracranial electrodes. Because of limited sensitivity, foramen ovale and epidural peg electrodes are rarely or no longer placed.

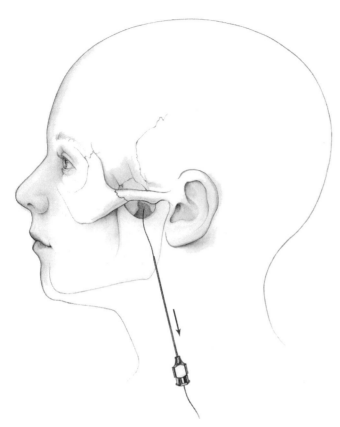

Figure 77.1   Placement of a sphenoidal electrode. A thin electrode wire is introduced into the subtemporal fossa within a 22-gauge lumbar puncture needle. After the needle is inserted to a depth of 3 to 5 cm, the cannula is withdrawn and the wire is left in place. The wire is looped and taped into place on the cheek, and the distal end I soldered to connectors for use in the electrode jackbox.

DEPTH ELECTRODES

Surgical Aspects

Depth electrodes are multiple-contact "needles" of polyurethane or other material that typically are inserted into the brain by way of twist-drill skull holes under stereotactic guidance (6–8). Modern computer-assisted image-based stereotaxy has greatly improved the ease and precision of depth electrode placement. A target is chosen on the MRI scan, and entry point, trajectory, and depth are calculated by the computer to result in precise placement of the electrode tip within 1 mm of the target.

A common approach for patients with suspected bitemporal epilepsy uses three electrodes, each with eight contacts that are advanced transversely through punctures in the middle or inferior temporal gyri into the amygdala and anterior and posterior hippocampus on each side (Fig. 77.2). These allow the survey of electrical activity from the mesial structures, from infolded gray matter of basal temporal gyri, and from the lateral temporal lobe.

An alternative trajectory for the evaluation of mesial temporal epilepsy is the longitudinal placement of depth electrodes by way of occipital burr holes (8–10). With this approach, the electrode traverses the course of the hippocampus along its axis, sampling electrical activity throughout its length. Extratemporal foci are surveyed by carefully locating the electrodes according to structural lesions or particular gyri with suspected involvement in the epileptogenic zone (11).

Depth electrodes may be placed under local or general anesthesia, with the latter preferred for lengthy procedures involving multiple insertions, and can be removed under local anesthesia. Previous insertion of depth electrodes does not significantly limit further options of epilepsy surgery, including the subsequent use of other electrode types.

Advantages

The main advantage is direct access to deep structures for EEG recording very close to potential generators (12–14). Electrodes can be left in place for days to weeks with minimal risk of infection, permitting extensive ictal recording. Ictal EEG onset with depth electrodes often precedes onset with scalp and sphenoidal electrodes by 20 or 30 seconds, and in some cases, especially auras ("simple partial seizures"), the EEG seizure pattern may be seen only with depth recording. Depth electrodes may clearly locate seizure onset when extracranial localization is unclear. In addition to seizure onset, seizure *termination* may also have localizing and prognostic value, with unilateral termination

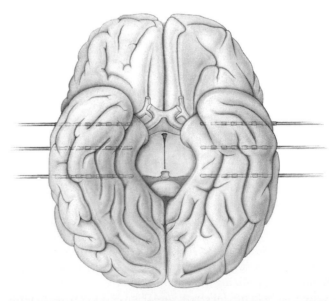

Figure 77.2   Bitemporal depth electrodes. In this array, three multicontact electrodes are inserted on each side so that the contacts distal to the insertion site lie within the amygdale, anterior hippocampus, and posterior hippocampus. The contacts most proximal to the insertion site lie within the lateral cortex of the middle temporal gyrus. Other arrays place electrodes in an anterior-posterior or superior-inferior orientation.

(as opposed to simultaneous bilateral, contralateral, or mixed termination) predicting better outcome after temporal lobectomy (15).

Disadvantages

Depth electrodes sample only a relatively small brain region, providing a very detailed but also very focused EEG sample. This focus may be inadequate when the issue is localization of seizure onset within a relatively large region such as the frontal lobe.

In addition, placement requires brain penetration. This raises theoretical concerns about damage to cortical areas outside the resection site and also makes depth electrodes inappropriate for the study of potential epileptogenic foci near vascular malformations. The examination of resected tissues has revealed gliosis, cystic degeneration, or microabscesses along the tracks of depth electrodes, but several studies (10) have failed to demonstrate any functional sequelae in the absence of clinically apparent bleeding or infection, and overall depth electrodes are safe (16).

The risk of bleeding or infection is only 0.5% to 5% (12,17). Routine imaging studies commonly reveal asymptomatic subdural collections of blood, but intraparenchymal hemorrhage is very rare [less than 1% in series (7,10) using modern stereotactic techniques]. The risk of significant hemorrhage is decreased by careful attention to electrode trajectories on preoperative planning studies so as to avoid major vascular structures.

SUBDURAL ELECTRODES (GRIDS AND STRIPS)

Surgical Aspects

Probably the most commonly used invasive electrodes, subdural electrodes are embedded in strips or sheets of polyurethane or other material and may be implanted subdurally over epileptogenic regions (Fig. 77.3) (18–25). These discs of stainless steel or platinum alloy, approximately 2 to 4 mm in diameter, are embedded in polyurethane at fixed interelectrode distances, typically 10 mm, in various arrays. The strips and grids include one or more cables with bundled insulated wires connecting to the individual electrodes. Cables can be connected by means of various interface blocks to conventional EEG equipment for recording and stimulation. Other subdural grids have been designed with electrode contacts on both sides of the polyurethane sheet for recording from both surfaces, as in interhemispheric locations.

Strips can be inserted under fluoroscopic guidance through individual burr holes or trephines for bilateral placement when the side of seizure onset must be determined. The cables exit through a stab wound separate from the main incision to assist with anchoring of the strip and to decrease cerebrospinal fluid leakage and infection.

Subdural strips may be placed under local or general anesthesia, although general anesthesia is preferred for multiple burr holes and multiple strip insertions. The risk of infection and hemorrhage with insertion of subdural strips has been reported to be less than 1% (9,21). Because mobility of implanted subdural strips may change the position of electrodes in relation to the intended recording target, serial skull roentgenograms should be performed to verify stability of position.

Grids are inserted by way of open craniotomy (Fig. 77.4). Flap design allows coverage of all regions of suspected epileptogenicity and subsequent access to any possible resection to the region of interest. Subdural plates may be "slid" beyond the edges of the craniotomy to cover adjacent areas, including basal temporal, basal frontal, and interhemispheric regions. Subdural grids are sutured to the overlying dura mater to prevent movement. A watertight dural closure around the electrode cables lessens the possibility of cerebrospinal fluid leakage. Whenever feasible, the overlying bone flap should be osteoplastic (attached to a vascularized muscle and periosteal pedicle) to prevent flap osteomyelitis. The electrode cable exits through a stab wound separate from the main incision, and watertight sutures are used at the exit site to reduce cerebrospinal fluid leakage. Despite these precautions, minor leakage frequently occurs without serious complications.

After completion of the evaluation with subdural electrodes, the patient is returned to the operating room for reopening of the craniotomy, removal of the subdural electrodes, and final resection of the mapped epileptogenic zone. This second operation typically is performed using general anesthesia, although local anesthesia is an option when further brain mapping is necessary. At reoperation, cultures are obtained from all layers of the wound, all electrode hardware, and the bone flap. If bacterial colonization of one or more wound layers is observed, the patient receives vigorous intravenous antibiotic therapy directed against the cultured organism(s) for two weeks following removal of the electrodes to reduce the risk of flap osteomyelitis.

With an overall rate of 26%, subdural grids present the greatest potential for complications (26). These include infection (12%), transient neurologic deficit (11%), epidural hematoma (2.5%), increased intracranial pressure (2.5%), infarction (1.5%), and death (0.5%). The occurrence of complications is associated with large numbers of grids/electrodes (more than 60 electrodes), lengthy monitoring (more than 10 days), older age, left-sided grid insertion, and burr holes in addition to the craniotomy. Improvements in grid technology, surgical technique, and postoperative care may reduce the rate of complications (26–28).

Functional Localization Studies

Functional localization techniques with subdural electrodes include cortical stimulation and evoked potential

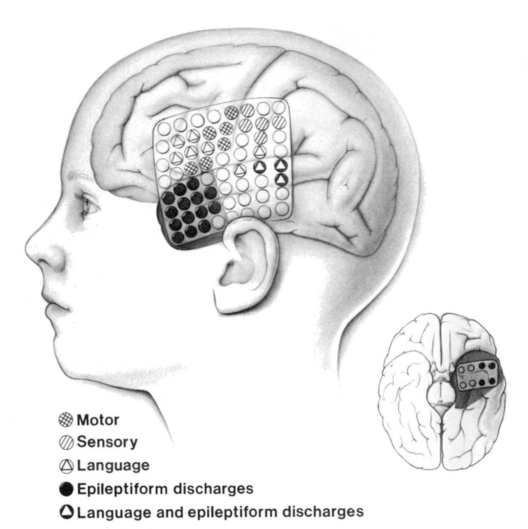

⊕ **Motor**

⊘ **Sensory**

△ **Language**

● **Epileptiform discharges**

◯ **Language and epileptiform discharges**

Figure 77.3 Results of electroencephalography (EEG) and cortical stimulation with subdural electrode grids. With scalp and sphenoidal EEG, this patient had epileptiform discharges from the anterior and posterior left temporal lobe. Extraoperative subdural EEG showed interictal sharp waves from anterolateral, posterolateral, and basal temporal areas. Seizures arose from anterior and basal temporal regions. The posterior temporal area with interictal sharp waves was within Wernicke language area, so this region was left untouched by the extensive left temporal lobectomy. Resection extended 7.5 cm posteriorly from the anterior temporal tip. Histopathologic examination of resected tissue showed cortical dysplasia; the magnetic resonance imaging techniques at that time were not adequate to reveal the subtle malformation. The patient remains seizure free on medication 12 years after surgery but has had seizures when medications were withdrawn.

studies. Cortical stimulation involves passage of a small electrical current through individual electrodes, with close observation for symptoms or interference with cortical function (20,29). An alternating current is applied for 5 to 10 seconds, with subsequent stepwise advancement from 1 mA to a maximum of 15 mA or until symptoms or afterdischarges on EEG develop. Symptoms during stimulation may include positive motor phenomena (tonic or clonic contraction of a muscle group), negative motor phenomena (inhibition of voluntary movements of the tongue, fingers, or toes), somatosensory phenomena (tingling, tightness, or numbness of a part of the body), or language impairment (speech hesitation or arrest, anomia, or recep-

tive difficulties). To screen for negative motor or language impairment during stimulation, the patient may be challenged to read or perform rapid alternating movements of the fingers, toes, or tongue. Signs or symptoms during stimulation of an electrode are interpreted to mean that the underlying cortex has importance for the affected function.

In addition to mapping eloquent cortex, stimulation may also help to localize epileptogenic cortex. After single pulse stimulation, "early responses" (starting within 100 ms) are found in all areas of cortex. Delayed responses (spikes or sharp waves occurring between 100 ms and 1 second after stimulation) appear to be significantly associated with the epileptogenic zone (30).

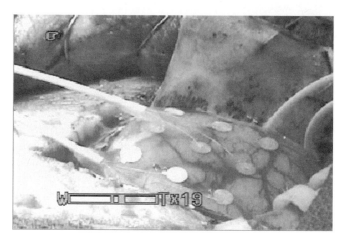

Figure 77.4 Temporal craniotomy with intraoperative placement of a subdural grid. Note the cable connecting the contacts to the EEG amplifier and the retracted dura mater in the upper portion (Courtesy of Fernando Vale, MD, University of South Florida and Tampa General Hospital).

Advantages

Subdural electrodes permit detailed definition of the epileptogenic zone in relation to eloquent cortex. Epileptiform discharges may be recorded during wakefulness, sleep, and seizures and then mapped (20) to define the safest, most

complete resection of epileptogenic zones (24,25). Ictal EEG patterns are usually well defined if electrodes are over the epileptogenic zone. At least for temporal lobe seizures, the time from EEG onset to clinical onset may have a prognostic value (31). Subdural electrodes can be visualized on and combined with imaging in order to localize EEG findings with respect to normal anatomy or lesions (Fig. 77.5).

In another method of functional localization (32), median or posterior tibial evoked potentials may be recorded directly from the cortical surface by means of subdural electrodes, with maximum amplitudes over the postcentral gyrus. Results may confirm rolandic sensorimotor localization by cortical stimulation.

In infants and young children, cortical stimulation studies are more challenging. Sensory, negative motor, and language function cannot be assessed reliably during stimulation in infants. Special stimulation paradigms are required to elicit positive motor effects in children younger than three or four years (32,33). Evoked potential studies with subdural electrodes may help to identify the postcentral gyrus at any age.

Disadvantages

The risks of wound infection and flap osteomyelitis are the main disadvantages of chronically implanted subdural

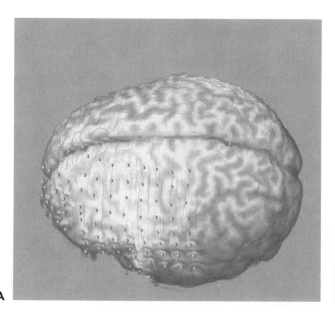

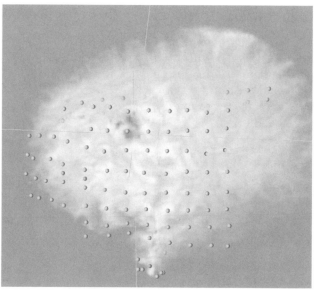

A

B

Figure 77.5 This 12-year-old girl with a 2-year history of left frontal lobe epilepsy underwent invasive evaluation with subdural grid electrodes. Preoperative MRI showed a hyperintense lesion on the fluid attenuated inversion recovery (FLAIR) and T2-weighted images in the left superior frontal gyrus extending to the ependymal surface of the lateral ventricle. **A** shows a volume-rendered brain image of the patient constructed from the postoperative three-dimensional T1-weighted MRI. Electrode location was identified by flow-void artifacts and coregistered on the image (*dots*). The lateral convexity of the frontal lobe is covered by an 8 × 8 array with 1-cm interelectrode spacing. **B** shows the relationship of the lesion (*dark area*) to the electrode. The FLAIR images were linearly overlaid on the same MRI, and the hyperintense lesion was highlighted after the T1 volume was made translucent. The lesion is located beneath the first two electrodes in the third column from the anterosuperior edge. The EEG onset of her habitual seizure (aura and right arm tonic seizure) was recorded from these as well as from the mesial frontal electrodes. The patient underwent resection of the superior and middle frontal gyri including the lesion. The pathologic diagnosis was consistent with cortical dysplasia.

electrode grids. The incidence of 5% to 15% (24,25) about a decade ago has decreased in recent years, but occasional infections have occurred despite compulsive intraoperative culturing of all wound layers and vigorous prophylactic use of antibiotics. Infection may be less frequent with subdural strips (22,33) than with grids.

Other complications of subdural electrodes—acute meningitis, cerebral edema, and hemorrhage—are rare. Meningitis necessitates immediate electrode removal and vigorous antibiotic therapy. Brain edema can, rarely, be symptomatic, requiring early removal of electrodes, but usually it can be successfully combated with judicious fluid and electrolyte management. Occurring in approximately 2% of patients (19), subdural or epidural hemorrhage may prompt premature removal of electrodes and evacuation of hemorrhage.

Concerns about intracranial pressure limit the number of subdural electrodes, so that only restricted unilateral cortical areas can be covered with grids. Strips can cover widespread areas through multiple burr holes, but mobility of the strips can be a problem and blind insertion of the strips may be impeded by subdural scarring or other structural lesions.

NEW OR INVESTIGATIONAL TECHNIQUES

Intraventricular Electrodes

In this newly proposed technique, frameless image guidance can be used to place a 10-contact depth electrode through a rigid neuroendoscope within the atrium of the lateral ventricle. Invasiveness is lessened and complications may be fewer than with transcortical depth electrode placement (34,35).

Cavernous Sinus Electrodes

This newer semi-invasive technique may be useful for lateralization of temporal lobe epilepsy (36,37). Wire electrodes can be placed in the cavernous sinus and the superior petrosal sinus by way of the jugular vein.

INTRAOPERATIVE ELECTROCORTICOGRAPHY AND FUNCTIONAL MAPPING

Surgical Aspects

Intraoperative electrocorticography (ECoG), the recording from electrodes laid directly over exposed cortex after craniotomy (29,38–40), can be performed with the patient under either local anesthesia (fully awake) or general anesthesia. Because general anesthetic agents may affect ECoG,

all inhalation agents are discontinued approximately 30 minutes before the recording. Paralytic agents, nitrous oxide, and intravenous narcotics are continued to maintain manageable general anesthesia without potential effects of inhalation agents.

Intraoperative ECoG may (occasionally) include the recording of evoked potentials to localize the rolandic fissure and orient the surgeon toward gyral anatomy so as to avoid resections in functional motor or sensory areas. Interictal epileptiform activity can be recorded for a stated period to define a zone of frequent interictal spiking, thereby helping the surgeon tailor the resection for maximal excision of these areas. Surgical manipulation itself, however, may create some spike activity ("injury spikes"), and the practice of "chasing spikes" to maximize resection has not been shown convincingly to improve the outcome of resective epilepsy procedures. Most investigators have found that spikes on postresection ECoG do not reliably predict a less favorable outcome in temporal lobe resections (24,41–47). Preexcision spikes on three or more gyri that persist after resection, especially at a distance from the resection border, carry a poor prognosis, at least in nontumoral frontal lobe epilepsy (47).

Intraoperative cortical stimulation can delineate areas of primary motor, sensory, and speech function with the patient under local anesthesia. Even with light general anesthesia (without paralytic agents), this technique can reliably identify primary motor areas by allowing direct observation of clonic or tonic movement in respective muscle groups and facilitating tailored resections close to motor regions (39).

Advantages

Intraoperative techniques permit definition of functional cortex in relation to the epileptogenic zone while avoiding the potential complications of long-term invasive electrodes. The procedure lengthens the operating time but otherwise imparts no added risk to the patient. Detailed intraoperative cortical stimulation under local anesthesia is readily performed in cooperative adolescents and adults (40) but is more difficult in young children or uncooperative adults. Even in young or difficult patients, however, it is usually possible to identify primary motor cortex intraoperatively with cortical stimulation and evoked potential studies using light general anesthesia (48).

Disadvantages

Because the total recording time of intraoperative techniques is limited to a few hours, recording during seizures is almost never obtained. Another limitation to intraoperative techniques is the stressful nature of the conditions for cortical stimulation while the patient is awake.

INDICATIONS AND CLINICAL USE

Suspected Bilateral Mesial Temporal Lobe Epilepsy

The need for invasive EEG in temporal lobe epilepsy has diminished as more powerful MRI has enhanced identification of hippocampal pathology. Nevertheless, bilateral mesial temporal lobe epilepsy is the most common indication for depth electrodes implanted into the amygdala and anterior and posterior hippocampus on both sides (8,14,49,50).

Bitemporal strips may also be used in this setting. Some authors (43) have found that subdural and depth electrodes are comparably sensitive for detection of interictal spikes in both mesial and neocortical temporal lobe epilepsy. Depth electrodes, however, are the only ones to lie within the mesial epileptogenic cortex and thus may better allow detection of mesial-onset seizures than do subdural strips, which can reach only the parahippocampal gyrus (51,52). For example, studies that used both methods simultaneously reported cases in which bitemporal strips failed to provide adequate information to proceed with surgery (52–54). Occasionally, subdural strips can even be falsely lateralizing (55). Only depth electrodes reliably record faster frequencies at onset (56,57), suggesting closer proximity to the generator. Although depth electrodes probably remain the gold standard for recording hippocampal onset, subdural strips are probably adequate when the issue is only lateralization of temporal lobe epilepsy (58). When extratemporal onset is a concern (e.g., in the setting of an extratemporal lesion of uncertain relevance), a combination of depth and subdural electrodes is appropriate (9,11,59).

Epileptogenic Zone Near Eloquent Cortex

Subdural electrodes are the method of choice whenever eloquent cortex must be clearly separated from the epileptogenic zone. For example, subdural electrodes may be used to define a frontal or parietal focus in relation to rolandic sensorimotor areas, a left lateral temporal focus in relation to Wernicke's language area, or a mesial frontal or parietal focus in relation to the supplementary motor area and primary motor cortex for the leg.

Although either extraoperative or intraoperative techniques can be used to resolve such localization problems, the considerable variability in preferred methods depends largely on the familiarity of the surgery team with each approach. In general, intraoperative techniques may be preferable when the primary objective is localization of rolandic motor areas, for example, in preparation for anatomic frontal lobectomy or lesionectomy. In fact, intraoperative mapping is often used before resection in patients without seizures. Extraoperative techniques may be preferable if ictal recording is required to define the epileptogenic zone. The two techniques can also be combined, with extraoperative seizure recording followed by intraoperative mapping just before resection.

Poor Localization of Epileptogenic Zone

Hemisphere Known but Exact Localization Uncertain

Relatively often, the results of the noninvasive evaluation unequivocally point to a hemisphere, but the lobe cannot be confidently identified. In these patients, prognosis for surgical outcome is typically guarded, but an attempt to better define the epileptogenic zone with invasive techniques may be appropriate in some patients, and outcome can be excellent (60). Because this requires coverage of large areas on one side, grids can be combined with strips or depth electrodes. Depth EEG has been used, with good results, to resolve other discrete localization issues such as mesial temporal versus orbitofrontal or cingulate seizure onset. In these cases, depth and subdural electrodes may be used together (53,59), especially for a presumed extratemporal onset, such as orbitofrontal (9) or occipital (11).

In the presence of a lesion apparent on MRI, even such subtle anomalies as a suspected cortical dysplasia, invasive EEG may not be necessary (61). However, any lesion should not be assumed to be the source of the seizures ("dual pathology"), as some lesions are often incidental (e.g., arachnoid cysts). If an extratemporal lesion is present but electroclinical data (EEG-video) suggest temporal onset, or if MRI evidence supports mesiotemporal sclerosis but electroclinical data suggest extratemporal onset, then invasive EEG (strips or grids) is needed.

Lobar Localization Known but Side Uncertain

Although most cases of extratemporal onset involve difficult *intrahemispheric* localization, lateralization is occasionally at issue. This is particularly common in seizures arising from the supplementary sensorimotor area, where symptomatology and midline epileptiform discharges indicate mesial frontal onset, but lateralization is unclear in the absence of imaging abnormalities or clinical lateralizing signs (62). These highly challenging cases may be difficult to clarify even with invasive EEG.

When the noninvasive presurgical evaluation does not sufficiently narrow the possibilities for localization, invasive studies may be of limited benefit.

CONCLUSIONS

With the advent of modern neuroimaging, the use of invasive electrodes has diminished. Presurgical evaluation in patients with localization-related epilepsy remains variable and controversial. No universal scheme is accepted by all epilepsy surgery centers. Techniques improve, and strategic approaches continue to evolve (63). In each case, the decisions whether or not to use an invasive technique and, if so, which one should be based on results of an extensive noninvasive evaluation including extracranial EEG, video and seizure semiology analysis, structural and functional neuroimaging, and neuropsychological testing. Appreciating the brain coverage, strengths, and weaknesses of each invasive technique will help in this choice. In addition, the risk of invasive techniques varies among surgeons; as with other types of surgical procedures, experience and successful practice are important. The lowest complication rates can be expected from experienced epilepsy neurosurgeons at high-volume epilepsy surgery centers.

ACKNOWLEDGMENT

The drawings in this chapter are original art by Elaine Bammerlin.

REFERENCES

1. Lüders H, Dinner DS, Morris HH, et al. EEG evaluation for epilepsy surgery in children. *Cleve Clin J Med* 1989;56:S53–S61.
2. Lüders HO, Engel J Jr, Munari C. Noninvasive preoperative evaluation: general principles. In: Engel J Jr, ed. *Surgical treatment of the epilepsies*, 2nd ed. New York: Raven Press, 1993:137–155.
3. Quesney LF, Risinger MW, Shewmon DA. Extracranial EEG evaluation. In: Engel J Jr, ed. *Surgical treatment of the epilepsies*, 2nd ed. New York: Raven Press, 1993:173–196.
4. Benbadis SR. Invasive EEG. In: Lüders HO, ed. *The epileptic seizure: pathophysiology and semiology*. Philadelphia: WB Saunders, 2000: 49–53.
5. Risinger MW. Invasive EEG. In: Lüders HO, ed. *The epileptic seizure: pathophysiology and semiology*. Philadelphia: WB Saunders, 2000: 32–48.
6. McCarthy G, Spencer DD, Riker RJ. The stereotaxic placement of depth electrodes in epilepsy. In: Lüders H, ed. *Epilepsy surgery*. New York: Raven Press, 1991:385–393.
7. Pillay PK, Barnett GH, Awad IA, et al. MRI-guided placement of depth electrodes in temporal lobe epilepsy: a comparison of the CRW and BRW arc systems. *Br J Neurosurg* 1992;6:47–53.
8. Spencer SS, So NK, Engel J Jr, et al. Depth electrodes. In: Engel J Jr, ed. *Surgical treatment of the epilepsies*, 2nd ed. New York: Raven Press, 1993:359–376.
9. Blatt DR, Roper SN, Friedman WA. Invasive monitoring of limbic epilepsy using stereotactic depth and subdural strip electrodes: surgical technique. *Surg Neurol* 1997;48:74–79.
10. Spencer DD. Stereotactic methods in the management of epilepsy. In: Heilbrun MP, ed. *Stereotactic neurosurgery*. Baltimore: Williams & Wilkins, 1988:161–178.
11. Palmini A, Andermann F, Dubeau F, et al. Occipitotemporal epilepsies: evaluation of selected patients requiring depth electrode studies and rationale for surgical approaches. *Epilepsia* 1993; 34:84–96.
12. So NK, Gloor P, Quesney F, et al. Depth electrode investigations in patients with bitemporal epileptiform abnormalities. *Ann Neurol* 1989;25:423–431.
13. Spencer SS. Depth electroencephalography in selection of refractory epilepsy for surgery. *Ann Neurol* 1981;9:207–214.
14. Spencer SS, Spencer DD, Williamson PD, et al. The localizing value of depth electroencephalography in 32 patients with refractory epilepsy. *Ann Neurol* 1982;12:248–253.
15. Fernandez G, Hufnagel A, Van Roost D, et al. Safety of intrahippocampal depth electrodes for presurgical evaluation of patients with intractable epilepsy. *Epilepsia* 1997;38:922–929.
16. Verma A, Lewis D, VanLandingham KE, et al. Lateralized seizure termination: relationship to outcome following anterior temporal lobectomy. *Epilepsy Res* 2001;47:9–15.
17. Spencer SS. Controversies in epileptology. Depth vs. subdural electrode studies for unlocalized epilepsy. *J Epilepsy* 1989;2: 123–127.
18. Arroyo S, Lesser RP, Awad IA, et al. Subdural and epidural grids and strips. In: Engel J Jr, ed. *Surgical treatment of the epilepsies*, 2nd ed. New York: Raven Press, 1993:377–386.
19. Lesser RP, Gordon B, Fisher R, et al. Subdural grid electrodes in surgery of epilepsy. In: Lüders H, ed. *Epilepsy surgery*. New York: Raven Press, 1991:399–408.
20. Lüders H, Lesser RP, Dinner DS, et al. Chronic intracranial recording and stimulation with subdural electrodes. In: Engel J Jr, ed. *Surgical treatment of the epilepsies*. New York: Raven Press, 1987:297–321.
21. Wyler AR. Subdural strip electrodes in surgery of epilepsy. In: Lüders H, ed. *Epilepsy surgery*. New York: Raven Press, 1991: 395–398.
22. Wyler AR, Walker G, Somes G. The morbidity of long-term seizure monitoring using subdural strip electrodes. *J Neurosurg* 1991;74: 734–737.
23. Wyler AR, Wilkus RJ, Blume WT. Strip electrodes. In: Engel J Jr, ed. *Surgical treatment of the epilepsies*, 2nd ed. New York: Raven Press, 1993:387–398.
24. Wyllie E, Lüders H, Morris HH, et al. Clinical outcome after complete or partial cortical resection for intractable epilepsy. *Neurology* 1987;37:1634–1641.
25. Wyllie E, Lüders H, Morris HH, et al. Subdural electrodes in the evaluation for epilepsy surgery in children and adults. *Neuropediatrics* 1988;19:80–86.
26. Hamer HM, Morris HH, Mascha EJ, et al. Complications of invasive video-EEG monitoring with subdural grid electrodes. *Neurology* 2002;58:97–103.
27. Onal C, Otsubo H, Araki T, et al. Complications of invasive subdural grid monitoring in children with epilepsy. *J Neurosurg* 2003; 98:1017–1026.
28. Simon SL, Telfeian A, Duhaime AC. Complications of invasive monitoring used in intractable pediatric epilepsy. *Pediatr Neurosurg* 2003;38:47–52.
29. Ojemann GA, Sutherling WW, Lesser RP, et al. Cortical stimulation. In: Engel J Jr, ed. *Surgical treatment of the epilepsies*, 2nd ed. New York: Raven Press, 1993:399–414.
30. Valentin A, Anderson M, Alarcon G, et al. Responses to single pulse electrical stimulation identify epileptogenesis in the human brain in vivo. *Brain* 2002;125(Pt 8):1709–1718.
31. Weinand ME, Kester MM, Labiner DM, et al. Time from ictal subdural EEG seizure onset to clinical seizure onset: prognostic value for selecting temporal lobectomy candidates. *Neurol Res* 2001;23: 599–604.
32. Nespeca M, Wyllie E, Lüders H, et al. Subdural electrodes in infants and young children. *J Epilepsy* 1990;3(Suppl 1):107–124.
33. Jayakar P, Alvarez LA, Duchowny MS, et al. A safe and effective paradigm to functionally map the cortex in childhood. *J Clin Neurophysiol* 1992;9:288–293.
34. Song JK, Abou-Khalil B, Konrad PE. Intraventricular monitoring for temporal lobe epilepsy: report on technique and initial results in eight patients. *J Neurol Neurosurg Psychiatry* 2003;74:561–565.
35. Jimenez O, Leal R, Nagore N. Minimally invasive electrodiagnostic monitoring in epilepsy surgery. *Br J Neurosurg* 2002;16:498–500.
36. Kunieda T, Ikeda A, Mikuni N, et al. Use of cavernous sinus EEG in the detection of seizure onset and spread in mesial temporal lobe epilepsy. *Epilepsia* 2000;41:1411–1419.
37. Mikuni N, Ikeda A, Murao K, et al. "Cavernous sinus EEG": a new method for the preoperative evaluation of temporal lobe epilepsy. *Epilepsia* 1997;38:472–482.
38. Ojemann GA. Intraoperative tailoring of temporal lobe resection. In: Engel J Jr, ed. *Surgical treatment of the epilepsies*, 2nd ed. New York: Raven Press, 1993:481–488.
39. Ojemann GA, Engel J Jr. Acute and chronic intracranial recording and stimulation. In: Engel J Jr, ed. *Surgical treatment of the epilepsies*. New York: Raven Press, 1987:263–296.
40. Penfield W, Jasper H. *Epilepsy and the functional anatomy of the human brain*. Boston, Mass: Little, Brown & Co, 1954.
41. Cascino GD, Trenerry MR, Jack CR, et al. Electrocorticography and temporal lobe epilepsy: relationship to quantitative MRI and operative outcome. *Epilepsia* 1995;36:692.

42. Kanazawa O, Blume WT, Girvin JP. Significance of spikes at temporal lobe electrocorticography. *Epilepsia* 1996;37:50–55.
43. Schwartz TH, Bazil CW, Walczak TS, et al. The predictive value of intraoperative electrocorticography in resections for limbic epilepsy associated with mesial temporal sclerosis. *Neurosurgery* 1997;40:302–309.
44. Tran TA, Spencer SS, Javidan M, et al. Significance of spikes recorded on intraoperative electrocorticography in patients with brain tumor and epilepsy. *Epilepsia* 1997;38:1132–1139.
45. Tran TA, Spencer SS, Marks D, et al. Significance of spikes recorded on electrocorticography in nonlesional medial temporal lobe epilepsy. *Ann Neurol* 1995;38:763–770.
46. Tuunainen A, Nousiainen U, Mervaala E, et al. Postoperative EEG and electrocorticography: relation to clinical outcome in patients with temporal lobe surgery. *Epilepsia* 1994;35:1165–1173.
47. Wennberg R, Quesney F, Olivier A, et al. Electrocorticography and outcome in frontal lobe epilepsy. *Electroencephalogr Clin Neurophysiol* 1998;106:357–368.
48. Rasmussen TB. Surgical aspects. In: Wise G, ed. *Topics in child neurology.* Englewood Cliffs, NJ: Spectrum Publications, 1977:143–153.
49. So NK. Depth electrode studies in mesial temporal epilepsy. In: Lüders H, ed. *Epilepsy surgery.* New York: Raven Press, 1991:371–384.
50. So NK, Olivier A, Andermann F, et al. Results of surgical treatment in patients with bitemporal epileptiform abnormalities. *Ann Neurol* 1989;25:432–439.
51. Spencer SS, Spencer DD, Williamson PD, et al. Combined depth and subdural electrode investigation in uncontrolled epilepsy. *Neurology* 1990;40:74–79.
52. Sperling MR, O'Connor MJ. Comparison of depth and subdural electrodes in recording temporal lobe seizures. *Neurology* 1989;39:1497–1504.
53. Brekelmans GJ, van Emde Boas W, Velis DN, et al. Comparison of combined versus subdural or intracerebral electrodes alone in presurgical focus localization. *Epilepsia* 1998;39:1290–1301.
54. Eisenschenk S, Gilmore RL, Cibula JE, et al. Lateralization of temporal lobe foci: depth versus subdural electrodes. *Clin Neurophysiol* 2001;112:836–844.
55. Alsaadi TM, Laxer KD, Barbaro NM, et al. False lateralization by subdural electrodes in two patients with temporal lobe epilepsy. *Neurology* 2001;57:532–534.
56. Spencer SS, Guimaraes P, Katz A, et al. Morphological patterns of seizures recorded intracranially. *Epilepsia* 1992;33:537–545.
57. van Veelen CW, Debets RM, van Huffelen AC, et al. Combined use of subdural and intracerebral electrodes in preoperative evaluation of epilepsy. *Neurosurgery* 1990;26:93–101.
58. Risinger MW, Gumnit RJ. Intracranial electrophysiologic studies. *Neuroimaging Clin N Am* 1995;5:559–573.
59. Privitera MD, Quinlan JG, Yeh H. Interictal spike detection comparing subdural and depth electrodes during electrocorticography. *Electroencephalogr Clin Neurophysiol* 1990;76:379–387.
60. Cukiert A, Buratini JA, Machado E, et al. Results of surgery in patients with refractory extratemporal epilepsy with normal or nonlocalizing magnetic resonance findings investigated with subdural grids. *Epilepsia* 2001;42:889–894.
61. Mariottini A, Lombroso CT, DeGirolami U, et al. Operative results without invasive monitoring in patients with frontal lobe epileptogenic lesions. *Epilepsia* 2001;42:1308–1315.
62. Laich E, Kuzniecky R, Mountz J, et al. Supplementary sensorimotor area epilepsy. Seizure localization, cortical propagation and subcortical activation pathways using ictal SPECT. *Brain* 1997;120:855–864.
63. Benbadis SR, Tatum WO IV, Vale FL. When drugs don't work: an algorithmic approach to medically intractable epilepsy. *Neurology* 2000;55:1780–1784.

Hippocampal Sclerosis and Dual Pathology

78

Evan J. Fertig   *Susan S. Spencer*

Over the past several decades, technical advances have revolutionized the surgical treatment of medically refractory epilepsy, allowing precise localization and resection with higher rates of success and less morbidity. As a result, epilepsy surgery is increasing worldwide; however, estimates of the number of appropriate candidates far exceed actual referrals to epilepsy centers (1).

Mesial temporal lobe epilepsy (MTLE) associated with hippocampal sclerosis (HS) has served as a model for this treatment. The most common localization-related epilepsy, MTLE has well-known clinical, electrographic, and radiographic characteristics, is usually medically refractory, and is amenable to surgical correction (2,3). In the past 15 years, major epilepsy centers have published at least 25 studies, including the first randomized, controlled trial of surgical therapy (4,5), in which approximately two thirds of patients achieved control of disabling seizures, with low rates of morbidity and mortality. In properly selected patients with MTLE, therefore, surgery is superior to pharmacotherapy. Long-term outcomes for seizure control, neuropsychologic function, and quality of life, however, remain poorly characterized (6).

This chapter describes the current practice of surgical management for MTLE, beginning with its pathologic definition and including hypotheses of its significance and etiology, medical treatment and response, diagnostic evaluation, selection of candidates, surgical approaches and outcomes, and approach to bitemporal epilepsy. Modern imaging techniques have identified extrahippocampal lesions in association with HS, and surgery for this so-called dual pathology is also reviewed.

HIPPOCAMPAL SCLEROSIS

Pathologic Findings

Hippocampal sclerosis (HS), also known as mesial temporal sclerosis or Ammon horn sclerosis, is the most common pathologic finding in MTLE. Neoplastic, vascular, developmental, or traumatic abnormalities are found less frequently (2). Neuronal loss, gliosis, and reorganization classically define HS (7,8). Neuronal loss and gliosis primarily involve hippocampal sectors CA1, CA3, and CA4, with relative sparing of CA2 (2). Cell loss can extend into adjacent entorhinal cortex and amygdala (9). MTL neoplasms can also cause neuronal loss in the hippocampus, but usually less extensively than in classic HS (10).

A high proportion of astrocytes with a high density of sodium channels account for the gliosis. Although found in regions of cell loss, these astrocytes are not significantly correlated with neuronal loss. They, too, are abnormal and can generate neuron-like action potentials (8,11).

Resected hippocampi reveal neuronal reorganization in and around the "sclerotic" hippocampus. Selective loss of somatostatin and neuropeptide Y interneurons is seen, with sprouting of neuropeptide Y interneurons and dynorphin-staining granule cells into the inner third of the dentate molecular layer (8,12,13). Mossy fiber reorganization has also been found in human hippocampi removed for uncontrolled seizures (14).

Overall, this pattern is unique to MTLE with HS. The role of any of these pathologic changes in seizure generation, however, remains undefined.

Etiology

The high correlation of pathologic HS with ipsilateral epileptiform features on electroencephalography (EEG), together with excellent outcome after temporal resection, suggests that HS might cause, rather than only coexist with, MTLE. Its genesis is still unexplained.

Patients with HS often give a history of an early risk factor, such as a febrile seizure, trauma, or infection before age 4. Febrile seizures have long been proposed as the cause of HS, because retrospective studies have consistently linked them, especially if complex or prolonged febrile seizures (15–18), with MTLE (19–21). Prospective studies of children with even prolonged febrile seizures have not, however, shown subsequent TLE (22,23). Nevertheless, the earlier the onset of seizures, the longer the seizure remission before emergence of intractable epilepsy (20).

Other evidence for HS as an acquired lesion comes from animal studies of sustained limbic seizures by intermittent stimulation of limbic pathways. Selective neuronal loss in CA1 and CA3 as well as gliosis and neuronal reorganization was observed; however, no spontaneous seizures occurred. Case studies in humans have found the development of HS after acquired lesions (24). However, many patients with chronic, uncontrolled epilepsy, including frequent generalized seizures, do not show features of HS (7,25), and patients who undergo electroconvulsive therapy are not at increased risk of epilepsy (26).

Another theory regards HS as the result of a developmental lesion, with febrile seizures the consequence of an underlying abnormality. Developmental migrational abnormalities are associated with HS (dual pathology) in 15% to 25% of cases; conversely, 10% to 15% of patients with HS also have cortical developmental abnormalities (2,27–29). HS can coexist with tumors, but usually only when they approximate the hippocampus; even then hippocampal cell loss is milder than with developmental lesions, suggesting a different mechanism (such as damage from local electrical propagation) (30). Overall, the severity of hippocampal cell loss is not proportional to the number of seizures or the duration of epilepsy. HS may thus be a preexisting lesion, rather than a sequela of damage from cumulative seizures (29–31).

Further evidence for a developmental cause of HS comes from three reports of children with MTLE who underwent surgical resection. Magnetic resonance imaging (MRI) demonstrated hippocampal atrophy, a known correlate of hippocampal cell loss, at the time of the first seizure before age 2 years. Increased T2 signal has not been seen before age 4 (27) and may reflect a secondary process, with hippocampal atrophy preexisting. Children over age 12 had pathologic hippocampal findings identical to those in adults. Children under 12 had cell loss confined to CA1 and the hilus, and no reorganization or sprouting. Sprouting age at surgery, and duration of epilepsy, but not degree of cell loss, were significantly correlated. The implication is that the 50% cell loss in CA1 and the hilus, together with gliosis, is an essential underlying element of HS at all ages. Sprouting and neuronal reorganization may be secondary and progressive, related to the duration of epilepsy. Increased T2 signal on MRI may be a correlate of the later-appearing neuronal sprouting or reorganization and is not necessary for development of MTLE. Indeed, hippocampal atrophy without T2 signal change is known to correlate with the typical clinical syndrome, electrographic characteristics, the classic pathologic features of HS, and a good surgical outcome.

It may not be possible to generalize the mechanism of HS in children and in patients of all ages. In one study (32), the incidence of dual pathology in children was 80%, far higher than in adults. This may explain the short delay between the initial insult and spontaneous unprovoked seizures in these patients. In later-onset MTLE, which has a longer latent period before spontaneous unprovoked seizures, epileptogenesis may occur more slowly by a different mechanism.

More evidence for a developmental model comes from families with MTLE and febrile seizures. Hippocampal volumes were measured in 23 members of two families, each including one member with MTLE, several members with only febrile seizures, and other individuals without febrile seizures or epilepsy (33). Both left hippocampal atrophy and T2 signal change were demonstrated in the person with MTLE. Left hippocampal atrophy but a normal signal was seen in all individuals with febrile seizures (but not MTLE) and in many of the seizure free family members. Unusual hippocampal architecture was consistent in each family but differed between the two families. These observations support the view of hippocampal atrophy as a developmental abnormality that facilitates febrile seizures and is sometimes associated with MTLE, perhaps related to other factors.

MEDICAL TREATMENT

Initial therapy for MTLE associated with HS is medical. Of all etiologies for partial epilepsy, partial epilepsy caused by HS has the worst prognosis for medical control, with only 10% to 42% of patients becoming seizure free (34,35). Moreover, an initial positive response does not necessarily predict a good long-term outcome. One-fourth of patients with medically refractory localization-related epilepsy have a significant period of seizure control and even remission before intractability is evident (20).

Greater success with newer antiepileptic drugs as monotherapy or in combination has not been documented (3,36).

A few patients may become seizure free after extended drug trials, but when to switch to a surgical approach remains unclear. Although medically refractory epilepsy has no standard definition, there is some evidence that complete control is highly unlikely after two antiepileptic drugs have failed (37). Surgical therapy is safe and efficacious; continued medical therapy poses risks of recurrent seizures, lost productive years, and higher mortality.

Clearly an argument exists for early surgical therapy. A multicenter prospective study is examining this issue (38).

SURGICAL TREATMENT OF HIPPOCAMPAL SCLEROSIS

Techniques for Patient Selection

The preoperative definition of HS depends on a combination of indirect methods. No single study alone is sufficient for demonstration of epileptogenicity. The use of MRI, positron emission tomography (PET), single-photon-emission computed tomography (SPECT), neuropsychological assessment, and continuous ictal and interictal video and EEG recording has resulted in 90% or better accuracy (39).

Scalp EEG (Including Spheroidal Electrodes)

MTLE with HS has a characteristic set of findings on EEG. Non-invasive scalp EEG is always performed initially. Anterior temporal spikes and sharp waves are the most common EEG, ending in patients with pathologically proven HS (40–42). Posterior and extratemporal sharp waves, if frequent or regular, suggest other pathologies (43). Bilateral independent anterior temporal spikes are not a contraindication to surgery, because most of these seizures still begin unilaterally in the medial temporal lobe (see bitemporal epilepsy below) (44,45).

Sphenoidal electrodes, though reportedly sensitive and specific for interictal activity from the mesial temporal region (40), can also record interictal activity from epileptogenic lateral temporal and orbital frontal regions (46).

Ictal discharges recorded with scalp EEG in MTLE are morphologically variable, frequently contaminated by artifact, and often delayed following clinical seizure onset. Interobserver reliability and accuracy of localization are poor, except for lateralization in patients with temporal lobe seizures (47). Temporal lobe seizures with HS can sometimes be lateralized and localized by the distinctive EEG pattern. Rhythmic theta or alpha activity within 30 seconds of the first subjective or objective indication of a seizure is strongly associated with HS and with control after resection. This pattern correctly lateralized onset in 80% of patients, as verified by intracranial recording (41) and interobserver reliability in its detection is high (48,49). Ictal onset may be bilateral and independent in up to 20% of patients (41,48,50) (see section on Bitemporal Epilepsy).

To test their use for localizing temporal lobe epileptic regions, sphenoidal electrodes were placed fluoroscopically to ensure that the recording tips were immediately below the foramen ovale (51). In a previous study (52), blindly placed sphenoidal electrodes were no better than anterior temporal electrodes in localizing yield.

Fluoroscopically placed sphenoidal electrodes were only slightly superior to anterior temporal electrodes in patients who reached class I or II Engel outcome but produced greater interrater agreement and earlier detection of ictal onset. This, the authors believed, might lead to fewer intracranial studies and less costly presurgical evaluation.

In 70% to 80% of patients with MTLE, scalp EEG, combined with other studies, will provide adequate electrical localization to accurately predict HS. Surgery is justified when there are lateralization, even without localization, of seizure onset on scalp EEG and hippocampal atrophy on MRI, with concordant unilateral temporal spikes, as long as some functional deficit confirms the mesial temporal localization and no studies provide discordant information (3).

Intracranial EEG

When localization from scalp EEG (or lateralization with other sufficient data) is lacking and other electrical documentation is needed, invasive recordings are used.

The decision to implant intracranial electrodes is not taken lightly because of the risk of hemorrhage and infection (53). The minimum number of implanted electrodes, often a combination of strip and depth electrodes, to detect the zone of seizure onset and the epileptogenic region is used (54). MRI guides stereotactic implantation of depth electrodes (55).

Before the advent of newer imaging techniques, intracranial electrodes were commonly used to evaluate MTLE. MRI can now reliably and noninvasively demonstrate HS, is highly predictive of epileptogenicity and excellent surgical outcome, and in most cases of MTLE and HS is concordant with ictal onset on scalp EEG. In light of these findings, intracranial EEG and its attendant risks can be avoided in most such patients (3).

Intracranial EEG may nevertheless be required if (i) atrophy is present on MRI without documentation of lateralized seizure onset, or with conflicting lateralization on scalp EEG, and (ii) if there is bilateral and independent temporal seizure onset.

The goals of intracranial studies for suspected MTLE are to determine lateralization (see bitemporal HS below) and to differentiate orbitofrontal, medial parietal, medial occipital, or neocortical temporal from hippocampal seizure onset. Hippocampal depth electrodes are most sensitive for documenting seizure onset in this location (Fig. 78.1) (56). These electrodes, which may be implanted from posterior to anterior to sample the length of the hippocampus, are accompanied by bilateral anterior, middle, and posterior temporal neocortical recording with either orthogonal depth electrodes or multiple subdural strips (Fig. 78.2). The electrode array is based on the clinical scenario and findings from functional imaging, scalp EEG, and MRI. A temporal grid with medial subdural strip placement is used when language mapping is needed. Because medial or orbitofrontal, parietal, or occipital seizures can mimic medial temporal seizures, additional depth or subdural electrodes may be placed in these regions when any information suggests those possibilities (53).

Recognition of normal intracranial background rhythms is essential, especially in hippocampal studies, to avoid erroneous localization (50). Physiologic electrographic activity can be seen that is not apparent on scalp EEG. Hippocampal spindles and the "third rhythm" (as

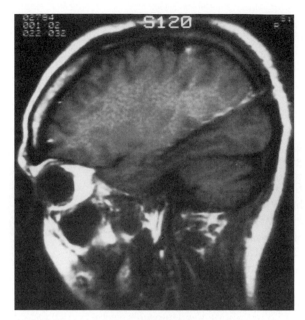

Figure 78.1 Sagittal magnetic resonance image demonstrates medial posterior depth electrode targeted to record along the length of the hippocampus with 12 individual contacts.

coined by Niedermeyer, an α-like pattern recorded directly over the temporal neocortex predominantly in the waking and drowsy states) are unusual but normal. The absence of blocking response helps differentiate this rhythm from posterior α and μ rhythms (57).

In general, interictal spikes are more widespread on intracranial EEG than on scalp EEG (53,58). Multifocal spikes are common in both temporal and extratemporal epilepsy, even with a single ictal-onset region (53). Medial temporal spikes, present in more than 95% of patients

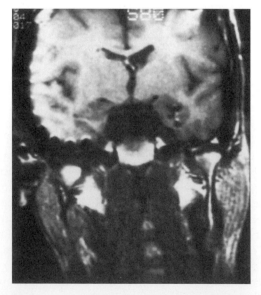

Figure 78.2 Coronal magnetic resonance image shows subdural strip (left) placed to record along lateral and mesial basal temporal lobe structures. The contralateral side shows the termination of two depth electrodes in hippocampus and entorhinal cortex.

with MTLE, are bilateral and independent in up to 80% (50,53,59). Although unilateral hippocampal interictal spiking (recorded from depth electrodes) has been associated with HS and good surgical outcome (60), bilateral spikes can be seen with both unilateral and bilateral HS. Ictal onset is more useful for localization.

Two patterns of seizure onset in the hippocampus have been characterized with intrahippocampal depth electrodes: an initial, periodic, high-voltage spike discharge at 1 to 2 Hz (Fig. 78.3) and a low-voltage β discharge (Fig. 78.4) (3). Seen almost exclusively in the hippocampus, the periodic pattern is related to pathologic markers of HS: it is inversely correlated with CA1 cell loss (61) and increased glial density in CA2 and CA3 (53,62). Ictal-onset morphologic features in MTLE may vary between these patterns within a single patient (63).

Seizure onset in pathologically proven HS also varies in a given patient between medial temporal locations, including hippocampus and entorhinal cortex (64), and regions of hippocampus (54). An examination of regional hippocampal atrophy by MRI found that the region of seizure onset within the hippocampus was not predicted by the distribution of maximal atrophy (54). The variability in initial seizure location and pattern suggests that MTLE (and presumably other partial epilepsies) is the product of a network of related regions rather than a single "focus."

Evolution of the electrical activity from initial ictal changes in the hippocampus follows predictable patterns. Typically, after more than 5 seconds of the initial periodic high-voltage spike, a low-voltage rhythmic discharge of approximately 13 Hz develops in the same electrodes, decreasing in frequency as it propagates. In 60% of seizures, initial propagation is to the ipsilateral temporal neocortex, in 30% to the contralateral hippocampus, and in 10% to both structures simultaneously. Involvement of the contralateral temporal neocortex has *not* been seen before contralateral hippocampal onset (50). Prolonged propagation time to the contralateral hippocampus is associated with HS (65), greater neuronal loss in CA4 (66), where the main interhippocampal commissural connection begins, and there is good surgical outcome (65,67).

Frequency differences in the initial discharge can also help to distinguish hippocampal from temporal neocortical onset. Seizures beginning in the temporal neocortex have slower (4 to 10 Hz) and faster frequencies (40 to 200 Hz) than hippocampal onsets (typically 13 to 20 Hz initially or after the 1- to 3-Hz periodic pattern) (50,63,68,69), which also show more variable ictal onset frequencies.

Structural Neuroimaging

Before MRI was available, presurgical assessment frequently required intracranial EEG. HS now can be usually diagnosed by MRI non-invasively, and in combination with concordant lateralized ictal onset on scalp EEG, favorable candidates for resection are selected.

MRI protocols with coronal sections perpendicular to the long axis of the hippocampus are most effective for detecting

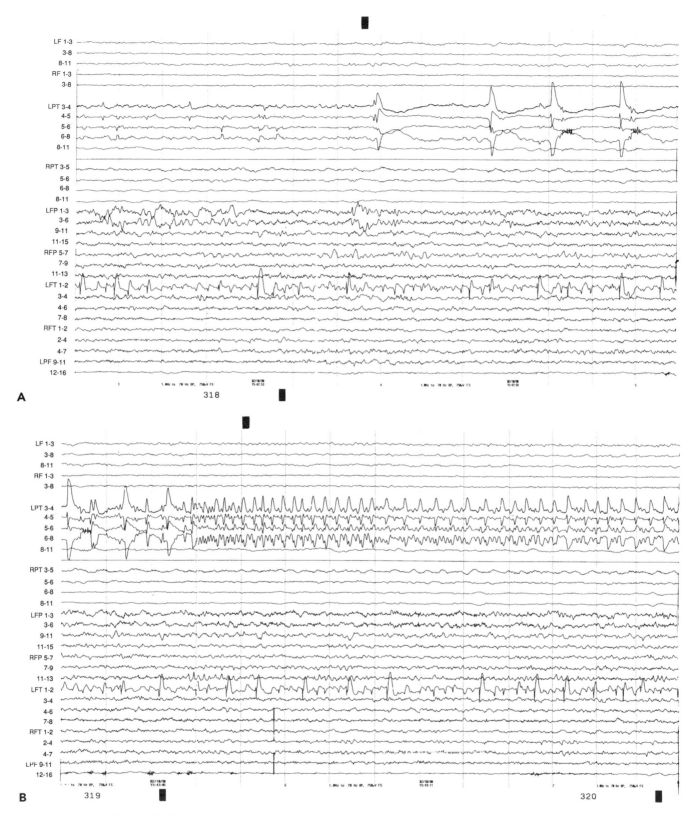

Figure 78.3 **A** and **B.** Continuous electroencephalographic segments show periodic spike discharge at onset of seizure in the left anteromedial temporal lobe. LPT and RPT, left and right hippocampal depth electrodes; LF and RF, left and right medial frontal depth electrodes; LFP and RFP, left and right frontoparietal subdural strips; LPF, left posterior frontal subdural strip. Contacts on all electrodes are numbered from deep (1) to superficial.

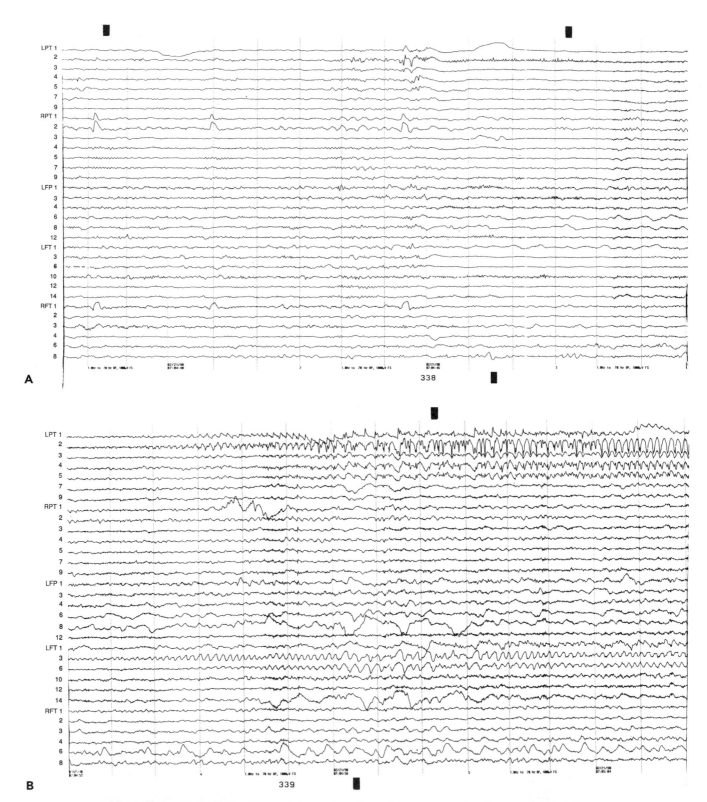

Figure 78.4   A and **B.** Continuous electroencephalographic segments show low-voltage fast discharge at the onset of a spontaneous seizure in the left medial temporal lobe. LPT and RPT, left and right hippocampal depth electrodes; LFP, left frontoparietal subdural strip; LFT and RFT, left and right frontotemporal subdural strips. Contacts on all electrodes are numbered from deep (1) to superficial.

HS (39), which appears as an increased T2-weighted signal or fluid-attenuated inversion recovery (FLAIR) in mesial temporal lobe structures (Fig. 78.5) and decreased size of the hippocampal formation, best assessed with coronal T1-weighted sequences (Fig. 78.6) (41,70–73). Neuronal counts from the resected hippocampus correlate directly and significantly with quantitative measures of decreased hippocampal size (74). When neuronal cell loss is at least 50%, MRI can reliably detect HS with a sensitivity of 90% (39). Volumetric studies of atrophy and T2 relaxometry may increase the diagnostic yield and aid in detecting bilateral HS.

Concordantly localized ictal onset on scalp EEG and hippocampal atrophy on MRI predict seizure control in more than 90% of patients undergoing temporal lobectomy (71,75–77). MRI provides the highest yield of accurate noninvasive localization for MTLE (72,73), and even by itself, hippocampal atrophy predicts excellent postoperative control in 86% of patients (71). Hippocampal atrophy on MRI is also very specific for HS (78).

The absence of hippocampal atrophy on MRI is *not* synonymous with the absence of HS, and in these situations, T2 signal changes can increase the yield (79). Surgical outcome without MRI-identified hippocampal atrophy is worse.

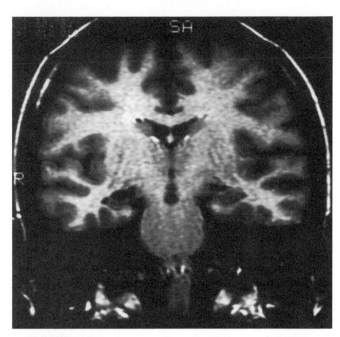

Figure 78.6 Coronal magnetic resonance image at same level as in Figure 78.5 shows focal hippocampal atrophy.

Clinical Seizure

Patients with HS have a well-described clinical syndrome. French and colleagues (21) retrospectively reviewed the clinical characteristics of seizures from patients with MTLE. Inclusion criteria were medial temporal seizure onset on depth EEG and medial temporal lobectomy/hippocampectomy with subsequent seizure freedom for at least two years. A pathologic diagnosis of HS was not required, but patients with circumscribed tumors or vascular malformations identified on pathologic specimens or neuroimaging were excluded. Complex partial seizures were the most common type of seizure. Secondary generalized seizures were reported in 57% as an infrequent type and were never the exclusive or predominant type. Ninety-six percent of patients had an aura. An abdominal visceral sensation, such as nausea, pressure, butterflies, or a rising epigastric sensation, were most often reported; fear was next in frequency. Olfactory auras, light-headedness, and déjà vu also occurred less commonly. Oral automatisms and impaired consciousness were noted during video-EEG monitoring (80). Appendicular automatisms were frequent ipsilateral to the lesion, while dystonia and Todd's hemiparesis were most frequent contralateral to the lesion. Head deviation was ipsilateral early and contralateral late in the seizure. Postictal aphasia was seen with dominant-hemisphere lesions.

These signs and symptoms, while suggestive of HS, are neither diagnostic nor exclusive. Seizures of lateral temporal, occipital, or parietal origin can have the same clinical characteristics if they spread to medial temporal structures and may give no overt clues to their lobe of origin. Conversely, seizures beginning in the medial temporal lobe may spread elsewhere, sometimes rapidly, and assume other clinical patterns. For these reasons, clinical manifestations cannot be considered primary criteria for localization except perhaps for the very earliest manifestations and for the aura.

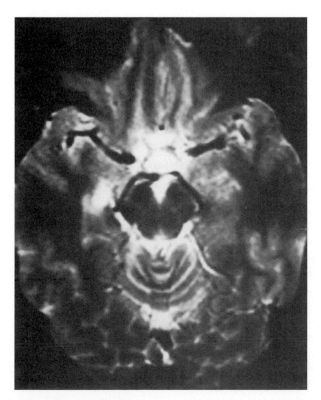

Figure 78.5 Magnetic resonance image demonstrates focal increased signal in hippocampus.

Neuropsychological Assessment (Including Intracarotid Amobarbital Test)

Neuropsychological testing and the intracarotid amobarbital test serve two purposes: (1) the testing itself can help demonstrate the abnormal hippocampal substrate, and (2) neuropsychological assessment identifies the degree of cognitive function in the epileptogenic hippocampi, preventing serious cognitive defect with resection. In the temporal lobe more than anywhere else, because hippocampal structures are important in memory, assessment may help to predict affected cerebral areas and avoid resection of functional ones. Results of standardized neuropsychological assessment of memory and language are used to infer lateralized temporal lobe dysfunction. The intracarotid amobarbital test assesses memory and language in each hemisphere independently (81). Lack of adequate unilateral memory often is taken as evidence of functional impairment of the involved hippocampus and is a contraindication to removal of the contralateral hippocampus (81).

Impaired verbal memory was directly and significantly correlated with cell counts in the dominant hippocampus, and an impaired memory score (measured by the intracarotid amobarbital test) was directly correlated with neuronal cell counts in the CA3 hippocampal subfield (82,83). These results provide increased confidence in the use of neuropsychological assessment for documenting the abnormal substrate in MTLE.

Functional Neuroimaging

Most epilepsy surgery centers use imaging of cerebral blood flow and metabolism to localize the epileptogenic temporal lobe.

PET performed with 2-deoxy-2-(^{18}F)fluoro-D-glucose (FDG) to map cerebral metabolism has demonstrated a 60% to 90% incidence of unilateral temporal lobe hypometabolism in patients with medically refractory MTLE (84,85) and reportedly has 100% sensitivity for HS (86). PET is useful when MRI findings are normal with similar implications. Temporal hypometabolism correlates with surgical success after temporal lobectomy (85,87,88).

PET has poor spatial resolution, however. Interictal hypometabolism encompasses much of the temporal lobe of seizure onset and is not limited to the mesial temporal structures. Changes can involve the ipsilateral frontal and parietal cortex, thalamus, and basal ganglia (39,89). Qualitative analysis of interictal FDG-PET frequently demonstrates greater hypometabolism of lateral than mesial temporal lobe in patients with MTLE (85,90). The wide hypometabolic area in MTLE may account for limited interobserver reliability (91).

Moreover, the mechanism underlying the hypometabolism in MTLE has not been elucidated. The degree of hypometabolism does not predict the pathologic finding in MTLE, i.e., tumor versus HS (87,92), and, unlike the degree of hippocampal atrophy with MRI, has not been correlated with severity of hippocampal neuronal loss (93,94). Hypometabolism is not seen in patients with controlled seizures (95) and hypometabolism on PET can be reversed with successful surgery (96). Reductions in metabolism may therefore reflect reversible dysfunction rather than an anatomic abnormality.

Perhaps 20% of drug-resistant TLE patients will not have glucose hypometabolism on PET or hippocampal atrophy. Tracers detecting novel biochemical alterations in the temporal lobe may provide a new way to localize epileptic foci. One small study (97) noted increased α[^{11}C]methyl-L-tryptophan (AMT) uptake on PET imaging in the hippocampus ipsilateral to the seizure focus in TLE patients with normal hippocampal volumes but *not* in those with hippocampal atrophy.

Usually performed to image cerebral perfusion, SPECT has become widely used in the presurgical evaluation of epilepsy patients. Tracers include technetium-99m-hexamethylpropylene amine oxime (99mTc-HMPAO or 99mTc-exametazime) or technetium-99m-ethyl cysteinate diethylester (99mTc-ECD or 99mTc-bicisate). Interictal SPECT in isolation does not localize HS well: temporal hypoperfusion is seen in 50% of cases or fewer with proven MTLE (39,98). Reports of greater than 60% yield used the stable agent ECD instead of HMPAO (99), were done in children (100–105), or involved quantitative analyses (50). The interictal yield is increased with more frequent seizure activity and with lesional substrates and is decreased with bilateral EEG findings or normal MRI (95,102).

Unlike other diagnostic imaging modalities, a SPECT injection can be made during ictus and the scan performed hours later when the patient is cooperative. The ictal scan is analyzed for regions of increased and decreased perfusion by subtracting the interictal perfusion scan to create a difference image, which is then superimposed on coregistered MRI for anatomic detail. Similar to interictal PET, ictal SPECT has an overall sensitivity of approximately 80% to 90%, with few false-positive results (98,106–109).

Selection of Patients for Intracranial EEG

Localization of epileptic activity by scalp or intracranial EEG is necessary but not sufficient for surgery. MRI, with its ability to noninvasively detect HS and many migrational disorders, has made previous evaluation protocols obsolete. Concordant localization to one temporal lobe by MRI and scalp ictal or interictal EEG, without any other contradictory information and with some confirmation by demonstration of focal *functional* impairment (SPECT, PET, neuropsychological profile, amytal test), allows resection to proceed (with due respect for functional areas as measured by neuropsychological assessment). MRI findings that fulfill this requirement include tumors, focal cortical dysplasia, hippocampal atrophy, or T2 signal change. PET may be similarly compelling in MTLE. Cases lacking these criteria require consideration for intracranial electrode recording the results of which are used to plan resection.

Procedures and Outcome

Procedures

Jasper and Kershman (110) were the first to note electrical localization of psychomotor seizures in the medial temporal lobe. Gibbs and colleagues (111), were the first to recommend surgery for medically refractory cases. Penfield and Flanigin (112,113) pioneered in recommending surgery for medically refractory cases.

The classic, and still most commonly performed procedure for MTLE, is the anterior temporal lobectomy (ATL) (114) in which a portion of the anterior lateral temporal neocortex is resected. To spare language, the most anterior 3.5 cm of the middle and inferior temporal gyri of the language-dominant hemisphere is resected; in the nondominant hemisphere, 4 to 5 cm is resected. Partial resection of the lateral temporal cortex allows access to the medial temporal lobe structures, which are then resected (115).

Over time, the importance of complete resection of the hippocampus emerged. The most common reason for failed surgery was retained epileptogenic tissue in the mesial structures, and resection of this residual tissue resulted in seizure freedom (116). The first and only randomized prospective study of surgery for MTLE found that a more radical hippocampal resection led to better seizure control, with no additional neuropsychological deficit.

Resection of lateral structures was therefore believed to be unnecessary and a possible cause of neuropsychological morbidity. In a 1984 modification, the mesial structures were removed through a limited temporal pole resection (119). In the selective amygdalohippocampectomy (AH), the amygdala, parahippocampal gyrus, and hippocampus are resected and the lateral neocortex is *completely* spared (120). This procedure initially required microdissection through the sylvian fissure; later modifications used MR frameless stereotactic image guidance systems to facilitate access to the temporal horn of the lateral ventricle from which the mesial structures are resected (115).

Whether AH has a true advantage over ATL is still debated. A report presented at the second International Conference on Epilepsy Surgery showed that 67.9% of the 3579 patients who underwent ATL were seizure free, 24% were improved, and 8.1% were unchanged. Respective results for the 413 patients who underwent AH were 68.8%, 22.3%, and 9%. No difference in seizure control emerged in a study that assigned patients to each procedure (121).

Evidence that sparing lateral temporal structures leads to less neuropsychological morbidity is also not convincing. Learning and memory specific for the nonoperated hemisphere improved postoperatively in patients with good seizure control, but detailed neuropsychological data were not reported (122). A similar lack of memory decline after AH emerged in another study (123), although verbal memory decreased significantly when AH was performed in the dominant hemisphere (124–126).

Declines in nonverbal memory after nondominant hemisphere resection is not usual (124,125). A comparison of neuropsychological outcomes in 23 patients undergoing AH or ATL found no major differences in cognitive outcome except for specific measures of paired associate learning and immediate recall of visuospatial material (123,124). It has been hypothesized that disruption of the mesial structures results in "disconnection" of the lateral structures, perhaps explaining the similar neuropsychological outcomes with the two procedures. In fact, FDG-PET demonstrated hypoperfusion of the temporal pole after AH (127).

Outcome

In the past 15 years, at least 25 studies have examined seizure outcome after anteromesial temporal resection for MTLE (not exclusively for HS, but most likely the majority) (4), including the first randomized controlled study of epilepsy surgery (5). Of the 1988 patients treated surgically, 1308 (66%) were free of disabling seizures; approximately 377 (19%) were improved; and about 252 (13%) showed no improvement. Surgical morbidity and mortality rates were low.

HS in resected tissue predicts a positive outcome. In an actuarial analysis according to pathologic substrates (128), the probability of becoming seizure free for 2 years, determined at 5-year follow up, was 62% with HS, 80% with foreign-tissue lesions (tumors, cavernous malformations), and 36% with normal tissue. A multivariable analysis (129) identified HS as the strongest independent predictor of good outcome (no seizures for 1 year after surgery).

International conferences have revealed increased use and success of surgery to control MTLE (89,130). As of 1987, more than 2000 patients underwent temporal lobectomy and 55% became seizure free. Six years later, more than 4000 temporal lobe resections freed nearly 70% of seizures.

It must be kept in mind though, that the majority of data on seizure outcome is from relatively short-term follow up. Follow-up lasted only 1 year in the only randomized controlled trial (5) and in most published series did not exceed 2 years. Outcome data at 5, 10, and 15 years after surgery are limited.

Also insufficiently documented is the risk of relapse after temporal lobectomy for mesial temporal sclerosis. In patients who had been seizure free for at least 1 year, Spencer reported a relapse rate of 15% over long-term follow-up (6). Another report noted that 62% of such patients were seizure free for 2 years at 5-year follow-up, but only 50% remained controlled for 5 years continuously (128); the highest relapse rate occurred with MTLE compared with tumors and cavernous malformations. Yoon and associates (131) expanded Spencer sample to 175 patients who were seizure free for 1 year and were followed up for 3 to 20 years (mean 8 years). Sixty-three percent never experienced a relapse, and those who did had very infrequent seizures. A longer seizure-free interval predicted fewer seizures after relapse. This study did not confirm the higher relapse rate for temporal compared with extratemporal resection.

Additional data are needed to determine the cause of relapse after an extended seizure-free interval, but seizures arising in the vicinity of the resection, bitemporal disease, or HS coexistent with other pathologic conditions are possible explanations.

Quality of Life

It is difficult to synthesize quality-of-life findings in the literature because this issue has been examined in different ways (4). Retrospective studies demonstrate a correlation with seizure outcome (132–135). The only prospective, randomized controlled study of ATL for TLE (5) documented better quality of life for patients treated surgically than medically after 1 year but did not stratify for seizure control.

A common flaw of quality-of-life studies is the lack of baseline data. Initial results of an ongoing prospective multicenter study in which 85% of the cohort had temporal lobe surgery show that quality-of-life measures improve slowly and only in seizure-free patients (136).

Predictors of Surgical Outcome

Individual studies have identified the following independent predictors of seizure control after surgery: hippocampal atrophy on MRI (alone and even more so with concordant EEG localization) (72); temporal lobe hypometabolism on PET (130,137); lateralization of memory function; an early risk factor; and absence of generalized or immediate postoperative seizures (41,73,129). Age of onset or preoperative seizure frequency, which both predict medical responsiveness, had no predictive value after surgery. Other factors studied in different groups of patients, with varying methods, have yielded conflicting results. Generalized tonic-clonic seizures predicted poor outcome, as did head trauma (41,73,81,129). Febrile seizures were sometimes associated with a good outcome (81). Duration of epilepsy generally did not predict response (41,137,138).

Bitemporal Epilepsy

A subset of patients with MTLE have bilateral independent ictal onset on scalp EEG or bilateral hippocampal atrophy (or both). Incidence can be determined by volumetric MRI and, depending on the definition used, ranges from 9.4% to 42% (139–141). Perhaps this is not surprising, as pathologic studies of HS reveal a high degree of bilaterality (2). Whether unilateral and bilateral MTLE involve true clinical differences in history is not clear. Patients with a history of encephalitis or meningitis were more likely than those

with febrile convulsions to have bilateral hippocampal atrophy on normalized volumetric MRI (142). Bitemporal epilepsy, as defined by depth EEG ictal onset, was significantly less likely to involve antecedent febrile seizures (143). In contrast, another study found that bilateral hippocampal atrophy on volumetric MRI was *more* common in patients with past febrile seizures (144). A third study (145) uncovered no difference in frequency of febrile seizures between the two groups as defined by intracranial EEG.

How bilateral medial temporal findings on noninvasive studies affect clinical practice is under discussion. Many of these patients undergo intracranial EEG. Previous reports asserted the need for most temporal lobe seizures to begin unilaterally in order to be controlled surgically (143,146). Comparing surgical outcome of patients with unilateral MTLE and a carefully selected group with bitemporal independent seizure onset (recorded by depth electrodes), Spencer and colleagues (143,146) found equivalent results in the two groups *regardless* of the distribution of seizures between sides. In this series, 11 of the 23 patients with bitemporal onset were selected for surgery by the following minimal criteria: (1) at least 50% of seizures began in the lobe to be resected; (2) memory (by intracarotid amobarbital test) was adequately sustained by the contralateral hemisphere; and (3) there was no evidence of extratemporal epilepsy. The results were interpreted to show the need for rigorous selection criteria for patients with bitemporal epilepsy, such that "silent" extratemporal seizure onset with variable propagation was excluded, but a specific percentage of lateralized distribution of seizure onset was not necessary and could even be equal between the two sides.

Because the predominance of ictal onset on intracranial EEG may not predict outcome in individuals with bitemporal epilepsy as well as once thought, ancillary studies must be used. Spencer series did not include MRI assessment of hippocampal atrophy, because the study was completed before qualitative (or quantitative) MRI was established as a sensitive and nearly specific indication of HS. Sirven and colleagues (147) examined how noninvasive presurgical data related to prognosis in patients with independent bitemporal onset in a contemporary scenario. Of 28 patients identified consecutively by intracranial EEG, 15 were offered surgery, and 10 became seizure free. The degree of seizure-onset laterality did not predict control. Seven of the 10 seizure-free patients had lateralized intracarotid amobarbital test results or unilateral hippocampal atrophy on MRI; none of the individuals with poorer outcome had either finding.

The prognostic significance of bilateral hippocampal atrophy is still undefined. One could assume that its presence would mean bitemporal epilepsy and poor surgical outcome. In one study (148), no correlation emerged between predominance of ictal onset and degree of hippocampal atrophy on MRI. Another study (141) found concordance between lateralization by MRI volumetry and by both interictal and ictal scalp EEG, but surgical outcome was not reported. When 74 consecutive patients who had undergone resection for MTLE were separated by volumetric MRI findings, the unilateral-atrophy group (63.5%) had a significantly better outcome than either the bilateral-atrophy (23%) or no-atrophy (13.5%) group (121). No extensive EEG correlates were provided. On the other hand, 10% of patients studied by invasive EEG had bilateral hippocampal atrophy that was not always associated with bilateral seizure onset (140). Excellent outcome was obtained with removal of the medial temporal lobe with predominant depth EEG–recorded onset.

The real pitfall is confusing "apparent" bitemporal epilepsy with true bilateral independent hippocampal onset (149). Bilateral independent onset, as found on scalp EEG, is common with HS but can also be seen with neocortical lesions, with variable propagation. This most commonly occurs from an occipital lobe lesion by way of the occipitotemporal fasciculus and splenium (150). The intracranial results must therefore be interpreted in the context of guidelines for intracranial EEG in mesial temporal–onset seizures and all other localizing information for confirmation.

Dual Pathology

Although most cases of MTLE with HS respond to unilateral resection of mesial temporal structures, the disorder also involves widespread changes in ipsilateral and contralateral cortical and subcortical structures, as shown by volumetric MRI and functional studies (151–156). HS is associated with an additional, usually developmental, lesion in approximately 15% to 30% of cases (Fig. 78.7) (28–30,42), a phenomenon called dual pathology. The lesions are not necessarily adjacent to atrophic hippocampus; they may be extratemporal and even contralateral (temporal and extratemporal) (30).

Dual pathology challenges the clinician to determine the source of the epilepsy: the extrahippocampal lesion or the atrophic hippocampus, or both. Frequently, the (more conspicuous) lesion on MRI is resected, while the atrophic hippocampus is overlooked (157). Alternatively, the atrophic hippocampus is resected, while other, sometimes subtle, cortical abnormalities are overlooked (151,157). The result in both cases is poor seizure outcome.

Retrospective studies indicate that resection of both the hippocampus and extrahippocampal lesion leads to better seizure outcome than resection of either structure alone (158,159). Removal of both structures produced complete control in 11 of 15 patients; two of 10 patients responded to resection of only the atrophic hippocampus and two of 16 patients to cortical lesionectomy (159). In an uncontrolled case series, reoperation with resection of the atrophic hippocampus improved seizure outcome (157). Neuropsychological or quality-of-life measures were not reported and surgical candidates were studied only with surface EEG. Intracranial EEG documentation of seizure

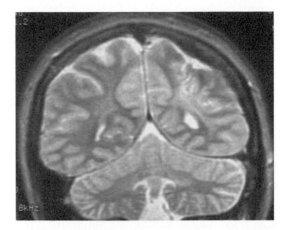

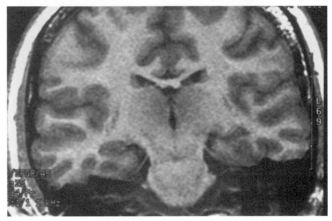

Figure 78.7 MR images from the same patient with dual pathology. Coronal T2-weighted image shows cortical atrophy likely consistent with a developmental abnormality (top). Coronal fast spoiled gradient echo image shows left focal hippocampal atrophy (bottom).

onset might have provided better guidance, and histopathologic studies could give insight into the proper surgical approach. Hippocampal cell loss in conjunction with gliomas and hamartomas tends to be less severe than with developmental lesions (10,30). Moreover, dual pathology with neoplasms usually occurs when they approximate the hippocampus, suggesting several pathophysiologic mechanisms of dual pathology, with the mechanism for nondevelopmental lesions being direct local seizure propagation. In those cases, resection of the tumor, with sparing of the hippocampus, may achieve seizure freedom with a potential for less neuropsychological morbidity than with resection of the hippocampus. Among patients who had only lesions resected, however (159), severity of hippocampal atrophy or type of lesion did not predict surgical outcome. The number of individuals with tumors in this study was not large enough to warrant the conclusion that dual resection is always necessary.

In conclusion, a careful review of neuroimaging findings in preparation for epilepsy surgery is necessary to exclude dual pathology. When dual pathology is common (i.e., developmental lesions), quantitative analysis of the hippocampus may be indicated. Intracranial recording may help to determine which lesion is epileptogenic. Other factors such as malignancy will also dictate the need for lesionectomy. The role of magnetic resonance spectroscopy is still emerging. Determination of the best surgical strategy (single versus combined resection, staged approach), will depend on results of prospective, randomized studies. In any event, resection of both the lesion and the atrophic hippocampus will produce excellent results.

ILLUSTRATIVE CASE REPORTS

Selecting patients for surgical therapy is complicated. Even if the prevailing principles are clear and the techniques standard, how they are combined often depends on the individual patient, historical data, and the primary and secondary characteristics of the evaluation. The permutations are myriad, and there is no substitute for experience. Three case reports illustrate the principles.

Patient 1

After a febrile seizure at age of one, this 32-year-old man remained seizure free until high-school years when complex partial seizures began and increased in frequency despite various combinations of phenytoin, carbamazepine, valproic acid, and gabapentin. At referral, he was having several seizures a day.

Intensive audiovisual EEG monitoring demonstrated left temporal slowing and no interictal epileptiform abnormalities. Four spontaneous seizures were characterized by oral and bilateral upper-extremity automatism and postictal dysphasia. An abdominal aura preceded each seizure. Left temporal Θ discharge on scalp EEG was followed by high-amplitude faster rhythmic activity and then profound slowing in the left temporal region. Interictal SPECT showed reduced perfusion in the left temporal region; left temporal hypometabolism was evident on PET. On MRI, the left hippocampus was shortened and small, with significant T2 signal change. Verbal IQ was 100, performance IQ, 95, and verbal and visual memory were mildly impaired; the profile was not well localized or lateralized. Intracarotid amobarbital testing documented left-hemisphere dominance for speech, with marginal left-hemisphere memory and excellent right-hemisphere memory.

Despite the absence of interictal surface EEG abnormalities, the diagnosis of MTLE was supported by the well-localized ictal discharge concordant with MRI, PET, and SPECT localization to the left medial temporal lobe, in the setting of a history of febrile seizures. Left anteromesial temporal lobectomy with hippocampectomy was performed, and the patient has been seizure free in the ensuing 60 months. Pathologic analysis of the resected tissue demonstrated neuronal loss and gliosis in the hippocampus consistent with HS.

This patient illustrates the classic history and findings of HS and associated MTLE.

Patient 2

This 33-year-old right-handed woman had her first seizure at 5 months after an anaphylactic reaction to penicillin. She was well until age 14 years, when penicillin led to status epilepticus; complex partial seizures continued despite multiple anticonvulsant drugs. At 21, intensive audiovisual EEG monitoring suggested both complex partial seizures, characterized by right-arm flexion and posturing, vocalization, automatisms, and loss of contact, and psychogenic nonepileptic seizures. Interictal EEG demonstrated left anterior temporal spikes; arrhythmic diffuse slowing was evident on the ictal recording. Computed tomography scan showed normal findings. Intracarotid amobarbital test at age 22 showed right-hemisphere dominance for language, intact right-hemisphere memory, and impaired left-hemisphere memory (two of six objects recalled). The patient also had a mixed personality disorder. Because of confusion about the nonepileptic and actual seizures, medical treatment continued, ineffectively, for 10 years. Upon reevaluation, seizures were occurring one to two times per week despite high serum blood levels of carbamazepine and primidone. Neurologic examination yielded normal results. Intensive audiovisual EEG monitoring again documented stereotyped seizures involving an aura of dizziness followed by right-arm tonic activity, groaning, gestural automatisms, and, half the time, loss of consciousness. Although clinically similar, the six recorded seizures varied on EEG. Three were associated with only bilateral rhythmic slowing without localization; one seizure demonstrated right temporal rhythmic activity; and the last two seizures showed left temporal rhythmic δ activity. Left anterior temporal sharp waves were again seen on interictal scalp EEG monitoring. Verbal IQ was 92 and performance IQ, 97, representing a decline from previous values. Verbal memory was now decreased, whereas visual memory was intact. MRI showed left temporal and left hippocampal atrophy. A second intracarotid amobarbital test confirmed previous right-hemisphere language memory findings, but now completely absent left-hemisphere memory.

Four depth electrodes and two subdural strip electrodes, implanted to sample hippocampus and amygdala, orbitofrontal regions, and lateral temporal areas bilaterally, demonstrated interictal spiking at an average frequency of one per minute from the midhippocampus to posterior hippocampus on the right. Eight seizures were recorded, all beginning with an aura that prompted the patient to alert the nurses. Consciousness was preserved, but she could not speak. Later, loss of contact, automatisms of both upper extremities, and tonic contraction of the right arm occurred. In one seizure, low-voltage desynchronization and subsequent fast activity began in the right midhippocampal region to anterior hippocampus.

Six seizures with a similar pattern of activity began in the left hippocampus. The last seizure appeared to start with rhythmic low-amplitude fast activity in the most medial contacts of the left temporal subdural strip electrode. Clinical activity in all these seizures followed electrical onset by 1 to 3 seconds.

Because of the predominantly left hippocampal onset, the left anterior temporal sharp waves on interictal scalp recording, total absence of left-hemisphere memory confirming functional impairment of the left medial temporal lobe, and left hippocampal atrophy demonstrated on MRI—and despite independent seizure origin in the right hippocampus and prominent right temporal spike focus on interictal depth EEG—left anteromedial temporal lobectomy and hippocampectomy were performed. The resected hippocampus demonstrated severe neuronal loss. The patient is seizure free on carbamazepine.

This patient illustrates the satisfactory response to temporal lobectomy, even when seizures arise in both temporal lobes, and the similarity of many findings in bitemporal and unitemporal epilepsy. Primary criteria were not fulfilled because of the multifocal seizure onset, but all others suggested left TLE. The predominantly right-sided hippocampal spiking on interictal depth-electrode study emphasized both the bilateral nature of TLE and the inconsistency of interictal (intracranial) spike localization with ictal onset localization.

Patient 3

This 25-year-old woman had complex febrile seizures starting at 11 months of age, followed soon after by afebrile seizures with eye deviation to the right preceding secondary generalization. Seizures were well controlled with phenobarbital monotherapy, which was tapered at 9 years. After 2 years of seizure freedom, episodes of staring, verbal unresponsiveness, and occasional secondary generalization without aura gradually increased in frequency despite valproic acid, phenobarbital, carbamazepine, and clonazepam alone and in various combinations. MRI was normal.

Audiovisual EEG monitoring interictally demonstrated bizarre frontal polyspikes, left greater than right. Four spontaneous seizures were characterized by verbal unresponsiveness, grunting, and bilateral leg kicking with left frontal ictal onset. MRI revealed qualitatively normal hippocampi with a left anteromedial frontal cystic lesion. Volumetric MRI revealed mild left hippocampal atrophy. Verbal IQ was 95, and performance IQ was 75, with deficits in language and memory, left greater than right. Intracarotid amobarbital testing documented left-hemisphere language dominance and impaired memory (left, three of six objects recalled; right, two of six). Left frontal craniotomy was performed with excision of a $2 \times 3 \times 4$ cm mass that revealed nonspecific vascular changes.

After antiepileptic medications were tapered, the patient remained seizure free for 4 years but then developed new complex partial seizures consisting of staring and unresponsiveness preceded by an aura of hot and cold in her chest. Despite treatment with phenytoin, gabapentin, and lamotrigine, she was having two to three seizures per week at the time of re-evaluation. Audiovisual EEG monitoring demonstrated left anterior temporal and midtemporal spikes interictally. The four spontaneous seizures recorded featured periodic sharp, high-amplitude left temporal discharges, followed by left-hemisphere slowing and left mid- to posterior temporal rhythmic Θ activity. All seizures involved staring and lip smacking at onset and right upper-extremity pronation postictally. Neuropsychological assessment was largely unchanged. PET revealed a focal region of hypometabolism in the left frontal lobe and marked hypometabolism of the left temporal lobe. Subtraction of interictal and ictal SPECT revealed left posterior temporoparietal hypoperfusion. MRI was unchanged except for postsurgical changes in the left frontal lobe. Because clinical semiology, ictal scalp EEG, MRI, and functional imaging were unable to distinguish a left temporal neocortical from a mesial temporal onset, intracranial EEG recording was performed with a grid over the left temporoparietal area and frontal cortex surrounding the previous resection, with strips along the mesial hemisphere, and hippocampal depth electrodes. Small spike discharges were noted from the left hippocampal and lateral frontal regions. Four complex partial seizures all began in the left hippocampus and entorhinal cortex.

Four years after left anteromedial temporal lobectomy with hippocampectomy, the patient continues to have rare complex partial seizures. The resected tissue demonstrated neuronal loss and gliosis in the hippocampus consistent with HS.

This patient illustrates the history and findings of dual pathology. Two independent epileptic foci were present but were manifested at different stages of the history. The first focus was a frontal lesion of probable developmental etiology; surgery produced 4 years of control. Left HS emerged as a second independent and newly intractable epileptic focus that proved amenable to surgery but required continued antiepileptic medication.

REFERENCES

1. Engel J Jr. A greater role for surgical treatment of epilepsy: why and when? *Epilepsy Currents* 2003;3:37–40.
2. Babb T, Brown W. Pathological findings in epilepsy. In: Engel JJ, ed. *Surgical treatment of the epilepsies*. New York: Raven Press, 1987:511–540.
3. Spencer SS. When should temporal-lobe epilepsy be treated surgically? *Lancet Neurol* 2002;1:375–382.
4. Engel J Jr, Wiebe S, French J, et al. Practice parameter: temporal lobe and localized neocortical resections for epilepsy: report of the Quality Standards Subcommittee of the American Academy of Neurology, in association with the American Epilepsy Society and the American Association of Neurological Surgeons. *Neurology* 2003;60:538–547.
5. Wiebe S, Blume WT, Girvin JP, et al. A randomized, controlled trial of surgery for temporal-lobe epilepsy. *N Engl J Med* 2001; 345:311–318.

6. Spencer SS. Long-term outcome after epilepsy surgery. *Epilepsia* 1996;37:807–813.

7. Gloor P. Mesial temporal sclerosis: historical background and an overview from a modern perspective. In: Luders H, ed. *Epilepsy surgery*. New York: Raven Press, 1991:689–703.

8. De Lanerolle NC, Kim JH, Brines ML. Cellular and molecular alterations in partial epilepsy. *Clin Neurosci* 1994;2:64–81.

9. Margerison JH, Corsellis JA. Epilepsy and the temporal lobes. A clinical, electroencephalographic and neuropathological study of the brain in epilepsy, with particular reference to the temporal lobes. *Brain* 1966;89:499–530.

10. De Lanerolle NC, Kim JH, Williamson A, et al. A retrospective analysis of hippocampal pathology in human temporal lobe epilepsy: evidence for distinctive patient subcategories. *Epilepsia* 2003;44:677–687.

11. O'Connor ER, Sontheimer H, Spencer DD, et al. Astrocytes from human hippocampal epileptogenic foci exhibit action potential-like responses. *Epilepsia* 1998;39:347–354.

12. de Lanerolle NC, Brines ML, Kim JH, et al. Neurochemical remodelling of the hippocampus in human temporal lobe epilepsy. *Epilepsy Res Suppl* 1992;9:205–219; discussion 220.

13. de Lanerolle NC, Kim JH, Robbins RJ, et al. Hippocampal interneuron loss and plasticity in human temporal lobe epilepsy. *Brain Res* 1989;495:387–395.

14. Sutula T, Cascino G, Cavazos J, et al. Mossy fiber synaptic reorganization in the epileptic human temporal lobe. *Ann Neurol* 1989;26:321–330.

15. Saltik S, Angay A, Ozkara C, et al. A retrospective analysis of patients with febrile seizures followed by epilepsy. *Seizure* 2003;12:211–216.

16. Trinka E, Unterrainer J, Haberlandt E, et al. Childhood febrile convulsions—which factors determine the subsequent epilepsy syndrome? A retrospective study. *Epilepsy Res* 2002; 50:283–292.

17. Hamati-Haddad A, Abou-Khalil B. Epilepsy diagnosis and localization in patients with antecedent childhood febrile convulsions. *Neurology* 1998;50:917–922.

18. Maher J, McLachlan RS. Febrile convulsions. Is seizure duration the most important predictor of temporal lobe epilepsy? *Brain* 1995;118(pt 6):1521–1528.

19. Janszky J, Woermann FG, Barsi P, et al. Right hippocampal sclerosis is more common than left after febrile seizures. *Neurology* 2003;60:1209–1210.

20. Berg AT, Langfitt J, Shinnar S, et al. How long does it take for partial epilepsy to become intractable? *Neurology* 2003;60:186–190.

21. French JA, Williamson PD, Thadani VM, et al. Characteristics of medial temporal lobe epilepsy, I: results of history and physical examination. *Ann Neurol* 1993;34:774–780.

22. Nelson KB, Ellenberg JH. Prognosis in children with febrile seizures. *Pediatrics* 1978;61:720–727.

23. Tarkka R, Paakko E, Pyhtinen J, et al. Febrile seizures and mesial temporal sclerosis: no association in a long-term follow-up study. *Neurology* 2003;60:215–218.

24. Worrell GA, Sencakova D, Jack CR, et al. Rapidly progressive hippocampal atrophy: evidence for a seizure-induced mechanism. *Neurology* 2002;58:1553–1556.

25. Mathern GW, Kuhlman PA, Mendoza D, et al. Human fascia dentata anatomy and hippocampal neuron densities differ depending on the epileptic syndrome and age at first seizure. *J Neuropathol Exp Neurol* 1997;56:199–212.

26. Blackwood DH, Cull RE, Freeman CP, et al. A study of the incidence of epilepsy following ECT. *J Neurol Neurosurg Psychiatry* 1980;43:1098–1102.

27. Spencer S, Novotny E, de Lanerolle N, et al. Mesial temporal sclerosis: electroclinical and pathological correlations and applications to limbic epilepsy in children. In: Avanzini G, Beaumanoir A, Mira L, eds. *Limbic seizures in children*. London: John Libbey & Company, 2001:44–54.

28. Raymond AA, Fish DR, Stevens JM, et al. Association of hippocampal sclerosis with cortical dysgenesis in patients with epilepsy. *Neurology* 1994;44:1841–1845.

29. Cendes F, Cook MJ, Watson C, et al. Frequency and characteristics of dual pathology in patients with lesional epilepsy. *Neurology* 1995;45:2058–2064.

30. Levesque MF, Nakasato N, Vinters HV, et al. Surgical treatment of limbic epilepsy associated with extrahippocampal lesions: the problem of dual pathology. *J Neurosurg* 1991;75:364–370.

31. Ho SS, Kuznecky RI, Gilliam F, et al. Congenital porencephaly and hippocampal sclerosis. Clinical features and epileptic spectrum. *Neurology* 1997;49:1382–1388.

32. Bocti C, Robitaille Y, Diadori P, et al. The pathological basis of temporal lobe epilepsy in childhood. *Neurology* 2003;60:191–195.

33. Fernandez G, Effenberger O, Vinz B, et al. Hippocampal malformation as a cause of familial febrile convulsions and subsequent hippocampal sclerosis. *Neurology* 1998;50:909–917.

34. Semah F, Picot MC, Adam C, et al. Is the underlying cause of epilepsy a major prognostic factor for recurrence? *Neurology* 1998;51:1256–1262.

35. Stephen LJ, Kwan P, Brodie MJ. Does the cause of localisation-related epilepsy influence the response to antiepileptic drug treatment? *Epilepsia* 2001;42:357–362.

36. Kwan P, Brodie MJ. Clinical trials of antiepileptic medications in newly diagnosed patients with epilepsy. *Neurology* 2003;60:S2–S12.

37. Kwan P, Brodie MJ. Early identification of refractory epilepsy. *N Engl J Med* 2000;342:314–319.

38. Engel JJ. Early randomized surgical epilepsy trial (ERSET). National Institute of Neurological Disorders and Stroke, Study ID Number R01NS42372, 2002.

39. Kuznecky RI, Knowlton RC. Neuroimaging of epilepsy. *Semin Neurol* 2002;22:279–288.

40. Ebner A, Hoppe M. Noninvasive electroencephalography and mesial temporal sclerosis. *J Clin Neurophysiol* 1995;12:23–31.

41. Williamson PD, French JA, Thadani VM, et al. Characteristics of medial temporal lobe epilepsy, II: interictal and ictal scalp electroencephalography, neuropsychological testing, neuroimaging, surgical results, and pathology. *Ann Neurol* 1993; 34:781–787.

42. Diehl B, Najm I, Mohamed A, et al. Interictal EEG, hippocampal atrophy, and cell densities in hippocampal sclerosis and hippocampal sclerosis associated with microscopic cortical dysplasia. *J Clin Neurophysiol* 2002;19:157–162.

43. Hamer HM, Najm I, Mohamed A, et al. Interictal epileptiform discharges in temporal lobe epilepsy due to hippocampal sclerosis versus medial temporal lobe tumors. *Epilepsia* 1999;40: 1261–1268.

44. Spencer S. Intracranial recording. In: Spencer S, Spencer D, eds. *Surgery for epilepsy*. Cambridge: Blackwell Scientific Publications, 1991:54–64.

45. Thadani VM, Williamson PD, Berger R, et al. Successful epilepsy surgery without intracranial EEG recording: criteria for patient selection. *Epilepsia* 1995;36:7–15.

46. Marks DA, Katz A, Booke J, et al. Comparison and correlation of surface and sphenoidal electrodes with simultaneous intracranial recording: an interictal study. *Electroencephalogr Clin Neurophysiol* 1992;82:23–29.

47. Spencer SS, Williamson PD, Bridgers SL, et al. Reliability and accuracy of localization by scalp ictal EEG. *Neurology* 1985;35: 1567–1575.

48. Risinger MW, Engel J Jr, Van Ness PC, et al. Ictal localization of temporal lobe seizures with scalp/sphenoidal recordings. *Neurology* 1989;39:1288–1293.

49. Sperling MR, O'Connor MJ, Saykin AJ, et al. A noninvasive protocol for anterior temporal lobectomy. *Neurology* 1992;42:416–422.

50. King D, Spencer S. Invasive electroencephalography in mesial temporal lobe epilepsy. *J Clin Neurophysiol* 1995;12:32–45.

51. Kanner AM, Parra J, Gil-Nagel A, et al. The localizing yield of sphenoidal and anterior temporal electrodes in ictal recordings: a comparison study. *Epilepsia* 2002;43:1189–1196.

52. Kanner AM, Jones JC. When do sphenoidal electrodes yield additional data to that obtained with antero-temporal electrodes? *Electroencephalogr Clin Neurophysiol* 1997;102:12–19.

53. Spencer SS, Sperling MR, Shewmon DA. Intracranial electrodes. In: Engel J Jr, Pedley TA, eds. *Epilepsy: a comprehensive textbook*. Philadelphia: Lippincott-Raven, 1997:1719–1747.

54. King D, Bronen RA, Spencer DD, et al. Topographic distribution of seizure onset and hippocampal atrophy: relationship between MRI and depth EEG. *Electroencephalogr Clin Neurophysiol* 1997; 103:692–697.

55. Davis LM, Spencer DD, Spencer SS, et al. MR imaging of implanted depth and subdural electrodes: is it safe? *Epilepsy Res* 1999;35:95–98.
56. Spencer SS, Spencer DD, Williamson PD, et al. Combined depth and subdural electrode investigation in uncontrolled epilepsy. *Neurology* 1990;40:74–79.
57. Niedermeyer E. The "third rhythm:" further observations. *Clin Electroencephalogr* 1991;22:83–96.
58. So NK. Depth electrode studies in mesial temporal lobe epilepsy. In: Luders H, ed. *Epilepsy surgery*. New York: Raven Press, 1992: 371–384.
59. Wieser HG, Williamson PD, Babb TL, et al. Surgically remediable temporal lobe syndromes. In: Engel JJ, ed. *Surgical treatment of the epilepsies*. New York: Raven Press, 1993:49–63.
60. Schuh LA, Henry TR, Ross DA, et al. Ictal spiking patterns recorded from temporal depth electrodes predict good outcome after anterior temporal lobectomy. *Epilepsia* 2000;41:316–319.
61. Spencer SS, Kim J, Spencer DD. Ictal spikes: a marker of specific hippocampal cell loss. *Electroencephalogr Clin Neurophysiol* 1992; 83:104–111.
62. Spencer SS, Kim J, deLanerolle N, et al. Differential neuronal and glial relations with parameters of ictal discharge in mesial temporal lobe epilepsy. *Epilepsia* 1999;40:708–712.
63. Spencer SS, Guimaraes P, Katz A, et al. Morphological patterns of seizures recorded intracranially. *Epilepsia* 1992;33:537–545.
64. Spencer SS, Spencer DD. Entorhinal–hippocampal interactions in medial temporal lobe epilepsy. *Epilepsia* 1994;35:721–727.
65. Lieb JP, Babb TL. Interhemispheric propagation time of human hippocampal seizures, II: relationship to pathology and cell density. *Epilepsia* 1986;27:294–300.
66. Spencer SS, Marks D, Katz A, et al. Anatomic correlates of interhippocampal seizure propagation time. *Epilepsia* 1992;33:862–873.
67. Cascino GD, Trenerry MR, Sharbrough FW, et al. Depth electrode studies in temporal lobe epilepsy: relation to quantitative magnetic resonance imaging and operative outcome. *Epilepsia*. 1995; 36:230–235.
68. Allen PJ, Fish DR, Smith SJ. Very high-frequency rhythmic activity during SEEG suppression in frontal lobe epilepsy. *Electroencephalogr Clin Neurophysiol* 1992;82:155–159.
69. Javidan MKA, Tran T, Pacia S, et al. Frequency characteristics of neocortical and hippocampal onset seizures. *Epilepsia* 1992;33 (Suppl 3):58.
70. Cascino GD, Jack CR Jr, Parisi JE, et al. Magnetic resonance imaging-based volume studies in temporal lobe epilepsy: pathological correlations. *Ann Neurol* 1991;30:31–36.
71. Kuznicky R, Burgard S, Faught E, et al. Predictive value of magnetic resonance imaging in temporal lobe epilepsy surgery. *Arch Neurol* 1993;50:65–69.
72. Spencer SS. The relative contributions of MRI, SPECT, and PET imaging in epilepsy. *Epilepsia* 1994;35(Suppl 6):S72–S89.
73. Spencer SS, McCarthy G, Spencer DD. Diagnosis of medial temporal lobe seizure onset: relative specificity and sensitivity of quantitative MRI. *Neurology* 1993;43:2117–2124.
74. Lencz T, McCarthy G, Bronen RA, et al. Quantitative magnetic resonance imaging in temporal lobe epilepsy: relationship to neuropathology and neuropsychological function. *Ann Neurol* 1992;31:629–637.
75. Jack CR Jr, Sharbrough FW, Cascino GD, et al. Magnetic resonance image-based hippocampal volumetry: correlation with outcome after temporal lobectomy. *Ann Neurol* 1992;31:138–146.
76. Radhakrishnan K, So EL, Silbert PL, et al. Predictors of outcome of anterior temporal lobectomy for intractable epilepsy: a multivariate study. *Neurology* 1998;51:465–471.
77. Armon C, Radtke RA, Friedman AH, et al. Predictors of outcome of epilepsy surgery: multivariate analysis with validation. *Epilepsia* 1996;37:814–821.
78. Watson C, Cendes F, Fuerst D, et al. Specificity of volumetric magnetic resonance imaging in detecting hippocampal sclerosis. *Arch Neurol* 1997;54:67–73.
79. King D, Bouthillier A, Kim J, et al. Medial temporal lobe epilepsy without hippocampal atrophy. *J Epilepsy* 1996;9:291–297.
80. Williamson PD, Thadani VM, French JA, et al. Medial temporal lobe epilepsy: videotape analysis of objective clinical seizure characteristics. *Epilepsia* 1998;39:1182–1188.
81. Spencer SS, Katz A. Arriving at the surgical options for intractable seizures. *Semin Neurol* 1990;10:422–430.
82. Sass KJ, Spencer DD, Kim JH, et al. Verbal memory impairment correlates with hippocampal pyramidal cell density. *Neurology* 1990;40:1694–1697.
83. Sass KJ, Lencz T, Westerveld M, et al. The neural substrate of memory impairment demonstrated by the intracarotid amobarbital procedure. *Arch Neurol* 1991;48:48–52.
84. Engel J Jr, Henry TR, Risinger MW, et al. Presurgical evaluation for partial epilepsy: relative contributions of chronic depth-electrode recordings versus FDG-PET and scalp-sphenoidal ictal EEG. *Neurology* 1990;40:1670–1677.
85. Theodore WH, Sato S, Kufta C, et al. Temporal lobectomy for uncontrolled seizures: the role of positron emission tomography. *Ann Neurol* 1992;32:789–794.
86. Spencer SS, Theodore WH, Berkovic SF. Clinical applications: MRI, SPECT, and PET. *Magn Reson Imaging* 1995;13:1119–1124.
87. Radtke RA, Hanson MW, Hoffman JM, et al. Temporal lobe hypometabolism on PET: predictor of seizure control after temporal lobectomy. *Neurology* 1993;43:1088–1092.
88. Manno EM, Sperling MR, Ding X, et al. Predictors of outcome after anterior temporal lobectomy: positron emission tomography. *Neurology* 1994;44:2331–2336.
89. Engel J Jr. Update on surgical treatment of the epilepsies. Summary of the Second International Palm Desert Conference on the Surgical Treatment of the Epilepsies (1992). *Neurology* 1993;43:1612–1617.
90. Sackellares JC, Siegel GJ, Abou-Khalil BW, et al. Differences between lateral and mesial temporal metabolism interictally in epilepsy of mesial temporal origin. *Neurology* 1990;40:1420–1426.
91. Drzezga A, Arnold S, Minoshima S, et al. 18F-FDG PET studies in patients with extratemporal and temporal epilepsy: evaluation of an observer-independent analysis. *J Nucl Med* 1999;40:737–746.
92. Debets RM, Sadzot B, van Isselt JW, et al. Is 11C-flumazenil PET superior to 18FDG PET and 123I-iomazenil SPECT in presurgical evaluation of temporal lobe epilepsy? *J Neurol Neurosurg Psychiatry* 1997;62:141–150.
93. Foldvary N, Lee N, Hanson MW, et al. Correlation of hippocampal neuronal density and FDG-PET in mesial temporal lobe epilepsy. *Epilepsia* 1999;40:26–29.
94. Henry TR, Babb TL, Engel J Jr, et al. Hippocampal neuronal loss and regional hypometabolism in temporal lobe epilepsy. *Ann Neurol* 1994;36:925–927.
95. Franceschi M, Messa C, Ferini-Strambi L, et al. SPET imaging of cerebral perfusion in patients with non-refractory temporal lobe epilepsy. *Acta Neurol Scand* 1993;87:268–274.
96. Hajek M, Wieser HG, Khan N, et al. Preoperative and postoperative glucose consumption in mesiobasal and lateral temporal lobe epilepsy. *Neurology* 1994;44:2125–2132.
97. Natsume J, Kumakura Y, Bernasconi N, et al. Alpha-[11C] methyl-L-tryptophan and glucose metabolism in patients with temporal lobe epilepsy. *Neurology* 2003;60:756–761.
98. Devous MD, Thisted RA, Morgan GF, et al. SPECT brain imaging in epilepsy: a meta-analysis. *J Nucl Med* 1998;39:285–293.
99. Grunwald F, Menzel C, Pavics L, et al. Ictal and interictal brain SPECT imaging in epilepsy using technetium-99m-ECD. *J Nucl Med* 1994;35:1896–1901.
100. Cross JH, Gordon I, Jackson GD, et al. Children with intractable focal epilepsy: ictal and interictal 99TcM HMPAO single photon emission computed tomography. *Dev Med Child Neurol* 1995;37: 673–681.
101. Harvey AS, Bowe JM, Hopkins IJ, et al. Ictal 99mTc HMPAO single photon emission computed tomography in children with temporal lobe epilepsy. *Epilepsia* 1993;34:869–877.
102. Heiskala H, Launes J, Pihko H, et al. Brain perfusion SPECT in children with frequent fits. *Brain Dev* 1993;15:214–218.
103. Menzel C, Steidele S, Grunwald F, et al. Evaluation of technetium-99m-ECD in childhood epilepsy. *J Nucl Med* 1996;37:1106–1112.
104. Miyazaki M, Hashimoto T, Omura H, et al. Infantile spasms with localized cerebral lesion detected by 99mTcHMPAO-SPECT. *No To Hattatsu* 1994;26:251–256. Japanese.
105. Packard AB, Roach PJ, Davis RT, et al. Ictal and interictal technetium-99m-bicisate brain SPECT in children with refractory epilepsy. *J Nucl Med* 1996;37:1101–1106.

106. Velasco TR, Wichert-Ana L, Leite JP, et al. Accuracy of ictal SPECT in mesial temporal lobe epilepsy with bilateral interictal spikes. *Neurology* 2002;59:266–271.

107. Newton MR, Berkovic SF, Austin MC, et al. Postictal switch in blood flow distribution and temporal lobe seizures. *J Neurol Neurosurg Psychiatry* 1992;55:891–894.

108. Rowe CC, Berkovic SF, Sia ST, et al. Localization of epileptic foci with postictal single photon emission computed tomography. *Ann Neurol* 1989;26:660–668.

109. Spanaki MV, Spencer SS, Corsi M, et al. Sensitivity and specificity of quantitative difference SPECT analysis in seizure localization. *J Nucl Med* 1999;40:730–736.

110. Jasper H, Kershman J. Electroencephalographic classification of the epilepsies. *Arch Neurol Psychiatry* 1941;45:903–943.

111. Gibbs EL, Gibbs FA, Fuster B. Psychomotor epilepsy. *Arch Neurol Psychiatry* 1948;60:331–339.

112. Penfield W, Flanigin FH. Surgical therapy of temporal lobe seizures. *Arch Neurol Psychiatry* 1950;64:491–500.

113. Meador KJ. Emergence of temporal lobe surgery for epilepsy. *Arch Neurol* 2001;58:1011–1012.

114. Engel JJ, Shewmon A. Who should be considered a surgical candidate? In: Engel JJ, ed. *Surgical treatment of the epilepsies.* New York: Raven Press, 1993:23–24.

115. McKhann GM 2nd, Bourgeois BF, Goodman RR. Epilepsy surgery: indications, approaches, and results. *Semin Neurol* 2002;22:269–278.

116. Awad IA, Nayel MH, Luders H. Second operation after the failure of previous resection for epilepsy. *Neurosurgery* 1991;28: 510–518.

117. Nayel MH, Awad IA, Luders H. Extent of mesiobasal resection determines outcome after temporal lobectomy for intractable complex partial seizures. *Neurosurgery* 1991;29:55–60; discussion 60–61.

118. Wyler AR, Hermann BP, Somes G. Extent of medial temporal resection on outcome from anterior temporal lobectomy: a randomized prospective study. *Neurosurgery* 1995;37:982–990; discussion 990–991.

119. Spencer DD, Spencer SS, Mattson RH, et al. Access to the posterior medial temporal lobe structures in the surgical treatment of temporal lobe epilepsy. *Neurosurgery* 1984;15:667–671.

120. Wieser HG, Yasargil MG. Selective amygdalohippocampectomy as a surgical treatment of mesiobasal limbic epilepsy. *Surg Neurol* 1982;17:445–457.

121. Arruda F, Cendes F, Andermann F, et al. Mesial atrophy and outcome after amygdalohippocampectomy or temporal lobe removal. *Ann Neurol* 1996;40:446–450.

122. Wieser HG. Selective amygdalo-hippocampectomy for temporal lobe epilepsy. *Epilepsia* 1988;29(Suppl 2):S100–S113.

123. Pauli E, Pickel S, Schulemann H, et al. Neuropsychologic findings depending on the type of the resection in temporal lobe epilepsy. *Adv Neurol* 1999;81:371–377.

124. Goldstein LH, Polkey CE. Short-term cognitive changes after unilateral temporal lobectomy or unilateral amygdalo-hippocampectomy for the relief of temporal lobe epilepsy. *J Neurol Neurosurg Psychiatry* 1993;56:135–140.

125. Gleissner U, Helmstaedter C, Schramm J, et al. Memory outcome after selective amygdalohippocampectomy: a study in 140 patients with temporal lobe epilepsy. *Epilepsia* 2002;43:87–95.

126. Helmstaedter C, Grunwald T, Lehnertz K, et al. Differential involvement of left temporolateral and temporomesial structures in verbal declarative learning and memory: evidence from temporal lobe epilepsy. *Brain Cogn* 1997;35:110–131.

127. Dupont S, Croize AC, Semah F, et al. Is amygdalohippocampectomy really selective in medial temporal lobe epilepsy? A study using positron emission tomography with (18)fluorodeoxyglucose. *Epilepsia* 2001;42:731–740.

128. Berkovic SF, McIntosh AM, Kalnins RM, et al. Preoperative MRI predicts outcome of temporal lobectomy: an actuarial analysis. *Neurology* 1995;45:1358–1363.

129. Berg AT, Walczak T, Hirsch LJ, et al. Multivariable prediction of seizure outcome one year after resective epilepsy surgery: development of a model with independent validation. *Epilepsy Res* 1998;29:185–194.

130. Engel JJ. Outcome with respect to epileptic seizures. In: Engel JJ, ed. *Surgical treatment of the epilepsies.* New York: Raven Press, 1987:553–570.

131. Yoon HH, Kwon HL, Mattson RH, et al. Long-term seizure outcome in patients initially seizure-free after resective epilepsy surgery. *Neurology* 2003;61:445–450.

132. Chovaz CJ, McLachlan RS, Derry PA, Cummings AL. Psychosocial function following temporal lobectomy: influence of seizure control and learned helplessness. *Seizure* 1994;3:171–176.

133. Wheelock I, Peterson C, Buchtel HA. Presurgery expectations, postsurgery satisfaction, and psychosocial adjustment after epilepsy surgery. *Epilepsia* 1998;39:487–494.

134. Kellett MW, Smith DF, Baker GA, et al. Quality of life after epilepsy surgery. *J Neurol Neurosurg Psychiatry* 1997;63:52–58.

135. Mihara T, Inoue Y, Watanabe Y, et al. Improvement of quality-of-life following resective surgery for temporal lobe epilepsy: results of patient and family assessments. *Jpn J Psychiatry Neurol* 1994;48:221–229.

136. Spencer SS, Berg AT, Vickrey BG, et al. Initial outcomes in the Multicenter Study of Epilepsy Surgery. *Neurology* 2003;61: 1680–1685.

137. McIntosh AM, Wilson SJ, Berkovic SF. Seizure outcome after temporal lobectomy: current research practice and findings. *Epilepsia* 2001;42:1288–1307.

138. Salanova V, Markand O, Worth R, et al. FDG-PET and MRI in temporal lobe epilepsy: relationship to febrile seizures, hippocampal sclerosis and outcome. *Acta Neurol Scand* 1998;97:146–153.

139. Quigg M, Bertram EH, Jackson T, et al. Volumetric magnetic resonance imaging evidence of bilateral hippocampal atrophy in mesial temporal lobe epilepsy. *Epilepsia* 1997;38:588–594.

140. King D, Spencer SS, McCarthy G, et al. Bilateral hippocampal atrophy in medial temporal lobe epilepsy. *Epilepsia* 1995;36: 905–910.

141. Cendes F, Li LM, Watson C, et al. Is ictal recording mandatory in temporal lobe epilepsy? Not when the interictal electroencephalogram and hippocampal atrophy coincide. *Arch Neurol* 2000;57:497–500.

142. Free SL, Li LM, Fish DR, et al. Bilateral hippocampal volume loss in patients with a history of encephalitis or meningitis. *Epilepsia* 1996;37:400–405.

143. Hirsch LJ, Spencer SS, Williamson PD, et al. Comparison of bitemporal and unitemporal epilepsy defined by depth electroencephalography. *Ann Neurol* 1991;30:340–346.

144. Barr WB, Ashtari M, Schaul N. Bilateral reductions in hippocampal volume in adults with epilepsy and a history of febrile seizures. *J Neurol Neurosurg Psychiatry* 1997;63:461–467.

145. So N, Gloor P, Quesney LF, et al. Depth electrode investigations in patients with bitemporal epileptiform abnormalities. *Ann Neurol* 1989;25:423–431.

146. Hirsch LJ, Spencer SS, Spencer DD, et al. Temporal lobectomy in patients with bitemporal epilepsy defined by depth electroencephalography. *Ann Neurol* 1991;30:347–356.

147. Sirven JI, Malamut BL, Liporace JD, et al. Outcome after temporal lobectomy in bilateral temporal lobe epilepsy. *Ann Neurol* 1997;42:873–878.

148. Spanedda F, Cendes F, Gotman J. Relations between EEG seizure morphology, interhemispheric spread, and mesial temporal atrophy in bitemporal epilepsy. *Epilepsia* 1997;38:1300–1314.

149. Spencer S, Spencer D. Apparent bitemporal epileptogenicity. In: Elisevich K, Smith B, eds. *Epilepsy surgery: case rounds.* Philadelphia: Lippincott-Raven, 2002:186–198.

150. Williamson PD, Thadani VM, Darcey TM, et al. Occipital lobe epilepsy: clinical characteristics, seizure spread patterns, and results of surgery. *Ann Neurol* 1992;31:3–13.

151. Sisodiya SM, Moran N, Free SL, et al. Correlation of widespread preoperative magnetic resonance imaging changes with unsuccessful surgery for hippocampal sclerosis. *Ann Neurol* 1997;41:490–496.

152. Lee JW, Andermann F, Dubeau F, et al. Morphometric analysis of the temporal lobe in temporal lobe epilepsy. *Epilepsia* 1998;39: 727–736.

153. DeCarli C, Hatta J, Fazilat S, et al. Extratemporal atrophy in patients with complex partial seizures of left temporal origin. *Ann Neurol* 1998;43:41–45.

154. Dreifuss S, Vingerhoets FJ, Lazeyras F, et al. Volumetric measurements of subcortical nuclei in patients with temporal lobe epilepsy. *Neurology* 2001;57:1636–1641.

155. Chugani DC, Chugani HT. Does serotonin have trophic effects in temporal lobe epilepsy? *Neurology* 2003;60:736–737.

156. Dupont S, Semah F, Baulac M, Samson Y. The underlying patho-physiology of ictal dystonia in temporal lobe epilepsy: an FDG-PET study. *Neurology* 1998;51:1289–1292.

157. Cascino GD, Jack CR Jr, Parisi JE, et al. Operative strategy in patients with MRI-identified dual pathology and temporal lobe epilepsy. *Epilepsy Res* 1993;14:175–182.

158. Li LM, Cendes F, Watson C, et al. Surgical treatment of patients with single and dual pathology: relevance of lesion and of hippocampal atrophy to seizure outcome. *Neurology* 1997;48:437–444.

159. Li LM, Cendes F, Andermann F, et al. Surgical outcome in patients with epilepsy and dual pathology. *Brain* 1999;122(Pt 5):799–805.

Resection for Uncontrolled Epilepsy in the Setting of Focal Lesions on MRI: Tumor, Vascular Malformation, Trauma, and Infarction

79

Dennis D. Spencer   *Alexandre C. Carpentier*

Advances in neuroimaging techniques, particularly high-resolution magnetic resonance imaging (MRI), have proved invaluable in identifying structural brain lesions in patients with epilepsy. Identification of focal lesions is particularly important when patients with medically refractory partial seizures are considered for epilepsy surgery, because the best outcomes after surgery are usually seen when focal MRI lesions can be identified and are concordant with electrographic findings. The assumption that all such focal lesions invariably predict the site of seizure origin may not be correct, however. Because the electroencephalogram (EEG) is the only readily available clinical method of assessing epileptogenic function, the identification of structural lesions in epilepsy often requires correlation with electrographic studies.

Guidelines for neuroimaging evaluation of patients with uncontrolled epilepsy (1) suggest obtaining T1, T2, three-dimensional volume acquisition, gadolinium contrast enhancement, fluid-attenuated inversion recovery (FLAIR), hippocampal volumetry, and fast spin-echo inversion recovery sequences and computed tomography (CT) for calcified lesions. Ictal single-photon-emission computed tomography (SPECT) and interictal [18F]fluoro-2-deoxyglucose ([18F]FDG) positron emission tomography (PET) also appear to be sensitive to epileptogenic regions. Using three-dimensional postprocessing software for coregistration of images from different modalities with those obtained on MRI can provide more precise information regarding localization.

Beside developmental abnormalities and mesial temporal sclerosis (discussed in another chapter), adult epileptogenic lesions can be distinguished by their histology and encompass the following:

1. Neoplasms (oligodendroglioma, oligoastrocytoma, astrocytoma, epidermoid cyst, astroblastoma, dysembryoplastic neuroepithelial tumor [DNET], gangliioglioma, xanthoastrocytoma)
2. Vascular abnormalities ("angiographically visible" or "occult" arteriovenous malformations [AVMs], cavernous angiomas)
3. Acquired gliosis and encephalomalacia: posttraumatic gliosis and hemosiderin deposition, inflammatory diseases, and ischemic lesions

Different lesions leading to intractable epilepsy have individual histologic, physiopathologic, and EEG properties that may be important to know about when a surgical treatment is planned.

When a lesion is proved to be the epileptogenic region by concordant data from scalp EEG, MRI, neuropsychological findings, and, if needed, PET and SPECT, surgical resection is often proposed. The volume of the resection, however, is still controversial. Should interictal spikes seen on electrocorticography direct the extent of the resection? Should the surrounding marginal cortex be excised along with the lesion? Should visual evidence of abnormal tissue be the only criterion for focus resection, or should preoperative imaging abnormalities guide the resection? If MRI is concordant with standard preoperative evaluations, can surgery be performed directly, or is there a need for a cortical mapping to avoid appreciable functional loss? Should resection be accompanied by multiple subpial transections in functional areas?

Surgical management is challenging, because it often requires separating resectable epileptogenic regions from cortex with appreciable function. The location of the functional cortex in relation to epileptogenic activity can interfere with a complete resection. However, many patients show worthwhile improvement or become seizure free after this "functionally limited" surgery.

Even when MRI studies document structural brain lesions, these are not invariably the sites of seizure origin. In fact, some patients' ictal onsets seen on scalp EEG recordings arise from a different location from the focal structural lesion seen on MRI. Epilepsy is, after all, fundamentally a problem of abnormal physiology. When noninvasive evaluations are discordant, intracranial monitoring is required. The invasive evaluation may or may not correlate the lesion with the epileptic focus. If not, the study may reveal dual pathology (2,3).

This chapter will describe the evaluation of adult epileptogenic lesions visible on MRI (except developmental abnormalities and mesial temporal sclerosis) and will provide a decision tree for invasive monitoring.

NEW MAGNETIC RESONANCE IMAGING AND FUNCTIONAL IMAGING TECHNIQUES FOR LESIONAL EPILEPSY

In patients undergoing presurgical evaluation, neuroimaging should provide data on the putative epileptogenic region, especially delineation of structural and functional abnormalities, prediction of the nature of the structural pathology, and detection of abnormalities distant from the epileptogenic zone. Emerging goals include functional magnetic resonance imaging (fMRI) identification of such brain regions as the primary sensorimotor, vision, and language and memory areas and the relation of these to the epileptogenic region.

In 1998, the Commission on Neuroimaging of the International League Against Epilepsy provided guidelines for neuroimaging evaluation of patients with uncontrolled epilepsy considered for surgery (1). However, minimal requirements for the number and type of tests have not yet been established.

CT scanning can detect certain structural lesions with calcification (e.g., cysticercosis); however, MRI has largely replaced its use. Even when a CT scan reveals an epileptogenic lesion, MRI often adds new and important data.

MRI examination is integral to presurgical planning. T1- and T2-weighted images, with thin contiguous slices and no interslice gap, should be obtained. Coronal and axial slices along with a three-dimensional volume acquisition constitute the standard protocol in most epilepsy centers. In some instances, gadolinium contrast enhancement may provide useful additional information. Other sequences such as FLAIR and fast spin-echo inversion recovery may have a role in selected cases (e.g., if standard imaging is normal or to clarify the significance of a possible focal abnormality). A careful qualitative and volumetric quantitative side-to-side ratios evaluation of the hippocampus corrected for intracranial volume may show evidence of dual pathology and/or bilateral disease.

In addition to static anatomic acquisitions, functional imaging has a crucial role in presurgical evaluations. Ictal and interictal SPECT, PET, fMRI, magnetic resonance spectroscopy (MRS), and diffusion MRI for fiber tracking are techniques that can help to define abnormal function, which may add correlative data in defining the epileptic region.

ELECTROENCEPHALOGRAPHIC FEATURES OF SYMPTOMATIC EPILEPSIES

A potential epileptogenic lesion may be identified far from where scalp ictal discharges seem to arise. False localization can be caused by propagation of ictal discharges, for example, from a parietal focus through the limbic system (4). Spread of epileptic activity from neocortical to medial temporal structures was proposed by Ajmone-Marsan and Gumnit (5) as being responsible for generation of seizures. Several subsequent observations were made regarding spread of seizures from temporal neocortex to the hippocampus (6,7). Walczak and colleagues (8) found that the majority of seizures originating in the temporal neocortex spread to mesiobasal temporal regions before behavioral expression.

For example, somatosensory auras followed by unilateral clonic and tonic motor seizures are well-recognized features of parietal lobe foci, especially of the perirolandic area (9). Many clinical findings have been linked with parietal lobe seizures, including epigastric sensations, vestibular and visual hallucinations, automatisms, and arrest reactions (9–11). These may be produced by the spread of discharges to surrounding areas. Ictal discharges can originate in the posterior cingulate gyrus and precuneus of the medial parietal lobe, but it is only when the ictal discharges propagate into the temporal lobes that symptoms of complex partial seizures of temporal lobe type occur (11).

The cingulum (which shares fibers with the limbic system) and the corpus callosum participate in propagation of ictal discharges to both temporal lobes and can offer a complex electrical spread pattern (4). This may complicate identification of a focal epileptogenic zone in the cingulum in cases with unremarkable MRI findings.

CORRELATION OF MAGNETIC RESONANCE IMAGING CHARACTERISTICS WITH COMMONLY IDENTIFIED PATHOLOGIES

Eriksson and coworkers (12) reported that a blinded review of MRI scans in their surgical series showed correlation with histopathologic findings in all cases of vascular malformation, in more than 75% cases of tumor or hippocampal sclerosis, and in 28.6% of major cortical malformations. A detailed description of the epileptogenic lesions most often identified on MRI is provided in the following sections.

Neoplasms

Epilepsy is a common presentation in patients with cerebral tumors. Low-grade cerebral neoplasms, including astrocytoma, mixed glioma, oligodendroglioma, and DNET, constitute the pathologic substrates in some 10% to 30% of patients with chronic intractable partial epilepsy (13,14). Epilepsy is the first symptom in 50% of astroglial neoplasms at presentation, and ganglioglioma may be the most common cause of tumor-related chronic epilepsy, with the highest incidence of seizures (88%) (15–17).

Oligodendroglioma

The morphologic spectrum of oligodendrogliomas includes tumors that are traditionally misinterpreted as "diffuse fibrillary astrocytomas." These consist of isolated neoplastic oligodendrocytes that are entrapped in a background composed of axons and fibrillary reactive gliosis. In some cases, a genetic deletion is present in the 1p19q locus. A series of 153 "pure" supratentorial oligodendrogliomas composed of "classic" or pseudo-"diffuse fibrillary oligodendrogliomas" showed that two-thirds of the tumors were exclusively isolated tumor cells (type III) and that only one-third exhibited both isolated tumor cells and solid tumor tissue components (type II). The type II tumor destroys brain parenchyma and forms new micro-blood vessels, whereas isolated tumor cells do not destroy the parenchyma and are not associated with microangiogenesis. Clinically, a neurologic deficit occurs in about 57% of type II but in only 8% of type III oligodendrogliomas. On MRI, contrast enhancement is observed in type II oligodendrogliomas (64%) but is

usually not seen in type III. The biologic behavior of these tumors seems to be closely related to the pattern of tumor growth. Emergence of microangiogenesis within a tumor that at first grows slowly with a type III pattern signals more aggressive behavior (18).

MRI typically reveals oligodendrogliomas to be hyperintense on spin density and T2-weighted images. Their signal is often heterogeneous owing to small cysts, calcification, or prior hemorrhage. Calcification is especially common and may be seen best on CT.

Statistics show anaplastic transformation in 50% of patients 10 years after diagnosis. Anaplastic transformation may be suspected on the basis of PET studies, because anaplastic oligodendrogliomas show a higher methionine and [^{18}F]FDG fixation than low-grade oligodendrogliomas. Radiotherapy and chemotherapy with gadolinium enhancement are usually indicated for recurrences (19). Survival for patients with anaplastic oligodendroglioma is about 3 years.

Low-Grade Astrocytoma

Low-grade astrocytomas associated with chronic seizures constitute a distinct clinicopathologic group of tumors that arise in young hosts (20 to 40 years old). These low-grade gliomas usually have an indolent course. An important factor in achieving long-term seizure control is complete removal of the lesion to tumor-free margins. In addition, complete resection of the tumor may be the most effective treatment for control of low-grade glioma growth. Margins may be limited by functional cortex, leading to partial tumor excision. For low-grade gliomas in the temporal lobe, additional medial temporal resection may be required. This is most often predicted preoperatively by MRI that shows the lesion infiltrating the hippocampus or hippocampal atrophy. Decisions about extralesional hippocampal resection should be based on evaluation of this presumed dual pathology using several variables in addition to hippocampal atrophy, including seizure history, video-EEG, semiology, proximity of the tumor to the hippocampus, and the neuropsychological profile of the patient, especially with regard to memory function (20).

On MRI, low-grade astrocytomas usually appear homogeneous, although some tumors have cystic components. The signal is hyperintense on double-echo sequence and hypointense on T1-weighted images. Calcification is seen on CT in the minority of low-grade astrocytomas, compared with the strong majority of oligodendrogliomas; however, because astrocytomas are the most common overall, any tumor with calcification is most likely to be of this type.

There appears to be a significant decrease in the risk of tumor recurrence in patients who undergo aggressive resection (100% 10-year survival) compared with patients who have anything less than gross-total resection (21). Gender, type of symptoms, length of preoperative symptoms, and timing of radiation therapy (immediate postoperative versus delayed radiotherapy) are not known to be significant in determining outcome, length of survival, recurrence, and/or incidence of transition to more malignant tumors. Within the population of patients with low-grade astrocytomas, those with chronic epilepsy usually have the best prognosis. Tumors associated with chronic epilepsy are much less likely to become more malignant over time (21). Irradiation can be used to reduce intractable seizure frequency in some patients with unresectable (biopsy-proven) low-grade astrocytoma (19). Focal radiation treatment may reduce seizures by more than 75% in 80% of cases, and the MRI often shows a tumor response to radiation that correlates with reduced seizure frequency (19). In patients who became seizure free, seizure recurrence is usually associated with tumor progression (14).

Ganglioglioma

Ganglioglioma may be the most common cause of tumor-related chronic epilepsy (22,23). The current World Health Organization (WHO) classification defines ganglioglioma as a neoplasm composed of neoplastic neural (ganglion cells) and glial elements (24). Ganglioglioma accounts for 0.4% to 9% (17) of primary brain tumors diagnosed at different institutions. It has been described in many parts of the central nervous system but is most commonly found in the temporal lobe (25,26).

The tumor has been localized by MRI or CT scans in the temporal (70%), frontal (10%), parietal (8%), and occipital (3%) lobes. MRI is able to detect the tumor with a very high degree of sensitivity, but findings are infrequently specific for ganglioglioma. On MRI, a wide variety of signals may be found (23), such as gadolinium enhancement in 60%, mass effect in 45%, cystic change in 30%, and cerebral edema in 5%. CT scan, suggested by Tampieri and colleagues (23), shows abnormality in 70%, with calcification in 35% of these, but is reported as normal in the other 30%.

Histologically, the tumors are composed of large polymorphic ganglion cells (pyramidal-like neurons), with vesicular nuclei and prominent nucleoli admixed with a neoplastic glial element, most often astrocytic. Mild perivascular chronic inflammation and vascular endothelial proliferation are usually found. Cortical dysplasia—generally adjacent to but separate from the tumor—is present in 40% of the cases described in the literature (22).

Good seizure control is seen in patients with resected ganglioglioma, despite years of medically resistant seizures: 80% of patients are seizure free (Engel class I) at 6 months, 72% at 1 year, and 63% at 2 years (22). Good outcome may be achieved, despite scalp EEG findings that may conflict with tumor location, and is more likely when surgery is performed relatively soon after epilepsy onset. MRI features such as presence or absence of gadolinium enhancement, mass effect, and cystic change had no measurable influence on the seizure outcome after tumor resection. Malignant degeneration is a rare consequence of these tumors, but the glial component can become anaplastic. No strong statistical data are available to indicate the frequency of such transformations.

Dysembryoplastic Neuroepithelial Tumor

DNETs are a group of supratentorial cortically based lesions that superficially resemble mixed oligoastrocytomas, oligodendrogliomas, and astrocytomas. Clinically, these tumors are associated with complex partial seizures beginning before the age of 20 years, with no neurologic deficit and no stigmata of phakomatosis (27). In the revised WHO classification, DNETs have been incorporated into the category of neuronal and mixed neuronoglial tumors. This classification describes a histologic variant characterized by the following criteria: cortical location, multinodular architecture (the nodule consisting of astrocytoma-like variants, oligodendrogliomas, or oligoastrocytomas), and foci of dysplastic cortical disorganization, showing a columnar structure perpendicular to the cortical surface. Daumas-Duport (28) described a glioneuronal element that was demonstrated to be specific and sufficient for diagnosing DNETs. Even if some of these tumors show a high MIB-1 labeling index, the spectrum of DNETs includes a simple form with a unique glioneuronal element. DNET is a surgically curable tumor of young patients with intractable partial seizures (29).

Daumas-Duport and colleagues (29) reported a series of 39 cases of neuroepithelial tumors associated with medically intractable complex partial seizures. The age at onset of symptoms ranged from 1 to 19 years (mean, 9 years). In addition to the chronic nature of the seizures (range, 2 to 18 years; mean, 9 years), one third of the patients showed radiologic features such as focal cranial deformity, indicating that the tumors had an early onset and were long-standing. In most cases, CT scans showed a "pseudo-cystic," well-demarcated, low-density appearance, associated in some cases with focal contrast enhancement (18%) or calcified hyperdensity (23%). MRI signals are hypo and hyper on T1 and T2 sequences, respectively. No edema, but possible gadolinium enhancement, can be seen. In a few cases, DNET was associated with neurofibromatosis type 1. The tumor involved primarily the temporal lobe (62%) but also occurred in the frontal lobe (31%). Although tumor removal was considered incomplete or subtotal in 17 patients (44%), long-term follow up (range, 1 to 18 years; mean, 9 years) showed neither clinical nor radiologic evidence of progression in any patient. Comparison of the survival data of the 13 subjects who had undergone postoperative radiotherapy with the 26 who had not indicated that radiation therapy was of no obvious benefit. The identification of DNET has therapeutic and prognostic implications because aggressive therapy can be avoided, thus sparing these young patients the deleterious long-term effects of radiotherapy or chemotherapy.

Pleomorphic Xanthoastrocytoma

Pleomorphic xanthoastrocytoma is a relatively rare brain tumor of adolescents and young adults, characterized by its superficial location, sometimes associated with a cyst, and by frequent involvement of the meninges. Temporal lobe localization helps explain why epilepsy predominates as a presenting symptom. Histology shows intracellular lipid inclusions, hypervascularization, and in all cases an arachnoidal component. The tumor is slow-growing, despite features of histologic atypia that place it in WHO grade II or III on the basis of elevated mitotic counts and the presence of punctiform necrosis. Immunostaining with the proliferation marker MIB-1 is present in only 2% of cells in the grade II group, whereas 5% show labeling in grade III. All pleomorphic xanthoastrocytomas express some amount of glial fibrillary acidic protein and are shown to elaborate a characteristic pericellular reticulin network. Surgical treatment is considered to offer the best survival outcome. Tumor recurrence with confirmed anaplasia still occurs in about 20% of cases at a mean postoperative follow up of 5 years, and survival for patients with recurring anaplastic xanthoastrocytomas is about 2 years.

Vascular Abnormalities

The term *occult* or *cryptic* cerebrovascular malformation has been used to describe any vascular malformation that cannot be detected angiographically (30,31). Angiographically occult vascular malformations (AOVMs) have been subclassified into four groups: AVMs, venous angiomas, cavernous angiomas, and telangiectasias. Lobato and coworkers (32) reported that 43.8% of AOVMs were thrombosed AVMs. Hematoma can obscure the underlying lesion, and CT and MRI may fail to identify specific pathologic subtypes of AOVMs (33). Seizures are the most common clinical presentation of occult AVMs (34). Wharen and colleagues (34) reported that 72% of patients with occult AVMs have seizures; the most common presentation is in the temporal lobe, producing complex partial seizures (35). In contrast, simple partial seizures can occur when occult AVM lesions are located in other neocortical areas (4,36). MRI of a lesion shows a serpiginous cluster of low-signal-intensity flow voids with areas of mixed signal intensity where the blood flow is slower or turbulent. Relation of feeding arteries and draining venous channels can be further appreciated by MR angiography. Arterial flow is visualized by three-dimensional time-of-flight techniques; the slower flow in areas of venous drainage is best seen by two-dimensional time of flight (37).

Intracranial hemorrhage is the most significant clinical manifestation of an AVM. An unruptured AVM carries a 4% yearly risk of hemorrhage; after a bleed the likelihood of recurrent hemorrhage is 6% in the first year and 4% in subsequent years (38–40). Morbidity caused by AVMs may also result from repeated minor hemorrhages or ischemia of surrounding brain as a result of cerebral steal. Therefore, consideration of treatment should be given to most patients with a diagnosed AVM.

Cavernous angiomas are frequently encountered in patients with intractable epilepsy. They are highly epileptogenic as a result of hemosiderin-induced gliosis. Histology shows fine vascular walls with no musculosa or elastin. Vascular growth factors are usually highly represented (Ki67,

vascular endothelial growth factor, proliferating cell nuclear antigen). Cavernous angiomas have been implicated in inducing secondary epileptogenic foci, leading to dual pathology (41). The MRI appearance is characteristic and shows a central core of increased intensity with a surrounding rim of decreased intensity on T2-weighted sequences, and multiloculated rounded areas of increased signal on T1-weighted sequences (37). There is no edema and little mass effect. The small size of afferent vessels, presence of thrombosis, and relative paucity of flow through these lesions make them difficult to detect on angiography.

Multiple lesions are seen in the familial form of cavernous angiomas with autosomal dominant inheritance pattern. When sporadic, multiple lesions are seen in fewer than one third of patients. Yearly risk of hemorrhage is estimated to be up to 2.7% per lesion per year, and risk of rebleeding after an initial bleeding episode is estimated to be between 20% and 85% (42).

Venous angiomas and telangiectasias rarely give rise to symptoms and are often incidental findings.

Lesionectomy, with removal of surrounding hemosiderin-stained brain, is considered the procedure of choice in carefully selected patients with epilepsy and AOVMs. Most series in the literature report that about 75% of patients are seizure free after lesionectomy. Age at onset, duration of seizures, age at resection, and gender do not affect outcome. Patients with neocortical AOVMs, in whom EEG findings correlated with the site of the lesion, are generally seizure free after resection, whereas treatment failures are generally associated with the presence of multiple intracranial lesions, poorly localized or diffuse EEG findings, discordant PET imaging, or a lesion in close proximity to the limbic system (43).

Epilepsy represents only 25% of onset symptoms in angiographically evident AVMs (44). AVMs have a very reasonable seizure outcome prognosis (76.9% seizure free) (35). Therapeutic protocols for AVMs depend on available techniques in each center. Usually, intra-arterial embolization is the first choice for high-flow arteriographically visible AVMs. Surgery can then be performed for seizure control (hemosiderin reactional gliosis), mass effect reduction, and residual nidus resection. Radiosurgery is often performed for lesions under 2.5 cm.

Symptomatic cavernous angiomas should be considered for surgical resection, including removal of the abnormal surrounding brain parenchyma whenever possible. Compared with AVMs, cavernous angiomas show a less favorable clinical response and higher complication rate when subjected to radiosurgery with comparable doses (45).

Acquired Gliosis and Encephalomalacia

Posttraumatic Epilepsy

Wilder Penfield, while working with Otfried Foerster in Breslau, Poland, studied a series of patients with posttraumatic frontal lesions. Their 1930 article (46) was the first to illustrate the point, recently reiterated by Kazemi and colleagues (47), that resection of frontal encephalomalacia may relieve intractable epilepsy.

In 1998, Andermann and colleagues (48) presented excellent surgical results (100% of patients became seizure free) in cases in which depressed frontal fractures led to encephalomalacia and intractable seizures. Many patients with posttraumatic epilepsy have bilateral or diffuse electrographic abnormalities. These patients have usually suffered high-velocity injuries with diffuse cortical damage. They require invasive electrode study, and there is less chance that one focal epileptogenic region will be isolated. Patients with focal injury, as discussed in the reports above, may be considered for focal resection guided by pathology shown on MRI and often supported by intracranial grid monitoring to confirm regional ictal onset and to map indispensable function. Image-guided surgery should be considered only if the injury was very focal and all supporting noninvasive evaluation was concordant, particularly cognitive testing and scalp and video-EEG electroclinical correlation (49).

Posttraumatic brain histology usually shows meningoencephalocicatrix, scar formation in brain parenchyma, meningoencephalocele, and porencephaly.

Inflammatory Diseases

Inflammatory diseases, such as postinfection (encephalitis, cysticercosis) or autoimmune (neurolupus, neurosarcoidosis) diseases, may induce diffuse or focal cortical lesions responsible for epilepsy. The overall frequency of neurologic involvement in sarcoidosis is estimated to be 5%, and within that percentage epilepsy occurs with a frequency of 5% to 18% (50). There are few MRI descriptions of neurosarcoidosis with histologic biopsy confirmation (51,52). Therefore, one can easily mistake neurosarcoidosis for low-grade tumors, lymphomas, encephalitis sequelae, or other inflammatory processes (53). MRI shows a contrast-enhancing mass lesion with surrounding T2 signal change and a high signal in the FLAIR sequence. Mass effect and surrounding edema are typically absent but have been described in some cases. PET studies can be performed to help differentiate neurosarcoidosis from high-grade gliomas. Sarcoid lesions show nonspecific hypometabolism (53). However, one can easily mistake neurosarcoidosis for low-grade tumors. Six surgical cases were described before 1974, showing reasonably good long-term outcome: All patients were seizure free after surgery for a mean period of 46 months. Epilepsy seems to be the first cause of death in patients with epileptogenic neurosarcoidosis. Radiotherapy for intra-axial neurosarcoid has been performed since 1985 with reasonable results (52). Seven patients have been reported, usually after all medication had failed to elicit a good clinical or radiologic response (52,54–56). Surgical removal of active cerebral granulomas in nonfunctional locations should still be seriously taken into consideration for intractable sarcoid lesions, especially those in a temporal

location. Early resection in such cases seems to prevent further cognitive impairments and control intractable epilepsy.

Surgical resection should be reserved for single active granulomas that are concordant with the video-EEG and other noninvasive evaluations. Otherwise, intracranial electrodes may be necessary to confirm ictal onset and provide functional mapping.

Meningitis or encephalitis in older children or adults infrequently results in MRI changes that can be used to guide surgery. In fact, few of these individuals have single localizable epileptogenic regions. They most frequently have diffuse regional or multifocal disease. The exception to this is epilepsy related to meningitis or encephalitis in children 5 years of age, in which hippocampal atrophy and unilateral medial temporal lobe epilepsy may result and may respond to anteromedial temporal resection.

Postischemic Epilepsy

Postischemic epilepsy may occur after arterial obliteration but mostly follows venous ischemia. In all cases, MRI abnormalities are evident. Patients require surgical intervention very rarely, as the epilepsy is often drug sensitive.

MAGNETIC RESONANCE IMAGING AND THE EPILEPTOGENIC REGION

The principal role of high-resolution MRI is definition of structural abnormalities that underlie seizure disorders. A range of tumors, vascular abnormalities, and acquired gliosis may be identified. Among patients with refractory partial seizures, most have an identifiable relevant abnormality on MRI. In those who do not, it is likely that the epileptogenic region may be defined by correlation between electrographic studies and functional neuroimaging studies. PET, providing data on regional cerebral blood flow, glucose metabolism, and ligand binding to specific receptors, also discloses occasional discordance between electrographic and imaging findings (57–59). It is possible, however, that other neuroimaging modalities such as ictal SPECT may be useful in evaluating difficult patients who present with discordant MRI and EEG findings by identifying functional changes in brain regions, especially at the time of a seizure (60–63). Subtraction ictal SPECT studies may prove particularly useful when coregistered with MRI (64,65).

fMRI is already used to identify cerebral areas responsible for specific functional processes. There may be a future role for fMRI in localizing seizure onsets (66) and interictal spikes. Similarly, potentially promising techniques that use EEG-triggered fMRI and electromagnetic tomography (67) may also be useful.

MRS provides a means of investigating cerebral metabolites and some neurotransmitters noninvasively. The concentrations of N-acetylaspartate, creatine, and choline-containing and other compounds may be estimated using proton MRS and may reveal focal neurochemical abnormalities that coincide with the epileptogenic region (68–70).

We will explore each of these modalities in the following sections.

Magnetic Resonance Imaging and Electroencephalography

Scalp Electroencephalography

Limitations of scalp-recorded EEG in patients with extratemporal seizures have been observed (71,72), as described above. Routine EEG studies may reveal variable findings (80), including persistently normal EEG recordings that may occur in patients with central cortical seizures (71,72). In other cases, extracranial EEG alone may be sufficient to establish a relationship between an MRI-identified structural abnormality and the epileptogenic zone. However, the importance of ictal EEG monitoring remains controversial in patients with lesional epilepsy (71,73). For example, lateralized epileptiform alterations in patients with a somatosensory or somatomotor aura and a perirolandic lesion are usually sufficient to localize a lesional epileptic syndrome.

Subdural Electroencephalography

Subdural EEG, with or without depth electrodes, is still indicated in some cases of lesional epilepsy. Subdural recordings can define the ictal zone in lesions commonly associated with more diffuse epileptogenic zones, such as developmental abnormalities and the acquired MRI-positive injuries of ischemia, infection, and trauma. Grids are also useful for mapping functional cortex near the lesions.

When a surgical procedure puts language cortex at risk, language mapping using cortical stimulation is frequently performed (74). Cortical stimulation mapping usually attempts to identify the location and extent of inferior frontal (Broca area), posterior temporal (Wernicke area), and basal temporal language regions as well as motor areas. Evoked potentials are performed to map sensory areas. The inferior frontal language region is readily identified by stimulation-induced arrest of speech. Stimulation of posterior temporal regions is often more subtle and usually causes deficits in naming and/or auditory comprehension. The basal temporal language area (posterior fusiform gyrus), when stimulated, often shows problems with object naming or reading. Cortical stimulation (bipolar stimulation from 2 to 10 mA to 50 Hz for 5 seconds, with a 200-microsecond biphasic spike duration) can be performed either during surgery on an awake and cooperative patient, or during an epilepsy unit study with implanted subdural electrodes.

Functional Magnetic Resonance Imaging and Single-Photon-Emission Computed Tomography

Functional neuroimaging of the brain has important clinical and research applications for patients with lesions associated with medically refractory seizures (62,75). Two important innovations, fMRI and subtraction ictal SPECT coregistered with structural MRI, have been introduced and may significantly alter the preoperative evaluation of patients, as well as the operative strategy. fMRI may identify functional cerebral cortex and thus may guide a more precise and coregistered placement of intracranial electrodes for video-EEG monitoring. It also provides reliable localization of the sensorimotor cortex in patients with perirolandic lesions and may demonstrate functional plasticity when lesions are developmental in origin (75,76). fMRI has been used successfully in research settings to identify language areas. Extraoperative or intraoperative electrical stimulation has shown fMRI to be reliably concordant with stimulation (75). Attempts are now being made to identify seizure foci by showing abnormal interictal signals. The main limitation of this procedure, at present, is related to patient motion.

SPECT, using the ^{99m}Tc radiotracer, is being increasingly used in the investigation of all the intractable symptomatic epilepsies, with or without MRI lesions. Interictal scans alone, using cerebral blood flow agents, are unreliable in identifying an epileptogenic region but may be ictally accurate if the tracer is injected when the seizure is first detected (no longer than 60 seconds after the end of the seizure). Structural MRI coregistration is then performed, with the interictal scan subtracted from the ictal scans (positive difference). The structural MRI can provide more precise information regarding localization of blood flow changes (64). The coregistered SPECT studies provide multimodality imaging demonstrating the area of cerebral hyperfusion in patients with lesions who are being considered for surgery (62,65,77). The sensitivity and specificity of such studies in patients with extratemporal seizures have been confirmed (62,77). O'Brien and colleagues (77) have recently completed a blinded study comparing coregistered SPECT techniques with the traditional "side-by-side" interictal and ictal SPECT images in 51 patients with intractable partial epilepsy. Coregistered SPECT demonstrated a significantly higher rate of localization (88.2% versus 39.2%; $p < 0.0001$) and better interobserver agreement (84.3% versus. 41.2%; $p < 0.0001$) than visual inspection of the interictal and ictal SPECT scans. The reconstructed images have also been shown to be of prognostic importance in patients undergoing epilepsy surgery (62,77). Patients whose SPECT localization was concordant with the epileptic brain tissue were more likely to have an excellent operative outcome than those with nonconcordant or nonlocalizing findings (62.5% versus. 20%; $p < 0.05$) (77).

Positron Emission Tomography and Magnetic Resonance Spectroscopy

PET is the only methodology in use today for noninvasive investigation of brain receptor function. PET can measure a wide range of neurotransmitter systems and metabolism. Although FDG-PET can provide absolute values for glucose metabolic rates, it is more frequently used to measure relative glucose utilization in regions suspected of being epileptogenic compared with contralateral regions. It is helpful to monitor the EEG during PET studies because unrecognized ictal activity could lead to otherwise unexplained increases in regional metabolism. Other tracers are appropriate for research purposes: ^{15}O-labeled water has been used to map cognitive functions, including speech. Lesional epilepsies usually do not require such exploration. In ongoing research with PET, investigators are attempting to identify individual signatures for the wide variety of epileptogenic tumors and developmental abnormalities.

MRS has been used to detect chemical changes in all types of brain lesions. For example, proton MRS imaging, used for developmental malformations, detects significant abnormalities in ratios of creatine to *N*-acetylated compounds and of choline to *N*-acetylated compounds (68). The results can be correlated with clinical, EEG, and histologic findings. MRS has been explored predominantly in the evaluation of patients with focal cortical dysplasia (78) and has shown some consistency in predicting tumor histology and tumor grading. Even if MRS remains a research technique and is not applicable to routine clinical work, it is an important advance that will be used more frequently to unravel the neurochemical substrates of epilepsy (Fig. 79.1).

Minimizing Surgical Risk with Functional Localization Studies

Extraoperative and intraoperative cortical stimulation studies remain the most widely used techniques for localization

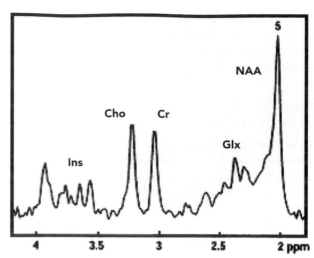

Figure 79.1   A normal spectroscopic MRI spectrum. NAA, *N*-acetyl-L-aspartate; Cr, total creatine and phosphocreatine; Cho, choline; Glx, total glutamate and glutamine; Ins, myoinositol.

of functional cortex before epilepsy surgery. However, functional neuroimaging of the brain has important clinical and research applications for patients with lesions associated with medically refractory seizures (62,75). Two important innovations, fMRI and diffusion MRI coregistered with structural MRI, have been introduced recently in clinical practice and may significantly modify the operative strategy and then improve the postoperative functional outcome of patients. fMRI may identify functional cerebral cortex and thus may guide a more precise and coregistered placement of intracranial electrodes for video-EEG monitoring. It also provides reliable localization of the sensorimotor cortex in patients with perirolandic lesions and may demonstrate

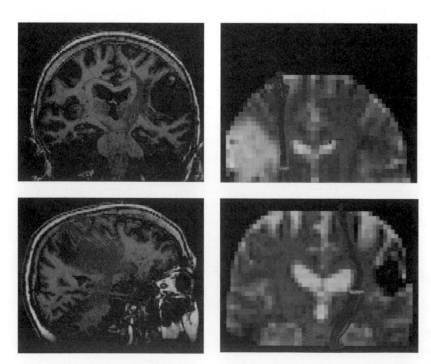

Figure 79.2   Fiber tracking with diffusion tensor MRI acquisition. Please see color insert.

functional plasticity when lesions are developmental in origin (75,76,79,80). fMRI has been used successfully in research settings to identify language areas. Extraoperative or intraoperative electrical stimulation has shown fMRI to be reliably concordant with stimulation (75,76), even during awake surgery around language areas (74).

Frameless techniques have been shown to reliably help the surgeon localize and delimit tissue resection, especially when various anatomic and functional/diffusion MRI sequences are coregistered in the neuronavigation device (81).

Diffusion MRI techniques allow analysis of water diffusion along fibers and permit the visualization of functional tract (Fig. 79.2). Such explorations are more and more commonly used to prevent the surgeon from destroying fibers during a deep parenchymal resection.

Magnetic Resonance Imaging and Dual Pathology

There are three subtypes of dual pathology: (1) incidental dual pathology, such as an epileptic focus in the hemisphere opposite an incidental MRI lesion (82); (2) true dual pathology, that is, multiple imaged substrates, such as congenital cavernomas or tubers in tuberous sclerosis [as noted earlier, a developmental abnormality (cortical dysplasia) or a tumor (ganglioglioma) may coexist, and particularly when the noninvasive evaluation is discordant, only invasive recordings will solve the problem]; and (3) secondary dual pathology, occurring when ipsilateral mesial temporal sclerosis is found to coexist with a lesion (such as a vascular malformation or cortical dysplasia). Some authors feel that hippocampal sclerosis is the consequence of an epileptogenic lesion. Secondary epileptogenic foci may be produced in the medial temporal lobe by frequent, chronic activation by the primary focus, as suggested by Yeh and Privitera (44). On the other hand, the lesion and hippocampal sclerosis may be different expressions of a single genetic aberration.

MRI is important for identifying "true" or "secondary" dual pathology, even when one of the lesions is subtle, for example, blurring of the grey-white junction in the temporal pole in association with more obvious hippocampal sclerosis. Invasive study may be required to define the strategy for surgical resection. Removal of both lesions may be important for postoperative seizure-free outcome.

SURGICAL STRATEGIES FOR MAGNETIC RESONANCE–IMAGED LESIONS

The major categories of MR-imaged epileptogenic substrates have been outlined above. In determining a reasonable surgical strategy, it is helpful to use a decision tree (described below) as a general guide. The first issue is to provide as accurate an MRI diagnosis as possible. For example, distinguishing cortical dysplasia from a glioma has two important

implications. First, if the lesion is a tumor, it may have serious consequences for the patient if it becomes more aggressive over time. Thus, depending on location, the presence of a tumor, regardless of epilepsy, may prompt surgical excision. The dual problem of medically intractable epilepsy and a tumor often motivates a more aggressive approach; a careful discussion with the patient and family is necessary when the lesions are in a cortical region with appreciable function. Second, MRI-detected tumors and some vascular abnormalities such as cavernomas are likely to be concordant with the results of other noninvasive evaluations and can frequently be approached surgically without intracranial recording. Other MRI substrates, which include developmental abnormalities, infection, trauma, and atrophy, may be associated with more diffuse seizure onset and more frequently necessitate an invasive study, when ictal localization is sought.

Some surgeons depend on intraoperative electrocorticography when deciding about the volume of tissue to be removed in cases of tumor or cavernoma excision. Our experience does not support using interictal spikes as markers of epileptogenesis adjacent to these lesions. Our basic strategy uses preoperative three-dimensional MRI planning coupled with frameless stereotactic localization of margins and confirmed by intraoperative frozen sections to ensure complete lesion resection, plus a 5- to 10-mm margin when it is not adjacent to cortex with appreciable function.

For the less well-circumscribed lesions, other than tumors and vascular abnormalities, intracranial recording is performed using a strategy that blankets the lesion, surrounding region, and projection paths with electrodes. For example, Figure 79.3A shows the MRI of a patient with a superior temporal cortex glioma; a noninvasive evaluation suggested a possible diffuse onset involving Heschl's gyrus and perhaps the hippocampus. The patient also had bilateral language representation on intracarotid amobarbital testing. The intracranial study (Fig. 79.3B and 79.3C) therefore provided for a right temporal inferior parietal grid and depth electrodes, both adjacent to the tumor and in the hippocampus. Lesion localization and depth electrode placement were accomplished using the Access frameless stereotactic device. Interictal spikes were abundant in the inferior parietal region and superior temporal gyrus. Ictal localization was adjacent to the tumor; it encroached on Heschl's gyrus but did not involve the hippocampus, which was preserved during an operation that resected the superior and middle gyrus, sparing the inferior parietal lobe. Language function was not found within the planned resection volume. The patient has been seizure free for 1 year since surgery.

Figure 79.4 illustrates a lesion in a right-handed 12-year-old boy whose preoperative evaluation was concordant with the presumed right frontal tumor. Direct surgery was therefore possible. Intraoperative stimulation localized the motor areas for the face and hand. The grade 1 astrocytoma could then be resected with comfortable 1-cm margins. The patient has been free of seizures for 5 years since surgery.

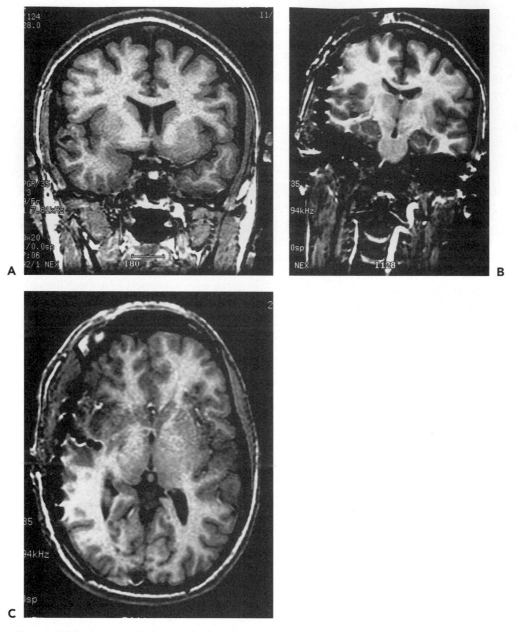

Figure 79.3   Temporal lobe ganglioglioma. **A:** Coronal T1-weighted magnetic resonance image (MRI) of a right-handed, right-hemisphere–dominant 22-year-old woman shows a ganglioglioma in the right superior temporal gyrus. **B:** Coronal T1-weighted MRI of the same patient is shown, after placement of an 8 × 8 contact Ad Tech grid covering the lesion and adjacent temporal, parietal, and frontal lobes for the purpose of ictal localization and language mapping. **C:** T1 axial MRI of the same patient depicts the grid's anteroposterior coverage and the proximal contacts of a depth electrode directed to the anterior hippocampus. Ictal events came from the tissue immediately posterior to the tumor.

Finally, the low-grade astrocytoma in Figure 79.5 was responsible for frequent medically intractable seizures in this right-handed, high-functioning, 31-year-old professional woman. The preoperative MRI diagnosis was glioma, but despite concordance of her preoperative testing, two major questions remained unanswered. First, was her hippocampus epileptogenic, as she had mild verbal memory compromise and slight hippocampal atrophy? Second, what was the precise localization of her language?

Basal language areas are very difficult to stimulate intraoperatively, and the patient had a prolonged fluent aphasia after each seizure. Grid and depth electrode mapping revealed no basal language areas, a language-free corridor to tumor resection, and no hippocampal involvement in the ictal events. At surgery, the hippocampus was spared. The patient had a mild decrease in short-term verbal memory but has been seizure free for 6 years and very functional.

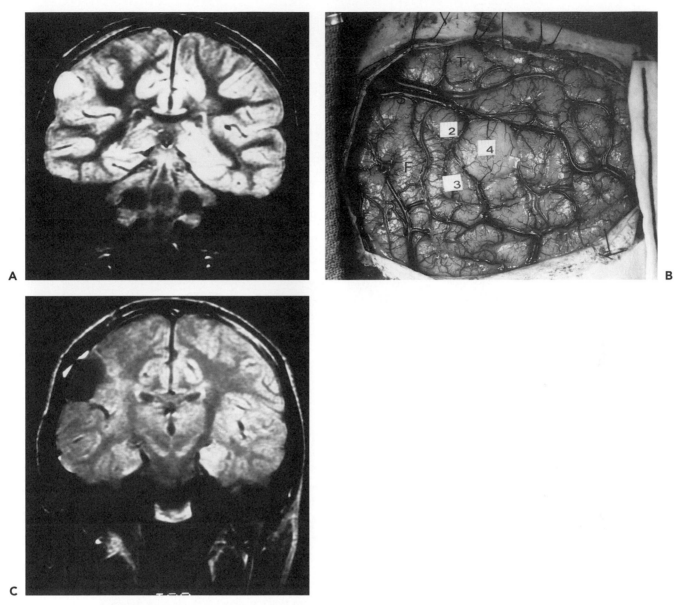

Figure 79.4   Right frontal lobe astrocytoma. **A:** T2-weighted magnetic resonance image (MRI) of a 12-year-old boy with intractable seizures shows a right frontal cortically based high-signal exophytic lesion. **B:** Intraoperative exposure is shown. S, sylvian vein; T, temporal lobe; F, frontal lobe; 2, restricted interictal spikes; 3, motor face area; 4, tumor. **C:** Postoperative T1 coronal MRI is shown.

The decision tree in Figure 79.6 summarizes these brief case reports with generalizable rules. It illustrates that the usual phase 1 and phase 2 evaluations are still used for the purpose of establishing concordance when an MRI lesion is found. When tumor and cavernoma are suspected and phases 1 and 2 are concordant, directed surgery is recommended, with a resection to normal nonpathologic cortex and always constrained by surrounding brain with appreciable function. The next division of the tree, which directs one to an intracranial study, is the same for suspected tumors and vascular lesions, in cases when noninvasive testing is nonconcordant, such as variable ictal localization or contradictory results on cognitive testing. It also includes developmental abnormalities; acquired injuries such as

infection, trauma, and ischemia; and nonspecific atrophy and gliosis, which often harbor developmental changes such as heterotopic neurons. Dual pathology also most often demands an intracranial study: Examples include a neocortical ganglioglioma plus cortical dysplasia or a temporal lobe tumor associated with hippocampal atrophy but borderline memory function. Resection of even a portion of a normally functioning dominant hippocampus will result in significant verbal learning impairment.

Intracranial study, as illustrated in the case histories, is most often recommended with dual pathology, and the MRI abnormality is used as one marker for electrode placement. All other facets of the noninvasive evaluation may also be used to direct electrodes, for example, in areas of

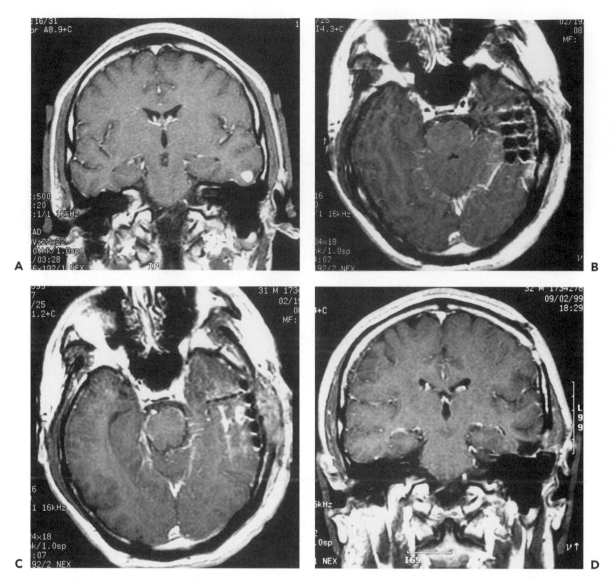

Figure 79.5 Inferior temporal lobe astrocytoma. **A:** Coronal T1 magnetic resonance image (MRI) with gadolinium contrast in a right-handed 31-year-old woman with medically intractable seizures characterized by fluent aphasia and secondary generalization. A lesion is noted in the inferior temporal gyrus that enhances and is associated with mild ipsilateral hippocampal atrophy. Verbal memory is only mildly affected on neuropsychological testing. **B:** Axial MRI of the same patient after placement of an 8 × 8 contact grid, cut to be molded around the vein of Labbé, so that potential basal language areas adjacent to the lesion might be mapped. **C:** Another T1-weighted contrast-enhanced scan after electrode placement illustrates a depth electrode introduced with the frameless stereotactic apparatus just anterior to the enhancing lesion and placed to determine hippocampal involvement with ictal events. **D:** Seven-month postoperative coronal enhanced image illustrates the limited resection based on focal ictal onsets over the tumor, with resection guided by the frameless system to frozen-section normal margins, sparing the hippocampus. The patient has been seizure free for 1 year after surgery.

PET hypometabolism or regions of severe cognitive deficit. An invasive phase 3 study may be followed by resection during the same hospitalization. Resection is guided by the best ictal volume, constrained by functional brain.

SUMMARY

MRI has had the most profound influence on epilepsy surgery programs of any technical advance in the past 20 years. It continues to be refined, and neuroradiologists are increasingly aware of subtle abnormalities that may represent biologically quiescent gliomas or developmental abnormalities. The importance of a thoughtful and properly ordered differential diagnosis cannot be overemphasized, and functional imaging adjuvants such as fMRI, PET, and SPECT have become more significant as the tools for coregistration with anatomic MRI have become more available. The incorporation of coregistered images into frameless stereotactic devices is currently revolutionizing how

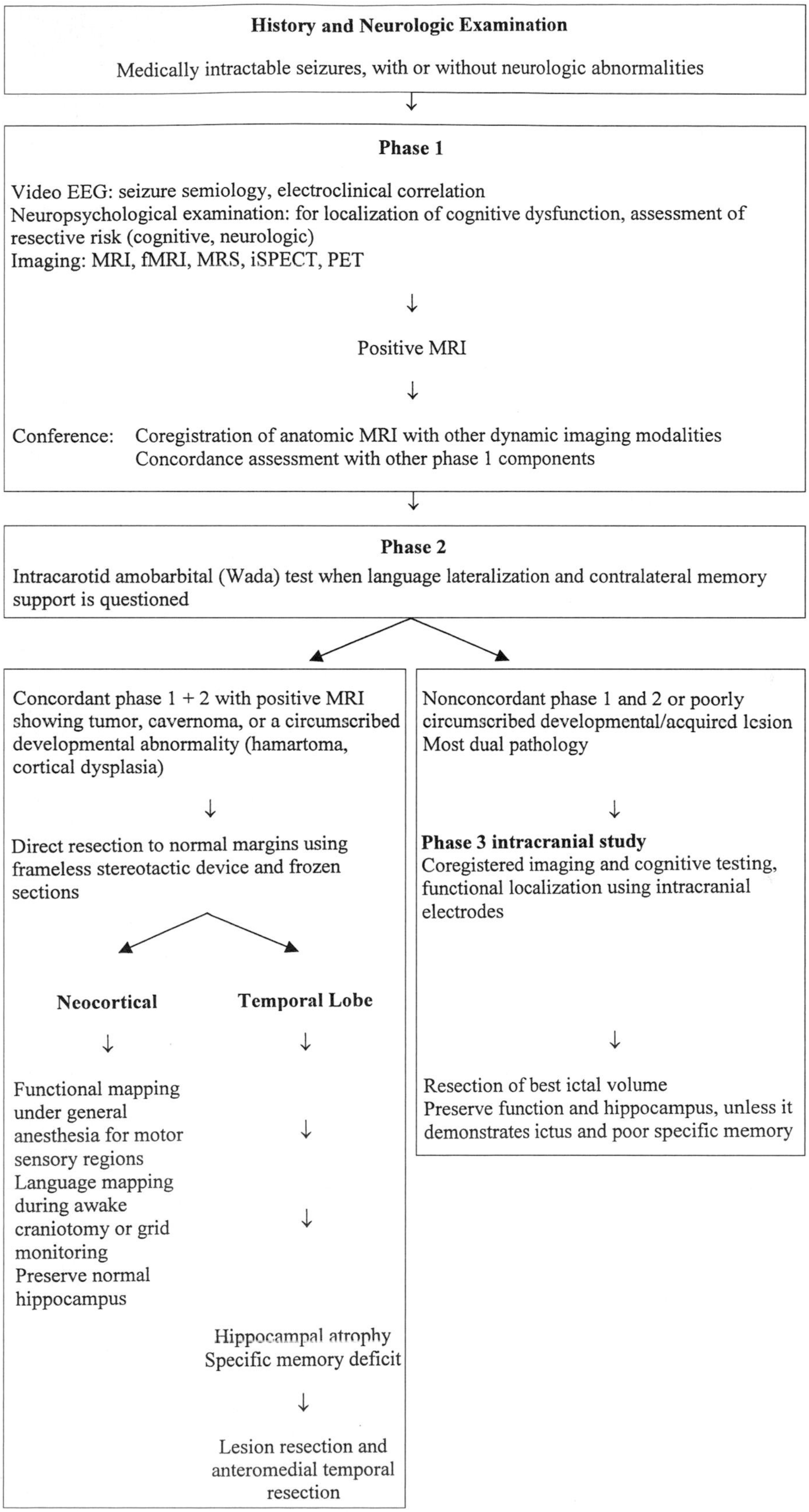

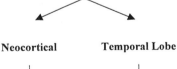

History and Neurologic Examination

Medically intractable seizures, with or without neurologic abnormalities

↓

Phase 1

Video EEG: seizure semiology, electroclinical correlation
Neuropsychological examination: for localization of cognitive dysfunction, assessment of resective risk (cognitive, neurologic)
Imaging: MRI, fMRI, MRS, iSPECT, PET

↓

Positive MRI

↓

Conference: Coregistration of anatomic MRI with other dynamic imaging modalities
Concordance assessment with other phase 1 components

↓

Phase 2

Intracarotid amobarbital (Wada) test when language lateralization and contralateral memory support is questioned

Concordant phase 1 + 2 with positive MRI showing tumor, cavernoma, or a circumscribed developmental abnormality (hamartoma, cortical dysplasia)	Nonconcordant phase 1 and 2 or poorly circumscribed developmental/acquired lesion Most dual pathology
↓	↓
Direct resection to normal margins using frameless stereotactic device and frozen sections	**Phase 3 intracranial study** Coregistered imaging and cognitive testing, functional localization using intracranial electrodes

Neocortical   **Temporal Lobe**

↓   ↓

Functional mapping under general anesthesia for motor sensory regions
Language mapping during awake craniotomy or grid monitoring
Preserve normal hippocampus

↓

Hippocampal atrophy
Specific memory deficit

↓

Lesion resection and anteromedial temporal resection

Resection of best ictal volume
Preserve function and hippocampus, unless it demonstrates ictus and poor specific memory

Figure 79.6   Decision tree for surgically treatable epilepsies with a magnetic resonance imaging (MRI)–detected lesion. EEG, electroencephalography; fMRI, functional magnetic resonance imaging; MRS, magnetic resonance spectroscopy; iSPECT, ictal single-photon-emission computed tomography; PET, positron emission tomography.

the critical preoperative data, including the EEG, are translated into the operative field, making surgery for lesional epilepsy safer and more accurate.

Surgery for uncontrolled epilepsy in the setting of MRI-detectable lesions offers excellent results in terms of epilepsy release. In discordant features between MRI and clinical data, electrophysiologic explorations are necessary to ensure good clinical outcome.

REFERENCES

1. Commission on Neuroimaging of the International League Against Epilepsy. Guidelines for neuroimaging evaluation of patients with uncontrolled epilepsy considered for surgery. *Epilepsia* 1998;39:1375–1376.
2. Ho H, Kuzniecky R, Gilliam F, et al. Temporal lobe developmental malformations and epilepsy: dual pathology and bilateral hippocampal abnormalities. *Neurology* 1998;50:748–754.
3. Li L, Cendes F, Watson C, et al. Surgical treatment of patients with single and dual pathology: relevance of lesion and of hippocampal atrophy to seizure outcome. *Neurology* 1997;48:437–444.
4. Fujii M, Akimura T, Ozaki S, et al. An angiographically occult arteriovenous malformation in the medial parietal lobe presenting as seizures of medial temporal lobe origin. *Epilepsia* 1999;40:377–381.
5. Ajmone-Marsan C, Gumnit R. Neurophysiological aspects of epilepsy. In: Vinken P, Bruyn G, eds. *Handbook of clinical neurology.* Amsterdam: North-Holland, 1974;15:30–59.
6. Stefan H, Schneider S, Abraham-Fuchs K, et al. The neocortico to mesio-basal propagation of focal epileptic activity during the spike-wave complex. *Electroencephalogr Clin Neurophysiol* 1991;79:1–10.
7. Wieser HG, Müller RU. Neocortical temporal seizures. In: Wieser HG, Elger CE, eds. *Presurgical evaluation of epileptics.* Berlin: Springer-Verlag, 1987:252–266.
8. Walczak T, Goodman R, Resor S, et al. Intracranial ictal electroencephalogram in nonlesional temporal neocortical seizures. *Neurology* 1996;46:A121–A122.
9. Ajmone-Marsan C, Goldhammer L. Clinical ictal patterns and electrographic data in cases of parietal seizures of fronto-central-parietal origin. In: Brazier MAB, ed. *Epilepsy: its phenomena in man.* New York: Academic Press, 1973:235–258.
10. Williamson PD, Boon PA, Thadani VM, et al. Parietal lobe epilepsy: diagnostic considerations and results of surgery. *Ann Neurol* 1992;31:193–201.
11. Williamson PD, Wieser H-G, Delgado-Escueta AV. Clinical characteristics of partial seizures. In: Engel J Jr, ed. *Surgical treatment of the epilepsies.* New York: Raven Press, 1987:101–120.
12. Eriksson S, Malmgren K, Rydenhag B, et al. Surgical treatment of epilepsy—clinical, radiological and histopathological findings in 139 children and adults. *Acta Neurol Scand* 1999;99:8–15.
13. Babb TL, Brown WJ. Pathological findings in epilepsy. In: Engel J Jr, ed. *Surgical treatment of the epilepsies.* New York: Raven Press, 1987:511–540.
14. Spencer DD, Spencer SS, Mattson RH, et al. Intracerebral masses in patients with intractable partial epilepsy. *Neurology* 1984;34:432–436.
15. Morris HH, Estes ML, Gilmore R, et al. Chronic intractable epilepsy as the only symptom of primary brain tumor. *Epilepsia* 1993;34:1038–1043.
16. Shady JA, Black PM, Kupsky WJ, et al. Seizures in children with supratentorial astroglial neoplasms. *Pediatr Neurosurg* 1994;21:23–30.
17. Zulch KJ. *Brain tumors: their biology and pathology,* 2nd ed. Berlin, Germany: Springer-Verlag, 1965:184.
18. Daumas-Duport C, Varlet P, Tucker ML, et al. Oligodendrogliomas. Part I: patterns of growth, histological diagnosis, clinical and imaging correlations: a study of 153 cases. *J Neurooncol* 1997;34:37–59.
19. Rogers LR, Morris HH, Lupica K. Effect of cranial irradiation on seizure frequency in adults with low-grade astrocytoma and medically intractable epilepsy. *Neurology* 1993;43:1599–1601.
20. Fried I. Management of low-grade gliomas: results of resections without electrocorticography. *Clin Neurosurg* 1995;42:453–463.
21. Piepmeier J, Christopher S, Spencer D, et al. Variations in the natural history and survival of patients with supratentorial low-grade astrocytomas. *Neurosurgery* 1996;38:872–879.
22. Morris HH, Matkovic Z, Estes ML, et al. Ganglioglioma and intractable epilepsy: clinical and neurophysiologic features and predictors of outcome after surgery. *Epilepsia* 1998;39:307–313.
23. Tampieri D, Moumdjian R, Melanson D, et al. Intracerebral gangliogliomas in patients with partial complex seizures: CT and MR imaging findings. *Am J Neuroradiol* 1991;12:749–755.
24. Kleihues P, Burger PC, Scheithauer BW. The new WHO classification of brain tumours. *Brain Pathol* 1993;3:255–268.
25. Celli P, Scarpinati M, Nardacci B, et al. Gangliogliomas of the cerebral hemispheres. Report of 14 cases with long-term follow-up and review of the literature. *Acta Neurochir* 1993;125:52–57.
26. Lang FF, Epstein FJ, Ransohoff J, et al. Central nervous system gangliogliomas. Part 2: clinical outcome. *J Neurosurg* 1993;79:867–873.
27. Prayson RA, Morris HH, Estes ML, et al. Dysembryoplastic neuroepithelial tumor: a clinicopathologic and immunohistochemical study of 11 tumors including MIB1 immunoreactivity. *Clin Neuropathol* 1996;15:47–53.
28. Daumas-Duport C. Dysembryoplastic neuroepithelial tumours. *Brain Pathol* 1993;3:283–295.
29. Daumas-Duport C, Scheithauer BWW, Chodkiewicz JP, et al. Dysembryoplastic neuroepithelial tumor: a surgically curable tumor of young patients with intractable partial seizures. Report of thirty-nine cases. *Neurosurgery* 1988;23:545–556.
30. Becker DH, Townsend JJ, Kramer RA, et al. Occult cerebrovascular malformations: a series of 18 histologically verified cases with negative angiography. *Brain* 1979;102:249–287.
31. Ogilvy CS, Heros RC, Ojemann RG, et al. Angiographically occult arteriovenous malformations. *J Neurosurg* 1988;69:350–355.
32. Lobato RD, Perez C, Rivas JJ, et al. Clinical, radiological, and pathological spectrum of angiographically occult intracranial vascular malformations: analysis of 21 cases and review of the literature. *J Neurosurg* 1988;68:518–531.
33. Robinson JR Jr, Awad IA, Masaryk TJ, et al. Pathological heterogeneity of angiographically occult vascular malformations of the brain. *Neurosurgery* 1993;33:547–555.
34. Wharen RE Jr, Scheithauer BW, Laws ER Jr. Thrombosed arteriovenous malformations of the brain: an important entity in the differential diagnosis of intractable focal seizure disorders. *J Neurosurg* 1982;57:520–526.
35. Edgar R, Baldwin M. Vascular malformation associated with temporal lobe epilepsy. *J Neurosurg* 1960;17:638–656.
36. Hashim ASM, Asakura T, Koichi U, et al. Angiographically occult arteriovenous malformations. *Surg Neurol* 1985;23:431–439.
37. Kesava PP, Turski PA. Magnetic resonance angiography of vascular malformations. *Magn Reson Imag Clin North Am* 1998;6:811–833.
38. Brown RD Jr, Wiebers DO, Forbes G, et al. The natural history of unruptured intracranial arteriovenous malformations. *J Neurosurg* 1988;68:352–357.
39. Ondra SL, Troupp H, George ED, et al. The natural history of symptomatic arteriovenous malformations of the brain: a 24-year follow-up assessment. *J Neurosurg* 1990;73:387–391.
40. Wilkins RH. Natural history of intracranial vascular malformations: a review. *Neurosurgery* 1985;16:421–430.
41. Lee HW, Seo DW, Hong SB, et al. Electroclinicopathologic relationship of epileptogenic foci in cavernous angioma. *Epilepsia* 1998;39:230–231.
42. Maraire Nozipo J, Awad Issam A. Cavernous malformations: natural history and indications for treatment. In: Hunt Batjer H, ed. *Cerebrovascular disease.* New York: Lippincott-Raven, 2004:669–677.
43. Kraemer DL, Griebel ML, Lee N, et al. Surgical outcome in patients with epilepsy with occult vascular malformations treated with lesionectomy. *Epilepsia* 1998;39:600–607.
44. Yeh H, Privitera MD. Secondary epileptogenesis in cerebral arteriovenous malformations. *Arch Neurol* 1991;48:1122–1124.

45. Pollock BE, Garces YI, Stafford SL, et al. Stereotactic radiosurgery for cavernous malformations. *J Neurosurg* 2000;93:987–991.
46. Foerster O, Penfield W. The structural basis of traumatic epilepsy and results of radical operation. *Brain* 1930;53:99–119.
47. Kazemi NJ, So EL, Mosewich RK, et al. Resection of frontal encephalomalacias for intractable epilepsy: outcome and prognostic factors. *Epilepsia* 1997;38:670–677.
48. Andermann F, Cukiert A, Olivier A. Excellent surgical results obtained in patients with a depressed frontal fracture leading to frontal encephalomalacia and intractable frontal seizures. *Epilepsia* 1998;39:108.
49. Cukiert A, Olivier A, Andermann F. Posttraumatic frontal lobe epilepsy with structural changes: excellent results after cortical resection. *Can J Neurol Sci* 1996;23:114–117.
50. Delaney P. Neurologic manifestations in sarcoidosis: review of the literature with a report of 23 cases. *Ann Intern Med* 1977;87:336–345.
51. Lexa FJ, Grossman RI. MR of sarcoidosis in the brain and spine: spectrum of manifestations and radiographic response to steroid therapy. *Am J Neuroradiol* 1994;15:973–982.
52. Stelzer KJ, Thomas CR, Berger MS, et al. Radiation therapy for sarcoid of the thalamus/posterior third ventricle: case report. *Neurosurgery* 1995;36:1188–1191.
53. Powers VJ, Micler FM. Sarcoidosis mimicking glioma: case report and review of intracranial mass lesions. *Neurology* 1981;31:907–910.
54. Agbogu BN, Stern BJ, Sewell C, et al. Therapeutic considerations in patients with refractory neurosarcoidosis. *Arch Neurol* 1995;52:875–879.
55. Bejar JM, Kerby GR, Ziegler DK, et al. Treatment of central nervous system sarcoidosis with radiotherapy. *Ann Neurol* 1985;18:258–260.
56. Chapelon C, Ziza JM, Piette JC, et al. Neurosarcoidosis: signs, course and treatment in 35 confirmed cases. *Medicine* 1990;69:261–276.
57. Engel J Jr, Kuhl D, Phelps M, et al. Comparative localization of epileptic foci in partial epilepsy by PET and EEG. *Ann Neurol* 1982;12:529–537.
58. Richardson M, Koepp M, Brooks D, et al. 11C-flumazenil PET reveals central benzodiazepine receptor binding abnormalities in partial epilepsy with normal MRI. *Neurology* 1996;46: S122–S123.
59. Richardson M, Koepp M, Brooks D, et al. 11C-flumazenil PET in neocortical epilepsy. *Neurology* 1998;51:485–492.
60. Duncan JS. Imaging and epilepsy. *Brain* 1997;120:339–377.
61. Ho S, Berkovic S, Berlangieri S, et al. Comparison of ictal SPECT and interictal PET in the presurgical evaluation of temporal lobe epilepsy. *Ann Neurol* 1995;37:738–745.
62. Sjoholm H, Rosen I, Elmquist D. Role of 123I-iomazenil SPECT imaging in drug resistant epilepsy with complex partial seizures. *Acta Neurol Scand* 1995;92:41–48.
63. Weis M, Feistal H, Stefan H. Utility of ictal SPECT: peri-ictal, post-ictal. *Acta Neurol Scand* 1994;152:145–147.
64. O'Brien T, So E, Mullan B, et al. Subtraction ictal SPECT co-registered with MRI improves clinical usefulness of SPECT in localizing the surgical seizure focus. *Neurology* 1998;50:445–454.
65. So EL, O'Brien TJ, Mullan BP, et al. Seizure localization in intractable partial epilepsy by subtraction SPECT co-registered to MRI: a study of 47 consecutive patients. *Epilepsia* 1996;37:S124.
66. Jackson G, Connelly A, Cross J, et al. Functional magnetic resonance imaging of focal seizures. *Neurology* 1994;44:850–856.
67. Seeck M, Lazeyras C, Michel C, et al. Non-invasive epileptic focus localization using EEG-triggered functional MRI and electromagnetic tomography. *Electroencephalogr Clin Neurophysiol* 1998;106: 522–534.
68. Carpentier A, Dupont S, Clemenceau S. Apport de la spectroscopie par résonance magnétique (SRM) dans les épilepsies partielles complexes. *Lett Neurol* 2001;10:423–426.
69. Cendes F, Andermann F, Preul M, et al. Lateralization of temporal lobe epilepsy based on regional metabolic abnormalities in proton magnetic resonance spectroscopic images. *Ann Neurol* 1994;35: 211–216.
70. Chu W, Hetherington H, Kuzniecky R, et al. Lateralization of human temporal lobe epilepsy by 31P NMR spectroscopic imaging at 4.1 T. *Neurology* 1998;51:472–479.
71. Cascino GD, Hulihan JF, Sharbrough FW, et al. Parietal lobe lesional epilepsy: electroclinical correlation and operative outcome. *Epilepsia* 1993;34:522–527.
72. Cascino GD, Kelly PJ, Sharbrough FW, et al. Long-term follow-up of stereotactic lesionectomy in partial epilepsy: predictive factors and electroencephalographic results. *Epilepsia* 1992;33: 639–644.
73. Cascino GD, Boon PAJM, Fish DR. Surgically remediable lesional epilepsy. In: Engel J Jr, ed. *Surgical treatment of the epilepsies*, 2nd ed. New York: Raven Press, 1993:77–86.
74. Ojemann GA, Ojemann J, Lettich E, et al. Cortical language localization in left, dominant hemisphere. An electrical stimulation mapping investigation in 117 patients. *J Neurosurg* 1989;71: 316–336.
75. Jack CR Jr, Lee CR, Riederer SJ. Functional magnetic resonance imaging. In: Cascino GD, Jack CR Jr, eds. *Neuroimaging in epilepsy: principles and practice*. Boston: Butterworth-Heinemann, 1995: 151–164.
76. Puce A, Constable RT, Luby ML, et al. Functional magnetic resonance imaging of sensory and motor cortex: comparison with electrophysiological localization. *J Neurosurg* 1995;83:262–270.
77. O'Brien TJ, So EL, Mullan BP, et al. Extent of resection of ictal subtraction SPECT focus is an important determinant of epilepsy surgery outcome. *Epilepsia* 1996;37:S182.
78. Kuzniecky R, Hetherington H, Pan J, et al. Proton spectroscopic imaging at 4.1 tesla in patients with malformations of cortical development and epilepsy. *Neurology* 1997;48:1018–1024.
79. Carpentier A, Constable RT, Schlosser M, et al. Patterns of fMRI activations in association with structural lesions in the central sulcus: a classification of plasticity. *J Neurosurg* 2001;94:946–954.
80. Carpentier A, Pugh KR, Westerveld M, et al. Language processing for different input modalities. Evidence of language plasticity in epilepsy. *Epilepsia* 2001;42:1241–1254.
81. Olivier A, Germano IM, Cukiert A, et al. Frameless stereotaxy for surgery of the epilepsies: preliminary experiences. Technical note. *J Neurosurg* 1994;81:629–633.
82. Holmes MD, Wilensky AJ, Ojemann GA, et al. Hippocampal or neocortical lesions on magnetic resonance imaging do not necessarily indicate site of ictal onsets in partial epilepsy. *Ann Neurol* 1999;45:461–465.

Epilepsy Surgery in Focal Malformations of Cortical Development

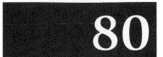

Jorge A. González-Martínez   *Imad M. Najm*   *William E. Bingaman*
Paul Ruggieri

Focal malformations caused by abnormal cortical development (MCD) are the pathologic substrates in an increasing number of patients with chronic epilepsy (1,2) and are even more common in children referred for surgical treatment (3,4). Among the histopathologic abnormalities included under this rubric are abnormalities of the architectural organization (laminar and columnar disorganization) of the cortex and the presence of dysmorphic (dysplastic) neurons, large neurons (meganeurons), and balloon cells (Fig. 80.1). Focal MCD may be restricted to the cortical mantle or may encompass the subcortical white matter and periventricular regions. As the sensitivity of neuroimaging techniques increases, even more patients with "cryptogenic" epilepsy will be found to have subtle alterations in cortical architecture (1,5,6) that may extend well beyond the abnormalities now visible on magnetic resonance imaging (MRI) scans (7). In surgical series, focal MCD tend to carry an unfavorable prognosis for seizure-free outcome (4,8).

As resective surgery depends on accurate preoperative localization of the epileptogenic zone, various clinical, electroencephalographic (EEG), anatomic, functional, metabolic, and neuropsychological techniques are enlisted to elucidate the pathologic cause and the relationships between the ictal onset zone and eloquent (functional) areas of the brain. Epilepsy surgery aims for the complete resection (or disconnection) of the cortical and subcortical areas responsible for the generation of seizures (epileptogenic zone) (9,10). Some epileptogenic areas may overlap with functional (eloquent) cortex, which must be preserved. An array of noninvasive and invasive diagnostic tools are available: analysis of seizure semiology, video-scalp electroencephalographic recordings, invasive subdural electrocorticographic (ECoG) recordings (intraoperative or extraoperative), extraoperative depth electrode recordings (stereo-encephalography [SEEG]), magnetoencephalography (MEG), and MRI. Neuroimaging techniques may provide functional (ictal single-photon-emission computed tomography [fSPECT] and fMRI), as well as metabolic (magnetic resonance spectroscopy [MRS] and positron emission tomography [PET]) information. These methods are usually complementary and will define cortical zones of interest: symptomatogenic, irritative, ictal onset, and functional deficit in addition to eloquent cortex and the epileptogenic lesion (for a detailed review, see refs. 9 and 10).

This chapter discusses methods to confirm the diagnosis of epilepsy in focal MCD; techniques to identify of the epileptogenic lesion; the role of subdural electrodes in localizing the epileptogenic zone and mapping the functional cortex and its relationships with the anatomic lesion; and surgical strategies and postresective seizure outcome.

DIAGNOSIS OF FOCAL EPILEPSY

Prolonged video-scalp EEG monitoring, analysis of clinical semiology, remains the gold standard for diagnosis of focal epilepsy (10). This noninvasive sampling technique gives an excellent overview of the location and extent of the epileptogenic areas but only approximates the boundaries of both the irritative and epileptogenic zones. Scalp electroencephalography detects only epileptiform activity

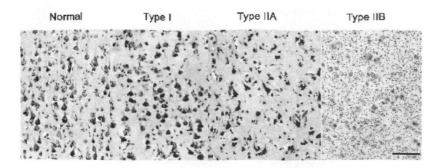

Figure 80.1 Histopathologic subtypes of malformations of cortical development compared with normal tissue. Note the architectural disorganization (type I), dysmorphic neurons (type IIA), and balloon cells (type IIB). Scale bar: 100 μm.

that results from EEG synchronization of large areas of cortex, estimated in some studies to be between 6 and 8 cm² (11), and recordings are disturbed by the smearing effect of bone and other high-resistance structures (e.g., meninges and scalp) between the cortical generators and the recording electrodes (12–14). MEG may overcome some of these problems (11). Between 85% and 100% of patients with MCD exhibit epileptiform discharges on interictal scalp EEG recordings (15,16), ranging from lobar to lateralized, nonlocalizing to diffuse (including generalized spike-wave patterns in some cases of subependymal heterotopia [16]). The spatial distribution of interictal spikes is usually more extensive than the structural abnormality as assessed by intraoperative inspection or visual analysis of MRI findings (16–19).

IDENTIFICATION OF THE ANATOMIC (POTENTIALLY EPILEPTOGENIC) LESION

MRI anatomic and signal abnormalities have been described in MCD (Fig. 80.2). An abnormal gyral anatomy or increased cortical thickness, or both, is common in some types of MCD (17,18). The underlying white matter is thin, with an increased signal on T2-weighted images. Other cases show variable changes that include short and indistinct white-matter digitations with asymmetric cortical thickening. Variable degrees of white-matter signal abnormalities may be evident on T2-weighted (or fluid attenuated inversion recovery [FLAIR]) images (20). The combination of overt gyral abnormalities and signal changes make the diagnosis of some dysplastic lesions obvious; however, subtle unilateral focal cortical abnormalities that are difficult to assess on conventional T1-weighted two-dimensional images may be the only finding. Despite significant MRI abnormalities in most cases of MCD, up to 25% of patients with "normal" MRIs had histopathologic changes in focal lesions (21). Milder forms of MCD characterized by cortical laminar and columnar disorganization in the absence of balloon cells may not be seen on high-resolution MRI (22). A recent review of patients treated surgically at the Cleveland Clinic between 1991 and 2001 noted normal results on visual analysis of high-resolution MRI studies in approximately 20% of patients with pathologically confirmed MCD (P. Widdess-Walsh and I. Najm, unpublished data, 2002).

MRI-based three-dimensional volume reconstructions have been used in an attempt to uncover sulcal or gyral abnormalities that may have gone undetected on visual analyses of the two-dimensional images (23–27). The utility of these postprocessing techniques has yet to be validated

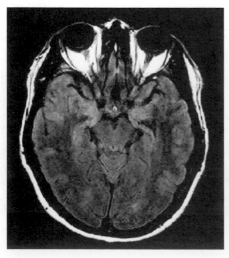

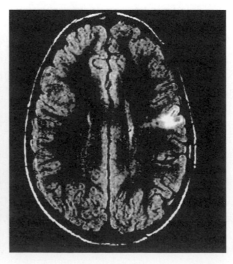

Figure 80.2 Magnetic resonance image. Characteristics of malformation of cortical development identified on axial fluid-attenuated inversion recovery images. **A:** "Mild" blurring of the gray-white matter junction and increased signal in the right temporal pole. **B:** "Severe" and characteristic abnormalities of some types of malformations caused by abnormal cortical development. Note the significant signal increase in the left perirolandic area and a track pointing toward the ventricular surface.

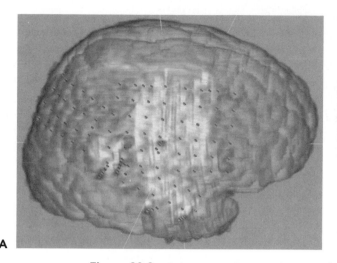
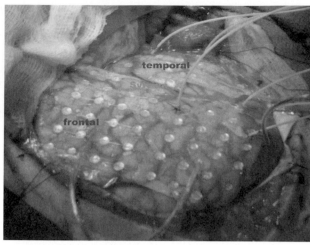

Figure 80.3   A: Intraoperative coregistration of subdural grids and depth electrodes on magnetic resonance imaging-based three-dimensional reconstruction of the brain. **B:** Corresponding intraoperative view of subdural grids and depths electrodes in their final position in the same patient. Frontal and temporal lobes and sylvian fissures are indicated. Please see color insert.

through careful outcome analyses and direct ECoG and histopathologic correlations. Novel magnetic resonance sequences such as diffusion tensor imaging (28) and magnetization transfer neuroimaging (29) may demonstrate abnormalities not visualized on conventional MRI, but as yet clinical experience with these methods is limited.

A sizable number of patients with MCD do not achieve a good outcome even after "complete" resection of the lesion. Of the adult patients operated on at the Cleveland Clinic between 1991 and 2001, 57% were seizure free at least 6 months after surgical resection (compared with 78% who underwent surgery for drug-resistant temporal lobe epilepsy caused by hippocampal sclerosis) (P. Widdess-Walsh and I. Najm, unpublished data, 2002). These results suggest that current imaging (and evaluation) techniques do not accurately map the extent of dysplastic and epileptogenic regions in MCD. In other words, the topographic and functional relationships between MRI-revealed focal MCD and the epileptogenic zone are far from clear and unequivocal: neither all focal MCD nor all components of a focal MCD are necessarily epileptogenic. For these reasons, additional techniques that directly record *in situ* epileptogenicity from the cortex and map the exact extent of the abnormalities, such as the placement of subdural grids or depth electrodes and prolonged extraoperative recordings, may be needed.

Subdural Electrodes (Strips and Grids)

Subdural electrodes (stainless steel or magnetic resonance-compatible platinum) electrodes, embedded in strips or sheets of polyurethane or other synthetic material, are implanted over the suspected epileptogenic or functional dysplastic regions (30–35). Subdural grids are inserted through either open craniotomy incisions or burrholes and registered stereotactically for extraoperative mapping (Fig.

80.3). The cortical covering may extend beyond the visualized cortical area, as grids may be slid over the edges of the craniotomy to cover adjacent areas for better ECoG or functional sampling. Besides the ECoG recordings and direct electrical stimulation studies, grids can be used to record somatosensory evoked potentials after stimulation of the trigeminal (lip) or median nerves for central sulcus localization.

Chronic extraoperative subdural techniques can record cortical ictal events and determine the functionality of the underlying cortex. Additionally, these recordings are performed on a relaxed, cooperative patient in the controlled environment of the epilepsy monitoring unit without the time constraints of the operating room.

Because foreign bodies are inserted into the cranial vault, the risks of the procedure include wound infection, flap osteomyelitis, acute meningitis, cerebral edema, and hemorrhage (36,37). Concerns about increased intracranial pressure may reduce the maximal number of electrodes that can be inserted and therefore produce incomplete epileptic mapping from large cortical areas. Other limitations may include the anatomic location of the proposed area of sampling (e.g., mesial orbitofrontal) and "re-do" surgeries with cortical adhesions. Where surgical access is difficult, as in the mesial surface of the hemispheres or in deep regions of the brain, SEEG, alone or combined with subdural grids, allows adequate coverage and precise targeting of the desired areas.

Implantation of Invasive Electrodes

When noninvasive studies produce nonconcordant or inconclusive information on the localization and extent of the seizure onset zone or the eloquent cortex, invasive studies involving subdural grids or depth electrodes may be needed (9,38,39). Jayakar (38) proposed the following relative indications for the use of subdural grids: normal results on structural imaging, extratemporal location, divergent noninvasive data, encroachment on eloquent cortex, tuberous sclerosis, and cortical dysplasia. Rosenow and Lüders (10) recommended subdural electrodes for patients with focal epilepsy (single focus) only when there is a reasonable hypothesis on the location of the epileptogenic zone (derived from noninvasive studies).

In patients with focal MCD, invasive electrode recordings are used to define the epileptogenic region and map eloquent areas.

Definition of the Epileptogenic Zone

In most cases of focal MCD, data generated from noninvasive EEG recordings and other electrophysiologic/neuroimaging techniques are sufficient to approximate the location of the epileptogenic zone.

Studies using direct ECoG recordings show that focal MCD lesions are intrinsically epileptogenic (17,19,40,41). Nevertheless, invasive monitoring to define the location and extent of epileptogenicity in focal MCD is warranted, because the epileptogenic area in these patients is frequently larger than the visually identified MCD (Fig. 80.4) (21,42–45). Moreover, in MCD lesions with a significant increase in FLAIR signal (balloon cell-containing dysplastic lesions), epileptogenicity arises mainly from the surrounding dysplastic cortex that is devoid of balloon cells (24,46).

Localization of Eloquent Cortical Regions

Because most MCD lesions are often localized in the frontal lobe (therefore in potentially eloquent cortex), an understanding of the functional status of the involved region(s) and its anatomic and pathologic correlates is important. We recently assessed the functional status (identified by direct cortical electrical stimulation) of focal MCD and its

relationship with imaging and *in situ* ECoG characteristics in patients who underwent focal neocortical resection for medically intractable epilepsy (46). Some focal MCD lesions characterized by significant FLAIR signal increase on MRI and located in anatomically functional areas (e.g., primary motor, Broca area) are not functional on direct electrical stimulation, and the same lesions showed no evidence of intrinsic epileptogenicity as assessed through mapping of the ictal onset zones. On the other hand, MCD lesions with mild or no FLAIR signal increase were functional and at times epileptogenic. These results agree with previous observations that eloquent function persisted in MCD devoid of balloon cells (47,48). Similar ECoG patterns were reported in patients with low-grade glial tumors (e.g., dysembryoplastic neuroepithelial tumor and ganglioglioma), whereas dysplastic and epileptic cortical areas were found immediately surrounding these lesions (49–51). Functional cortex may therefore be displaced within the same hemisphere and have direct implications on the options for epilepsy surgery.

Proposed Indications for Use of Subdural Grids

Because the limited success of surgical resection in patients with MCD likely reflects the lack of an accurate definition of the epileptogenic lesion's "true margins," direct ECoG recordings with subdural grids are needed.

Subdural electrodes should be used to evaluate patients with suspected focal MCD after the diagnosis of focal epilepsy is confirmed through careful analysis of the seizure semiology, noninvasive scalp electroencephalogram recordings, and other anatomic and functional neuroimaging studies. The goals (mapping of epileptogenicity and function) and limitations and risks should be clearly understood.

Electroencephalography-triggered fMRI and the awaited development of microimaging techniques to map molecular

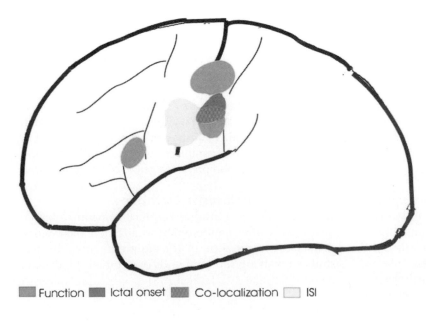

■ Function ■ Ictal onset ▨ Co-localization ☐ ISI

Figure 80.4 Illustration showing a case of malformations caused by abnormal cortical development with significant signal fluid attenuated inversion recovery increase (*yellow*). Note the lack of overlap of the epileptic area (*red*) and the lesion (*yellow*). Please see color insert.

markers of epileptogenicity will obviate the need for invasive recordings.

SURGICAL STRATEGY

Resection (or at least disconnection) of focal MCD remains the treatment of choice for patients with pharmacoresistent focal epilepsy. Several investigators have claimed that complete resection of the lesion evident on MRI is the most important factor in seizure control (18,25) and emphasize that because the epileptogenic region frequently exceeds the boundaries of the obvious dysplastic cortex, lesionectomy alone may be insufficient. The age of the patient, severity of epilepsy, preoperative deficit, and goals of surgery warrant an individualized approach.

Once the epileptogenic zone has been defined, the functional status of the cortex in and around the MCD must be determined (52–55) with either invasive electroencephalograph evaluation or awake craniotomy, chosen when the MCD involves eloquent cortex. Extraoperative mapping with subdural grids or depth electrodes identifies functional cortex and epileptogenic tissue and allows histologic analysis of cortex surrounding electroencephalograph-identified abnormal sites. Seizures are recorded to provide ictal onset information.

Intraoperative frameless stereotactic MRI localization coregistered with PET, ictal SPECT, three-dimensional MRI, and fMRI aid in identification of lesion boundaries, metabolic boundaries, and surrounding cortical anatomy. This information can be analyzed on neuronavigational stereotactic displays. ECoG, identification of the central sulcus by somatosensory evoked potential, and direct electrical cortical stimulation require a neurologist and a neurophysiology team experienced in intraoperative mapping techniques.

Resection of dysplastic cortex and surrounding electrically abnormal cortex involves correlation with findings from preoperative imaging, intraoperative electrical recordings, and tactile surgical feedback. Dysplastic cortex is firm or "rubbery" and may have a distinct color. It often extends deeper than normal cortex to the underlying periventricular zone. Generous margins of resection are advocated whenever possible; eloquent locations dictate a more restricted approach and may be one reason for unsatisfactory outcomes.

SURGICAL OUTCOME

The efficacy of surgery for the management of MCD remains unknown. Several series in the literature (Table 80.1) generally report a less-favorable response compared

TABLE 80.1

OUTCOME IN SURGICAL TREATMENT OF MALFORMATIONS OF CORTICAL DEVELOPMENT (SELECTED SERIES)

Study	No. of Patients	Outcome	Follow-up (years)	Pathologic Lesion
Taylor et al. (45)	10	70% seizure free or >90% reduction	5.5	Focal cortical dysplasia (8), vascular malformation (1), inconclusive (1)
Palmini et al. (18)	26	42% "excellent or good"	5.0	Focal cortical dysplasia (12), tuberous sclerosis (8), inconclusive (4)
Hirabayashi et al. (40)	17	35% seizure free or greatly reduced	5.0	Not available
Otsubo et al. (56)	9	33% seizure free	2	Focal cortical dysplasia (8)
Chugani et al. (57)	23	78% seizure free or >90% reduction	1.3	Focal cortical dysplasia (18), gliotic cysts (4), normal (1)
Wyllie et al. (58)	30	62% seizure free, 17% with >90% reduction	2.25	Focal cortical dysplasia (30)
Palmini et al. (55)	32	55% seizure free or >90% reduction	At least 1	Grade III dysplasia[a] (64%)
Raymond et al. (21)	35	60% seizure free or >90% reduction	3	Dysembryoplastic neuroepithelial tumor (60%)
Kuzniecky et al. (47)	11	78% seizure free or >90% reduction	16–48 months	Focal cortical dysplasia (11)
Lo Russo et al. (59)	126	69% seizure free	At least 1	Focal cortical dysplasia (81)

[a]Based on grading scheme of Palmini and colleagues (55).

with hippocampal sclerosis and epileptic low-grade tumors (18,21,40,45,47,55–59).

The 20-year series of Taylor and colleagues (45) involved 10 patients with pathologically identified focal MCD, none of whom underwent preoperative computed tomography (CT) scans. Seven patients (70%) were seizure free or dramatically improved after surgery, with a mean follow-up of 5.5 years. One patient had an arteriovenous malformation; in another, pathologic examination yielded inconclusive results. If these patients are excluded, a seizure-free outcome occurred in 6 of 8 patients (75%). This result may be explained in part by the predominance of temporal lobe involvement, which may allow for a more complete resection.

Twenty years later, Palmini and associates (18) described 26 patients with "focal neuronal migration disorders," diagnosed by pathologic analysis and imaging results, who were treated surgically from 1975 to 1989. Twenty-four patients had an adequate follow-up (mean, 5 years). Only 12 patients had focal MCD; the remainder had tuberous sclerosis or inconclusive diagnosis. Overall, 42% had an excellent or good outcome; two patients were seizure free. Complete resection of the lesion defined by preoperative MRI or intraoperative visualization was possible in only four patients. Resection of the epileptogenic zone demonstrated by scalp or invasive electroencephalography did not correlate with surgical outcome. The authors identified the extent of resection as the most important prognostic indicator.

Hirabayashi and coworkers (40) reported on 17 patients with MCD treated surgically between 1980 and 1990. Scalp EEG and ECoG did not correlate positively with outcome. Six patients were seizure free or almost so (35%), and three were improved (18%). Pathologic details were reported in five patients; three with extensive lesions had poor outcomes, and two with focal lesions had good outcomes. Correlation of resection with outcome was not performed. The authors concluded that a temporal lobe location and the presence of focal lesions were correlated with better outcome after resective surgery.

The nine children with MCD reported by Otsubo and colleagues (56) were treated surgically between 1987 and 1991. MRI showed abnormalities in eight patients; seven (78%) had a multilobar focus on the scalp interictal electroencephalogram; in six patients (77%), ictal electroencephalography was nonlocalizable. The entire cohort had "characteristic spike activity" on intraoperative ECoG; however, seven children demonstrated multilobar or widespread electrical activity. Three patients underwent temporal lobectomy; four, multilobar resections; one patient had a frontal resection; and one, an occipital lobectomy. Three patients (33%) were seizure free; the remaining six patients (66%) had more than a 50% reduction in seizure frequency at a mean follow-up of 24 months. No conclusions were drawn regarding the extent of resection of the anatomic or epileptogenic lesion and outcome.

Chugani and associates (57) reported on 23 children with infantile spasms, evaluated with MRI and PET studies, who had surgery between 1987 and 1992 (15 resections, 8 hemispherectomies). CT or MRI studies were abnormal in nine patients (39%), whereas the entire study population showed abnormalities on PET. Scalp and intraoperative electroencephalography correlated well with PET localization; both were used to guide surgical resection. Excluding the patients who underwent hemispherectomy (8) and the two patients with normal findings and a gliotic cyst, a seizure-free outcome of 62% was achieved. The authors concluded that PET is an effective method for localizing epileptogenic zones that correlate with cortical malformations on pathologic analysis. Bilateral PET changes correlated with poor postoperative outcome.

From 1980 through 1992, 30 patients, described by Wyllie and associates (58), underwent surgery for pathologically verified MCD. Seventeen extratemporal and 13 temporal sites were identified through imaging, electroencephalography, and surgical inspection. Of the patients with extratemporal sites, seven of 16 had positive MRI findings, and all 7 had positive PET results. Surgery consisted of a frontal or parietal resection (11 patients), a multilobar resection (2 patients), and 4 hemispherectomies. Preoperatively, 10 patients had chronic subdural electrode recordings. After an average 27-month follow-up, 53% were seizure free, and 29% had more than a 90% reduction in seizure frequency. Thirteen patients had temporal lobe epilepsy. Normal MRI findings preoperatively raised no suspicion of dysplasia, which was found, without hippocampal sclerosis, in all patients on pathologic examination. Seventy-seven percent of patients were seizure free after 25 months of follow-up. The authors proposed a better outcome for MCD involving the temporal lobe, noting, however, dramatic improvement in the extratemporal group.

In 1994 and 1995, Palmini and associates (18,55) updated their series of 34 patients with focal dysplastic lesions. Sixty-seven percent demonstrated a repetitive ictal spiking pattern from restricted areas of the cortex. When this pattern was seen during ECoG, the region correlated with the lesion in 82% of patients. Interictal activity continued to be more widespread than the lesion itself. Three fourths of patients whose epileptic areas were excised had a good outcome. In contrast, when the areas that exhibited rhythmic activity remained in place, outcome was universally poor. Complete or major removal of the anatomic lesion together with the continuous ictal activity (when present) during ECoG, the author surmised, is necessary for good outcomes.

Of the 100 patients with MCD and epilepsy reported by Raymond and coworkers in 1994 (21), 35 underwent surgery. Only five patients had focal dysplastic lesions, and of these, one patient is seizure free, and another achieved a reduction in seizures exceeding 90%. (Twenty-two patients were found to have a dysembryoplastic neuroepithelial tumor.)

Kuzniecky and colleagues (47) reported their experience with 11 patients with frontocentral malformation, nine of whom underwent surgical resection. Subdural grid evaluation preoperatively in six patients helped to regionalize but not localize the ictal onset zone. MRI identified the lesion in 10 of 11 patients; in the sole exception, the lesion was demonstrated by an ictal SPECT study. In the frontal lobe group of five patients, four underwent resection, and only one was seizure free, although all had significant reductions. In the central lobe group (six patients), surgery in five produced three improvements and two failures.

In the 2003 series of 126 patients reported by Lo Russo and associates (59), 81 had a diagnosis of focal MCD. Seventy-five patients (59.5%) underwent stereoelectroencephalography to define eloquent or epileptogenic areas. After at least 1 year of follow-up, 49% were seizure free.

On the basis of these reports, results of surgery for MCD are disappointing, compared with results for other lesional epilepsies; however, several points about the literature are worth mentioning. Most of these studies are retrospective, involving patients from the past five decades and not adequately representing the advances in imaging and surgical techniques realized in the past 5 years alone. Many MCD lesions were discovered incidentally on pathologic examination and were not the "target" of the surgery. The series also included a large variety of MCD lesions with different characteristics, sizes, locations, and treatments. Details of surgical techniques and complications are mostly lacking. Finally, surgical selection bias and relatively short follow-up may not reflect the true natural history. Taken together, these factors make it difficult to draw definite conclusions about the efficacy of surgery.

Despite these limitations, however, the literature supports the role of surgery in managing focal MCD associated with intractable epilepsy. Removal of the anatomic lesion, though important, may not be sufficient for seizure-free outcome (19,55,58,59). In addition, certain electrographic features are highly distinctive for MCD and should be resected. Lesions within eloquent brain can be approached aggressively with functional mapping techniques. Importantly, the entire MRI-defined lesion cannot be considered epileptogenic, and partial resections, especially when eloquent cortex overlaps with focal MCD, may lead to seizure-free outcome. When these strategies define the surgical plan, success may approach that of other lesional epilepsies.

To evaluate current treatment, we reviewed the Cleveland Clinic experience since 1997. A single-surgeon series (by W.E.B.) of 330 craniotomies performed for medical intractable epilepsy between 1997 and 2000 identified 105 pathologically verified cases of MCD. In 26 patients, MCD was the primary target of the surgery (anatomic substrate of the epilepsy). The remaining cases were associated with neoplasm and hemispheric dysplasia or were incidental. Of the 26 patients with focal MCD,

77% were resected completely, guided by stereotactic imaging or invasive monitoring, or both. Complete resection of the MCD led to cessation of seizure activity in all these patients at a mean follow-up of 3.4 years (personal observations).

CONCLUSIONS

Focal MCD constitute a large group of histopathologic cortical malformations with distinct architectural/cellular abnormalities, variable, MRI characteristics, and differing degrees of *in situ* epileptogenicity and functional representation.

Surgery is the treatment of choice for selected patients. The extent of the structural lesion and its correlation with the epileptogenic area must be determined to achieve a good outcome; however, presurgical management is complicated by the lack of a noninvasive technique that can accomplish all of these goals. The best surgical approach, we believe, is the complete resection of the MRI-defined lesion and the epileptogenic zone when they are concordant and do not involve eloquent cortex.

ACKNOWLEDGMENT

This work was supported by grants K08 NS02046 and R21 NS42354 from the National Institute of Neurological Disorders and Stroke (NINDS) to Imad M. Najm.

REFERENCES

1. Bartolomei F, Gavaret M, Dravet C, et al. Late onset epilepsy associated with regional brain cortical dysplasia. *Eur Neurol* 1999; 42:11–16.
2. Li L, Fish D, Sisodiya S, et al. High resolution magnetic resonance imaging in adults with partial or secondary generalised epilepsy attending a tertiary referral unit. *J Neurol Neurosurg Psychiatry* 1995;59:384–387.
3. Kuzniecky R, Murro A, King D, et al. Magnetic resonance imaging in childhood intractable partial epilepsies: pathologic correlations. *Neurology* 1993;43:681–687.
4. Wyllie E, Comair YG, Kotagal P, et al. Seizure outcome after epilepsy surgery in children and adolescents. *Ann Neurology* 1998;44: 740–748.
5. Ruggieri P. MRI techniques for the identification of neuronal migration disorders: practical considerations. In: Kotagal P, ed. *The epilepsies: etiologies and prevention.* New York: Academic Press, 1999:45–59.
6. Shorvon S. MRI of cortical dysplasias. *Epilepsia* 1997;38(Suppl 10):13–18.
7. Sisodiya S, Free S, Stevens J, et al. Widespread cerebral structural changes in patients with cortical dysgenesis and epilepsy. *Brain* 1995;118:1039–1050.
8. Engel JJ. Surgery for seizures. *N Engl J Med* 1996;334:647–652.
9. Lüders H, Engel JJ, Munari C. Noninvasive preoperative evaluation: general principles. In: Engel J, ed. *Surgical treatment of the epilepsies.* New York: Raven Press, 1993:137–155.
10. Rosenow F, Luders H. Presurgical evaluation of epilepsy. *Brain* 2001;124:1683–1700.
11. Ebersole J. EEG and MEG dipole source modeling. In: Engel J, Pedley T, eds. *Epilepsy: a comprehensive textbook.* Philadelphia: Lippincott-Raven, 1998:919–939.
12. Benbadis S. Invasive EEG. In: Lüders H, ed. *The epileptic seizure: pathophysiology and semiology.* New York: WB Saunders, 2000:49–53.

13. Risinger M. Invasive EEG. In: Lüders H, ed. *The epileptic seizure: pathophysiology and semiology.* New York: WB Saunders, 2000:32–48.
14. Risinger M, Gumnit R. Intracranial electrophysiologic studies. *Neuroimag Clin North Am* 1995;5:559–573.
15. Aicardi J. The place of neuronal migration abnormalities in child neurology. *Can J Neurol Sci* 1994;21:185–193.
16. Raymond A, Fish D, Boyd S, et al. Cortical dysgenesis: serial EEG findings in children and adults. *Electroencephalogr Clin Neurophysiol* 1995;94:389–397.
17. Palmini A, Andermann F, Olivier A, et al. Focal neuronal migration disorders and intractable partial epilepsy: a study of 30 patients. *Ann Neurol* 1991;30:741–749.
18. Palmini A, Andermann F, Olivier A, et al. Focal neuronal migration disorders and intractable partial epilepsy: results of surgical treatment. *Ann Neurol* 1991;30:750–757.
19. Palmini A, Gambardella A, Andermann F, et al. Intrinsic epileptogenicity of human dysplastic cortex as suggested by corticography and surgical results. *Ann Neurol* 1995;37:476–487.
20. Berg M, Ketonen L, Erbe G, et al. Anterior temporal lobe gray white matter differentiation correlates with side of seizure onset in temporal lobe epilepsy. *Neurology* 1993;43:364.
21. Raymond A, Fish D, Sisodiya S, et al. Abnormalities of gyration, heterotopias, tuberous sclerosis, focal cortical dysplasia, microdysgenesis, dysembryoplastic neuroepithelial tumour and dysgenesis of the archicortex in epilepsy. Clinical, EEG and neuroimaging features in 100 adult patients. *Brain* 1995;118(Pt 3): 629–660.
22. Kuzniecky R, Garcia J, Faught E, et al. Cortical dysplasia in temporal lobe epilepsy: magnetic resonance imaging correlations. *Ann Neurol* 1991;29:293–298.
23. Lapresto E, Mohamed A, Najm I, et al. The clinical utility of 3D reconstructed MRI in patients with cortical dysplasia. *Epilepsia* 1999;40(Suppl 7):191.
24. Rona S, Najm I, Ying Z, et al. MRI correlates of focal cortical dysplasia: a study with multimodal image analyses. *Epilepsia* 2000; 41(Suppl 7):63.
25. Sisodiya S, Free S. Disproportion of cerebral surface areas and volumes in cerebral dysgenesis. MRI-based evidence for connectional abnormalities. *Brain* 1997;120:271–281.
26. Sisodiya S, Stevens J, Fish D, et al. The demonstration of gyral abnormalities in patients with cryptogenic partial epilepsy using three-dimensional MRI. *Arch Neurol* 1996;53:28–34.
27. Winkler P, Vollmar C, Krishnan K, et al. Usefulness of 3-D reconstructed images of the human cerebral cortex for localization of subdural electrodes in epilepsy surgery. *Epilepsy Res* 2000;41:169–178.
28. Eriksson SH, Symms MR, Rugg-Gunn FJ, et al. Diffusion tension imaging in patients with epilepsy and malformations of cortical development. *Brain* 2001;124:617–626.
29. Rugg-Gunn F, Eriksson SH, Boulby PA, et al. Magnetization transfer imaging in focal epilepsy. *Neurology* 2003;60:1638–1645.
30. Lesser R, Gordon B, Fisher E, et al. Subdural grid electrodes in surgery for epilepsy. In: Lüders H, ed. *Epilepsy surgery.* New York: Raven Press, 1991:399–408.
31. Lüders H, Lesser R, Dinner D. Chronic intracranial recording and stimulation with subdural electrodes. In: Engel JJ, ed. *Surgical treatment of the epilepsies.* New York: Raven Press, 1987:297–321.
32. Wyler A. Subdural strip electrodes in surgery of epilepsy. In: Lüders H, ed. *Epilepsy surgery.* New York: Raven Press, 1991:395–398.
33. Wyler A, Wilkus R, Blume W. Strip electrodes. In: Engel JJ, ed. *Surgical treatment of the epilepsies.* New York: Raven Press, 1993:387–398.
34. Wyllie E, Lüders H, Morris H, et al. Clinical outcome after complete or partial cortical resection for intractable epilepsy. *Neurology* 1987;37:1634–1641.
35. Wyllie E, Lüders H, Morris H, et al. Subdural electrodes in the evaluation for epilepsy surgery in children and adults. *Neuropediatrics* 1988;19:80–86.
36. Benbadis S, Wyllie E, Bingaman W. Intracranial electroencephalography and localization studies. In: Wyllie E, ed. *The treatment of epilepsy: principles and practice.* Philadelphia: Lippincott Williams & Wilkins, 2000:1067–1075.
37. Lee W, Lee J, Lee S, et al. Complications and results of subdural grid electrode implantation in epilepsy surgery. *Surg Neurol* 2000;54:346–351.
38. Jayakar P. Invasive EEG monitoring in children: when, where and what? *J Clin Neurophysiol* 1999;16:408–418.
39. Lüders H, Lesser R, Dinner D, et al. Commentary: chronic intracranial recording and stimulation with subdural electrodes. In: Engel JJ, ed. *Surgical treatment of the epilepsies.* New York: Raven Press, 1987:297–321.
40. Hirabayashi S, Binnie C, Janota I, et al. Surgical treatment of epilepsy due to cortical dysplasia: clinical and EEG findings. *J Neurol Neurosurg Psychiatry* 1993;56:765–770.
41. Najm I, Ying Z, Babb T, et al. NMDA receptor 2A/B subtype differential expression in human cortical dysplasia: correlation with in situ epileptogenicity. *Epilepsia* 2000;41:971–976.
42. Awad I, Assirati J, Burgess R, et al. A new class of electrodes of "intermediate invasiveness:" preliminary experience with epidural pegs and foramen ovale electrodes in the mapping of seizure foci. *Neurol Res* 1991;13:177–183.
43. Raymond A, Fish D. EEG features of focal malformations of cortical development. *J Clin Neurophysiol* 1996;13:495–506.
44. Richardson M, Koepp M, Brooks D, et al. Benzodiazepine receptors in focal epilepsy with cortical dysgenesis: an ^{11}C-flumazenil PET study. *Ann Neurol* 1996;40:188–198.
45. Taylor DFM, Bruton C, Corsellis J. Focal dysplasia of the cerebral cortex in epilepsy. *J Neurol Neurosurg Psychiatry* 1971;34:369–387.
46. Marusic P, Najm I, Ying Z, et al. Focal cortical dysplasias in eloquent cortex: functional characteristics and correlation with MRI and histopathological changes. *Epilepsia* 2002;43:27–32.
47. Kuzniecky R, Morawetz R, Faught E, et al. Frontal and central lobe focal dysplasia: clinical, EEG and imaging features. *Dev Med Child Neurol* 1995;37:159–166.
48. Preul MC, Leblanc R, Cendes F, et al. Function and organization in dysgenic cortex. Case report. *J Neurosurg* 1997;87:113–121.
49. Diehl B, Najm I, Ruggieri P, et al. Postictal diffusion weighted imaging in a case with lesional epilepsy. *Epilepsia* 1999;40:1667–1671.
50. Prayson RA, Estes ML, Morris HH. Coexistence of neoplasia and cortical dysplasia in patients presenting with seizures. *Epilepsia* 1993;34:609–615.
51. Wolf HK, Müller MB, Spanle M, et al. Ganglioglioma: a detailed histopathological and immunocytochemical analysis of 61 cases. *Acta Neuropathol* 1994;88:166–173.
52. Gambardella A, Palmini A, Andermann F, et al. Usefulness of focal rhythmic discharges on scalp EEG of patients with focal cortical dysplasia and intractable epilepsy. *Electroencephalogr Clin Neurophysiol* 1996;98:243–249.
53. Kuzniecky R, Mountz J, Wheatley G, et al. Ictal single photon emission computed tomography demonstrated localized epileptogenesis in cortical dysplasia. *Ann Neurol* 1993;34:627–631.
54. Lee N, Radke R, Gray L, et al. Neuronal migration disorders: positron emission tomography correlations. *Ann Neurol* 1994;35:290–297.
55. Palmini A, Gambardella A, Andermann F, et al. Operative strategies for patients with cortical dysplastic lesions and intractable epilepsy. *Epilepsia* 1994;35:S57–S71.
56. Otsubo H, Hwang PA, Jay V, et al. Focal cortical dysplasia in children with localization-related epilepsy: EEG, MRI, and SPECT findings. *Pediatr Neurol* 1993;9:101–107.
57. Chugani HT, Shewmon A, Shields D, et al. Surgery for intractable infantile spasms: neuroimaging perspectives. *Epilepsia* 1993;34: 764–771.
58. Wyllie E, Baumgartner C, Prayson R, et al. The clinical spectrum of focal cortical dysplasia and epilepsy. *J Epilepsy* 1994;7:303–312.
59. Lo Russo G, Tassi L, Cossu M, et al. Focal cortical resection in malformations of cortical development. *Epileptic Disord* 2003;5 (Suppl 2):S115–S123.

Hemispherectomy: Medications, Technical Approaches, and Results

José Luis Montes   *Jean-Pierre Farmer*   *Frederick Andermann*   *Chantal Poulin*

HISTORICAL AND BACKGROUND CONSIDERATIONS

Walter Dandy first described hemispherectomy as a surgical technique in 1928 for the management of glioblastoma (1). Ten years later, MacKenzie reported its use in a patient with epilepsy. It was not until 1950 (2,3), when Krynauw recounted the performance of hemispherectomy in patients with infantile hemiplegia, intractable seizures, and behavioral disorder, that the technique gained acceptance in the management of severely handicapped patients. Optimal results, wrote Krynauw, depended on proper case selection. A number of his criteria have withstood the test of time: good basic personality, parental collaboration, and predominantly unilateral cerebral involvement.

In 1966, Oppenheimer and Griffith (4) described a delayed complication, usually appearing after a trouble-free period lasting an average of 8 years. A suspected sequel of episodes of repeated minute intracranial bleeding over years resulted in obstructive hydrocephalus. Postmortem findings were consistent with what Noetzel had called superficial hemosiderosis of the central nervous system (5,6).

To prevent this complication, subtotal hemispherectomy or multilobar excision (1,7,8) was devised, in which the major epileptogenic area was resected and some parts of the abnormal hemisphere were left in place. These procedures were adequate to prevent the long-term complications; however, the results for seizure control were clearly less effective than those of anatomic hemispherectomy. In the mid-1970s, modifications to anatomic hemispherectomy were introduced to prevent delayed complications and improve seizure

control. Rasmussen (9) devised the anatomically subtotal, but functionally complete, hemispherectomy. The Oxford variant (10) recommended completing the anatomic hemispherectomy and then tacking the dura to the falx and tentorium to collapse the subdural space at the expense of the epidural space. Hemidecortication and hemicorticectomy (11) have also been used. The hemispherotomy technique of Delalande, the peri-insular hemispherotomy of Villemure (12), and the transsylvian functional hemispherectomy of Schramm (12) represent attempts to perform a complete disconnection with minimal removal of brain.

IMPACT OF SEVERE EPILEPSY IN CHILDHOOD

The past two decades have witnessed an increased awareness of the nature of childhood epilepsy, especially the deleterious effects of seizures and of long-term anticonvulsant therapy on intellectual and behavioral development. These factors, combined with an improved understanding of the maturation and plasticity of the growing brain, have led to a shift in emphasis and to a trend for earlier surgical treatment of intractable epilepsy, particularly the use of hemispherectomy (13–16).

The extensive dendritic arborization, providing the primary postsynaptic receptors for axonal connections and synapse formation, and the evolution of myelination that occurs in the first few years of life have an enormous impact on the acquisition of both intellectual and social skills. This period of optimal brain plasticity allows the best functional recovery of any deficit the epilepsy, or the surgery, may cause in specific functions. Experimental work in animals has shown that functional recovery after hemispherectomy is nearly complete when it is done in young animals compared to adults. Extensive reorganization of cortical and subcortical projection fibers has been observed, as well as return of almost normal metabolic rates in basal nuclei after surgery, all suggesting valuable recovery (17–23).

Increasingly, the impact of ictal and interictal epileptic discharges on the functioning of the maturing brain has been a source of concern. Normal synaptogenesis depends on normal surrounding electrical fields, appropriate environmental stimuli, and physiologic stability (24). The ictal and interictal discharges alter the homeostatic electric fields and the release of neurotransmitters, as well as synaptic maturation and transmission. The deleterious effect of hypoxia also contributes to interference with normal brain maturation and development.

DIAGNOSTIC EVALUATIONS

History and Neurologic Findings

The history and clinical findings in candidates for hemispherectomy (1,7,8,25–29) usually reveal a severe hemispheric encephalopathy. Common etiologies include malformations of cortical development involving multiple lobes or the entire hemisphere with hemimegalencephaly or without hemispheric enlargement, ischemic stroke, and predominantly unilateral perinatal ischemic injury mimicking periventricular leukomalacia. Less common are Sturge-Weber and Rasmussen syndromes. Patients may have a facial port-wine stain as in Sturge-Weber syndrome. Patients with hemimegalencephaly may show ipsilateral somatic overgrowth or the cutaneous findings of epidermal nevus syndrome or hypomelanosis of Ito. They usually have hemiparesis associated with a hemisensory deficit that is often difficult to assess in small children. Most patients have a homonymous hemianopsia or, in the case of progressive syndromes, will acquire one. In many patients with congenital hemiplegia, body asymmetry will be obvious, at times complicated by sympathetic dysfunction on the affected side.

The type and frequency of seizures in these patients are variable, but the onset usually dates from early infancy, often from the first few days of life. Most of these patients have different types of seizures, such as partial motor, absences, or complex partial attacks. A number of patients, particularly infants, have seizures that by definition are nonlocalizing, such as generalized tonic and atonic seizures, myoclonic seizures, or infantile spasms. The clinical detection of the focal origin and onset of seizures continues to be a challenge in infants. Clinical semiology generally does not help localize or lateralize seizure onset in children younger than 2 years (28).

As in all surgical candidates, a careful evaluation to establish seizure intractability should be undertaken. This is usually not a problem, given the often catastrophic presentation in most of these children (28,30). A careful review of pharmacologic management with optimal doses of anticonvulsant medication (1), both as monotherapy and in combination therapy, should be carried out. If previous pharmacologic management has been less than ideal, additional drug trials should be undertaken. However, surgery should not be delayed in a child with daily or frequent prolonged seizures with a low likelihood of response, as in hemimegalencephaly or other malformations of cortical development.

No surgical procedure arouses as much initial disbelief as hemispherectomy. Repeated discussions with the family are essential and should include interpretations of the operative procedure. The possibility of surgical treatment should be broached early, with emphasis on the extent of the procedure and its potential results. The risks of operative complications, as well as the possibility of aggravating incomplete deficits, such as a mild hemiparesis or an incomplete hemianopsia, should be mentioned. On the other hand, the high chance of seizure freedom after surgery compared with nonsurgical options, as well as potential postsurgical benefits in behavior and development should be explored.

Structural Imaging

Optimal visualization of both hemispheres is mandatory with high-resolution magnetic resonance imaging (MRI), which has helped define many associated structural anomalies, such as gliotic changes with encephaloclastic porencephalies or Rasmussen encephalitis (31), progressive atrophic changes with Sturge-Weber syndrome or Rasmussen encephalitis, and changes seen in migrational hemispheric syndromes, such as increased gray-matter thickness, poor gray-white differentiation, abnormal gyral and sulcal patterns, and the abnormal clefts characteristic of widespread cortical dysplasia and hemimegalencephaly (32). MRI with gadolinium enhancement can define pial angiomatosis. Venous magnetic resonance angiography can identify the vascular changes associated with venous drainage in patients with Sturge-Weber syndrome, cortical dysplasia, or hemimegalencephaly, precluding the need for an arteriogram. Computed tomography (CT) scans often show large porencephalic lesions, particularly if calcifications are present, and atrophic changes.

Functional Imaging

Indirect measurement of cerebral blood flow by single-photon-emission computed tomography (SPECT) has become an important tool in the evaluation of children with epilepsy (33). In patients with active epileptogenic abnormalities, such as those with epilepsia partialis continua, the areas of highest perfusion may help define the most epileptogenic tissue. In one study (34), interictal hypoperfusion was superior to MRI with gadolinium in establishing the extent of brain damage from pial angiomatosis in Sturge-Weber syndrome. Hypoperfusion of the contralateral cerebellar hemisphere, reflecting corticopontocerebellar pathways, may be another helpful lateralizing sign. Unilateral hypoperfusion in brain SPECT correlated with good results in patients whose electroencephalographic (EEG) findings point to involvement of the contralateral hemisphere (34). Return of regional cerebral blood flow to normal in the nonaffected hemisphere may indicate more normal functioning and maturation after seizures are controlled (35).

Positron emission tomography (PET) provides an indication of the metabolic state of the hemisphere (36). Hypometabolism in the abnormal hemisphere is a helpful lateralizing sign. In children with Sturge-Weber syndrome (37), PET frequently shows a markedly depressed metabolic rate in the affected hemisphere, extending beyond the abnormalities seen on brain MRI or CT. Cortical hypometabolism in the opposite hemisphere in patients with hemimegalencephaly has indicated bilateral abnormalities with a higher chance of partial or no seizure control after surgery. Ipsilateral hypometabolic changes or ipsilateral areas of hypermetabolism surrounded by hypometabolic changes, usually related to intense epileptic activity, have been found in children with lateralized scalp EEG but normal MRI results (38,39); this may aid in deciding whether to perform hemispherectomy, hemispherotomy, or multiple lobar resections and in predicting whether good postoperative results will be achieved. Metabolic recovery of the ipsilateral caudate nucleus (40) and other brain regions, such as the lateral premotor, caudal sensory motor, and inferior parietal cortices (41), often years after hemispherectomy, may be an indication of functional reorganization (40) and may parallel functional improvement (42).

Proton magnetic resonance spectroscopy (43,44) reveals decreased N-acetylaspartate (NAA) levels in patients with Rasmussen encephalitis; this involves the entire hemisphere and correlates with brain atrophy. Elevated levels of glutamine and glutamate may be significant, highlighting the potential role of abnormal excitatory neurotransmitters in the generation of seizures (43). A marked decrease in the size of spectral peaks, centered at 0.98 and 1.3 parts per million (ppm) coupled with an increased choline level, may indicate concurrent active demyelination and cell death (43).

Functional MRI has been used to study reorganization of sensorimotor function. In some patients, activation of premotor, supplementary motor, and inferior parietal cortices with passive movement of the hemiplegic hand have been found in the ipsilateral hemisphere (45,46). Sensory evoked responses of lower amplitude and increased latency compared with those on the normal side (47) have been

recorded. Transcranial magnetic stimulation and motor-evoked potentials have shown that the reorganization of motor function follows a diverse pattern and does not correlate with the degree of neurologic impairment (48,49).

Video Electroencephalographic Studies

Scalp video-EEG monitoring is essential in the evaluation of hemispheric syndromes (1,50,51), from both diagnostic and prognostic standpoints. Well-localized or -lateralized interictal and ictal EEG abnormalities correlating with the clinical and imaging findings usually predict excellent postsurgical results, although bilateral epileptogenic abnormalities, including hypsarrhythmia, may be seen. In these instances, subtle clues such as continuous regional slowing; predominance of epileptiform abnormalities in one region; absence of background or physiologic rhythms such as spindles; vertex waves over one hemisphere; or focal ictal EEG onset may help localize or lateralize the epileptogenic zone(s).

Sometimes the scalp electroencephalogram shows bilateral independent discharges, suggesting epileptogenicity in both hemispheres, particularly in postmeningitic, posttraumatic, or posthemorrhagic encephalopathies. This finding may also represent the development of secondary epileptogenesis in the contralateral hemisphere. When good clinical, functional, and MRI lateralization is associated with large encephaloclastic porencephaly, a review of previous electroencephalogram recordings may help to clarify the significance of the contralateral findings (28).

Ipsilateral burst suppression, particularly during sleep, has been reported in patients with hemimegalencephaly (52,53) and represents a good lateralizing finding.

The following findings on scalp electroencephalography (considered independently) are indicative of a good outcome: the presence of (a) ipsilateral suppression of physiologic rhythms in the abnormal hemisphere; (b) multifocal epileptic activity confined to the damaged hemisphere; or (c) bilateral but synchronous discharges maximum in the abnormal hemisphere (54); and the absence of (d) contralateral slowing; (e) generalized or bilateral independent spiking (55); and (f) abnormalities in background activity over the "good hemisphere." Increasingly, however, evidence shows that the prognosis depends on multiple factors like the etiology, unilateral or bilateral MRI findings, and the completeness of the resection rather than on the presence of specific EEG patterns (56,57).

Neuropsychological Evaluations

Early psychological evaluation is important to establish the level of cognitive function. Serial testing can ascertain whether improvement or deterioration has taken place. In children younger than age 5 years, periodic application of Griffith's developmental scales is usually sufficient for assessment. Older children, adolescents, and adults require formal psychological testing to assess all aspects of neuropsychological function. Intellectual function in patients with diffuse hemispheric syndromes varies (58–61). Children with early static injury to one hemisphere and timely control of seizures may have intelligence approaching the low-normal range. Severe intellectual impairment may indicate bilateral diffuse hemispheric involvement or chronic interference caused by frequent seizures or by frequent or continuous EEG epileptic activity (62).

The best development is often seen in children who began with a better neuropsychological profile, even if they deteriorated after the onset of seizures. Children with profound mental retardation tend to do less well as far as global development is concerned, even if hemispherectomy completely eliminates the seizures. Another important factor is the presence of migration disorders, particularly hemimegalencephaly. As a group, these children seem to respond less well to hemispherectomy, both in seizure control and in developmental gains. With early severe hemispheric lesions, usually associated with a profound hemiparesis, shift of language to the other hemisphere is to be expected. Results of dichotic listening testing (63) point to complete lateralization of speech by age 5 years. When this technique is used in children able to understand it, contralateral paradoxical ear extinction is usually noted. Some preservation of auditory spatial localization has been noted in hemispherectomized patients, some of whom perform at normal or near-normal levels, particularly if early damage occurred (64). Some children, especially those with Rasmussen encephalitis or other progressive hemispheric syndromes affecting the dominant hemisphere, may need speech assessment with the intracarotid amobarbital test to determine lateralization or shift of speech. Functional MRI and PET language activation show promise in the assessment of speech localization.

Integrity of both hemispheres appears to greatly facilitate the acquisition of new knowledge and functions in the developing brain. However, the importance of language development, or language shift in children with progressive encephalopathy of the dominant hemisphere, cannot be overemphasized. According to Taylor (61) and other researchers, the left hemisphere appears to be phylogenetically superior to the right in language acquisition. Some shift of language seems to occur even in patients with disease onset in later childhood. Most investigators agree that right hemispherectomy patients perform syntactic comprehension tests consistent with their estimated mental age (60), whereas only a few patients with left hemispherectomy achieve this level. The same can be said for speech perception, although studies have failed to show a difference in overall speech production between the two groups. It seems that once speech is acquired (60), it can be maintained by an intact cerebral hemisphere on the right or the left side. Two other important considerations in language development or shifting are the common association of nonverbal cognitive deficits in these children and the different capacity of the two hemispheres in relation to language acquisition across individuals.

Clearly, however, transferred speech, irrespective of how early the insult, is never as well developed as naturally acquired speech. Language after dominant-hemisphere disconnection, especially in older children with Rasmussen syndrome, remains abnormal.

Neuropsychological assessments (65) of posthemispherectomy patients suggest that in infancy the two hemispheres are equally capable of supporting the development of reading skills, both an orthographic input lexicon and phonologic output lexicon, and can access a semantic system based on these. However, the left hemisphere seems to be superior for the development of spelling. Generally, the left hemisphere after right hemispherectomy is better able to perform grapheme to-phoneme transformations under simple conditions but still shows some degree of phonologic dyslexia. Neither hemisphere seems to support the development of phoneme-to-grapheme transformation (phonologic dysgraphia) to assist in spelling.

Impairment in the development of nonverbal communication, social interaction, and attention gestures has been found in children with early onset intractable seizures (66). PET studies show that glucose metabolic rates in the prefrontal cortex of the normal hemisphere are decreased irrespective of the side of the hemispherectomy.

Curtiss and associates (67) found that clinical variables predicted language outcome only when considered within distinct etiologic groups. Their review of 43 patients showed that children with developmental etiologies had lower spoken language rank than those with acquired pathologic conditions and that higher spoken language rank was more likely after surgery in children with acquired etiologies who underwent right hemispherectomy. In children with Rasmussen encephalitis treated with left hemispherectomy, gains in expressive functions usually lag behind receptive functions, mimicking, to some extent, a normal pattern of speech development (67,68).

Assessments of the development or transfer of language clearly demonstrate that a number of factors influence the final results, including the site of the hemispheric insult, etiology, age at injury, and the presence or absence of seizure disorder, as well as the presence or absence of progression of the illness. Neither hemisphere is independently capable of developing normal language functions when one hemisphere is affected by a congenital or acquired pathologic condition (69–71).

Abnormal behavior, consisting of impulsiveness, inattentiveness, aggressiveness, hyperactivity, and poor judgment, is frequently seen in patients with diffuse hemispheric syndromes (32,45,62,72). These behaviors have no specific localizing value and appear to be related to pathologic substrate, burden of epilepsy, and anticonvulsant medications. Behavioral disorders are not a contraindication to surgical treatment. Many parents report improved behavior after surgery when decreases in or cessation of seizures permits reductions in the number and doses of antiepileptic medications.

SYNDROMES

Porencephaly

Patients with prenatal and perinatal insults associated with large encephaloclastic porencephalic cysts are good candidates for hemispherectomy. The etiologic factors are variable. Although some cysts are a result of trauma, usually they are caused by vascular occlusions secondary to prenatal thrombotic events, meningitis, or cardiac surgery. If the insult occurs early in fetal development, migrational disorders or cortical disorganization (e.g., polymicrogyria) may occur. Intracerebral hemorrhage associated with prenatal or perinatal thrombocytopenia, as well as bleeding secondary to rupture of vascular malformations, can cause large porencephalic cysts that typically do not follow a vascular distribution. If seizures are intractable and the clinical, imaging, and EEG findings are well correlated, surgical results are generally excellent.

Hemimegalencephaly

Hemimegalencephaly is a neuronal migration disorder with enlargement and dysplasia that affects one hemisphere predominantly. The abnormality may be an isolated finding or may be associated with one of the neurocutaneous syndromes, such as neurofibromatosis, Klippel-Trénaunay syndrome, hypomelanosis of Ito, linear nevus sebaceous of Jadassohn, and Proteus syndrome (32). The MRI shows a dysplastic and enlarged hemisphere with variable findings, such as (a) thickening of the gray matter; (b) pachygyria; (c) enlarged or smaller ventricle compared with the unaffected side; (d) calcifications; (e) hypoplasia of the corpus callosum; and (f) occasionally, schizencephalic clefts (Fig. 81.1). Histopathologic examination usually shows severe cortical migrational disorders in the affected hemisphere (73). A number of autopsies, however, have detected subtle migrational disorders in the so-called normal side (74), consisting of irregular cortical lamination and abundant single scattered neurons in subcortical white matter. Electron microscopy has shown hyperplasia of glial cells with giant astrocytes often containing several nuclei and proliferation of Rosenthal fibers. The Golgi stain shows

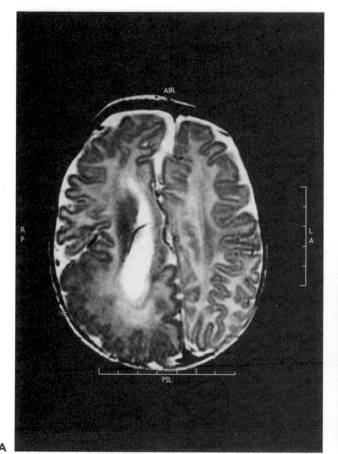

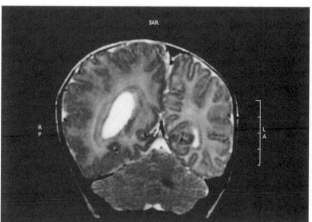

A

B

Figure 81.1 An axial (**A**) and coronal (**B**) T2-weighted images in a patient with hemimegalencephaly shows thick gray matter with abnormal gyration. There are abnormal signal and distribution of the white matter in the parietal lobe, ventricular asymmetry (the right being smaller), and mild contralateral cerebellar atrophy.

giant neurons with a perikaryon covered by perisomatic processes and complex dendritic proliferation (75). The epilepsy varies in severity, but is usually intractable.

Extensive Unilateral Cortical Dysplasia

Another lateralized migrational disorder, extensive unilateral cortical dysplasia, may be best treated with hemispherectomy. Contralateral hemiparesis is often found but in many instances is not as profound as that seen with encephaloclastic central-region porencephaly. The associated seizure disorder varies in severity, and MRI can detect most of these lesions. PET scanning often shows focal hypometabolic changes (39) corresponding to the pathologic substrate or to the often continuous EEG seizure activity.

Staged procedures may be considered in the surgical management of these patients, particularly when there is little or no motor deficit, although the best results of surgical treatment depend on complete resection of the abnormality visible on MRI (76). Excisions guided by MRI may be effective in seizure control; however, more subtle abnormalities in the remaining brain may continue or begin to cause seizures once the primary generator has been excised. Another consideration is that dysplastic cortical brain may harbor some motor-sensory or speech function. In patients with bilateral cortical dysplasia, resective surgery is generally not feasible, and callosotomy or vagal nerve stimulation remain the only options.

Sturge-Weber Syndrome

Sturge-Weber syndrome presents with a facial port-wine stain located in the territory of the trigeminal nerve, associated with ipsilateral leptomeningeal angiomatosis. The cutaneous angioma is absent in fewer than 10% of patients. Ipsilateral ophthalmic abnormalities, principally glaucoma, are often present. Cerebral calcifications and venous abnormalities develop progressively. In 20% of patients, the lesions are bilateral; however, even in these patients hemispherectomy can be an option if there is good clinical and EEG lateralization (77). When seizures begin in infancy, the prognosis is guarded. Pathologic analysis in this group has shown a four-layer microgyric cortex below the angiomatosis (78). MRI with gadolinium demonstrates the extent of pial angiomatosis, but SPECT and PET may be more sensitive (37), showing the extent of the associated cerebral hypoperfusion (Fig. 81.2). In children with severe epileptic syndromes and progressive neurologic dysfunction (79), hemispherectomy may be considered even before maximal hemiparesis is established. The differential diagnosis includes other calcified occipital cortical lesions, such as those associated with celiac disease and folic acid deficiency.

Rasmussen Syndrome

Rasmussen syndrome (80), or chronic encephalitis and epilepsy, is a specific progressive disease in children, primarily affecting one hemisphere. The illness is active for several years and is nearly always self-limited. Half of all patients have an infectious or inflammatory episode before the epilepsy begins. Multiple seizure types are usually present, and epilepsia partialis continua, a characteristic feature, occurs in more than half the patients. Mental deterioration usually develops.

The electroencephalogram findings are not specific (51). Slow-wave abnormalities are frequently bilateral but asymmetric. Independent foci of epileptic discharge over the opposite hemisphere occur in about one third of patients, and bilateral synchronous discharges are found in half. There is radiologic evidence of slowly progressive ipsilateral brain atrophy (31). Early changes identified on MRI in some patients include high signal on T2-weighted images in the cortex and white matter, cortical atrophy in the frontoinsular region, and moderate atrophy of the head of the caudate nucleus (81) (Fig. 81.3). PET scanning shows hypometabolism over the affected hemisphere (33), and SPECT studies show reduced perfusion. Proton magnetic resonance spectroscopy demonstrates focal lactate accumulation in the area of epilepsia partialis continua (44). Low levels of NAA are found diffusely in the affected hemisphere and are suggestive of neuronal loss and demyelination (43,44). Increased glutamate levels may play a role in epileptogenesis. Pathologic findings consist of perivascular lymphocytic cuffs with microglial nodules predominantly in the cortex. The inflammatory elements also may be present in the leptomeninges (82). Examination of the cerebrospinal fluid may show elevations in lymphocyte count and protein levels ranging from 50 to 98 mg/dL. Glutamate receptor 3 subunit (GluR3) antibodies have been described in some patients (83), but the technique has been difficult to reproduce. Several medical treatments, such as gamma globulin (84), high-dose steroids (85), plasmapheresis (83), and intraventricular interferon alfa (86), have been tried with variable, but usually transient, responses. Progression of the disease, even after hemispherectomy, has been described in the ipsilateral caudate nucleus and hippocampus, contralateral cerebellar hemisphere, and brainstem as demonstrated by MRI changes, persistence of ictal activity, and focal hyperperfusion on SPECT (87).

SURGICAL PROCEDURES

The preparation of any patient for hemispherectomy requires special considerations. The child's weight, nutritional status, and estimated blood volume from the planned resection, burden of seizures, morbidity and mortality consequences if surgery is withheld, and social circumstances all affect the timing of surgery. Some anticonvulsant medications, specifically valproic acid, may interfere with clotting mechanisms by reducing platelet counts. An adequate amount of blood should be cross-matched for replacement. Planning the patient's postoperative anticonvulsant medications with the neurologist and the possibility of transient coverage with intravenous or rectal medications should be discussed. Parents should be prepared

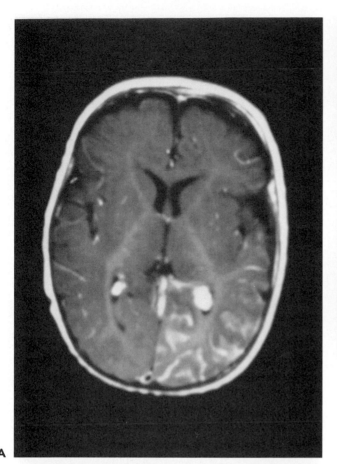

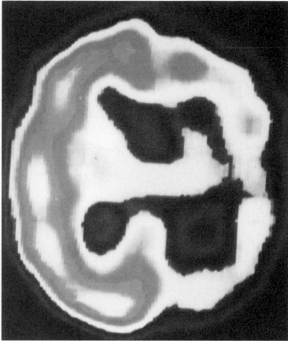

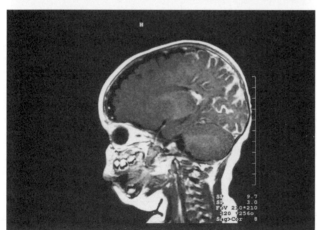

Figure 81.2 On magnetic resonance imaging, axial and sagittal-cuts T1-weighted images with gadolinium, in a patient with Sturge-Weber syndrome, show cortical atrophy of the left hemisphere secondary to ischemia and the enhancement associated with the subpial angiomatosis (**A** and **B**). ^{99m}Technetium hexamethylpropyleneamineoxime single-photon-emission computed tomography, axial cut, demonstrates the area of hypoperfusion; at surgery, the subpial angiomatosis extended to the frontal pole (**C**).

for the expected postoperative symptoms, the possibility of increased deficit, the need for intensive care management, and the chances of complete seizure freedom.

Special consideration must be given to intraoperative and postoperative management if the patient is a young child (88). Preparation for the possibility of massive and sudden blood loss has to be made. In children weighing less than 20 kg, rapid external blood replacement with old blood may lead to severe hyperkalemia; consequently, donor blood should be less than 10 days old. Arterial and central venous pressure monitoring is essential. Coagulopathies related to massive blood replacement, sometimes exceeding the child's blood volume, are a possibility; replacement with fresh-frozen plasma, coagulation factors, and platelets

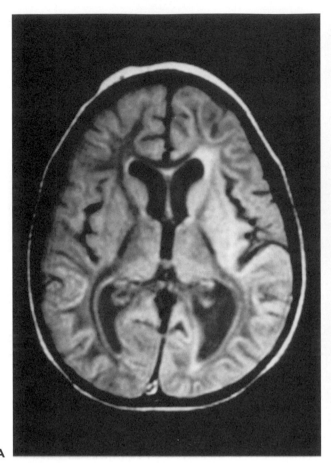
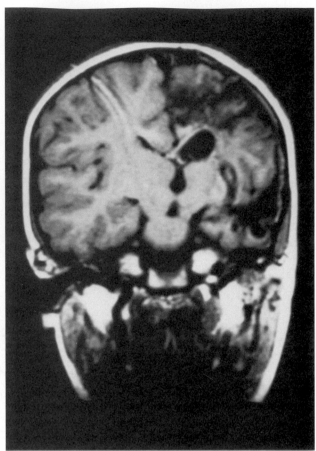

A   B

Figure 81.3 Magnetic resonance imaging axial cut T1-weighted image in a patient with Rasmussen encephalitis shows increased signal in the insula and parietooccipital cortex; associated periventricular gliosis is also seen on the left hemisphere (**A**). Six months later the same patient shows diffuse hemispheric atrophic changes, with severe cortical damage and ventricular asymmetry (**B**).

should be available. The patient should be monitored for hypothermia, which may occur because of a large surface to volume ratio, limited amounts of insulating body fat, increased metabolic rate related to the surgical trauma, and extensive fluid replacement at room temperature. Hypokalemia is related to dilutional effects.

In the immediate postoperative period, hemodynamic stability may sometimes be affected and necessitate continued resuscitation measures in the intensive care unit. Fever is common. Seizures raise concern for acute encephalopathy, infection, or failure of surgery and may be difficult to diagnose in a child who is intubated, sedated, and perhaps paralyzed. Postoperative judicious use of EEG monitoring should be considered if seizures are suspected. Massive hemorrhage into the resection cavity has been reported, with initial minimal symptoms owing to the presence of expected hemiparesis.

A rehabilitation program should be well established. This includes physiotherapy and occupational therapy to assess changing motor deficits and to optimize the development of daily living skills, speech therapy to stimulate the establishment or shift of speech, and psychological evaluation to assess cognitive function and the presence of

behavioral or maladaptive social problems. Postoperative MRI, electroencephalography, and assessment by the entire team are imperative.

Anatomic Hemispherectomy

Anatomic hemispherectomy was the original technique used in a number of centers until the late 1960s. Techniques depended on (89) whether surgery involved multiple lobar excisions or *en bloc* resection, and whether caudate nucleus, putamen, globus pallidus, amygdala, and hippocampus, as well as insular cortex, were resected or left in place. The report of delayed complications such as cerebral hemosiderosis after anatomic hemispherectomy prompted a number of modifications. In the past 10 years, there has been a resurgence in the use of anatomic hemispherectomy, followed by shunting of the cavity after an initial period of external drainage to remove serosanguineous cerebrospinal fluid (14). Such precautions, it is hoped, will avert the formation of subdural membranes that may become potential sites for recurrent hemorrhage. Others who perform complete anatomic hemispherectomy opt for close clinical and radiologic observation to detect the development of hydrocephalus and only then proceed with shunting.

A number of factors must be taken into account in the selection of anatomic over functional hemispherectomy (90), including safety because of the risk of hemorrhage, efficacy in seizure control, size of the lateral ventricles, presence of atrophy, previous surgery, age of the child, and consistency of the cerebral tissue. Anatomic hemispherectomy is recommended in patients with a small lateral ventricle, in those with dysplastic syndromes because of the risk of hemorrhage and firmness of the tissue, and in very young children.

Anatomic hemispherectomy has also been performed in patients in whom functional hemispherectomy has failed, with mixed results. Its use in patients with hemimegalencephaly has yielded promising results for postoperative seizure control (91,92).

Oxford Modification

In 1970, Wilson (93) devised a method designed to prevent subacute cerebral hemosiderosis and hydrocephalus that was based on tacking the dura to the falx and tentorium to collapse the subdural space at the expense of the epidural space. In 1983, Adams (9) described the technique and established its principles (10,94), which include immaculate hemostasis at operation and reduction in the subdural space, in terms of both the surface area of the dura and the volume of the subdural cavity, to discourage formation of subdural hematoma. In addition, the subdural cavity must be isolated from the ventricular system by obstruction of the ipsilateral foramen of Monro with a muscle plug and removal of the choroid plexus. Further modifications of this technique have been introduced (95).

Hemidecortication and Hemicorticectomy

In 1979, Hoffman described a number of children with Sturge-Weber syndrome who had undergone hemidecortication, a technique first proposed in 1968 by Ignelzi and Bucy. The rationale was to leave the diencephalon with enough white matter to cover the ventricular system, allowing the cavity to be gradually filled by brain growth during childhood. This would avoid the hemorrhagic complications seen in older children and adults. Hoffman reasoned that removal of the cortex with preservation of the white matter and basal ganglia should have equivalent results in seizure control (10,79).

Functional Hemispherectomy

In 1983, Rasmussen proposed functional hemispherectomy (anatomically subtotal but physiologically complete). Using this procedure in eight patients, he obtained the full advantages in seizure control and behavioral improvement

provided by anatomic hemispherectomy, but without the complications (8).

The technique involves a temporal lobectomy, including mesiotemporal structures, followed by a suprasylvian central corticectomy extending to the level of the falx. Corpus callosotomy and disconnection of the parietooccipital and temporal lobes are performed posterior to the splenium; the frontal lobe is disconnected on a plane corresponding to the level of the sphenoid wing (Fig. 81.4). It is not unusual in postresection corticography for continuous spiking or electrographic seizures to be recorded from the isolated cortex, but disconnection from the rest of the brain prevents the occurrence of clinical seizures (96).

Hemispherotomy

In 1992, Delalande coined the term *hemispherotomy* to describe a technique in which disconnection predominates over excision. The lateral ventricle is entered by way of a posterior frontal vertex approach. A callosotomy is performed from within the ventricle, followed by transection at the basal ganglia from the trigone to the inferomesial frontal region.

In 1995, Villemure and Mascott (11) described periinsular hemispherotomy as a modification of classic functional hemispherectomy. In this procedure, suprainsular and infrainsular windows are opened after removal of the frontal, parietal, and temporal opercula. From within the ventricle, a parasagittal callosotomy is completed. The frontal lobe is disconnected in the coronal plane at the level of the greater wing of the sphenoid, and a posterior splenial callosotomy is continued with subpial aspiration anteriorly across the fimbria fornix at the level of the trigone. The amygdala and the insula are then excised.

In 1995, and later in 2001, Schramm explained his transsylvian-functional approach in which transsylvian exposure of the circular sulcus allowed transcortical exposure of the ventricular system. The circumferential disconnection is followed by an amygdalohippocampectomy (12).

RESULTS

A number of hemispherectomy series have been published in the past decade (10,11,16,89,90,97,98). In one series (98), 17 patients underwent classic anatomic hemispherectomy and were followed up for a mean of 28 years. Three unrelated deaths occurred, and one patient was lost to follow-up. Of the remaining 13 patients, 47% had no seizures. Two patients developed hydrocephalus 13 and 16 years after surgery and responded well to shunting.

Another series (97) included 52 hemispherectomies carried out over 20 years in which most patients underwent hemidecortication. Fifty-four percent were seizure free, and the majority required no medication. Another 38% had fewer seizures, for an overall good result of 92%. Among a

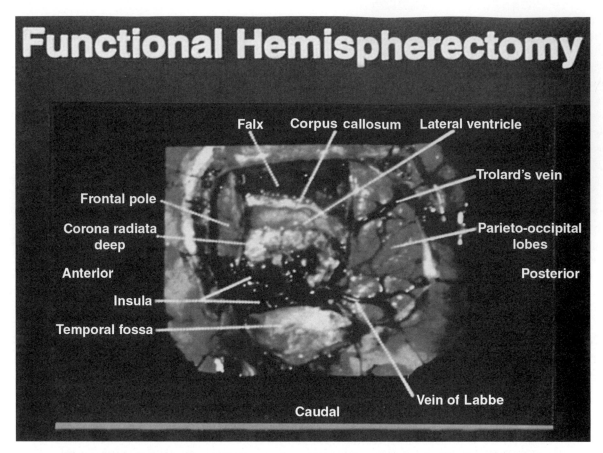

Figure 81.4 Functional hemispherectomy in a child age 3 years 8 months. The frontal and parietooccipital lobes are left in place, and the blood supply remains intact. The temporal and central areas are removed. A complete callosotomy is performed.

subgroup of patients with longer follow-up (average, 7.4 years), 11 (42%) led an independent life.

In a pediatric series (90) whose participants had a median age of 3.3 years at the time of surgery, and a follow-up lasting at least 1 year, 88% of patients had more than a 90% reduction in seizure frequency; 60% were seizure free.

A review of the McGill University experience from 1978 to 1998 includes 68 patients; 55 underwent functional hemispherectomy and 13, peri-insular hemispherotomy. Of the 25 encephaloclastic porencephalies, 20 were secondary to a vascular accident, 3 were posttraumatic, and 2 were postmeningitic. There were 21 cases of Rasmussen encephalitis, 8 of Sturge-Weber syndrome, 9 of diffuse cortical dysplasias, and 5 of hemimegalencephaly. The mean age at surgery was 12.2 years, and follow-up ranged from 1 to 21 years (average, 9.1 years). Fifty-two patients (80%) were seizure free, more than half without medication; 14% had the number of seizures reduced by more than 90%; four patients showed moderate improvement or no change. Improvement in mental function and behavior was frequently observed. The preoperative functional level was an important predictor of the overall result. Intellectual improvement was significantly better in children who originally functioned at a high level, even if the onset of seizures had caused significant regression preoperatively. Adaptive behavior, social skills, and sleeping habits also improved.

Postoperative seizure outcome was best for vascular etiologies such as congenital middle-cerebral-artery-territory infarcts, followed by progressive disorders, such as Rasmussen encephalitis and Sturge-Weber syndrome. Developmental etiologies, including hemimegalencephaly and diffuse hemispheric migrational disorders, led to the least successful outcome. The group with dysplastic developmental malformations also consistently had severe cognitive and developmental delays, even when seizure control was good. Within this group, patients who have preservation of normal architecture in one lobe may have better seizure control (57).

COMPLICATIONS

Before the operative procedure, the family should be informed of the possible outcomes of hemispherectomy. For patients with an incomplete neurologic deficit, the expected worsening of the motor and sensory (47,48) deficit or anticipated changes to the visual fields (99–103) should be clearly explained. A number of patients, particularly those with incomplete motor deficit, exhibit flaccid hemiplegia initially after surgery that usually improves within a month. After hemispherectomy, patients should be able to walk and to use their arm, but finger movements, hand function, and foot tapping, usually already absent preoperatively, will not return. In the McGill University series, 14 patients (22%) showed improvement in motor function after hemispherectomy, mainly related to a reduction in spasticity; most of these patients had Rasmussen encephalitis or encephaloclastic porencephaly. Ten patients (15%) showed some degree of worsening postoperatively.

Mortality is between 1% and 5% in most series (18,30,82,86,90,94,97,104). Many deaths are related to hemorrhage during surgery, particularly in children with low circulating blood volume; others occur in the early postoperative period.

During surgery, meticulous anesthetic technique is essential (88). Careful planning of the skin and bone flap, aided by neuronavigational technology, if available, provides invaluable assistance. Either neuronavigational technology or ultrasonography (105) can be used to identify the midline at gyrus rectus, the extent of the callosotomy, and the anterior and posterior disconnections. Even in encephaloclastic cases, in which the surface intraoperative shift is significant, the midline structure does not shift as the navigational system remains reliable. Meticulous implementation of neurosurgical and microsurgical technique is paramount. Avoidance of involvement of the contralateral hemisphere, as well as avoidance of damage to the brainstem, posterior circulation, and cranial nerves, is essential. Preservation of arteries and veins in functional hemispherectomy can prevent infarction and swelling in the immediate postoperative period, as well as later progressive atrophy.

Early postoperative complications are usually related to hemodynamic instability, hypokalemia or hyperkalemia, and hypothermia and can be prevented by appropriate intensive care management. Seizures at this time may be serious if prolonged and may arise in the opposite hemisphere. Low levels of anticonvulsant drugs related to blood loss and surgical trauma may be observed. Monitoring of possible epileptic activity, coupled with intravenous anticonvulsant therapy and surveillance of blood levels, is usually sufficient. Hydrocephalus can present soon after surgery. External drainage for removal of blood products and monitoring of intracranial pressure are adequate measures. CT scan monitoring after removal of the ventricular drain is required, particularly if a patient presents with signs of increased intracranial pressure. In the McGill University series, four patients (7.5%) developed hydrocephalus requiring shunting.

Infection is rare and may involve the wound, cerebrospinal fluid, bone flap, or remaining parenchyma. Most infections respond to adequate antibiotic coverage, occasionally to debridement, or to removal of the bone flap. Most patients with infection develop aseptic meningitis, characterized by low-grade fever, severe headache, irritability, and lethargy. The judicious use of external drainage to remove blood products may be required to decrease this complication.

Residual nondisconnected tissue causing EEG epileptic activity with corresponding clinical seizures may be observed after technically difficult hemispherectomies, such as those associated with hemimegalencephaly. Electrocorticography after acute disconnection has shown burst suppression in the remaining cortex. EEG epileptic activity without clinical seizures may be observed postoperatively over areas of brain that have been disconnected (54) but remain viable.

Infection and hydrocephalus may also be late postoperative complications, so far reported only with anatomic hemispherectomy. Hydrocephalus with superficial cerebral hemosiderosis (106,107) has been described in patients more than 30 years after anatomic hemispherectomy. Other rare complications, such as dystonic attacks or bilateral ballistic movements (108), have occurred years after the surgical procedure. Bipolar illness (109) manifesting years after hemispherectomy is unlikely to be directly related to the procedure.

SUMMARY

Hemispherectomy is a radical surgical procedure that can be invaluable in the management of hemispheric syndromes involving intractable epilepsy. The adverse effects on the development and maturation of the brain of infants and young children that may be caused by these often catastrophic epilepsies should lead to careful, critical, and timely evaluation and consideration of early surgery. When the disconnection is complete, hemispherectomy, performed with any of the different techniques available, will have similar, excellent results on the control of seizures and will lead to intellectual and behavioral improvements. Hemispherectomy carries a significantly higher risk of mortality than other surgical procedures used to manage intractable epilepsy. An experienced team capable of accurate diagnosis and medical and surgical management, as well as pediatric anesthetic and intensive care support, are crucial for good outcome in these patients.

REFERENCES

1. Andermann F, Freeman JM, Vigevano F, et al. Surgical remediable diffuse hemispheric syndromes. In: Engel J Jr, ed. *Surgical treatment of epilepsies*, 2nd ed. New York: Raven Press, 1993:87–101.
2. Törmä T, Donner M. Hemispherectomy in early hemiplegia and intractable epilepsy. *Acta Paediatr Scand* 1971;60:545–552.
3. Villemure JG. Anatomical to functional hemispherectomy from Krynauw to Rasmussen. *Epilepsy Res Suppl* 1992;5:209–215.
4. Oppenheimer DR, Griffith HB. Persistent intracranial bleeding as a complication of hemispherectomy. *J Neurol Neurosurg Psychiatry* 1966;29:229–240.
5. Falconer MA. Delayed complications associated with ventricular dilatation following hemispherectomy. In: *Proceedings of the 1st Mexican Congress of Neurological Surgery*. 1969:96–97.
6. Falconer MA, Wilson PJE. Complications related to delayed hemorrhage after hemispherectomy. *J Neurosurg* 1969;30:413–426.

7. Andermann F. Clinical indications for hemispherectomy and callosotomy. *Epilepsy Res* 1992;5(Suppl):189–199.

8. Rasmussen T. Hemispherectomy for seizures revisited. *Can J Neurol Sci* 1983;10:71–78.

9. Adams CBT. Hemispherectomy —a modification. *J Neurol Neurosurg Psychiatry* 1983;46:617–619.

10. Villemure JG, Adams CBT, Hoffman HJ, et al. Hemispherectomy. In: Engel J Jr, ed. *Surgical treatment of epilepsies,* 2nd ed. New York: Raven Press, 1993:511–518.

11. Villemure JG, Mascott CR. Peri-insular hemispherotomy: surgical principles and anatomy. *Neurosurgery* 1995;37:975–981.

12. Schramm J, Kral T, Clusmann H. Transsylvian keyhole functional hemispherectomy. *Neurosurgery* 2001;49:891–901.

13. Humbertclaude VT, Coubes PA, Robain O, et al. Early hemispherectomy in a case of hemimegalencephaly. *Pediatr Neurosurg* 1997;27:268–271.

14. Peacock WJ. Hemispherectomy for the treatment of intractable seizures in childhood. *Neurosurg Clin North Am* 1995;6:3680–3695.

15. Villemure JG, Rasmussen T. Functional hemispherectomy in children. *Neuropediatrics* 1993;24:53–55.

16. Vining EPG, Freeman JM, Brandt J, et al. Progressive unilateral encephalopathy of childhood (Rasmussen's syndrome): a reappraisal. *Epilepsia* 1993;34:639–650.

17. Burgess JW, Villablanca JR, Levine MS. Recovery of function after neonatal or adult hemispherectomy in cats: II, limb bias and development, paw usage, locomotion, and rehabilitative effects of exercise. *Behav Brain Res* 1986;20:1–18.

18. Burgess JW, Villablanca JR, Levine MS. Recovery of function after neonatal or adult hemispherectomy in cats: III, complex functions: open field exploration, social interactions, maze and hole-board performance. *Behav Brain Res* 1986;20:217–230.

19. Gomez-Pinilla F, Villablanca JR, Sonmier BJ, et al. Reorganization of pericruciate cortical projections to the spinal cord and dorsal column nuclei after neonatal or adult cerebral hemispherectomy. *Brain Res* 1986;385:343–355.

20. Hovda DA, Villablanca JR. Differential brain stem nuclei. Generation after neonatal or adult cerebral hemispherectomy in cats. *Anat Res* 1986;214:56A.

21. Hovda DA, Villablanca JR. Sparing of visual field perception in neonatal, but not adult hemispherectomized cats: relationship with oxidative metabolism of superior colliculus. *Behav Brain Res* 1990;37:119–132.

22. Villablanca JR, Burgess JW, Benedetti F. There is less thalamic degeneration in neonatal-lesioned than in adult-lesioned cats after cerebral hemispherectomy. *Brain Res* 1986;368:211–225.

23. Villablanca JR, Burgess JW, Olmstead CE. Recovery of function after neonatal or adult hemispherectomy in cats: I, time course, movement, posture and sensory motor tests. *Behav Brain Res* 1986;19:205–226.

24. Kellaway P. Afferent input: a critical factor in the ontogenesis of brain electrical activity. In: Burch N, Altshuber HL, eds. *Behavior and brain electrical activity.* New York: Plenum, 1975:391–420.

25. Duchowny M, Jayakar P, Resnick T, et al. Epilepsy surgery in the first three years of life. *Epilepsia* 1998;39:737–743.

26. Tinuper P, Andermann F, Villemure JG, et al. Functional hemispherectomy for treatment of epilepsy associated with hemiplegia: rationale, indications, results, and comparison with callosotomy. *Ann Neurol* 1988;24:27–34.

27. Vining EPG, Freeman JM, Pillas DJ, et al. Why would you remove half a brain? The outcome of 58 children after hemispherectomy—the Johns Hopkins experience: 1968 to 1996. *Pediatrics* 1997;100:163–171.

28. Wyllie E. Surgery for catastrophic localization-related epilepsy in infants. *Epilepsia* 1996;37(Suppl 1):S22–S25.

29. Wyllie E, Comair YG, Kotagal P, et al. Epilepsy surgery in infants. *Epilepsia* 1996;37:625–637.

30. Wyllie E, Comair YG, Kotagal P, et al. Seizure outcome after epilepsy surgery in children and adolescents. *Ann Neurol* 1998;44:740–748.

31. Tampieri D, Melanson D, Ethier R. Imaging of chronic encephalitis. In: Andermann F, ed. *Chronic encephalitis and epilepsy: Rasmussen's syndrome.* Boston: Butterworth-Heinemann, 1991:47–60.

32. Griffith PD, Welch RJ, Gardner-Medwin D, et al. The radiological features of hemimegalencephaly including three cases associated with proteus syndrome. *Neuropediatrics* 1994;25:140–144.

33. Hwang PA, Gilday DL, Spire JP, et al. In: Andermann F, ed. *Chronic encephalitis and epilepsy: Rasmussen's syndrome.* Boston: Butterworth-Heinemann, 1991:61–72.

34. Carmant L, O'Tuama LA, Roach PJ, et al. Technetium-99m HmPAO brain SPECT and outcome of hemispherectomy for intractable seizures. *Pediatr Neurol* 1994;11:203–207.

35. Chiron C, Raynaud C, Jambaqué I, et al. A serial study of regional cerebral blood flow before and after hemispherectomy in a child. *Epilepsy Res* 1991;8:232–240.

36. Rintahaka PJ, Chugani HT, Messa C, et al. Hemimegalencephaly: evaluation with positron emission tomography. *Pediatr Neurol* 1993;9:21–28.

37. Chugani HT, Mazziotta JC, Phelps ME. Sturge-Weber syndrome: a study of cerebral glucose utilization with positron emission tomography. *J Pediatr* 1989;114:244–253.

38. Chugani HT, Shewmon DA, Peacock WJ, et al. Surgical treatment of intractable neonatal-onset seizure: the role of positron emission tomography. *Neurology* 1988;38:1178–1188.

39. Chugani HT, Shewmon DA, Shields WD, et al. Surgery for intractable infantile spasms: neuroimaging perspectives. *Epilepsia* 1993;34:764–771.

40. Chugani HT, Jacobs B. Metabolic recovery in caudate nucleus of children following cerebral hemispherectomy. *Ann Neurol* 1994; 36:794–797.

41. Leonhardt G, Bingel U, Spiekermann G, et al. Cortical activation in patients with functional hemispherectomy. *J Neurol* 2001;248: 881–888.

42. Müller RA, Chugani HT, Muzik O, et al. Brain organization of motor and language functions following hemispherectomy: a [^{15}O]-water positron emission tomography study. *Child Neurol* 1998;13:16–22.

43. Geller E, Faerber EN, Legido A, et al. Rasmussen encephalitis: complementary role of multitechnique neuroimaging. *Am J Neuroradiol* 1998;19:445–449.

44. Matthews PM, Andermann F, Arnold DL. Proton magnetic resonance spectroscopy study of chronic encephalitis and epilepsy. In: Andermann F, ed. *Chronic encephalitis and epilepsy: Rasmussen's syndrome.* Boston: Butterworth-Heinemann, 1991: 73–77.

45. Graveline CJ, Mikolis DJ, Crawley AP, et al. Regionalized sensorimotor plasticity after hemispherectomy fMRI evaluation. *Pediatr Neurol* 1998;19:337–342.

46. Bittar RG, Ptito A, Reutens DS. Somatosensory representation in patients who have undergone hemispherectomy: a functional magnetic resonance imaging study. *J Neurosurg* 2000;92:45–51.

47. Müller F, Kunesch E, Binkofski F, et al. Residual sensorimotor functions in a patient after right-sided hemispherectomy. *Neuropsychologia* 1991;29:125–145.

48. Benecke R, Meyer BU, Freund HJ. Reorganisation of descending motor pathways in patients after hemispherectomy and severe hemispheric lesions demonstrated by magnetic brain stimulation. *Exp Brain Res* 1991;83:419–426.

49. Kastrup O, Leonhardt G, Korthen M, et al. Cortinal motor reorganization following early brain damage and hemispherectomy demonstrated by transcranial magnetic stimulation. *Clin Neurophysiol* 2000:111:1346–1356.

50. Holmes GL. Intractable epilepsy in children. *Epilepsia* 1996;37 (Suppl 3):14–27.

51. So NK, Gloor P. Electroencephalographic and electrocorticographic findings in chronic encephalitis of the Rasmussen type. In: Andermann F, ed. *Chronic encephalitis and epilepsy: Rasmussen's syndrome.* Boston: Butterworth-Heinemann, 1991:37–45.

52. Konkol RJ, Maister BH, Wells RG, et al. Hemimegalencephaly: clinical, EEG, neuroimaging, and IMP-SPECT correlation. *Pediatr Neurol* 1990;6:414–418.

53. Vigevano F, Bertini E, Boldrini R, et al. Hemimegalencephaly and intractable epilepsy: benefits of hemispherectomy. *Epilepsia* 1989;30:833–843.

54. Smith SJM, Andermann F, Villemure JG, et al. Functional hemispherectomy: EEG findings, spiking from isolated brain postoperatively and prediction of outcome. *Neurology* 1991;41: 1790–1794.

55. Carmant L, Kramer U, Riviello JJ, et al. EEG prior to hemispherectomy: correlation with outcome and pathology. *Electroencephalogr Clin Neurophysiol* 1995;4:265–270.

56. Doring S, Cross H, Boyd S, et al. The significance of bilateral EEG abnormalities before and after hemispherectomy in children with unilateral major hemisphere lesions. *Epilepsy Res* 1999;34:65–73.

57. Devlin AM, Cross JS, Harkness W, et al. Clinical outcomes of hemispherectomy for epilepsy in childhood and adolescence. *Brain* 2003;126:556–566.

58. Gott PS. Cognitive abilities following right and left hemispherectomy. *Cortex* 1973;9:266–274.

59. Smith A, Sugar O. Development of above normal language and intelligence 21 years after left hemispherectomy. *Neurology* 1975;25:813–818.

60. Stark RE, Bleile K, Brandt J, et al. Speech–language outcomes of hemispherectomy in children and young adults. *Brain Lang* 1995;51:406–421.

61. Taylor LB. Neuropsychologic assessment of patients with chronic encephalitis. In: Andermann F, ed. *Chronic encephalitis and epilepsy: Rasmussen's syndrome.* Boston: Butterworth-Heinemann, 1991:111–121.

62. Rosenblatt B, Vernet O, Montes JL, et al. Continuous unilateral epileptiform discharge and language delay: effect of functional hemispherectomy on language acquisition. *Epilepsia* 1998;39:787–792.

63. Wester K, Hugdahl K, Asbjørnsen A. Dichotic listening during forced-attention in a patient with left hemispherectomy. *Percept Motor Skills* 1991;72:151–159.

64. Zatorre RJ, Ptito A, Villemure JG. Preserved auditory spatial localization following cerebral hemispherectomy. *Brain* 1995;118:879–889.

65. Ogden JA. Phonological dyslexia and phonological dysgraphia following left and right hemispherectomy. *Neuropsychologia* 1996;34:905–918.

66. Caplan R, Curtis S, Chugani HT, et al. Pediatric Rasmussen encephalitis: social communication, language, PET, and pathology before and after hemispherectomy. *Brain Cogn* 1996;32:45–66.

67. Curtiss S, de Bode S, Mathern GW. Spoken language outcomes after hemispherectomy: factoring in etiology. *Brain Lang* 2001;79:379–396.

68. Boatman D, Freeman J, Vining E, et al. Language recovery after left hemispherectomy in children with late-onset seizures. *Ann Neurol* 1999;46:579–586.

69. Gott PS. Language after dominant hemispherectomy. *J Neurol Neurosurg Psychiatry* 1973;36:1082–1088.

70. Vargha-Khadem F, Carr LJ, Isaacs E, et al. Onset of speech after left hemispherectomy in a nine-year-old boy. *Brain* 1997;120:159–182.

71. Vargha-Khadem F, Isaacs EB, Papaleloudi H, et al. Development of language in six hemispherectomized patients. *Brain* 1991;114:473–495.

72. Ameli NO. Hemispherectomy for the treatment of epilepsy and behavior disturbance. *Can J Neurol Sci* 1980;7:33–38.

73. Farrell MA, DeRosa MJ, Curran JG, et al. Neuropathologic findings in cortical resections (including hemispherectomies) performed for the treatment of intractable childhood epilepsy. *Acta Neuropathol* 1992;83:246–259.

74. Jahan R, Mischel PS, Curran JG, et al. Bilateral neuropathologic changes in a child with hemimegalencephaly. *Pediatr Neurol* 1997;17:344–349.

75. Robain O, Chiroa C, Dulac O. Electron microscopic and Golgi study in a case of hemimegalencephaly. *Acta Neuropathol* 1989;77:664–666.

76. Palmini A, Gambardella A, Andermann F, et al. Operative strategies for patients with cortical dysplastic lesions and intractable epilepsy. *Epilepsia* 1994;35:S57–S71.

77. Tuxhorn IE, Pannek HW. Epilepsy in bilateral Sturge-Weber syndrome. *Pediatr Neurol* 2002;26:394–397.

78. Simonati A, Colamaria V, Bricolo A, et al. Microgyria associated with Sturge-Weber angiomatosis. *Childs Nerv Syst* 1994;10:392–395.

79. Ogunmekan AO, Hwang PA, Hoffman JH. Sturge-Weber-Dimitri disease: role of hemispherectomy in prognosis. *Can J Neurol Sci* 1989;16:78–80.

80. Oguni H, Andermann F, Rasmussen TB. The natural history of the syndrome of chronic encephalitis and epilepsy: a study of the MNI series of forty-eight cases. In: Andermann F, ed. *Chronic encephalitis and epilepsy: Rasmussen's syndrome.* Boston: Butterworth-Heinemann, 1991:7–35.

81. Chiapparini L, Granata T, Farina L, et al. Diagnostic imaging in 13 cases of Rasmussen's encephalitis: can early MRI suggest the diagnosis? *Neuroradiology* 2003;45:171–183.

82. Robitaille Y. Neuropathologic aspects of chronic encephalitis. In: Andermann F, ed. *Chronic encephalitis and epilepsy: Rasmussen's syndrome.* Boston: Butterworth-Heinemann, 1991;7:79–110.

83. Antozzi C, Granata T, Aurisano N, et al. Long-term selective IgG immuno-adsorption improves Rasmussen's encephalitis. *Neurology* 1998;51:302–305.

84. Walsh PJ. Treatment of Rasmussen's syndrome with intravenous gammaglobulin. In: Andermann F, ed. *Chronic encephalitis and epilepsy: Rasmussen's syndrome.* Boston: Butterworth-Heinemann, 1991:201–204.

85. Dulac O, Robain O, Chiron C, et al. High-dose steroid treatment of epilepsia partialis continua due to chronic focal encephalitis. In: Andermann F, ed. *Chronic encephalitis and epilepsy: Rasmussen's syndrome.* Boston: Butterworth-Heinemann, 1991:193–199.

86. Maria BL, Ringdahl DM, Mickle JP, et al. Intraventricular alpha interferon therapy for Rasmussen's syndrome. *Can J Neurol Sci* 1993;20:333–336.

87. Thomas P, Zifkin B, Ghetau G, et al. Persistence of ictal activity after functional hemispherectomy in Rasmussen syndrome. *Neurology* 2003;60:140–142.

88. Brian JE Jr, Deshpande JK, McPherson RW. Management of cerebral hemispherectomy in children. *J Clin Anesth* 1990;2:91–95.

89. Villemure JG. Hemispherectomy techniques. In: Luders H, ed. *Epilepsy surgery.* New York: Raven Press, 1991:569–578.

90. Peacock WJ, Wehby-Grant MC, Shields WD, et al. Hemispherectomy for intractable seizures in children: a report of 58 cases. *Childs Nerv Syst* 1996;12:376–384.

91. Battaglia D, DiRocco C, Iuvone L, et al. Neuro-cognitive development and epilepsy outcome in children with surgically treated hemimegalencephaly. *Neuropediatrics* 1999;30:307–313.

92. DiRocco C, Ianelli A. Hemimegalencephaly and intractable epilepsy: complications of hemispherectomy and their correlations with the surgical technique. *Pediatr Neurosurg* 2000;33:198–207.

93. Wilson PJE. More "second thoughts" on hemispherectomy in infantile hemiplegia. *Dev Med Child Neurol* 1970;12:799–800.

94. Beardsworth E, Adams CBT. Modified hemispherectomy for epilepsy: early results in 10 cases. *Br J Neurosurg* 1988;2:73–84.

95. Dunn LT, Miles JB, May PL. Hemispherectomy for intractable seizures: a further modification and early experience. *Br J Neurosurg* 1995;9:775–783.

96. Wennberg RA, Quesney LF, Villemure JG. Epileptiform and non-epileptiform paroxysmal activity from isolated cortex after functional hemispherectomy. *Electroencephalogr Clin Neurophysiol* 1997;102:437–442.

97. Carson BS, Javedan SP, Freeman JM, et al. Hemispherectomy: a hemidecortication approach and review of 52 cases. *J Neurosurg* 1996;84:903–911.

98. Davies KG, Maxwell RE, French LA. Hemispherectomy for intractable seizures: long-term results in 17 patients followed for up to 38 years. *J Neurosurg* 1993;78:733–740.

99. Estañol B, Romero R, Sáenz de Viteri M, et al. Oculomotor and oculovestibular functions in a hemispherectomy patient. *Arch Neurol* 1980;37:365–368.

100. Troost BT, Daroff RB, Weber RB, et al. Hemispheric control of eye movements: II, quantitative analysis of smooth pursuit in a hemispherectomy patient. *Arch Neurol* 1972;27:449–452.

101. Troost BT, Weber RB, Daroff RB. Hemispheric control of eye movements: I, quantitative analysis of refixation saccades in a hemispherectomy patient. *Arch Neurol* 1972;27:441–448.

102. Wessinger CM, Fendrich R, Gazzaniga MS, et al. Extrageniculostriate vision in humans: investigations with hemispherectomy patients. *Prog Brain Res* 1996;112:405–413.

103. Wessinger CM, Fendrich R, Gazzaniga MS, et al. Residual vision with awareness in the field contralateral to a partial or complete functional hemispherectomy. *Neuropsychologia* 1996;34:1129–1137.

104. Villemure JG. Hemispherectomy: techniques and complications. In: Wyllie E, ed. *The treatment of epilepsy: principles and practice,* 2nd ed. Baltimore, MD: Williams & Wilkins, 1997:1081–1086.

105. Kanev PM, Foley CM, Miles D. Ultrasound-tailored functional hemispherectomy for surgical control of seizures in children. *J Neurosurg* 1997;86:762–767.

106. Kalkanis SN, Blumenfeld H, Sherman JC, et al. Delayed complications thirty-six years after hemispherectomy: a case report. *Epilepsia* 1996;37:758–762.

107. Strowitzki M, Kiefer M, Steudel WI. Acute hydrocephalus as a late complication of hemispherectomy. *Acta Neurochir Wien* 1994; 131:253–259.

108. Wroe S, Richens A, Compston A. Bilateral ballistic movements occurring as a late complication of hemispherectomy and responding to sulpiride. *J Neurol* 1986;233:315–316.

109. Forrest DV. Bipolar illness after right hemispherectomy: a response to lithium carbonate and carbamazepine. *Arch Gen Psychiatry* 1982;39:817–819.

Epilepsy Surgery in the Absence of a Lesion on Magnetic Resonance Imaging

82

Elson L. So

Magnetic resonance imaging (MRI) is a prerequisite in the evaluation of patients for epilepsy surgery. It is well known that epilepsy surgery involving a focal MRI lesion generally confers the best prognosis for postsurgical seizure control (1,2). Complete resection of the lesion is associated with the probability of excellent postsurgical outcome that ranges from 70% to 90%, depending on the location and nature of the MRI lesion. In fact, patients with an MRI lesion that has concordant interictal and ictal electroencephalographic (EEG) discharges are the most privileged epilepsy surgery candidates, as they have approximately a 95% probability of successful seizure control following surgery (3,4).

In the absence of an MRI lesion, evaluation for epilepsy surgery becomes more challenging and complex. The location of the surgical focus and the extent of its resection are not as apparent in patients with nonlesional epilepsy as they are in those with lesional epilepsy. Additionally, the prognosis for postsurgical seizure control is not as favorable in patients with nonlesional epilepsy as it is in those with lesional epilepsy. This chapter discusses the challenges involved in epilepsy surgery evaluation when no lesion is present on MRI, and will describe a diagnostic approach and surgical strategy for optimizing the outcome of resective surgery in patients with nonlesional intractable focal epilepsy.

DEFINING MAGNETIC RESONANCE IMAGING-NEGATIVE EPILEPSY (NONLESIONAL EPILEPSY)

In the absence of an MRI lesion, epilepsy is referred to as *nonlesional epilepsy*. The term nonlesional epilepsy is sometimes used only when histologic examination of resected brain tissue does not reveal a well-recognized pathologic abnormality, such as a tumor or vascular malformation. Because this chapter discusses presurgical diagnosis and surgical strategy with a negative MRI, nonlesional epilepsy refers to the *absence of a potentially epileptogenic lesion on MRI*, regardless of what the postsurgical histopathologic examination may eventually reveal. The diagnostic and therapeutic issues covered in this chapter relate to resective surgery in patients with intractable focal epilepsy.

Before MRI is said to be "negative" and epilepsy is considered "nonlesional," it is necessary to verify that the MRI was performed with techniques that optimize the ability to detect potentially epileptogenic lesions (5,6). Standard MRI studies are insufficient for the evaluation of patients for epilepsy surgery. Sensitivity in detecting a lesion was only 50% with expert review of standard MRI studies, but it increased to 91% with expert review of epilepsy-protocol MRI studies of the same patients (7). Specific MRI imaging techniques and sequences must be used to minimize the risk of missing an epileptogenic lesion that would have facilitated presurgical localization and subsequent resection of the seizure focus. The requisite imaging techniques and sequences are described in the literature (5) and are affirmed by the Commission on Neuroimaging of the International League Against Epilepsy (8). The basic requirements are that (a) field strength of the MRI magnet must be 1.5 tesla or greater; (b) image slice thickness should be 1.5 mm or thinner, with no interslice gap; (c) images should be displayed in coronal, axial, and sagittal views; (d) T1-weighted, T2-weighted, and fluid attenuated inversion recovery (FLAIR) images should be obtained; (e) temporal lobe images should be obtained at oblique coronal planes that are perpendicular to the long axis of the hippocampal formation; and (f) quantitative volumetric measurement of the amygdala–hippocampal complex should be available.

Ideally, three-dimensional rendition of the brain surface must be possible when needed, along with the capability for accurate coregistration of images from other diagnostic procedures. Finally, physicians who review the MRI images must be highly skilled in detecting and interpreting the structural alterations associated with epileptic seizure disorders.

Despite absence of an MRI lesion, pathologic examination of cerebral tissue removed during surgery for nonlesional intractable epilepsy invariably reveals abnormal findings (9). Nonspecific gliosis, the most common finding, consists of varying degrees of glial proliferation and reduced neuronal population, or altered neuronal morphology (10). Varying degrees of malformation of cortical development are also observed, ranging from typical cortical dysplasia (11) to microdysgenesis. Microdysgenesis consists of abnormal clustering of neurons in amount or location, or minute cortical/subcortical foci of disorganized mature but nonneoplastic elements of neuronal and glial origins (glioneuronal hamartia) (12). Occult tumors and vascular malformations are reported to be present in 15% of the nonlesional epilepsy surgical specimens (9). Furthermore, nonlesional temporal lobe epilepsy is often considered putatively as lateral neocortical in seizure origin, but such an assumption should be made with caution because pathologic evidence of mesial temporal sclerosis is encountered in some patients whose MRI shows no amygdala–hippocampal atrophic or signal changes (13,14).

Regardless of the histologic basis of nonlesional epilepsy, the ultimate relevance of focal nonlesional epilepsy surgery is seizure control leading to satisfactory quality of life. Such a definitive outcome should be the gold standard for determining the accuracy of preoperative diagnostic tests in delineating the epileptogenic zone. Unfortunately, most published reports do not use this standard, relying instead on extracranial or intracranial ictal EEG-onset zone or focus (ictal onset zone) as the standard for comparison.

IMPLICATIONS OF NONLESIONAL INTRACTABLE EPILEPSY

The absence of MRI lesion is not uncommon in patients who undergo evaluation for intractable epilepsy. The proportion of intractable focal epilepsy patients with nonlesional MRI varies between centers, but the rate has been estimated at 10% to 15% of surgical series (9). Much of the variation in the rates reported is determined by the type of patients evaluated and the MRI techniques used. In the absence of a potentially epileptogenic lesion on MRI, localization of the site for epilepsy surgery is more complex, surgical resection is more difficult, and postoperative outcome is generally less favorable than that in lesional epilepsy surgery.

Limitations of Noninvasive Presurgical Evaluation in Patients with Nonlesional Epilepsy

Although the importance of a complete and accurate medical history in the evaluation of epilepsy cannot be overemphasized, seizure description provided by witnesses can be inadequate or inaccurate for the purpose of localizing seizure onset. A prospective study involving patients' close friends and relatives demonstrated that their median accuracy for recalling features of convulsive seizures that they had observed was only 45%, compared with 70% for nonconvulsive seizures (15). Therefore, seizure semiology in each patient must be confirmed by analysis of video recordings of habitual seizures. Although several clinical manifestations of seizures correctly lateralize seizure onset to a hemisphere in 80% to 90% of patients (16), semiologic features are not as helpful in localizing seizure onset to a specific area or region within the hemisphere (17).

MRI and extracranial electroencephalography are the two major laboratory tests used in the initial phase of presurgical evaluation of candidates for epilepsy surgery. When the MRI is negative, greater reliance is placed on extracranial electroencephalography to determine the location of the epileptogenic zone (i.e., the focus that, when resected, results in seizure control). Both interictal and ictal extracranial EEG discharges have been valuable in identifying candidates who may benefit from epilepsy surgery, especially from anterior temporal lobectomy (4,18–20). In general, the location of the interictal epileptiform discharges (IEDs) on the scalp suggests the location of the seizure focus on the brain (21), but the association between the two varies with different IED locations (22). The association is best with temporal lobe IED. Caution should still be exercised when imputing temporal lobe IED to temporal lobe epilepsy, because temporal lobe location of extracranial IEDs is encountered in patients with frontal lobe, parietal lobe, or occipital lobe epilepsy (23–25).

In temporal lobectomy candidates, the IED location on the scalp and the presence of an MRI lesion are independently and equally predictive of postsurgical seizure control (4). The presence of temporal lobe IEDs that are all concordant with temporal lobe ictal discharges is associated with a three to four times greater probability of excellent postsurgical seizure control than when IEDs are absent or nonconcordant. This odds ratio is similar to that between the presence and the absence of a focal MRI lesion. Moreover, in patients with lesional epilepsy, exclusively concordant scalp IEDs improve the surgical prognosis beyond that conferred by the presence of an MRI lesion. The rate of excellent postsurgical outcome in these patients is 94% when exclusively concordant IEDs are present versus 60% when they are absent. Conversely, the presence of exclusively concordant IEDs is not associated with a better prognosis for seizure control in patients undergoing nonlesional temporal lobe surgery. The probability of excellent postsurgical outcome is approximately 60% to 65%, regardless of the presence or absence of concordant IEDs in patients with nonlesional epilepsy.

IEDs are often absent or widespread in patients with frontal lobe epilepsy (26). In one study, nearly 20% of patients with frontal lobe epilepsy do not have scalp-recorded IEDs and, when present, IEDs were discordant with the frontal epileptogenic zone in 45% of patients (25). In patients undergoing frontal lobe surgery, the value of extracranial IED in localizing the epileptogenic zone and in predicting the postsurgical outcome is limited. The presence and location of scalp-recorded IED are not independently associated with the outcome of frontal lobe epilepsy surgery, which is the most common type of extratemporal epilepsy surgery (18).

Extracranial ictal EEG has certain inherent limitations, even in those with intractable epilepsy whose MRI had revealed a potentially epileptogenic lesion. Between 25% and 30% of all seizures recorded in patients with unilateral mesial temporal lobe epilepsy (27) or MRI-detected hippocampal atrophy (19) could not be lateralized to the diseased temporal lobe. In addition, a similar proportion of seizures could not be lateralized in patients who underwent successful temporal lobectomy (28). As many as 60% of extracranially recorded seizures in temporal lobectomy candidates had no localizing features at seizure onset (29). Of temporal lobectomy candidates, 10% had extracranial seizures with conflicting features (30) and 18% had falsely localizing seizures (31). The situation is no better in patients with extratemporal epilepsy. Approximately 35% to 50% of seizures recorded extracranially in extratemporal epilepsy are nonlateralizing (28). Epileptogenic foci in the mesial frontal region are frequently devoid of detectable IEDs or ictal discharges on the scalp (32,33). In one study, false lateralization or localization occurred in 28% of occipital and 16% of parietal seizures (33). Moreover, scalp-recorded seizure onset may not be obvious at extratemporal epileptogenic sites, but ictal discharges may appear instead at a temporal region to which it has spread (34–36).

In many of the above situations, invasive ictal electroencephalogram recordings can still be obviated when MRI shows a relevant lesion and other concordant clinical or interictal EEG features are also present (37). However, when MRI shows no lesion, insufficiently localizing EEG seizures complicate the task of delineating the epileptogenic focus for surgical resection. Furthermore, the finding of temporal lobe seizure onset on scalp electroencephalogram recordings cannot be relied on solely for localization of the ictal focus in patients with nonlesional epilepsy. In one study, 11 of 33 intractable epilepsy patients with negative MRIs had proven extratemporal seizure onset despite apparent onset of scalp-recorded EEG seizures at the temporal lobe region (38).

Complexity of Invasive Electroencephalogram Recordings and Surgical Resection in Patients with Nonlesional Epilepsy

In the absence of an MRI lesion, the adequacy of the extent of intracranial electrode implantation or surgical resection is not as apparent as when a lesion is present. The situation often calls for extensive intracranial electrode implantation over large regions in one or both hemispheres. Unfortunately, serious neurologic complications have been reported in 4% to 5% of patients with depth electrode implantation (39) and in as many as 20% of those with subdural electrode implantation (40). The number of intracranial electrodes required for sufficient coverage is difficult to determine when there is no structural abnormality on MRI. It is not unusual that additional electrodes need to be implanted when initial implantation yields insufficient information. Unfortunately, the risk for complications rises with the extent of intracranial electrode implantation. It is estimated that the risk for major complications increases by 40% for every 20 additional subdural electrodes implanted, with the risk as high as 82% with bilateral hemisphere implantations (41).

In lesional epilepsy surgery, surgical resection is guided mainly by the location and extent of the cerebral structural abnormality and its associated EEG abnormalities. In many patients, surgical resection that is restricted to the MRI lesion and its immediate surrounding tissues (lesionectomy) is sufficient for achieving seizure control (42). One study showed that the probability of seizure control is high when the MRI lesion is resected, but seizure outcome is poor when the resection involves mainly the abnormal electroencephalogram focus, not the MRI lesion (43).

In nonlesional epilepsy surgery, clinicians and surgeons are deprived of neuroanatomic landmarks to guide the extent of resection. In such cases, resection is then based on the extent of electroencephalogram abnormalities, but extensive resection based on abnormal EEG discharges raises the risk of perioperative morbidity. Conversely, restricted resection that spares electrophysiologically abnormal tissues may reduce the probability of postsurgical seizure control, especially in patients with extratemporal neocortical epilepsy (44).

Less Favorable Prognosis in Patients with Nonlesional Epilepsy Surgery

It has been known for some time that a remarkable discrepancy exists between the outcomes of lesional and nonlesional surgeries in patients with intractable focal epilepsy. The probability of excellent postsurgical outcome following nonlesional surgery is uniformly lower across many studies in the literature (45). In one series of 157 consecutive patients who underwent anterior temporal lobotomy, 62% of those with no MRI lesion versus 85% of those with an MRI lesion had an excellent outcome (i.e., no seizures, auras only, or rare nocturnal seizures) (4). The outcome in patients undergoing nonlesional frontal lobe surgery is even less favorable. In a study of 68 patients who underwent frontal lobe epilepsy surgery, only 40% of those without an MRI lesion had an excellent postsurgical outcome, whereas 72% of those with an MRI lesion experienced an excellent outcome (18). Moreover, the value of the intracranial electroencephalogram recording is limited in patients whose MRI detects no lesions. Only 22% of such patients became seizure free following epilepsy surgery, despite the presurgical localization of seizure onset by the intracranial electroencephalogram recording (46).

DIAGNOSTIC APPROACH IN NONLESIONAL EPILEPSY SURGERY

When MRI detects no lesion in patients undergoing evaluation for epilepsy surgery, the surgical focus has to be determined by detecting the abnormal functions associated with epileptic seizure activities or with epileptogenic properties. Abnormal functions of the seizure focus can be detected clinically by observing the seizure semiology, electrographically by analyzing the electroencephalogram recording, and topographically by assessing functional imaging results. Intracranial electrode implantation is required in many patients with nonlesional intractable epilepsy. In the absence of a structural lesion on MRI, functional imaging becomes essential for guiding intracranial electrode implantation and for limiting the extent of the implantation. In some cases, functional imaging results can obviate the need for intracranial electrode implantation. Functional imaging tests that are commonly used in epilepsy surgery evaluation include positron emission tomography (PET), single-photon-emission computed tomography (SPECT), magnetic resonance spectroscopy (MRS), and magnetoencephalography (MEG). The following sections discuss the application of noninvasive tests that are useful in the evaluation of patients for nonlesional epilepsy surgery.

Video with Extracranial Electroencephalographic Recordings

Despite their limitations, seizure semiology and extracranial electroencephalography must still be fully explored for clues that help lateralize or localize seizure onset. Some seizure auras have localizing value (47). Auras involving the perirolandic or occipital regions are especially useful in localizing seizure onset (23,24). Seizure semiology adds lateralizing information to that obtained from extracranial ictal EEG recordings. Without semiology, seizure onset can be adequately lateralized by noninvasive EEG recordings in only 65% of temporal lobectomy candidates (48). When seizure semiology is added, seizure onset is adequately lateralized in almost 95% of the candidates (48).

Some types of extracranial IEDs and ictal discharges have value in determining the location of a seizure focus and in guiding intracranial electrode implantation. Exclusively unifocal IEDs are strong predictors of the site of the ictal onset zone in both lesional and nonlesional temporal and extratemporal epilepsy (4,49). Resection of an extratemporal focus that is the sole location of IEDs is associated with a 77% probability of seizure-free outcome, regardless of the presence or absence of an MRI lesion (49). In temporal lobe epilepsy, the preponderance of scalp or sphenoidal IEDs at one temporal lobe strongly suggests that the ictal onset zone resides within that lobe. Ninety-five percent of the patients with a greater than 95% preponderance of IEDs at one anterior temporal region had intracranially recorded seizures originating at the same region (50).

It has been reported that epilepsies involving certain parts of the cerebral hemispheres have distinct EEG discharge patterns at ictal onset (33). For instance, a repetitive epileptiform pattern is more frequently encountered in seizures arising from the lateral frontal convexity, whereas a rhythmic temporal theta discharge pattern is exclusively seen in temporal lobe seizures. However, the majority of patients in whom these observations were made had MRI lesions, and it is not clear whether the findings are consistently observed in patients with nonlesional epilepsy. More recently, it was found that the presence of a fast discharge in the beta-frequency range at the onset of a frontal seizure is highly indicative of the location of the epileptogenic zone (20) (Figs. 82.1 and 82.2). Approximately 90% of patients with this focal ictal beta-discharge pattern at seizure onset became seizure free following resection of the frontal lobe focus, even when the MRI was negative. In comparison, postsurgical seizure freedom occurred in only 16.7% of nonlesional frontal lobe epilepsy patients who did not have a focal ictal beta-discharge pattern.

Positron Emission Tomography in Patients with Nonlesional Epilepsy

The most commonly used radioactive ligand in PET studies of patients with epilepsy is 2-[^{18}F]fluoro-2-deoxy-D-glucose (FDG). Because of the short half-life and long cerebral uptake of FDG, FDG-PET studies are performed during the interictal period. The following discussion of FDG-PET findings refers to the well-known feature of interictally reduced

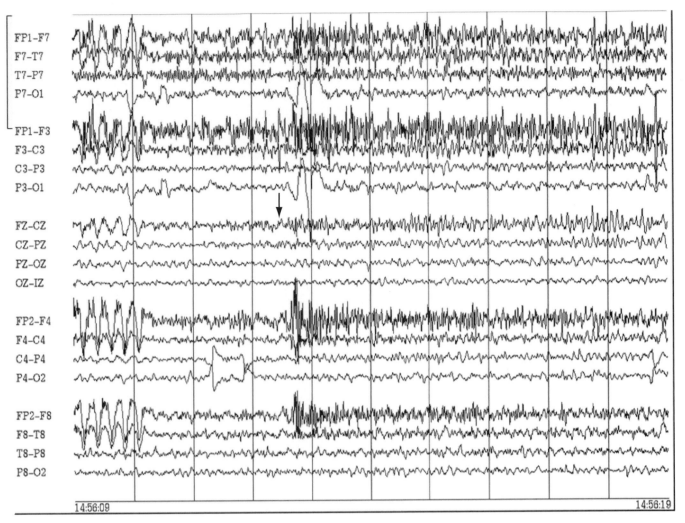

Figure 82.1 Scalp electroencephalogram shows beta-frequency discharge at seizure onset. The discharge is best seen at F_z-C_z (*arrow*) because the channel is less affected by muscle artefact than F_3-C_3 or F_4-C_4. The beta-frequency discharge precedes a higher amplitude and lower frequency rhythmic activity that subsequently builds up and spreads. (From Worrell G, So E, Kazemi J, et al. Focal ictal beta discharge on scalp EEG predicts excellent outcome of frontal lobe epilepsy surgery. *Epilepsia* 2002;43:277–282, with permission.)

glucose uptake (i.e., hypometabolism) that is suggestive of an underlying potentially epileptogenic focus or region.

A review of the literature in 1994 found that approximately 70% of temporal lobe epilepsy patients have temporal lobe hypometabolic abnormalities on their interictal FDG-PETs (51). However, most patients in the studies reviewed had MRI lesions, and most PET images were assessed by visual inspection. Quantitative measurements of FDG uptake increase the sensitivity of PET studies in patients with focal epilepsy (52,53). Using quantitative measurements, a study of mostly temporal lobe epilepsy and some extratemporal lobe epilepsy patients demonstrated that the interictal hypometabolic zone was concordant with the intracranial ictal EEG onset zone in all patients (54). In another study, 75% of patients who had reduced lateral temporal FDG uptake of 15% or more, as compared with the other side, became seizure free after temporal lobectomy (52). This finding is particularly important

because 67% of the patients in the study did not have a relevant MRI lesion. The study also showed that the finding of a hypometabolic temporal lobe is particularly useful when the extracranial ictal electroencephalogram is not localizing.

In contrast to the usefulness of interictal FDG-PET in patients with nonlesional temporal lobe epilepsy, the technique is not as useful in those with extratemporal lobe epilepsy. Whereas the yield of FDG-PET in lesional extratemporal epilepsy is modest (51), the yield declines when MRI is normal or when ictal EEG is indeterminate for seizure onset (55,56). Studies of FDG-PET in patients with nonlesional extratemporal epilepsy have generally reported a low yield. Only 9% of nonlesional extratemporal epilepsy patients have a localized FDG-PET abnormality (51). An exception was a study that reported that 85% of nonlesional frontal lobe epilepsy patients had a unilateral frontal hypometabolic region (57). However, the location of the hypometabolic region observed in that study

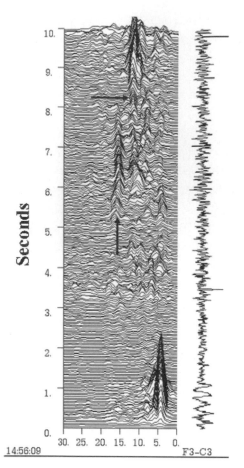

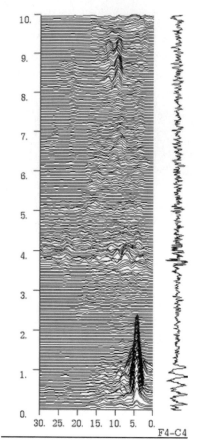

Figure 82.2 Time-frequency analysis of two channels: F_3-C_3 (*left*) and F_4-C_4 (*right*). The graph shows the spectral power (z axis [V^2/m^2]) as a function of time (y axis [seconds]) and frequency (x axis [Hertz]). At seizure onset, there is a 17-Hz discharge at the F_3-C_3 channel (*vertical arrow*). The beta-frequency discharge precedes the buildup of lower-frequency and higher-amplitude activity (*horizontal arrow*). (Adapted from Worrell G, So E, Kazemi J, et al. Focal ictal beta discharge on scalp EEG predicts excellent outcome of frontal lobe epilepsy surgery. *Epilepsia* 2002;43: 277–282, with permission.)

did not correspond to the ictal EEG onset zone in 20% of the patients.

Caution must be exercised when using FDG-PET for localizing the focus for either temporal or extratemporal epilepsy surgery. In temporal lobe epilepsy, the hypometabolic PET defect frequently involves the lateral or inferior neocortical region, even in patients with mesial temporal sclerosis or with mesial temporal ictal onset (58). Furthermore, the abnormal FDG-PET focus is not confined to the temporal lobe in 30% of patients with proven mesial temporal lobe epilepsy. In these patients, the abnormal PET focus extends into the ipsilateral frontal lobe region (59). Similarly, the region of FDG-PET abnormality in patients with suspected frontal lobe epilepsy is often diffuse and poorly localized (55,60). In one study, the size of the hypometabolic region exceeded the ictal EEG onset zone in nearly 40% of patients with nonlesional frontal lobe epilepsy (57).

Despite the low yield of FDG-PET in extratemporal epilepsy, its clinical application is not limited to patients with suspected temporal lobe epilepsy. The clinical and EEG profiles, of many patients with MRI-negative intractable epilepsy are insufficient for classifying with confidence the epilepsy as either temporal or extratemporal, or

for lateralizing with a certainty the seizure onset to one hemisphere. In those situations, the use of such functional imaging tests as PET should be considered as a means of detecting additional evidence for distinguishing between the two main types of focal epilepsy or for lateralizing seizure onset to one hemisphere. The PET abnormality is then used to guide the location and to limit the extent of intracranial electrode implantation. A wide region of PET abnormality that affects both temporal and extratemporal areas can be still be implanted with intracranial electrodes to detect a more discrete focus of ictal EEG onset. PET abnormalities confined to one hemisphere can obviate the need for bilateral hemispheric implantation of intracranial electrodes.

Some PET studies using the central benzodiazepine-receptor binding radiotracer [^{11}C]flumazenil (FMZ) have shown promising results in nonlesional epilepsy surgery patients. Comparison of the extent of reduced FMZ binding defect with the extent of reduced FDG uptake defect shows that in patients with intractable partial epilepsy, the FMZ-PET defect is smaller than the FDG-PET defect (61,62) (Fig. 82.3). The size of the FMZ-PET defect, but not of the FDG-PET defect, is predictive of postsurgical seizure outcome (62). A large FMZ-PET defect is associated with a

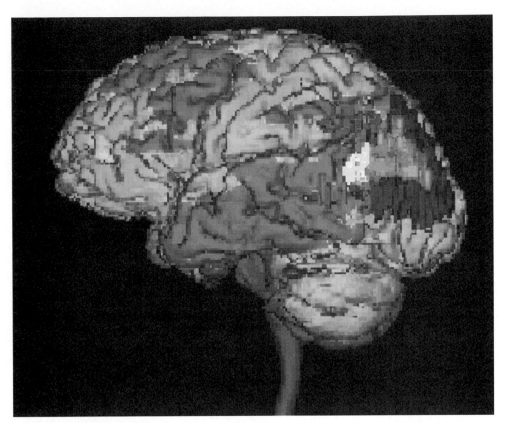

Figure 82.3 Surface distribution of marked 2-deoxy-2-[^{18}F] fluoro-2-deoxy-D-glucose (FDG)-positron emission tomography (PET) (red) and [^{11}C]flumazenil (FMZ)-PET (white) abnormalities, as well as the region of cortical resection (black), in a patient with left posterior parietal seizure focus. The bulk of the cortex with decreased FMZ binding was removed, whereas the majority of the hypometabolic cortex was not resected. The patient has been seizure free for 40 months. (From Juhasz C, Chugani D, Muzik O, et al. Relationship of flumazenil and glucose PET abnormalities to neocortical epilepsy surgery outcome. *Neurology* 2001;56:1650–1658, with permission.) Please see color insert.

poor postsurgical outcome. Patients who became seizure free following epilepsy surgery have a smaller area of FMZ-PET defect remaining after surgical resection. However, several studies using different techniques and criteria for defining FMZ-PET abnormality have found overall low sensitivity of the test in nonlesional partial epilepsy. In a group of patients with either temporal or extratemporal lobe epilepsy, FMZ-PET was reported to be abnormal in only 44% of the patients (63). The rate was even lower, at 23%, in patients with nonlesional extratemporal epilepsy (64). Moreover, FMZ-PET has been reported to have a high rate of false localization of seizure onset focus (63,65). The technique incorrectly localized the seizure onset focus in 2 of 6 patients with nonlesional temporal lobe epilepsy and in 3 of 6 patients with nonlesional frontal lobe epilepsy (63). The disparity in the degree of specificity of FMZ-PET between studies may be a result of differences in techniques used in image acquisition and coregistration to the MRI.

A recent study using the radiotracer α-[^{11}C]methyl-L-tryptophan (AMT) to assess aberrant serotonin synthesis has also yielded encouraging results in patients with nonlesional partial epilepsy (66,67). The study compared AMT-PET with FDG-PET in 27 patients, 19 of whom had normal MRI. The sensitivity of AMT-PET in terms of agreement with intracranial ictal EEG onset was lower than that of FDG-PET (39% versus 73%, respectively), but specificity of AMT-PET was better than that of FDG-PET (100% versus

63%, respectively). Only 9 (47%) of the 19 MRI-negative patients had an abnormal AMT-PET. Another study reports even lower sensitivity of AMT-PET in patients with nonlesional neocortical epilepsy (68). Only 3 (27%) of the 11 nonlesional neocortical epilepsy patients in that study had an AMT-PET abnormality that agreed with the abnormal focus based on electroclinical data. Additional data are needed to determine how AMT-PET relates to outcome of nonlesional epilepsy surgery.

Subtraction Ictal Single-Photon-Emission Computed Tomography Coregistered to Magnetic Resonance Imaging

SPECT radiotracers, such as technetium-hexamethyl propyleneamine oxime (^{99m}Tc-HMPAO) and technetium-ethyl cysteinate dimer (^{99m}Tc-ECD), have properties of rapid cerebral uptake and long half-lives, permitting their intravenous injection soon after seizure onset in order to detect the phenomenon of hyperperfusion associated with seizure activity (i.e., ictal SPECT). The radiotracer can also be injected interictally to detect a hypoperfusion focus that is observed with some seizure foci. However, a meta-analysis of the literature on interictal SPECT concluded that its sensitivity and reliability are very inconsistent, and that ictal SPECT studies are preferred for seizure localization (69). Ictal SPECT is more sensitive than interictal PET in detecting an abnormal focus in MRI-negative patients with epilepsy (70). In addition, the rate of false localization is lower with ictal SPECT than with interictal PET.

The conventional method of interpreting ictal SPECT studies is based on the subjective visual appreciation of differences in perfusion patterns between the ictal and the interictal images. The method has several limitations, however. The overall intensity of the ictal and the interictal images frequently varies because of differences between the two studies in such factors as the amount of radiotracer injected and the time between injection and image acquisition. The subjective visual comparison of the two studies is also limited by differences in the level of image slices, and by the absence of anatomical landmarks in the images of both interictal and ictal studies.

To overcome the shortcomings of the conventional method of reviewing ictal and interictal SPECT images, concepts of digital subtraction of SPECT images and coregistration of the difference images with MRI were proposed and demonstrated (71,72). The subtraction ictal single-photon-emission computed tomography coregistered to magnetic resonance imaging (SISCOM) technique was subsequently developed so that ictal images can be subtracted digitally from interictal images to derive images of the difference in perfusion intensity between the two studies (73) (Fig. 82.4). The technique thresholds the difference image to display only pixels with intensities of perfusion that are more than two standard deviations from the mean. This peak intensity image is then registered on the MRI. The SISCOM technique is superior to the conventional method in detecting a hyperperfusion focus

(sensitivity rates of 88% versus 39%, respectively) (74). Furthermore, the results of SISCOM studies are independently predictive of epilepsy surgery outcome, whereas the results of the conventional method of SPECT reviews are not. Consequently, the following discussion on the use of SPECT in patients with MRI-negative epilepsy is devoted to the SISCOM technique.

SISCOM is useful in individuals with nonlesional epilepsy (74). In a group of 24 patients with either nonlesional temporal lobe or nonlesional extratemporal epilepsy, SISCOM revealed a hyperperfusion focus in 22 patients (91%). Furthermore, the predictive value of SISCOM for surgical outcome was independent of MRI, even when MRI-positive patients were included in the analysis. The rate of excellent postsurgical outcome was nearly 70% when the SISCOM focus was included in the surgical resection, but the rate was only 20% when the SISCOM focus was absent or excluded from the resection.

Despite the best efforts in attempting to inject the SPECT radioligand during seizure activity, the radioligand is often injected postictally instead, especially when seizures are brief in duration. When the seizure activity ends, the initially hyperperfused focus becomes progressively, but transiently, hypoperfused relative to the interictal state (i.e., postictal hypoperfusion) (75,76). Although the prototypical peri-ictal SPECT abnormality is a hyperperfusion focus, the SISCOM method can be adjusted to enhance the detection of postictal hypoperfusion (77). The rate of detecting a hypoperfusion focus using the SISCOM technique is 76%, whereas the rate with the conventional

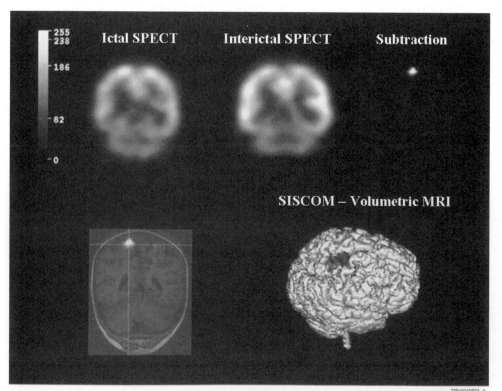

Figure 82.4 Steps to obtaining subtraction ictal SPECT (single-photon emission computed tomography) coregistered to MRI (magnetic resonance imaging) (SISCOM) image. Ictal (*upper left*) and interictal (*upper middle*) SPECT images are obtained. After normalization of their mean intensities and coregistration with each other, subtraction is performed to obtain a "difference" image (*upper right*). The difference image is then coregistered with MRI images at specific planes (*lower left*) or on the surface of a three-dimensional MRI image (*lower right*). (From So E. Role of neuroimaging in the management of seizure disorders. *Mayo Clin Proc* 2002;77:1251–1264, with permission.) Please see color insert.

visual comparison of peri-ictal and ictal images is only 36%.

Although most positive postictal SISCOM studies consist of a hypoperfused region or focus, one-third of positive postictal SISCOM studies still show a hyperperfusion focus. Moreover, ictal SISCOM studies rarely reveal a hypoperfused focus or region instead of a hyperperfusion focus. Therefore, we routinely use the SISCOM technique to assess both hyperperfusion and hypoperfusion changes, regardless of whether the injection was ictal or postictal in timing. This dual method of SISCOM image review is useful specifically in the presurgical evaluation of those with nonlesional extratemporal epilepsy, with SISCOM revealing an abnormal focus in 77% of patients with the disorder (78). When surgical resection involved the SISCOM focus, 55% of the patients had an excellent outcome (78). In contrast, none of the patients had an excellent outcome when surgical resection did not involve the SISCOM focus or when a SISCOM focus was absent (78). The modest rate of 55% excellent outcome in SISCOM-inclusive surgery must be viewed from the historical perspective of only 40% of nonlesional frontal lobe epilepsy patients at the same center having an excellent surgical outcome prior to development and use of the SISCOM technique (18). Of patients in the SISCOM series, 35% had no localized ictal EEG discharges. The intracranial ictal onset of patients in the series often involved the parietal or occipital regions, which harbored eloquent cortex that had restricted the extent of surgical resection. On the other hand, the majority of patients in the earlier non-SISCOM series had wide resection of the frontal lobe, largely unconstrained by the absence of eloquent cortex.

Magnetic Resonance Spectroscopy in Patients with Nonlesional Epilepsy

MRS measures unique magnetic signals induced from specific chemical compounds in the living brain. Cerebral metabolites that are commonly assessed with proton MRS (^{1}H-MRS) include N-acetylaspartate (NAA), creatine (Cr), and choline (Cho) (79). NAA signals reflect neuronal activity or function, whereas Cr and Cho signals originate from glial cells. The most frequently reported MRS abnormality associated with a potentially epileptogenic focus is reduced NAA signal relative to the Cr signal (reduced NAA:Cr ratio). In patients with temporal lobe epilepsy, lateralization of an ^{1}H-MRS abnormality is usually made by detecting an asymmetry between the temporal lobes in the signals of these metabolites. A lower NAA:Cr ratio at one temporal lobe suggests that the seizure focus is located within that lobe (Fig. 82.5).

The yield of ^{1}H-MRS is good in lesional temporal lobe epilepsy. In patients with MRI-detected loss of amygdala-hippocampal volume, the sensitivity of ^{1}H-MRS in revealing a lateralized abnormality is 85%, with nearly all agreeing with the MRI abnormality or the ictal EEG focus (80). However, the yield of ^{1}H-MRS is inconsistent among series of nonlesional temporal lobe epilepsy patients. The proportion of nonlesional temporal lobe epilepsy patients with an ^{1}H-MRS abnormality that lateralized to the ictal EEG focus ranged from 27% to 92% in several different studies (80–83). This wide variation may be a result of differences in the MRS techniques used and to the small number of patients in each reported series. There is still no evidence that an ^{1}H-MRS abnormality involving a nonlesional temporal lobe independently predicts seizure control after surgical resection of the lobe.

Bitemporal ^{1}H-MRS abnormalities are frequently observed in patients with both lesional and nonlesional temporal lobe epilepsy (84,85). As many as 60% of the patients have been reported to have bilateral MRS abnormalities (84). Care must be exercised in treating these patients, in order to ascertain that the temporal lobe to be surgically resected is more severely abnormal than the contralateral temporal lobe. Prognosis for postsurgical seizure freedom is poor when the ^{1}H-MRS at the nonresected temporal lobe is more severely abnormal than the resected temporal lobe (86,87). Moreover, an abnormal ^{1}H-MRS in the language-dominant temporal lobe is associated with verbal memory deficits following contralateral temporal lobectomy (88). Therefore, an important use of MRS is to assess the status of the temporal lobe contralateral to the side of contemplated temporal lobectomy.

Figure 82.5 ^{1}H spectra measured at the temporal lobes (*boxes in middle figure*) of a 40-year-old patient with intractable epilepsy and normal epilepsy-protocol magnetic resonance image. Graphs of the spectra show major peaks of signal intensity corresponding to N-acetylaspartate (NAA) and creatine (Cr). The NAA:Cr ratio at the right temporal region is significantly lower than the control values (*left figure*). The left temporal lobe NAA:Cr ratio is normal (*right figure*). Seizure onset occurred at the right temporal region. The patient has been seizure free following right temporal lobectomy.

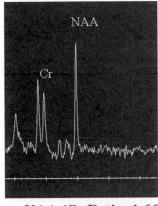

NAA /Cr Ratio=1.66

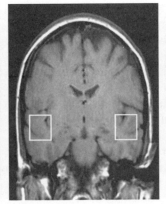

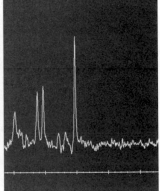

NAA /Cr ratio=1.99

The usefulness of MRS in nonlesional extratemporal epilepsy surgery remains to be proven. In a study of six patients with nonlesional frontal lobe seizure, each of whom had a well-localized ictal EEG focus, the ictal EEG focus had a low NAA:Cr ratio (89). In this study, the localized ictal EEG focus was used to guide placement of the region of interest for ^{1}H-MRS measurement. Otherwise, ^{1}H-MRS measurements could not be efficiently conducted, because the frontal lobes comprise a much larger volume of brain parenchyma than do the temporal lobes. The findings in this study are not applicable to the majority of patients with nonlesional frontal lobe epilepsy, because most of the individuals do not have a well-localized EEG focus to serve as a target for ^{1}H-MRS measurement (26). Patients who do not have an identifiable ictal EEG focus have a greater need for ^{1}H-MRS localization than those who have an ictal EEG focus.

A technique using large regions of interest, with segmentation of the regions into subdivisions, has been used in 20 patients with nonlesional extratemporal epilepsy (90). The sensitivity of the technique in detecting MRS abnormalities was 42%, which corresponded to the localization by other clinical and EEG data. Thus far, this technique has not been shown to influence surgical outcome. MRS abnormalities often extend well beyond the ictal EEG focus in patients with either temporal or extratemporal epilepsy (91,92). This occurred in 35% of patients in one series of temporal lobe and extratemporal epilepsy (91).

Magnetoencephalography in Patients with Nonlesional Epilepsy

MEG is used to localize the magnetic source of spike discharges that are associated with the epileptic focus (93). Because of technical requirements and limitations, MEG recording sessions are typically a few hours in duration; consequently, this technique is limited to the detection and analysis of interictal spike discharges. Ictal recordings can be achieved in a few selected patients whose seizures are very frequent or inducible (94–96).

The localization of magnetoencephalographic interictal spikes in lesional epilepsy correlates well with location of the MRI lesion. MEG further identifies irritative tissues in the proximity of the lesion (97,98). Although EEG spikes are usually more abundant than magnetoencephalographic spikes (99), magnetoencephalographic spikes are still detectable in 73% to 84% of epilepsy surgery candidates with either lesional or nonlesional MRI (100,101). However, in one study of lesional and nonlesional patients with either temporal or extratemporal epilepsy, only 52% of MEG procedures were concordant, and 14% were discordant, with the epileptogenic focus (102).

Thus far, data on the experience of MEG in nonlesional epilepsy surgery involve only a small number of patients in each reported series (100,101,103–109). In one study, MEG was able to localize the source of spikes in 11 (91%) of 12 patients with MRI-negative temporal or extratemporal epilepsy (101). The location of the magnetoencephalographic spikes corresponded to the localization by electroclinical data. The sensitivity of MEG in detecting interictal spikes was only 32% in another study limited to patients with nonlesional mesial temporal lobe epilepsy (109). The correlation between magnetoencephalographic localization and electrocorticographic findings was only partial in these patients (109). The discrepancy in the yield of MEG between these two studies may be because the latter study did not include patients with lateral neocortical epilepsy. The sensitivity of MEG in detecting spikes is not uniform between regions of the brain. Spike discharges that are restricted to the mesial temporal regions are not as easily detected by MEG as are discharges occurring at the lateral neocortical regions (101,110–112). Accordingly, MEG studies in extratemporal neocortical epilepsy have higher yields than do studies in patients with temporal lobe epilepsy (104,113). In one report on 11 children with nonlesional extratemporal neocortical epilepsy, MEG localization of interictal spikes in 10 patients (91%) corresponded to the ictal onset zone as defined by intracranial EEG recording (104). Nine patients (82%) became seizure free or had greater than 90% seizure reduction following surgical resection or multiple subpial transection of the ictal onset zone and the surrounding irritative cortex. Another study demonstrated that the extent of resection of the magnetoencephalographic abnormality in patients with nonlesional extratemporal epilepsy is significantly associated with the rate of postsurgical seizure freedom (107). Eight (89%) of 9 patients who had complete resection of the magnetoencephalographic abnormality became seizure free, compared with only 1 (9%) of 11 patients whose magnetoencephalographic abnormality was either incompletely resected or not resected.

In both lesional and nonlesional temporal lobe epilepsy, there is a good but not absolute correspondence between dipole orientation of magnetoencephalographic spikes and the location of seizure onset within the temporal lobe (114). Intracranial EEG seizures occurred at the lateral neocortical region in 82% of patients with posterior temporal vertical orientation of magnetoencephalographic dipoles, but in no patients with anterior temporal vertical dipole orientation. Nonetheless, 15% of patients with anterior temporal horizontal dipoles also had EEG seizure onsets at the lateral neocortical region (103). In patients with nonlesional epilepsy, MEG cannot be relied on solely for surgical resection of selective areas of the brain (115). Magnetoencephalographic spikes indicate the probable location of the center of epileptiform activity, but they do not represent the entire extent of the irritative zone (106). Intracranial EEG recordings need to be considered to delineate the full extent of the irritative and the ictal onset zones prior to surgery. MEG localization is useful in guiding the location and the extent of the intracranial electrode implantation in patients with nonlesional epilepsy (100).

The complementary roles of MEG and electroencephalography must be recognized (116,117). MEG records tangentially oriented magnetic fields generated by spike discharges, whereas electroencephalography preferentially records radially oriented electrical fields of spike discharges. The superiority of MEG in spatial resolution complements the benefit of electroencephalography in temporal resolution. One advantage of MEG over electroencephalography in the clinical setting is in the evaluation of patients with prior craniotomy or cranial injury (118). In these patients, magnetoencephalographic signals are less distorted by skull or dural defects than are EEG signals.

OPERATIVE STRATEGY IN NONLESIONAL EPILEPSY SURGERY

Intracranial Electrode Implantation

Intracranial electrode implantation and recording are required in most cases of nonlesional epilepsy surgery, especially when the suspected focus is in the extratemporal region. Intracranial electrode implantation should be performed to delineate fully the location and the extent of the ictal onset zone and its associated irritative zones, as well as to identify any neighboring eloquent cortex that needs to be spared of the surgery. Intracranial electrode implantation can be obviated in some patients who possess sufficient noninvasive electroclinical and functional imaging abnormalities that are concordant in identifying an abnormal focus that is distant from eloquent cortex. Such a situation is more obvious when a standard anterior temporal lobectomy is already the preferred surgical technique, especially in epilepsy involving the nondominant temporal lobe (52,119). Otherwise, to optimize postsurgical seizure control and to minimize perioperative complications intracranial electrodes have to be implanted for tailoring the extent of surgical resection or transection.

Ideally, the location and extent of electrode implantation in patients with nonlesional epilepsy should not be dictated exclusively by the results of a single diagnostic modality. False localization has occurred with each of the diagnostic modalities discussed in the previous sections (30,115,120–122). Concordance of the results from clinical, electrophysiologic, and functional imaging evaluation enhances confidence in selecting the site for intracranial electrode implantation or surgical treatment (Fig. 82.6).

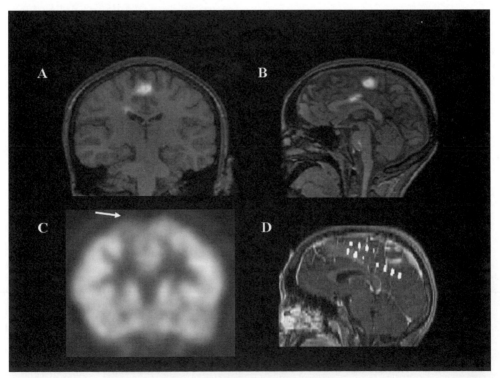

Figure 82.6 A: Coronal view of subtraction ictal SPECT (single-photon emission computed tomography) coregistered to magnetic resonance imaging (MRI) (SISCOM) showing an apparently midline hyperperfusion focus in a 13-year-old male who had between 1 and 10 attacks per night of bilateral extremity movements and facial grimacing. Epilepsy-protocol MRI was normal and scalp ictal electroencephalogram was nonlocalizing. **B:** Sagittal view of SISCOM shows that the hyperperfusion focus was at the right posterior mesial frontal region. **C:** 2-[18F]fluoro-2-deoxy-D-glucose (FDG)-positron emission tomography (PET) shows a hypometabolic focus corresponding to the SISCOM hyperperfusion focus. **D:** MRI with coregistered CT (computed tomography)-derived images of subdural electrode contacts (white marks) on the SISCOM and PET abnormalities. The intracranial EEG recording confirmed ictal onset at the SISCOM and PET abnormalities. Surgical resection of the region rendered the patient free of seizures, with minimal weakness in the left toes. Pathologic examination of the specimen revealed cortical dysplasia. Please see color insert.

Electrode implantation should be guided by consistent results from the various diagnostic modalities. If the modalities reveal conflicting findings or if only one modality has localizing features, more extensive implantation may have to be considered to ensure that ictal onset and irritative zones are not overlooked.

There are patients whose electroclinical data and functional imaging studies are all devoid of clues as to the potential location of the seizure focus. These patients are generally considered to be poor surgical candidates. Continued pursuit of seizure localization would require extensive bilateral hemisphere implantation with subdural electrodes, or selective implantation of both hemispheres with strip and depth electrodes. The risk-to-benefit ratio of these approaches should be carefully weighed in each patient. Every effort must be made to note any lateralizing feature in the diagnostic modalities, which, when present, may warrant the concentration of electrodes in one hemisphere or at one region. For instance, a combination of neuropsychological test and intracarotid amobarbital test (Wada test) results has been shown to lateralize correctly the epileptogenic temporal lobe in 81% of patients whose temporal lobes did not show mesial temporal sclerosis (123).

The previous discussion on noninvasive diagnostic modalities demonstrates that the abnormality revealed by each modality does not always match the ictal EEG onset zone or the irritative zone (91,92,121,124,125). Currently, no evidence in nonlesional epilepsy favors resection of the functional imaging abnormality over resection of the abnormal EEG focus, or vice versa. To date, the extent of resection has prognostic implications in three functional imaging modalities: SISCOM, MEG, and the FMZ-PET.

Nonetheless, EEG abnormalities were not completely disregarded in the studies that evaluated these three modalities. Therefore, the putative principle and practice in nonlesional epilepsy surgery is to resect both functional imaging and EEG abnormalities, whenever this can be safely accomplished. A FDG-PET abnormality can appear very diffuse, such that complete resection of the abnormality may be impractical or unsafe. In planning the extent of surgical resection in such a situation, the relationship between the diffuse functional imaging abnormality and the EEG abnormality must be fully elucidated in each patient. For this purpose, intracranial electrode coverage should encompass as much as possible the functional imaging abnormality and also extend beyond its dimensions. The extent of the coverage is also dictated by the proximity of the abnormalities to anatomical structures that serve critical cortical functions, such as cognitive, speech, or motor functions. For this purpose, the integration of images of functional imaging, electroencephalography, and cortical functions into the patient's MRI is essential when planning electrode implantation and surgical resection or transection.

Integration of Multimodality Images for Surgical Planning

The spatial concordance of abnormalities of different diagnostic modalities can be assessed by coregistering the abnormalities on the background of the patient's brain MRI (71,126) (Fig. 82.7). The coregistration makes it possible to study the spatial relationship of the abnormalities to each other, and also to appreciate their relationship to neuroanatomical structures. Computed tomography (CT)- or

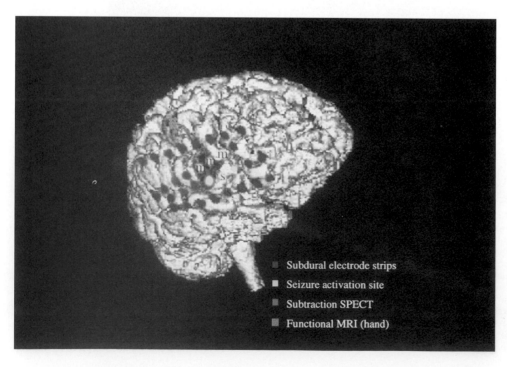

■ Subdural electrode strips
■ Seizure activation site
■ Subtraction SPECT
■ Functional MRI (hand)

Figure 82.7 Three-dimensional rendition of MRI (magnetic resonance imaging) of brain with coregistration of sensory area of the hand identified with functional MRI (green), subtraction ictal SPECT (single-photon emission computed tomography) coregistered to MRI (SISCOM) hyperperfusion focus (red), subdural electrodes (blue), and electrodes where electroencephalograph-detected seizures commenced (yellow). m = electrode sites where facial motor activity was elicited with electrocortical stimulation; s = electrode site where sensory function was elicited. (From So E. Role of neuroimaging in the management of seizure disorders. *Mayo Clin Proc* 2002;77: 1251–1264, with permission.) Please see color insert.

Figure 82.8 A: Three-dimensional reconstruction of the patient's head from frameless stereotactic MRI (magnetic resonance imaging) procedure showing scalp fiduciary markers (*lower arrow*) and the surface-rendered subtraction ictal SPECT (single-photon emission computed tomography) coregistered to MRI (SISCOM) focus (*upper arrow*). **B:** Scalp fiduciary markers are then registered into a computer to create a transformational matrix, so that the MRI image space can be related to the physical space of the patient's head. **C:** During surgery, the surgeon uses a probe to point at the location in the operative field. **D:** The surgeon views the computer screen where the crosshairs indicate how close the tip of the probe is to the SISCOM-detected abnormality. This observation is used to guide implantation of intracranial electrodes or surgical resection or transection of the abnormal focus. (Adapted from So E, O'Brien T, Brinkmann B, et al. The EEG evaluation of single photon emission computed tomography: abnormalities in epilepsy. *J Clin Neurophysiol* 2000;17:10–28 and So E. Integration of EEG, MRI, and SPECT in the evaluation of patients for epilepsy surgery. *Epilepsia* 2000; 41 (Suppl 3):S48–S54, with permission.)

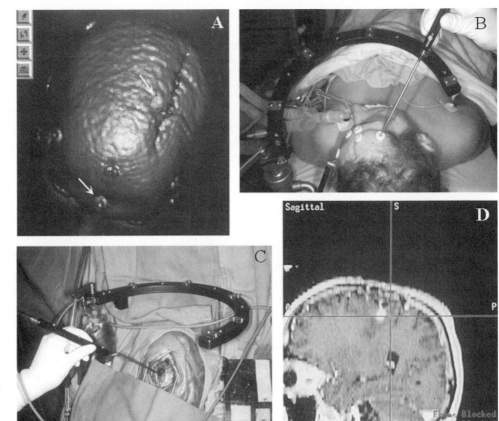

MRI-derived images of intracranial electrodes also can be registered on the patient's brain MRI. At the conclusion of the prolonged video-EEG monitoring session, the location of the ictal onset and interictal discharges can be noted on the coregistered intracranial electrodes. Through this method, the irritative and the ictal onset zones are related topographically to the functional imaging abnormalities. The risk of surgery in compromising eloquent functions of the brain can be inferred by recognizing the underlying and surrounding MRI anatomy, then subsequently confirmed by using the implanted electrodes to electrically stimulate the cortical surface.

The resultant MRI image, with coregistered images of physiologic and pathologic functions, serves as a map for planning and guiding surgical treatment in patients with nonlesional epilepsy. However, allowances must be made for a small, inherent degree of error when coregistering images on the MRI. Therefore, the coregistration technique used must be validated to determine the "worst case" degree of error (71,73).

Image-Guided Navigational Surgical Technique

During surgery for nonlesional epilepsy, the surgeon has to be able to determine how the images of different diagnostic modalities correspond to the surgically exposed brain surface (126,127). The Stealth Image Guided System (128) can be used to relate the MRI graphic space to the physical space of the operative field (Fig. 82.8). The technology requires the presurgical performance of a frameless stereotactic MRI procedure that registers 10 fiduciary scalp markers into an MRI matrix. After this procedure, the positions of these fiduciary scalp markers are manually registered by an infrared probe into a transformational matrix. With the use of the transformational matrix during surgery, the surgeon can see how a spot on the patient's exposed brain relates to the location of the functional imaging abnormality on the MRI. This is accomplished by pointing the tip of a probe at the spot of interest on the exposed brain. The tip of the probe is represented by crosshairs on the computer screen that illustrate the MRI containing the functional imaging abnormality. The cursor guides the surgeon's movement of the probe in locating the functional imaging abnormality on the exposed brain surface. This technology makes it possible to locate the functional imaging abnormality on a normal-appearing brain surface. The technology is especially useful when a discrete functional imaging abnormality, such as a SISCOM focus, is the target of electrode implantation. After the electrodes are implanted, a CT scan or MRI is performed to derive images of the electrode contacts, in order for these images to be segmented and registered on the patient's MRI, along with the SISCOM focus. When ictal or interictal EEG abnormalities are recorded during the long-term video-EEG monitoring, the active electrode contacts can be identified on the MRI, and their relationship to the SISCOM focus can be assessed.

This image-guided navigational technology is also used for surgically resecting or transecting areas of functional imaging and electrophysiologic abnormalities. This technique makes it possible to identify the location of the electrode contacts that recorded abnormal EEG activity or critical cortical functions, even when the electrodes have been removed to allow surgical resection or transection of underlying brain tissue.

SUMMARY

Epilepsy surgery in the absence of an MRI lesion presents special challenges in the presurgical identification and the surgical treatment of the epileptogenic focus. Evidence of lateralizing or localizing abnormalities must be sought from noninvasive sources and tests, specifically from the results of clinical, electrophysiologic, neuropsychologic, and functional imaging studies. The limitations and drawbacks of each noninvasive or minimally invasive modality must be considered. Concordance of the results serves as an important basis for further evaluation with invasive EEG recording, or, in some cases, for obviating the need for invasive recording.

The absence of a visible abnormality on the surgically exposed brain makes it essential to use the technology of image-guided navigational surgery. This technique makes it possible to accurately implant, resect, or transect parts of the brain that correspond to areas of functional imaging and electrophysiologic abnormalities. As much as possible, intracranial electrodes should cover the cortical tissue that immediately surrounds the functional imaging abnormality. The electrodes should also cover neighboring structures that can potentially serve important brain functions, so that mapping of these functions can be performed. Patients should understand that the outcome of nonlesional epilepsy surgery is generally not as favorable as that of lesional surgery.

REFERENCES

1. Boon P, Williamson P, Fried I, et al. Intracranial, intraaxial, space-occupying lesions in patients with intractable partial epilepsy: an anatomoclinical, neuropsychological, and surgical correlation. *Epilepsia* 1991;32:467–476.
2. Cascino G, Boon P, Fish D. Surgically remediable lesional syndromes. In: Engel JJ, ed. *Surgical treatment of the epilepsies*. New York: Raven Press, 1993:77–86.
3. Garcia P, Laxer K, Barbaro N, et al. Prognostic value of magnetic resonance imaging hippocampal abnormalities in patients undergoing temporal lobectomy for medically refractory seizures. *Epilepsia* 1994;35:520–524.
4. Radahkrishnan K, So E, Silbert P, et al. Predictors of outcome of anterior temporal lobectomy for intractable epilepsy. A multivariate study. *Neurology* 1998;51:465–471.
5. Jack C Jr, Theodore W, Cook M, et al. MRI-based hippocampal volumetrics: data acquisition, normal ranges, and optimal protocol. *Magn Reson Imag* 1995;13:1057–1064.
6. Bergin P, Fish D, Shorvon E, et al. Magnetic resonance imaging in partial epilepsy: Additional abnormalities shown with fluid attenuated inversion recovery (FLAIR) pulse sequence. *J Neurol Neurosurg Psychiatr* 1995;58:439–443.
7. Von Oertzen J, Urbach H, Jungbluth S, et al. Standard magnetic resonance imaging is inadequate for patients with refractory focal epilepsy. *J Neurol Neurosurg Pyschiatr* 2002;73:643–647.
8. Guidelines for neuroimaging evaluation of patients with uncontrolled epilepsy considered for surgery. Commission on Neuroimaging of the International League Against Epilepsy. *Epilepsia* 1998;39:1375–1376.
9. Spencer S, Lee SA. Nonlesional neocortical epilepsy: invasive evaluation. In: Luders H, Comair Y, eds. *Epilepsy surgery*. Philadelphia: Lippincott Williams & Wilkins, 2001:1026–1033.
10. Hughes J, Adams C. Pathological findings in 50 cases of temporal lobe epilepsy (partial complex seizures) treated by anterior temporal lobectomy. In: Proter R, ed. *Advances in epileptology. XV International Epilepsy Symposium*. New York: Raven Press, 1984:457–462.
11. Porter B, Judkins A, Clancey R, et al. Dysplasia. A common finding in intractable pediatric temporal lobe epilepsy. *Neurology* 2003;61:365–368.
12. Kasper B, Stefan H, Buchfelder M, et al. Temporal lobe microdysgenesis in epilepsy versus control brains. *J Neuropathol Exp Neurol* 1999;58:22–28.
13. Lencz T, McCarthy G, Bronen R, et al. Quantitative magnetic resonance imaging in temporal lobe epilepsy: relationship to neuropathology and neuropsychological function. *Ann Neurol* 1992;31:629–637.
14. Jackson G, Kuzniecky R, Cascino G. Hippocampal sclerosis without detectable hippocampal atrophy. *Neurology* 1994;44:42–46.
15. Rugg-Gunn F, Harrison N, Duncan J. Evaluation of the accuracies of seizure description by relatives of patients with epilepsy. *Epilepsy Res* 2001;443:193–199.
16. Chee M, Kotagal P, Van Ness P, et al. Lateralizing signs in intractable partial epilepsy: blinded multiple-observer analysis. *Neurology* 1993;43:2519–2525.
17. Manford M, Fish D, Shorvon S. An analysis of clinical seizure patterns and their localizing value in frontal and temporal lobe epilepsies. *Brain* 1996;119:17–40.
18. Mosewich R, So E, O'Brien T, et al. Factors predictive of the outcome of frontal lobe epilepsy surgery. *Epilepsia* 2000;41:843–849.
19. Cambier D, Cascino G, So E, et al. Video-EEG monitoring in patients with hippocampal atrophy. *Acta Neurol Scand* 2001;103:1–7.
20. Worrell G, So E, Kazemi J, et al. Focal ictal beta discharge on scalp EEG predicts excellent outcome of frontal lobe epilepsy surgery. *Epilepsia* 2002;43:277–282.
21. Dodrill C, Wilkus R, Ojemann G, et al. Multi-disciplinary prediction of seizure relief from cortical resection surgery. *Ann Neurol* 1986;20:2–12.
22. Kellaway P. The incidence, significance, and natural history of spike foci in children. In: Henry C, ed. *Current clinical neurophysiology: update on EEG and evoked potentials*. Amsterdam: Elsevier, 1980:171–175.
23. Williamson P, Boon P, Thadani V, et al. Parietal lobe epilepsy: diagnostic considerations and results of surgery. *Ann Neurol* 1992;31:193–201.
24. Williamson P, Thadani V, Darcey T, et al. Occipital lobe epilepsy: clinical characteristics, seizure spread patterns and results of surgery. *Ann Neurol* 1992;31:3.
25. Vadlamudi L, So E, Worrell G, et al. Factors underlying scalp interictal discharges in intractable frontal lobe epilepsy. *Epilepsia* 2001;42(Suppl 7):28.
26. Quesney L, Constain M, Rasmussen T, et al. Presurgical EEG investigation in frontal lobe epilepsy. *Epilepsy Res* 1992;5(Suppl):55–69.
27. Pataraia E, Lurger S, Serles W, et al. Ictal EEG in unilateral mesial temporal lobe epilepsy. *Epilepsia* 1998;39:608–614.
28. Walczak T, Radtke R, Lewis D. Accuracy and interobserver reliability of scalp ictal EEG. *Neurology* 1992;42:2279–2285.
29. Blume W, Ravindran J, Lowry N. Late lateralizing and localizing features of scalp-recorded temporal lobe seizures. *J Clin Neurophysiol* 1998;15:514–520.

30. Sirven J, Liporace J, French J, et al. Seizures in temporal epilepsy: reliability of scalp/sphenoidal ictal reading. *Neurology* 1997;48: 1041–1046.
31. Risinger M, Engel J Jr, Van Ness P, et al. Ictal localization of temporal lobe seizures with scalp/sphenoidal recordings. *Neurology* 1989;39:1288–1293.
32. Bautista E, Spencer D, Spencer S. EEG findings in frontal lobe epilepsies. *Neurology* 1998;50:1765–1771.
33. Foldvary N, Klem G, Hammel M, et al. The localizing value of ictal EEG in focal epilepsy. *Neurology* 2001;57:2022–2028.
34. Cascino G, Andermann F, Berkovic S. Gelastic seizures and hypothalamic hamartomas: evaluation of patients undergoing chronic intracranial EEG monitoring and outcome of surgical treatment. *Neurology* 1993;43:747–750.
35. Palmini A, Andermann F, Dubeau F, et al. Occipitotemporal epilepsies: evaluation of selected patients requiring depth electrode studies and surgical approaches. *Epilepsia* 1993;34: 84–96.
36. Isnard J, Guenot M, Ostrowsky K, et al. The role of insular cortex in temporal lobe epilepsy. *Ann Neurol* 2000;48:614–623.
37. Sammaritano M, de Lotbiniere A, Andermann F, et al. False lateralization by surface EEG of seizure onset in patients with temporal lobe epilepsy and gross focal cerebral lesions. *Ann Neurol* 1987;21:361–369.
38. Lee S, Yun C, Oh J, et al. Intracranial ictal onset zone in nonlesional lateral temporal lobe epilepsy on scalp ictal EEG. *Neurology* 2003;61:757–764.
39. Fernandez G, Hufnagel A, Van Roost D, et al. Safety of intrahippocampal depth electrodes for presurgical evaluation of patients with intractable epilepsy. *Epilepsia* 1997;38:922–929.
40. Swartz B, Rich J, Dwan P, et al. The safety and efficacy of chronically implanted subdural electrodes: a prospective study. *Surg Neurol* 1996;46:87–93.
41. Hamer H, Morris H, Mascha E, et al. Complications of invasive video-EEG monitoring with subdural grids. *Neurology* 2002;58: 98–103.
42. Cascino G, Kelly P, Sharbrough F, et al. Long-term follow-up of stereotactic lesionectomy in partial epilepsy: predictive factors and electroencephalographic results. *Epilepsia* 1992;33: 639–644.
43. Clarke D, Olivier A, Andermann F, et al. Surgical treatment of epilepsy: the problem of lesion/focus incongruence. *Surg Neurol* 1996;46:585–586.
44. Bautista R, Cobbs M, Spencer D, et al. Prediction of surgical outcome by interictal epileptiform abnormalities during intracranial EEG monitoring in patients with extrahippocampal seizures. *Epilepsia* 1999;40:880–890.
45. Engel JJ, Shewmon A. Who should be considered a surgical candidate? In: Engel JJ, ed. *Surgical treatment of the epilepsies.* New York: Raven Press, 1993:23–34.
46. Schiller Y, Cascino G, Sharbrough F. Chronic intracranial EEG monitoring for localizing the epileptogenic zone: an electroclinical correlation. *Epilepsia* 1998;39:1302–1308.
47. Palmini A, Gloor P. The localizing value of auras in partial seizures: a prospective and retrospective study. *Neurology* 1992;42: 801–808.
48. Serles W, Caramanos Z, Lindinger E, et al. Combining ictal surface-electroencephalography and seizure semiology improves lateralization in temporal lobe epilepsy. *Epilepsia* 2000;41: 1567–1573.
49. Holmes M, Kutsky R, Ojemann G, et al. Interictal, unifocal spikes in refractory extratemporal epilepsy predict ictal origin and postsurgical outcome. *Epilepsy Res* 2000;111:1802–1808.
50. Kanner A, Morris H, Luders H, et al. Usefulness of unilateral interictal sharp waves of temporal lobe origin in prolonged video-EEG monitoring studies. *Epilepsia* 1993;34:884–889.
51. Spencer S. The relative contributions of MRI, SPECT, and PET imaging in epilepsy. *Epilepsia* 1994;35(Suppl 6):S72–S89.
52. Theodore W, Sato S, Kufta C, et al. Temporal lobectomy for uncontrolled seizures: the role for positron emission tomography. *Ann Neurol* 1992;32:789–794.
53. Manno E, Sperling M, Ding X, et al. Predictors of outcome after anterior temporal lobectomy: positron emission tomography. *Neurology* 1994;44:2331–2336.

54. Theodore W, Sato S, Kufta C, et al. FDG-positron emission tomography and invasive EEG: seizure focus detection and surgical outcome. *Epilepsia* 1997;38:81–86.
55. Henry T, Sutherling W, Engel J, et al. Interictal cerebral metabolism in partial epilepsies of neocortical origin. *Epilepsy Res* 1991;10:174–182.
56. Abou-Khalil B, Kuzniecky R, Kessler R, et al. Positron emission tomography in extratemporal epilepsy. *Epilepsia* 1993;34:121.
57. da Silva E, Chugani D, Muzik O, et al. Identification of frontal lobe epileptic foci in children using positron emission tomography. *Epilepsia* 1997;38:1198–1208.
58. Hajek M, Antonini A, Leenders K, et al. Mesiobasal versus lateral temporal lobe epilepsy: metabolic differences in the temporal lobe shown by interictal ^{18}F-FDG positron emission tomography. *Neurology* 1993;43:79.
59. Engel JJ, Henry T, Swartz B. Positron emission tomography in frontal lobe epilepsy. In: Jasper H, Riggio S, Goldman-Rakic S, eds. *Epilepsy and the functional anatomy of the frontal lobe.* New York: Raven Press, 1995:223–238.
60. Swartz B, Halgren E, Delgado-Escueta A, et al. Neuroimaging in patients with seizures of probable frontal lobe origin. *Epilepsia* 1989;30:547–558.
61. Henry T. Functional neuroimaging with positron emission tomography. *Epilepsia* 1996;37:1141–1154.
62. Juhasz C, Chugani D, Muzik O, et al. Relationship of flumazenil and glucose PET abnormalities to neocortical epilepsy surgery outcome. *Neurology* 2001;56:1650–1658.
63. Ryvlin R, Bouvard S, Le Bars D, et al. Clinical utility of flumazenil-PET versus [^{18}F]fluorodeoxyglucose-PET and MRI in refractory partial epilepsy: a prospective study in 100 patients. *Brain* 1998;121:2067–2081.
64. Richardson MP, Keopp M, Brooks D, et al. ^{11}C-flumazenil PET in neocortical epilepsy. *Neurology* 1998;51:485–492.
65. Keopp M, Hammers A, Labbe C, et al. ^{11}C-flumazenil PET in patients with refractory temporal lobe epilepsy and normal MRI. *Neurology* 2000;54:332–339.
66. Chugani D, Chugani H. PET mapping of serotonin synthesis. In: Henry T, Duncan J, Berkovic S, eds. *Functional imaging in the epilepsies.* Philadelphia: Lippincott Williams & Wilkins, 2000:165–171.
67. Juhasz C, Chugani D, Muzik O, et al. Alpha-methyl-L-tryptophan PET detects epileptogenic cortex in children with intractable epilepsy. *Neurology* 2003;60:960–968.
68. Fedi M, Reutens D, Okazawa H, et al. Localizing value of alpha-methyl-L-tryptophan PET in intractable epilepsy of neocortical origin. *Neurology* 2001;57:1629–1636.
69. Devous M Sr, Thisted R, Morgan G, et al. SPECT imaging in epilepsy: a meta-analysis. *J Nucl Med* 1998;39:285–293.
70. Ho S, Berkovic S, Berlangieri S, et al. Comparison of ictal SPECT and interictal PET in the presurgical evaluation of temporal lobe epilepsy. *Ann Neurol* 1995;37:738–774.
71. Erickson B, Jack CJ. Correlation of single photon emission CT with MR image data. *AJNR Am J Neuroradiol* 1993;14:713–720.
72. Zubal G, Spencer S, Imam K, et al. Difference images calculated from ictal and interictal technetium-99m-HMPAO SPECT scans of epilepsy. *J Nucl Med* 1995;36:684–689.
73. O'Brien T, O'Connor MK, Mullan BP, et al. Subtraction ictal SPECT co-registered to MRI in partial epilepsy: description and technical validation of the method with phantom and patient studies. *Nucl Med Commun* 1998;19:31–45.
74. O'Brien T, So EL, Mullan BP, et al. Subtraction ictal SPECT co-registered to MRI improves clinical usefulness of SPECT in localizing the surgical seizure focus. *Neurology* 1998;50:445–454.
75. Rowe C, Berkovic S, Austin M, et al. Patterns of postictal cerebral blood flow in temporal lobe epilepsy: qualitative and quantitative analysis. *Neurology* 1991;41:1096–1103.
76. Ho S, Berkovic S, Newton M, et al. Parietal lobe epilepsy: clinical features and seizure localization by ictal SPECT. *Neurology* 1994;44:2277–2284.
77. O'Brien T, So E, Mullan B, et al. Subtraction SPECT co-registered to MRI improves postictal SPECT localization of seizure foci. *Neurology* 1999;52:137–146.
78. O'Brien T, So E, Mullan P, et al. Subtraction peri-ictal SPECT is predictive of extratemporal epilepsy surgery outcome. *Neurology* 2000;55:1668–1676.

79. Garcia P, Laxer K. Magnetic resonance spectroscopy. In: Latchaw R, Jack CJ, eds. *Epilepsy.* Philadelphia: WB Saunders, 1995:675–682.

80. Cendes F, Caramanos Z, Andermann F, et al. Proton magnetic resonance spectroscopic imaging and magnetic resonance imaging volumetry in the lateralization of temporal lobe epilepsy: a series of 100 patients. *Ann Neurol* 1997;42:737–746.

81. Woermann F, McLean M, Bartlett P, et al. Short echo time single-voxel ^{1}H magnetic resonance spectroscopy in magnetic resonance imaging-negative temporal lobe epilepsy: different biochemical profile compared with hippocampal sclerosis. *Ann Neurol* 1999;45:369–376.

82. Ng T, Comair Y, Xue M, et al. Temporal lobe epilepsy: presurgical localisation with proton chemical shift imaging. *Radiology* 1994;193:465–472.

83. Connelly A, Van Paesschen W, Porter D, et al. Proton magnetic resonance spectroscopy in MRI-negative epilepsy. *Neurology* 1998;51:61–66.

84. Maton B, Gilliam F, Sawrie S, et al. Correlation of scalp EEG and ^{1}H-MRS metabolic abnormalities in temporal lobe epilepsy. *Epilepsia* 2001;42:417–422.

85. Conelly A, Jackson G, Duncan J, et al. Magnetic resonance spectroscopy in temporal lobe epilepsy. *Neurology* 1994;4:1411–1417.

86. Kuzniecky R, Hugg J, Hetherington H, et al. Predictive value of ^{1}H MRSI outcome in temporal lobectomy. *Neurology* 1999;53:694–698.

87. Suhy J, Laxer K, Capizzano A, et al. ^{1}H-MRSI predicts surgical outcome in MRI-negative temporal lobe epilepsy. *Neurology* 2002;58:821–823.

88. Incisa della Rochetta A, Gadian D, Connelly A, et al. Verbal memory impairment after right temporal lobe surgery: the role of contralateral damage as revealed by ^{1}H magnetic resonance spectroscopy and T_2 relaxometry. *Neurology* 1995;45:797–802.

89. Garcia P, Laxer K, van der Grond J, et al. Proton magnetic resonance spectroscopic imaging in patients with frontal lobe epilepsy. *Ann Neurol* 1995;37:279.

90. Stanley J, Cendes F, Dubeau F, et al. Proton magnetic resonance spectroscopic imaging in patients with extratemporal epilepsy. *Epilepsia* 1998;39:267–273.

91. Li L, Andermann F, Dubeau F, et al. Spatial extent of neuronal metabolic dysfunction measured by proton MR spectroscopic imaging in patients with localization-related epilepsy. *Epilepsia* 2000;41:666–674.

92. Mueller S, Suhy J, Laxer K, et al. Reduced extrahippocampal NAA in mesial temporal lobe epilepsy. *Epilepsia* 2002;43:1210–1216.

93. Ebersole J, Squires K, Eliashiv S, et al. Applications of magnetic source imaging in evaluation of candidates for epilepsy surgery. *Neuroimaging Clin N Am* 1995;5:267–288.

94. Sutherling WW, Crandall PH, Engel J Jr, et al. The magnetic field of complex partial seizures agrees with intracranial localizations. *Ann Neurol* 1987;21:548–558.

95. Eliashiv D, Elsas M, Squires K, et al. Ictal magnetic source imaging as a localizing tool in partial epilepsy. *Neurology* 2002;59:1600–1610.

96. Assaf B, Karkar K, Laxer K, et al. Ictal magnetoencephalography in temporal and extratemporal lobe epilepsy. *Epilepsia* 2003;44:1320–1327.

97. Stefan H, Schuler P, Abraham-Fuchs K, et al. Magnetic source localization and morphological changes in temporal lobe epilepsy: comparison of MEG/EEG, ECoG and volumetric MRI in presurgical evaluation of operated patients. *Acta Neurol Scand Suppl* 1994;152:83–88.

98. Otsubo H, Ochi A, Elliott I, et al. MEG predicts epileptic zone in lesional extrahippocampal epilepsy: 12 pediatric surgery cases. *Epilepsia* 2001;42:1523–1530.

99. Sutherling W, Crandall P, Cahan L, et al. The magnetic field of epileptic spikes agrees with intracranial localizations in complex partial epilepsy. *Neurology* 1988;38:778–786.

100. Smith JR, Schwartz B, Gallen C, et al. Utilization of multichannel magnetoencephalography in the guidance of ablative seizure surgery. *J Epilepsy* 1995;8:119–130.

101. Knowlton R, Laxer K, Aminoff M, et al. Magnetoencephalography in partial epilepsy: clinical yield and localization accuracy. *Ann Neurol* 1997;42:622–631.

102. Wheless JW, Willmore LJ, Breier JI, et al. A comparison of magnetoencephalography, MRI, and V-EEG in patients evaluated for epilepsy surgery. *Epilepsia* 1999;40:931–941.

103. Ebersole J. Classification of MEG spikes in temporal lobe epilepsy. In: Yoshimoto T, Kotani, M, Kuriki S, et al., eds. *Recent advances in biomagnetism.* Sendai, Japan: Tohuku University Press, 1999:758–761.

104. Minassian B, Otsubo H, Weiss S, et al. Magnetoencephalographic localization in pediatric epilepsy surgery: comparison with invasive intracranial electroencephalography. *Epilepsia* 1999;46:627–633.

105. Lamusuo S, Fross N, Ruottinen H, et al. [^{18}F] FDG-PET and whole-scalp MEG localization of epileptogenic cortex. *Epilepsia* 1999;40:921–930.

106. Baumgartner C, Pataraia E, Lindinger G, et al. Neuromagnetic recordings in temporal lobe epilepsy. *J Clin Neurophysiol* 2000;17:177–189.

107. Smith JR, King DW, Park YD, et al. Magnetic source imaging guidance of gamma knife radiosurgery for the treatment of epilepsy. *J Neurosurg* 2000;93(Suppl 3):136–140.

108. Iwasaki M, Nakasoto N, Shamoto H, et al. Surgical implications of neuromagnetic spike localization in temporal lobe epilepsy. *Epilepsia* 2002;43:415–424.

109. Leijten F, Huiskamp GJM, Hilgerson I, et al. High-resolution source imaging in mesiotemporal lobe epilepsy: a comparison between MEG and simultaneous EEG. *J Clin Neurophysiol* 2003;20:227–238.

110. Baumgartner C, Barth DS, Levesque M, et al. Detection of epileptiform discharges on magnetoencephalography in comparison to invasive measurements. In: Hoke M, Evne SM, Okada YC, et al., eds. *Biomagnetism. Clinical aspects.* Amsterdam: Elsevier, 1992:7–71.

111. Mikuni N, Nagamine T, Ikeda A, et al. Simultaneous recording of epileptiform discharges by MEG and subdural electrodes in temporal lobe epilepsy. *Neuroimage* 1997;5:298–306.

112. Oishi M, Otsubo H, Kameyama S, et al. Epileptic spikes: magnetoencephalography versus simultaneous electrocorticography. *Epilepsia* 2002;43:1390–1395.

113. Smith JR, Schwartz B, Gallen C, et al. Multichannel magnetoencephalography in ablative seizure surgery outside the anteromesial temporal lobe. *Stereotact Funct Neurosurg* 1995;65:81–85.

114. Ebersole J, Smith J. MEG spike modeling differentiates basomesial from lateral cortical temporal epilepsy [abstract]. *Electroencephalogr Clin Neurophysiol* 1995;95:20.

115. Goldman A, Wheless JW, Venkataraman V, et al. Magnetoencephalography mislocalizes interictal epileptogenic activity in mesial temporal epilepsy [abstract]. *Epilepsia* 2001;42:97.

116. Yoshinaga H, Nakahori T, Ohtsuka Y, et al. Benefit of simultaneous recording of EEG and MEG in dipole localization. *Epilepsia* 2002;43:924–928.

117. Barkley G, Baumgartner C. MEG and EEG in epilepsy. *J Clin Neurophysiol* 2003;20:163–178.

118. Kirchberger K, Hummel C, Stefan H. Postoperative multichannel magnetoencephalography in patients with recurrent seizures after epilepsy surgery. *Acta Neurol Scand* 1998;98:1–7.

119. Engel JJ, Henry T, Rissinger M. Presurgical evaluation for partial epilepsy: relative contributions of chronic depth-electrode recordings versus FDG-PET and scalp-sphenoidal ictal EEG. *Neurology* 1990;40:1670–1677.

120. Sperling M, Alavi A, Reivich M, et al. False lateralization of temporal lobe epilepsy with FDG positron emission tomography. *Epilepsia* 1995;36:722–727.

121. So E, O'Brien T, Brinkmann B, et al. The EEG evaluation of single photon emission computed tomography: abnormalities in epilepsy. *J Clin Neurophysiol* 2000;17:10–28.

122. Kantarci K, Shin C, Britton J, et al. Comparative diagnostic utility of ^{1}H MRS and DWI in evaluation of temporal lobe epilepsy. *Neurology* 2002;58:1553–1556.

123. Akanuma N, Alarcon G, Lum F, et al. Lateralising value of neuropsychological protocols for presurgical assessment of temporal lobe epilepsy. *Epilepsia* 2003;44:408–418.

124. Lucignani G, Tassi L, Fazio F, et al. Double-blinded stereo-EEG and FDG PET study in severe partial epilepsies: are the electrical and metabolic findings related? *Eur J Nucl Med* 1996;23: 1498–1507.

125. Juhasz C, Chugani D, Muzik O, et al. Is epileptogenic cortex truly hypometabolic on interictal positron emission tomography? *Ann Neurol* 2000;48:88–96.

126. So E. Integration of EEG, MRI, and SPECT in the evaluation of patients for epilepsy surgery. *Epilepsia* 2000;41(Suppl 3): S48–S54.

127. Gross RE, Dean A, Lewine J, et al. The relationship of magnetic source imaging to ictal electrocorticography in a neuro-navigational workspace. *Stereotact Funct Neurosurg* 1999;73: 109–114.

128. Smith K, Frank K, Bucholz R. The NeuroStation—a highly accurate, minimally invasive solution to frameless stereotactic neurosurgery. *Comput Med Imaging Graph* 1994;18:247–256.

129. So E. Role of neuroimaging in the management of seizure disorders. *Mayo Clin Proc* 2002;77:1251–1264.

Epilepsy Surgery in Infants and Children

83

Ajay Gupta   Elaine Wyllie   William E. Bingaman

Surgery is now a well-established treatment for adults and children with medically intractable seizures (1–5). Several centers around the world have published their surgical experience and seizure outcome data after surgery in children, and results are encouraging from pediatric series involving infants and young children (1,3,6–14) and adolescents (10,15–21). However, identification of appropriate pediatric surgical candidates, especially infants and children, remains a challenge because of complex interactions of several unique and age-related factors (4,22).

This chapter focuses on these unique and age-related differences that interplay in the management of children who are likely to benefit from the surgical treatment of epilepsy. The step critical to surgical strategy in children as well as adults is the identification of a focal, resectable epileptogenic zone. Clues to the epileptogenic zone are found in seizure symptomatology, electroencephalography(EEG), and neuroimaging results. Some aspects of these features are similar to those in adult candidates, whereas others are unique to infants and children. Table 83.1 compares common findings during diagnostic evaluation of pediatric and adult patients for epilepsy surgery.

SEIZURE SEMIOLOGY DURING VIDEO-ELECTROENCEPHALOGRAPHY IN INFANTS AND CHILDREN

Clinical features of focal seizures may differ in pediatric and adult surgical candidates. Independent studies (23–25) of videotaped seizures from patients at separate institutions indicated that the classification of epileptic seizures of the International League Against Epilepsy (26),

originally reflecting experience in older patients, was not applicable to infants younger than 3 years of age. In the study by Acharya and colleagues (23), only 3 of 21 patients had unmistakable characteristics of localized seizure onset, including clonic jerking of one extremity. In the remaining patients, seizures consisted of a decrease in behavioral motor activity with indeterminate level of consciousness and minimal or no automatisms, arising from temporal or temporoparietal regions, or bilateral tonic stiffening sometimes preceded by bilateral eyelid blinking, arising from frontal or frontoparietal regions. Other authors (24,27) have also noted bilateral motor phenomena during partial seizures in infants. The mechanism is unknown but may include ictal activation of subcortical regions or of the supplementary sensorimotor area. A localized electroencephalographic seizure pattern clarifies the focal nature of the epileptogenic process.

Seizure characteristics signaling localized onset in older patients may be absent or unidentifiable in infants. For example, an aura is an important clue to focal onset in older children and adults, but sensory phenomena are difficult to detect and are rarely observed during video-EEG studies in infants (23). Clinical seizure onset may be difficult to notice, especially in mentally impaired young children, and this may create a challenge during diagnostic evaluation like video-EEG and ictal single-photon-emission computer tomography (SPECT) (28,29). Complex gestural automatisms and altered awareness are hallmarks of many partial seizures in older patients, but assessment of the ictal level of consciousness in infants is fraught with problems, and automatisms, when present, tend to be simple, bland, and predominantly oral. In infants, distinguishing automatisms from normal background behavioral activity can be difficult (23,24).

TABLE 83.1

COMMONLY ENCOUNTERED DIFFERENCES DURING DIAGNOSTIC EVALUATION AND SURGICAL DECISION MAKING IN PEDIATRIC AND ADULT PATIENTS

Characteristic Findings	Infants/Young Children	Adult Patients
History, seizure semiology, and examination		
Specific auras	Rare (unable to communicate)	Common
Seizure semiology	Stereotypic (like "epileptic spasms" or "bland stare")	May indicate symptomatogenic zone
Clinical seizure onset, ictal examination, postseizure recall	Unable or difficult to confirm	Easier
Ictal lateralizing features	Uncommon or unreliable	Common and reliable
Neurologic deficit on examination	Difficult to elicit (mild hemiparesis, visual fields)	Easy to elicit
Neuropsychological testing for surgical risk	Less objective (because of age, severe cognitive and behavior difficulties)	Helpful in pointing to specific deficits
Scalp EEG patterns		
Confounding factor of developmental EEG evolution	Present	Absent
Stereotypic and nonlocalizing interictal and ictal patterns	Common (hypsarrhythmia, generalized discharges)	Absent
Imaging and pathologic substrates		
Confounding factor of developmental brain MRI changes	Present	Absent
Ictal SPECT	Difficult (brief frequent seizures, clusters, difficult ictal onset)	Easier
Common location and extent of lesions	Extratemporal large lesions	Temporal, smaller lesions
Common etiologies	Congenital (cortical dysplasia, malformation, tumor, perinatal stroke)	Hippocampal sclerosis, focal cortical dysplasia
Surgical considerations		
Morbidity and mortality	Higher (because of age, weight, larger resections, coexisting disabilities)	Lower
Timing and best techniques for surgery	More controversial and require planning and experience	Less controversial
Invasive mapping (intracranial grids or depth electrodes)	Not practical in most infants and young children	Possible
Intraoperative neurophysiologic techniques	Limited utility, more challenging in infants	Very useful
Goals of surgery/successful seizure control	Cognitive improvement, schooling, behavior, productive adult life	Job, driving, independence

Abbreviations: EEG, electroencephalographic; MRI, magnetic resonance imaging; SPECT, single-photon-emission computed tomography.

SCALP ELECTROENCEPHALOGRAPHY PATTERNS, INFANTILE SPASMS, AND FOCAL CORTICAL LESIONS

Within the first 2 years of life, focal cortical lesions may manifest as infantile spasms and hypsarrhythmia (7,14,30,32). The spasms may be intermixed with partial seizures (Fig. 83.1) or may replace a previous partial seizure type altogether, becoming the only active seizure type (Fig. 83.4). The mechanism is unknown, but a clue may be the relationship between age of onset of spasms and location of the lesion. Koo and Hwang (33) found that spasms began earliest in patients with occipital lesions (mean age, 3 months), appeared later in patients with centrotemporoparietal lesions (mean age, 6 months), and occurred latest in patients with frontal lesions (mean age, 10 months). This timing coincides with maturation in those regions; rapid increases in synaptic density and sequential myelination that proceed from the back to the front of the brain. Infantile spasms appear to result from an age-related pathologic interaction between a focal cortical lesion and normal developmental processes.

Chugani and colleagues (8,32–34) first emphasized the role of positron emission tomography (PET) and magnetic resonance imaging (MRI) in identifying focal cortical lesions in children with infantile spasms and hypsarrhythmia, describing several patients with cessation or dramatic reduction of seizures after cortical resection or hemispherectomy. Their experience has been replicated elsewhere (3,31). In that 65% of affected children are free of seizures after surgery (7), infantile spasms are not predictive of poor outcome. However, the identification of

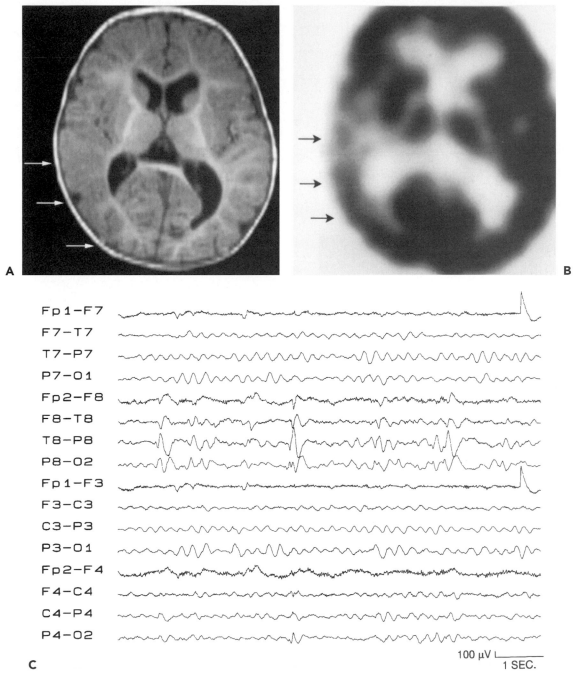

Figure 83.1 *Case 1.* (All images are of the same patient.) **A:** Axial magnetic resonance image from an 8-month-old boy, showing focal malformation of cortical development in the right temporo-occipital region (*arrows*). Findings were subtle and included decreased arborization of the white matter and thickened, poorly sulcated cortex. Seizures began 14 hours after an unremarkable term birth and occurred 20 to 30 times per day. The boy was otherwise normal except for developmental delay. **B:** 2-[^{18}F]fluoro-2-deoxy-D-glucose positron emission tomography scan at age 8 months, showing glucose hypometabolism in the right temporo-occipital region (*arrows*). **C:** Interictal electroencephalogram at age 8 months, showing right posterior temporal sharp waves (maximum at the T8 and P8 electrodes), slowing, and decreased background activity. **D:** Ictal electroencephalogram at age 8 months with seizure pattern maximum in the right posterior temporal region (T8 electrode). Seizures involved bilateral clonic eyelid blinking, rhythmic interruption of crying, and bilateral clonic arm twitching. **E:** Ictal electroencephalogram at age 8 months, showing diffuse electrodecrement (*arrow,* preceded and followed by movement artifact) during an asymmetric spasm with extension and elevation of both arms (left more than right) and tonic closure of the left eyelid. **F:** Magnetic resonance image showing the right temporo-occipital resection performed at age 22 months. Fourteen months later, the child still has developmental delay but remains free of seizures off all antiepileptic medication. (A and C–F are from Wyllie E. Surgical treatment of epilepsy in infants and children. *Can J Neurol Sci* 2000;27:106–110, with permission.)

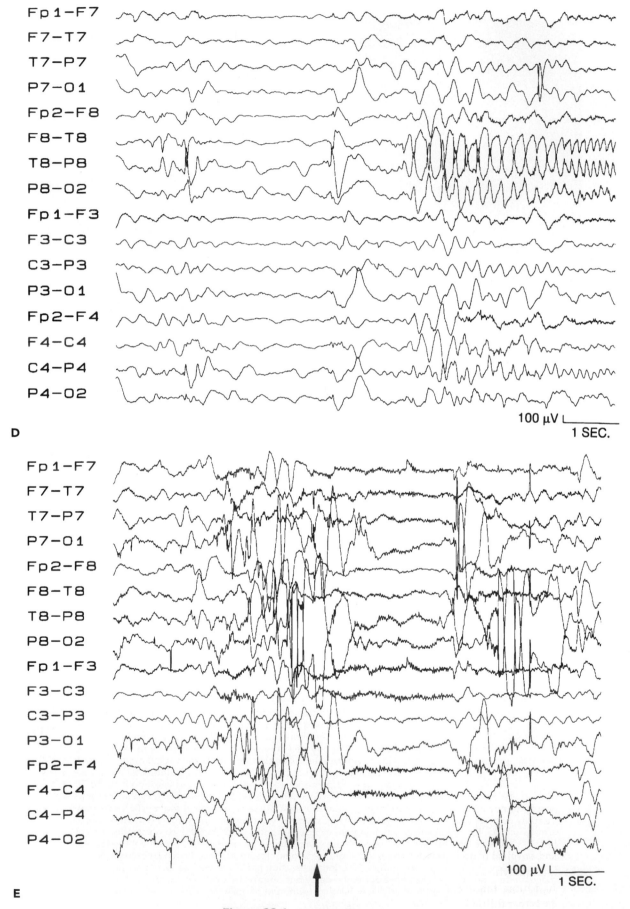

Figure 83.1 (continued)

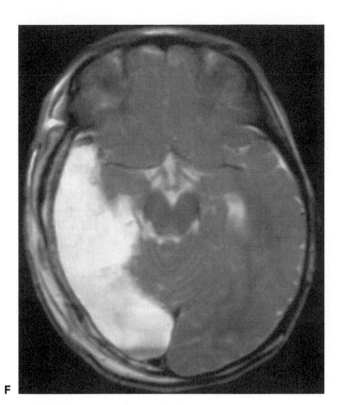

F

Figure 83.1   *(continued)*

appropriate surgical candidates may be complicated by the absence of focal EEG seizure patterns in the setting of spasms with diffuse electrodecrements.

The goal of the presurgical evaluation in patients with infantile spasms is to identify a region of cortical abnormality. Helpful EEG findings can include a predominance of interictal sharp waves over one region; localized slowing, decreased background activity, or absent sleep spindles over the affected region or hemisphere; unilateral electrodecremental events; asymmetric EEG seizures; or a history of partial seizures (4,14). Neurologic examination may show evidence of unilateral hemispheric dysfunction with decreased spontaneous movement of one arm (hemiparesis) or gaze preference to one side (homonymous hemianopia) (4,14). The generalized scalp EEG patterns in the presence of a focal lesion may not be limited to infants. Recently, Gupta and Wyllie (unpublished data, presented at the American Academy of Neurology meeting, 2004) described older children with a unilateral focal or hemispheric abnormality that presented with exclusively generalized interictal and ictal EEG patterns. Initially, these children were rejected for surgical treatment owing to the presence of exclusively generalized EEG findings. Because of a desperate situation with daily dreadful seizures, failure of all treatment modalities, and minimal risk of new postoperative side effects, surgical treatment was offered as a last resort. Of eight patients who underwent surgery, six were seizure free; one had more than 90% and one had a 50% seizure reduction at 1-year follow-up. However, in children, as in older patients, the location of the focal epileptogenic

lesion must be defined, whenever possible, by a convergence of results from clinical examination, EEG, anatomic, and functional neuroimaging, and other testing (4).

ANATOMIC AND FUNCTIONAL NEUROIMAGING

Neuroimaging is a critical component of surgical strategy at every patient age. A focal epileptogenic lesion on the MRI seems to indicate a better prognosis for seizure-free outcome. In the Cleveland Clinic pediatric series from 1990 to 1996 (3), 54% of patients were seizure free and 19% had only rare seizures after extratemporal or multilobar resections. In contrast, in the Montreal Neurological Institute pediatric series (35) (excluding tumor cases) during the pre-MRI era between 1940 and 1980, only 27% had few or no seizures after frontal resection. The more favorable results from the Cleveland Clinic may be a result of identification of a focal epileptogenic lesion on preoperative MRI in 85% of patients. Almost identical results were reported in an adult series (36) of extratemporal resections performed in Bonn, Germany, from 1987 to 1993, with 54% of patients free of seizures after surgery. Seizure-free outcome in that series was significantly more common in lesional than nonlesional cases, with 82% of lesions identified preoperatively by MRI. The absence of MRI localization appears to be an unfavorable prognostic sign, although some patients may have good outcome after electroencephalogram-guided cortical resection. The yield of brain MRI, particularly in neocortical frontal and temporal lobe epilepsy, could be enhanced by use of high-resolution imaging, specialized protocols with thin sections, and experience of the reader (see Chapter 74) (37).

PET is also an important neuroimaging tool for pediatric epilepsy surgery. Chugani and colleagues (7) found that a localized region of hypometabolism may identify focal cortical dysplasia even without abnormal features on MRI. This is especially helpful in infants because immature myelination challenges identification of subtle dysgenetic abnormalities of the gray-white junction on routine brain MRI protocols. PET scans using special tracers have been reported to be useful in some children with tuberous sclerosis (38,39). Ictal SPECT remains a challenging modality to use in children; however, it has been increasingly used in many centers in selected pediatric cases (28,40–42). Acquisition and interpretation of ictal SPECT in children are complicated as a result of several factors (28). First, interictal SPECT may be difficult to obtain owing to multiple daily seizures in this group of patients. Second, difficulty in promptly recognizing the clinical onset of ictal behavioral changes because of age and coexistent mental retardation may result in a late injection for an ictal SPECT. Third, some extratemporal seizures may be brief and spread rapidly. Fourth, children may require sedation on two occasions to obtain interictal and ictal scans. Magnetic resonance spectroscopy (MRS), magnetoencephalography

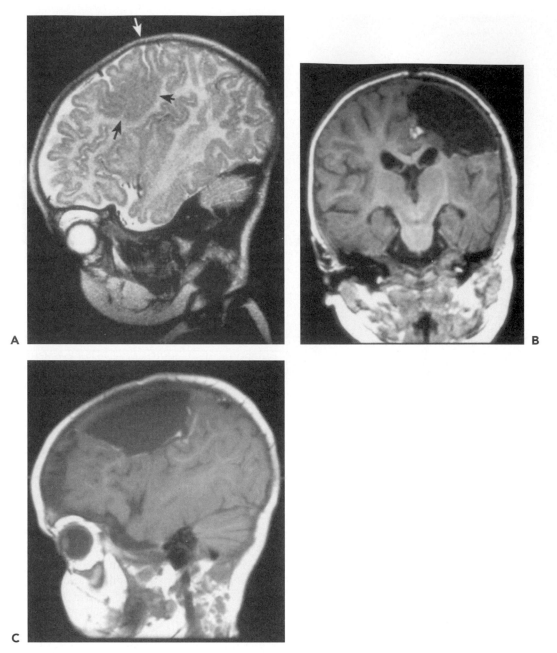

Figure 83.2 *Case 2.* **A:** Sagittal magnetic resonance image showing focal malformation of cortical development cerebral dysgenesis (*black arrow*) in the left posterior frontal lobe extending across the central sulcus (*white arrow*) into the anterior portion of the postcentral gyrus. The boy was 4 months old at the time of the magnetic resonance imaging, with intractable daily seizures since the first day of life after an uncomplicated full-term delivery. Seizures involved clonic jerking of the right arm and leg, with eye deviation toward the left, or opisthotonic posturing with stiffening and extension of all extremities. Ictal and interictal epileptiform discharges were localized to the left central region. Moderately severe right hemiparesis and mild developmental delay were also present. (From Wyllie E. Surgical treatment of epilepsy in children. *Pediatr Neurol* 1998;19:179–188, with permission.) **B:** Coronal and **(C)** sagittal scans performed 2 days after cortical resection at age 9 months. Prior to resection, electroencephalographic seizure was recorded over the lesion with intraoperative electrocorticography, and primary hand motor cortex was identified in the same area by intraoperative cortical stimulation. Postoperatively, the hemiparesis was transiently minimally worse, returning to preoperative baseline within days. Twenty-two months later, the child is making developmental progress and has had no seizures on a reduced dose of antiepileptic medication.

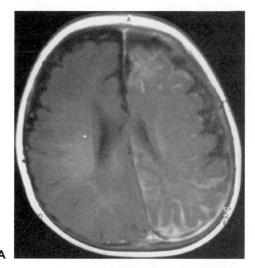
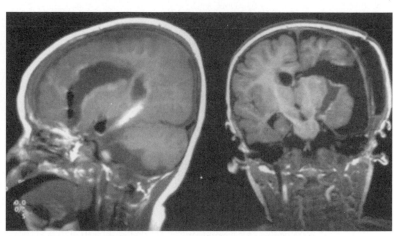

Figure 83.3 *Case 3.* **A:** Axial magnetic resonance image at age 12 months, showing Sturge-Weber malformation with left hemispheric atrophy and pial angiomatosis. Starting at age 2 months, seizures occurred once or twice per day characterized by jerking of the right arm or decreased behavioral activity with bilateral eye blinking and lip smacking. Physical examination revealed right hemiparesis, right hemianopia, and developmental delay. Ictal and interictal epileptiform abnormalities were seen in multiple areas of the left hemisphere. **B:** Sagittal (*left*) and coronal (*right*) magnetic resonance images showing the left hemispheric disconnection performed at age 12 months. No seizures occurred during the 8 months since surgery on a reduced dose of antiepileptic medications. Surgery did not worsen neurologic deficits, and the child has progressed developmentally.

(MEG), and other innovative neuroimaging procedures have not yet been extensively studied in infants (4,43).

ETIOLOGIES AND PATHOLOGIC SUBSTRATES OF EPILEPSY IN PEDIATRIC PATIENTS

Causes of epilepsy differ in children and adults. Hippocampal sclerosis, the most common etiologic factor in adult candidates for epilepsy surgery, is uncommon in children. In a multicenter, predominantly adult series (2), 73% of 5,446 epilepsy surgeries (excluding corpus callosotomies) were performed for nonlesional temporal lobe epilepsy, including hippocampal sclerosis. In contrast, in a pediatric epilepsy surgery series (3) from the Cleveland Clinic Foundation, hippocampal sclerosis was the cause in only 12% of 62 children (3 months to 12 years of age) and in 15% of 74 adolescents (13 to 20 years of age). Although hippocampal sclerosis may begin in childhood, the typical presentation for surgical evaluation is in early adulthood. When hippocampal sclerosis occurs in pediatric candidates for epilepsy surgery, the clinical and EEG features may be similar to those in adults (44). However, pediatric patients appear to have an especially high incidence of dual pathology with cortical dysplasia in addition to the hippocampal sclerosis (44).

In pediatric candidates, the predominant etiologic factors are focal, multilobar or extensive hemispheric malformation of cortical development (cortical dysplasia) (Figs. 83.1, 83.2, and 83.5), and low-grade tumor (3,45). These were the cause

of the epilepsy in 57% of adolescents, 70% of children, 90% of infants younger than age 3 years in the Cleveland Clinic series (3), and 90% of infants treated surgically in the series of Duchowny and colleagues (1). Less common causes are vascular malformation, arachnoid cyst, and localized injury caused by infarction, trauma, or infection (1,3).

Hemispheric syndromes are also important etiologies in children undergoing epilepsy surgery in the form of hemispherectomy (45). Hemispheric malformations of cortical development like hemimegalencephaly (Fig. 83.5), Sturge-Weber syndrome (Fig. 83.3), and perinatal unilateral cerebral ischemic insults are the most common etiologic factors in children and adolescents who had hemispheric ablation procedures, with Rasmussen chronic focal encephalitis occurring less frequently (3,45).

The age-related differences in etiology result in an age-related spectrum of surgical procedures. Anteromesial temporal resections predominate in adults (2) but not in children. In pediatric series, extratemporal or multilobar resections or hemispherectomies composed 44% of the surgeries in adolescents, 50% in children, and 90% in infants (1,3).

SURGICAL CONSIDERATIONS IN PEDIATRIC PATIENTS

Identification of Candidates: The Timing of Surgery

Critical features of surgical candidacy at any age include intractable epilepsy interfering with quality of life or

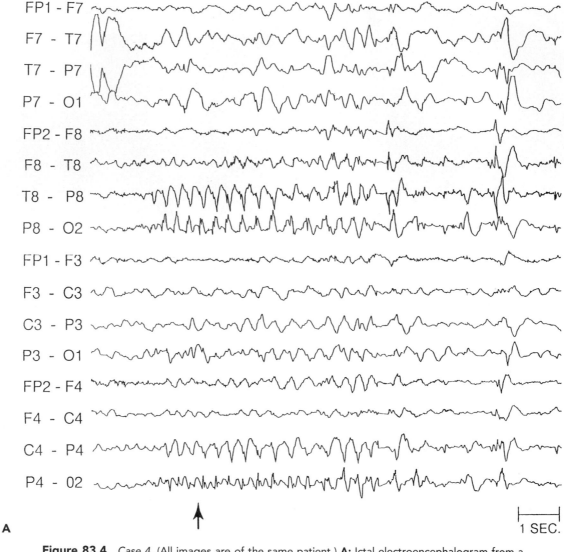

FP1 - F7

F7 - T7

T7 - P7

P7 - O1

FP2 - F8

F8 - T8

T8 - P8

P8 - O2

FP1 - F3

F3 - C3

C3 - P3

P3 - O1

FP2 - F4

F4 - C4

C4 - P4

P4 - 02

A

1 SEC.

Figure 83.4 *Case 4.* (All images are of the same patient.) **A:** Ictal electroencephalogram from a 4.5-month-old infant (patient 2,089) showing right parietal onset of a partial seizure (*arrow*). Seizures began at age 2 months and occurred several times a day. **B:** Ictal electroencephalogram at age 13 months, showing hypsarrhythmia with diffuse electrodecrement at the onset of an infantile spasm (*arrow*). Evolution from partial seizures to infantile spasms occurred at age 7 months. The infant had delayed cognitive development and reduced visual attentiveness but no motor deficits. **C:** Sleep spindles were consistently reduced over the right hemisphere, providing further evidence of right hemisphere dysfunction. **D:** This carefully selected segment of the interictal electroencephalogram shows that spikes were sometimes predominant over the right parietal region, despite the diffuse hypsarrhythmic pattern during most of the recording. Normal faster frequencies were reduced in that area. **E:** Magnetic resonance imaging (MRI) at 13 months showed bilateral periventricular leukomalacia, worse in the right parietal region. The findings could have resulted from intrauterine right germinal matrix hemorrhage several weeks before the uneventful term birth. No cortical dysplasia or gyral abnormality was evident on MRI. **F:** Interictal 2-[18F]fluoro-2-deoxy-D-glucose positron emission tomography at 13 months showing right parieto-occipitotemporal hypometabolism. **G:** Postoperative MRI showing the right parieto-occipitotemporal resection performed at age 15 months. Histopathologic analysis of resected tissue revealed microscopic cortical dysplasia, possibly as a result of disturbance of late neuronal migration at the time of the intrauterine intraventricular hemorrhage. The infant remains free of seizures 17 months after operation and has made "catch-up" developmental progress. (A, B, E, and F are from Wyllie E, Comair Y, Ruggieri P, et al. Epilepsy surgery in the setting of periventricular leukomalacia and focal cortical dysplasia. *Neurology* 1996;46:839–841, with permission; A and G are from Wyllie E, Comair YG, Kotagal P, et al. Epilepsy surgery in infants. *Epilepsia* 1996;37:625–637, with permission.)

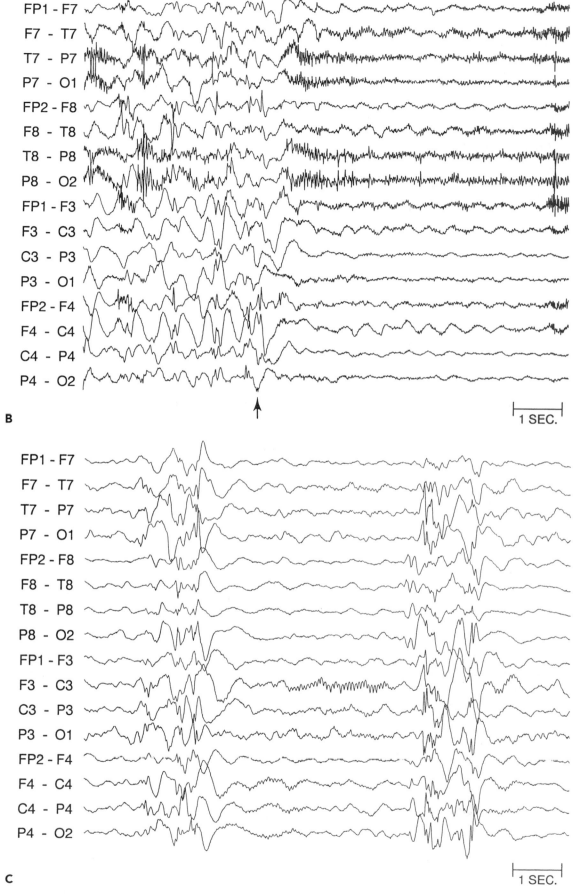

Figure 83.4 (continued)

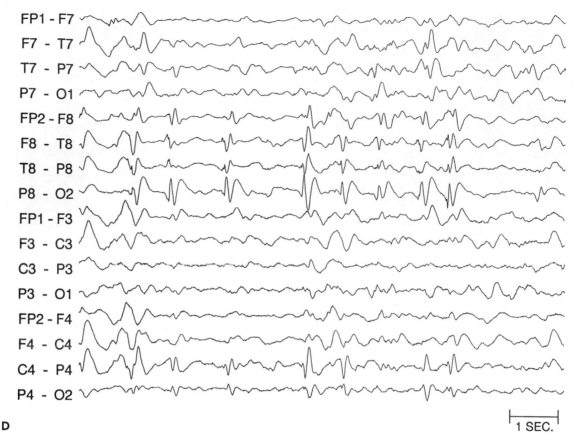

D

1 SEC.

Figure 83.4 (continued)

development, clear identification of a localized epileptogenic zone, and low risk for new postoperative neurologic deficits. However, for each of these factors, age-related issues must be considered in light of results from an extensive presurgical evaluation. The risk of proceeding with surgery must be weighed against the risk of continuing with uncontrolled seizures treated medically. If careful analysis yields a favorable risk-to-benefit ratio for surgery, the available data suggest that it is appropriate to proceed regardless of age.

The usual delay from onset of seizure intractability to surgery is still in the range of 12 to 15 years at most centers, reflecting a reluctance to consider surgery during childhood. Results from pediatric series do not justify this reluctance but instead suggest that children should be referred for surgical evaluation at whatever age they present with severe focal epilepsy. Complicated cases warrant referral to specialized centers with extensive pediatric experience.

Goals of Epilepsy Surgery in Children and Adolescents

The goals of epilepsy surgery can vary according to age. In adolescents and adults, the main goals are usually related to driving, independence, and employment, and their

achievement requires complete postoperative freedom from seizures (46). For infants and children, the goals often center on relief of catastrophic epilepsy, resumption of developmental progression, and improvement in behavior. These goals may sometimes be reached even in the absence of complete freedom from seizures. For infants and young children with many daily seizures and developmental stagnation or regression, a postoperative outcome with rare or infrequent seizures and resumption of developmental progression may be gratifying. Even in the less-favorable-outcome group with malformation of cortical development, 68% of patients in the Cleveland Clinic series had few or no seizures after surgery (3).

In pediatric practice, developmental outcome is of paramount importance. Developmental delay is common in pediatric epilepsy surgery candidates, especially infants. Duchowny and associates (1) noted normal preoperative development in only 20% of infant candidates for epilepsy surgery, whereas the remainder had moderate (52%) or severe (28%) delay. Postoperatively, the developmentally normal infants remained normal after surgery, whereas the severely delayed infants remained severely delayed. Parents reported cognitive and social gains in children with seizure-free outcome, although these were difficult to appreciate on examination (1). Other researchers have made similar observations (7,14).

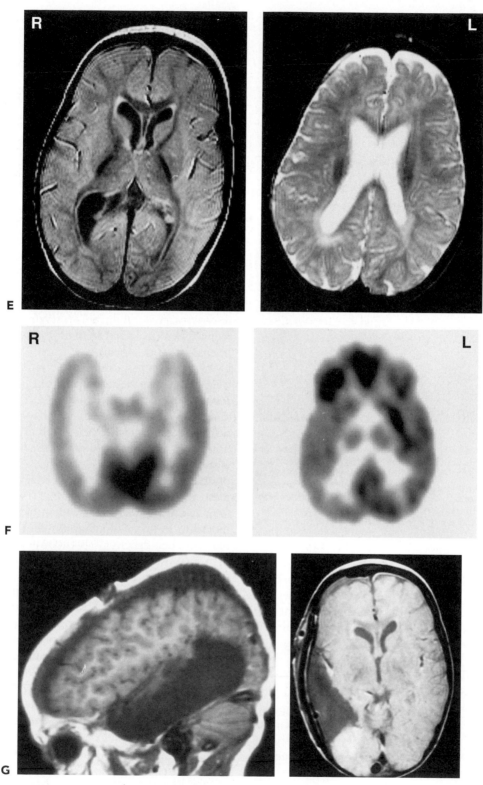

Figure 83.4 (continued)

Seizures that begin in the first few years of life, regardless of etiology, constitute a risk factor for mental retardation (47–49). Early surgical intervention may reduce this risk, but quantitative and prospectively collected data are scant. Asarnow and colleagues (50) studied results of the Vineland assessment in 24 patients with infantile spasms who underwent focal cortical resection or hemispherectomy at a mean age of 21 months. Raw scores 2 years after surgery increased significantly compared with preoperative levels, although only four children had a normal rate of

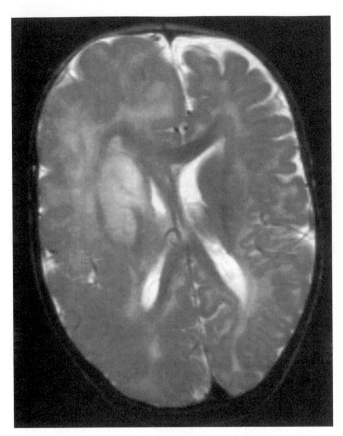

Figure 83.5 T2-weighted sagittal image of "typical" hemimegalencephaly showing diffuse right hemispheric enlargement and dysplasia. Midline shift with bulging of anterior falx to the left and compression of the right lateral ventricle suggest a mass effect as a result of increased volume of the brain parenchyma. Dysplastic changes are diffuse, with thick and disorganized cortex, poor gray-white matter differentiation, and abnormal signal in the white matter. Note that the basal ganglia are also dysplastic with abnormal increased signal.

development. The Adjusted Behavioral Composite scores were significantly higher for children who had higher preoperative scores or earlier surgery. Surgery within the first year of life may therefore maximize developmental outcome by allowing resumption of developmental progression during critical stages of brain maturation (50). A more recent study (51) on cognitive outcome of hemispherectomy in 53 children who underwent presurgical and postsurgical testing reported moderate cognitive and behavioral improvement in most patients. The most significant predictor of cognitive skills after surgery was etiology, with dysplasia patients scoring lowest in intelligence and language but not in visual-motor skills (51). Other studies have also reported similar improvements in the cognitive and behavior spheres after hemispherectomy (52–54).

Psychosocial outcome may also be better after earlier surgery. At the advent of epilepsy surgery, Falconer (16) urged that adolescents be considered for operative treatment before the end of secondary school so that they could pass more normally through the maturational stages of early adulthood. In patients who had temporal resection for childhood-onset epilepsy and were studied after a mean interval of 15 years, Mizrahi and colleagues (19) noted that later surgery was associated with greater permanent psychosocial, behavioral, and educational problems. Delaying surgery for childhood-onset epilepsy may have disadvantages.

Age-Related Risks of Epilepsy Surgery

The extensive multilobar and hemispheric surgeries performed in children and adolescents may carry some risk. In the Cleveland Clinic series (3), 2 of 149 patients (1.3%) died immediately after surgery, and Paolicchi and colleagues (11) reported 1 postoperative death among 83 patients (1.2%) in a pediatric series from Miami Children's Hospital. Mortality may be slightly higher for infants, in part because of their small blood volumes. One or two infant deaths were reported in surgery series from the University of California at Los Angeles (34), Johns Hopkins Medical Center (55,56), and Miami Children's Hospital (1,11). These results emphasize the need to reserve surgery for infants with severe epilepsy. Risk may be reduced by a dedicated team of pediatric anesthesiologists, intensivists, and surgeons.

At any age, the mortality from epilepsy surgery must be weighed against the mortality from uncontrolled seizures treated medically. Nashef and associates (57) found this risk to be 1:295 per year in children and adolescents with severe epilepsy and learning disabilities. In a population-based cohort study in children (58) (1 to 16 years of age) who developed epilepsy between 1977 and 1985, 26 (3.8%) of 692 children died 1999. The majority (13 of 26) who died had secondarily generalized seizures. Neurologic deficit was the only independent factor that determined mortality. In this study, mortality in children with comorbid neurologic deficits (15 per 1000 person-years) was higher than in those without any deficits (0.7 per 1000 person-years). Mortality in the children with seizures and no neurologic deficits was no different from that in the reference nonepileptic population. A Dutch study (59,60) reported similar results. These epidemiologic data reinforce consideration for early surgical intervention, as children with catastrophic partial epilepsy who are candidates for surgery often have neurologic deficits and secondarily generalized seizures. The increased long-term mortality from epilepsy in children can also be seen in outcome studies of epilepsy surgery. During long-term follow-up, late death occurred in 2% of the Cleveland Clinic series (3) and in 11% of a series from Guldvog and associates involving patients with persistent seizures (17).

Other risks of epilepsy surgery, including new postoperative neurologic deficits (e.g., hemiparesis or language impairment), may be reduced in pediatric patients as a result of developmental plasticity. Language may transfer to the right hemisphere during the course of destructive processes such as Rasmussen chronic focal encephalitis or may develop in an unusual region of the left hemisphere in a congenital left frontal or posterotemporal tumor (43,61). In these cases, the epileptogenic lesion may be resected or

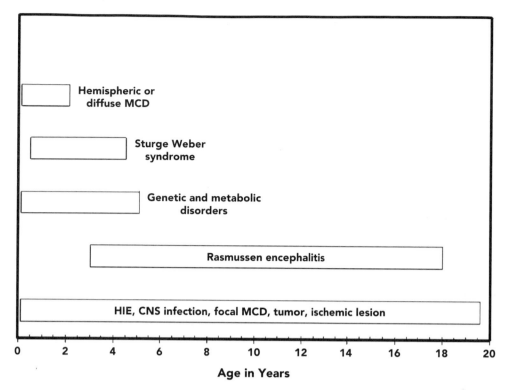

Figure 83.6   Usual age of seizure onset and common etiologies/pathologic substrates often encountered in children with epilepsy. (Modified from Gupta A, Wyllie E. Presurgical evaluation in children with catastrophic epilepsy. In: Luders H, Rosenow F, eds. *Presurgical assessment of the epilepsies with clinical neurophysiology and functional imaging.* Amsterdam: Elsevier, 2004:451–459.)

disconnected without producing new language deficits. Motor function may also partially develop outside a damaged or malformed rolandic region, so that resection of a perirolandic lesion results in little or no additional postoperative motor deficit (Fig. 83.2). Factors favoring developmental plasticity include early onset of the lesion (e.g., perinatal infarction or congenital malformation) and surgery performed within the first few years of life.

Decrements in postoperative verbal memory scores may follow left mesial temporal resection in adults, especially in individuals with high preoperative scores (62,63). Little is known about this potential complication in children, although similar risk factors were identified in a small pediatric series examining cognitive outcome after temporal lobe resection (64). It is not known whether the intracarotid amobarbital procedure can accurately predict this complication in children. Low memory retention scores may occur during this testing in a significant proportion of children (65), and withholding mesial temporal resection from otherwise favorable candidates on the basis of this finding alone may not be appropriate.

Seizure Outcome After Epilepsy Surgery

Published studies on surgical outcome are reliable but difficult to compare owing to the inclusion of patients with diverse pathologic conditions, use of different evaluation and surgical techniques, and variable definitions of post-

operative outcome and follow-up. Good postoperative outcomes with rare or no seizures occur with similar frequencies at all ages, according to recent series in infants, children, adolescents, and adults, despite age-related differences in causes and surgery types (1,3,11,14,66,67). The likelihood of a favorable seizure outcome postoperatively does not diminish significantly, even in infancy. These results compare favorably with those achieved during controlled trials of new antiepileptic drugs, in which the rate of "responders" (at least 50% improvement in seizure frequency) was 20% to 40% and seizure freedom was fairly rare (68). More recent studies (69) show only modest chances of seizure freedom (less than 5%) after failure of two antiepileptic medications and report no difference between established and newer antiepileptic drugs used as initial monotherapy.

Certain subgroups appear especially likely to be free of seizures after surgery. In the Cleveland Clinic pediatric series (3), this outcome was significantly more common in patients who had temporal resection (78%) than in those who had extratemporal or multilobar resection (54%). However, this difference based on surgery type disappeared when results were analyzed by etiologic factors. Significantly more patients with low-grade tumor (82%) than patients with malformation of cortical development (52%) were seizure free, regardless of whether the surgery was temporal (86% for tumor versus 56% for dysplasia) or extratemporal/multilobar (75% for tumor versus 50% for dysplasia) (3).

Duchowny and colleagues (1) noted that it is relatively meaningless to consider pediatric patients treated with temporal resection as a special-outcome subgroup because of the varied etiologic factors in younger patients. In children, surgically managed temporal lobe epilepsy is not synonymous with hippocampal sclerosis. However, in the pediatric patients who have hippocampal sclerosis, postoperative seizure outcome appears similar to that in adults. In a series of 34 children and adolescents with hippocampal sclerosis who had anteromesial temporal resection at the Cleveland Clinic for intractable temporal lobe epilepsy, 78% of patients were free of seizures after surgery (44).

Published series (52,53,70,71) in children who underwent hemispherectomy for any indication report seizure freedom rates in the range of 50% to 65% after a postoperative follow-up of 3 months to 22 years. Rates of seizure freedom were consistently lower in children who underwent hemispherectomy for congenital malformations than in children who had the procedure for acquired diseases like Rasmussen encephalitis and ischemic stroke (45). From 30% to 50% of children with hemispheric malformations of cortical development and 55% to 80% of those with acquired causes were seizure free after hemispherectomy. Few reports that analyzed seizure outcome in subgroups of patients with hemispheric malformations of cortical development showed higher rates (68% to 80%) of seizure freedom in partial (sparing anterior or posterior brain regions) or nonhemimegalencephalic (without excessive growth of the affected hemisphere) types compared with classic hemimegalencephaly (45).

CONCLUSIONS

All children with catastrophic epilepsy, regardless of age, must be promptly evaluated for diagnosis and surgical candidacy. The risk-to-benefit ratio should then be cautiously weighed for every child in light of several complex age-related issues, which are discussed in this chapter. Young age entails special challenges for presurgical evaluation, but it also provides a great opportunity to attain early freedom from daily seizures and to achieve the maximum cognitive potential. Evaluation and treatment of complex cases are best done at specialized centers with extensive experience in pediatric epilepsy surgery.

REFERENCES

1. Duchowny M, Jayakar P, Resnick T, et al. Epilepsy surgery in the first three years of life. *Epilepsia* 1998;39:737–743.
2. Engel J Jr. Surgery for seizures. *N Engl J Med* 1996;334:647–652.
3. Wyllie E, Comair YG, Kotagal P, et al. Seizure outcome after epilepsy surgery in children and adolescents. *Ann Neurol* 1998;44:740–748.
4. Gupta A, Wyllie E. Presurgical evaluation in children with catastrophic epilepsy. In: Luders H, Rosenow F, eds. *Presurgical assessment of the epilepsies with clinical neurophysiology and functional imaging.* Amsterdam: Elsevier, 2004:451–459.
5. Wiebe S, Blume WT, Girvin JP, et al. A randomized, controlled trial of surgery for temporal-lobe epilepsy. *N Engl J Med* 2001;345:311–318.
6. Adelson PD, Peacock WJ, Chugani HT, et al. Temporal and extended temporal resections for the treatment of intractable seizures in early childhood. *Pediatr Neurosurg* 1992;18:169–178.
7. Chugani HT, Shewmon DA, Shields WD, et al. Surgery for intractable infantile spasms: neuroimaging perspectives. *Epilepsia* 1993;34:764–771.
8. Chugani HT, Shields WD, Shewmon DA, et al. Infantile spasms: I. PET identifies focal cortical dysgenesis in cryptogenic cases for surgical treatment. *Ann Neurol* 1990;27:406–413.
9. Duchowny MS, Resnick TJ, Alvarez LA, et al. Focal resection for malignant partial seizures in infancy. *Neurology* 1990;40:980–984.
10. Green JR, Pootrakul A. Surgical aspects of the treatment of epilepsy during childhood and adolescence. *Ariz Med* 1982;39:35–38.
11. Paolicchi JM, Jayakar P, Dean P, et al. Predictors of outcome in pediatric epilepsy surgery. *Neurology* 2000;54:642–647.
12. Peacock WJ, Wehby-Grant MC, Shields WD, et al. Hemispherectomy for intractable seizures in children: a report of 58 cases. *Childs Nerv Syst* 1996;12:376–384.
13. Wyllie E, Chee M, Granstrom ML, et al. Temporal lobe epilepsy in early childhood. *Epilepsia* 1993;34:859–868.
14. Wyllie E, Comair YG, Kotagal P, et al. Epilepsy surgery in infants. *Epilepsia* 1996;37:625–637.
15. Davidson S, Falconer MA. Outcome of surgery in 40 children with temporal-lobe epilepsy. *Lancet* 1975;1:1260–1263.
16. Falconer MA. Significance of surgery for temporal lobe epilepsy in childhood and adolescence. *J Neurosurg* 1970;33:233–252.
17. Guldvog B, Loyning Y, Hauglie-Hanssen E, et al. Surgical treatment for partial epilepsy among Norwegian children and adolescents. *Epilepsia* 1994;35:554–565.
18. Meyer FB, Marsh WR, Laws ER Jr, et al. Temporal lobectomy in children with epilepsy. *J Neurosurg* 1986;64:371–376.
19. Mizrahi EM, Kellaway P, Grossman RG, et al. Anterior temporal lobectomy and medically refractory temporal lobe epilepsy of childhood. *Epilepsia* 1990;31:302–312.
20. Polkey CE. Selection of patients with intractable epilepsy for resective surgery. *Arch Dis Child* 1980;55:841–844.
21. Whittle IR, Ellis HJ, Simpson DA. The surgical treatment of intractable childhood and adolescent epilepsy. *Aust N Z J Surg* 1981;51:190–196.
22. Wyllie E. Surgical treatment of epilepsy in children. *Pediatr Neurol* 1998;19:179–188.
23. Acharya JN, Wyllie E, Luders HO, et al. Seizure symptomatology in infants with localization-related epilepsy. *Neurology* 1997;48:189–196.
24. Nordli DR Jr, Bazil CW, Scheuer ML, et al. Recognition and classification of seizures in infants. *Epilepsia* 1997;38:553–560.
25. Hamer HM, Wyllie E, Luders HO, et al. Symptomatology of epileptic seizures in the first three years of life. *Epilepsia* 1999;40:837–844.
26. Commission on Classification and Terminology of the International League Against Epilepsy. Proposal for revised clinical and electroencephalographic classification of epileptic seizures. *Epilepsia* 1981;22:489–501.
27. Dravet C, Catani C, Bureau M, et al. Partial epilepsies in infancy: a study of 40 cases. *Epilepsia* 1989;30:807–812.
28. Gupta A, Raja S, Kotagal P, et al. Ictal SPECT in children with partial epilepsy due to focal cortical dysplasia. *Pediatr Neurol* 2004;31:89–95.
29. Lawson JA, O'Brien TJ, Bleasel AF, et al. Evaluation of SPECT in the assessment and treatment of intractable childhood epilepsy. *Neurology* 2000;55:1391–1393.
30. Asanuma H, Wakai S, Tanaka T, et al. Brain tumors associated with infantile spasms. *Pediatr Neurol* 1995;12:361–364.
31. Brockhaus A, Elger CE. Complex partial seizures of temporal lobe origin in children of different age groups. *Epilepsia* 1995;36:1173–1181.
32. Chugani HT, Shewmon DA, Sankar R, et al. Infantile spasms: II. Lenticular nuclei and brain stem activation on positron emission tomography. *Ann Neurol* 1992;31:212–219.
33. Koo B, Hwang P. Localization of focal cortical lesions influences age of onset of infantile spasms. *Epilepsia* 1996;37:1068–1071.
34. Chugani HT, Shewmon DA, Peacock WJ, et al. Surgical treatment of intractable neonatal-onset seizures: the role of positron emission tomography. *Neurology* 1988;38:1178–1188.

35. Fish DR, Smith SJ, Quesney LF, et al. Surgical treatment of children with medically intractable frontal or temporal lobe epilepsy: results and highlights of 40 years' experience. *Epilepsia* 1993;34: 244–247.
36. Zentner J, Hufnagel A, Ostertun B, et al. Surgical treatment of extratemporal epilepsy: clinical, radiologic, and histopathologic findings in 60 patients. *Epilepsia* 1996;37:1072–1080.
37. Grant PE, Barkovich AJ, Wald LL, et al. High-resolution surface-coil MR of cortical lesions in medically refractory epilepsy: a prospective study. *AJNR Am J Neuroradiol* 1997;18:291–301.
38. Chugani DC, Chugani HT, Muzik O, et al. Imaging epileptogenic tubers in children with tuberous sclerosis complex using alpha-[^{11}C]methyl-L-tryptophan positron emission tomography. *Ann Neurol* 1998;44:858–866.
39. Rintahaka PJ, Chugani HT. Clinical role of positron emission tomography in children with tuberous sclerosis complex. *J Child Neurol* 1997;12:42–52.
40. Chiron C, Vera P, Kaminska A, et al. Single-photon emission computed tomography: ictal perfusion in childhood epilepsies. *Brain Dev* 1999;21:444–446.
41. Koh S, Jayakar P, Resnick T, et al. The localizing value of ictal SPECT in children with tuberous sclerosis complex and refractory partial epilepsy. *Epileptic Disord* 1999;1:41–46.
42. Vera P, Kaminska A, Cieuta C, et al. Use of subtraction ictal SPECT co-registered to MRI for optimizing the localization of seizure foci in children. *J Nucl Med* 1999;40:786–792.
43. Janszky J, Ebner A, Kruse B, et al. Functional organization of the brain with malformations of cortical development. *Ann Neurol* 2003;53:759–767.
44. Mohamed A, Wyllie E, Ruggieri P, et al. Temporal lobe epilepsy due to hippocampal sclerosis in pediatric candidates for epilepsy surgery. *Neurology* 2001;56:1643–1649.
45. Gupta A, Carreno M, Wyllie E, et al. Hemispheric malformations of cortical development. *Neurology* 2004;62(6 Suppl 3): S20–S26.
46. Sperling MR, Saykin AJ, Roberts FD, et al. Occupational outcome after temporal lobectomy for refractory epilepsy. *Neurology* 1995; 45:970–977.
47. Dikmen S, Matthews CG, Harley JP. Effect of early versus late onset of major motor epilepsy on cognitive-intellectual performance: further considerations. *Epilepsia* 1977;18:31–36.
48. Huttenlocher PR, Hapke RJ. A follow-up study of intractable seizures in childhood. *Ann Neurol* 1990;28:699–705.
49. Klove H, Matthews CG. Neuropsychological evaluation of the epileptic patient. *Wis Med J* 1969;68:296–301.
50. Asarnow RF, LoPresti C, Guthrie D, et al. Developmental outcomes in children receiving resection surgery for medically intractable infantile spasms. *Dev Med Child Neurol* 1997;39: 430–440.
51. Pulsifer MB, Brandt J, Salorio CF, et al. The cognitive outcome of hemispherectomy in 71 children. *Epilepsia* 2004;45:243–254.
52. Taha JM, Crone KR, Berger TS. The role of hemispherectomy in the treatment of holohemispheric hemimegalencephaly. *J Neurosurg* 1994;81:37–42.
53. Kossoff EH, Vining EP, Pillas DJ, et al. Hemispherectomy for intractable unihemispheric epilepsy: etiology vs outcome. *Neurology* 2003;61:887–890.
54. Maehara T, Shimizu H, Kawai K, et al. Postoperative development of children after hemispherotomy. *Brain Dev* 2002;24:155–160.
55. Kossoff EH, Vining EP, Pyzik PL, et al. The postoperative course and management of 106 hemidecortications. *Pediatr Neurosurg* 2002;37:298–303.
56. Vining EP, Freeman JM, Pillas DJ, et al. Why would you remove half a brain? The outcome of 58 children after hemispherectomy—the Johns Hopkins experience: 1968 to 1996. *Pediatrics* 1997;100(2 Pt 1):163–171.
57. Nashef L, Fish DR, Garner S, et al. Sudden death in epilepsy: a study of incidence in a young cohort with epilepsy and learning difficulty. *Epilepsia* 1995;36:1187–1194.
58. Camfield CS, Camfield PR, Veugelers PJ. Death in children with epilepsy: a population-based study. *Lancet* 2002;359:1891–1895.
59. Appleton RE. Mortality in paediatric epilepsy. *Arch Dis Child* 2003;88:1091–1094.
60. Callenbach PM, Westendorp RG, Geerts AT, et al. Mortality risk in children with epilepsy: the Dutch study of epilepsy in childhood. *Pediatrics* 2001;107:1259–1263.
61. DeVos KJ, Wyllie E, Geckler C, et al. Language dominance in patients with early childhood tumors near left hemisphere language areas. *Neurology* 1995; 45:349–356.
62. Chelune GJ, Naugle RI, Luders H, et al. Prediction of cognitive change as a function of preoperative ability status among temporal lobectomy patients seen at 6-month follow-up. *Neurology* 1991;41:399–404.
63. Seidenberg M, Hermann B, Wyler AR, et al. Neuropsychological outcome following anterior temporal lobectomy in patients with and without the syndrome of mesial temporal lobe epilepsy. *Neuropsychology* 1998;12:303–316.
64. Szabo CA, Wyllie E, Stanford LD, et al. Neuropsychological effect of temporal lobe resection in preadolescent children with epilepsy. *Epilepsia* 1998;39:814–819.
65. Hamer HM, Wyllie E, Stanford L, et al. Risk factors for unsuccessful testing during the intracarotid amobarbital procedure in preadolescent children. *Epilepsia* 2000;41:554–563.
66. Duchowny M, Levin B, Jayakar P, et al. Temporal lobectomy in early childhood. *Epilepsia* 1992;33:298–303.
67. Wyllie E, Comair Y, Ruggieri P, et al. Epilepsy surgery in the setting of periventricular leukomalacia and focal cortical dysplasia. *Neurology* 1996; 46:839–841.
68. Marson AG, Kadir ZA, Chadwick DW. New antiepileptic drugs: a systematic review of their efficacy and tolerability. *BMJ* 1996;313: 1169–1174.
69. Kwan P, Brodie MJ. Early identification of refractory epilepsy. *N Engl J Med* 2000;342:314–319.
70. Morino M, Shimizu H, Ohata K, et al. Anatomical analysis of different hemispherotomy procedures based on dissection of cadaveric brains. *J Neurosurg* 2002;97:423–431.
71. Schramm J. Hemispherectomy techniques. *Neurosurg Clin N Am* 2002;13:113–134, ix.

Corpus Callosotomy and Multiple Subpial Transections

84

Michael C. Smith   *Richard Byrne*   *Andres M. Kanner*

CORPUS CALLOSOTOMY

Corpus callosotomy was first introduced as a surgical treatment for medically intractable epilepsy by Van Wagenen and Herren in 1939 (1). The ultimate goal of callosal section is to abolish the bilateral synchrony (or near synchrony) of cortical epileptiform activity, which can result in seizures with bilateral motor manifestations, such as atonic, tonic, myoclonic, and tonic-clonic seizures. However, synchronous corticofugal epileptic discharges can also disrupt brainstem mechanisms that affect posture and tone of proximal limb and axial muscles, leading to atonic or akinetic seizures (2). The following section briefly reviews some of the more relevant studies that have played an important role in the development and refinement of the techniques used in corpus callosotomy.

Neurophysiologic Basis

The corpus callosum is the most important interhemispheric commissural connection in the brain, with approximately 180 million axons in humans (3). These axons connect homotopic as well as heterotopic cortical regions (4), and exert inhibitory as well as excitatory effects (5). This latter property of the corpus callosum has been suggested as an explanation for the clinical reports of increased partial seizures following callosotomy in humans (6,7) and in animals (8). Studies in rhesus monkeys show that section of the two-thirds anterior corpus callosum results in the development of partial seizures five times faster than in nonbisected animals (9). In the amygdala kindling model of the cat, Wada and Sato (10)

reported that section of the corpus callosum accelerated the final stages of generalized convulsions.

The corpus callosum provides interhemispheric connection, unifying certain motor functions and sensory perceptions of the axial or midline visual and somatosensory world. Axons connecting the frontal lobes occupy a rostral position, whereas those connecting parietal, temporal, and occipital cortices are positioned more caudally, in that order.

The role of the corpus callosum in epileptogenesis is evident from various studies in animals. In the feline model of generalized epilepsy, Musgrave and Gloor (11) demonstrated the loss of bilateral synchrony of spike and slow-wave discharges following total section of the corpus callosum, and anterior commissure. Callosal section in the photosensitive baboon *Papio papio* resulted in a decrement in the synchronization of epileptiform discharges and of seizures triggered by photic stimulation (12,13). In a 1950 study of four monkeys by Kopeloff and colleagues (8), seizures generated by unilateral application of aluminum oxide cream had a bilateral motor expression. Following callosal section, the clinical manifestations were restricted to a distribution contralateral to the seizure focus.

It must be remembered that although the corpus callosum may be the most important anatomic structure for the interhemispheric spread of epileptic activity, it is not the only one. Anterior and posterior commissures and thalamus and brainstem structures may all play a role in the spread of discharge from one hemisphere to the other. Suppression of synchronized epileptic activity is routinely and repeatedly seen in acute models of generalized seizures. However, in most models of chronic epilepsy, synchronized epileptic activity returns over months following callosotomy. This suggests that the epileptic activity uses alternate pathways over time. In patients who demonstrate lateralized epileptic activity postoperatively, there is a general tendency for these discharges to synchronize again over the first postoperative year.

Studies in Humans

The first series of 10 patients was published in 1940 by Van Wagenen and Herren (1). However, the real interest in this procedure developed almost 30 years later, when Wilson reported on the Dartmouth series of callosotomies (14). In general, the clinical series have repeated the animal studies, demonstrating the efficacy of callosotomy in treating seizures requiring bilateral synchrony for their clinical expression. In 1985, Spencer and associates (15) reported the abolition of a bilaterally synchronous ictal onset in all 5 patients who underwent a complete section of the corpus callosum, but in only 5 of 10 patients who underwent a two-thirds anterior section. In contrast, interictal bisynchronous discharges persisted even after a complete section, albeit with a significantly lower frequency. A significant reduction in bisynchronous discharges has been reported in several other patient series (14,16–19). However, as with animal studies, there are a number of reports of an increase in partial seizures (2,20–24) and Spencer and coworkers described them as being more intense as well (25). Other researchers report a conversion of generalized to partial seizures following callosotomy.

Indications

In 1985, Williamson suggested the use of corpus callosotomy to treat infantile hemiplegia, Rasmussen syndrome, Lennox-Gastaut syndrome, and frontal lobe epilepsy. Hemispherectomy is the treatment of choice for such hemispheric syndromes as Rasmussen syndrome and perinatal infarction with hemiplegia, whereas cortical resection is performed in patients with frontal lobe epilepsy. The primary use of corpus callosotomy has been for the treatment of patients with Lennox-Gastaut syndrome. As new medications, the ketogenic diet, and vagus nerve stimulation have become available for these patients, corpus callosotomy has been reserved as a later therapy for patients with severe refractory epilepsy with frequent injurious drop attacks.

Efficacy

In general, the purpose of corpus callosotomy is to palliate a patient's intractable seizure condition by decreasing or abolishing the most incapacitating of the generalized seizures and thus improving the patient's quality of life (QOL). Overall, 50% to 77% of patients with Lennox-Gastaut syndrome have been reported to have a satisfactory

outcome, defined as a seizure reduction of 50% to 80% or more in the different series. The best response has been observed in patients with drop attacks presenting as tonic and atonic seizures. However, there is evidence that patients with atonic seizures derived a greater benefit from the procedure than did those with tonic seizures (18,19,22,26–28). In 1996, Phillips and Sakas (29) reported the results of anterior callosotomy in 20 patients. They divided outcome into freedom from seizures and significant reduction (70%) of seizures. Using these criteria, 16 of 20 patients (80%) experienced significant improvement of a 70% or greater decrease in seizure frequency. Eleven of 13 patients with atonic seizures had the best outcome, and favorable results were found in 14 of 18 patients with generalized tonic-clonic seizures. Gates and colleagues (30) reported that tonic seizures in the presence of an ictal electroencephalographic pattern consisting of an electrodecremental response were associated with a very good outcome in 92% of patients 10 years of age or older. However, this association of seizure type and ictal electroencephalographic pattern was not predictive of outcome in younger patients (16,30).

Corpus callosotomy yields a significant reduction in generalized tonic-clonic seizures in 50% to 80% of several patient series (6). Oguni and coworkers (28) and Spencer and associates (7) suggest that patients with secondarily generalized tonic-clonic seizures in the presence of electroencephalographic evidence of secondary bilateral synchrony and clinical or neuroradiologic evidence of focality derive greater benefit than those with generalized tonic-clonic seizures without these characteristics. This view is not universally accepted; Phillips and Sakas do not consider neuroimaging or electroencephalographic findings to be predictive of outcome (29).

Patients with complex partial seizures are less likely to respond to this procedure; approximately 40% derive a significant reduction in seizures. Simple partial seizures are rarely affected by callosotomy. Corpus callosotomy had been used in patients with frontal lobe seizures in whom the seizure focus could not be lateralized because of very rapid spread of epileptiform activity. However, Purves and colleagues (31) reported on six such patients who underwent a two-thirds anterior callosotomy without favorable results.

Corpus callosotomy may be performed as a partial resection involving the anterior two thirds of the corpus callosum (the majority of cases) or as a complete section. The decision to use one technique over the other remains controversial. Studies by Cendes and coworkers (32), Harbaugh and associates (27), and Reutens and colleagues (33) showed no difference in seizure control between complete and partial sections. Spencer and associates (7), on the other hand, reported the elimination of generalized tonic-clonic seizures in 77% of patients who underwent a complete section of the corpus callosum, compared with 35% of patients who underwent a two-thirds anterior

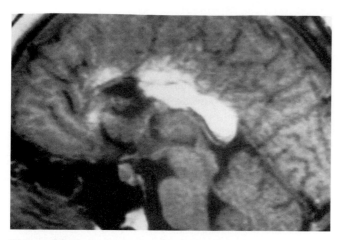

Figure 84.1 Sagittal magnetic resonance image showing the effects of the posterior completion of a corpus callosotomy. High signal, representing acute blood, is seen extending to the posterior extent of the corpus callosotomy, documenting a complete callosotomy.

callosotomy. Following a reanalysis of 50 callosotomy patients, Spencer and coworkers (24) concluded that a two-thirds anterior section should be considered for patients with tonic, atonic, or myoclonic seizures, whereas a complete section should be reserved for those with an incomplete response to the two-thirds anterior section. Maehara and Shimizu (34) advocate a complete callosotomy, especially in children and adults with widespread epilepsy. In any event, when a complete section is considered, it should be carried out as a two-stage procedure in order to minimize neuropsychological complications (Fig. 84.1).

Impact of Seizure Reduction on Quality of Life

In 1997, Rougier and associates reviewed the literature on the efficacy of corpus callosotomy and its effect on QOL (35). They found a favorable outcome, defined as a 50% seizure reduction in 60% to 80% of all patients with atonic seizures and tonic seizures resulting in falls. Favorable outcomes in patients with tonic-clonic seizures varied from 40% to 80%. Patients with complex or simple partial seizures experienced significant improvement less often. Improvements in QOL indices and social adjustment did not always coincide with reduction in seizure frequency. The length of time that a patient had had intractable epilepsy and its deleterious effect on the patient's cognitive and social function were important variables in predicting QOL improvements. In a study conducted at the Cleveland Clinic in Cleveland, Ohio, 9 of 17 patients experienced a greater than 80% reduction in their targeted seizures, and 15 of 17 reported satisfaction with the surgical outcome. However, improvement in alertness and responsiveness, not necessarily reduction in seizure frequency, was most closely associated with satisfaction with surgical outcome. Papo and colleagues (36) reviewed the records of 36 patients with intractable seizures of mixed types. Twenty-seven had

had an anterior callosotomy, 8 had had a complete callosotomy in two stages, and 1 had had a posterior callosotomy. Of the 36 patients, 30 had adequate follow-up to report meaningful results. Fourteen had excellent results (defined as a greater than 90% reduction in targeted seizure type), five had good results (greater than 50% reduction), six had poor results (less than 50% reduction), and five showed no change. Global QOL measures did not always coincide with improvement in seizure frequency. In some patients with excellent seizure results, no clear change in QOL was reported. The authors suggest that this might be related to the long duration of uncontrolled seizures and their effect on cognitive function. Gilliam and coworkers (37) have also noted that overall clinical improvement did not always correlate with seizure reduction.

Surgical Technique

Under general anesthesia, the patient is placed in the supine position with pressure points padded. The head is placed in pin fixation in neutral position, with the neck slightly flexed. The hair is clipped and the skin prepped. A lumbar drain may be placed to aid in retraction of the midline. A variety of skin incisions may be used for anterior callosal sectioning, all of which provide access to the anterior midline. A coronally oriented skin incision 2 cm anterior to the coronal suture, exposing both sides of the midline, will afford the needed exposure. This incision will usually expose more of the right side than the left, because approach from the right allows retraction of the nondominant hemisphere. Hodaie and associates propose the use of image guidance, in part to analyze the parasagittal veins and thus determine the side of entry (38). A craniotomy is performed just anterior to the coronal suture, crossing midline to expose the sagittal sinus. The procedure can be performed without exposing the sinus, but retraction of the sinus is then not possible and sinus bleeding is more difficult to control if encountered. The dural flap is based on the sinus, and retraction of the dura allows retraction of the sinus. Although the exposure is anterior to the coronal suture, all but the most insignificant bridging veins should be spared. Planning the approach and exposure may thus be aided by examining preoperative magnetic resonance imaging (MRI) or magnetic resonance angiography (MRA) scans (Fig. 84.1). If a bridging vein complex does not allow retraction because of a far lateral entry of the vein into the sagittal sinus, a dural incision may be made in the form of a triangle around the laterally entering vein to allow retraction of the dural flap without disturbing the vein.

Once an unencumbered view of the intrahemispheric fissure is obtained, the medial aspect of the exposed frontal lobe is covered with moist cottonoids and self-retaining retractors are gently advanced. The falx is followed down the midline until the cingulated gyri are encountered. An error that is sometimes made is to mistake this view of the adherent cingulate gyri for the corpus callosum. The cingulated gyri are separated under magnification in the midline, exposing the corpus callosum and the pericallosal arteries. Once this view is obtained and the retractors are set, a final check of the anterior exposure confirms the exposure of the anterior corpus callosum if the genu is visible.

The actual division of the anterior corpus callosum is performed with a microdissection instrument and gentle suction. This should begin in the midline of the callosum just posterior to the genu. Great care is taken to separate, but not disturb, the pericallosal arteries. At this level, certain landmarks, such as the cavum septum pellucidum, are visible beneath the corpus callosum, even if the landmark is only a potential space in the individual patient. This midline landmark is valuable, if found, because it confirms the complete transection of the callosal fibers and allows one to stay out of the lateral ventricles. If the lateral ventricle is entered, intraoperative or postoperative bleeding may result in hydrocephalus. The transection is then carried forward into the genu and the rostrum of the corpus callosum. The disconnection is carried out downward following the A2 branches as they approach the anterior communicating artery complex.

The extent of posterior callosal sectioning is determined preoperatively. Some surgeons advise a simple one-half callosal sectioning, which can be measured by comparing the intraoperative transection to the length of the callosum on the preoperative sagittal MRI. This and other techniques, such as intraoperative plain films and stereotaxy, have been used to confirm the length of the callosotomy (39). Other authors advocate a three-quarter sectioning, as there is some indication that seizure control may be more complete. If a complete corpus callosotomy is to be performed, the sectioning may be done with a microdissector or suction aspiration to the splenium. A complete posterior sectioning is confirmed by viewing the arachnoid-covered vein of Galen in the posterior midline. If only an anterior transection is planned, an MRI-compatible marker should be placed at the posterior border of the anterior transection in order to view on imaging studies and to note on reoperation, if necessary, the extent of the first procedure. Hemostasis is obtained, and any entry into a lateral ventricle is covered with Gelfoam. A standard craniotomy closure is performed.

Complications

Complications unique to corpus callosotomy as a surgical procedure are neuropsychological in nature. Well-described acute and chronic neuropsychological sequelae are possible following callosotomy (40,41). Varying degrees of the acute disconnection syndrome, characterized by a lethargic, apathetic mutism during the first few days after surgery, are commonly seen. In our experience and that of other investigators, this syndrome is always transient in nature. The predictors of this transient state are related to the extent of callosal sectioning, baseline cognitive impairment, and the amount of traction necessary to gain access to the corpus callosum. Other observed early manifestations of the acute disconnection syndrome include incontinence, bilateral Babinski sign, and apraxia.

The chronic disconnection syndrome was not well recognized when callosotomy was initially described (1). Detailed neuropsychological testing reveals deficits that are common after callosotomy but are not usually clinically significant. Other than mutism, the majority of neuropsychological alterations occur with posterior callosotomy. This is caused by disruption of communication between visual and tactile cortical sensory functions and verbal expression. Because of the disconnection between the hemispheres, an object placed only in the left visual field of a left-hemisphere-dominant patient will be seen by the right hemisphere, but the information will not be transferred to the left hemisphere for speech production. Thus, the patient recognizes the object but cannot name it. Similarly, an object placed in the left hand but not seen may be recognized by its shape and size, but will not be named. This is interesting but not clinically disabling to the patient, because objects are normally seen by both hemispheres and can be felt with either hand. If a patient has bilateral speech representation, dysphasia may be a postoperative complication. This should be considered before complete callosotomy is undertaken in a patient with mixed speech dominance.

A disturbing complication known as alien hand syndrome has been reported (41). In this condition, poor cooperation or even antagonistic behavior between the left and right hand is noted. The verbal dominant hemisphere may express displeasure with the actions of the ipsilateral extremities. This phenomenon is usually short-lived and is generally observed only in the immediate postoperative period; however, on rare occasions it may persist. Initially performing only an anterior callosotomy can minimize the likelihood and the extent of these neuropsychological sequelae. If the anterior callosotomy is unsuccessful in controlling seizures, a completion of the callosotomy may be performed at a later time.

Other complications that have been observed are related to frontal lobe retraction: cingulate gyrus injury; injury to the pericallosal arteries, bridging veins, or superior sagittal sinus; and hydrocephalus following entry into the lateral ventricle. Incidence of postoperative hydrocephalus secondary to entry into the ventricular system and subsequent ventriculitis is dramatically reduced by using an operative microscope and carefully respecting ventricular boundaries. Transient mutism may be reduced by minimizing retraction of the frontal cortex and retracting the nondominant frontal lobe, if possible. Despite this, mutism may occur transiently in up to 30% of patients.

Spencer and colleagues reported a meta-analysis of long-term neurologic sequelae of both anterior and complete corpus callosotomy (7). They found that motor sequelae were reported in 56% of complete and 8% of anterior callosotomy patients; language impairments in 14% and 8%, respectively; and both cognitive impairment and behavioral impairment in 11% and 8%, respectively.

Some authors have suggested certain contraindications to corpus callosotomy. Spencer and associates (7,15) found that patients with severe mental retardation (intelligence quotient [IQ] less than 45) did not derive any benefit from the procedure. Other studies, however, have not found any relationship between IQ and outcome (32,33,42–44). A relative contraindication has been proposed concerning patients whose hemisphere of language dominance is not that of hand dominance (45). Speech difficulties, with sparing of writing, has been identified in patients who are right-hemisphere-dominant for speech and are right-handed, and dysgraphia with intact speech has been identified in left-handed patients with a left-dominant hemisphere.

Conclusion

Corpus callosotomy is an effective surgical technique for the treatment of selected pharmacoresistant epileptic syndromes, particularly those characterized by epileptic drop attacks, such as atonic seizures. Over the past 10 years, use of corpus callosotomy has decreased as a result of the introduction of new antiepileptic drugs, especially lamotrigine and topiramate, and a rekindling of interest in the ketogenic diet. The vagal nerve stimulator and cortical stimulation may be beneficial in patients with atonic seizures, but no conclusive date are yet available; in fact, certain epilepsy centers in the United States are now considering treatment with vagal nerve stimulation before performing corpus callosotomy. In general, anterior corpus callosotomy may still be an underutilized procedure, especially for patients with intractable atonic seizures associated with recurrent falls and subsequent head injury. Radiosurgery has been proposed as an alternative to surgical callosotomy by Pendl and coworkers (46). Although this is a promising approach, several questions about volume–dose analysis and long-term efficacy have to be answered.

MULTIPLE SUBPIAL TRANSECTION

Focal-onset medically intractable epilepsy has been surgically treated for 70 years by location of the seizure focus and resection of the involved cortex. A certain proportion of patients who undergo evaluation for possible surgical resection are found to have an epileptogenic zone originating in, or overlapping with, eloquent cortex. Traditionally, some of these patients were denied surgery because resection of primary speech, motor, sensory, or visual cortex would result in unacceptable deficits. Multiple subpial transection (MST) was developed specifically to address this problem. This technique disrupts the intracortical horizontal fiber system while preserving the columnar organization of the cortex (i.e., its vertically oriented input and output systems and vascular supply) (47). The transection of horizontal fibers is aimed at preventing the propagation of epileptic discharges, thus averting the synchronous neuronal activation that ultimately results in the development of clinical seizures. The preservation of the columnar organization of the cortex prevents or minimizes disruption of the functional state of the transected cortex.

The development of this technique was derived from three sets of experiments, each unrelated to the others or to the field of epilepsy surgery. The first set of experiments by Asanuma and Sakata (48), by Hubel and Wiesel (49), and by Mountcastle (50) demonstrated that the vertically oriented micro and macro columns (with their vertically oriented input, output, and vascular supply) are the organizational unit of functional cortical architecture. The functional role of the intracortical horizontal fiber system is yet to be firmly established, however. In the second set of experiments, Sperry (51) demonstrated that surgical disruption of the horizontal fiber system in the visual cortex of the cat, while sparing the columnar organization, does not affect the testable functional status. The third set of experiments was related to the importance of the horizontal fiber system as a "critical component in cortical circuit necessary for generation and elaboration of paroxysmal discharges." Epileptic activity in the form of spikes or sharp waves requires a synchronous neuronal activation of a contiguous cortical surface area of at least 12 to 25 mm^2 (52–54). Tharp (54) found that epileptic foci would synchronize their activity if the distance between them was 5 mm or less, and that disrupting the neuropil between the foci would desynchronize the epileptic activity.

With this information, Morrell and colleagues hypothesized that sectioning of the intracortical horizontal fibers at 5-mm intervals, while preserving the columnar organization of the cortex, could abolish epileptic activity yet preserve the functional status of the transected cortex (47). Testing this hypothesis in the monkey, Morrell produced an epileptic focus with aluminum gel lesions in the left precentral motor cortex, which resulted in the development of focal motor seizures. Using a small wire, he disconnected the horizontal fibers at 5-mm intervals throughout the epileptogenic zone. This procedure, the first subpial transection for epilepsy, stopped the seizures, and the monkey sustained no motor deficits. To confirm that what he had transected was motor cortex, 1 year later Morrell surgically removed the transected area, resulting in the expected hemiparesis. With this experimental evidence, Morrell and colleagues moved forward into the treatment of intractable human neocortical epilepsy arising in or overlapping eloquent cortex. Most of their work was carried out at the Rush Epilepsy Center, Chicago, Illinois, with Walter W. Whisler, MD, PhD (55). MST has now been performed at our epilepsy center in more than 100 patients with seizure foci in or overlapping eloquent cortex. The procedure and its results are described below.

Indications

MST may be considered in patients in whom the epileptic zone arises from or overlaps with eloquent cortex, such that resection would be expected to result in an unacceptable deficit. The procedure is performed after a detailed presurgical evaluation, which includes closed-circuit television/electroencephalographic recording of habitual seizures using scalp and intracranial electrodes, mainly subdural grids. In addition, detailed functional mapping to identify eloquent cortex by electrical cortical stimulation and evoked potentials is performed. Neuropsychological testing and intracarotid amobarbital tests, as well as functional neuroimaging studies, all assist in defining the baseline function and risks of the procedure. Magnetoencephalography studies are also useful in the evaluation of children with an acquired epileptic aphasia or Landau-Kleffner syndrome (56), as they allow more accurate identification of the source of the dipole, especially its depth within a sulcus.

MST can be performed as the sole procedure or in conjunction with resection of noneloquent cortex, depending on the extent to which the epileptogenic zone involves eloquent cortex. In fact, the latter scenario is the most common form in which MST is used at our center. Candidates are typically patients with dominant temporal neocortical epilepsy, dominant frontal lobe epilepsy, or primary sensory, motor, or visual cortex involvement. In patients undergoing resection/transection, resection of noneloquent cortex is performed at within 1.5 cm of the identified eloquent cortex. We recognize that this patient group is problematic for the evaluation of the clinical effectiveness of MST.

Cortical Surgical Anatomy

Human cortex is arranged in a gyral pattern, which is fairly constant between individuals. However, the microgyral patterns of individual gyri may be considerably variable. These cortical variations must be taken into account in any procedure in which transections are being made perpendicular to the long axis of a gyrus. Thus, careful inspection of each gyrus prior to the procedure is important. Gray matter is, on average, 5 mm thick over the crown of a gyrus. However, the depth of each sulcus varies.

These points are critical in subpial transection procedures because the objective is to divide the neuropil at 5-mm intervals perpendicular to the long axis of the gyrus, while preserving the overlying pia with its blood vessels and the underlying white matter tracts and U fibers.

About one-third of our patients have undergone MST as their primary procedure. These patients mainly had either epilepsia partialis continua because of Rasmussen encephalitis or a Landau-Kleffner syndrome. In the patients

with Rasmussen syndrome, the epileptogenic zone arose from primary language and/or motor cortex, whereas in patients with Landau-Kleffner syndrome, it involved posterior language cortex.

Operative Procedure

Patients are given preoperative antibiotics and steroids, and are positioned so that the surgical site is at the highest point in the operative field. This makes intraoperative electrocorticography (ECoG), resection, and transection easier. The head is held in Mayfield head fixation and all pressure points are padded. If the operation is performed with the patient awake, comfort is an important issue.

Anesthesia is accomplished with intravenous methohexital and a generous amount of local anesthetics. Although methohexital activates interictal epileptiform activity, such activation does not extend beyond the epileptogenic zone (57). Furthermore, the degree of activation can be minimized by lowering the infusion rate of methohexital. At our center, we perform intraoperative ECoG in all cases, even when mapping with subdural grids has been done, to ensure that the initial transections result in the desired abolition of epileptic activity.

Transections

Before performing the transections, careful inspection of the gyri, microgyral pattern, sulci, and vascular supply is carried out. Transections are first performed in the more dependent areas to avoid the problem of subarachnoid blood obscuring the other areas. At the edge of the visible gyrus, in an avascular area, a 20-gauge needle is used to open a hole in the pia. The tip of the subpial transection hook is introduced into the gray matter layer and advanced to the next sulcus in a direction perpendicular to the long axis of the gyrus. The tip of the hook is held upward and is visible immediately beneath the pia. It is important that the pia be left undisturbed to minimize vascular injury and scarring. The transection hook is designed with a handle, a malleable shaft, and a tip that is 4 mm in length (paralleling the cortical width) and 1 mm in width. If the 4-mm tip is introduced just below the pia, it should remain in the gray matter layer, leaving the white matter undisturbed. The tip is angled at 105 degrees and is blunt. These two features make snagging or injuring a vessel unlikely. However, it is important to avoid crossing a sulcus where buried vessels are unprotected.

After the first transection is completed, bleeding from the pial opening is controlled with small pieces of Gelfoam and a cottonoid. The 4-mm tip is then placed up against the cortex next to the transection, so as to select the next transection site 5 mm from the first. This is repeated until the identified epileptogenic zone is transected. Over a few minutes, the transection lines take on a striped appearance from the petechial hemorrhages along the way.

Minimal bleeding is encountered if the transections are performed properly. ECoG is repeated at the conclusion of the transections. The transected area displays a significant attenuation of the background activity, with elimination of the spikes. In cases of persistent epileptiform activity, the possibility that activity is coming from the depth of a sulcus or from remote areas must be considered. On rare occasions, when persistent activity is clearly identified as originating in an area that has been transected, transecting down into the sulcus may be performed. To do this safely, the tip of the probe should be turned away from the sulcus as the instrument is advanced.

Favorable outcomes using alternative instruments and methods of transection have been described by other neurosurgeons (58).

Seizure Outcome

To eliminate resection as a confounding variable, evaluation of seizure outcome following MST should be carried out only in those patients who underwent MST. Sixteen patients with partial epilepsy have had pure transections at our center, with at least 2 years' follow-up (Table 84.1). Six patients (37.5%) have remained seizure free or have had only auras (Engel class I outcome [59]), six (37.5%) have had rare seizures or greater than 90% seizure reduction (Engel classes II and III), and four patients have had no benefit (Engel class IV). Thus, 75% of the patients have derived significant benefit from surgery. Among the 68 patients who underwent resection plus transection, 48.5% had an Engel class I outcome, 33.5% had an Engel class II or III outcome, and 18% had no benefit. It should be kept in mind that the patients who underwent pure transection would have been uniformly rejected for surgery in the past. Also, six of those patients had Rasmussen encephalitis, a progressive disorder in which MST is expected to provide only temporary relief. Many of the patients who underwent transection and resection also had been previously rejected for surgery. In all of these cases, a minimum of 2 years' follow-up was obtained.

Patients treated with MST for Landau-Kleffner syndrome are analyzed separately because control of clinically overt seizures is often achieved with drug therapy. The most important outcome is recovery of language function. To date, we have performed MST in 22 patients with Landau-Kleffner syndrome at our center. Transection has included intrasylvian and perisylvian cortex and, in some patients, transection of the Broca area. In 14 children, we obtained neuropsychological data comparing preoperative and postoperative language profiles. These data show that 50% of the children experienced significant language recovery (60), whereas in the remaining patients, partial or no recovery was reported.

Surgical Morbidity

Acute Postoperative Morbidity
Cerebral edema is expected following MST, peaking on the third to fourth postoperative day. Consequently, patients are expected to experience transient dysfunction of transected cortex, with ensuing neurologic deficits lasting 2 to 3 weeks. Sometimes mild deficits may persist for several months. Similar observations have been made at the other centers where MST is performed (Table 84.2).

Chronic Morbidity
In the first 100 patients who underwent MST at our center, neurologic complications occurred in 15, resulting in a permanent neurologic deficit in 7 and a transient deficit in 8. Among the seven patients with a permanent deficit, six deficits resulted directly from complications related to the transection; two patients had a footdrop caused by a subcortical venous hemorrhage, documented on neuroradiologic studies; two patients had language deficits; one patient developed a parietal sensory loss; and one patient experienced a visual deficit. In interpreting these results, it is useful to consider the number of patients who had MST in each of the eloquent cortical areas. Thus, 23 underwent transection of the Broca area, 52 of motor cortex, and 57 of

---

TABLE 84.1
POSTSURGICAL OUTCOME

| | | Engel Classification | | | | Neurologic Complications | |
| | | Significant Worthwhile Improvement | | | No Significant Improvement | | |
Surgical Procedure	No. of Patients	Class I	Class II	Class III	Class IV	Transient	Permanent
MST only partial seizures	16	6 (37.5%)	4 (25%)	2 (12.5%)	4 (25%)	1 (6%)	3 (19%)
MST only LKS	16	9 (57.7%)	2 (12.5%)	2 (12.5%)	3 (18%)	2 (12.5%)	—
MST/resection	68	33 (48.5%)	7 (10%)	16 (23.5%)	12 (18%)	7 (10%)	4 (6%)
TOTALS	**100**	**48**	**13**	**20**	**19**	**10**	**7**

Abbreviations: LKS, Landau-Kleffner syndrome; MST, multiple subpial transection.

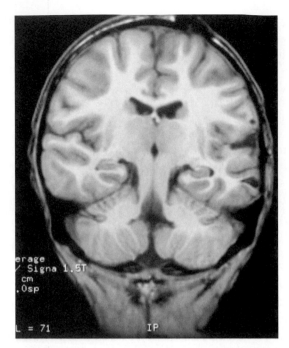

Figure 84.2 Coronal magnetic resonance image of a patient who underwent extensive multiple subpial transaction (MST) of the left frontotemporoparietal cortex. Often the effects of MST are not visible, but if there is snagging of vessels and minor hemorrhage, focal areas of encephalomalacia are seen.

primary somatosensory cortex; of note, a mild but definite diminution in rapid, skilled finger movement was identified in 29 of the 57 patients. Finally, MST was carried out in the Wernicke area and the angular and supramarginal

gyri in 45 patients. Some patients had transection in more than one area (Fig. 84.2).

Multiple Subpial Transection at Other Centers

MST is being performed today in epilepsy centers around the world. Table 84.2 summarizes the outcome and complications reported in 8 patient series (excluding our own series), totaling 158 patients (61–67). Outcome data were classified in different ways by the nine centers; however, we summarized the data by grouping it into two categories: significantly improved (equivalent to Engel class I, II, or III) and no meaningful improvement (equivalent to Engel class IV). A total of 210 patients (81%) fell into the category of significant improvement. Not all centers have reported such favorable outcomes (63–67). In addition, there are reports of recurrence of late seizures following MST (63–67). Thirty-four patients (13.2%) were reported to have experienced a neurologic deficit (Fig. 84.3).

CONCLUSIONS

Corpus callosotomy and MST are different surgical techniques in which the basic modus operandi is a disconnection procedure. The efficacy of corpus callosotomy has now been demonstrated in multiple centers around the world, although other therapies are usually exhausted first. Although MST is being used with increasing frequency in epilepsy centers worldwide, the procedure has yet to gain

TABLE 84.2

POSTSURGICAL OUTCOME FOLLOWING MULTIPLE SUBPIAL TRANSECTION AT EPILEPSY CENTERS

| Author, Year (Ref. No.) | No. of Patients | Significant Improvement | | No Worthwhile Improvement | | Neurologic Complications | |
		Only MST	MST & RES	MST Only	MST & RES	No. of Patients	Type (No. of Patients)
Shimizu et al., 1991 (65)	12	12	—	0	0	0	—
Sawhney et al., 1995 (66)	21	8	12	1	0	0	—
Zonghui, 1995	50	32[a]	—	18[a]	—	0	—
Wyler et al., 1995 (67)	6	6	—	0	—	1	Mild motor (1)
Hufnagel et al., 1997 (62)	22	4	15	2	1	7	Mild speech deficits (2); mild motor deficits (3); overt speech deficits (2)
Pacia, 1997 (64)	21	3	18	0	1	9	Mild dysnomia (7); moderate dysphasia (1); loss of proprioception in hand (1)
Rougier et al., 1934 (35)	7	2	0	5	0	0	
Patil et al., 1997[b]	19	4	13	1	1	0	
Rush Epilepsy Center	100	25	56	7	12	17	Permanent (7); transient (8); sensorimotor (13)
TOTAL	**258**	**96**	**114**	**34**	**15**	**34**	

Abbreviations: MST, multiple subpial transection; RES, resection.
[a]In this study, it was not clear whether MST alone versus MST-resection was performed.
[b]Patil AA, Andrews RV, Torkelson R. Surgical treatment of intractable seizures with multilobar or bihemispheric seizure foci. *Surg Neurol* 1997;47:72–78.

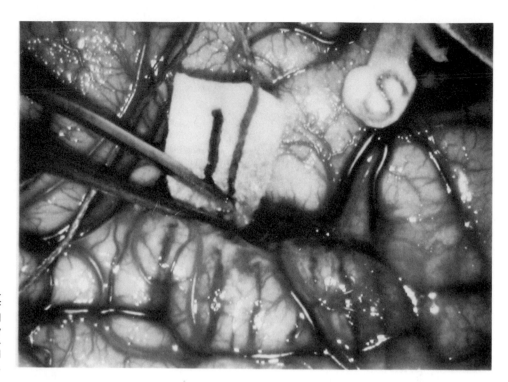

Figure 84.3 Example of extensive multiple subpial transection of multiple gyri in the frontoparietal cortex. Note the fine capillary bleeding, marking the site of transection, and the transient neocortical swelling produced by the procedure.

universal acceptance. Additional experimental and clinical studies are needed before this surgical technique is integrated into the therapeutic armamentarium at all major epilepsy centers. Much of the success of both procedures depends on the proper selection of patients and the experience of the neurologic and neurosurgical teams. A learning curve should be expected whenever these procedures are newly implemented at any epilepsy center.

ACKNOWLEDGMENT

We thank Irene O'Connor for her editorial assistance and encouragement.

REFERENCES

1. Van Wagenen WP, Herren RY. Surgical division of commissural pathways in the corpus callosum: relation to spread of an epileptic attack. *Arch Neurol Psychiatry* 1940;44:740–759.
2. Blume WT. Corpus callosotomy: a critical review. In: Tuxhom I, Holthausen H, Boenigk H, eds. *Pediatric epilepsy syndromes and their surgical treatment.* London: John Libbey, 1997:815–829.
3. Tomasch J. Size, distribution, and number of fibres in the human corpus callosum. *Anat Rec* 1954;119:119–135.
4. Pandya DN, Seltzer B. The topography of commissural fibers. In: Lepore F, Ptito M, Jaspar HH, eds. *Two hemispheres—one brain: functions of the corpus callosum.* New York: Alan R. Liss, 1986:47–73.
5. Asanuma H, Okuda O. Effects of transcallosal volleys on pyramidal tract cell activity of cat. *J Neurophysiol* 1962;25:198–208.
6. Gates JR, dePaola L. Corpus callosum section. In: Sliovon S, Dreifuss F, Fish D, et al., eds. *The treatment of epilepsy.* London: Blackwell Scientific, 1996:722–738.
7. Spencer SS, Spencer DD, Williamson PD, et al. Corpus callosotomy for epilepsy. I: seizure effects. *Neurology* 1988;38:19–24.
8. Kopeloff N, Kennard MA, Pacalla BL, et al. Section of corpus callosum in experimental epilepsy in the monkey. *Arch Neurol Psychiatry* 1950;63:719–727.
9. DePaola L, Gates LR, Ritter FJ, et al. Persistence of generalized ictal electroencephalographic onset after corpus callosotomy. *Neurology* 1996.
10. Wada JA, Sata M. The generalized convulsive seizures induced by daily electrical stimulation of the amygdala in split brain cats. *Epilepsia* 1975;16:417–430.
11. Musgrave J, Gloor P. The role of the corpus callosum in bilateral interhemispheric synchrony of spike and wave discharge in feline generalized penicillin epilepsy. *Epilepsia* 1980;21:369–378.
12. Naquet R, Wada JA. Role of the corpus callosum in photosensitive seizures of epileptic baboon *Papio papio. Adv Neurol* 1992;57:579–587.
13. Wada JA, Jomai S. Effect of anterior two-thirds callosal bisection upon bisymmetrical and bisynchronous generalized convulsions kindled from amygdala in epileptic baboon, *Papio papio.* In: Reeves AG, ed. *Epilepsy and the corpus callosum.* New York: Plenum Press, 1985:75–97.
14. Wilson DH, Reeves AG, Gazzaniga MS, et al. Cerebral commissurotomy for control of intractable seizures. *Neurology* 1977;27:708–715.
15. Spencer SS, Spencer DD, Williamson PD, et al. Effects of corpus callosum section on secondary bilaterally synchronous interictal EEG discharges. *Neurology* 1985;35:1689–1694.
16. Courtney W, Gates JR, Ritter F, et al. Prediction of seizure outcome after corpus callosotomy in patients ten years or older. *Epilepsia* 1993;34(Suppl):43.
17. Huck FR, Radvany J, Avila JO, et al. Anterior callosotomy in epileptics with multiform seizures and bilateral synchronous spike and wave EEG pattern. *Acta Neurochir Suppl (Wein)* 1980;30:127–135.
18. Nordgren RE, Reeves AG, Viguera AC, et al. Corpus callosotomy for intractable seizures in the pediatric age group. *Arch Neurol* 1991;48:364–372.
19. Wilson DH, Reeves A, Gazzaniga MS. "Central" commissurotomy for intractable generalized epilepsy: series two. *Neurology* 1982;32:687–697.
20. Gates Jr. Candidacy for corpus callosotomy. In: Luders H, ed. *Epilepsy surgery.* New York: Raven Press, 1991:140–150.
21. Gates JR. Presurgical evaluation for epileptic surgery in the era of long-term monitoring for epilepsy. In: Apuzzo MLJ, ed. *Neurosurgical aspects of epilepsy.* Chicago: AANS Publications, 1991:59–72.
22. Gates JR, Maxwell R, Leppik IE, et al. Electroencephalographic and clinical effects of total corpus callosotomy. In: Reeves AG, ed.

Epilepsia and the corpus callosum. New York: Plenum Press, 1986: 315–328.

23. Gates JR, Mireles R, Maxwell RE, et al. Magnetic resonance imaging, electroencephalogram and selected neuropsychological testing in staged corpus callosotomy. *Arch Neurol* 1986;43:1188–1191.
24. Spencer SS, Katz A, Ebersole J, et al. Ictal EEG changes with corpus callosum section. *Epilepsia* 1993;34:568–573.
25. Spencer SS, Spencer DD, Glaser GH, et al. More intense focal seizure types after callosal section; the role of inhibition. *Ann Neurol* 1984;16:686–693.
26. Fuiks KS, Wylfer AR, Hermann BP, et al. Seizure outcome from anterior and complete corpus callosotomy. *J Neurosurg* 1991;74: 573–578.
27. Harbaugh RE, Wilson DH, Reeves AG, et al. Forebrain commissurotomy for epilepsy: review of 20 consecutive cases. *Acta Neurochir (Wien)* 1983;68:263–275.
28. Oguni H, Olivier A, Andermann F, et al. Anterior callosotomy in the treatment of medically intractable epilepsies: a study of 43 patients with a mean follow-up of 39 months. *Ann Neurol* 1991;30:357–364.
29. Philips J, Sakas DE. Anterior callosotomy for intractable epilepsy: outcome in a series of twenty patients. *Br J Neurosurg* 1996;10: 351–356.
30. Gates JR, Courtney W, Ritter F, et al. Prediction of seizure outcome after corpus callosotomy among young children. *Epilepsia* 1993;34(Suppl):111.
31. Purves SJ, Wada JA, Woodhurst WB. Anterior callosotomy for complex partial seizures. Paper presented at the Second Dartmouth International Conference on Epilepsy and the Corpus Callosum; August 12, 1991; Hanover, New Hampshire.
32. Cendes F, Ragazzo PC, da Costa V, et al. Corpus callosotomy in treatment of medically resistant epilepsy: preliminary results in a pediatric population. *Epilepsia* 1993;34:910–917.
33. Reutens DC, Bye AM, Hopkins IJ, et al. Corpus callosotomy for intractable epilepsy: seizure outcome and prognostic factors. *Epilepsia* 1993;34:904–909.
34. Machara T, Shimizu H. Surgical outcome of corpus callosotomy in patients with drop attacks. *Epilepsia* 2001;42:67–71.
35. Rougier A, Claverie B, Pedespan JM, et al. Callosotomy for intractable epilepsy: overall outcome. *J Neurosurg Sci* 1997;41: 51–57.
36. Papo I, Quattrini A, Ortenzi A, et al. Predictive factors of callosotomy in drug-resistant epileptic patients with a long follow-up. *J Neurosurg Sci* 1997;41:31–36.
37. Gilliam F, Wyllie E, Kotagal P, et al. Parental assessment of functional outcome after corpus callosotomy. *Epilepsia* 1996;37: 753–757.
38. Hodaie M, Musharbash A, Otsubo H, et al. Image-guided, frameless stereotactic sectioning of the corpus callosum in children with intractable epilepsy. *Pediatr Neurosurg* 2000;34:286–294.
39. Awad IA, Wyllie E, Luders H, et al. Intraoperative determination of the extent of the corpus callosotomy for epilepsy: two simple techniques. *Neurosurgery* 1990;25:102–106.
40. Black PM, Holmes G, Lombroso CT. Corpus callosum section for intractable epilepsy in children. *Pediatr Neurosurg* 1992;18: 298–304.
41. Ferguson SM, Rayport M, Corrie WS. Neuropsychiatric observations on behavioral consequences of corpus callosum section for seizure control. In: Reeves AG, ed. *Epilepsy and the corpus callosum.* New York: Plenum Press, 1985:501–514.
42. Sass KJ, Spencer SS, Novelly RA, et al. Amnestic and attention impairments following corpus callosum section for epilepsy. *J Epilepsy* 1988;1:61–66.
43. Gates JR, Rosenfeld WE, Maxwell RE, et al. Response of multiple seizure types to corpus callosum section. *Epilepsia* 1987;28:28–34.
44. Gates JR, Ritter FJ, Ragazzo PC, et al. Corpus callosum section in children: seizure response. *J Epilepsy* 1990;3:271–278.
45. Spencer SS, Gates JR, Reeves AG, et al. Corpus callosum section. In: Engel J Jr, ed. *Surgical treatment of the epilepsies.* New York: Raven Press, 1987:425–444.
46. Pendl G, Eder H, Schroettner O, et al. Corpus callosotomy with radiosurgery. *Neurosurgery* 1999;45:303–308.
47. Morrell F, Whisler WW, Bleck T. Multiple subpial transection: a new approach to the surgical treatment of focal epilepsy. *J Neurosurg* 1989;70:231–239.
48. Asanuma H, Sakata H. Functional organization of a cortical efferent system examined with focal depth stimulation in cats. *J Neurophysiol* 1967;30(Suppl):35–54.
49. Hubel DH, Wiesel TN. Receptive fields, binocular interaction and functional architecture in the cat's visual cortex. *J Physiol* 1962; 160:106–154.
50. Mountcastle VB. Modality and topographic properties of single neurons of cat's somatic sensory cortex. *J Neurophysiol* 1957;20:408–434.
51. Sperry RW. Physiological plasticity and brain circuit theory. In: Harlow HF, Woolsey CN, eds. *Biological and biochemical bases of behavior.* Madison: University of Wisconsin Press, 1958:401–418.
52. Lueders H, Bustamante I, Zablow L, et al. The independence of closely spaced discrete experimental spike foci. *Neurology* 1981;31:846–851.
53. Reichenthal E, Hocherman S. The critical cortical areas for development of penicillin-induced epilepsy. *Electroencephalogr Clin Neurophysiol* 1977;42:248–251.
54. Tharp BR. The penicillin focus: a study of field characteristics using cross-correlation analysis. *Electroencephalogr Clin Neurophysiol* 1971;31:45–55.
55. Morrell F, Whisler W. Multiple subpial transection: technique, results and pitfalls. *Jpn J Neurosurg* 1993;12:101–107.
56. Morrell F. Electrophysiology of CSWS in Landau-Kleffner syndrome. In: Majno E, ed. *Continuous spikes and waves during slow sleep. Electrical status epilepticus during slow sleep acquired epileptic aphasia and related conditions.* Milan, Italy: Mraiani Foundation, 1995:77–90.
57. Kanner AM, Kaydanova Y, de Toledo-Morrell L, et al. Tailored anterior temporal lobectomy: relation between effect of resection of mesial structures and post-surgical seizure outcome. *Arch Neurol* 1995;52:173–178.
58. Wyler AR, Wilkus RJ, Rotard SW, et al. Multiple subpial transection for partial seizures in sensorimotor cortex. *Neurosurgery* 1995;37:1122–1128.
59. Engel J. Outcome with respect to epileptic seizures. In: Engel J Jr, ed. *Surgical treatment of the epilepsies.* New York: Raven Press, 1987:553–571.
60. Grote CL, VanSlyke P, Hoeppner JB. Language outcome following multiple subpial transection for Landau-Kleffner syndrome. *Brain* 1999;122:561–566.
61. Devinsky O, Perrine K, Vazquez B, et al. Multiple subpial transections in the language cortex. *Brain* 1994;117:255–265.
62. Hufnagel A, Zentner J, Fernandez G, et al. Multiple subpial transection for control of epileptic seizures: effectiveness and safety. *Epilepsia* 1997;38:678–688.
63. Lui L, Zhao Q, Li S, et al. Multiple subpial transection for treatment of intractable epilepsy. *Chin Med J* 1995;108:539–541.
64. Pacia SV, Devinsky O, Perrine K, et al. Multiple subpial transection for intractable partial seizures: seizure outcome. *J Epilepsy* 1997;10:86–91.
65. Shimizu H, Suzuki I, Ishima B, et al. Multiple subpial transection (MST) for the control of seizures that originated in unresectable cortical foci. *Jpn J Psychiatry Neurol* 1991;45:354–356.
66. Sawhney IMS, Robertson IJA, Polkey CE, et al. Multiple subpial transection: a review of 21 cases. *J Neurol Neurosurg Psychiatry* 1995;58:344–349.
67. Wyler AR, Wilkus RJ, Rotard SW, et al. Multiple subpial transection for partial seizures in sensorimotor cortex. *Neurosurgery* 1995;37:1122–1128.

Newer Operative and Stereotactic Techniques and Their Application to Hypothalamic Hamartoma

85

A. Simon Harvey   *Jeremy L. Freeman*

Hypothalamic hamartomas (HHs), or hamartomata, are congenital, tumor-like malformations of the tuber cinereum that are associated with precocious puberty, epilepsy, intellectual disability, and behavioral disturbances. The common seizure type seen in individuals with HH is the gelastic seizure in which patients have uncontrollable laughter. Such seizures often present from the first year of life. In many patients with HH, there is evolution of the epilepsy overtime, with appearance of complex partial, focal motor, atonic and convulsive seizures (1). Such epileptic progression is usually associated with behavioral deterioration, cognitive arrest or decline, and the appearance of generalized spike-waves on scalp electroencephalogram (EEG) (2–4). Epileptic seizures associated with HH are typically refractory to treatment (1–3), although some patients experience only minor gelastic attacks without the aforementioned progression (5,6). Patients undergoing surgical evaluation have usually failed treatment with antiepileptic drugs, vagal nerve stimulation, and the ketogenic diet.

HHs are unique epileptogenic lesions that pose challenges for the epileptologist in the course of presurgical evaluation. Because of the deep location, amorphous structure, and complex connectivity of HHs, it is not possible to record interictal or ictal epileptiform activity using scalp electroencephalography. Ictal single-photon-emission com-

puted tomography (SPECT) may show HH hyperperfusion in some patients (7,8), but if seizures are brief or the HH is small, this may not be present. Clinical seizure characteristics and scalp electroencephalography during partial seizures may suggest focal frontal or temporal involvement (1,9), often lateralized in patients with asymmetrically attached HH. Similarly, generalized seizures and spike-wave EEG patterns may suggest a widespread epileptic disturbance of the cerebrum (1,9). Depth EEG recordings may reveal interictal epileptiform activity in the HH, and ictal activity arising in the HH during gelastic seizures has been reported (3,7,10–12). However, depth EEG recordings do not reveal ictal origin of tonic seizures in the HH (10), nor do they show HH origin of generalized slow spike-waves in patients with SGE (4). Thus, demonstration of seizure origin from the HH may be difficult or impossible, and associated focal or generalized electroclinical features may suggest localized or diffuse cortical origin of seizures.

In recent surgical series, seizure origin in the HH was generally assumed, without confirmation from depth recordings, and focal or lateralized clinical or EEG findings were ignored (3,13–16). The key elements in the presurgical evaluation of patients with HH and intractable epilepsy should be to (a) determine the type of seizures, the presence of SGE, and the impact of epilepsy on the patient; (b) demonstrate the anatomy of the HH and exclude any associated cortical malformation; (c) characterize the patient's cognitive, behavioral, and psychiatric profile; and (d) assess the patient's preoperative endocrine and visual status (17–19).

HHs also pose considerable challenges for the epilepsy surgeon, requiring expertise with third ventricular microsurgical, endoscopic, or stereotactic techniques. The postoperative course of patients with HH is different from that of other epilepsy surgery patients, in that many have transient diabetes insipidus and require close attention to fluid management (14,16,17,20); nocturnal tonic seizures may persist for weeks after surgery before gradually "running down" (4,16,21,22); and transient or permanent short-term memory impairment (12,16,23), appetite stimulation (4,12,14,16), hemiparesis (3,12,14,16), and ocular palsy (3,12,14,20) are not uncommon complications of surgery.

The disappointing early results from cortical resection (9), corpus callosotomy (9,24), and attempted hamartoma removal (25–28), as well as concern about widespread cerebral dysgenesis (29) or epileptogenesis (1,9), dissuaded many clinicians from surgery in patients with HH, despite the disabling and often progressive nature of the seizure disorder. It was not until data was amassed from depth electroencephalography (7,10,11) and ictal SPECT (7,8) supporting the HH origin of at least gelastic seizures, and reports emerged of successful surgical amelioration of seizures with minimal morbidity (7,8,15,21,30–32), that surgical treatment of HH became more widely adopted (2,33). Currently, several operative techniques are described using open craniotomy (pterional, frontotemporal, frontal, or paramedian) and either microsurgical or endoscopic resection, disconnection, or ablation of the HH. Minimally invasive stereotactic approaches with image-guided endoscopy, radiofrequency thermocoagulation, and radiosurgery are also reported. In 2003, approximately 120 patients with HH undergoing more than 150 operations for epilepsy were reported in the literature, with surgery performed from early infancy (14,23) to young adulthood (mean age at surgery, 11 years). The following is a review of surgical approaches for the treatment of intractable epilepsy associated with HH; some of these novel approaches also have been applied to other epileptogenic lesions.

PTERIONAL AND FRONTOTEMPORAL OPERATIVE APPROACHES

Early approaches to the resection of HH associated with epilepsy (26,27,34–36) drew on neurosurgical experience with resection of craniopharyngiomas, other suprasellar tumors, and HH associated with precocious puberty. These lateral approaches from below are performed with a pterional or large frontotemporal craniotomy, accessing the HH via a transsylvian, transfrontal, subtemporal, or subfrontal approach (3,14,21,23,30,31), in some cases following

removal of the temporal pole and/or orbital cortex. HHs associated with precocious puberty are treatable in this fashion (23,37), as these lesions tend to be pedunculated and lack much of an intraventricular attachment (4,31,38). However, such approaches to epileptogenic HH may be ineffective, as only the subventricular component of the HH can be removed, leaving the intraventricular component attached to the mammillary bodies—a connection that seems to be important for epileptogenesis (2–4,33). Furthermore, the neurosurgeon encounters pituitary and neurovascular structures, which significantly increase the risk for endocrine complications, stroke, and oculomotor paresis (3,14). In the multicenter series reported by Palmini and colleagues (3), of 12 patients with HH ages 3 to 33 years (mean age, 8 years) undergoing surgery using a pterional or frontotemporal approach, complete resection was achieved in only 2, thalamocapsular stroke occurred in 4, and third nerve palsy was reported in 4, with the neurologic deficits improving or resolving in all patients. Three patients were seizure free, six had a greater than 90% reduction in seizures, and four had a 50% or less reduction in seizures (mean follow-up, 3.3 years). Improvements in behavior, cognition, and development were reported in all patients, regardless of seizure outcome.

The technical challenges, inadequacy of intraventricular resection, and operative complications associated with pterional and frontotemporal approaches forced some surgeons to adopt alternative strategies (8,14). Delalande and Fohlen now advocate disconnection as a safer alternative to resection, with comparable seizure outcome (14). Their approach is to disconnect the infraventricular component of the HH via a pterional craniotomy. Of 14 patients ages 1 to 19 years (mean age, 11 years) who underwent pterional disconnection, 2 developed a stroke and 1 developed panhypopituitarism. Seven patients required subsequent endoscopic disconnection of the intraventricular component of their HH (see Endoscopic Approaches), with the resultant seizure outcome in the 12 patients with more than 1-year follow-up being seizure freedom in 5 and 80% to 90% seizure reduction in 7. Behavioral improvements were reported in 10 patients.

TRANSCALLOSAL OPERATIVE APPROACH

Recognizing the technical challenges and suboptimal results with classic pterional and frontotemporal approaches to epileptogenic HH, as well as the likely importance of resecting the intraventricular component of the HH attached posteriorly to the mammillary body, Rosenfeld and associates adopted a transcallosal approach to intraventricular resection of HHs (8). This approach is interhemispheric, passing through a 2- to 3-cm opening in the anterior corpus callosum, between the columns of the fornices, to access the HH within the third ventricle. The technique allows clear and direct vision of the intraventricular

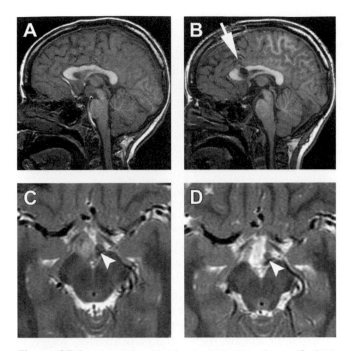

Figure 85.1 T1-weighted midsagittal (**A, B**) and magnified T2-weighted axial (**C, D**) images at the level of the hypothalamus in an 8-year-old boy with multiple daily gelastic and complex partial seizures, before (**A, C**) and after (**B, D**) transcallosal resection of his hypothalamic hamartoma (HH). The operative trajectory is shown on the postoperative midsagittal image (*large white arrow*). Preservation of the myelinated left mamillary body at the margin of the HH resection is shown on the axial images (*white arrowheads*). The procedure was associated with transient postoperative hypernatremia without diuresis, appetite stimulation, and mild nonverbal short-term memory disturbance that subsequently improved. The patient is seizure free at 16 months' follow-up.

component of the HH under the operating microscope, and complete or near-complete resection or disconnection of the intraventricular HH with the ultrasonic aspirator, using the third ventricular walls and pial floor as surgical margins (Fig. 85.1). Furthermore, this approach avoids injury to the circle of Willis, oculomotor nerve, optic chiasm, and pituitary stalk, as the resection is performed from entirely within the HH in the third ventricle. In a series of 29 consecutive patients ages 4 to 23 years (mean age, 10 years) undergoing transcallosal surgery for HH (19 with SGE), complete or near-complete resection (with or without disconnection) was achieved in 22 patients. The HH varied considerably in size, symmetry of hypothalamic attachment, and interpeduncular extension, but all had an intraventricular component with mammillary attachment (16,18). The broadly attached, inferior component of some large HHs that extended laterally could not be resected or disconnected, but this did not seem to correlate with seizure outcome.

In this series, seizure freedom was achieved in 15 patients, greater than 90% seizure reduction in 7 patients, 55% to 85% seizure reduction in 3 patients, and less than 40% seizure reduction in 4 patients, follow-up being from 1 to 6 years (mean, 2.5 years) (16). Most striking in this

series was the improvement in patients with SGE, in whom tonic seizures were frequently abolished, the scalp EEG improved, and better language and behavior were observed (4,16), dispelling the notion that these patients have diffuse and irreversible cerebral dysfunction or dysplasia(1,9,29). In six patients, the phenomenon of "running down" of generalized seizures was observed (4,16).

Small thalamic strokes were seen in only two patients in this series, none of which resulted in permanent neurologic deficits. Morbidity consisted of memory impairment in four patients, weight gain in five patients, and the need for thyroxine replacement in five patients. Transient hypernatremia and other biochemical disturbances of endocrine dysfunction occurred more often in this than in other surgical series (4,16). Short-term memory dysfunction occurred presumably as a result of forniceal or mammillary body injury sustained during intraventricular resection of the HH. In a young child with SGE, short-term memory disturbance may not be noticeable, and might even be masked by improvements in speech and behavior, but in an older patient with milder epilepsy and intact cognition, transcallosal surgery poses some risk to memory.

STEREOTACTIC RADIOFREQUENCY THERMOCOAGULATION

Radiofrequency thermocoagulation, a means of producing a localized lesion in a deep cerebral structure, is typically used in the treatment of movement disorders (39,40). A depth probe inserted stereotactically into the brain via a small frontal craniotomy or burr hole, usually under local anesthesia, is heated at its tip to approximately 80°C (176°F) for about 1 minute to produce a destructive lesion. Stereotactic radiofrequency ablation of HH was first reported by Kuzniecky and colleagues following recording of seizures with EEG monitoring and production of laughter with electrical stimulation of a depth electrode in the HH of one patient (7). Further reports followed (22,41), and Kuzniecky and Guthrie further developed their technique (12) to incorporate radiofrequency ablation with endoscopy (see Endoscopic Approaches). Multiple lesions may be produced and repeat procedures are not uncommon (Fig. 85.2). Stereotactic ablation of the mammillothalamic tract was reported in one patient with a HH who had continued seizures following pterional resection (3)

Sixteen patients with HH who underwent stereotactic radiofrequency ablation are reported in the literature, with eight requiring further ablations or surgical procedures (3,7,12,22,41). In a series of nine patients ages 2 to 30 years (mean age, 16 years) who underwent stereotactic radiofrequency ablation of HH, six required further stereotactic or endoscopic procedures (12). Ultimately, three patients became seizure free or had auras only, four had an 80% to 90% seizure reduction, and four had a 50% or less reduction in seizures. Morbidity included

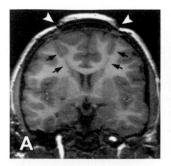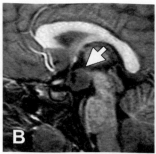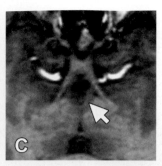

Figure 85.2   T1-weighted tilted coronal (**A**), midsagittal (**B**), and magnified axial (**C**) images at the level of the hypothalamus in a 9-year-old girl who underwent stereotactic radiofrequency thermocoagulation of her hypothalamic hamartoma (*large white arrows*) on two separate occasions at age 7 years. The coronal image shows the position of bilateral burr holes (*white arrowheads*) and the tracts created by placement of the depth electrodes (*black arrows*). The extent of the lesions created and their proximity to the optic tracts can be appreciated best on the axial image. The procedure was complicated by hyperphagia with sustained weight gain, and the patient continued to have frequent disabling seizures.

transient oculomotor palsy in one patient and appetite stimulation in another. The need for repeat procedures and the lower seizure-free rates most likely reflect the limited impact of the small lesions induced. Stereotactic radiofrequency thermocoagulation is probably suitable for small HHs only, or perhaps for large HHs in the area of hypothalamic attachment of the lesion. Potential problems with stereotactic radiofrequency thermocoagulation include small errors in stereotactic localization and the inability to confirm HH insertion with prior stimulation in an anesthetized patient. Relatively low morbidity and short hospital stay are clear advantages of stereotactic radiofrequency ablation compared with open craniotomy approaches.

ENDOSCOPIC APPROACHES

Ventricular neuroendoscopy has found a place in epilepsy surgery in the treatment of HH. Delalande and Fohlen use stereotactically guided endoscopy to disconnect the intraventricular HH or its component, often following pterional resection or disconnection of the infraventricular component (14). Access to the third ventricle is obtained via a transcortical approach through the frontal horn of the lateral ventricle and the foramen of Monro. In Delalande and Fohlen's series of nine patients undergoing endoscopic disconnection, seven had had prior pterional disconnection; one of two patients undergoing only endoscopic disconnection required a repeat procedure. No complications were observed following endoscopic disconnection. The one patient with more than 1-year follow-up after endoscopic surgery is seizure free.

Guthrie and Kuzniecky have moved from stereotactic radiofrequency ablation to endoscopic resection and endoscopic radiofrequency ablation (12). In 2 of 3 patients, surgery was uncomplicated and the patients became seizure free; a third patient experienced a brainstem infarct

and had only modest seizure improvement. Other reports of endoscopy are few (3,25), and larger series are required to determine whether such "minimally invasive" surgery is safe and effective. The nonpterional approach with avoidance of suprasellar neurovascular structures may be the important factor associated with reduced complications in these patients.

STEREOTACTIC RADIOSURGERY

Stereotactic radiosurgery is a means of delivering high-dose, ionizing radiation to a stereotactically defined intracranial target, with a steep radiation fall-off outside of the treated volume. The aim is to bring about delayed radiation necrosis, injury, or functional change to a lesion or brain site, with minimal effect on surrounding tissues. This is achieved by stereotactic definition of the target, collimation of a radiation beam to the size of the target, and dose averaging of multiple intersecting radiation beams. Currently, three radiation delivery systems are used for radiosurgery: (a) cyclotron-based, particle-beam systems for delivery of electrons, protons, neutrons, and alpha particles; (b) linear accelerator-based, photon-beam systems for delivery of x-rays (LINAC systems; www.linac.com); and (c) radioisotope-based, photon-beam systems for delivery of gamma rays (Leksell Gamma Knife systems; www.elekta.com). The Gamma Knife uses 201 ^{60}Co sources evenly distributed on the surface of a sphere, which produce photons of gamma radiation collimated to produce multiple beams of radiation that intersect at the same focal point. Adjustable, secondary collimators on a helmet fixed to the patient's head focus the radiation on the target, guided by sophisticated three-dimensional computerized dose planning (42,43).

The aim of radiosurgery depends on the pathology, with tissue necrosis (desired in tumors) and endothelial degeneration (desired in vascular malformations) requiring doses of 20 to 50 Gy. In patients with epilepsy, it is suggested that lower-dose radiation (<20 Gy) will bring about change in synaptic connectivity and neurotransmitters, leading to a rise in seizure threshold without neurologic deficit (44,45). Gamma Knife surgery is often recommended for the treatment of epilepsy associated with small, discrete lesions in deep, inaccessible locations or close to critical vascular or neural structures, but it may also play a role in the treatment of seizures involving eloquent cortex, if seizure remission can be induced without functional deficit. Potential disadvantages of radiosurgery are the inability to perform intraoperative electroencephalography, lack of histopathology, delay in seizure improvement, risk of delayed radionecrosis with large regional treatments, and theoretical risk of secondary tumors.

Gamma Knife radiosurgery has been used for the treatment of epilepsy associated with arteriovenous malformations (46), tumors (47), and cavernous angiomas (48), with 50% to 85% of patients in these series becoming seizure free or having significant seizure reductions when followed for 2 to 4 years. Gamma Knife surgery has been used as a minimally invasive approach for the treatment of corpus callosotomy (49) and anterior temporal lobectomy (50,51). Regis and colleagues reported on 16 patients with mesial temporal lobe epilepsy and hippocampal sclerosis who had Gamma Knife radiation to the affected temporal lobe, with 80% of them becoming seizure free over 6 to 21 months (50).

Gamma Knife surgery is well suited for the treatment of HHs, with use of the technique reported in 13 patients ages 1 to 32 years (mean age, 11 years) (13,15,32,52,53). Typical doses administered were 12 to 20 Gy (median marginal dose, 15.25 Gy) per 40% to 60% isodose, with two reported patients having second treatments of 35 Gy and 23 Gy (15). Five patients became seizure free over 3 months to 3 years, with significant improvement observed in the remainder, in whom follow-up was 1 to 6 years (mean, 3 years). No complications were reported. Like stereotactic radiofrequency ablation, Gamma Knife surgery is probably best suited for small HHs or for the hypothalamic attachment of larger HHs. Minimal morbidity and short hospital stays are clear advantages.

SUMMARY

The last decade has seen a resurgence of interest and improved outcomes in epilepsy surgery for HH. The technical challenges provided by these lesions have led to novel operative and stereotactic approaches to removal, disconnection, and ablation of HHs.

Comparing approaches is difficult because of relatively small patient numbers in most published series, differences in techniques between centers, patients undergoing multiple different procedures, and variable reporting of outcomes. If seizure outcomes are compared in patients undergoing only one surgical technique, and analysis is confined to series with adequate reporting and minimum 1-year follow-up, Engel class I or II outcome (seizure freedom, auras only, rare seizures only) resulted in 19 of 29 patients (66%) undergoing transcallosal resection (8,16); 3 of 5 patients (60%) undergoing endoscopic procedures (12,14); 5 of 13 patients (38%) undergoing Gamma Knife surgery (15,38,53); 9 of 25 patients (36%) undergoing pterional or frontotemporal approaches to resection or disconnection (3,14,26,31); and 3 of 11 patients (27%) undergoing stereotactic radiofrequency ablation (7,12,22,41).

Seizure outcome does not seem to be related to patient age, epilepsy factors such as presence of SGE, or HH characteristics such as size and extent of resection (16). Poor outcomes with pterional and frontotemporal approaches likely result from the inability to resect the intraventricular portion of the HH, whereas poor outcomes with stereotactic radiofrequency ablation and radiosurgery may reflect the small size of the lesions created. Neurovascular complications are significantly greater for operative compared with stereotactic approaches, more so with pterional and frontotemporal approaches than with transcallosal approaches. Endocrine and memory disturbances appear to be more common with the transcallosal approach. Endoscopic techniques hold promise, but there is limited experience at this stage.

Challenges for the future include the long-term follow-up of large series of treated patients, comparison of different operative and stereotactic approaches, and study of the impact of early surgery in patients with HH and refractory seizures. If the proposal that HH and gelastic epilepsy represent a model of epileptic deterioration through secondary epileptogenesis (2,3,4,54), then early surgery in patients with this condition may prevent the disabling neurobehavioral disturbances seen in many affected individuals. Finally, if the intrinsic epileptogenicity of HH is shown to be caused by an integral central connection, such as the mammillary bodies and mammillothalamic tract, then perhaps limited stereotactic approaches directed at such targets may provide the safest and most effective treatment.

REFERENCES

1. Berkovic SF, Andermann F, Melanson D, et al. Hypothalamic hamartomas and ictal laughter: evolution of a characteristic epileptic syndrome and diagnostic value of magnetic resonance imaging. *Ann Neurol* 1988;23:429–439.
2. Berkovic SF, Kuzniecky RI, Andermann F. Human epileptogenesis and hypothalamic hamartomas: new lessons from an experiment of nature. *Epilepsia* 1997;38:1–3.
3. Palmini A, Chandler C, Andermann F, et al. Resection of the lesion in patients with hypothalamic hamartomas and catastrophic epilepsy. *Neurology* 2002;58:1338–1347.
4. Freeman JL, Harvey AS, Rosenfeld JV, et al. Generalized epilepsy in hypothalamic hamartoma: evolution and postoperative resolution. *Neurology* 2003;60:762–767.
5. Sturm JW, Andermann F, Berkovic SF. "Pressure to laugh": an unusual epileptic symptom associated with small hypothalamic hamartomas. *Neurology* 2000;54:971–973.

6. Striano S, Striano P, Cirillo S, et al. Small hypothalamic hamartomas and gelastic seizures. *Epileptic Disord* 2002;4:129–133.

7. Kuzniecky R, Guthrie B, Mountz J, et al. Intrinsic epileptogenesis of hypothalamic hamartomas in gelastic epilepsy. *Ann Neurol* 1997;42:60–67.

8. Rosenfeld JV, Harvey AS, Wrennall J, et al. Transcallosal resection of hypothalamic hamartomas, with control of seizures, in children with gelastic epilepsy. *Neurosurgery* 2001;48:108–118.

9. Cascino GD, Andermann F, Berkovic SF, et al. Gelastic seizures and hypothalamic hamartomas: evaluation of patients undergoing chronic intracranial EEG monitoring and outcome of surgical treatment. *Neurology* 1993;43:747–750.

10. Kahane P, Munari C, Minotti L, et al. The role of the hypothalamic hamartoma in the genesis of gelastic and dacrystic seizures. In: Tuxhorn I, Hothausen H, Boenigk H, eds. *Paediatric epilepsy syndromes and their surgical treatment.* London: John Libbey; 1997: 447–461.

11. Munari C, Kahane P, Francione S, et al. Role of the hypothalamic hamartoma in the genesis of gelastic fits (a video-stereo-EEG study). *Electroencephalogr Clin Neurophysiol* 1995;95:154–160.

12. Kuzniecky R, Guthrie B. Stereotactic surgical approach to hypothalamic hamartomas. *Epileptic Disord* 2003;5:275–280.

13. Dunoyer C, Ragheb J, Resnick T, et al. The use of stereotactic radiosurgery to treat intractable childhood partial epilepsy. *Epilepsia* 2002;43:292–300.

14. Delalande O, Fohlen M. Disconnecting surgical treatment of hypothalamic hamartoma in children and adults with refractory epilepsy and proposal of a new classification. *Neurol Med Chir (Tokyo)* 2003;43:61–68.

15. Régis J, Bartolomei F, de Toffol B, et al. Gamma knife surgery for epilepsy related to hypothalamic hamartomas. *Neurosurgery* 2000;47:1343–1351.

16. Harvey AS, Freeman JL, Rosenfeld JV, Berkovic SF. Transcallosal resection of hypothalamic hamartomas in patients with intractable epilepsy. *Epileptic Disord* 2003;5:257–265.

17. Freeman JL, Zacharin M, Rosenfeld JV, Harvey AS. The endocrinology of hypothalamic hamartoma surgery for intractable epilepsy. *Epileptic Disord* 2003;5:239–247.

18. Freeman JL, Coleman LT, Wellard RM, et al. MR imaging and spectroscopic study of epileptogenic hypothalamic hamartomas: analysis of 72 cases. *AJNR Am J Neuroradiol* 2004;25:460–462.

19. Harvey AS, Freeman JL, Berkovic SF. Presurgical evaluation in patients with hypothalamic hamartomas. In: Rosenow F, Lüders HO, eds. *Presurgical assessment of the epilepsies with clinical neurophysiology and functional imaging.* Elsevier, 2004:441–450.

20. Striano S, Meo R, Bilo L, et al. Gelastic epilepsy: symptomatic and cryptogenic cases. *Epilepsia* 1999;40:294–302.

21. Nishio S, Morioka T, Fukui M, Goto Y. Surgical treatment of intractable seizures due to hypothalamic hamartoma. *Epilepsia* 1994;35:514–519.

22. Fukuda M, Kameyama S, Wachi M, Tanaka R. Stereotaxy for hypothalamic hamartoma with intractable gelastic seizures: technical case report. *Neurosurgery* 1999;44:1347–1350.

23. Mottolese C, Stan H, Bret P, et al. Hypothalamic hamartoma: the role of surgery in a series of eight patients. *Childs Nerv Syst* 2001;17:229–236.

24. Pallini R, Bozzini V, Colicchio G, et al. Callosotomy for generalized seizures associated with hypothalamic hamartoma. *Neurol Res* 1993;15:139–141.

25. Breningstall GN. Gelastic seizures, precocious puberty, and hypothalamic hamartoma. *Neurology* 1985;35:1180–1183.

26. Sato M, Ushio Y, Arita N, Mogami H. Hypothalamic hamartoma: report of two cases. *Neurosurgery* 1985;16:198–206.

27. Sher PK, Brown SB. Gelastic epilepsy. Onset in neonatal period. *Am J Dis Child* 1976;130:1126–1131.

28. Ponsot G, Diebler C, Plouin P, et al. Hypothalamic hamartoma and gelastic crises: Apropos of 7 cases [French]. *Arch Fr Pediatr* 1983;40:757–761.

29. Sisodiya SM, Free SL, Stevens JM, et al. Widespread cerebral structural changes in two patients with gelastic seizures and hypothalamic hamartomata. *Epilepsia* 1997;38:1008–1010.

30. Machado HR, Hoffman HJ, Hwang PA. Gelastic seizures treated by resection of a hypothalamic hamartoma. *Childs Nerv Syst* 1991;7:462–465.

31. Valdueza JM, Cristante L, Dammann O, et al. Hypothalamic hamartomas: with special reference to gelastic epilepsy and surgery. *Neurosurgery* 1994;34:949–958.

32. Arita K, Kurisu K, Iida K, et al. Subsidence of seizure induced by stereotactic radiation in a patient with hypothalamic hamartoma. Case report. *J Neurosurg* 1998;89:645–648.

33. Berkovic SF, Arzimanoglou A, Kuzniecky R, et al. Hypothalamic hamartoma and seizures: a treatable epileptic encephalopathy. *Epilepsia* 2003;44:969–973.

34. Northfield DW, Russell DS. Pubertas praecox due to hypothalamic hamartoma: report of two cases surviving surgical removal of the tumour. *J Neurol Neurosurg Psychiatry* 1967;30:166–173.

35. Pendl G. Gelastic epilepsy in tumours of the hypothalamic region. *Adv Neurosurgery* 1975;3:442–449.

36. Takeuchi J, Handa H, Miki Y, et al. Precocious puberty due to a hypothalamic hamartoma. *Surg Neurol* 1979;11:456–460.

37. Stewart L, Steinbok P, Daaboul J. Role of surgical resection in the treatment of hypothalamic hamartomas causing precocious puberty. Report of six cases. *J Neurosurg* 1998;88:340–345.

38. Arita K, Ikawa F, Kurisu K, et al. The relationship between magnetic resonance imaging findings and clinical manifestations of hypothalamic hamartoma. *J Neurosurg* 1999;91:212–220.

39. Lozano A, Hutchison W, Kiss Z, et al. Methods for microelectrode-guided posteroventral pallidotomy. *J Neurosurg* 1996;84:194–202.

40. Vitek JL, Bakay RA, Hashimoto T, et al. Microelectrode-guided pallidotomy: technical approach and its application in medically intractable Parkinson's disease. *J Neurosurg* 1998;88:1027–1043.

41. Parrent AG. Stereotactic radiofrequency ablation for the treatment of gelastic seizures associated with hypothalamic hamartoma. Case report. *J Neurosurg* 1999;91:881–884.

42. Friedman WA, Bova FJ. Stereotactic radiosurgery. In: Crockard A, Hayward R, Hoff JT, eds. *Neurosurgery: the scientific basis and clinical practice,* 3rd ed. Oxford, UK: Blackwell Science, 2000:3317–3339.

43. Spiegelmann R, Friedman WA. Principles of stereotaxis. In: Tindall GT, Cooper PR, Barrow DL, eds. *The practice of neurosurgery.* Baltimore, MD: Lippincott Williams & Wilkins, 1996:887–895.

44. Chen ZF, Kamiryo T, Henson SL, et al. Anticonvulsant effects of gamma surgery in a model of chronic spontaneous limbic epilepsy in rats. *J Neurosurg* 2001;94:270–280.

45. Régis J, Kerkerian-Legoff L, Rey M, et al. First biochemical evidence of differential functional effects following gamma knife surgery. *Stereotact Funct Neurosurg* 1996;66(Suppl 1):29–38.

46. Gerszten PC, Adelson PD, Kondziolka D, et al. Seizure outcome in children treated for arteriovenous malformations using gamma knife radiosurgery. *Pediatr Neurosurg* 1996;24:139–144.

47. Schrottner O, Eder HG, Unger F, et al. Radiosurgery in lesional epilepsy: brain tumors. *Stereotact Funct Neurosurg* 1998;70(Suppl 1):50–56.

48. Régis J, Bartolomei F, Kida Y, et al. Radiosurgery for epilepsy associated with cavernous malformation: retrospective study in 49 patients. *Neurosurgery* 2000;47:1091–1097.

49. Pendl G, Eder HG, Schroettner O, Leber KA. Corpus callosotomy with radiosurgery. *Neurosurgery* 1999;45:303–307.

50. Régis J, Bartolomei F, Rey M, et al. Gamma knife surgery for mesial temporal lobe epilepsy. *J Neurosurg* 2000;93(Suppl 3):141–146.

51. Kawai K, Suzuki I, Kurita H, et al. Failure of low-dose radiosurgery to control temporal lobe epilepsy. *J Neurosurg* 2001;95: 883–887.

52. Unger F, Schrottner O, Haselsberger K, et al. Gamma knife radiosurgery for hypothalamic hamartomas in patients with medically intractable epilepsy and precocious puberty. Report of two cases. *J Neurosurg* 2000;92:726–731.

53. Unger F, Schrottner O, Feichtinger M, et al. Stereotactic radiosurgery for hypothalamic hamartomas. *Acta Neurochir Suppl* 2002; 84:57–63.

54. Morrell F. Varieties of human secondary epileptogenesis. *J Clin Neurophysiol* 1989;6:227–275.

Outcome and Complications of Epilepsy Surgery

86

Deepak K. Lachhwani   *Elaine Wyllie*

The past decade has seen epilepsy surgery rise favorably in the ranks of treatment options for medically refractory seizures. Numerous factors have contributed to this reality, foremost among them being improved diagnostic and surgical techniques. Equally important are an increased understanding of medical refractoriness, the natural course of epilepsy specific to etiology, and developmental plasticity influencing timing of surgery, along with mounting evidence regarding effectiveness of epilepsy surgery in controlling seizures and exerting a positive impact on quality of life. These factors in concert have catapulted epilepsy surgery from the last resort in a relatively hopeless situation of intractable seizures to a treatment of choice in carefully selected candidates with refractory focal epilepsy who have a favorable risk-to-benefit ratio for operation.

As with most solutions, epilepsy surgery has its share of shortcomings. While aiming for relief from epilepsy, one must also take into account the potential for complications directly related to surgery as well as for impairment in existing neurologic function. Accumulating experience from specialized epilepsy centers makes the equation of risk versus benefit a dynamic one. For example, postoperative seizure outcome may be favorable in selected patients with focal epileptogenic lesions on magnetic resonance imaging (MRI), even in the setting of epileptic spasms and hypsarrhythmia or other generalized seizure types and a poorly localizing electroencephalographic (EEG) record. At the same time, the face of perceived risk involved in epilepsy surgery is changed by the ability of selected centers to safely offer a wide range of procedures, such as mesial temporal resection for hippocampal sclerosis, multilobar resections for malformations of cortical development, hemispherectomy or cortical resection for catastrophic epilepsy in early infancy, and resective surgery during medically refractory status epilepticus (RSE). The evolving assessment for risk versus benefit must be weighed individually for every patient and be based on many factors.

POTENTIAL BENEFITS OF EPILEPSY SURGERY: SEIZURE OUTCOME

The likelihood of a favorable postsurgical seizure outcome is based primarily on data suggesting that seizures are arising from a resectable cortical region, as evidenced by convergent localizing information from seizure semiology, surface EEG recording, and neuroimaging. Detection of a focal epileptogenic lesion relies heavily on MRI, which has maintained its superiority among the neuroimaging modalities as the most accurate technique for visualizing anatomic detail *in vivo*. A clean convergence of data from all three domains is desirable for a good outcome. Because the EEG and semiology are less likely to indicate a restricted brain region with crisp margins, and may even implicate a more diffuse process, prognosis often depends heavily on the presence of a *lesion* on MRI with well-defined margins, its *location*, and its underlying *etiology*.

Presence or Absence of a Focal Lesion on Magnetic Resonance Imaging

Nonlesional MRI findings in patients who have focal epilepsy based on semiology and a surface EEG record may indicate a lower chance for seizure-free postoperative outcome (1). In contrast, patients with focal epilepsy as a consequence of a circumscribed lesion, such as mesial temporal sclerosis, low-grade neoplasm, vascular malformation, or focal malformation of cortical development, appear to have a better chance of seizure-free outcome (2,3). Use of adjunctive tests such as 2-[^{18}F]fluoro-2-deoxy-D-glucose-positron emission tomography (FDG-PET), and ictal and interictal single-photon-emission computed tomography may also contribute to identification of the ictal onset zone in nonlesional cases, but identification of an MRI lesion is still more desirable for delineating the potential epileptogenic zone and facilitating subsequent surgical planning.

Location of the Epileptogenic Zone

Location of the epileptogenic zone in a region that can be safely removed compared with proximity of the epileptogenic zone to eloquent cortical areas has obvious implications in surgical planning. If surgical resection is limited as a result of an unacceptable trade-off in acquiring new neurologic deficit, a less optimistic seizure-free outcome is to be expected. Extraoperative invasive recording with eloquent cortical mapping as well as intraoperative electrocorticography may be used to maximize resection without compromising neurologic function, but ultimately success will depend on the completeness of resection of the epileptogenic zone. Perhaps at least partially because of these issues, patients with mesial temporal epilepsy have a better chance for a seizure-free surgical outcome than those with neocortical temporal epilepsy, and patients with temporal lobe epilepsy have a better surgical outcome than those with extratemporal epilepsy (3–5). Significant limitations on the size of resection arise in perirolandic epilepsy and neocortical frontal or temporal lobe epilepsy in the language-dominant hemisphere.

Etiology

Of the different etiologies, results of epilepsy surgery in patients with *hippocampal sclerosis* are most gratifying, with centers consistently reporting more than 80% seizure-free outcomes. Early experience suggests that both selective amygdalohippocampectomies and less-selective temporal resections (including the mesial structures) are equally likely to produce a good surgical outcome (6,7). Memory findings on preoperative neuropsychological testing may ascribe function to the hippocampus on the side of resection, and in such instances a tailored resection that spares the hippocampus (corticoamygdalectomy) has been performed. However, the seizure-free rates drop to 51% after a hippocampus-sparing resection (8), and whether there is a definite benefit in memory outcome if a somewhat "deaf-ferentated" hippocampus is left behind is debatable. More data are required to realize the merits of such a selective surgical procedure.

Surgery in patients with epilepsy due to *low-grade neoplasm* is also viewed optimistically, and seizure freedom may be realized in a majority of them. In a pediatric series, 86% of patients in whom gross total resection of the neoplasm was accomplished were seizure free at follow-up (9). In an adult series from the same institution involving patients with ganglioglioma and intractable epilepsy, 63% were seizure free at follow-up overall, and a good outcome was likely with a lower age at operation and a shorter duration of epilepsy (10).

Cortical dysplasia results in seizure-free outcome rates ranging from 40% to 60% (5,11). This may be, in part, because MRI can underestimate the extent of a histologic abnormality and, in part, because of the inclusion of patients with diffuse multilobar or hemispheric malformations together with discrete focal cortical dysplasias in surgical series (12,13). Patients with focal cortical dysplasia are more amenable to a complete resection and as a subgroup of all dysplasia patients tend to have a seizure-free outcome comparable to that of patients with hippocampal sclerosis or low-grade neoplasm (2,14,15). In a study including 22 patients with focal cortical dysplasia, resection of the epileptogenic zone guided by histopathologically proven clear margins was significantly associated with an improved seizure outcome (92% seizure free versus 43% when resection was histopathologically proved to be subtotal) (2).

Multilobar or hemispheric malformations of cortical development form the other end of the spectrum of cortical malformations. Surgical treatment is very effective, and the method of choice is usually an extensive multilobar resection or hemispherectomy. In 12 children who underwent functional hemispherectomy for diffuse cortical malformation involving most or all of one hemisphere, seizure freedom or greater than 90% reduction in seizure burden was achieved in more than 80% of patients; 50% of patients were seizure free (13). In this series, patients with hemimegalencephaly were less likely to achieve seizure freedom (40% seizure free) compared with patients with hemispheric atrophy or relative sparing of one or part of a lobe as evident on MRI (83% seizure free). Possible explanations for this observation include likelihood of epileptogenic potential from abnormal subcortical structures of the removed hemisphere or the presence of contralateral epileptogenicity caused by microscopic abnormalities. Despite these challenges, surgery significantly lessened the burden of disease and must therefore be considered in patients with refractory epilepsy.

Approximately 15% of patients with hippocampal sclerosis evident on MRI also have evidence of cortical dysgenesis. Such "dual pathology" is also well recognized in neuronal migration disorders, low-grade neoplasms such as gliomas or dysembryoplastic neuroepithelial tumors, porencephalic cysts, vascular malformations, and reactive gliosis (16). A less favorable postoperative seizure outcome is more likely with coexisting dual pathology when only one abnormality is removed; therefore, surgical planning should be appropriately modified to include both lesions when possible (17,18). Removal of mesial temporal structures in addition to a temporal neoplasm was noted to result in a better outcome (92.8% seizure free) compared with that seen in patients who underwent resection of the tumor only (18.8% seizure free) (19). As with localization-related epilepsies in general, large resections are likely to be associated with a better outcome. Equally important, reoperation to extend the surgical resection should be considered if the initial resection is ineffective (18,20). In one series, more than 60% of patients with initial surgical failures (after lesionectomy alone) became seizure free after subsequent reoperation to remove the remaining epileptogenic tissue (19).

Special Situations

Medically Refractory Status Epilepticus (RSE) of focal origin, a medical emergency that may be encountered when seizures cannot be controlled despite high-dose suppressive therapy (HDST) to pharmacologic coma (21,22), is associated with significant morbidity and mortality. Studies report universal morbidity in survivors (23) and mortality ranging between 16% and 43.5% (24–26). If status epilepticus is deemed to be of focal origin, resective surgery may be an option. Scattered case reports have suggested that multiple subpial transections, cortical resection, corpus callosotomy, or implantation of a vagus nerve stimulator may be effective for controlling seizures in RSE (27–30). The concern of compounding risks of neurosurgery together with those of status epilepticus is a genuine one and may be one reason for underuse of a surgical approach in RSE of focal origin. However, uncontrolled status epilepticus and prolonged maintenance of pharmacologic coma are themselves not without risks, and these may even outweigh the risks of neurosurgical intervention (23–26). At tertiary epilepsy surgery centers with sufficient surgical experience and specially trained personnel, the surgical risk may be even lower and must be balanced against the risks of prolonged HDST. In a surgical series of 10 pediatric patients with RSE of focal origin in whom at least 2 weeks of HDST had failed, resective surgery was able to stop seizures acutely in the entire group (31). These patients had experienced morbidity during the prolonged phase of medical management in the intensive care unit. In contrast, no mortality and no substantial morbidity as a consequence of surgery occurred. After a median follow-up of 7 months, 7 of the 10 patients were seizure free, and 3 had a significant improvement in their epilepsy. These initial data highlight a potential role for resective surgery in a clinical situation of very limited therapeutic options and substantial risks for prolonged RSE and pharmacologic coma (31).

Diffuse EEG abnormalities in the presence of a focal MRI lesion constitute another special situation when epilepsy surgery may occasionally be an appropriate option. The presence of generalized interictal and ictal abnormalities on surface electroencephalography, with only a few exceptions, is considered an unfavorable sign for surgical candidacy. However, in the early 1990s, it was first recognized that selected infants with diffuse hypsarrhythmia and nonlocalizable scalp ictal EEG patterns during spasms became seizure free after resection of congenital lesions seen on PET and MRI scans (32). The immaturity of networks is felt to be the basis of such a diffuse EEG phenotype in the presence of a focal lesion during infancy. The interaction between focal epileptogenesis and a developing brain beyond the first year of life is not well known. It is widely appreciated that the developing brain undergoes dynamic changes and that there is an overabundance of synapses, which peak by about 2 years of age and remain high for most of the first 10 years of life, before decreasing to adult levels between 15 and 20 years of age (33,34). It is therefore conceivable that owing to the presence of a focal insult during early life, a diffuse EEG phenotype may be encountered beyond infancy.

We studied eight patients (mean age, 8 years at surgery and 2 years at seizure onset) with desperately severe epilepsy in the setting of a focal or hemispheric brain lesion and generalized features on EEG and seizure semiology (Gupta A, Wyllie E, Lachhwani DK, et al. Children with generalized scalp EEG discharges and focal brain lesions—could they be surgical candidates? Personal communication. 2004.). Adequate trials of multiple antiepileptic drugs (AEDs) had failed in these patients, who continued to have a significant seizure burden (several seizures per day and many episodes of status epilepticus). Surgery (cortical resection or functional hemispherectomy) was offered as a last resort after considerable deliberation, bioethics consultation, and informed parental consent. At the time of last follow-up (median, 11 months), seven of the eight patients were seizure free, and one patient had a greater than 90% reduction in seizure burden. All eight families also reported a brighter affect and overall improvement in quality of life for these patients after surgery. Although the numbers are small and follow-up is limited, these preliminary results show promise and provide clues to understanding the interacting forces of pathologic (epileptogenic) and physiologic networks of a young and developing brain that may result in a particular phenotype.

Prognostic Implications of Acute Postoperative Seizures

Acute postoperative seizures (APOS) occur within 1 week of resective surgery and are further classified as "early" (within 24 hours after surgery) or late (more than 24 hours and less than 1 week after surgery) (35–37). Seizures after resective surgery are of concern not only because they are emotionally devastating to patients and their families but also because they imply an incomplete resection of the epileptogenic zone or the presence of a more diffuse epileptogenic process than was determined preoperatively. Factors pertaining to acute surgical complications, such as hemorrhage, raised intracranial pressure, low AED levels, and infection, also may result in postoperative seizures.

The available literature suggests that APOS may have an impact on overall outcome. It is important to bear in mind, however, that studies to evaluate APOS have certain limitations that are difficult to overcome. The account of seizures is often based on history obtained from a family member or care provider who may not have proper experience and training to classify seizure type. Moreover, because video-EEG monitoring is not routinely performed after surgery, nonepileptic paroxysmal movements may be misinterpreted as seizures, or subtle epileptic seizures may be overlooked. Therefore, careful documentation is required.

APOS following temporal lobe resections were found to result in poor long-term seizure-free outcome, especially if they were noted beyond the first postoperative day (between days 1 and 7) (36). Patients with a single postoperative seizure or seizures restricted to the first postoperative day did not have a worse prognosis (36). Another study found no difference in prognosis between early versus late APOS; however, patients with APOS similar to their habitual preoperative seizures did poorly compared with patients whose APOS were auras or focal motor and/or generalized tonic-clonic seizures (35). No significant predictive factors were found that predisposed patients to APOS (35).

APOS after extratemporal resections are of particular concern because as a group these patients do less well than do patients who have temporal lobe resections (1,38). In a study of 65 patients who underwent frontal lobe resections, APOS were noted in up to 25% (39). At the 1-year follow-up, seizure-free outcome was similar in the two groups of patients (47.1% of those with versus 50.0% of those without a history of APOS). The study found that more patients without than with APOS had a decrease in seizure activity (70.8% versus 58.8%), but the difference was not significant.

In another study of 148 pediatric patients, 25% experienced APOS (37). This study also found a significant negative impact of APOS on seizure-free outcome rates (50.1% seizure free versus 80% seizure free). Patients with extratemporal epilepsy undergoing extratemporal resections were at significantly greater risk of experiencing APOS.

Discontinuation of Antiepileptic Drugs After Successful Epilepsy Surgery

There is a paucity of systematic data evaluating withdrawal of AEDs after varying periods of seizure remission in medically managed patients. The only randomized, controlled trials involve pediatric patients, and their results support waiting for 2 or more seizure-free years before discontinuing AEDs (40). The widely accepted 2-year mark may reflect a time during which spontaneous remission or "outgrowing" of the epilepsy could have occurred. It is not known whether this same timeframe applies after a focal epileptogenic cortical region has been surgically resected.

How long AED therapy should be continued after successful epilepsy surgery is unclear. In practice, AEDs are continued arbitrarily for varying periods or indefinitely, even though a patient is completely seizure free. Because of an absence of systematic data, the decision to discontinue medications often depends on the patient's or the family's wishes as well as on the treating physician's comfort level.

In a study involving 210 epilepsy surgery patients, AED therapy was changed in 180 patients during postsurgical follow-up: tapered and discontinued in 84, simplified but continued in 96 (41). At the 5-year follow-up, more than 60% (n = 62) of the patients remained seizure free after AED discontinuation. Of the 22 patients who had a seizure breakthrough, 20 were successfully controlled after the AED was restarted. Furthermore, the duration of postoperative seizure-free AED continuation did not have a bearing on the risk of seizure breakthrough, indicating that patients interested in discontinuing AED treatment can do so early (41). Experience with pediatric patients suggests an optimistic outlook for successful discontinuation of AEDs in seizure-free postoperative patients (Lachhwani DK, Loddenkemper T, Holland K, et al. Discontinuation of antiepileptic medications after epilepsy surgery in children. Personal communication. 2004.). AEDs were withdrawn in 68 of 97 pediatric patients who were seizure free for at least 6 months postsurgery; 57 (84%) remained seizure free, while 11 (16%) had seizure recurrence during a median follow-up of 68 months. Reinstatement of AEDs controlled seizures in 7 of 11 patients; 3 continued to have rare seizures; and 1 patient had frequent auras. The risk for seizure recurrence was significantly increased if AED discontinuation occurred at less than 6 months than at less than 12 or 24 months (respective odds ratios 4.9, 1.9, 1.9). No additional benefit was gained by waiting longer than 1 year (Lachhwani DK, Loddenkemper T, Holland K, et al. Discontinuation of antiepileptic medications after epilepsy surgery in children. Personal communication. 2004.). Therefore, it seems that the paradigm of waiting for 2 or more seizure-free years before attempting AED withdrawal may not be entirely applicable to patients who have undergone surgical removal of the epileptogenic substrate as a specific intervention for the cure of their epilepsy. Such patients may not need to remain on medications for several seizure-free years.

The decision for AED withdrawal may be complicated in adults by a reluctance to risk even a single seizure recurrence because of psychosocial consequences for driving and employment. Other concerns about postoperative

AED withdrawal may include the risk of status epilepticus as the first recurrent seizure episode or reemergence of medically refractory epilepsy that fails to come under control despite resumption of AEDs. However, results from available studies discussed above indicate that these risks are low.

RISKS OF EPILEPSY SURGERY: NEW POSTOPERATIVE DEFICITS

At experienced epilepsy centers, few unanticipated complications are related to the neurosurgical procedure. These include hemorrhagic or ischemic problems resulting in permanent neurologic sequelae, intracranial hematoma, infection, hydrocephalus, and surgical injury to nearby structures important to neurologic function. In a series of 708 consecutive patients over 6.5 years, less than 3% had any surgical complications, and less than 1% had neurologic complications (42). Although there was no mortality in this series, it is occasionally encountered and as an exception may remain inevitable (43).

The most common example of operative neurologic morbidity is an expected deficit, incurred to accomplish efficient removal of epileptogenic tissue. Asymptomatic visual-field deficits are seen in more than 50% of patients as a consequence of anterior temporal resections. Sectioning of the Meyer loop during removal of temporal lobe structures results in an upper homonymous quadrantanopsia. The patient is usually unaware of this deficit, which may be elicited only on visual-field testing. More severe visual-field cuts including homonymous hemianopia result from large temporo-occipital lobe resection or hemispherectomy. This clearly undesirable, permanent neurologic deficit may have long-term implications, including an inability to obtain driving privileges. A chance to remove a severe seizure burden and its adverse effect on quality of life may outweigh the setback of an anticipated visual-field deficit and should be contemplated in this light.

Primary Motor and Sensory Function

Surgical resection involving the perirolandic area carries a substantial risk of permanent deficit in neurologic function. Extensive mapping of function in relation to the epileptogenic zone is warranted and may be accomplished with the aid of extra- or intraoperative studies using subdural electrodes. Functional deficit can be avoided or minimized by preferential sparing of eloquent cortical areas. Resection in the primary face motor area of the nondominant hemisphere is usually tolerable, as it typically results in mild or transient facial weakness (44). This outcome is in contrast to similar resection in the dominant hemisphere, where motor speech control is also at risk,

although in one case series involving three patients, the dysarthria was transient and resolved after 1 to 2 weeks (45). Motor weakness after resection of cortical areas responsible for proximal large muscle groups in the upper and lower extremities is transient and resolves to a large extent over time. This is helpful in counseling families, because such recovery bodes well for a regained ability to ambulate independently after the acute postoperative period of worsened motor function.

Sensory deficits after resections in primary sensory cortex responsible for proximal limbs are also rarely disabling. However, the cortical sensory motor hand area should be spared whenever possible, as resection is likely to result in a disabling loss in fine finger movements or lead to a permanent impairment in important sensory hand functions such as tactile object recognition and two-point discrimination (46–48).

In a progressive epilepsy syndrome such as Rasmussen encephalitis, medical management typically fails to halt the disease and relieve epilepsy, and results with immunomodulatory therapy are variable. Surgery is currently the only definitive treatment, and the method of choice is a functional hemispherectomy. The timing of hemispherectomy depends heavily on the onset of motor deficit during the illness. When further worsening as a result of the disease itself is imminent, surgical intervention to stop seizures may appear desirable, even in the face of acute postsurgical worsening of the hemiparesis and incurrence of a new homonymous hemifield cut.

Memory

Impairment in memory function after temporal lobectomy is a major cause for concern owing to its attendant morbidity. The difficulty in identifying patients at greatest risk for such a decline only compounds the problem. Several variables are implicated in the likelihood and severity of verbal memory deficits after a dominant temporal lobe resection including the hippocampus. Patients rendered seizure free after epilepsy surgery are less likely to have a significant memory deficit than are patients with continued postoperative seizures (49,50). Memory decline may correlate with the extent of lateral temporal resection, but not with the extent of mesial resection (50). Another study of 47 patients did not find a correlation between memory outcome and extent of mesial or lateral cortical resection (51).

Under physiologic conditions, the two hippocampi are essential components of the memory network responsible for acquiring and retaining new and old information. In a disease state such as mesial temporal epilepsy, knowledge of the functional reserve of the preserved hippocampus (to be able to independently support memory function after surgery), as well as the functional adequacy of the pathologic hippocampus (slated to be removed), would assist in predicting the likelihood of memory decline in any given patient (52). This approach to evaluation has gained widespread acceptance owing to its apparently logical basis and reproducible reliability (53). A high preoperative neuropsychological testing score (functionally adequate hippocampus) is predictive of a poorer outcome on memory functioning after surgery (54–56). This is validated at the microscopic level, where statistically significant correlations between hippocampal neuron loss and impaired memory suggest that surgical removal of a hippocampus with minimal neuronal cell loss is more likely to result in a significant decline in memory (57). It may be inferred that the patients who face the maximum risk of postoperative memory impairment after dominant temporal lobe surgery are those with high baseline memory performance and absence of hippocampal atrophy on MRI.

Speech and Language

Residing within the inferior and middle frontal gyrus of the dominant cerebral hemisphere, the Broca area is responsible for motor speech output as well as comprehension (58). The Wernicke area, within the posterior aspect of the superior and middle temporal gyrus, angular gyrus, and supramarginal gyrus, functions predominantly in the comprehension of auditory and visual stimuli (59). In adults with epilepsy, sparing of these eloquent cortical areas is crucial to prevent severely disabling deficits in communicating skills (60), as mature networks of the adult brain possess only limited potential for reorganization after an injury. In patients with dominant temporal resection, subtle decrements in naming and language function may be noted despite careful attempts to spare language areas (61,62).

Dominant temporal resections are more forgiving and are associated with a better functional outcome in younger patients. Developmental plasticity during the first 5 to 7 years of life allows for reorganization of language networks in the presence of acquired pathology, as well as after surgical intervention. Language transfer to the right hemisphere is known to occur with an early left-sided injury, so that development of language function in the right hemisphere can be expected for infants facing left hemispherectomy or left frontal or posterior temporal resection. In these cases, the eventual quality of language development will reflect the child's overall cognitive development, which varies depending on the underlying etiology of the epileptogenic process and the extent of its impact on the right hemisphere. Similarly, new postoperative language deficits are not a concern for older patients with congenital hemiparesis who are facing left hemispherectomy for refractory epilepsy caused by pre- or perinatal hemispheric injury such as middle cerebral artery infarction. In these patients, language dominance in the right hemisphere can be assumed or documented by intracarotid amobarbital testing.

Rare cases of language transfer are also reported to occur as late as 10 to 15 years (63,64). One report included two adolescents with early left hemispheric language domi-

nance proven by intracarotid amobarbital testing, followed by subsequent transfer of language to the right hemisphere between 9 and 15 years later (65). These patients had developed language impairment following Rasmussen chronic encephalitis beginning at 8 to 11 years of age that led to left hemispherectomy at 14 and 15 years of age, followed by postoperative improvement in language functions (65). These cases illustrate that some plasticity for language recovery may exist even into later childhood.

POTENTIAL BENEFITS OF EPILEPSY SURGERY: QUALITY-OF-LIFE OUTCOME

Freedom from seizures should be a stepping-stone toward the ultimate goal of epilepsy surgery, an improvement in overall quality of life. The 1990 National Institutes of Health Consensus Conference Panel on Epilepsy Surgery was one of the first attempts to address the issue of quality-of-life measures in epilepsy surgery outcome studies (66). Developed at this conference, the Epilepsy Surgery Inventory (ESI-55) is a self-reported measure of 11 dimensions of health-related quality of life (66). As patients' perception of their own well-being became central to assessment of quality-of-life outcome, several comprehensive tools were devised since the ESI-55 to quantify this global aspect (66–69). Most of these are suitable for epilepsy patients who are beyond the first decade of life.

While these comprehensive tools continue to evolve toward ease of implementation and reliability of outcome assessment, it behooves us not to lose sight of some basic differences in the way we perceive successful outcome after epilepsy surgery in an adult patient as opposed to a pediatric or an adolescent patient. In simple terms, the major milestones that an adult epilepsy patient hopes to realize after successful epilepsy surgery are driving, independent living, and employment (70). Earlier in life, other goals apply. In an infant with catastrophic epilepsy leading to a prolonged hospital stay for aggressive seizure management, a marked reduction in seizure frequency and severity enabling discharge from the hospital may be the first and foremost milestone on the road to improvement in quality of life—for both the patient and the family. In a young child, improving behavioral interaction with peers and surroundings, attaining motor and cognitive milestones, and succeeding in school are key measures of outcome. These are unique to different chronologic ages and are therefore difficult to incorporate into a single measurement tool relevant across all pediatric age groups. On the basis of the scant pediatric data available, it appears that early intervention provides the best chance to optimize developmental outcome in young patients (71–73). Inadvertent delay in surgical intervention and continued seizures may result in a lost window of opportunity. Timing of epilepsy surgery is therefore critical.

Only when outcome measures are sensitive to these unique features during childhood and adolescence will we be closer to an accurate assessment of results after early intervention with epilepsy surgery.

REFERENCES

1. Mosewich RK, So EL, O'Brien TJ, et al. Factors predictive of the outcome of frontal lobe epilepsy surgery. *Epilepsia* 2000;41:843–849.
2. Cohen-Gadol AA, Ozduman K, Bronen RA, et al. Long-term outcome after epilepsy surgery for focal cortical dysplasia. *J Neurosurg* 2004;101:55–65.
3. Spencer SS, Berg AT, Vickrey BG, et al. Initial outcomes in the Multicenter Study of Epilepsy Surgery. *Neurology* 2003;61: 1680–1685.
4. Berg AT, Walczak T, Hirsch LJ, et al. Multivariable prediction of seizure outcome one year after resective epilepsy surgery: development of a model with independent validation. *Epilepsy Res* 1998;29:185–194.
5. Wyllie E, Comair YG, Kotagal P, et al. Seizure outcome after epilepsy surgery in children and adolescents. *Ann Neurol* 1998;44: 740–748.
6. Engel J Jr, Van Ness PC, Rasmussen TB, et al. Outcome with respect to epileptic seizures. In: Engel J Jr, ed. *Surgical treatment of the epilepsies.* New York: Raven Press, 1993:609–621.
7. Wieser HG, Ortega M, Friedman A, et al. Long-term seizure outcomes following amygdalohippocampectomy. *J Neurosurg* 2003; 98:751–763.
8. Kim HI, Olivier A, Jones-Gotman M, et al. Corticoamygdalectomy in memory-impaired patients. *Stereotact Funct Neurosurg* 1992;58: 162–167.
9. Khajavi K, Comair YG, Prayson RA, et al. Childhood ganglioglioma and medically intractable epilepsy. A clinicopathological study of 15 patients and a review of the literature. *Pediatr Neurosurg* 1995;22:181–188.
10. Morris HH, Matkovic Z, Estes ML, et al. Ganglioglioma and intractable epilepsy: clinical and neurophysiologic features and predictors of outcome after surgery. *Epilepsia* 1998;39:307–313.
11. Aykut-Bingol C, Bronen RA, Kim JH, et al. Surgical outcome in occipital lobe epilepsy: implications for pathophysiology. *Ann Neurol* 1998;44:60–69.
12. Edwards JC, Wyllie E, Ruggeri PM, et al. Seizure outcome after surgery for epilepsy due to malformation of cortical development. *Neurology* 2000;55:1110–1114.
13. Carreno M, Wyllie E, Bingaman W, et al. Seizure outcome after functional hemispherectomy for malformations of cortical development. *Neurology* 2001;57:331–333.
14. Bautista JF, Foldvary-Schaefer N, Bingaman WE, et al. Focal cortical dysplasia and intractable epilepsy in adults: clinical, EEG, imaging, and surgical features. *Epilepsy Res* 2003;55:131–136.
15. Britton JW, Cascino GD, Sharbrough FW, et al. Low-grade glial neoplasms and intractable partial epilepsy: efficacy of surgical treatment. *Epilepsia* 1994;35:1130–1135.
16. Cendes F, Cook MJ, Watson C, et al. Frequency and characteristics of dual pathology in patients with lesional epilepsy. *Neurology* 1995;45:2058–2064.
17. Li LM, Cendes F, Watson C, et al. Surgical treatment of patients with single and dual pathology: relevance of lesion and of hippocampal atrophy to seizure outcome. *Neurology* 1997;48:437–444.
18. Li LM, Cendes F, Andermann F, et al. Surgical outcome in patients with epilepsy and dual pathology. *Brain* 1999;122(Pt 5):799–805.
19. Jooma R, Yeh HS, Privitera MD, et al. Lesionectomy versus electrophysiologically guided resection for temporal lobe tumors manifesting with complex partial seizures. *J Neurosurg* 1995;83:231–236.
20. Awad IA, Nayel MH, Luders H. Second operation after the failure of previous resection for epilepsy. *Neurosurgery* 1991;28: 510–518.
21. Bleck TP. Advances in the management of refractory status epilepticus. *Crit Care Med* 1993;21:955–957.
22. Claassen J, Hirsch LJ, Emerson RG, et al. Treatment of refractory status epilepticus with pentobarbital, propofol, or midazolam: a systematic review. *Epilepsia* 2002;43:146–153.
23. Sahin M, Menache CC, Holmes GL, et al. Prolonged treatment for acute symptomatic refractory status epilepticus: outcome in children. *Neurology* 2003;61:398–401.
24. Gilbert DL, Gartside PS, Glauser TA. Efficacy and mortality in treatment of refractory generalized convulsive status epilepticus in children: a meta-analysis. *J Child Neurol* 1999;14:602–609.
25. Kim SJ, Lee DY, Kim JS. Neurologic outcomes of pediatric epileptic patients with pentobarbital coma. *Pediatr Neurol* 2001;25:217–220.
26. Sahin M, Menache CC, Holmes GL, et al. Outcome of severe refractory status epilepticus in children. *Epilepsia* 2001;42:1461–1467.
27. D'Giano CH, Del CG, Pomata H, et al. Treatment of refractory partial status epilepticus with multiple subpial transection: case report. *Seizure* 2001;10:382–385.
28. Fenyes G. Therapy of status epilepticus by cortical excisions [Hungarian]. *Ideggyogy Sz* 1957;10:105–107.
29. Ma X, Liporace J, O'Connor MJ, et al. Neurosurgical treatment of medically intractable status epilepticus. *Epilepsy Res* 2001;46:33–38.
30. Winston KR, Levisohn P, Miller BR, et al. Vagal nerve stimulation for status epilepticus. *Pediatr Neurosurg* 2001;34:190–192.
31. Alexopoulos A, Deepak K, Lachhwani M, et al. Resective surgery to treat refractory status epilepticus in children with focal epileptogenesis. *Neurology* 2005;64:567–570.
32. Chugani HT, Shields WD, Shewmon DA, et al. Infantile spasms, I: PET identifies focal cortical dysgenesis in cryptogenic cases for surgical treatment. *Ann Neurol* 1990;27:406–413.
33. Lagercrantz H, Ringstedt T. Organization of the neuronal circuits in the central nervous system during development. *Acta Paediatr* 2001;90:707–715.
34. Chugani HT. A critical period of brain development: studies of cerebral glucose utilization with PET. *Prev Med* 1998;27:184–188.
35. Malla BR, O'Brien TJ, Cascino GD, et al. Acute postoperative seizures following anterior temporal lobectomy for intractable partial epilepsy. *J Neurosurg* 1998;89:177–182.
36. Garcia PA, Barbaro NM, Laxer KD. The prognostic value of postoperative seizures following epilepsy surgery. *Neurology* 1991;41: 1511–1512.
37. Park K, Buchhalter J, McClelland R, et al. Frequency and significance of acute postoperative seizures following epilepsy surgery in children and adolescents. *Epilepsia* 2002;43:874–881.
38. Wiebe S, Blume WT, Girvin JP, et al. A randomized, controlled trial of surgery for temporal-lobe epilepsy. *N Engl J Med* 2001;345: 311–318.
39. Tigaran S, Cascino GD, McClelland RL, et al. Acute postoperative seizures after frontal lobe cortical resection for intractable partial epilepsy. *Epilepsia* 2003;44:831–835.
40. Sirven JI, Sperling M, Wingerchuk DM. Early versus late antiepileptic drug withdrawal for people with epilepsy in remission. *Cochrane Database Syst Rev* 2001;3:CD001902.
41. Schiller Y, Cascino GD, So EL, et al. Discontinuation of antiepileptic drugs after successful epilepsy surgery. *Neurology* 2000;54: 346–349.
42. Behrens E, Schramm J, Zentner J, et al. Surgical and neurological complications in a series of 708 epilepsy surgery procedures. *Neurosurgery* 1997;41:1–9.
43. Buchhalter JR, Jarrar RG. Therapeutics in pediatric epilepsy, part 2: epilepsy surgery and vagus nerve stimulation. *Mayo Clin Proc* 2003;78:371–378.
44. Cukiert A, Buratini JA, Machado E, et al. Results of surgery in patients with refractory extratemporal epilepsy with normal or nonlocalizing magnetic resonance findings investigated with subdural grids. *Epilepsia* 2001;42:889–894.
45. Cukiert A, Buratini JA, Machado E, et al. Seizure's outcome after cortical resections including the face and tongue rolandic areas in patients with refractory epilepsy and normal MRI submitted to subdural grids' implantation. *Arq Neuropsiquiatr* 2001;59: 717–721.
46. Corkin S, Milner B, Rasmussen T. Effects of different cortical excisions on sensory thresholds in man. *Trans Am Neurol Assoc* 1964;89:112–116.
47. Corkin S, Milner B, Rasmussen T. Somatosensory thresholds—contrasting effects of postcentral-gyrus and posterior parietal-lobe excisions. *Arch Neurol* 1970;23:41–58.
48. Corkin S, Milner B, Taylor L. Bilateral sensory loss after unilateral cerebral lesion in man. *Trans Am Neurol Assoc* 1973;98:118–122.

49. Novelly RA, Augustine EA, Mattson RH, et al. Selective memory improvement and impairment in temporal lobectomy for epilepsy. *Ann Neurol* 1984;15:64–67.

50. Ojemann GA, Dodrill CB. Verbal memory deficits after left temporal lobectomy for epilepsy. Mechanism and intraoperative prediction. *J Neurosurg* 1985;62:101–107.

51. Wolf RL, Ivnik RJ, Hirschorn KA, et al. Neurocognitive efficiency following left temporal lobectomy: standard versus limited resection. *J Neurosurg* 1993;79:76–83.

52. Chelune GJ. Hippocampal adequacy versus functional reserve: predicting memory functions following temporal lobectomy. *Arch Clin Neuropsychol* 1995;10:413–432.

53. Jokeit H, Ebner A, Holthausen H, et al. Individual prediction of change in delayed recall of prose passages after left-sided anterior temporal lobectomy. *Neurology* 1997;49:481–487.

54. Chelune GJ, Naugle RI, Luders H, et al. Prediction of cognitive change as a function of preoperative ability status among temporal lobectomy patients seen at 6-month follow-up. *Neurology* 1991;41:399–404.

55. Chelune GJ, Naugle RI, Hermann BP, et al. Does presurgical IQ predict seizure outcome after temporal lobectomy? Evidence from the Bozeman Epilepsy Consortium. *Epilepsia* 1998;39:314–318.

56. Kneebone AC, Chelune GJ, Dinner DS, et al. Intracarotid amobarbital procedure as a predictor of material-specific memory change after anterior temporal lobectomy. *Epilepsia* 1995;36:857–865.

57. Sass KJ, Sass A, Westerveld M, et al. Specificity in the correlation of verbal memory and hippocampal neuron loss: dissociation of memory, language, and verbal intellectual ability. *J Clin Exp Neuropsychol* 1992;14:662–672.

58. Schaffler L, Luders HO, Dinner DS, et al. Comprehension deficits elicited by electrical stimulation of Broca's area. *Brain* 1993;116(Pt 3):695–715.

59. Schaffler L, Luders HO, Beck GJ. Quantitative comparison of language deficits produced by extraoperative electrical stimulation of Broca's, Wernicke's, and basal temporal language areas. *Epilepsia* 1996;37:463–475.

60. Pilcher WH, Rusyniak WG. Complications of epilepsy surgery. *Neurosurg Clin North Am* 1993;4:311–325.

61. Saykin AJ, Stafiniak P, Robinson LJ, et al. Language before and after temporal lobectomy: specificity of acute changes and relation to early risk factors. *Epilepsia* 1995;36:1071–1077.

62. Stafiniak P, Saykin AJ, Sperling MR, et al. Acute naming deficits following dominant temporal lobectomy: prediction by age at 1st risk for seizures. *Neurology* 1990;40:1509–1512.

63. Boatman D, Freeman J, Vining E, et al. Language recovery after left hemispherectomy in children with late-onset seizures. *Ann Neurol* 1999;46:579–586.

64. Hertz-Pannier L, Chiron C, Jambaque I, et al. Late plasticity for language in a child's non-dominant hemisphere: a pre- and post-surgery fMRI study. *Brain* 2002;125(Pt 2):361–372.

65. Loddenkemper T, Wyllie E, Lardizabal D, et al. Late language transfer in patients with Rasmussen encephalitis. *Epilepsia* 2003;44:870–871.

66. Vickrey BG. A procedure for developing a quality-of-life measure for epilepsy surgery patients. *Epilepsia* 1993;34(Suppl 4):S22–S27.

67. Devinsky O, Vickrey BG, Cramer J, et al. Development of the quality of life in epilepsy inventory. *Epilepsia* 1995;36:1089–1104.

68. Wiebe S, Eliasziw M, Matijevic S. Changes in quality of life in epilepsy: how large must they be to be real? *Epilepsia* 2001;42:113–118.

69. Cramer JA, Westbrook LE, Devinsky O, et al. Development of the Quality of Life in Epilepsy Inventory for Adolescents: the QOLIE-AD-48. *Epilepsia* 1999;40:1114–1121.

70. Wass CT, Rajala MM, Hughes JM, et al. Long-term follow-up of patients treated surgically for medically intractable epilepsy: results in 291 patients treated at Mayo Clinic Rochester between July 1972 and March 1985. *Mayo Clin Proc* 1996;71:1105–1113.

71. Bittar RG, Rosenfeld JV, Klug GL, et al. Resective surgery in infants and young children with intractable epilepsy. *J Clin Neurosci* 2002;9:142–146.

72. Gilliam F, Wyllie E, Kashden J, et al. Epilepsy surgery outcome: comprehensive assessment in children. *Neurology* 1997;48:1368–1374.

73. Wyllie E, Comair YG, Kotagal P, et al. Epilepsy surgery in infants. *Epilepsia* 1996;37:625–637.

Part VI

Psychosocial Aspects of Epilepsy

87. Cognitive Effects of Epilepsy and of Antiepileptic Medications   1185
88. Psychiatric Comorbidity of Epilepsy   1197
89. Driving and Social Issues in Epilepsy   1201

Cognitive Effects of Epilepsy and of Antiepileptic Medications

Kimford J. Meador

COGNITIVE DEFICITS IN EPILEPSY

As a group, individuals with epilepsy have impaired cognitive performance in comparison to healthy subjects matched for age and education (1); however, considerable intersubject variability does exist. Most persons with epilepsy have intelligence in the normal range, and some have superior cognitive abilities. Various factors can have a detrimental effect on cognition in epilepsy, including (a) the cause of seizures; (b) cerebral lesions acquired prior to onset of seizures; (c) seizure type; (d) age at onset of epilepsy; (e) seizure frequency; (f) duration and severity of seizures; (g) physiologic dysfunction (intraictal, interictal, or postictal) resulting from seizures; (h) structural cerebral damage as a consequence of repetitive or prolonged seizures; (i) hereditary factors; (j) psychosocial factors; (k) sequelae of epilepsy surgery; and (l) untoward effects of antiepileptic drugs (AEDs) (2,3).

The etiology of seizures may be one of the strongest factors influencing cognitive abilities (4). Patients with seizures attributable to progressive cerebral degeneration usually exhibit dementia, those with mental retardation have an increased incidence of epilepsy, and those with seizures caused by a focal brain lesion may exhibit a specific neuropsychological pattern of deficits. In contrast, patients with idiopathic epilepsy are more likely to have normal intelligence (4). Seizure type may be strongly associated with cognition (5). Patients with juvenile myoclonic epilepsy usually have normal intelligence, but children with infantile spasms have a poor prognosis. In general, the earlier the age of seizure onset, the more likely it is that a patient will have cognitive impairment. Additionally, patients with mental retardation are more likely to have refractory epilepsy (5,6).

Seizure frequency, duration, and severity may affect cognition in several ways (3,7). Obviously, cognition is impaired intraictally when consciousness is altered during generalized or complex partial seizures. Epileptiform discharges and postictal suppression may impair cognition interictally (8,9). Recent temporal lobe seizures impair consolidation of memory (10). Classic postictal Todd paralysis lasts less than 24 hours, but postictal cognitive dysfunction, such as dysphasia, may persist for several days. Chronic physiologic dysfunction may also exist beyond the area of epileptogenesis. For example, positron emission tomography scans reveal interictal hypometabolism extending to the lateral temporal cortex in patients with epilepsy caused by mesial temporal lobe sclerosis (11). Repetitive or prolonged seizures may permanently damage the cerebral substrate via anoxia, lactic acidosis, or excessive excitatory neurotransmitters. Even temporal lobe seizures of relatively modest frequency over several decades can increase the severity of hippocampal atrophy and reduce cognitive abilities (12,13).

Factors indirectly related to epilepsy may also affect cognition. Hereditary factors strongly influence intelligence. In fact, maternal intelligence quotient (IQ) is the most influential factor overall in predicting a child's intelligence (14).

Psychosocial factors may adversely affect cognition through such mechanisms as depression or restriction of environmental influences (15). Finally, surgical or pharmacologic treatment of seizures may produce adverse cognitive effects.

EPILEPSY SURGERY

Epilepsy surgery does not usually cause any general cognitive decline because dysfunctional tissue is primarily removed (16). Surgery may even result in improved cognition because of the reduction in seizures and AEDs. However, clinically significant postoperative cognitive deficits may occur. For example, left temporal lobectomy may lead to declines in naming and in verbal memory. However, the risks are largely predictable (17,18). Risks are greater if age of epilepsy onset is later or if hippocampal gliosis/atrophy is not present. Verbal memory is at greater risk following left temporal lobectomy if baseline verbal memory is high or functional assessments suggest greater residual preoperative function of the left temporal lobe. Thus, a patient undergoing left temporal lobectomy is at increased risk if the patient has high baseline verbal memory and high memory performance with right intracarotid amobarbital injection and low with left injection. In contrast, a decline in visuospatial memory is inconsistent following right temporal lobectomy. Rarely, unilateral temporal lobectomy has resulted in a severe global anterograde memory disorder. Fortunately, modern advances in preoperative evaluation techniques have minimized this risk. In addition, selective amygdalohippocampectomy may reduce the risk for memory loss compared with standard anterior two-thirds temporal lobectomy (19). In contrast to risks, patients who become seizure free from epilepsy surgery have a significant improvement in their emotional well-being and perceived quality of life (QOL) (20).

Vagal Nerve Stimulation

Some studies have reported mild cognitive or behavioral improvement following vagus nerve stimulation (VNS) (21,22), but this may be the result of reduced seizures. Other studies have shown no positive or negative effects of VNS on cognition or behavior in patients with epilepsy (23,24).

ANTIEPILEPTIC DRUGS

AEDs reduce neuronal irritability and thus may reduce neuronal excitability and impair cognition. Because AEDs are the major therapeutic intervention in epilepsy, their cognitive effects are of particular concern to physicians, who must consider the risk-to-benefit ratio of any treatment. Therefore, differentiating the cognitive effects of AEDs and placing them in the proper perspective are important.

Although all AEDs may impair cognition, such side effects are usually modest, as assessed by neuropsychological tests in patients on monotherapy in whom anticonvulsant blood levels are within standard therapeutic ranges (25). Furthermore, the cognitive effects may be partially offset by the reduction in seizures. It is clear that the risk of cognitive side effects rises with polypharmacy and with increasing AED dosages and anticonvulsant blood levels (26). Decreasing the number of AEDs frequently improves cognition and may reduce the number of seizures (27). However, the best drug regimen for an individual patient is the one that best controls seizures with the fewest side effects, and for some patients this regimen may involve polytherapy. Despite the modest cognitive effects of AEDs on formal neuropsychological testing, these effects can be clinically pertinent, as evidenced by the highly significant inverse correlation of neurotoxicity symptoms and QOL scores (28). Despite the absence of overt toxicity on examination, patients who exhibit more symptoms of neurotoxicity have lower perceived QOL.

The differential cognitive effects of AEDs are controversial and certain agents are promoted as being superior in this regard. For the older AEDs, more consistent adverse effects are observed with barbiturates and benzodiazepines, but results are mixed for carbamazepine, phenytoin, and valproate (25,26). Several of the newer AEDs appear to have fewer cognitive side effects than the older AEDs, but the effects of the newer AEDs relative to each other and to older AEDs are not yet fully determined.

Historical Perspective

AED-induced cognitive deficits actually led to the discovery of the first effective AED. In 1850, Huette (29) noted that bromide produces general sedation, mental slowing, and depression of sexuality. The anticonvulsant effects of bromide were discovered in 1857 after Locock (30) suggested that the agent might be efficacious for patients with hysterical epilepsy, which was believed to result from excessive masturbation. The first systematic investigation of the cognitive effects of AEDs was conducted in 1940. Somerfeld-Ziskind and Ziskind (31) randomized 100 patients with epilepsy to phenobarbital or ketogenic diet. Phenobarbital controlled seizures better, but there were no differences on neuropsychological testing. Numerous studies (25,26,32) have subsequently examined the cognitive side effects of AEDs. Although there is agreement on the effects of polytherapy and dosage/blood levels, the differential AED cognitive effects remain controversial (33).

Methodological Issues

The literature examining the cognitive effects of AEDs must be viewed critically, because flaws in experimental design, analysis, and interpretation occur frequently (26,32). Errors in experimental design include subject selection bias, nonequivalence of clinical variables, and nonequivalence of dependent variables. Selection bias is a problem when subjects are not randomly assigned to a treatment group or inadequately matched, or if the sample size is inadequate for a parallel-group design. Examples of nonequivalence of clinical variables include the failure to control for anticonvulsant blood levels or seizure frequency. Nonequivalence of dependent measures may occur when there is no assurance that treatment groups performed similarly on dependent measures prior to treatment. Additional design issues include sample size, test–retest effects, and the characteristics of behavioral tests. Issues related to statistical analysis and interpretation include type I error, use of inappropriate statistics, nonorthogonal contrasts, and comparison of studies with nonequivalent designs/statistics. Even when statistically significant findings are apparent, the magnitude and impact of the findings have to be interpreted in terms of clinical significance, taking into account the overall risk-to-benefit ratio of the AED and the severity of the seizure disorder in question. The magnitude of AED effects on standard neuropsychological measures is generally modest and may be missed if appropriate study designs are not used (34).

Review of Selected Studies of Older Antiepileptic Drugs

Using a double-blind, randomized, crossover, monotherapy study, Dodrill and Troupin (35) compared the cognitive effects of carbamazepine and phenytoin in patients with epilepsy. When they reanalyzed their data, controlling for anticonvulsant blood levels, no differences were observed (36). Consistent with these results, Meador and associates (37) found no cognitive differences between carbamazepine and phenytoin in patients with epilepsy, but evidence of worse performance with phenobarbital was revealed.

Meador and colleagues examined the effects of several AEDs using randomized, double-blind, crossover designs in healthy volunteers to control for the confounding effects of seizures and preexisting brain abnormalities. The investigators found no overall difference between carbamazepine and phenytoin (38,39), but 52% of the variables were significantly worse with AEDs than with nondrugs. In another study (40), 32% of the variables were significantly worse with phenobarbital than with phenytoin or valproate, with the latter two agents being similar to each other. Again, about half of all variables were significantly worse with AEDs compared with nondrugs. Overall, these results suggest greater untoward cognitive effects with phenobarbital, but no clinically significant differences in cognitive side effects among carbamazepine, phenytoin, and valproate. The magnitude of effect with these three agents appears to be less than that with acute-dose over-the-counter antihistamines (41), but their effects can be clinically significant.

Consistent with these findings, the large Veterans Administration (VA) Cooperative Study (42), comparing the cognitive effects of carbamazepine, phenobarbital, phenytoin, and primidone in patients with new-onset epilepsy, found "no consistent pattern" across AEDs and little change in cognition from pre- to post-AED treatment conditions. In addition, the second VA Cooperative Study (43) found no cognitive differences between carbamazepine and valproate. Other studies comparing carbamazepine and phenytoin have described modest negative effects on cognition with both agents, but few differential effects (44,45).

A possible criticism of some of the crossover studies described above might be the relatively short duration of treatment. Dodrill and Wilensky (46) addressed this issue in a study that examined neuropsychological performance over 5 years in patients with epilepsy. The patients were on stable regimens consisting of phenytoin alone, phenytoin with other AEDs, or AED regimens exclusive of phenytoin. No differences in cognitive performance were observed over the 5-year follow-up.

Newer Antiepileptic Drugs

Several newer AEDs are available. Although a number of studies offer some insight into the profiles and magnitude of neurobehavioral effects associated with the use of these agents, many questions remain unanswered. The available published data are reviewed here, and additional information is expected future investigations.

Felbamate

Well-controlled systematic investigations of the cognitive effects associated with felbamate use are unlikely, given the restrictions imposed by the systemic toxic effects of the agent. Anecdotally, felbamate is reported to be alerting, in contrast to older AEDs, and even produces insomnia. This effect is beneficial to the behavior of some patients but detrimental to that of others.

Gabapentin

Several studies of gabapentin as add-on therapy in patients with epilepsy report subjective improvements in well-being (47). Although generally well tolerated, gabapentin has produced behavioral side effects in children, including irritability, hyperactivity, and agitation (48,49). When comparing gabapentin with placebo in patients with partial epilepsy, using a double-blind, dose-ranging (1200 to 2400 mg per day), add-on, crossover design, Leach and coworkers (50) found one positive effect and no negative effects, except for more subjective drowsiness. A double-blind, randomized, crossover study of healthy volunteers (51) compared gabapentin and carbamazepine during two 5-week treatment periods. Significantly better performance was seen with gabapentin versus carbamazepine on 26% of the variables, carbamazepine was worse than nondrug on 48%

of the variables, and gabapentin was worse than nondrug on 19% of the variables. Although both agents produced some effects, significantly fewer untoward cognitive effects were seen with gabapentin compared with carbamazepine. These results have been supported by two subsequent double-blind studies in healthy volunteers comparing treatment with carbamazepine and gabapentin. Greater electroencephalographic slowing and more frequent cognitive complaints were reported with carbamazepine in adults (52), and better overall tolerability was seen with gabapentin in healthy elderly adults (53).

Lamotrigine

One study of patients with epilepsy found no cognitive effects with lamotrigine compared with placebo on a limited neuropsychological battery (54). A double-blind, randomized, crossover design, with two 10-week treatment periods, in healthy adults revealed significantly better performance on more than half of the variables (e.g., cognitive speed, memory, mood factors, sedation, perception of cognitive performance, and other QOL perceptions) with lamotrigine versus carbamazepine (55). Other studies with healthy adults demonstrated fewer cognitive side effects with lamotrigine compared with carbamazepine, diazepam, phenytoin, placebo, and valproate (56–58). In clinical trials, lamotrigine was better tolerated than carbamazepine and phenytoin (59–61). Several studies (54,59,62) using QOL measures demonstrated beneficial effects with lamotrigine compared with placebo or carbamazepine. Lamotrigine has psychotropic properties, as evidenced by positive effects in patients with bipolar disorder and in those with epilepsy who have severe cognitive impairment (63–65).

Levetiracetam

Although the overall side-effect profile of levetiracetam has been quite favorable in clinical trials, a paucity of formal neuropsychological data is available on the subject. A preliminary study by Neyens and colleagues (66) showed no significant changes in cognitive performance in patients with chronic epilepsy who were treated with levetiracetam, but the study was single-blind, with only 10 patients and no control group. An acute reversible adverse behavioral syndrome has been reported in children treated with levetiracetam (67), but the incidence of behavioral events in adult patients is reported to be lower than with other AEDs overall (68).

Oxcarbazepine

Few published cognitive studies with oxcarbazepine are available. Oxcarbazepine has been tolerated slightly better than carbamazepine, phenytoin, and valproate in clinical studies. No differences in cognitive effects were found with oxcarbazepine and phenytoin in a small randomized, monotherapy, double-blind, parallel-group study (69) of patients with new-onset epilepsy. Mixed results were reported in a randomized, double-blind, placebo-controlled, crossover study (70) in 12 healthy volunteers treated for 2 weeks with low-dose (150 or 300 mg twice daily) oxcarbazepine; reaction time slowed, but participants had slightly better subjective alertness and improved on a cancellation task.

Tiagabine

Tiagabine inhibits the reuptake of the inhibitory neurotransmitter γ-aminobutyric acid (GABA). No significant cognitive effects were reported in a small, low-dose, add-on study (71) and in a large, randomized, double-blind, add-on, placebo-controlled, parallel-group, dose–response study in patients with epilepsy (72).

Topiramate

In clinical trials, topiramate produced somnolence, psychomotor slowing, language problems, and difficulty with memory. The word-finding difficulty seen in some patients is unique to topiramate. A single-blind, randomized, parallel-group study (73) in 17 healthy volunteers compared gabapentin, lamotrigine, and topiramate. Topiramate was associated with significantly greater effects than the other two AEDs at 1 month; however, the titration rate for topiramate was faster than that recommended. In a study of 38 patients with epilepsy tested on/off or off/on topiramate, declines in verbal fluency, attention, processing speed, and working memory, but not retention, were associated with topiramate use (74). In contrast, two randomized, multicenter, double-blind studies of topiramate versus valproate as adjunctive therapy to carbamazepine in patients with epilepsy found less-profound effects. Valproate was slightly better tolerated in terms of dropouts, but few differences were found on neuropsychological testing after slow titration and 8 weeks' maintenance. Only 1 of 17 variables (i.e., verbal memory) in one study (75) and 2 of 30 variables (i.e., verbal fluency and a graphomotor task) in another study (76) were worse with topiramate compared with valproate. Although most patients will tolerate topiramate, there is a subset of individuals at risk for clinically significant cognitive side effects. Factors affecting these adverse effects include titration rate, maintenance time, dose, polytherapy, and individual susceptibility.

Vigabatrin

In four double-blind, randomized, add-on studies of patients with epilepsy (78–81), vigabatrin had few adverse effects on cognition or QOL compared with placebo, despite elevated brain levels of GABA. A single-dose study in healthy volunteers showed less impairment than lorazepam (81), and vigabatrin produced fewer adverse effects than carbamazepine in a small, open-label, randomized, parallel-group study of patients with epilepsy (82). Abnormal behaviors, including depression and psychosis, have been reported in 3.4% of adults in controlled clinical trials, but vigabatrin has not been shown to be associated with a greater risk for these effects than other AEDs (83).

Zonisamide

Zonisamide appears to have a wide therapeutic index but can cause sedation. The agent was reported to impair cognition (e.g., learning), but some tolerance appeared to develop over 24 weeks in a small, preliminary add-on study in patients (84). Further investigation is warranted.

Effects of Antiepileptic Drugs at Age Extremes

Fewer AED studies have been conducted at the extremes of the age spectrum. The increased susceptibility of the elderly to the cognitive effects of a variety of agents is attributable to both pharmacokinetic and pharmacodynamic factors. For example, it is well established that the elderly are at increased risk for untoward cognitive effects from benzodiazepines (85). Similar to studies in younger adults, one study (86) reported comparable cognitive effects of phenytoin and valproate in elderly patients. Reanalysis of the original VA Cooperative Study comparing carbamazepine, phenobarbital, phenytoin, and primidone revealed that elderly patients were easier to control but had greater cognitive side effects (87). The initial results from a new VA Cooperative Study of three AEDs in elderly patients with new-onset epilepsy revealed that patients are more likely to remain on gabapentin or lamotrigine compared to carbamazepine (88). This finding was predominately a result of side effects that were least likely with lamotrigine, intermediate with gabapentin, and worse with carbamazepine. The results of formal neuropsychological testing will be available soon.

Because the modest effects of AEDs on attention and memory might be additive over the long-term during neurodevelopment, children may be at higher risk for developing cognitive side effects from AEDs. An additional concern raised by an animal study (89) is that the detrimental effects of AEDs might interact with the epilepsy and the underlying cerebral abnormalities to produce even greater impairments in neurodevelopment. Unfortunately, fewer studies have been conducted in children, and no studies with the newer AEDs have been completed. Only one double-blind, randomized, crossover, monotherapy study (90) has been conducted in children with epilepsy; the performance in children taking phenobarbital was poorer than that of children taking valproate on several measures. Adverse cognitive effects of phenobarbital have also been found in placebo-controlled, parallel-group studies of children with febrile convulsions (91,92). Similar to the outcomes of adult studies, comparisons of carbamazepine, phenytoin, and valproate in children have yielded few differences (93–96).

NEURODEVELOPMENTAL EFFECTS OF *IN UTERO* ANTIEPILEPTIC DRUG EXPOSURE

A variety of factors may contribute to the observed neurodevelopmental deficits in children of mothers with epilepsy, including AEDs, seizures during pregnancy, seizure type, heredity, maternal age/parity, and socioeconomic status (97,98). Data from animals and humans suggest that AEDs have an important role in this regard. However, the magnitude of the effects and the differential effects of *in utero* AED exposure on neurodevelopment remain unresolved.

Animal Studies

AED-induced dysmorphogenesis has been observed in animals, with many of the malformations corresponding to clinical reports (99–101). The behavioral consequences of prenatal AED exposure have not been investigated as extensively as AED-induced somatic abnormalities but have been noted to occur at dosages lower than those associated with somatic malformations (102).

Phenobarbital at maternal levels of 40 to 200 mg/mL produces neuronal deficits and reduced brain weight in mice (103,104). *In utero* phenobarbital also impairs the development of several reflexes, open-field activity, schedule-controlled behavior, and brain levels of catecholamines in mice (105–107). Prenatal phenytoin at maternal plasma levels of 10 to 25 mg/mL produces dose-dependent, long-lasting behavioral abnormalities (e.g., impaired coordination and learning) in rats (108–115). Vorhees (110,114,116,117) found significant, but less striking, neurobehavioral effects with trimethadione (250 mg/kg) and valproate (150 to 200 mg/kg), and demonstrated that phenytoin and valproate alter neuronal membranes in the hippocampus (118,119).

Animal studies of prenatal AED treatment support a teratogenic role for AEDs and suggest that *in utero* AEDs may produce neurobehavioral deficits. However, interspecies differences preclude direct extrapolation of animal results to humans.

Human Studies

A number of investigations have examined the somatic and functional development of children of mothers with epilepsy (100,101,120–123). Although it is clear that the risks for birth defects and neurodevelopmental deficits are increased in these children, recent consensus guidelines could not delineate, based on available data, which of the AEDs is the most teratogenic (120). Furthermore, the consensus statement pointed out the controversy concerning the relative risks associated with prenatal exposure to different AEDs for producing impairments in postnatal psychomotor development.

The majority of investigations report an increased risk for developmental delay in children of mothers with epilepsy (2,122–134). However, a few studies (135–137) report no significant developmental delays in AED-exposed offspring. The incidence of mental retardation is increased in children of mothers with epilepsy versus children of mothers without epilepsy, but not in children of fathers with epilepsy versus controls (130,138). A recent retrospective population-based study found that 19% of children exposed *in utero* to AEDs had developmental delay versus 3% of unexposed children (139). Multiple factors could contribute to the observed differences, but animal studies suggest that AEDs play at least a partial role. Few data are available for AED effects in children of nonepileptic women, but one study suggests that the risk for somatic malformations is similar in children of mothers without epilepsy who take AEDs (140). In children of mothers with epilepsy, the risk for mental retardation is related to intrauterine growth retardation, major malformations, numerous (nine or more) minor malformations, and *in utero* AED exposure (127). Reduced head circumference has been reported in newborns exposed to a variety of AEDs and is associated with impaired psychomotor development (126,134,138,141–143). However, several other studies (130,136,144–146) found no microcephaly or attributed reduced head circumference to factors other than AED exposure. Fujioka and associates (124) suggested complex interrelationships, finding an increased risk with increased dose and numbers of AEDs, decreased maternal education, impaired maternal-child relationship, and maternal partial seizure disorder. Gaily and coworkers (125) related risk for cognitive dysfunction to seizures during pregnancy, maternal partial seizure disorder, and low paternal education, but not to AED exposure. Hattig and colleagues (147) reported greater cognitive impairment with polytherapy compared with monotherapy and with valproate as monotherapy.

Two studies from Denmark (148) examined the effects of *in utero* phenobarbital exposure on intelligence in adult men of mothers without epilepsy. Men exposed prenatally to phenobarbital had significantly lower verbal IQ scores than predicted (approximately seven IQ points) in both studies. Lower socioeconomic status and being the offspring of an "unwanted" pregnancy markedly increased the magnitude of the negative effects (approximately 20 IQ points). One weakness of the studies is that phenobarbital was prescribed primarily for hypertension, but the effects of hypertension and preeclampsia were not controlled for in the analyses. Nevertheless, the findings are important because they suggest that behavioral teratogenic sequelae of prenatal phenobarbital exposure in humans can continue into adulthood, and that socioeconomic and psychological factors may interact with drug exposure to exacerbate the cognitive deficits.

A retrospective study of 594 school-age children exposed *in utero* to AEDs suggests that valproate may have greater detrimental effects on neurodevelopment than carbamazepine, other monotherapy, or no drug on neurodevelopment (149). Special education was required in 30% of children exposed to valproate monotherapy, compared with 3% for carbamazepine, 6% with other monotherapy, and 11% with no drug. Preliminary results from a prospective study support this observation (150). The mean IQ of children exposed *in utero* to valproate was 83, compared with 95 for children exposed to other AEDs, but the monotherapy valproate group was small in size. These two studies suggest that valproate may pose a special risk, but additional research is needed to confirm this conclusion.

Disparities across studies are partly a result of differences in methodology and patient populations. Formal assessments of mental performance were made in most studies, but in many it is unclear whether investigators were blind as to AED exposure when assessments were made. In many prospective studies, follow-up began postnatally rather than during pregnancy. That the influences of other disease and non–disease-related factors have not been addressed in an empirical fashion, including genetic and environmental factors (e.g., parental IQ and education, seizure type and frequency during pregnancy, AED dose and anticonvulsant blood levels, maternal age/parity, socioeconomic status, and home environment), is critically important. For example, formal IQ measures of parents have rarely been used, and IQ values of both parents are almost never included. The critical question of whether there are differential effects across AEDs remains unanswered.

Possible Mechanisms of Antiepileptic Drug Effects on Neurodevelopment

A teratogen operates on a susceptible genotype, and this process may involve the interaction of multiple-liability genes (151). For example, discordant outcomes have been observed for dizygotic twin fetuses exposed to phenytoin (152). Functional deficits can occur at dosages lower than those required to produce somatic abnormalities, and it is unclear whether similar mechanisms may be involved in both functional and anatomical defects. Proposed possible mechanisms underlying functional teratogenicity of AEDs include folate, reactive intermediates (e.g., epoxides or free radicals), ischemia, apoptosis related mechanisms, and neuronal suppression.

Reactive Intermediates

The fetotoxicity of some AEDs may be mediated not by the parent compound, but by toxic intermediary metabolites (153). Oxide intermediates (epoxides) are highly reactive and can covalently bond nucleic acids. Arene oxides are detoxified by epoxide hydrolase, and inhibition of this enzyme in an animal model leads to an increase in malformations (154). Low epoxide hydrolase activity in amniocytes correlates with subsequent dysmorphic features at term in children exposed to phenytoin (153,155). However, conversion of an AED to an epoxide requires cytochrome P450 enzymes, which are not expressed in embryonic tissues (156). Therefore, the viability of the epoxide mechanism is questionable, because the epoxide would have to be formed by the maternal enzymes and would likely react and bind to maternal tissues before reaching the fetus.

Alternatively, AEDs may be bioactivated to free-radical reactive intermediates by means of embryonic prostaglandin H synthetase or lipoxygenases (157–159). Once generated, these reactive oxygen species may bind to DNA, protein, or lipids, resulting in teratogenesis. Phenytoin-induced oxidative macromolecular lesions and teratogenic defects are reduced by prostaglandin H synthetase inhibitors, free-radical–trapping agents, antioxidants (e.g., vitamin E), and antioxidative enzymes (e.g., superoxide dismutase).

Ischemia/Hypoxia

Ischemia-induced embryopathy in animals resembles phenytoin-induced defects, and hyperoxic chamber treatment reduces malformations caused by phenytoin (160). However, the resemblance to AED defects may be due to free-radical–induced ischemia.

Folate

During pregnancy, folate demands are increased because of the involvement of this vitamin in DNA and RNA synthesis. Phenobarbital, phenytoin, and primidone, but not carbamazepine, deplete folate (161–164), and valproate affects folate-dependent one-carbon metabolism (165). Blood folate concentrations are significantly lower in women with epilepsy who have abnormal pregnancy outcomes (166). In addition, Biale and Lewenthal (167) found that infants of mothers with epilepsy who received no folate supplementation had a 15% rate of malformation, but no congenital abnormalities were identified in 33 folate-supplemented children.

Apoptosis Related Mechanisms

In utero ethanol exposure can result in widespread apoptotic neurodegeneration, reduced brain mass, and neurobehavioral deficits. The effect is primarily the result of third-trimester exposure and is a result of the combined effects of NMDA glutamate receptor blockade and $GABA_A$ receptor activation (168). A study in neonatal rats revealed widespread apoptosis in the developing brain as a result of exposure to clonazepam, diazepam, phenobarbital, phenytoin, vigabatrin, or valproate (169). The effect appeared to be caused by reduced expression of neurotrophins and levels of protein kinases that promote neuronal growth and survival. Of note, the adverse effects were ameliorated by (β-estradiol, which has neurotrophic effects.

Neuronal Suppression

AEDs suppress neuronal irritability and, as a consequence, impair neuronal excitation. Reduction of neuronal excitation

in utero might alter synaptic growth and connectivity during these early stages of neurodevelopment, resulting in long-term deficits in cognition and behavior.

CONCLUSIONS

Patients with epilepsy are at increased risk for cognitive impairment, and a variety of factors may adversely affect cognition in this population. As the major therapeutic modality for epilepsy, AEDs are of special concern to physicians. All AEDs can produce some cognitive side effects, which are increased with polypharmacy and higher dosage/anticonvulsant blood levels. With polypharmacy, the effects are additive and may be dramatic, even when all the anticonvulsant blood levels are within "standard therapeutic ranges." However, the treatment goal in each patient is to achieve the best control of seizures while producing the fewest side effects. For an individual patient, the best risk-to-benefit ratio may be obtained with the judicious use of polypharmacy or with the anticonvulsant blood level above the "standard therapeutic range" in monotherapy. However, the physician should be alert to the increased risk for cognitive side effects in these circumstances.

AEDs may also produce positive or negative behavioral alterations (e.g., mood stabilization, irritability/agitation, psychosis). Carbamazepine, lamotrigine, and valproate have established positive psychotropic effects. Several of the other AEDs may also have positive psychotropic effects.

The magnitude of AED effect on cognition is commonly much smaller than the effects of epilepsy-related factors. When AEDs are used in monotherapy with anticonvulsant blood levels within standard therapeutic ranges, their cognitive effects on formal neuropsychological tests of cognition are modest. However, AED effects can frequently be clinically significant, as evidenced by the adverse effects of subtle neurotoxic symptoms on patient QOL. The major cognitive effects of AEDs are on psychomotor processing speed and sustained attention (i.e., vigilance). Secondarily, these effects may have an impact on learning and memory. Cognitive impairments induced by AEDs may be of particular concern for adults with jobs requiring speed or sustained vigilance and for children in whom the additive effects during neurodevelopment may have long-lasting consequences.

Although the database is incomplete, there is evidence of clinically significant differential cognitive effects for some AEDs (e.g., poorer performance with phenobarbital and benzodiazepines). However, individual patients may tolerate one AED better than another. Studies are needed to examine more thoroughly the relative cognitive effects of the new AEDs and to delineate the cognitive effects of all AEDs at age extremes, especially in the fetus and in children.

REFERENCES

1. Smith DB, Craft BR, Collins J, et al. VA Cooperative Study Group 118. Behavioral characteristics of epilepsy patients compared with normal controls. *Epilepsia* 1986;27:760–768.
2. Lennox WG. Brain injury, drugs and environment as causes of mental decay in epilepsy. *Am J Psychiatry* 1942;99:174–180.
3. Lesser RP, Lüders H, Wyllie E, et al. Mental deterioration in epilepsy. *Epilepsia* 1986;27(Suppl 2):S105–S123.
4. Perrine K, Gershengorm J, Brown ER. Interictal neuropsychological function in epilepsy. In: Devinsky O, Theodore WH, eds. *Epilepsy and behavior.* New York: Wiley-Liss, 1991:181–193.
5. Huttenlocher PR, Hapke RJ. A follow-up study of intractable seizures in childhood. *Ann Neurol* 1990;28:699–705.
6. Dodrill CB. Neuropsychological aspects of epilepsy. *Psychiatr Clin North Am* 1992;15:383–394.
7. Dikmen S, Matthews CG. Effect of major motor seizure frequency upon cognitive-intellectual functions in adults. *Epilepsia* 1977;18:21–29.
8. Kasteleijn-Nolst Trenite DGA, Riemersma JBJ, Binnie CD, et al. The influence of subclinical epileptiform EEG discharges on driving behaviour. *Electroencephalogr Clin Neurophysiol* 1987;67:167–170.
9. Shewmon DA, Erwin RJ. The effect of focal interictal spikes on perception and reaction time. I. General considerations. *Electroencephalogr Clin Neurophysiol* 1988;69:319–337.
10. Jokeit H, Daamen M, Zang H, et al. Seizures accelerate forgetting in patients with left-sided temporal lobe epilepsy. *Neurology* 2001;57:125–126.
11. Henry TR, Chugani HT, Abou-Khalil BW, et al. Positron emission tomography. In: Engel J, ed. *Surgical treatment of the epilepsies.* New York: Raven Press, 1993:211–232.
12. Theodore WH, Bhatia S, Hatta J, et al. Hippocampal atrophy, epilepsy duration, and febrile seizures in patients with partial seizures. *Neurology* 1999; 52:132–136.
13. Jokeit H, Ebner A. Long term effects of refractory temporal lobe epilepsy on cognitive abilities: a cross sectional study. *J Neurol Neurosurg Psychiatry* 1999;67:44–50.
14. Sattler JM. *Assessment of children,* 3rd ed. San Diego: Jerome M Sattler, 1992.
15. Hermann BP. Quality of life in epilepsy. *J Epilepsy* 1992;5:153–165.
16. Dodrill CB, Hermann BP, Rausch R, et al. Neuropsychological testing for assessing prognosis following surgery for epilepsy. In: Engel J, ed. *Surgical treatment of the epilepsies.* New York: Raven Press, 1993:263–271.
17. Loring DW, Meador KJ. Neuropsychological aspects of epilepsy surgery. In: Feinberg TE, Farah MJ, eds. *Behavioral Neurology and Neuropsychology.* New York: McGraw-Hill, 1997:657–666.
18. Clusman H, Schramm J, Kral T, et al. Prognostic factors and outcome after different types of resection for temporal lobe epilepsy. *J Neurosurg* 2002; 97:1131–1141.
19. Helmstaedter C, Reuber M, Elger CC. Interaction of cognitive aging and memory deficits related to epilepsy surgery. *Ann Neurol* 2002;52:89–94.
20. Markand ON, Salanova V, Whelihan E, et al. Health-related quality of life outcome in medically refractory epilepsy treated with anterior temporal lobectomy. *Epilepsia* 2000;41:749–759.
21. Hoppe C, Helmstaedter C, Scherrmann J, et al. Self-Reported Mood Changes following 6 Months of Vagus Nerve Stimulation in Epilepsy Patients. *Epilepsy Behav* 2001;2:335–342.
22. Majoie HJ, Berfelo MW, Aldenkamp AP, et al. Vagus nerve stimulation in children with therapy-resistant epilepsy diagnosed as Lennox-Gastaut syndrome: clinical results, neuropsychological effects, and cost-effectiveness. *J Clin Neurophysiol* 2001;18:419–428.
23. Hoppe C, Helmstaedter C, Scherrmann J, et al. No evidence for cognitive side effects after 6 months of vagus nerve stimulation in epilepsy patients. *Epilepsy Behav* 2001;2:351–356.
24. Aldenkamp AP, Majoie HJ, Berfelo MW, et al. Long-term effects of 24-month treatment with vagus nerve stimulation on behaviour in children with Lennox-Gastaut syndrome. *Epilepsy Behav* 2002;3:475–479.
25. Meador KJ. Cognitive side effects of antiepileptic drugs. *Can J Neurol Sci* 1994;21(Suppl 3):S12–S16.
26. Meador KJ, Loring DW. Cognitive effects of antiepileptic drugs. In: Devinsky O, Theodore WH, eds. *Epilepsy and behavior.* New York: Wiley-Liss, 1991:151–170.
27. Shorvon SD, Reynolds EH. Reduction in polypharmacy for epilepsy. *Br Med J* 1979;2:1023–1025.
28. Gilliam F, Kuzniecky R, Faught E, et al. Impact of adverse antiepileptic drug effects on quality of life in refractory epilepsy. *Epilepsia* 1999;40(Suppl):64–65.
29. Huette C. Recherches sur les proprietes physiologiques et thérapeutiques de bromure de potassium. *Memoirs de la Societe de Biologie* 1850;2:19.
30. Locock C. Discussion of paper by EH Seiveking. Analysis of 42 cases of epilepsy observed by the author. *Lancet* 1857;1:527–528.
31. Somerfeld-Ziskind E, Ziskind E. Effect of phenobarbital on the mentality of epileptic patients. *Arch Neurol Psychiatry* 1940;43:70–79.
32. Vermeulen J, Aldenkamp AP. Cognitive side-effects of chronic antiepileptic drug treatment: a review of 25 years of research. *Epilepsy Res* 1995;22:65–95.
33. Aldenkamp AP, Vermeulen J. Phenytoin and carbamazepine: differential effects on cognitive function. *Seizure* 1995;4:95–104.
34. Meador KJ. Cognitive and behavioral assessments in antiepileptic drug trials. In: French J, Dichter M, Leppik I, eds. *Antiepileptic drug development. Advances in neurology series,* vol 76. Philadelphia: Lippincott-Raven Publishers, 1998:231–238.
35. Dodrill CB, Troupin AS. Psychotropic effects of carbamazepine in epilepsy: a double-blind comparison with phenytoin. *Neurology* 1977;27:1023–1028.
36. Dodrill CB, Troupin AS. Neuropsychological effects of carbamazepine and phenytoin: a reanalysis. *Neurology* 1991;41:141–143.
37. Meador KJ, Loring DW, Huh K, et al. Comparative cognitive effects of anticonvulsants. *Neurology* 1990;40:391–394.
38. Meador KJ, Loring DW, Abney OL, et al. Effects of carbamazepine and phenytoin on EEG and memory in healthy adults. *Epilepsia* 1993;34:153–157.
39. Meador KJ, Loring DW, Allen ME, et al. Comparative cognitive effects of carbamazepine and phenytoin in healthy adults. *Neurology* 1991;41:1537–1540.
40. Meador KJ, Loring DW, Moore EE, et al. Comparative cognitive effects of phenobarbital, phenytoin and valproate in healthy subjects. *Neurology* 1995;45:1494–1499.
41. Meador KJ, Loring DW, Thompson EE, et al. Differential cognitive effects of terfenadine and chlorpheniramine. *J Allergy Clin Immunol* 1989;84:322–325.
42. Smith DB, Mattson RH, Cramer JA, et al. Results of a nationwide Veterans Administration Cooperative Study comparing the efficacy and toxicity of carbamazepine, phenobarbital, phenytoin, and primidone. *Epilepsia* 1987;28(Suppl 3):S50–S58.
43. Prevey ML, Delaney RC, Cramer JA, et al. Effect of valproate on cognitive functioning. Comparison with carbamazepine. The Department of Veterans Affairs Epilepsy Cooperative Study 264 Group. *Arch Neurol* 1996;53:1008–1016.
44. Pulliainen V, Jokelainen M. Effects of phenytoin and carbamazepine on cognitive functions in newly diagnosed epileptic patients. *Acta Neurol Scand* 1994;89:81–86.
45. Smith KR, Goulding PM, Wilderman D, et al. Neurobehavioral effects of phenytoin and carbamazepine in patients recovering from brain trauma: a comparative study. *Arch Neurol* 1994;51:653–660.
46. Dodrill CB, Wilensky AJ. Neuropsychological abilities before and after 5 years of stable antiepileptic drug therapy. *Epilepsia* 1992;33:327–334.
47. Dimond KR, Pande AC, Lamoreaux L, et al. Effect of gabapentin (Neurontin) [corrected] on mood and well-being in patients with epilepsy. *Prog Neuropsychopharmacol Biol Psychiatry* 1996;20:407–417.
48. Lee DO, Steingard RJ, Cesena M, et al. Behavioral side effects of gabapentin in children. *Epilepsia* 1996;37:87–90.
49. Wolf SM, Shinnar S, Kang H, et al. Gabapentin toxicity in children manifesting as behavioral changes. *Epilepsia* 1995;36:1203–1205.
50. Leach JP, Girvan J, Paul A, et al. Gabapentin and cognition: a double-blind, dose-ranging, placebo-controlled study in refractory epilepsy. *J Neurol Neurosurg Psychiatry* 1997;62:372–376.

51. Meador KJ, Loring DW, Ray PG, et al. Differential cognitive effects of carbamazepine and gabapentin. *Epilepsia* 1999;40:1279–1285.

52. Salinsky MC, Binder LM, Oken BS, et al. Effects of gabapentin and carbamazepine on the EEG and cognition in healthy volunteers. *Epilepsia* 2002;43:482–490.

53. Martin R, Meador K, Turrentine L, et al. Comparative cognitive effects of carbamazepine and gabapentin in healthy senior adults. *Epilepsia* 2001;42:764–771.

54. Smith D, Baker G, Davies G, et al. Outcomes of add-on treatment with lamotrigine in partial epilepsy. *Epilepsia* 1993;34:312–322.

55. Meador KJ, Loring DW, Ray PG, et al. Differential cognitive and behavioral effects of carbamazepine and lamotrigine. *Neurology* 2001;56:1177–1182.

56. Aldenkamp AP, Arends J, Bootsma HP, et al. Randomized double-blind parallel-group study comparing cognitive effects of a low-dose lamotrigine with valproate and placebo in healthy volunteers. *Epilepsia* 2002;43:19–26.

57. Cohen AF, Ashby L, Crowley D, et al. Lamotrigine (BW430C), a potential anticonvulsant. Effects on the central nervous system in comparison with phenytoin and diazepam. *Br J Clin Pharmacol* 1985;20:619–629.

58. Hamilton MJ, Cohen AF, Yuen AW, et al. Carbamazepine and lamotrigine in healthy volunteers: relevance to early tolerance and clinical trial dosage. *Epilepsia* 1993;34:166–173.

59. Gillham R, Baker G, Thompson P, et al. Standardization of self-report questionnaire for use in evaluating cognitive, affective and behavioural side-effects of anti-epileptic drug treatments. *Epilepsy Res* 1996;24:47–55.

60. Brodie MJ, Overstall PW, Giorgi L, for the UK Lamotrigine Elderly Study Group. Multicentre, double-blind, randomised comparison between lamotrigine and carbamazepine in elderly patients with newly diagnosed epilepsy. *Epilepsy Res* 1999;37:81–87.

61. Steiner TJ, Dellaportas CI, Findley LJ, et al. Lamotrigine monotherapy in newly diagnosed untreated epilepsy: a double-blind comparison with phenytoin. *Epilepsia* 1999;40:601–607.

62. Brodie M, Richens A, Yuen AWC, for the UK Lamotrigine/Carbamazepine Monotherapy Trial Group. Double-blind comparison of lamotrigine and carbamazepine in newly diagnosed epilepsy. *Lancet* 1995;345:476–479.

63. Buchanan N. The efficacy of lamotrigine on seizure control in 34 children, adolescents and young adults with intellectual and physical disability. *Seizure* 1995;4:233–236.

64. Meador KJ, Baker GA. Behavioral and cognitive effects of lamotrigine. *J Child Neurol* 1997;12(Suppl 1):S44–S47.

65. Uvebrant P, Bauziene R. Intractable epilepsy in children. The efficacy of lamotrigine treatment, including non-seizure-related benefits. *Neuropediatrics* 1994;25:284–289.

66. Neyens LG, Alpherts WC, Aldenkamp AP. Cognitive effects of a new pyrrolidine derivative (levetiracetam) in patients with epilepsy. *Prog Neuropsychopharmacol Biol Psychiatry* 1995;19:411–419.

67. Kossoff EH, Bergey GK, Freeman JM, et al. Levetiracetam psychosis in children with epilepsy. *Epilepsia* 2001;42:1611–1613.

68. Cramer JA, De Rue K, Devinsky O, et al. A systematic review of the behavioral effects of levetiracetam in adults with epilepsy, cognitive disorders, or an anxiety disorder during clinical trials. *Epilepsy Behav* 2003;4:124–32.

69. Aikia M, Kalviainen R, Sivenius J, et al. Cognitive effects of oxcarbazepine and phenytoin monotherapy in newly diagnosed epilepsy: one year follow-up. *Epilepsy Res* 1992;11:199–203.

70. Curran HV, Java R. Memory and psychomotor effects of oxcarbazepine in healthy human volunteers. *Eur J Clin Pharmacol* 1993;44:529–533.

71. Sveinbjornsdottir S, Sander JW, Patsalos PN, et al. Neuropsychological effects of tiagabine, a potential new antiepileptic drug. *Seizure* 1994;3:29–35.

72. Dodrill CB, Arnett JL, Sommerville K, et al. Cognitive and quality of life effects of differing dosages of tiagabine in epilepsy. *Neurology* 1997;48:1025–1031.

73. Martin R, Kuzniecky R, Ho S, et al. Cognitive effects of topiramate, gabapentin, and lamotrigine in healthy young adults. *Neurology* 1999;52:321–326.

74. Lee S, Sziklas V, Andermann F, et al. The effects of adjunctive topiramate on cognitive function in patients with epilepsy. *Epilepsia* 2003;44:339–347.

75. Aldenkamp AP, Baker G, Mulder OG, et al. A multicenter, randomized clinical study to evaluate the effect on cognitive function of topiramate compared with valproate as add-on therapy to carbamazepine in patients with partial-onset seizures. *Epilepsia* 2000;41:1167–1178.

76. Meador KJ, Loring DW, Hulihan JF, et al. Differential cognitive and behavioral effects of topiramate and valproate. *Neurology* 2003;60:1483–1488.

77. Dodrill CB, Arnett JL, Sommerville KW, et al. Evaluation of the effects of vigabatrin on cognitive abilities and quality of life in epilepsy. *Neurology* 1993;43:2501–2507.

78. Dodrill CB, Arnett JL, Sommerville KW, et al. Effects of differing dosages of vigabatrin (Sabril) on cognitive abilities and quality of life in epilepsy. *Epilepsy* 1995;36:164–173.

79. Gillham RA, Blacklaw J, McKee PJW, et al. Effect of vigabatrin on sedation and cognitive function in patients with refractory epilepsy. *J Neurol Neurosurg Psychiatry* 1993;56:1271–1275.

80. Grunewald RA, Thompson PJ, Corcoran R, et al. Effects of vigabatrin on partial seizures and cognitive function. *Neurol Neurosurg Psychiatry* 1994;57:1057–1063.

81. Saletu B, Grunberger J, Linzmayer L, et al. Psychophysiological and psychometric studies after manipulating the GABA system by vigabatrin, a GABA-transaminase inhibitor. *Int J Psychophysiol* 1986;4:63–80.

82. Kalviainen R, Aikia M, Saukkonen AM, et al. Vigabatrin versus carbamazepine monotherapy in patients with newly diagnosed epilepsy: a randomized controlled study. *Arch Neurol* 1995;52:989–996.

83. Ferrie CD, Robinson RO, Panayiotopoulos CP. Psychotic and severe behavioural reactions with vigabatrin: a review. *Acta Neurol Scand* 1996;93:1–8.

84. Berent S, Sackellares JC, Giordani B, et al. Zonisamide (CI-912) and cognition: results from preliminary study. *Epilepsia* 1987;28:61–67.

85. Taylor JL, Tinklenberg JR. Cognitive impairment and benzodiazepines. In: Meltzer HY, ed. *Psychopharmacology: the third generation of progress.* New York: Raven Press, 1987:1449–1454.

86. Craig I, Tallis R. The impact of sodium valproate and phenytoin on cognitive function in elderly patients: results of a single-blind randomized comparative study. *Epilepsia* 1994;35:381–390.

87. Ramsey RE, Pryor F. Epilepsy in the elderly. *Neurology* 2000;55(Suppl 1):S9–S14.

88. Rowan AJ, Ramsay RE, Collins JF, et al. New onset geriatric epilepsy: a randomized study of gabapentin, lamotrigine, and carbamazepine. *Neurology* 2005;64:1868–1873.

89. Mikati MA, Holmes GL, Chronopoulos A, et al. Phenobarbital modifies seizure-related brain injury in the developing brain. *Ann Neurol* 1994;36:425–433.

90. Vining EPG, Mellitis ED, Dorsen MM, et al. Psychologic and behavioral effects of antiepileptic drugs in children: a double-blind comparison between phenobarbital and valproic acid. *Pediatrics* 1987;80:165–174.

91. Camfield CS, Chaplin S, Doyle AB, et al. Side effects of phenobarbital in toddlers: behavioral and cognitive aspects. *J Pediatr* 1979;95:361–365.

92. Farwell JR, Lee YJ, Hirtz DG, et al. Phenobarbital for febrile seizures—effects on intelligence and on seizure recurrence. *N Engl J Med* 1990;322:364–369.

93. Aldenkamp AP, Alpherts WCJ, Blennow G, et al. Withdrawal of antiepileptic medication in children—effects on cognitive function: the multicenter Holmfrid study. *Neurology* 1993;43:41–50.

94. Forsythe I, Butler R, Berg I, et al. Cognitive impairment in new cases of epilepsy randomly assigned to carbamazepine, phenytoin, and sodium valproate. *Dev Med Child Neurol* 1991;33:524–534.

95. Forsythe WI, Sills MA. One drug for childhood grand mal: medical audit for three-year remissions. *Dev Med Child Neurol* 1984;26:742–748.

96. Tonnby B, Nilsson HL, Aldenkamp AP, et al. Withdrawal of antiepileptic medication in children. Correlation of cognitive

function and plasma concentration—the multicentre "Holmfrid" study. *Epilepsy Res* 1994;19:141–152.

97. Leavitt AM, Yerby MS, Robinson N, et al. Epilepsy in pregnancy: developmental outcome of offspring at 12 months. *Neurology* 1992;42(Suppl 5):141–143.

98. Yerby MS. Pregnancy and epilepsy. *Epilepsia* 1991;32(Suppl 6):S51–S59.

99. Dansky LV, Finnell RH. Parental epilepsy, anticonvulsant drugs, and reproductive outcome: epidemiologic and experimental findings spanning three decades; 2: human studies. *Reprod Toxicol* 1991;5;301–335.

100. Finnell RH, Dansky LV. Parental epilepsy, anticonvulsant drugs, and reproductive outcome: epidemiologic and experimental findings spanning three decades; 1: animal studies. *Reprod Toxicol Rev* 1991;5;281–299.

101. Fisher JE, Vorhees C. Developmental toxicity of antiepileptic drugs: relationship to postnatal dysfunction. *Pharm Res* 1992;26:207–221.

102. Adams J, Vorhees CV, Middaugh LD. Developmental neurotoxicity of anticonvulsants: human and animal evidence on phenytoin. *Neurotoxicol Teratol* 1990;12:203–214.

103. Fishman RHB, Gaathon A, Yanai J. Early barbiturate treatment eliminates peak serum thyroxide levels in neonatal mice and produces ultrastructural damage in brain of adults. *Dev Brain Res* 1982;5:202–205.

104. Yanai J, Rosselli-Austin L, Tabakoff B. Neuronal deficits in mice following prenatal exposure to phenobarbital. *Exp Neurol* 1979;64:237–244.

105. Middaugh LD, Santos CA III, Zemp JW. Effects of phenobarbital given to pregnant mice on behavior of mature offspring. *Dev Psychobiol* 1975;8:305–313.

106. Middaugh LD, Santos CA III, Zemp JW. Phenobarbital during pregnancy alters operant behavior of offspring in C57BL/6J mice. *Pharmacol Biochem Behav* 1975;3:1137–1139.

107. Middaugh LD, Thomas TN, Simpson LW, et al. Effects of prenatal maternal injections of phenobarbital on brain neurotransmitters and behavior of young C57 mice. *Neurobehav Toxicol Teratol* 1981;3:271–275.

108. Elmazar MMA, Sullivan FM. Effect of prenatal phenytoin administration on postnatal development of the rat: a behavioral teratology study. *Teratology* 1981;24:115–124.

109. Mullenix P, Tassinari MS, Keith DA. Behavioral outcome after prenatal exposure to phenytoin in rats. *Teratology* 1983;27:149–157.

110. Vorhees CV. Fetal anticonvulsant syndrome in rats: dose- and period-response relationships of prenatal diphenylhydantoin, trimethadione and phenobarbital exposure on the structural and functional development of the offspring. *J Pharmacol Exp Ther* 1983:227:274–287.

111. Vorhees CV. Fetal anticonvulsant syndrome in rats: effects on postnatal behavior and brain amino acid content. *Neurobehav Toxicol Teratol* 1985;7:471–482.

112. Vorhees CV. Fetal anticonvulsant exposure: effects of behavioral and physical development. *Ann N Y Acad Sci* 1986;477:49–62.

113. Vorhees CV. Fetal hydantoin syndrome in rats: dose–effect relationships of prenatal phenytoin on postnatal development and behavior. *Teratology* 1987;35:287–303.

114. Vorhees CV, Minck DR. Long-term effects of prenatal phenytoin exposure on offspring behavior in rats. *Neurotoxicol Teratol* 1989;11:295–305.

115. Vorhees CV, Rindler JM, Minck DR. Effects of exposure period and nutrition on the developmental neurotoxicity of anticonvulsants in rats: short and long-term effects. *Neurotoxicology* 1990;11:273–283.

116. Vorhees CV. Behavioral teratogenicity of valproic acid: selective effects on behavior after prenatal exposure to rats. *Psychopharmacology* 1987;92:173–179.

117. Vorhees CV. Teratogenicity and developmental toxicity of valproic acid. *Teratology* 1987;35:195–202.

118. Vorhees CV, Rauch SL, Hitzemann RJ. Prenatal phenytoin exposure decreases neuronal membrane order in rat offspring hippocampus. *Int J Dev Neurosci* 1990;8:283–288.

119. Vorhees CV, Rauch SL, Hitzemann RJ. Prenatal valproic acid exposure decreases neuronal membrane order in rat offspring hippocampus and cortex. *Neurotoxicol Teratol* 1991;13:471–474.

120. Delgado-Escueta AV, Janz D. Consensus guidelines: preconception counseling, management, and care of the pregnant woman with epilepsy. *Neurology* 1992;42(Suppl 5):149–160.

121. Dressens AB, Boer K, Koppe JG, et al. Studies on long-lasting consequences of prenatal exposure to anticonvulsant drugs. *Acta Paediatr* 1994;83(Suppl 404):54–64.

122. Granström ML, Gaily E. Psychomotor development in children of mothers with epilepsy. *Neurology* 1992;42:144–148.

123. Janz D. On major malformations and minor anomalies in the offspring of parents with epilepsy: review of the literature. In: Janz D, Dam M, Richens A, et al, eds. *Epilepsy, pregnancy, and the child.* New York: Raven Press, 1982:211–222.

124. Fujioka K, Kaneko S, Hirano T, et al. A study of the psychomotor development of the offspring of epileptic mothers. In: Sato T, Shinagawa S, eds. *Antiepileptic drugs and pregnancy.* Amsterdam: Excerpta Medica, 1984:415–424.

125. Gaily E, Kantola-Sorsa E, Granström ML. Specific cognitive dysfunction in children with epileptic mothers. *Dev Med Child Neurol* 1990;32:403–414.

126. Hanson JW, Myrianthopoulos NC, Harvey MAS, et al. Risks to the offspring of women treated with hydantoin anticonvulsants, with emphasis on the fetal hydantoin syndrome. *J Pediatrics* 1976;89:662–668.

127. Hill RM, Tennyson LM. Maternal drug therapy: effect on fetal and neonatal growth and neurobehavior. *Neurotoxicology* 1986;7:121–140.

128. Jones KL, Lacro RV, Johnson KA, et al. Pattern of malformations in the children of women treated with carbamazepine during pregnancy. *N Engl J Med* 1989;320:1661–1666.

129. Losche G, Steinhausen HC, Koch S, et al. The psychological development of children of epileptic parents. II. The differential impact of intrauterine exposure to anticonvulsant drugs and further influential factors. *Acta Paediatr* 1994;83:961–966.

130. Nelson KB, Ellenberg DH. Maternal seizure disorder, outcome of pregnancy, and neurologic abnormalities in the children. *Neurology* 1982;32:1247–1254.

131. Speidel BD, Meadow SR. Maternal epilepsy and abnormalities of the fetus and newborn. *Lancet* 1972;2:839–843.

132. Steinhausen HC, Losche G, Koch S, et al. The psychological development of children of epileptic parents. I. Study design and comparative findings. *Acta Paediatr* 1994;83:955–960.

133. Vanoverloop D, Schnell RR, Harvey EA, et al. The effects of prenatal exposure to phenytoin and other anticonvulsants on intellectual function at 4 to 8 years of age. *Neurotoxicol Teratol* 1992;14:329–335.

134. Vert P, Deblay MF, Andre M. Follow-up study on growth and neurological development of children born to epileptic mothers. In: Janz D, Dam M, Richens A, et al, eds. *Epilepsy, pregnancy, and the child.* New York: Raven Press, 1982:433–436.

135. Andermann E. Development in offspring of epileptic parents. In: Akimoto H, Kazamatsuri H, Seino M, et al., eds. *Advances in epileptology: XIIIth Epilepsy International Symposium.* New York: Raven Press, 1982:415–424.

136. Dieterich E, Steveling A, Lukas A, et al. Congenital anomalies in children of epileptic mothers and fathers. *Neuropediatrics* 1980;11:274–283.

137. Granström ML, Hiilesmaa VK. Physical growth of the children of epileptic mothers: preliminary results from the prospective Helsinki study. In: Janz D, Dam M, Richens A, et al., eds. *Epilepsy, pregnancy, and the child.* New York: Raven Press, 1982:397–401.

138. Majewski F, Steger M, Richter B, et al. The teratogenicity of hydantoins and barbiturates in humans, with considerations on the etiology of malformations and cerebral disturbances in the children of epileptic parents. *Int J Biol Res Pregnancy* 1981;2:37–45.

139. Dean JC, Hailey H, Moore SJ, et al. Long-term health and neurodevelopment in children exposed to antiepileptic drugs before birth. *J Med Genet* 2002;39:251–259.

140. Holmes LB, Harvey EA, Coull BA, et al. The teratogenicity of anticonvulsant drugs. *N Engl J Med* 2001;344:1132–1138.

141. Bertollini R, Kallen B, Mastroiacova P, et al. Anticonvulsant drugs in monotherapy. Effect on the fetus. *Eur J Epidemiol* 1987;3:164–171.

142. Jäger-Roman E, Rating D, Koch S, et al. Somatic parameters, diseases and psychomotor development in the offspring of epileptic

parents. In: Janz D, Dam M, Richens A, et al., eds. *Epilepsy, pregnancy and the child.* New York: Raven Press, 1982:425–432.

143. Majewski F, Steger M. Fetal head growth retardation associated with maternal phenobarbitone/primidone and/or phenytoin therapy [letter]. *Eur J Pediatr* 1984;141:188–189.

144. Dieterich E. Antiepileptika embryopathien. *Ergeb Inn Med Kinderheilkd* 1980;43:93–107.

145. Gaily EK, Granström ML, Hiilesmaa VK, et al. Head circumference in children of epileptic mothers: contributions of drug exposure and genetic background. *Epilepsy Res* 1990;5:217–222.

146. Kelly TE, Edwards P, Rein M, et al. Teratogenicity of anticonvulsant drugs, II: a prospective study. *Am J Med Genet* 1984;19:435–443.

147. Hattig H, Helge H, Steinhausen HC. Infants of epileptic mothers: developmental scores at 18 months. In: Wolf P, Dam M, Janz D, et al., eds. *Advances in Epileptology: XVIth Epilepsy International Symposium.* New York: Raven Press, 1987:579–582.

148. Reinisch JM, Sanders SA, Mortensen EL, et al. In utero exposure to phenobarbital and intelligence deficits in adult men. *JAMA* 1995;274:1518–1525.

149. Adab N, Jacoby A, Smith D, et al. Additional educational needs in children born to mothers with epilepsy. *J Neurol Neurosurg Psychiatry* 2001;70:15–21.

150. Gailey E, Kantola-Sorsa E, Hiilesmaa V, et al. Intelligence in children of mothers with epilepsy [abstract]. *Epilepsia* 2002;43 (Suppl 8):56.

151. Finnell RH, Chernoff GF. Gene-teratogen interactions. An approach to understanding the metabolic basis of birth defects. In: Nau H, Scott WJ, eds. *Pharmacokinetics in teratogenesis.* Boca Raton, FL: CRC Press, 1987:97–109.

152. Phelan MC, Pellock JM, Nance WE. Discordant expression of fetal hydantoin syndrome in heteropaternal dizygotic twins. *N Engl J Med* 1982;307:99–101.

153. Buehler BA, Delimont D, Waes MV, et al. Prenatal prediction of risk of the fetal hydantoin syndrome. *N Engl J Med* 1990;322:1567–1572.

154. Martz F, Failinger C, Blake D. Phenytoin teratogenesis: correlation between embryopathic effect and covalent binding of putative arene oxide metabolite in gestational tissue. *J Pharm Exp Ther* 1977;203:231–239.

155. Finnell RH, Buehler BA, Kerr BM, et al. Clinical and experimental studies linking oxidative metabolism to phenytoin-induced teratogenesis. *Neurology* 1992;42:25–31.

156. Juchau MR. Chemical teratogenesis in humans: biochemical and molecular mechanisms. In: Jucker E, ed. *Progress in drug research.* Basel: Birkhauser Verlag, 1997:25–92.

157. Wells PG, Zubovits JT, Wong ST, et al. Modulation of phenytoin teratogenicity and embryonic covalent binding by acetylsalicylic acid, caffeic acid, and alpha-phenyl-N-t-butylnitrone: implications for bioactivation by prostaglandin synthetase. *Toxicol Appl Pharmacol* 1989;97:192–202.

158. Wells PG, Kim PM, Laposa RR, et al. Oxidative damage in chemical teratogenesis. *Mutat Res* 1997;396:65–78.

159. Wong M, Wells PG. Modulation of embryonic glutathione reductase and phenytoin teratogenicity by 1,3-bis(2-chloroethyl)-1-nitrosourea (BCNU). *J Pharmacol Exp Ther* 1989;250:336–342.

160. Danielsson B, Skold AC, Azarbayjani F, et al. Pharmacokinetic data support pharmacologically induced embryonic dysrhythmia as explanation to fetal hydantoin syndrome in rats. *Toxicol Appl Pharmacol* 2000;163:164–175.

161. Carl GF, Smith DB. Interaction of phenytoin and folate in the rat. *Epilepsia* 1983;24:494–501.

162. Carl GF, Smith DB. Effect of chronic phenobarbital treatment on folates and one-carbon enzymes in the rat. *Biochem Pharm* 1984;21:3457–3463.

163. Carl GF, Smith ML. Chronic primidone treatment in the rat: an animal model of primidone therapy. *Res Commun Chem Path Pharmacol* 1988;61:365–376.

164. Carl GF, Smith ML. Chronic carbamazepine treatment in the rat: efficacy, toxicity, and effect on plasma and tissue folate concentrations. *Epilepsia* 1989;30:217–224.

165. Carl GF, DeLoach C, Patterson J. Chronic sodium valproate treatment in the rat: toxicity versus protection against seizures induced by Indoklon. *Neurochem Int* 1986;8:41–45.

166. Danksy LV, Andermann E, Rosenblatt D, et al. Anticonvulsants, folate levels and pregnancy outcome: a prospective study. *Ann Neurol* 1987;21:176–182.

167. Biale Y, Lewenthal H. Effect of folic acid supplementation on congenital malformations due to anticonvulsant drugs. *Eur J Obstet Gynecol Reprod Biol* 1984;18:211–216.

168. Ikonomidou C, Bittigau P, Ishimaru MJ, et al. Ethanol-induced apoptotic neurodegeneration in fetal alcohol syndrome. *Science* 2000;287:1056–1060.

169. Bittigau P, Sifringer M, Ikonomidou C. Antiepileptic drugs and apoptosis in the developing brain. *Ann N Y Acad Sci* 2003;993:103–114.

Psychiatric Comorbidity of Epilepsy

88

Steven C. Schachter

Epilepsy is a model for brain-behavior relationships. Seizures affect behavior, and behavior affects seizures. Psychiatric comorbidity is common among patients with epilepsy, the clinical presentation is frequently atypical, and there is often a temporal relationship to seizures. This chapter reviews four of the most commonly encountered psychiatric disorders in patients with epilepsy: depression, psychosis, anxiety, and aggression.

DEPRESSION

Depression is the most frequently occurring comorbid psychiatric disorder in patients with epilepsy, with prevalence rates of 10% to 20% among patients with controlled seizures and 20% to 60% among those with refractory epilepsy (1,2). Suicide accounts for one of the highest standardized mortality rates of all causes of death in persons with epilepsy and is 10 times more common in patients with epilepsy than in the general population (3).

Studies of depression and health-related quality of life have shown that depression is a better predictor of quality of life than are verbal memory, psychomotor function, cognition, seizure frequency, and seizure severity (4–7).

Depressive symptoms vary according to the temporal relation to seizure occurrence. Symptoms may arise prior to seizure onset (preictal), as an expression of the seizure (ictal), following seizures (postictal), or unrelated to seizure occurrence (interictal). The clinical presentation in up to 50% of depressed patients with epilepsy does not meet any of the *Diagnostic and Statistical Manual of Mental Disorders* (DSM) Axis I categories (8,9).

Interictal depression is the most common presentation. It mimics a dysthymic disorder, with endogenous features and an intermittent course, and has been termed interictal dysphoric disorder by Blumer (9). Prominent symptoms include irritability, anhedonia, feelings of hopelessness and helplessness, fear, and anxiety.

Ictal depression manifests as the clinical expression of a simple partial seizure (SPS) in which depression is the sole symptom. The most common ictal psychiatric symptoms are anhedonia, guilt, and suicidal ideation. Preictal depression is characterized by a dysphoric mood that precedes a seizure by hours or days (10) and that usually ends with the seizure. Postictal depression has long been recognized but its frequency of occurrence is unknown. Symptoms often persist for hours to several days.

Depression is both underrecognized and undertreated in patients with epilepsy. A number of reasons have been proposed, including lack of clinical recognition, the consideration that depression is an expected, or "normal," reaction to having epilepsy and therefore not necessary to treat separately, and concern that all antidepressants may exacerbate seizures. A further limiting factor is the lack of controlled trials for depression in patients with epilepsy.

Before treatment is begun, iatrogenic factors should be considered, such as the recent discontinuation of an antiepileptic therapy with mood-stabilizing properties (e.g., carbamazepine, lamotrigine, valproate, and vagus nerve stimulation); the recent introduction or dosage increase of an antiepileptic drug (AED) with potential negative psychotropic properties (e.g., primidone, phenobarbital, topiramate, vigabatrin, and tiagabine); or the recent remission of seizures (i.e., "forced normalization").

In the absence of controlled trials, the choice of an antidepressant should be based on safety, tolerability, and ease of use (i.e., frequency of dosage, likelihood of drug–drug interactions). It is prudent to avoid bupropion, maprotiline, and amoxapine because of their potential for exacerbating seizures (11). By contrast, selective serotonin reuptake inhibitors (SSRIs) are unlikely to worsen seizure frequency or severity, and are generally effective for dysthymic disorders, symptoms of irritability, and poor frustration tolerance. Furthermore, an overdose of an SSRI is unlikely to be fatal, interactions with AEDs are minimal, and side effects are manageable.

Among the SSRIs, sertraline has been best studied. Kanner and associates used sertraline to treat depression in 100 patients with epilepsy. Depressive symptoms improved in the majority of patients, with seizures definitely worsening in only one patient (12). Sertraline can be initiated at 25 to 50 mg per day and increased every 3 weeks as needed, to 200 mg per day or the maximum tolerated dose.

Other pharmacologic options include venlafaxine, tricyclic antidepressants (TCAs), and antiepileptic therapies with mood-stabilizing properties. Monoamine oxidase (MAO) inhibitors require dietary vigilance to minimize the risk for hypertension, and lithium is a proconvulsant in nonepileptic patients and is associated with electroencephalographic changes. Electroconvulsive therapy is not contraindicated and should be considered for patients with pharmacologically refractory depression.

Psychotherapy can help patients cope with limitations imposed by epilepsy and may result in significant improvements in rating scales of depression and anxiety, as well as seizure frequency (13).

PSYCHOSIS

A bidirectional relationship between epilepsy and psychosis was proposed during the 19th century. The likelihood of an episode of psychosis occurring in patients with epilepsy varies according to the epilepsy syndrome, seizure severity, and seizure frequency. Consequently, the frequency of psychosis among patients with epilepsy is 14%, compared with 3% in patients with idiopathic generalized epilepsy. In addition, psychosis is reported in 0.6% to 7% of patients with epilepsy in the community versus 19% to 27% of hospital-derived populations (14).

Psychotic symptoms present according to the temporal relation to seizures. The most common form of psychosis in patients with epilepsy occurs between seizures (interictal). Postictal psychosis is less common, and ictal psychotic ideation is rare.

Hill and colleagues observed that patients with interictal psychosis did not display lack of affect, or "asocial or withdrawn attitude" (15). Slater and colleagues confirmed these atypical features, while noting that psychotic episodes included paranoid delusions with visual and auditory hallucinations (16). Consequently, he coined the term "schizophrenia-like psychosis." Compared with the psychosis of schizophrenia, patients with interictal psychosis have an absence of negative symptoms, better premorbid state, less deterioration of personality, and better response to pharmacotherapy. Possible contributing factors include postictal psychosis, AED toxicity, and AED withdrawal (17).

Postictal psychosis typically begins within several days of a cluster of complex partial or secondarily generalized seizures and includes hallucinations, paranoia, and delusions (18–22).

In general, psychotropic agents that are associated with a high incidence of seizures in nonepileptic patients should be avoided. These include certain antipsychotics (i.e., clozapine, chlorpromazine, and loxapine) and certain antidepressants (i.e., clomipramine, amoxapine, maprotiline, and bupropion).

Therapies that are less likely to exacerbate seizures include olanzapine 5 to 25 mg per day (major side effects are somnolence, weight gain, and glucose intolerance); risperidone 0.5 to 6 mg per day (associated with weight gain and extrapyramidal side effects); molindone 50 to 200 mg per day; haloperidol (particularly if intramuscular or intravenous administration is needed); and lorazepam 0.5 to 2 mg per day (in conjunction with an antipsychotic to reinforce a sleep schedule) (23).

ANXIETY

Anxiety disorders are generally subdivided into panic disorder, obsessive-compulsive disorder, and generalized anxiety disorder (GAD). The comorbidity of epilepsy and anxiety is less-well studied than are the comorbidities of depression and psychosis; studies suggest that the prevalence of anxiety disorders in patients with epilepsy ranges from 3% to 50%.

Anxiety may occur prior to seizure onset (preictal), as an expression of a seizure (ictal), during the postictal period, or between seizures (interictal). Anxiety disorders most commonly present interictally and usually as a GAD. Contributing factors include the unpredictability of seizures, psychosocial difficulties, and iatrogenic factors (use of felbamate, vigabatrin, or topiramate, or withdrawal of benzodiazepines or phenobarbital).

Interestingly, interictal anxiety does not necessarily correlate with seizure frequency (24) and may develop paradoxically with seizure freedom (e.g., postoperative).

Panic attacks should be differentiated from partial seizures. Factors favoring the diagnosis of panic attacks include gradual onset of symptoms, duration from minutes to hours, and lack of postepisode confusion.

To date, no controlled studies of anxiolytic therapy in patients with epilepsy have been conducted. Pharmacologic treatments used empirically include SSRIs, TCAs (e.g., imipramine), benzodiazepines, venlafaxine, buspirone, and AEDs, including valproic acid, gabapentin, and oxcarbazepine.

Nonpharmacologic treatment may be helpful in individual cases, including family and supportive psychotherapy and self-help groups.

AGGRESSION

The relationship between epilepsy and aggressive behavior is controversial. Studies implicate traumatic brain damage, psychosis, and mild to severe cognitive deficits as contributing factors to violent behavior in patients with epilepsy (25–32).

Aggressive behavior is probably underdiagnosed because of underreporting to physicians because of embarrassment or lack of appreciation that the behavior may constitute a treatable disorder.

Aggressive and violent behavior may occur with a temporal relationship to seizures. Some patients exhibit irritability and aggression in the minutes, hours, or days leading up to a seizure (preictal) (10,33). Directed, purposeful, aggressive, or violent behavior during seizures (ictal) is generally considered rare (34–37). Postictal aggression is well recognized. Violent behavior may result from attempts at physical restraint, termed "resistive violence" (34,38). Violent behavior may also occur in association with a postictal psychosis (39).

Interictal aggression has been studied in selected groups of patients and prisoners with epilepsy. In these populations, impulsive, aggressive behavior is seen between seizures in up to 56% of patients with temporal lobe epilepsy (40–46). Conversely, Rodin found evidence of "destructive-assaultive" behavior in 4.8% of patients with epilepsy seen at a tertiary referral center over a 5-year period (37).

Because AEDs may indirectly cause aggressive behavior as a consequence of a forced normalization (47), or as a consequence of sedative and disinhibiting side effects, iatrogenic causes should first be considered.

Treatment depends on the severity of the behavior and the temporal relationship to seizures. Ictal aggression should respond to AEDs. Postictal resistive violence is best treated by avoiding or limiting physical restraint during the postictal period (48,49). Aggression associated with postictal psychosis is treated by reducing seizure clusters and by the acute administration of benzodiazepines and psychotropic agents such as haloperidol (22,50). Psychiatric hospitalization should be considered for patients at risk for impulsive, potentially self-injurious behavior.

The treatment of interictal aggression is less certain, because it does not necessarily improve with complete seizure control (51,52) and controlled studies are lacking. AEDs (particularly carbamazepine and valproate) and antidepressants have been used empirically.

SUMMARY

Psychiatric comorbidities are common in patients with epilepsy, significantly impact quality of life independent of seizures, and have a variable clinical presentation depending on the temporal relation to seizures.

Depression occurs most frequently, but is underdiagnosed and undertreated. Pharmacologic and interpersonal therapies for depression, psychosis, anxiety, and aggressive behavior should be individualized. Controlled therapeutic trials are needed to better define the efficacy and safety of psychotropic agents in patients with epilepsy.

REFERENCES

1. Mendez MF, Cummings JL, Benson DF. Depression in epilepsy. Significance and phenomenology. *Arch Neurol* 1986;43:766–770.
2. O'Donoghue MF, Goodridge DM, Redhead K, et al. Assessing the psychosocial consequences of epilepsy: a community-based study. *Br J Gen Pract* 1999;49:211–214.
3. Harden CL, Goldstein MA. Mood disorders in patients with epilepsy: epidemiology and management. *CNS Drugs* 2002;16:291–302.
4. Perrine K, Hermann BP, Meador KJ, et al. The relationship of neuropsychological functioning to quality of life in epilepsy. *Arch Neurol* 1995;52:997–1003.
5. Lehrner J, Kalchmayr R, Serles W, et al. Health-related quality of life (HRQOL), activity of daily living (ADL) and depressive mood disorder in temporal lobe epilepsy patients. *Seizure* 1999;8:88–92.
6. Attarian H, Dowling J, Carter J, Gilliam F. Video EEG monitoring prior to vagal nerve stimulator implantation. *Neurology* 2003;61:402–403.
7. Gilliam F. Optimizing health outcomes in active epilepsy. *Neurology* 2002;58(8 Suppl 5):S9–S20.
8. Kanner AM, Palac S. Depression in epilepsy: a common but often unrecognized comorbid malady. *Epilepsy Behav* 2000;1:37–51.
9. Blumer D. Antidepressant and double antidepressant treatment for the affective disorder of epilepsy. *J Clin Psychiatry* 1997;58:3–11.
10. Blanchet P, Frommer GP. Mood change preceding epileptic seizures. *J Nerv Ment Dis* 1986;174:471–476.
11. Pisani F, Spina E, Oteri G. Antidepressant drugs and seizure susceptibility: from *in vitro* data to clinical practice. *Epilepsia* 1999;40(Suppl 10):S48–S56.
12. Kanner AM, Kozak AM, Frey M. The use of sertraline in patients with epilepsy: is it safe? *Epilepsy Behav* 2000;1:100–105.
13. Gillham RA. Refractory epilepsy: an evaluation of psychological methods in outpatient management. *Epilepsia* 1990;31:427–432.
14. Torta R, Keller R. Behavioral, psychotic, and anxiety disorders in epilepsy: etiology, clinical features, and therapeutic implications. *Epilepsia* 1999;40(Suppl 10):S2–S20.
15. Hill D, Pond DA, Mitchell W, Falconer MA. Personality changes following temporal lobectomy for epilepsy. *J Ment Sci* 1957;103:18–27.
16. Slater E, Beard AW, Glithero E. The schizophrenialike psychoses of epilepsy. *Br J Psychiatry* 1963;109:95–150.
17. Ketter TA, Malow BA, Flamini R, et al. Anticonvulsant withdrawal-emergent psychopathology. *Neurology* 1994;44:55–61.
18. Logsdail SJ, Toone BK. Postictal psychoses. *Br J Psychiatry* 1988;152:246–252.
19. Savard G, Andermann F, Olivier A, Remillard GM. Postictal psychosis after partial complex seizures: a multiple case study. *Epilepsia* 1991;32:225–231.
20. Torta R, Keller R. Behavioral, psychotic, and anxiety disorders in epilepsy: etiology, clinical features, and therapeutic implications. *Epilepsia* 1999;40(Suppl 10):S2–S20.
21. Levine DN, Finklestein S. Delayed psychosis after right temporoparietal stroke or trauma: relation to epilepsy. *Neurology* 1982;32:267–273.
22. Lancman M. Psychosis and peri-ictal confusional states. *Neurology* 1999;53(Suppl 2):S33–S38.
23. Kanner AM. Psychosis of epilepsy: a neurologist's perspective. *Epilepsy Behav* 2000;1:219–227.
24. Goldstein MA, Harden CL. Epilepsy and anxiety. *Epilepsy Behav* 2000;1:228–234.

25. Elliott FA. Violence. The neurologic contribution: an overview. *Arch Neurol* 1992;49:595–603.
26. Fenwick P. Aggression and epilepsy. In: Trimble MR, Bolwig TG, eds. *Aspects of epilepsy and psychiatry.* Chichester, UK: John Wiley, 1986:31–60.
27. Lewis DO, Pincus JH, Shanok SS, Glaser GH. Psychomotor epilepsy and violence in a group of incarcerated adolescent boys. *Am J Psychiatry* 1982;139:882–887.
28. Hodgins S. Mental disorder, intellectual deficiency, and crime. Evidence from a birth cohort. *Arch Gen Psychiatry* 1992;49: 476–483.
29. Mouridsen SE, Tolstrup K. Children who kill: a case study of matricide. *J Child Psychol Psychiatry* 1988;29:511–515.
30. Trimble MR. *Psychoses of epilepsy.* New York: Raven Press; 1991.
31. Herzberg JL, Fenwick PBC. The aetiology of aggression in temporal-lobe epilepsy. *Br J Psychiatry* 1988;153:50–55.
32. Mendez MF, Doss RC, Taylor JL. Interictal violence in epilepsy. Relationship to behavior and seizure variables. *J Nerv Ment Dis* 1993;181:566–569.
33. Fenwick P. Psychiatric disorders in epilepsy. In: Hopkins A, ed. *Epilepsy.* London: Chapman and Hall, 1987:511–553.
34. Delgado Escueta AV, Mattson RH, King L, et al. Special report. The nature of aggression during epileptic seizures. *N Engl J Med* 1981;305:711–716.
35. King D, Ajmone Marsan C. Clinical features and ictal patterns in epileptic patients with EEG temporal lobe foci. *Ann Neurol* 1977;2:138–147.
36. Ramani V, Gumnit RJ. Intensive monitoring of epileptic patients with a history of episodic aggression. *Arch Neurol* 1981;38: 570–571.
37. Rodin EA. Psychomotor epilepsy and aggressive behavior. *Arch Gen Psychiatry* 1973;28:210–213.
38. Treiman MR, Delgado-Escueta V. Aggression during fear and fight in complex partial seizures: a CCTV-EEG analysis. *Epilepsia* 1981;22:243.
39. Kanemoto K, Kawasaki J, Mori E. Violence and epilepsy: a close relation between violence and postictal psychosis. *Epilepsia* 1999;40:107–109.
40. Moyer KE. *The psychobiology of aggression.* New York: Harper & Row, 1976.
41. Devinsky O, Bear D. Varieties of aggressive behavior in temporal lobe epilepsy. *Am J Psychiatry* 1984;141:651–656.
42. Mungas D. An empirical analysis of specific syndromes of violent behavior. *J Nerv Ment Dis* 1983;171:354–361.
43. Currie S, Heathfield KWG, Henson RA, Scott DF. Clinical course and prognosis of temporal lobe epilepsy. A survey of 666 patients. *Brain* 1971;94:173–190.
44. Falconer MA. Reversibility by temporal-lobe resection of the behavioral abnormalities of temporal-lobe epilepsy. *N Engl J Med* 1973;289:451–455.
45. Glaser GH. Limbic epilepsy in childhood. *J Nerv Ment Dis* 1967;144:391–397.
46. Serafetinides EA. Aggressiveness in temporal lobe epileptics and its relation to cerebral dysfunction and environmental factors. *Epilepsia* 1965;6:33–42.
47. Pakalnis A, Drake ME, John K, Kellum JB. Forced normalization. Acute psychosis after seizure control in seven patients. *Arch Neurol* 1987;44:289–292.
48. Keats MM, Mukherjee S. Antiaggressive effect of adjunctive clonazepam in schizophrenia associated with seizure disorder. *J Clin Psychiatry* 1988;49:117–118.
49. Ashford JW, Schulz SC, Walsh GO. Violent automatism in a partial complex seizure. Report of a case. *Arch Neurol* 1980;37: 120–122.
50. Fenwick P. Aggression and epilepsy. In: Devinsky O, Theodore WH, eds. *Epilepsy and behavior.* New York: Wiley-Liss, 1991:85–96.
51. Taylor DC. Aggression and epilepsy. *J Psychosom Res* 1969;13: 229–236.
52. Bear DM, Fedio P. Quantitative analysis of interictal behavior in temporal lobe epilepsy. *Arch Neurol* 1977;34:454–467.

89

Driving and Social Issues in Epilepsy

Joseph F. Drazkowski   *Joseph I. Sirven*

A person with epilepsy faces many social concerns that are taken for granted by those without the disorder (1,2). A recent quality-of-life (QOL) survey identified driving a motor vehicle as the number one concern for a person with epilepsy (1). In addition to driving, other important social issues for a person with epilepsy include obtaining and maintaining employment, and participating in athletic and recreational activities (2). This chapter explores important social issues that can influence the QOL of a person with epilepsy.

EVALUATION OF THE RISK OF ENGAGING IN A DESIRED ACTIVITY

Although on some level everyone must balance the risks of engaging in a desired activity against the potential benefits derived from that activity, this cost-to-benefit analysis assumes added significance for the person with epilepsy. A person with epilepsy must conduct the analysis in the context of a specific situation, with the consideration that a seizure-related injury might occur during the specific activity. To determine potential risk, a person with epilepsy needs to understand all aspects of the specific activity and must try to predict the potential exposure to injury should a seizure occur during participation. The risk of seizure recurrence will determine, at least in part, how safe it is to participate in a desired activity. Factors that influence seizure recurrence have been reported (3) and may provide important insight into determining the risks associated with a desired activity. These factors include the presence of an abnormal electroencephalogram (EEG), initial seizure type, and etiology of the seizure. Symptomatic seizures are twice as likely as idiopathic seizures to recur (4–6). Partial seizures are also more likely to recur compared

with an initial major motor seizure (4,7). If the etiology of a seizure disorder is head injury, the risk for recurrence may be higher. In patients with severe head injury, the recurrence rates for seizures are 7.1% and 11.5% at 1 and 5 years, respectively, (8) with severe head injury defined as amnesia and/or loss of consciousness for more than 24 hours, or the presence of an intracranial hematoma. Structural lesions, such as brain tumors, stroke, abscesses, and penetrating head wounds, all carry an increased risk for recurrent seizures. Seizures caused by alcohol use, on the other hand, are unlikely to recur if abstinence is maintained. After a new-onset major motor seizure in a patient with a normal examination and work-up, including magnetic resonance imaging (MRI), electroencephalography, and blood tests, seizure recurrence is estimated to range between 25% (5) and approximately 70% (9) at 3 years. Another review suggested a recurrence risk of 50%, also at 3 years (7). If one remains in remission (i.e., seizure free) for 2 years or longer, a good prognosis is possible (10).

The danger period for a particular activity should also be considered when evaluating potential risk. The person with epilepsy is exposed to less risk when the danger period for an activity is brief. For example, target shooting with a lethal weapon likely poses little risk to the shooter or people in close proximity except for that very short period of time when squeezing the trigger. In contrast, such activities as motorbike riding or hang gliding might present a relatively high risk for the person with epilepsy as danger periods encompass the entire time they are involved in the activity. Activities with inherent danger must also be factored into the decision of whether to participate. For example, table tennis is certainly less dangerous than bullfighting. Finally, other factors, such as medication compliance, medication side effects, age, concomitant medical problems, use of safety equipment, and a prolonged and consistent aura, can all influence the risks faced by a person with epilepsy when engaging in a specific activity.

DRIVING AND THE PERSON WITH EPILEPSY

The Risks

A person with epilepsy faces a risk of injury and a risk of causing injury if a seizure should occur while operating a motor vehicle. Driving is a privilege, not a right. This privilege is governed by individual country, state, or territorial governments (11). There are approximately 225 million registered vehicles in the United States. In 2002, an estimated 6.7 million motor vehicle crashes occurred in the United States (12). These crashes resulted in approximately 3 million injuries and more than 42,000 deaths (12). It is estimated that approximately 0.5% to 1.0% of the U.S. population has epilepsy (3), potentially placing more than 2.5 million drivers with epilepsy on the roads of the United States. However, the actual number of persons with epilepsy who drive with or without a valid license is unknown. Applicants for a motor vehicle license must answer questions about their medical status and affirm that they are healthy and fit to drive before they are allowed to operate a motor vehicle. One study suggested that only 14% of individuals had answered truthfully on their driving application when asked about the presence of epilepsy (13). In a

prospective survey of 367 patients with localization-related epilepsy pooled from a consortium of comprehensive epilepsy programs, approximately 30% of the respondents had operated a motor vehicle in the previous 12 months (14). The paucity of available data makes it difficult to definitively establish the number of automobile crashes caused by persons with epilepsy who have a seizure while driving. Reports suggest that persons with epilepsy account for approximately 0.02% to 0.04% of all reported automobile car crashes (15,16). In contrast, alcohol-related crashes comprise approximately 7% of car crashes but account for approximately 40% of all fatalities nationwide (17).

Seizures are unpredictable, and the presumption is that longer seizure-free intervals translate into a decreased likelihood of seizure-related crashes. Verifying this is difficult, however, as individual driving records are generally not available for review. A recent retrospective survey of patients in several Maryland outpatient epilepsy clinics suggested that the risk of motor vehicle crashes was reduced by 85% and 93% if the patient did not have a seizure at 6 months and 12 months, respectively (18). This survey relied on self-reported crashes.

It has been suggested that self-reporting of crashes by respondents in surveys is unreliable (19,20). Drazkowski and colleagues (16) reviewed actual accident reports in Arizona from crashes caused by seizures before and after the seizure-free interval was reduced from 12 to 3 months (Table 89.1). Although no significant increases in seizure-related crashes were reported, the retrospective study provided some objective

TABLE 89.1

CHANGES IN THE INCIDENCE RATES OF CRASHES (/10^9 MILES DRIVEN) AFTER REDUCING THE RESTRICTION ON DRIVERS WITH EPILEPSY FROM 12 TO 3 MONTHS, 3 YEARS BEFORE AND AFTER LAW CHANGE

Type/Cause	Before 95% CI	After	Incidence[a] Rate	95% CI		RR[b]
Total						
Seizure	1.1	1.1	−0.028	−0.30–0.24	0.98	0.77–1.24
Other medical	2.6	2.6	−0.092	−0.51–0.33	0.97	0.82–1.13
Not seizure (103)	2.6	2.8	0.20	0.19–0.22	1.08	1.07–1.08
Injury						
seizure	0.58	0.76	0.18	−0.03–0.39	1.31	0.95–1.80
Other medical	1.6	1.3	−0.21	−0.52–0.10	0.87	0.70–1.07
Not seizure (103)	1.0	1.1	0.045	0.037–0.053	1.04	1.04–1.05
Fatal[c]						
Seizure	0.046	0.016	−0.029	−0.076–0.017	0.36	0.07–1.85
Other medical	0.055	0.099	0.043	−0.027–0.11	1.79	0.67–4.8
Not seizure	20	21	1.6	0.39–2.7	1.08	1.02–1.14

Abbreviations: CI, confidence interval; RR, relative risk.
[a]Incidence rate difference (before versus after).
[b]Relative risk (before versus after).
[c]Fatal crashes are a subset of the injury category and are segregated for separate analysis.
Modified from Drazkowski JF, Fisher RS, Sirven JI, et al. Seizure-related motor vehicle crashes in Arizona before and after reducing the driving restriction from 12 to 3 months. *Mayo Clin Proc* 2003;78:819–825, with permission.

data on these crashes. To date, no controlled prospective data are available to guide regulating authorities as to the optimum seizure-free interval for the protection of both the person with epilepsy and the public.

The Regulatory Requirements

The first seizure-related car crash was reported near the turn of the 19th century. Since then, regulatory authorities have placed restrictions on driving for the person with epilepsy. Almost a decade ago, the American Academy of Neurology, the American Epilepsy Society, and the Epilepsy Foundation of America convened a conference of thought leaders to issue guidelines on the topic of driving and the person with epilepsy (21). Recommendations from the conference included (a) a seizure-free interval of 3 months, (b) allowances for purely nocturnal seizures, and (c) a provision allowing driving when there is an established pattern of a prolonged and consistent aura (21).

Determining the risk of a crash caused by the driver with epilepsy is difficult. Traditionally, the duration of seizure freedom is used by authorities to determine when it is safe for a person with epilepsy to drive. Seizure-free intervals adopted by jurisdictions vary widely and have many unique exceptions (22) (Tables 89.2 and 89.3). State regulatory agencies and the Epilepsy Foundation of America website (www.efa.org) can be contacted for current laws governing driving and epilepsy (23). In an editorial, Krumholz suggested that it is time to consider uniform laws governing epilepsy and driving throughout the United States (24). International rules on driving have been reviewed, and because of the high variability among individual countries, it has been suggested that the appropriate national authority be consulted to determine current local laws regarding driving before traveling to these nations (25).

Six states currently have laws that require health care providers to report persons with epilepsy to the appropriate state driving authorities. The rationale behind the reporting requirement is that a person with epilepsy will not reliably self-report the presence of active or recurrent seizures to the proper authority. Laws that require a health care provider to report a person with epilepsy to authorities are criticized as impairing the physician–patient relationship and thus compromising optimal medical care. The premise is that when physicians are required to report epilepsy to driving authorities, persons with epilepsy may conceal information about their seizures to avoid being reported and potentially losing their license (19). Of persons with epilepsy who had been counseled about driving laws, only 27% reported their condition to the appropriate authorities (26). This is assuming that the health care professional knows the proper laws, but in one survey, only 13% of providers knew the appropriate requirements (27). In California, which is the most populous state requiring physician reporting, a survey again suggested that the physician reporting requirement impaired medical care

and the doctor–patient relationship (28). There are no available studies showing that physician reporting reduces seizure-related automobile crashes. In Canada, a conference of invited experts concluded that the laws requiring health care professionals to report persons with epilepsy to authorities should be abolished and suggested that driving laws be uniform across Canada (29). An editorial by emergency department physicians suggested that mandatory reporting of seizures be abolished in the United States (30). This editorial highlighted several other medical conditions and situations that are associated with a similar or higher relative risk of a car crash compared with epilepsy, such as sleep, apnea, diabetes, dementia, and cell phone use (distraction) (30).

EMPLOYMENT AND THE PERSON WITH EPILEPSY

QOL surveys have identified employment issues and concerns of persons with epilepsy as significant (1,2). The economic impact that epilepsy has on society is huge (more than $10.8 billion per year) and is largely attributable to indirect employment-related costs, which account for 85% of all epilepsy costs (31). Persons with epilepsy are reported to have lower household incomes, which are estimated to be 93% of the U.S. median income (32), compared with the general population.

In the United States, the rate of unemployment for persons with epilepsy is reported to be between 25% and 69% (32,33). The overall nationwide rate of graduation from high school is approximately 82%; for persons with epilepsy, that rate is approximately 64% (32). Although many factors are likely to contribute to the high rate of unemployment among persons with epilepsy, poorly controlled epilepsy is associated with a high level of unemployment (33). Age of epilepsy onset also impacts employment status, with an earlier age of onset correlating with work difficulties later in life (34). In patients with adult-onset epilepsy, initial seizure control or lack of control does affect work status. Newly diagnosed, unprovoked seizures in adults do not seem to negatively impact employment rates. The same study associated the development of refractory seizures in adults with reduced income (35).

Many persons with epilepsy have to deal with the reality of employment discrimination. A survey of young persons with epilepsy enrolled in a job-training program in Ireland indicated that 50% of the participants believed they were being actively discriminated against when seeking employment (36).

The Americans with Disabilities Act (ADA) was enacted in 1990 to combat job discrimination against individuals with illnesses. The law was intended to help persons with epilepsy and persons with other disabilities obtain and retain employment. A prominent feature of the ADA is that a person with a covered malady cannot be discriminated

TABLE 89.2

DRIVING AND EPILEPSY: REGULATIONS AND PRACTICES OF U.S. STATES

State	Legal Seizure-Free Restriction (mo)[a] Recommendation[c]	Rare Exceptions to SFI Considered Based on Mitigating Factors (e.g., Daytime Driving if Nocturnal Seizures Only)[b]	Required MVA Medical Review (Interval in y)	Mandatory Physician Reporting	MVA License Appeal	Physician Liab for Driving
Alabama	6	No	Annually for 5 y from last seizure	No	Yes	No
Alaska	6	No	Individual	No	Yes	Yes
Arizona	3	Nocturnal, aura, and AED revision	Individual	No	Yes	No
Arkansas	12	No	Individual	No	Yes	Yes
California	3, 6, or 12	Nocturnal, breakthrough, and AED revision	Individual	Yes	Yes	Yes
Colorado	None	No	Individual	No	Yes	No
Connecticut	3[a]	No	Individual	No	Yes	Yes
Delaware	None	No	Individual	Yes	Yes	No
District of Columbia	12	Nocturnal, AED revision, and solitary seizure	1 (until seizure-free for 5 y)	No	Yes	Yes
Florida	24[a]	Nocturnal (must supply EEG)	Individual	No	Yes	No
Georgia	6	First seizure and nocturnal	Individual	No	Yes	No
Hawaii	None	No	Individual	No	Yes	Yes
Idaho	None	MD recommendation	1 (or semiannually)	No	Yes	No
Illinois	None	No	Individual	No	Yes	No
Indiana	None	No	Individual	No	Yes	Yes
Iowa	6	Nocturnal	6 mo, then at every renewal	No	Yes	No
Kansas	6	Nocturnal and solitary seizure	1 (until 3 y seizure-free)	No	Yes	No
Kentucky	3	No	1	No	Yes	No
Louisiana	6	AED revision	Individual	No	No	No
Maine	3[a]	Seizure "breakthrough"	Individual	No	Yes	No
Maryland	3	AED revision	Individual	No	Yes	No
Massachusetts	6[a]	MAB recommendation	Individual	No	Yes	Yes
Michigan	6	AED revision	Individual	No	Yes	Yes
Minnesota	6	Acute illness, AED revision, and first seizure	Every 6 mo (until 1 y seizure-free)	No	Yes	No
Mississippi	12	No	Individual	No	No	No
Missouri	6	MD recommendation	Individual	No	No	No
Montana	None	No	No (MVA may require)	No	Yes	No
Nebraska	3	No	No	No	Yes	Yes
Nevada	3	MD recommendation	1 (for 3 y)	Yes	Yes	Yes
New Hampshire	12[a]	MD recommendation	No	No	Yes	Yes
New Jersey	12	Neurologic MAB recommendation	Every 6 mo for 2 y	Yes	Yes	Yes
New Mexico	12[a]	Nocturnal	Individual	No	Yes	No
New York	12[a]	AED revisions or MD recommendation	Individual	No	Yes	No
North Carolina	6–12	Nocturnal, auras, and AED revision	1	No	Yes	No
North Dakota	6[a]	No	1 (at least 3 y)	No	Yes	No
Ohio	None	No	6 and 12 mo, then annually	No	Yes	No
Oklahoma	12	Nocturnal	MVA determines	No	Yes	No
Oregon	6[a]	Nocturnal, auras, AED revision, and acute illness	Individual	Yes	Yes	Yes

TABLE 89.2
(continued)

State	Legal Seizure-Free Restriction (mo)[a] Recommendation[c]	Rare Exceptions to SFI Considered Based on Mitigating Factors (e.g., Daytime Driving if Nocturnal Seizures Only)[b]	Required MVA Medical Review (Interval in y)	Mandatory Physician Reporting	MVA License Appeal	Physician Liab for Driving
Pennsylvania	6	Nocturnal, auras, AED revision, and acute illness	Individual	Yes	Yes	No
Rhode Island	None	MAB recommendation	Yes	No	Yes	No
South Carolina	6	No	6 mo, then 3 y annually	No	Yes	No
South Dakota	12[a]	No	Every 6 mo (until seizure-free)	No	Yes	Yes
Tennessee	6	No	At discretion of MAB	No	Yes	Yes
Texas	6	AED revision	1	No	Yes	No
Utah	3[a]	Yes	6 mo (until seizure-free 1 y)	No	Yes	No
Vermont	None	No	Individual	Yes	Yes	Yes
Virginia	6	Nocturnal, aura, AED revision, and acute illness	Individual	No	Yes	No
Washington	6	MD recommendation	Individual	No	Yes	Yes
West Virginia	12	Nocturnal, aura, AED revision, and acute illness	Individual	No	Yes	No
Wisconsin	3	No	6 mo for 2 y	No	Yes	No
Wyoming	3	Nocturnal	1	No	Yes	Yes

Abbreviations: AED, antiepileptic drug; EEG, electroencephalogram; MAB, medical advisory board; MVA, motor vehicle administration; SFI, seizure-free interval.
[a]Seizure-free restriction frequently adjusted by MVA, MAB, and treating physicians.
[b]Mitigating factors considered in permitting some patients to drive despite less-than-minimum seizure-free period include auras, nocturnal seizures only, seizure breakthrough during physician-directed AED change, and solitary or first seizure.
[c]No = physicians legally immune or indemnified; yes = physician possibly liable for driving recommendation.
From Krauss GL, Ampaw L, Krumholz A. Individual state driving restrictions for people with epilepsy in the U.S. *Neurology* 2001;57:1780–1785, with permission.

against if "reasonable accommodations" can be made that would allow the covered individual to obtain or remain in a specific job. But the ADA exempts employers with 15 or fewer employees, thereby eliminating many small businesses. Furthermore, what constitutes a reasonable accommodation was left open to interpretation. The standard may be based on the actual cost of any modifications required that allow a person to keep a specific job. Finally, the employee must be able to perform the "essential" tasks of the job. Administrative and court rulings have made it clear that the protection sought has not been achieved (37). In a unanimous U.S. Supreme Court opinion, Justice O'Connor wrote that for an individual to be considered disabled, the person's disability must be "permanent or long-term," and the impairment must "prevent or severely restrict the individual from doing activities that are of central importance to most people's daily lives" (38). The following

statement summarizes the court's opinion: "Merely having an impairment does not make one disabled for the purposes of the ADA." This ruling and others like it have changed the thinking on what defines disability for many patients. Determinations about disability are fraught with complexities and should be considered on a case-by-case basis, taking into account the unique facts involved. Individual cases may require specialized legal advice.

Certain jobs may be perfectly safe for many persons with epilepsy but other jobs may impose unacceptable risk. A person with epilepsy must carefully evaluate jobs involving dangerous machinery, or equipment heights, or situations in which there is a possibility for injury or death because of potentially dangerous conditions in the event of a seizure. Persons with epilepsy also face regulatory-imposed restrictions for some jobs. For example, a person with epilepsy's pursuit of a commercial pilot's license is severely

TABLE 89.3

SUMMARY OF DRIVING REGULATIONS IN STATES WITH FLEXIBLE DRIVING RESTRICTIONS FOR PATIENTS WITH EPILEPSY

State	Flexible Driving Restrictions
California	6 mo seizure-free; 3 mo if seizure during physician-directed AED reduction or previously seizure-free 6 mo; 12 mo if repetitive seizure (several in 1–2 mo) after 6–12 mo seizure-free period
Colorado	Treating physician determines restriction; 2-y restriction if not under medical care
Connecticut	Minimum 3-mo seizure-free period, with restriction determined by MAB and treating physician; 6 mo without recommendation
Delaware	Treating physician determines restriction; must have been under physician's care for 3 mo
Florida	MAB usually shortens seizure-free period from 24 mo to 6 mo if under adequate medical treatment
Hawaii	MAB determines, usually 6 mo seizure-free; treating physician indicates stable prognosis
Idaho	Treating physician recommends restriction
Illinois	MAB determines, treating physician certifies patient is safe to drive; usually requires 6 mo seizure-free
Indiana	Treating physician determines restriction; 12-mo seizure-free restriction without physician recommendation
Maine	Functional ability profile: driving generally permitted if >3 mo seizure-free or 2 y seizure-free and off AED >3 mo
Massachusetts	6 mo seizure-free; MAB may reduce interval if recommended by treating physician; MAB may increase seizure-free restriction
Montana	Treating physician recommends restriction; must attest that condition is stable and would not interfere with safe driving
New Hampshire	12-mo seizure-free restriction; MVA frequently shortens interval on recommendation of treating physician
New Mexico	12 mo seizure-free; MAB frequently shortens to 6 mo
New York	12 mo seizure-free; MVA frequently shortens to 6 mo based on recommendation of treating physician
North Carolina	6–12 mo seizure-free; determined by medical advisor
North Dakota	6 mo seizure-free; temporary license for commuting to work or school frequently authorized by MAB if >3 mo seizure-free with recommendation from treating physician
Ohio	Treating physician recommends restriction
Oregon	6-mo seizure-free period usual; shorter intervals considered on recommendation of treating physician
Rhode Island	MAB determines restriction
South Dakota	12 mo seizure-free; MAB may issue temporary license earlier with 6-mo reviews if physician verifies patient's statement that seizures are under control.
Utah	Functional profile and treating physician recommendation (commonly 3 mo seizure-free); may recommend limited driving (<40 mph, local roads, daytime only)
Vermont	MAB determines restriction, usually 6 mo seizure-free

Abbreviations: AED, antiepileptic drug; MAB, medical advisory board; MVA, motor vehicle administration; mph, miles per hour.
From Krauss FL, Ampaw L, Krumholz A. Individual state driving restrictions for people with epilepsy in the US. *Neurology* 2001;57:1780–1785, with permission.

limited by the Federal Aviation Administration (FAA) (39). Similarly, a person with epilepsy wishing to obtain a commercial driver's license (CDL) to operate a truck in interstate commerce must overcome significant hurdles imposed by the federal Department of Transportation. The diagnosis of epilepsy and the use of antiepileptic drugs (AEDs) generally disqualify an applicant or current driver from obtaining a CDL. A CDL is required to operate a truck with a gross weight greater than 24,000 pounds. Although many states have mirrored the federal regulations with regard to state commercial driving laws, individual state regulations should be reviewed for accuracy. Commercial and military scuba diving is similarly restricted for the person with epilepsy (38). Tailoring the specific job to the person with

TABLE 89.4

FACTORS REQUIRED FOR CONSIDERATION OF SOCIAL SECURITY ADMINISTRATION DISABILITY BENEFITS

- Four partial seizures per month
- One major motor seizure per month
- Continued seizures despite adequate use of medication for 3 months
- Electroencephalograph results
- Detailed description of the events documented in the medical record

epilepsy, based on the person's unique, individual situation, should be emphasized.

Under Social Security Administration (SSA) regulations, epilepsy is covered by specific listings (40). These listings, which define what constitutes a disability for the person with epilepsy, are used in determining who is eligible to receive disability payments. Persons with epilepsy are required to provide specific evidence, through medical records documenting that they "meet the listing," as featured in Table 89.4. Other factors, such as postictal effects of seizures and side effects of prescribed medications, may be considered in determining disability, especially during a hearing or an appeals process for a denied claim. The specific listings for epilepsy are sections 11.03 and 11.02 for minor motor and major motor seizures, respectively (40). The diagnosis of pseudoseizure or nonepileptic seizure (NES) may also be covered by SSA regulations under section 12.07. This listing is in the psychiatry section of the code that covers conversion disorder/somatoform disorders. Although NES is not epilepsy, many of the patients evaluated in epilepsy centers around the country are ultimately diagnosed with this condition, which can be as debilitating as epilepsy.

SPORTS AND RECREATIONAL ACTIVITIES

Persons with epilepsy are often excluded or discouraged from participation in sports and recreational activities because of fear of what might occur during the activity. When making decisions about participating in any activity, a person with epilepsy must consider the consequences of a seizure that may occur at any moment during that particular activity.

Epilepsy and Recreational Vehicles

Motorized vehicles can potentially cause serious injury or death even in persons without epilepsy. The unpredictability of uncontrolled seizures might pose a serious threat should a seizure occur at the wrong time. Operating motorized vehicles is associated with a prolonged danger period.

A seizure that occurs while a person is piloting a private plane is likely to have disastrous consequences. Noncommercial aviation is at least partially regulated by the FAA. A third-class pilot's license is required for all general noncommercial aviation (39). If an individual has experienced a single unprovoked seizure with no EEG abnormalities, normal brain imaging, and no additional risk factors, that person can be considered for a third-class license if he or she has not taken an AED for 4 consecutive years. Uncomplicated childhood febrile seizures may not disqualify a person from obtaining a third-class license. The FAA uses certified examiners to assist in the decision-making process for granting licenses when there is a potential medical problem. Piloting ultralight aircraft, hang gliders, and other small aircraft may not require a license, but these are unlikely to be any safer than a private plane should a mishap occur.

Other motorized vehicles, such as motorcycles, personal watercraft, all terrian vehicle (4 wheel) and boats may pose less of a threat to a person with epilepsy than does flying. If the person with epilepsy operating the vehicle has a prolonged and consistent aura, it may allow that person the opportunity to stop and protect himself or herself. However, other factors should be considered by a person with epilepsy when contemplating engaging in some of these activities. For example, drowning is a common accident among persons with epilepsy (41). The use of a personal flotation device at all times when operating or riding in any watercraft should be considered. When operating off-road vehicles, safety equipment should also be considered, especially the use of boots, shoulder pads, protective clothing, and helmets. Although a person operating such a vehicle does not require a license, specific training courses are available and are highly recommended.

In contrast, organized motor sports generally require some form of medical clearance before participation (38). The different motor sport sanctioning bodies, such as the Sports Car Club of America (SCCA), the National Association of Stock Car Racers, and the IndyCar Series all have specific requirements for a person to be allowed to drive in sanctioned events. Each series requires approval from a qualified health care professional before driving, and therefore specific rules should be reviewed.

The Person with Epilepsy and Athletics

The decision to participate in individual (i.e., one-on-one) and team sports should follow those principles outlined above in order to ensure maximum benefits (and thus satisfaction) and safety. The extent to which a person with epilepsy wishes to pursue athletics is an individual decision that should be based on individual circumstances. Each team or individual sport presents different challenges that may affect a person with epilepsy in different ways. Many one-on-one sports are less likely to pose a threat to a person with epilepsy. For example, the potential injury a person with epilepsy might sustain during golf, tennis, or running track is likely to be low, whereas a seizure sustained during boxing, hang gliding, ski flying, or waterskiing would pose a much higher risk. Table 89.5 classifies risks to the person with epilepsy according to the sport.

Participation in team sports should also be determined on an individual basis. Football could be dangerous if a player is unable to protect him- or herself during a play, whereas basketball is less likely to be dangerous. Noncommercial scuba diving is also not regulated from a medical standpoint, but good judgment is required on the part of the participant. Hyperventilation techniques and the high concentration of inspired oxygen used during scuba diving have the potential to provoke seizures. The person with epilepsy should also inform his or her dive buddy, instructor, and dive master of the potential risk should a seizure occur during diving. Water sports and drowning pose a likely threat to the person with epilepsy. A review of drowning deaths found that 40% of seizure-related drownings occurred during recreational activities (41). Among persons with epilepsy, 83% of deaths during drowning occurred in those with subtherapeutic levels of AEDs, with the remainder of such drownings occurring where bathing was unsupervised. A study by Gotze found

no increase in seizure occurrence during strenuous swimming (42).

Exercise-provoked seizures are a controversial issue. The available data on such seizures is limited, suggesting that sports participation does not provoke seizure recurrence (43) and in some cases may even reduce seizure occurrence (44). Recent opinion has encouraged sports participation for the person with epilepsy despite the potential risks (45). The decision regarding person with epilepsy participation in sporting activities must be made on an individual basis.

Often overlooked are the possible AED-associated side effects that may interfere with participation in sports. For example, zonisamide reduces sweating in children and could potentially lead to heat-related injury in hot climates. Tremor associated with the use of valproic acid could be dangerous when shooting target pistols. And phenytoin-induced ataxia could potentially be deadly while riding a motorbike (46). Individualizing the specific drug side-effect profile, patient characteristics, and particular recreational activity generally should all be considered when advising the person with epilepsy about participation in recreational and sporting activities.

CONCLUSIONS

The patient with epilepsy poses many challenges to the health care professional. In addition to the usual concerns persons with epilepsy have about seizure control and medication effects, social issues play an important role in their everyday lives. An understanding of the unique difficulties with respect to driving, employment, and recreational/sporting activities that confront the person with epilepsy can be used to improve the QOL of many of these patients. It must be emphasized that each patient has individual characteristics requiring knowledge of the specific activity in which the person with epilepsy wishes to participate.

TABLE 89.5

SPORTING ACTIVITIES CLASSIFIED ACCORDING TO POSSIBLE RISK FOR THE PERSON WITH EPILEPSY

Low risk
  Track
  Cross-country skiing
  Golf
  Bowling
  Ping-Pong
  Baseball
  Weight training (machines)
Moderate risk
  Football
  Biking
  Soccer
  Gymnastics
  Horseback riding
  Basketball
  Boating/sailing
High risk
  Scuba diving
  Hang gliding
  Motor sports
  Boxing
  Downhill skiing/ski flying
  Long-distance swimming
  Hockey
  Boxing

Modified from Mesad SM, Devinsky O. Epilepsy and the athlete. In: Jordan BD, Tsairis P, Warren PF, eds. *Sport neurology*, 2nd ed. Philadelphia: Lippincott-Raven Publishers, 1998, p. 285 with permission.

REFERENCES

1. Gilliam F, Kuzniecky R, Faught E, et al. Patient-validated content of epilepsy-specific quality-of-life measurement. *Epilepsia* 1997;38: 233–236.
2. Fisher RS, Vickrey BG, Gibson P, et al. The impact of epilepsy from the patient's perspective I. Descriptions and subjective perceptions. *Epilepsy Res* 2000;41:39–51.
3. Hauser WA, Hesdorffer DC, eds. *Epilepsy: frequency, causes, and consequences.* New York: Demos, 1990.
4. Camfield PR, Camfield CS, Dooley JM, et al. Epilepsy after a first unprovoked seizure in childhood. *Neurology* 1985;35:1657–1660.
5. Hauser WA, Anderson VE, Loewenson RB, McRoberts SM. Seizure recurrence after a first unprovoked seizure. *N Engl J Med* 1982; 307:522–528.
6. Annegers JF, Shirts SB, Hauser WA, et al. Risk of recurrence after an initial unprovoked seizure. *Epilepsia* 1986;27:43–50.
7. Hopkins A, Garman A, Clarke C. The first seizure in adult life: value of clinical features, electroencephalography, and computerised tomographic scanning in prediction of seizure recurrence. *Lancet* 1988;1:721–726.

8. Annegers JF, Grabow JD, Groover RV, et al. Seizures after head trauma: a population study. *Neurology* 1980;30(7 Pt 1):683–689.
9. Elwes RD, Johnson AL, Shorvon SD, et al. The prognosis for seizure control in newly diagnosed epilepsy. *N Engl J Med* 1984;311:944–947.
10. Sander JWAS, Shorvon SD. Remission periods in epilepsy and their relations to long-term prognosis. In: Wolf P, Dam M, Janz D, et al., eds. *Advances in epileptology: XVIth Epilepsy International Symposium.* New York: Raven Press, 1987:353–356.
11. Fisher RS, Parsonage M, Beaussart, M. Epilepsy and driving: an international perspective. Joint Commission on Drivers' Licensing of the International Bureau for Epilepsy and the International League Against Epilepsy. *Epilepsia* 1994;35:675–684.
12. National Highway Traffic Safety Administration, National Center for Statistics and Analysis. Available at: http://www-nrd.nhtsa.dot.gov/pdf/nrd-30/NCSA/Rpts/2003/2002EARelease.pdf. Last accessed on June 28, 2003.
13. van der Lugt PJ. Is an application form useful to select patients with epilepsy who may drive? *Epilepsia* 1975;16:743–746.
14. Berg AT, Vickrey BG, Sperling MR, et al. Driving in adults with refractory localization-related epilepsy. *Neurology* 2000;54:625–630.
15. Millengen KS. Epilepsy and driving. *Proc Aust Assoc Neurol* 1976;13:67–72.
16. Drazkowski JF, Fisher RS, Sirven JI, et al. Seizure-related motor vehicle crashes in Arizona before and after reducing the driving restriction from 12 to 3 months. *Mayo Clin Proc* 2003;78:819–825.
17. *Arizona motor vehicle crash facts 1997.* Available at: http://www.dot.state.az.us/roads/crash/index.htm. Last accessed on March 24, 2003.
18. Krauss GL, Krumholz A, Carter RC, et al. Risk factors for seizure-related motor vehicle crashes in patients with epilepsy. *Neurology* 1999;52:1324–1329.
19. Salinsky MC, Wegener K, Sinnema F. Epilepsy, driving laws, and patient disclosure to physicians. *Epilepsia* 1992;33:469–472.
20. Taylor J, Chadwick DW, Johnson T. Accident experience and notification rates in people with recent seizures, epilepsy or undiagnosed episodes of loss of consciousness. *QJM* 1995;88:730–740.
21. Consensus conference on driver licensing and epilepsy: American Academy of Neurology, American Epilepsy Society, and Epilepsy Foundation of America. Washington, DC, May 31–June 2, 1991. Proceedings. *Epilepsia* 1994;35:662–705.
22. Krauss GL, Ampaw L, Krumholz A. Individual state driving restrictions for people with epilepsy in the US. *Neurology* 2001;57:1780–1785.
23. Epilepsy Foundation of America website: www.efa.org. Last accessed on June 20, 2003.
24. Krumholz A. To drive or not to drive: the 3-month seizure-free interval for people with epilepsy [editorial]. *Mayo Clin Proc* 2003;78:817–818.
25. Ooi WW, Gutrecht JA. International regulations for automobile driving and epilepsy. *J Travel Med* 2000;7:1–4.
26. Taylor J, Chadwick DW, Johnson T. Accident experience and notification rates in people with recent seizures, epilepsy or undiagnosed episodes of loss of consciousness. *QJM* 1995;88:733–740.
27. Long L, Reeves AL, Moore JL, et al. An assessment of epilepsy patients' knowledge of their disorder. *Epilepsia* 2000;41:727–731.
28. Rodrigues KM, Callanan MA, Risinger MW, et al. *Should physicians be responsible for reporting their patients to the DMV?* Available at: http://www.cma.org. Last accessed June 26, 2003.
29. Remillard GM, Zifkin BG, Andermann F. Epilepsy and motor vehicle driving—a symposium held in Quebec City, November 1998. *Can J Neurol Sci* 2002;29:315–325.
30. Lee W, Wolfe T, Shreeve S. Reporting epileptic drivers to licensing authorities is unnecessary and counterproductive. *Ann Emerg Med* 2002;39:656–659.
31. Begley CE, Annegers JF, Lairson DR, et al. Methodological issues in estimating the cost of epilepsy. *Epilepsy Res* 1999;33:39–55.
32. Fisher RS, Vickrey BG, Gibson P, et al. The impact of epilepsy from the patient's perspective II. Views about therapy and health care. *Epilepsy Res* 2000;41:53–61.
33. Salgado PC, Souza EA. Impact of epilepsy at work: evaluation of quality of life. *Arq Neuropsiquiatr* 2002;60:442–445.
34. Chaplin JE, Wester A, Tomson T. Factors associated with the employment problems of people with established epilepsy. *Seizure* 1998;7:299–303.
35. Lindsten H, Stenlund H, Edlund C, et al. Socioeconomic prognosis after a newly diagnosed unprovoked epileptic seizure in adults: a population-based case-control study. *Epilepsia* 2002;43:1239–1250.
36. Carroll D. Employment among young people with epilepsy. *Seizure* 1992;1:127–131.
37. Epilepsy Foundation of America. *Civil rights.* Available at: http://www.epilepsyfoundation.org/Advocacy/rights/rights.html. Last accessed on August 22, 2002.
38. Drazkowski JF. Management of the social consequences of seizures. *Mayo Clin Proc* 2003;78:641–649.
39. Federal Aviation Administration Regulations Title 14 parts 67.109, 67.09, and 67.309. Available at: http://www.faa.gov. Last accessed on June 30, 2003.
40. Social Security Administration. *Disability evaluation under social security.* Publication 64–039. Baltimore, MD: Author, 1999.
41. Ryan CA, Dowling G. Drowning deaths in people with epilepsy. *CMAJ* 1993;148:781–784.
42. Gotze W, Kubicki S, Munter M, et al. Effect of physical exercise on seizure threshold (investigated by electroencephalographic telemetry). *Dis Nerv Syst* 1967;28:664–667.
43. Committee on the Medical Aspects of Sports. *Medical evaluation of the athlete: a guide.* Chicago: American Medical Association, 1979.
44. Livingston S, Berman W. Participation of epileptic patients in sports. *JAMA* 1973;224:236–238.
45. van Linschoten R, Backx FJ, Mulder OG, et al. Epilepsy and sports. *Sports Med* 1990;10:9–19.
46. Mesad SM, Devinsky O. Epilepsy and the athlete. In: Jordan BD, Tsairis P, Warren PF, eds. *Sport neurology,* 2nd ed. Philadelphia: Lippincott-Raven Publishers, 1998.

Indications for Antiepileptic Drugs Sanctioned by the United States Food and Drug Administration

Kay C. Kyllonen

Authors in this text have described uses of antiepileptic drugs based on clinical experience and results of clinical trials. In some cases, these clinical indications are broader than those sanctioned by the U.S. Food and Drug Administration (FDA) for product labeling.

To obtain specific FDA-sanctioned indications, pharmaceutical companies present efficacy data from controlled clinical trials. If the data are judged scientifically sound, then the FDA may approve use of the drug for the specific types of patients and seizures studied in the trials. The approved indications are based only on the data presented by the pharmaceutical manufacturer and may not reflect all of the available research information. Once the indications are authorized by the FDA, the pharmaceutical manufacturers may not promote use of the drug for indications other than those specifically delineated in the labeling. However, this does not preclude the "off-label" use of these medications for other indications, including those discussed in this clinical text. By necessity, certain patient populations—most notably, children—are routinely treated outside of the labeled indications, because prior to recent FDA regulations, they were rarely included in controlled clinical trials.

Antiepileptic medications mentioned in this text are listed in the following table with their FDA-approved epilepsy-related indications from the 2004 online edition of the *DrugDex System* (1) or the 2004 online edition of *Drug Facts and Comparisons* (2), standard references for pharmacists. Some of the listed indications use archaic terminology because they were designated prior to the adoption of international standards for seizure and epilepsy classification. Some drugs not included in *DrugDex System* or *Drug Facts and Comparisons* are listed as investigational in the United States in the 2004 online *NDA Pipeline* (3) or "Facts and Comparisons Investigational Drugs" section, which lists all new drug applications filed during 2003. Others are not yet in any part of the federal approval process and have been marked as "not listed" in the table.

Only four antiepileptics had specific FDA-approved pediatric indications listed in the 1999 *Physicians' Desk Reference* (4) or *Drug Facts and Comparisons* (5). At this writing 15 medications carry specific FDA approval for pediatric indications. For many other antiepileptic drugs, pediatric use is implied in the approved product information by mentioning use in specific pediatric syndromes (e.g., infantile spasms or febrile seizures), by listing pediatric formulations (chewable tablets or elixirs), or by describing dosage schedules based on pediatric ages or body weights. The table notes whether pediatric doses are listed in the *DrugDex System* (1), *The Pediatric Dosage Handbook* (6), or *Drug Facts and Comparisons* (2), regardless of whether or not the drug carries a specific FDA-approved pediatric

Drug	Listed Indications: Seizure or Epilepsy Type	Pediatric Dose	Pediatric Labeling Indication
Acetazolamide	Centrencephalic epilepsies (petit mal, unlocalized seizures)	Yes	
ACTH	Infantile spasms	Yes	Yes (age ≥6 years)
Carbamazepine	Epilepsy—partial seizures with complex symptomatology (psychomotor, temporal lobe), generalized tonic-clonic seizures (grand mal), mixed seizures	Yes	
Clobazam	Investigational in the United States	Yes	
Clonazepam	Lennox-Gastaut syndrome (petit mal variant), akinetic and myoclonic seizures	Yes	
Diazepam	Status epilepticus, severe recurrent convulsive disorders	Yes	Yes (age >6 months)
Ethosuximide	Absence (petit mal) epilepsy	Yes	Yes
Ethotoin	Tonic-clonic (grand mal) and complex partial seizures	Yes	Yes
Felbamate	Adjunctive therapy in Lennox-Gastaut syndrome, monotherapy for partial seizures in adults with epilepsy	Yes	Yes (age >2 years)
Fosphenytoin	Short-term treatment of acute seizures, including status epilepticus; prevention of seizures during and after neurosurgery; substitute for oral phenytoin	Yes	
Gabapentin	Adjunctive treatment of partial seizures with or without generalization	Yes	Yes (age >3 years)
Lamotrigine	Adjunctive treatment of partial seizures and Lennox-Gastaut syndrome	Yes	Yes
Levetiracetam	Treatment of partial seizures and primary generalized epilepsy	Yes	Yes
Lorazepam	FDA indication for status epilepticus	Yes	
Loreclezole	Not listed	Yes	
Mephenytoin	Withdrawn from market		
Mephobarbital	Grand mal and petit mal epilepsy	Yes	Yes
Metharbital	Not listed		
Methsuximide	Absence seizures refractory to other drugs	Yes	
Midazolam	No FDA indication for seizure disorders		
Nitrazepam	Investigational in the United States		
Oxcarbamazepine	Partial seizures	Yes	Yes (age ≥4 years)
Paraldehyde	Withdrawn from human use		
Paramethadione	Withdrawn from market	Yes	
Phenacemide	Severe epilepsy, mixed forms of complex partial (psychomotor) seizures refractory to other drugs	Yes	
Phenobarbital	Generalized and partial seizures, febrile seizures	Yes	Yes
Phenytoin	Generalized tonic-clonic (grand mal) and complex partial (psychomotor, temporal lobe) seizures, prevention and treatment of seizures occurring during or following neurosurgery	Yes	Yes
Primidone	Grand mal, psychomotor, and focal epileptic seizures	Yes	Yes (age >8 years)
Pyridoxine	Pyridoxine-dependent seizures	Yes	
Remacemide	Investigational in the United States		
Stiripentol	Adjunctive therapy for partial and generalized epilepsy, investigational in the United States		
Tiagabine	Adjunctive therapy for partial seizures	Yes	Yes (age ≥12 years)
Topiramate	Adjunctive therapy for partial seizures	Yes	Yes (age >2 years)
Trimethadione	Absence seizures refractory to other medications	Yes	
Valproate	Simple and complex absence seizures, adjunctive therapy in multiple seizure types, including absence and complex partial seizures	Yes	
Vigabatrin	Adjunctive therapy for complex partial seizures, investigational in the United States		
Zonisamide	Adjunctive therapy for partial seizures	Yes	

Abbreviations: ACTH, adrenocorticotropic hormone (corticotropin); FDA, U.S. Food and Drug Administration.

indication. Dosing schedules are further discussed in "Part IV: Antiepileptic Medications" of this textbook; however, it is advisable to consult full prescribing information before clinical use.

REFERENCES

1. Klasco RK, ed. *DrugDex System*. Greenwood Village, CO: Thomson MICROMEDEX, edition expires June 2004.

2. CNS agents: anticonvulsants, and investigational drugs. In: *Drug Facts and Comparisons*, eFacts [database online], 2004. Available from Wolters Kluwer Health, Inc. Last accessed May 20, 2004.

3. Silverman B, Goodfellow B, Frederick C, et al., eds. NDA PIPELINE [database online]. FDC Reports. Available at: http://www.ndapipeline.com. Last accessed May 20, 2004.

4. Arky R (consultant). *Physicians' desk reference*, 53rd ed. Montvale, NJ: Medical Economics, 1999.

5. Olin BR, Hagemann RC, eds. *Drug facts and comparisons, 1999*. June update. St. Louis: Facts and Comparisons, 1999.

6. Taketomo CK, Hodding JH, Kraus DM, eds. *The pediatric dosage handbook*, 10th ed. Hudson, OH: Lexicomp, 2003.

Index

Page numbers followed by f indicate a figure; t following a page number indicates tabular material.

A

A current, 77
ABCB1, 751–752, 752f
ABCB1 C3435T polymorphism, 755
ABCC1, 751–752, 752f
ABCC2, 751–752, 752f
Abdominal auras, 230t, 232t, 233t, 235
Abdominal pain, recurrent, in children, 637
Absence epilepsy
  childhood, 359, 396–399
    clinical features of, 397
    EEG findings in, 397
      absence seizure, 192f
      absence status epilepticus, 193f
    epidemiology of, 396–397
    etiology and genetics of, 397–398
    history of, 396
    outcome and prognosis in, 398–399
    seizure semiology in, 397
    topiramate for, 881
    treatment of, 398
  eyelid myoclonia with/without, 416
  juvenile, 359, 399–400
  myoclonic, 393
  myoclonic or clonic, 393, 414–415
Absence seizures, 305–312. *See also*
      Generalized epilepsies;
      Generalized seizures
  with atonic components, 227
  atypical, 317–319, 318f
    in Lennox-Gastaut syndrome, 430
  with automatisms, 227
  causes of, 310
  cerebral blood flow and metabolism in,
      312
  clinical features of, 305–306
    with atypical absences, 306
    with myoclonic absence, 306
    photosensitivity in, 306
    with typical absences, 305–306
  definition of, 227
  diagnosis of, 309–310
  EEG features of, 307–309
    in atypical absences
      ictal discharges, 308, 308f
      interictal, 308
    in childhood, 192f
    delta activity in, generalized
      rhythmic, 308
    low-voltage fast rhythms in, 308
    mixed patterns in, 309, 309f
    in typical absences
      ictal discharges, 307, 307f
      interictal, 307–308, 310f

functional MRI of, 312
genetics and acquired factors in,
      310–311, 311f
with impairment of consciousness only,
      227
with mild clonic components, 227
neurochemistry of, 312
pathogenesis of, 310–312, 311f
with tonic components, 227
Absence status epilepticus, childhood,
      EEG of, 193f
Absorption, of antiepileptic drugs,
      655–657. *See also specific drugs*
  bioavailability in, 655–656, 656t
  rate of, 656–657, 657f
Accuracy, diagnostic, 112
Acetazolamide, 949f, 953–954
  for catamenial-associated seizures, 698
  indications for, 1212t
Acetylcholine receptors, 95, 106
N-Acetylcysteine, for progressive
      myoclonic epilepsies, 422
N-Acetylglutamate synthetase deficiency,
      550
Acidemia, neonatal seizures from
  arginosuccinic, 500
  methylmalonic, 551
  propionic, 551
Aciduria
  γ-hydroxybutyric, 556
  isovaleric, 550–551
  neonatal seizures from, 550–551
  organic, 550–551, 555
Acquired factors, in absence seizures,
      310–311, 311f
Acquired immunodeficiency syndrome
      (AIDS), 114, 576–577
ACTH. *See* Adrenocorticotropic hormone
      (ACTH)
Action potential, 73, 73f, 127–129, 128f
  calcium, 92
  sodium, 92
Activation paralysis, in focal seizures, 245
Activation procedures, 625
Active control, 650
Acycloenzyme A oxidase deficiency,
      549–550
Adenosine, 95
Adenosine receptors, 95
Adrenal disorders, 573
Adrenal insufficiency, 573
Adrenocorticotropic hormone (ACTH),
      931–936
  historical background on, 931

indications for, 1212t
for infantile spasms, 931–934, 933t
  adverse effects of, 933–934
  brain-adrenal axis in, 932
  efficacy and dosing of, 932–933, 933t
  mechanism of action of, 932
  recommended protocols for, 934,
      935t
  vs. vigabatrin, 934
for Landau-Kleffner syndrome and
      related disorders, 936
for Lennox-Gastaut syndrome, 437,
      934–936
for Ohtahara syndrome, 934–936
for other myoclonic disorders, 935–936
Adrenocorticotropin. *See*
      Adrenocorticotropic hormone
      (ACTH)
Adrenoleukodystrophy
  neonatal seizures from, 549
  X-linked, 558
Adverse effects, of antiepileptic drugs,
      688–690, 689t. *See also specific
      drugs*
  barbiturates, neonatal, 507
  carbamazepine, 739, 764–765
  in drug approval process, 735–736
  ethosuximide, 739
  felbamate, 740
  fosphenytoin, 797
  gabapentin, 740
  lamotrigine, 740, 741t
  monitoring for, 735–743 (*See also
      specific agents*)
    at-risk profiles in, 737–738, 738t
    clinical, 738–739, 739t
    drug approval process and, 735–736
    effectiveness of, 735
    idiosyncratic reactions in, 737, 737t
    legal and medical disclaimer on, 743
    malpractice/negligence cases on,
        736–737, 736t
    screening tests in, 739, 739t
    standards of care in, 736
  oxcarbazepine, 740, 767–768
  phenobarbital, 507, 740–741
  phenytoin, 741, 795–797
  screening tests for, 739, 739t
  tiagabine, 741
  topiramate, 741
  valproate (valproic acid), 741–742,
      778–779
  vigabatrin, 742
  zonisamide, 742

Affective symptomatology, 225–226
  benign partial epilepsy with, 386
Afferents, motor cortex, 259
Age, 112–113
  on recurrence risk, 685
Agenesis, of corpus callosum, 30
Aggression, 1199
Agyria, 4f
Agyria-pachygyria. See Lissencephaly
Aicardi syndrome, 361
AIDS
  CNS infections in, 576–577
  epilepsy in, 114
Akinetic seizures. See Atonic seizures
Albumin, age on, 672f
Alcohol abuse, 984
Alcohol withdrawal, 576
Alpers disease, 557–558
Alternating hemiplegia, of childhood, 634
Aluminum hydroxide model, 99
Alveus, 57, 60f, 61f
Amino acid disorders, 555–556
Ammon horn (cornu ammonis), 56, 57,
    58f, 60f, 62f
Amnesia, 242
  in focal seizures, 242
  transient global, vs. epilepsy, 640
Amobarbital procedure, intracarotid,
    1031–1038, 1076. See also
    Intracarotid amobarbital
    procedure
AMPA glutamate receptors, 92–94, 93f
Amphetamines, 579–580
  neonatal seizures from, 501
Amplifiers, differential, in localization
    with EEG, 146, 146f
Amplitude measurement, in electrical
    fields, 147
Amygdala, 55
Amygdalo-hippocampal seizures, 355
Analgesics, 578t, 579
Analysis of results, 651–652
Anatomic hemispherectomy, 1118–1119
Anesthetics, 578t
  general, 578t, 579
  inhalational
    halogenated, 580
    for refractory status epilepticus, 615
  local, 578t
Angelman syndrome, 417, 418f, 481–482,
    481f
  antiepileptic drugs for seizures in,
    422–423, 423f
  vs. Lennox-Gastaut syndrome, 436
Angioglioma, 9f
Angioma, cavernous, 8f
  MRI of, 1014, 1016f
Animal models, of epilepsy, 98–99
Anoxia
  adult, 575–576
  perinatal, 575
Anterior frontopolar epilepsy, 368
Anterior frontopolar seizures, 355
Anterolateral dorsal convexity seizures, in
    focal seizures, 243
Antibiotics, 578t, 579
Antidepressants, 570, 578t

Antiepileptic drug–metabolizing enzymes,
    747–748
  genes for, 748–751, 748f, 749t (See also
      under Pharmacogenetics, of
      antiepileptic drugs)
    CYP (cytochrome P450), 748–750,
      748f, 749t
    CYP2C9, 749
    CYP2C19, 749
    CYP3A4 and CYP3A5, 750
    EPHX1, 750
    UGT1 and UGT2, 750–751
Antiepileptic drugs (AEDs), 948, 948t. See
    also specific drugs
  absorption of, 655–657
    bioavailability in, 655–656, 656t
    rate of, 656–657, 657f
  adverse effects of, 688–690, 689t (See
      also under Adverse effects, of
      antiepileptic drugs; specific drugs)
    monitoring for, 735–743
  age-specific dosing of, 676–677, 677t
  analysis of results in, 651–652
  on bone health, 700
  in breast milk, 708–709
  clearance of, 659–661, 660f
    in hepatic disease, 721–722, 721t, 722t
    in renal disease, 719–721, 720t
  cognitive effects of, 1186–1189
    at age extremes, 1189
    historical perspective on, 1186
    methodological issues in, 1186–1187
    in newer AEDs, 1187–1189
    in older AEDs, 1187
  continuation of, risk of, 688–690, 689t
  discontinuation of
    counseling families on, 690
    medication taper in, 687
    after resective surgery, 687–688
    risk of, 688
    in seizure free, 684–685, 687
    after surgery, 1178–1179
  drug interactions of, non-AED, 665,
    666t–669t
  efficacy and safety trials on, 648–649
  in elderly, 593–601 (See also specific drugs)
    choice of, 594–595
    clinical pharmacology of, 594, 595t
    comedications with, 594, 595t
  elimination of, 658–659, 658f
    in hepatic disease, 721–722, 721t, 722t
    in renal disease, 719–721, 720t
  experimental trial design for, 649–651,
    649f
    as adjunctive therapy vs.
      monotherapy, 650–651
    blinding in, 649
    control groups in, 649–650
    parallel vs. crossover design in, 649f,
      650
  for febrile seizures, 516–517
  on fertility, 700
  for generalized tonic-clonic seizures,
    296–297
  in hepatic disease, 721–722, 721t, 722t
    (See also specific drugs)
  human testing of, 647–648

  with immunosuppressive therapy,
    730–731
  indications for, 1211–1213, 1212t
  infants born to mothers on, 709
  initiation of
    in adults, 691
    in children, 690–691
    counseling families on, 690
    risk of, 688–690, 689t
  interactions among
    pharmacodynamic, 663–664, 663t
    pharmacokinetic, 661–663, 661f, 662t
  length of treatment with, 687
  for Lennox-Gastaut syndrome, 436
  less commonly used, 947–957
    acetazolamide, 949f, 953–954
    background on, 947
    barbiturates, 949f, 951–953 (See also
      Barbiturates; specific agents)
    bromides, 956
    ethotoin, 947–949, 949f
    methsuximide, 655–663, 656t,
      949–951, 949f
    pyridoxine, 954–956
  for multiple handicaps, epilepsy with,
    589–591, 590f
  myoclonic seizures from, 422
  for neonatal seizures, 504–507, 506f
    potential deleterious CNS effects of,
      507
  newer, 939–944 (See also specific agents)
    carabersat, 940, 940t
    chemistry and mechanism of action
      of, 939, 940t
    fluorofelbamate, 940t, 941
    future directions in, 943–944
    for generalized tonic-clonic seizures,
      298–300
    harkoseride, 940t, 941
    pharmacokinetics of, 939, 940t
    retigabine, 940t, 941–942
    rufinamide, 940t, 942
    safinamide, 940t, 942
    talampanel, 940t, 942–943
    UCB 34714, 943
    valproate derivatives, 940t, 943
  not treating with, risk of, 688
  on oral contraceptive efficacy, 705–706
  osteopenia from, 700
  PET and, 1046 (See also Positron
    emission tomography (PET))
  pharmacogenetics of, 747–756 (See also
    Pharmacogenetics, of
    antiepileptic drugs)
  pharmacokinetics of, 647, 655–663,
    656t (See also Pharmacokinetics,
    of antiepileptic drugs)
  in pregnancy, 707–709, 708t
  on plasma concentrations of other
    drugs, 667t–669t
  for poststroke patients with seizures,
    530
  for posttraumatic epilepsy, 523–524
  preclinical development of, 645–647
    drug discovery in, 645
    mechanism of action in,
      differentiating, 646

primary screening models in, 646
tolerance and pharmacokinetics of, 647, 833
toxicity of, 647
in pregnancy, 705–714 (*See also* Pregnancy)
neonatal outcome with, 709–711, 710t
for Rasmussen encephalitis, 449
recurrence risk and
factors in, 685–686
after first unprovoked seizure, 681–683
after two seizures, 683
relapse and, prognosis after, 687
in renal disease, 719–721, 720t (*See also specific drugs*)
on sexual function, 699–700
teratogenicity of, 711–712
in utero, neurodevelopmental effects of, 1189–1191
animal studies of, 1189
human studies of, 1189–1190
possible mechanisms of, 1190–1191
withdrawal of, 691–692
Antiestrogen, for catamenial-associated seizures, 698
Antineoplastic agents, 578t, 580
Antipsychotics, 578t, 579
Anxiety, 1198
Aphasia, acquired epileptic, 361
Aplastic anemia, from felbamate, 917
Apnea, infant, 634
Apoptosis, 15–16
Apoptosis disorders, 24, 24f
Apparent life-threatening events, in infants, 634
Area under the curve (AUC), 655–656, 660, 660f
Arginase deficiency, 550, 556
Arginine:glycine aminotransferase deficiency, 554
Argininosuccinate lysase deficiency, 550
Argininosuccinate synthetase deficiency, 550
Arginosuccinic acidemia, 500
Aristaless-related homeobox (ARX) gene mutations, 503
Arterial spin labeling (ASL) perfusion magnetic resonance imaging, 1013
Artifacts, EEG, 155, 157f, 158f
ARX gene mutation, 503
Ascertainment bias, 111–112
Aspiration pneumonia, from generalized tonic-clonic seizures, 287–288
Astrocytoma
foramen of Monro, 7f
giant cell, 7f
low-grade
diffuse fibrillary, 10f
MRI features and pathology of, 1089–1090
Ataxia, 84
Athletics, 1207–1208, 1208t
Atlas of epileptiform abnormalities, 183–214. *See also*

Electroencephalographic atlas of epileptiform abnormalities
Atonic components, in absence seizures, 227
Atonic seizures
atypical, 324–326, 325f
definition of, 228
in Lennox-Gastaut syndrome, 430–431
EEG of, 197f, 325f
in myoclonic epilepsies, 408, 408f
Attention deficit hyperactivity disorder, staring spells in, 636
Attenuation factor, 143
Atypical seizures, 317–327
absence, 317–319, 318f
atonic, 324–326, 325f
myoclonic, 319–321, 320f
pathophysiology of, 326
tonic, 321–324
clinical correlation of, 323–324
clinical features of, 321–322, 321f
electrophysiology of, 322–323, 322f, 323f
treatment of, 326–327
Auditory auras, 230t, 232t, 233t, 234
Auditory seizures, 225
Auras, 229–237
auditory, 230t, 232t, 233t, 234
autonomic, 237
cephalic, 230t, 232t, 233t, 235
cold shivering as, 237
combinations of, and march, 229–230
content of, 231
definition of, 226–227, 229
depression as, 236
dizziness as, 234
elation as, 236
emotional, 232t, 233t, 236
epigastric or abdominal, 230t, 232t, 233t, 235
fear as, 236
in focal seizures, 244–245
gustatory, 230t, 232t, 233t, 235
individual determinants of, 231
in localization
clinical, 231–232, 232t, 233t
EEG, 232–233
olfactory, 230t, 232t, 233t, 234–235
piloerection as, 237
pleasure as, 236
premonitions in, 229
presence and absence of, 230–231, 230t
in prodromes, 229
psychic, 230t, 232t, 233t, 236–237, 236t
seizure with, 226–227
sexual, 237
somatosensory, 230t, 232t, 233t, 233–234, 233t
urinary urgency as, 237
vertiginous, 230t, 232t, 233t, 234
visceral (viscerosensory), 230t, 232t, 233t, 235
visual, 230t, 232t, 233t, 234
and focal clonic seizure, 206f–207f
Autism, 587–588, 588t
Automatic behavior, 245

Automatisms, 226
absence seizures with, 227
in focal seizures, 245
Automobile driving, 1202–1203, 1202t, 1204t–1206t
Automotor, 242
Autonomic auras, 237
Autonomic symptoms, 225
in focal seizures, 248
Autosomal dominant cortical reflex myoclonus and epilepsy (ADCME), 417
Average reference, in field determination, 154
Awareness, 225
Axes, in syndrome-oriented epilepsy classification, 348, 348t
Axons
callosal, 22
growth of, 17
pioneer, 21
Azathioprine, with antiepileptic drugs, 730–731

B
Balloon cells, 5f
Baltic myoclonus, 560
Band heterotopia, 28–29, 28f, 1019, 1020f. *See also* Subcortical-band (laminar) heterotopia
Barbiturates, 578t, 579, 949f, 951–953. *See also* Mephobarbital; Phenobarbital; Primidone
absorption, distribution, and metabolism of, 952
chemistry and mechanism of action of, 949f, 951–952
drug interactions and adverse effects of, 952–953
efficacy and clinical use of, 952
historical background on, 951
impotence from, 700
for Lennox-Gastaut syndrome, 436–437
for neonatal seizures, 505–507
other medications on plasma concentration of, 666t
on plasma concentrations of other drugs, 668t
Baseline shifts, EEG, 129f, 131f, 132–134, 133f, 134f
epileptic, 137, 137f
Basilar migraine, 639
Batten disease, late-onset, 559–560
Benign childhood epilepsy with centrotemporal spikes (BCECTS), 270–271, 358, 374–382
clinical manifestations of, 375–376
EEG manifestations of, 376–377, 376f–380f
epidemiology of, 374–375
genetics of, 375
historical perspective on, 374
investigations on, 380–381
neuropsychological aspects of, 377–380
pathophysiology of, 375
prognosis in, 381–382, 382f
treatment of, 381

Benign familial autosomal dominant myoclonic epilepsy (BFAME), 417

Benign familial infantile convulsion (BFIC), 328

Benign familial infantile seizures, 503

Benign familial neonatal convulsion (BFNC), 358, 503
KCNQ2/3 K+ channels and, 84, 503

Benign focal epilepsy of childhood, 270–271

Benign focal epileptiform discharges of childhood, 271
EEG of
centrotemporal sharp waves in, 198f, 271
dipole potentials in, 199f
left and right central sharp waves in, 200f
occipital sharp waves in, 200f

Benign frontal epilepsy, 386

Benign myoclonic epilepsy of infancy (BMEI), 328, 359, 409–411, 413, 479–480

Benign myoclonus of early infancy, 632–633

Benign neonatal convulsion, 358, 503

Benign neonatal myoclonus, 631
in infants, asleep, 631

Benign occipital epilepsy (BOE) of childhood, 382–385
early-onset, 382–383
EEG of, 383–384, 383f, 384f
epidemiology of, 382
genetics of, 382
investigations of, 384
late-onset, 383
neuropsychology of, 384
prognosis in, 385
treatment of, 385

Benign paroxysmal vertigo, in children, 637

Benign partial epilepsies syndromes, childhood, 373–386
benign childhood epilepsy with centrotemporal spikes (BCECTS), 374–382 (See also Benign childhood epilepsy with centrotemporal spikes (BCECTS))
benign occipital epilepsy of childhood, 382–385, 383f, 384f (See also Benign occipital epilepsy (BOE) of childhood)
general features of, 374t
proposed, not yet recognized by ILAE
benign frontal epilepsy, 386
benign partial epilepsy in infancy (BPEI), 385
benign partial epilepsy of adolescence, 385
benign partial epilepsy with affective symptoms (BPEAS), 386
benign partial epilepsy with extreme somatosensory evoked potentials (BPE-ESEP), 386

Benign partial epilepsy of adolescence, 385

Benign partial epilepsy of infancy (BPEI), 385, 479

Benign partial epilepsy with affective symptoms (BPEAS), 386

Benign partial epilepsy with extreme somatosensory evoked potentials (BPE-ESEP), 386

Benign rolandic epilepsy, 270–271

Benzodiazepines, 829–846. See also specific agents
absorption, distribution, and metabolism of, 834, 835f
adverse effects of, 837
for atypical tonic seizures, 327
for benign myoclonic epilepsy of infancy, 413
for benign occipital epilepsy of childhood, 385
chemistry and mechanism of action of, 829–834
anticonvulsant activity in, 830
efficacy in, 829–830
excitatory GABA_A currents in, 831–832
in flumazenil, 834
GABA_A receptor complex in, 830–831, 832f
GABA_A receptor molecular biology in, 832, 832f
GABA_A receptor plasticity and tolerance in, 833
GABA_A receptor subunits in, 833
peripheral benzodiazepine receptor in, 831
potency in, 829, 830t
structure in, 829, 830f
clinical pharmacology of, 836t
drug interactions of, 834–835
efficacy of, antiepileptic, 835–837
for acute seizures, 836, 836t
for long-term chronic treatment, 836–837
for status epilepticus, 835–836
in elderly, 595t, 600
for epileptic spasms, 342
for Lennox-Gastaut syndrome, 436
for multiple handicaps, epilepsy with, 589
for myoclonus in atypical seizures, 327
for myotonic-astatic epilepsy, 413
for neonatal seizures, 506
new strategies for, 846
pharmacogenetics of, 754–755
pharmacokinetics of, 657t
in infants and children, 672–673
for poststroke patients, 530
in renal and liver disease, 726
for severe myoclonic epilepsy of infants, 414
teratogenicity of, 711

Bias
ascertainment, 111–112
prevalence, 111, 111f
referral center, 112

Bicuculline-induced seizures, 99

Bilateral asymmetric tonic seizure, 268

Bioavailability, of antiepileptic drugs, 655–656, 656t. See also specific drugs

Bioelectric activity, of neuronal and glial cells, 127, 128f

Biotinidase deficiency, 500, 553

Bipolar montage
field identification with, 151–152, 151t, 152f
longitudinal, 184f
with maximum negativity at end of chain, 155, 155f
with no phase reversal, 148, 151f, 151t, 152f
with phase reversal, 151t, 152, 152f, 157, 158f
transverse, 184f

Bitemporal epilepsy, surgery for, 1078–1079

Bitemporal sharp waves, in temporal lobe epilepsy, 201f, 202f

Blast, 13

Blinding, in antiepileptic drug trials, 649

Blitz-Nick-Salaam Krämpfe, 359. See also Spasms, epileptic

Bobble-head doll syndrome, 639

Body movements, in focal seizures, 246

Body rocking, in infants, 632

Bone health, 700

Boundary problems, in electrical fields, 145–146

Bourneville disease. See Tuberous sclerosis

Brain mapping, [15O] water PET in, 1048

Brainstem motor efferents, 258

Breach rhythm, in EEG, 191f

Breast milk, antiepileptic drugs in, 708–709

Breath-holding spell, cyanotic
EEG of, 213f
in infants, 634

Bromides, 956
pharmacokinetics of, 655–659, 656t (See also Pharmacokinetics, of antiepileptic drugs)

Bronchial agents, 578t

Bundle of Probst, 30

C

CA1 neurons, 57, 60f, 63f

Ca2+-dependent potassium channels, 75f, 77–78

CA2 neurons, 57, 60f, 63f

CA3 neurons, 57, 60f, 63f

CA4 neurons, 57, 60f, 63f

CACNA1G, 752–753

CACNA1H, 752–753

CACNA1I, 752–753

Calcium action potential, 92

Calcium (Ca2+) channels, 76t, 79–81
epilepsies linked to, 105–106
P/Q-type, 84

Calcium-channel blockers, 578t, 579

Callosal axons, 22

Callosotomy, corpus, 1159–1163. See also Corpus callosotomy

Candidate genes, in antiepileptic drug pharmacogenetics, 747–753. *See also* Pharmacogenetics, of antiepileptic drugs

Carabersat, 940, 940t

Carbamazepine, 761–766
    absorption and distribution of, 761
    adverse effects of, 739, 764–765
    age-specific dosing of, 677t
    for Angelman syndrome, seizures in, 422–423, 423f
    for atypical tonic seizures, 327
    for benign childhood epilepsy with centrotemporal spikes, 381
    for benign occipital epilepsy of childhood, 385
    chemistry and mechanism of action of, 761, 762f
    clinical use of, 765–766
    drug interactions of, 763, 763t
        other medications on plasma concentration of, 666t
        plasma concentrations of other drugs with, 667t–668t
    efficacy of, 763–764
    in elderly, 595t, 596t, 598–599
    felbamate on, 915–916, 916t
    for focal epilepsies, symptomatic, 370
    for generalized tonic-clonic seizures, 297–298
    indications for, 1212t
    for juvenile absence epilepsy, 400
    for juvenile myoclonic epilepsy, 396, 422
    metabolism of, 761–762
    on myoclonic epilepsy, 422
    vs. oxcarbazepine, 769
    pharmacogenetics of, 752f, 754–755
    pharmacokinetics of, 655–659, 656t, 762t (*See also* Pharmacokinetics, of antiepileptic drugs)
        in infants and children, 673–674
        in pregnancy, 706–708, 707t
    precautions and contraindications with, 766
    in renal and liver disease, 725–726
    steady state and clearance of, 656t, 660, 660f
    teratogenicity of, 765

Carbamoyl phosphate synthetase deficiency, 500, 550

Carbohydrate metabolism disorders, 552

Carbonic anhydrase, 953

Carbonic anhydrase inhibitor. *See also* Acetazolamide
    for catamenial-associated seizures, 698
    topiramate as, 884–885

Carboxylase deficiency, multiple early onset, 552

Cardiovascular disease, 528
    epilepsy with, 527–534 (*See also* Stroke, epilepsy after)

Carnitine palmitoyltransferase I/II deficiencies, 551

Catamenial-associated seizures, 698

Cataplexy, 638–639

Cavernous angioma, 8f, 1014, 1016f

Cavernous sinus electrodes, 1064

Celiac disease, 578

Cell membrane, electrical polarity of, 17

Cellular neurophysiology, 69–85
    ion channels and intrinsic membrane properties in, 69–74
        action potential in, 73, 73f
        electrical activity in, 69–70, 70f
        general properties of ion channels in, 70–73, 70f–73f
        Hodgkin-Huxley experiments and model in, 72f–74f, 73–74
        voltage-dependent ion channels in, 74–84 (*See also* Voltage-dependent (-gated) ion channels)

Central anticholinergic syndrome, 580

Central nervous system infections, 576–577
    parasitic, 577

Central sharp waves, in benign focal epileptiform discharges of childhood, 200f

Centrotemporal distribution, in EEG, 155, 158f

Centrotemporal sharp waves, in benign focal epileptiform discharges of childhood, 198f

Cephalic auras, 230t, 232t, 233t, 235

Cephalosporins, 578t, 579

Cerebellar hypoplasia, genes in, 25t

Cerebral blood flow studies, SPECT, 1046–1047, 1047f

Cerebral cortex
    in 22-week fetus, 19, 21f
    architecture of, 18–19
    gyration in, 21–22, 25

Cerebral development, 13–23
    of cortex, 18–22 (*See also* Cortical development)
    ontogenesis in, 13–18 (*See also* Ontogenesis)
        genetic programming of, 22–23

Cerebral dysgenesis, 13, 23–32
    classification of, 31t, 32
    corpus callosum, 30
    focal cortical dysplasias, 30
    gastrulation and neurulation disorders, 23
    hemimegalencephaly, 30–32
    heterotopia
        periventricular nodular, 27–28
        subcortical laminar, 28–29, 28f
    holoprosencephaly, 23, 25t, 26–27
    lissencephaly type 1 (Miller-Dieker syndrome), 29
    mitotic proliferation and apoptosis disorders, 24, 24f
    myelination disorders, 26
    neonatal seizures from, 501–502, 503f
    neural crest separation and migration disorders, 23
    neurite growth disorders, 26
    neuroblast migration disorders, 24–26, 25t
    schizencephaly, 29–30
    segmentation disorders, 23

septooptic-pituitary dysplasia, 27
    tuberous sclerosis, 30
    X-linked hydrocephalus with pachygyria/polymicrogyria, 30

Cerebral embolism, *vs.* epilepsy, 640

Cerebral malformations. *See* Cerebral dysgenesis

Cerebral neocortex ontogeny, 19–20, 20f, 21f

Cerebral palsy, 587

Cerebrohepatorenal (Zellweger) syndrome, 26

Cerebrovascular disease
    epilepsy *vs.*, 639
    epilepsy with, 527–534 (*See also* Cardiovascular disease, epilepsy with)

Ceroid lipofuscinosis, 361
    adult, 362
    juvenile, 362
    late infantile, 361

Cesarean section, 706

Channel gating, mechanisms of, 70–73, 70f–73f

Channelopathies, 76t, 83–84

Cherry-red spot myoclonus syndrome, 362, 558–559

Childhood absence epilepsy, 359, 396–399. *See also* Absence epilepsy, childhood

Childhood epilepsy, 1143–1156. *See also* *specific disorders*
    anatomic and functional neuroimaging in, 1147–1149, 1148f
    diagnostic evaluation of, *vs.* adults, 1143, 1144t
    EEG of
        in absence epilepsy
            absence seizure, 192f
            absence status epilepticus, 193f
        in benign focal epileptiform discharges
            centrotemporal sharp waves, 199f
            dipole potentials, 199f
            left and right central sharp waves, 200f
            occipital sharp waves, 200f
        video, seizure semiology in, 1143
    etiologies and pathologic substrates in, 1145f–1147f, 1149, 1149f–1155f
    occipital, 270–271
    with occipital paroxysms, 358
    PET evaluation of, 1045–1046, 1045f, 1046f
    scalp EEG patterns, infantile spasms, and focal cortical lesions in, 1144–1147, 1145f–1147f
    severe, 1111–1112
    surgery for, 1149–1156
        age-related risks in, 1150f–1154f, 1154–1155
        goals of, 1152–1154
        identification of candidates for, 1149–1152
        seizures outcome after, 1155–1156

Childhood occipital epilepsy (COE), 270–271

Chloral hydrate, for refractory status epilepticus, 615

Chlorambucil, 580

Chloride channels, epilepsies linked to, 106

Chlormethiazole, for refractory status epilepticus, 615

Cholera, 577

Chorea, in children, 635

Chromosomal anomalies, epilepsies with, 480–483
  Angelman syndrome, 481–482, 481f
  Down syndrome (trisomy 21), 482
    epilepsy in adults with, 482
    epilepsy in children with, 482
  fragile X, 482–483
  Klinefelter syndrome (47, XXY), 483
  Rett syndrome, 482
  ring chromosome 14 in, 480–481
  ring chromosome 20 in, 480, 480f

Chronic focal encephalitis, 441–451. See also Rasmussen encephalitis (syndrome)

Cimetidine, 580

Cingulate gyrus epilepsy, 369

Cingulate gyrus seizures, 243

Cingulate seizures, 355

Citrullinemia, 500

Classification, of epilepsies, 347–353. See also specific disorders
  1989 ILAE, 347–348
  2001 ILAE proposal, syndrome-oriented, 348–349, 348t
  five-dimensional patient-oriented proposal, 349–353, 350t–352t
    advantages of, 352–353
    epileptogenic zone in, 350, 350t
    etiology in, 351, 351t
    limitations of, 353
    related medical information in, 351–352
    seizure classification in, 350–351
    seizure frequency in, 351, 352t

Classification, of epilepsies and epileptic syndromes, proposed revised, 354–363
  definitions, 357–461
    epilepsies and syndromes undetermined as to whether focal or generalized, 358, 360–361
    generalized cryptogenic or symptomatic (age-related), 359–360
    generalized epilepsies and syndromes, 358
    generalized symptomatic of nonspecific etiology (age-related), 360
    idiopathic generalized (age-related), 358–359
    idiopathic localization-related, 358
    localization-related epilepsies and syndromes, 357–358
    international classification of epilepsies and epileptic syndromes, 354–357
    frontal lobe, 355–356
    occipital lobe, 357

parietal lobe, 356
temporal lobe, 354–355
precipitated seizures, 362–363
symptomatic generalized epilepsies of specific etiologies, 361–362

Classification, of seizures, 217–220
  comments on, 220
  electroclinical approach to, limitations of, 217–218
  evolution of current system of, 217
  proposal on, 218–219, 219t
  proposed revised, 222–228
    addendum on, 223–224
    definition of terms in, 224–228
    generalized seizures (convulsive or nonconvulsive), 222–223, 224t
    partial (focal, local) seizures, 222, 223t
    unclassified epileptic seizures, 223
  symptomatology alone in, 219t
    advantages of, 218

Clearance, of antiepileptic drugs, 659–661, 660f. See also specific drugs
  in hepatic disease, 721–722, 721t, 722t
  in renal disease, 719–721, 720t

Clinical use, of antiepileptic drugs. See specific drugs

Clobazam, 844–845, 844f. See also Benzodiazepines
  for benign childhood epilepsy with centrotemporal spikes, 381
  indications for, 1212t
  for juvenile myoclonic epilepsy, 416
  for myoclonic epilepsies, progressive, 422
  pharmacokinetics of, 657t
    in infants and children, 672–673
  for severe myoclonic epilepsy of infants, 414

Clonazepam, 842–843. See also Benzodiazepines
  adverse effects and drug interactions of, 842
  for benign childhood epilepsy with centrotemporal spikes, 381
  clinical applications of, 842–843
  clinical pharmacology of, 836t
  in elderly, 595t, 600
  indications for, 1212t
  for juvenile myoclonic epilepsy, 396, 416
  for myoclonic epilepsies, progressive, 422
  pharmacokinetics of, 657t, 842
    in infants and children, 673
  for refractory status epilepticus, 615
  structure of, 842, 842f

Clonic absence epilepsy, 414–415

Clonic seizures
  absence, 227
  definition of, 227–228
  focal motor, 262–263
  in focal seizures, 243

Clonus, prominent rhythmic distal, 417, 418f

Clorazepate, 843–844, 843f. See also Benzodiazepines
  in elderly, 595t, 600

Clozapine, 578t, 579

Cobblestone brain malformations, 45, 48. See also Lissencephaly type 2

Cobblestone lissencephaly, 1017

Cocaine, 501, 579–580

Cognitive deficits, 225
  of epilepsy surgery, 1186
  after prolonged status epilepticus, 289

Cognitive effects
  of antiepileptic drugs, 1186–1189 (See also Antiepileptic drugs (AEDs), cognitive effects of)
  of epilepsy, 1185–1186
  of vagal nerve stimulation, 1186

Cold shivering, as aura, 237

Combinatorial system, 184f

Commissure development, forebrain, 22

Comorbidity, 122

Complex partial seizure, 241–251. See also Focal seizures with impaired consciousness
  with automatisms, in temporal lobe epilepsy, 203f
  definition of, 241–242
  video-EEG of, 997f–1001f, 999

Compliance, imperfect, 984

Confusional migraine, in children, 637

Congenital disorders of glycosylation, 558

Congenital folate malabsorption, 554

Congenital malformations, in infants of mothers on antiepileptic drugs, 709–710, 710t, 738

Consciousness
  definition of, 224–225
  impairment of, with absence seizures, 227
  loss of, 242 (See also Focal seizures with impaired consciousness)

Constipation, in children, 637

Constitutive androstane receptor (CAR), 753

Continuous seizure types, 265

Continuous spike waves of slow sleep (CSWS), 455–458
  clinical presentation of, 456–457
  definition of, 455–456
  diagnosis of, 456, 457f
  etiologic factors in, 457
  outcome in, 458
  treatment of, 459–460

Contraception, 698–699, 705–706

Contraceptives, antiepileptic drugs on, 705–706, 738

Control groups
  active, 650
  dose, 650
  historical, 649–650
  placebo, 650

Contusion, electrode-related, 11f

Convulsive seizures. See Tonic seizures

Cornu ammonis (Ammon horn), 22, 56, 57, 58f, 60f, 62f

Corpus callosotomy, 1159–1163
  complications of, 1162–1163
  efficacy of, 1160–1161, 1161f
  human studies of, 1160
  indications for, 1160
  neurophysiologic basis of, 1159–1160
  seizure reduction on quality of life
      with, 1161
  surgical technique in, 1161–1162
Corpus callosum
  agenesis and dysgenesis of, 30
  development of, 22
Cortex, 18–19
  "double," 28–29, 28f, 43
Cortical atrophy, 9f
Cortical-band heterotopia, 48. *See also*
      Subcortical-band (laminar)
      heterotopia
Cortical development, 18–22
  cerebral cortex gyration in, 21–22
  cerebral neocortex ontogeny in, 19–20,
      20f, 21f
  cortex architecture in, 18–19
  forebrain commissure development in,
      22
  paleocortex (hippocampus) ontogeny
      in, 22
  subplate neurons in, 21
Cortical developmental malformations,
      37–45
  classification of, 37, 38t
  cobblestone brain malformations, 45–46
  cortical dysplasia with neoplastic
      changes, 40
  epidemiology of, 37
  excessive single ectopic white-matter
      neurons, 46
  focal cortical dysplasia, 39t, 40, 40f
  genetic testing and counseling for,
      48–49
  hemimegalencephaly, 38–40, 38f, 38t,
      39t
  heterotopia, 39t, 42–45
      periventricular nodular, 39t, 43,
          42f
      subcortical-band, 39t, 43–44, 44f
  lissencephaly, 44–45, 44f, 45t
  megalencephaly syndromes, 39t, 41, 41f
  microcephaly syndromes, 39t, 41–42,
      41f
  MRI of, 1016–1019, 1016t, 1017f–1021f
  neuronal and glial proliferation
      with abnormal cell types, 38, 38t
      with normal cell types, 39t, 41–42,
          41f
  of neuronal migration, 39t, 42–46, 42f,
      44f, 45t (*See also specific
      malformations*)
  transmantle dysplasia with abnormal
      but nonneoplastic cells, 39t, 40
Cortical developmental malformations,
      focal
  epilepsy surgery for, 1103–1109
      diagnosis of focal epilepsy in,
          1103–1104
      identifying anatomic lesion in,
          1104–1107

defining epileptogenic zone in,
      1106, 1106f
  localizing eloquent cortical regions
      in, 1106
  subdural electrodes (strips and
      grids) in, 1105–1107, 1105f
  MRI abnormalities in, 1104–1105,
      1104f
  outcome of, 1107–1109, 1107t
  strategy for, 1107
  histopathology of, 1103, 1104f
Cortical dysplasia, 4f, 5f, 7f
  animal models of, 99
  extensive unilateral, hemispherectomy
      for, 1116
  focal, 30
  MRI of, 1018, 1020f
  neurocutaneous syndromes and, 543
Cortical function, fMRI and [^{15}O] water
      PET in mapping of, 1048
Cortical microdysgenesis, 47–48
Cortical organization, 19
  malformations of, 46–47
      cortical microdysgenesis, 47–48
      focal cortical dysplasia without
          balloon cells, 47–48
      polymicrogyria, 47, 46f
Cortical reflex myoclonus, 319
Cortical tuber, 7f
Corticobulbar tract, 258–259
Corticospinal tract, 258–259
Corticosteroids. *See* Steroid hormones
Corticotropin, for epileptic spasms, 341
Crashes, auto, 1202–1203, 1202t
Creatine metabolism, inborn errors of,
      554
Crohn disease, 578
Crossover design, 649f, 650
Cryptococcal meningitis, 576–577
Curvilinear reconstructions, 1024
Cyanotic breath-holding spells
  EEG of, 212f–213f
  in infants, 634
Cyclophosphamide, for Rasmussen
      encephalitis, 450
Cyclosporine, with antiepileptic drugs,
      730
CYP2C9, 749
CYP2C19, 749
CYP3A4, 750
CYP3A5, 750
Cytochrome P (CYP) 450 system
  genes for, 748–750, 748f, 749t
  in infants and children, 672
Cytokines, proinflammatory, in febrile
      seizures, 512
Cytomegalovirus retinitis, 577
Cytomegaly, neuronal, 5f

D
De Morsier syndrome, 27
Death, sudden, from generalized tonic-
      clonic seizures, 289
Definitions, 109–110. *See also*
      Classification; *specific terms*
Degenerative progressive myoclonic
      epilepsy, Lundborg type, 362

Delayed rectifiers, 76–77
Delta activity, in generalized tonic-clonic
      seizures, 289–290, 290f
Dendrite growth, 17
Dendrite growth disorders, 26
Dentate gyrus, 56, 57–58, 58f, 59f, 61f
  development of, 22
  in hippocampus excitability, 62
Dentatorubral-pallidoluysian atropha
      (DRPLA), 561
Depression, 1197–1198
  as aura, 236
Depth electrodes, 1060–1061, 1060f
Derivations, in localization with EEG,
      146–147
Dermatologic disorders, from generalized
      tonic-clonic seizures, 289
Desipramine, 579
Devalproex sodium. *See* Valproate
      (valproic acid)
Development, 13. *See also specific areas*
  in offspring of mothers on antiepileptic
      drugs, 709
Diabetes mellitus, epilepsy with, 558
Diagnosis. *See also specific disorders*
  accuracy of, 112
  EEG in, 169–180 (*See also*
      Electroencephalography (EEG),
      in epilepsy diagnosis)
  incorrect, 983
Dialeptic, 242
Dialeptic seizures. *See* Absence seizures
Dialysis disequilibrium, 573–574
Diaphragmatic herniation, from general-
      ized tonic-clonic seizures, 288
Diazepam, 837–839. *See also*
      Benzodiazepines
  absorption, distribution, and
      metabolism of, 837–838
  adverse effects and drug interactions of,
      838
  clinical applications of, 838–839
  clinical pharmacology of, 836t
  in elderly, 595t, 600
  for febrile seizures, 517
  indications for, 1212t
  for multiple handicaps, epilepsy with,
      589
  for neonatal seizures, 506
  pharmacogenetics of, 754
  pharmacokinetics of, 657t
      in infants and children, 673
  for status epilepticus, 612, 613t,
      614–615
      prehospital, 617
      refractory, 615
  structure of, 837, 837f
Differential amplifiers, in localization,
      146, 146f
Diffusion tensor imaging (DTI), 1022, 1023f
Diffusion-weighted imaging, 1013
DiGeorge syndrome, 503
Dipole modeling, source localization and,
      159–160
Dipole potentials, in benign focal
      epileptiform discharges of
      childhood, 199f

Direct intrahippocampal pathway, 59, 64f
Disability, 1207, 1207t
Distribution
of antiepileptic drugs, 657–658 (*See also specific drugs*)
EEG, centrotemporal, 155, 158f
volume of, 657–658
Dizziness, as aura, 234
Dorsolateral seizures, 356
Dose control, 650
Dosing. *See also specific drugs*
of antiepileptic drugs, age-specific, 676–677, 677t
inadequate, 984
loading dose and volume of distribution in, 657–658
maximum tolerated dose in, 647
pharmacodynamic interactions between antiepileptic drugs on, 663, 663t
"Double cortex," 28–29, 28f, 43
Double dentate, 4f
Down syndrome (trisomy 21), 482
epilepsy in adults with, 482
epilepsy in children with, 482
Downregulation, in developmental defects, 23
Dravet syndrome, 360, 413–414
epilepsy with, 516
GEFS+ and, 516
Driving, 1202–1203, 1202t, 1204t–1206t
Drop attacks, 324–326, 325f. *See also* Atonic seizures
Drowsiness
rhythmical temporal theta bursts of, 188f
with seizure, 226
Drug abuse, 984
Drug approval process, adverse effects of antiepileptic drugs and, 735–736
Drug choice, incorrect, 983–984
Drug concentrations, plasma. *See specific drugs*
Drug development, antiepileptic drug, 645–654
analysis of results in, 651–652
discovery in, 645
efficacy and safety trials on, 648–649
experimental trial design for, 649–651, 649f (*See also* Experimental trial design, in antiepileptic drug development)
human testing of, 647–648
preclinical development of, 645–647
Drug dosage. *See* Dosing; *specific agents*
Drug-induced seizures, 578–579, 578t
myoclonic, 422–423, 423t
Drug interactions among antiepileptic drugs. *See also specific drugs*
and other medications, 665, 666t–669t
pharmacodynamic, 663–664, 663t
pharmacokinetic, 661–663, 661f, 662t
Drug receptors. *See also specific drugs*
genes for, 752–753
Drug transporters, genes for, 751–752, 752f

Dual pathology
epilepsy surgery and, 1079–1080
epileptogenic regions on MRI, 1095
Duration of epilepsy, recurrence risk and, 683, 686
Dyscontrol syndrome, episodic, 637
Dysembryoplastic neuroepithelial tumor, 9f, 10f
MRI of, 1014, 1016f, 1090
Dysgenesis, cerebral. *See* Cerebral dysgenesis
Dyskinesias. *See also specific disorders*
paroxysmal, in children, 636
Dysmnesic symptoms, 225
Dysmorphic neurons, 5f
Dysphasia, 225
Dysplasia. *See also specific disorders*
focal cortical, 30
Dyssynergia cerebellaris myoclonia with epilepsy, 362
Dystonia, 639
Dystonic posturing, in focal seizures, 247
Dystrophies, neuroaxonal, 559

E
Early infantile epileptic encephalopathy (EIEE), 478, 504
with suppression burst, 360
Early myoclonic encephalopathy (EME), 360, 409, 477–478, 478f, 503–504, 505f
Early onset multiple carboxylase deficiency, 552
Eating epilepsy, 470
Echinococcal infections, of CNS, 577
Eclampsia, 580–581
Ectopia, 24
Edema
progressive encephalopathy with, 556–557
pulmonary, from generalized tonic-clonic seizures, 288, 288f
Efferents
brainstem motor, 258
motor cortex, 258–259
Efficacy, of antiepileptic drugs, 648–649. *See also specific drugs* and disorders
EJM 1, 394–395
EJM 2, 395
EJM 3, 395
Elation, as aura, 236
Elderly, epilepsy in, 593–601
antiepileptic drugs for, 594–601, 595t–597t
benzodiazepines, 595t, 600
carbamazepine, 595t, 596t, 598–599
choice of, 594–595
clinical pharmacology of, 594, 595t–597t
comedication interactions with, 594, 595t
felbamate, 595t, 596t, 599
gabapentin, 595t, 596t, 599
lamotrigine, 595t, 596t, 599
levetiracetam, 595t, 596t, 599–600
non-antiepileptic drug interactions of, 600–601

oxcarbazepine, 595t, 596t, 600
phenobarbital, 595t, 596t, 599
phenytoin, 595–598, 595t–597t
tiagabine, 595t, 597t, 600
topiramate, 595t, 597t, 600
valproate (valproic acid), 595t, 597t, 599
epidemiology of, 593–594
Electrical fields
brain generators and, 142–146
boundary problems in, 145–146
electrode placement as spatial sampling in, 145
sources of, 142–143
surface electrical manifestations in, 143f, 144–145, 145f
volume conduction in, 143–144, 143f
scalp determination of, 147–154
amplitude measurement in, 147
choice of reference in, 154
mapping in, 147–150, 149f–151f
peak identification in, 147, 148f
rules for field identification in, 150–153, 151t
with bipolar montage, 151–152, 151t, 152f
with referential montage, 151t, 153, 153f
Electrical polarity, of cell membranes, 17
Electrocorticography, intraoperative, 1064
Electrodecremental response, 178, 178f, 337f
Electrodes
cavernous sinus, 1064
depth, 1060–1061, 1060f
infarcts and contusions related to, 11f
intraventricular, 1064
position of
in combinatorial system, 184f
as spatial sampling, 145
sphenoidal, 1059, 1060f
subdural (grids and strips), 1061–1064, 1062f (*See also* Subdural electrodes (grids and strips))
advantages of, 1063
disadvantages of, 1063–1064, 1063f
for focal cortical developmental malformations, 1105–1106, 1105f
identification of, 1105–1107, 1105f
proposed indications for, 1106–1107
functional localization studies with, 1061–1062
Electroencephalographic atlas of epileptiform abnormalities, 183–214
bipolar montage, 184f
electrode position and nomenclature of combinatorial system, 184f
focal epilepsies, 185, 199f–211f
benign focal epileptiform discharges of childhood
centrotemporal sharp waves, 199f
dipole potentials, 199f
left and right central sharp waves, 200f
occipital sharp waves, 200f

frontal lobe epilepsy
  frontal sharp waves, 204f
  frontal sharp waves with 2-degree
    bilateral synchrony, 205f
  subclinical EEG seizure, +50
    seconds, 206f
  subclinical EEG seizure, onset, 206f
occipital lobe epilepsy
  visual aura and focal clonic seizure,
    -10 seconds, 207f
  visual aura and focal clonic seizure,
    clinical onset, 207f
perirolandic epilepsy
  epilepsia partialis continua, 211f
  focal clonic seizure, +10 seconds,
    209f
  focal clonic seizure, clinical onset,
    209f
  left arm tonic seizure, 210f
  right frontocentral sharp waves,
    210f
supplemental motor area epilepsy
  sharp waves at vertex, 208f
  tonic seizure, 208f
temporal lobe epilepsy
  bitemporal sharp waves, 202f
  complex partial seizure with
    automatisms, 203f
  partial ("hypomotor") seizure, 201f
  temporal sharp wave, 201f
generalized epilepsies, 183–184,
    192f–198f
  childhood absence epilepsy
    absence seizure, 192f
    absence status epilepticus, 193f
  infantile spasms
    hypsarrhythmia, 195f
    seizure, 195f
  intractable epilepsy with multifocal
    spikes, 197f
  juvenile myoclonic epilepsy
    cluster of myoclonic jerks, 194f
    myoclonic jerk with photic
      stimulation, 194f
  Lennox-Gastaut syndrome
    atonic seizures, 197f, 325f
    generalized paroxysmal fast and
      polyspikes in sleep, 196f
    generalized sharp- and slow-wave
      complexes, 196f
    stimulation-related epilepsy, reading-
      induced spike-and-wave
      complexes, 198f
methods, 183, 184f
nonepileptic paroxysmal disorders,
    185–186, 211f–214f
  cyanotic breath-holding spell,
    213f
  narcolepsy, 214f
  pallid infantile syncope, ocular
    compression test of, 212f
normal patterns, 183, 184f–191f
  6-Hz "phantom" spike and wave,
    187f
  14-Hz and 6-Hz positive spikes, 186f
  breach rhythm, 191f
  hyperventilation effect, 190f

hypnagogic hypersynchrony, 189f
photic driving, 191f
rhythmical temporal theta bursts of
  drowsiness, 188f
sleep spindle, 190f
small sharp spike, 186f
subclinical rhythmical electrographic
  discharges of adults, 188f
V-waves and positive occipital sharp
  transients (POSTS), 189f
wicket spikes, 187f
Electroencephalography (EEG). *See also*
    Electrical fields, brain generators
    and; *specific disorders*
of absence epilepsy
  childhood, 397
  juvenile, 398
  myoclonic or clonic, 414
of absence seizures, 307–309
  in atypical absences
    ictal discharges, 308, 308f
    interictal, 308
  in childhood, 192f
  delta activity, generalized rhythmic,
    308
  low-voltage fast rhythms, 308
  mixed patterns, 309, 309f
  in typical absences
    ictal discharges, 307, 307f
    interictal, 307–308, 310f
ambulatory, of psychogenic
    nonepileptic seizures, 624
of Angelman syndrome, 417, 418f
of atypical tonic seizures, 322–323,
    322f, 323f
of autism, 587
of benign childhood epilepsy with
    centrotemporal spikes, 376–377,
    376f–380f
of benign myoclonic epilepsy of
    infancy, 410
of benign occipital epilepsy of
    childhood, 383–384, 383f, 384f
cavernous sinus electrodes in, 1064
of continuous spike waves of slow
    sleep, 456, 457f
electrical fields in (*See also* Electrical
    fields)
  brain generators and, 142–146
  scalp determination of, 147–154
of epilepsia partialis continua, 268
of epilepsies with prominent rhythmic
    distal clonus, 417, 418f
in epilepsy diagnosis, 169–180
  3-Hz spike and wave pattern in, 176,
    176f, 289–291
  electrodecremental response in, 178,
    178f
  extracranial recordings in, limitations
    of, 170–171
  for generalized epilepsies, primary,
    175–176
  historical perspective on, 169
  hypsarrhythmia in, 179f, 180
  interictal and ictal recording in, 170
  interpretation pitfalls in, 171, 186f,
    187f

methods in, 170
multiple spike and wave pattern in,
    176–177, 177f
in newborns and infants, 179f, 180
paroxysmal or rhythmic fast activity
    in, 177–178, 178f, 318f
in partial epilepsies, clinical use of,
    172–175
  frontal lobe, 174
  occipital lobe, 174–175, 175f
  perirolandic, 175, 175f
  temporal lobe, 173–174, 173f
in partial epilepsies, interictal
    epileptiform patterns in,
    171–172, 171f, 172f
photoparoxysmal response in, 179
rationale for, 169–170
slow spike and wave pattern in, 177,
    196f, 308f, 320f
of epilepsy with generalized tonic-
    clonic seizures only, in children,
    400
of epileptic spasms, 336–338, 337f
extracranial, 1059
of focal motor seizures, 264–265,
    265f–267f
of focal seizures with impaired
    consciousness, 248–250,
    248f–251f
  ictal, 249–250, 250f, 251f
  interictal, 248–249, 248f, 249f
of Gaucher disease, type III, 419f
of generalized epilepsy with febrile
    seizures plus, 401–402
of generalized tonic-clonic seizures,
    289–295
  ictal findings, 294–295, 295f–297f
  incidental interictal epileptiform
    activity, 294
  interictal epileptiform activity,
    290–291, 292f, 293f
  nonepileptiform activity, 285f,
    289–290, 290f, 291f
  photoparoxysmal response, 291, 293f
  secondary generalized interictal
    epileptiform activity, 291–293,
    293f, 294f
interictal, limitations of, 995f, 996
intracranial, 1059–1064
  electrodes in, depth, 1060–1061,
    1060f
  electrodes in, overview of, 1059
  electrodes in, subdural (grids and
    strips), 1061–1064, 1062f, 1063f
    for focal cortical developmental
      malformations, 1105–1107, 1105f
    for epileptogenic zone localization,
      1065
    for epileptogenic zone near eloquent
      cortex, 1065
    for hippocampal sclerosis surgery,
      1071–1072, 1072f–1074f
    indications and clinical use of, 1065
    for mesial temporal lobe epilepsy,
      suspected bilateral, 1065
intraventricular electrodes in, 1064
invasive, with nonlesional epilepsy, 1126

Electroencephalography (EEG) *(Continued)*
of juvenile myoclonic epilepsy, 393, 394f
of Landau-Kleffner syndrome, 459
of Lennox-Gastaut syndrome, 431–434, 432f, 433f
mapping with, 141–142
of metabolic and mitochondrial diseases, inherited, 562–563, 563t
of myoclonic epilepsies, 407–408, 408f juvenile, 415
of myotonic-astatic epilepsy, 411–412, 412f
neurophysiologic basis of, 127–138
baseline shifts (EEG, direct current), 129f, 131f, 132–134, 133f, 134f
epileptic, 137, 137f
bioelectric activity of neuronal and glial cells, 127, 128f
epileptic field potential basics, 133f–135f, 134–135
field potentials
changes in, 132
with focal epileptic activity, 135–136, 135f
with generalized tonic-clonic activity, 136, 136f
generation of, 130–131, 130f, 131f
in neuronal networks, 131, 131f
glial cells, 129–130, 129f
neurons, 127–129, 128f
wave generation (conventional EEG), 132, 132f
epileptic, 137, 138f
of psychogenic nonepileptic seizures, 624–625, 629
previous abnormal, 625–626
of Rasmussen encephalitis (syndrome), 445
recurrence risk and, 685–686
scalp
for epilepsy surgery in infants and children, 1144–1147, 1145f–1146f
subdural, 1093
of seizures, recurrence risk and, 682
of severe myoclonic epilepsy of infants, 413–414
source localization with, 141–142, 154–157 *(See also* Localization, EEG in)
computer-aided methodology for, 157–160, 159f
of status epilepticus, 606, 606f–608f, 612f–613f
in stroke, 529
subdural, of epileptogenic regions, 1093
of supplementary sensorimotor seizures, 269–270, 269f–271f
of symptomatic epilepsies, 1088–1089
of temporal lobe epilepsies, 355
video *(See* Video-electroencephalogram monitoring)
of vigabatrin-induced myoclonic jerks, 423, 423f
Electronic screens, photosensitive seizures from, 467–468

Electroshock model, 99
Elimination, of antiepileptic drugs, 658–659, 658f. *See also specific drugs*
in hepatic disease, 721–722, 721t, 722t
in renal disease, 719–721, 720t
Eloquent cortical regions
in focal malformations of cortical development, localizing, 1106
intracranial EEG for epileptogenic zone near, 1065
Embolism, cerebral, *vs.* epilepsy, 640
Emotion, intracarotid amobarbital procedure on, 1036
Emotional auras, 232t, 233t, 236
Employment, 1203–1207, 1207t
Encephalitis, 576
limbic, 581
Rasmussen, 9f, 441–451 *(See also* Rasmussen encephalitis (syndrome))
Encephalomalacia, MRI of, 1015
and pathology, 1091–1092
Encephalopathic generalized epilepsy, 429–438
differential diagnosis of, 435–436, 435t
EEG features in, 431–434, 432f, 433f
etiology of, 434, 434t
in Lennox-Gastaut syndrome, 429–430 *(See also* Lennox-Gastaut syndrome)
neuroimaging of, 435
neurologic dysfunction in, 434
neuropathology of, 434–435
other syndromes in, 430
prognosis in, 437–438
seizure types in, 430–431
treatment of, 436–437
Encephalopathy
early infantile epileptic, 478, 504
early myoclonic, 360, 409, 477–478, 478f, 503–504, 505f
epileptic, 455 *(See also* Encephalopathic generalized epilepsy; *specific disorders)*
glycine, 500
hepatic, 578
myoclonic infantile, 581
Enflurane, 578t, 579
EPHX1, 750
Epidemiology, 110–115. *See also specific disorders*
age in, 112–113
ascertaining cases of, 111–112, 111f
diagnostic accuracy *vs.* representativeness in, 112
diagnostic technology and expertise in, 110–111
etiology in, 113–114
history of, 110
incidence and prevalence of, 112, 113t, 114t
Epidermal nevus syndrome, 11f, 542, 542f
epilepsy with, 542
neurocristopathies in, 23
vascular dysplasias and, 543
Epigastric auras, 230t, 232t, 233t, 235, 237

Epilepsia partialis continua, 228, 265–268. *See also* Motor cortex
clinical semiology of, 266–268
definition of, 225, 265–266
EEG findings in, 268
in perirolandic epilepsy, 211f
Epilepsia partialis continua of Kojevnikov, 266
Epilepsies and syndromes undetermined as to whether focal or generalized, 358, 360–361
Epilepsy
classification of, 347–353 *(See also* Classification, of epilepsies; Classification, of epilepsies and epileptic syndromes)
proposed revised, 354–363
definition of, 110, 487
diagnosis of, 110
eating, 470
etiology of, 110
after febrile seizures, 515–516
GABA$_A$ receptors and, 831
hot water, 471
language-induced, 469
misdiagnosis of, 623
musicogenic, 469–470
with prominent rhythmic distal clonus, 417, 418f
reading, 468–469
with reflex seizures, 463–472
startle, 471
Epilepsy surgery. *See* Surgery
Epilepsy syndromes. *See also specific syndromes*
antiepileptic drug testing and, 648
classification of generalized tonic-clonic seizures in, 280–282
concept of, 349
definition of, 110
of early infantile onset, 503–504, 504f
as function of age, 349
recurrence risk with, 686
Epilepsy with continuous spike-waves during slow-wave sleep, 360–361
Epilepsy with generalized tonic-clonic seizures only, 400–401
Epilepsy with GTCS on awakening, 359. *See also* Juvenile myoclonic epilepsy
Epilepsy with myoclonic absences, 360
Epilepsy with myoclonic-astatic seizures, 359–360
Epilepsy with reflex seizures. *See* Reflex epilepsy
Epileptic auras. *See* Auras
Epileptic encephalopathy, 455–456. *See also* Encephalopathic generalized epilepsy; *specific disorders*
Epileptic field potentials, 133f–135f, 134–135
Epileptic march, 225, 229–230
Epileptic myoclonus, 407. *See also* Myoclonic epilepsies
Epileptic seizures. *See* Seizure(s)
Epileptic spasms. *See* Spasms, epileptic

Epileptiform patterns. *See* Electroencephalographic atlas of epileptiform abnormalities; Electroencephalography (EEG)

Epileptogenesis
definition of, 91
glial cells in, 95–98, 96f, 97f
hyperexcitability in, 91–98 (*See also* Hyperexcitability)

Epileptogenic lesions. *See also* Focal lesions on MRI; *specific lesions*
classification of, 1087–1088
MRI of, 1022

Epileptogenic region in focal lesions on MRI, 1092–1095
functional localization studies on surgical risk in, 1094–1095, 1094f
functional MRI and SPECT of, 1093
MRI and dual pathology in, 1095
PET and MR spectroscopy of, 1093–1094, 1094f
scalp EEG of, 1093
subdural EEG of, 1093

Epileptogenic zone, 350, 350t
dipoles in, 144 (*See also* Electrical fields, brain generators and)
in focal malformations of cortical development, 1106, 1106f
intracranial EEG for localization of, 1065
MRI of, 1022
near eloquent cortex, EEG for, 1065

Episodic ataxia type 1, 84
Episodic ataxia type 2, 84
Episodic dyscontrol syndrome, 637
Estrogen, 697, 697f
changes in, on seizures, 698
on neuronal excitability, 695–696

Ethosuximide, 817–824
for absence epilepsy, childhood, 398
absorption of, 818
adverse effects of, 822–823
monitoring for, 739
age-specific dosing of, 677t
for atypical seizures, 326–327
for benign myoclonic epilepsy of infancy, 413
chemistry and mechanism of action of, 817, 818f
clinical use of, 823–824
distribution of, 819
drug interactions of, 820
on plasma concentration, 666t
efficacy of, 820–822
historical background on, 817
indications for, 823–824, 1212t
for juvenile myoclonic epilepsy, 396
for Lennox-Gastaut syndrome, 437
metabolism and excretion of, 818f, 819–820
monitoring with, 824
for myotonic-astatic epilepsy, 413
pharmacokinetics of, 655–659, 656t, 817–818 (*See also* Pharmacokinetics, of antiepileptic drugs)
in infants and children, 674

in pregnancy, 706–708, 707t
racemic mixture in, 817–818
in renal and liver disease, 726

Ethotoin, 947–949, 949f, 1212t

Etiology, 113–114. *See also specific disorders*
of epilepsy, 110
of seizures, 682
on recurrence risk, 685

Etomidate, 580, 615

Excessive single ectopic white-matter neurons, 45

Excitatory postsynaptic potentials, 127–129, 128f

Excretion, of antiepileptic drugs. *See specific drugs*

Experimental trial design, in antiepileptic drug development, 649–651, 649f
for adjunctive therapy *vs.* monotherapy, 650–651
blinding in, 649
control groups in, 649–650
parallel *vs.* crossover design in, 649f, 650

Extratemporal lobe epilepsy, PET in, 1044–1045

Eye blinking, in focal seizures, 246
Eye closure–induced seizures, 467
Eye fluttering, in focal seizures, 246
Eyelid myoclonia, with/without absences, 416

F

[¹⁸F] FDG-PET, temporal lobe epilepsy and, 1042–1043, 1042f
Factitious disorder, 637–638, 638t
Familial autosomal dominant myoclonic epilepsy (FAME), 417
Familial hemiplegic migraine, 84
Familial incontinentia pigmenti, 502
Fatty acid oxidation defects, 551
Fear, as aura, 236
Febrile convulsions, 361
Febrile seizures, 511–517
definition of, 110
historical perspective on, 511
neuropsychological status after, later, 516
predisposing factors in
age, 512
associated factors, 512–513
fever, 512
genetics, 511–512
risk assessment in
epilepsy risk in, 515–516
generalized epilepsy with febrile seizures plus in, 516
hippocampal sclerosis association in, 515
recurrence risk in, 514–515
therapy for, 516–517
types of
complex febrile seizures, 513–514
febrile status epilepticus, 514
simple febrile convulsions, 513
Febrile seizures plus, generalized epilepsy with (GEFS+), 320, 401–402

Felbamate, 913–919
absorption, distribution, and metabolism of, 914–915
adverse effects of, 916–917
monitoring for, 740, 918–919
age-specific dosing of, 677t
for atypical tonic seizures, 327
on carbamazepine, 915–916, 916t
chemistry of, 913, 914f
clinical use of, 917–919, 918t
cognitive effects of, 1187
drug interactions of, 915, 916t
efficacy of, 915
in elderly, 595t, 596t, 599
for generalized tonic-clonic seizures, 297, 298–299
historical background on, 913
indications for, 1212t
for Lennox-Gastaut syndrome, 437
mechanism of action of, 913–914
pharmacokinetics of, 655–659, 656t (*See also* Pharmacokinetics, of antiepileptic drugs)
in infants and children, 674
in pregnancy, 706–708, 707t
on phenytoin, 916, 916t
on plasma concentrations of other drugs, 667t
in renal and liver disease, 727
teratogenicity of, 712
on valproate, 916, 916t
on warfarin requirement, 916
withdrawal from, 919

Fertility, 699
Fetal hydantoin syndrome, 796
Fibromas, ungual, 6f
Field determination, 142
brain generators in, 142–146 (*See also* Electrical fields)
rules for, 150–153, 151t
with bipolar montage, 151–152, 151t, 152f
with referential montage, 151t, 153, 153f
scalp determination of, 147–154 (*See also* Electrical fields)

Field patterns, in EEG *vs.* MEG, 162, 162f
with current dipole generator, 160, 161f
with vertically oriented dipole, 162, 163f

Field potentials
changes in, 132
with focal epileptic activity, 135–136, 135f
with generalized tonic-clonic activity, 136, 136f
generation of, 130–131, 130f, 131f
in neuronal networks, 131, 131f

"Fifth-day fits," 503

Five-dimensional patient-oriented epilepsy classification proposal, 349–353, 350t–352t
advantages of, 352–353
epileptogenic zone in, 350, 350t
etiology in, 351, 351t
limitations of, 353
related medical information in, 351–352
seizure classification in, 350–351
seizure frequency in, 351, 352t

Flicker
self-induced, 466
visually evoked seizures not induced by, 466–467
Flumazenil, 834
Fluorofelbamate, 940t, 941
Fluoxetine, 578t, 579
fMRI. *See* Functional magnetic resonance imaging (fMRI)
Focal clonic seizure
in perirolandic epilepsy
+10 seconds, 209f
clinical onset, 209f
visual aura and, in occipital lobe epilepsy
-10 seconds, 207f
clinical onset, 207f
Focal cortical dysplasia, 30, 39t, 40, 40f
MRI of, 1019f, 1020–1022
with white-matter signal abnormalities, 1018, 1019f
without balloon cells, 47
Focal cortical lesions, epilepsy surgery in infants and children and, 1144–1147, 1145f–1148f
Focal encephalitis, chronic, 441–451. *See also* Rasmussen encephalitis (syndrome)
Focal epilepsies, 242. *See also* Focal seizures with impaired consciousness
diagnosis of, 1103–1104
Focal epilepsies, EEG atlas of, 185, 198f–211f
benign focal epileptiform discharges of childhood
centrotemporal sharp waves, 199f
dipole potentials, 199f
left and right central sharp waves, 200f
occipital sharp waves, 200f
frontal lobe epilepsy
frontal sharp waves, 204f, 205f
subclinical EEG seizure, 206f
occipital lobe epilepsy, visual aura and focal clonic seizure, 207f
perirolandic epilepsy
epilepsia partialis continua, 211f
focal clonic seizure, 209f
left arm tonic seizure, 210f
right frontocentral sharp waves, 210f
supplemental motor area epilepsy
sharp waves at vertex, 208f
tonic seizure, 208f
temporal lobe epilepsy
bitemporal sharp waves, 202f
complex partial seizure with automatisms, 203f
partial ("hypomotor") seizure, 201f
temporal sharp wave, 201f
Focal epilepsies, symptomatic, 365–371
etiologic factors in, 370
frontal lobe, 367–369
anterior frontopolar, 368
cingulate gyrus, 369
dorsolateral, 368–369
orbitofrontal, 368

supplementary sensorimotor area, 368
management of, 370–371
motor area, 369
occipital lobe, 370
parietal lobe, 369–370
temporal lobe, 365–367
mesial, 365–366
neocortical, 366–367
Focal lesions on MRI
correlation of MRI features with common pathologies in, 1089–1092
astrocytoma, low-grade, 1089–1090
dysembryoplastic neuroepithelial tumor, 1090
ganglioglioma, 1090, 1095, 1096f
gliosis and encephalomalacia, acquired, 1091–1092
inflammatory diseases, 1092
oligodendroglioma, 1089
pleomorphic xanthoastrocytoma, 1090–1091
postischemic epilepsy, 1092
posttraumatic epilepsy, 1091–1092
vascular abnormalities, 1091
diffuse EEG abnormalities with, surgical outcomes with, 1177
EEG features of, 1088–1089
epileptogenic region in, 1092–1095
functional localization studies on surgical risk in, 1094–1095, 1094f
functional MRI and SPECT of, 1093
MRI and dual pathology in, 1095
PET and MR spectroscopy of, 1093–1094, 1094f
scalp EEG of, 1093
subdural EEG of, 1093
new MRI and functional imaging techniques for, 1088
on postsurgical seizure outcome, 1175–1176
resection for, 1087–1100
surgical strategies for, 1095–1098, 1096f–1099f
decision tree in, 1097, 1099f
dual pathology in, 1097–1098
with inferior temporal lobe astrocytoma, 1096, 1098f
with right frontal lobe astrocytoma, 1095, 1097f
with temporal lobe ganglioglioma, 1095, 1096f
Focal malformations of cortical development, epilepsy surgery in, 1103–1109. *See also* Cortical developmental malformations, focal
Focal motor seizures, 261–265. *See also* Epilepsia partialis continua; Motor cortex; Supplementary sensorimotor area (SSMA) seizures
benign focal epilepsy of childhood, 270–271
classification of, 262 (*See also* Classification, of seizures)

clinical semiology of, 262
clonic, 262–263
definition of, 225, 261–262
differential diagnosis of, 272–273
EEG findings in, 264–265, 265f–267f
hemiconvulsion-hemiplegia-epilepsy syndrome in, 272
hemispheric epilepsy in, 272
history of, 257
oculocephalic deviation in, 264
Rasmussen syndrome in, 271–272
tonic, 263–264
versive, 264
vocalization or arrest of vocalization in, 264
Focal motor status epilepticus, 266
Focal neocortical epilepsies, MRI for, 1013–1022, 1014t, 1015f–1021f, 1016t
epileptogenic zone and lesion in, 1022
with initial negative MRI, 1019–1022, 1019f
negative mass effect in, 1015–1016
no mass effect/cortical development malformations in, 1016–1019, 1016t, 1017f–1021f
positive mass effect/mass lesion in, 1013–1015, 1014t, 1015f, 1016f
protocol for, 1010t, 1013
role of, 1013
Focal seizures with impaired consciousness, 241–251
amnesia in, 242
from different locations, 242–244
EEG features of, 248–250
ictal, 249–250, 250f, 251f
interictal, 248–249, 248f, 249f
focal epilepsy in, 242
of frontal lobe origin, 243
historical background on, 241
loss of consciousness in, 242
of occipital lobe origin, 244
of parietal lobe origin, 244
semiologic features of, 244–248
auras, 244–245
automatisms, 245–246, 246t
autonomic phenomena, 248
language disturbances, 247–248
motor phenomena, 246–247
of temporal lobe origin, 243–244
terminology for, 241–242
treatment of, 250–251
unresponsiveness in, 242
Folate malabsorption, congenital, 554
Folic acid, for neural tube defect prevention, 713
Folinic acid–responsive neonatal seizures, 500–501
Follicle-stimulating hormone (FSH), 696, 697f
Foramen of Monro giant cell astrocytomas, 7f
Forced thinking, 237
Forebrain commissure development, 22
Fosphenytoin, 785–798. *See also* Phenytoin
absorption and bioavailability of, 789
adverse effects of, 797

chemistry and mechanism of action of, 786, 786f
clinical use of, 798
distribution of, 789
drug interactions of, 791, 791t–793t
efficacy of, 795 (*See also* Phenytoin, efficacy of)
excretion of, 790
formulations of, 786t
historical background on, 785
indications for, 1212t
metabolism of, 789–790, 790f
plasma concentrations of, 790
other medications on, 666t–667t
on plasma concentrations of other drugs, 668t–669t
for poststroke patients, 530
for status epilepticus, 615
Fragile X, 483
Frequency measures, of epilepsy, 14t, 112, 113t
Frontal lobe epilepsy, 367–369
anterior frontopolar, 368
benign, 386
cingulate gyrus, 369
dorsolateral, 368–369
EEG of, 174
frontal sharp waves, 204f, 205f
subclinical EEG seizure, 206f
international classification of, 355–356
orbitofrontal, 368
supplementary sensorimotor area, 368
Frontal lobe seizures
focal, with impaired consciousness, 243
right, video-EEG of, 999, 1003f–1004f
right mesial, SISCOM study of, 1005, 1005f, 1006
Frontopolar epilepsy, anterior, 368
Fructose-1,6-bisphosphatase aldolase deficiency, 552
Fructose-1,6-bisphosphatase deficiency, 552
Fructose intolerance, hereditary, 552
Fukuyama muscular dystrophy (lissencephaly type 2), 25, 25t, 29, 45
Functional hemispherectomy, 1119, 1120f
Functional localization studies
of epileptogenic regions, 1094–1095, 1094f
for lesional epilepsy, 1088
with subdural electrodes, 1061–1062
Functional magnetic resonance imaging (fMRI), 1047–1048
[^{15}O] water PET and, 1047–1048
advantages and limitations of, 1053
of epileptogenic regions, 1093
ictal and interictal localization with, 1053
language lateralization and localization with, 1049–1051, 1050f–1052f
memory studies with, 1051–1052
motor and sensory mapping with, 1048–1049, 1049f
principles of, 1048–1049
Functional mapping, intraoperative, 1064

Functional neuroimaging, 1041–1058. *See also* Neuroimaging, metabolic and functional

G
G protein signaling pathways, 83
GABA (γ-aminobutyric acid). *See also* GABA
in absence seizures, 312
in neonatal seizures, 490, 490f
GABA receptors, 94–95
epilepsies linked to, 106
GABA$_A$ receptors, 94–95, 831
neonatal seizures on, 490, 490f
studies of, 1043–1044, 1044t
GABA$_B$ receptors, 95, 312
Gabapentin, 855–865
adverse effects of, monitoring for, 740
age-specific dosing of, 677t
for benign childhood epilepsy with centrotemporal spikes, 381
chemistry of, 855, 856f
cognitive effects of, 1187–1188
concentration–effect relationship of, 859
drug interactions of, 858
efficacy and safety of, clinical studies of, 859–863
as adjunctive, open-label, 860–861
as adjunctive, placebo-controlled, 859–860, 859t
as monotherapy, 862–863
pediatric, 863
in elderly, 595t, 596t, 599
for focal epilepsies, symptomatic, 371
for generalized tonic-clonic seizures, 298, 300
indications for, 1212t
for juvenile myoclonic epilepsy, 396
mechanisms of action of, 856–857, 856t
optimizing therapy with, 865
pharmacokinetics of, 655–659, 656t (*See also* Pharmacokinetics, of antiepileptic drugs)
absorption in, 857, 857t
distribution in, 858
elimination in, 858
in infants and children, 674
in pregnancy, 706–708, 707t
for poststroke patients with seizures, 530
in renal and liver disease, 727
safety and toxicity of, 863–865, 864t
teratogenicity of, 712
Galactosialidosis, 559
γ-hydroxybutyric acid (GHB), 580
in absence seizures, 312
γ-hydroxybutyric acid (GHB) metabolism disorders, 556
γ-hydroxybutyric aciduria, 556
Ganglioglioma, MRI of, 1014, 1015f, 1090, 1095, 1096f
and pathology, 1090, 1095, 1096f
Ganglionic eminence, 20, 21f
Gastaut-type benign occipital epilepsy of childhood, 383–384, 383f, 384f

Gastrointestinal disease, 578
Gastrulation, 14
Gastrulation disorders, 23
Gating, channel
mechanisms of, 70–73, 70f–73f
of voltage-dependent ion channels, 71f, 72f, 81–82, 82f (*See also* Voltage-dependent (-gated) ion channels)
Gaucher disease, juvenile, 362
Gaucher disease type II, 559
Gaucher disease type III, EEG of, 419f
GEFS+. *See* Generalized epilepsy with febrile seizures plus (GEFS+)
General anesthetics, 578t, 579
Generalized cryptogenic or symptomatic (age-related) epilepsies, 359–360
Generalized epilepsies, 358. *See also* Absence seizures
cryptogenic, 347–348
encephalopathic, 429–438 (*See also* Encephalopathic generalized epilepsy)
idiopathic and symptomatic, 347
PET in evaluation of, 1045
primary and secondary, 347
probably symptomatic, 349
Generalized epilepsies, EEG atlas of, 183–184, 192f–198f
childhood absence epilepsy
absence seizure, 192f
absence status epilepticus, 193f
infantile spasms
hypsarrhythmia, 195f
seizure, 195f
intractable epilepsy with multifocal spikes, 197f
juvenile myoclonic epilepsy, 194f
Lennox-Gastaut syndrome
atonic seizures, 197f, 325f
generalized paroxysmal fast and polyspikes in sleep, 196f
generalized sharp- and slow-wave complexes, 196f
stimulation-related epilepsy, reading-induced spike-and-wave complexes, 198f
Generalized epilepsy with febrile seizures plus (GEFS+), 320, 401–402, 516
Generalized seizures, 227. *See also* Absence seizures
Generalized symptomatic of nonspecific etiology epilepsies (age-related), 360
Generalized tonic-clonic seizures (GTCSs), 227, 279–300
classification of, 279–282
epilepsy syndrome classification in, 280–282
historical overview of, 279
terminology in, 280
clinical and physiologic manifestations of, 282–289
complications in, 287–289, 288f
immediate postictal phase, 285, 285f
immediate pre–tonic-clonic phase, 283–284

Generalized tonic-clonic seizures
(GTCSs), *(Continued)*
postictal recovery phase, 285–287,
285f, 286f, 286t
premonitory symptoms and
precipitating factors in, 283, 283t
tonic-clonic phase, 284–285, 284f,
285f
EEG manifestations of, 289–295
ictal findings, 294–295, 295f–297f
incidental interictal epileptiform
activity, 294
interictal epileptiform activity,
290–291, 292f, 293f
nonepileptiform activity, 285f,
289–290, 290f, 291f
photoparoxysmal response, 291, 293f
secondary generalized interictal
epileptiform activity, 291–293,
293f, 294f
epidemiologic factors in, 282
genetics and inheritance in, 281–282
idiopathic, 280–282
in juvenile myoclonic epilepsy, 393
prognosis in, 295–296, 299f
therapy in, 296–300
antiepileptic drug, monotherapy,
296–297
antiepileptic drug, newer, 298–300
carbamazepine, 297–298
felbamate, 297, 298–299
gabapentin, 298, 300
lamotrigine, 297, 298, 299
levetiracetam, 300
oxcarbazepine, 300
phenobarbital, phenytoin, and
valproate (valproic acid),
297–298
polytherapy and polypharmacy,
rational, 297
tiagabine, 298, 299
topiramate, 298, 299
valproate, 297–299
vigabatrin, 298, 300
zonisamide, 298, 299–300
Generalized tonic-clonic seizures only,
epilepsy with, 400–401
Genes, in pharmacogenetics of
antiepileptic drugs, 747–753. *See
also* Pharmacogenetics, of
antiepileptic drugs
Genetic testing
for cobblestone brain malformations, 48
for cortical-band heterotopia, 48
for hemimegalencephaly, 47
for heterotopia, 48
for lissencephaly, 48
for megalencephaly syndromes, 48
for microcephaly, primary, 48
for perisylvian polymicrogyria, 49
for periventricular nodular heterotopia,
48
for schizencephaly, 49
for subcortical-band (laminar)
heterotopia, 48
for tuberous sclerosis, 48
for X-linked lissencephaly, 48

Genetics, 103–106
of absence epilepsy, childhood,
397–398
of absence seizures, 310–311, 311f
of benign childhood epilepsy with
centrotemporal spikes, 375
of benign occipital epilepsy of
childhood, 382
in brain malformations, 31t, 32
of febrile seizures, 511–512
of idiopathic generalized epilepsies,
105–106
indications of, 104
of juvenile myoclonic epilepsy,
393–395
of neonatal seizures, chronic, 503
in ontogenesis programming, 22–23
in posttraumatic epilepsy, 522
of progressive myoclonus epilepsies,
419, 420t
mapping of, 281
rationale for evaluation for, 104–105
of tuberous sclerosis, 537–538
Genital automatisms, in focal seizures,
246
Gestural automatisms, in focal seizures,
246
Giant cell astrocytomas, 7f
Glial cells
in EEG, 129–130, 129f
bioelectric activity of, 127, 128f
in epileptogenicity, 95–98, 96f, 97f
Glial proliferation malformations, with
normal cell types, 39t, 41–42,
41f
Glioblastoma multiforme, 10f
Gliosis, 3f, 9f
MRI features and pathology of,
1091–1092
Global tonic seizures, 321
Globoid cell leukodystrophy, 553
Glucose metabolism disturbances,
572–573
Glut-1 deficiency syndrome, 552, 554
Glutamate receptors
AMPA and NMDA, 92–94, 93f
metabotropic, 94
Glycine encephalopathy, 500
Glycosylation, congenital disorders of,
558
G_{M1} gangliosidosis types I and II, 553
Gonadotropin-releasing hormone
(GnRH), 696, 697, 697f
Gradiometers, 160
Grand mal seizures. *See* Tonic-clonic
seizures
Granulomatous vasculitis, 581
Grids (subdural electrode), 1061–1064,
1062f, 1063f
for focal cortical developmental
malformations, 1105–1106, 1105f
identification of, 1105–1107, 1105f
proposed indications for, 1106–1107
functional localization studies with,
1061–1062
Growth, 13
Growth cone, 17

Growth factors, in apoptosis, 16
Growth hormone, epilepsy on, 697
Guanidinoacetate *N*-methyltransferase
deficiency, 554
Gustatory auras, 225, 230t, 232t, 233t,
235
Gyration, cerebral cortex, 21–22, 25

H
H_2-blockers, 580
Hallervorden-Spatz disease, 559
Hallucinations, structured, 226, 236–237,
236t
Halogenated inhalational anesthetics, 580
Hamamartomatosis, congenital. *See*
Tuberous sclerosis
Hamartia, 7f
Hamartomas
hypothalamic (*See* Hypothalamic
hamartomas)
retinal, 6f, 7f
Hand automatisms, in focal seizures, 246
Handicaps, multiple, epilepsy with,
585–591
autism, 587–588, 588t
cerebral palsy, 587
diagnostic evaluation of, 589
Landau-Kleffner syndrome, 588–589,
589t
mental retardation, 585–587, 586t
therapy for, 589–591, 590f
Harkoseride, 940t, 941
Hashimoto encephalopathy, 573
Hashimoto thyroiditis, 573
Head banging in infants
asleep, 631
awake, 632
Head drops, in children, 636
Head nodding, in children, 636
Head rolling, in infancy, 632
Head tilt, 639
Head trauma
from generalized tonic-clonic seizures,
287
posttraumatic epilepsy from, 521–524
(*See also* Posttraumatic epilepsy)
Head turning. *See* Version
Head version. *See* Version
Headaches
in children, 635–636
ictal, 232t, 233t, 235–236, 636
Heavy metal intoxication, 580
Hemiconvulsion, 263, 272
Hemiconvulsion–hemiplegia–epilepsy
(HHE) syndrome, 272, 483–484,
484f
Hemicorticectomy, 1119
Hemidecortication, 1119
Hemimegalencephaly, 30–32, 38–40, 38f,
38t, 39t
genetic testing and counseling for, 48
hemispherectomy for, 1115–1116, 1115f
MRI of, 1016, 1017f
Hemiplegia
alternating, of childhood, 634
in hemiconvulsion-hemiplegia-epilepsy
syndrome, 272, 483–484, 483f

Hemiplegia-hemiatrophy-epilepsy (HHE) syndrome, 361
Hemispherectomy, 1111–1121
  complications of, 1120–1121
  diagnostic evaluations in, 1112–1115
    functional imaging, 1112–1113
    history, 1112
    neurologic, 1112
    neuropsychological, 1113–1115
    structural imaging, 1112
    video EEG studies, 1113
  for hemimegalencephaly, 1115–1116, 1115f
  historical and background considerations in, 1111
  for porencephaly, 1115
  for Rasmussen syndrome, 1116
  results with, 1119–1120
  for Sturge-Weber syndrome, 1116, 1117f
  surgical procedures in, 1116–1119
    anatomic hemispherectomy in, 1118–1119
    functional hemispherectomy in, 1119, 1120f
    hemidecortication and hemicorticectomy in, 1119
    hemispherotomy in, 1119
    Oxford modification in, 1119
  for unilateral cortical dysplasia, extensive, 1116
Hemispheric epilepsy, 272
Hemispherotomy, 1119
Hemodialysis patient, 574
Hepatic disease. See Liver disease
Hepatic encephalopathy, 578
Hepatic metabolism, age on, 672, 672f
Hereditary fructose intolerance, 552
Herniation, diaphragmatic, from generalized tonic-clonic seizures, 288
Heroin, seizures from, 501, 579–580
Heterotopia, 24, 39t, 42–45
  band, 28–29, 28f
    MRI of, 1019, 1020f
  cortical-band, genetic testing and counseling for, 48
  genes in, 25t
  genetic testing and counseling for, 48
  nodular, 4f
  periventricular nodular, 27–28, 39t, 42–43, 42f
  subcortical-band (laminar), 28–29, 28f, 39t, 43–44, 44f
    genes in, 25t
    genetic testing and counseling for, 48
Heterotopic gray matter, 5f
High-field MRI, 1024
Hippocampal changes, MRI and video-EEG of, 1005, 1005f
Hippocampal gyrus calcification, epilepsy with, 543
Hippocampal sclerosis, 3f, 59–66, 1069–1081
  anatomic pathology of, 60
  epileptogenesis mechanisms in, 61–65, 65f, 66f
  etiology of, 1070

febrile seizures and, 515
history of, 59
medical treatment for, 1070–1071
neurophysiology of, 65–66
pathogenesis of, 61–62
pathologic findings in, 1069
surgery for, 1071–1080
  with bitemporal epilepsy, 1078–1079
  case reports on, 1080–1081
  with clinical seizures, 1075
  dual pathology in, 1079–1080
  functional neuroimaging for, 1076
  neuropsychological assessment in, 1076
  patient selection for, 1071–1073, 1072f–1075f, 1076–1077
  predictors of outcome in, 1078
  procedures and outcome in, 1077–1078
  quality of life in, 1078
Hippocampal shape analysis, 1013
Hippocampus
  anatomy of, 55–56, 56f, 57f
  connections of, 58–59, 62f
  direct intrahippocampal pathway in, 59, 64f
  histology of, 56–58, 58f–63f
  layers of, 57, 60f–62f
  ontogeny of, 22
  polysynaptic pathway in, 58–59, 61f–63f
  subfields of, 57, 63f
Hirschsprung disease, neurocristopathies in, 23
Histamine ligand studies, 1044, 1044t
Histidase deficiency, 556
Histidinemia, 556
Historical control, 649–650
HIV, CNS infections in, 576–577
Hodgkin-Huxley experiments and model, 72f–74f, 73–74, 81
Holocarboxylase synthetase deficiency, 552
Holoprosencephaly, 23, 25t, 26–27
Homeobox genes, 503
Homocystinuria, 558
Homonymous hemianopsia, vs. epilepsy, 639–640
Homunculus, motor, 260f
Hormones
  in apoptosis, 16
  disturbances of, in epilepsy, 697–698
  reproductive (See also specific hormones)
    changes in, on seizures, 698
    on neuronal excitability, 695–696
    seizures on, 696–697, 697f
Hot water epilepsy, 471
Human immunodeficiency virus (HIV), CNS infections in, 576–577
Human microsomal epoxide hydrolase (mEH), 750
Huntington's disease, infantile, 361
Hydatid disease, of CNS, 577
Hydrocephalic attacks, 639
Hydrocephalus, 7f
  shunted, 639
  X-linked, with pachygyria/polymicrogyria, 25t, 30

5-Hydroxy-L-tryptophan, for progressive myoclonic epilepsies, 422
Hyperammonemia, 578
  from valproate, 779
Hyperbaric oxygenation, 580
Hyperexcitability, 91–98
  acetylcholine receptors in, 95
  adenosine receptors in, 95
  AMPA and NMDA glutamate receptors in, 92–94, 93f
  chemical and electrical interactions in, 95
  extracellular space changes in, 95
  GABA receptors in, 94–95
  glial cells in epileptogenicity and, 95–98, 96f, 97f
  hypersynchrony in, 95
  ion concentration changes in, 95
  metabotropic glutamate receptors in, 94
Hyperexplexia, in infants, 633
Hyperglycemia, nonketotic, seizures with, 572–573
  neonatal, 500, 548
Hyperornithinemia-hyperammonemia-homocitrullinuria syndrome, 555
Hyperphenylalaninemias, 555
Hypersynchrony, 95
  hypnagogic, 189f
Hyperthyroidism, 573
Hyperventilation effect, on EEG, 190f
Hypnagogic hypersynchrony, 189f
Hypnagogic paroxysmal dystonia, in sleeping children, 635
Hypnic jerks, 635
Hypocalcemia, 572
Hypoglycemia, 572–573, 578
Hypomagnesemia, 572
Hypomelanosis of Ito
  epilepsy with, 543
  neonatal seizures in, 502
Hypomotor, 242
Hyponatremia, 571–572, 768
Hypoparathyroidism, 573
Hypophosphatemia, 572
Hypopigmented macules, 6f
Hypothalamic hamartomas, 361, 1169–1170
  MRI of, 1019, 1021f
  newer operative techniques for
    pterional and frontotemporative approaches in, 1170
    transcallosal approach in, 1170–1171, 1171f
  stereotactic techniques for
    endoscopic approaches in, 1172
    stereotactic radiofrequency ablation in, 1171–1172, 1172f
    stereotactic radiosurgery in, 1172–1173
Hypothalamic–pituitary axis, 696, 697f
Hypothalamic–pituitary–gonadal axis, epilepsy on, 697
Hypothalamus, 696
Hypothyroidism, myelination disorders in, 26
Hypoxia
  adult, 575–576
  perinatal, 575

Hypsarrhythmia, 179f, 180, 931
  EEG of, 179f, 180, 336, 337f
  in infants and children, 195f, 1144
Hysterical seizures. *See* Psychogenic
    nonepileptic seizures (PNES)

I

Ictal headaches, 232t, 233t, 235–236, 636
Ictal patterns, in partial epilepsies, 172
Ictal recording, 170
Ictal vomiting, in focal seizures, 248
Idiopathic, 391
Idiopathic generalized epilepsies
  age-related, 358–359
  of childhood and adolescence, 391–402
    childhood absence epilepsy, 396–399
      (*See also* Absence epilepsy,
        childhood)
    epilepsy with generalized tonic-clonic
        seizures only, 400–401
    generalized epilepsy with febrile
        seizures plus, 320, 401–402
    juvenile absence epilepsy, 399–400
    juvenile myoclonic epilepsy, 392–396
      (*See also* Juvenile myoclonic
        epilepsy)
    as part of generalized epilepsy
        spectrum, 402
  definition of, 391
  genetics of, 105–106
  specific syndromes as continuum in,
      391–392
  terminology in, 391
Idiopathic localization-related epilepsies,
    358
Idiopathic partial epilepsies of childhood,
    373–386. *See also* Benign
    childhood epilepsy with
    centrotemporal spikes
    (BCECTS); Benign occipital
    epilepsy (BOE); Benign partial
    epilepsies syndromes, childhood
Idiosyncratic reactions, 737, 737t. *See also*
    Adverse effects, of antiepileptic
    drugs
  to antiepileptic drugs, monitoring for,
      737, 737t
  to fosphenytoin, 796
  to phenytoin, 796
ILAE classification. *See also* Classification,
    of epilepsies
  1989, 347–348
ILAE proposal (syndrome-oriented
    classification). *See also*
    Classification, of epilepsies
  2001, 348–349, 348t
Illusions, 226, 236–237, 236t
Image-guided navigational surgical
    technique, for nonlesional
    epilepsy, 1137–1138, 1137f
Immediate seizures, posttraumatic, 522
Immune therapy, for Rasmussen
    encephalitis, 449
Immunocompromised, CNS infections in,
    576–577
Immunoglobulin (Ig). *See* Intravenous
    gammaglobulin (IVIG)

Immunoglobulin (Ig) G
    immunoadsorption, for
    Rasmussen encephalitis, 449, 450
Immunosuppressive therapy
  antiepileptic drugs with, 730–731
  for Rasmussen encephalitis, 450
Impact seizures, posttraumatic, 522
Impotence, 700
Impulsive petit mal, 359. *See also* Juvenile
    myoclonic epilepsy
Inborn errors of creatine metabolism, 554
Inborn errors of metabolism. *See also*
    specific disorders
  in adults, 362
  in children and adolescents, 362
  in infants and children, 361
  neonatal seizures from, 499–501
Incidence, 112, 113t, 114t
Incontinentia pigmenti, epilepsy with,
    542–543
Inductions, 625
Indusium griseum, 22
Infant apnea, 634
Infantile neuroaxonal dystrophy, 559
Infantile spasms. *See also* Spasms, epileptic
  ACTH for, 931–934, 933t
    adverse effects of, 933–934
    brain-adrenal axis in, 932
    efficacy and dosing of, 932–933, 933t
    mechanism of action of, 932
    recommended protocols for, 934,
        935t
    vs. vigabatrin, 934
  definition and classification of, 359
  differential diagnosis of, 338–340,
      339t, 340t
  EEG of
    hypsarrhythmia in, 195f
    seizure in, 195f
  epilepsy surgery in infants and children
      and, 1144–1147, 1145f–1148f
  general considerations in, 931–932
  prednisone for, 934
Infants, epilepsies in, 477–480,
    1143–1156. *See also specific*
    epilepsies
  anatomic and functional neuroimaging
      in, 1147–1149, 1148f
  benign, 479–480
    benign myoclonic epilepsy of infancy,
        328, 359, 409–411, 413,
        479–480
    benign partial epilepsy of infancy,
        385, 479
  diagnostic evaluation of, *vs.* adults,
      1143, 1144t
  EEG recording of, 179f, 180
  etiologies and pathologic substrates in,
      1145f–1147f, 1149, 1149f–1155f
  scalp EEG patterns, infantile spasms,
      and focal cortical lesions in,
      1144–1147, 1145f–1148f
  seizure semiology in video EEG for, 1143
  severe myoclonic, 413–414
  surgery for, 1149–1156
    age-related risks in, 1150f–1154f,
        1154–1155

goals of, 1152–1154
identification of candidates in,
    1149–1152
seizure outcome after, 1155–1156
symptomatic generalized, 477–479
  early infantile epileptic
      encephalopathy in, 478, 504
  early myoclonic encephalopathy in,
      360, 409, 477–478, 478f,
      503–504, 505f
  migrating partial seizures of infancy
      in, 478–479, 479f, 503, 504f
Infarct
  electrode-related, 11f
  remote, 8f
Infections, 576–577
  after liver and renal transplantation, 731
  systemic, 577
Infertility, 699
Inflammatory bowel disease, 578
Inflammatory diseases, 1092
Inhalational anesthetics, for refractory
    status epilepticus, 615
Inheritance, 103–106. *See also* Genetics;
    specific disorders
  indications of, 104
  rationale for evaluation for, 104–105
Inherited metabolic and mitochondrial
    disorders, 547–566. *See also*
    Metabolic and mitochondrial
    disorders, inherited
Inhibitory postsynaptic potentials,
    128–129, 128f
Interactions, drug. *See* Drug interactions;
    specific drugs
Interferon-alpha, for Rasmussen
    encephalitis, 449
Interictal EEG, limitations of, 995f, 996
Interictal epileptiform patterns, in partial
    epilepsies, 171–172, 171f, 172f
Interictal imaging, 1022, 1022f
Interictal recording, 170
Intermediate zone, 19, 20f
International classification of epilepsies
    and epileptic syndromes,
    354–357. *See also* Classification,
    of epilepsies
  frontal lobe, 355–356
  occipital lobe, 357
Interstitiospinal tract, 258
Intoxication, 578–580, 578t
  heavy metal, 580
Intracarotid amobarbital procedure,
    1031–1038
  attention and emotion in, 1036
  criticism of, 1034
  for hippocampal sclerosis, 1076
  history of, 1031
  language assessment in, 1032–1033
  methodology for, 1031–1032
  predicting memory and seizure control
      outcomes from, 1035
  Wada memory testing in, 1033
    with children, 1035
    criticism of, 1033–1034
    Medical College of Georgia protocol
        for, 1036–1038

Intracranial electrode implantation, for nonlesional epilepsy, 1135–1136, 1135f
Intracranial electroencephalography, 1059–1066. *See also* Electroencephalography (EEG), intracranial
Intractability, medical, 983–989. *See also* Medical intractability
Intractable epilepsy, 993–994
  with multifocal spikes, 197f
Intrahippocampal pathway, direct, 59, 64f
Intraoperative electrocorticography, 1064
Intravenous gammaglobulin (IVIG)
  for epileptic spasms, 342–343
  for Rasmussen encephalitis, 449, 450
Intraventricular electrodes, 1064
Inward rectifier K$^+$ channels, 77
Ion channels
  general properties of, 70–73, 70f–73f
  identification of, 75
Ion channels and intrinsic membrane properties, 69–74
  action potential in, 73, 73f
  basis of electrical activity in, 69–70, 70f
  general properties of ion channels in, 70–73, 70f–73f (*See also specific channels*)
  Hodgkin-Huxley experiments and model in, 72f–74f, 73–74
Isoniazid, 578t, 579
Isopotential contour map, 148–150, 149f
Isovaleric aciduria, 550–551

J
Jacksonian epilepsy, 263
Jacksonian seizure, 225
Jansky Bielschowsky disease, 361
Jerks. *See* Chorea; Myoclonic jerks
Jitteriness, in infants, 631–632
Juvenile absence epilepsy, 359, 399–400
Juvenile myoclonic epilepsy, 359, 392–396, 394f, 415–416
  clinical features of, 392
  EEG of, 393, 394f
    cluster of myoclonic jerks in, 194f
    myoclonic jerk with photic stimulation in, 194f
  genetics and etiology of, 393–395
  history and epidemiology of, 392
  outcome and prognosis in, 396
  pharmacologic treatment of, 395–396
    in pregnancy, 396
  seizure semiology in, 392–393, 394f
  topiramate for, 880–881

K
K$^+$ channels. *See* Potassium (K$^+$) channels
Kainic acid–induced seizures, 99
Kallman syndrome, genes in, 25t
KCNQ2/3 K$^+$ channels, and benign familial neonatal convulsions, 84, 503
Kearns-Sayre syndrome, 638
Keratan sulfate, 17
Ketamine, 578t, 579, 580
  for refractory status epilepticus, 615

Ketogenic diet, 961–966
  administration of, 963–964
  adverse effects of, 964–965
  clinical indications and effectiveness of, 965–966
  for epileptic spasms, 342
  historical background on, 961
  for Lennox-Gastaut syndrome, 437
  for myoclonus in atypical seizures, 327
  scientific basis of, 962–963
Ketone bodies, 961–962
Ketosis, 572–573
Ketotic hyperglycemia, 500
Kidney disease. *See* Renal disease
Kidney transplantation
  antiepileptic drugs in, 730–731
  seizures after, 731
Kindling model, 98–99
Kinky hair disease, 556
Klinefelter syndrome (47, XXY), 483
Kojewnikow syndrome, 228, 265–268, 356. *See also* Epilepsia partialis continua; Rasmussen encephalitis (syndrome)
Kozhevnikov syndrome. *See* Epilepsia partialis continua
Krabbe disease, 553
Kuf's disease, 362
Kv1.1 K$^+$ channel, and episodic ataxia type 1, 84

L
Lafora bodies, 10f
Lafora body disease, 420–421, 420t, 421t
Lafora disease, 10f, 362, 560
Laminated architecture, 19
Lamotrigine, 869–873
  for absence epilepsy
    childhood, 398
    juvenile, 400
  absorption, distribution, and metabolism of, 869–870
  adverse effects of, monitoring for, 740, 741t
  for atypical seizures, 326–327
  chemistry and mechanism of action of, 869, 870f
  cognitive effects of, 1188
  dosing of
    age-specific, 677t
    strategies for, 872–873
  drug interactions of, 870–871
  efficacy of, 871
  in elderly, 595t, 596t, 599
  for epileptic spasms, 342
  for focal epilepsies, symptomatic, 370–371
  for generalized tonic-clonic seizures, 297, 298, 299
  indications for, 1212t
  for juvenile myoclonic epilepsy, 395–396, 422
  for Lennox-Gastaut syndrome, 436
    myoclonic jerks from, 423
    myoclonic seizures from, 422
  other medications on plasma concentration of, 666t

pharmacokinetics of, 655–659, 656t (*See also* Pharmacokinetics, of antiepileptic drugs)
  in infants and children, 674
  in pregnancy, 706–708, 707t
  for poststroke patients, 530
  in renal and liver disease, 726–727
  teratogenicity of, 711–712
  tolerability and adverse events with, 871–872, 872t
Landau-Kleffner syndrome, 361, 458–460, 588–589, 589t
  ACTH and steroids for, 936
Language assessment. *See also* Wada memory testing
  in intracarotid amobarbital procedure, 1032–1033
  in Medical College of Georgia Wada protocol, 1036–1037
Language disturbances, in focal seizures, 247–248
Language-induced epilepsy, 469
Language lateralization and localization, with fMRI, 1049–1051, 1050f–1052f
Late-onset Batten disease, 559–560
Late-onset multiple carboxylase deficiency, 553
Late-onset myoclonic epilepsy in Down syndrome (LOMEDS), 482
Lateral temporal seizures, 355
Lead intoxication, 580
Left arm tonic seizure, in perirolandic epilepsy, 210f
Leigh syndrome, 551–552
Lennox-Gastaut syndrome, 429–438
  ACTH and steroids for, 934–936
  definition and classification of, 359
  differential diagnosis of, 435–436, 435t
  from early infantile epileptic encephalopathy, 478
  EEG of, 431–434, 432f, 433f
    atonic seizures in, 197f, 325f
    generalized paroxysmal fast and polyspikes in sleep in, 196f
    generalized sharp- and slow-wave complexes in, 196f
  etiology of, 434, 434t
  from lamotrigine, in children, 871
  neuroimaging of, 435
  neurologic dysfunction in, 434
  neuropathology of, 434–435
  prognosis in, 437–438
  seizure types in, 430–431
  with severe myoclonic epilepsy of infants, 414
  topiramate for, 880
  treatment of, 436–437
  vigabatrin in, 925
Leptomeninges, 4f
Lesional epilepsy
  MRI for, 1088
  surgery for, 994
Leukodystrophy
  globoid cell, 553
  metachromatic, 557

Levetiracetam, 901–904
 absorption, distribution, and
  metabolism of, 902
 adverse effects of, 903–904, 904t
 age-specific dosing of, 677t
 for atypical tonic seizures, 327
 chemistry of, 901, 902f
 clinical use of, 904
 cognitive effects of, 1188
 drug interactions of, 902
 efficacy of, 903
 in elderly, 595t, 596t, 599–600
 for focal epilepsies, symptomatic, 371
 for generalized tonic-clonic seizures,
  300
 indications for, 1212t
 for juvenile myoclonic epilepsy, 396
 for Lennox-Gastaut syndrome, 437
 mechanism of action of, 901–902
 for myoclonus in atypical seizures, 327
 pharmacokinetics of, 655–659, 656t
  (See also Pharmacokinetics, of
  antiepileptic drugs)
  in infants and children, 674–675
  in pregnancy, 706–708, 707t
 for poststroke patients, 530
 in renal and liver disease, 729–730
 teratogenicity of, 712
Lidocaine, 578t, 579
 neonatal seizures from, 501
 for refractory status epilepticus, 615
Life-threatening events, apparent, in
  infants, 634
Ligand-gated channels, 71, 72f
Limbic encephalitis, 581
Limbic system, 55–56, 56f
Lindane, 578t, 579
Linear sebaceous nevi, 503
Linezolid, 579
Lissencephaly, 4f, 25, 43–45, 44f, 45t
 genes in, 25, 25t
 genetic testing and counseling for, 48
 MRI of
  classic, 1016
  cobblestone, 1017
  lissencephaly/pachygyria, 1017
 X-linked, 44–45, 45t
Lissencephaly-pachygyria, 361
Lissencephaly type 1 (Miller-Dieker
  syndrome), 29
 genes in, 25, 25t
 genetic testing and counseling for, 48
Lissencephaly type 2 (Walker-Warburg
  syndrome, Fukuyama muscular
  dystrophy, muscle-eye-brain
  disease of Santavuori, Meckel-
  Gruber syndrome), 29, 32, 45–46
 genes in, 25, 25t
Listeria monocytogenes infection, 576–577
Lithium, 578t, 579
Liver disease, antiepileptic drugs in,
  721–730
 benzodiazepines, 726
 carbamazepine, 725–726
 ethosuximide, 726
 felbamate, 727, 917
 gabapentin, 727

levetiracetam, 729–730
 overview of, 721–722, 721t, 722t
 oxcarbazepine, 727–728
 phenobarbital, 724
 phenytoin, 722–724, 723f
 primidone, 724
 tiagabine, 728–729
 topiramate, 728
 valproate (valproic acid), 724–725
 vigabatrin, 729
 zonisamide, 728
Liver transplantation
 antiepileptic drugs in, 730–731
 seizures after, 731
Loading dose, volume of distribution and,
  657–658
Local anesthetics, 578t
Localization, EEG in, 141–142, 154–157
 artifacts in, 155, 157f, 158f
 assumptions in, 154
 bipolar montage in
  with maximum negativity at end of
   chain, 155, 155f
  with phase reversal, 157, 158f
 centrotemporal distribution in, 155,
  158f
 choosing between two possibilities in,
  150f, 154–155, 155f–158f
 computer-aided methodology for,
  157–160
  dipole modeling in, 159–160
  topographic mapping in, 157–159,
   159f
 derivations and montages in, 146–147
 differential amplifiers in, 146, 146f
 instrumentation in, 146–147, 146f,
  147f
 localization rules in, 155–157, 158f
 polarity conventions in, 146, 147f
 rolandic spikes in, 155, 158f
 sharply contoured waveforms in, 155,
  156f
Localization-related epilepsies and
  syndromes, 357–358
Localization-related seizures. *See* Focal
  motor seizures
Long-term potentiation, 92–93
Longitudinal bipolar montage, 184f
Lorazepam, 839–840. *See also*
  Benzodiazepines
 adverse effects and drug interactions of,
  840
 clinical applications of, 840
 clinical pharmacology of, 836t
 in elderly, 595t, 600
 for febrile seizures, 517
 indications for, 1212t
 for neonatal seizures, 506
 pharmacokinetics of, 657t, 839
  in infants and children, 673
 for status epilepticus, 612–613, 613t,
  614–615
  emergency department or inpatient,
   616t, 617
  prehospital, 617
  refractory, 615
 structure of, 839, 839f

Loreclezole, 1212t
Luteinizing hormone (LH), 696, 697f
 epilepsy on, 697
Lyme disease, 576
Lysosomal disorders, 552–553, 558–559
 of early infancy, 552–553

M
M current, 77
Macules, hypopigmented, 6f
Magnetic resonance imaging (MRI).
  See also Functional magnetic
  resonance imaging (fMRI)
 arterial spin labeling (ASL), 1013
 of head with left occipital
  malformation, 999, 1003f
 of hippocampal changes, 1005, 1005f
 for lesional epilepsy, 1088
Magnetic resonance imaging (MRI), in
  epilepsy surgery evaluation,
  1009–1025
 for focal neocortical epilepsies,
  1013–1022, 1014t, 1015f–1021f,
  1016t (*See also* Focal neocortical
  epilepsies)
 future imaging perspectives and trends
  in, 1022–1025, 1022f–1024f
 curvilinear reconstructions/3D
  rendering in, 1024
 diffusion tensor imaging in, 1022,
  1023f
 high-field MRI in, 1024
 magnetization transfer imaging in,
  1022–1023
 multimodal imaging in, 1024–1025,
  1024f
 postictal and interictal imaging in,
  1022, 1022f
 semiautomated voxel-based
  morphometry in, 1023–1024,
  1023f
 for mesial temporal lobe epilepsy,
  1010–1013, 1011f, 1011t (*See also*
  Mesial temporal lobe epilepsy,
  MRI for)
 patient selection for, 1009
 type of MRI in, 1009–1010, 1010t
Magnetic resonance imaging (MRI)-
  negative epilepsy, 1125–1126
Magnetic resonance spectroscopy (MRS)
 of epileptogenic regions, 1093–1094,
  1094f
 for medial temporal lobe epilepsy, 1012
 for nonlesional epilepsy, 1133–1134,
  1133f
Magnetization transfer imaging,
  1022–1023
Magnetoencephalography (MEG),
  160–165, 1024–1025, 1024f
 field determination in, 161–162, 162f,
  163f
 localization in, 141–142, 162–165, 164f
 magnetometers and gradiometers in,
  160
 for nonlesional epilepsy, 1134–1135
 volume conduction in, 161
 waveforms in, 160–161, 161f

Magnetometers, 160
Malaria, cerebral, 577
Malformations
  cerebral (*See* Cerebral dysgenesis; *specific malformations*)
  congenital, in infants of mothers on antiepileptic drugs, 709–710, 710t, 738
  cortical developmental, 37–45 (*See also* Cortical developmental malformations)
    MRI of, 1016–1019, 1016t, 1017f–1021f
  in epilepsy, 361
Malignancy, 581
Malpractice cases, on antiepileptic drugs, 736–737, 736t
MAO-B ligand studies, 1044, 1044t
Maple syrup urine disease, 499–500, 550
Mapping, 141–142
  brain, [^{15}O] water PET in, 1048
  EEG in, 141–142
  of electrical fields, 147–150, 149f–151f
  fMRI in, 1048–1049, 1049f
  functional intraoperative, 1064
  genetic, of progressive myoclonic epilepsies, 281–282
  in scalp determination of electrical fields, 147–150, 149f–151f
  topographic, computer-aided, 157–159, 159f
March
  aura combinations and, 229–230
  epileptic, 225
Marginal zone, 19, 20f
Massive epileptic myoclonus, 319
Masturbation, infantile, 632
Maturation, 13
Maximum tolerated dose (MTD), 647, 663, 663t
MDR1 (ABCB1, PGY1), 751–752, 752f
Mechanism of action, of antiepileptic drugs. *See also specific drugs*
  differentiating, 646
Meckel-Gruber syndrome (lissencephaly type 2), 29
Medical intractability
  in children, 988
  definitions in, 983, 985–988, 985t
    drugs failed and treatment course in, 985–987, 986f, 986t
    intended context of, 984
    seizure frequency in, 985t, 987
    treatment duration in, 987–988
  future research on, 988–989
  imperfect compliance or inappropriate lifestyle in, 984
  inadequate dosage in, 984
  incorrect diagnosis in, 983
  incorrect drug choice in, 983–984
  pseudoresistance in, 983–984
Medically refractory status epilepticus of focal origin, surgical outcomes with, 1177
Medication-induced seizures, 578–579, 578t
  myoclonic, 422–423, 423t

Medroxyprogesterone, 698, 705
MEG. *See* Magnetoencephalography (MEG)
Megalencephaly syndromes, 39t, 41, 41f, 47
Membrane potential, 69–70, 70f
Membrane properties, intrinsic, 69–74. *See also* Ion channels and intrinsic membrane properties
Memory testing, Wada, 1033
  in children, 1035
  criticism of, 1033–1034
  Medical College of Georgia protocol for, 1036–1038
Meningitis, 576–577
Menkes disease, 556
Menkes kinky-hair disease, myelination disorders in, 26
Menopause, epilepsy at, 698
Menstrual cycle, seizures and, 698
Mental automatisms, in focal seizures, 245
Mental retardation
  causes of, 585, 586t
  epilepsy with, 585–587
Meperidine, 578t, 579
Mephenytoin
  indications for, 1212t
  pharmacokinetics of, 655–659, 656t (*See also* Pharmacokinetics, of antiepileptic drugs)
Mephobarbital, 949f, 951–953
  indications for, 1212t
Mepivacaine, 501
Mercury intoxication, 580
MERRF, 417–422, 420t, 421t, 560
Mesial temporal lobe epilepsy (MTLE), 365–366, 1065. *See also* Hippocampal sclerosis
  case report on, 1080
  MRI for, 1010–1013
    MR spectroscopy in, 1012
    new techniques in, 1013
    protocol in, 1010, 1011t
    qualitative assessment in, 1010–1012, 1011f
    quantitative assessment in, 1012
  surgery for, 994
  suspected bilateral, intracranial EEG for, 1065
Mesiobasal limbic seizures, 355
Metabolic and mitochondrial disorders, inherited, 547–566. *See also specific disorders*
  of childhood and adolescence, 558–561
    adrenoleukodystrophy (X-linked), 558
    dentatorubral-pallidoluysian atropha (DRPLA), 561
    diabetes mellitus, 558
    Gaucher disease type II, 559
    homocystinuria, 558
    Lafora disease, 560
    lysosomal disorders, 558–559
    mitochondrial encephalopathy with lactic acidosis and stroke-like episodes (MELAS), 560–561

    myoclonic epilepsy with ragged-red fibers (MERRF), 417–422, 420t, 421t, 560
    neuroaxonal dystrophies, 559
    neuronal ceroid lipofuscinosis type III, 559–560
    progressive myoclonus epilepsies, 560–561
    screening tests for, 564t–565t
    sialidosis type I, 558–559
    sialidosis type II, 559
    Unverricht-Lundborg progressive familial myoclonic epilepsy, 560
  diagnostic investigation of, 561–563, 562t, 563t
  of early infancy, 552–557
    3-phosphoglycerate dehydrogenase deficiency, 556
    amino acid disorders, 555–556
    arginase deficiency, 556
    biotinidase deficiency, 553
    congenital folate malabsorption, 554
    γ-hydroxybutyric acid metabolism disorders, 556
    glut-1 deficiency syndrome, 554
    G_{M1} gangliosidosis types I and II, 553
    histidinemia (histidase deficiency), 556
    hyperornithinemia-hyperammonemia-homocitrullinuria syndrome, 555
    hyperphenylalaninemias, 555
    inborn errors of creatine metabolism, 554
    Krabbe disease, 553
    late-onset multiple carboxylase deficiency, 553
    lysosomal disorders, 552–553
    Menkes disease (kinky hair disease), 556
    methylenetetrahydrofolate reductase deficiency, 554
    organic acidurias, 555
    phenylketonuria, 555
    progressive encephalopathy with edema, hypsarrhythmia, and optic neuropathy, 556–557
    Sandhoff disease, 553
    screening tests for, 564t
    Tay-Sachs disease, 552–553
    tyrosinemia type III, 555
    urea cycle defects, 556
    vitamin metabolism disorders, 553–554
  of late infancy, 557–558
    Alpers disease (progressive infantile poliodystrophy), 557–558
    congenital disorders of glycosylation, 558
    metachromatic leukodystrophy, 557
    mucopolysaccharidoses, 557
    neuronal ceroid lipofuscinoses, 557
    Schindler disease, 557
    screening tests for, 564t
  in newborn, 548–552
    acycloenzyme A oxidase deficiency, 549–550

Metabolic and mitochondrial disorders, inherited *(Continued)*
carbohydrate metabolism disorders, 552
early onset multiple carboxylase deficiency (holocarboxylase synthetase deficiency), 552
fatty acid oxidation defects, 551
fructose-1,6-biphosphatase deficiency, 552
glut-1 deficiency syndrome, 552
hereditary fructose intolerance (fructose-1,6-biphosphatase aldolase deficiency), 552
Leigh syndrome, 551–552
maple syrup urine disease, 550
molybdenum cofactor deficiency, 548–549
neonatal adrenoleukodystrophy, 549
nonketotic hyperglycinemia, 548
organic acidurias, 550–551
peroxisomal disorders, 549–550
pyridoxine dependency, 548
pyruvate carboxylase deficiency, 551
pyruvate dehydrogenase deficiency, 551
screening tests for, 564t
sulfite oxidase deficiency, 548–549
urea cycle disorders, 550
Zellweger syndrome, 549
screening tests for, 564t–565t
treatment of, 563, 565
Metabolic disorders, seizures with, 571–574, 575t
adrenal, 573
glucose metabolism, 572–573
hypocalcemia, 572
hypomagnesemia, 572
hyponatremia, 571–572
hypoparathyroidism, 573
hypophosphatemia, 572
ketosis, 572–573
thyroid, 573
uremia, 573–574
Metabolic neuroimaging, 1041–1058. *See also* Neuroimaging, metabolic and functional
Metabolism, of antiepileptic drugs. *See specific drugs*
Metabotropic glutamate receptors, 94
Metachromatic leukodystrophy, 557
Methamphetamine, 579–580
Metharbital, 1212t
Methotrexate, 580
Methsuximide, 949–951
absorption, distribution, and metabolism of, 950
chemical structure of, 949f
chemistry and mechanism of action of, 949–950
drug interactions of, 951
efficacy and clinical use of, 950–951
historical background on, 949
indications for, 1212t
for juvenile myoclonic epilepsy, 416
pharmacokinetics of, 655–663, 656t (*See also* Pharmacokinetics, of antiepileptic drugs)

Methylenetetrahydrofolate reductase deficiency, 554
Methylmalonic acidemia, 500, 551
Methylxanthines, 578t, 579
Microcalcifications, 7f
Microcephaly, primary
genes in, 25t
genetic testing and counseling for, 48
Microcephaly syndromes, 39t, 41–42, 41f
Microdysgenesis, cortical, 46–47
Micropolygyria, 4f
Microsomal epoxide hydrolase (mEH), 750
Midazolam, 840–842. *See also* Benzodiazepines
adverse effects and drug interactions of, 841
clinical applications of, 841–842
clinical pharmacology of, 836t
indications for, 1212t
pharmacokinetics of, 840–841
for status epilepticus, 613
prehospital, 617
refractory, 615–616
structure of, 840, 841f
Midbrain agenesis, genes in, 25t
Migraine
in children, 636–637
basilar, 639
confusional, 637
familial hemiplegic, 84
Migrating partial seizures of infancy, 478–479, 503, 504f
Milk, breast, antiepileptic drugs in, 708–709
Miller-Dieker syndrome (lissencephaly 1), 29, 44, 45t
genes in, 25, 25t
genetic testing and counseling for, 48
neuroblast migration disorders in, 25
Mimetic automatisms, in focal seizures, 246
Minimum-norm estimation (MNE), 164–165, 164f
Mitochondrial disorders, inherited. *See* Metabolic and mitochondrial disorders, inherited; *specific disorders*
Mitochondrial encephalopathy with lactic acidosis and stroke-like episodes (MELAS), 560–561
Mitotic proliferation
disorders of, 24, 24f
of neuroblasts, 15
Molecular layer, 19, 20f
Molybdenum cofactor deficiency, 501, 548–549
Monitoring, for adverse effects of antiepileptic drugs, 735–743. *See also under* Adverse effects, of antiepileptic drugs
Monoamine oxidase inhibitors, 578t, 579
Montage
bipolar
longitudinal, 184f
with maximum negativity at end of chain, 155, 155f

with no phase reversal, 148, 151f, 151t, 152f
with phase reversal, 151t, 152, 152f, 157, 158f
transverse, 184f
field identification with
bipolar, 151–152, 151t, 152f
referential, 151t, 153, 153f
in localization with EEG, 146–147
Mortality, 121–122
Motor area, primary, 259–260, 260f
Motor area epilepsy, 369
Motor cortex
functional anatomy of, 257–261
efferent and afferent connections of, 258–259
major areas in, 257–258, 258f
premotor cortex in, 258f, 261
primary motor area in, 258f, 259–260, 260f
stimulation studies of, 259
supplementary sensorimotor area in, 260–261
historical work on, 257
Motor cortex afferents, 259
Motor cortex efferents, 258–259
Motor cortex epilepsies, 356
Motor homunculus, 260f
Motor phenomena, in focal seizures, 246–247
Motor signs, 225
Movement-induced seizures. *See* Proprioceptive-induced seizures
MRI-negative epilepsy, 1125–1126
MRP1 (ABCC1), 751–752, 752f
MRP2 (ABCC2), 751–752, 752f
Mucopolysaccharidoses, 557
Multidrug resistance-associated protein 1 (MRP1), 751
Multifocal myoclonus, in children, 635
Multifocal partial seizures, neonatal, 503, 504f
Multifocal spikes, EEG of intractable epilepsy with, 197f
Multimodal imaging, 1024–1025, 1024f
Multimodality image integration, for nonlesional epilepsy surgery, 1136–1137, 1136f
Multinucleation, 5f
Multiple carboxylase deficiency, early onset, 552
Multiple spike and wave, 176–177, 177f
Multiple subpial transection, 1163–1166
cortical surgical anatomy in, 1164
historical background on, 1163–1164
indications for, 1164
operative procedure in, 1164
at other centers, 1166, 1166t, 1167f
seizure outcome with, 1165, 1165t
surgical morbidity of, 1165–1166, 1166f
transections in, 1164–1165
Munchausen syndrome by proxy, 637–638, 638t
Muscle-eye-brain disease of Santavuori (lissencephaly type 2), 25, 25t, 29, 45–46
Musicogenic epilepsy, 469–470

Myelin, 18
Myelination, 18
Myelination disorders, 26
Myoclonic encephalopathy, early, 360
Myoclonic epilepsies, 319, 407–423
    absence, 414–415, 881
    classification by age of onset of, 409t
    clinical and EEG features of, 407–408,
        408f
    definition of, 407
    differential diagnosis of, 408, 408f
    drug-induced, 422–423, 423t
    etiology of, 408–409
    of infancy and early childhood,
        409–414
        benign myoclonic epilepsy of infancy,
            328, 359, 409–411, 413,
            479–480
        myotonic-astatic epilepsy, 411–413,
            412f
        severe myoclonic epilepsy of infants
            (Dravet syndrome), 413–414
    juvenile, 359, 392–396, 394f, 415–416
        clinical features of, 392
        EEG of, 393, 394f
            cluster of myoclonic jerks in, 194f
            myoclonic jerk with photic
                stimulation in, 194f
        genetics and etiology of, 393–395
        history and epidemiology of, 392
        outcome and prognosis in, 396
        pharmacologic treatment of, 395–396
            in pregnancy, 396
        seizure semiology in, 392–393, 394f
    of late childhood and adolescence,
        414–417
        juvenile myoclonic epilepsy, 415–416
        myoclonic (or clonic) absence
            epilepsy, 414–415
    in newborn, 409
        topiramate for, 881
    progressive, 560–561
    undefined epilepsies with myoclonic
        seizures, in late childhood and
        adolescence, 416–417
    with variable age of onset, 417–423
        Angelman syndrome, 417, 418f
        autosomal dominant cortical reflex
            myoclonus and epilepsy, 417
        (benign) familial autosomal dominant
            myoclonic epilepsy, 417
        epilepsies with prominent rhythmic
            distal clonus, 417, 418f
        progressive myoclonus epilepsies,
            417–422, 419f, 420t, 421t
            classification of, 420t
            EEG of, 418, 419f
            epidemiology of, 417–419
            genetic mapping of, 281
            Lafora body disease in, 420–421,
                420t, 421t
            molecular genetics of, 419, 420t
            neuronal ceroid lipofuscinoses in,
                420t, 421–422, 421t
            treatment of, 422
            Unverricht-Lunborg disease in,
                419–420, 420t, 421t

Myoclonic epilepsy with ragged-red fibers
    (MERRF), 417–422, 420t, 421t,
    560
Myoclonic infantile encephalopathy, 581
Myoclonic jerks, 319
    vs. clonic focal motor seizures, 263
    definition of, 227
    EEG of
        cluster of, 194f
        with photic stimulation, 194f
Myoclonic seizures
    atypical, 319–321, 320f
    in atypical tonic seizures, 323, 323f
    definition of, 227, 263
    drug-induced, 422–423, 423t
    in Lennox-Gastaut syndrome, 431
    photic stimuli–induced, 416–417
    undefined epilepsies with, in late child-
        hood and adolescence, 416–417
Myoclonus, 319
    benign, of early infancy, 632–633
    in children, 635
    cortical reflex, 319
    definition of, 392, 407
    etymology of, 392
    negative, 263
    reticular reflex, 319
Myotonic-astatic epilepsy, 411–413, 412f
Myxedema, 573

N

N-acetylcysteine, for progressive
    myoclonic epilepsies, 422
N-acetylglutamate synthetase deficiency,
    550
N current, 80
Narcolepsy, 214f, 638
Natural history, of seizures, 117–122
    comorbidity in, 122
    mortality in, 121–122
    predictors of intractable disease in,
        120–121
    prognostic predictors in, 119
    remission in
        predictors of successful medication
            withdrawal after, 119–120, 120f
        relapse after, 120
        from time of diagnosis, predictors of,
            118–119, 119f
        from time of first seizure, likelihood
            of, 117–118, 118t
Necrotizing vasculitis, 581
Negative myoclonus, 263
Negligence cases, on antiepileptic drugs,
    736–737, 736t
Neocortex, cerebral, ontogeny of, 19–20,
    20f, 21f
Neocortical epilepsies, focal, MRI for,
    1013–1022, 1014t, 1015f–1021f,
    1016t. See also Focal neocortical
    epilepsies
Neocortical temporal lobe epilepsy
    (NTLE), 366–367
Neonatal adrenoleukodystrophy, 549
Neonatal convulsions
    benign familial, KCNQ2/3 K+ channels
        and, 84

chronic postnatal epilepsy in, 506–507,
    506f
Neonatal outcome, 709–711, 710t
Neonatal seizures, 360, 487–510
    classification and clinical features of,
        487, 488f, 490–495, 492t
        clinical classification in, 491, 492t
        electroclinical associations in, 491
        electrographic seizures in, 491
        etiologic factors in, 495–504, 499t
        interictal background and prediction
            value in, 491–495
        measures of electrographic seizure
            "burden" in, 494–495,
            496f–499f
        morphology in, 493, 494f–495f
        spatial distribution in, 493, 497f
        special ictal EEG morphologies in,
            493–494
        temporal profile in, 493, 496f
        seizure pathophysiology in, 491, 493t
    definition of, 110
    EEG of, 179f, 180
    etiologic factors in
        acute, 495–501, 501t
            hypoxic-ischemic, 495–499, 500f,
                502f
            inborn errors of metabolism,
                499–501
            metabolic, 499, 499t
            neonatal intoxications, 501
        chronic, 501–504, 501t
            cerebral dysgenesis, 501–502, 503f
            epilepsy syndromes of early
                infantile onset, 503–504, 504f
            genetic conditions, 503
            neurocutaneous syndromes,
                502–503
            TORCH infections, 502
    etiology and mechanisms of, 487–488,
        488f
    historical background on, 487
    incidence of, 487
    inherent harm from, 489–490, 490f
    prognostic significance of, 488–489,
        489f
    treatment of, 504–507
        for chronic postnatal epilepsy,
            506–507, 506f
        deleterious effects of, on immature
            CNS, 507
Neonates
    EEG recording in, 179f, 180
    myoclonic epilepsies in, 409
    vitamin K deficiency in, with mothers
        on antiepileptic drugs, 710–711
Neoral, with antiepileptic drugs, 730
Neural crest, separation and migration of,
    15, 23
Neural induction, 13
Neural placode formulation, 14
Neural tube
    gradients of genetic expression in, 23
    segmentation of, 14–15, 23
Neurite, growth disorders of, 26
Neuroaxonal dystrophies, 559
Neuroblast, 13, 15

Neuroblast migration, 14, 16, 16f
Neuroblast migration disorders, 24–26, 25t
Neurocristopathies, 23
Neurocutaneous melanosis, epilepsy with, 543
Neurocutaneous syndromes
 cortical dysplasias and, 543
 epilepsy with, 537–543
  epidermal nevus syndrome, 542, 542f
  hippocampal gyrus calcification, 543
  hypomelanosis of Ito, 543
  incontinentia pigmenti, 542–543
  neurocutaneous melanosis, 543
  neurofibromatosis type I, 542
  Sturge-Weber syndrome, 540–541, 541f
  tuberous sclerosis, 537–540, 538f
  Urbach-Wieth disease, 543
 neonatal seizures from, 502–503
Neurocysticercosis, 113–114, 577
Neurodevelopmental effects, of antiepileptic drugs in utero, 1189–1191
 animal studies of, 1189
 human studies of, 1189–1190
 possible mechanisms of, 1190–1191
Neuroepithelial cell, 13
Neuroepithelial tumor, dysembryoplastic, 9f, 10f
 MRI of, 1014, 1016f, 1090
Neurofibromatosis type I, epilepsy with, 542
Neuroimaging. See also specific types
 with uncontrolled epilepsy, 1087
Neuroimaging, metabolic and functional, 1041–1058. See also specific imaging techniques
 [15O] water PET and brain mapping in, 1048
 clinical recommendations for use of, with partial epilepsy, 1053
 fMRI
  and [15O] water PET, 1047–1048
  advantages and limitations of, 1053
  ictal and interictal localization with, 1053
  language lateralization and localization with, 1049–1051, 1050f–1052f
  memory studies with, 1051–1052
  motor and sensory mapping with, 1048–1049, 1049f
  principles of, 1048–1049
 for hippocampal sclerosis surgery, 1076
 PET, 1042–1046 (See also Positron emission tomography (PET))
  antiepileptic drugs and, 1046
  of childhood epilepsy, 1045–1046, 1045f, 1046f
  of extratemporal lobe epilepsy, 1044–1045
  of generalized epilepsy, 1045
  principles of, 1041
  of temporal lobe epilepsy
   [18F] FDG-PET, 1042–1043, 1042f
   other PET ligands, 1043–1044, 1044t

SPECT (See also Single-photon emission computed tomography (SPECT))
 cerebral blood flow studies in, 1046–1047, 1047f
 principles of, 1041
Neurologic status, on recurrence risk, 685
Neuromeres, 14
Neuromodulating chemical, synthesis of, 18
Neuronal cells, bioelectric activity of, in EEG, 127, 128f
Neuronal ceroid lipofuscinoses, 420t, 421–422, 421t, 557
Neuronal ceroid lipofuscinosis type III, 559–560
Neuronal cytomegaly, 5f
Neuronal excitability, steroid hormones on, 695–696
Neuronal migration disorders, 282. See also specific disorders
Neuronal migration malformations, 39t, 42–45, 42f, 43f, 44t. See also specific malformations
Neuronal proliferation malformations, with normal cell types, 39t, 41–42, 41f
Neuronogenesis, 15
Neurons, 127
 dysmorphic, 5f
 in EEG, 127–129, 128f
 subplate, 21
Neuropeptides, in apoptosis, 16
Neurosyphilis, 576
Neurotransmitters. See also specific neurotransmitters
 biosynthesis and release of, 18
 on voltage-dependent channels, 83
Neurotrophins, in axon and dendrite growth, 17
Neurulation, 14
Neurulation disorders, 23
Nevus flammeus, 7f
Newborn. See Neonates
Night terrors, 635
Nightmares, in children, 635
Nitrazepam, 845–846, 845f. See also Benzodiazepines
 indications for, 1212t
 pharmacokinetics of, 657t
Nitrous oxide, 580
NMDA glutamate receptors, 92–94, 93f
NMDA ligand studies, 1044, 1044t
Nodular heterotopia, 4f
Nomenclature. See also Classification, of epilepsies
 of combinatorial system, 184f
Nonconvulsive status epilepticus
 EEG in, 431–434, 432f, 433f
 in Lennox-Gastaut syndrome, 431
Nonepileptic events. See Psychogenic nonepileptic seizures (PNES)
Nonepileptic paroxysmal disorders, 631–640. See also Paroxysmal disorders, nonepileptic
 in children, 635–638
 EEG atlas of, 185–186, 211f–214f
 in infancy, 631–635

in late childhood, adolescence, and adulthood, 638–640
Nonepileptic seizures. See Psychogenic nonepileptic seizures (PNES)
Nonketotic hyperglycemia, 572–573
 neonatal, 500, 548
Nonlesional epilepsy, 1125–1138
 defined, 1125–1126
 intractable, 1126–1128
 invasive EEG in, 1127
 prognosis in, 1128
Nonlesional epilepsy, surgery for
 definitions in, 1125–1126
 diagnostic approach in, 1128–1135
  magnetoencephalography in, 1134–1135
  MR spectroscopy in, 1133–1134, 1133f
  PET in, 1128–1131, 1131f
  subtractional ictal SPECT coregistered to MRI in, 1131–1133, 1132f
  video with extracranial EEG in, 1128, 1129f, 1130f
 noninvasive presurgical evaluation for, 1126–1127
 operative strategy in, 1135–1138
  image-guided navigational surgical technique in, 1137–1138, 1137f
  integration of multimodality images for surgical planning in, 1136–1137, 1136f
  intracranial electrode implantation in, 1135–1136, 1135f
Nonneurologic medical conditions, seizures with, 571–582. See also specific conditions
 agents, 578t, 580
 alcohol, 576
 antineoplastic agents, 578t, 580
 central anticholinergic syndrome, 580
 eclampsia, 580–581
 gastrointestinal disease, 578
 heavy metal intoxication, 580
 hyperbaric oxygenation, 580
 infections, 576–577
 intoxication, 578–580, 578t
 malignancy, 581
 metabolic disorders, 571–574, 575t
 oxygen deprivation, 575–576
 transplantation, organ, 581–582
 vasculitis, 581
Norclobazam, 657t
Normephenytoin, 655–663, 656t. See also Pharmacokinetics, of antiepileptic drugs
Normethsuximide, 655–659, 656t
NPS 1776, 943
NR1I2, 753
NR1I3, 753
Nuclear organization, 18–19
Nuclear-receptor subfamily 1, group 1, members 2 and 3, 753
Number of seizures, recurrence risk with, 686

O
[15O] water PET, 1047–1048
Obstetric complications, 706, 706t

Occipital lobe epilepsy, 370
  childhood, 270–271
    EEG of, 174–175, 175f
      visual aura and focal clonic seizure,
        -10 seconds, 207f
      visual aura and focal clonic seizure,
        clinical onset, 207f
    focal seizures in, 244
    international classification of, 357
Occipital sharp waves, in benign focal
    epileptiform discharges of
    childhood, 200f
Ocular compression test, EEG of, in
    infants, 212f
Oculocephalic deviation, 264
Ohtahara syndrome, 478, 504, 934–935
Olfactory auras, 230t, 232t, 233t,
    234–235
Olfactory sensations, 225
Oligodendroglioma, 1089
Ontogenesis, 13–18
  apoptosis in, 15–16
  axon and dendrite growth in, 17
  cell membrane electrical polarity in, 17
  of cerebral neocortex, 19–20, 20f, 21f
  gastrulation and neural placode
    formulation in, 14
  genetic programming of, 22–23
  mitotic proliferation of neuroblasts
    (neuronogenesis) in, 15
  myelination in, 18
  neural crest separation and migration
    in, 15
  neural tube segmentation in, 14–15
  neuroblast migration in, 16, 16f
  neurotransmitter biosynthesis and
    release in, 18
  neurulation in, 14
  of paleocortex (hippocampus), 22
  synaptogenesis in, 17
  transmitter receptor formation in, 18
Opercular seizures, 356
Opiate-receptor–binding studies, 1044,
    1044t
Opiates, 580
Opportunistic central nervous system
    infections, 576–577
Opsoclonus, in infants, 633
Opsoclonus-myoclonus syndrome, 581
Oral contraceptives, antiepileptic drugs on
    efficacy of, 705–706, 738
Oral trauma, from generalized tonic-
    clonic seizures, 287
Orbitofrontal epilepsy, 368
Orbitofrontal seizures, 243, 355
Organ transplantation, 581–582
Organic acidurias, 555
  neonatal seizures from, 550–551
Organizer genes, 22–23
Ornithine carbamyl transferase deficiency,
    500
Ornithine transcarbamoylase deficiency,
    550
Ornithine transport deficiency,
    intramitochondrial, 555
Oroalimentary automatisms, in focal
    seizures, 245–246, 246t

Orthopedic injury, from generalized tonic-
    clonic seizures, 287
Orthostatic syncope, 638
Osteopenia, from antiepileptic drugs,
    700
Outcome variable, in antiepileptic drug
    trials, 651–652
Overexpression, in developmental defects,
    23
Oxcarbazepine
  absorption, distribution, and
    metabolism of, 766
  adverse effects of, 767–768
    monitoring for, 740
  age-specific dosing of, 677t
  for Angelman syndrome, seizures in,
    423
  vs. carbamazepine, 769
  chemistry and mechanism of action of,
    761, 762f
  clinical use of, 768–769
  cognitive effects of, 1188
  drug interactions of, 763t, 766
    other medications on plasma
      concentration of, 666t
    on plasma concentrations of other
      drugs, 667t
  efficacy of, 766–767
  in elderly, 595t, 596t, 600
  for focal epilepsies, symptomatic,
    370–371
  for generalized tonic-clonic seizures,
    300
  indications for, 1212t
  pharmacokinetics of, 655–659, 656t,
    762t (See also Pharmacokinetics,
    of antiepileptic drugs)
    in infants and children, 675
    in pregnancy, 706–708, 707t
  for poststroke patients, 530
  in renal and liver disease, 727–728
  teratogenicity of, 712, 768
Oxford modification, of
    hemispherectomy, 1119
Oxygen deprivation, 575–576

P

P-glycoprotein, 751
P/Q-type Ca^{2+} channels, 84
Pachygyria, 26
  MRI of, 1017
  neurocutaneous syndromes with, 29
  X-linked hydrocephalus with, 30
Paired homeobox (PAX) families, 22
Paleocortex, ontogeny of, 22
Pallid syncope, infantile, 634–635
  EEG of ocular compression test for,
    211f–212f
Palpitations, as autonomic auras, 237
Panayiotopoulos syndrome, 383–384,
    383f, 384f. See also Benign
    occipital epilepsy (BOE) of
    childhood
Panic attacks, 639
Panic disorders, 639
Pantothenate kinase-associated
    neurodegeneration, 559

Paraldehyde
  indications for, 1212t
  for status epilepticus
    prehospital, 617
    refractory, 615
Parallel design, 649f, 650
Paralysis
  activation, in focal seizures, 245
  periodic, 639
  sleep, 638
Paramethadione, 1212t
Parasitic central nervous system infections,
    577
Parietal lobe epilepsy, 369–370
  international classification of, 356
Parietal lobe focal seizures, 244
Paroxysmal disorders, nonepileptic,
    631–640
  classification of, 631, 632t
  disease-related behaviors in, 639–640
  EEG atlas of, 185–186, 211f–214f
    cyanotic breath-holding spell,
      213f
    narcolepsy, 214f
    pallid infantile syncope, ocular
      compression test of, 212f
  in infancy, 631–635
    respiratory derangements and
      syncope
      cyanotic breath-holding spells, 634
      infant apnea or apparent life-
        threatening events, 634
      pallid syncope, 634–635
    of sleep
      benign neonatal myoclonus, 631
      head banging, 631
    of wakefulness
      alternating hemiplegia, 634
      benign myoclonus of early infancy,
        632–633
      head banging or rolling and body
        rocking, 632
      jitteriness, 631–632
      masturbation, 632
      opsoclonus, 633
      rumination, 633
      shuddering attacks, 633
      spasmodic torticollis, 633
      spasmus nutans, 633
      startle disease or hyperexplexia,
        633
  in late childhood, adolescence, and
    adulthood, 638–640
    of wakefulness
      basilar migraine, 639
      cataplexy, 638–639
      narcolepsy, 638
      panic disorders, 639
      syncope, 638, 638t
      tremor, 639
Paroxysmal disorders in children,
    nonepileptic, 635–638
  dyskinesias, 636
  of sleep
    hypnagogic paroxysmal dystonia, 635
    myoclonus, 635
    night terrors (pavor nocturnus), 635

Paroxysmal disorders in children,
  nonepileptic (*Continued*)
  nightmares, 635
  sleepwalking, 635
  of wakefulness
    benign paroxysmal vertigo, 637
    chorea, 635
    confusional migraine, 637
    head nodding, 636
    headaches, 636–637
    migraine, 636–637
    Munchausen syndrome by proxy,
      637–638, 638t
    myoclonus, 635
    paroxysmal dyskinesias, 636
    rage attacks, 637
    recurrent abdominal pain, 637
    staring spells, 636
    stereotypic movements, 636
    stool-withholding activity and
      constipation, 637
    tics, 635–636
Paroxysmal event, 349
Paroxysmal fast activity, EEG, 177–178,
  178f
  in atypical myoclonic seizures, 318,
    318f
  in atypical tonic seizures, 322–323,
    322f
  in sleep, in Lennox-Gastaut syndrome,
    196f, 431, 433f
Partial continuous epilepsy. *See* Epilepsia
  partialis continua
Partial epilepsy, benign
  with affective symptoms, 386
  with extreme somatosensory evoked
    potentials, 386
Partial epilepsy in infancy, benign, 385
Partial epilepsy of adolescence, benign,
  385
Partial ("hypomotor") seizure, in
  temporal lobe epilepsy, 201f
Partial seizures, 224. *See also* Focal motor
  seizures
Partial seizures of infancy, migrating,
  478–479, 479f
Patch clamp technique, 70, 70f
Pathologic substrates, 3–11
  angioglioma, 9f
  astrocytomas
    foramen of Monro, 7f
    giant cell, 7f
  balloon cells, 5f
  cavernous angioma, 8f
  cortical atrophy, 9f
  cortical tuber, 7f
  double dentate, 4f
  dysembryoplastic neuroepithelial
    tumor, 9f, 10f
  dysmorphic neurons, 5f
  dysplasia, cortical, 4f, 5f, 7f
  electrode-related infarcts and
    contusions, 11f
  epidermal nevus syndrome, 11f
  glioblastoma multiforme, 10f
  gliosis, 9f
  hamartia, 7f

heterotopic gray matter, 5f
hippocampal sclerosis and gliosis, 3f
hydrocephalus, 7f
hypopigmented macules, 6f
Lafora bodies and Lafora disease, 10f
leptomeninges, 4f
lissencephaly (agyria), 4f
low-grade diffuse fibrillary astrocytoma,
  10f
microcalcifications, 7f
multinucleation, 5f
neuronal cytomegaly, 5f
nevus flammeus, 7f
nodular heterotopia, 4f
perisylvian polymicrogyria
  (micropolygyria), 4f
pleomorphic xanthoastrocytomas, 10f
Rasmussen encephalitis, 9f
remote infarct, 8f
retinal hamartomas, 6f, 7f
Sturge-Weber syndrome, 7f, 8f
subependymal nodular, 5f
tuberous sclerosis, 6f, 7f
ungual fibromas, 6f
Pattern-sensitive seizures, 466–467
Patterns, of EEG. *See*
  Electroencephalographic atlas of
  epileptiform abnormalities
Pavor nocturnus, 635
Peak identification, in electrical fields,
  147, 148f
Penicillin model, 99
Penicillins, 578t, 579
Pentazocine, 578t, 579
Pentobarbital, for refractory status
  epilepticus, 615–616
Pentylenetetrazol-induced seizures, 99
Perforant pathway, 58–59, 61f–63f
Periodic lateralized epileptiform
  discharges (PLEDs), 172, 172f
Periodic paralysis, 639
Perirolandic epilepsy
  EEG diagnosis of, 175, 175f
  EEG of, 175, 175f
    epilepsia partialis continua, 211f
    focal clonic seizure, +10 seconds,
      209f
    focal clonic seizure, clinical onset,
      209f
    left arm tonic seizure, 210f
    right frontocentral sharp waves,
      210f
Perisylvian polymicrogyria, 4f, 47
  genetic testing and counseling for,
    48–49
Periventricular nodular heterotopia,
  27–28, 39t, 42–43, 42f
  genes in, 25t
  genetic testing and counseling for, 48
  MRI of, 1019, 1021f
  X-linked, 39t, 43
Peroxisomal disorders, 549–550
Petit mal. *See* Absence seizures
PGY1, 751–752, 752f
Pharmacodynamic interactions, among
  antiepileptic drugs, 663–664,
  663t

Pharmacogenetics, of antiepileptic drugs,
  747–756
  benzodiazepines, 754–755
  candidate genes in, 747–753
    for AED-metabolizing enzymes,
      747–751, 748f, 749t
      CYP (cytochrome P450), 748–750,
        748f, 749t
      CYP2C9, 749
      CYP2C19, 749
      CYP3A4 and *CYP3A5*, 750
      EPHX1, 750
      UGT1 and *UGT2*, 750–751
    for drug receptors, 752–753
      CACNA1G, *CACNA1H*, and
        CACNA1I, 752–753
      NR1I2 and *NR1I3*, 753
      SCN1A, *SCN2A*, *SCN3A*, and
        SCN8A, 752
    for drug transporters: *MDR1 (ABCB1,
      PGY1)*, *MRP1 (ABCC1)*, and
      MRP2 (ABCC2), 751–752, 752f
  definition of, 747
  future research on, 755–756
  other drugs, 755
  phenobarbital, 754
  phenytoin, 753–754
Pharmacogenomics, 747
Pharmacokinetics, of antiepileptic drugs,
  647, 655–663, 656t
  absorption in, 655–657
    absorption rate, 656–657, 657f
    bioavailability, 655–656, 656t
  distribution in, 657–658
  drug interactions in, 661–663, 661f,
    662t
  elimination in, 658–659, 658f
  in infants and children, 671–677
    age-specific dosing in, 676–677, 677t
    benzodiazepines, 672–673
    carbamazepine, 673–674
    developmental, 671–672
    ethosuximide, 674
    felbamate, 674
    gabapentin, 674
    lamotrigine, 674
    oxcarbazepine, 675
    phenobarbital, 675
    phenytoin, 675
    tiagabine, 675
    topiramate, 675–676
    valproate, 676
    vigabatrin, 676
    zonisamide, 676
  interactions among antiepileptic drugs
    in, 661–663, 661f, 662t
  in pregnancy, 707–709, 708t
  steady state and clearance in, 659–661,
    660f, 661f
Pharmacoresistance, 983
Phase reversals, 147, 148f. *See also specific
  montages*
Phenacemide, 1212t
Phencyclidine, 579–580
Phenobarbital, 805–812, 951
  absorption, distribution and
    metabolism of, 807

adverse effects of, 810–811
  monitoring for, 740–741
age-specific dosing of, 677t
for benign childhood epilepsy with
    centrotemporal spikes, 381
chemistry and mechanism of action of,
    805–807, 806f
clinical use of, 811–812, 812f
drug interactions of, 808–809, 809t
efficacy of, 809–810
in elderly, 595t, 596t, 599
for febrile seizures, 517
for generalized tonic-clonic seizures,
    297–298
historical background on, 805
indications for, 1212t
for juvenile myoclonic epilepsy, 396,
    416
for Lennox-Gastaut syndrome, 436–437
for myoclonic epilepsies, progressive,
    422
for neonatal seizures, 505–506
  adverse effects of, 507
pharmacogenetics of, 754
pharmacokinetics of, 655–659, 656t
    (See also Pharmacokinetics, of
      antiepileptic drugs)
  in infants and children, 675
  in pregnancy, 706–708, 707t
for poststroke patients, 530
for posttraumatic epilepsy prophylaxis,
    524
in renal and liver disease, 724
for status epilepticus, 612, 613t, 614
  refractory, 615–616
teratogenicity of, 711
Phenothiazines, 578t, 579
Phenylketonuria, 361, 555
Phenytoin, 785–798
  absorption of, 786–787
  adverse effects of, 795–797
    monitoring for, 741
  age-specific dosing of, 677t
  on Angelman syndrome, seizures in,
      423
  for atypical tonic seizures and tonic
      status epilepticus, 327
  for benign childhood epilepsy with
      centrotemporal spikes, 381
  chemistry and mechanism of action of,
      785, 786f
  clinical use of, 797–798
  distribution of, 787
  drug interactions of, 790–791,
      791t–793t
  efficacy of, 791–795, 794f
  in elderly, 595–598, 595t–597t
  excretion of, 789
  felbamate on, 916, 916t
  for focal epilepsies, symptomatic, 370
  formulations of, 786t
  for generalized tonic-clonic seizures,
      297–298
  historical background on, 785
  indications for, 1212t
  for juvenile myoclonic epilepsy, 396,
      422

in liver disease, 722–724, 723f
metabolism of, 787–789, 789f, 790f
for neonatal seizures, 506
pharmacogenetics of, 753–754
pharmacokinetics of, 655–659, 656t
    (See also Pharmacokinetics, of
      antiepileptic drugs)
  in infants and children, 675
  in pregnancy, 706–708, 707t
  plasma concentrations of, 790
    other medications on, 666t–667t
  on plasma concentrations of other
      drugs, 668t–669t
  for posttraumatic epilepsy
    early, 523
    prophylaxis against, 524
  in renal disease, 722–723, 723f
  for status epilepticus, 612–614, 613t
  steady state and clearance of, 660–661
  teratogenicity of, 711
  for uremia, 573
Pheochromocytoma, 573
3-Phosphoglycerate dehydrogenase
    deficiency, 556
Photic driving, in EEG, 191f
Photic stimulation
  myoclonic jerks with, EEG of, 194f
  myoclonic seizures from, in late
      childhood and adolescence,
      416–417
Photoparoxysmal response, in EEG, 179
Photosensitive epilepsy, pure, 465–466
Photosensitive seizures, from television
    and other electronic screens,
    467–468
Photosensitivity, with spontaneous
    seizures, 466
Pilocarpine model, 99
Piloerection, as aura, 237
Pioneer axons, 21
Piracetam, for progressive myoclonic
    epilepsies, 422
Placebo control, 650
Plasma drug concentrations. See specific
    drugs
Plasmapheresis, for Rasmussen
    encephalitis, 449, 450
Pleasure, as aura, 236
Pleomorphic xanthoastrocytoma, 10f,
    1090–1091
Pneumonia, aspiration, from generalized
    tonic-clonic seizures, 287–288
Polarity, electrical, of cell membrane, 17
Polarity conventions, in localization with
    EEG, 146, 147f
Poliodystrophy, progressive infantile,
    557–558
Polycystic ovary syndrome, 699
Polymicrogyria, 26, 46–47, 46f
  genetic, 47
  genetic testing and counseling for, 48
  MRI of, 1017–1018, 1017f
  perisylvian, 4f, 47
    genetic testing and counseling for,
        48–49
  syndromes of, 47
  X-linked hydrocephalus with, 30

Polypharmacy, rational, for generalized
    tonic-clonic seizures, 297
Polyspike-and-wave complexes, 193f
  in atypical myoclonic seizures, 318,
      318f
  in atypical tonic seizures, 323, 323f
Polyspikes, EEG, in Lennox-Gastaut
    syndrome in sleep, 196f
Polysynaptic excitatory postsynaptic
    potential, 128f, 129
Polysynaptic pathway, 58–59, 61f–63f
Polytherapy
  rational, for generalized tonic-clonic
      seizures, 297
  teratogenicity of, 712
Porencephaly, hemispherectomy for, 1115
Porphyria, 574, 575t
Positive occipital sharp transients
    (POSTS), 189f
Positron emission tomography (PET)
    [^{15}O] water, 1047–1048
  antiepileptic drugs and, 1046
  of childhood epilepsy, 1045–1046,
      1045f, 1046f
  of epileptogenic region in focal lesions
      on MRI, 1093–1094, 1094f
  of extratemporal lobe epilepsy,
      1044–1045
  of generalized epilepsy, 1045
  of nonlesional epilepsy, 1128–1131, 1131f
  principles of, 1041
  of temporal lobe epilepsy
    with [^{18}F] FDG, 1042–1043, 1042f
    with other ligands, 1043–1044, 1044t
Postanesthetic syndrome, 580
Postictal imaging, 1022, 1022f
Postictal paralysis, 228
Postischemic epilepsy, 1092
Postnatal epilepsy, chronic, 506–507, 506f
Postoperative seizures, acute, prognostic
    implications of, 1177–1178
Poststroke epilepsy, 527–534. See also
    Stroke, epilepsy after
Postsynaptic potentials, 127
Posttraumatic epilepsy, 521–524
  clinical features of, 523
  diagnostic studies of, 523
  future directions in, 524
  incidence of, 521
  MRI features and pathology of,
      1091–1092
  pathology and pathophysiology of,
      522–523
  preventing seizures in, 524
  prevention of, 524
  risk factors for, 521–522
  seizures in, early vs. late, 521
  terminology in, 521
  treatment of, 523–524
Posttraumatic seizure, 521
Potassium (K$^+$) channels, 74f, 76–78, 76t
  Ca^{2+}-dependent, 75f, 77–78
  epilepsies linked to, 105
  inward rectifier K, 77
  KCNQ2/3, and benign familial
      neonatal convulsions, 84, 503
  Kv1.1, and episodic ataxia type 1, 84

Potassium (K$^+$)-selective membrane, 69, 70f
Potentiation, long-term, 92
Praxis-induced seizures, 468
Precipitated seizures, epileptic, 362–363
Predictors
 of intractable disease, 120–121
 prognostic, during epilepsy, 119
Prednisone
 with antiepileptic drugs, 730
 for infantile spasms, 934
Prefrontal cortex, functional anatomy of, 257, 258f
Pregabalin, 855–865
 chemistry of, 855, 856f
 clinical studies of efficacy and safety of, 859–863
  as adjunctive, open-label, 861–862
  as adjunctive, placebo-controlled, 859–860, 860t
  concentration–effect relationship of, 859
 drug interactions of, 858
 mechanisms of action of, 856–857, 856t
 pharmacokinetics of
  absorption in, 857–858, 857t
  distribution in, 858
  elimination in, 858
 safety and toxicity of, 863–865, 864t
Pregnancy, 705–714
 antiepileptic drugs in
  on contraceptive effectiveness, 705–706
  pharmacokinetics of, 707–709, 708t
  teratogenicity of, 711–712
 complications of, 706, 706t
 generalized tonic-clonic seizures and, 287
 management strategies in, 713–714
 neonatal outcome in, 709–711, 710t
 obstetric complications in, 706
 seizure control in, 706–707, 707t, 738
 teratogenicity in, 711–713
  of antiepileptic drugs, 711–712
  folic acid in, 713
  genetic predisposition in, 712–713
Pregnane X receptor (PXR), 753
Premonitions, aura in, 229
Premotor cortex, 258f, 261
Prescription medication–induced seizures, 578–579, 578t
Prevalence, 112, 113t, 114t
Prevalence bias, 111, 111f
Primary motor area, 258f, 259–260, 260f
Primary reading epilepsy, 363
Primidone, 805–812, 951
 absorption, distribution and metabolism of, 807–808
 adverse effects of, 810–811
 chemistry and mechanism of action of, 805–807, 806f
 clinical use of, 812
 drug interactions of, 808–809, 809t
 efficacy of, 810
 historical background on, 805
 indications for, 1212t

for juvenile myoclonic epilepsy, 396, 416
 for Lennox-Gastaut syndrome, 436–437
 pharmacokinetics of, 655–659, 656t (See also Pharmacokinetics, of antiepileptic drugs)
  in pregnancy, 706–708, 707t
  in renal and liver disease, 724
  teratogenicity of, 711
Prodromes, aura in, 229
Progesterone, 697, 697f
 antiepileptic drugs on, 705
 for catamenial-associated seizures, 698
 on neuronal excitability, 695–696
Programmed cell death. See Apoptosis
Progressive encephalopathy with edema, hypsarrhythmia, and optic neuropathy (PEHO syndrome), 556–557
Progressive familial myoclonic epilepsy, Unverricht-Lundborg, 560
Progressive infantile poliodystrophy, 557–558
Progressive myoclonus epilepsies, 417–422, 419f, 420t, 421t, 560–561
 classification of, 420t
 EEG of, 418, 419f
 epidemiology of, 417–419
 genetic mapping of, 281–282
 Lafora body disease in, 420–421, 420t, 421t
 molecular genetics of, 419, 420t
 neuronal ceroid lipofuscinoses in, 420t, 421–422, 421t
 treatment of, 422
 Unverricht-Lunborg disease in, 419–420, 420t, 421t
Prolactin, 696, 697f
 epilepsy on, 697
Prolonged tonic seizures, 321
Proof of principle, 647
Propionic acidemia, 500, 551
Propofol, 580
 for refractory status epilepticus, 615–616
Proposed revised classification of epilepsies and epileptic syndromes, 354–363. See also Classification, of epilepsies and epileptic syndromes
Propoxyphene, 578t, 579
 neonatal seizures from, 501
Proprioceptive-induced seizures, 470–471
Prosomeres, 14
Provoked seizure, acute, 110
Pseudoresistance, 983–984
Pseudoseizures, 983. See also Psychogenic nonepileptic seizures (PNES)
Pseudo–steady-state phenomenon, 661
Psychiatric comorbidity, 1197–1199
 aggression in, 1199
 anxiety in, 1198
 depression in, 1197–1198
 psychosis in, 1198
Psychic auras, 230t, 232t, 233t, 236–237, 236t

Psychic symptoms, 225–226
Psychogenic nonepileptic seizures (PNES), 623–629
 in children, 628
 diagnosis of
  confirming, 624–625
  difficult and special issues in, 625–626
  suspecting, 623–624
 after epilepsy surgery, 626
 epilepsy surgery in patients with, 626
 management of, 627–628
 misdiagnosis of epilepsy and, 623
 overview of, 623
 in perspective, 628
 prognosis in, 627
 psychopathology of, 626–627
 terminology for, 623
Psychogenic seizures, 623. See also Psychogenic nonepileptic seizures (PNES)
 nonepileptic, 983
Psychosis, 1198
Puberty, seizures arising in, 698
Pulmonary edema, from generalized tonic-clonic seizures, 288, 288f
Pure photosensitive epilepsy, 465–466
Pyknolepsy, 359
Pyridoxine, 954–956, 1212t
Pyridoxine dependency, 361
 neonatal seizures from, 548
Pyridoxine-dependent seizures, neonatal, 500
Pyruvate carboxylase deficiency, 551
Pyruvate dehydrogenase deficiency, 551

R
Radiofrequency ablation, stereotactic, for hypothalamic hamartomas, 1171–1172, 1172f
Rage attacks, in children, 637
Ramsay-Hunt syndrome, 362
Rasmussen encephalitis (syndrome), 271–272, 356, 441–451. See also Kojewnikow syndrome
 clinical presentations of, 442–445
  basal ganglia involvement in, 443–444
  bilateral hemispheric involvement in, 443
  brainstem variant in, 444
  clinical variants in, 442–443
  double pathology in, 444–445
  focal and chronic protracted variants in, 443
  late-onset adolescent and adult variants in, 443
  multifocal variant in, 444
  typical course of, 442
 diagnosis of, early, 447t, 448–449
 EEG of, 445
 etiology and pathogenesis of, 446–449
 future perspectives on, 450–451
 hemispherectomy for, 1116
 history of, 441–442
 imaging of, 445–446
 MRI of, 1015
 treatment of, 449–450

Rational polypharmacy, for generalized
tonic-clonic seizures, 297
Rational polytherapy, for generalized
tonic-clonic seizures, 297
Reading epilepsy, 468–469
primary, 363
Reading-induced spike-and-wave
complexes, 198f
EEG of, 198f
Receptors
acetylcholine, 95
epilepsies linked to, 106
adenosine, 95
formation of, 18
GABA, 94–95
epilepsies linked to, 106
glutamate, AMPA and NMDA, 92–94,
93f
metabotropic, 94
Recreational activities, 1207–1208, 1208t
Recreational drugs, 984
seizures from, 579–580
Recreational vehicles, 1207
Rectifiers
delayed, 76–77
slow, delayed, 77
Recurrence risk
factors in, 685–686
after first unprovoked seizure, 681–683
after two seizures, 683
Reference, choice of, in scalp determination
of electrical fields, 154
Referential montage
field identification with, 151t, 153, 153f
with and without phase reversal, 151t,
153, 153f
Referral center bias, 112
Reflex epilepsy, 463–472
basic mechanisms of, 463–465
with complex nonvisual activity,
468–472
eating epilepsy, 470
hot water epilepsy, 471
language-induced epilepsy, 469
miscellaneous reflex seizures, 471
musicogenic epilepsy, 469–470
praxis, 468
proprioceptive-induced seizures,
470–471
reading epilepsy, 468–469
startle epilepsy, 471
thinking, 468
touch-evoked seizures, 471
definition and classification of, 463
with visual triggers, 465–466
not induced by flicker, 466–467
television and other electronic
screens, 467–468
Reflex syncope, 638
Regulator genes, 22–23
Relapse
prognosis after, 687
after remission, 120
Remacemide, 1212t
Remission
predictors of successful medication
withdrawal after, 119–120, 120f

relapse after, 120
from time of diagnosis, predictors of,
118–119, 119f
from time of first seizure, likelihood of,
117–118, 119t
Renal disease, antiepileptic drugs in,
719–730
benzodiazepines, 726
carbamazepine, 725–726
ethosuximide, 726
felbamate, 727
gabapentin, 727
levetiracetam, 729
overview of, 719–721, 720t
oxcarbazepine, 727–728
phenobarbital, 724
phenytoin, 722–723, 723f
primidone, 724
tiagabine, 728–729
topiramate, 728
valproate (valproic acid), 724–725
vigabatrin, 729
zonisamide, 728
Renal function, age on, 672, 672f
Renal transplantation
antiepileptic drugs in, 730–731
seizures after, 731
Repolarization, 73, 73f, 92
Representativeness, 112
Reproductive health, 699–700
Resective surgery, antiepileptic drug
withdrawal after, 687–688
Respiratory derangements, in infants
cyanotic breath-holding spells, 634
infant apnea or apparent life-
threatening events, 634
pallid syncope, 634–635
Responsiveness, 225
Resting leakage current, 75f, 78
Reticular reflex myoclonus, 319
Reticulospinal tract, 258
Retigabine, 940t, 941–942
Retinal hamartomas, 6f, 7f
Retinitis, cytomegalovirus, 577
Rett syndrome, 482, 636
genes in, 25t
Revised classification of epilepsies and
epileptic syndromes, proposed,
354–363. See also Classification,
of epilepsies and epileptic
syndromes
Rhinencephalic seizures, 355
Rhombomeres, 14
Rhythmic distal clonus, prominent,
epilepsies with, 417, 418f
Rhythmic fast activity, in EEG, 177–178,
178f
Rhythmic movement disorder, 631
Rhythmical temporal theta bursts of
drowsiness, 188f
Right frontal lobe seizures, video-EEG of,
999, 1003f–1004f
Right frontocentral sharp waves, in
perirolandic epilepsy, 210f
Right mesial frontal lobe seizures,
SISCOM study of, 1005, 1005f,
1006

Riley-Day syndrome, neurocristopathies
in, 23
Risk, of engaging in desired activities,
1201–1202
Rocking, body, in infants, 632
Rolandic epilepsy
benign, 270–271
EEG diagnosis of, 175, 175f
Rolandic seizures, in benign childhood
epilepsy with centrotemporal
spikes, 377, 378f–380f
Rolandic spikes
in benign childhood epilepsy with
centrotemporal spikes, 376,
376f–377f
in localization, 155, 158f
Rubrospinal tract, 258
Rufinamide, 940t, 942
Rumination, in infants, 633

S
Safety, of antiepileptic drugs, 648–649.
See also specific drugs and
disorders
Safinamide, 940t, 942
Sandhoff disease, 361, 553
Sandifer syndrome, 633
Santavuori-Haltia-Hagbery disease, 361
Schindler disease, 557
Schizencephaly, 29–30, 47
genes in, 25t
genetic testing and counseling for, 49
MRI of, 1018, 1018f
Sclerosis, hippocampal, 3f
SCN1A, 752
SCN2A, 752
SCN3A, 752
SCN8A, 752
Screening models, for antiepileptic drugs,
646
Screening tests, for adverse effects with
antiepileptic drugs, 739, 739t
Sebaceous nevi, linear, 503
Segmentation, neural tube, 14–15
disorders of, 23
Seizure(s). *See also specific types*
acute provoked, 110
with affective symptomatology,
225–226
atonic, 228
with aura, 226–227
with automatisms, 226
with autonomic symptoms, 225
bicuculline-induced, 99
clonic, 227–228
with cognitive disturbances, 225
from complex nonvisual activity,
468–472
complex partial, 241–251 (*See also* Focal
seizures with impaired
consciousness)
with complex symptomatology,
226–227
definition of, 487
with drowsiness or somnolence, 226
with dysmnesic symptoms, 225
with dysphasia, 225

Seizure(s) *(Continued)*
  eating-induced, 470
  epilepsia partialis continua (*See*
        Epilepsia partialis continua)
  epileptic, 109 (*See also specific seizures*)
        precipitated, 362–363
  eye closure–induced, 467
  febrile, 110
  frequency of, in five-dimensional
        patient-oriented epilepsy
        classification proposal, 351, 352t
  generalized, 227
  with hallucinations, structured, 226
  with higher cerebral function
        disturbances, 225–226
  hormonally sensitive, treatment of, 698
  with illusions, 226
  in infantile spasms, EEG of, 195f
  jacksonian, 225
  kainic acid–induced, 99
  language-induced, 469
  after liver transplantation, 731
  with motor signs, 225
  movement-induced (*See* Proprioceptive-
        induced seizures)
  musicogenic, 469–470
  myoclonic, 227
  natural history of, 117–122 (*See also*
        Natural history, of seizures)
  neonatal, 110
  partial, 224
  pattern-sensitive, 466–467
  pentylenetetrazol-induced, 99
  praxis-induced, 468
  precipitated, 362–363
  proprioceptive-induced, 470–471
  with psychic symptoms, 225–226
  from reading, 468–469
  reflex, 463–472 (*See also* Reflex
        epilepsy)
  after renal transplantation, 731
  on reproductive hormones, 696–697
  self-induced, in photosensitive, 467
  with self-induced flicker, 466
  with sensory symptoms, 225
  with somatosensory symptoms, 225
  subclinical EEG, in frontal lobe epilepsy
        +50 seconds, 206f
        onset, 205f
  thinking-induced, 468
  tonic, 228
  tonic-clonic, 227
  touch-evoked, 471
  unclassified epileptic, 228
  unprovoked, 110
  visually evoked
        not induced by flicker, 466–467
        in reflex epilepsy, 465–466
Seizure classification, 217–220
  antiepileptic drug testing and, 648
  comments on, 220
  electroclinical approach to, limitations
        of, 217–218
  evolution of current system of, 217
  in five-dimensional patient-oriented
        epilepsy classification proposal,
        350–351

proposal on, 218–219, 219t
  proposed revised, 222–228
        addendum on, 223–224
        definition of terms in, 224–228
        generalized seizures (convulsive or
              nonconvulsive), 222–223, 224t
        partial (focal, local) seizures, 222,
              223t
        unclassified epileptic seizures, 223
  recurrence risk and, 683, 686
  symptomatology alone in, 219t
        advantages of, 218
Seizure control, in pregnancy, 706–707,
        707t, 738
Seizure focus identification, SPECT in,
        1046–1047, 1047f
Seizure recurrence, factors in, 685–686,
        1201
        after first unprovoked seizure, 681–683
        after two seizures, 683
Seizure risk, in offspring of parents with
        epilepsy, 711
Selective IgG immunoadsorption, for
        Rasmussen encephalitis, 449,
        450
Selective serotonin reuptake inhibitors
        (SSRIs), 578t, 579
Self-induced flicker, 466
Semiautomated voxel-based
        morphometry, 1023–1024, 1023f
Sensory mapping, fMRI, 1048–1049,
        1049f
Sensory symptoms, 225
Septo-optic-pituitary dysplasia, genes in,
        25t
Septohippocampal nucleus, 22
Septooptic-pituitary dysplasia, 27
Serine biosynthesis defect, 556
Serotonin receptor and synthesis studies,
        1044, 1044t
Serotonin syndrome, 579
Sertraline, 578t, 579
Severe epilepsy, in childhood, 1111–1112
Severe myoclonic epilepsy of infants, 360,
        413–414
Sex-hormone binding globulin (SHBG)
        antiepileptic drugs on, 705
        epilepsy on, 697
Sexual auras, 237
Sexual automatisms, in focal seizures, 246
Sexual function, 699–700
Sharp waves, EEG
        in benign focal epileptiform discharges
              of childhood
              centrotemporal, 199f
              occipital left and right, 200f
        bitemporal, in temporal lobe epilepsy,
              202f
        in epilepsy diagnosis, 171
        in epileptic spasms, 336–337, 337f
        frontal, in frontal lobe epilepsy, 204f
              with 2-degree bilateral synchrony,
                    205f
        frontocentral, right, in perirolandic
              epilepsy, 210f
        in Lennox-Gastaut syndrome, 196f, 431,
              432f

temporal, in temporal lobe epilepsy,
        201f
        at vertex, in supplemental motor area
              epilepsy, 208f
Shigellosis, 577
Shivering, cold, as aura, 237
Short tonic seizures, 321
Shuddering attacks, in infants, 633
Sialidosis, with isolated deficit in
        neuraminidase, 362
Sialidosis type I, 558–559
Sialidosis type II, 559
Side effects. *See* Adverse effects, of
        antiepileptic drugs; *specific agents*
Single-photon emission computed
        tomography (SPECT)
        cerebral blood flow studies with,
              1046–1047, 1047f
        of epileptogenic regions, 1093
        principles of, 1041
        subtractional ictal coregistered to MRI,
              for nonlesional epilepsy,
              1131–1133, 1132f
Single-photon emission computed
        tomography (SPECT)
        coregistered to MRI (SISCOM),
              1004–1005, 1005f
SISCOM, 1004–1005, 1005f
Sleep
        generalized paroxysmal fast and
              polyspikes in, 196f, 431, 433f
        nonepileptic paroxysmal disorders in
              children of
              hypnagogic paroxysmal dystonia, 635
              myoclonus, 635
              night terrors (pavor nocturnus), 635
              nightmares, 635
              sleepwalking, 635
        nonepileptic paroxysmal disorders in
              infancy of
              benign neonatal myoclonus, 631
              head banging, 631
        slow, continuous spike waves of,
              455–458 (*See also* Continuous
              spike waves of slow sleep)
Sleep paralysis, 638
Sleep spindle, 190f
Sleep starts, 635
Sleep state, at time of first seizure,
        recurrence risk and, 682–683
Sleepwalking, in children, 635
Slow spike and wave, 177
        in absence seizures, 308f
        in atypical myoclonic seizures, 318,
              318f, 319, 320f
        in Lennox-Gastaut syndrome, 196f
Slow-wave complexes, in Lennox-Gastaut
        syndrome, 196f, 431, 432f
Small sharp spike, 186f
Smearing effect, 144
Smith-Lemli-Opitz syndrome,
        holoprosencephaly in, 27
Social Security Administration disability
        benefits, 1207, 1207t
Sodium action potential, 92
Sodium (Na$^+$) channels, 75f, 76t, 78–79
        epilepsies linked to, 105

Sodium valproate. *See* Valproate (valproic acid)
Solid-angle rule, 144, 145f
Somatosensory auras, 230t, 232t, 233–234, 233t
Somatosensory evoked potentials, extreme, benign partial epilepsy with, 386
Somatosensory symptoms, 225
Somnolence, with seizure, 226
Spasmodic torticollis, in infants, 633
Spasms, epileptic, 333–343
   clinical presentation of, 333–334
   definition and classification of, 359
   differential diagnosis of, in infants, 338–340, 339t, 340t
   electrophysiology of, 336–338, 337f
   epidemiology of, 333
   etiology of, 335–336
   history of, 333
   pathophysiology of, 334–335
   prognosis in, 343
   treatment of, 340–343
      benzodiazepines in, 342
      corticotropin in, 341
      other antiepileptic drugs in, 342–343
      pyridoxine in, 342
      valproate (valproic acid) in, 342
      vigabatrin in, 341–342
Spasmus nutans, in infants, 633
Spatial perception disorders, 225
Spatial sampling, electrode placement as, 145
SPD 421 (DP16, DP-VPA), 943
Speech arrest, 264
Speech disturbances, in focal seizures, 247–248
Sphenoidal electrodes, 1059, 1060f
Spielmeyer-Vogt-Sjögren disease, 362, 559–560
Spike and wave, EEG
   3-Hz, 176, 176f, 289–291
   6-Hz "phantom," 187f
   in generalized tonic-clonic seizures
      3-Hz, 289–291
      4-Hz, 290
      5-Hz, 290
      irregular, 290, 292f
   multiple, 176–177, 177f
   slow, 177
      in absence seizures, 308f
      in atypical myoclonic seizures, 318, 318f, 319, 320f
      in Lennox-Gastaut syndrome, 196f
Spike complexes, multiple, in generalized tonic-clonic seizures, 290, 292f
Spikes, EEG
   6-Hz positive, 186f
   14-Hz positive, 186f
   in epilepsy diagnosis, 171
   in Lennox-Gastaut syndrome
      generalized paroxysmal fast and polyspikes in sleep, 196f, 431, 433f
      polyspikes in sleep, 196f
   multifocal, intractable epilepsy with, 197f

rolandic, in localization, 155, 158f
   small sharp, 186f
   surface-negative, 146, 146f
   surface-positive, 146, 146f
   wicket, 187f
Spinocerebellar ataxia type 6, 84
Sports, 1207–1208, 1208t
Sprue, nontropical, 578
St. John's wort, 579
Staring spells, in children, 636
Startle disease, in infants, 633
Startle epilepsy, 471
Status epilepticus, 605–617
   antiepileptic drug therapy for, 611–617
      emergency department or inpatient, 616t, 617
      prehospital, 617
      primary (first-line agents), 612–614, 613t
      refractory disease, 615–617, 615t
      second-line agents, 614–615
      timetable for, 616t
   benzodiazepines for, 835
   classification of, 265–266
   definition of, 265–266, 605
   epidemiology of, 609
   etiology of, 609, 609t
   focal motor, 266
   management of, 610–611, 611t, 612f–613f
   MRI of, 1022, 1022f
   nonconvulsive, in Lennox Gastaut syndrome, 431
   pathophysiology of, 607–609
   posttraumatic, 523
   prognosis with, 610
   refractory
      of focal origin, outcomes of surgery for, 1177
      topiramate for, 881
   stages of, 605–606, 606f–608f, 606t
   trends in patients with, 606–607
Steady-state concentrations (C_{SS}), 655, 659–661, 660f, 661f
Stereotactic radiofrequency ablation, for hypothalamic hamartomas, 1171–1172, 1172f
Stereotactic radiosurgery, for hypothalamic hamartomas, 1172–1173
Stereotypic movements, in children, 636
Steroid hormones. *See also specific hormones*
   with antiepileptic drugs, 730
   antiepileptic drugs on, 705–706
   epilepsy on, 697
   historical background on, 931
   for infantile spasms, 931–934
   for Lennox-Gastaut syndrome, 437
   on neuronal excitability, 695–696
   for Ohtahara and Lennox-Gastaut syndromes, 934–936
   for other myoclonic disorders, 935–936
   for Rasmussen encephalitis, 449–450
Stevens-Johnson syndrome, from antiepileptic drugs, malpractice/negligence cases on, 736t, 737

Stimulation-related epilepsy, EEG of, 198f
Stiripentol
   indications for, 1212t
   for severe myoclonic epilepsy of infants, 414
Stool-withholding activity, in children, 637
Stratum lacunosum, 57, 60f–62f
Stratum moleculare, 57, 60f–62f
Stratum oriens, 57, 60f, 61f
Stratum pyramidale, 57, 60f–62f
Stratum radiatum, 57, 60f–62f
Strips (subdural electrode), 1061–1064, 1062f, 1063f. *See also* Subdural electrodes (grids and strips)
   for focal cortical developmental malformations
      identification of, 1105–1107, 1105f
      proposed indications for, 1106–1107
Stroke
   neonatal, 528
   pediatric, 527–528
Stroke, epilepsy after, 527–534
   adult patients with, 528–530, 529f
   incidence of, 527
   pediatric patients with, 527–528
   pharmacotherapy for seizures in, 530
   surgery for refractory seizures in, 530–534
      clinical features and seizure semiology in, 531
      interictal and ictal epileptiform abnormalities in, 531, 531f–532f
      neuroimaging in, 531–532, 533f–534f
      procedure in, 532–534
Sturge-Weber syndrome, 7f, 8f, 361, 540–541
   clinical features and neuroimaging of, 540–541, 541f
   cortical dysplasias and, 543
   epilepsy with, 541
   hemispherectomy for, 1116, 1117f
   MRI of, 1015–1016
   neonatal seizures in, 503
Subclinical EEG seizure, in frontal lobe epilepsy
   +50 seconds, 206f
   onset, 206f
Subclinical rhythmical electrographic discharges of adults, 188f
Subcortical-band (laminar) heterotopia, 28–29, 28f, 39t, 43–44, 44f. *See also* Cortical-band heterotopia
   genes in, 25t
   genetic testing and counseling for, 49
Subcortical laminar heterotopia, 28–29, 28f
Subdural electrodes (grids and strips), 1061–1064, 1062f, 1063f
   advantages of, 1063
   disadvantages of, 1063–1064, 1063f
   for focal cortical developmental malformations, 1105–1106, 1105f
   identification of, 1105–1107, 1105f
   proposed indications for, 1106–1107
   functional localization studies with, 1061–1062

Subdural electroencephalography, of
    epileptogenic regions, 1093
Subependymal nodular heterotopic gray
    matter, 5f
Subiculum, 22, 58, 58f
Subpial transection, multiple, 1163–1166
    see also Multiple subpial
    transection
Subplate neurons, 21
Subplate zone, 19, 20f
Substrate-directed epilepsy, surgery for,
    994
Substrates, pathologic, 3–11. See also
    Pathologic substrates
Subtractional ictal SPECT, coregistered to
    MRI, for nonlesional epilepsy,
    1131–1133, 1132f
Subventricular zone, 19, 20f
Succinic semialdehyde dehydrogenase
    deficiency, 556
Succinimides. See also Ethosuximide
    other medications on plasma
        concentration of, 666t
Sudden death, from generalized tonic-
    clonic seizures, 289
Sudden infant death syndrome, 634
Sulfite oxidase deficiency, 501
    neonatal seizures from, 548–549
Sulthiame, for benign childhood
    epilepsy with centrotemporal
    spikes, 381
Superconducting quantum interference
    device (SQUID), 160
Supplemental motor area, 260–261
Supplemental motor area epilepsy, EEG of
    sharp waves at vertex, 207f
    tonic seizure, 208f
Supplementary motor cortex, 259
Supplementary motor seizures, 243, 355
Supplementary negative motor area, 259
Supplementary sensorimotor area
    (SSMA), 257, 260–261
Supplementary sensorimotor area (SSMA)
    epilepsy, 368
Supplementary sensorimotor area (SSMA)
    seizures, 268–270. See also Motor
    cortex
    clinical semiology of, 268–269
    EEG findings in, 269–270, 269f–271f
Surface electrical manifestations, 143f,
    144–145, 145f
Surface-negative spike, 146, 146f
Surface-positive spike, 146, 146f
Surgery, 994. See also specific disorders;
    specific surgeries
    complications of, 1179–1180
    discontinuation of antiepileptic drugs
        after, 1178–1179
    for focal malformations of cortical
        development, 1103–1109
        (See also Cortical developmental
        malformations, focal)
    for hippocampal sclerosis, 1071–1080
        (See also Hippocampal sclerosis,
        surgery for)
    identification of patients for, 994
        (See also Surgical candidacy)

in infants and children, 1143–1156
    (See also Childhood epilepsy,
    surgery for; Infants, epilepsies in,
    surgery for)
for medial temporal lobe epilepsy,
    994
memory deficits after, 1179–1180
motor and sensory functional deficits
    after, 1179
MRI in evaluation for, 1009–1025
    (See also Magnetic resonance
    imaging (MRI), in epilepsy
    surgery evaluation)
outcomes of, 1175–1181
quality-of-life outcomes of, 1180–1181
for refractory seizures in epilepsy after
    stroke, 530–534 (See also Stroke,
    epilepsy after)
seizure outcomes of, 1175–1179
    with acute postoperative seizures,
        1177–1178
    with diffuse EEG abnormalities with
        focal MRI lesion, 1177
    etiology in, 1176–1177
    focal lesion on MRI in, 1175–1176
    with medically refractory status
        epilepticus of focal origin, 1177
speech and language deficits after, 1180
for substrate-directed or lesional
    epilepsy, 994
without lesion on MRI, 1125–1138
    (See also Nonlesional epilepsy,
    surgery for)
Surgical candidacy, medical intractability
    for, 983–989. See also Medical
    intractability
Surgical candidacy, recognition of,
    993–1006
    case reports of, 996f, 998f–1005f,
        1005–1006
    epidemiology of, 993
    intractable epilepsy in, 993–994
    SISCOM of, 1003–1005, 1005f
    video-EEG evaluation of, 994–1002,
        995f–1003f (See also Video-
        electroencephalogram
        monitoring)
Sympathomimetics, 578t
Symptomatic focal epilepsies. See Focal
    epilepsies, symptomatic
Symptomatic generalized epilepsies and
    syndromes, 360
Symptomatic generalized epilepsies of
    specific etiologies, 361–362
Synaptogenesis, 17
Syncope
    in older children and adolescents, 638,
        638t
    orthostatic, 638
    pallid infantile, 634–635
        EEG of ocular compression test for,
            212f
    reflex, 638
Syndrome-oriented epilepsy classification,
    348–349, 348t
Systemic infections, 577
Systemic necrotizing vasculitis, 581

T

Tachycardia, as autonomic auras, 237
Tacrolimus (FK506), with antiepileptic
    drugs, 730
Talampanel, 940t, 942–943
Tay-Sachs disease, 361, 552–553
Tectospinal tract, 258
Television-induced seizures, 467–468
Temporal intermittent rhythmic delta
    activity (TIRDA), 171–172, 171f
Temporal lobe epilepsy, 365–367, 366t
    case report on, 1080–1081
    EEG of, 173–174, 173f
        bitemporal sharp waves, 202f
        complex partial seizure with
            automatisms, 203f
        partial ("hypomotor") seizure, 201f
        temporal sharp wave, 200f
    focal seizures in, 243–244
    international classification of, 354–355
    left temporal spike discharges in, 996,
        996f
    mesial, 365–366, 1065 (See also Mesial
        temporal lobe epilepsy (MTLE))
    case report on, 1080
    MRI for, 1010–1013, 1011f, 1011t (See
        also under Mesial temporal lobe
        epilepsy (MTLE))
    surgery for, 994
    suspected bilateral, intracranial EEG
        for, 1065
    MRI for, new techniques in, 1013
    neocortical, 366–367
    PET in
        with [^{18}F] FDG, 1042–1043, 1042f
        with other ligands, 1043–1044, 1044t
Temporal sharp wave, in temporal lobe
    epilepsy, 201f
Teratogenicity, 711–713. See also specific
    drugs
    of carbamazepine, 765
    of fosphenytoin, 797
    of oxcarbazepine, 768
    of phenytoin, 796
Testosterone, 697, 697f
"Tet" spells, 639
Theophylline, 578t, 579
    neonatal seizures from, 501
Theta bursts, of drowsiness, rhythmical
    temporal, 188f
Thinking, forced, 237
Thinking-induced seizures, 468
Thiopental, for refractory status
    epilepticus, 615–616
Three-dimensional (3D) rendering, 1024
Thyroid disorders, 573
Thyroid hormones, on neuronal
    excitability, 695–696
Thyrotoxicosis, 573
Tiagabine, 907–909
    adverse effects of, 908–909
        monitoring for, 741
    age-specific dosing of, 677t
    chemistry of, 907, 908f
    clinical use of, 909
    cognitive effects of, 1188
    drug interactions of, 908

efficacy of, 908
in elderly, 595t, 597t, 600
for focal epilepsies, symptomatic, 371
for generalized tonic-clonic seizures, 298, 299
historical background on, 907
indications for, 1212t
mechanism of action of, 907
pharmacokinetics of, 655–659, 656t, 907–908 (*See also* Pharmacokinetics, of antiepileptic drugs)
   in infants and children, 675
   in pregnancy, 706–708, 707t
   in renal and liver disease, 728–729
teratogenicity of, 712
Tics, in children, 635–636
Todd's (postictal) paralysis, 225, 228
Tolerance, of antiepileptic drugs, 647
Tonic axial seizures, 321
Tonic axorhizomelic seizures, 321
Tonic-clonic seizures
   definition of, 227
   generalized, 227, 279–300 (*See also* Generalized tonic-clonic seizures)
      epilepsy with, 400–401
      in juvenile myoclonic epilepsy, 393
Tonic components, with absence seizures, 227
Tonic focal motor seizures, 263–264
Tonic postural seizures, 321
Tonic posturing, in focal seizures, 246–247
Tonic seizures
   atypical, 321–324
      clinical correlation of, 323–324
      clinical features of, 321–322, 321f
      electrophysiology of, 322–323, 322f, 323f
   definition of, 228
   left arm, in perirolandic epilepsy, 210f
   in Lennox-Gastaut syndrome, 430
   in myoclonic epilepsies, 408, 408f
   in supplemental motor area epilepsy, 208f
Tonic spasms, 321
Topiramate, 877–886
   adverse effects of, 883–886
      carbonic anhydrase inhibition in, 884–885
      on central nervous system, 883–884
      in children, 885
      idiosyncratic toxicity in, 885–886
      monitoring for, 741
      weight loss in, 885
   age-specific dosing of, 677t
   for atypical tonic seizures, 327
   chemistry of, 877, 878f
   clinical use of, 886
   cognitive effects of, 1188
   drug interactions of, 878–879
   efficacy of, 879–883
      as adjunctive therapy, 879–881
      as monotherapy, 881–883
      in other clinical uses, 883
   in elderly, 595t, 597t, 600
   for epileptic spasms, 342

for focal epilepsies, symptomatic, 371
for generalized tonic-clonic seizures, 298, 299
historical background on, 877
indications for, 1212t
for Lennox-Gastaut syndrome, 436
mechanisms of action of, 877
monitoring of, 878
for myoclonus in atypical seizures, 327
pharmacokinetics of, 655–659, 656t, 877–878 (*See also* Pharmacokinetics, of antiepileptic drugs)
   in infants and children, 675–676
   in pregnancy, 706–708, 707t
   on plasma concentrations of other drugs, 667t
   for poststroke patients, 530
   in pregnancy, 886
   in renal and liver disease, 728
   teratogenicity of, 712
Topographic EEG mapping, 157–159, 159f
TORCH infections, 502
Torticollis, spasmodic, in infants, 633
Touch-evoked seizures, 471
Tourette syndrome, 636
Toxicity. *See also* Adverse effects, of antiepileptic drugs; *specific drugs*
   of antiepileptic drugs, 647
Toxoplasmosis
   cerebral, 576–577
   of CNS, 577
Toxoplasmosis, other infections, rubella, cytomegalovirus, and herpes virus (TORCH infections), 502
Transient global amnesia, *vs.* epilepsy, 640
Transient ischemia attacks, *vs.* epilepsy, 639
Transmantle dysplasia, with abnormal but nonneoplastic cells, 39t, 40
Transplantation, organ, 581–582
Transporters, pharmacogenetics of, 755
Transverse bipolar montage, 184f
Trauma, epilepsy after, 521–524, 1091–1092. *See also* Posttraumatic epilepsy
Treatment. *See specific disorders*
Tremor, 639
Trials, experimental, on antiepileptic drugs, 649–651, 649f. *See also* Experimental trial design, in antiepileptic drug development; *specific drugs*
Trichinosis, of CNS, 577
Tricyclic antidepressants, 578t, 579
Trimethadione, 1212t
Trisomy 21 (Down syndrome), 482–483
   epilepsy in adults with, 482–483
   epilepsy in children with, 482
Truncal movements, in focal seizures, 246
Tuber, cortical, 7f
Tuberin, 537
Tuberous sclerosis, 6f, 30, 537–540
   clinical features of, 538–539, 538f
   epilepsy with, 539–540
   forme fruste of, cortical dysplasias and, 543

genetics of, 537–538
   genes and loci in, 25t
   testing and counseling in, 48
neonatal seizures with, 502
neurite growth in, 26
parenchyma in, 7f
West syndrome in, 361
Tumors. *See specific tumors*
Two seizures, recurrence risk after, 683
Tyrosinemia type III, 555

U
UCB 34714, 943
UDP-glucuronosyltransferase (UGT), 750–751
Ulcerative colitis, 578
Undefined epilepsies, with myoclonic seizures, 416–417
Underexpression, in developmental defects, 23
Ungual fibromas, 6f
Unprovoked seizure, 110
Unresponsiveness, in focal seizures, 242
Unverricht-Lunborg disease, 419–420, 420t, 421t
Unverricht-Lundborg progressive familial myoclonic epilepsy, 560
Upregulation, in developmental defects, 23
Urbach-Wieth disease, epilepsy with, 543
Urea-cycle abnormalities, 500
Urea cycle defects, 550, 556
Uremia, 573–574
Urinary urgency, as aura, 237

V
V-waves, 189f
Vagus nerve stimulation therapy, 969–977
   advantages and disadvantages of, 976
   for atypical tonic seizures, 327
   clinical studies on, 973–974
   cognitive effects of, 1186
   complications and adverse effects of, 975–976, 975t
   efficacy of, 970–972, 970t, 972t
   experimental studies on, 972–973
   future developments in, 976–977
   history of, 969–970, 970t, 971f
   initiation and maintenance of, 974–975, 974f, 975t
   for Lennox-Gastaut syndrome, 437
   mechanism of action of, 972
   parameters of, 972, 972t
   selection of candidates for, 974
Valproate (valproic acid), 775–780
   for absence epilepsy
      childhood, 398
      juvenile, 400
   absorption of, 656t, 657, 657f, 775–776
   adverse effects of, 778–779
      monitoring for, 741–742
   age-specific dosing of, 677t
   at-risk patients treated with, 737–738, 738t
   for atypical absence seizures, 326–327
   for atypical seizures, 326

Valproate (valproic acid) *(Continued)*
for atypical tonic seizures, 327
for benign childhood epilepsy with
centrotemporal spikes, 381
for benign myoclonic epilepsy of
infancy, 413
chemistry and mechanism of action of,
775, 776f
clinical use of, 779–780
distribution and metabolism of, 656t,
775–776
drug interactions of, 776–777
efficacy of, 777–778
in elderly, 595t, 597t, 599
for epileptic spasms, 342
felbamate on, 916, 916t
for focal epilepsies, symptomatic, 370
for generalized tonic-clonic seizures,
297–299
historical background on, 775
indications for, 1212t
for juvenile myoclonic epilepsy, 395,
416
for Lennox-Gastaut syndrome, 436
for myoclonic epilepsies, progressive,
422
for myoclonus in atypical seizures, 327
for myotonic-astatic epilepsy, 413
pharmacokinetics of, 655–659, 656t
(*See also* Pharmacokinetics, of
antiepileptic drugs)
in infants and children, 676
in pregnancy, 706–708, 707t
plasma concentration of, other
medications on, 666t
on plasma concentrations of other
drugs, 667t–669t
for poststroke patients, 530
in pregnancy, for juvenile myoclonic
epilepsy, 396
in renal and liver disease, 724–725
for severe myoclonic epilepsy of infants,
414
for status epilepticus, 614–616
teratogenicity of, 711
for tonic status epilepticus, 327
Valproate (valproic acid) derivatives, 940t,
943
Valrocemide, 940t, 943
Vascular abnormalities, 1091
Vasculitis, 581
Ventricular zone, 19, 20f
Ventromedial system, 258
Verapamil, 578t, 579
Version (head turning), 264
definition of, 264
in focal motor seizures, 264
in focal seizures with impaired
consciousness, 247
Versive seizures, focal motor, 264
Vertebrobasilar syndromes, *vs.* epilepsy,
639
Vertiginous auras, 230t, 232t, 233t, 234
Vertiginous symptoms, 225
Vertigo, benign paroxysmal, in children,
637
Vestibulospinal tract, 258

Video-electroencephalogram monitoring
case reports of, 996f, 998f–1005f,
1005–1006
of hippocampal changes, 1005, 1005f
in intractable epilepsy, 994–1002,
995f–1003f
benign sporadic sleep spike (small
sharp spike) in, 995f, 996
in complex partial seizure,
997f–1001f, 999
interictal EEG limitations and, 995f,
996
left temporal spike discharges in,
996, 996f
left temporal wicket waves in, 995f,
996
limitations of, 996, 999
in partial seizure, 999, 1002f
in right frontal lobe seizures, 999,
1003f–1004f
for surgical localization, 997f–1003f,
999–1003
for nonlesional epilepsy, 1128, 1129f,
1130f
of psychogenic nonepileptic seizures,
624–625, 629
for seizure semiology in infants and
children, 1143
Video game–induced seizures, 467
Vigabatrin, 921–927
absorption, distribution, and
metabolism of, 923–924
adverse effects of, 925–926
monitoring for, 742
age-specific dosing of, 677t
for Angelman syndrome, seizures in,
423
chemistry of, 921, 922f
in children, 924–925
clinical use and monitoring of,
926–927
cognitive effects of, 1188–1189
drug interactions of, 925
efficacy of, 924–925
for epileptic spasms, 341–342
for generalized tonic-clonic seizures,
298, 300
historical background on, 921
indications for, 1212t
for juvenile myoclonic epilepsy, 396
mechanisms of action of, 921–923
for myoclonic epilepsies, progressive, 422
myoclonic jerks from, 423, 423f
pharmacokinetics of, 655–659, 656t
(*See also* Pharmacokinetics, of
antiepileptic drugs)
in infants and children, 676
in renal and liver disease, 729
teratogenicity of, 712
Visceral (viscerosensory) auras, 230t,
232t, 233t, 235
Visual auras, 230t, 232t, 233t, 234
and focal clonic seizure, in occipital
lobe epilepsy, 206f–207f
Visually evoked seizures, 225
not induced by flicker, 466–467
in reflex epilepsy, 465–466

Vitamin K deficiency, in infants of
mothers on antiepileptic drugs,
710–711
Vitamin metabolism disorders,
553–554
Vocalization, in focal motor seizures,
264
Voltage-dependent (-gated) ion channels,
71–84, 72f–73f
calcium, 76t, 79–81
diseases and electrical activity patterns
of, 76t, 83–84
gating of, 71f, 72f, 81–82, 82f
identification of, 75
modulation of, 82–83
neurons in, 74–75
potassium, 74f, 76–78, 76t
sodium, 75f, 76t, 78–79
structure of, 75–76, 75f
Voltage/electrode map, 148–150, 150f
Voltage-gated calcium channels. *See*
Calcium (Ca^{2+}) channels
Voltage-gated potassium channels. *See*
Potassium (K$^+$) channels
Voltage-gated sodium channels. *See*
Sodium (Na$^+$) channels
Volume conduction
in electroencephalography, 143–144,
143f
in magnetoencephalography, 161
Volume of distribution (V$_d$), of
antiepileptic drugs, 657–658
in infants and children, 671–672

W
Waardenburg syndrome,
neurocristopathies in, 23
Wada memory testing, 1033
in children, 1035
criticism of, 1033–1034
Medical College of Georgia protocol
for, 1036–1038
Walker-Warburg syndrome (lissencephaly
type 2), 29, 32, 45
genes in, 25t
neuroblast migration disorders in,
25
Warfarin, felbamate on, 916
Wave generation, EEG, 132, 132f
epileptic, 137, 138f
Waveforms
in epilepsy diagnosis (*See*
Electroencephalography (EEG),
in epilepsy diagnosis)
in magnetoencephalography, 160–161,
161f
sharp, in epileptic spasms, 337f
sharply contoured, 155, 156f
West syndrome, 333–343, 931. *See also*
Infantile spasms; Spasms,
epileptic
definition and classification of, 359
topiramate for, 881
in tuberous sclerosis, 361
Whipple disease, 578
White-matter neurons, excessive single
ectopic, 45

Wicket spikes, 187f
Wilson disease, "wing-beating tremor" of, 639
Withdrawal, of antiepileptic drugs
    medication taper in, 687
    in seizure free, 684–685, 687

X

X-linked hydrocephalus with pachygyria/
    polymicrogyria, 25t, 30
X-linked lissencephaly, 44–45, 45t, 48
X-linked periventricular nodular
    heterotopia, 39t, 42
Xanthoastrocytoma, pleomorphic, 10f,
    1090–1091

Z

Zellweger syndrome, 549
Zonisamide, 891–897
    adverse effects of, 896–897, 896t
        monitoring for, 742
    age-specific dosing of, 677t
    for atypical tonic seizures, 327
    chemistry of, 891, 892f
    clinical trials on, 894–896
    cognitive effects of, 1189
    drug-food interactions of, 893–894
    drug interactions of, 893, 893t
    for epileptic spasms, 342
    for focal epilepsies, symptomatic, 371
    for generalized tonic-clonic seizures,
        298, 299–300
    historical background on, 891
    indications for, 1212t
    for Lennox-Gastaut syndrome, 437
    mechanism of action of, 891
    for myoclonic epilepsies, progressive,
        422
    for myoclonus in atypical seizures,
        327
    pharmacokinetics of, 655–659, 656t,
        891–893, 892t, 893t (*See also*
        Pharmacokinetics, of
        antiepileptic drugs)
    in infants and children, 676, 892
    in pregnancy, 706–708, 707t
    in renal and liver disease, 728, 893
    teratogenicity of, 712